Fields
VIROLOGY

VOLUME 3: RNA Viruses

SEVENTH
EDITION

Fields
VIROLOGY
VOLUME 3: RNA Viruses

EDITORS-IN-CHIEF

Peter M. Howley, MD

Shattuck Professor of Pathological Anatomy
Departments of Immunology and Pathology
Harvard Medical School
Boston, Massachusetts

David M. Knipe, PhD

Higgins Professor of Microbiology and Molecular Genetics
Head, Harvard Program in Virology
Department of Microbiology
Blavatnik Institute
Harvard Medical School
Boston, Massachusetts

ASSOCIATE VOLUME EDITORS

Blossom Damania, PhD

Boshamer Distinguished Professor
Vice Dean for Research, School of Medicine
Department of Microbiology and Immunology
University of North Carolina at Chapel Hill
Chapel Hill, North Carolina

Sean P. J. Whelan, PhD

Marvin A. Brennecke Distinguished Professor
Chair, Molecular Microbiology
School of Medicine
Washington University in St. Louis
St. Louis, Missouri

Jeffrey I. Cohen, MD

Chief, Laboratory of Infectious Diseases
National Institute of Allergy and Infectious Diseases
National Institutes of Health
Bethesda, Maryland

Eric O. Freed, PhD

HIV Dynamics and Replication Program
Center for Cancer Research
National Cancer Institute
Frederick, Maryland

ASSOCIATE EDITOR

Lynn Enquist, PhD

Henry L. Hillman Professor of Molecular Biology
Department of Molecular Biology
Princeton University
Princeton, New Jersey

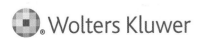

Philadelphia • Baltimore • New York • London
Buenos Aires • Hong Kong • Sydney • Tokyo

Acquisitions Editor: Nicole Dernoski
Development Editor: Ariel S. Winter
Editorial Coordinator: Oliver Raj
Editorial Assistant: Kristen Kardoley
Marketing Manager: Kirsten Watrud
Production Project Manager: Kirstin Johnson
Manager, Graphic Arts & Design: Stephen Druding
Manufacturing Coordinator: Beth Welsh
Prepress Vendor: Straive

Copyright © 2023 Wolters Kluwer

9 8 7 6 5 4 3 2 1

Printed in Mexico

Cataloging in Publication data available on request from publisher

ISBN: 978-1-9751-1260-8

shop.lww.com

QUADM0822

Contributors

Larry J. Anderson, MD
Professor of Infectious Diseases
Department of Pediatrics
Emory University School of Medicine and Children's Healthcare of
    Atlanta
Atlanta, Georgia

Udeni B. R. Balasuriya, BVSc, MS, PhD, FSLCVS
Professor of Virology and Director
Louisiana Animal Disease Diagnostic Laboratory
Department of Pathobiological Science
School of Veterinary Medicine
Louisiana State University
Baton Rouge, Louisiana

Charles R. M. Bangham, ScD, FRS, FMedSci
Co-director
Institute of Infection
Imperial College, United Kingdom

John H. Beigel, MD
Associate Director for Clinical Research
Division of Microbiology and Infectious Diseases
National Institute of Allergy and Infectious Diseases
National Institutes of Health
Bethesda, Maryland

Louis-Marie Bloyet, PhD
Instructor
Department of Molecular Microbiology
School of Medicine
Washington University in St. Louis
St. Louis, Missouri

Thomas Briese, PhD
Associate Professor
Department of Epidemiology
Associate Director
Center for Infection and Immunity
Mailman School of Public Health
Columbia University
New York, New York

Ursula J. Buchholz, PhD
Chief
RNA Viruses Section
Laboratory of Infectious Diseases
National Institute of Allergy and Infectious Diseases
National Institutes of Health
Bethesda, Maryland

Peter L. Collins, PhD
Principal Investigator (Retired)
RNA Viruses Section
Laboratory of Infectious Diseases
National Institute of Allergy and Infectious Diseases
National Institutes of Health
Bethesda, Maryland

Valerie Cortez, PhD, MS
Assistant Professor
Department of Molecular, Cell & Developmental Biology
University of California, Santa Cruz
Santa Cruz, California

Sue E. Crawford, PhD
Assistant Professor
Department of Molecular Virology and Microbiology
Baylor College of Medicine
Houston, Texas

Terence S. Dermody, MD
Vira I. Heinz Distinguished Professor and Chair of Pediatrics
Professor of Microbiology and Molecular Genetics
University of Pittsburgh School of Medicine
Physician-in-Chief and Scientific Director
UPMC Children's Hospital of Pittsburgh
Pittsburgh, Pennsylvania

Ronald C. Desrosiers, PhD
Professor
University of Miami Miller School of Medicine
Miami, Florida

Siyuan Ding, PhD
Assistant Professor
Department of Molecular Microbiology
School of Medicine
Washington University in St. Louis
St. Louis, Missouri

W. Paul Duprex, PhD
Director, Center for Vaccine Research
Professor of Microbiology and Molecular Genetics
Center for Vaccine Research
University of Pittsburgh
Pittsburgh, Pennsylvania

Mary K. Estes, PhD
Distinguished Service Professor
Molecular Virology and Microbiology and Medicine
Baylor College of Medicine
Houston, Texas

David T. Evans, PhD
Professor
Pathology and Laboratory Medicine
University of Wisconsin-Madison
Madison, Wisconsin

Ying Fang, PhD
Professor
Department of Pathobiology
University of Illinois at Urbana-Champaign
Urbana, Illinois

Eric O. Freed, PhD
HIV Dynamics and Replication Program
Center for Cancer Research
National Cancer Institute
Frederick, Maryland

James E. Gern, MD
Professor of Pediatrics and Medicine
University of Wisconsin School of Medicine and Public Health
Madison, Wisconsin

Stephen P. Goff, PhD
Higgins Professor of Biochemistry
Department of Biochemistry and Molecular Biophysics
Department of Microbiology and Immunology
Columbia University Medical Center
New York, New York

Stephen A. Goldstein, PhD
Postdoctoral Research Associate
Department of Human Genetics
University of Utah School of Medicine
Salt Lake City, Utah

Harry B. Greenberg, MD
Professor and Associate Dean of Research
Professor of Medicine and Microbiology and Immunology
Stanford University
Stanford, California

Diane E. Griffin, MD, PhD
University Distinguished Service Professor
W. Harry Feinstone Department of Molecular Microbiology and
    Immunology
Johns Hopkins Bloomberg School of Public Health
Baltimore, Maryland

Ottmar Herchenröder, PhD
Research Scientist
Institute of Experimental Gene Therapy and Cancer Research
Rostock University Medical Center
Rostock, Germany

Christiane Herden, Prof Dr habil
Full Professor
Institute of Veterinary Pathology
Justus-Liebig-University Giessen
Giessen, Germany

Tom C. Hobman, PhD, FCAHS
Professor
Department of Cell Biology
University of Alberta
Edmonton, Canada

Brenda G. Hogue, MEd, PhD
Professor
Biodesign Institute
School of Life Sciences
Arizona State University
Tempe, Arizona

Daniel R. Kuritzkes, MD
Chief, Division of Infectious Diseases; Harriet Ryan Albee Professor
of Medicine
Division of Infectious Diseases
Brigham and Women's Hospital and Harvard Medical School
Boston, Massachusetts

Robert LeDesma, PhD
Department of Molecular Biology
Princeton University
Princeton, New Jersey

Julian L. Leibowitz, MD, PhD
Professor and MD/PhD Program Director
Department of Microbial Pathogenesis and Immunology
Texas A&M University College of Medicine
Bryan, Texas

Stanley M. Lemon, MD
Professor
Departments of Medicine and Microbiology & Immunology
UNC Lineberger Comprehensive Cancer Center
The University of North Carolina at Chapel Hill
Chapel Hill, North Carolina

Dirk Lindemann, PhD
Professor of Molecular Virology
Institute of Medical Microbiology and Virology
Medical Faculty Carl Gustav Carus
University Hospital Carl Gustav Carus
Technische Universität Dresden
Dresden, Germany

W. Ian Lipkin, MD
John Snow Professor of Epidemiology and Director
Center for Infection and Immunity
Mailman School of Public Health
Professor of Pathology and Neurology
College of Physicians & Surgeons
Columbia University
New York, New York

Masao Matsuoka, MD, PhD
Professor
Department of Hematology, Rheumatology, and Infectious
    Diseases
Faculty of Life Sciences, Kumamoto University
Kumamoto, Japan

Asuncion Mejias, MD, PhD, MsCS
Associate Professor of Pediatrics
The Ohio State University College of Medicine
Pediatrics, Division of Infectious Diseases
Abigail Wexner Research Institute at Nationwide Children's
    Hospital
Columbus, Ohio

Melanie Ott, MD, PhD
Director, Senior Investigator
Gladstone Institute of Virology
Senior Vice President
Gladstone Institutes
University of California San Francisco
San Francisco, California

Ann C. Palmenberg, PhD
Professor
Department of Biochemistry
Institute for Molecular Virology
University of Wisconsin-Madison
Madison, Wisconsin

John S. L. Parker, BVMS, PhD
Associate Professor of Virology
Baker Institute for Animal Health
Cornell University
Ithaca, New York

Alexander Ploss, PhD
Associate Professor of Molecular Biology
Department of Molecular Biology
Princeton University
Princeton, New Jersey

Linda J. Rennick, PhD
Research Assistant Professor of Microbiology and
    Molecular Genetics
Center for Vaccine Research
University of Pittsburgh
Pittsburgh, Pennsylvania

Jürgen A. Richt, DVM, PhD
Regents Distinguished Professor
Department of Diagnostic Medicine/Pathology
College of Veterinary Medicine
Kansas State University
Manhattan, Kansas

Monica J. Roth, PhD
Merck Research Laboratory Professor in Clinical
    Pharmacology
Department of Pharmacology
Rutgers-Robert Wood Johnson Medical School
Piscataway, New Jersey

Polly Roy, OBE, FMedSci, FRSB, PhD, MSc
Professor of Virology
Department of Infection Biology
London School of Hygiene and Tropical Medicine
London, United Kingdom

Steven A. Rubin, PhD
Sr. Director, Global Regulatory Affairs
GSK
Rockville, Maryland

Stacey Schultz-Cherry, PhD
Full Member
Department of Infectious Diseases
St. Jude Children's Research Hospital
Senior Associate Dean
St. Jude Children's Research Hospital Graduate School of Biomedical
    Sciences
Memphis, Tennessee

Eileen P. Scully, MD, PhD
Assistant Professor of Medicine
Department of Medicine, Division of Infectious Diseases
Johns Hopkins University
Baltimore, Maryland

Barbara Sherry, PhD
Professor and Department Head
Department of Molecular Biomedical Sciences
College of Veterinary Medicine
North Carolina State University
Raleigh, North Carolina

Eric J. Snijder, PhD
Professor of Molecular Virology
Department of Medical Microbiology
Leiden University Medical Center
Leiden, The Netherlands

Timothy M. Uyeki, MD, MPH, MPP
Chief Medical Officer
Influenza Division, National Center for Immunization and
    Respiratory Diseases
Centers for Disease Control and Prevention
Atlanta, Georgia

Susan R. Weiss, PhD
Professor and Vice Chair
Department of Microbiology
Perelman School of Medicine
University of Pennsylvania
Philadelphia, Pennsylvania

Sean P. J. Whelan, PhD
Marvin A. Brennecke Distinguished Professor
Chair, Molecular Microbiology
School of Medicine
Washington University in St. Louis
St. Louis, Missouri

Preface

In the early 1980s, Bernie Fields originated the idea of a virology reference textbook that combined the molecular aspects of viral replication with the medical features of viral infections. This broad view of virology reflected Bernie's own research, which applied molecular and genetic analyses to the study of viral pathogenesis, providing an important part of the foundation for the field of molecular pathogenesis. Bernie led the publication of the first three editions of Virology, but he unfortunately died soon after the third edition went into production. The third edition became *Fields Virology* in his memory, and it is fitting that the book continues to carry his name. A number of changes and enhancements have now been introduced with the seventh edition of *Fields Virology*. The publication format of *Fields Virology* has been changed from a two-volume book published every 5 to 6 years to an annual publication that comprises approximately one-fourth of the chapters organized by category. The annual publication provides both a physical book volume and importantly an eBook with an improved platform. Using an eBook format, our expectation is that individual chapters can be easily updated when major advances, outbreaks, etc., occur. The editorial board organized the four-volume series for the seventh edition to consist of volumes on Emerging Viruses, DNA Viruses, RNA Viruses, and Fundamental Virology, to be published on an annual basis, with the expectation that the topics will cycle approximately every 4 years creating an annualized, up-to-date publication. Each volume will contain approximately 20 chapters. The first volume of this seventh edition of *Fields Virology*, entitled Emerging Viruses, was published in 2020, and the second volume, DNA Viruses, was published in 2021. This third volume, RNA Viruses, has been principally edited by Eric O. Freed, Jeffrey I. Cohen, Blossom Damania, Peter M. Howley, David M. Knipe, and Sean P. J. Whelan. There have been continued rapid advances in virology since the previous edition, and all of the chapters in the RNA Viruses volume are either completely new or have been significantly updated to reflect these advances. In this seventh edition, we have chosen to highlight important references published since the last edition while maintaining older classics. The main emphasis continues to be on viruses of medical importance and interest, but other viruses are described in specific cases where more is known about their mechanisms of replication or pathogenesis. We wish to thank Patrick Waters of Harvard Medical School and all of the editorial staff members of Wolters Kluwer for all their important contributions to the preparation of this book.

David M. Knipe, PhD
Peter M. Howley, MD
Jeffrey I. Cohen, MD
Blossom Damania, PhD
Lynn Enquist, PhD
Eric O. Freed, PhD
Sean P. J. Whelan, PhD

RNA Viruses is the third volume of the seventh edition of *Fields Virology*. The first two volumes, Emerging Viruses and DNA Viruses, were published in 2020 and 2021, respectively. The next volume, Fundamental Virology, will be published in 2023. There have been continued rapid advances in virology since the sixth edition that was published in 2013, and all of the chapters in the RNA Viruses volume are either completely new or have been significantly updated to reflect these advances. In this seventh edition, we have chosen to highlight important references published since the last edition while maintaining older classics.

This volume covers all the RNA viruses of medical importance, including viruses that infect humans and animals. RNA viruses of plants, insects, and bacteria will be included in the fourth volume of the seventh edition, Fundamental Virology. In addition to RNA virus families, several thematic issues arise in the consideration of the RNA viruses in this volume. Similar to the DNA viruses, several of the RNA viruses are associated with persistent infections and as a consequence are associated directly or indirectly with cancer. This volume includes chapters that detail the major advances in our understanding of the molecular biology and disease pathogenesis associated with human immunodeficiency virus (HIV). Chapters on a number of RNA viruses were included in the first volume, Emerg-

ing Viruses, which with the exception of two new chapters on SARS-CoV-2, the emerging viruses in Volume 1 are not included in this third volume. We note that the *Coronaviridae* chapter in the Emerging Viruses volume was published just months prior to the current pandemic and therefore did not include SARS-CoV-2.

The organization of the chapters in this edition is similar to that of the previous editions. For most of the viruses, there is a single chapter that combines both the basic and clinical aspects of the virus. For several of the viruses, the basic virology related to viral replication and the viral pathogenesis are split between two chapters. In the RNA volume, this includes the retroviruses, the human immunodeficiency viruses, and SARS-CoV-2. We are grateful to Eric O. Freed, Jeffrey I. Cohen, Blossom Damania, and Sean S. P. Whelan, who joined us to participate in putting this volume together. We also are thankful to the chapter authors who have updated their chapters for this volume and to the new authors who have joined us in this continued endeavor to provide a comprehensive resource in virology.

Peter M. Howley
David M. Knipe

Contents

Contributors   v
Preface   viii

Introduction   ix

1   Rhinoviruses   1
James E. Gern • Ann C. Palmenberg

2   Hepatoviruses   22
Stanley M. Lemon

3   Astroviruses   59
Valerie Cortez • Stacey Schultz-Cherry

4   Rubella Virus   75
Tom C. Hobman

5   Arteriviruses   104
Ying Fang • Eric J. Snijder • Udeni B. R. Balasuriya

6   Bornaviridae   131
W. Ian Lipkin • Christiane Herden • Jürgen A. Richt • Thomas Briese

7   Rhabdoviridae   161
Sean P. J. Whelan • Louis-Marie Bloyet

8   Mumps Virus   206
Steven A. Rubin • Linda J. Rennick • W. Paul Duprex

9   Measles Virus   228
Diane E. Griffin

10   Respiratory Syncytial Virus and Metapneumovirus   267
Ursula J. Buchholz • Larry J. Anderson • Peter L. Collins • Asuncion Mejias

11   Orthoreoviruses   318
Terence S. Dermody • John S. L. Parker • Barbara Sherry

12   Rotaviruses   362
Sue E. Crawford • Siyuan Ding • Harry B. Greenberg • Mary K. Estes

13   Orbiviruses   414
Polly Roy

14   Hepatitis E Virus   443
Robert LeDesma • Alexander Ploss

15   Retroviridae   465
Stephen P. Goff • Monica J. Roth

16   Human T-Cell Leukemia Virus Types 1 and 2   527
Charles R. M. Bangham • Masao Matsuoka

17   Human Immunodeficiency Viruses: Replication   558
Melanie Ott • Eric O. Freed

18   HIV-1: Pathogenesis, Clinical Manifestations, and Treatment   618
Eileen P. Scully • Daniel R. Kuritzkes

19   Nonhuman Lentiviruses   648
Ronald C. Desrosiers • David T. Evans

20   Foamy Viruses   679
Dirk Lindemann • Ottmar Herchenröder

21 **Severe Acute Respiratory Syndrome Coronavirus 2 (SARS-CoV-2)** 706

Stephen A. Goldstein • Brenda G. Hogue • Julian L. Leibowitz • Susan R. Weiss

22 **SARS-CoV-2/COVID-19: Clinical Characteristics, Prevention, and Treatment** 741

John H. Beigel • Timothy M. Uyeki

Index 785

Rhinoviruses

James E. Gern • Ann C. Palmenberg

History
Infectious Agent
  Classification
  Physical Characteristics
Pathogenesis and Pathology
  Entry into the Host
  Site of Primary Replication
  Spread
  Cell and Tissue Tropism
  Immune Response
  Release from Host and Mode of Transmission
  Virulence
  Persistence
Epidemiology
  Age
  Morbidity
  Origin and Spread of RV Infections
  Prevalence and Seroepidemiology
  Genetic Diversity of Virus
Clinical Features
Diagnosis
  Differential
  Laboratory
Prevention and Control
Perspective

HISTORY

The common cold has been recognized for millennia, and both the illness and prescribed remedies have been influenced by and engendered a broad body of folklore. In fact, the name of the illness stems from the belief that being chilled caused the illness, a concept which studies using experimental inoculation techniques have been unable to verify.[61] In Chinese traditional medicine, colds were considered an illness of wind and cold, and the Roman physician Galen wrote *"The white-colored substance (the phlegma) collects mostly … in those who have been chilled in some way"*.[14] Through the ages, ideas about pathogenesis varied widely, and suggestions for common cold cures were creative, occasionally bizarre, and seldom helpful. Yet, enthusiasm for a cure for the common cold remains quite high today; a recent web-based search yielded 211,000,000 hits in response to the terms *"common cold cure."*

In 1914, Kruse demonstrated that cell-free filtrates of nasal secretions from affected individuals could transmit colds.[149] Dochez et al. confirmed these findings in 1930 by transmitting colds to volunteers and apes using filtered nasal secretions that were free of bacteria, indicating a viral etiology.[58] Progress in finding the underlying cause for colds was accelerated immediately after World War II by the establishment of the Common Cold Unit (CCU) by the UK Medical Research Council in 1946.[256] Housed in an hospital unit founded by Harvard University and the American Red Cross to support Great Britain during the war, the building was eventually donated to the British government. At that time, it was presumed the cold-causing virus was different from influenza.[256] The goals of the CCU, as led by Christopher Andrewes and later David Tyrrell, were to identify the common cold virus, its means of transmission, and describe the host characteristics that sometimes promoted more severe illness. Between 1946 and 1989, when the unit closed, over 20,000 volunteers had participated in those studies.

The first rhinoviruses (RVs) were isolated by two independent groups,[201,210] starting around 1956. It was not long before researchers realized that several different virus families actually contributed to common cold illnesses, and that among these the RV included numerous serotypes. A collaborative program in 1967 classified all then-known isolates into 55 different serotypes.[218] Serotypes 56 to 89 were added in 1971,[1] and the remainder of the classic 101 RV-A&B in 1987.[97] More recent molecular sequencing techniques led to the description of the genetically distinct RV-C species whose isolates do not grow in standard tissue culture.[155] These viruses, along with several previously unknown RV-A&B genotypes, initiated a renewed period of discovery related to RV epidemiology, their extended classification, and many additional insights into the role of specific RV not only in common colds but also otitis, sinusitis, lower respiratory infections, and acute exacerbations of chronic respiratory diseases such as asthma.

INFECTIOUS AGENT

Classification

The RVs (formerly *Human Rhinoviruses*, HRVs) comprise the RV-A, RV-B, and RV-C species of the *Enterovirus* genus in the *Picornaviridae* family. Present classification is based on overt similarities in genome organization, capsid properties, and primary sequence conservation.[195] Viruses are assigned to a species if they share greater than 70% amino acid identity in the P1, 2C, and 3CD regions with other members. Within species, isolates are subdivided into numeric genotypes (Fig. 1.1). For the RV-A&B, the foundation assignments included the historic clinical panels archived by the American Type Culture Collection, which were indexed into the 101 original serotypes after assessment of antigenic cross-reactivity in rabbits or guinea pigs. RV-A87 was subsequently reassigned to the *Enterovirus D* (EV-D68) after reevaluation of genetic, immunogenic, and receptor use (decay-accelerating factor as a receptor) properties.[225] Ultimately, the difficulty of testing clinical viruses for immunogenicity made serotyping obsolete, and such cataloging was never actively employed for any RV-C. Instead, current genotype assignments respect the historic RV-A&B index system, but now rely heavily on sequence comparisons, primarily of the VP1 region or VP4/VP2. Strains in a common genotype, including most of the historic serotypes, share a general threshold of approximately 11% nucleotide divergence in their VP1 genes.[233] Full genome sequencing showed that some original types were more closely related than this and warranted reassignment (e.g., A44, A95, and A98 were abolished and the isolates combined into A29, A8, and A54, respectively), while others such as A8 and A45 defining "clade D" may be sufficiently different for eventual designation as a fourth species (Fig. 1.1). Many newly described RV-C genomes are not yet fully sequenced, so isolate genotyping is based primarily on VP1 genetic threshold data. To prevent ambiguity, RV-A (80 types), RV-B (32 types), and RV-C (57 types) nomenclature conventions require both the species letter and genotype assignment (e.g., A16, B14, C15). The RV designation (e.g., RV-A16) may be included for clarity.

Physical Characteristics

As enteroviruses, the RV have genome organizations (Fig. 1.2) and capsid structures (Fig. 1.3) similar to those of polioviruses, coxsackieviruses, and ECHO viruses. But unlike other enteroviruses that remain viable at pH 3.0, RV particles are unstable below pH 5 to 6. The icosahedral capsid (~30 nm diameter) has

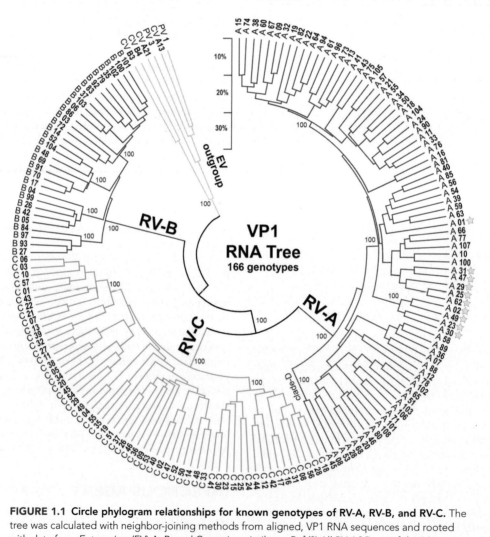

FIGURE 1.1 Circle phylogram relationships for known genotypes of RV-A, RV-B, and RV-C. The tree was calculated with neighbor-joining methods from aligned, VP1 RNA sequences and rooted with data from *Enterovirus* (EV) A, B, and C species, similar to Ref.[196] All RV-A&B are of the Major (ICAM-1) receptor group except those 10 labeled with stars (Minor receptor group, LDLR). The RV-C receptor is CDHR3. Bootstrap values (percent of 2,000 replicates) are indicated at key nodes. Genbank accession numbers for this dataset are in eTable 1.1.

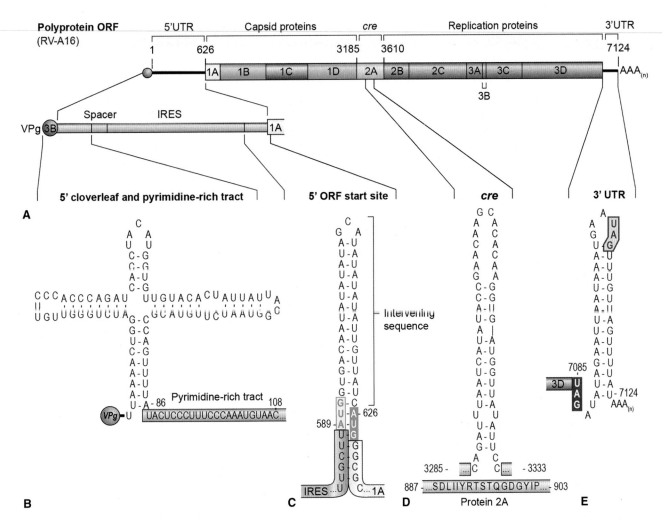

FIGURE 1.2 The genome of an RV encodes a single polyprotein open reading frame **(A)**. Important RNA structural motifs include a 5′ cloverleaf **(B)**, ORF start-site stem **(C)**, a cis-acting replication (*cre*) element **(D)**, and 3′ stem motif.

60 copies each of proteins VP1, VP2, VP3, and VP4, named in order of descending electrophoretic mobility. The four proteins derived from a common P1 precursor stay together during assemble as a biological subunit, or protomer. The protein shell surrounds a densely packed, single-stranded, positive-sense, RNA genome of 7,079 (C1) to 7,233 (B92) bases, a count which does not include the variable length 3′ poly(A) tail. Several RV capsids have been resolved atomic resolution, including A1 (*1r1a*), A2 (*1fpn*), A16 (*1ayn*), B3 (*1rhi*), B14 (*4RV*), and C15 (*5k0u*), with multiple other determinations showing receptor interactions (e.g., A16 with ICAM-1, *1d3e*; C15 with CDHR3, *6psf*) or antiviral drug interactions (e.g., A16 with pleconaril, *1c8m*). Like poliovirus, the surfaces of RV capsids are dominated by the three largest proteins (Fig. 1.3). VP4 is internal to the structure, centered near the fivefold axis. Around the 12 raised exterior fivefold VP1 "plateaus," a symmetrical "canyon" provides receptor binding sites and discontinuous immunogenic surfaces[230] to each RV-A&B. The C15 structure has a different surface topology, including three major VP1 deletions, which lower the fivefold plateau and remove most of the surrounding canyon features. Individual RV-C genotypes compensate for this loss of mass with characteristic unique-sequence, highly immunogenic "finger-like" surface loops contributed by

a relative insertion near the C-terminus of VP1.[163] Common to all RV, the VP1 cores surround a hydrophobic "pocket" or cavity. Type-1 long (e.g., B14) or type-2 short (e.g., A16) pocket shapes are defined for most RV-A&B and determine whether a particular virus is susceptible to drugs like pleconaril or WIN compounds aimed at inhibiting the uncoating process.[7] The RV-C VP1 pockets have partially collapsed shapes, inaccessible to drug diffusion, rendering these isolates refractive to similar antiviral therapies.[163]

All RV genomes are messenger-sense, encoding the polyprotein reading frame (ORF) and multiple important RNA structural motifs (Fig. 1.2). Adjacent to the 5′ cloverleaf, a regulatory feature for translation and replication, each RV encodes a strain-specific pyrimidine-rich tract that may be involved in suppressing innate immunity triggers.[196] The type-1 IRES 3′ to this tract includes a variable-length stem structure pairing the ORF start site (AUG) with an upstream AUG. Unlike poliovirus, intervening sequences between these AUGs are probably not scanned by initiating ribosomes.[121] The picornavirus VPg uridylylation reaction, required for RNA synthesis, is templated by a secondary structure called the *cre* (cis-acting replication element) whose location varies in every species of picornavirus. For the RV-A, the *cre* is in the 2A gene.[243] For the RV-B, the

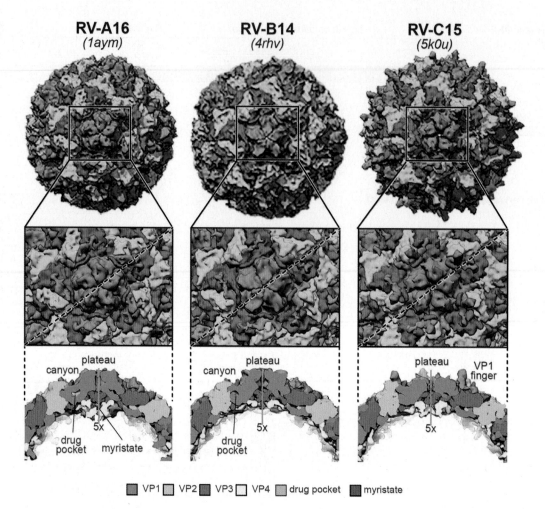

RV-A16
(1aym)

RV-B14
(4rhv)

RV-C15
(5k0u)

| ■ VP1 | □ VP2 | ■ VP3 | □ VP4 | ▤ drug pocket | ■ myristate |

FIGURE 1.3 Comparative capsids A16 (*1aym*), B14 (*4rhv*), and C15 (*5k0u*) illustrate the icosahedral surface topography of VP1 (*blue*), VP2 (*green*), and VP3 (*red*) proteins. The VP4 is internal to the capsid. Antiviral capsid drugs (RV-A&B) bind in a pocket, internal to VP1. All VP4 proteins have N-terminal myristate modifications, although these are rarely characterized in structure determinations. Throughout this chapter, imaged or referenced Protein Database (PDB) structure identification numbers are indicated parenthetically. Images courtesy of Dr. Jean-Yves Sgro (University of Wisconsin-Madison).

cre is in the 2C gene.[243] The RV-C *cre* is in the 1B gene.[24] The short, 3′ untranslated sequences (UTR) are of highly variable sequence. Invariably, they configure as an inclusive stem motif displaying at least one bogus termination codon in the terminal loop. This codon may be in-frame or out-of-frame with the authentic ORF stop site and has been proposed to play a role in the recruitment of translation termination factors.[196]

In general, the RV lifecycle after infection is that of canonical enteroviruses, requiring 14 to 24 hours for cell death and lytic progeny release. The 2A and 3C proteases embedded in the polyprotein undergo monomolecular and/or bimolecular reactions to release mature enzymes or their precursors, both for further polyprotein cleavage, and for a variety of cellular proteolytic events to inactivate innate immunity functions, aid IRES-dependent translation, and rearrange cell processes advantageous to the virus. Among these, RV strain-dependent, 2A-catalyzed cleavage of multiple Phe/Gly-containing nucleoporin proteins (Nups) and eIFG translation factors may elicit different cell responses and cellular translational shutoff that directly or indirectly leads to distinct disease phenotypes.[270] Also like other enteroviruses, RV infection induces significant rearrangements in cellular membranes and their lipid components, including the ER and trans-golgi network as they establish protective compartments favorable to RNA replication, genome translation, and progeny assembly.[220] Proposed interference in these pathways, as essential viral replication requirements, may suggest possible novel antiviral targets.

PATHOGENESIS AND PATHOLOGY

Entry Into the Host

The primary portal of entry for RV infections is through inoculation of either the eyes or nose. Studies of seronegative infected volunteers have shown that very low doses of RV, substantially less than the amount needed to infect cells *in vitro* (1 tissue culture infectious dose$_{50}$ [TCID50]), can cause infection when introduced via the conjunctiva or nasal mucosa. In contrast, approximately 10,000 times as much virus is needed to cause productive infection when the inoculation site is the tongue or external nares.[50]

Site of Primary Replication

The primary site of infection is the airway epithelium. In studies of airway tissues from either natural or experimentally induced colds, detection of viral protein or RNA is largely confined to the epithelial layer, along with an occasional cell in the subepithelial layer.[11,26,185] The RV-A and RV-C mainly replicate in ciliated epithelial cells[89,125] (Fig. 1.4). RV-A&B may also replicate in specialized nonciliated epithelial cells in the adenoids that express high levels of ICAM-1.[277]

Spread

For years it was assumed that RV infection was confined to the upper airway and did not affect the chest except under unusual circumstances. Early experiments in cell culture systems indicated that RV replicate best at 33°C to 35°C, and it was assumed that warmer temperatures in the lower airways (37°C) could limit RV infections to the cooler upper airways. Contrary to these initial assumptions, direct measurements in the lower airways have shown that large and medium size airways are at the ideal temperature for RV replication (Fig. 1.5).[175] More recent replication studies demonstrate that RV-C and many RV-A types can replicate very well at 37°C.[13,198] In addition, cultured lower airway epithelial cells support RV replication *in vitro* at least as well, and perhaps even better, than cells derived from the upper airways.[167,184] Interestingly, cooler temperatures can inhibit cellular antiviral responses such as apoptosis and RNAseL, which could permit greater viral replication in the cooler temperatures of the upper airways.[76]

Following experimental inoculation of the upper airway, RV has been detected in the lower airways of individuals with a variety of techniques. Secretions from the lower airways sampled by bronchoscopy and bronchial lavage were analyzed by RT-PCR, and more than half of the lower airway specimens tested positive for RV.[81,229] These findings were extended by subsequent studies demonstrating the presence of intracellular RV RNA and protein using *in situ* hybridization and immunohistochemistry.[185,197] Analysis of cells in sputum has been used to provide an estimate of the quantity and kinetics of viral shedding from the large lower airways. After experimental inoculation of seronegative volunteers, viral shedding from the upper

Distance from Nares (cm)	Temp. (insp/exp)
18.2	32/33
31.4	33/34
37.3	34/35
39.4	34.5/35.2
41.2	36/37

FIGURE 1.5 Temperatures in the large lower airways are ideal for RV replication. Direct measurements of temperature in lower airways have been recorded at measured distances from the nares using a bronchoscope equipped with a small thermistor.[175] Even when the inspired air is at room temperature (20.7°C), airway temperatures in the medium and large airways are in the range of 33°C to 35°C. In contrast, small airway temperatures approach core temperature (37°C). Abbreviations: insp, inspiration; exp, expiration.

airway peaks 2 to 4 days later. In contrast, peak levels of virus in the sputum occurs 3 to 7 days after inoculation.[185] In addition, about half of the volunteers have viral shedding in the sputum that is equal to or exceeds that found in the nasal secretions. Notably, only small amounts of virus are detected in bronchial lavage specimens, which originate from distal airways and alveoli.[185] These findings suggest that RV infections likely begin in the upper airway and can spread to the large and medium-sized airways during some illnesses.

Natural cold studies also confirm that RV can replicate in the lower airways. Viral recovery from sputum during colds can exceed that obtained from upper airway samples.[113,266] In epidemiologic studies, RV is frequently detected in children and adults with lower airway illnesses such as bronchiolitis, exacerbations of asthma, and pneumonia.[122,123,179,180,204] In wheezing

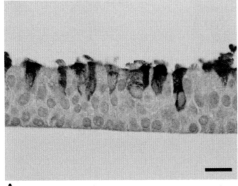
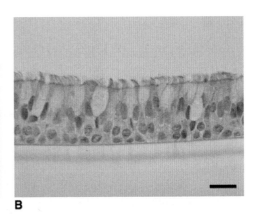

FIGURE 1.4 RV-C15 replication within ciliated epithelial cells in tissue culture. Primary human bronchial epithelial cells were differentiated at air–liquid interface that then inoculated either RV-C15 **(A)** or medium alone **(B)**. The cells were stained for C15 capsid and imaged by light microscopy. C15 capsid is represented by brown-staining cells. Scale bars indicate 20 μm. (Reprinted from Griggs TF, Bochkov YA, Basnet S, et al. Rhinovirus C targets ciliated airway epithelial cells. *Respir Res* 2017;18(1):84. https://creativecommons.org/licenses/by/4.0/.)

infants, RV has been detected in lower airway biopsies, and RV detection was associated with reduced lung function in these infants.[170] In children with tracheostomies, samples of nasal mucus can be obtained directly from the lower airway without contamination from nasal secretions, and RV detection rates from upper versus lower airway specimens are similar.[235]

In addition to infecting the nasopharynx, conjunctiva, and lower airways, RV can be recovered in specimens obtained from the middle ear and sinuses.[38,205] The respiratory epithelium in these locations is contiguous with that of the nasopharynx, and the virus presumably spreads via local extension. Rhinovirus viremia has been detected in infected children by PCR and appears to be more common during RV-C illnesses.[168,281] A study of experimentally infected adults showed no evidence of circulating RV RNA (45). RVs are inactivated at pH < 6, thus preventing swallowed virus from replicating in the gastrointestinal tract.[90]

Cell and Tissue Tropism

Biopsies of the upper airway from infected volunteers show a patchy pattern of epithelial infection with small foci of infected cells.[10,206] Point cultures of the airway have demonstrated high levels of RV shedding in the nasopharynx and especially in the adenoidal region.[278] Examination of biopsies obtained during experimentally induced colds suggests that a specific type of nonciliated adenoidal epithelial cell expresses high levels of ICAM-1 and supports high-level viral replication.[277] It is

possible that these cells play a sentinel role in the detection of viral respiratory infections.

The receptors used by RV are also expressed by airway cells other than epithelial cells. Besides epithelial cells, RV can bind to macrophages, monocytes, B cells, eosinophils, and fibroblasts.[80,84,98] Macrophages and monocytes are good sources of type I and type III interferons, which may explain why there is little or no RV replication in these cells.[146] Airway fibroblasts[84] support RV replication in tissue culture, but it has not been established whether these cells, which are located several cell layers under the epithelial surface, are infected *in vivo*.

Receptors

All RV-A&B use intercellular adhesion molecule–1 (ICAM-1, 101 "major" types) or alternatively, low, or very low-density lipoprotein receptor (LDLR, VLDLR, 10 "minor" types) for recognition and attachment to cells[88,263] (Fig. 1.6). The RV-C instead require interactions with CDHR3, cadherin-related family member 3.[27] This protein is coexpressed with FOX-J1, a transcription factor that regulates the differentiation of ciliated cells,[20] but the precise native function of CDHR3 remains unknown. While the *ICAM-1* gene is ubiquitous to all humans, the CDHR3 display density on the apical surfaces of ciliated pulmonary epithelial cells is dependent upon a nucleotide polymorphism (rs6967330) encoding a Tyr529 to Cys529 substitution in the protein's extracellular repeat domain 5 (EC5), an allele change, which is also among the strongest known genetic

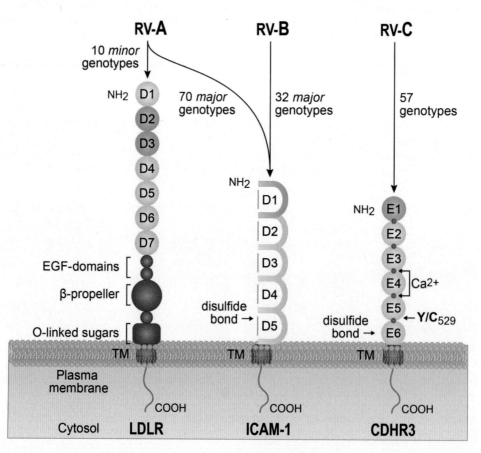

FIGURE 1.6 The RV receptors. Comparative schematics of human ICAM-1, LDLR, and CDHR3 show the virus interactive domains among the various extracellular repeat units.

correlates for childhood virus-induced asthma susceptibility.[20,30] The asthmatic risk sequence (Tyr529), ancestral to all human and primate lineages, confers a 5- to 50-fold RV-C enhanced infection susceptibility to cultured or primary cells.[20,29,271] The asthma-protective allele (Cys529), by far the dominant geno-type in world-wide modern human populations, is maintained by balancing selection[193] and prevents the encoded protein from properly exiting the ER after synthesis, reducing the cell surface concentration and availability to virus.

Biochemistry and structure determinations show all recep-tor interactions with their respective RV are through N-prox-imal protein domain contacts with discrete virion binding footprints (Fig. 1.7). Structure examples include B14 with solu-ble ICAM-1 domains 1 to 2 (*1d3i*), A2 with domain 3 VLDLR (*3dpr*), and C15 with CDHR3 EC1 (*6psf*). In addition, the major group virus A89 can bind to heparin sulfate in cultured cells, in the absence of ICAM-1[262] as can C15 if adapted to do so through a single VP1 capsid mutation (Thr125Lys) near the fivefold axis.[28] Studies utilizing atopic force spectroscopy indicate that after initial RV binding, multiple receptor pro-teins (i.e., ICAM-1) are rapidly recruited (within 200 millisec-onds).[217]

Species Tropism

RV primarily infect humans. Chimpanzees can be experi-mentally infected with RV-A&B, but while viral shedding is detected, there are few symptoms of illness.[115] In contrast, a recent RV-C outbreak in a wild chimpanzee population pro-duced severe illness in almost 100% of the individuals, sev-eral of which died.[226] Given that all nonhuman primates share the susceptible Tyr529 CDHR3 receptor allele, such epizoot-ics are presumably triggered through human contact, as these viruses are not known to circulate naturally in nonhuman pop-ulations. RV-A&B do not bind to murine ICAM-1, but the minor group viruses can bind to murine LDLR[283] and replicate in murine epithelial cells.[32,255] Certain RV strains have been spe-cifically selected for this property by serial passage in murine cell lines.[17,100] Epithelial cells from transgenic mice engineered to express human ICAM-1 also support replication of major group viruses.[17] There are no current equivalent transgenic mice displaying human CDHR3 (Tyr529).

The demonstration that any RV-A&B can grow even mar-ginally in murine epithelial cells has led to the development of murine models for those RV infection. The models resem-ble some features of human infections, including replication in the respiratory epithelium, induction of type I interferons and neutrophil chemokines, and neutrophilic airway inflam-mation.[17,112] In addition, RV infection of mice increases inflam-mation in response to allergen exposure, suggesting that these models could be informative for asthma.[17] Experimental limita-tions include the requirement for a large inoculating dose, and short duration (<24 hours) of significant viral replication and shedding.

Immune Response

Immunohistochemistry

RV infections produce relatively little cytopathology. Findings on biopsy during the peak of the illness include tissue edema and a sparse infiltration of neutrophils and mononuclear cells in the nasal mucosa.[275,276] Similar changes occur in bronchial biopsies, and RV-induced cellular infiltration may be more

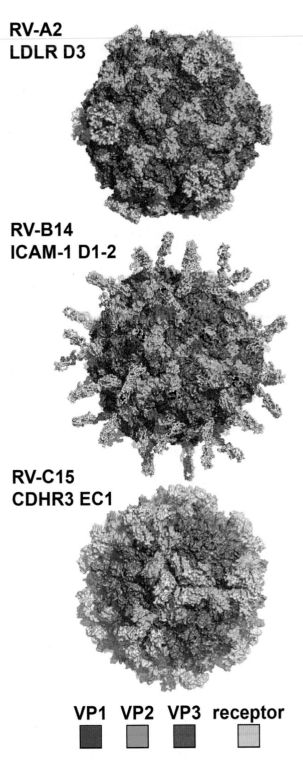

RV-A2
LDLR D3

RV-B14
ICAM-1 D1-2

RV-C15
CDHR3 EC1

VP1　VP2　VP3　receptor

FIGURE 1.7 Virus–receptor interactions. Crystallography or cryo-EM structure determinations for A2 (minor) and LDLR domain 3 (*1v9u*), C15 and CDHR3 EC1 domain (*6psf*), and B14 with ICAM-1 D1-2 (*1d3i* alpha carbon only, superimposed on *4hrv*) show the different receptor contact footprints, generally representative of all such analogous bindings.

pronounced in patients with asthma.[288] The mild pathology together with the small number of infected cells suggests that the immune response to RV rather than direct virus-induced injury contributes most to respiratory symptoms.

Mediators of Inflammation

RV infection induced a variety of proinflammatory cytokines and mediators (Table 1.1). Most of these factors are present in peak concentrations during the acute cold and correlate with illness severity and viral shedding.[16] A number of studies have focused on whether blocking these mediators can relieve symptoms of RV illnesses. Kinins and leukotrienes are of special interest due to their effects on vasodilation and edema, which are prominent findings during acute colds.[116,285] RV infection of volunteers with asthma induced increased mRNA and activity of human kallikrein, a critical enzyme for the release of kinins, in the lower airways.[42] These mediators can also cause smooth muscle contraction as well as edema and thus could promote airway obstruction in patients with asthma. Kinins are increased early in the course of a cold,[212] but testing their role in pathogenesis awaits the development of safe and effective kinin inhibitors. Leukotrienes (LTs) are overproduced during viral respiratory infections,[79] but the cysteinyl leukotriene receptor antagonist montelukast did not affect cold symptoms in experimentally infected volunteers.[143] In addition, intranasal administration of LTB4 before experimental inoculation had no significant effects on either viral replication or symptoms.[273]

RV-induced cytokines may also promote vascular permeability; experiments conducted *in vitro* demonstrate that TNF-α, IL-1β, and IFN-γ can each increase vascular permeability.[227] Notably, common colds have little effect on concentrations of histamine in the nose,[68] and second-generation antihistamines (which are specific H1 receptor antagonists) have no effect on cold symptoms.[188]

Analysis of nasal secretions after experimental inoculation demonstrate that the thin rhinorrhea during the early stages of a cold contains serum proteins (e.g., IgG, albumin), and as the cold progresses, the composition shifts to mucin proteins.[116,285] This progression suggests that the pathophysiology of rhinorrhea is time-dependent and shifts from early vascular leakage to local secretion of mucus during the mid to latter stages of a cold.

Epithelium

The airway epithelium is the first line of defense against RV infections and initiates and orchestrates downstream responses of other airway cells (Fig. 1.8). Epithelial-derived mucins, antimicrobial peptides, and surfactant proteins in the mucus layer nonspecifically deter infection.[110] In addition, well-differentiated epithelial cells are relatively resistant to RV infection.[166] The epithelium may serve as a barrier against RV infection; RV-A replication is enhanced when apical cells of well-differentiated epithelial cell cultures are either damaged or stripped away.[124] This property may help to explain how exposure to factors such as pollutants and allergic inflammation that can damage epithelium also increase the risk and/or severity of RV illnesses. RV infection itself can disrupt the barrier function of the epithelium[164,221] and delay repair processes,[138] which may amplify harmful effects of bacterial pathogens, allergens, or irritants.

In addition to being the principal host cells for RV infections, airway epithelial cells initiate antiviral and proinflammatory immune responses. Attachment of RV to ICAM-1 activates signaling cascades that increase expression of chemokine genes such as CXCL10.[78,146] RV can also bind to and activate TLR2, which stimulates NFκV.[250] Once RV particles uncoat in the endosome, the release of single-stranded RNA activates additional innate immune sensors. These include toll-like receptors such as TLR3 and TLR7 that are expressed on endosomal membranes, and the double-stranded RNA-dependent protein kinase (PKR) and RNA helicases (retinoic acid–induced gene I [RIG-I] and melanoma-differentiation–associated gene-5 [MDA5]). TLR3 is constitutively expressed on airway epithelial cells, and RV activation of TLR3 leads to induction of RIG-I and MDA5.[237] All three of these molecules help to upregulate innate interferon responses.[237,264] The clinical importance of MDA5 is supported by a case report of a patient with severe recurrent RV illnesses associated with a genetic abnormality that reduced expression of MDA5.[152] Blockade of TLR3 in clinical trials produced mixed results in that upper airway symptoms in normal individuals were attenuated, but volun-

---

TABLE 1.1   Examples of RV-Induced Mediators and Cytokines

Category	Examples	Comments	References
Mediators	Kinins	Vasodilation and edema	116,212,285
	Leukotrienes	↑Vascular permeability and bronchoconstriction	79
	Nitric oxide	Vasodilation, bronchoconstriction	52,73,222
	Prostaglandins	Regulate inflammation	153
Antivirals	IFNα	Low concentrations in nasal secretions[a]	137,147
	IFNβ	Possibly deficient in asthma	137,268
	IFNλ (IL28, IL29)	Possibly deficient in asthma	44, 137
	β-Defensins	Activity against bacteria and enveloped viruses	63,213
Chemokines	CXCL10	Attracts Th1 cells	147,241,267
	CXCL8	Attracts neutrophils	82,248,254
	CCL2	Attracts monocytes, T cells, and dendritic cells	96
Cytokines	IL-1	Proinflammatory	211
	IL-6	Proinflammatory	166
	IL-17	Neutrophilic inflammation	126
Growth factors and tissue repair	G-CSF	↑Production of neutrophils in bone marrow	127
	TGF-β	↑Collagen synthesis, immunoregulation	60
	VEGF	Angiogenesis and airway remodeling	51

[a]True for all interferons.

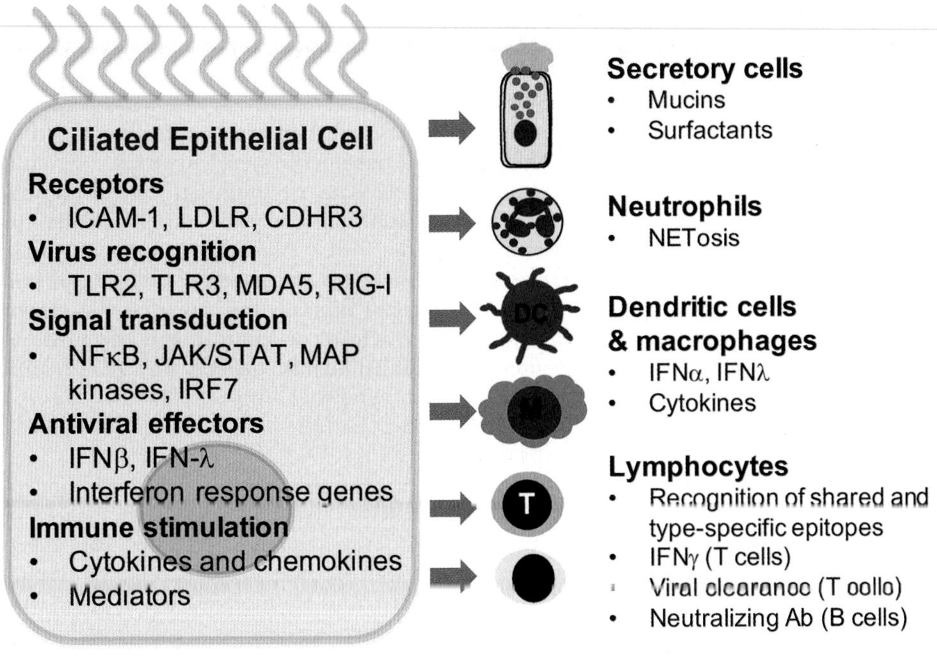

Ciliated Epithelial Cell

Receptors
- ICAM-1, LDLR, CDHR3

Virus recognition
- TLR2, TLR3, MDA5, RIG-I

Signal transduction
- NFκB, JAK/STAT, MAP kinases, IRF7

Antiviral effectors
- IFNβ, IFN-λ
- Interferon response genes

Immune stimulation
- Cytokines and chemokines
- Mediators

Secretory cells
- Mucins
- Surfactants

Neutrophils
- NETosis

Dendritic cells & macrophages
- IFNα, IFNλ
- Cytokines

Lymphocytes
- Recognition of shared and type-specific epitopes
- IFNγ (T cells)
- Viral clearance (T cells)
- Neutralizing Ab (B cells)

FIGURE 1.8 Airway epithelial cells initiate the immune response to RV. RVs primarily infect ciliated airway epithelial cells, and virus recognition triggers signaling pathways that activate antiviral effectors and initiates the synthesis of proinflammatory cytokines and chemokines. Secretion of these factors together with release of viral progeny then recruit and activate other airway cells including secretory cells, airway macrophages (M), dendritic cells (DC), neutrophils (PMN), T cells, and B cells Abbreviation: NET, neutrophil extracellular traps.

teers with asthma had no improvement in lower airway symptoms following experimental inoculation.[232]

Engagement of cell surface receptors and RNA sensing molecules leads to activation of signaling cascades including NFκB, JAK/STAT pathways, MAP kinases, and IRF7.[31,67,107,140,154,265,287] The net result of these actions is activation of viral sensing and antiviral effector pathways, interferons, and a variety of proinflammatory cytokines and chemokines (Table 1.1). Type I interferons inhibit RV replication by inducing multiple antiviral pathways, and also prime epithelial cell chemokine responses.[5,147] Interferon-γ has several effects on viral replication and inflammatory responses. It is a potent inducer of ICAM-1[145] and soluble ICAM-1.[272] IFN-γ also enhances the RV-induced secretion of chemokines such as CCL5.[145] RV-induced chemokines from epithelial cells and other sources attract a variety of cells into the airway, including dendritic cells, monocytes, macrophages, epithelial cells, and lymphocytes. The ensuing cellular response promotes antiviral effects and killing of infected cells, but interferon and cellular responses can also contribute to airway pathology and clinical symptoms.

Cellular Immune Responses

Macrophages are the principal cells in lower airway secretions, and these cells are important contributors to the innate antiviral response. Little to no replication of RV has been observed in airway macrophages or blood monocytes. As in epithelial cells, RVs activate NF-κB and STAT-1-dependent pathways in monocytes and macrophages.[96,146,156] Monocytes and macrophages are important sources of cytokines (e.g., TNF-α), chemokines (e.g., CXCL8, CXCL10, CCL2), and type I and type III interferons during RV infections.[96,137] Airway dendritic cells are interdigitated into the epithelium, and as major producers of type I interferons,[231,282] are likely to be important in orchestrating the early innate response to RV infection. Mononuclear cell secretion of IFN-α potentiates RV-induced epithelial cell chemokine secretion and antiviral responses.[147]

Neutrophils are the most numerous cells in airway secretions during an RV cold.[127,276] While neutrophilic inflammation correlates with respiratory symptoms, the role of these cells in the antiviral response is unclear. Following experimental RV inoculation, G-CSF is secreted into the nasal secretions within 24 hours, followed closely by increased in circulating G-CSF that could boost the production of neutrophil precursors in the bone marrow.[127] Neutrophils increase in the blood 1 to 2 days postinoculation and are then recruited to upper and lower airway secretions. The P2X$_7$ receptor is a cation channel expressed on epithelial cells and leukocytes that is activated after binding ATP and can, therefore, initiate inflammatory responses secondary to virus-induced cellular damage and other stimuli that release ATP. In volunteers who were experimentally inoculated with RV, P2X$_7$ pore activity measured in blood cells correlated with the influx of neutrophils into upper airway secretions during the acute cold.[54] In a mouse model, RV can activate neutrophils to release double-stranded RNA in neutrophil extracellular traps (NETosis).[249] The released DNA can modulate airway inflammation to promote type-2 responses, potentially adding to disease severity.

Lymphocyte numbers dip briefly in the blood during an acute cold and rise in nasal secretions, but to a lesser extent than neutrophils.[161,162] T-cell responses are critical for resolution of RV infections, as indicated by reports of prolonged and sometimes severe symptoms in immunosuppressed individuals or those with primary immune deficiencies.[117] T-cell responses can be directed at either serotype-specific or shared antigens.[6,186] Stimulation of peripheral blood mononuclear cells with peptide pools derived from RV capsids induces a broad-based immune response that is characterized by increased expression of genes for IL-1β TNF, IFNγ, and down-regulation of anti-inflammatory cytokine IL-10.[6] These responses may differ by species, as T memory responses to RV-A were more pronounced that those to RV-C *in vitro*. Experimental infection increases circulating cross-reactive T cells with a memory effector phenotype and T-helper-1 polarization during the acute infection.[186] There is some evidence that RV-specific T-cell responses preinfection could contribute to viral clearance[187] and milder clinical symptoms response,[199] suggesting a potential role for cross-reactive lymphocytes in the initial antiviral response. RV-specific epitopes for CD8+ T cells have recently been identified.[86]

Gene Expression and Metabolomics Studies

Several studies have evaluated how RV infections modify gene expression *in vivo* and in experimental models. Analysis of samples obtained during experimentally induced or natural infections have verified and extended the results of targeted analyses and demonstrate up-regulation of signaling molecules, antiviral pathways, chemokines, interferon-responsive genes, and other immunoregulatory genes.[214] Genetic variation influences RV-induced expression of multiple antiviral genes in peripheral blood mononuclear cells (PBMCs).[35] A few studies have compared responses of RVs to those of other respiratory viruses. Nasal cells from children hospitalized for acute respiratory illness demonstrated unique gene signatures for RSV versus RV.[284] Patterns of PBMC gene expression also differ by virus, and these patterns are distinct enough accurately identify the viral pathogen.[286] In cell lines, RV and influenza infections induce many overlapping responses.[141] Compared to influenza, RV infection induced a greater activation of cellular repair mechanisms, which could relate to the more benign clinical course of RV infections.

Gene expression studies have also tested how chronic diseases such as asthma influence RV-induced responses. Chronic airway inflammation is one of the hallmarks in asthma and type-2 inflammatory responses (e.g., IL-33, IL-4, IL-5) are most often predominant. The ratio of type-2 responses to type I interferon gene expression in nasal cells is related to the subsequent risk for a virus-induced wheezing illness.[4] During wheezing illnesses, several gene networks are induced that regulate ciliated epithelial cells, type I interferon, macrophage responses, and type 2 inflammation.[4] In cultured airway epithelial cells from patients with asthma and COPD, RV-induced antiviral responses were delayed.[260]

Role of Antibody

Experimental RV infections can induce antibody responses within 7 to 14 days. These responses can be either serotype-specific or cross-reactive[118] and epitopes may or may not be neutralizing. Whether RV species influence the quantity of antibody responses is uncertain. Compared to RV-A&B, children were reported to have lower antibody responses to recombinant VP1,[119] but an array that included representatives of all three species measured greater responses RV-C proteins and peptides.[192]

Both IgG and IgA responses to RV can be associated with protection from reinfection.[2,50,203] In addition, serial challenges with heterotypic viruses can sometimes also reduce frequency of infection to the second virus. This finding suggests either that some types can induce cross-neutralizing antibody or else there are other protective mechanisms not involving antibody.[74] Patterns of limited antibody-mediated cross-neutralization were demonstrated in studies using inoculation of rabbits.[45]

Release From Host and Mode of Transmission

The transmission of RV infections has been the subject of a number of creative and innovative studies. Dick and colleagues compared the RV transmission rates from experimentally infected donors to seronegative recipients under controlled conditions.[57] Some volunteers wore arm restraints or plastic collars designed to prevent hand to face contact;

rates of transmission were similar for these volunteers compared to those with no restraints. On the other hand, Gwaltney et al. found that contact with coffee cups or plastic tiles contaminated with wet secretions could transmit RV infections to volunteers who handled the fomites and then rubbed their eyes and nares with their fingertips.[77] In addition, transmission of RV can be inhibited by cleaning the hands with virucidal solutions or by the use of virucidal tissues when blowing the nose.[56] Notably, articles with dried secretions contain little virus and were not able to transmit colds. Collectively, these findings indicate that RV can be transmitted by either aerosol or fomites, and the predominant mode of transmission may depend on age, personal hygiene, and degree of viral shedding.

Virulence

While all rhinoviruses can cause asymptomatic infection or mild colds, RV-A and RV-C types are more likely than RV-B to be detected during lower respiratory illnesses. Age affects the relative contribution of RV-A versus RV-C to lower respiratory illnesses. RV-C infections are more often associated with bronchiolitis and other wheezing illnesses in infants and young children[8,40] and in children with asthma.[22] Compared to other RV species, RV-C infections in children with asthma are more often associated with hospitalization and readmission and are more frequently detected in children who require admission to an intensive care unit.[47,48] RV-C infections are also more likely than the other species to cause viremia in children.[168] In older children and adults with lower respiratory symptoms, RV-A is more commonly detected than RV-C.[289] Many different RV-A and RV-C types have been detected during acute wheezing illnesses or other lower respiratory illnesses, but the multitude of RV types has made it difficult to determine whether specific types are more virulent within a species.

Persistence

Several studies have observed that following acute RV infections, virus can sometimes be detected for weeks,[128,280] and this has led to speculation that RV might cause chronic infection. However, studies that have performed RV typing following either natural or experimentally induced infections document that most RV infections are cleared after 1 to 2 weeks.[173,194] Prolonged detection of RV is usually explained by serial infections with different RV types, and shedding of a singly inoculated viruses for 4 weeks or longer is a rare event in immune competent individuals.[130,173] In contrast, immunodeficient children and immunosuppressed adults can develop prolonged illnesses with shedding of the same RV type for months.[117,135]

RV is commonly detected in the absence of respiratory symptoms in young children (25% to 44%),[150,160,259] while rates of RV detection in asymptomatic adults are less than 5%.[289] In surveillance studies of infants, 10% to 20% of these "asymptomatic infections" reflect viral shedding following recovery from a cold or a prodromal period just before the onset of respiratory illness.[128] Studies that have performed serial sampling of respiratory secretions have found no evidence that RV can establish a "carrier state" characterized by persistent low-level viral shedding.[130,202] Immune responses to asymptomatic infections are muted.[105] These findings indicate that asymptomatic infections are common and need to be considered in epidemiologic studies linking infection to illness outcomes.

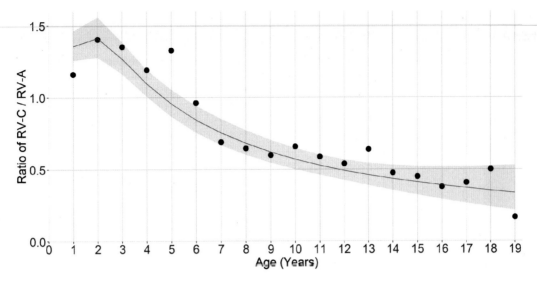

FIGURE 1.9 Age is strongly related to the relative prevalence of RVA versus RV-C illnesses. RV detection data from 14 different studies were pooled, and the type and species of RV was available for 6,613 specimens collected during illnesses. Individual points represent the RV-C to RV-A detection ratio for each year of age. The line and shaded area represent the logistic regression model fitted to the sample-level data and the associated 95% confidence intervals, respectively. (From Choi T, Devries M, Bacharier LB, et al. Enhanced neutralizing antibody responses to rhinovirus C and age-dependent patterns of infection. *Am J Respir Crit Care Med* 2021;203:822–830. Reprinted with permission of the American Thoracic Society. Copyright © 2021 American Thoracic Society. All rights reserved. The American Journal of Respiratory and Critical Care Medicine is an official journal of the American Thoracic Society.)

EPIDEMIOLOGY

Age

RV infections are most common in infants and young children. Infection rates are somewhat lower in the first 6 months of life, possibly due to transplacentally acquired neutralizing antibody, and then rates are relatively high throughout infancy and early childhood.[55,75,120] Age differentially affects infections with RV species; RV-C infections are more common until age 6 years, and then RV-A infections become increasingly predominant[40] (Fig. 1.9). Accordingly, in a large European study of adults with cough, RV-A types were most commonly detected.[289] Among young adults, infection rates are greater in mothers and women of similar age compared to men. In older adults, this relationship is reversed and illness rates are higher in men.[92]

Morbidity

RVs cause a broad spectrum of illness including asymptomatic infections, common colds and other upper respiratory illnesses, bronchitis and wheezing illnesses, and lower respiratory tract infections including bronchiolitis, bronchitis, wheezing, and pneumonia (Fig. 1.10). The wide range of illness suggests that in addition to species-related virulence, there are host and environment factors that contribute to the risk of more severe disease.

Host factors include extremes in age (infants, the elderly) and chronic respiratory diseases such as asthma,[134,191] chronic

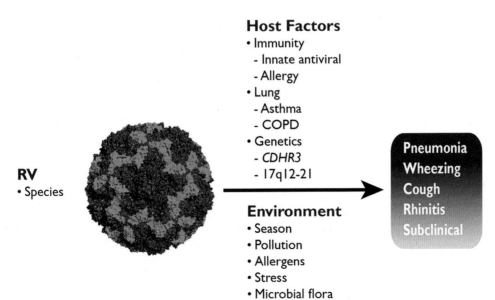

FIGURE 1.10 The spectrum of RV illness (see text).

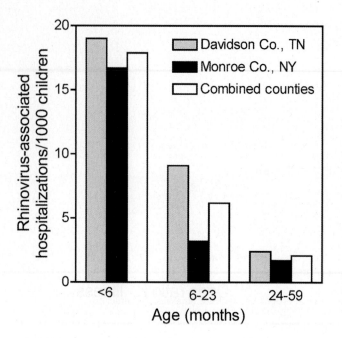

FIGURE 1.11 Age-related hospitalization rates for rhinovirus lower respiratory infection. (From Miller EK, Lu X, Erdman DD, et al. Rhinovirus-associated hospitalizations in young children. *J Infect Dis* 2007;195:773–781. Reproduced by permission of the Infectious Diseases Society of America.)

group and progressively diminished though age 6 years. RV is the second leading cause of bronchiolitis, and RV bronchiolitis has distinct features related to the airway microbiome, the mucosal immune response, and metabolites in airway secretions.[64,101,244] Among children, risk factors for RV wheezing illnesses in early life include reduced lung function,[258] asthma, and genetic polymorphisms. For example, genetic variation in MDA-5 has been associated with recurrent severe RV illnesses,[152] the 17q12-21 locus is associated with increased RV wheezing and asthma,[36] and a *CDHR3* SNP has been linked to increased risk of RV-C illnesses and recurrent wheezing.[29,30] In the elderly and in chronic care facilities, RV infections can cause influenza-like illnesses.[190,257]

RV infections have been closely linked to the inception and exacerbation of asthma (Fig. 1.12). While most infants who wheeze with respiratory viruses outgrow this tendency, a subset subsequently develop recurrent wheezing illnesses and asthma. Wheezing with RV infections during infancy and early childhood is one of the strongest indicators of risk for recurrent wheezing[53,160] and subsequent childhood asthma.[120,148] This relationship is strongest in children with allergic features such as airway or blood eosinophilia or allergen-specific IgE (allergic sensitization).[120,151]

In children and adults with established asthma, viral respiratory illnesses RV infections remain strongly associated with acute exacerbations of asthma. The relationship between RV infections and acute asthma is especially close in childhood. RV infection contributes to up to 85% of asthma exacerbations in children compared to about half of exacerbations in adults.[108,134,191] There is a remarkable similarity in the seasonal patterns of RV infections and exacerbations of asthma, especially in school-aged children for whom hospitalizations due to asthma have a strong fall and spring preponderance year after year.[132,133] As in preschoolers, the risk of acute wheeze is greatest for children and adults with the combination of RV infection

obstructive lung disease,[34,228] and cystic fibrosis.[139,239] Population-based hospitalization rates were calculated for children hospitalized in Rochester NY and Nashville TN (Fig. 1.11); one major children's hospital serves the population in each of these communities.[180] Hospitalization rates were highest (18 hospitalizations/1,000 children) for the 0- to 6-month age

Inception

Healthy Infant

RSV
RV
Other
viruses

↓ *Lung function*
Dysbiosis
Tobacco smoke

Wheezing illnesses

Resolution   Asthma

Exacerbation

Child or adult with asthma

RV
Influenza
Other
viruses

Allergy
↓ *Lung function*
Dysbiosis
Allergen exposure
Pollutants

Asthma exacerbations

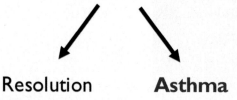

FIGURE 1.12 RV infections and asthma (see text).

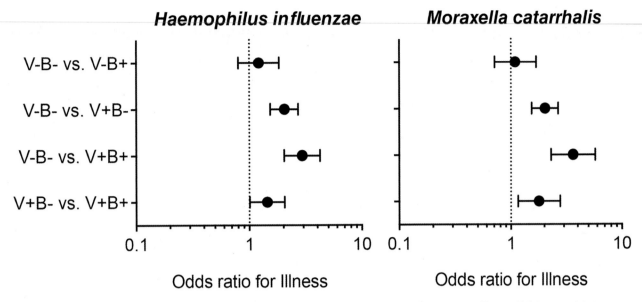

FIGURE 1.13 Detection of RV and bacterial pathogens both contribute to the risk of respiratory illness. Children provided weekly nasal mucus samples that were analyzed for RV and bacterial pathogens by PCR. The odds ratios represent the probability of experiencing illness symptoms according to patterns of pathogen detection. Each illness was matched with an asymptomatic period of the same length, and the probability of pathogen detection was compared. Abbreviations: V-, no virus detected; V+ RV detected; B-, no bacterial pathogen detected; B+ bacterial pathogen detected. (Graphs drawn from data in Bashir H, Grindle K, Vrtis R, et al. Association of rhinovirus species with common cold and asthma symptoms and bacterial pathogens. *J Allergy Clin Immunol* 2018;141:822–824 e829.)

and allergic features.[240] For allergic individuals, exposure to allergens further increases the risk of RV-induced wheeze.[189]

The strong association between RV infection, allergy, and wheeze was investigated in two studies of children with moderate to severe asthma who were treated with omalizumab, a monoclonal antibody that prevents circulating IgE from binding to its receptor, thus inhibiting IgE-mediated allergic responses. Treatment with omalizumab reduced the rates of acute virus-induced wheezing illnesses, most of which were associated with RV infection.[33,247] These findings were especially prominent during the spring and fall RV (and asthma exacerbation) seasons. Surveillance for RV and respiratory symptoms were conducted weekly throughout the trial and demonstrated that omalizumab reduced RV detection and symptomatic colds by about one-third. In addition, omalizumab increased blood mononuclear cell RV-induced interferon responses and reduced the peak and duration of viral shedding.[69,83] These findings are in agreement with experimental models that had identified reduced antiviral responses in study subjects with allergic asthma,[44,268] and in cultured cells from individuals with asthma.[83,138]

RV infections are associated with an increase in the prevalence of bacterial pathogens such as *Moraxella catarrhalis*, *Streptococcus pneumoniae*, and *Haemophilus influenzae*. Detection of bacterial pathogens together with RVs is a risk factor for respiratory illness (Fig. 1.13), and in children with asthma, acute exacerbations.[19,144] Notably, these bacterial pathogens are also associated with sinusitis, otitis media, bronchitis, pneumonia, and exacerbations of COPD. Thus, RV and bacterial pathogens may synergize to promote a variety of upper and lower respiratory illnesses.

Other risk factors for RV-induced wheezing include exposure to indoor or outdoor pollutants, and failure to use asthma control medications.[39,62,261] Psychosocial stress has also been related to the frequency and severity of natural and experimentally induced respiratory illnesses.[43,216] While spring and fall are the peak seasons for RV prevalence, RV is more likely to cause lower respiratory ill-

nesses in the winter.[159] Notably, vitamin D status has been shown to be associated with the prevalence of upper respiratory illnesses, although specific links to RV infections have not been established.[87] In patient with COPD, RV infections can promote long-lasting overgrowth of bacterial pathogens.[169]

Origin and Spread of RV Infections

In general, transmission of RV infections is relatively inefficient. Young children have the highest rates of RV illnesses and also appear to transmit infections most effectively. In family surveillance studies, transmission from children to other children and adults was much more common than transmission from adult to children or other adults.[136,202] Epidemics with RV are uncommon, although they have been reported to occur associated with "flu-like" illnesses in nursing homes.[70,109] Secondary attack rates within families vary between 30% and 70%.

Conditions that affect transmission of RV infections were identified in studies of experimentally inoculated RV "donors" and seronegative adult "recipients." Short-term (15 minutes to 3 hours) contact led to transmission rates of less than 10%, even in the presence of loud vocalization, card playing, and kissing.[50,93] Higher rates of transmission were observed among donor and recipients married couples (38% transmission rate),[49] and in a crowded research hut in Antarctica (88% to 100% transmission rate).[111] Transmission of natural colds in a more spacious Antarctic hut occurred at a relatively low rate (~1% per day among 200 inhabitants), and it was notable that transmission rates were similar among long-term residents and recent arrivals to the research station.[269] In clinical studies that reproduced the close contact of the studies in Antarctica, the best predictor of transmission of a cold from a donor to a seronegative recipient was the duration of exposure (Fig. 1.14).[178] In general, factors that promote transmission include young age, symptomatic illness, crowding, high-level viral shedding from the index case, and seronegativity of the recipient.[131,183]

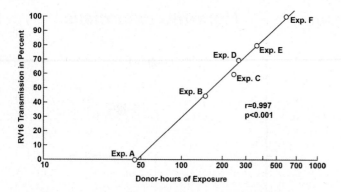

FIGURE 1.14 Relationship between the exposure and transmission of A16. A series of experiments (A-F) was conducted in which donors with severe experimentally induced colds (A16) were housed with seronegative recipients for varying lengths of time. The groups were housed in a clinical research unit from 5 to 79 hours, and samples of nasal lavage fluid were obtained for 10 days and analyzed for viral shedding. One donor-hour of exposure (DHE) was defined as exposure to one infected donor for an hour. There was a straight line relationship between the logarithm of DHE and the risk of RV transmission. (From Meschievitz CK, Schultz SB, Dick EC. A model for obtaining predictable natural transmission of rhinoviruses in human volunteers. *J Infect Dis* 1984;150(2):195–201. Reproduced by permission of Oxford University Press.)

Prevalence and Seroepidemiology

Epidemiologic studies of RV prevalence are best conducted with molecular diagnostics because of difficulties in culturing these viruses (especially the RV-C types). RV infections occur year round, with increased prevalence in the fall and spring in temperate climates,[75,182,279] while in tropical climates peak prevalence can occur during dry seasons[9,165] or infections can be distributed throughout the year.[8] The increased prevalence in the fall has led to speculation that school-based transmission among children may drive this trend.[133] This is supported by a RV surveillance study conducted in the United Kingdom during the COVID-19 pandemic.[207] The national lockdown was associated with a marked reduction in RV infections, and when the lockdown was eased, infection rates initially remained low. However, when children returned to school, RV detection in adults quickly rebounded to prepandemic levels. RV infections continue during the wintertime but account for less than 50% of infections during this period of time due to the plethora of other respiratory viruses found at this time of year. Overall, RV infections account for about half of common cold infections over the entire year, and more than 80% of infections during peak seasons in the spring and fall RV.

Over 20 types of RV can circulate within a community at any given period of time, and the composition of RV types in a single community changes almost completely from season to season and year to year.[181,194] Despite the complex and evanescent patterns of RV epidemiology, an international survey of RV detection over a 20-year time period suggests that some types have a consistently high prevalence (e.g., A78, C2) or a consistently low prevalence over time.[40] Some studies have reported species-specific patterns of RV seasonal prevalence,[179,194] but because the range of viruses differs markedly with season and location, additional data are needed to confirm these patterns.

Neutralizing antibody responses to RV have been measured in experimental inoculation studies[94,253] and in a limited number of natural infection studies. Serologic responses

to the RV-A&B serotypes can be detected in infants, and the number of serotypes to which antibodies are present increases throughout childhood and adolescence.[91,183] The prevalence of serotype-specific antibodies peaks in young adults (mean percent positive = 60% for RV-A&B types) and remains at 40% to 50% throughout adulthood. Type-specific antibody in the same individual can persist at relatively stable levels for several years.[246] More recently, neutralizing antibody responses to RV-C types have been measured using a PCR-based assay, since these viruses generally do not form plaques in cell lines.[40] Throughout childhood, neutralizing antibody responses to RV-C are more prevalent than responses to other RV species.[40] These findings suggest that RV-C–specific responses may be of greater magnitude or duration compared to other RV species.

Genetic Diversity of Virus

As might be predicted expected from the original RV typing system, much of the RV sequence diversity manifests as amino acid changes in capsid surface regions mapped as neutralizing immunogenic epitopes (Nims). Completion of the full cohort of RV-A&B sequences along with many RV-C identified extensive evidence for historic recombination among species clades.[196] Surprisingly, these recombinants did not exchange capsid regions. The most commonly trades included the 5′ UTR, primarily upstream of the IRES, or less frequently, fragments from P2 to P3 regions. Sequencing from multiple field isolates has confirmed this idea, showing the RV-A and RV-C frequently recombine, and when they do, they exchange not the expected capsid Nims, but 5′ UTR regions, including the pyrimidine-rich tracts, and their respective 2A protease genes.[114,176] It is not clear why evolution apparently favors these particular recombinants although strict adherence to spontaneous protomer assembly requirements may be involved. Alternatively, divergent recombinant protease specificities may help these viruses regulate the overall cell response to infection.

Picornavirus polymerases have a high error rate, estimated at 10^{-3} to 10^{-4} errors/nucleotide/cycle of replication. As a result, all RV genotypes exist as quasispecies populations. Analysis of 34 full RV sequences of prototype strains demonstrated that the RV genome as a whole is under purifying selective pressure, with focal areas of diversifying pressure at antigenic sites in the structural genes, and in the 3C protease and 3D polymerase.[142] Mutation rates have also been determined for A39 after experimental inoculation.[46] The calculated mutation rate after 5 days of replication *in vivo* was 3.4×10^{-4} mutations/nucleotides over the whole ORF, and specific hypervariable mutation sites were located within VP1, VP2, VP3, 2C, and 2C sequences.

CLINICAL FEATURES

Experimental inoculation studies have enabled detailed observations of the time course of clinical manifestations of RV infection.[23,49,57,178] Following inoculation with virus, the first signs of illness are usually sore or scratchy throat with an onset as soon as 16 hours postinoculation, followed by malaise and rhinitis. The first nasal symptoms are rhinorrhea, which usually begins with a watery discharge. During the peak of the cold, the discharge becomes mucoid or purulent and is accompanied by nasal congestion, cough, and headache. Low-grade fevers can occur in infected children and are uncommon among adults with RV infections. The latent period after infection is generally 1 to 2 days, and peak symptoms generally occur between 2 and 4 days following inoculation. Most colds are either over or are clearly subsiding within 1 week; cough and nasal symptoms that persist for 10 days or longer without improvement suggest either secondary bacterial sinusitis,[219] or else a second infection with a different virus.[130] Symptom patterns do not reliably differentiate RV illnesses from those caused from other viruses. Studies of adults indicate that RV may be more likely to present with sore throat, have prominent nasal symptoms in most individuals, and are less likely to be associated with fever.[12]

RV can also cause infections of the middle ear, sinuses, and lower airways. Eustation tube dysfunction occurs in about half of experimentally induced or naturally occurring RV infections.[174] Studies of natural colds also link detection of RVs in the nasal secretions or middle ear fluid to otitis media (OM).[41,224,274] A prospective 1-year study of the role of viral URI in OM enrolled 294 children between the ages of 6 months and 3 years, and the viruses most often detected were RV and adenoviruses (27% of OM for each virus).[41] Approximately one third of RV infections were complicated by acute OM, and another 20% of cases had asymptomatic middle ear effusions. Another longitudinal study prospectively sampled nasal secretions of 1- to 5-year-old children and siblings at the onset of either cold or otologic symptoms.[3] RV infection was detected at least once in 70% of the children, and 44% of these infections were associated with either OM with effusion or acute OM.

To investigate effects of RV on the paranasal sinuses, Gwaltney and colleagues performed sinus computerized tomography (CT) scans during the peak symptom period following experimental RV inoculation of 31 adults. During the acute cold, 27 subjects (87%) had swelling and or mucosal thickening and fluid collection in one or both of the maxillary sinuses.[95] A subset of the study subjects had repeat scans 2 weeks later, and these abnormalities had spontaneously subsided in 79%. Likewise, Puhakka et al. tracked findings on serial plain radiographs in individuals with naturally acquired common colds and found that 38% developed mucosal thickening and either air–fluid levels or opacification of the sinuses on day 7 of the cold.[215] These abnormalities resolved without treatment on follow-up films obtained on day 21. Whether sinusitis is caused by RV or a combination or RV plus bacteria has not been resolved, but an important clinical point is that the illness subsided without antibiotic treatment. In addition to being associated with acute sinusitis, RV infections are more common in patients with chronic rhinosinusitis.[18]

In infants, RV can cause bronchiolitis, which is a syndrome consisting of upper airway symptoms that progress to severe cough, wheezing, and tachypnea. In severe cases, significant air trapping and hypoventilation can lead to hypoxia and need for hospitalization for supportive care. RV is second only to RSV as a cause for bronchiolitis in infants.[37,129] In patients with chronic asthma, RV infections often begin with typical cold symptoms and then progress to asthma exacerbations that include severe cough, wheezing, shortness of breath, and in severe cases, hypoxia. Similar exacerbations of chronic respiratory symptoms also occur in patients with cystic fibrosis or COPD.[34,139]

DIAGNOSIS

Differential

RV infections cause respiratory symptoms that are quite similar to those caused by other respiratory viruses. Compared to influenza, RV is less likely to cause fever, myalgia, and headache. In general, signs and symptoms of rhinitis are prominent, but there are no true differentiating features. The spring and fall peaks in RV epidemiology follow the same general pattern as hay fever in many geographic locations. Differentiation of common cold and allergy symptoms can be difficult, but there are some differences in symptom profiles. Compared to respiratory allergies, RV infections are of shorter duration, are more likely to cause sore throat, and are less likely to cause nasal and ocular pruritus.

Laboratory

Virus isolation and identification. Tissue culture is a relatively insensitive method for RV detection. Fetal lung fibroblast cells (WI-38, MRC-5, and Wis.L cells) or RV-sensitive lines of HeLa cells are commonly used for RV detection. Notably, RV-C viruses cannot be cultured in standard cell lines, which lack the receptor to bind RV-C, but have been propagated in HeLa cells transduced to express CDHR3,[27] and in organ cultures or differentiated cultures of upper or lower airway epithelium.[13,26,99] While typing of RV-A&B species isolates is possible using specific antisera, these reagents are not available for RV-C. At present, molecular identification is generally used to identify RV species and type.[25,234]

RV detection is greatly improved through the use of RT-PCR[25] or other molecular techniques.[59,142] The 5′ untranslated region contains several highly conserved regions that are usually targeted for primer design (Fig. 1.15). The regions usually targeted for genotyping are the 5′UTR, VP2-4, or VP1. Sequences in the capsid protein coding region are more variable, which helps to distinguish genotypes but also complicates

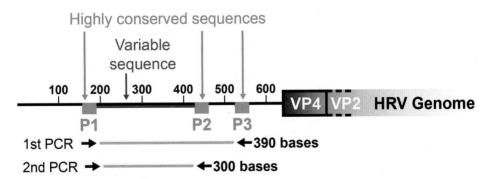

FIGURE 1.15 Selection of primers for PCR-based diagnostic tests for RV infection. The most conserved sites in the RV genome are in the 5′ untranslated region in the area of stem loop structures that bind ribosomal proteins. These sites are targeted for primer design (P1, P2, P3) that can be used for single or nested reverse-transcriptase PCR. (Figure courtesy of Wai Ming Lee [University of Wisconsin-Madison].)

the design of broadly applicable primers. Higher rates of success (close to 100%) have been achieved by targeting the 5′UTR.[158] Classification based on partial sequences must be considered as tentative, since recombination among RV can occur.[196]

Nasopharyngeal aspirates or nasal swabs are the best specimens for RV detection, and yields are lower from throat swabs.[242,266] A "nose-blow" technique has been used to obtain nasal secretions for clinical research protocols utilizing PCR-based diagnostics with good recovery rates.[103,194,209] Viral transport medium containing a protein source such as gelatin or albumin helps to stabilize the viral capsid for best results with tissue culture or molecular techniques. Nasal swabs obtained at home and mailed to the laboratory also provide specimens suitable for analysis by molecular techniques.[202,266]

PREVENTION AND CONTROL

The cure for the common cold remains enigmatic. Many approaches have been explored, including nutritional supplements, immune modulators, antiviral agents, and mediator antagonists to block specific common cold symptoms. Vitamin C has long been touted for common cold treatment; however, a meta-analysis of common cold treatment studies found no consistent effects on either preventing colds or reducing their duration.[106] A Cochrane review of clinical studies found evidence that zinc lozenges reduce common cold duration but have significant side effects including bad taste and nausea.[236] Topical zinc was marketed as a homeopathic treatment for colds but was taken off the market due to association with anosmia.[72] Large-scale trials of Echinacea have provided no evidence of efficacy.[15,252]

Medications targeting specific symptoms can be helpful in relieving some aspects of the common cold. Examples include use of decongestants and topical ipratropium for relief of congestion and rhinorrhea, respectively.[65] Vapor rub (petroleum jelly with aromatic oils) may relieve some common cold symptoms, perhaps by stimulation of ion channels.[200] Cough syrups are ineffective. Notably, marketing of combination cough and cold medications to children has been stopped by the FDA due to reports of toxicity with overdoses, and even a small number of children receiving standard doses of these medications. There is evidence that warm drinks, as recommended for generations, can provide symptomatic relief from malaise and nasal symptoms without troublesome side effects.[223]

Improved knowledge of RV molecular virology and host responses has led to several attempts to develop antivirals. Interferon-α has antiviral effects *in vitro* and shortens the duration and severity of colds, but topical application led to nasal irritation and bleeding.[71,102] Soluble ICAM-1 prevents binding of major group viruses to their receptor,[172] and recombinant CDHR3 subproteins inhibit RV-C binding and replication.[271] Capsid binding agents that bind to the VP1 pocket and inhibit viral binding and/or uncoating have shown modest antiviral effects and efficacy in clinical trials.[103] RV-C are resistant to capsid binding agents because their VP1 pocket is inaccessible,[21] which may account for the modest efficacy of these antivirals against natural RV infections. An inhibitor to the 3C protease (rupintrivir) also showed broad anti-RV (including RV-C) activity *in vitro* and modest efficacy in clinical trials.[99,104] Unfortunately, these antiviral approaches have not so far led to development of a clinically useful medication.

The molecules tested to date have been limited by combinations of modest efficacy, side effects, and/or drug interactions.[251] New molecular approaches are being investigated, such as the development of DNAzymes to cleave conserved regions of the RV genome.[208]

One limitation to RV-specific antiviral approaches is that many respiratory viruses contribute to respiratory morbidity in children and other high-risk individuals. To meet this challenge, treatments are being developed to boost mucosal immune responses to enhance broad resistance to viral pathogens. These approaches include oral or topical administration of bacterial extracts or other TLR agonists that prime mucosal antiviral responses.[238] Another potential approach to improve mucosal antiviral responses is to reduce allergic inflammation, which can inhibit virus-induced interferon production.[69,83] Finally, there is evidence that the balance of commensal to pathogenic bacteria in airway secretions is related to the probability and severity of RV illness,[144,171] raising hopes that manipulation of the airway microbiota with either probiotics or prebiotics could enhance resistance to viral respiratory illnesses.

Once considered implausible due to the plethora of RV types, there is renewed interest in developing vaccines targeting RV.[177] One strategy for vaccine development is based on identification of conserved B-cell epitopes that are shared among different RV types and species.[66,85,118] These epitopes can elicit cross-neutralizing immune responses. However, so far cross-protection has been limited. Similar efforts are underway to determine whether shared T-cell epitopes could induce cross-protection against multiple viruses.[186] Finally, a prototype multiplex vaccine containing 50 different RV-A types induced protective antibody responses to 49 of the included viruses in mice and macaques.[157] The ceiling for the number of antigens is unknown, but even after excluding the nonvirulent RV-B types, this approach still faces major immunologic and logistical challenges given the approximately 140 RV-A and RV-C types.

PERSPECTIVE

The development of molecular diagnostic tests for RV has led to a better appreciation of their role in respiratory illnesses, especially with respect to lower respiratory illness in young children and patients with chronic lung diseases. Findings from recent studies underscore the ubiquitous nature of RV infections and at the same time have led to some caution in interpretation of RV detection during illnesses due to high rates of asymptomatic illness. That RV is linked to a full spectrum of respiratory illness also raises questions about the nature of factors that modify illness severity. Identification of environmental and personal determinants of illness severity could provide new preventive strategies, and this is especially important for high-risk populations.

Another revelation for common cold researchers was the discovery of the RV-C species in 2006. After a hiatus of almost 20 years following the cataloguing of what most virologists considered to be the final RV serotypes, clinical studies utilizing molecular diagnostics led to the discovery of more than 70 additional RV types. There is growing evidence that RV-C viruses may be more likely than other species to cause lower respiratory illness in infants and children, and acute exacerbations of asthma.

The cure for the common cold remains elusive. After some initial failures took the wind out of the sails of these efforts, the recognition that RV infections are an important cause of lower respiratory illnesses has generated renewed interest in RV antivirals. Recent advances in understanding the molecular pathogenesis of RV illnesses, including RV-C, provide renewed optimism that this goal will be achieved. Finally, social distancing during the COVID-19 pandemic led to a dramatic reduction in RV-related illnesses,[245] and understanding the mechanisms of this phenomenon could lead to some practical recommendations to prevent RV transmission to susceptible individuals.

REFERENCES

1. A collaborative report: rhinoviruses—extension of the numbering system. *Virology* 1971;43:524–526.
2. Alper CM, Doyle WJ, Skoner DP, et al. Prechallenge antibodies: moderators of infection rate, signs, and symptoms in adults experimentally challenged with rhinovirus type 39. *Laryngoscope* 1996;106:1298–1305.
3. Alper CM, Winther B, Mandel EM, et al. Rate of concurrent otitis media in upper respiratory tract infections with specific viruses. *Arch Otolaryngol Head Neck Surg* 2009;135:17–21.
4. Altman MC, Gill MA, Whalen E, et al. Transcriptome networks identify mechanisms of viral and nonviral asthma exacerbations in children. *Nat Immunol* 2019;20:637–651.
5. Amineva SP, Aminev AG, Palmenberg AC, et al. Rhinovirus 3C protease precursors 3CD and 3CD' localize to the nuclei of infected cells. *J Gen Virol* 2004;85:2969–2979.
6. Anderson D, Jones AC, Gaido CM, et al. Differential gene expression of lymphocytes stimulated with rhinovirus A and C in children with asthma. *Am J Respir Crit Care Med* 2020;202:202–209.
7. Andries K, Dewindt B, Snoeks J, et al. Two groups of rhinoviruses revealed by a panel of antiviral compounds present sequence divergence and differential pathogenicity. *J Virol* 1990;64:1117–1123.
8. Annamalay AA, Jroundi I, Bizzintino J, et al. Rhinovirus C is associated with wheezing and rhinovirus A is associated with pneumonia in hospitalized children in Morocco. *J Med Virol* 2016;89(4):582–588. doi: 10.1002/jmv.24684.
9. Annamalay AA, Lanaspa M, Khoo SK, et al. Rhinovirus species and clinical features in children hospitalised with pneumonia from Mozambique. *Trop Med Int Health* 2016;21:1171–1180.
10. Arruda E, Boyle TR, Winther B, et al. Localization of human rhinovirus replication in the upper respiratory tract by in situ hybridization. *J Infect Dis* 1995;171:1329–1333.
11. Arruda E, Mifflia TE, Gwaltney JMJ, et al. Localization of rhinovirus replication in vitro with in situ hybridization. *J Med Virol* 1991;54:634–638.
12. Arruda E, Pitkaranta A, Witek TJJ, et al. Frequency and natural history of rhinovirus infections in adults during autumn. *J Clin Microbiol* 1997;35:2864–2868.
13. Ashraf S, Brockman-Schneider R, Bochkov YA, et al. Biological characteristics and propagation of human rhinovirus-C in differentiated sinus epithelial cells. *Virology* 2013;436:143–149.
14. Atzl I, Helms R. Common cold. In: *A Short History of the Common Cold.* Basel, Switzerland: Birkhauser Verlag; 2009.
15. Barrett B, Brown R, Rakel D, et al. Echinacea for treating the common cold: a randomized trial. *Ann Intern Med* 2010;153:769–777.
16. Barrett B, Brown R, Voland R, et al. Relations among questionnaire and laboratory measures of rhinovirus infection. *Eur Respir J* 2006;28:357–363.
17. Bartlett NW, Walton RP, Edwards MR, et al. Mouse models of rhinovirus-induced disease and exacerbation of allergic airway inflammation. *Nat Med* 2008;14:199–204.
18. Basharat U, Aiche MM, Kim MM, et al. Are rhinoviruses implicated in the pathogenesis of sinusitis and chronic rhinosinusitis exacerbations? A comprehensive review. *Int Forum Allergy Rhinol* 2019;9:1159–1188.
19. Bashir H, Grindle K, Vrtis R, et al. Association of rhinovirus species with common cold and asthma symptoms and bacterial pathogens. *J Allergy Clin Immunol* 2018;141:822–824 e829.
20. Basnet S, Bochkov YA, Brockman-Schneider RA, et al. CDHR3 asthma-risk genotype affects susceptibility of airway epithelium to rhinovirus C infections. *Am J Respir Cell Mol Biol* 2019;61(4):450–458. doi: 10.1165/rcmb.2018-0220OC.
21. Basta HA, Ashraf S, Sgro JY, et al. Modeling of the human rhinovirus C capsid suggests possible causes for antiviral drug resistance. *Virology* 2014;448:82–90.
22. Bizzintino J, Lee WM, Laing IA, et al. Association between human rhinovirus C and severity of acute asthma in children. *Eur Respir J* 2011;37:1037–1042.
23. Blair HT, Greenberg SB, Stevens PM, et al. Effects of rhinovirus infection on pulmonary function of healthy human volunteers. *Am Rev Respir Dis* 1976;114:95–102.
24. Bochkov YA, Gern JE. Clinical and molecular features of human rhinovirus C. *Microbes Infect* 2012;14:485–494.
25. Bochkov YA, Grindle K, Vang F, et al. Improved molecular typing assay for rhinovirus species A, B, and C. *J Clin Microbiol* 2014;52:2461–2471.
26. Bochkov YA, Palmenberg AC, Lee WM, et al. Molecular modeling, organ culture and reverse genetics for the emerging respiratory pathogen human rhinovirus C. *Nat Med* 2011;17:627–632.
27. Bochkov YA, Watters K, Ashraf S, et al. Cadherin-related family member 3, a childhood asthma susceptibility gene product, mediates rhinovirus C binding and replication. *Proc Natl Acad Sci U S A* 2015;112:5485–5490.
28. Bochkov YA, Watters KE, Basnet S, et al. Mutations in VP1 and 3A proteins improve binding and replication of rhinovirus C15 in HeLa-E8 cells. *Virol J* 2016;499:350–360.
29. Bonnelykke K, Coleman AT, Evans MD, et al. Cadherin-related family member 3 genetics and rhinovirus C respiratory illnesses. *Am J Respir Crit Care Med* 2018;197:589–594.
30. Bonnelykke K, Sleiman P, Nielsen K, et al. A genome-wide association study identifies CDHR3 as a susceptibility locus for early childhood asthma with severe exacerbations. *Nat Genet* 2014;46:51–55.
31. Bosco A, Wiehler S, Proud D. Interferon regulatory factor 7 regulates airway epithelial cell responses to human rhinovirus infection. *BMC Genomics* 2016;17:76.
32. Brockman-Schneider RA, Amineva SP, Bulat MV, et al. Nasal and otologic effects of experimental respiratory syncytial virus infection in adults. *Am J Otolaryngol* 2002;23:70–75.
33. Busse WW, Morgan WJ, Gergen PJ, et al. Randomized trial of omalizumab (anti-IgE) for asthma in inner-city children. *N Engl J Med* 2011;364:1005–1015.
34. Cafferkey J, Coultas JA, Mallia P. Human rhinovirus infection and COPD: role in exacerbations and potential for therapeutic targets. *Expert Rev Respir Med* 2020;14:777–789.
35. Caliskan M, Baker SW, Gilad Y, et al. Host genetic variation influences gene expression response to rhinovirus infection. *PLoS Genet* 2015;11:e1005111.
36. Caliskan M, Bochkov YA, Kreiner-Moller E, et al. Rhinovirus wheezing illness and genetic risk of childhood-onset asthma. *N Engl J Med* 2013;368:1398–1407.
37. Calvo C, Pozo F, García-García ML, et al. Detection of new respiratory viruses in hospitalized infants with bronchiolitis: a thee year prospective study. *Acta Paediatr* 2010;99:883–887.
38. Chantzi FM, Papadopoulos NG, Bairamis T, et al. Human rhinoviruses in otitis media with effusion. *Pediatr Allergy Immunol* 2006;17:514–518.
39. Chauhan AJ, Inskip HM, Linaker CH, et al. Personal exposure to nitrogen dioxide (NO2) and the severity of virus-induced asthma in children. *Lancet* 2003;361:1939–1944.
40. Choi T, Devries M, Bacharier LB, et al. Enhanced neutralizing antibody responses to rhinovirus C and age-dependent patterns of infection. *Am J Respir Crit Care Med* 2021;203:822–830.
41. Chonmaitree T, Revai K, Grady JJ, et al. Viral upper respiratory tract infection and otitis media complication in young children. *Clin Infect Dis* 2008;46:815–823.
42. Christiansen SC, Eddleston J, Bengtson SH, et al. Experimental rhinovirus infection increases human tissue kallikrein activation in allergic subjects. *Int Arch Allergy Immunol* 2008;147:299–304.
43. Cohen S. Psychological stress and susceptibility to upper respiratory infections. *Am J Respir Crit Care Med* 1995;152:s53–s58.
44. Contoli M, Message SD, Laza-Stanca V, et al. Role of deficient type III interferon-lambda production in asthma exacerbations. *Nat Med* 2006;12:1023–1026.
45. Cooney MK, Kenny GE, Tam R, et al. Cross relationships among 37 rhinoviruses demonstrated by virus neutralization with potent monotypic rabbit antisera. *Infect Immun* 1973;7:335–340.
46. Cordey S, Junier T, Gerlach D, et al. Rhinovirus genome evolution during experimental human infection. *PLoS One* 2010;5:e10588.
47. Cox DW, Bizzintino J, Ferrari G, et al. Human rhinovirus species C infection in young children with acute wheeze is associated with increased acute respiratory hospital admissions. *Am J Respir Crit Care Med* 2013;188:1358–1364.
48. Cox DW, Khoo SK, Zhang G, et al. Rhinovirus is the most common virus and rhinovirus-C is the most common species in paediatric intensive care respiratory admissions. *Eur Respir J* 2018;52:1800207.
49. D'Alessio DJ, Meschievitz CK, Peterson JA, et al. Transmission of experimental rhinovirus colds in volunteer married couples. *J Infect Dis* 1976;133:28–36.
50. D'Alessio DJ, Meschievitz CK, Peterson JA, et al. Short-duration exposure and the transmission of rhinoviral colds. *J Infect Dis* 1984;150:189–194.
51. De SD, Dagher H, Ghildyal R, et al. Vascular endothelial growth factor induction by rhinovirus infection. *J Med Virol* 2006;78:666–672.
52. de Gouw HW, Grünberg K, Schot R, et al. Relationship between exhaled nitric oxide and airway hyperresponsiveness following experimental rhinovirus infection in asthmatic subjects. *Eur Respir J* 1998;11:126–132.
53. de Winter JJ, Bont L, Wilbrink B, et al. Rhinovirus wheezing illness in infancy is associated with medically attended third year wheezing in low risk infants: results of a healthy birth cohort study. *Immun Inflamm Dis* 2015;3:398–405.
54. Denlinger LC, Shi L, Guadarrama A, et al. Attenuated P2X7 pore function as a risk factor for virus-induced loss of asthma control. *Am J Respir Crit Care Med* 2009;179:265–270.
55. Dick EC, Blumer CR, Evans AS. Epidemiology of infections with rhinoviruses type 43 and 5 in a group of University of Wisconsin student families. *Am J Epidemiol* 1967;86:386–400.
56. Dick EC, Hossain SU, Mink KA, et al. Interruption of transmission of rhinovirus colds among human volunteers using virucidal paper handkerchiefs. *J Infect Dis* 1986;153:352–356.
57. Dick EC, Jennings LC, Mink KA, et al. Aerosol transmission of rhinovirus colds. *J Infect Dis* 1987;156:442–448.
58. Dochez AR, Shibley GS, Mills KC. Studies in the common cold : IV. Experimental transmission of the comon cold to anthropoid apes and human beings by means of a filtrable agent. *J Exp Med* 1930;52:701–716.
59. Dominguez SR, Briese T, Palacios G, et al. Multiplex MassTag-PCR for respiratory pathogens in pediatric nasopharyngeal washes negative by conventional diagnostic testing shows a high prevalence of viruses belonging to a newly recognized rhinovirus clade. *J Clin Virol* 2008;43:219–222.
60. Dosanjh A. Transforming growth factor-beta expression induced by rhinovirus infection in respiratory epithelial cells. *Acta Biochim Biophys Sin (Shanghai)* 2006;38:911–914.
61. Douglas RCJ, Couch RB, Lindgren KM. Cold doesn't affect the "common cold" in study of rhinovirus infections. *JAMA* 1967;199:29–30.
62. Duff AL, Pomeranz ES, Gelber LE, et al. Risk factors for acute wheezing in infants in infants and children: viruses, passive smoke, and IgE antibodies to inhalant allergens. *Pediatrics* 1993;93:535–540.
63. Duits LA, Nibbering PH, van Strijen E, et al. Rhinovirus increases human beta-defensin-2 and -3 mRNA expression in cultured bronchial epithelial cells. *FEMS Immunol Med Microbiol* 2003;38:59–64.
64. Dumas O, Mansbach JM, Jartti T, et al. A clustering approach to identify severe bronchiolitis profiles in children. *Thorax* 2016;71:712–718.
65. Eccles R, Eriksson M, Garreffa S, et al. The nasal decongestant effect of xylometazoline in the common cold. *Am J Rhinol* 2008;22:491–496.

66. Edlmayr J, Niespodziana K, Popow-Kraupp T, et al. Antibodies induced with recombinant VP1 from human rhinovirus exhibit cross-neutralisation. *Eur Respir J* 2011;37:44–52.

67. Edwards MR, Hewson CA, Laza-Stanca V, et al. Protein kinase R, IKB kinase-beta and NF-KB are required for human rhinovirus induced pro-inflammatory cytokine production in bronchial epithelial cells. *Mol Immunol* 2007;44:1587–1597.

68. Eggleston PA, Hendley JO, Gwaltney JMJ. Mediators of immediate hypersensitivity in nasal secretions during natural colds and rhinovirus infection. *Acta Otolaryngol Suppl* 1984;413:25–35.

69. Esquivel A, Busse WW, Calatroni A, et al. Effects of omalizumab on rhinovirus infections, illnesses, and exacerbations of asthma. *Am J Respir Crit Care Med* 2017;196:985–992.

70. Falsey AR, Treanor JJ, Betts RF, et al. Viral respiratory infections in the institutionalized elderly: clinical and epidemiologic findings. *J Am Geriatr Soc* 1992;40:115–119.

71. Farr BM, Gwaltney JMJ, Adams KF, et al. Intranasal interferon-alpha 2 for prevention of natural rhinovirus colds. *Antimicrob Agents Chemother* 1984;26:31–34.

72. Food and Drug Administration, US Department of Health and Human Services. Drug Products Labeled as Homeopathic: Guidance for FDA Staff and Industry (Revision 1). October 2019. https://www.fda.gov/media/131978/download.

73. Ferguson EA, Eccles R. Changes in nasal nitric oxide concentration associated with symptoms of common cold and treatment with a topical nasal decongestant. *Acta Otolaryngol* 1997;117:614–617.

74. Fleet WF, Couch RB, Cate TR, et al. Homologous and heterologous resistance to rhinovirus common cold. *Am J Epidemiol* 1965;82:185–196.

75. Fox JP, Cooney MK, Hall CE, et al. Rhinoviruses in Seattle families, 1975-1979. *Am J Epidemiol* 1985;122:830–846.

76. Foxman EF, Storer JA, Vanaja K, et al. Two interferon-independent double-stranded RNA-induced host defense strategies suppress the common cold virus at warm temperature. *Proc Natl Acad Sci U S A* 2016;113:8496–8501.

77. Gama RE, Horsnell PR, Hughes PJ, et al. Amplification of rhinovirus specific nucleic acids from clinical samples using the polymerase chain reaction. *J Med Virol* 1989;28:73–77.

78. Gentile DA, Fireman P, Skoner DP. Elevations of local leukotriene C4 levels during viral upper respiratory tract infections. *Ann Allergy Asthma Immunol* 2003;91:270–274.

79. Gern JE, Dick EC, Kelly EAB, et al. Rhinovirus-specific T cells recognize both shared and serotype-restricted viral epitopes. *J Infect Dis* 1997;175:1108–1114.

80. Gern JE, Galagan DM, Jarjour NN, et al. Detection of rhinovirus RNA in lower airway cells during experimentally-induced infection. *Am J Respir Crit Care Med* 1997;155:1159–1161.

81. Gern JE, Vrtis RF, Grindle KA, et al. Relationship of upper and lower airway cytokines to outcome of experimental rhinovirus infection. *Am J Respir Crit Care Med* 2000;162:2226–2231.

82. Ghildyal R, Dagher H, Donninger H, et al. Rhinovirus infects primary human airway fibroblasts and induces a neutrophil chemokine and a permeability factor. *J Med Virol* 2005;75:608–615.

83. Gill MA, Liu AH, Calatroni A, et al. Enhanced plasmacytoid dendritic cell antiviral responses after omalizumab. *J Allergy Clin Immunol* 2018;141:1735–1743 e1739.

84. Ginde AA, Mansbach JM, Camargo CAJ. Association between serum 25-hydroxyvitamin D level and upper respiratory tract infection in the Third National Health and Nutrition Examination Survey. *Arch Intern Med* 2009;169:384–390.

85. Glanville N, McLean GR, Guy B, et al. Cross-serotype immunity induced by immunization with a conserved rhinovirus capsid protein. *PLoS Pathog* 2013;9:e1003669.

86. Gomez-Perosanz M, Sanchez-Trincado JL, Fernandez-Arquero M, et al. Human rhinovirus-specific CD8 T cell responses target conserved and unusual epitopes. *FASEB J* 2021;35:e21208.

87. Green RM, Cusotvic A, Sanderson G, et al. Synergism between allergens and viruses and risk of hospital admission with asthma: case-control study. *Br Med J* 2002;324:763.

88. Greve JM, Davis G, Meyer AM, et al. The major human rhinovirus receptor is ICAM-1. *Cell* 1989;56:839–847.

89. Griggs TF, Bochkov YA, Basnet S, et al. Rhinovirus C targets ciliated airway epithelial cells. *Respir Res* 2017;18:84.

90. Griggs TF, Bochkov YA, Nakagome K, et al. Production, purification, and capsid stability of rhinovirus C types. *J Virol Methods* 2015;217:18–23.

91. Gwaltney JM Jr, Hendley JO. Transmission of experimental rhinovirus infection by contaminated surfaces. *Am J Epidemiol* 1982;116:828–833.

92. Gwaltney JM Jr, Hendley JO, Simon G, et al. Rhinovirus infections in an industrial population. I. The occurrence of illness. *N Engl J Med* 1966;275:1261–1268.

93. Gwaltney JM Jr, Moskalski PB, Hendley JO. Hand-to-hand transmission of rhinovirus colds. *Ann Intern Med* 1978;88:463–467.

94. Gwaltney JM Jr, Park J, Paul RA, et al. Randomized controlled trial of clemastine fumarate for treatment of experimental rhinovirus colds. *Clin Infect Dis* 1996;22:656–662.

95. Gwaltney JM Jr, Phillips CD, Miller RD, et al. Computed tomographic study of the common cold. *N Engl J Med* 1994;330:25–30.

96. Hall DJ, Bates ME, Guar L, et al. The role of p38 MAPK in rhinovirus-induced monocyte chemoattractant protein-1 production by monocytic-lineage cells. *J Immunol* 2005;174:8056–8063.

97. Hamparian VV, Colonno RJ, Cooney MK, et al. A collaborative report: rhinoviruses-extension of the numbering system from 89 to 100. *Virology* 1987;159:191–192.

98. Handzel ZT, Busse WW, Sedgwick JB, et al. Eosinophils bind rhinovirus and activate virus-specific T cells. *J Immunol* 1998;160:1279–1284.

99. Hao W, Bernard K, Patel N, et al. Infection and propagation of human rhinovirus C in human airway epithelial cells. *J Virol* 2012;86:13524–13532.

100. Harris JR, Racaniello VR. Changes in rhinovirus protein 2C allow efficient replication in mouse cells. *J Virol* 2003;77:4773–4780.

101. Hasegawa K, Perez-Losada M, Hoptay CE, et al. RSV vs. rhinovirus bronchiolitis: difference in nasal airway microRNA profiles and NFkappaB signaling. *Pediatr Res* 2018;83:606–614.

102. Hayden FG, Albrecht JK, Kaiser DL, et al. Revention of natural colds by contact prophylaxis with intranasal alpha2-interferon. *N Engl J Med* 1986;314:71–75.

103. Hayden FG, Herrington DT, Coats TL, et al. Efficacy and safety of oral pleconaril for treatment of colds due to picornaviruses in adults: results of 2 double-blind, randomized, placebo-controlled trials. *Clin Infect Dis* 2003;36:1523–1532.

104. Hayden FG, Turner RB, Gwaltney JM, et al. Phase II, randomized, double-blind, placebo-controlled studies of ruprintrivir nasal spray 2-percent suspension for prevention and treatment of experimentally induced rhinovirus colds in healthy volunteers. *Antimicrob Agents Chemother* 2003;47:3907–3916.

105. Heinonen S, Jartti T, Garcia C, et al. Rhinovirus detection in symptomatic and asymptomatic children: value of hosttranscriptome analysis. *Am J Respir Crit Care Med* 2016;193:772–782.

106. Hemila H, Chalker E. Vitamin C for preventing and treating the common cold. *Cochrane Database Syst Rev* 2013;2013(1):CD000980. 10.1002/14651858.CD000980.pub4.

107. Hewson CA, Haas JJ, Bartlett NW, et al. Rhinovirus induces MUC5AC in a human infection model and in vitro via NF-KB and EGFR pathways. *Eur Respir J* 2010;36:1425–1435.

108. Heymann PW, Carper HT, Murphy DD, et al. Viral infections in relation to age, atopy, and season of admission among children hospitalized for wheezing. *J Allergy Clin Immunol* 2004;114:239–247.

109. Hicks LA, Shepard CW, Britz PH, et al. Two outbreaks of severe respiratory disease in nursing homes associated with rhinovirus. *J Am Geriatr Soc* 2006;54:284–289.

110. Holgate ST. Epithelium dysfunction in asthma. *J Allergy Clin Immunol* 2007;120:1233–1244.

111. Holmes MJ, Reed SE, Stott EJ, et al. Studies of experimental rhinovirus type 2 infections in polar isolation and in England. *J Hyg (Lond)* 1976;76:379–393.

112. Hong JY, Chung Y, Steenrod J, et al. Macrophage activation state determines the response to rhinovirus infection in a mouse model of allergic asthma. *Respir Res* 2014;15:63.

113. Horn MEC, Reed SE, Taylor P. Role of viruses and bacteria in acute wheezy bronchitis in childhood: a study of sputum. *Arch Dis Child* 1979;54:587–592.

114. Huang T, Wang W, Bessaud M, et al. Evidence of recombination and genetic diversity in human rhinoviruses in children with acute respiratory infection. *PLoS One* 2009;4:e6355.

115. Huguenel ED, Cohn D, Dockum DP, et al. Prevention of rhinovirus infection in chimpanzees by soluble intercellular adhesion molecule-1. *Am J Respir Crit Care Med* 1997;155:1206–1210.

116. Igarashi Y, Skoner DP, Doyle WJ, et al. Analysis of nasal secretions during experimental rhinovirus upper respiratory infections. *J Allergy Clin Immunol* 1993;92:722–731.

117. Ison MG, Hayden FG, Kaiser L, et al. Rhinovirus infections in hematopoietic stem cell transplant recipients with pneumonia. *Clin Infect Dis* 2003;36:1139–1143.

118. Iwasaki J, Smith WA, Stone SR, et al. Species-specific and cross-reactive IgG1 antibody binding to viral capsid protein 1 (VP1) antigens of human rhinovirus species A, B and C. *PLoS One* 2013;8:e70552.

119. Iwasaki J, Smith WA, Khoo SK, et al. Comparison of rhinovirus antibody titers in children with asthma exacerbations and species-specific rhinovirus infection. *J Allergy Clin Immunol* 2014;134:25–32.

120. Jackson DJ, Gangnon RE, Evans MD, et al. Wheezing rhinovirus illnesses in early life predict asthma development in high-risk children. *Am J Respir Crit Care Med* 2008;178:667–672.

121. Jackson RJ. A comparative view of initiation site selection mechanisms. In: Hershey JWB, Matthews MB, Sonenberg N, eds. *Translational Control*. New York: Cold Spring Harbor Laboratory Press; 1996:71–112.

122. Jain S, Self WH, Wunderink RG, et al.; CDC EPIC Study Team. Community-acquired pneumonia requiring hospitalization. *N Engl J Med* 2015;373:2382.

123. Jain S, Williams DJ, Arnold SR, et al.; CDC EPIC Study Team. Community-acquired pneumonia requiring hospitalization among U.S. children. *N Engl J Med* 2015;372:835–845.

124. Jakiela B, Brockman-Schneider RA, Amineva SP, et al. Basal cells of differentiated bronchial epithelium are more susceptible to rhinovirus infection. *Am J Respir Cell Mol Biol* 2008;38:517–523.

125. Jakiela B, Gielicz A, Plutecka H, et al. Th2-type cytokine-induced mucus metaplasia decreases susceptibility of human bronchial epithelium to rhinovirus infection. *Am J Respir Cell Mol Biol* 2014;51:229–241.

126. Jamieson KC, Wiehler S, Michi AN, et al. Rhinovirus induces basolateral release of IL-17C in highly differentiated airway epithelial cells. *Front Cell Infect Microbiol* 2020;10:103.

127. Jarjour NN, Gern JE, Kelly EAB, et al. The effect of an experimental rhinovirus 16 infection on bronchial lavage neutrophils. *J Allergy Clin Immunol* 2000;105:1169–1177.

128. Jartti T, Lehtinen P, Vuorinen T, et al. Persistence of rhinovirus and enterovirus RNA after acute respiratory illness in children. *J Med Virol* 2004;72:695–699.

129. Jartti T, Lehtinen P, Vuorinen T, et al. Respiratory picornaviruses and respiratory syncytial virus as causative agents of acute expiratory wheezing in children. *Emerg Infect Dis* 2004;10:1095–1101.

130. Jartti T, Lee WM, Pappas T, et al. Serial viral infections in infants with recurrent respiratory illnesses. *Eur Respir J* 2008;32:314–320.

131. Jennings LC, Dick EC. Transmission and control of rhinovirus colds. *Eur J Epidemiol* 1987;3:327–335.

132. Johnston NW, Johnston SL, Duncan JM, et al. The September epidemic of asthma exacerbations in children: a search for etiology. *J Allergy Clin Immunol* 2005;115:132–138.

133. Johnston NW, Johnston SL, Norman GR, et al. The September epidemic of asthma hospitalization: school children as disease vectors. *J Allergy Clin Immunol* 2006;117:557–562.

134. Johnston SL, Pattemore PK, Sanderson G, et al. Community study of role of viral infections in exacerbations of asthma in 9-11 year old children. *BMJ* 1995;310:1225–1229.

135. Kainulainen L, Vuorinen T, Rantakokko-Jalava K, et al. Recurrent and persistent respiratory tract viral infections in patients with primary hypogammaglobulinemia. *J Allergy Clin Immunol* 2010;126:120–126.

136. Kamau E, Onyango CO, Otieno GP, et al. An intensive, active surveillance reveals continuous invasion and high diversity of rhinovirus in households. *J Infect Dis* 2019;219:1049–1057.

137. Khaitov MR, Laza-Stanca V, Edwards MR, et al. Respiratory virus induction of alpha-, beta- and lambda-interferons in bronchial epithelial cells and peripheral blood mononuclear cells. *Allergy* 2009;64:375–386.

138. Kicic A, Stevens PT, Sutanto EN, et al. Impaired airway epithelial cell responses from children with asthma to rhinoviral infection. *Clin Exp Allergy* 2016;46:1441–1455.

139. Kiedrowski MR, Bomberger JM. Viral-bacterial co-infections in the cystic fibrosis respiratory tract. *Front Immunol* 2018;9:3067.
140. Kim J, Sanders SP, Siekierski ES, et al. Role of NF-KB in cytokine production induced from human airway epithelial cells by rhinovirus infection. *J Immunol* 2000;165: 3384–3392.
141. Kim TK, Bheda-Malge A, Lin Y, et al. A systems approach to understanding human rhinovirus and influenza virus infection. *Virology* 2015;486:146–157.
142. Kistler AL, Webster DR, Rouskin S, et al. Genome-wide diversity and selective pressure in the human rhinovirus. *Virol J* 2007;4:40.
143. Kloepfer KM, DeMore JP, Vrtis RF, et al. Effects of montelukast on patients with asthma after experimental inoculation with human rhinovirus 16. *Ann Allergy Asthma Immunol* 2011;106:252–257.
144. Kloepfer KM, Lee WM, Pappas TE, et al. Detection of pathogenic bacteria during rhinovirus infection is associated with increased respiratory symptoms and asthma exacerbations. *J Allergy Clin Immunol* 2014;133:1301–1307 e1303.
145. Konno S, Grindle KA, Lee WM, et al. Interferon-γ enhances rhinovirus-induced RANTES secretion in human airway epithelial cells. *Am J Respir Cell Mol Biol* 2002;26:594–601.
146. Korpi-Steiner NL, Bates ME, Lee WM, et al. Human rhinovirus induces robust IP-10 release by monocytic cells, which is independent of viral replication but linked to type I interferon receptor ligation and STAT1 activation. *J Leukoc Biol* 2006;80:1364–1374.
147. Korpi-Steiner NL, Valkenaar SM, Bates ME, et al. Human monocytic cells direct the robust release of CXCL10 by bronchial epithelial cells during rhinovirus infection. *Clin Exp Allergy* 2010;40:1203–1213.
148. Kotaniemi-Syrjanen A, Vainionpaa R, Reijonen TM, et al. Rhinovirus-induced wheezing in infancy the first sign of childhood asthma? J Allergy Clin Immunol 2003;111:66–71.
149. Kruse W. The etiology of cough and nasal catarrh. *MMW Munch Med Wochenschr* 1914;61:1574.
150. Kusel MM, de Klerk NH, Holt PG, et al. Role of respiratory viruses in acute upper and lower respiratory tract illness in the first year of life: a birth cohort study. *Pediatr Infect Dis J* 2006;119:680–686.
151. Kusel MM, de Klerk NH, Kebadze T, et al. Early-life respiratory viral infections, atopic sensitization, and risk of subsequent development of persistent asthma. *J Allergy Clin Immunol* 2007;119:1105–1110.
152. Lamborn IT, Jing H, Zhang Y, et al. Recurrent rhinovirus infections in a child with inherited MDA5 deficiency. *J Exp Med* 2017;214:1949–1972.
153. Lane Starr NM, Evans MD, Lee KE, et al. Ensemble analysis identifies nasal 15-keto-PGE2 as a predictor of recovery in experimental rhinovirus colds. *J Infect Dis* 2021;224(5): 839–849. doi: 10.1093/infdis/jiab015.
154. Lau C, Wang X, Song L, et al. Syk associates with clathrin and mediates phosphatidylinositol 3-kinase activation during human rhinovirus internalization. *J Immunol* 2008;180:870–880.
155. Lau SK, Yip CC, Tsoi HW, et al. Clinical features and complete genome characterization of a distinct human rhinovirus (HRV) genetic cluster, probably representing a previously undetected HRV species, HRV-C, associated with acute respiratory illness in children. *J Clin Microbiol* 2007;45:3655–3664.
156. Laza-Stanca V, Stanciu LA, Message SD, et al. Rhinovirus replication in human macrophages induces NF-KB-dependent tumor necrosis factor alpha production. *J Virol* 2006;80:8248–8258.
157. Lee S, Nguyen MT, Currier MG, et al. A polyvalent inactivated rhinovirus vaccine is broadly immunogenic in rhesus macaques. *Nat Commun* 2016;7:12838.
158. Lee WM, Kiesner C, Pappas T, et al. A diverse group of previously unrecognized human rhinoviruses are common causes of respiratory illnesses in infants. *PLoS One* 2007;2:e966.
159. Lee WM, Lemanske RF Jr, Evans MD, et al. Human rhinovirus species and season of infection determine illness severity. *Am J Respir Crit Care Med* 2012;186:886–891.
160. Lemanske RFJ, Jackson DJ, Gangnon RE, et al. Rhinovirus illnesses during infancy predict subsequent childhood wheezing. *J Allergy Clin Immunol* 2005;116:571–577.
161. Levandowski RA, Ou DW, Jackson GG. Acute-phase decrease of T lymphocyte subsets in rhinovirus infection. *J Infect Dis* 1986;153:743–748.
162. Levandowski RA, Pachucki CT, Rubenis M. Specific mononuclear cell response to rhinovirus. *J Infect Dis* 1983;148:1125.
163. Liu Y, Hill M, Klose T, et al. Atomic structure of a rhinovirus C, a virus linked to severe childhood asthma. *Proc Natl Acad Sci U S A* 2016;113:8997–9002.
164. Looi K, Buckley AG, Rigby PJ, et al. Effects of human rhinovirus on epithelial barrier integrity and function in children with asthma. *Clin Exp Allergy* 2018;48:513–524.
165. Lopes GP, Amorim IPS, Melo BO, et al. Identification and seasonality of rhinovirus and respiratory syncytial virus in asthmatic children in tropical climate. *Biosci Rep* 2020;40:BSR20200634.
166. Lopez-Souza N, Dolganov G, Dubin R, et al. Resistance of differentiated human airway epithelium to infection by rhinovirus. *Am J Physiol Lung Cell Mol Physiol* 2004;286:L373–L381.
167. Lopez-Souza N, Favoreto S, Wong H, et al. In vitro susceptibility to rhinovirus infection is greater for bronchial than for nasal airway epithelial cells in human subjects. *J Allergy Clin Immunol* 2009;123:1384–1390.
168. Lu X, Schneider E, Jain S, et al. Rhinovirus viremia inpatients hospitalized with community-acquired pneumonia. *J Infect Dis* 2017;216:1104–1111.
169. Mallia P, Footitt J, Sotero R, et al. Rhinovirus infection induces degradation of antimicrobial peptides and secondary bacterial infection in chronic obstructive pulmonary disease. *Am J Respir Crit Care Med* 2012;186:1117–1124.
170. Malmstrom K, Pitkaranta A, Carpen O, et al. Human rhinovirus in bronchial epithelium of infants with recurrent respiratory symptoms. *J Allergy Clin Immunol* 2006;118: 591–596.
171. Mansbach JM, Luna PN, Shaw CA, et al. Increased Moraxella and Streptococcus species abundance after severe bronchiolitis is associated with recurrent wheezing. *J Allergy Clin Immunol* 2020;145:518–527 e518.
172. Marlin SD, Staunton DE, Springer TA, et al. A soluble form of intercellular adhesion molecule-1 inhibits rhinovirus infection. *Nature* 1990;344:70–72.
173. Martin ET, Kuypers J, Chu HY, et al. Heterotypic infection and spread of rhinovirus A, B, and C among childcare attendees. *J Infect Dis* 2018;218:848–855.
174. McBride TP, Doyle WJ, Hayden FG, et al. Alterations of the eustachian tube, middle ear, and nose in rhinovirus infection. *Arch Otolaryngol Head Neck Surg* 1989;115:1054–1059.
175. McFadden ERJ, Pichurko BM, Bowman HF, et al. Thermal mapping of the airways in humans. *J Appl Physiol* 1985;58:564–570.
176. McIntyre CL, McWilliam Leitch EC, Savolainen-Kopra C, et al. Analysis of genetic diversity and sites of recombination in human rhinovirus species C. *J Virol* 2010;84: 10297–10310.
177. McLean GR. Vaccine strategies to induce broadly protective immunity to rhinoviruses. *Hum Vaccin Immunother* 2020;16:684–686.
178. Meschievitz CK, Schultz SB, Dick EC. A model for obtaining predictable natural transmission of rhinoviruses in human volunteers. *J Infect Dis* 1984;150:195–201.
179. Miller EK, Edwards KM, Weinberg GA, et al. A novel group of rhinoviruses is associated with asthma hospitalizations. *J Allergy Clin Immunol* 2009;123:98–104.
180. Miller EK, Lu X, Erdman DD, et al. Rhinovirus-associated hospitalizations in young children. *J Infect Dis* 2007;195:773–781.
181. Monto AS, Bryan ER, Ohmit S. Rhinovirus infections in Tecumseh, Michigan: Frequency of illness and number of serotypes. *J Infect Dis* 1987;156:43–49.
182. Monto AS, Cavallaro JJ. The Tecumseh study of respiratory illness. IV. Prevalence of rhinovirus serotypes, 1966-1969. *Am J Epidemiol* 1972;96:352–360.
183. Monto AS, Johnson KM. A community study of respiratory infections in the tropics. II. The spread of six rhinovirus isolates within the community. *Am J Epidemiol* 1968;88: 55–68.
184. Mosser AG, Brockman-Schneider RA, Amineva SP, et al. Similar frequency of rhinovirus-infectable cells in upper and lower airway epithelium. *J Infect Dis* 2002;185:734–743.
185. Mosser AG, Vrtis RF, Burchell L, et al. Quantitative and qualitative analysis of rhinovirus infection in bronchial tissues. *Am J Respir Crit Care Med* 2005;171:645–651.
186. Muehling LM, Mai DT, Kwok WW, et al. Circulating memory CD4+ T cells target conserved epitopes of rhinovirus capsid proteins and respond rapidly to experimental infection in humans. *J Immunol* 2016;197:3214–3224.
187. Muehling LM, Turner RB, Brown KB, et al. Single-cell tracking reveals a role for pre-existing CCR5+ memory Th1 cells in the control of rhinovirus-A39 after experimental challenge in humans. *J Infect Dis* 2018;217:381–392.
188. Muether PS, Gwaltney JMJ. Variant effect of first- and second-generation antihistamines as clues to their mechanism of action on the sneeze reflex in the common cold. *Clin Infect Dis* 2001;33:1438–1488.
189. Murray CS, Poletti G, Kebadze T, et al. Study of modifiable risk factors for asthma exacerbations: virus infection and allergen exposure increase the risk of asthma hospital admissions in children. *Thorax* 2006;61:376–382.
190. Nicholson KG, Kent J, Hammersley V, et al. Risk factors for lower respiratory complications of rhinovirus infections in elderly people living in the community: prospective cohort study. *BMJ* 1996;313:1119–1123.
191. Nicholson KG, Kent J, Ireland DC. Respiratory viruses and exacerbations of asthma in adults. *BMJ* 1993;307:982–986.
192. Niespodziana K, Stenberg-Hammar K, Megremis S, et al. PreDicta chip-based high resolution diagnosis of rhinovirus-induced wheeze. *Nat Commun* 2018;9:2382.
193. O'Neill MB, Laval G, Texeria JC, et al. Genetic susceptibility to severe childhood asthma and rhinovirus-C maintained by balancing selection in humans for 150,000 years. *Hum Mol Genet* 2020;29:736–744.
194. Olenec JP, Kim WK, Lee WM, et al. Weekly monitoring of children with asthma for infections and illness during common cold seasons. *J Allergy Clin Immunol* 2010;125:1001–1006.
195. Palmenberg AC, Rathe JA, Liggett SB. Analysis of the complete genome sequences of human rhinovirus. *J Allergy Clin Immunol* 2010;125:1190–1199.
196. Palmenberg AC, Spiro D, Kuzmickas R, et al. Sequencing and analyses of all known human rhinovirus genomes reveals structure and evolution. *Science* 2009;324:55–59.
197. Papadopoulos NG, Bates PJ, Bardin PG, et al. Rhinoviruses infect the lower airways. *J Infect Dis* 2000;181:1875–1884.
198. Papadopoulos NG, Sanderson G, Hunter J, et al. Rhinoviruses replicate effectively at lower airway temperatures. *J Med Virol* 1999;58:100–104.
199. Parry DE, Busse WW, Sukow KA, et al. Rhinovirus-induced peripheral blood mononuclear cell responses and outcome of experimental infection in allergic subjects. *J Allergy Clin Immunol* 2000;105:692–698.
200. Paul IM, Beiler JS, King TS, et al. Vapor rub, petrolatum, and no treatment for children with nocturnal cough and cold symptoms. *Pediatrics* 2010;126:1092–1099.
201. Pelon W, Mogabgab WJ, Phillips IA, et al. A cytopathogenic agent isolated from naval recruits with mild respiratory illnesses. *Proc Soc Exp Biol Med* 1957;94:262–267.
202. Peltola V, Waris M, Osterback R, et al. Rhinovirus transmission within families with children: incidence of symptomatic and asymptomatic infections. *J Infect Dis* 2008;197:382–389.
203. Perkins JC, Tucker DN, Knopf HL, et al. Comparison of protective effect of neutralizing antibody in serum and nasal secretions in experimental rhinovirus type 13 illness. *Am J Epidemiol* 1969;90:519–526.
204. Piralla A, Rovida F, Campanini G, et al. Clinical severity and molecular typing of human rhinovirus C strains during a fall outbreak affecting hospitalized patients. *J Clin Virol* 2009;45:311–317.
205. Pitkaranta A, Arruda E, Malmberg H, et al. Detection of rhinovirus in sinus brushings of patients with acute community-acquired sinusitis by reverse transcription-PCR. *J Clin Microbiol* 1997;35:1791–1793.
206. Pitkaranta A, Puhakka T, Makela MJ, et al. Detection of rhinovirus RNA in middle turbinate of patients with common colds by in situ hybridization. *J Med Virol* 2003;70: 319–323.
207. Poole S, Brendish NJ, Tanner AR, et al. Physical distancing in schools for SARS-CoV-2 and the resurgence of rhinovirus. *Lancet Respir Med* 2020;8:e92-e93.
208. Potaczek DP, Unger SD, Zhang N, et al. Development and characterization of DNAzyme candidates demonstrating significant efficiency against human rhinoviruses. *J Allergy Clin Immunol* 2019;143:1403–1415.

209. Powell KR, Shorr R, Cherry JD, et al. Improved method for collection of nasal mucus. *J Infect Dis* 1977;136:109–111.

210. Price WH. The isolation of a new virus associated with respiratory clinical disease in humans. *Proc Natl Acad Sci U S A* 1956;42:892–896.

211. Proud D, Gwaltney JMJ, Hendley JO, et al. Increased levels of interleukin-1 are detected in nasal secretions of volunteers during experimental rhinovirus colds. *J Infect Dis* 1994;169:1007–1013.

212. Proud D, Naclerio RM, Gwaltney JM, et al. Kinins are generated in nasal secretions during natural rhinovirus colds. *J Infect Dis* 1990;161:120–123.

213. Proud D, Sanders SP, Wiehler S. Human rhinovirus infection induces airway epithelial cell production of human beta-defensin 2 both in vitro and in vivo. *J Immunol* 2004;172:4637–4645.

214. Proud D, Turner RB, Winther B, et al. Gene expression profiles during *in vivo* human rhinovirus infection: insights into the host response. *Am J Respir Crit Care Med* 2008;178:962–968.

215. Puhakka T, Makela MJ, Alanen A, et al. Sinusitis in the common cold. *J Allergy Clin Immunol* 1998;102:304–408.

216. Ramratnam S, Lockhart A, Visness CM, et al.; Inner City Asthma Consortium. Maternal stress and depression are associated with respiratory phenotypes in urban children. *J Allergy Clin Immunol* 2021;148(1):120–127. 10.1016/j.jaci.2021.03.005.

217. Rankl C, Kienberger F, Wildling L, et al. Multiple receptors involved in human rhinovirus attachment to live cells. *Proc Natl Acad Sci U S A* 2008;105:17778–17783.

218. Rhinoviruses: a numbering system. *Nature* 1967;213:761–762.

219. Rosenfeld RM, Piccirillo JF, Chandrasekhar SS, et al. Clinical practice guideline (update): adult sinusitis. *Otolaryngol Head Neck Surg* 2015;152:S1–S39.

220. Roulin PS, Lötzerich M, Torta F, et al. Rhinovirus uses a phosphatidylinositol 4-phosphate/cholesterol counter-current for the formation of replication compartments at the ER-golgi interface. *Cell Host Microbe* 2014;16:677–690.

221. Sajjan US, Wang Q, Zhao Y, et al. Rhinovirus disrupts the barrier function of polarized airway epithelial cells. *Am J Respir Crit Care Med* 2008;178:1271–1281.

222. Sanders SP, Siekierski ES, Porter JD, et al. Nitric oxide inhibits rhinovirus-induced cytokine production and viral replication in a human respiratory epithelial cell line. *J Virol* 1998;72:934–942.

223. Sanu A, Eccles R. The effects of a hot drink on nasal airflow and symptoms of common cold and flu. *Rhinology* 2008;46:271–275.

224. Savolainen-Kopra C, Blomqvist S, Kilpi T, et al. Novel species of human rhinoviruses in acute otitis media. *Pediatr Infect Dis J* 2009;28:59–61.

225. Savolainen C, Blomqvist S, Mulders MN, et al. Genetic clustering of all 102 human rhinovirus prototype strains: serotype 87 is close to human enterovirus 70. *J Gen Virol* 2002;83:333–340.

226. Scully EJ, Basnet S, Wrangham RW, et al. Lethal respiratory epidemic in wild chimpanzees associated with human rhinovirus C. *Emerg Infect Dis* 2018;24:267–274.

227. Sedgwick JB, Menon I, Gern JE, et al. Effects of inflammatory cytokines on the permeability of human lung microvascular endothelial cell monolayers and differential eosinophil transmigration. *J Allergy Clin Immunol* 2002;110:752–756.

228. Seemungal T, Harper-Owen R, Bhowmik A, et al. Respiratory viruses, symptoms, and inflammatory markers in acute exacerbations and stable chronic obstructive pulmonary disease. *Am J Respir Crit Care Med* 2001;164:1618–1623.

229. Sheppard D, Rizk NW, Boushey HA, et al. Mechanism of cough and bronchoconstriction induced by distilled water aerosol. *Am Rev Respir Dis* 1983;127:691–694.

230. Sherry B, Mosser AG, Colonno RJ, et al. Use of monoclonal antibodies to identify four neutralization immunogens on a common cold picornavirus, human rhinovirus 14. *J Virol* 1985;57:246–257.

231. Siegal FP, Kadowaki N, Shodell M, et al. The nature of the principal type 1 interferon-producing cells in human blood. *Science* 1999;284:1835–1837.

232. Silkoff PE, Flavin S, Gordon R, et al. Toll-like receptor 3 blockade in rhinovirus-induced experimental asthma exacerbations: a randomized controlled study. *J Allergy Clin Immunol* 2018;141:1220–1230.

233. Simmonds P, Gorbalenya AE, Harvala H, et al. Recommendations for the nomenclature of enteroviruses and rhinoviruses. *Arch Virol* 2020;165:793–797.

234. Simmonds P, McIntyre CL, Savolainen-Kopra C, et al. Proposals for the classification of human rhinovirus species C into genotypically assigned types. *J Gen Virol* 2010;91:2409–2419.

235. Simons E, Schroth MK, Gern JE. Analysis of tracheal secretions for rhinovirus during natural colds. *Pediatr Allergy Immunol* 2005;16:276–278.

236. Singh M, Das RR. Zinc for the common cold. *Cochrane Database Syst Rev* 2013;(6):CD001364.

237. Slater L, Bartlett NW, Haas JJ, et al. Co-ordinated role of TLR3, RIG-I and MDA5 in the innate response to rhinovirus in bronchial epithelium. *PLoS Pathog* 2010;6:e1001178.

238. Sly PD, Galbraith S, Islam Z, et al. Primary prevention of severe lower respiratory illnesses in at-risk infants using the immunomodulator OM-85. *J Allergy Clin Immunol* 2019;144:870–872 e811.

239. Smyth AR, Smyth RL, Tong CYW, et al. Effect of respiratory virus infections including rhinovirus on clinical status in cystic fibrosis. *Arch Dis Child* 1995;73:117–120.

240. Soto-Quiros M, Avila L, Platts-Mills TA, et al. High titers of IgE antibody to dust mite allergen and risk for wheezing among asthmatic children infected with rhinovirus. *J Allergy Clin Immunol* 2012;129:1499–1505 e1495.

241. Spurrell JC, Wiehler S, Zaheer RS, et al. Human airway epithelial cells produce IP-10 (CXCL10) in vitro and in vivo upon rhinovirus infection. *Am J Physiol Lung Cell Mol Physiol* 2005;289:L85–L95.

242. Spyridaki IS, Christodoulou I, de Beer L, et al. Comparison of four nasal sampling methods for the detection of viral pathogens by RT-PCR-A GA(2)LEN project. *J Virol Methods* 2009;156:102–106.

243. Steil BP, Barton DJ. Cis-active RNA elements (CREs) and picornavirus RNA replication. *Virus Res* 2009;139:240–252.

244. Stewart CJ, Hasegawa K, Wong MC, et al. Respiratory syncytial virus and rhinovirus bronchiolitis are associated with distinct metabolic pathways. *J Infect Dis* 2018;217:1160–1169.

245. Taquechel K, Diwadkar AR, Sayed S, et al. Pediatric asthma health care utilization, viral Testing, and air pollution changes during the COVID-19 pandemic. *J Allergy Clin Immunol Pract* 2020;8:3378–3387 e3311.

246. Taylor-Robinson D. Studies on some viruses (rhinoviruses) isolated from common colds. *Arch Gesamte Virusforsch* 1963;13:281–293.

247. Teach SJ, Gill MA, Togias A, et al. Pre-seasonal treatment with either omalizumab an inhaled corticosteroid boost to prevent fall asthma exacerbations. *J Allergy Clin Immunol* 2015;136:1476–1485.

248. Teran LM, Johnston SL, Schroder JM, et al. Role of nasal interleukin-8 in neutrophil recruitment and activation in children with virus-induced asthma. *Am J Respir Crit Care Med* 1997;155:1362–1366.

249. Toussaint M, Jackson DJ, Swieboda D, et al. Host DNA released by NETosis promotes rhinovirus-induced type-2 allergic asthma exacerbation. *Nat Med* 2017;23:681–691.

250. Triantafilou K, Vakakis E, Richer EA, et al. Human rhinovirus recognition in non-immune cells is mediated by Toll-like receptors and MDA-5, which trigger a synergetic pro-inflammatory immune response. *Virulence* 2011;2:22–29.

251. Turner RB. New considerations in the treatment and prevention of rhinovirus infections. *Pediatr Ann* 2005;34:53–57.

252. Turner RB, Bauer R, Woelkart K, et al. An evaluation of *Echinacea angustifolia* in experimental rhinovirus infections. *N Engl J Med* 2005;353:341–348.

253. Turner RB, Dutko FJ, Goldstein NH, et al. Efficacy of oral WIN 54954 for prophylaxis of experimental rhinovirus infection. *Antimicrob Agents Chemother* 1993;37:297–300.

254. Turner RB, Weingand KW, Yeh CH, et al. Association between interleukin-8 concentration in nasal secretions and severity of symptoms of experimental rhinovirus colds. *Clin Infect Dis* 1998;26:840–846.

255. Tuthill TJ, Papadopoulos NG, Jourdan P, et al. Mouse respiratory epithelial cells support efficient replication of human rhinovirus. *J Gen Virol* 2003;84:2829–2836.

256. Tyrrell DA. The common cold—my favourite infection. The eighteenth Majority Stephenson memorial lecture. *J Gen Virol* 1987;68:2053–2061.

257. van Beek J, Veenhoven RH, Bruin JP, et al. Influenza-like illness incidence is not reduced by influenza vaccination in a cohort of older adults, despite effectively reducing laboratory-confirmed influenza virus infections. *J Infect Dis* 2017;216:415–424.

258. van der Zalm MM, Uiterwaal CS, Wilbrink B, et al. The influence of neonatal lung function on rhinovirus-associated wheeze. *Am J Respir Crit Care Med* 2011;183:262–267.

259. van der Zalm MM, van Ewijk BE, Wilbrink B, et al. Respiratory pathogens in children with and without respiratory symptoms. *J Pediatr* 2009;154:396–400.

260. Veerati PC, Troy NM, Reid AT, et al. Airway epithelial cell immunity is delayed during rhinovirus infection in asthma and COPD. *Front Immunol* 2020;11:974.

261. Venarske DL, Busse WW, Griffin MR, et al. The relationship of rhinovirus-associated asthma hospitalizations with inhaled corticosteroids and smoking. *J Infect Dis* 2006;193:1536–1543.

262. Vlasak M, Goesler I, Blaas D. Human rhinovirus type 89 variants use heparan sulfate proteoglycan for cell attachment. *J Virol* 2005;79:5963–5970.

263. Vlasak M, Roivainen M, Reithmayer M, et al. The minor receptor group of human rhinovirus (HRV) includes HRV23 and HRV25, but the presence of a lysine in the VP1 HI loop is not sufficient for receptor binding. *J Virol* 2005;79:7389–7395.

264. Wang Q, Nagarkar DR, Bowman ER, et al. Role of double-stranded RNA pattern recognition receptors in rhinovirus-induced airway epithelial cell responses. *J Immunol* 2009;183:6989–6997.

265. Wang X, Lau C, Wiehler S, et al. Syk is downstream of intercellular adhesion molecule-1 and mediates human rhinovirus activation of p38 MAPK in airway epithelial cells. *J Immunol* 2006;177:6859–6870.

266. Waris M, Osterback R, Lahti E, et al. Comparison of sampling methods for the detection of human rhinovirus RNA. *J Clin Virol* 2013;58:200–204.

267. Wark PA, Bucchieri F, Johnston SL, et al. IFN-gamma-induced protein 10 is a novel biomarker of rhinovirus-induced asthma exacerbations. *J Allergy Clin Immunol* 2007;120:586–593.

268. Wark PA, Johnston SL, Bucchieri F, et al. Asthmatic bronchial epithelial cells have a deficient innate immune response to infection with rhinovirus. *J Exp Med* 2005;201:937–947.

269. Warshauer DM, Dick EC, Mandel AD, et al. Rhinovirus infections in an isolated Antarctic station: Transmission of the viruses and susceptibility of the population. *Am J Epidemiol* 1989;129:319–340.

270. Watters K, Inankur B, Gardiner JC, et al. Differential disruption of nucleocytoplasmic trafficking pathways by rhinovirus 2A proteases. *J Virol* 2017;91:e02472-02416.

271. Watters K, Palmenberg AC. CDHR3 extracellular domains EC1-3 mediate rhinovirus C interaction with cells and as recombinant derivatives, are inhibitory to virus infection. *PLoS Pathog* 2018;14:e1007477.

272. Whiteman SC, Spiteri MA. IFN-gamma regulation of ICAM-1 receptors in bronchial epithelial cells: soluble ICAM-1 release inhibits human rhinovirus infection. *J Inflamm (Lond)* 2008;5:8.

273. Widegren H, Andersson M, Borgeat P, et al. LTB4 increases nasal neutrophil activity and conditions neutrophils to exert antiviral effects. *Respir Med* 2011;105:9971006.

274. Winther B, Alper CM, Mandel EM, et al. Temporal relationships between colds, upper respiratory viruses detected by polymerase chain reaction, and otitis media in young children followed through a typical cold season. *Pediatrics* 2007;119:1069–1075.

275. Winther B, Brofeldt S, Christensen B, et al. Light and scanning electron microscopy of nasal biopsy material from patients with naturally acquired common colds. *Acta Otolaryngol* 1984;97:309–318.

276. Winther B, Farr BM, Thoner RB, et al. Histopathologic examination and enumeration of polymorphonuclear leukocytes in the nasal mucosa during experimental rhinovirus colds. *Acta Otolaryngol Suppl* 1984;413:19–24.

277. Winther B, Greve JM, Gwaltney JMJ, et al. Surface expression of intercellular adhesion molecule 1 on epithelial cells in the human adenoid. *J Infect Dis* 1997;176:523–525.

278. Winther B, Gwaltney JMJ, Mygind M, et al. Sites of rhinovirus recovery after point inoculation of the upper airway. *JAMA* 1986;256:1763–1767.

279. Winther B, Hayden FG, Hendley JO. Picornavirus infections in children diagnosed by RT-PCR during longitudinal surveillance with weekly sampling: Association with symptomatic illness and effect of season. *J Med Virol* 2006;78:644–650.

280. Wood LG, Powell H, Grissell TV, et al. Persistence of rhinovirus RNA and IP-10 gene expression after acute asthma. *Respirology* 2011;16:291–299.

281. Xatzipsalti M, Kyrana S, Tsolia M, et al. Rhinovirus viremia in children with respiratory infections. *Am J Respir Crit Care Med* 2005;172:1037–1040.

282. Xi Y, Troy NM, Anderson D, et al. Critical role of plasmacytoid dendritic cells in regulating gene expression and innate immune responses to human rhinovirus-16. *Front Immunol* 2017;8:1351.

283. Yin FH, Lomax NB. Establishment of a mouse model for human rhinovirus infection. *J Gen Virol* 1986;67:2335–2340.

284. Yu J, Peterson DR, Baran AM, et al. Host gene expression in nose and blood for the diagnosis of viral respiratory infection. *J Infect Dis* 2019;219:1151–1161.

285. Yuta A, Doyle WJ, Gaumond E, et al. Rhinovirus infection induces mucus hypersecretion. *Am J Physiol Lung Cell Mol Physiol* 1998;274:L1017–L1023.

286. Zaas AK, Chen M, Varkey J, et al. Gene expression signatures diagnose influenza and other symptomatic respiratory viral infections in humans. *Cell Host Microbe* 2009;6:207–217.

287. Zaheer RS, Proud D. Human rhinovirus-induced epithelial production of CXCL10 is dependent upon IFN regulatory factor-1. *Am J Respir Cell Mol Biol* 2010;43:413–421.

288. Zhu J, Message SD, Qiu Y, et al. Airway inflammation and illness severity in response to experimental rhinovirus infection in asthma. *Chest* 2014;145:1219–1229.

289. Zlateva KT, van Rijn AL, Simmonds P, et al.; GRACE Study Group. Molecular epidemiology and clinical impact of rhinovirus infections in adults during three epidemic seasons in 11 European countries (2007-2010). *Thorax* 2020;75:882–890.

Hepatoviruses

Stanley M. Lemon

History
Hepatovirus Classification and Diversity
Genome Structure
   Genome Organization
   5′ UTR Structure and Function
   Polyprotein-Coding RNA
   3′ UTR Structure and Function
HAV Proteins
   Nomenclature
   P1 Capsid Proteins
   P2 Proteins: 2B and 2C
   P3 Proteins: 3A, 3B (VPg), 3C^{pro}, and 3D^{pol}
Morphology and Properties of Hepatovirus Virions
   Infectious Extracellular Virions
   Naked Nonenveloped Virions (nHAV)
   Quasi-enveloped Virions (eHAV)
Replication Cycle
   Attachment, Entry, and Uncoating
   Hepatovirus Translation
   Polyprotein Processing
   RNA Replication
   Capsid Assembly
   RNA Packaging
   Quasi-envelopment and Release
Pathogenesis
   Host Range
   Tropism
   Animal Models
   Steps in HAV Pathogenesis
   Cell-Intrinsic and Innate Immune Host Responses to HAV
   Humoral Immune Responses to HAV Infection
   Cellular Immune Responses to HAV Infection
   Immunity
   Mechanisms of Liver Injury
Epidemiology
   Transmission
   Incidence and Geographic Distribution of HAV Infection
Clinical Manifestations of HAV Infection
Diagnosis
Management of Hepatitis A
Prevention and Control
   General Measures
   Passive Immunoprophylaxis
   Hepatitis A Vaccines
Perspectives
Acknowledgments

HISTORY

Descriptions of sporadic and epidemic jaundice, the most evident outward clinical sign of infection with hepatitis A virus (HAV), extend back through antiquity to the times of Hippocrates of Kos in the 5th century BC.[443] Whether such descriptions reflect hepatitis A or other infectious causes of jaundice is unknown, and they have been a source of speculation by medical historians for over a century.[58] However, both large and small outbreaks of disease that seem very likely to have been hepatitis A were common by the 18th century in Europe and the middle of the 19th century in the United States.[58,371] Epidemics of jaundice, known as *jaunisse des camps*, were often linked to military campaigns and plagued both federal and rebel troops in the American Civil War as well as soldiers on both sides of the Franco-Prussian war. By the last third of the 19th century, family-based and community-wide outbreaks of a generally benign, febrile illness associated with jaundice, typically involving children under the age of 16 and consistent with acute hepatitis A, were widely reported throughout the United States, suggesting that HAV was endemic among Americans and that most adults were immune due to prior exposure.[371]

An infectious cause of what was known as "sporadic or epidemic catarrhal jaundice" was widely suspected by the beginning of the 20th century.[76] Multiple studies carried out in human subjects around the time of World War II confirmed the presence of an infectious agent in duodenal secretions and other body fluids,[395] and led to the first clear recognition of distinct forms of transmissible hepatitis, one which was transmitted by ingestion of contaminated food or water (short incubation or "infectious jaundice") and another associated with the administration of blood or blood products (long incubation or "homologous serum jaundice").[19,156,273] Following the war, F. O. MacCallum[239] classified these as "type A" and "type B" hepatitis, establishing a classification scheme that exists to the present. The distinguishing epidemiologic features of these two distinct types of hepatitis, and the absence of cross-protection conferred by infection with each, were confirmed in studies carried out by Saul Krugman and associates involving the experimental infection of children institutionalized at the Willowbrook State School in Staten Island, NY.[201] The ethics of these studies, carried out in vulnerable children in the absence of informed consent, have been broadly criticized and remain the subject of debate.[258] An infectious inoculum generated during the Willowbrook studies, known as MS-1, was subsequently used to infect volunteer inmates held at the Joliet State Prison in Joliet, IL.[36] A fecal sample from one of the subjects in this study was the source of virus in which HAV particles were first identified using the then novel technique of immune electron microscopy by Stephen Feinstone, Albert Kapikian, and Robert Purcell at the U.S. National Institutes of Health in 1973[109,111] (Fig. 2.1B). Similar HAV particles were identified in human fecal material independently and almost simultaneously by Stephen Locarnini and Alan Ferris working at Monash University in Melbourne, Australia.[109,236]

Discovery of the HAV particle ushered in the modern era of HAV virology and was followed in relatively rapid succession by successful propagation of HAV in cell culture by Phillip Provost working at Merck,[299] molecular cloning of the viral genome,[270,377] the development of infectious molecular clones

paving the way for reverse molecular genetic studies,[61] and a prototype formalin-inactivated HAV vaccine produced in cell culture.[30] By the early 1990s, large clinical trials had confirmed the efficacy of similarly produced commercial HAV vaccines.[170,413] The utilization of these vaccines in universal immunization programs targeting young children in Israel and in the southwestern United States resulted in dramatic decreases in the community-wide incidence of acute hepatitis A.[3,78] Widespread use of these vaccines in high-income countries, and growing wealth and improved public health infrastructure in other regions, has subsequently altered the global epidemiology of hepatitis A.[172] Nonetheless, while rates of disease fell rapidly in all age groups following introduction of the vaccine in the United States in 1995, HAV has re-emerged as a public health threat in recent years with widespread outbreaks associated with homelessness and opioid addiction causing over 23,000 hospitalizations and 376 deaths between 2016 and 2021.[49,123]

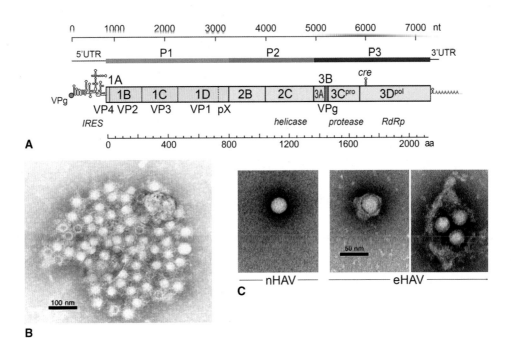

FIGURE 2.1 Hepatitis A virus (HAV). A: Organization of the HAV genome showing the single long open reading frame (ORF) encoding the viral polyprotein, divided into three major segments, P1 (capsid protein) and P2 and P3 (nonstructural proteins), and flanked by 5′ and 3′ untranslated RNA (UTR). A small virally encoded protein (3B or VPg) is covalently linked to the 5′ terminal uridylic acid in the RNA. RNA structures critical for replication exist within both 5′ and 3′ UTRs as well as within the ORF (*cre*, cis-acting replication element). An IRES (internal ribosome entry site) with complex secondary and tertiary RNA structure located within the 5′ UTR directs cap-independent translation of the polyprotein. Primary proteolytic cleavage of the polyprotein occurs at the P1/P2 junction and is mediated in *cis* by proteinase activity associated with 3C^pro. The P1 segment is ultimately processed into three major capsid proteins, 1B (VP2), 1C (VP3), and 1D (VP1pX) and a fourth much smaller capsid polypeptide, 1A (VP4). Enzymatic activities associated with the P2 and P3 nonstructural proteins include the 2C ATPase/helicase, 3C^pro cysteine protease, and 3D^pol RNA-dependent RNA polymerase (RdRp). **B:** Aggregates of naked HAV particles (nHAV) identified in a human fecal specimen by immune electron microscopy. (Reproduced from Feinstone SM. History of the discovery of hepatitis A virus. *Cold Spring Harb Perspect Med* 2019;9(5):a031740.) Both empty and full capsids are evident. **C:** Transmission electron microscopy images of nHAV and quasi-enveloped eHAV particles produced in cell culture and purified by banding in an isopycnic iodixanol gradient. Membranes can be seen surrounding full capsids in the eHAV virions. (Adapted by permission from Nature: Feng Z, Hensley L, McKnight KL, et al. A pathogenic picornavirus acquires an envelope by hijacking cellular membranes. *Nature* 2013;496(7445):367–371. Copyright © 2013 Springer Nature.)

Previously considered to infect only primates, hepatoviruses are now known to be widely distributed in nature, infecting numerous mammalian species, with clear phylogenetic evidence of having undergone multiple past interspecies jumps.[96] Ancestral reconstructions of HAV suggest that it entered human populations from a rodent source, and perhaps ultimately originated in bats.[96] Since continuous chains of transmission are required for HAV to maintain its presence in human populations,[352,420] this seems likely to have occurred only in the past 6,000 to 8,000 years, coincident with the development of agriculture and the shift from humans living a hunter-gatherer existence to settling in increasingly large centers of population. Consistent with this, molecular clock models based on the rate of evolution of the HAV genome estimate entry of the virus into human populations about 3,500 years ago.[203]

HEPATOVIRUS CLASSIFICATION AND DIVERSITY

Initially classified provisionally as "enterovirus 72," HAV was recognized soon after the molecular cloning of its genome to be a distinct member of the *Picornaviridae* family. It is currently classified within the genus *Hepatovirus*, one of 68 genera in the family *Picornaviridae*.[309,435] The classification of HAV within a separate genus, distinct from other picornaviruses, rests largely on phylogenetic comparisons (Fig. 2.2). However, HAV has been recognized historically to be distinct from other well-studied mammalian picornaviruses, including enteroviruses, cardioviruses, and aphthoviruses, by its (a) tropism for hepatocytes, the major cell type present in mammalian liver; (b) unusual physical resistance to high temperatures and low pH; (c) slow and generally noncytopathic replication in cell culture; and (d) unique features of its genome, including the short length and lack of myristoylation of its VP4 capsid protein and the absence of a 2A protease.[248] Beyond these differences, more recently recognized points of distinction include the nonlytic cellular release of newly replicated virus as "quasi-enveloped" virions ("eHAV"), fully assembled capsids completely enclosed within infectious extracellular vesicles resembling exosomes[112] (Fig. 2.1C), and unusual features of the capsid structure found also in parechoviruses and the capsids of picorna-like cripaviruses of insects.[362,405] Avian encephalomyocarditis virus is closely related to HAV and was previously classified within the genus *Hepatovirus*. However, it is now considered sufficiently distinct to be placed within its own genus, the genus *Tremovirus*. Duck HAV is also classified within a distinct genus, *Avihepatovirus*.

Prior to 2015, hepatoviruses were identified only in humans and a relatively small number of nonhuman primate species. That changed dramatically in 2015 with the identification of hepatoviruses infecting seals, woodchucks, and multiple species of rodents as well as bats and other small mammals.[11,85,96,432] Based on phylogenetic comparisons, these viruses are grouped at present into nine distinct species recognized by the International Committee on the Taxonomy of Viruses, named *Hepatovirus A* to *Hepatovirus I*[434,435] (Fig. 2.3A). Within these species, there is 3.8% (*Hepatovirus A*) to 29% (*Hepatovirus G*) nucleotide sequence divergence (mean 16%)[353] (Fig. 2.3B). Interspecies divergence ranges from 30% to 42% (mean 38%). Viruses

recovered from humans and nonhuman primates are closely related to members of the *Hepatovirus A* species, which has been further grouped into six genotypes (genotypes I to VI). Genotypes I to III have been recovered from infected humans, whereas genotypes IV to VI are based on a small number of *Hepatovirus A* sequences recovered only from nonhuman primates[176,313,353] (Fig. 2.3A). Genotypes I and III have a worldwide distribution, whereas genotype II strains have been identified in Europe (France) and Africa (Sierra Leone). No significant differences have been recognized in the pathogenicity of different human HAV genotypes.

Although there may be minor antigenic differences between viruses recovered from humans and nonhuman primates,[104,269,383] all *Hepatovirus A* strains appear to belong to a single serotype.[44,70,218] Limited evidence suggests that *Hepatovirus H* viruses from bats and *Hepatovirus F* virus from a marsupial opossum may be antigenically related to *Hepatovirus A*.[85,96] Sera from these hepatovirus host species are reactive with human HAV antigen. However, only *Hepatovirus A* has been isolated in cell culture, and little is known about the antigenic characteristics of other hepatovirus species.

GENOME STRUCTURE

Genome Organization

Similar to other picornaviruses, the HAV genome is a single-stranded, nonsegmented, plus-sense RNA molecule approximately 7,487 nucleotides in length (Fig. 2.1A). It contains a single large open reading frame encoding a polyprotein of approximately 2,230 amino acids, flanked by a relatively lengthy approximately 734 nucleotide 5' untranslated region (UTR) and a short 3' UTR of approximately 63 nucleotides followed by a poly(A) tail approximately 40 to 60 nucleotides long. Compared to other picornaviruses, the G+C content of the HAV genome is relatively low (37% vs. 46% for poliovirus).[291] RNA structure critical for RNA translation and/or replication exists within the 5' UTR, near the 3' end of the polyprotein-coding region, and likely also within the 3' UTR. The 5' end of the genome is uncapped and covalently linked to a small, virally encoded peptide, VPg (also known as 3B),[411] which by analogy with poliovirus is likely to be the primer for RNA synthesis. Although never demonstrated for hepatoviruses, studies with other plus-strand RNA viruses suggest that the genome may assume a circular structure at some point in its replication cycle, possibly by being bridged by RNA-binding proteins interacting with the 5' and 3' UTRs.[157,404]

5' UTR Structure and Function

The 5' UTR is approximately 734 nucleotides in length and contains extensive secondary and tertiary structures required for efficient translation and/or viral RNA synthesis (Fig. 2.4). Major structural features have been predicted by thermodynamic modeling constrained by covariant base pairing identified in phylogenetic comparative sequence analyses and confirmed by mapping sites at which synthetic RNA transcripts are cleaved by single- or double-strand–specific ribonucleases (RNases).[43,212,332] Direct biophysical analysis has been limited to NMR studies of a short, pyrimidine-rich sequence (pY1) between nucleotides 99 and 140 in the prototype HM175

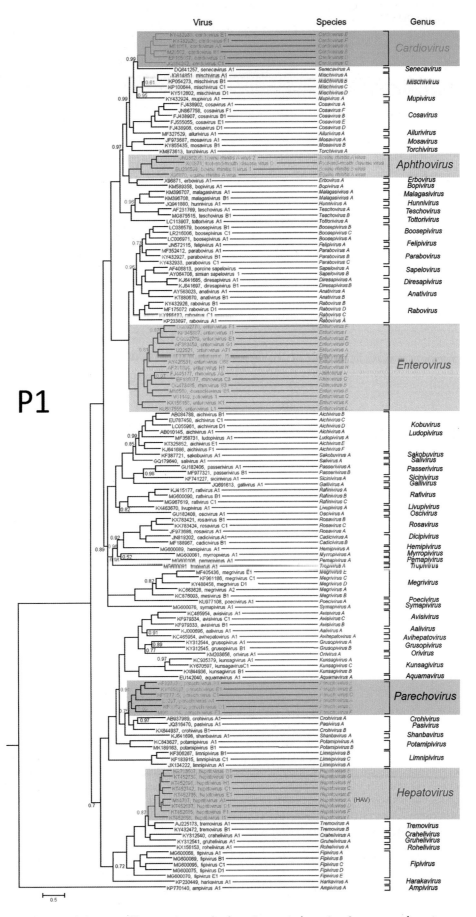

FIGURE 2.2 Phylogeny of hepatovirus and other picornaviral species. Sequences of species cluster by genus. Phylogeny based on P1 (capsid-coding) nucleotide sequences. (Modified from Report ICTV. Picornaviridae. https://talk.ictvonline.org/ictv-reports/ictv_online_report/positive-sense-rna-viruses/w/picornaviridae. Accessed May 30, 2021. Ref.[309])

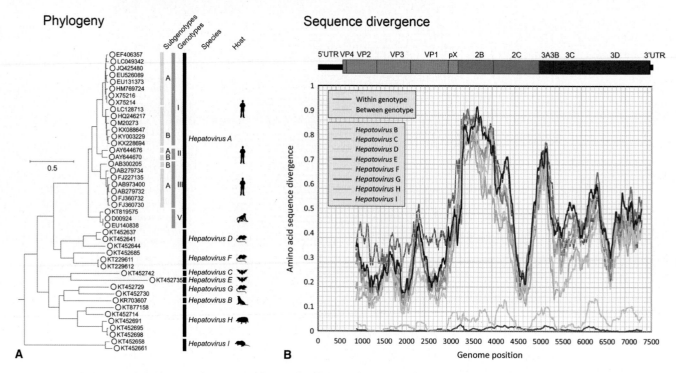

FIGURE 2.3 Phylogeny and sequence divergence of hepatoviruses. A: Phylogeny based on available complete coding sequences from representative strains determined by maximum likelihood using an optimized substitution model. **B:** Sequence divergence was calculated from windows of greater than 90 codons. (Reprinted with permission from Smith DB, Simmonds P. Classification and genomic diversity of enterically transmitted hepatitis viruses. *Cold Spring Harb Perspect Med* 2018;8(9):a031880. Copyright © 2018 Cold Spring Harbor Laboratory Press.)

Hepatovirus A strain.[151] Functional correlates have been determined by mutational analyses and reverse molecular genetic studies examining the impact of deletions and/or substitutions within the 5′ UTR on translation of synthetic RNA transcripts or replication of the virus.[45,332,334] Much of this work was accomplished decades ago.

The 5′ UTR is composed of three major domains, each with distinct structure and function. The 5′ terminal 98 nucleotides form a complex series of three stem–loop structures containing two putative pseudoknots that act as strong stops to primer extension (Fig. 2.4). Sequence in this region of the 5′ UTR is highly conserved, with greater than 94% identity among *Hepatovirus* A strains. While unexplored experimentally, these structures likely contribute functionally to viral RNA synthesis in a manner similar to the 5′ terminal cloverleaf structure in poliovirus RNA. Downstream of this element is a pyrimidine-rich track (pY1) (Fig. 2.4), which varies in length from approximately 20 to 40 nucleotides among *Hepatovirus* A strains and contains multiple cytidylic acid and uridylic acid triplets.[332,334] NMR studies suggest that this region forms a condensed, stacked structure with extensive noncanonical U•U base pairing.[151,332] Surprisingly, most of the pY1 sequence can be deleted with no apparent consequence on virus yield in cell culture or replication within the liver in nonhuman primates.[333] Small deletions at its 3′ end (nts 136 to 144 in HM175 virus) result in temperature-sensitive replication phenotypes with as much as a 3.6 $\log_{10}$ difference in virus yield at 37°C versus 31°C due to impaired viral RNA synthesis.[334]

The third distinct functional element within the 5′ UTR is an internal ribosome entry site (IRES) that directs the cap-independent initiation of translation of the viral RNA (Fig. 2.4).

The location of the IRES (nucleotides 154 to 735) was mapped by analyzing the impact of deletions on the translational activity of monocistronic and dicistronic RNA transcripts in which the 5′ UTR sequence was placed in the intercistronic space between RNA encoding different reporter proteins.[43,45,135] The *Hepatovirus* A IRES is composed of four major complex RNA stem–loops (Fig. 2.4). This higher-ordered RNA structure is unique among the *Picornaviridae*, resulting in the IRES being classified as a type III IRES among five structurally distinct IRES types recognized to exist in different picornaviruses.[277] There are, however, shared features with the type II IRES found in aphthoviruses and cardioviruses, including a putative pseudoknot and a second, short pyrimidine-rich sequence (pY2) located just upstream of the initiator AUG codon[45,212] (Fig. 2.4). The IRES structure is similar in other hepatovirus species, with the exception of *Hepatovirus* C and *Hepatovirus* E, which have type IV IRES elements similar to those found in tremoviruses and sapeloviruses, distinct picornaviral genera, and hepatitis C virus (HCV), a member of the *Flaviviridae*.[11,96,353]

Several host cell RNA-binding proteins have been shown to interact with the 5′ UTR of HAV and to modulate the efficiency of virus translation, including poly(rC)-binding protein 2 (PCBP2),[145] polypyrimidine tract–binding protein 1 (PTBP1),[143] and glyceraldehyde-3-phosphate dehydrogenase (GAPDH).[329,428] Specific binding of the 3C^{pro} protease has also been reported and may play a role in RNA replication.[205]

Polyprotein-Coding RNA

Only a single open reading frame (ORF) within the HAV genome is known to be translated into protein. This ORF extends from nucleotide 735 to 7,415 in the HM175 virus

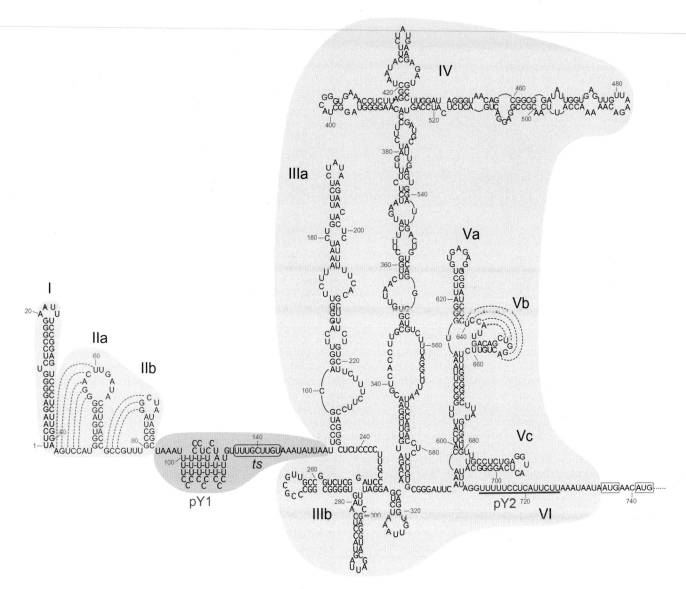

FIGURE 2.4 Secondary RNA structure within the HAV 5′ UTR. The model was devised by a combination of thermodynamic modeling constrained by base-pairing identified by covariant sequence analysis and sites of cleavage by single- and double-stranded RNA-specific ribonucleases.[43] Putative pseudoknots at the 5′ terminus (shaded in *yellow*) are likely important for recognition of the RNA by the viral replicase complex. A lengthy polypyrimidine track (pY1, *gray*) with a stacked structure formed by extensive noncanonical U-U base pairing is of unknown function.[151] Deletion mutations near its 3′ end result in a temperature-sensitive (*ts*) phenotype. The IRES (internal ribosome entry site, *blue*) directs internal initiation of translation at either of two downstream AUGs (*red boxes*) and contains a second pyrimidine-rich track (pY2) similar to that found in some other picornaviral IRES elements. Nucleotides are numbered from the 5′ end of the genome. Model based on wild-type HM175 virus (GenBank M14707). (Adapted by permission from Springer: Martin A, Lemon SM. The molecular biology of hepatitis A virus. In: Ou J, ed. *Hepatitis Viruses*. Boston, MA: Kluwer Academic Publishers; 2002:23–50. Copyright © 2002 Springer Science+Business Media New York.)

genome, encoding a polyprotein of 2,227 amino acids with a predicted molecular mass of 251.5 kDa (Fig. 2.1A). Codon usage throughout the ORF is exceptionally divergent from human codon usage and strongly biased (Fig. 2.5A). Codon bias can be assessed by calculating a measure known as the "effective number of codons" (Nc), which can range from 61 (all possible codons used without preference) downward to approximately 20 (extremely biased).[421] The Nc of the HAV ORF is 39, compared to 54 for poliovirus.[291] In part, this extreme codon bias may have resulted from evolutionary pressure to reduce CpG dinucleotide frequency to escape restriction by the zinc-finger

antiviral protein (ZAP).[16] In support of that argument, the percent CpG dinucleotides present in HAV is 0.36% versus 2.68% for poliovirus.[291] Alternatively, the atypical codon usage of HAV has been suggested to be an evolutionary adaptation that slows the kinetics of protein synthesis in order to promote cotranslational folding of the capsid proteins that assemble into an exceptionally stable capsid.[12,67,79] However, this hypothesis fails to explain why codon bias extends throughout the ORF, including sequence encoding nonstructural proteins required for viral RNA synthesis. Hepatovirus codon usage closely matches that of triatoma virus and cricket paralysis virus and

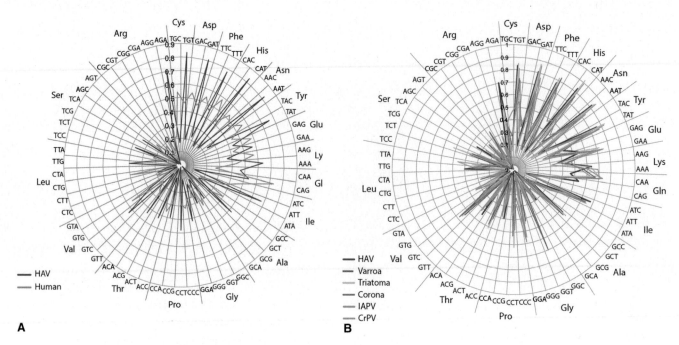

FIGURE 2.5 Hepatovirus codon usage wheel plots. A: Comparison of HAV versus human codon usage shows a marked difference and heavily biased codon use by HAV. HAV codon use is based on an average of six different genotypes. **B:** Codon usage wheel plots showing a high level of similarity between HAV codon usage and codon use by multiple insect viruses. *Triatoma* codon usage matches that of its insect triatomine host. *Varroa*, *Varroa* destructor virus of mites (*Iflaviridae*); Corona, 229E human alpha coronavirus (*Coronaviridae*); IAPV, Israeli acute paralysis virus (*Dicistroviridae*); CrPV, cricket paralysis virus (*Dicistroviridae*). (From Wassenaar TM, Jun SR, Robeson M, et al. Comparative genomics of hepatitis A virus, hepatitis C virus, and hepatitis E virus provides insights into the evolutionary history of Hepatovirus species. *Microbiologyopen* 2020;9(2):e973. Reprinted by permission of John Wiley & Sons, Inc.)

their invertebrate insect hosts[79,410] (Fig. 2.5B). Similarities have also been noted in the capsid structures of these picorna-like viruses of insects and HAV,[405] and it is likely that the codon bias in HAV is a vestige of an ancient common ancestor. Human alpha coronaviruses, which like hepatoviruses may have an evolutionary origin in bats, share a similar codon usage bias[96,410] (Fig. 2.5B).

In addition to encoding the proteins of HAV, the ORF contains secondary RNA structure essential for replication of the virus.[425] Nucleotides 5,948 to 6,057 in the HM175 virus genome, which are located within the segment encoding the 3D^pol RNA-dependent RNA polymerase, folds into an elongated stem–loop structure with an AAACA/G motif present within the 5′ proximal portion of the terminal loop that is typical of *cre* elements found within the genomes of other picornaviruses.[139,424,425] Replication of a subgenomic HAV replicon was ablated by mutations that disrupted either the secondary RNA structure or the AAACA/G motif of the putative *cre* element without changing the amino acid sequence of the polymerase.[425] Replication could be rescued by reinserting the stem–loop at an alternative position within the replicon, indicating that its position within the genome is not critical to its function. The secondary structure and location of the putative *cre* element is conserved in multiple hepatovirus species.[96] Based on studies with other picornaviruses,[281] the *cre* sequence is likely to template uridylation of the protein primer for viral RNA synthesis, VPg.

3′ UTR Structure and Function

The 3′ UTR is approximately 63 nucleotides in length and well conserved among *Hepatovirus A* strains. Shorter 3′ UTRs reported for some strains seem likely to represent incomplete genomes. Thermodynamic modeling and nuclease sensitivity studies suggest that the 3′ UTR contains conserved secondary RNA structure, including a potential pseudoknot.[91] Both nonstructural viral proteins (3ABC) and host cell RNA-binding proteins, including GAPDH, have been reported to interact specifically with the 3′ UTR.[91,208,209] The functional significance of these interactions is not well characterized, but they are likely to be important for viral RNA synthesis. The 3′ UTR terminates in a poly(A) tail of up to approximately 60 nucleotides, the length of which appears to influence the stability and replication potential of the RNA genome.[207]

HAV PROTEINS

Nomenclature

Four structural and six nonstructural mature proteins are expressed by HAV. All are derived from proteolytic processing of the polyprotein encoded by the single large ORF (Fig. 2.6C). Nomenclature for these proteins is based on the L-4-3-4 scheme proposed for picornaviruses by Rueckert and Wimmer,[319] which divides the polyprotein into three segments: P1, P2, and P3. The N-terminal P1 segment is processed into the structural proteins that form the capsid: 1A (otherwise known as VP4), 1B (VP2), 1C (VP3), and 1D (VP1pX). The middle P2 segment is processed into the nonstructural 2B and 2C (helicase) proteins and the C-terminal P3 segment into the remaining nonstructural proteins: 3A, 3B (the genome-linked protein, VPg), 3C^pro (a cysteine protease), and 3D^pol (RNA-dependent RNA polymerase) (Fig. 2.1A).

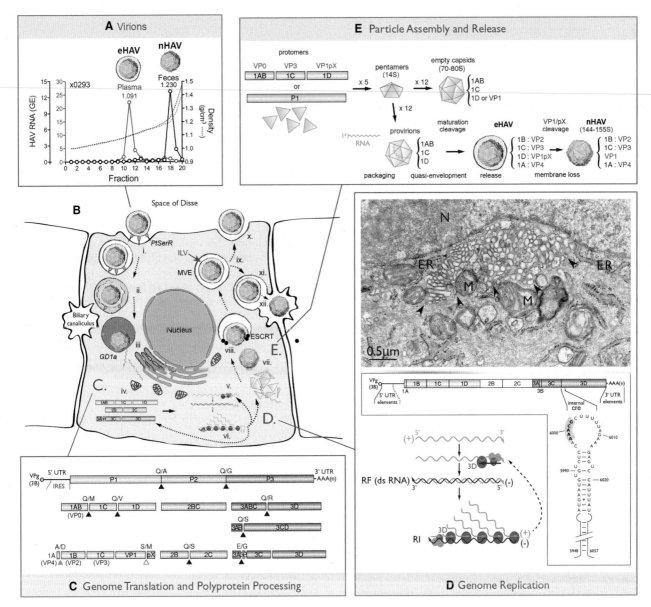

FIGURE 2.6 HAV replication cycle. A: Infectious nonenveloped virions (nHAV) are shed in feces of infected persons, whereas quasi-enveloped (eHAV) are found in the blood. These virion types have different buoyant densities and can be separated by isopycnic gradient centrifugation. **B:** Cell entry and release of quasi-enveloped eHAV. (i) eHAV enters cells by clathrin-mediated endocytosis mediated in part by phosphatidylserine receptors (PtSerR) like TIM-1 and dependent upon integrin β1. nHAV also enters by clathrin-dependent endocytosis, likely mediated by attachment to both proteins and gangliosides. (ii) Both virion types traffic through Rab5A+ early and Rab7a+ late endosomes, with the eHAV membrane degraded by lysosomal acid lipase (LAL) and Niemann-Pick C1 protein (NPC1) in late endolysosomes. (iii) Capsid binding to gangliosides such as GD1a is essential for subsequent steps in entry. Whether uncoating occurs within the endolysosome or within the cytoplasm after traversing the endolysosomal membrane is not known. (iv) HAV RNA released into the cytoplasm acts as template for cap-independent translation of the viral polyprotein, which is subsequently processed by 3Cpro at the junctions indicated by *black triangles*, by an unknown cellular protease(s) at the VP1/pX junction in 1D (*open triangle*), or following packaging of the RNA at the 1A/1B junction in an RNA-dependent cleavage reaction (*gray triangle*) (see panel **C**). Dipeptide cleavage sites are shown for stable processing intermediates and mature proteins. (v) Genome replication proceeds in replication organelles comprised of virus-induced tubular–vesicular membranes forming in close proximity to the endoplasmic reticulum (ER) and mitochondria (M) (see panel **D**; N, nucleus). A replicase complex comprised of 3Dpol and other nonstructural proteins assembles at the 3′ end of the positive-strand genomic RNA and drives transcription of a minus-strand RNA copy, thereby generating double-stranded replicating form (RF) RNA. RNA synthesis is primed by VPg-pUpU following uridylation of 3B (VPg) in a reaction templated by a short sequence within the terminal loop of the cis-active RNA element (*cre*), a complex stem–loop structure located within the 3Dpol-coding RNA. Additional RNA structures within 5′ and 3′ untranslated RNA (UTR) are required for RNA replication. (vi) Multiple rounds of positive-strand RNA synthesis are templated by the RF minus-strand, producing replication intermediate (RI) RNA, in a reaction also primed by VPg-pUpU. (vii) Nascent positive-strand RNA is directed to the ER to template subsequent translation of more viral proteins, serves as template within replication organelles for additional rounds of minus-strand RNA synthesis, or is packaged into nascent capsids assembling from P1 polypeptides (see panel **E**). (viii) Fully assembled capsids containing viral RNA recruit ALIX and other components of the endosomal sorting system required for transport (ESCRT) to bud into multivesicular endosomes (MVE), thereby forming intralumenal vesicles (ILV) containing capsids. (ix) MVEs traffic either (x) to the basolateral hepatocyte membrane where MVE and plasma membrane fusion releases ILVs as eHAV into hepatic sinusoids through which blood flows or (xi) to the apical hepatocyte membrane where fusion releases eHAV into biliary canaliculi. (xii) High concentrations of unbuffered bile salts in the proximal biliary track strip membranes from eHAV particles, resulting in gastrointestinal shedding of naked nHAV. (Modified from Martin and Hollinger, Field's 6th ed. Chapter 19. Panel A adapted by permission from Nature: Feng Z, Hensley L, McKnight KL, et al. A pathogenic picornavirus acquires an envelope by hijacking cellular membranes. *Nature* 2013;496(7445):367–371. Copyright © 2013 Springer Nature.; Electron micrograph in panel **D** courtesy of Dr. Rainer Gosert, Institute for Medical Microbiology, Basel, Switzerland.)

HAV deviates from the L-4-3-4 scheme applicable to most picornaviruses in lacking a nonstructural 2A protein, which in many picornaviruses directs the primary cleavage of the polyprotein. Primary cleavage of the HAV polyprotein occurs at the P1/P2 junction and is mediated by 3C^pro, acting in *cis* and possibly also in *trans*.[153,328] The 1D protein found in extracellular quasi-enveloped virions is 345 amino acids in length.[112] Its C-terminal 71 amino acid segment is referred to variably as "2A" or "pX"[8] and has major roles in capsid assembly[152,247] and quasi-enveloped virion biogenesis.[182] It is cleaved from the capsid following degradation of the eHAV membrane, resulting in a 274 amino acid VP1 protein in naked virions, and has no subsequent known function (Fig. 2.6E). To avoid confusion, this segment of 1D is referred to herein as pX. Recent x-ray crystallography studies suggest that a β-barrel formed by the N terminus of 2B may be a vestigial remnant of a nonstructural 2A protein expressed by an ancestral virus.[393]

P1 Capsid Proteins

Almost all processing of the polyprotein is carried out by protease activity associated with 3C[328] (Fig. 2.6C). Primary cleavage at the 1D/2B (P1/P2) junction (amino acid 836 in HM175 virus), followed by secondary cleavage at 1B/C, and 1C/1D produces three large structural proteins, 1AB (otherwise known as VP0, ~25.5 kDa), 1C (VP3, 27.8 kDa), and 1D (VP1pX, 38.5 kDa) (Fig. 2.6C).[142,247,328] Sixty copies of each of these assemble to form the viral capsid, with 1AB (VP0) undergoing a late "maturation" cleavage following packaging of the RNA that results in a very small 1A (VP4) protein (21 to 23 amino acids, or 2.2 to 2.5 kDa depending on the AUG codon at which translation initiates) and mature 1B (VP2, 24.9 kDa). 1A (VP4) is N-terminally myristoylated in enteroviruses but not in hepatoviruses.[372] Full-length 1D (VP1pX) is found in early morphogenesis intermediates and in quasi-enveloped eHAV virions released from cells[8,112] but undergoes additional processing with release of the C-terminal 8.3-kDa pX fragment upon disruption of the eHAV membrane[112,147,246] (see Nomenclature). This results in a 31.2-kDa VP1 protein in naked, nonenveloped virions shed from infected individuals (Fig. 2.6C). The protease responsible for this late 1D cleavage event is uncertain, but *in vitro* studies show that it can be mediated by either trypsin or cathepsin L and siRNA knockdown of cathepsin L impedes VP1pX proteolysis in infected cells.[266,331] The cleavage is efficient but leaves VP1 with a heterogeneous carboxy terminus.[147] Individual capsid proteins expressed from recombinant RNA in bacterial systems have little antigenic relatedness to the assembled HAV capsid.

P2 Proteins: 2B and 2C

The P2P3 segment released by the primary polyprotein cleavage is further processed by the 3C protease into P2 (2BC) and P3 (3ABCD) intermediates. 2BC is subsequently processed into 2B and 2C, possibly by 3ABC rather than mature 3C^pro.[177] Both 2B and 2C are closely associated with intracellular membranes.[144,342] Overexpression studies suggest that the 2B and 2BC proteins may be responsible for induction of an extended tubular–vesicular membrane network forming in close proximity to the rough endoplasmic reticulum in infected cells.[144,374] Such membrane rearrangements are common to all positive-strand RNA viruses and provide an essential structural framework for the assembly of the RNA replication machinery.

2B Protein

At 251 amino acids in length, the 28.7-kDa HAV 2B protein is among the largest 2B proteins expressed by any member of the *Picornaviridae* and is over twice the length of the enterovirus 2B protein. This likely reflects the inclusion of vestigial 2A sequence at its amino terminus.[393] The crystal structure of a recombinant protein representing the pX segment of 1D ("2A") fused to the N-terminal 146 amino acids of 2B revealed that the N terminus of 2B contains a curved five-stranded antiparallel β-sheet structurally similar to the β-barrel domain of enteroviral 2A proteins, followed by a C-terminal helical bundle.[393] In solution, this segment of the 2B protein self-assembles into higher-order amyloid-like fibrillar structures. This fibrillar polymerization could play a key role in reorganization of host membranes, as 2B is anchored to host membranes by a helical segment near its carboxy terminus.[131,342] Another study showed that a 60-residue synthetic peptide from the C-terminal region of 2B associated with synthetic membranes and formed small pores, suggesting that 2B may have viroporin activity.[342] Unlike the 2B proteins of enteroviruses, however, HAV 2B does not appear to alter host cell Ca^++ homeostasis.[84]

2C Protein

The 38.5-kDa 2C protein has received less attention experimentally. Like the 2C protein of other picornaviruses, HAV 2C contains a superfamily 2 helicase with classic Walker A and B sequence motifs.[141] The protein has been reported to have RNA-binding activity with preference for the 3′ end of HAV negative-strand RNA.[18] These activities are likely to be required for replication of the viral RNA and possibly also packaging of newly replicated RNA.[181] Like many other picornaviruses, HAV RNA synthesis is inhibited by low concentrations of guanidine, which targets the 2C protein of enteroviruses.[53,427] Cell culture–adaptive mutations in both 2B and 2C have been associated with enhanced replication of HAV and subgenomic HAV replicons in cell culture.[100,102,226,427]

P3 Proteins: 3A, 3B (VPg), 3C^pro, and 3D^pol

3AB and Vpg

Processing of 3ABCD results in at least six mature proteins with distinct activities: 3A, which serves to anchor the 3ABCD polypeptide to membranes[23,423]; 3B, the small genome-linked protein that likely serves as primer for RNA synthesis[411]; 3ABC, 3C^pro, and 3CD, all catalytically active proteases with distinct cellular localization and substrate cleavage specificities[241,306,423]; and 3D^pol, an RNA-dependent RNA polymerase[373] (Fig. 2.6C). The short 8.0-kDa 3A protein contains a transmembrane domain that directs 3ABC to membranes associated with mitochondria where it cleaves the mitochondrial antiviral signaling protein (MAVS).[23,24,423] Recombinant His-tagged 3AB protein has been shown to form stable dimers, interact with 3CD, and associate specifically with HAV RNA.[23] 3B, otherwise known as VPg, the genome-linked protein, is 23 amino acids in length and linked covalently through a tyrosine in the third position to the 5′ terminal uridylic acid of the positive-strand viral RNA.[411] The first two bases in the HAV genome are U-U, as in other picornaviruses, consistent with 3B being uridylated to VPg-pUpU and serving as the protein primer for new viral RNA synthesis.[280,281]

3C^pro Protease

The 24.1-kDa 3C^pro protease was among the first viral proteases to have its structure solved by x-ray crystallography.[6] A cysteine protease, 3Cpro assumes a two-domain structure with two antiparallel β-barrel domains characteristic of chymotrypsin-like serine proteinases.[6,27] The substrate-binding domain is located in a narrow groove between the two β-barrel domains. The active site residues are Cys172 and His44; catalysis is not dependent upon a catalytic triad.[27] An RNA-binding domain marked by the motif KFRDI, conserved in all picornaviruses,[140] is located on the side of the molecule opposite the substrate-binding domain.[27] An Asp-to-Asn substitution in this motif ablates replication of the virus.[133] Binding of recombinant 3C^pro to RNA was significantly enhanced by dimerization of the protein via a disulfide bond involving Cys24 and by the presence of a peptide substrate.[283] The protease is active both in cis and trans and capable of cleaving itself out of the polyprotein.[153,373] Cleavage is dependent upon substrate residues P4 through P'2, with a strong preference for Gln in the P1 position, and a hydrophobic residue, Leu, Ile, or Val at P4.[178,285,328] Gly, Ala, or Ser are preferred at the P'1 position, although other P'1 residues in the polyprotein include Val, Met, and Arg. The cleavage specificity of the *Hepatovirus A* protease appears to be conserved among other hepatovirus species.[11,96,117]

An irreversible peptidyl monofluoromethyl ketone inhibitor of 3C^pro has been shown to inhibit the production of virus in cell culture.[267] The crystal structure of a dipeptide inhibitor bound to 3C^pro has also been reported.[26] In addition to mediating most polyprotein processing events, 3C^pro cleaves NF-kB essential modulator (IKKg or NEMO), the regulatory subunit of the IKK inhibitor complex, and the stable precursor polypeptide, 3ABC, cleaves MAVS, two host proteins involved in activation of antiviral interferon responses.[117,402,423] MAVS cleavage is dependent upon the transmembrane domain in 3A that directs 3ABC to mitochondria-associated membranes.[423] An additional polyprotein processing intermediate, 3CD, that represents unprocessed protease–polymerase (Fig. 2.6C), cleaves a third innate immune signaling molecule, TIR domain–containing adaptor inducing interferon-β (TICAM1 or TRIF).[306] TRIF cleavage is dependent upon the fusion with 3D and very inefficient with mature 3C^pro. The fusion with 3D alters substrate specificity, allowing for cleavage at TRIF sites with acidic P4 residues, reflecting some flexibility in the substrate-binding domain.[27,306] 3C^pro cleavage of the host RNA-binding proteins PCBP2 and poly(A)-binding protein (PABP1) has also been described.[438,439] Overexpression of 3C^pro leads to vacuolization and caspase-independent cell death.[341]

3D^pol Polymerase

Much less is known about the structure and function of the 56.3-kDa HAV 3D^pol RNA-dependent RNA polymerase, as efforts to express it in active form have uniformly failed due to extreme insolubility.[373] The polymerase contains the active-site YGDD motif common to all picornaviral polymerases and viral RNA in which these Asp residues are substituted with Ala fails to replicate.[81] The 3D^pol proteins of *Hepatovirus A* viruses have a C-terminal CXXX motif, suggesting that C-terminal prenylation may contribute to membrane association, but this motif is not present in other hepatovirus species. A Phe42-to-Leu substitution in HAV 3D^pol was reported to increase the rate of replication of the virus,[199] but little more is known about the protein. 3C^pro and 3D^pol are expressed only at low levels in infected cells and may be subject to ubiquitination and proteasome-mediated degradation.[237] The nucleoside analog, sofosbuvir, used clinically for treatment of hepatitis C, has modest activity against 3D^pol and inhibits HAV replication with an IC$_{50}$ of 6.3 to 9.9 µM.[183]

MORPHOLOGY AND PROPERTIES OF HEPATOVIRUS VIRIONS

Infectious Extracellular Virions

There are two types of extracellular hepatovirus virions: naked, nonenveloped virions (nHAV) approximately 30 nm in diameter, found in bile and feces, that have morphology similar to other picornaviral virions, and quasi-enveloped virions (eHAV), found in the blood, that consist of small extracellular vesicles containing 1 to 3 capsids.[112,405] Both virus types are infectious and found in cell cultures. eHAV is released from infected cells in a nonlytic manner. This is likely the major if not the only mechanism of virus release *in vivo*. Naked particles comprise a minor fraction of the virus found in supernatant fluids of infected cell cultures.[112,162] They likely result from the cytopathic effects of cell culture–adapted viruses.[162,226,436] Most evidence suggests that the virus is noncytolytic *in vivo*, and only quasi-enveloped eHAV is detectable in the blood of acutely infected humans or chimpanzees[112] (Fig. 2.6A). Nonenveloped virions shed in feces are largely if not entirely produced within the liver.[15,111,112,161,251] These naked virions are generated by the detergent action of bile salts, which strip membranes from eHAV during its passage to the gut through the biliary tract[111,112,162] (Fig. 2.6B).

Naked Nonenveloped Virions (nHAV)

The HAV capsid is assembled from 60 copies each of the three major structural proteins produced by 3C^pro processing of the P1 segment: 1AB (VP0), 1C (VP3), and 1D (VP1pX) (Fig. 2.6E). Both empty and full capsids are found in infected cells, with 1AB (VP0) processed to 1A (VP4) and 1B (VP2) in full particles containing the viral genome.[405] This maturation cleavage has been reported to occur slowly, over days, in virus recovered from infected cell lysates.[34] VP1pX also undergoes additional processing, with the pX segment trimmed from the capsid following its release from eHAV vesicles into the extracellular environment.[8,112] Thus, mature nHAV capsids shed in feces or found in supernatant fluids of infected cells contain four proteins, three of which are exposed on the surface of the particle (VP2, VP3, and VP1).[405] The capsids are significantly more stable than enterovirus capsids at low pH and high temperature.[324,348] HAV remains infectious for up to 8 hours at pH 1.0 at room temperature.[324] At neutral pH, approximately 2.0 log$_{10}$ infectivity is lost from crude virus preparations after 10 minutes at 60°C.[226] Stability is increased significantly in the presence of 1 M Mg^{++}, such that a comparable loss of infectivity requires incubation for 10 minutes at 80°C.[226,348] When suspended in milk, 0.1% to 1.0% infectivity survives statutory pasteurization conditions.[279] Heat inactivation results from the loss of capsid integrity and release of the RNA genome.[405] Interestingly, thermostability in the absence of excess Mg^{++} is greatest at pH approximately 5.0.[405] In ThermoFluor assays with purified virus under conditions in which the temperature was ramped up from 4°C to 99°C at 10 seconds 0.5°C intervals, genome release and loss of particle integrity were coincident at 76°C to 77°C.[405] In similar assays with poliovirus, RNA release occurred at approximately 45°C.[401] Multiple studies show that nHAV is highly resistant to drying, various organic solvents and detergents.[220,223,227]

Infectious naked virus particles band at a density of approximately 1.33 g/cm^3 in isopycnic CsCl gradients, with a minor fraction banding at approximately 1.42 g/cm^3 that likely has greater capsid permeability to Cs$^+$ cations.[224,347] Banding is at a density of 1.28 to 1.31 g/cm^3 in nonionic medium.[112] Full capsids containing RNA sediment at approximately 144S and empty capsids at approximately 80S.[346,405] A 3Å atomic model of the capsid generated by x-ray crystallography of formaldehyde-fixed particles reveals all three major capsid proteins to be folded as eight-stranded antiparallel β-barrels, forming a pseudo $T = 3$ icosahedron approximately 30 nm in diameter[362,405] (Fig. 2.7A). The small VP4 protein is not visible in the model, and VP1 terminates at the VP1/pX cleavage site near the surface. The surface of the capsid is relatively smooth and featureless, substantially negatively charged, and lacks both the deep canyon surrounding the fivefold axis of symmetry and the hydrophobic pocket of VP1 found in enteroviruses[362,405]

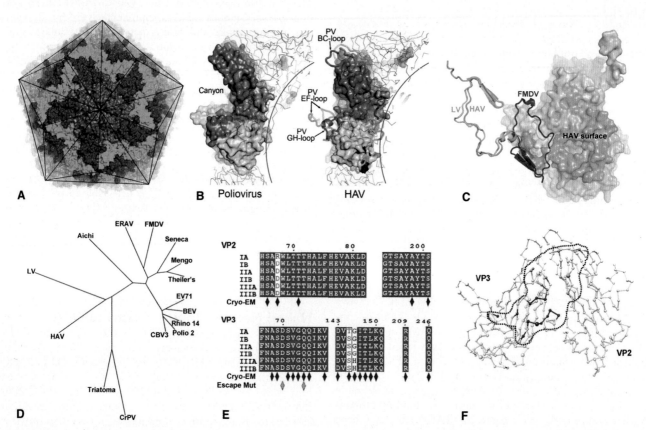

FIGURE 2.7 Structure of the HAV capsid. A: Accessible surface in an atomic structure of HAV determined by x-ray crystallography (VP1, *blue*; VP2, *green*; VP3, *red*).[405] *Black lines* represent particle facets. **B:** Comparative views of the surfaces of the biological protomers of HAV and poliovirus, showing HAV lacks the deep "canyon" surrounding the fivefold axis of symmetry in poliovirus. **C:** VP2 domain swap. A surface-rendered biological protomer of HAV is depicted with the amino terminus of VP2 shown in cartoon representation (*green*) and with the amino termini of Ljungan virus (LV, a parechovirus, *cyan*) and foot-and-mouth disease virus (FMDV, an aphthovirus, *magenta*) superimposed. The amino termini of HAV and LV share a structural conformation distinct from FMDV (and enteroviruses) and similar to what is found in insect cripaviruses. **D:** Structure-based phylogenetic tree of representative picornaviruses and cripaviruses. CrPV, cricket paralysis virus. **E:** Amino acid sequences of VP2 and VP3 conserved in each genotype form the conformationally defined major neutralizing antigenic site of HAV. *Blue diamonds* indicate residues within the cryo-EM footprints of monoclonal neutralizing antibodies.[46] *Green diamonds* represent residues at which neutralization-escape mutations have been identified.[288] **F:** Conserved amino acid residues of the major HAV neutralizing antigenic site mapped onto the VP2 and VP3 structures in the HAV protomer. (Panels **A** and **B** adapted by permission from Nature: Wang X, Ren J, Gao Q, et al. Hepatitis A virus and the origins of picornaviruses. *Nature* 2015;517(7532):85–88. Copyright © 2015 Springer Nature.; panels **C** and **D** adapted with permission from Stuart DI, Ren J, Wang X, et al. Hepatitis A virus capsid structure. *Cold Spring Harb Perspect Med* 2019;9(5):a031807. Copyright © 2019 Cold Spring Harbor Laboratory Press.; panels **E** and **F** modified from Cao L, Liu P, Yang P, et al. Structural basis for neutralization of hepatitis A virus informs a rational design of highly potent inhibitors. *PLoS Biol* 2019;17(4):e3000229. https://creativecommons.org/licenses/by/4.0/.)

(Fig. 2.7B). In comparison with enteroviruses, a domain swap at the N terminus of VP2 near the twofold axis of symmetry strengthens the connectivity between adjacent HAV pentamer subunits (Fig. 2.7C). A similar domain swap is found in the VP0 protein of parechoviruses,[442] which cluster phylogenetically with hepatoviruses (Fig. 2.2), suggesting that these genera represent a structurally and genetically distinct clade of picornaviruses.[362] This domain swap is also present in insect cripaviruses, which share codon usage with HAV,[410] suggesting an ancient evolutionary link (Fig. 2.7D).[362,405] The general structure of empty capsids is very similar, although the amino termini of VP0 and VP1 are more disordered than in RNA-containing particles.[362]

The crystal structure of the capsid provides little insight into where receptor binding occurs, or how the capsid disassembles during infection.[362,405] Capsid thermostability is lessened by binding of an Fab fragment of a potent monoclonal neutralizing antibody, R10, suggesting that it might be acting as a receptor mimic.[407] In contrast, stability is enhanced by divalent binding of the intact antibody, which was shown to block virus binding to cells.[407] A 3.4 Å cryo-EM structure of the capsid in complex with this antibody shows that it binds at the pentamer interface near the twofold axis of symmetry, interacting with residues from VP2 and VP3.

The antigenic structure of the capsid has been explored in studies characterizing viral neutralization escape mutants and by cryo-EM mapping of antibody footprints on the capsid surface.[46,288,357,362,407] The results of these studies are largely consistent and suggest that most neutralizing antibodies, including R10, bind a single, highly conserved, conformationally defined immunodominant antigenic site composed of residues from VP3 and to a lesser extent VP2[46,288,357] (Fig. 2.7E and F). However, escape from neutralization by some antibodies is afforded by amino acid substitutions at VP1 residues outside the footprint of this immunodominant site.[288] This suggests the existence of a second, minor antigenic site, or possibly a novel mechanism of neutralization escape.[362] Empty and full capsids are antigenically indistinguishable.[405]

Quasi-enveloped Virions (eHAV)

Most progeny virions released from cell cultures infected with low passage, noncytopathic HAV are quasi-enveloped.[162,175] Quasi-enveloped virions are small vesicles ranging from 50 to 110 nm diameter that contain one to three, rarely four, HAV capsids.[112] These infectious virions band in isopycnic iodixanol gradients at a density of 1.08 to 1.12 g/cm^3,[112] and have many of the attributes of exosomes, small extracellular vesicles that mediate the transfer of cargo between cells to promote intercellular communication. The 1D (VP1pX) protein in these capsids is unprocessed VP1pX, in contrast to the processed VP1 present in naked particles.[112,256] VP1pX is resistant to proteinase K in the absence of detergents, but rapidly processed to VP1 with loss of the pX segment following detergent disruption of the eHAV membrane.[112] The capsids contain more 1B (VP2) than 1AB (VP0), indicating that most VP0 has undergone the late maturation cleavage (Fig. 2.6E). eHAV capsids are presumed to be antigenically and structurally identical to the naked capsid, but they are occluded by membranes and do not bind anticapsid antibodies in the absence of detergent.[112]

Quantitative proteomic studies using stable amino acid labeling (SILAC) show that eHAV vesicles released by infected Huh-7.5 cells contain only the structural (capsid) proteins of the virus and no nonstructural proteins.[256] This indicates that the capsids are sorted for export from the cell by a highly specific process. The host proteins associated with eHAV are similar to those found in exosomes.[256] However, when compared with exosomes released by uninfected Huh-7.5 cells, eHAV is relatively enriched for a number of endolysosomal proteins, including LAMP1 (lysosome-associated membrane glycoprotein 1), DPP4 (dipeptidyl peptidase-4), CD9, and proteins associated with endosomal sorting complexes required for transport (ESCRT), such as ALIX (ALG-2–interacting protein X or programmed cell death 6–interacting protein) and CHMP4B (charged multivesicular body protein 4B).[256] Immunoprecipitation experiments show that DPP4 is associated with the eHAV membrane, whereas ALIX is more tightly bound to the capsid, reflecting its critical role in eHAV biogenesis (see "Quasi-envelopment and Release"). None of the HAV capsid proteins are predicted to have transmembrane domains, and the inability of high titer convalescent antibody to immunoprecipitate eHAV confirms the absence of viral proteins on its surface.[256] eHAV membranes are enriched in sphingomyelins and ceramides compared with host cell membranes (unpublished data) and display phosphatidylserine on their surface.[116]

REPLICATION CYCLE

Attachment, Entry, and Uncoating

Multiple unique features of hepatoviruses, including a novel capsid assembly mechanism involving 1D protein–dependent formation of pentamer subunits[59,293] (see "Capsid Assembly"), exceptional thermostability of the capsid that is greatest at the low pH of endolysosomes,[405] and a lack of a requirement for the phospholipase PLA2G16 during entry,[312] suggest that the mechanism by which HAV enters, uncoats, and transfers its genome to the cytoplasm differs from other well-studied picornaviruses that enter and uncoat within endosomal compartments.[405,441] Mechanisms of attachment and entry are only partially understood for hepatoviruses and are complicated by the fact that there are two types of extracellular infectious particles requiring different attachment and to some extent entry pathways. Available data suggest that both virion types are taken up into cells by clathrin-dependent endocytosis and subsequently traffic to LAMP1$^+$ late endolysosomes[312] (Fig. 2.6B). The membrane surrounding the capsid in eHAV is degraded in the late endolysosome, releasing the capsid that (like the nHAV capsid) binds endosomal gangliosides in a step essential for entry.[81,312] Events beyond the endolysosome and specific mechanisms leading to the release of the RNA genome into the cytoplasm are unknown but are likely to be similar for both the nHAV-derived and the eHAV-derived capsids.

Naked Virus Entry

The receptor(s) driving endocytosis of the nHAV particle are obscure. Attachment and entry requires Ca^{++} and is reduced in cell culture by treatment with trypsin, β-galactosidase, phospholipase A2 or C, or sialidase,[81,330,355,433] suggesting the involvement of multiple types of cell surface molecules. Studies carried out in the 1990s by Kaplan and colleagues, prior to the discovery of quasi-enveloped virions, suggested that TIM1 (T-cell immunoglobulin mucin receptor 1, CD365) acts as a receptor for HAV, leading to its alternate name, "hepatitis A virus cellular receptor 1" (HAVCR1).[107,108,187,376] TIM1 is a type 1 membrane glycoprotein with an N-terminal, cysteine-rich immunoglobulin-like domain separated from the cell surface by an extended mucin-like domain.[187] Monoclonal antibody raised to an African green monkey kidney cell line (GL37), selected for being highly permissive for HAV infection,[381] blocked infection of these cells by interacting with simian TIM1. Subsequent studies identified the human TIM1 homolog and suggested that it similarly functions as a receptor for HAV.[108]

However, the role of TIM1 in HAV infection remains controversial. Incubating HAV with high concentrations (100 μg/mL) of the combined TIM1 immunoglobulin and mucin-like domains resulted in an approximately 40-fold loss of infectivity, as well as the loss of detectable virus in sucrose gradients.[350] This was interpreted as evidence for uncoating (capsid disassembly), but this was not demonstrated directly. More recent studies show that the extracellular immunoglobulin-like V domain of TIM1 binds the purified HAV capsid with low affinity and does not trigger uncoating or reduce its thermostability in ThermoFluor assays.[376,407] Costafreda and Kaplan[66] reported that CRISPR knockout of TIM1 rendered GL37 cells resistant to both nHAV and eHAV infection. However, two other groups of investigators have reported contradictory data, both showing that CRISPR-mediated TIM1 knockout restricts neither entry nor infection in a variety of cell types.[82,83,204] Das et al.[82,83] found that the loss of TIM1 had no impact on nHAV infection of Huh-7.5, Vero, or GL37 cells and only slightly slowed entry of quasi-enveloped eHAV. These latter data are consistent with TIM1 acting as an accessory attachment factor for eHAV by binding phosphatidylserine displayed on its surface,[82,83,116] much as TIM1 augments the entry of many canonical enveloped viruses.[265] Further supporting the conclusion that TIM1 is not an essential receptor, double-knockout $Tim1^{-/-}Ifnar1^{-/-}$ mice are readily infected with HAV and show little difference in permissiveness from $Ifnar1^{-/-}$ mice lacking only the type I interferon receptor.[82] Thus, an essential protein receptor has yet to be identified for HAV.

The endocytosis of naked virions is both clathrin and dynamin dependent, and incoming particles colocalize sequentially with the small GTPases Rab5a and Rab7A, as they traffic through early to late endosomes where the capsid dissembles.[312] Endocytosis is blocked by siRNA-mediated depletion of integrin β1,[312] but no specific α-integrin–binding partner has been identified. nHAV entry is relatively resistant to chloroquine.[112]

Recent genome-wide CRISPR screens carried out in search of a receptor have revealed that gangliosides (sphingolipids with carbohydrate headgroups containing one or more sialic acid moieties) are essential for HAV entry and infection.[81,204] Hepatoma cells made deficient in gangliosides by genetic knockout of ceramide glucosyltransferase (UGCG), the enzyme catalyzing the first step in ganglioside synthesis, or treatment with the iminosugar UGCG inhibitor miglustat (N-butyl-1-deoxynojirimycin), are refractory to infection with either nHAV or eHAV due to a failure of the viral genome to gain entry to the cytoplasm and undergo translation.[81,262] nHAV was shown to undergo endocytosis in such cells, followed by trafficking to LAMP1[+] late endolysosomes, where trafficking was arrested without uncoating of the genome.[81] Productive infection could be rescued by adding gangliosides to the culture medium, even hours after inoculation of the cells with virus. This reflects the ability of exogenously added gangliosides to become embedded in the plasma membrane and traffic to endolysosomes.[80] Naked nHAV was shown to bind gangliosides coating a solid-phase support, whereas preincubating nHAV with gangliosides blocked infection.[81] Thus, gangliosides appear to act as endolysosomal receptors for HAV and are essential for successful entry of the virus.

Solid-phase ELISA assays suggest that the capsid binds gangliosides with relatively little specificity for the glycan head group.[81] This is consistent with the interaction being driven primarily by electrostatic interactions between negatively charged glycans and positively charged regions of the capsid surface.[405] Nonetheless, disialogangliosides appear to bind the capsid with greater affinity than monosialogangliosides. The disialoganglioside GD1a was most active in blocking infection when preincubated with virus, with a 50% inhibitory concentration (IC$_{50}$) of 1.25 μM.[81] This may reflect the spatial positioning of the two α2,3-linked sialic acid residues in GD1a and suggests a specific role for GD1a in HAV entry. GD1a comprises only a small percentage of the gangliosides present in Huh-7.5 cells but represents approximately 10% of the gangliosides present in the murine liver in vivo.[81,262] These recent findings are consistent with HAV infection being blocked partially by pretreating cells with sialidase[81] and with earlier observations showing that the HAV capsid hemagglutinates human erythrocytes and binds glycophorin A.[68,99,321] Hemagglutination is reduced by a Gly-to-Asp substitution at VP1 residue 217 (HM175 virus), suggesting a possible site of ganglioside interaction on the capsid surface.[68]

Events in entry beyond the binding of GD1a to the capsid within the late endolysosome are unknown. In vitro studies indicate that the thermostability of the capsid is not altered by the binding of disialylated gangliosides, suggesting that gangliosides do not trigger uncoating of the genome.[81] Binding to GD1a is a signal for sorting of murine polyomavirus from the endolysosome to the ER, where the virus usurps components of the cytosolic extraction machinery to penetrate the membrane and enter the cytoplasm largely intact.[98,305,308] It is possible that HAV follows a similar path and that uncoating of the genome is triggered subsequently by interactions of the capsid with an unknown cytosolic protein.[405] How membrane penetration occurs is unknown. Pores form in endosomal membranes during the entry of other picornaviruses,[126] and the VP4 protein of HAV has been reported to have pore-forming activity.[343] However, the position of VP4 within the capsid is uncertain,[405] and it is not known whether it is externalized during the entry process. Breaches in endosomal membranes consistent with pore formation were not observed during nHAV entry.[312]

Quasi-enveloped Virion Entry

The entry of canonical enveloped viruses typically involves membrane fusion mediated by a virally encoded surface glycoprotein (a "peplomer").[154] No such proteins exist within the quasi-envelope of eHAV.[256] Like nHAV, these virions are taken up into cells via endocytosis. eHAV endocytosis is clathrin dependent and to a lesser degree caveolin dependent, and as with the naked nHAV particle, it results in trafficking through Rab5a⁺ early and Rab7A⁺ late endosomes to LAMP1⁺ endolysosomes.[312] Like the naked virion, endocytosis of eHAV is dependent upon integrin β1. However, in contrast to nHAV, eHAV entry is strongly inhibited by the lysosomal poison chloroquine.[112] Given the absence of viral proteins on its surface, the initial attachment and endocytosis of quasi-enveloped virus is most likely mediated by nonspecific interactions, including the binding of phosphatidylserine receptors such as TIM1 to phosphatidylserine on the eHAV surface.[82,83] TIM1 is widely expressed, particularly in the kidney, and similarly facilitates the attachment and entry of a variety of conventional enveloped viruses.[265] The density of such receptors may determine the relative efficiency with which naked and quasi-enveloped viruses initially bind to cells. For example, eHAV binding to GL37 green monkey kidney cells, which express very high levels of TIM1, is more efficient than binding of nHAV at 4°C, whereas the binding efficiencies are reversed in Huh-7.5 cells, which express much less TIM1.[83] In the absence of TIM1, it is likely that other phosphatidylserine receptors, such as TIM4 or AXL, may facilitate endocytosis.

Experiments with purified eHAV virions labeled with an irreversible membrane dye indicate that the eHAV membrane is degraded within LAMP1⁺ endolysosomes.[312] The acidic compartment of the lysosome plays an important role in the constitutive degradation of membrane lipids,[198] and proteins involved in this process, including lysosomal acid lipase (LAL)[312] and Niemann-Pick C1 protein (NPC1),[65,312] contribute to the degradation of the eHAV membrane. Degradation of the quasi-envelope is rate limiting in the entry of eHAV and is slowed by RNAi-mediated knockdown or chemical inhibitors of LAL.[312] The process requires several hours, rendering the entry kinetics of eHAV significantly slower than naked virus.[82,112,312] While the lysosomal NPC1 protein acts as a conventional receptor for filoviruses, interacting directly with the Ebola virus glycoprotein,[47,406] its role in HAV entry reflects its normal physiologic activity as a cholesterol transporter and likely involves scavenging cholesterol from the quasi-envelope membrane. The end result of this process is the release of the naked capsid into the endolysosomal lumen. Although lysosomal cathepsins have been suggested to process 1D (VP1pX) to VP1,[266] it is not known whether this cleavage is essential for subsequent steps in the entry process.

Like nHAV, eHAV is not able to infect cells deficient in gangliosides.[81] eHAV undergoes endocytosis and trafficking through early endosomes in such cells but stalls in the late LAMP1⁺ endolysosome, failing to uncoat the genome. It seems likely that the eHAV capsid interacts with endosomal gangliosides receptors in a manner similar to the nHAV capsid and that subsequent events in entry are identical for the two particle types.[81] However, in contrast to nHAV entry, uncoating of the eHAV capsid is associated with a loss of lysosomal membrane integrity suggestive of pore formation.[312] The significance of this difference is uncertain. It could reflect a mechanistic difference in how the capsids penetrate the membrane, or perhaps more rapid membrane repair in endolysosomal compartments breached by nHAV.

Hepatovirus Translation

Following disassembly of the capsid and its release into the cytosol, the HAV RNA genome associates with ribosomes and directs the synthesis of the viral polyprotein. Unlike enteroviruses, successful engagement of the ribosome by the RNA is not dependent upon the phospholipase, PLA2G16.[312] Like all picornaviruses, there is no 5′ m⁷G cap on the positive-strand viral RNA, and translation is initiated internally under control of an IRES located within the 5′ UTR (Fig. 2.4). Only the *Hepatovirus A* IRES has been characterized functionally. IRES elements in other *Hepatovirus* species, some of which are structurally distinct, have not been studied. *Hepatovirus A* translation is slow and inefficient, and rate-limiting for replication in cultured cells.[130,415] This appears to reflect specific features of the HAV IRES coupled with the extreme codon bias present in the ORF (see "Polyprotein-Coding RNA") that results in a need to recruit low abundance tRNAs.[12,67,291,410] The secondary RNA structure of the type III HAV IRES is unique to hepatoviruses, although it shares some features with the type II IRES elements of aphthoviruses and cardioviruses[45,212] (see "5′ UTR Structure and Function"). Translation initiates at the first or third codon (second in frame Met codon) in the ORF, 735 to 741 nucleotides from the 5′ end of the RNA, with the second in-frame Met codon being favored.[43,45] There is no evidence for scanning of the RNA by ribosomes prior to the initiation of translation.

The HAV IRES has unique host factor requirements. Biochemical studies reveal a surprising need for the cap-binding eukaryotic initiation factor 4F (eIF4F) component, eIF4E.[5,38] The eIF4F complex is crucial for cap-dependent host translation as it recruits 40S ribosome subunits and other initiation factors to the 5′ m⁷G cap on cellular mRNAs.[335] It consists of the cap-binding protein (eIF4E), a scaffold protein (eIF4G), an RNA helicase (eIF4A), and eIF4B. Biochemical studies indicate that the HAV IRES requires the cap-binding eIF4E component to initiate translation, as well as the binding site for eIF4E within the eIF4G scaffold.[5,37,38] HAV translation is thus inhibited by recombinant 4E-binding protein 1 (4E-BP1).[38] HAV IRES activity is also inhibited by the poliovirus 2A protease, which cleaves the eIF4G scaffold subunit of the eIF4F complex.[415] Also consistent with this unusual requirement of the IRES for eIF4E, HAV replication is blocked by inhibition of the mammalian target of rapamycin (mTOR),[422] which results in sequestration of eIF4E by hypophosphorylated 4E-BP1.[5] Why cap-independent HAV translation requires the cap-binding eIF4E subunit of eIF4F is perplexing, as there is no cap on HAV RNAs. eIF4E binding to eIF4G has been shown recently to enhance the binding affinity of the eIF4F complex for the HAV IRES and increase the helicase activity of eIF4A in unwinding duplex RNA within the IRES.[17] However, a similar effect was observed also with the poliovirus IRES, which requires neither eIF4E nor the integrity of eIF4G.

Like other viral and cellular IRES elements,[137,276] the translation-initiating activity of the HAV IRES is significantly modulated by several host RNA-binding proteins that act as IRES-transactivating factors (ITAFs). PCBP2 binds to RNA immediately upstream of the IRES and is required for efficient HAV IRES activity in HeLa cell lysates.[145] PTBP1 binds to stem–loop IIIa, near the 5′ border of the IRES (Fig. 2.4) and strongly stimulates HAV translation when overexpressed in monkey kidney cells.[51,143] The glycolytic enzyme, GAPDH, has substantial RNA-binding activity, particularly for AU-rich elements, and binds to a site overlapping the PTBP1-binding site within the IRES.[329,416] Overexpression of GAPDH significantly suppressed IRES activity in monkey kidney cell cultures.[428] This was not observed in human hepatoma (Huh-7) cells, which express higher levels of PTB. Interestingly, translation directed by the wild-type HAV IRES was more efficiently suppressed by GAPDH than translation directed by the IRES from a cell culture–adapted virus (HM175/p16) with greater basal translational activity and reduced affinity for GAPDH.[428] Thus, although mutations in 2B and 2C are paramount for adaptation of wild-type HAV to efficient replication in cultured cells,[100,102] adaptive mutations within the IRES are also selected during passage of HAV in cell culture.[130,428]

Recent genome-wide CRISPR screens for HAV host factors have highlighted the critical role of translation in replication of HAV. Among candidate essential host factors, independent screens in two different laboratories identified several translation-related proteins, including PTBP1, multiple components of eIF3, and eIF4B.[81,204] One screen also identified host cell proteins known to function in UFMylation, a ubiquitin-like posttranslational modification of proteins, in which UFM1 is conjugated to proteins and UBA5, UFL1, UFC1, and UFSP2 serve as essential host factors for this process.[204] Targeted knockout of UBA5 (ubiquitin-like modifier-activating enzyme 5) suppressed HAV replication and limited translation of a subgenomic HAV RNA. The defect in HAV translation was linked to a lack of UFMylation of the 60S ribosome-associated protein L26 (RPL26),[204] a major cellular target of UFMylation.[398]

CRISPR host factor screens have also identified the zinc-finger RNA-binding protein ZCCHC14 to be essential for HAV replication.[81,204] ZCCHC14 associates with the terminal nucleotidyltransferases, TENT4A and TENT4B (also known as PAPD7 and PAPD5), forming a complex that acts to maintain the stability of cellular and some viral mRNAs by introducing occasional nonadenosine residues into the poly-(A) tail.[195,232] These noncanonical polymerases were also identified as candidate host factors in one of the screens, and CRISPR knockout of either ZCCHC14 or the TENT4A/B polymerases was found to substantially impair HAV replication.[204] A small molecule dihydroquinolizinone inhibitor of the TENT4A/B proteins, RG7834,[150,364] was shown to have striking antiviral activity against HAV replication in liver organoids (EC$_{50}$ = 12.8 nM).[204] Additional experiments showed that knocking out both TENT4A and TENTB had no effect on the length of the HAV poly-(A) tail or the stability of HAV RNA. Preliminary data pointed to a defect in HAV translation in ZCCHC14-deficient cells,[204] but the underlying mechanism remains obscure.

Polyprotein Processing

Proteolytic processing of the polyprotein occurs cotranslationally, in close proximity to the rough ER, with initial cleavage occurring at the 1D/2B junction upon synthesis of the 3C protease (Fig. 2.6C).[142,247] With the exception of the RNA-dependent 1AB maturation cleavage that follows packaging of the genome,[34] and the trimming of pX from VP1 following the release of capsids from eHAV into the extracellular milieu,[147,246] each of the subsequent processing events is mediated by 3C^{pro}.[153,178,327,328,373] Secondary cleavages in the P1 and P2P3 intermediate products produced by the primary cleavage likely occur in a fixed temporal sequence that is optimized for replication of the virus and dependent upon substrate concentrations, cellular localization, and cleavage specificities of 3C^{pro} and the stable proteolytically active, processing intermediate 3ABC.[327,423]

RNA Replication

Like all picornaviruses, the first step in replication of the positive-strand RNA genome is the synthesis of a negative-strand complement (Fig. 2.6D). This results in double-stranded replicative form RNA that serves as template for the synthesis of new positive-strand RNAs. Replication proceeds in a nonconservative manner, with more positive-strand RNA molecules produced than negative-strand copies. As a result, the negative strand is always present in lesser abundance than the positive-strand RNA and likely is always in a duplex and never single stranded. Relatively, little is known about hepatoviral RNA synthesis at a molecular level, and current concepts of this process are based largely on inferences from much more detailed studies of enteroviruses.

RNA synthesis is presumed to occur in replication organelles consisting of tubular–vesicular membranous structures forming in close association with the rough ER in infected cells[144] (Fig. 2.6D). At an ultrastructural level, these membranous structures differ minimally from the replication organelles of enteroviruses.[144] Enteroviral RNAs are synthesized on the cytosolic surface of these membranes,[29,169,316] and this seems likely to be the case for HAV RNA as well. Similar membranes can be induced by overexpression of the HAV 2B and 2BC proteins, and immune electron microscopy of infected cell cultures shows both 2B and 2C are associated with these membranes.[144,374] 2B is thought to bind membranes via a helical transmembrane segment near its C terminus. Subsequent amyloid-like fibrillar aggregation of the protein has been proposed to lead to the reorganization of cellular membranes around 2B fibers.[131,393] The membranes provide a scaffold for assembly of replication complexes containing most if not all of the nonstructural viral proteins and may also shield dsRNA replication intermediates from detection by innate immune pathogen-associated molecular pattern receptors.

The source of the membranes induced by hepatoviruses is uncertain. An N-terminal transmembrane domain in the hepatovirus 3A protein targets 3ABC to membranes associated with mitochondria.[423] In contrast, the enterovirus 3A protein is targeted to the ER or post-ER compartment, consistent with the origin of membranes associated with enteroviral replication organelles.[414] This suggests the interesting possibility that HAV replication might occur on mitochondrial-associated membranes. Replacing the HAV 3A transmembrane domain with the analogous poliovirus 3A sequence resulted in a loss of replication competence.[114] Enteroviruses induce a substantial rewiring of cellular lipid synthesis to facilitate the formation of replication organelles derived from remodeled ER or Golgi membranes.[257] Phosphatidylinositol 4-kinase-IIIβ (PI4K-IIIβ) plays a key role in the formation of enteroviral replication organelles and is recruited to membranes by the enterovirus 3A protein acting in concert with host acyl-coenzyme A binding domain containing 3 (ACBD3).[169,238,318] A mammalian two-hybrid screen suggested that HAV 3A may also bind ACBD3,[148] but ACBD3 has not been shown to be important for replication. Both chemical inhibition and genetic depletion experiments using luciferase reporter replicons indicate that HAV RNA replication proceeds independently of both PI4K-IIIβ and PI4K-IIIα, which is co-opted by hepaciviruses to facilitate similar membrane rearrangements.[105]

Lipid metabolic pathways are nonetheless important in HAV RNA replication. A CRISPR screen identified both acetyl-CoA carboxylase (ACACA) and very-long-chain 3-oxoacyl-CoA reductase (HSD17B12, 17-betahydroxysteroid dehydrogenase type 12) as essential host factors.[81] Both enzymes are required for synthesis of very-long-chain fatty acids (VLCFA) containing ≥22 carbons in the acyl tail.[159,190] Sphingolipids with VLCFA tails can modulate membrane function by spanning both inner and outer leaflets, stabilizing regions of high curvature such as at the neck of budding vesicles or in very small vesicles.[190,315] How VLCFA contributes to the HAV life cycle has yet to be defined, but HSD17B12 is required for both hepacivirus RNA replication and virion assembly.[264] Other host factors identified in genome-wide CRISPR screens include PDAP1 (28-kDa heat- and acid-stable phosphoprotein) and AXIN (axis inhibition protein 1).[81,204] Their roles in the virus life cycle have yet to be defined.

The replication of some enteroviruses is dependent upon components of host autophagic signaling, including the autophagy-related LC3 protein that associates with the membranes of replication organelles in a nonlipidated form.[2,171] While the role of autophagy in hepatovirus replication has not been studied in detail, siRNA depletion of the key autophagy protein beclin-1 has no impact on HAV replication,[112] and rapamycin, a potent inducer of autophagy, has strong antiviral activity against HAV.[422]

As in enteroviruses, HAV RNA synthesis is likely protein primed. An early step in the replication of poliovirus RNAs is the uridylation of the small poliovirus 3B (VPg) protein, resulting in VPg-pUpU, which subsequently primes both negative- and positive-strand RNA synthesis.[280] Uridylation is mediated by the $3D^{pol}$ and 3CD proteins of poliovirus and occurs via a slide-back mechanism templated by an adenylic acid triplet located within the terminal loop of the *cre*, a stable stem–loop structure located within polyprotein-coding RNA[139,281] (Fig. 2.6D). HAV possesses all of these elements: a conserved, stable *cre* stem–loop located within the $3D^{pol}$ coding sequence with an AAACA/G motif in its top loop,[425] and the covalent linkage of its small 3B (VPg) protein to the 5′ terminal uridylic acid of HAV RNA,[411] which like all picornaviruses begins with two uridylic acid residues. Stable RNA structures at both ends of the genome, including the 5′ terminal stem–loop and putative pseudoknots (Fig. 2.4), and RNA structure within and possibly upstream of the 3′ UTR, likely coordinate the positioning of a multiprotein replicase complex on the RNA with $3D^{pol}$ as its catalytic core.[23,180,205,207,209,283] In addition to the mTOR inhibitors rapamycin and Torin 1, HAV RNA synthesis is sensitive to a variety of inhibitors, including the nucleoside analog sofosbuvir, cyclosporin A, tacrolimus, and inhibitors of ATP-binding cassette transporters.[105,183,422]

Capsid Assembly

Assembly of the HAV capsid proceeds in a general manner similar to other picornaviruses, but with some distinct differences, and is dependent upon processing of the P1 segment of the polyprotein. The proteolytically active 3ABC processing intermediate may be more active than the mature $3C^{pro}$ protein in mediating these processing events.[206] The 1AB (VP0), 1C (VP3), and 1D (VP1pX) proteins released from the P1 segment form a single "protomer," the basic building block of the capsid. Five protomers assemble into a 14S "pentamer" (Fig. 2.6E).[39] These pentamer subunits react with some but not all monoclonal antibodies recognizing conformational neutralization

epitopes displayed on the surface of the fully assembled capsid.[358] In other well-studied picornaviruses, pentamer assembly is nucleated by the N-terminally myristoylated VP4 (1A) component of 1AB.[181] By contrast, the assembly of HAV pentamers is dependent upon a discreet segment of the pX sequence located near the C terminus of 1D (VP1pX).[59,293] Whether this reflects a direct scaffolding function of pX, or the influence of the pX segment on folding of the P1 proteins into a conformation optimized for proteolytic processing by $3C^{pro}$, is uncertain.[59] The lack of involvement of 1A (VP4) in HAV pentamer assembly is consistent with the very small size of VP4 and the lack of myristoylation of the protein.[372] It also allows for foreign protein sequences to be fused to the N terminus of VP4 in recombinant viruses without loss of viability.[437] In the final step in assembly, 12 pentamer subunits assemble to form the viral capsid[405] (Fig. 2.6E). Capsid assembly does not require replication of the virus and is recapitulated in cells infected with recombinant vaccinia viruses expressing the P1 and P2P3 polyprotein segments.[59,418]

RNA Packaging

The mechanism by which RNA is packaged into the capsid is not understood. Both 70-80S "empty" capsids and 144-150S "full" capsids containing RNA are found in lysates of infected cells.[8,405] It remains unclear as to whether these particles represent sequential stages in assembly of the complete virus or, alternatively, whether empty capsids represent a dead end in morphogenesis. Most evidence favors an encapsidation model in which pentamers condense around an RNA molecule, driven either by electrostatic charge or by iterative capsid protein interactions with multiple packaging signals distributed across the genome.[360,442] Details for HAV are uncertain, but cryo-EM models of the structure of the complete virus particle show that the RNA exists in a layered fashion, contacting the capsid proteins at multiple points,[407] A role for the 2C ATPase has been identified in packaging of enteroviral RNAs into capsids,[14,234] but this possibility has not been explored for hepatoviruses. RNA packaging is highly efficient in HAV-infected cell cultures, with greater than 95% of the positive-strand viral RNA packaged in capsids.[9]

RNA packaging results in cleavage of 1AB (VP0) into 1A (VP4) and 1B (VP2), likely by an autocatalytic mechanism broadly conserved among picornaviruses[160] (Fig. 2.6E). This "maturation" cleavage appears to proceed more slowly with HAV than in other picornaviruses,[34] and x-ray crystallography studies suggest that a greater fraction of 1AB (VP0) remains unprocessed in HAV particles containing RNA.[405] Capsids that have packaged RNA and contain mostly cleaved 1AB (VP0), 1C (VP3), and intact 1D (VP1pX) are subsequently sorted for export from the cell as quasi-enveloped virions.[112]

Quasi-envelopment and Release

Electron microscopy of liver tissue and infected cell cultures has demonstrated the presence of HAV capsids within cytoplasmic vesicles resembling multivesicular endosomes (MVE).[72,338,369] Additional evidence suggests that HAV particles accumulate within lysosome-associated membrane protein 2 (LAMP2)⁺ endolysosomes in infected cell cultures.[331] These observations are consistent with other data suggesting that quasi-enveloped virions are generated by budding of assembled viral capsids into MVEs in an ESCRT-dependent process mirroring the biogenesis of exosomes[158] (Fig. 2.6B). Quantitative proteomics studies of purified eHAV virions show that HAV capsids are sorted for export in a highly selective fashion, as extracellular eHAV vesicles contain no detectable HAV nonstructural proteins.[256]

Two factors are required for budding of the capsid into MVEs: membrane association and ESCRT recruitment.[396] While it is uncertain how capsids are sorted to the surface of endosomes, HAV capsid proteins contain specific adaptor sequences resembling the "late domains" of canonical enveloped viruses that mediate interactions with the ESCRT-associated protein ALIX.[124,215] The C-terminal pX sequence, downstream of the segment required for pentamer assembly,[59] forms a complex with ALIX.[182] Deletion of the C-terminal half of pX eliminated the release of quasi-enveloped virions from cells, whereas fusing this sequence to the C terminus of green fluorescent protein (GFP) resulted in the export of GFP from cells in exosomes.[182] Tandem YPX$_{1-3}$L late domain motifs also exist within the 1B (VP2) capsid protein that interact with ALIX.[112,138] Mutations ablating the VP2 motifs not only impair eHAV release but also interfere with capsid assembly, making these peptide motifs difficult to study.[138] In contrast to pX, which is on the surface of the capsid, x-ray crystallography shows these putative VP2 late domains are largely buried in the structure of the mature capsid.[405] How they could interact with ALIX is uncertain, but "breathing" has been shown to occur in the structures of other picornaviral capsids, resulting in externalization of otherwise internal VP4 and VP1 polypeptide sequences.[233]

Interactions with ALIX feed the capsid into the ESCRT system, resulting in the recruitment of ESCRT-III components that sculpt the membrane, promoting budding of the capsid and finally mediating membrane scission.[397] This results in the formation of capsid-laden intraluminal vesicles (ILVs) that are subsequently released into the extracellular environment as quasi-enveloped virions upon fusion of the limiting membrane of the MVE with the plasma membrane of the cell (Fig. 2.6B). RNAi-mediated depletion of ALIX, as well as the ESCRT-III complex proteins, charged multivesicular protein 2A (CHMP2A) and IST1 homolog (IST), or the ESCRT accessory protein VPS4B, inhibits the release of eHAV from infected cells.[112,256] ALIX, IST1, and CHMP1A, CHMP1B, and CHMP4B, components of ESCRT-III, are also physically associated with extracellular eHAV produced in cell culture.[256]

Hepatocytes are highly polarized cells of epithelial origin with basolateral membranes facing onto the space of Disse, which communicates with blood flowing through hepatic sinusoids, and a smaller apical membrane abutting the lumen of the biliary canaliculus, which communicates ultimately with the gut[40,382] (Fig. 2.6B). *In vivo*, copious amounts of virus are released into the bile across the apical membrane of hepatocytes and subsequently shed in feces.[162,325] Functional cell culture models of polarized hepatocytes are limited, but HAV release has been studied in polarized cultures of various cell types using permeable transwell systems. Early studies showed that HAV release occurred in a vectorial fashion, predominantly from the apical surface of polarized CaCo-2 colonic epithelial cells, and that release was inhibited by brefeldin A.[35] On the other hand, release from polarized HepG2-N6 cells of hepatocyte origin was found to be primarily from the basolateral membrane.[354] More recent studies show that the virus released across both

basolateral and apical membranes is predominantly (if not exclusively) quasi-enveloped in polarized cultures of both cell types.[162] Although basolateral-to-apical transcytosis is very inefficient in transwell experiments,[69,162] a small fraction of naked virions inoculated intravenously into mice undergo transcytosis across hepatocytes and are released into bile.[69] This release is significantly enhanced by IgA anti-HAV, which facilitates transcytosis via the epithelial polymeric immunoglobulin receptor (pIgR).[69] The biological significance of these findings is uncertain, since the virus present in blood is quasi-enveloped.[112]

While nonlytic release of quasi-enveloped virus is the major mechanism of viral egress in cell culture, a variable proportion of new viral progeny may be found in the supernatant fluids of infected cell cultures unassociated with membranes.[112,162] These particles are likely released from dying cells or derived from extracellular eHAV virions that have lost their membrane. In these extracellular naked virions, 1D has been processed to VP1 with loss of the pX polypeptide from the particle, leaving VP1 with a heterogeneous C terminus[147,307] (Fig. 2.6E, see "P1 Capsid Proteins").

PATHOGENESIS

Host Range

As a genus, hepatoviruses infect a wide range of mammalian species, including opossums, members of the order Marsupialia that diverged genetically from other mammals approximately 170 mya.[11,85,96,260,432] Phylogenetic analyses show discordance in the topologies of virus and host phylogenies suggestive of frequent cross-species and cross-order host shifts during the evolution of hepatoviruses.[85,96] Statistically significant virus–host phylogenic concordance is greatest in the P1 segment of the genome encoding the capsid protein and less in the P2P3 segment encoding nonstructural proteins.[85] At the level of viral species, the natural host range of *Hepatovirus A* is restricted to primates, with some evidence for host species specificity linked to virus genotype. Viruses in genotypes I to III have been recovered from humans, whereas viruses in genotypes IV to VI have been recovered only from nonhuman primates (see Fig. 2.3A). Viruses isolated from Old World monkeys that cluster in genotype V have minor antigenic differences from human HAV.[104,269,383] The genotype V AGM-27 virus, which was isolated from an African green monkey, causes severe hepatitis in this species but is substantially less virulent in chimpanzees.[104] On the other hand, the genotype 1a MS-1 virus, recovered from infected children in the Willowbrook studies, gained virulence in tamarins upon serial passage but became relatively attenuated for chimpanzees.[42]

Infections are possible outside the natural host range of *Hepatovirus A*. Dunkin-Hartley guinea pigs were reported to be susceptible to infection, although few quantitative data were provided to support this claim.[168] More definitively, mice can be infected if they are genetically deficient in type I interferon responses[161] (see "Animal Models"). This indicates host species restriction is related to the capacity of *Hepatovirus A* to evade innate immune responses,[161,163] not a requirement for a specific cellular receptor. Consistent with this, a variety of cultured cell lines of primate and nonprimate origin are permissive for HAV infection.[32,93,106]

Tropism

Hepatovirus A is highly hepatotropic with hepatocytes the cell type most prominently infected in the liver. Viral RNA levels are highest in liver tissue, and HAV RNA and virus-specific antigen have been localized to hepatocytes both in humans and experimentally infected nonhuman primates.[200,251,290,338,367,368] *In situ* hybridization has also confirmed the presence of *Hepatovirus A* RNA in hepatocytes of infected *Ifnar1*[−/−] and *Mavs*[−/−] mice.[161] However, other cell types may also be infected within the liver. HAV antigen and RNA have been identified within Kupffer cells, tissue-resident macrophages in the liver, as well as sinusoidal endothelial cells.[337,338,368] Other species of hepatoviruses appear to be equally hepatotropic. *Hepatovirus B* ("phopivirus") RNA was identified in hepatocytes of infected harbor seals (*Phoca vitulina*)[11] and *Hepatovirus H* RNA in hepatocytes of an infected bat (*Eidolon helvum*).[96] *Hepatovirus F* RNA levels were highest in the liver of infected woodchucks (*Marmota himalayana*),[431,432] but appreciable quantities of RNA were also present in the spleen. This likely reflects scavenging of the virus from blood, as negative-strand *Hepatovirus F* RNA was found only in liver tissue. The molecular basis of hepatotropism is not understood.

Given that HAV is typically transmitted in a fecal–oral manner, several studies have sought evidence for replication within cells of the gastrointestinal tract. HAV-specific immunofluorescence was identified in a small number of epithelial cells lining crypts of the small intestine of orally infected owl monkeys (*Aotus trivirgatus*),[15] but a detailed search for viral antigen in tissues from the gastrointestinal tract of infected tamarins (*Saguinus mystax*) revealed no evidence for replication in the gut.[250] On the other hand, negative-strand *Hepatovirus A* RNA replication intermediates were identified in salivary gland tissues of infected cynomolgus monkeys (*Macaca fascicularis*) using a validated, strand-specific RT-PCR assay,[7] and virus has been found in tonsillar tissue, saliva, and throat washings from infected chimpanzees (*Pan troglodytes*) and owl monkeys (*Aotus trivirgatus*).[15,60] Immunocompromised Alb-urokinase–type plasminogen activator (Alb/uPA) SCID beige mice with chimeric human livers were also found to be infectable by intranasal inoculation of virus but not oral gavage.[163]

Animal Models

Nonhuman Primate Models of Infection

A variety of Old World and New World nonhuman primate species are susceptible to *Hepatovirus A*.[302] Many of these species have been used to model human infection, including chimpanzees (*Pan troglodytes*),[89,252] rhesus and cynomolgus macaques (*Macaca mulatta* and *M. fascicularis*),[7,336] green monkeys (*Cercopithecus aethiops*),[336] tamarins (*Saguinus mystax* and *S. labiatus*),[253,300] and owl monkeys (*Aotus trivirgatus*).[214] In general, infection in each of these species is consistent with observations in humans in which the liver is generally not accessible for studies, suggesting that pathogenesis is very similar in humans and nonhuman primates.[36,111,155,202]

Tamarins were recognized to be susceptible to hepatitis A prior to discovery of the virus.[165] Subsequent studies in chimpanzees, tamarins, and owl monkeys were critical in demonstrating HAV hepatotropism and defining the virologic events in hepatitis A[90,189,210,252,322,325] (Fig. 2.8). Acute inflammatory liver injury, marked by the sudden appearance of elevated serum levels of liver-specific enzymes, especially alanine aminotransferase (ALT), typically occurs coincident with the appearance of anti-HAV antibodies, about 2 to 3 weeks after virus challenge. The onset of acute liver injury is preceded by increasing fecal shedding of virus and is associated with a low magnitude viremia[60,369] (Fig. 2.8E). Viral antigen is found within hepatocytes and in hepatic Kupffer cells, with lesser amounts located within germinal centers of the spleen and lymph nodes and along the glomerular basement membrane in the kidney.[250,337]

Studies in chimpanzees were particularly informative because of their large size and close genetic relatedness to humans.[89,210,252] Such studies are no longer permissible due to ethical considerations. Pathologic findings in the chimpanzee liver closely recapitulate those seen in humans, although chimpanzees are in general less severely affected than adult humans.[89,252,268,292,370] This may reflect the influence of age on viral pathogenesis, as young children typically have milder disease than adults, and many of the chimpanzees studied were relatively young. In chimpanzees, the earliest elevations of serum ALT levels are associated temporally with focal hepatic necrosis and the appearance of periportal infiltrates consisting primarily of lymphocytes and macrophages[75,292] (Fig. 2.8G). At later stages of the infection, there is more aggressive piecemeal necrosis, characterized by disruption of the limiting plate of the portal tract and portal-to-portal bridging necrosis. Necrotic and apoptotic, caspase-3+ hepatocytes are evident throughout much of the parenchyma, although the centrilobular zone may be relatively spared. Histologic evidence of inflammation and hepatocellular apoptosis recede slowly over weeks, with serum enzyme levels returning to normal prior to resolution of the histologic lesions[75,292] (Fig. 2.8E). HAV is incapable of establishing long-term persistent infections, either in humans or in nonhuman primates, and fecal shedding of virus declines rapidly following the appearance of anti-HAV antibodies.[210] Nonetheless, viral RNA persists within the liver for many months, most likely in a nonreplicative state as fecal shedding of virus is not detected.[210] Despite the tendency to mild disease, fulminant hepatitis has been reported in an HAV-infected chimpanzee.[1,375] Innate immune responses to HAV infection are generally muted and of low magnitude in chimpanzees compared to responses observed in HCV-infected chimpanzees (Fig. 2.8A) (see "Cell Intrinsic and Innate Immune Host Responses to HAV"). Virus-specific CD4+ and CD8+ T-cell responses have been detected in chimpanzees (Fig. 2.8A) (see "Cellular Immune Responses to HAV Infection").

Large amounts of virus are found in the bile of chimpanzees,[325] consistent with the notion that virus shed in feces is derived primarily from the liver. Extensive efforts to document an enteric site of virus replication in orally and intravenously infected primates generated generally negative results[15,250,251] (see "Tropism").

Murine Models of Human Hepatitis A

Genetically modified mice provide a useful model of hepatitis A, recapitulate many aspects of the infection in nonhuman primates and humans, and are much more accessible than nonhuman primate models. Normal mice are not susceptible to infection with HAV, but *Ifnar1*[−/−] mice that lack expression of

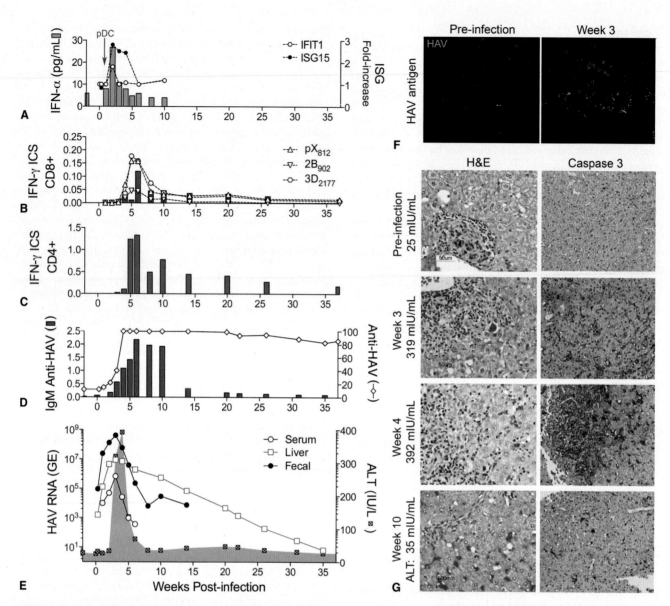

FIGURE 2.8 HAV infection in experimentally infected chimpanzees. A: Serum interferon (IFN)-α levels and relative intrahepatic abundance of interferon-stimulated IFIT1 and ISG15 mRNAs measured by reverse transcription–polymerase chain reaction. **B and C:** Circulating virus-specific CD8+ and CD4+ T cells detected by intracellular cytokine staining (ICS) for IFN-γ (also shown in **B** are virus-specific CD8+ T cells identified by staining with three different tetramers). **D:** Serum IgM–specific and total anti-HAV activities measured by ELISA. **E:** Serum, liver, and fecal HAV RNA measured by RT-PCR and serum alanine transaminase (ALT) activities by enzymatic assay. GE, genome equivalent. **F:** Fluorescent antibody staining for HAV antigen in liver (*green*) of an infected chimpanzee. Nuclei visualized by DAPI co-stain (*red*). **G:** (*left*) Hematoxylin and eosin (H&E) staining and immunohistochemical staining for cleaved caspase-3 in sequential liver sections of a chimpanzee postinfection. At 3 and 4 weeks, the normal hepatic architecture is moderately disordered and there is piecemeal necrosis with extensive periportal inflammatory infiltrates extending into the parenchyma with diffuse hepatocellular swelling. By week 10, inflammatory infiltrates are resolving and the normal architecture of the liver has been largely restored. Cleaved caspase-3 staining indicative of hepatocellular apoptosis is prominent at week 3. (Panels **A-E** reprinted from Walker CM, Feng Z, Lemon SM. Reassessing immune control of hepatitis A virus. *Curr Opin Virol* 2015;11:7–13. Copyright © 2015 Elsevier. With permission; Panels **F** and **G** adapted with permission from Lanford RE, Feng Z, Chavez D, et al. Acute hepatitis A virus infection is associated with a limited type I interferon response and persistence of intrahepatic viral RNA. *Proc Natl Acad Sci U S A* 2011;108(27):11223–11228.)

the type I interferon receptor can be infected either by intravenous or intraperitoneal inoculation[161] (Fig. 2.9). Viral RNA is found at very low levels in many organs, but replication is confined to the liver and associated with viremia, fecal shedding of virus via the biliary tract, serum ALT elevations, and impressive inflammatory changes in the liver.[161,162] Apoptotic

hepatocytes with cleaved caspase-3 are scattered throughout the parenchyma, surrounded by aggregates of lymphocytes and macrophages (Fig. 2.9C). The normal liver architecture may be completely destroyed, with large, confluent areas of inflammation, in mice inoculated with large amounts of virus. F4/80+CD11B+ macrophages and CD3−NK1.1+ natural killer

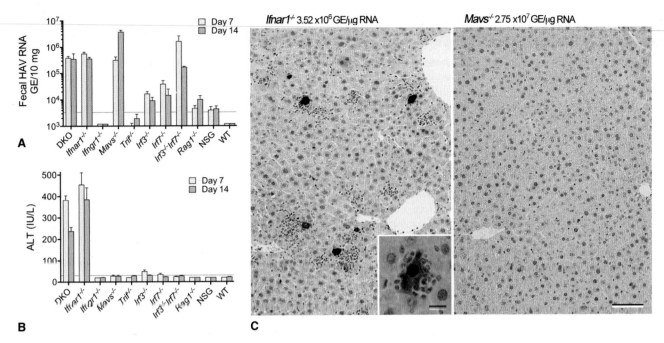

FIGURE 2.9 HAV infection in genetically modified mice. Fecal HAV shedding (A) and serum alanine aminotransferase (ALT) (B) activities 7 and 14 days after intravenous inoculation of genetically modified mice with HAV.[161] Mice with genetic knockout of the type I interferon receptor (IFNAR1), or key components of RIG-I–like helicase-induced signaling pathways leading to type I interferon synthesis are susceptible to infection, but no disease (ALT elevations) is observed in infected animals lacking mitochondrial antiviral signaling protein (MAVS) or interferon regulatory factor (IRF)3/7 expression. Double knockout (DKO): $Ifnar1^{-/-}Ifngr1^{-/-}$. **C:** Histopathology with immunohistochemical staining for cleaved caspase-3 in liver sections from infected $Ifnar1^{-/-}$ and $Mavs^{-/-}$ animals. Multiple apoptotic, caspase-3+ hepatocytes are evident in infected $Ifnar1^{-/-}$ liver (see **inset**), most surrounded by mixed inflammatory cell infiltrates. There are no pathologic changes in the infected $Mavs^{-/-}$ tissue, which contained greater amounts of viral RNA. Bar = 100 μm (inset bar = 12.5 μm). (Adapted from Hirai-Yuki A, Hensley L, McGivern DR, et al. MAVS-dependent host species range and pathogenicity of human hepatitis A virus. *Science* 2016;353(6307):1541–1545. Reprinted with permission from AAAS.)

cells are sharply increased in number within the liver, and both CD4+ and CD8+ T lymphocytes are found in infiltrates.[161,162,262] Mice lacking expression of mitochondrial antiviral signaling protein ($Mavs^{-/-}$ mice) or IRFs ($Irf3^{-/-}Irf7^{-/-}$ double-knockout mice) are also susceptible to infection but develop no ALT elevation and have no inflammatory response to the infection within the liver[161] (Fig. 2.9A and B). Prechallenge T-cell and NK cell depletion does not diminish the severity of the hepatitis in $Ifnar1^{-/-}$ mice, and liver injury in these animals appears to result from MAVS-dependent transcriptional activation of IRF3 and subsequent IRF3-dependent induction of proapoptotic interferon-stimulated genes (ISGs).[161] Only wild-type HAV is capable of infecting $Ifnar1^{-/-}$ mice, as no infection was observed with cell culture–adapted virus (unpublished data).

Efforts have also been made to model HAV infection in Alb-urokinase–type plasminogen activator (Alb-uPA) SCID beige mice with chimeric human livers.[163] Following intravenous or intraperitoneal inoculation with wild-type virus, these mice became viremic and shed virus in feces. Immunohistochemical studies revealed the presence of viral RNA in human hepatocytes costained with antibody to human cytokeratin 18 but not in resident murine hepatocytes.[163] Virus found in the blood banded in iodixanol at a density consistent with quasi-enveloped eHAV, while virus in bile or shed in feces was nonenveloped. Both types of particles were infectious when used to challenge naive animals.[163] Interestingly, these mice could not be infected by oral gavage but were infected by intranasal exposure to the virus.

Animal Models of Other Hepatovirus Species

Experimental infections of animals with hepatovirus species other than *Hepatovirus A* are limited thus far to *Hepatovirus F*. Woodchucks (*Marmota monax*) inoculated intravenously with woodchuck hepatovirus developed fever, became viremic, shed virus in feces, and had histologic evidence of hepatitis.[431] High levels of positive-strand viral RNA were detected in the liver and spleen, but negative-strand RNA was found only in the liver.

Steps in HAV Pathogenesis

Infection typically results from oral exposure to naked nHAV particles contaminating food or otherwise present in the environment. Less commonly, infection is initiated from parenteral exposure to the virus (see "Transmission"). How the virus reaches the liver from the gut is not known. Viral antigen has been detected in epithelial cells lining crypts of the small intestines a few days after oral inoculation of owl monkeys,[15] but there is no other direct evidence for a gastrointestinal site of replication (see "Tropism"). The minimal dose of virus to achieve infection is approximately 10,000-fold greater when given orally instead of intravenously to chimpanzees or tamarins.[304] Thus, passage from the gut to the liver is very inefficient. One possibility is that the virus undergoes apical-to-basolateral transcytosis across specialized microfold ("M") cells overlying mucosal-associated lymphoid tissues, allowing it to breach the gastrointestinal epithelial barrier, as proposed for poliovirus.[278,344,366] Transport from the gut to the liver by the binding of virus to HAV-specific

IgA, followed by apical-to-basolateral transport across the gastrointestinal epithelium via pIgR, and subsequent infection of the liver by HAV-IgA complexes via the asialoglycoprotein receptor, has also been suggested.[92,94] This seems unlikely to be important in primary infection but could result in an enterohepatic circulation of HAV once IgA antibodies have developed and could play a role in relapsing hepatitis A infections (see "Clinical Manifestations of HAV Infection").[95]

Once in the liver, the virus establishes a productive infection in hepatocytes (and possibly also liver sinusoidal endothelial cells).[251,338,368] Most evidence, including the robust infection of hepatocytes in *Mavs*[−/−] mice in the absence of hepatocyte injury (Fig. 2.9C),[161] suggests that replication is noncytolytic. Virus is released as quasi-enveloped eHAV virions from the basolateral membrane of the hepatocyte into blood flowing through the hepatic sinusoids (Fig. 2.6B), resulting in viremia and leading to infection of additional hepatocytes and spread within the liver.[112,162] eHAV is similarly released from the smaller apical hepatocyte membrane into the biliary canaliculus (Fig. 2.6B), where it is stripped of membranes by high concentrations of unbuffered bile salts.[162,163,325] Naked, nonenveloped virus is then shed in feces. Infection remains clinically silent for 2 to 3 weeks after exposure during which there are multiple rounds of infection and a growing mass of infected hepatocytes.

Between 3 and 5 weeks after initial exposure, this subclinical phase of the infection is terminated, often abruptly, by the onset of liver injury coincident with the first manifestations of adaptive immune responses: virus-specific IgM antibodies and inflammatory intrahepatic cell infiltrates.[210,222,386,440] Liver injury is immunopathologically mediated and not due to viral cytolysis (see "Mechanisms of Liver Injury"). What triggers this sudden change in tolerance for the infection is unclear, but it could be the number of hepatocytes infected and/or the size of the antigenic mass. Consistent with this hypothesis, there is a strong inverse correlation between the titer of an inoculum and the time to first elevation of ALT in tamarins.[303]

Virulence (i.e., liver injury) is linked to the replicative capacity of the virus in the liver and is typically attenuated during cell culture passage of the virus. Wild-type virus can be isolated in a variety of mammalian cell lines, but replication is typically inefficient and slow.[32] Upon serial passage in cell culture, HAV replicates more rapidly and to higher titer and in some cases with cytopathic effect.[77,226] Adaptation to cell culture results in a progressive loss of fitness in nonhuman primates.[110,188,296] Enhanced replication in cell culture is associated with key changes in the 2B protein and, to a lesser extent, within the 5′ UTR, whereas mutations in 2C and 1D have been linked to virulence in tamarins.[101,102,128,175] A candidate attenuated vaccine derived by cell culture passage of virus demonstrated very poor immunogenicity in humans,[259] yet such vaccines are used in some countries (see "Hepatitis A Vaccines").

Cell-Intrinsic and Innate Immune Host Responses to HAV

Cell culture–based studies show that HAV replication is restricted by both basal and induced expression of multiple ISGs, with IRF1 playing a key role.[118,422] Experiments involving RNAi-mediated depletion of antiviral factors linked to retinoic acid–induced gene I (RIG-I)-like receptor (RLR) and Toll-like receptor (TLR) signaling identified key roles for IRF1 and to a lesser extent RIG-I,

LGP2 (also known as RLR-3 or DHX58), and both type I and type III interferon receptors in restricting HAV replication in PH5CH8 immortalized human hepatocytes.[422] Important IRF1-regulated effector genes included RARRES3 (phospholipase A and acyltransferase 4), ERAP2 (ER aminopeptidase 2), NMI (N-myc-interactors), and the canonical ISG, MX1 (interferon-induced GTP-binding protein Mx1). IRF1 was shown to act independently of MAVS, IRF3, and STAT1 (signal transducer and activator of transcription 1)-dependent signaling pathways and to be required for basal protection against HAV that does not require transcription.[422] Consistent with this, *Irf1*[−/−] mice lacking IRF1 expression were capable of supporting limited replication of the virus. Protein kinase R (PKR) has also been shown to sense HAV infection and to restrict replication in PH5CH8 cells by mediating a global shutdown of translation.[115] This activity is inhibited by the nucleotide-binding domain and leucine-rich repeat (NLR) protein NLRX1, which competes with PKR for binding to HAV RNA, thereby allowing synthesis of critical IRF1-regulated innate immune effector genes.[115] Thus, host cell intrinsic responses to HAV infection are complex, multilayered, and nuanced by competing interactions and overlapping signaling pathways.

HAV replication is sensitive to type I interferons in cell culture. The IC_{50} of recombinant IFN-a2b is approximately 1 unit/mL.[28,385,423] However, studies in chimpanzees have shown that acute HAV infection evokes only minimal intrahepatic type I IFN responses, much less than HCV infection[210] (Fig. 2.8A). Plasmacytoid dendritic cells (pDCs), which typically produce large amounts of type 1 interferon in response to virus infections, respond robustly when placed in coculture with HAV-infected cells or exposed to quasi-enveloped eHAV but not naked virions.[116] pDCs can be detected within hepatic sinusoids by the end of the first week of infection in chimpanzees but subsequently disappear and are not present at the peak of virus replication[116] (Fig. 2.8A).

Interferon responses are disrupted by the 3C[pro] processing intermediates, 3ABC and 3CD, which proteolytically cleave and functionally eliminate MAVS and TRIF, respectively, key signaling adaptor molecules involved in the induction of interferon responses[119,306,423] (Fig. 2.10) (see "3C[pro] Protease"). Interestingly, these same adaptor proteins are targeted for cleavage by the unrelated HCV serine protease, NS3/4A.[230,231] The mature HAV protease, 3C[pro], also cleaves NEMO, a bridging adaptor required for NF-κB activation and IFN-β expression, which may contribute to the differences observed between HAV and HCV.[402] The 2B protein also has been suggested to act cooperatively with 3ABC in suppressing MAVS-dependent activation of IRF3.[282]

In addition to exerting antiviral effects, interferon-induced genes may contribute to the pathogenesis of HAV infection. HAV infection is transcriptionally silent in *Mavs*[−/−] mice in which there is no evidence of hepatitis (Fig. 2.9B), whereas there are profound changes in the RNA transcriptome associated with the inflammatory liver injury in infected *Ifnar1*[−/−] mice.[161,363] High-throughput sequencing demonstrated the up-regulation of hundreds of genes in *Ifnar1*[−/−] mice, including pattern recognition receptors, interferons, chemokines, cytokines, and other ISGs.[363] These genes were induced by direct transcriptional activity of IRF3 in the absence of signaling through the type I interferon receptor and include some

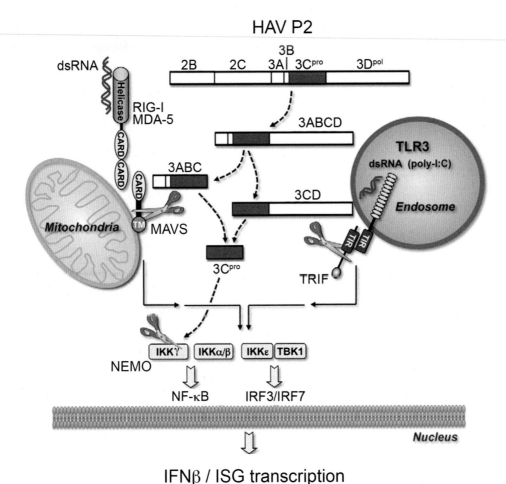

HAV P2

IFNβ / ISG transcription

FIGURE 2.10 Disruption of virus-induced interferon induction signaling pathways by the HAV 3Cᵖʳᵉ protease. 3Cᵖʳᵒ and its stable precursor processing intermediates, 3ABC and 3CD, cleave key signaling molecules involved in transcriptional induction of interferon-β. A transmembrane domain near its amino terminus results in the mitochondrial localization of 3ABC, which then cleaves the mitochondrial antiviral signaling protein (MAVS), a crucial adaptor for RIG-I–like receptor (RLR)-mediated interferon responses. 3CD cleaves TIR domain–containing adaptor inducing interferon-β (TICAM1 or TRIF), a key adaptor of Toll-like receptor 3 (TLR3) signaling, whereas mature 3Cᵖʳᵒ protein cleaves NF-kB essential modulator (IKKg or NEMO), a regulatory subunit of the IKK inhibitor complex. The degradation of these host signaling proteins impedes the activation of transcription factors, NF-κB, and interferon regulatory factors (IRF) 3 and 7, that are essential for induction of an interferon-mediated antiviral state. (Modified from Qu L, Feng Z, Yamane D, et al. Disruption of TLR3 signaling due to cleavage of TRIF by the hepatitis A virus protease-polymerase processing intermediate, 3CD. *PLoS Pathog* 2011;7(9):e1002169. https://creativecommons.org/licenses/by/3.0/.)

with proapoptotic activity that may contribute to the inflammatory response to infection in mice. Chemokines, including CXCL10, are similarly robustly expressed in an IRF3-dependent, interferon-independent manner in infected hepatocytes within the liver of human subjects with acute hepatitis A.[365] These cytokines and chemokines may have pleiotropic effects on immune cell recruitment and T-cell activation.

Humoral Immune Responses to HAV Infection

HAV infection evokes a strong humoral immune response that persists for life and provides a high level of protection against reinfection. Neutralizing antibodies directed against the capsid appear in the serum shortly before or coincident with elevations of ALT activity.[219] This early antibody response is primarily IgM and is supplanted within several weeks by a strong and lasting IgG antibody response[97,120,216,222] (Fig. 2.11A). IgM antibodies may be detected for up to 6 to 12 months after the onset of disease, depending on the sensitivity of the test employed, and provide a useful serologic marker for diagnosis of hepatitis A. IgA anti-HAV can also be detected in serum and persists for up to 2 years, but secretory IgA anti-HAV is uncommon in saliva or fecal suspensions[10,235,349,356] (Fig. 2.11A).

Studies in chimpanzees demonstrated that the appearance of anti-HAV in serum is matched by striking up-regulation of genes involved in B-cell development and immunoglobulin (Ig) synthesis within the liver, including genes encoding both heavy and light chain Ig components and the chemokine CXCL13

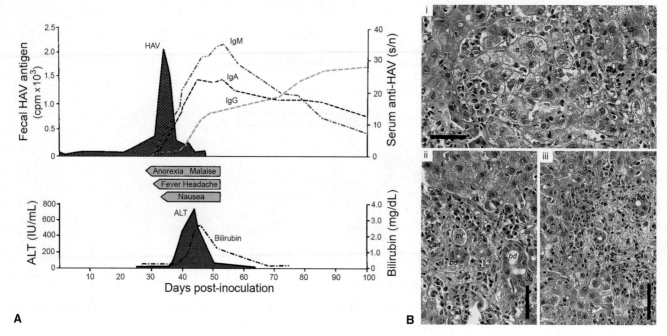

FIGURE 2.11 Clinical findings in acute hepatitis A in humans. A: Virologic and serologic findings during acute HAV infection in a human subject who was infected experimentally by oral inoculation of serum containing MS-1 virus.[36] Fecal HAV antigen and serum antibody responses were measured by solid-phase radioimmunoassays. **B:** Hematoxylin and eosin-stained liver tissue from a 37-year-old male with naturally occurring hepatitis A complicated by prolonged cholestasis and autoimmune hemolytic anemia.[194] The biopsy was taken shortly after the patient was begun on prednisolone therapy. (i) The normal architecture of the liver has been disrupted. The hepatic plates are disordered by swelling of hepatocytes and parenchymal inflammatory infiltrates causing lobular disarray. Hepatocytes are swollen (a) with a lacey appearance to the cytoplasm. Clusters of plasma cells (b) are present within the parenchyma. (ii) Periportal piecemeal necrosis: (c) an inflammatory infiltrate comprised of lymphocytes and macrophages has disrupted the limiting plate. (iii) Piecemeal necrosis (c) associated with adjacent remnants of necrotic or eosinophilic apoptotic (d) hepatocytes. *bd*, bile ducts; *pv*, portal vein; *art*, hepatic artery branch. Bars = 50 μm. (Panel **A** modified from Lemon SM. 1985. Type A viral hepatitis: new developments in an old disease. *N Engl J Med* 313(17):1059–1067. Copyright © 1985 Massachusetts Medical Society. Reprinted with permission from Massachusetts Medical Society; Panel **B** reprinted with permission from Cullen JM, Lemon SM. Comparative pathology of hepatitis A virus and hepatitis E virus infection. *Cold Spring Harb Perspect Med* 2019;9(4):a033456. Copyright © 2019 Cold Spring Harbor Laboratory Press. Stained liver section kindly provided by Sook Hyang-Jeong, Seoul National University Bundang Hospital, Seoul, Korea.)

that recruits B cells to the liver.[210] Circulating CD27(hi) CD38(hi) HAV-specific IgM-secreting plasmablasts are present in the blood of infected humans and can be identified by labeling with fluorescently tagged VP1 capsid protein.[167] Increased numbers of plasma cells are typically evident within the liver (Fig. 2.11B).[75] Plasmablasts secreting non–HAV-specific IgM antibodies are also increased in blood, likely mobilized from the bone marrow or spleen.[167]

The analysis of viral neutralization escape mutants generated with monoclonal antibodies, and more recent cryo-EM studies of antibody footprints on the capsid surface, indicates that most neutralizing antibodies target a single, conserved, conformational antigenic site formed by residues from VP3 and VP2[46,287,357,407] (Fig. 2.7E and F) (see "Naked Nonenveloped Virions [nHAV]"). Coupled with limited cross-genotype neutralization studies,[221] these data support the existence of a single *Hepatovirus A* serotype. Thus, infection with any strain of HAV results in protection against reinfection by all genotypes of the virus (see "Immunity"). Antibodies targeting the nonstructural P2 and P3 proteins of HAV are also elicited by infection.[179,314,359] These antibodies likely play little role in protection against infection or disease but offer the potential to discriminate antibody responses resulting from infection versus

immunization with inactivated vaccines that do not express these proteins.

Mechanisms of Antibody-Mediated Neutralization

Immunofocus reduction assays analogous to plaque reduction neutralization assays of cytopathic viruses show that nHAV particles are highly susceptible to neutralization and that most monoclonal antibodies directed against the capsid have neutralizing activity[219,288] (Fig. 2.12A). Potent neutralizing antibodies only minimally destabilize the capsid structure, and cryo-EM structures of virus–antibody complexes suggest that such antibodies neutralize the virus by blocking interactions with cellular receptors.[46,405] *In silico* docking studies identified a small molecule, golvatinib, that binds to the major antigenic site recognized by antibodies on the capsid and inhibits infection with an IC_{50} of approximately 1 μg/mL.[46] How the capsid disassembles is not understood, however, and it remains possible that antibodies that bridge across pentamer subunits[358] might stabilize the virus and prevent uncoating.

In contrast to nHAV, quasi-enveloped eHAV particles show no evidence of neutralization in immunofocus reduction assays when incubated with potent neutralizing antibodies prior to

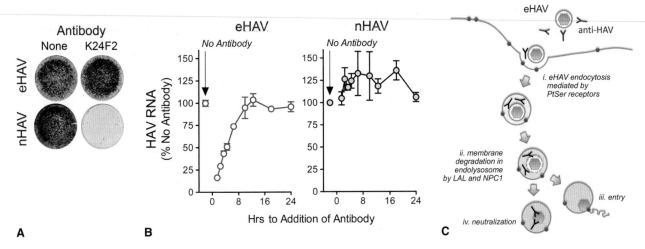

FIGURE 2.12 Antibody-mediated neutralization of quasi-enveloped virus. A: A quantal immunofocus assay reveals robust neutralization of nHAV following incubation with a murine monoclonal anticapsid antibody (K24F2) versus complete resistance to neutralization of quasi-enveloped eHAV virions isolated from the same isopycnic gradient. **B:** Postendocytosis neutralization of eHAV. Viral replication (shown as percent RNA in the absence of antibody) is blocked by antibody added to cell cultures as late as 6 to 8 hours after adsorption and removal of an eHAV inoculum. Similar treatment of nHAV-infected cultures has no effect on viral outgrowth. **C:** Mechanism proposed for postendocytosis neutralization of eHAV within an endolysosomal compartment. IgG and IgA antibodies can neutralize eHAV in this fashion but not IgM antibody with potent neutralizing activity against nHAV in the immunofocus assay.[112] (Panels **A** and **B** adapted by permission from Nature: Feng Z, Hensley L, McKnight KL, et al. A pathogenic picornavirus acquires an envelope by hijacking cellular membranes. *Nature* 2013;496(7445):367–371. Copyright © 2013 Springer Nature; Panel C modified with permission of Annual Reviews, Inc. from Feng Z, Hirai-Yuki A, McKnight KL, et al. Naked viruses that aren't always naked: quasi-enveloped agents of acute hepatitis. *Annu Rev Virol* 2014;1(1):539–560; permission conveyed through Copyright Clearance Center, Inc. Copyright © 2014 by Annual Reviews, https://www.annualreviews.org. Ref.113)

inoculation onto cells[112] (Fig. 2.12B). This explains why infectious virus can be found in sera from nonhuman primates that also contain antibody.[15,60] However, the infectivity of eHAV can be neutralized following endocytosis of both virus and antibody, and degradation of the quasi-envelope within late endolysosomes.[112] Trafficking of eHAV to endolysosomes and degradation of the quasi-envelope occur slowly, and viral replication can be inhibited by antibody added to cell cultures as late as 4 to 6 hours following inoculation and removal of the virus inoculum (Fig. 2.12.B,C).[112,312] No immunoglobulin receptor or transporter has shown to be required for this. The length of time during which eHAV remains susceptible to neutralization in endosomes following its endocytosis can be extended by treating cells with lalistat-2, an inhibitor of LAL that slows degradation of the viral quasi-envelope.[312] Similar experiments with nHAV show no reduction in viral replication when antibody is added to cultures even immediately after endocytosis of the virus,[112] presumably because these particles either uncoat or reach an essential receptor before sufficient antibody is endocytosed and reaches the virus.

Postendocytosis neutralization of eHAV has been demonstrated with multiple IgG isotypes and IgA but not IgM anti-HAV.[112] Unlike IgG anti-HAV, IgM antibody with potent neutralizing activity against nHAV was unable to neutralize eHAV when added to cell cultures following removal of an eHAV inoculum, either because the antibody was unstable or not taken up by the cell into endolysosomes. This suggests that the early antibody response to HAV, which is composed primarily of IgM antibody (Fig. 2.11A), may have limited capacity to restrict the spread of eHAV within the liver.[97,120,216,222]

Cellular Immune Responses to HAV Infection

T-Cell Responses in Nonhuman Primates

The T-cell response to HAV is not well understood because of difficulties accessing the liver compartment and the lack, until

recently, of a tractable small animal model for hepatitis A. Studies in the late 1980s showed that virus-specific cytotoxic CD8+ T cells are present in both the blood and liver of humans with acute hepatitis A and produce type II interferon-γ (IFN-γ) that both up-regulates HLA class I expression and has antiviral activity against HAV.[121,240,384,386] 51Cr release assays demonstrated that CD8+ T-cell clones derived from the liver were capable of killing autologous fibroblasts in an infection-dependent manner. These seminal studies led to the concept that CD8+ T cells control the infection and that the liver injury in acute hepatitis A results from an immunopathologic attack on hepatocytes by cytotoxic T cells.[121]

More recent studies provide limited support for this hypothesis.[399,400] Twenty years after the identification of virus-specific CD8+ T cells, specific class I epitopes were identified in several HAV proteins using predictive algorithms and testing of a panel of viral peptides in intracellular cytokine staining assays.[326] CD8+ cells targeting one immunodominant class I epitope in 3D[pol] were shown to be present in peripheral blood by HLA-A2 tetramer staining during the acute phase of the infection and to have a CD38(hi)CD127(lo) activation phenotype.[326] Class I epitopes were broadly conserved among different *Hepatovirus A* genotypes, suggesting that T-cell escape may be uncommon. These results suggested that HAV elicits a broad, multi-specific CD8+ T-cell response and are consistent with the view that CD8+ T cells control the infection. Since virus-specific CD8+ T cells were found to express IFNg, it was suggested that virus replication might be limited by noncytolytic as well as cytolytic activity of these cells.[326]

A subsequent study, in which T-cell responses were investigated in experimentally infected chimpanzees, offers a somewhat different view.[440] This study had the advantage of following the kinetics of the CD8+ and CD4+ T-cell responses under tightly controlled conditions not possible in human studies, but it also examined only circulating lymphocytes and not T cells within the liver at the site of infection. A CD4+ T helper cell response was shown to dominate the T-cell response to the virus and to target multiple class II epitopes located in different parts of the polyprotein.[440] Virus-specific CD4+ T cells appeared coincident with ALT elevations, and their abundance correlated kinetically with subsequent declines in fecal virus shedding and intrahepatic HAV RNA.[440] These CD4+ T cells were multifunctional, producing IFN-γ, TNF-α, IL-2, and IL-21 and thus could play a central role in control of the infection. HAV-specific CD8+ T cells were also identified in the blood during the acute phase of the infection by tetramer staining when ALT levels were elevated, but most lacked cytotoxic activity and IFN-γ production at the point of virus control.[440] Improved CD8+ effector functions were observed only late in the infection, when virus replication was well controlled. CD4+CD25+Foxp3+ regulatory T cells (Treg cells) have been studied in humans. These cells are reduced in number and have diminished suppressor activity in patients with severe liver injury due to HAV.[54,55] This was attributed to virus binding TIM-1 expressed on the surface of Treg cells.[242] Taken collectively, these studies are consistent with T cells playing a major role in controlling the virus and suggest noncytolytic immune control by virus-specific CD4+ T cells may be especially important.

T-Cell Responses to HAV Infection in Mice

The intrahepatic T-cell response to infection has also been studied in *Ifnar1*[−/−] mice. These mice are immunocompromised by the global absence of type I interferon signaling, yet infection of these animals recapitulates many features of hepatitis A in humans and is associated with large increases in the numbers of intrahepatic CD4+ and CD8+ T cells expressing the activation marker CD44.[161,262] These cells include a large population of virus-specific CD8+ T cells identified by tetramer staining for several class I epitopes and intracellular cytokine staining.[263] Depleting mice of either CD8+ or CD4+ T cells prior to virus challenge did not modify the subsequent course of the infection or the severity of HAV-associated liver injury,[161] but depleting either CD4+ or CD8+ T cells in mice with established infection led in both cases to increases in HAV replication and fecal virus shedding, as well as a concomitant worsening of the liver injury.[262] By contrast, immunization with an HAV peptide vaccine increased the abundance of virus-specific CD8+ T cells in the liver, reduced viral loads in the liver, and lessened liver injury.[262] Thus, in this murine model of HAV infection, T cells have a role in control of the infection, but contrary to commonly held tenets, they protect against HAV-associated liver injury, not contribute to it. These data provide support for liver injury being mediated primarily by IRF3-induced gene expression in this model[161,363] (see "Mechanisms of Liver Injury").

Immunity

Early studies demonstrating that symptomatic infectious hepatitis (presumably hepatitis A) could be prevented by preexposure administration of pooled human serum immune globulin[134] provide clear evidence of the potent protection against disease afforded by antibodies. More recent studies, applying different assays for anti-HAV antibodies to sera from recipients of immune globulin and participants in vaccine efficacy trials, have established correlates of protection.[33,225] Seven days after receiving a single intramuscular dose of immune globulin (0.6 mg/kg), when protection against symptomatic infection is very high, the reciprocal geometric mean titer (serum dilution) of neutralizing anti-HAV was 27.5 when measured by an immunofocus reduction assay (RIFIT, radioimmunofocus inhibition test) and 146 when measured in an HAV antigen reduction assay (HAVARNA).[219,225] The geometric mean titer determined by a commercial ELISA test was 46.1 mIU/mL when measured against a World Health Organization standard. Levels of HAV-specific antibodies were similar in children 4 weeks after immunization with a formalin-inactivated vaccine (VAQTA*),[225] a point in time postimmunization at which recipients were approximately 100% protected against symptomatic infection.[413] A level of 10 mIU/mL is generally considered protective,[228] but this is probably true for any level of detectable antibody.

These relatively low antibody levels may not protect against subclinical infection, and serologic studies suggest that subclinical infections occur in some recipients of immune globulin.[286] Much higher levels of antibody are present after booster vaccination, or following natural infection.[86,225] Experiments in nonhuman primates suggest that these high levels of antibody may provide sterilizing immunity to the virus.[87,301,399] Immunity is lifelong. However, waning levels of antibodies in older individuals may allow for subclinical reinfections that boost HAV-specific IgG responses.[392]

Virus-specific CD4+ and CD8+ T cells may contribute to protection against disease (see "Cellular Immune Responses to HAV Infection"), but this has been demonstrated only in the *Ifnar1*[−/−] mouse model of hepatitis A.[263]

Mechanisms of Liver Injury

Multiple mechanisms likely contribute to the liver injury associated with acute HAV infection.[403] However, cytotoxic damage resulting directly from virus replication in hepatocytes is unlikely to be involved. Virus variants that are highly adapted to growth in cell culture such as HM175/18f can induce strong cytopathic effects,[71,226] but wild-type and early cell culture passage variants typically replicate without either cytopathic effect[32,77,125,297,299] or shut-off of host protein synthesis.[132] Moreover, fecal shedding of virus replicated in the liver is typically maximal just prior to ALT elevation and does not correlate with liver injury.[15,60,210,302] HAV also replicates robustly in *Mavs*[−/−] mice without evidence of liver injury.[161]

Several immunopathogenic mechanisms of liver injury have been proposed. These include (a) killing of hepatocytes by activated virus-specific CD8+ T cells,[121,386] (b) innate-like cytotoxicity of nonspecific "bystander" CD8+ T cell and mucosal-associated invariant T (MAIT) cells activated by IL-15,[191,311] and (c) proapoptotic activity of IRF3-regulated genes induced through RLR/MAVS signaling pathways.[161,363] While cytotoxic virus-specific CD8+ T cells were widely assumed to be responsible for liver injury following their discovery in the 1980s, more recent studies indicate that most circulating virus-specific CD8+ T cells do not acquire effector functions until after the ALT has normalized in chimpanzees,[440] and studies in humans suggest that HAV-specific CD8+ T-cell activation correlates inversely with liver injury.[191] These observations cast doubt on the role of virus-specific CD8+ T cells in liver injury (see "Cellular Immune Responses to HAV Infection").

On the other hand, T-cell receptor–independent activation of non–HAV-specific memory CD8+ T cells was found to correlate with ALT levels in hospitalized patients with severe hepatitis A.[191] Bystander memory CD8+ cells with specificity for other viruses were activated by interleukin-15 (IL-15) released from infected hepatocytes and exerted innate-like NKG2D- and NKp30-dependent cytotoxicity. Mucosal-associated invariant T (MAIT) cells are abundant within the liver and have also been shown to be activated, possibly by IL-15, and to exert increased innate-like granzyme B-dependent cytotoxicity in patients with acute hepatitis A.[311] Bystander T cell and MAIT cell activation has been associated with liver injury in patients with severe disease, but may play lesser roles in less severe infection. IL-15 was not induced in HAV-infected chimpanzees or Ifnar1[−/−] mice with modest ALT elevations.[210,363]

Studies in Ifnar1[−/−] mice implicate cell-intrinsic host responses to HAV as a cause of liver injury. Although the specific ISG(s) responsible for hepatocellular apoptosis and inflammation associated with HAV infection have not been identified, liver injury is dependent upon IRF3-mediated transcriptional responses and requires phosphorylation of IRF3 at Ser388/399 induced by MAVS signaling.[161,363] These various mechanisms of immune-mediated liver damage are not mutually exclusive and may be operative collectively.[403]

Fulminant Hepatitis A

Why some persons develop fulminant and potentially fatal liver disease when acutely infected with HAV is unknown. There is no compelling epidemiologic or virologic evidence linking fulminant hepatitis to particular strains of the virus. In one study, patients with fulminant hepatitis A, defined by either encephalopathy or serum factor V levels less than 50% of normal, were more likely to have low or undetectable levels of viral RNA in serum than patients with less severe hepatitis A, suggesting that liver failure resulted from an overexuberant immune response rather than excessive virus replication.[310] Another study found that serum HAV RNA levels were higher on admission to hospital but declined more rapidly in patients with fulminant hepatitis A than in those with less severe disease.[127] Enhanced Th1-biased immune responses have been documented in patients with fulminant disease, including high IL-12/IL-10 ratios, increased TNF-α, and an inverse correlation between CXCL5 (RANTES) expression and viremia.[20] In some instances, fulminant hepatitis A may have an underlying genetic basis.[184] Fulminant infection has been linked in one case to a loss of function mutation in IL-18-binding protein (IL18BP), which could have led to excessive IL-18–stimulated NK cell killing of hepatocytes.[21] A case–control study also found an association between a six-amino acid insertion in TIM1 and severe hepatitis A.[193] This insertion enhanced binding of TIM1 to the virus and increased natural killer T (NKT) cell killing of infected hepatocytes.

EPIDEMIOLOGY

Transmission

HAV is transmitted predominantly from person-to-person via the fecal–oral route. Fecal excretion of infectious virus is highest during the 2 weeks preceding and a few days following the onset of symptoms[210,378] (Fig. 2.11A). Shedding of virus detectable by reverse transcription–polymerase chain reaction (RT-PCR) may continue for weeks thereafter, but whether this reflects shedding of infectious virus is uncertain. Large amounts of virus are found in feces at the peak of infection, enhancing the potential for contamination of food, and leading to common-source, foodborne hepatitis A outbreaks.[88] The high physical stability of the naked virus particle contributes to this potential (see "Naked Nonenveloped Virions [nHAV]"). Furthermore, HAV can be concentrated by filter-feeding bivalve shellfish, which pose a risk for transmission when collected from contaminated waters.[22,289]

Parenteral transmission of HAV is less common but well documented. Viremia is detectable for a median of 42 days in patients with acute hepatitis A, and like fecal shedding is highest in magnitude prior to the onset of symptoms.[210,378] Thus, blood or plasma donation, or potentially the shared use of injection devices during the early, asymptomatic phase of the infection, may result in blood-borne transmission of HAV and rare instances of transfusion-transmitted hepatitis A.[196] Particularly prominent examples of blood-borne HAV transmission include an outbreak in a neonatal intensive care unit in which two infants were transfused with a contaminated donor unit of blood,[317] and infections in recipients of early high-purity, solvent/detergent-treated factor VIII concentrates that were not subjected to additional heat inactivation.[243]

In addition to common-source foodborne outbreaks, community-wide outbreaks of hepatitis A occur that often disproportionately involve men who have sex with men (MSM).[64,272,320] Community-wide outbreaks of hepatitis A have also been increasingly associated with homelessness and illicit injection drug use in the United States.[122] These outbreaks likely result from a combination of both parenteral and fecal–oral transmission of the virus. Risk factors for infection were identified in only 35.2% of hepatitis A cases reported to the U.S. Centers for Disease Control and Prevention in 2019.[48] The most frequently identified risk factor was injection drug use (46%), followed much less frequently by sexual or household contact with a case of hepatitis A, or international travel. MSM comprised only 5% of cases.

Incidence and Geographic Distribution of HAV Infection

The incidence of HAV infection varies widely among different geographic regions and is strongly dependent upon economic factors and social structure. Infection rates are generally high in low-income countries with poor public health sanitation and low in wealthier nations with better infrastructure (Fig. 2.13). As economies have become increasingly globalized and interdependent, and the economic wealth of some low- and middle-income countries has increased, marked changes have occurred in the epidemiology of hepatitis A.[172] The global burden of HAV infection has decreased in recent decades due to improvements in public health and sanitation that have lessened the spread of the virus.[172] Many low- and middle-income countries have transitioned from high to low or intermediate HAV endemicity, leading to increases in the average age at which an individual becomes infected.[174] This results in higher proportions of older persons who are HAV seronegative and thus susceptible to infection.[173] Since infection is more likely to be symptomatic

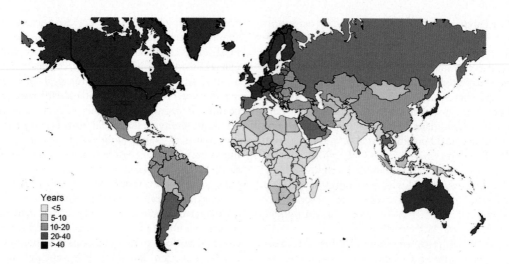

FIGURE 2.13 Global hepatitis A prevalence. Map showing the estimated age in years at midpoint of population immunity (AMPI, point at which 50% of the population is seropositive) for HAV by country in 2015. (Reprinted with permission from Jacobsen KH. Globalization and the changing epidemiology of hepatitis A virus. *Cold Spring Harb Perspect Med* 2018;8(10):a031716. Copyright © 2018 Cold Spring Harbor Laboratory Press.)

in older individuals, this results in greater proportions of acute HAV infections being symptomatic and can potentially increase the overall disease burden.[4,388,429]

Immunization is being increasingly used to control the spread and public health impact of the virus. Efforts to universally immunize children have had a profound effect on the spread of virus and the community-wide incidence of symptomatic disease in some countries.[4,340,408] Yet, the incidence of HAV infections remains high in many regions of the world, including sub-Saharan Africa and the Indian subcontinent, where in most recent surveys the age at the midpoint of population immunity (AMPI, the age by which 50% of the population is seropositive) remains less than 5 years[172,174] (Fig. 2.13).

Globalization has also impacted the epidemiology of HAV in high-income countries. Increasing international food trade has resulted in outbreaks of infection related to foodstuff imported from lower-income regions with higher HAV endemicity.[172] A case in point is a recent multistate outbreak of hepatitis A in the United States caused by contaminated frozen pomegranate arils imported from Turkey.[63] Increases in homelessness and opioid abuse have also fueled recent changes in the epidemiology of HAV in the United States.[122,164] Vaccination led to marked reductions in the incidence of hepatitis A, with reported cases falling from an average of 26,000 cases/year (9.2 to 29/100,000) prior to introduction of vaccines in 1995 to 3,579 cases (1.2/100,000) by 2010[409] (Fig. 2.14A). This downward trend reversed beginning in 2016 with 18,846 cases (5.7/100,000) reported in 2019[3], erasing much of the previous gains from immunization.[122] Most of these cases were associated with community-wide outbreaks among individuals reporting

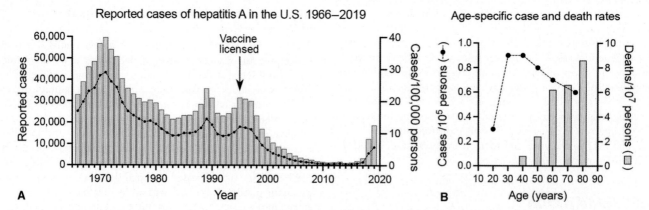

FIGURE 2.14 Reported hepatitis A cases and hepatitis A–related deaths in the United States. A: Cases of hepatitis A reported to the National Notifiable Diseases Surveillance System, U.S. Centers for Disease Control and Prevention from 1966 to 2019. Reported cases represent an uncertain fraction of all cases and underestimate the actual incidence of infection. Recent increases in the rate of infection have reversed much of the reduction in incidence achieved by the introduction of vaccines in the United States in 1995. **B:** Age-specific rates of hepatitis A (cases per 100,000 persons reported in 2017) and hepatitis A–related deaths (deaths per 10,000,000 persons during the period 2012–2016). [Data compiled from CDC Hepatitis Surveillance reports].

drug use or homelessness. Overall, 24,000 hospitalizations (61% of reported cases) and 376 deaths (0.94%) were attributed to hepatitis A between 2016 and mid-2021.[49]

The National Health and Nutrition Examination Survey (NHANES), conducted by the U.S. Centers for Disease Control and Prevention found the prevalence of anti-HAV among adults aged greater than 20 years to be 24.2% during 2007–2012, a significant decline from 29.5% during 1999–2006.[197] Thus, a large majority of adult Americans are susceptible to infection.

CLINICAL MANIFESTATIONS OF HAV INFECTION

The clinical manifestations of HAV infection range from a complete lack of symptoms, to mild anicteric hepatitis, acute icteric hepatitis, and fulminant hepatic failure. The most important factor influencing disease severity is age.[13,339] In very young children, most infections are asymptomatic and not associated with jaundice. Less than 16% of children involved in day care–associated outbreaks who transmitted virus to older household contacts were symptomatic.[25,149] By contrast, infection results in clinical illness in the majority of older children and adults, and overt jaundice occurs in as many as two-thirds.[213] The risk of fulminant hepatitis and death, although rare at all ages, is also much higher in older patients, rising progressively above the age of 40[52] (Fig. 2.14B).

The incubation period from exposure to onset of symptoms ranges from 15 to 50 days, with a mean of approximately 30 days (Fig. 2.11A). Onset may be abrupt, with fatigue, malaise, nausea, vomiting, diarrhea, anorexia, fever, and abdominal pain, followed after a few days by dark ("Coca-Cola colored") urine, scleral icterus, and clay-colored stools.[217,426] Arthralgias may be reported. Physical findings include jaundice, tender hepatomegaly, and occasionally splenomegaly. An evanescent skin rash is seen in some patients. Laboratory findings include elevated serum ALT and aspartate aminotransferase (AST)

activities, with ALT elevations greater than AST and peaking at less than 4,000 IU/L (often much less), but occasionally exceeding 10,000 IU/L. Alkaline phosphatase levels are usually moderately elevated (mean ~350 IU/L), as is total serum bilirubin (mean ~5 mg/dL).[339,379] Radiographic abnormalities include perihepatic lymph node enlargement and thickening of the gallbladder wall.[339] Liver biopsy is rarely done but shows primarily centrilobular hepatitis with periportal inflammatory infiltrates rich in plasma cells and, in some cases, eroding the limiting plate[370] (Fig. 2.11B). Cholestasis may be prominent. Symptoms and signs typically regress over 2 to 3 weeks, with biochemical abnormalities usually returning to normal within 2 to 4 months.

Atypical manifestations of hepatitis A include acute renal injury, prolonged hepatic cholestasis, and relapsing disease. Acute kidney injury was reported in 2% to 7% of hospitalized patients in two large series from Korea, with half of these patients requiring dialysis.[56,185] Prolonged cholestasis occurred in 4.7% and was associated with preexisting chronic HBV infection and pruritus.[185] Serum bilirubin levels may reach 40 mg/dL in patients with persistent cholestasis, but the outcome is invariably benign with spontaneous resolution.[323] Relapsing hepatitis A occurs in 10% to 20% of patients, typically several weeks after apparent recovery from a primary episode of acute hepatitis A and is marked by a recrudescence of the symptoms and signs of the disease.[136,323] The underlying pathogenesis of relapsing hepatitis is not understood, but the presence of virus in the feces of some patients with clinical relapse suggests transient virus escape from immune control.[351] Other rare manifestations of HAV infection include optic neuritis, transverse myelitis, aplastic anemia, hemolytic anemia, thrombocytopenia, and pancreatitis.[261,323]

Overall, the prognosis for patients with acute hepatitis A is excellent, with the vast majority experiencing complete recovery leading to lifelong immunity against reinfection (Fig. 2.15). Pregnancy does not enhance disease severity, although preterm labor and premature rupture of membranes have been reported.[379,380] Progression to chronic viral hepatitis,

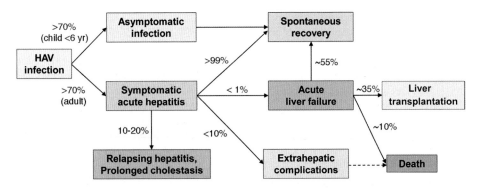

FIGURE 2.15 HAV infection outcome. Clinical outcome of acute HAV infection. The majority of infections in adults are symptomatic, whereas most infections in young children are asymptomatic. Symptoms and signs of hepatitis resolve spontaneously in almost all patients eventually, but recovery can be slow and in a substantial fraction of all patients associated with prolonged cholestasis. Acute liver failure associated with submassive hepatic necrosis occurs in an unfortunate, small percentage of patients. The risk of fulminant hepatitis is increased in individuals over 40 to 50 years of age and in persons with underlying chronic hepatitis C. (Reprinted with permission from Shin EC, Jeong SH. Natural history, clinical manifestations, and pathogenesis of hepatitis A. *Cold Spring Harb Perspect Med* 2018;8(9):a031708. Copyright © 2018 Cold Spring Harbor Laboratory Press.)

as seen in acute HBV and HCV infection, does not occur. Rarely, however, acute HAV infection may trigger the development of chronic autoimmune hepatitis.[389] The most serious complication, fulminant hepatitis A, occurs in 0.2% to 0.9% of cases and is marked by submassive hepatic necrosis with liver failure manifested by low serum factor V levels and hepatic encephalopathy. Risk factors include infection at greater than 40 to 50 years of age (Fig. 2.14), male sex, and underlying chronic hepatitis C.[52,390] Fulminant hepatitis A is life threatening, resulting in liver transplantation or death in approximately 40% of affected patients. A large, multicenter study of patients with acute liver failure associated with HAV infection identified patient age, serum bilirubin, prothrombin time international normalized ratio (INR), ammonia, creatinine, and hemoglobin levels as independent predictors of death or the need for transplantation.[192]

DIAGNOSIS

The symptoms and signs of hepatitis A are nonspecific and cannot be distinguished clinically from other types of acute viral hepatitis. A diagnosis of hepatitis A may be suggested by the epidemiologic setting, but a specific diagnosis requires detection of the virus or serologic confirmation. This is usually achieved clinically by detection of serum IgM antibody, which can be detected for approximately 4 to 6 months following acute infection using commercially available enzyme-linked immunosorbent (ELISA) assays[222,417] (Fig. 2.11A). Seroconversion can be delayed occasionally, and if negative on first testing, patients should be retested for IgM anti-HAV in 1 to 2 weeks if the diagnosis is strongly suspected. While very useful in the setting of acute hepatitis, IgM anti-HAV assays have low positive predictive value in the absence of clinical or epidemiologic evidence suggesting infection due to false-positive results.[50]

Many types of tests have been developed to detect IgG anti-HAV, which appears more slowly than IgM anti-HAV following infection but persists for life (Fig. 2.11A). While it is not a useful marker of acute infection, IgG anti-HAV tests can be used to assess vaccine responses and immunity. Levels in excess of 10 mIU/mL are generally considered indicative of immunity, but any level of detectable IgG anti-HAV is probably protective against disease.[225,228] Assays for antibodies to nonstructural viral proteins can distinguish serologic responses to infection from those due to immunization with inactivated vaccines, which do not produce such antibodies,[179,359] but these tests are not generally available. Nucleic acid tests using RT-PCR will usually reveal the presence of HAV in fecal samples at the time of clinical presentation. While this represents the most specific approach to diagnosis, it is costly and generally not used clinically. Cell culture is not a reliable means of diagnosis due to the slow and variable replication of wild-type HAV in cultured cells.[32,77,297]

MANAGEMENT OF HEPATITIS A

There are no specific therapies available for the treatment of acute hepatitis A. Patients should be made comfortable and managed conservatively. Hospitalization may be considered depending on the need to control nausea and to provide intravenous hydration, but it is usually not indicated. Bed rest offers no specific advantage. Corticosteroids can be considered for patients with prolonged cholestasis[323] but are usually not necessary and have no role in the management of the typical patient. IgM anti-HAV–positive patients with acute liver failure marked by worsening assays of hepatic synthetic function and encephalopathy should be considered for liver transplantation.[271]

PREVENTION AND CONTROL

General Measures

Given that most infections result from fecal–oral transmission of the virus, good personal hygiene including handwashing, clean drinking water, and public health sanitation have important roles in prevention of HAV infection. Handwashing is particularly important, as HAV survives well on human hands, and infectious virus is readily transmitted to inanimate surfaces.[254] Commonly used institutional handwashing agents containing triclosan or chlorhexidine provide superior removal of virus compared with washing with tap water alone.[255,345] Good hygiene may be difficult to maintain in crowded institutional settings, particularly preschool day care centers caring for diapered children, and is not a substitute for immunization against hepatitis A.

HAV is somewhat resistant to chlorination, but treatment with greater than 2.0 mg/L residual free chlorine for 15 minutes has been shown to render the virus noninfectious in nonhuman primate challenge experiments.[284] Uncooked food, contaminated either at its source or during preparation, is an important vehicle for transmission of the infection, particularly for international travelers to regions of high HAV endemicity. Bivalve shellfish concentrate the virus from seawater and are responsible for outbreaks of hepatitis A. Heating simply to the point of opening of the shell is likely to be inadequate for inactivating the virus.[41] Kinetic inactivation experiments suggest that a 6-log reduction of infectivity in contaminated blue mussels requires exposure to boiling water for 2.7 to 3.2 minutes and much longer at lower temperatures.[41]

Passive Immunoprophylaxis

Passive immunization with polyclonal human immune globulin was shown to provide 80% to 90% protection against symptomatic infectious hepatitis in studies carried out during and shortly after World War II.[134,361,419] More recent studies in epidemic settings and in household contacts of persons with acute hepatitis A have shown that immune globulin (IG), prepared from pooled human plasma by cold ethanol fractionation,[62] provides high level protection against symptomatic HAV infection when administered both prior to and within 2 weeks of exposure.[391,419] The prevention of symptomatic infection by IG in postexposure settings likely results from postendocytosis neutralization (Fig. 2.12C) of circulating quasi-enveloped virus,[112] decreasing the mass of replicating virus and thereby limiting immunopathologic host responses. Sufficient antigen may yet be produced to evoke protective endogenous antibody responses, resulting in what has been termed "passive–active" immunoprophylaxis.[419] Serious adverse reactions to IG administration are rare, but anaphylaxis has been reported in persons with immunoglobulin A deficiency.

Decreases in the incidence of hepatitis A with related declines in population antibody prevalence have raised concerns regarding the antibody content of contemporary lots of IG and have resulted in recent changes in specific recommendations for the use of IG promulgated by various national authorities.[274,430] However, a recent open-label trial demonstrated that administration of a single intramuscular 0.2 mg/kg dose of IG resulted in a mean C_{max} of 118 mIU/mL with a mean $t_{1/2}$ of 47.1 days.[186] Levels above 10 mIU/mL persisted for over 60 days. Nonetheless, inactivated HAV vaccine has been shown to be equivalently protective against symptomatic infection if administered within 2 weeks of exposure, diminishing the role of IG in postexposure prophylaxis.[391] Vaccine is generally preferred over the use of IG due to the length of protection afforded, ease of administration, lower incidence of pain at the injection site, and generally greater availability and acceptability.[274]

Hepatitis A Vaccines

Inactivated HAV Vaccines

Two general types of hepatitis A vaccines are in use globally: formalin-inactivated whole virus vaccines and live virus vaccines containing virus attenuated by serial passage in cell culture.[228,340] Inactivated vaccines produced by multiple manufacturers are widely used in Western countries and have compiled an outstanding record of safety and effectiveness following early randomized clinical trials in children demonstrating their clinical efficacy.[57,170,413] Inactivated vaccines are produced by formaldehyde inactivation of attenuated viruses produced in cell culture.[229] They are usually adjuvanted with aluminum hydroxide, although one vaccine uses a virosome formulation to enhance immunogenicity.[166] Two inactivated, alum-adjuvanted HAV vaccines are licensed in the United States for use in adults and children over 12 months of age: VAQTA® (Merck) and HAVRIX® (GlaxoSmithKline). Both are produced from attenuated virus strains grown in MRC-5 human diploid fibroblasts. A two-dose regimen of either of these vaccines provides greater than 95% protection against symptomatic hepatitis A.[170,412,413] HAVRIX® is also available formulated in combination with recombinant HBV vaccine as TWINRIX® (GlaxoSmithKline).

The Advisory Committee on Immunization Practices of the U.S. Centers for Disease Control and Prevention has recommended routine immunization of all children aged 12 to 23 months with inactivated hepatitis A vaccine since 2006. More recent recommendations for preexposure prophylaxis include the immunization of all children and adolescents aged 2 to 18 years who have not previously been immunized ("catch-up vaccination"), persons with chronic liver disease of any type, persons infected with human immunodeficiency virus, persons who use illicit drugs or who are homeless, international travelers (including children >6 months of age) going to regions of high HAV endemicity, persons who will have close contact with children adopted from countries with high rates of hepatitis A, and those who live in group settings where a high proportion of individuals have risk factors for HAV infection.[274,275] As discussed above (see "Passive Immunoprophylaxis"), immunization with hepatitis A vaccine is also recommended for postexposure prophylaxis.[275] Vaccine should be administered as soon as possible after exposure and is protective if given within 2 weeks of exposure.[391] Because immune response to the vaccine may be blunted in older individuals, IG may also be administered at a different anatomic site to those over the age of 40 at the discretion of the provider.[275]

Protection is evident within 2 weeks of primary immunization and has been demonstrated in persons immunized as late as 2 weeks after exposure to the virus.[391,413] Mathematical modeling suggests that protective levels of antibody will be present in greater than 99% of persons 25 to 50 years after immunization.[249] It is thus likely that vaccine immunity will persist for life without the need for booster immunization.[387] Universal childhood immunization is recommended in many high-income, low-endemicity countries, and increasingly considered in middle-income countries transitioning from high-to-low endemicity with paradoxical increases in the incidence of symptomatic infection[172,228,340] (see "Epidemiology"). A one-dose regimen has been used successfully for universal childhood immunization in Argentina.[394] A combined hepatitis A and typhoid vaccine has been approved for use in some countries.[211]

Live Attenuated HAV Vaccine

Cell culture passage reduces the capacity of HAV to replicate and to induce both disease and immunity to infection in nonhuman primates and humans.[128,129,259,294,295] This change in the virus phenotype is associated with mutations in 2B and other nonstructural proteins.[102,103,146] Poor immunogenicity of a candidate attenuated vaccine, coupled with early evidence of high immunogenicity of formaldehyde-inactivated HAV led to the abandonment of most efforts to develop attenuated vaccines.[30,298] However, attenuated HAV vaccines have been successfully developed in China from cell culture–passaged virus variants[31,244,245] and are used in multiple countries.[73,74,228] These attenuated HAV vaccines have not been studied in the same detail as inactivated vaccines. They are somewhat less immunogenic than formalin-inactivated HAV vaccines, yet appear to have similar efficacy and to be safe.[74] Reversion of these attenuated vaccines to virulence has not been noted clinically.

PERSPECTIVES

Few viruses have undergone such a major change in our understanding of their biology as has HAV over the past decade. Recognition of the role played by quasi-envelopment in the pathogenesis of hepatitis A,[112] the marked differences existing between hepatoviruses and enteroviruses in both capsid structure and mechanisms of assembly and cell entry,[81,405] and the discovery of multiple hepatovirus species infecting a wide range of mammals[96] have dramatically altered our perspectives on HAV. However, many aspects of the HAV life cycle remain to be discovered, and there are certain to be additional surprises lying ahead of us. Perhaps the biggest unknown is the potential for non-*Hepatovirus A* viruses to infect humans. Hepatoviruses circulating in bat populations appear to share not only antigenicity with human HAV but also similar capacities to disrupt innate immune antiviral responses in human cells.[96,117] Hepatovirus phylogeny shows stark evidence of multiple trans-species jumps in the past, and this should perhaps be a warning to us for the future. Yet, the challenges are not all scientific. Recent increases in the rates of infection and numbers of HAV-associated deaths linked to homelessness and drug use in the United States (Fig. 2.14)[122] highlight an urgent need to intensify efforts to immunize vulnerable populations against this vaccine-preventable disease.

ACKNOWLEDGMENTS

The author gratefully acknowledges Zongdi Feng, Chris Walker, Jason Whitmire, and Kevin McKnight for critical review of the manuscript. Recent hepatovirus research in the author's laboratory has been supported by the National Institute of Allergy and Infectious Diseases under grants R01-AI131685, R01-AI103083, and R01-AI150095.

REFERENCES

1. Abe K, Shikata T. Fulminant type A viral hepatitis in a chimpanzee. *Acta Pathol Jpn* 1982;32:143–148.
2. Abernathy E, Mateo R, Majzoub K, et al. Differential and convergent utilization of autophagy components by positive-strand RNA viruses. *PLoS Biol* 2019;17:e2006926.
3. Advisory Committee on Immunization Practices. Prevention of hepatitis A through active or passive immunization: recommendations of the Advisory Committee on Immunization Practices (ACIP). *MMWR Recomm Rep* 2006;55:1–23.
4. Aggarwal R, Goel A. Hepatitis A: epidemiology in resource-poor countries. *Curr Opin Infect Dis* 2015;28:488–496.
5. Ali IK, McKendrick L, Morley SJ, et al. Activity of the hepatitis A virus IRES requires association between the cap-binding translation initiation factor (eIF4E) and eIF4G. *J Virol* 2001;75:7854–7863.
6. Allaire M, Chernala MM, Malcolm BA, et al. Picornaviral 3C cysteine proteinases have a fold similar to chymotrypsin-like serine proteinases. *Nature* 1994;369:72–76.
7. Amado LA, Marchevsky RS, de Paula VS, et al. Experimental hepatitis A virus (HAV) infection in cynomolgus monkeys (*Macaca fascicularis*): evidence of active extrahepatic site of HAV replication. *Int J Exp Pathol* 2010;91:87–97.
8. Anderson DA, Ross BC. Morphogenesis of hepatitis A virus: isolation and characterization of subviral particles. *J Virol* 1990;64:5284–5289.
9. Anderson DA, Ross BC, Locarnini SA. Restricted replication of hepatitis A virus in cell culture: encapsidation of viral RNA depletes the pool of RNA available for replication. *J Virol* 1988;62:4201–4206.
10. Angarano G, Trotta F, Monno L, et al. Serum IgA anti-hepatitis A virus as detected by enzyme-linked immunosorbent assay. Diagnostic significance in patients with acute and protracted hepatitis A. *Diagn Microbiol Infect Dis* 1985;3:521–523.
11. Anthony SJ, St Leger JA, Liang E, et al. Discovery of a novel Hepatovirus (phopivirus of seals) related to human hepatitis A virus. *mBio* 2015;6(4):e01180-15.
12. Aragones L, Guix S, Ribes E, et al. Fine-tuning translation kinetics selection as the driving force of codon usage bias in the hepatitis A virus capsid. *PLoS Pathog* 2010;6:e1000797.
13. Armstrong GL, Bell BP. Hepatitis A virus infections in the United States: model-based estimates and implications for childhood immunization. *Pediatrics* 2002;109:839–845.
14. Asare E, Mugavero J, Jiang P, et al. A single amino acid substitution in poliovirus nonstructural protein 2CATPase causes conditional defects in encapsidation and uncoating. *J Virol* 2016;90:6174–6186.
15. Asher LVS, Binn LN, Mensing TL, et al. Pathogenesis of hepatitis A in orally inoculated owl monkeys (*Aotus trivirgatus*). *J Med Virol* 1995;47:260–268.
16. Atkinson NJ, Witteveldt J, Evans DJ, et al. The influence of CpG and UpA dinucleotide frequencies on RNA virus replication and characterization of the innate cellular pathways underlying virus attenuation and enhanced replication. *Nucleic Acids Res* 2014;42:4527–4545.
17. Avanzino BC, Fuchs G, Fraser CS. Cellular cap-binding protein, eIF4E, promotes picornavirus genome restructuring and translation. *Proc Natl Acad Sci U S A* 2017;114: 9611–9616.
18. Banerjee R, Dasgupta A. Interaction of picornavirus 2C polypeptide with the viral negative-strand RNA. *J Gen Virol* 2001;82:2621–2627.
19. Barker MH, Capps RB, Allen FW. Acute infectious hepatitis in the Mediterranean theater: including acute hepatitis without jaundice. *JAMA* 1945;128:997–1003.
20. Baruah V, Tiwari D, Hazam RK, et al. Prognostic, clinical, and therapeutic importance of RANTES-CCR5 axis in hepatitis A infection: a multiapproach study. *J Med Virol* 2021;93:3656–3665.
21. Belkaya S, Michailidis E, Korol CB, et al. Inherited IL-18BP deficiency in human fulminant viral hepatitis. *J Exp Med* 2019;216:1777–1790.
22. Bellou M, Kokkinos P, Vantarakis A. Shellfish-borne viral outbreaks: a systematic review. *Food Environ Virol* 2013;5:13–23.
23. Beneduce F, Ciervo A, Kusov Y, et al. Mapping of protein domains of hepatitis A virus 3AB essential for interaction with 3CD and viral RNA. *Virology* 1999;264:410–421.
24. Beneduce F, Ciervo A, Morace G. Site-directed mutagenesis of hepatitis A virus protein 3A: effects on membrane interaction. *Biochim Biophys Acta* 1997;1326:157–165.
25. Benenson MW, Takafuji ET, Bancroft WH, et al. A military community outbreak of hepatitis type A related to transmission in a child care facility. *Am J Epidemiol* 1980;112:471–481.
26. Bergmann EM, Cherney MM, McKendrick J, et al. Crystal structure of an inhibitor complex of the 3C proteinase from hepatitis A virus (HAV) and implications for the polyprotein processing in HAV. *Virology* 1999;265:153–163.
27. Bergmann EM, Mosimann SC, Chernaia MM, et al. The refined crystal structure of the 3C gene product from hepatitis A virus: Specific proteinase activity and RNA recognition. *J Virol* 1997;71:2436–2448.
28. Berthillon P, Crance JM, Leveque F, et al. Inhibition of the expression of hepatitis A and B viruses (HAV and HBV) proteins by interferon in a human hepatocarcinoma cell line (PLC/PRF/5). *J Hepatol* 1996;25:15–19.
29. Bienz K, Egger D, Pasamontes L. Association of polioviral proteins of the P2 genomic region with the viral replication complex and virus-induced membrane synthesis as visualized by electron microscopic immunocytochemistry and autoradiography. *Virology* 1987;160:220–226.
30. Binn LN, Bancroft WH, Lemon SM, et al. Preparation of a prototype inactivated hepatitis A virus vaccine from infected cell cultures. *J Infect Dis* 1986;153:749–756.
31. Binn LN, Lemon SM. Hepatitis A. In: Artenstein AW, ed. *Vaccines, a Biography*. New York: Springer-Verlag; 2010:335–346.
32. Binn LN, Lemon SM, Marchwicki RH, et al. Primary isolation and serial passage of hepatitis A virus strains in primate cell cultures. *J Clin Microbiol* 1984;20:28–33.
33. Binn LN, Macarthy PO, Marchwicki RH, et al. Laboratory tests and reference reagents employed in studies of inactivated hepatitis A vaccine. *Vaccine* 1992;10(Suppl 1): S102–S105.
34. Bishop NE, Anderson DA. RNA-dependent cleavage of VPO capsid protein in provirions of hepatitis A virus. *Virology* 1993;197:616–623.
35. Blank CA, Anderson DA, Beard M, et al. Infection of polarized cultures of human intestinal epithelial cells with hepatitis A virus: vectorial release of progeny virions through apical cellar membranes. *J Virol* 2000;74:6476–6484.
36. Boggs JD, Melnick JL, Conrad ME, et al. Viral hepatitis: clinical and tissue culture studies. *JAMA* 1970;214:1041–1046.
37. Borman AM, Kean KM. Intact eukaryotic initiation factor 4G is required for hepatitis A virus internal initiation of translation. *Virology* 1997;237:129–136.
38. Borman AM, Michel YM, Kean KM. Detailed analysis of the requirements of hepatitis A virus internal ribosome entry segment for the eukaryotic initiation factor complex eIF4F. *J Virol* 2001;75:7864–7871.
39. Borovec SV, Anderson DA. Synthesis and assembly of hepatitis A virus-specific proteins in BS-C-1 cells. *J Virol* 1993;67:3095–3102.
40. Boyer JL. Bile formation and secretion. *Compr Physiol* 2013;3:1035–1078.
41. Bozkurt H, D'Souza DH, Davidson PM. Determination of thermal inactivation kinetics of hepatitis A virus in blue mussel (*Mytilus edulis*) homogenate. *Appl Environ Microbiol* 2014;80:3191–3197.
42. Bradley DW, Schable CA, McCaustland KA, et al. Hepatitis A virus: growth characteristics of in vivo and in vitro propagated wild and attenuated virus strains. *J Med Virol* 1984;14:373–386.
43. Brown EA, Day SP, Jansen RW, et al. The 5′ nontranslated region of hepatitis A virus: secondary structure and elements required for translation in vitro. *J Virol* 1991;65: 5828–5838.
44. Brown EA, Jansen RW, Lemon SM. Characterization of a simian hepatitis A virus (HAV): antigenic and genetic comparison with human HAV. *J Virol* 1989;63:4932–4937.
45. Brown EA, Zajac AJ, Lemon SM. In vitro characterization of an internal ribosomal entry site (IRES) present within the 5′ nontranslated region of hepatitis A virus RNA: Comparison with the IRES of encephalomyocarditis virus. *J Virol* 1994;68:1066–1074.
46. Cao L, Liu P, Yang P, et al. Structural basis for neutralization of hepatitis A virus informs a rational design of highly potent inhibitors. *PLoS Biol* 2019;17:e3000229.
47. Carette JE, Raaben M, Wong AC, et al. Ebola virus entry requires the cholesterol transporter Niemann-Pick C1. *Nature* 2011;477:340–343.
48. Centers for Disease Control and Prevention. Hepatitis Surveillance Statistics. 2019. https://www.cdc.gov/hepatitis/statistics/2019surveillance/index.htm. Accessed July 4, 2021.
49. Centers for Disease Control and Prevention. Hepatitis Outbreaks. https://www.cdc.gov/hepatitis/outbreaks/2017March-HepatitisA.htm. Accessed March 9.
50. Centers for Disease Control and Prevention (CDC). Positive test results for acute hepatitis A virus infection among persons with no recent history of acute hepatitis—United States, 2002–2004. *MMWR Morb Mortal Wkly Rep* 2005;54:453–456.
51. Chang KH, Brown EA, Lemon SM. Cell type-specific proteins which interact with the 5′ nontranslated region of hepatitis A virus RNA. *J Virol* 1993;67:6716–6725.
52. Chen CM, Chen SC, Yang HY, et al. Hospitalization and mortality due to hepatitis A in Taiwan: a 15-year nationwide cohort study. *J Viral Hepat* 2016;23:940–945.
53. Cho MW, Ehrenfeld E. Rapid completion of the replication cycle of hepatitis A virus subsequent to reversal of guanidine inhibition. *Virology* 1991;180:770–780.
54. Choi YS, Jung MK, Lee J, et al. Tumor necrosis factor-producing T-regulatory cells are associated with severe liver injury in patients with acute hepatitis A. *Gastroenterology* 2018;154:1047–1060.
55. Choi YS, Lee J, Lee HW, et al. Liver injury in acute hepatitis A is associated with decreased frequency of regulatory T cells caused by Fas-mediated apoptosis. *Gut* 2015;64: 1303–1313.
56. Choi HK, Song YG, Han SH, et al. Clinical features and outcomes of acute kidney injury among patients with acute hepatitis A. *J Clin Virol* 2011;52:192–197.
57. Clemens R, Safary A, Hepburn A, et al. Clinical experience with an inactivated hepatitis A vaccine. *J Infect Dis* 1995;171(Suppl 1):S44–S49.
58. Cockayne EA. Catarrhal jaundice, sporadic and epidemic, and its relation to acute yellow atrophy of the liver. *Q J Med* 1912;6:1–29.
59. Cohen L, Benichou D, Martin A. Analysis of deletion mutants indicates that the 2A polypeptide of hepatitis A virus participates in virion morphogenesis. *J Virol* 2002;76: 7495–7505.
60. Cohen JI, Feinstone S, Purcell RH. Hepatitis A virus infection in a chimpanzee: duration of viremia and detection of virus in saliva and throat swabs. *J Infect Dis* 1989;160:887–890.
61. Cohen JI, Ticehurst JR, Feinstone SM, et al. Hepatitis A virus cDNA and its RNA transcripts are infectious in cell culture. *J Virol* 1987;61:3035–3039.
62. Cohn EJ, Oncley JL, Strong LE, et al. Chemical, clinical, and immunological studies on the products of human plasma fractionation. I. The characterization of the protein fractions of human plasma. *J Clin Invest* 1944;23:417–432.
63. Collier MG, Khudyakov YE, Selvage D, et al. Outbreak of hepatitis A in the USA associated with frozen pomegranate arils imported from Turkey: an epidemiological case study. *Lancet Infect Dis* 2014;14:976–981.
64. Corey L, Holmes KK. Sexual transmission of hepatitis A in homosexual men: incidence and mechanism. *N Engl J Med* 1980;302:435–438.
65. Costafreda MI, Abbasi A, Lu H, et al. Exosome mimicry by a HAVCR1-NPC1 pathway of endosomal fusion mediates hepatitis A virus infection. *Nat Microbiol* 2020;5:1096–1106.

66. Costafreda MI, Kaplan G. HAVCR1 (CD365) and its mouse ortholog are functional hepatitis A virus (HAV) cellular receptors that mediate HAV infection. *J Virol* 2018;92(9):e02065-17.
67. Costafreda MI, Pérez-Rodriguez FJ, D'Andrea L, et al. Hepatitis A virus adaptation to cellular shutoff is driven by dynamic adjustments of codon usage and results in the selection of populations with altered capsids. *J Virol* 2014;88:5029–5041.
68. Costafreda MI, Ribes E, Franch A, et al. A single mutation in the glycophorin A binding site of hepatitis A virus enhances virus clearance from the blood and results in a lower fitness variant. *J Virol* 2012;86:7887–7895.
69. Counihan NA, Anderson DA. Specific IgA enhances the transcytosis and excretion of hepatitis A virus. *Sci Rep* 2016;6:21855.
70. Crevat D, Crance JM, Chevrinais AM, et al. Monoclonal antibodies against an immunodominant and neutralizing epitope on hepatitis A virus antigen. *Arch Virol* 1990;113:95–98.
71. Cromeans T, Fields HA, Sobsey MD. Replication kinetics and cytopathic effect of hepatitis A virus. *J Gen Virol* 1989;70:2051–2062.
72. Cromeans T, Humphrey C, Sobsey M, et al. Use of immunogold preembedding technique to detect hepatitis A viral antigen in infected cells. *Am J Anat* 1989;185:314–320.
73. Cui F, Hadler SC, Zheng H, et al. Hepatitis A surveillance and vaccine use in China from 1990 through 2007. *J Epidemiol* 2009;19:189–195.
74. Cui F, Liang X, Wang F, et al. Development, production, and postmarketing surveillance of hepatitis A vaccines in China. *J Epidemiol* 2014;24:169–177.
75. Cullen JM, Lemon SM. Comparative pathology of hepatitis A virus and hepatitis E virus infection. *Cold Spring Harb Perspect Med* 2019;9(4):a033456.
76. Cuthbert JA. Hepatitis A: old and new. *Clin Microbiol Rev* 2001;14:38–58.
77. Daemer RJ, Feinstone SM, Gust ID, et al. Propagation of human hepatitis A virus in African Green Monkey kidney cell culture: primary isolation and serial passage. *Infect Immun* 1981;32:388–393.
78. Dagan R, Leventhal A, Anis E, et al. Incidence of hepatitis A in Israel following universal immunization of toddlers. *JAMA* 2005;294:202–210.
79. D'Andrea L, Pérez-Rodríguez FJ, de Castellarnau M, et al. The critical role of codon composition on the translation efficiency robustness of the hepatitis A virus capsid. *Genome Biol Evol* 2019;11:2439–2456.
80. Daniotti JL, Iglesias-Bartolome R. Metabolic pathways and intracellular trafficking of gangliosides. *IUBMB Life* 2011;63:513–520.
81. Das A, Barrientos RC, Shiota T, et al. Gangliosides are essential endosomal receptors for quasi-enveloped and naked hepatitis A virus. *Nat Microbiol* 2020;5:1069–1078.
82. Das A, Hirai-Yuki A, Gonzalez-Lopez O, et al. TIM1 (HAVCR1) is not essential for cellular entry of either quasi-enveloped or naked hepatitis A virions. *mBio* 2017;8(5):e00969-17. doi: 10.1128/mBio.00969-00917.
83. Das A, Maury W, Lemon SM. TIM1 (HAVCR1): an essential "receptor" or an "accessory attachment factor" for hepatitis A virus? *J Virol* 2019;93:e01793-01718.
84. de Jong AS, de Mattia F, Van Dommelen MM, et al. Functional analysis of picornavirus 2B proteins: effects on calcium homeostasis and intracellular protein trafficking. *J Virol* 2008;82:3782–3790.
85. de Oliveira Carneiro I, Sander AL, Silva N, et al. A novel marsupial hepatitis A virus corroborates complex evolutionary patterns shaping the genus hepatovirus. *J Virol* 2018;92(13):e00082-18.
86. Delem A, Safary A, De Namur F, et al. Characterization of the immune response of volunteers vaccinated with a killed vaccine against hepatitis A. *Vaccine* 1993;11:479–484.
87. D'Hondt E, Purcell RH, Emerson SU, et al. Efficacy of an inactivated hepatitis A vaccine in pre- and postexposure conditions in marmosets. *J Infect Dis* 1995;171(Suppl 1):S40–S43.
88. Di Cola G, Fantilli AC, Pisano MB, et al. Foodborne transmission of hepatitis A and hepatitis E viruses: A literature review. *Int J Food Microbiol* 2021;338:108986.
89. Dienstag JL, Feinstone SM, Purcell RH, et al. Experimental infection of chimpanzees with hepatitis A virus. *J Infect Dis* 1975;132:532–545.
90. Dienstag JL, Popper H, Purcell RH. The pathology of viral hepatitis types A and B in chimpanzees. *Am J Pathol* 1976;85:131–144.
91. Dollenmaier G, Weitz M. Interaction of glyceraldehyde-3-phosphate dehydrogenase with secondary and tertiary RNA structural elements of the hepatitis A virus 3′ translated and non-translated regions. *J Gen Virol* 2003;84:403–414.
92. Dotzauer A, Brenner M, Gebhardt U, et al. IgA-coated particles of hepatitis A virus are translocalized antivectorially from the apical to the basolateral site of polarized epithelial cells via the polymeric immunoglobulin receptor. *J Gen Virol* 2005;86:2747–2751.
93. Dotzauer A, Feinstone SM, Kaplan G. Susceptibility of nonprimate cell lines to hepatitis A virus infection. *J Virol* 1994;68:6064–6068.
94. Dotzauer A, Gebhardt U, Bieback K, et al. Hepatitis A virus-specific immunoglobulin A mediates infection of hepatocytes with hepatitis A virus via the asialoglycoprotein receptor. *J Virol* 2000;74:10950–10957.
95. Dotzauer A, Heitmann A, Laue T, et al. The role of immunoglobulin A in prolonged and relapsing hepatitis A virus infections. *J Gen Virol* 2012;93:754–760.
96. Drexler JF, Corman VM, Lukashev AN, et al.; Hepatovirus Ecology Consortium. Evolutionary origins of hepatitis A virus in small mammals. *Proc Natl Acad Sci U S A* 2015;112:15190–15195.
97. Duermeyer W, van der Veen J. Specific detection of IgM-antibodies by ELISA, applied in hepatitis-A. *Lancet* 1978;ii:684–685.
98. Dupzyk A, Tsai B. Bag2 is a component of a cytosolic extraction machinery that promotes membrane penetration of a nonenveloped virus. *J Virol* 2018;92:e00607-18.
99. Eckels KH, Summers PL, Dubois DR. Hepatitis A virus hemagglutination and a test for hemagglutination inhibition antibodies. *J Clin Microbiol* 1989;27:1375–1376.
100. Emerson SU, Huang YK, McRill C, et al. Mutations in both the 2B and 2C genes of hepatitis A virus are involved in adaptation to growth in cell culture. *J Virol* 1992;66:650–654.
101. Emerson SU, Huang YK, Nguyen H, et al. Identification of VP1/2A and 2C as virulence genes of hepatitis A virus and demonstration of genetic instability of 2C. *J Virol* 2002;76:8551–8559.
102. Emerson SU, Huang YK, Purcell RH. 2B and 2C mutations are essential but mutations throughout the genome of HAV contribute to adaptation to cell culture. *Virology* 1993;194:475–480.
103. Emerson SU, Rosenblum B, Feinstone S, et al. Identification of the hepatitis A virus genes involved in adaptation to tissue-culture growth and attenuation. In: R.A. Lerner, H. Ginsberg, R.M. Chanock, (eds). *Vaccines 89: Modern Approaches to New Vaccines Including Prevention of AIDS*. Cold Spring Harbor, NY: Cold Spring Harbor Laboratory Press; 1989:427–430.
104. Emerson SU, Tsarev SA, Govindarajan S, et al. A simian strain of hepatitis a virus, AGM-27, functions as an attenuated vaccine for chimpanzees. *J Infect Dis* 1996;173:592–597.
105. Esser-Nobis K, Harak C, Schult P, et al. Novel perspectives for hepatitis A virus therapy revealed by comparative analysis of hepatitis C virus and hepatitis A virus RNA replication. *Hepatology* 2015;62:397–408.
106. Feigelstock DA, Thompson P, Kaplan GG. Growth of hepatitis A virus in a mouse liver cell line. *J Virol* 2005;79:2950–2955.
107. Feigelstock D, Thompson P, Mattoo P, et al. Polymorphisms of the hepatitis A virus cellular receptor 1 in African green monkey kidney cells result in antigenic variants that do not react with protective monoclonal antibody 190/4. *J Virol* 1998;72:6218–6222.
108. Feigelstock D, Thompson P, Mattoo P, et al. The human homolog of HAVcr-1 codes for a hepatitis A virus cellular receptor. *J Virol* 1998;72:6621–6628.
109. Feinstone SM. History of the discovery of hepatitis A virus. *Cold Spring Harb Perspect Med* 2018;9(5):a031740.
110. Feinstone SM, Daemer RJ, Gust ID, et al. Live attenuated vaccine for hepatitis A. *Dev Biol Stand* 1983;54:429–432.
111. Feinstone SM, Kapikian AZ, Purcell RH. Hepatitis A: detection by immune electron microscopy of a viruslike antigen associated with acute illness. *Science* 1973;182:1026–1028.
112. Feng Z, Hensley L, McKnight KL, et al. A pathogenic picornavirus acquires an envelope by hijacking cellular membranes. *Nature* 2013;496:367–371.
113. Feng Z, Hirai-Yuki A, McKnight KL, et al. Naked viruses that aren't always naked: quasi-enveloped agents of acute hepatitis. *Annu Rev Virol* 2014;1:539–560.
114. Feng Z, Lemon SM. Hepatitis A virus. In: Ehrenfeld E, Domingo E, Roos RP, eds. *The Picornaviruses*. Washington, DC: ASM Press; 2010:383–396.
115. Feng H, Lenarcic EM, Yamane D, et al. NLRX1 promotes immediate IRF1-directed antiviral responses by limiting dsRNA-activated translational inhibition mediated by PKR. *Nat Immunol* 2017;18:1299–1309.
116. Feng Z, Li Y, McKnight KL, et al. Human pDCs preferentially sense enveloped hepatitis A virions. *J Clin Invest* 2015;125:169–176.
117. Feng H, Sander AL, Moreira-Soto A, et al. Hepatovirus 3ABC proteases and evolution of mitochondrial antiviral signaling protein (MAVS). *J Hepatol* 2019;71:25–34.
118. Feng H, Zhang Y-B, Gui J-F, et al. Interferon regulatory factor 1 (IRF1) and anti-pathogen innate immune responses. *PLoS Pathog*. 2021:17(1):e1009220.
119. Fensterl V, Grotheer D, Berk I, et al. Hepatitis A virus suppresses RIG-I-mediated IRF-3 activation to block induction of beta interferon. *J Virol* 2005;79:10968–10977.
120. Flehmig B, Ranke M, Berthold H, et al. A solid-phase radioimmunoassay for detection of IgM antibodies to hepatitis A virus. *J Infect Dis* 1979;140:169–175.
121. Fleischer B, Fleischer S, Maier K, et al. Clonal analysis of infiltrating T lymphocytes in liver tissue in viral hepatitis A. *Immunology* 1990;69:14–19.
122. Foster MA, Hofmeister MG, Kupronis BA, et al. Increase in hepatitis A virus infections—United States, 2013–2018. *MMWR Morb Mortal Wkly Rep* 2019;68:413–415.
123. Foster M, Ramachandran S, Myatt K, et al. Hepatitis A virus outbreaks associated with drug use and homelessness—California, Kentucky, Michigan, and Utah, 2017. *MMWR Morb Mortal Wkly Rep* 2018;67:1208–1210.
124. Freed EO. Viral late domains. *J Virol* 2002;76:4679–4687.
125. Frösner GG, Deinhardt F, Scheid R, et al. Propagation of human hepatitis A virus in a hepatoma cell line. *Infection* 1979;7:303–305.
126. Fuchs R, Blaas D. Uncoating of human rhinoviruses. *Rev Med Virol* 2010;20:281–297.
127. Fujiwara K, Kojima H, Yasui S, et al. Hepatitis A viral load in relation to severity of the infection. *J Med Virol* 2011;83:201–207.
128. Funkhouser AW, Purcell RH, D'Hondt E, et al. Attenuated hepatitis A virus: genetic determinants of adaptation to growth in MRC-5 cells. *J Virol* 1994;68:148–157.
129. Funkhouser AW, Raychaudhuri G, Purcell RH, et al. Progress toward the development of a genetically engineered attenuated hepatitis a virus vaccine. *J Virol* 1996;70:7948–7957.
130. Funkhouser AW, Schultz DE, Lemon SM, et al. Hepatitis A virus translation is rate-limiting for virus replication in MRC-5 cells. *Virology* 1999;254:268–278.
131. Garriga D, Vives-Adrián L, Buxaderas M, et al. Cloning, purification and preliminary crystallographic studies of the 2AB protein from hepatitis A virus. *Acta Crystallogr Sect F Struct Biol Cryst Commun* 2011;67:1224–1227.
132. Gauss-Muller V, Deinhardt F. Effect of hepatitis A virus infection on cell metabolism in vitro. *Proc Soc Exp Biol Med* 1984;175:10–15.
133. Gauss-Muller V, Kusov YY. Replication of a hepatitis A virus replicon detected by genetic recombination in vivo. *J Gen Virol* 2002;83:2183–2192.
134. Gellis SS, Stokes J Jr, Brother GM, et al. The use of human immune serum globulin (gamma globulin) in infectious (epidemic) hepatitis in the Mediterranean theater of operations. I. Studies on prophylaxis in two epidemics of infectious hepatitis. *JAMA* 1945;128:1062–1063.
135. Glass MJ, Jia XY, Summers DF. Identification of the hepatitis A virus internal ribosome entry site: in vivo and in vitro analysis of bicistronic RNAs containing the HAV 5′ noncoding region. *Virology* 1993;193:842–852.
136. Glikson M, Galun E, Oren R, et al. Relapsing hepatitis A. Review of 14 cases and literature survey. *Medicine (Baltimore)* 1992;71:14–23.
137. Godet AC, David F, Hantelys F, et al. IRES trans-acting factors, key actors of the stress response. *Int J Mol Sci* 2019;20(4):924.
138. Gonzalez-Lopez O, Rivera-Serrano EE, Hu F, et al. Redundant late domain functions of tandem VP2 YPX3L motifs in nonlytic cellular egress of quasi-enveloped hepatitis A virus. *J Virol* 2018;92:1308–1318.
139. Goodfellow I, Chaudhry Y, Richardson A, et al. Identification of a cis-acting replication element within the poliovirus coding region. *J Virol* 2000;74:4590–4600.
140. Gorbalenya AE, Donchenko AP, Blinov VM, et al. Cysteine proteases of positive strand RNA viruses and chymotrypsin-like serine proteases. A distinct protein superfamily with a common structural fold. *FEBS Lett* 1989;243:103–114.

141. Gorbalenya AE, Koonin EV. Helicases: amino acid sequence comparisons and structure-function relationships. *Curr Opin Struct Biol* 1993;3:419–429.
142. Gosert R, Cassinotti P, Siegl G, et al. Identification of hepatitis A virus non-structural protein 2B and its release by the major virus protease 3C. *J Gen Virol* 1996;77:247–255.
143. Gosert R, Chang KH, Rijnbrand R, et al. Transient expression of cellular polypyrimidine-tract binding protein stimulates cap-independent translation directed by both picornaviral and flaviviral internal ribosome entry sites in vivo. *Mol Cell Biol* 2000;20:1583–1595.
144. Gosert R, Egger D, Bienz K. A cytopathic and a cell culture adapted hepatitis A virus strain differ in cell killing but not in intracellular membrane rearrangements. *Virology* 2000;266:157–169.
145. Graff J, Cha J, Blyn LB, et al. Interaction of poly(rC) binding protein 2 with the 5′ noncoding region of hepatitis A virus RNA and its effects on translation. *J Virol* 1998;72:9668–9675.
146. Graff J, Emerson SU. Importance of amino acid 216 in nonstructural protein 2B for replication of hepatitis A virus in cell culture and in vivo. *J Med Virol* 2003;71:7–17.
147. Graff J, Richards OC, Swiderek KM, et al. Hepatitis A virus capsid protein VP1 has a heterogeneous C terminus. *J Virol* 1999;73:6015–6023.
148. Greninger AL, Knudsen GM, Betegon M, et al. ACBD3 interaction with TBC1 domain 22 protein is differentially affected by enteroviral and kobuviral 3A protein binding. *mBio* 2013;4:e00098-00013.
149. Hadler SC, Webster HM, Erben JJ, et al. Hepatitis A in day-care centers: a community-wide assessment. *N Engl J Med* 1980;302:1222–1227.
150. Han X, Zhou C, Jiang M, et al. Discovery of RG7834: the first-in-class selective and orally available small molecule hepatitis B virus expression inhibitor with novel mechanism of action. *J Med Chem* 2018;61:10619–10634.
151. Hardin CC, Sneeden JL, Lemon SM, et al. Folding of pyrimidine-enriched RNA fragments from the vicinity of the internal ribosomal entry site of hepatitis A virus. *Nucleic Acids Res* 1999;27:665–673.
152. Harmon SA, Emerson SU, Huang YK, et al. Hepatitis A viruses with deletions in the 2A gene are infectious in cultured cells and marmosets. *J Virol* 1995;69:5576–5581.
153. Harmon SA, Updike W, Jia XY, et al. Polyprotein processing in cis and in trans by hepatitis A virus 3C protease cloned and expressed in *Escherichia coli*. *J Virol* 1992;66:5242–5247.
154. Harrison SC. Viral membrane fusion. *Nat Struct Mol Biol* 2008;15:690–698.
155. Havens WP Jr. Period of infectivity of patients with experimentally induced infectious hepatitis. *J Exp Med* 1946;83:251–258.
156. Havens WP Jr, Ward R, Drill VA, et al. Experimental production of hepatitis by feeding icterogenic materials. *Proc Soc Exp Biol Med* 1944;57:206–208.
157. Herold J, Andino R. Poliovirus RNA replication requires genome circularization through a protein-protein bridge. *Mol Cell* 2001;7:581–591.
158. Hessvik NP, Llorente A. Current knowledge on exosome biogenesis and release. *Cell Mol Life Sci* 2018;75:193–208.
159. Hiltunen JK, Kastaniotis AJ, Autio KJ, et al. 17B-hydroxysteroid dehydrogenases as acyl thioester metabolizing enzymes. *Mol Cell Endocrinol* 2019;489:107–118.
160. Hindiyeh M, Li QH, Basavappa R, et al. Poliovirus mutants at histidine 195 of VP2 do not cleave VP0 into VP2 and VP4. *J Virol* 1999;73:9072–9079.
161. Hirai-Yuki A, Hensley L, McGivern DR, et al. MAVS-dependent host species range and pathogenicity of human hepatitis A virus. *Science* 2016;353:1541–1545.
162. Hirai-Yuki A, Hensley L, Whitmire JK, et al. Biliary secretion of quasi-enveloped human hepatitis A virus. *mBio* 2016;7:e01998-01916.
163. Hirai-Yuki A, Whitmire JK, Joyce M, et al. Murine models of hepatitis A virus infection. *Cold Spring Harb Perspect Med* 2019;9(1):a031674.
164. Hofmeister MG, Foster MA, Teshale EH. Epidemiology and transmission of hepatitis A virus and hepatitis E virus infections in the United States. *Cold Spring Harb Perspect Med* 2018;9(4):a033431.
165. Holmes AW, Wolfe L, Rosenblate H, et al. Hepatitis in marmosets: induction of disease with coded specimens from a human volunteer study. *Science* 1969;165:816–817.
166. Holzer BR, Hatz C, Schmidt-Sissolak D, et al. Immunogenicity and adverse effects of inactivated virosome versus alum-adsorbed hepatitis A vaccine: a randomized controlled trial. *Vaccine* 1996;14:982–986.
167. Hong S, Lee HW, Chang DY, et al. Antibody-secreting cells with a phenotype of Ki-67low, CD138high, CD31high, and CD38high secrete nonspecific IgM during primary hepatitis A virus infection. *J Immunol* 2013;191:127–134.
168. Hornei B, Kammerer R, Moubayed P, et al. Experimental hepatitis A virus infection in guinea pigs. *J Med Virol* 2001;64:402–409.
169. Hsu NY, Ilnytska O, Belov G, et al. Viral reorganization of the secretory pathway generates distinct organelles for RNA replication. *Cell* 2010;141:799–811.
170. Innis BL, Snitbhan R, Kunasol P, et al. Protection against hepatitis A by an inactivated vaccine. *JAMA* 1994;271:1328–1334.
171. Jackson WT, Giddings TH Jr, Taylor MP, et al. Subversion of cellular autophagosomal machinery by RNA viruses. *PLoS Biol* 2005;3:e156.
172. Jacobsen KH. Globalization and the changing epidemiology of hepatitis A virus. *Cold Spring Harb Perspect Med* 2018;8:a031716.
173. Jacobsen KH, Koopman JS. Declining hepatitis A seroprevalence: a global review and analysis. *Epidemiol Infect* 2004;132:1005–1022.
174. Jacobsen KH, Wiersma ST. Hepatitis A virus seroprevalence by age and world region, 1990 and 2005. *Vaccine* 2010;28:6653–6657.
175. Jansen RW, Newbold JE, Lemon SM. Complete nucleotide sequence of a cell culture-adapted variant of hepatitis A virus: comparison with wild-type virus with restricted capacity for in vitro replication. *Virology* 1988;163:299–307.
176. Jansen RW, Siegl G, Lemon SM. Molecular epidemiology of human hepatitis A virus defined by an antigen-capture polymerase chain reaction method. *Proc Natl Acad Sci U S A* 1990;87:2867–2871.
177. Jecht M, Probst C, Gauss-Muller V. Membrane permeability induced by hepatitis A virus proteins 2B and 2BC and proteolytic processing of HAV 2BC. *Virology* 1998;252:218–227.
178. Jewell DA, Swietnicki W, Dunn BM, et al. Hepatitis A virus 3C proteinase substrate specificity. *Biochemistry* 1992;31:7862–7869.
179. Jia XY, Summers DF, Ehrenfeld E. Host antibody response to viral structural and nonstructural proteins after hepatitis A virus infection. *J Infect Dis* 1992;165:273–280.
180. Jia XY, Tesar M, Summers DF, et al. Replication of hepatitis A viruses with chimeric 5′ nontranslated regions. *J Virol* 1996;70:2861–2868.
181. Jiang P, Liu Y, Ma HC, et al. Picornavirus morphogenesis. *Microbiol Mol Biol Rev* 2014;78:418–437.
182. Jiang W, Ma P, Deng L, et al. Hepatitis A virus structural protein pX interacts with ALIX and promotes the secretion of virions and foreign proteins through exosome-like vesicles. *J Extracell Vesicles* 2020;9:1716513.
183. Jiang W, Muhammad F, Ma P, et al. Sofosbuvir inhibits hepatitis A virus replication in vitro assessed by a cell-based fluorescent reporter system. *Antiviral Res* 2018;154:51–57.
184. Jouanguy E. Human genetic basis of fulminant viral hepatitis. *Hum Genet* 2020;139:877–884.
185. Jung YM, Park SJ, Kim JS, et al. Atypical manifestations of hepatitis A infection: a prospective, multicenter study in Korea. *J Med Virol* 2010;82:1318–1326.
186. Kankam M, Griffin R, Price J, et al. Polyvalent human immune globulin: a prospective, open-label study assessing anti-hepatitis A virus (HAV) antibody levels, pharmacokinetics, and safety in HAV-seronegative healthy subjects. *Adv Ther* 2020;37:2373–2389.
187. Kaplan G, Totsuka A, Thompson P, et al. Identification of a surface glycoprotein on African green monkey kidney cells as a receptor for hepatitis A virus. *EMBO J* 1996;15:4282–4296.
188. Karron RA, Daemer R, Ticehurst J, et al. Studies of prototype live hepatitis A virus vaccines in primate models. *J Infect Dis* 1988;157:338–345.
189. Keenan CM, Lemon SM, LeDuc JW, et al. Pathology of hepatitis A infection in the owl monkey (*Aotus trivirgatus*). *Am J Pathol* 1984;115:1–8.
190. Kihara A. Very long-chain fatty acids: elongation, physiology and related disorders. *J Biochem* 2012;152:387–395.
191. Kim J, Chang DY, Lee HW, et al. Innate-like cytotoxic function of bystander-activated CD8(+) T Cells is associated with liver injury in acute hepatitis A. *Immunity* 2018;48:161–173.e165.
192. Kim JD, Cho EJ, Ahn C, et al. A model to predict 1-month risk of transplant or death in hepatitis A-related acute liver failure. *Hepatology* 2019;70:621–629.
193. Kim HY, Eyheramonho MB, Pichavant M, et al. A polymorphism in TIM1 is associated with susceptibility to severe hepatitis A virus infection in humans. *J Clin Invest* 2011;121:1111–1118.
194. Kim HS, Jeong SH, Jang JH, et al. Coinfection of hepatitis A virus genotype IA and IIIA complicated with autoimmune hemolytic anemia, prolonged cholestasis, and false-positive immunoglobulin M anti-hepatitis E virus: a case report. *Korean J Hepatol* 2011;17:323–327.
195. Kim D, Lee YS, Jung SJ, et al. Viral hijacking of the TENT4-ZCCHC14 complex protects viral RNAs via mixed tailing. *Nat Struct Mol Biol* 2020;27:581–588.
196. Kim MJ, Shin JY, Oh JA, et al. Identification of transfusion-transmitted hepatitis A through postdonation information in Korea: results of an HAV lookback (2007–2012). *Vox Sang* 2018. https://doi.org/10.1111/vox.12672
197. Klevens RM, Denniston MM, Jiles-Chapman RB, et al. Decreasing immunity to hepatitis A virus infection among US adults: Findings from the National Health and Nutrition Examination Survey (NHANES), 1999–2012. *Vaccine* 2015;33:6192–6198.
198. Kolter T, Sandhoff K. Lysosomal degradation of membrane lipids. *FEBS Lett* 2010;584:1700–1712.
199. Konduru K, Kaplan GG. Determinants in 3Dpol modulate the rate of growth of hepatitis A virus. *J Virol* 2010;84:8342–8347.
200. Krawczynski KK, Bradley DW, Murphy BL, et al. Pathogenetic aspects of hepatitis A virus infection in enterally inoculated marmosets. *Am J Clin Pathol* 1981;76:698–706.
201. Krugman S, Giles JP, Hammond J. Infectious hepatitis: evidence for two distinctive clinical, epidemiological, and immunological types of infection. *JAMA* 1967;200:365–373.
202. Krugman S, Ward R, Giles JP, et al. Infectious hepatitis: detection of virus during the incubation period and in clinically inapparent infection. *N Engl J Med* 1959;261:729–734.
203. Kulkarni MA, Walimbe AM, Cherian S, et al. Full length genomes of genotype IIIA Hepatitis A Virus strains (1995–2008) from India and estimates of the evolutionary rates and ages. *Infect Genet Evol* 2009;9:1287–1294.
204. Kulsuptrakul J, Wang R, Meyers NL, et al. A genome-wide CRISPR screen identifies UFMylation and TRAMP-like complexes as host factors required for hepatitis A virus infection. *Cell Rep* 2021;34:108859.
205. Kusov YY, Gauss-Muller V. In vitro RNA binding of the hepatitis A virus proteinase 3C (HAV 3Cpro) to secondary structure elements within the 5′ terminus of the HAV genome. *RNA* 1997;3:291–302.
206. Kusov Y, Gauss-Muller V. Improving proteolytic cleavage at the 3A/3B site of the hepatitis A virus polyprotein impairs processing and particle formation, and the impairment can be complemented in trans by 3AB and 3ABC. *J Virol* 1999;73:9867–9878.
207. Kusov YY, Gosert R, Gauss-Muller V. Replication and in vivo repair of the hepatitis A virus genome lacking the poly(A) tail. *J Gen Virol* 2005;86:1363–1368.
208. Kusov YY, Morace G, Probst C, et al. Interaction of hepatitis A virus (HAV) precursor proteins 3AB and 3ABC with the 5′ and 3′ termini of the HAV RNA. *Virus Res* 1997;51:151–157.
209. Kusov Y, Weitz M, Dollenmeier G, et al. RNA-protein interactions at the 3′ end of the hepatitis A virus RNA. *J Virol* 1996;70:1890–1897.
210. Lanford RE, Feng Z, Chavez D, et al. Acute hepatitis A virus infection is associated with a limited type I interferon response and persistence of intrahepatic viral RNA. *Proc Natl Acad Sci U S A* 2011;108:11223–11228.
211. Lau CL, Streeton CL, David MC, et al. The tolerability of a combined hepatitis A and typhoid vaccine in children aged 2–16 years: an observational study. *J Travel Med* 2016;23:tav023.
212. Le SY, Chen JH, Sonenberg N, et al Conserved tertiary structural elements in the 5′ non-translated region of cardiovirus, aphthovirus and hepatitis A virus RNAs. *Nucleic Acids Res* 1993;21:2445–2451.

213. Lednar WM, Lemon SM, Kirkpatrick JW, et al. Frequency of illness associated with epidemic hepatitis A virus infections in adults. *Am J Epidemiol* 1985;122:226–233.
214. LeDuc JW, Escajadillo A, Lemon SM. Transmission of hepatitis A virus among captive Panamanian owl monkeys. *Lancet* 1981;2(8260-61):1427–1428.
215. Lee S, Joshi A, Nagashima K, et al. Structural basis for viral late-domain binding to Alix. *Nat Struct Mol Biol* 2007;14:194–199.
216. Lemon SM. IgM neutralizing antibody to hepatitis A virus. *J Infect Dis* 1985;152:1353–1354.
217. Lemon SM. Type A viral hepatitis: new developments in an old disease. *N Engl J Med* 1985;313:1059–1067.
218. Lemon SM, Binn LN. Antigenic relatedness of two strains of hepatitis A virus determined by cross-neutralization. *Infect Immun* 1983;42:418–420.
219. Lemon SM, Binn LN. Serum neutralizing antibody response to hepatitis A virus. *J Infect Dis* 1983;148:1033–1039.
220. Lemon SM, Binn LN. Incomplete neutralization of hepatitis A virus in vitro due to lipid-associated virions. *J Gen Virol* 1985;66:2501–2505.
221. Lemon SM, Binn LN, Marchwicki R, et al. In vivo replication and reversion to wild-type of a neutralization-resistant variant of hepatitis A virus. *J Infect Dis* 1990;161:7–13.
222. Lemon SM, Brown CD, Brooks DS, et al. Specific immunoglobulin M response to hepatitis A virus determined by solid-phase radioimmunoassay. *Infect Immun* 1980;28:927–936.
223. Lemon SM, Jansen RW. A simple method for clonal selection of hepatitis A virus based on recovery of virus from radioimmunofocus overlays. *J Virol Methods* 1985;11:171–176.
224. Lemon SM, Jansen RW, Newbold JE. Infectious hepatitis A virus particles produced in cell culture consist of three distinct types with different buoyant densities in CsCl. *J Virol* 1985;54:78–85.
225. Lemon SM, Murphy PC, Provost PJ, et al. Immunoprecipitation and virus neutralization assays demonstrate qualitative differences between protective antibody responses to inactivated hepatitis A vaccine and passive immunization with immune globulin. *J Infect Dis* 1997;176:9–19.
226. Lemon SM, Murphy PC, Shields PA, et al. Antigenic and genetic variation in cytopathic hepatitis A virus variants arising during persistent infection: evidence for genetic recombination. *J Virol* 1991;65:2056–2065.
227. Lemon SM, Murphy PC, Smith A, et al. Removal/neutralization of hepatitis A virus during manufacture of high purity, solvent/detergent factor VIII concentrate. *J Med Virol* 1994;43:44–49.
228. Lemon SM, Ott JJ, Van Damme P, et al. Type A viral hepatitis: a summary and update on the molecular virology, epidemiology, pathogenesis and prevention. *J Hepatol* 2018;68:167–184.
229. Lewis JA, Armstrong ME, Larson VM, et al. Use of a live attenuated hepatitis A vaccine to prepare a highly purified, formalin-inactivated hepatitis A vaccine. In: Hollinger FB, Lemon SM, Margolis HS, (eds). *Viral Hepatitis and Liver Disease.* Baltimore, MD: Williams & Wilkins; 1991:94–97.
230. Li K, Foy E, Ferreon JC, et al. Immune evasion by hepatitis C virus NS3/4A protease-mediated cleavage of the Toll-like receptor 3 adaptor protein TRIF. *Proc Natl Acad Sci U S A* 2005;102:2992–2997.
231. Li XD, Sun L, Seth RB, et al. Hepatitis C virus protease NS3/4A cleaves mitochondrial antiviral signaling protein off the mitochondria to evade innate immunity. *Proc Natl Acad Sci U S A* 2005;102:17717–17722.
232. Lim J, Kim D, Lee YS, et al. Mixed tailing by TENT4A and TENT4B shields mRNA from rapid deadenylation. *Science* 2018;361:701–704.
233. Lin J, Lee LY, Roivainen M, et al. Structure of the Fab-labeled "breathing" state of native poliovirus. *J Virol* 2012;86:5959–5962.
234. Liu Y, Wang C, Mueller S, et al. Direct interaction between two viral proteins, the non-structural protein 2C and the capsid protein VP3, is required for enterovirus morphogenesis. *PLoS Pathog* 2010;6:e1001066.
235. Locarnini SA, Coulepis AG, Kaldor J, et al. Coproantibodies in hepatitis A; detection of enzyme-linked immunosorbent assay and immune electron microscopy. *J Clin Microbiol* 1980;11:710–716.
236. Locarnini SA, Ferris AA, Stott AC, et al. Letter: pitfalls in hepatitis A? *Lancet* 1974;2:1007.
237. Losick VP, Schlax PE, Emmons RA, et al. Signals in hepatitis A virus P3 region proteins recognized by the ubiquitin-mediated proteolytic system. *Virology* 2003;309:306–319.
238. Lyoo H, van der Schaar HM, Dorobantu CM, et al. ACBD3 is an essential pan-enterovirus host factor that mediates the interaction between viral 3A protein and cellular protein PI4KB. *mBio* 2019;10:e02742-18.
239. MacCallum FO. Hepatitis. *Br Med Bull* 1953;9:221–225.
240. Maier K, Gabriel P, Koscielniak E, et al. Human gamma interferon production by cytotoxic T lymphocytes sensitized during hepatitis A virus infection. *J Virol* 1988;62:3756–3763.
241. Malcolm BA, Chin SM, Jewell DA, et al. Expression and characterization of recombinant hepatitis A virus 3C proteinase. *Biochemistry* 1992;31:3358–3363.
242. Manangeeswaran M, Jacques J, Tami C, et al. Binding of hepatitis A virus to its cellular receptor 1 inhibits T-regulatory cell functions in humans. *Gastroenterology* 2012;142:1516–1525.e1513.
243. Mannucci PM, Gdovin S, Gringeri A, et al. Transmission of hepatitis A to patients with hemophilia by factor VIII concentrates treated with organic solvent and detergent to inactivate viruses. *Ann Intern Med* 1994;120:1–7.
244. Mao JS, Dong DX, Zhang HY, et al. Primary study of attenuated live hepatitis A vaccine (H2 strain) in humans. *J Infect Dis* 1989;159:621–624.
245. Mao JS, Dong DX, Zhang SY, et al. Further studies of attenuated live hepatitis A vaccine (H2 strain) in humans. In: Hollinger FB, Lemon SM, Margolis HS, eds. *Viral Hepatitis and Liver Disease.* Baltimore, MD: Williams & Wilkins; 1991:110–111.
246. Martin A, Benichou D, Chao SF, et al. Maturation of the hepatitis A virus capsid protein VP1 is not dependent on processing by the 3Cpro proteinase. *J Virol* 1999;73:6220–6227.
247. Martin A, Escriou N, Chao SF, et al. Identification and site-direct mutagenesis of the primary (2A/2B) cleavage site of the hepatitis A virus polyprotein: functional impact on the infectivity of HAV transcripts. *Virology* 1995;213:213–222.
248. Martin A, Lemon SM. The molecular biology of hepatitis A virus. In: Ou J, ed. *Hepatitis Viruses.* Norwell, MA: Kluwer Academic Publishers; 2002:23–50.
249. Martin JC, Petrecz ML, Stek JE, et al. Using the power law model to predict the long-term persistence and duration of detectable hepatitis A antibody after receipt of hepatitis A Vaccine (VAQTA™). *Vaccine* 2021;39:2764–2771.
250. Mathiesen LR, Drucker J, Lorenz D, et al. Localization of hepatitis A antigen in marmoset organs during acute infection with hepatitis A virus. *J Infect Dis* 1978;138:369–377.
251. Mathiesen LR, Moller AM, Purcell RH, et al. Hepatitis A virus in the liver and intestine of marmosets after oral inoculation. *Infect Immun* 1980;28:45–48.
252. Maynard JE, Bradley DW, Gravelle CR, et al. Preliminary studies of hepatitis A in chimpanzees. *J Infect Dis* 1975;131:194–197.
253. Maynard JE, Krushak DH, Bradley DW, et al. Infectivity studies of hepatitis A and B in non-human primates. *Dev Biol Stand* 1975;30:229–235.
254. Mbithi JN, Springthorpe VS, Boulet JR, et al. Survival of hepatitis A virus on human hands and its transfer on contact with animate and inanimate surfaces. *J Clin Microbiol* 1992;30:757–763.
255. Mbithi JN, Springthorpe VS, Sattar SA. Comparative in vivo efficiencies of hand-washing agents against hepatitis A virus (HM-175) and poliovirus type 1 (Sabin). *Appl Environ Microbiol* 1993;59:3463–3469.
256. McKnight KL, Xie L, González-López O, et al. Protein composition of the hepatitis A virus quasi-envelope. *Proc Natl Acad Sci U S A* 2017;114:6587–6592.
257. Melia CE, Peddie CJ, de Jong AWM, et al. Origins of enterovirus replication organelles established by whole-cell electron microscopy. *mBio* 2019;10(3):e00951-19.
258. Metzger WG, Ehni HJ, Kremsner PG, et al. Experimental infections in humans—historical and ethical reflections. *Trop Med Int Health* 2019;24:1384–1390.
259. Midthun K, Ellerbeck E, Gershman K, et al. Safety and immunogenicity of a live attenuated hepatitis A virus vaccine in seronegative volunteers. *J Infect Dis* 1991;163:735–739.
260. Mishra N, Fagbo SF, Alagaili AN, et al. A viral metagenomic survey identifies known and novel mammalian viruses in bats from Saudi Arabia. *PLoS One* 2019;14:e0214227.
261. Mishra A, Saigal S, Gupta R, et al. Acute pancreatitis associated with viral hepatitis: a report of six cases with review of literature. *Am J Gastroenterol* 1999;94:2292–2295.
262. Misumi I, Li Z, Sun L, et al. Iminosugar glucosidase inhibitors reduce hepatic inflammation in HAV-infected Ifnar1(−/−) mice. *J Virol* 2021. doi: 10.1128/JVI.00058-21.
263. Misumi I, Mitchell JE, Lund MM, et al. T cells protect against hepatitis A virus infection and limit infection-induced liver injury. *J Hepatol* 2021;75:1323–1334.
264. Mohamed B, Mazeaud C, Baril M, et al. Very-long-chain fatty acid metabolic capacity of 17-beta-hydroxysteroid dehydrogenase type 12 (HSD17B12) promotes replication of hepatitis C virus and related flaviviruses. *Sci Rep* 2020;10:4040.
265. Moller-Tank S, Maury W. Phosphatidylserine receptors: enhancers of enveloped virus entry and infection. *Virology* 2014;468–470:565–580.
266. Morace G, Kusov Y, Dzagurov G, et al. The unique role of domain 2A of the hepatitis A virus precursor polypeptide P1-2A in viral morphogenesis. *BMB Rep* 2008;41:678–683.
267. Morris TS, Frormann S, Shechosky S, et al. In vitro and ex vivo inhibition of hepatitis A virus 3C proteinase by a peptidyl monofluoromethyl ketone. *Bioorg Med Chem* 1997;5:797–807.
268. Murphy BL, Maynard JE, Bradley DW, et al. Immunofluorescence of hepatitis A virus antigen in chimpanzees. *Infect Immun* 1978;21:663–665.
269. Nainan OV, Margolis HS, Robertson BH, et al. Sequence analysis of a new hepatitis A virus naturally infecting cynomolgus macaques (*Macaca fascicularis*). *J Gen Virol* 1991;72:1685–1689.
270. Najarian R, Caput D, Gee W, et al. Primary structure and gene organization of human hepatitis A virus. *Proc Natl Acad Sci U S A* 1985;82:2627–2631.
271. Navarro MED, Yao CC, Whiteley A, et al. Liver transplant evaluation for fulminant liver failure due to acute hepatitis A infection: case series and literature review. *Transpl Infect Dis* 2021;23:e13476.
272. Ndumbi P, Freidl GS, Williams CJ, et al. Hepatitis A outbreak disproportionately affecting men who have sex with men (MSM) in the European Union and European Economic Area, June 2016 to May 2017. *Euro Surveill* 2018;23(33):1700641. doi: 10.2807/1560-7917.
273. Neefe JR, Gellis SS, Stokes J Jr. Homologous serum hepatitis and infectious (epidemic) hepatitis: studies in volunteers bearing on immunological and other characteristics of the etiological agents. *Am J Med* 1946;1:3–22.
274. Nelson NP, Link-Gelles R, Hofmeister MG, et al. Update: recommendations of the Advisory Committee on Immunization Practices for use of hepatitis A vaccine for postexposure prophylaxis and for preexposure prophylaxis for international travel. *MMWR Morb Mortal Wkly Rep* 2018;67:1216–1220.
275. Nelson NP, Weng MK, Hofmeister MG, et al. Prevention of hepatitis A virus infection in the United States: recommendations of the Advisory Committee on Immunization Practices, 2020. *MMWR Recomm Rep* 2020;69:1–38.
276. Niepmann M. Internal translation initiation of picornaviruses and hepatitis C virus. *Biochim Biophys Acta* 2009;1789:529–541.
277. Nikonov OS, Chernykh ES, Garber MB, et al. Enteroviruses: classification, diseases they cause, and approaches to development of antiviral drugs. *Biochemistry (Mosc)* 2017;82:1615–1631.
278. Ouzilou L, Caliot E, Pelletier I, et al. Poliovirus transcytosis through M-like cells. *J Gen Virol* 2002;83:2177–2182.
279. Parry JV, Mortimer PP. The heat sensitivity of hepatitis A virus determined by a simple tissue culture method. *J Med Virol* 1984;14:277–283.
280. Paul AV, Van Boom JH, Filippov D, et al. Protein-primed RNA synthesis by purified poliovirus RNA polymerase. *Nature* 1998;393:280–284.
281. Paul AV, Yin J, Mugavero J, et al. A "slide-back" mechanism for the initiation of protein-primed RNA synthesis by the RNA polymerase of poliovirus. *J Biol Chem* 2003;278:43951–43960.
282. Paulmann D, Magulski T, Schwarz R, et al. Hepatitis A virus protein 2B suppresses beta interferon (IFN) gene transcription by interfering with IFN regulatory factor 3 activation. *J Gen Virol* 2008;89:1593–1604.

283. Peters H, Kusov YY, Meyer S, et al. Hepatitis A virus proteinase 3C binding to viral RNA: correlation with substrate binding and enzyme dimerization. *Biochem J* 2005;385: 363–370.
284. Peterson DA, Hurley TR, Hoff JC, et al. Effect of chlorine treatment on infectivity of hepatitis A virus. *Appl Environ Microbiol* 1983;45:223–227.
285. Petithory JR, Masiarz FR, Kirsch JF, et al. A rapid method for determination of endoproteinase substrate specificity: specificity of the 3C proteinase from hepatitis A virus. *Proc Natl Acad Sci U S A* 1991;88:11510–11514.
286. Pierce PF, Cappello M, Bernard KW. Subclinical infection with hepatitis A in Peace Corps volunteers following immune globulin prophylaxis. *Am J Trop Med Hyg* 1990;42:465–469.
287. Ping LH, Jansen RW, Stapleton JT, et al. Identification of an immunodominant antigenic site involving the capsid protein VP3 of hepatitis A virus. *Proc Natl Acad Sci U S A* 1988;85:8281–8285.
288. Ping LH, Lemon SM. Antigenic structure of human hepatitis A virus defined by analysis of escape mutants selected against murine monoclonal antibodies. *J Virol* 1992;66:2208–2216.
289. Pintó RM, Costafreda MI, Bosch A. Risk assessment in shellfish-borne outbreaks of hepatitis A. *Appl Environ Microbiol* 2009;75:7350–7355.
290. Pinto MA, Marchevsky RS, Baptista ML, et al. Experimental hepatitis A virus (HAV) infection in *Callithrix jacchus*: early detection of HAV antigen and viral fate. *Exp Toxicol Pathol* 2002;53:413–420.
291. Pinto RM, Perez-Rodriguez FJ, D'Andrea L, et al. Hepatitis A virus codon usage: implications for translation kinetics and capsid folding. *Cold Spring Harb Perspect Med* 2018;8(10):a031781.
292. Popper H, Dienstag JL, Feinstone SM, et al. The pathology of viral hepatitis in chimpanzees. *Virchows Arch A Pathol Anat Histol* 1980;387:91–106.
293. Probst C, Jecht M, Gauss-Muller V. Intrinsic signals for the assembly of hepatitis A virus particles. Role of structural proteins VP4 and 2A. *J Biol Chem* 1999;274:4527–4531.
294. Provost PJ, Banker FS, Wadsworth CW, et al. Further evaluation of a live hepatitis A vaccine in marmosets. *J Med Virol* 1991;34:227–231.
295. Provost PJ, Bishop RP, Gerety RJ, et al. New findings in live, attenuated hepatitis A vaccine development. *J Med Virol* 1986;20:165–175.
296. Provost PJ, Conti PA, Giesa PA, et al. Studies in chimpanzees of live, attenuated hepatitis A vaccine candidates. *Proc Soc Exp Biol Med* 1983;172:357–363.
297. Provost PJ, Giesa PA, McAleer WJ, et al. Isolation of hepatitis A virus in vitro in cell culture directly from human specimens. *Proc Soc Exp Biol Med* 1981;167:201–206.
298. Provost PJ, Hilleman MR. An inactivated hepatitis A virus vaccine prepared from infected marmoset liver. *Proc Soc Exp Biol Med* 1978;159:201–203.
299. Provost PJ, Hilleman MR. Propagation of human hepatitis A virus in cell culture in vitro. *Proc Soc Exp Biol Med* 1979;160:213–221.
300. Provost PJ, Villarejos VM, Hilleman MR. Tests in rufiventer and other marmosets of susceptibility to human hepatitis A virus. *Primates Med* 1978;10:288–294.
301. Purcell RH, D'Hondt E, Bradbury R, et al. Inactivated hepatitis A vaccine: active and passive immunoprophylaxis in chimpanzees. *Vaccine* 1992;10(Suppl 1):S148–S151.
302. Purcell RH, Emerson SU. Animal models of hepatitis A and E. *ILAR J* 2001;42:161–177.
303. Purcell RH, Feinstone SM, Ticehurst JR, et al. In: Vyas GN, Dienstag JL, Hoofnagle JH, eds. *Viral Hepatitis and Liver Disease*. Orlando, FL: Grune & Stratton; 1984.
304. Purcell RH, Wong DC, Shapiro M. Relative infectivity of hepatitis A virus by the oral and intravenous routes in 2 species of nonhuman primates. *J Infect Dis* 2002;185:1668–1671.
305. Qian M, Cai D, Verhey KJ, et al. A lipid receptor sorts polyomavirus from the endolysosome to the endoplasmic reticulum to cause infection. *PLoS Pathog* 2009;5:e1000465.
306. Qu L, Feng Z, Yamane D, et al. Disruption of TLR3 signaling due to cleavage of TRIF by the hepatitis A virus protease-polymerase processing intermediate, 3CD. *PLoS Pathog* 2011;7:e1002169.
307. Rachow A, Gauss-Muller V, Probst C. Homogeneous hepatitis A virus particles. Proteolytic release of the assembly signal 2A from procapsids by factor Xa. *J Biol Chem* 2003;278:29744–29751.
308. Ravindran MS, Bagchi P, Cunningham CN, et al. Opportunistic intruders: how viruses orchestrate ER functions to infect cells. *Nat Rev Microbiol* 2016;14:407–420.
309. Report ICTV. Picornaviridae. https://talk.ictvonline.org/ictv-reports/ictv_online_report/positive-sense-rna-viruses/w/picornaviridae. Accessed May 30, 2021.
310. Rezende G, Roque-Afonso AM, Samuel D, et al. Viral and clinical factors associated with the fulminant course of hepatitis A infection. *Hepatology* 2003;38:613–618.
311. Rha MS, Han JW, Kim JH, et al. Human liver CD8(+) MAIT cells exert TCR/MR1-independent innate-like cytotoxicity in response to IL-15. *J Hepatol* 2020;73:640–650.
312. Rivera-Serrano EE, Gonzalez-Lopez O, Das A, et al. Cellular entry and uncoating of naked and quasi-enveloped human hepatoviruses. *Elife* 2019;8:e43983.
313. Robertson BH, Jansen RW, Khanna B, et al. Genetic relatedness of hepatitis A virus strains recovered from different geographic regions. *J Gen Virol* 1992;73:1365–1377.
314. Robertson BH, Jia XY, Tian H, et al. Antibody response to nonstructural proteins of hepatitis A virus following infection. *J Med Virol* 1993;40:76–82.
315. Rog T, Orlowski A, Llorente A, et al. Interdigitation of long-chain sphingomyelin induces coupling of membrane leaflets in a cholesterol dependent manner. *Biochim Biophys Acta* 2016;1858:281–288.
316. Romero-Brey I, Bartenschlager R. Endoplasmic reticulum: the favorite intracellular niche for viral replication and assembly. *Viruses* 2016;8(6):160.
317. Rosenblum LS, Villarino ME, Nainan OV, et al. Hepatitis A outbreak in a neonatal intensive care unit: risk factors for transmission and evidence of prolonged viral excretion among preterm infants. *J Infect Dis* 1991;164:476–482.
318. Roulin PS, Lotzerich M, Torta F, et al. Rhinovirus uses a phosphatidylinositol 4-phosphate/cholesterol counter-current for the formation of replication compartments at the ER-Golgi interface. *Cell Host Microbe* 2014;16:677–690.
319. Rueckert RR, Wimmer E. Systematic nomenclature of picornavirus proteins. *J Virol* 1984;50:957–959.
320. Sachdeva H, Benusic M, Ota S, et al. Community outbreak of hepatitis A disproportionately affecting men who have sex with men in Toronto, Canada, January 2017–November 2018. *Can Commun Dis Rep* 2019;45:262–268.
321. Sanchez G, Aragones L, Costafreda MI, et al. Capsid region involved in hepatitis A virus binding to glycophorin A of the erythrocyte membrane. *J Virol* 2004;78:9807–9813.
322. Schaffner F, Dienstag JL, Purcell RH, et al. Chimpanzee livers after infection with human hepatitis viruses A and B: ultrastructural studies. *Arch Pathol Lab Med* 1977;101:113–117.
323. Schiff ER. Atypical clinical manifestations of hepatitis A. *Vaccine* 1992;10(Suppl 1): S18–S20.
324. Scholz E, Heinricy U, Flehmig B. Acid stability of hepatitis A virus. *J Gen Virol* 1989; 70(Pt 9):2481–2485.
325. Schulman AN, Dienstag JL, Jackson DR, et al. Hepatitis A antigen particles in liver, bile, and stool of chimpanzees. *J Infect Dis* 1976;134:80–84.
326. Schulte I, Hitziger T, Giugliano S, et al. Characterization of CD8+ T-cell response in acute and resolved hepatitis A virus infection. *J Hepatol* 2010;54:201–208.
327. Schultheiss T, Kusov YY, Gauss-Müller V. Proteinase 3C of hepatitis A virus (HAV) cleaves the HAV polyprotein P2-P3 at all sites including VP1/2A and 2A/2B. *Virology* 1994;198:275–281.
328. Schultheiss T, Sommergruber W, Kusov Y, Gauss-Müller V. Cleavage specificity of purified recombinant hepatitis A virus 3C proteinase on natural substrates. *J Virol* 1995;69: 1727–1733.
329. Schultz DE, Hardin CC, Lemon SM. Specific interaction of glyceraldehyde 3-phosphate dehydrogenase with the 5′ nontranslated RNA of hepatitis A virus. *J Biol Chem* 1996;271:14134–14142.
330. Seganti L, Superti F, Orsi N, et al. Study of the chemical nature of Frp/3 cell recognition units for hepatitis A virus. *Med Microbiol Immunol* 1987;176:21–26.
331. Seggewiß N, Paulmann D, Dotzauer A. Lysosomes serve as a platform for hepatitis A virus particle maturation and nonlytic release. *Arch Virol* 2016;161:43–52.
332. Shaffer DR, Brown EA, Lemon SM. Large deletion mutations involving the first pyrimidine-rich tract of the 5′ nontranslated RNA of human hepatitis A virus define two adjacent domains associated with distinct replication phenotypes. *J Virol* 1994;68:5568–5578.
333. Shaffer DR, Emerson SU, Murphy PC, et al. A hepatitis A virus deletion mutant which lacks the first pyrimidine-rich tract of the 5′ nontranslated RNA remains virulent in primates after direct intrahepatic nucleic acid transfection. *J Virol* 1995;69:6600–6604.
334. Shaffer DR, Lemon SM. Temperature-sensitive hepatitis A virus mutants with deletions downstream of the first pyrimidine-rich tract of the 5′ nontranslated RNA are impaired in RNA synthesis. *J Virol* 1995;69:6498–6506.
335. Shahbazian D, Parsyan A, Petroulakis E, et al. eIF4B controls survival and proliferation and is regulated by proto-oncogenic signaling pathways. *Cell Cycle* 2010;9:4106–4109.
336. Shevtsova ZV, Lapin BA, Doroshenko NV, et al. Spontaneous and experimental hepatitis A in Old World monkeys. *J Med Primatol* 1988;17:177–194.
337. Shimizu YK, Mathiesen LR, Lorenz D, et al. Localization of hepatitis A antigen in liver tissue by peroxidase-conjugated antibody method: light and electron microscopic studies. *J Immunol* 1978;121:1671–1679.
338. Shimizu YK, Shikata T, Beninger PR, et al. Detection of hepatitis A antigen in human liver. *Infect Immun* 1982;36:320–324.
339. Shin EC, Jeong SH. Natural history, clinical manifestations, and pathogenesis of hepatitis A. *Cold Spring Harb Perspect Med* 2018;8:a031708.
340. Shouval D. Immunization against Hepatitis A. *Cold Spring Harb Perspect Med* 2019;9(2):a031682.
341. Shubin AV, Demidyuk IV, Lunina NA, et al. Protease 3C of hepatitis A virus induces vacuolization of lysosomal/endosomal organelles and caspase-independent cell death. *BMC Cell Biol* 2015;16:4.
342. Shukla A, Dey D, Banerjee K, et al. The C-terminal region of the non-structural protein 2B from Hepatitis A Virus demonstrates lipid-specific viroporin-like activity. *Sci Rep* 2015;5:15884.
343. Shukla A, Padhi AK, Gomes J, et al. The VP4 peptide of hepatitis A virus ruptures membranes through formation of discrete pores. *J Virol* 2014;88:12409–12421.
344. Siciński P, Rowiński J, Warchoł JB, et al. Poliovirus type 1 enters the human host through intestinal M cells. *Gastroenterology* 1990;98:56–58.
345. Sickbert-Bennett EE, Weber DJ, Gergen-Teague MF, et al. Comparative efficacy of hand hygiene agents in the reduction of bacteria and viruses. *Am J Infect Control* 2005;33:67–77.
346. Siegl G, Frosner GG. Characterization and classification of virus particles associated with hepatitis A. I. Size, density and sedimentation. *J Virol* 1978;26:40–47.
347. Siegl G, Frosner GG, Gauss-Muller V, et al. The physicochemical properties of infectious hepatitis A virions. *J Gen Virol* 1981;57:331–341.
348. Siegl G, Weitz M, Kronauer G. Stability of hepatitis A virus. *Intervirology* 1984;22: 218–226.
349. Sikuler E, Keynan A, Hanuka N, et al. Detection and persistence of specific IgA antibodies in serum of patients with hepatitis A by capture radioimmunoassay. *J Med Virol* 1983;11:287–294.
350. Silberstein E, Xing L, van de Beek W, et al. Alteration of hepatitis A virus (HAV) particles by a soluble form of HAV cellular receptor 1 containing the immunoglobulin- and mucin-like regions. *J Virol* 2003;77:8765–8774.
351. Sjogren MH, Tanno H, Fay O, et al. Hepatitis A virus in stool during clinical relapse. *Ann Intern Med* 1987;106:221–226.
352. Skinhoj P, Mikkelsen F, Hollinger FB. Hepatitis Ain Greenland: importance of specific antibody testing in epidemiologic surveillance. *Am J Epidemiol* 1977;105:140–147.
353. Smith DB, Simmonds P. Classification and genomic diversity of enterically transmitted hepatitis viruses. *Cold Spring Harb Perspect Med* 2018;8:a031880.
354. Snooks MJ, Bhat P, Mackenzie J, et al. Vectorial entry and release of hepatitis A virus in polarized human hepatocytes. *J Virol* 2008;82:8733–8742.
355. Stapleton JT, Frederick J, Meyer B. Hepatitis A virus attachment to cultured cell lines. *J Infect Dis* 1991;164:1098–1103.
356. Stapleton JT, Lange DK, LeDuc JW, et al. The role of secretory immunity in hepatitis A virus infection. *J Infect Dis* 1991;163:7–11.
357. Stapleton JT, Lemon SM. Neutralization escape mutants define a dominant immunogenic neutralization site on hepatitis A virus. *J Virol* 1987;61:491–498.

358. Stapleton JT, Raina V, Winokur PL, et al. Antigenic and immunogenic properties of recombinant hepatitis A virus 14S and 70S subviral particles. *J Virol* 1993;67:1080–1085.
359. Stewart DR, Morris TS, Purcell RH, et al. Detection of antibodies to the nonstructural 3C proteinase of hepatitis A virus. *J Infect Dis* 1997;176:593–601.
360. Stockley PG, Twarock R, Bakker SE, et al. Packaging signals in single-stranded RNA viruses: nature's alternative to a purely electrostatic assembly mechanism. *J Biol Phys* 2013;39:277–287.
361. Stokes J, Jr., Farquhar JA, Drake ME, et al. Infectious hepatitis: length of protection by immune serum globulin (gamma globulin) during epidemics. *JAMA* 1951;147:714–719.
362. Stuart DI, Ren J, Wang X, et al. Hepatitis A virus capsid structure. *Cold Spring Harb Perspect Med* 2019;9(5):a031807.
363. Sun L, Li Y, Misumi I, et al. IRF3-mediated pathogenicity of human hepatitis A virus in mice. PLoS Pathog. 2021;17:e1009960.
364. Sun L, Zhang F, Guo F, et al. The dihydroquinolizinone compound RG7834 inhibits the polyadenylase function of PAPD5 and PAPD7 and accelerates the degradation of matured hepatitis B virus surface protein mRNA. *Antimicrob Agents Chemother* 2020;65:e00640-20.
365. Sung PS, Hong SH, Lee J, et al. CXCL10 is produced in hepatitis A virus-infected cells in an IRF3-dependent but IFN-independent manner. *Sci Rep* 2017;7:6387.
366. Takahashi Y, Misumi S, Muneoka A, et al. Nonhuman primate intestinal villous M-like cells: an effective poliovirus entry site. *Biochem Biophys Res Commun* 2008;368:501–507.
367. Taylor GM, Goldin RD, Karayiannis P, et al. In situ hybridization studies in hepatitis A infection. *Hepatology* 1992;16:642–648.
368. Taylor M, Goldin RD, Ladva S, et al. In situ hybridization studies of hepatitis A viral RNA in patients with acute hepatitis A. *J Hepatol* 1994;20:380–387.
369. Taylor KL, Murphy PC, Asher LVS, et al. Attenuation phenotype of a cell culture-adapted variant of hepatitis A virus (HM175/p16) in susceptible new world owl monkeys. *J Infect Dis* 1993;168:592–601.
370. Teixera MR Jr, Weller IVD, Murray A, et al. The pathology of hepatitis A in man. *Liver* 1982;2:53–60.
371. Teo CG. 19th century and early 20th-century jaundice outbreaks, the USA. *Epidemiol Infect* 2018;146:138–146.
372. Tesar M, Jia XY, Summers DF, et al. Analysis of a potential myristoylation site in hepatitis A virus capsid protein VP4. *Virology* 1993;194:616–626.
373. Tesar M, Pak I, Jia XY, et al. Expression of hepatitis A virus precursor protein P3 in vivo and in vitro: polyprotein processing of the 3CD cleavage site. *Virology* 1994;198:524–533.
374. Teterina NL, Bienz K, Egger D, et al. Induction of intracellular membrane rearrangements by HAV proteins 2C and 2BC. *Virology* 1997;237:66–77.
375. Theamboonlers A, Abe K, Thongmee C, et al. Complete coding sequence and molecular analysis of hepatitis A virus from a chimpanzee with fulminant hepatitis. *J Med Primatol* 2012;41:11–17.
376. Thompson P, Lu J, Kaplan GG. The Cys-rich region of hepatitis A virus cellular receptor 1 is required for binding of hepatitis A virus and protective monoclonal antibody 190/4. *J Virol* 1998;72:3751–3761.
377. Ticehurst JR, Racaniello VR, Baroudy BM, et al. Molecular cloning and characterization of hepatitis A virus cDNA. *Proc Natl Acad Sci U S A* 1983;80:5885–5889.
378. Tjon GM, Coutinho RA, van den Hoek A, et al. High and persistent excretion of hepatitis A virus in immunocompetent patients. *J Med Virol* 2006;78:1398–1405.
379. Tong MJ, El-Farra NS, Grew MI. Clinical manifestations of hepatitis A: Recent experience in a community teaching hospital. *J Infect Dis* 1995;171(Suppl 1):S15–S18
380. Tong MJ, Thursby M, Rakela J, et al. Studies on the maternal-infant transmission of the viruses which cause acute hepatitis. *Gastroenterology* 1981;80:999–1004.
381. Totsuka A, Moritsugu Y. Hepatitis A vaccine development in Japan. In: Nishioka K, Suzuki H, Mishiro S, et al., eds. *Viral Hepatitis and Liver Disease*. Tokyo, Japan: Springer-Verlag; 1994:509–513.
382. Treyer A, Musch A. Hepatocyte polarity. *Compr Physiol* 2013;3:243–287.
383. Tsarev SA, Emerson SU, Balayan MS, et al. Simian hepatitis A virus (HAV) strain AGM-27: comparison of genome structure and growth in cell culture with other HAV strains. *J Gen Virol* 1991;72:1677–1683.
384. Vallbracht A, Gabriel P, Maier K, et al. Cell-mediated cytotoxicity in hepatitis A virus infection. *Hepatology* 1986;6:1308–1314.
385. Vallbracht A, Hofmann L, Wurster KG, et al. Persistent infection of human fibroblasts by hepatitis A virus. *J Gen Virol* 1984;65:609–615.
386. Vallbracht A, Maier K, Stierhof YD, et al. Liver-derived cytotoxic T cells in hepatitis A virus infection. *J Infect Dis* 1989;160:209–217.
387. Van Damme P, Banatvala J, Fay O, et al. Hepatitis A booster vaccination: is there a need? *Lancet* 2003;362:1065–1071.
388. Van Effelterre T, Guignard A, Marano C, et al. Modeling the hepatitis A epidemiological transition in Brazil and Mexico. *Hum Vaccin Immunother* 2017;13:1942–1951.
389. Vento S, Garofano T, di Perri G, et al. Identification of hepatitis A virus as a trigger for autoimmune chronic hepatitis type 1 in susceptible individuals. *Lancet* 1991;337:1183–1187.
390. Vento S, Garofano T, Renzini C, et al. Fulminant hepatitis associated with hepatitis A virus superinfection in patients with chronic hepatitis C. *N Engl J Med* 1998;338:286–290.
391. Victor JC, Monto AS, Surdina TY, et al. Hepatitis A vaccine versus immune globulin for postexposure prophylaxis. *N Engl J Med* 2007;357:1685–1694.
392. Villarejos VM, Serra C J, Anderson-Visona K, et al. Hepatitis A virus infection in households. *Am J Epidemiol* 1982;115:577–586.
393. Vives-Adrian L, Garriga D, Buxaderas M, et al. Structural basis for host membrane remodeling induced by protein 2B of hepatitis A virus. *J Virol* 2015;89:3648–3658.
394. Vizzotti C, González J, Gentile A, et al. Impact of the single-dose immunization strategy against hepatitis A in Argentina. *Pediatr Infect Dis J* 2014;33:84–88.
395. Voegt H. Zur Aetiologie der Hepatitis epidemica. *MMW Munch Med Wochenschr* 1942;89:76–79.
396. Votteler J, Ogohara C, Yi S, et al. Designed proteins induce the formation of nanocage-containing extracellular vesicles. *Nature* 2016;540:292–295.
397. Votteler J, Sundquist WI. Virus budding and the ESCRT pathway. *Cell Host Microbe* 2013;14:232–241.
398. Walczak CP, Leto DE, Zhang L, et al. Ribosomal protein RPL26 is the principal target of UFMylation. *Proc Natl Acad Sci U S A* 2019;116:1299–1308.
399. Walker CM. Adaptive immune responses in hepatitis A virus and hepatitis E virus infections. *Cold Spring Harb Perspect Med* 2019;9(9):a033472.
400. Walker CM, Feng Z, Lemon SM. Reassessing immune control of hepatitis A virus. *Curr Opin Virol* 2015;11:7–13.
401. Walter TS, Ren J, Tuthill TJ, et al. A plate-based high-throughput assay for virus stability and vaccine formulation. *J Virol Methods* 2012;185:166–170.
402. Wang D, Fang L, Wei D, et al. Hepatitis A virus 3C protease cleaves NEMO to impair induction of beta interferon. *J Virol* 2014;88:10252–10258.
403. Wang M, Feng Z. Mechanisms of hepatocellular injury in hepatitis A. *Viruses* 2021;13(5):861.
404. Wang L, Jeng KS, Lai MM. Poly(C)-binding protein 2 interacts with sequences required for viral replication in the hepatitis C virus (HCV) 5′ untranslated region and directs HCV RNA replication through circularizing the viral genome. *J Virol* 2011;85:7954–7964.
405. Wang X, Ren J, Gao Q, et al. Hepatitis A virus and the origins of picornaviruses. *Nature* 2015;517:85–88.
406. Wang H, Shi Y, Song J, et al. Ebola viral glycoprotein bound to its endosomal receptor Niemann-Pick C1. *Cell* 2016;164:258–268.
407. Wang X, Zhu L, Dang M, et al. Potent neutralization of hepatitis A virus reveals a receptor mimic mechanism and the receptor recognition site. *Proc Natl Acad Sci U S A* 2017;114:770–775.
408. Wasley A, Miller JT, Finelli L. Surveillance for acute viral hepatitis—United States, 2005. *MMWR Surveill Summ* 2007;56:1–24.
409. Wasley A, Samandari T, Bell BP. Incidence of hepatitis A in the United States in the era of vaccination. *JAMA* 2005;294:194–201.
410. Wassenaar TM, Jun SR, Robeson M, et al. Comparative genomics of hepatitis A virus, hepatitis C virus, and hepatitis E virus provides insights into the evolutionary history of Hepatovirus species. *Microbiologyopen* 2020;9:e973.
411. Weitz M, Baroudy BM, Maloy WL, et al. Detection of a genome-linked protein (VPg) of hepatitis A virus and its comparison with other picornaviral VPgs. *J Virol* 1986;60:124–130.
412. Werzberger A, Kuter B, Nalin D. Six years' follow-up after hepatitis A vaccination. *N Engl J Med* 1998;338:1160.
413. Werzberger A, Mensch B, Kuter B, et al. A controlled trial of a formalin-inactivated hepatitis A vaccine in healthy children. *N Engl J Med* 1992;327:453–457.
414. Wessels E, Duijsings D, Lanke KH, et al. Effects of picornavirus 3A proteins on protein transport and GBF1-dependent COP-I recruitment. *J Virol* 2006;80:11852–11860.
415. Whetter LE, Day SP, Elroy-Stein O, et al. Low efficiency of the 5′ nontranslated region of hepatitis A virus RNA in directing cap-independent translation in permissive monkey kidney cells. *J Virol* 1994;68:5253–5263.
416. White MR, Khan MM, Deredge D, et al. A dimer interface mutation in glyceraldehyde-3-phosphate dehydrogenase regulates its binding to AU-rich RNA. *J Biol Chem* 2015;290:1770–1785.
417. Wiedmann M, Boehm S, Schumacher W, et al. Evaluation of three commercial assays for the detection of hepatitis a virus. *Eur J Clin Microbiol Infect Dis* 2003;22:129–130.
418. Winokur PL, McLinden JH, Stapleton JT. The hepatitis A virus polyprotein expressed by a recombinant vaccinia virus undergoes proteolytic processing and assembly into viruslike particles. *J Virol* 1991;65:5029–5036.
419. Winokur PL, Stapleton JT. Immunoglobulin prophylaxis for hepatitis A. *Clin Infect Dis* 1992;14:580–586.
420. Wong DC, Purcell RH, Rosen L. Prevalence of antibody to hepatitis A and hepatitis B viruses in selected populations of the South Pacific. *Am J Epidemiol* 1979;110:227–236.
421. Wright F. The 'effective number of codons' used in a gene. *Gene* 1990;87:23–29.
422. Yamane D, Feng H, Rivera-Serrano EE, et al. Constitutive expression of interferon regulatory factor 1 drives intrinsic hepatocyte resistance to multiple RNA viruses. *Nat Microbiol* 2019;4:1096–1104.
423. Yang Y, Liang Y, Qu L, et al. Disruption of innate immunity due to mitochondrial targeting of a picornaviral protease precursor. *Proc Natl Acad Sci U S A* 2007;104:7253–7258.
424. Yang Y, Rijnbrand R, McKnight KL, et al. Sequence requirements for viral RNA replication and VPg uridylylation directed by the internal cis-acting replication element (cre) of human rhinovirus type 14. *J Virol* 2002;76:7485–7494.
425. Yang Y, Yi M, Evans DJ, et al. Identification of a conserved RNA replication element (cre) within the 3Dpol-coding sequence of hepatoviruses. *J Virol* 2008;82:10118–10128.
426. Yao G. Clinical spectrum and natural history of viral hepatitis A in a 1988 Shanghai epidemic. In: Hollinger FB, Lemon SM, Margolis H, eds. *Viral Hepatitis and Liver Diseases*. New York: Williams & Wilkins; 1991:76–78.
427. Yi M, Lemon SM. Replication of subgenomic hepatitis A virus RNAs expressing firefly luciferase is enhanced by mutations associated with adaptation of virus to growth in cultured cells. *J Virol* 2002;76:1171–1180.
428. Yi M, Schultz DE, Lemon SM. Functional significance of the interaction of hepatitis A virus RNA with glyceraldehyde 3-phosphate dehydrogenase (GAPDH): opposing effects of GAPDH and polypyrimidine tract binding protein on internal ribosome entry site function. *J Virol* 2000;74:6459–6468.
429. Yoon EL, Sinn DH, Lee HW, et al. Current status and strategies for the control of viral hepatitis A in Korea. *Clin Mol Hepatol* 2017;23:196–204.
430. Young MK. The indications and safety of polyvalent immunoglobulin for post-exposure prophylaxis of hepatitis A, rubella and measles. *Hum Vaccin Immunother* 2019;15:2060–2065.
431. Yu JM, Li LL, Xie GC, et al. Experimental infection of Marmota monax with a novel hepatitis A virus. *Arch Virol* 2018;163(5):1187–1193.
432. Yu JM, Li LL, Zhang CY, et al. A novel hepatovirus identified in wild woodchuck Marmota himalayana. *Sci Rep* 2016;6:22361.
433. Zajac AJ, Amphlett EM, Rowlands DJ, et al. Parameters influencing the attachment of hepatitis A virus to a variety of continuous cell lines. *J Gen Virol* 1991;72:1667–1675.

434. Zell R. Picornaviridae—the ever-growing virus family. *Arch Virol* 2018;163:299–317.

435. Zell R, Delwart E, Gorbalenya AE, et al. ICTV Virus Taxonomy Profile: Picornaviridae. *J Gen Virol* 2017;98:2421–2422.

436. Zhang HC, Chao SF, Ping LH, et al. An infectious cDNA clone of a cytopathic hepatitis A virus: genomic regions associated with rapid replication and cytopathic effect. *Virology* 1995;212:686–697.

437. Zhang Y, Kaplan GG. Characterization of replication-competent hepatitis A virus constructs containing insertions at the N terminus of the polyprotein. *J Virol* 1998;72:349–357.

438. Zhang B, Morace G, Gauss-Muller V, et al. Poly(A) binding protein, C-terminally truncated by the hepatitis A virus proteinase 3C, inhibits viral translation. *Nucleic Acids Res* 2007;35:5975–5984.

439. Zhang B, Seitz S, Kusov Y, et al. RNA interaction and cleavage of poly(C)-binding protein 2 by hepatitis A virus protease. *Biochem Biophys Res Commun* 2007;364:725–730.

440. Zhou Y, Callendret B, Xu D, et al. Dominance of the CD4+ T helper cell response during acute resolving hepatitis A virus infection. *J Exp Med* 2012;209:1481–1492.

441. Zhou D, Zhao Y, Kotecha A, et al. Unexpected mode of engagement between enterovirus 71 and its receptor SCARB2. *Nat Microbiol* 2019;4:414–419.

442. Zhu L, Wang X, Ren J, et al. Structure of Ljungan virus provides insight into genome packaging of this picornavirus. *Nat Commun* 2015;6:8316.

443. Zuckerman AJ. The history of viral hepatitis from antiquity to the present. In: Deinhardt F, Deinhardt J, eds. *Viral Hepatitis: Laboratory and Clinical Science*. New York: Marcel Dekker; 1983:3–32.

Valerie Cortez • Stacey Schultz-Cherry

Introduction
History
Classification
Virion structure and composition
Genome structure and organization
    ORF1a and ORF1b
    ORF2
    ORFX
Stages of replication
    Attachment and entry
    Uncoating
    Translation
    Transcription/Replication
    Assembly and release
Pathogenesis and pathology
    Entry into the host and primary site of replication
    Cell and tissue tropism
    Immune response
    Release from host and transmission
    Virulence and persistence
Epidemiology
    Origin and spread of epidemics
    Prevalence and seroepidemiology
    Genetic diversity of virus
Clinical features
Diagnosis
    Differential
    Laboratory
Prevention and control
    Treatment
    Vaccines
Perspectives
Acknowledgments

INTRODUCTION

The family *Astroviridae* includes viruses with icosahedral morphology and is nonenveloped. Their genome is composed of positive-sense, single-stranded RNA (ssRNA) and is organized into three open reading frames (ORFs).

Astroviruses (AstVs) have been identified in many different animal species, with new strains isolated on a regular basis, highlighting their continued emergence and broad host range. Although they are classically known as enteric viruses associated with acute gastroenteritis, extra-gastrointestinal disease has become increasingly recognized. Human-infecting AstVs, in particular, are common causes of gastroenteritis in young children and contribute to sporadic outbreaks.

HISTORY

The term *astrovirus* was coined by Madeley and Cosgrove in 1975 to describe small, round viruses with a distinctive five- or six-pointed, star-like appearance (astron, *star* in Greek) of about 28 to 30 nm in diameter.[127,128] They were initially observed by negative-stain electron microscopy (EM) in the stools of infants hospitalized with diarrhea and in outbreaks of gastroenteritis in newborn nurseries (Fig. 3.1). Subsequently, viral particles of similar size and morphology were identified by EM in association with diarrhea in a wide variety of young mammals and birds.

An important milestone was achieved in 1981 when Lee and Kurtz reported the isolation and passage of a human isolate of astrovirus in primary cell cultures.[118] This led to the recognition of five serotypes in 1984,[114] collectively known as human astroviruses (HAstVs), development of an enzyme immunoassay to detect viral antigen in the late 1980s,[82] and confirmation of their clinical importance.[83] The molecular characterization of HAstV isolates subsequently permitted the recognition of eight serotypes based on their reactivity to hyperimmune sera and the design of molecular probes for use as diagnostic tools. Beginning in 2008, metagenomic and consensus sequencing approaches led to the identification of novel AstV from humans, commonly referred to as VA and MLB viruses, based on the location they were first identified (Virginia, United States, and Melbourne, Australia, respectively),[55–57,100] in addition to numerous AstVs from a broad range of animal hosts.[18,54,126,132,147,166,182,195,209] The efficient propagation of classical and novel human-infecting AstVs in cell lines[91,93,198] and the use of turkey[105,191,215] and murine isolates in animal models[33,40,213] has further advanced our knowledge of the molecular and structural biology, as well as the pathogenesis of these viruses. Still, there is a relative paucity of data available from the murine and turkey models, highlighting the need for expanded studies as well as the development of *in vivo* models for human-infecting AstV.

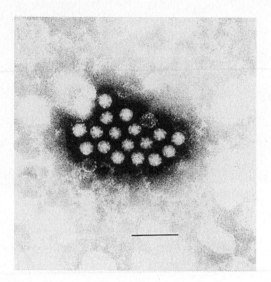

FIGURE 3.1 Electron micrograph of astrovirus in a human fecal specimen. Bar = 100 nm. (Courtesy of T. W. Lee and J. B. Kurtz.)

CLASSIFICATION

The genomic architecture of the AstV genome places the ORFs encoding the nonstructural proteins at the 5′ end and the ORF encoding the structural proteins at the 3′ end. Distinctive features of this family include their morphology,[168] the lack of an RNA helicase domain encoded in the genome, and the usage of a ribosomal frameshifting mechanism to translate the RNA-dependent RNA polymerase (RdRp).[96]

AstVs were originally classified into genera and species based solely on the host of origin; however, recent characterization of novel AstVs has shown that isolates from different animal species can be genetically similar, while genetically diverse viruses can be isolated from the same animal species.[100,126,218] In fact, AstVs that infect humans occupy four distinct phylogenetic clades and include viruses that are more similar to other animal isolates, such as those from mink and sheep, than the classical eight HAstV serotypes[100] (Fig. 3.2). These highly divergent viruses found among humans, as well as pigs[126] and bats,[32,218] represent polyphyly that is indicative of cross-species transmission, which has been further supported by the identification of recombinant AstVs from different host species.[44,46]

Together, these recent findings challenged the long-held dogma that AstVs were species-specific, leading to a new classification system based on the amino acid sequence of ORF2 (Astroviruses Study Group, 9th Report ICTV, 2010), which encodes the capsid polyprotein and represents the most variable region of the genome. Based on this naming system, two genera are distinguished within the *Astroviridae* family: *Mamastrovirus* and *Avastrovirus* (Fig. 3.3). Viruses belonging to the genus *Mamastrovirus* include isolates from a number of mammals, including humans, pigs, cats, mink, sheep, cows, dogs, bats, mice, rats, deer, and marine mammals, such as sea lions and bottlenose dolphins, among others. This genus includes two genogroups, GI and GII, that encompass 10 and 9 genotypes, respectively. The HAstV, MLB, VA2-5, and VA1-3 viruses are classified into *Mamastrovirus* genotypes 1, 6, 8, and 9, respectively.

Viruses from the genus *Avastrovirus* include isolates from many avian species, including turkeys, ducks, chickens, guinea

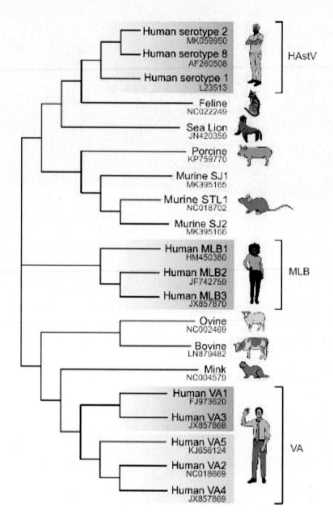

FIGURE 3.2 Human-infecting AstVs occupy four distinct clades. Phylogenetic analysis of ORF2 amino acid sequences highlight HAstV, MLB, VA1-3, and VA2-5 clades that have been identified in humans. Phylogenetic relationships inferred by maximum likelihood estimation (LG+F) and tree constructed based on 1,000 bootstrapped replicates using MEGA X 10.1.8.

fowl, and wild aquatic birds. This genus includes two proposed genotypes in genogroup GI and one in GII. Similarly to the HAstV serotypes, members of some of these species can be distinguished by serology, indicating the existence of viral serotypes within avastrovirus genotypes.[186,189]

Because the AstV nomenclature is currently in flux and has yet to assign a classification for all strains discussed in this chapter, host species and commonly used names will be used as references.

VIRION STRUCTURE AND COMPOSITION

Ultrastructural analysis of HAstVs propagated in cell culture by EM revealed icosahedral particles of 41 nm, with spikes protruding from the surface.[168] However, the star-like form of the particles was observed only after alkaline treatment. More recent studies by cryo-EM and image processing of immature and mature (infectious) HAstV particles not only confirmed the spiked icosahedral structure of virions[49] but also noted

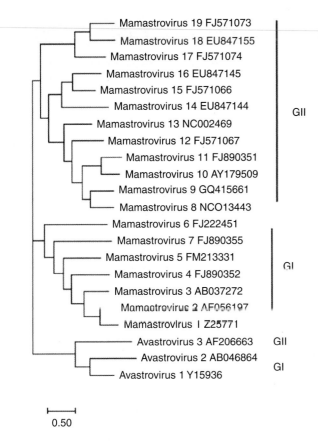

0.50

FIGURE 3.3 The *Astroviridae* family includes two genera with two genogroups each. Virus genotypes are classified based on the ORF2 amino acid sequence distances. (Classification proposed by the Astroviruses Study Group, 9th Report ICTV, 2010.)

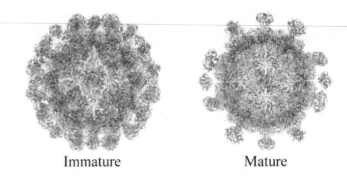

FIGURE 3.4 Three-dimensional reconstruction of HAstV. Immature and mature virus models made by fitting core and spike crystal structures into the cryo-electron microscopy. Models are colored according to structural domains: inner core (*purple*), outer core (*yellow*), and spike (*green*). (Courtesy of Dr. Rebecca DuBois, University of California, Santa Cruz.)

remains to be explored. In addition, it is becoming clearer that structural findings for the classical HAstV serotypes may not be generalizable to all AstV strains, as discussed in the next sections.

Nascent AstV particles are formed by its 90-kd capsid protein surrounding the viral genome.[141] Extracellular particles released from HAstV-infected cells are formed by protein VP70, which results from the intracellular processing of VP90. In cell culture, HAstV particles obtained after trypsin treatment consist of three proteins in the range of 32 to 34, 27 to 29, and 25 to 26 kd, with the last two proteins overlapping in sequence.[16,139] More recently, it was shown that fully infectious virions that undergo complete proteolytic processing consist of just two proteins: VP34 and VP27.[3] However, the composition of mature virions is highly dependent on the virus strain. For example, a porcine-infecting AstV was shown to contain five distinguishable proteins,[179] whereas an ovine-infecting AstV was found to have only two 33-kd proteins.[81] Moreover, the human-infecting strains VA1, MLB1, and MLB2 do not require trypsin treatment for infectivity.[91,198] Thus, there is likely considerable heterogeneity in virion structure and composition within this virus family.

GENOME STRUCTURE AND ORGANIZATION

AstVs have a positive-sense, polyadenylated ssRNA genome that varies in length from approximately 6 to 8 kilobases (kb), depending on the isolate (Fig. 3.5). The RNA extracted from

remarkable differences between the two types of particles, high lighting a maturation process. The immature virus, 46 nm in diameter, contains 180 copies of a single protein of 70 kd (VP70) arranged in a T = 3 icosahedral symmetry. Two kinds of spikes, localized at two- and fivefold vertices, can be observed in these particles. An internal protein layer forming the capsid core is almost identical in immature and mature particles, whereas the distal layer that forms the spikes shows dramatic changes after virion maturation via proteolysis (Fig. 3.4). In immature particles, the distal layer contains 90 globular spikes that are reduced to 30 spikes after proteolysis and is required for HAstV infectivity. To what extent these cleavage events mediate exposure of the receptor-binding site, promote internalization or uncoating

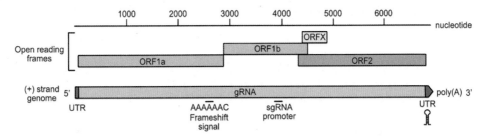

FIGURE 3.5 Genome organization of human astrovirus. The genomic RNA, approximately 6 to 8 kb, contains three main open reading frames (ORF1a, ORF1b, and ORF2). ORFX has also been described among many AstVs. Key genomic characteristics of this virus family include the frameshift signal, the sequence upstream of ORF2 that acts as promoter for synthesis of the sgRNA, and the stem–loop at the 3' end.

AstV particles, as well as RNA transcribed from a full-length genomic copy of complementary DNA (cDNA) clone, are able to initiate a productive infection in cultured cells, although with varying efficiencies.[66] Two positive-sense RNA species have been identified in AstV-infected cells: the full-length genomic RNA (gRNA) and a subgenomic RNA (sgRNA) of approximately 2.4 kb.[151]

The viral genome includes 5' and 3' untranslated regions (UTRs) and three main ORFs of variable length depending on the isolate. The two ORFs located toward the 5' end of the genome, designated ORF1a and ORF1b, encode several non-structural proteins that are involved in transcription and replication of the virus genome; however, many of their functions have not been fully characterized. ORF1a and ORF1b overlap in 10 to 148 nucleotides (nt) in the genome of mammalian viruses and between 10 and 45 nt in avian viruses. The overlapping region contains an essential signal for translation of the viral RNA polymerase encoded in ORF1b through a −1 nt frameshift mechanism at the conserved AAAAAAC motif.[96,130] The third main ORF, found at the 3' end of the genome and designated ORF2, encodes the capsid polyprotein and is expressed via a subgenomic promoter.[150]

Based on the transcription initiation site determined for the sgRNA in HAstV and other mammalian AstVs, ORF1b and ORF2 overlap by 6 to 11 nt. Conserved motifs within this region at the start of ORF2 shows partial identity with the 5' end of the gRNA, suggesting that it has an important role for the synthesis of both gRNA and sgRNA.[98] However, the existence, length, and homology of this ORF1b/ORF2 overlapping region vary in avian and mammalian viruses.[60,98,126] Importantly, analysis of recombinant AstV isolated from different host species has identified this region as a hot spot for recombination.[46,186,201]

Of note, the terminal end of ORF2 and the adjacent 3'-UTR are highly conserved among many AstVs. The sequence of this region and predicted secondary structure fit a stem–loop II-like motif that is also found in members of other RNA virus families, including *Coronaviridae* and *Caliciviridae*,[95,126,149] suggesting that it is relevant for AstV genome replication. However, exceptions exist, and the MLB clade of viruses lacks this conserved region of RNA secondary structure in the 3'-UTR.[95,126] *In silico* analyses have identified putative host protein binding at conserved sequence motifs at both the 5' and 3' UTRs that appear to be involved with replication,[45] including a polypyrimidine tract–binding protein, which was confirmed experimentally *in vitro*.[53]

ORF1a and ORF1b

The polypeptide encoded by ORF1a (nsp1a) can range from 787 to 1,240 amino acids (aa) in length in avian and mammalian viruses. Five to six helical transmembrane motifs have been identified at the amino terminus followed by a viral serine protease (Pro)[98] (Fig. 3.6), which has features consistent with trypsin-like proteases.[185] Two predicted coiled-coil structures are present in nsp1a, one just upstream of the first helical transmembrane motif and the second one downstream of Pro, suggesting that some protein products of nsp1a form oligomers.[98] A viral protein genome–linked (VPg) encoded downstream of Pro was first predicted based on its similarity with the VPg of caliciviruses,[4] and its synthesis later confirmed to be essential for infectivity.[61] Finally, a hypervariable region (HVR) located downstream of

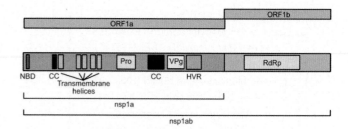

FIGURE 3.6 Nonstructural proteins predicted encoded by ORF1a and ORF1b. Polyproteins nsp1a and nsp1ab are translated from ORF1a and ORF1a/b. NBD, nucleotide-binding domain; CC, coiled-coil; Pro, viral protease; VPg, viral protein genome–linked; HVR, hypervariable region; RdRp, RNA-dependent RNA polymerase.

the VPg contains insertion/deletions that contribute to the variation of ORF1a length and is involved in replication efficiency of HAstV,[75] including adaptation to cultured cells.[206]

The polypeptide nsp1a/b translated via a frameshift mechanism at the junction of ORF1a/ORF1b produces a polypeptide of 515 to 539 aa that encodes an RdRp, which is similar to the RdRp of picornaviruses, caliciviruses, and certain plant viruses.[4,96]

Regions that could encode an RNA helicase have not been identified in the AstV genome.[96] The absence of an RNA helicase domain is unusual for a positive-strand RNA virus with a genome longer than 6 kb.[96,99] While the amino terminus of nsp1a contains a predicted nucleoside-binding domain (NBD) with similar features of a nucleoside triphosphate–binding motif in some helicases,[4] it lacks other motifs, such as the substrate-binding and hydrolysis domains present in these enzymes.[99] Thus, it is likely that AstVs utilize a host helicase to promote its replication cycle, and in support of this idea, a recent study showed that knockdown of the host helicase DDX23 reduces replication efficiency.[154]

ORF2

The largest sequence variability in the AstV genome is found in ORF2, which codes for the viral capsid. This polyprotein varies from 672 to 851 aa in length depending on the isolate. The N-terminal half of the protein forms the capsid core of the particle,[110] which is conserved among AstVs,[97,203] since it is thought to interact with the gRNA within the virion.[67,214] The C-terminal half of the protein contains the spike domain, which is predicted to participate in the early binding interactions of the virus with the host cell.[110] The spike domain shows considerable genetic heterogeneity among AstVs isolated from different host species and also defines the eight HAstV serotypes. High-resolution structures obtained by x-ray crystallography have shown that the HAstV capsid core (residues 80 to 411 of HAstV serotype 1) forms two linear subdomains consisting of a jelly-roll β-barrel inner core and a squashed β-barrel outer core that contains multiple trypsin cleavage sites[12,194,214] (Fig. 3.7). The HAstV spike domain (residues 430 to 648) in VP25 and VP27 forms the globular spikes that consist of dimeric structures containing a three-layered β-sandwich fold.[12,48,214] The structure of an avian AstV capsid spike has also been resolved and has demonstrated significant structural divergence compared to HAstV.[51]

ORFX

An alternative ORF (named ORFX) of 91 to 122 codons overlapping ORF2 in a +1 reading frame has been described in

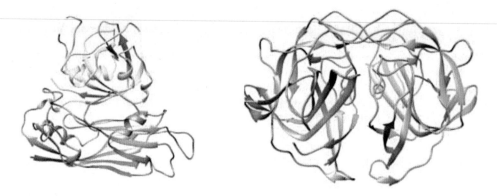

FIGURE 3.7 Crystal structures of the HAstV capsid core and spike domains. Dimeric spike domain. Models are colored according to structural domains: inner core (*purple*), outer core (*yellow*), and spike (*green*). (Courtesy of Dr. Rebecca DuBois, University of California, Santa Cruz.)

many mammalian AstVs.[50,58,124] Its start site, located 41 to 50 nt downstream of the ORF2 AUG, is placed in a better Kozak sequence than that of ORF2 and is translated through a leaky scanning mechanism. The precise mechanism and oligomeric state of the encoded protein, XP, is currently unknown, but it has been shown to play a functional role in virion assembly and/or release.[124] Comparative genomic analysis indicates that this alternative ORF is present in GI mamastroviruses (including all HAstV serotypes and MLB viruses), whereas it is typically absent in GII mamastroviruses (including VA viruses).[124] Instead, GII viruses have a predicted ORFY in the −1 frame and are thought to be accessed via a ribosomal frameshift.[124] Based on these differences in the phylogenetic topology of mamastroviruses, it is possible that these alternative ORFs evolved independently and therefore could perform different functions. It is notable that because ORFX overlaps ORF2 in a dispensable region of the capsid,[194] it represents a region of flexibility, which could support its independent evolutionary history.

STAGES OF REPLICATION

Studies directed toward understanding the early interactions of AstVs with their host cells have been limited and have primarily focused on HAstV serotypes 1, 2, and 8; however, more recent studies have extended our understanding to novel human-infecting viruses that have shown a much more delayed replication cycle in comparison to the typical 24-hour cycle for HAstV.[79,91,198] Thus, a general view of the replication cycle can be depicted (Fig. 3.8), although it is unclear whether the steps or timing outlined here can be ascribed to all AstVs or even to all human-infecting AstVs.

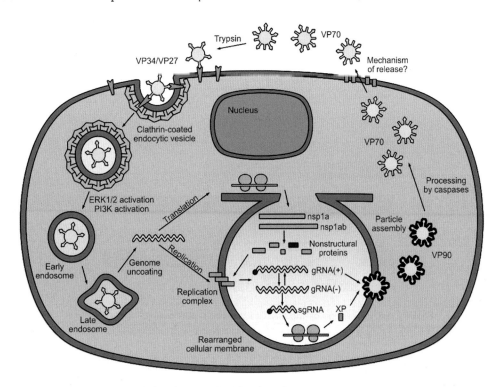

FIGURE 3.8 Replication cycle of HAstV. See details in the text.

Attachment and Entry

Cell receptor molecules for AstVs have not been identified. Since different human-infecting strains show distinct tropism in cultured cells,[24,91,93,198] it is likely that their initial binding interactions are different. For example, the commonly used human adenocarcinoma cell line, Caco-2, supports the replication of all HAstV serotypes and VA1 but is not permissive to MLB1 or MLB2.[24,91,198] Structural analysis of the HAstV capsid protein has identified a putative receptor binding site on the highly variable spike domain[48] and is supported by the fact that antibodies that bind region can block virus infectivity in Caco-2 cells.[13,19] Motifs within the spike have also been predicted to bind to oligosaccharide moieties[48,51]; however, specific binding partners have not yet been identified. What is increasingly clear for HAstV serotypes is that infectivity is greatly enhanced (3 to 5 logs) and largely dependent on trypsin proteolysis.[12,139,171] Because trypsin treatment of particles drastically changes its structure by pruning spike from the surface (Fig. 3.4), it is likely that this facilitates receptor interactions.

HAstV entry has been estimated to occur within a halftime of 10 minutes following inoculation,[140] and early studies showed that binding triggered endocytosis based on ultrastructural analysis and the use of endocytosis-blocking agents.[47] It was more recently shown that this endocytic pathway is clathrin dependent and that the virus uses early to late endosomes to begin the replication cycle.[140]

Within the first 15 minutes after HAstV inoculation, the ERK1/2 signaling pathway is activated and can be triggered during virus binding and/or entry into the cell.[153] Although the mechanism for this activation is unknown, it is also triggered after VA1 infection but not until 30 minutes postinoculation.[79] Accordingly, for both HAstV and VA1, ERK1/2 activation appears to be required to establish a productive infection, since inhibitors of this kinase significantly reduced virus yield. The early phosphoinositide 3-kinase pathway activation is also important for the HAstV replication, but the trigger and downstream signaling cascade is currently undefined.[190]

Uncoating

The mechanism through which the viral genome is released from the infecting virus particle into the cytoplasm for translation, the cell site where it occurs, and the cellular and viral factors involved in this event are currently unknown, but the process of uncoating occurs within 130 minutes postinoculation.[140] Host protein disulfide isomerase A4 was recently shown to be involved in HAstV uncoating and was identified by serotype-specific direct binding to the capsid spike domain,[3] indicating that there may be additional mechanisms that facilitate uncoating.

Translation

As do most cellular mRNAs, astroviral RNA contains a poly-A tail at the 3′ end but does not have a 5′ cap structure. Instead, a VPg is encoded in ORF1a,[61,96] and this protein is thought to modulate the translation of viral mRNAs by interacting with translation initiation factors, as has been described for caliciviruses.[30,43] At least 4 tyrosine residues, known for binding to ribonucleic acid, were shown to be important for HAstV replication, but the tyrosine at position 693 was found to be absolutely critical for replication to promote the covalent linkage between the VPg and viral RNA.[61]

Nonstructural Polyproteins Synthesis and Processing

After uncoating, the gRNA is translated into nonstructural proteins that are produced as polyprotein precursors and then proteolytically cleaved into smaller proteins. ORF1a directs the synthesis of nsp1a (~100 kd), whereas nsp1ab (160 kd) is translated from both ORF1a and ORF1b through a frameshift mechanism (Fig. 3.9). Both polyproteins are processed cotranslationally at their amino termini, so that the expected full-length proteins are not, or very rarely, observed in HAstV-infected cells. Information regarding processing of the nonstructural polyproteins has been obtained by *in vitro* translation, transient expression of cDNA clones, and analysis of HAstV-infected cells, using antibodies to different regions of nsp1a and nsp1ab.[65,68,142,207] No specific processing of nsp1a and nsp1ab was observed by *in vitro* translation of cDNA-derived transcripts,[68] indicating a requirement for cellular factors.

The processing of nsp1a occurs through iterative cleavage steps, including intermediate proteins, that ultimately generate at least five products ranging in size from 74 to 5.5 kd.[65,74,102,142,207]

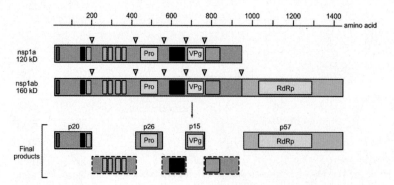

FIGURE 3.9 Processing of the HAstV nonstructural proteins. Nsp1a and nsp1ab are processed by cellular and viral proteases, with cleavage sites noted (*gray arrow heads*). The N terminus is cleaved by a cellular protease, whereas the others are thought to be mediated by Pro cleavage and are supported by indirect evidence of the observed final products, some of which remain unconfirmed and/or have uncharacterized functions (*dotted boxes*).

These include the viral Pro, which contains a basic S1 pocket that cleaves acidic residues (Glu and Asp) at position P1[185] and also the VPg, which aids in translation of the nonstructural and structural proteins as mentioned above. A 20-kd protein from the N terminus of nsp1a has been described as the sole product generated by cleavage from a cellular protease,[65] as it is only produced by *in vitro* translation in the presence of microsomes.[138] With exception of this cleavage event, all other processing of nsp1a and nsp1ab polyproteins are believed to depend on the Pro, and sites at residues 410 and 655 of nsp1a have been confirmed experimentally.[65] The other nsp1a products, including the HVR downstream of the VPg described earlier, likely serve other functions that have yet to be defined.

Translation of the RdRp (~57 kd) occurs through a −1 frameshift mechanism in the overlapping region between ORF1a and ORF1b.[142] The signal that modulates this event has two key features conserved among all astroviruses: a heptameric sequence (AAAAAAC) and the potential to form a downstream stem–loop structure.[96,130]

Structural Polyprotein Synthesis and Processing

The structural proteins of HAstV encoded in ORF2 are synthesized from the sgRNA as a polyprotein precursor of 87 to 90 kd (VP90) (Fig. 3.10). VP90 is then intracellularly cleaved at Asp-657 to yield VP70[10] through intermediates of 75 to 85 kd,[141] whose biological relevance, if any, is not known. Processing of VP90 to VP70 is carried out by cellular enzymes (caspases) that are involved in apoptotic processes.[102] Caspase activity is triggered during infection by an unknown mechanism, although nsp1a has been implicated.[10,73] Pro may also be a likely candidate since it can cleave Asp residues[185] and therefore could activate procaspases. The caspase recognition motifs present at the carboxy-terminal region of VP90 are conserved among AstV

strains, but it is likely that different caspases can be involved in the cleavage of VP90 since the motifs vary among isolates. While activity of initiator (caspase-8, -9, and -4) and executioner (caspase-3 and -7) caspases is clearly detected at 12 hours postinfection (hpi),[10] caspase-3 and caspase-9 seem particularly efficient at processing VP90. Of note, both VP90 and VP70 can assemble into viral particles.[10,138] Extracellular particles formed by VP70 are weakly infectious, but its infectivity is strongly enhanced by treatment with trypsin,[12,139] which is present in the intestinal lumen. It has even been shown that VP90-assembled particles generated in the presence of caspase inhibitors can be rendered infectious by trypsin treatment.[141] VP70 contains cleavage sites that yield VP41 (the N-terminal product) and VP28 (the C-terminal product) polypeptides. VP41 is subsequently cleaved at its carboxy terminus to yield VP34, which forms the capsid core. A single-point mutation in VP34 (Thr-227 to Ala or Ser) can block the production of nascent HAstV, but the precise mechanism is not defined.[135] VP28 is cleaved to the final products VP27 and VP25 that share their carboxy termini and form the spikes of the virion.[139] More recently, it was shown that fully matured, infectious HAstV particles actually lack VP25.[3] Thus, the final mature virion is composed of VP34 and VP27. Structural information on other human-infecting viruses from the VA and MLB clades as well as other mammalian AstVs remain to be determined, but it is notable that the maturation process via trypsin proteolysis may not play an essential role.

Transcription/Replication

Astrovirus RNA synthesis has not been well-studied. In general, the gRNA is first used as a template to synthesize a full-length negative-sense RNA (gRNA(−)) which in turn is used as a template to produce both the full-length gRNA and the sgRNA.

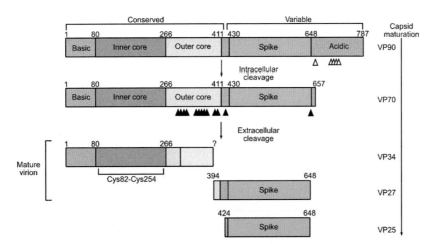

FIGURE 3.10 The HAstV structural protein VP90 domain structure and proteolytic processing. The primary ORF2 product, VP90, contains two domains that can be distinguished by their degree of conservation: the N-terminal domain is highly conserved and forms the core of the capsid; the hypervariable C-terminal domain forms the spikes of the virus particle. VP90 contains basic and acidic regions that are highly conserved. The primary product of ORF2 is sequentially processed at its carboxy terminus by caspases (*open arrow heads*) to generate VP70, the main protein present in extracellular particles. These particles are processed by trypsin (*closed arrow heads*) to generate protein intermediates and then the final products VP34, VP27, and VP25. Virion maturation is complete after VP25 disassociates from the particle.

These double-stranded RNA molecules can be detected by immunofluorescent staining by 6 hpi in HAstV-infected and 12 hpi in VA1-infected cells.[79,80] Nascent gRNA and sgRNA can be detected by PCR at 8 hpi, indicating that at this time gRNA(−) is already synthesized. The gRNA(−) can start to be detected at 9 hpi, and it accumulates to 0.7% to 4% of gRNA.[90] Similar to caliciviruses, the viral polymerase recognizes a cis-element that acts as a promoter on gRNA(−) to synthesize the sgRNA, which in the case of HAstV can reach 5- to 10-fold higher molar abundance than the full-length gRNA.[151]

Synthesis of gRNA(−) and accumulation of gRNA require protein synthesis but not cellular DNA transcription.[90] Pro, VPg, RdRp, VP90, gRNA(−), and viral particles have all been found to be associated with internal cell membranes.[62,74,138] This suggests that RNA replication and the first steps of morphogenesis are carried out associated with the observed membranous structures that probably derive from the ER[62] based on their localization[74] and the predicted hydrophobic transmembrane helixes in nsp1a may contribute to the targeting of replication complexes to these membranes. It is likely that rearrangement of internal membranes is induced by AstV infection, and this has been observed in the infected intestinal epithelial cells of lambs.[70]

Assembly and Release

The expression of ORF2 in cultured cells using recombinant vaccinia virus[42] or baculovirus[28] as vectors leads to the assembly of virus-like particles, indicating that the encoded protein is able to self-assemble in the absence of gRNA. However, these particles were unstable and show atypical morphology when purified, indicating a defective assembly.[28,152] Consistent with these data, virus assembly tolerates some deletion or changes in the 30 N-terminal basic amino acids of VP90/VP70, which are thought to interact with the gRNA in the particles.[67]

Assembly likely takes place within the same proximity of replication, but VP90-containing particles can also be detected in the cytosol.[138] After their initial assembly, viral particles are thought to separate from the membrane-associated structures, exposing their carboxy termini, which would then undergo caspase cleavage.[138] Proteolytic processing by caspases of VP90 to yield VP70 is required for cell egress of the virus, as caspase inhibitors can block this step, whereas proapoptotic factors, such as TRAIL, can promote it.[141] In addition to its role in cleaving VP90 to VP70, the activity of caspase-3 is required for efficient viral egress.[10] Despite caspase-3 activations and apoptotic markers detected at 12 hpi, cell death is typically not observed even at high multiplicities of infection.[10] A nonlytic mechanism appears to be involved in the release of HAstV and also for VA1 and MLB strains.[79,91,198] In support of this, XP, the viroporin coded by ORFX in a subset of mammalian AstVs, can mediate virion formation and/or release.[124] It remains to be seen whether XP does so through ion channel activity or if it has a role in trafficking of nascent particles from the ER to the trans-Golgi network to the plasma membrane, much like the Matrix-2 protein encoded by influenza viruses or Viral Protein U encoded by human immunodeficiency virus-1.[124] It was also recently described that a murine-infecting AstV may exit the cell through a nonlytic mechanism via the secretory pathway within goblet cells, the main epithelial cells that produce the intestinal mucous barrier, as perturbations in mucous production led to a decrease in virus replication.[38] However, it is likely

that AstVs use more than one mechanism to exit the cell, as a cytopathic effect has been observed upon infection with porcine[179] and chicken-infecting AstV strains.[14]

PATHOGENESIS AND PATHOLOGY

Entry Into the Host and Primary Site of Replication

As enteric pathogens, AstVs can transmit via the fecal–oral route, which was originally demonstrated by experimental inoculation of human volunteers with HAstV.[115,144] The virus can also transmit through fomites and contaminated food or water.[2,164] In the case of avian viruses, transmission occurs through the fecal–oral route, but it has also been proposed to occur by vertical transmission.[123,192] As discussed in greater detail in the following sections, extra-gastrointestinal disease associated with AstVs is becoming increasingly appreciated and may indicate alternate routes of infection and sites of replication.

Cell and Tissue Tropism

Mammalian AstVs primarily infect epithelial cells of the intestinal tract. Much of what we understand about the tissue tropism of human-infecting AstVs comes from a handful of case reports, *in vitro* models, and more recently, the use of epithelial only cultures derived from human intestinal epithelial crypt cells, known as enteroid and colonoids based on whether they are derived from the small intestine or colon, respectively. In 2004, a biopsy was obtained from an immunocompromised child with persistent diarrhea, which revealed HAstV present in the small intestine and within mature epithelial cells near the villus tips in the jejunum and duodenum but not in the stomach[175] (Fig. 3.11). A recent study in enteroids and colonoids demonstrated a multicellular tropism for VA1, with the highest proportion of infected cells identified among mature enterocytes, goblet cells, and CD44+ progenitor cells.[106] HAstV and MLB1 could also be propagated in enteroid and colonoid

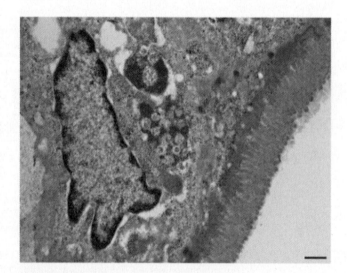

FIGURE 3.11 Electron micrograph of a jejunal enterocyte demonstrating cytoplasmic paracrystalline viral arrays of HAstV. Bar = 500 nm. (Courtesy of Glenn Anderson, Great Ormond Street Hospital for Children.)

cultures, although their specific cell tropisms remain undefined in these models. The only immortalized cell line identified thus far that is capable of propagating HAstV, VA, and MLB viruses are A549 cells, which were derived from human alveolar basal epithelial adenocarcinoma cells.[24,91,198] Consistent across these *in vitro* models is the lack of cell death and inflammation following infection with all human-infecting AstVs,[77,79,91,133,198] which was also observed in the biopsy sample from the immunocompromised child with persistent diarrhea.[175] The precise mechanism driving acute gastroenteritis after infection remains unclear. One potential mechanism may come from the ability of the HAstV capsid to increase the permeability of Caco-2 cells grown in a monolayer, disrupt the actin cytoskeleton, and reorganize occludin, a tight junction protein.[152] However, it was recently shown that VA1 inoculation does not disrupt barrier permeability or reorganize occludin in Caco-2 cells.[79] Thus, there may be distinct mechanism(s) of disease for human-infecting AstVs.

The spectrum of human enteric AstV disease is mirrored in other host species, ranging from nonpathogenic infections to severe gastroenteritis. Murine-infecting AstVs were discovered in research and commercial animal housing facilities across the globe[54,157] and were established as a small animal model of asymptomatic infection since animals do not exhibit signs of gastroenteritis.[33,40] Even in infected animals deficient in innate and adaptive immune responses, there is a lack of clinical disease despite detectable virus in multiple organs.[213] Like HAstV, the virus selectively infects the mouse small intestine and has shown a propensity for goblet cells in wild-type C56BL/6 animals (Fig. 3.12A) and both goblet cells and enterocytes in immunodeficient *Rag2^-/-Il2rg^-/-* animals that lack B, T, and NK cells.[38,40,86] Using single-cell transcriptional profiling, it was discovered that only a subset of goblet cells were infected in wild-type mice.[38] This subset included goblet cells that were actively secreting mucus. Consistent with these findings, murine enteroids grown as two-dimensional monolayers support AstV replication (Fig. 3.12B) and differentiated enteroids with an air–liquid interface produce even higher amounts of virus,[86] highlighting a propensity for actively secreting cells.[205]

Studies of other mamastroviruses indicate that ovine- and bovine-infecting AstV may have an expanded tropism beyond epithelial cells, including subepithelial cells[184] as well as M cells of the small intestine.[210] Infections of gnotobiotic lambs with ovine-infecting AstVs lead to diarrhea, transient villus atrophy, and crypt hypertrophy,[70,184] but the data are more mixed for bovine-infecting AstVs, and the lack of disease observed following experimental infection of gnotobiotic calves has led a subset of these viruses to be deemed nonpathogenic,[210] whereas others have been associated with enteritis.[131]

Avian AstVs primarily replicate in epithelial cells of the gut, but extra-gastrointestinal spread in the kidney, pancreas, lymphoid organs, and liver can lead to more severe diseases.[15,60,188] Turkey-infecting AstVs isolated from birds with poult enteritis mortality syndrome, characterized by enteritis, growth depression, and high mortality rates, have been used as a model to study AstV pathogenesis using turkey poults.[15,104] Like mammalian hosts, there are no drastic morphologic changes or cell death resulting from infection in poults. Instead, F-actin redistribution at the apical region of jejunum tight junctions, along with defects in Na+ absorption and changes in expression of sodium/hydrogen exchangers are thought to cause a secretory diarrhea.[137,138] Similar to HAstV, the capsid protein of turkey-infecting AstV was also shown to induce diarrhea, indicating a shared mechanism of disease.[137]

Since 2010, mammalian AstVs have been increasingly identified in cases of central nervous system (CNS) disease, highlighting a potential new site of replication and distinct pathogenesis for certain strains. Eleven cases of AstV CNS disease have been identified thus far in humans,[25,36,59,109,125,155,165,172,208,211] with the majority occurring in immunocompromised patients. While VA1, MLB1, MLB2, and HAstV serotypes 1 and 4 have been implicated as causative agents, VA1 was identified in five of these cases, indicating a potential propensity for the CNS. Postmortem analyses of brain tissue have indicated virus localized in astrocytes[165] and neurons[25,155,165] and are supported experimentally by the ability of VA1 to propagate in primary astrocytes and the immortalized neuronal cell line, SK-N-SH.[93] CNS disease has also been identified in cattle, sheep, muskox, alpaca, swine, and mink hosts with genetically related AstVs.[6,18,20–23,112,121,134,163,173,178] In particular, neuroinvasive bovine-infecting AstVs are frequently detected in cases of encephalitis by molecular screening, and ample histologic

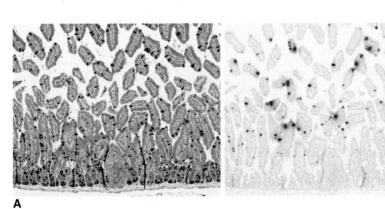
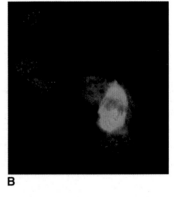

FIGURE 3.12 AstV infection in murine small intestinal goblet cells. A: Muc2 staining highlights goblet cells in *brown* (*left*) and AstV-infected cells in *red* (*right*) from a serial tissue sections collected from the duodenum of an infected C57BL/6 mouse. (Courtesy of Dr. Valerie Cortez, University of California, Santa Cruz.) **B:** AstV-infected cell (virus, *green*; nuclei, *blue*) within a two-dimensional murine enteroid culture. (Courtesy of Dr. Megan Baldridge, Washington University in St. Louis.)

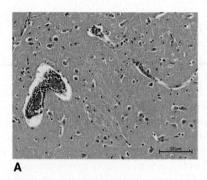 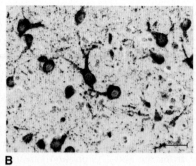 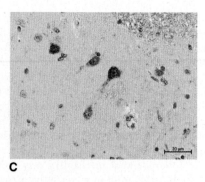

A   B   C

FIGURE 3.13 Bovine infection in the mesencephalon of a cow with neurological disease and nonsuppurative encephalitis.
A: Perivascular cuffs involving mononuclear cells are a hallmark of viral brain infection (hematoxylin and eosin stain). **B and C:** Demonstration of viral RNA by *in situ* hybridization (*brown*) and of viral antigen by immunohistochemistry (capsid protein, *red*) in neuronal cell bodies and processes. Magnifications are indicated by scale bars. (Courtesy of Nicole Wildi DVM and Dr. Torsten Seuberlich, University of Bern.)

evidence has identified viral RNA and antigen in the brain[176] (Fig. 3.13). Additionally, both mink-infecting and bovine-infecting AstVs can be transmitted to healthy animals via inoculation with infected brain homogenates, demonstrating a causal relationship. However, the mechanism by which AstVs either spread beyond the intestinal tract or if the virus enters through another anatomical site is currently unknown. Because viremia has been observed in many human cases,[35,36,85,117,172,196,211,212,216] it is possible that this would allow for extra-gastrointestinal spread. Alternatively, AstV detection in nasal and nasopharyngeal swabs[34,37,187,196,211,212] could implicate the respiratory tract as a potential portal of entry and dissemination. This is supported by the detection of a porcine-infecting AstV in the CNS, respiratory tract, and circulatory system but not feces of recently weaned pigs with neurologic disease.[20]

Immune Response

Determinants of immunity to AstV are not well understood. Symptomatic infection is primarily found in two age groups: young children and elderly patients in long-term care facilities. Indirect evidence suggests that AstV-specific antibodies could play a role in limiting infection in the host.[115] The biphasic age distribution of symptomatic infection indicates that antibody acquired early in life provides partial protection from illness through most of adult life and that immunity to AstV wanes, rendering the elderly at risk for reinfection. In wild-type mice, it was shown that animals were protected for 2 weeks following clearance of the initial infection, but reinfection could occur at 8 and 12 weeks postclearance, indicating that immunity is not long-lasting.[40] In a study of children in eight low-income sites across the globe, prior HAstV infection was associated with reduced risk of a second infection within the first 2 years of life, which also provides evidence of at least short-term protection.[169] Given the diversity of AstVs and serotype-specific immunity,[44,114,189] it is also unlikely that exposure to one strain affords much antibody protection against another. While mucosal T-cell responses remain largely unexplored, human leukocyte antigen (HLA)-restricted HAstV-specific T cells were identified in the lamina propria of duodenal biopsies collected from healthy adults,[148] but it is not known whether these cells mediate protection. In turkeys, it was also noted that total CD4+ and CD8+ T cells did not increase after infection in turkeys, but modest levels of AstV-specific antibodies were detected.[103] Together, these data highlight a role

for adaptive immune responses against these viruses, but it is unclear whether these responses are sustained and whether they offer cross-protection against different strains.

Multiple lines of evidence indicate that AstV elicits suboptimal innate immune responses, which likely precludes the induction of inflammation[33,40,104,175] and robust adaptive immunity. Type I and type III interferon (IFN) responses are made early after HAstV, VA1, MLB1, and MLB2 infections, but unlike exogenous IFN treatment, endogenous levels are unable to control viral replication.[77,106,133] Still, AstV drives sufficient levels of IFN-λ that mediate protection against murine norovirus coinfection in immunodeficient $Rag2^{-/-} Il2rg^{-/-}$ animals.[87] Collectively, these data suggest that IFNs are made in response to infection, but they are insufficient in controlling replication, and it is possible that AstVs have the means to subvert their induction and/or function. Minimal proinflammatory cytokine and chemokine production has been observed following HAstV and VA1 infection *in vitro*. However, VA1 infection induced notable exceptions, including IL-8 in Caco-2 cells and CXCL10 in primary astrocytes and neuronal cells,[79,93] indicating cell signaling that could recruit innate and adaptive immune cells. Indeed, AstV infection in turkeys can increase nitric oxide production in macrophages, and this could mediate virus inhibition.[103] It is also notable that TGF-β, an immunosuppressive cytokine,[104] is activated in turkeys following AstV infection and could play a role in dampening immune responses. The HAstV capsid protein has also been shown to block complement activation through the classical and lectin pathways by binding C1q and mannose-binding lectin, respectively.[72,78] By interfering with either the complement system and/or cytokine and chemokine induction, AstV can stymie its host from mounting a robust immune response.

Release From Host and Transmission

Following replication in the intestine, AstVs are shed in the feces. Adult human volunteer studies and systemic reviews have established the incubation period for HAstV to be approximately 3 to 4 days, although a shorter incubation period of 24 to 36 hours was noted after an outbreak at a kindergarten.[107,119,144] The highest viral shedding occurs by day 6, with levels proportional to symptom severity.[144] Large numbers of HAstV particles, equivalent to approximately 10^{10} to 10^{11} virus genomes per gram of feces, have been observed in patients with diarrhea.[75] In a recent study, HAstV, MLB, and VA virus was shed at a median range of 10^2 to 10^7 RNA copies/mL in children with and without diarrhea.[200] It remains unknown what proportion of virus shed in feces represents infectious particles and whether this differs across strains.

Virulence and Persistence

To date, there are not clear genetic demarcations that define virulent AstV strains. It is notable that CNS infections, in contrast to enteric infections, are associated with cell death and reactive gliosis.[25,155,165] Currently, it is unclear whether specific AstV strains can induce differential disease or whether within-host viral dynamics drive the dissemination of the virus outside the gut and to the brain. While the subset of CNS-associated mammalian strains that infect humans and other animal hosts cluster within the same clade, there are other divergent AstVs associated with CNS disease, indicating that both scenarios could be supported.

AstV persistence has been studied in mice and humans, with a common theme of prolonged infections identified in immunocompromised hosts. HAstV has been associated with chronic diarrhea among immunocompromised pediatric and adult patients, including reports of patients persistently shedding virus for over a year.[17,39,41,64] Similarly, it has been shown that animals deficient in adaptive and innate immune factors can become persistently infected and fail to clear the virus.[133,213] Even wild-type mice can exhibit prolonged virus shedding for 3 to 10 weeks, which is likely virus and mouse strain dependent.[33,40,133] Likewise, in a small study, persistent gastroenteritis was associated with HAstV serotype 3 in otherwise healthy children.[27] MLB1 and MLB2 were also recently found to persist in culture even after cell passaging.[198] Together, these data would suggest that there are likely viral and host factors that dictate virus persistence.

EPIDEMIOLOGY

Origin and Spread of Epidemics

The precise origins of human-infecting AstVs are unknown. The phylogenetic relationships for AstVs suggest that some human-infecting viruses, particularly VA and MLB viruses, may have originated in animals. A few lines of evidence could support bats and pigs as potential reservoirs due to the high diversity of AstVs identified within these host species.[126,218] As discussed in greater detail below, there is ample evidence of cross-species transmission of mammalian and avian AstVs.

AstV can spread person-to-person but also through contaminated food and water. Person-to-person spread is an important cause of nosocomial and community-acquired infections, including outbreaks of diarrhea in childcare settings[145,146] and sporadic outbreaks among elderly patients.[94,120] Epidemiologic data indicate that contaminated food is also a main source for HAstV infection. Large, food-borne outbreaks, affecting thousands of individuals, have occurred among school-aged children as well as adults.[159] HAstV has been found in bivalve mollusks and water from different origins.[29] The capsid affords the virus resistance against chlorination and normal disinfectants[116,174] and can therefore maintain its infectiousness for months.[1] AstV prevalence peaks during the winter months,[197] but most studies report year-round transmission.

Prevalence and Seroepidemiology

The lack of active surveillance networks for AstV and comprehensive diagnostics capable of detecting HAstV, VA, and MLB viruses[162] has led to an enormous underreporting and underdiagnosis of human infections. In addition, similar rates of infection in symptomatic and asymptomatic individuals have been observed across the world,[11,143,161,197] highlighting what is likely a massive underestimation of total viral burden. Worldwide, human-infecting AstVs have primarily been identified in young children, but the elderly and persons of all ages who are immunocompromised are also at risk for disease.[41,71,94,197] While the age distribution in the young can vary depending on several factors, such as underlying immune and nutritional status,[160] studies from high-, middle-, and low-income countries indicate that the initial exposure to AstV occurs within the first 3 years of life,[76,160] with the incidence highest in the first year of life.[63,129,156] Antibodies to HAstV serotypes have been shown to be acquired in early childhood, quickly reaching 90% by age 5.[108,111,113] Based on epidemiologic studies of AstV in humans that have primarily focused on HAstV, serotype 1 is the predominant strain found in children, but this can vary with age and geographic location.[197] In general, the positivity rate for HAstV is approximately 5% but has been reported to be over 30% in some cohorts.[197]

Less data are available for MLB and VA viruses,[26,84] but the positivity rate across cohorts is generally lower than HAstV at approximately 1.5%, although one study found over 10%.[197] They have been commonly identified in young children, although strain-specific associations with gastroenteritis are mixed.[88,101,143,181,199,217] Seroprevalence studies also indicate that exposure to MLB and VA viruses is more common than indicated by cohort studies of acute gastroenteritis, with positivity rates ranging from 65% to 100%.[26,84] This could indicate a much higher frequency of asymptomatic or nondiarrheal infections compared to HAstV.

Systemic spread has been identified among all ages and has most frequently been detected in patients with a number of immunocompromised conditions, such as cancer as well as primary immunodeficiencies.[39,41,64,71] Because this collective population is more at risk for severe disease, increased awareness and prioritization should be given to the surveillance of AstVs within this population, particularly in patients who exhibit neurologic symptoms.

Genetic Diversity of Virus

Even among RNA viruses, the *Astroviridae* family is characterized by an incredible level of diversity. For example, within the eight serotypes of HAstV, there is 64% to 84% homology within the capsid protein.[197] In comparison, there is only 23% to 24% homology between VA2-VA4, VA1-VA3, and VA5 viruses and approximately 27.5% homology within the MLB clade.[197] With new AstV strains frequently recognized, there is an ever-increasing appreciation for the diversity and broad host range of this virus family. Both the identification of recombinant strains in turkeys, guinea fowl, ducks, porcines, bovines, sea lions, and yaks as well as divergent strains observed within the same host species suggest low species barriers that would allow for interspecies transmission events.[44] As evidence of this, brown rats from urban settings were found to harbor strains with shared homology with MLB viruses,[31] and an MLB2-like virus was identified in a chimpanzee housed in a zoo.[204] Avian AstVs have even been identified in mink,[18] and there is serologic evidence of avian AstV-specific antibodies in poultry workers.[136]

CLINICAL FEATURES

Gastroenteritis caused by AstV infection primarily affects young children throughout the world but is typically milder than rotavirus infection and does not lead to significant dehydration or hospitalization.[202] Severe gastroenteritis resulting in death has been reported[180] but is thought to be extremely rare. Table 3.1 summarizes the clinical features associated with this disease; however, these features can vary depending on the population studied. For example, in a recent study of children less than 2 years of age in eight low- and middle-income countries, HAstV disease severity exceeded all enteropathogens except for rotavirus.[160] Complications such as dehydration can develop in patients with underlying gastrointestinal disease, poor nutritional status, as well as coinfections, which are incredibly common and can occur in over 30% of cases, depending on the study.[197] In a study of adult volunteers, the development of gastroenteritis was limited and dependent on the size of the inoculum.[144] Symptoms typically resolve within a few days and shedding ceases within a 2-week period, with longer durations for immunocompromised patients, as mentioned above. In other mammals, diarrhea as well as vomiting outbreaks have been observed, including in dogs,[193] cats,[122] and even cheetahs.[7]

In patients with neurologic involvement, clinical features include cognitive impairment, seizures, headache, uncontrolled dystonic movement, and limb weakness.[36,59,125,165,172,211] In contrast to AstV gastroenteritis, CNS infections have primarily been fatal.[25,36,125,155,165,211] On occasion, AstV has been associated with necrotizing enterocolitis in premature infants,[8,9] as well as other with intestinal diseases, such as intussusception[5,89] and celiac disease.[183] AstV was also found in feces from five children with nonpoliovirus acute flaccid paralysis,[100] although a direct causative association was not determined.

A spectrum of disease has also been noted in avian species infected with AstVs. Infections in chickens have been associated with stunting and acute interstitial nephritis,[177] whereas fatal hepatitis has been observed in ducklings.[69] AstV infection in turkeys is associated with diarrhea as well as poult enteritis mortality syndrome, which causes high mortality.[188] However, subclinical and mild infections have also been noted in turkeys, ducks, and chickens.[14,123,192] It is likely that there are virus strain–specific differences that contribute to this spectrum of disease. In addition, mixed infections could also play a significant role in AstV pathogenesis, especially in commercial farm settings with dense animal populations and a plethora of pathogens.[167]

DIAGNOSIS

Differential

Astrovirus should be suspected in cases of mild to severe gastrointestinal illness, particularly among young, elderly, and immunocompromised individuals. AstV infection should also be included in a differential diagnosis in immunocompromised patients with neurological symptoms.

Laboratory

After their discovery, AstVs were primarily detected by direct EM examination of negative-stained fecal specimens. Since then, technologies range from ELISA-based assays to identify virus from stool or to identify virus-specific antibodies.[162] As more sequence data on AstV genomes became available, detection techniques have since moved to molecular-based probes and RT-PCR assays. However, the high sequence variability within this virus family largely precludes the use of a universal molecular assay for all members. Instead, genotype-specific methods or multiplexed RT-PCR assays have been developed recently for diagnosis of multiple human and animal viruses.[162] These types of assays work well in the detection and screening process, but unbiased approaches are still widely used given the ever-expanding list of novel AstVs, and these technologies primarily employ endpoint PCR with degenerate primers or high-throughput metagenomic sequencing.

PREVENTION AND CONTROL

Treatment

Since the generally mild and self-limiting nature of gastroenteritis caused by AstVs, treatment is generally not needed unless a person becomes dehydrated and would need oral or intravenous fluid resuscitation. In rare instances, intravenous immunoglobulin has been successfully used to treat severely immunodeficient patients with either persistent gastroenteritis[17] or CNS disease,[59] but the data are mixed,[41] and larger studies are needed to determine its efficacy. Recent studies of HAstV and VA1 infection in Caco-2 cells have implicated that the broad-spectrum antimicrobial, nitazoxanide, as well as the antivirals, ribavirin and favipiravir, are effective against viral replication.[79,80,92] While the precise drug action is not yet known, the block for

TABLE 3.1	Clinical symptoms of HAstV infection
Diarrhea, average duration (2–3 days)	72%–100%
Abdominal pain	50%
Vomiting, average duration (1 day)	20%–70%
Fever	20%–25%
Dehydration to some degree	24%–30%
Severe dehydration	0%–5%
Hospitalization, average duration (6 days)	6%
Severity score[a] (1–20) (average)	5
Otitis	13%
Bronchiolitis	33%

[a]Twenty point scoring system based on Ruuska T, Vesikari T. Rotavirus disease in Finnish children: use of numerical scores for clinical severity of diarrhoeal episodes. *Scand J Infect Dis* 1990;22(3):259–267. Ref.[170]

Adapted with permission from Walter JE, Mitchell DK. Astrovirus infection in children. *Curr Opin Infect Dis* 2003;16(3):247–253.

nitazoxanide appears to be prior to the formation of replication complexes and was also shown to reduce virus levels in the turkey poult model.[80] These major advancements offer potential treatment options for AstV CNS disease, which are unfortunately lacking.

Vaccines

No vaccines have been developed for AstV infections in any host species; however, inoculation of the recombinant, baculovirus-expressed capsid protein into hens partially protected their offspring from gut lesions and weight depression after virus challenge.[177] The mechanism of protection remains unclear, but capsid-based antigens could be a useful approach for future vaccine design.[52]

PERSPECTIVES

The public health perception of AstVs has changed since the discovery of divergent viruses associated with severe CNS disease in humans. There is a clear need to characterize neuroInvasive AstVs in order to improve their detection and development of treatment strategies. *In vivo* and *in vitro* models will help to increase our appreciation of the broader spectrum of disease caused by AstVs, including host and viral factors that dictate disease outcomes. Expanded use of animal models for both mammalian and avian AstVs is greatly needed to study the elicitation of protective immunity and pathogenesis, including the interactions with coinfecting enteropathogens and commensal organisms. Increasing evidence indicates that interspecies transmission is common for this virus family, and additional study is needed to identify sources of emergent strains and investigate potential animal reservoirs. Aiding in this endeavor would be a refined understanding of the replication cycle, particularly the receptor and/or binding partners that initiate virus entry, as these can determine cellular and host tropisms. Additional structural and functional analyses of the viral proteins, particularly those that remain uncharacterized, will help to define this virus family. The cellular factors and mechanisms involved in viral replication are only beginning to be characterized, and future studies of host–virus interactions offer promising new directions.

ACKNOWLEDGMENTS

We apologize to our colleagues whose work has not been cited due to space constraints. We thank Dr. Rebekah Honce for graphic design, Dr. Shaoyuan Tan for phylogenetic analyses, and our colleagues for sharing unpublished images. Our laboratories acknowledge the financial support from St. Jude Children's Research Hospital Children's Infectious Defense Center, ALSAC, the Hartwell Foundation, and the National Institute of Allergy and Infectious Diseases.

REFERENCES

1. Abad FX, Pintó RM, Villena C, et al. Astrovirus survival in drinking water. *Appl Environ Microbiol* 1997;63(8):3119–3122.
2. Abad FX, Villena C, Guix S, et al. Potential role of fomites in the vehicular transmission of human astroviruses. *Appl Environ Microbiol* 2001;67(9):3904–3907.
3. Aguilar-Hernández N, López S, Arias CF. Minimal capsid composition of infectious human astrovirus. *Virology* 2018;521:58–61.
4. Al-Mutairy B, Walter JE, Pothen A, et al. Genome prediction of putative genome-linked viral protein (VPg) of astroviruses. *Virus Genes* 2005;31(1):21–30.
5. Aminu M, Ameh EA, Geyer A, et al. Role of astrovirus in intussusception in Nigerian infants. *J Trop Pediatr* 2009;55(3):192–194.
6. Arruda B, Arruda P, Hensch M, et al. Porcine Astrovirus type 3 in central nervous system of swine with polioencephalomyelitis. *Emerg Infect Dis* 2017;23(12):2097–2100.
7. Atkins A, Wellehan JFX, Childress AL, et al. Characterization of an outbreak of astroviral diarrhea in a group of cheetahs (Acinonyx jubatus). *Vet Microbiol* 2009;136(1–2):160–165.
8. Bagci S, Eis-Hübinger AM, Franz AR, et al. Detection of astrovirus in premature infants with necrotizing enterocolitis. *Pediatr Infect Dis J* 2008;27(4):347–350.
9. Bagci S, Eis-Hübinger AM, Yassin AF, et al. Clinical characteristics of viral intestinal infection in preterm and term neonates. *Eur J Clin Microbiol Infect Dis* 2010;29(9):1079–1084.
10. Banos-Lara Ma del R, Méndez E. Role of individual caspases induced by astrovirus on the processing of its structural protein and its release from the cell through a non-lytic mechanism. *Virology* 2010;401(2):322–332.
11. Barbosa G, Caetano A, Dábilla N, et al. Classical human astroviruses in symptomatic and asymptomatic children of Goiás, Brazil: positivity rates, viral loads, and molecular characterization. *J Med Virol* 2020;92(8):1053–1058.
12. Bass DM, Qiu S. Proteolytic processing of the astrovirus capsid. *J Virol* 2000;74(4):1810–1814.
13. Bass DM, Upadhyayula U. Characterization of human serotype 1 astrovirus-neutralizing epitopes. *J Virol* 1997;71(11):8666–8671.
14. Baxendale W, Mebatsion T. The isolation and characterisation of astroviruses from chickens. *Avian Pathol* 2004;33(3):364–370.
15. Behling-Kelly E, Schultz-Cherry S, Koci M, et al. Localization of astrovirus in experimentally infected turkeys as determined by in situ hybridization. *Vet Pathol* 2002;39(5):595–598.
16. Belliot G, Laveran H, Monroe SS. Capsid protein composition of reference strains and wild isolates of human astroviruses. *Virus Res* 1997;49(1):49–57.
17. Björkholm M, Celsing F, Runarsson G, et al. Successful intravenous immunoglobulin therapy for severe and persistent astrovirus gastroenteritis after fludarabine treatment in a patient with Waldenström's macroglobulinemia. *Int J Hematol* 1995;62(2):117–120.
18. Blomström A-L, Widén F, Hammer A-S, et al. Detection of a novel astrovirus in brain tissue of mink suffering from shaking mink syndrome by use of viral metagenomics. *J Clin Microbiol* 2010;48(12):4392–4396.
19. Bogdanoff WA, Campos J, Perez EI, et al. Structure of a human astrovirus capsid-antibody complex and mechanistic insights into virus neutralization. *J Virol* 2017;91(2).
20. Boros Á, Albert M, Pankovics P, et al. Outbreaks of neuroinvasive astrovirus associated with encephalomyelitis, weakness, and paralysis among weaned pigs, Hungary. *Emerg Infect Dis* 2017;23(12):1982–1993.
21. Boujon CL, Koch MC, Kauer RV, et al. Novel encephalomyelitis-associated astrovirus in a muskox (Ovibos moschatus): a surprise from the archives. *Acta Vet Scand* 2019;61(1):31.
22. Boujon CL, Koch MC, Wüthrich D, et al. Indication of cross-species transmission of astrovirus associated with encephalitis in sheep and cattle. *Emerg Infect Dis* 2017;23(9):1604–1608.
23. Bouzalas IG, Wüthrich D, Walland J, et al. Neurotropic astrovirus in cattle with nonsuppurative encephalitis in Europe. *J Clin Microbiol* 2014;52(9):3318–3324.
24. Brinker JP, Blacklow NR, Herrmann JE. Human astrovirus isolation and propagation in multiple cell lines. *Arch Virol* 2000;145(9):1847–1856.
25. Brown JR, Morfopoulou S, Hubb J, et al. Astrovirus VA1/HMO-C: an increasingly recognized neurotropic pathogen in immunocompromised patients. *Clin Infect Dis* 2015;60(6):881–888.
26. Burbelo PD, Ching KH, Esper F, et al. Serological studies confirm the novel astrovirus HMOAstV-C as a highly prevalent human infectious agent. *PLoS One* 2011;6(8):e22576.
27. Caballero S, Guix S, El-Senousy WM, et al. Persistent gastroenteritis in children infected with astrovirus: association with serotype-3 strains. *J Med Virol* 2003;71(2):245–250.
28. Caballero S, Guix S, Ribes E, et al. Structural requirements of astrovirus virus-like particles assembled in insect cells. *J Virol* 2004;78(23):13285–13292.
29. Carter MJ. Enterically infecting viruses: pathogenicity, transmission and significance for food and waterborne infection. *J Appl Microbiol* 2005;98(6):1354–1380.
30. Chaudhry Y, Nayak A, Bordeleau M-E, et al. Caliciviruses differ in their functional requirements for eIF4F components. *J Biol Chem* 2006;281(35):25315–25325.
31. Chu DKW, Chin AWH, Smith GJ, et al. Detection of novel astroviruses in urban brown rats and previously known astroviruses in humans. *J Gen Virol* 2010;91(Pt 10):2457–2462.
32. Chu DKW, Poon LLM, Guan Y, et al. Novel astroviruses in insectivorous bats. *J Virol* 2008;82(18):9107–9114.
33. Compton SR, Booth CJ, Macy JD. Murine astrovirus infection and transmission in neonatal CD1 mice. *J Am Assoc Lab Anim Sci* 2017;56(4):402–411.
34. Cordey S, Brito F, Vu D-L, et al. Astrovirus VA1 identified by next-generation sequencing in a nasopharyngeal specimen of a febrile Tanzanian child with acute respiratory disease of unknown etiology. *Emerg Microbes Infect* 2016;5(9):e99.
35. Cordey S, Hartley M-A, Keitel K, et al. Detection of novel astroviruses MLB1 and MLB2 in the sera of febrile Tanzanian children. *Emerg Microbes Infect* 2018;7(1):27.
36. Cordey S, Vu D-L, Schibler M, et al. Astrovirus MLB2, a new gastroenteric virus associated with meningitis and disseminated infection. *Emerg Infect Dis* 2016;22(5):846–853.
37. Cordey S, Zanella M-C, Wagner N, et al. Novel human astroviruses in pediatric respiratory samples: a one-year survey in a Swiss tertiary care hospital. *J Med Virol* 2018;90(11):1775–1778.
38. Cortez V, Boyd DF, Crawford JC, et al. Astrovirus infects actively secreting goblet cells and alters the gut mucus barrier. *Nat Commun* 2020;11(1):2097.
39. Cortez V, Freiden P, Gu Z, et al. Persistent infections with diverse co-circulating astroviruses in pediatric oncology patients, Memphis, Tennessee, USA. *Emerg Infect Dis* 2017;23(2):288–290.
40. Cortez V, Sharp B, Yao J, et al. Characterizing a murine model for astrovirus using viral isolates from persistently infected immunocompromised mice. *J Virol* 2019;93(13).

41. Cubitt WD, Mitchell DK, Carter MJ, et al. Application of electronmicroscopy, enzyme immunoassay, and RT-PCR to monitor an outbreak of astrovirus type 1 in a paediatric bone marrow transplant unit. *J Med Virol* 1999;57(3):313–321.
42. Dalton RM, Pastrana EP, Sánchez-Fauquier A. Vaccinia virus recombinant expressing an 87-kilodalton polyprotein that is sufficient to form astrovirus-like particles. *J Virol* 2003;77(16):9094–9098.
43. Daughenbaugh KF, Wobus CE, Hardy ME. VPg of murine norovirus binds translation initiation factors in infected cells. *Virol J* 2006;3:33.
44. De Benedictis P, Schultz-Cherry S, Burnham A, et al. Astrovirus infections in humans and animals - molecular biology, genetic diversity, and interspecies transmissions. *Infect Genet Evol* 2011;11(7):1529–1544.
45. De Nova-Ocampo M, Soliman MC, Espinosa-Hernández W, et al. Human astroviruses: in silico analysis of the untranslated region and putative binding sites of cellular proteins. *Mol Biol Rep* 2019;46(1):1413–1424.
46. Donato C, Vijaykrishna D. The broad host range and genetic diversity of mammalian and avian astroviruses. *Viruses* 2017;9(5).
47. Donelli G, Superti F, Tinari A, et al. Mechanism of astrovirus entry into Graham 293 cells. *J Med Virol* 1992;38(4):271–277.
48. Dong J, Dong L, Méndez E, et al. Crystal structure of the human astrovirus capsid spike. *Proc Natl Acad Sci U S A* 2011;108(31):12681–12686.
49. Dryden KA, Tihova M, Nowotny N, et al. Immature and mature human astrovirus: structure, conformational changes, and similarities to hepatitis E virus. *J Mol Biol* 2012;422(5):650–658.
50. Du Y, Ji C, Liu T, et al. Identification of a novel protein in porcine astrovirus that is important for virus replication. *Vet Microbiol* 2021;255:108984.
51. DuBois RM, Freiden P, Marvin S, et al. Crystal structure of the avian astrovirus capsid spike. *J Virol* 2013;87(14):7853–7863.
52. Espinosa R, López T, Bogdanoff WA, et al. Isolation of neutralizing monoclonal antibodies to human astrovirus and characterization of virus variants that escape neutralization. *J Virol* 2019;93(2).
53. Espinosa-Hernández W, Velez-Uriza D, Valdés J, et al. PTB binds to the 3′ untranslated region of the human astrovirus type 8: a possible role in viral replication. *PLoS One* 2014;9(11):e113113.
54. Farkas T, Fey B, Keller G, et al. Molecular detection of novel astroviruses in wild and laboratory mice. *Virus Genes* 2012;45(3):518–525.
55. Finkbeiner SR, Holtz LR, Jiang Y, et al. Human stool contains a previously unrecognized diversity of novel astroviruses. *Virol J* 2009;6:161.
56. Finkbeiner SR, Kirkwood CD, Wang D. Complete genome sequence of a highly divergent astrovirus isolated from a child with acute diarrhea. *Virol J* 2008;5:117.
57. Finkbeiner SR, Li Y, Ruone S, et al. Identification of a novel astrovirus (astrovirus VA1) associated with an outbreak of acute gastroenteritis. *J Virol* 2009;83(20):10836–10839.
58. Firth AE, Atkins JF. Candidates in astroviruses, seadornaviruses, cytorhabdoviruses and coronaviruses for +1 frame overlapping genes accessed by leaky scanning. *Virol J* 2010;7:17.
59. Frémond M-L, Pérot P, Muth E, et al. Next-generation sequencing for diagnosis and tailored therapy: a case report of astrovirus-associated progressive encephalitis. *J Pediatric Infect Dis Soc* 2015;4(3):e53–e57.
60. Fu Y, Pan M, Wang X, et al. Complete sequence of a duck astrovirus associated with fatal hepatitis in ducklings. *J Gen Virol* 2009;90(Pt 5):1104–1108.
61. Fuentes C, Bosch A, Pintó RM, et al. Identification of human astrovirus genome-linked protein (VPg) essential for virus infectivity. *J Virol* 2012;86(18):10070–10078.
62. Fuentes C, Guix S, Bosch A, et al. The C-terminal nsP1a protein of human astrovirus is a phosphoprotein that interacts with the viral polymerase. *J Virol* 2011;85(9):4470–4479.
63. Gabbay YB, da Luz CRNE, Costa IV, et al. Prevalence and genetic diversity of astroviruses in children with and without diarrhea in São Luís, Maranhão, Brazil. *Mem Inst Oswaldo Cruz* 2005;100(7):709–714.
64. Gallimore CI, Taylor C, Gennery AR, et al. Use of a heminested reverse transcriptase PCR assay for detection of astrovirus in environmental swabs from an outbreak of gastroenteritis in a pediatric primary immunodeficiency unit. *J Clin Microbiol* 2005;43(8):3890–3894.
65. Geigenmüller U, Chew T, Ginzton N, et al. Processing of nonstructural protein 1a of human astrovirus. *J Virol* 2002;76(4):2003–2008.
66. Geigenmüller U, Ginzton NH, Matsui SM. Construction of a genome-length cDNA clone for human astrovirus serotype 1 and synthesis of infectious RNA transcripts. *J Virol* 1997;71(2):1713–1717.
67. Geigenmüller U, Ginzton NH, Matsui SM. Studies on intracellular processing of the capsid protein of human astrovirus serotype 1 in infected cells. *J Gen Virol* 2002;83(Pt 7):1691–1695.
68. Gibson CA, Chen J, Monroe SA, et al. Expression and processing of nonstructural proteins of the human astroviruses. *Adv Exp Med Biol* 1998;440:387–391.
69. Gough RE, Collins MS, Borland E, et al. Astrovirus-like particles associated with hepatitis in ducklings. *Vet Rec* 1984;114(11):279.
70. Gray EW, Angus KW, Snodgrass DR. Ultrastructure of the small intestine in astrovirus-infected lambs. *J Gen Virol* 1980;49(1):71–82.
71. Grohmann GS, Glass RI, Pereira HG, et al. Enteric viruses and diarrhea in HIV-infected patients. Enteric opportunistic infections working group. *N Engl J Med* 1993;329(1):14–20.
72. Gronemus JQ, Hair PS, Crawford KB, et al. Potent inhibition of the classical pathway of complement by a novel C1q-binding peptide derived from the human astrovirus coat protein. *Mol Immunol* 2010;48(1–3):305–313.
73. Guix S, Bosch A, Ribes E, et al. Apoptosis in astrovirus-infected CaCo-2 cells. *Virology* 2004;319(2):249–261.
74. Guix S, Caballero S, Bosch A, et al. C-terminal nsP1a protein of human astrovirus colocalizes with the endoplasmic reticulum and viral RNA. *J Virol* 2004;78(24):13627–13636.
75. Guix S, Caballero S, Bosch A, et al. Human astrovirus C-terminal nsP1a protein is involved in RNA replication. *Virology* 2005;333(1):124–131.
76. Guix S, Caballero S, Villena C, et al. Molecular epidemiology of astrovirus infection in Barcelona, Spain. *J Clin Microbiol* 2002;40(1):133–139.
77. Guix S, Pérez-Bosque A, Miró L, et al. Type I interferon response is delayed in human astrovirus infections. *PLoS One* 2015;10(4):e0123087.
78. Hair PS, Gronemus JQ, Crawford KB, et al. Human astrovirus coat protein binds C1q and MBL and inhibits the classical and lectin pathways of complement activation. *Mol Immunol* 2010;47(4):792–798.
79. Hargest V, Davis AE, Tan S, et al. Human astroviruses: a tale of two strains. *Viruses* 2021;13(3).
80. Hargest V, Sharp B, Livingston B, et al. Astrovirus replication is inhibited by nitazoxanide in vitro and in vivo. *J Virol* 2020;94(5).
81. Herring AJ, Gray EW, Snodgrass DR. Purification and characterization of ovine astrovirus. *J Gen Virol* 1981;53(Pt 1):47–55.
82. Herrmann JE, Nowak NA, Perron-Henry DM, et al. Diagnosis of astrovirus gastroenteritis by antigen detection with monoclonal antibodies. *J Infect Dis* 1990;161(2):226–229.
83. Herrmann JE, Taylor DN, Echeverria P, et al. Astroviruses as a cause of gastroenteritis in children. *N Engl J Med* 1991;324(25):1757–1760.
84. Holtz LR, Bauer IK, Jiang H, et al. Seroepidemiology of astrovirus MLB1. *Clin Vaccine Immunol* 2014;21(6):908–911.
85. Holtz LR, Wylie KM, Sodergren E, et al. Astrovirus MLB2 viremia in febrile child. *Emerg Infect Dis* 2011;17(11):2050–2052.
86. Ingle H, Hassan E, Gawron J, et al. Murine astrovirus tropism for goblet cells and enterocytes facilitates an IFN-λ response in vivo and in enteroid cultures. *Mucosal Immunol* 2021;14:751–761.
87. Ingle H, Lee S, Ai T, et al. Viral complementation of immunodeficiency confers protection against enteric pathogens via IFN-lambda. *Nat Microbiol* 2019;4:1120–1128.
88. Jacobsen S, Höhne M, Marques AM, et al. Co-circulation of classic and novel astrovirus strains in patients with acute gastroenteritis in Germany. *J Infect* 2018;76(5):457–464.
89. Jakab F, Péterfai J, Verebély T, et al. Human astrovirus infection associated with childhood intussusception. *Pediatr Int* 2007;49(1):103–105.
90. Jang SY, Jeong WH, Kim MS, et al. Detection of replicating negative-sense RNAs in CaCo-2 cells infected with human astrovirus. *Arch Virol* 2010;155(9):1383–1389.
91. Janowski AB, Bauer IK, Holtz LR, et al. Propagation of astrovirus VA1, a neurotropic human astrovirus, in cell culture. *J Virol* 2017;91(19).
92. Janowski AB, Dudley H, Wang D. Antiviral activity of ribavirin and favipiravir against human astroviruses. *J Clin Virol* 2020;123:104247.
93. Janowski AB, Klein RS, Wang D. Differential in vitro infection of neural cells by astroviruses. *MBio* 2019;10(4).
94. Jarchow-Macdonald AA, Halley S, Chandler D, et al. First report of an astrovirus type 5 gastroenteritis outbreak in a residential elderly care home identified by sequencing. *J Clin Virol* 2015;73:115–119.
95. Jiang H, Holtz LR, Bauer I, et al. Comparison of novel MLB-clade, VA-clade and classic human astroviruses highlights constrained evolution of the classic human astrovirus nonstructural genes. *Virology* 2013;436(1):8–14.
96. Jiang B, Monroe SS, Koonin EV, et al. RNA sequence of astrovirus: distinctive genomic organization and a putative retrovirus-like ribosomal frameshifting signal that directs the viral replicase synthesis. *Proc Natl Acad Sci U S A* 1993;90(22):10539–10543.
97. Jonassen CM, Jonassen TØ, Saif YM, et al. Comparison of capsid sequences from human and animal astroviruses. *J Gen Virol* 2001;82(Pt 5):1061–1067.
98. Jonassen CM, Jonassen TØ, Sveen TM, et al. Complete genomic sequences of astroviruses from sheep and turkey: comparison with related viruses. *Virus Res* 2003;91(2):195–201.
99. Kadaré G, Haenni AL. Virus-encoded RNA helicases. *J Virol* 1997;71(4):2583–2590.
100. Kapoor A, Li L, Victoria J, et al. Multiple novel astrovirus species in human stool. *J Gen Virol* 2009;90(Pt 12):2965–2972.
101. Khamrin P, Thongprachum A, Okitsu S, et al. Multiple astrovirus MLB1, MLB2, VA2 clades, and classic human astrovirus in children with acute gastroenteritis in Japan. *J Med Virol* 2016;88(2):356–360.
102. Kiang D, Matsui SM. Proteolytic processing of a human astrovirus nonstructural protein. *J Gen Virol* 2002;83(Pt 1):25–34.
103. Koci MD, Kelley LA, Larsen D, et al. Astrovirus-induced synthesis of nitric oxide contributes to virus control during infection. *J Virol* 2004;78(3):1564–1574.
104. Koci MD, Moser LA, Kelley LA, et al. Astrovirus induces diarrhea in the absence of inflammation and cell death. *J Virol* 2003;77(21):11798–11808.
105. Koci MD, Seal BS, Schultz-Cherry S. Molecular characterization of an avian astrovirus. *J Virol* 2000;74(13):6173–6177.
106. Kolawole AO, Mirabelli C, Hill DR, et al. Astrovirus replication in human intestinal enteroids reveals multi-cellular tropism and an intricate host innate immune landscape. *PLoS Pathog* 2019;15(10):e1008057.
107. Konno T, Suzuki H, Ishida N, et al. Astrovirus-associated epidemic gastroenteritis in Japan. *J Med Virol* 1982;9(1):11–17.
108. Koopmans MP, Bijen MH, Monroe SS, et al. Age-stratified seroprevalence of neutralizing antibodies to astrovirus types 1 to 7 in humans in The Netherlands. *Clin Diagn Lab Immunol* 1998;5(1):33–37.
109. Koukou G, Niendorf S, Hornei B, et al. Human astrovirus infection associated with encephalitis in an immunocompetent child: a case report. *J Med Case Rep* 2019;13(1):341.
110. Krishna NK. Identification of structural domains involved in astrovirus capsid biology. *Viral Immunol* 2005;18(1):17–26.
111. Kriston S, Willcocks MM, Carter MJ, et al. Seroprevalence of astrovirus types 1 and 6 in London, determined using recombinant virus antigen. *Epidemiol Infect* 1996;117(1):159–164.
112. Küchler L, Rüfli I, Koch MC, et al. Astrovirus-associated polioencephalomyelitis in an alpaca. *Viruses* 2020;13(1).
113. Kurtz J, Lee T. Astrovirus gastroenteritis age distribution of antibody. *Med Microbiol Immunol* 1978;166(1–4):227–230.
114. Kurtz JB, Lee TW. Human astrovirus serotypes. *Lancet* 1984;2(8416):1405.
115. Kurtz JB, Lee TW, Craig JW, et al. Astrovirus infection in volunteers. *J Med Virol* 1979;3(3):221–230.
116. Kurtz JB, Lee TW, Parsons AJ. The action of alcohols on rotavirus, astrovirus and enterovirus. *J Hosp Infect* 1980;1(4):321–325.

117. Lau P, Cordey S, Brito F, et al. Metagenomics analysis of red blood cell and fresh-frozen plasma units. *Transfusion* 2017;57(7):1787–1800.
118. Lee TW, Kurtz JB. Serial propagation of astrovirus in tissue culture with the aid of trypsin. *J Gen Virol* 1981;57(Pt 2):421–424.
119. Lee RM, Lessler J, Lee RA, et al. Incubation periods of viral gastroenteritis: a systematic review. *BMC Infect Dis* 2013;13:446.
120. Lewis DC, Lightfoot NF, Cubitt WD, et al. Outbreaks of astrovirus type 1 and rotavirus gastroenteritis in a geriatric in-patient population. *J Hosp Infect* 1989;14(1):9–14.
121. Li L, Diab S, McGraw S, et al. Divergent astrovirus associated with neurologic disease in cattle. *Emerg Infect Dis* 2013;19(9):1385–1392.
122. Li Y, Gordon E, Idle A, et al. Astrovirus outbreak in an animal shelter associated with feline vomiting. *Front Vet Sci* 2021;8:628082.
123. Liu N, Jiang M, Wang M, et al. Isolation and detection of duck astrovirus CPH: implications for epidemiology and pathogenicity. *Avian Pathol* 2016;45(2):221–227.
124. Lulla V, Firth AE. A hidden gene in astroviruses encodes a viroporin. *Nat Commun* 2020;11(1):4070.
125. Lum SH, Turner A, Guiver M, et al. An emerging opportunistic infection: fatal astrovirus (VA1/HMO-C) encephalitis in a pediatric stem cell transplant recipient. *Transpl Infect Dis* 2016;18(6):960–964.
126. Luo Z, Roi S, Dastor M, et al. Multiple novel and prevalent astroviruses in pigs. *Vet Microbiol* 2011;149(3–4):316–323.
127. Madeley CR, Cosgrove BP. Letter: 28 nm particles in faeces in infantile gastroenteritis. *Lancet* 1975;2(7932):451–452.
128. Madeley CR, Cosgrove BP. Letter: viruses in infantile gastroenteritis. *Lancet* 1975;2(7925):124.
129. Maldonado Y, Cantwell M, Old M, et al. Population-based prevalence of symptomatic and asymptomatic astrovirus infection in rural Mayan infants. *J Infect Dis* 1998;178(2):334–339.
130. Marczinke B, Bloys AJ, Brown TD, et al. The human astrovirus RNA-dependent RNA polymerase coding region is expressed by ribosomal frameshifting. *J Virol* 1994;68(9):5588–5595.
131. Martella V, Catella C, Capozza P, et al. Identification of astroviruses in bovine and buffalo calves with enteritis. *Res Vet Sci* 2020;131:59–68.
132. Martella V, Moschidou P, Pinto P, et al. Astroviruses in rabbits. *Emerg Infect Dis* 2011;17(12):2287–2293.
133. Marvin SA, Huerta CT, Sharp B, et al. Type I interferon response limits astrovirus replication and protects against increased barrier permeability in vitro and in vivo. *J Virol* 2016;90(4):1988–1996.
134. Matias Ferreyra FS, Bradner LK, Burrough ER, et al. Polioencephalomyelitis in domestic swine associated with porcine astrovirus type 3. *Vet Pathol* 2020;57(1):82–89.
135. Matsui SM, Kiang D, Ginzton N, et al. Molecular biology of astroviruses: selected highlights. *Novartis Found Symp* 2001;238:219–233; discussion 233–236.
136. Meliopoulos VA, Kayali G, Burnham A, et al. Detection of antibodies against Turkey astrovirus in humans. *PLoS One* 2014;9(5):e96934.
137. Meliopoulos VA, Marvin SA, Freiden P, et al. Oral administration of astrovirus capsid protein is sufficient to induce acute diarrhea in vivo. *MBio* 2016;7(6).
138. Méndez E, Aguirre-Crespo G, Zavala G, et al. Association of the astrovirus structural protein VP90 with membranes plays a role in virus morphogenesis. *J Virol* 2007;81(19):10649–10658.
139. Méndez E, Fernández-Luna T, López S, et al. Proteolytic processing of a serotype 8 human astrovirus ORF2 polyprotein. *J Virol* 2002;76(16):7996–8002.
140. Méndez E, Muñoz-Yañez C, Martín CS-S, et al. Characterization of human astrovirus cell entry. *J Virol* 2014;88(5):2452–2460.
141. Méndez E, Salas-Ocampo E, Arias CF. Caspases mediate processing of the capsid precursor and cell release of human astroviruses. *J Virol* 2004;78(16):8601–8608.
142. Méndez E, Salas-Ocampo MPE, Munguía ME, et al. Protein products of the open reading frames encoding nonstructural proteins of human astrovirus serotype 8. *J Virol* 2003;77(21):11378–11384.
143. Meyer CT, Bauer IK, Antonio M, et al. Prevalence of classic, MLB-clade and VA-clade astroviruses in Kenya and the Gambia. *Virol J* 2015;12:78.
144. Midthun K, Greenberg HB, Kurtz JB, et al. Characterization and seroepidemiology of a type 5 astrovirus associated with an outbreak of gastroenteritis in Marin County, California. *J Clin Microbiol* 1993;31(4):955–962.
145. Mitchell DK, Matson DO, Jiang X, et al. Molecular epidemiology of childhood astrovirus infection in child care centers. *J Infect Dis* 1999;180(2):514–517.
146. Mitchell DK, Van R, Morrow AL, et al. Outbreaks of astrovirus gastroenteritis in day care centers. *J Pediatr* 1993;123(5):725–732.
147. Mittelholzer C, Hedlund K-O, Englund L, et al. Molecular characterization of a novel astrovirus associated with disease in mink. *J Gen Virol* 2003;84(Pt 11):3087–3094.
148. Molberg O, Nilsen EM, Sollid LM, et al. CD4+ T cells with specific reactivity against astrovirus isolated from normal human small intestine. *Gastroenterology* 1998;114(1):115–122.
149. Monceyron C, Grinde B, Jonassen TO. Molecular characterisation of the 3′-end of the astrovirus genome. *Arch Virol* 1997;142(4):699–706.
150. Monroe SS, Jiang B, Stine SE, et al. Subgenomic RNA sequence of human astrovirus supports classification of Astroviridae as a new family of RNA viruses. *J Virol* 1993;67(6):3611–3614.
151. Monroe SS, Stine SE, Gorelkin L, et al. Temporal synthesis of proteins and RNAs during human astrovirus infection of cultured cells. *J Virol* 1991;65(2):641–648.
152. Moser LA, Carter M, Schultz-Cherry S. Astrovirus increases epithelial barrier permeability independently of viral replication. *J Virol* 2007;81(21):11937–11945.
153. Moser LA, Schultz-Cherry S. Suppression of astrovirus replication by an ERK1/2 inhibitor. *J Virol* 2008;82(15):7475–7482.
154. Murillo A, Vera-Estrella R, Barkla BJ, et al. Identification of host cell factors associated with astrovirus replication in caco-2 cells. *J Virol* 2015;89(20):10359–10370.
155. Naccache SN, Peggs KS, Mattes FM, et al. Diagnosis of neuroinvasive astrovirus infection in an immunocompromised adult with encephalitis by unbiased next-generation sequencing. *Clin Infect Dis* 2015;60(6):919–923.
156. Naficy AB, Rao MR, Holmes JL, et al. Astrovirus diarrhea in Egyptian children. *J Infect Dis* 2000;182(3):685–690.
157. Ng TFF, Kondov NO, Hayashimoto N, et al. Identification of an astrovirus commonly infecting laboratory mice in the US and Japan. *PLoS One* 2013;8(6):e66937.
158. Nighot PK, Moeser A, Ali RA, et al. Astrovirus infection induces sodium malabsorption and redistributes sodium hydrogen exchanger expression. *Virology* 2010;401(2):146–154.
159. Oishi I, Yamazaki K, Kimoto T, et al. A large outbreak of acute gastroenteritis associated with astrovirus among students and teachers in Osaka, Japan. *J Infect Dis* 1994;170(2):439–443.
160. Olortegui MP, Rouhani S, Yori PP, et al. Astrovirus infection and diarrhea in 8 countries. *Pediatrics* 2018;141(1).
161. Pennap G, Pager CT, Peenze I, et al. Epidemiology of astrovirus infection in Zaria, Nigeria. *J Trop Pediatr* 2002;48(2):98–101.
162. Pérot P, Lecuit M, Eloit M. Astrovirus diagnostics. *Viruses* 2017;9(1).
163. Pfaff F, Schlottau K, Scholes S, et al. A novel astrovirus associated with encephalitis and ganglionitis in domestic sheep. *Transbound Emerg Dis* 2017;64(3):677–682.
164. Pinto RM, Abad FX, Gajardo R, et al. Detection of infectious astroviruses in water. *Appl Environ Microbiol* 1996;62(5):1811–1813.
165. Quan PL, Wagner TA, Briese T, et al. Astrovirus encephalitis in boy with X-linked agammaglobulinemia. *Emerg Infect Dis* 2010;16(6):918–925.
166. Reuter G, Pankovics P, Delwart E, et al. Identification of a novel astrovirus in domestic sheep in Hungary. *Arch Virol* 2012;157(2):323–327.
167. Reynolds DL, Saif YM, Theil KW. A survey of enteric viruses of turkey poults. *Avian Dis* 1987;31(1):89–98.
168. Risco C, Carrascosa JL, Pedregosa AM, et al. Ultrastructure of human astrovirus serotype 2. *J Gen Virol* 1995;76(Pt 8):2075–2080.
169. Rogawski McQuade ET, Liu J, Kang G, et al. Protection from natural immunity against enteric infections and etiology-specific diarrhea in a longitudinal birth cohort. *J Infect Dis* 2020;222(11):1858–1868.
170. Ruuska T, Vesikari T. Rotavirus disease in Finnish children: use of numerical scores for clinical severity of diarrhoeal episodes. *Scand J Infect Dis* 1990;22(3):259–267.
171. Sanchez-Fauquier A, Carrascosa AL, Carrascosa JL, et al. Characterization of a human astrovirus serotype 2 structural protein (VP26) that contains an epitope involved in virus neutralization. *Virology* 1994;201(2):312–320.
172. Sato M, Kuroda M, Kasai M, et al. Acute encephalopathy in an immunocompromised boy with astrovirus-MLB1 infection detected by next generation sequencing. *J Clin Virol* 2016;78:66–70.
173. Schlottau K, Schulze C, Bilk S, et al. Detection of a novel bovine astrovirus in a cow with encephalitis. *Transbound Emerg Dis* 2016;63(3):253–259.
174. Schultz-Cherry S, King DJ, Koci MD. Inactivation of an astrovirus associated with poult enteritis mortality syndrome. *Avian Dis* 2001;45(1):76–82.
175. Sebire NJ, Malone M, Shah N, et al. Pathology of astrovirus associated diarrhoea in a paediatric bone marrow transplant recipient. *J Clin Pathol* 2004;57(9):1001–1003.
176. Selimovic-Hamza S, Boujon CL, Hilbe M, et al. Frequency and pathological phenotype of bovine astrovirus CH13/NeuroS1 infection in neurologically-diseased cattle: towards assessment of causality. *Viruses* 2017;9(1).
177. Sellers H, Linneman E, Icard AH, et al. A purified recombinant baculovirus expressed capsid protein of a new astrovirus provides partial protection to runting-stunting syndrome in chickens. *Vaccine* 2010;28(5):1253–1263.
178. Seuberlich T, Wüthrich D, Selimovic-Hamza S, et al. Identification of a second encephalitis-associated astrovirus in cattle. *Emerg Microbes Infect* 2016;5:e71.
179. Shimizu M, Shirai J, Narita M, et al. Cytopathic astrovirus isolated from porcine acute gastroenteritis in an established cell line derived from porcine embryonic kidney. *J Clin Microbiol* 1990;28(2):201–206.
180. Singh PB, Sreenivasan MA, Pavri KM. Viruses in acute gastroenteritis in children in Pune, India. *Epidemiol Infect* 1989;102(2):345–353.
181. Siqueira JAM, de Souza Oliveira D, de Carvalho TCN, et al. Astrovirus infection in hospitalized children: molecular, clinical and epidemiological features. *J Clin Virol* 2017;94:79–85.
182. Smits SL, van Leeuwen M, Kuiken T, et al. Identification and characterization of deer astroviruses. *J Gen Virol* 2010;91(Pt 11):2719–2722.
183. Smits SL, van Leeuwen M, van der Eijk AA, et al. Human astrovirus infection in a patient with new-onset celiac disease. *J Clin Microbiol* 2010;48(9):3416–3418.
184. Snodgrass DR, Angus KW, Gray EW, et al. Pathogenesis of diarrhoea caused by astrovirus infections in lambs. *Arch Virol* 1979;60(3–4):217–226.
185. Speroni S, Rohayem J, Nenci S, et al. Structural and biochemical analysis of human pathogenic astrovirus serine protease at 2.0 A resolution. *J Mol Biol* 2009;387(5):1137–1152.
186. Strain E, Kelley LA, Schultz-Cherry S, et al. Genomic analysis of closely related astroviruses. *J Virol* 2008;82(10):5099–5103.
187. Taboada B, Espinoza MA, Isa P, et al. Is there still room for novel viral pathogens in pediatric respiratory tract infections? *PLoS One* 2014;9(11):e113570.
188. Tang Y, Murgia MV, Ward L, et al. Pathogenicity of turkey astroviruses in turkey embryos and poults. *Avian Dis* 2006;50(4):526–531.
189. Tang Y, Saif YM. Antigenicity of two turkey astrovirus isolates. *Avian Dis* 2004;48(4):896–901.
190. Tange S, Zhou Y, Nagakui-Noguchi Y, et al. Initiation of human astrovirus type 1 infection was blocked by inhibitors of phosphoinositide 3-kinase. *Virol J* 2013;10:153.
191. Thouvenelle ML, Haynes JS, Reynolds DL. Astrovirus infection in hatchling turkeys: histologic, morphometric, and ultrastructural findings. *Avian Dis* 1995;39(2):328–336.
192. Todd D, Wilkinson DS, Jewhurst HL, et al. A seroprevalence investigation of chicken astrovirus infections. *Avian Pathol* 2009;38(4):301–309.
193. Toffan A, Jonassen CM, De Battisti C, et al. Genetic characterization of a new astrovirus detected in dogs suffering from diarrhoea. *Vet Microbiol* 2009;139(1–2):147–152.
194. Toh Y, Harper J, Dryden KA, et al. Crystal Structure of the human astrovirus capsid protein. *J Virol* 2016;90(20):9008–9017.
195. Tse H, Chan W-M, Tsoi H-W, et al. Rediscovery and genomic characterization of bovine astroviruses. *J Gen Virol* 2011;92(Pt 8):1888–1898.
196. van der Doef HPJ, Bathoorn E, van der Linden MPM, et al. Astrovirus outbreak at a pediatric hematology and hematopoietic stem cell transplant unit despite strict hygiene rules. *Bone Marrow Transplant* 2016;51(5):747–750.

197. Vu D-L, Bosch A, Pintó RM, et al. Epidemiology of classic and novel human astrovirus: gastroenteritis and beyond. *Viruses* 2017;9(2):33.
198. Vu D-L, Bosch A, Pintó RM, et al. Human astrovirus MLB replication in vitro: persistence in extraintestinal cell lines. *J Virol* 2019;93(13).
199. Vu D-L, Sabrià A, Aregall N, et al. Novel human astroviruses: prevalence and association with common enteric viruses in undiagnosed gastroenteritis cases in Spain. *Viruses* 2019;11(7).
200. Vu D-L, Sabrià A, Aregall N, et al. A Spanish case–control study in <5 year-old children reveals the lack of association between MLB and VA astrovirus and diarrhea. *Sci Rep* 2020;10(1):1760.
201. Walter JE, Briggs J, Guerrero ML, et al. Molecular characterization of a novel recombinant strain of human astrovirus associated with gastroenteritis in children. *Arch Virol* 2001;146(12):2357–2367.
202. Walter JE, Mitchell DK. Astrovirus infection in children. *Curr Opin Infect Dis* 2003;16(3):247–253.
203. Wang QH, Kakizawa J, Wen LY, et al. Genetic analysis of the capsid region of astroviruses. *J Med Virol* 2001;64(3):245–255.
204. Wang X, Wang J, Zhou C, et al. Viral metagenomics of fecal samples from non-human primates revealed human astrovirus in a chimpanzee, China. *Gut Pathog* 2016;8:53.
205. Whitcutt MJ, Adler KB, Wu R. A biphasic chamber system for maintaining polarity of differentiation of cultured respiratory tract epithelial cells. *In Vitro Cell Dev Biol* 1988;24(5):420–428.
206. Willcocks MM, Ashton N, Kurtz JB, et al. Cell culture adaptation of astrovirus involves a deletion. *J Virol* 1994;68(9):6057–6058.
207. Willcocks MM, Boxall AS, Carter MJ. Processing and intracellular location of human astrovirus non-structural proteins. *J Gen Virol* 1999;80(Pt 10):2607–2611.
208. Wilson MR, Sample HA, Zorn KC, et al. Clinical metagenomic sequencing for diagnosis of meningitis and encephalitis. *N Engl J Med* 2019;380(24):2327–2340.
209. Woo PCY, Lau SKP, Teng JLL, et al. A novel astrovirus from dromedaries in the Middle East. *J Gen Virol* 2015;96(9):2697–2707.
210. Woode GN, Pohlenz JF, Gourley NE, et al. Astrovirus and Breda virus infections of dome cell epithelium of bovine ileum. *J Clin Microbiol* 1984;19(5):623–630.
211. Wunderli W, Meerbach A, Güngör T, et al. Astrovirus infection in hospitalized infants with severe combined immunodeficiency after allogeneic hematopoietic stem cell transplantation. *PLoS One* 2011;6(11):e27483.
212. Wylie KM, Mihindukulasuriya KA, Sodergren E, et al. Sequence analysis of the human virome in febrile and afebrile children. *PLoS One* 2012;7(6):e27735.
213. Yokoyama CC, Loh J, Zhao G, et al. Adaptive immunity restricts replication of novel murine astroviruses. *J Virol* 2012;86(22):12262–12270.
214. York RL, Yousefi PA, Bogdanoff W, et al. Structural, mechanistic, and antigenic characterization of the human astrovirus capsid. *J Virol* 2015;90(5):2254–2263.
215. Yu M, Tang Y, Guo M, et al. Characterization of a small round virus associated with the poult enteritis and mortality syndrome. *Avian Dis* 2000;44(3):600–610.
216. Zanella MC, Cordey S, Laubscher F, et al. Unmasking viral sequences by metagenomic next-generation sequencing in adult human blood samples during steroid-refractory/dependent graft-versus-host disease. *Microbiome* 2021;9(1):28.
217. Zaraket H, Abou-El-Hassan H, Kreidieh K, et al. Characterization of astrovirus-associated gastroenteritis in hospitalized children under five years of age. *Infect Genet Evol* 2017;53:94–99.
218. Zhu HC, Chu DKW, Liu W, et al. Detection of diverse astroviruses from bats in China. *J Gen Virol* 2009;90(Pt 4):883–887.

Tom C. Hobman

Introduction
Infectious Agent
  Morphology and physicochemical properties of the virion
  Biological characteristics
  Structure and organization of the genome
  Replication strategy
  Virus assembly and secretion
  RUBV persistence
  Animal models of rubella virus infection
  Antigenic composition and determinants
Epidemiology
  Incidence
  Origin and spread of epidemics
  Molecular epidemiology
Clinical Features
  Acute rubella
  Congenital rubella syndrome
Diagnosis
  Differential
  Laboratory
Prevention and Control
  Vaccines
Perspective

INTRODUCTION

Rubella virus (RUBV) is the etiologic agent of *rubella*, a mild exanthematous disease associated with low-grade fever, lymphadenopathy, and a short-lived morbilliform rash. Rubella was first described as a distinct disease in the early 1800s.[162] It was first called *Rötheln* by the German physician de Bergen,[77] leading to the common name of German measles, a milder form of the much more serious exanthem caused by the paramyxovirus, measles virus. Subsequently, in 1866, the disease name was anglicized to *rubella* by the British physician Veale 1866.[274]

A predominantly a childhood disease, rubella is still endemic in many parts of the world. However, the introduction of comprehensive vaccination programs through the world has drastically reduced the incidence of the disease. From 2007 to 2019, the incidence of RUBV infections decreased from 13.9 to 1.7 cases per million people.[206] Thus, as of 2019, 24% of the global population live in countries where rubella has been

eliminated or controlled. However, this leaves a significant number of developing nations, particularly in Africa, at risk for continuing rubella outbreaks (Fig. 4.1).

Until the keen observations of the ophthalmologist Norman Gregg, rubella was considered a relatively benign infection associated with considerably less morbidity than measles. In 1941, Gregg encountered a large number of children with cataracts, many of whom had additional serious congenital defects. He noted that an apparent epidemic of congenital cataracts was directly preceded by a large rubella outbreak. Gregg proposed that the cataracts as well as the often associated congenital cardiac abnormalities were the consequence of maternal infection during pregnancy.[95] Further studies by other investigators confirmed that the virus could have devastating effects on a developing fetus when acquired by the mother in early pregnancy.[288] The realization that viruses can act as teratogenic agents spurred the efforts to develop an attenuated vaccine.

A key step in vaccine development was isolation and growth of RUBV in cultured cells.[204,287] In 1969, the first rubella vaccine was licensed in the United States, 5 years after the last major epidemic in that country and shortly before the next significant outbreak was predicted to occur. Fortunately, no other major rubella epidemics occurred largely in part to the adoption of universal vaccination in infancy, which has been remarkably successful in controlling natural rubella and its devastating teratogenic effects.[242] Despite this, RUBV is still the leading vaccine-preventable cause of birth defects.

INFECTIOUS AGENT

RUBV is an enveloped positive-strand RNA virus of the genus *Rubivirus* within the newly established family *Matonaviridae*.[278] Prior to 2018, RUBV was classified within the family *Togaviridae*, which contains the large alphavirus genus whose members include the well-studied model pathogens Sindbis and Semliki Forest viruses. RUBV shares a common genome organization and replication strategy with alphaviruses (Fig. 4.2). Humans appear to be the only natural host and reservoir for RUBV. Of note, within the newly designated *Matonaviridae* family, some nonhuman rubiviruses such as Ruhugu and Rustrela viruses use bats and mice as reservoirs, respectively.[21] In addition, some matonaviruses can infect certain fish species including Pacific

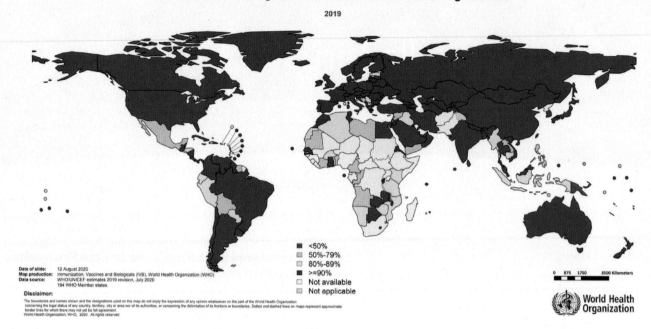

FIGURE 4.1 World map showing countries that employ rubella virus–containing vaccines. (From https://www.who.int/immunization/monitoring_surveillance/burden/vpd/surveillance_type/passive/rubella/en/)

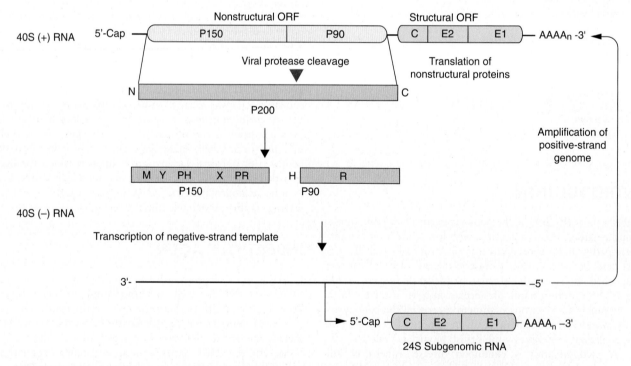

FIGURE 4.2 Organization and expression of the RUBV genome. The genome is a single-stranded 40S RNA containing two open reading frames (ORFs). The 5′ proximal ORF encodes the nonstructural proteins p150 and p90. The 40S genome serves as an mRNA for translation of the nonstructural protein precursor P200, which is cleaved by a virus-encoded protease to produce p150 and p90. The relative positions of methyltransferase (M), Y, proline hinge (PH), X, protease (PR), helicase (H), and RNA-dependent polymerase (R) domains within p150 and p90 proteins are shown. These two proteins form the viral replicase that synthesizes a negative-sense 40S RNA, which then serves as a template for synthesis of more genomic RNA and the 24S subgenomic RNA. Both the 40S and 24S positive-sense RNAs are capped and polyadenylated.

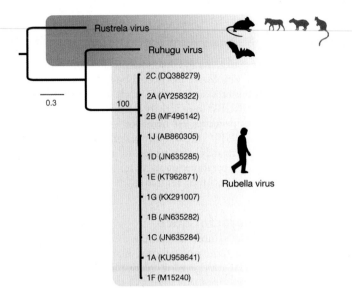

electric rays.[96] RUBV is most closely related to the bat-borne Ruhugu virus, which has led to speculation that RUBV may have evolved as a zoonotic pathogen. Although only one serotype exists, there are at least 11 genotypes of RUBV (Fig. 4.3), which can be grouped into 2 clades.[300] Circulation of clade 2 viruses, which contains three genotypes, is limited to Eurasia, while clade 1 viruses are more widely distributed. The genome of RUBV is a 5′capped positive-sense RNA molecule of approximately 10 kilobases (kb) with a poly (A) tail. There is no serological cross-reactivity between the alphaviruses and RUBV, and only limited genome sequence similarity, predominantly within the nonstructural genes in regions that encode functional domains such as the polymerase and protease activities. However, conservation of B-cell epitopes on certain *Rubivirus* E1 glycoproteins suggests that current serological assays to detect RUBV might also detect Ruhugu and Rustrela viruses.[21]

FIGURE 4.3 Phylogenetic tree showing 11 different genotypes of RUBV and their relationship to two mouse- and bat-borne rubiviruses (RUSV and RUHV). *Black* silhouettes represent the natural hosts of each virus, and *red* silhouettes represent spill-over hosts for RUSV. Numbers beside nodes indicate bootstrap values (as a percentage; only values for major branches are shown); the scale bar indicates the number of amino acid substitutions per site. (Adapted by permission from Nature: Bennett AJ, Paskey AC, Ebinger A, et al. Relatives of rubella virus in diverse mammals. *Nature* 2020;586(7829):424–428. Copyright © 2020 Springer Nature.)

Morphology and Physicochemical Properties of the Virion

Early transmission electron microscopy studies reported that RUBV virions are spherical particles[12,180] and the primary budding site in most cell types is the Golgi (Fig. 4.4). Subsequent high-resolution microscopy studies have revealed much more information regarding the structure of RUBV particles, which are heterogeneous in nature. While most virions are indeed spherical (average diameter ~70 nm), elongated tubular particles of up to 150 nm can also be observed in preparations[17,156] (Fig. 4.5). RUBV particles contain a nucleocapsid (30 to 40 nm diameter), which consists

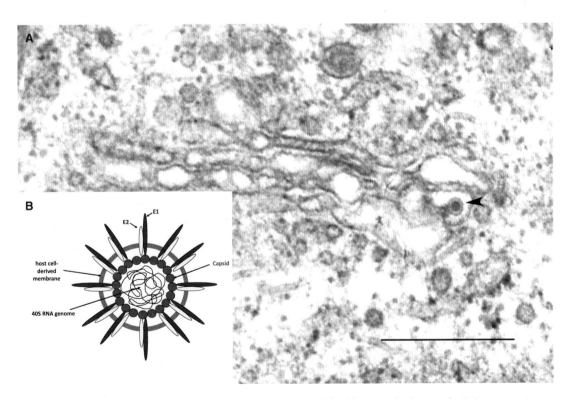

FIGURE 4.4 A: Electron micrograph of a rubella virion (*arrowhead*) budding into the lumen of a Golgi cisterna in an infected Vero cell. Note the electron-lucent halo that surrounds the electron-dense nucleocapsid. Bar = 0.5 μm. (Image kindly provided by Dr. John Law and Ms. Honey Chan). **B:** Schematic of an RUBV virion.

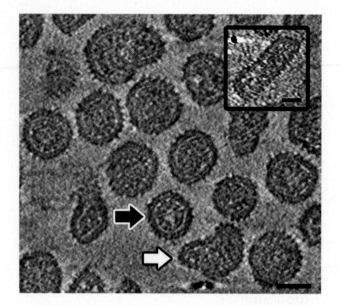

FIGURE 4.5 Rubella virions are heterogeneous. Tomographic reconstruction showing the cross section of several rubella virions near their center. The virions are variable in size and shape. The *black arrow* indicates an approximately spherical virion and the *white arrow* indicates a tear-drop-shaped virion. A nearly cylindrical virion is also shown (*inset right*). The images were generated by averaging four planes of voxels and represent a thickness of 6.0 nm. High density is black, and the scale bar represents 50 nm. (Adapted with permission of American Society for Microbiology from Battisti AJ, Yoder JD, Plevka P, et al. Cryo-electron tomography of rubella virus. *J Virol.* 2012;86(20):11078–11085; permission conveyed through Copyright Clearance Center, Inc.)

of a single molecule of genomic RNA complexed with approximately 300 copies of the capsid protein and has been described as "a sparsely populated region in the center of the virions." They nucleocapsid core is surrounded by a host-derived envelope.[179] Between the core and the envelope is an approximately 7-nm-thick electron-lucent region giving the virions the appearance of having a ring or "toga" surrounding the nucleocapsid.

Initial studies suggested that RUBV nucleocapsids had a T = 3 icosahedral symmetry[163] thereby distinguishing them from those of alphaviruses, which are arranged with a T = 4 symmetry. However, cyro-electron microscopy studies by Michael Rossmann's group revealed that RUBV particles do not in fact exhibit icosahedral symmetry.[17] The viral envelope that contains the glycoprotein spikes is 9 to 12 nm thick, and the two viral membrane proteins E2 and E1, which make up the spikes that project 6 to 8 nm from the envelope,[267] are organized in sets of four to six parallel rows that enwrap the virus particle surface in a helical manner.[17,156] This arrangement appears to be unique among enveloped RNA viruses.

The buoyant density of rubella virions in sucrose gradients is 1.18 to 1.19 g/mL.[118] In comparison, the buoyant density of alphavirus virions is 1.20 g/mL, a difference that may be attributable to a wider electron-lucent zone between the core and envelope in RUBV particles. The reported sedimentation coefficient of RUBV virions ranges from 240S to 350S.[11] The difficulty in obtaining highly purified homogenous preparations of RUBV virions was one of the numerous technical reasons that until recently impeded the progress of structural analysis.

The infectivity of RUBV virions is rapidly lost following exposure to protein denaturing agents (formaldehyde, ethylene oxide, and beta-propiolactone) or treatments/reagents that damage nucleic acids (ultraviolet light or photodynamic dyes). Moreover, because it is an enveloped virus, exposure of RUBV preparations to nonionic or ionic detergents and lipid solvents abrogates the infectivity of virions.[203] Virions are inactivated by incubation at 56°C for less than 20 minutes and even at much lower temperatures such as 37°C, and RUBV loses activity slowly ($t_{1/2}$ = 48 hours).[172] When stored at temperatures less than −60°C in the presence of protein stabilizers, RUBV preparations maintain their infectivity for many years. Fortunately, with respect to vaccine distribution, lyophilized RUBV preparations are stable for years and months at 4°C and ambient temperatures, respectively.[207]

Biological Characteristics

RUBV has a restricted host range (only humans) *in vivo* but replicates in a wide variety of cultured mammalian cell lines, including primary African green monkey kidney cells, BHK21, RK13, and Vero cell lines. All strains of the virus are slightly temperature sensitive, with higher yields of virus obtained when infected cells are cultured at 35°C rather than at 37°C. The vaccine strains RA27/3 and Cendehill are completely growth restricted at 39°C, while some wild-type isolates are still able to replicate at 41°C albeit at lower levels.[42]

In comparison to the rapid lytic infection of mammalian cells by alphaviruses, RUBV replicates more slowly with an eclipse phase of 10 to 12 hours (c.f. 4 hours for Sindbis or Semliki Forest viruses), and peak titers of secreted virus are not observed until 36 to 48 hours.[101,273] By comparison, peak viral titers for alphaviruses are observed within 8 hours. As well as exhibiting relatively slow replication kinetics, the amount of infectious RUBV progeny released per cell is estimated to be 1,000-fold less than for alphaviruses. Under optimal conditions, RUBV-infected BHK-21 and Vero cells can produce titers of 10^7 and 10^8 plaque-forming units (pfu) per mL, respectively.[12,272] The relatively poor replication of RUBV may be due to a number of factors including low uptake of virus and/or inefficiencies associated with the replicase/transcriptase complex or limitations of the assembly process. For example, RUBV buds into the Golgi complex, which is a much smaller membrane compartment than the endoplasmic reticulum or the plasma membrane. Another factor that may play a role is the high G+C content of the viral genome (69.5%), which predicted to form stable secondary and tertiary structures that may impede replication/transcription or translation.[80] Also related to the G+C content, the codon usage by RUBV is different from that of mammalian cells, requiring utilization of tRNAs that may be of low abundance, a factor that has been suggested to limit the rate of protein synthesis.[255]

Effects on Host Cell

Although RUBV can have devastating effects on the developing human fetus, infection of most cultured primate or rodent cell lines does not result in major cytopathology. However, in some cell lines (Vero, BHK-21, and RK13), when high multiplicities of infection (MOIs) are employed, the virus causes rounding and detachment of cells commencing at 24 hours postinfection and increasing over the next 72 hours. Much of the RUBV-induced cytopathic effect is likely the result of apoptosis.[73,169,217] Virons that are first inactivated by ultraviolet light do not induce apoptosis, indicating that viral replication is required to cause cell death.[73,114] The cytopathic determinants

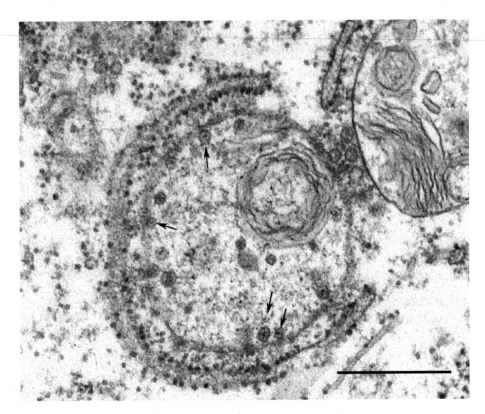

FIGURE 4.6 Electron micrograph of viral replication complex is associated with rough endoplasmic reticulum. Spherules are indicated by *arrows*. Bar = 0.5 μm. (Image kindly provided by Dr. John Law and Ms. Honey Chan.)

of RUBV have been mapped to the nonstructural genes,[215] and in agreement with this, expression of RUBV structural proteins alone in Vero cells does not induce apoptosis.[114] Paradoxically, primary human embryonic fibroblasts seem to be particularly immune to the effects of RUBV-induced apoptosis.[3]

At low (<1) or moderate (1 to 3) MOIs, little virus-cytopathic effect is observed in most cultured cells,[73,132] and chronic infections can readily be established (see "Replication Strategy"). Induction of apoptosis in response to RUBV infection is undoubtedly an important antiviral defense mechanism that is employed by cells against many RNA viruses. Because viruses are obligate parasites, they require a living cell for replication. Depending upon the apoptotic stimuli, cells can be killed in a matter of hours; a situation that would be seemingly problematic for RUBV, which has a long eclipse period and whose replication peak occurs between 2 and 4 days postinfection.[101] However, the maximum RUBV-induced apoptosis does not occur until after 5 days postinfection,[169] which is consistent with a scenario where the virus actively blocks apoptosis early in infection. Indeed, it has been shown that RUBV-infected cells can be highly resistant to apoptotic stimuli.[121] Mapping studies showed that the capsid protein is responsible for this process, which presumably provides a window of opportunity for the virus to replicate before apoptosis is initiated.

In most cell types, cellular macromolecular synthesis on a global level does not appear to be significantly affected, even following high-multiplicity infections (5 to 10 pfu per cell). For example, host cell RNA synthesis continues normally, and protein synthesis is only slightly reduced at 72 hours postinfection in several highly permissive cell lines.[101] However,

in mitogen-stimulated peripheral blood mononuclear cells (PBMCs), host cell protein synthesis was reportedly inhibited by more than 90% at 48 hours postinfection.[43] The capsid protein has been shown to block translation *in vitro*,[177] but it has yet to be determined whether this viral protein is responsible for inhibition of protein synthesis in PBMCs or other cell types.

A number of characteristic morphologic changes occur in RUBV-infected cells. Similar to other RNA viruses, RUBV infection is accompanied by drastic rearrangement of cellular membranes. The endoplasmic reticulum (ER), Golgi complex, and mitochondria are often closely arranged around the virus replication complexes (Fig. 4.6), which are derived from endosomes and/or lysosomes.[142,143] This arrangement of organelles could in theory facilitate the efficient transfer of virus genome from the site of RNA replication (endosomes) to the area of virus assembly (Golgi complex). Whereas organelle rearrangement is common in cells infected with RNA viruses, the formation of electron-dense plaques (22 to 25 nm in thickness) between organelles is unique to RUBV infection.[140] The plaques (Fig. 4.7) and associated organelles have been termed confronting membranes or confronting cisternae and commonly involve outer membranes of mitochondria and rough ER, adjacent mitochondria, and adjacent ER membranes, respectively. Expression of capsid protein in the absence of other viral proteins induces mitochondrial clustering and formation of plaques,[18] and immunoelectron microscopy revealed that capsid protein is a major component of the plaques.[123] A large pool of capsid protein is targeted to the surface of mitochondria,[19,144] and subsequently, it was reported that capsid affects

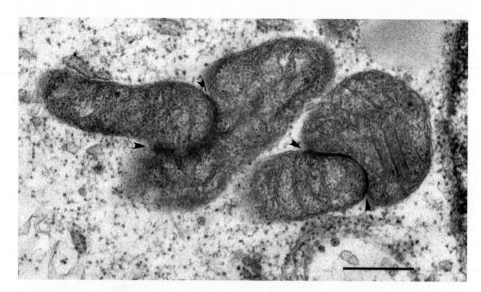

FIGURE 4.7 Aggregation of mitochondria and formation of electron-dense intermitochondrial plaques in RUBV-infected cells. Bar = 0.5 µm. (Image kindly provided by Dr. John Law and Ms. Honey Chan.)

mitochondrial import.[123] The latter may explain the loss of cristae and dysmorphic (club-shaped appearance) mitochondria in RUBV-infected cells.[139] Together, these observations reflect the close link between RUBV replication and mitochondrial physiology.

Phenotypic Variation

Although there are at least 11 genotypes of RUBV (Fig. 4.3), there is only one serotype, and infection with one strain provides protection against all others recognized to date. Despite the limited genetic differences seen (0.8% to 2.1% at the amino acid level)[250,299] among RUBV strains, significant differences in hemagglutination,[150] plaque morphology,[132] temperature sensitivity, virus yield, and cell tropism have been reported.[42] Compared to natural RUBV infection, administration of vaccine strains is associated with milder acute symptoms and a lower incidence of complications such as joint and[25,78,259]teratogenic effects.[15]

The major neutralization epitopes appear to be highly conserved among RUBV strains,[26,81] although differences have been noted in the kinetics of neutralization[93] and in reactivity to certain monoclonal antibodies.[42] However, both infection and immunization are believed to provide protection against all other strains for the duration of the immune response elicited, except in cases where incomplete immunity is induced.[260]

The vaccine strains, RA27/3 and Cendehill, display different tissue tropisms from wt+ strains, including growth restriction in both PBMCs and the B-cell lines, Raji and Cess cells.[42] These two strains also show limited replication in cells derived from human joint tissue,[172] with the Cendehill strain completely inhibited in synovial organ cultures and chondrocytes. In comparison, wt+ strains replicate to high titer (10^6 to 10^7 pfu/mL) in joint cells. The determinants that govern growth in joint tissue have been mapped to the 5′ end of the genome, which encodes the nonstructural proteins, and as such, it is likely that replication rather than binding and entry events determine tropism.[152]

Structure and Organization of the Genome

The genome of RUBV is a single molecule of positive-strand RNA of approximately 10 kb with a GC content of 69.5%; by far the highest of any RNA virus sequenced to date.[6] The 5′ end of the RNA has a 7-methyl-guanosine cap,[187] while at the 3′ end, there is a poly (A) tract with a mean length of 53 nucleotides.[279] The genome consists of two nonoverlapping polycistronic open reading frames (ORFs) separated by a nontranslated region of 123 nucleotides (Fig. 4.2).[216] The 5′ proximal ORF (~6,385 nucleotides) encodes the nonstructural proteins, while the 3′ proximal ORF (3,189 nucleotides) encodes the three structural proteins, capsid, E2, and E1. The structural proteins are translated from a 5′ capped and polyadenylated subgenomic RNA that is collinear with the 3′ one-third of the 40S genome.[187] The complete nucleotide sequences have been determined for the genomes of several wild-type and vaccine strains of RUBV[80] and are available in GenBank. In addition, infectious cDNA clones of several strains have been produced and used to map genetic elements involved in viral replication and attenuation.[152,219,279,295]

Cis-Acting Elements

The availability of infectious RUBV cDNA clones[152,219,295] and replicons[268] has enabled the application of reverse genetics to study the roles of cis-acting elements in genome replication. Both the 5′ and 3′ untranslated regions (UTRs) of the RUBV genome are predicted to form secondary structures that influence transcription and translation events. The predicted 5′ stem–loop (5′SL), which encompasses nucleotides 15 to 65, has a terminal loop as well as a bulge in the stem and a hinge region (Fig. 4.8). It likely forms a pseudoknot,[218] a structure that has been shown in a number of plant and animal viruses to enhance binding of proteins that function in RNA replication.[63,124] Within the single-stranded leader sequence (nucleotides 1 to 14) and the stem–loop, there are three AUG codons starting at nucleotides 3, 41, and 57. Translation of the long ORF encoding the nonstructural genes is initiated at AUG_{41}, while the first

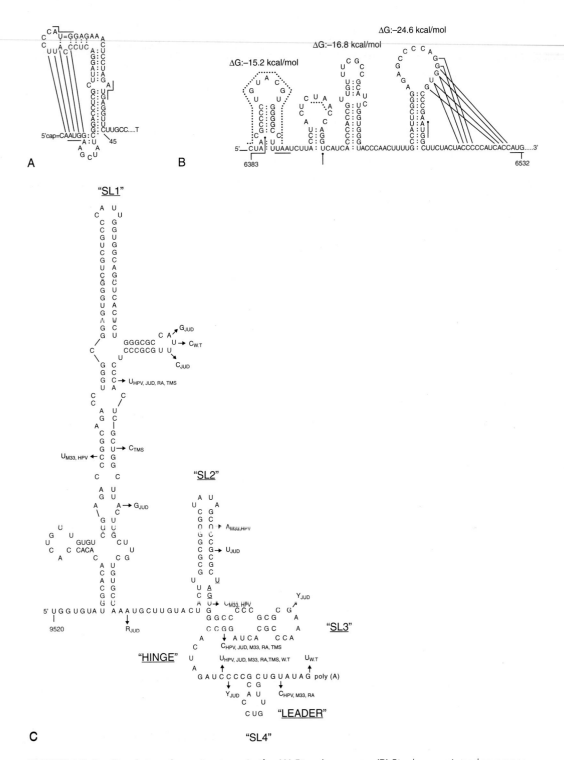

FIGURE 4.8 Predicted stem–loop structures in the (A) 5′ end sequence, **(B)** 5′ subgenomic end sequence, and **(C)** 3′ end sequence. Potential pairing of bases to form pseudoknots in structures **(A)** and **(B)** are shown with *dotted lines*. (**A** and **B** adapted from Frey TK. Molecular biology of rubella virus. *Adv Virus Res* 1994;44:69–160. Copyright © 1994 Elsevier. With permission; **C** adapted with permission of American Society for Microbiology from Chen MH, Frey TK. Mutagenic analysis of the 3′ cis-acting elements of the rubella virus genome. *J Virol* 1999;73(4):3386–3403; permission conveyed through Copyright Clearance Center, Inc.)

and third AUGs are in a different reading frame and are terminated at nucleotides 54 and 90, respectively. Indeed, site-specific mutagenesis studies suggest that AUG₃ is not essential for viral replication,[218] nor is it known whether short peptides that originate from either AUG₃ or AUG₅₇ play any role in virus biology. However, it is notable that the three AUG codons are conserved in all strains sequenced to date.[152,218] Analysis of the 5′ end sequences of a number of RUBV strains revealed that the stem–loop is largely conserved and that polymorphisms are restricted to the terminal loop or the hinge region.[124,218]

Mutations in the 5′SL are associated with differences in viral yield and plaque morphology[218] as well as tropism for joint tissue.[152]

Between the nonstructural and structural genes is a 123-bp region that is predicted to form a series of stem–loops (Fig. 4.8). This region shares 58% identity with the equivalent region in the Sindbis virus genome and may be important for regulating synthesis of the subgenomic RNA. In addition, translation of the structural genes is affected by mutations in this region, which forms the 5′ end of the subgenomic RNA.[202] In the 3′ UTR, there is a stretch of 59 nucleotides following the stop codon at nucleotide 9701. A complex secondary structure involving three major stem–loop structures[48] has been predicted for the 3′ terminal 240 nucleotides (Fig. 4.8). These 3′ UTR sequences function in *cis* to regulate transcription, specifically, synthesis of plus-strand viral RNAs but not negative-sense RNA.[49]

Encapsidation Signal

In vitro binding studies using radiolabeled viral RNA segments and nitrocellulose-immobilized capsid protein revealed that capsid protein binds with relatively high affinity to a 29-nucleotide segment located in the 5′NS gene region between nucleotides 347 and 375.[149]

Nonstructural ORF and Protein Products

The nonstructural (NS) genes are located in the 5′ end of the viral genome within a long ORF commencing at AUG_{41}. The NS ORF is translated as a single greater than 200-kd polyprotein, which is cleaved into two products, p150 and p90,[159] that function in replication and transcription of viral RNAs (Fig. 4.2). The gene order of the 5′ ORF is NH_2-p150-p90-COOH. The two nonstructural proteins have several enzymatic activities, including RNA polymerase, protease, and helicase, and together form the viral replicase. Proteolytic processing of the p200 polyprotein marks the switch from synthesis of negative-strand genomic RNA to synthesis of plus-strand RNA.[145]

P150 contains several domains that are conserved among other RNA virus–encoded proteins. A protease domain located in the carboxyl portion of p150 (Fig. 4.2) is responsible for cleavage of the nonstructural precursor protein p200 and is critical for virus replication.[51,296] Mutagenesis studies have shown that the RUBV protease is a metalloprotease that requires divalent cations for activity[147,148] and functions in both *cis* and *trans* modes.[146] Treatment of RUBV-infected cells with the Hsp90 inhibitor 17-allylamino-17-desmethoxygeldanamycin reduces viral titers by 100-fold.[239] Hsp90, a molecular chaperone, interacts with p150 and is thought to promote RUBV replication by facilitating processing of p200 and stabilizing p150. Replication of alphaviruses is also dependent on Hsp90, which interacts with NSP3 and NSP4[65,226] and also promotes stability of NSP2.[182]

A putative methyltransferase domain in the amino terminus of p150 is predicted to function in capping the viral RNA.[238] P150 also contains an X domain that has homology to the nonstructural proteins of alphaviruses, coronaviruses, and hepatitis E virus.[92] The function of the X domain is not well characterized, but it is required for *trans* cleavage by the RUBV protease and in alphaviruses at least and is important for replication.[99] Interestingly, the X domain is the region that is most highly conserved between RUBV and alphaviruses.[69] Two other domains of unknown function, Y and a proline hinge, are also present in P150. The order of these domains in p150 is NH_2-methyltransferase-Y domain-proline hinge domain-X domain-protease-COOH. The second nonstructural protein, p90, comprises 905 amino acid residues and contains the replicase and helicase motifs. Based on comparison with global RNA-dependent RNA polymerase consensus sequences,[125] the GDD tripeptide at amino acids 1965 to 1967 of p90 is the active site of the RUBV replicase. An RNA-stimulated NTPase that promotes unwinding of the template during RNA replication is associated with the helicase motif.[98] Finally, while not required for assembly of virus particles, interaction between p150 and the capsid protein is important for expression of viral genes and infectivity of virions.[164,240]

The localization of RUBV nonstructural proteins, p150 and p90, is less well studied than that of the structural proteins. This is in part because nonstructural proteins are present at relatively low concentrations in infected cells, and furthermore, attempts to produce useful antibodies against these antigens have met with limited success. However, it has been reported that p150 associates with long tubular structures that correspond to sites of viral RNA synthesis,[134] whereas P90 can be detected in discrete cytoplasmic puncta that form linear chains.[5] The identity of the p90-associated structures was not determined, but it is likely that they are replication complexes derived from endocytic vacuoles. Presumably, a large pool of p150 is also localized to the p90-positive foci. No information regarding sequences that target the nonstructural proteins to endocytic membranes has been reported.

Structural ORF and Protein Products

The structural genes are contained within the 3′ ORF of the 40S genomic RNA; however, they are actually translated from a subgenomic 24S RNA that is produced in infected cells. There are two in-frame AUG initiation codons in the subgenomic RNA separated by 21 nucleotides. The downstream AUG is in the more favorable context for translation initiation, but *in vitro* mutagenesis experiments indicate that both codons can be used.[53] The 24S subgenomic RNA encodes three structural proteins, which are translated in the order NH2-C-E2-E1-COOH.[186] Unlike alphavirus structural proteins, which require both host cell signal peptidase and a capsid-associated protease for complete processing,[170] processing of the RUBV structural polyprotein (Fig. 4.9) into C, E2, and E1 only requires signal peptidase, which is encoded by the host cell.[158,253]

In the absence of genomic RNA, coordinated expression of the RUBV structural proteins in mammalian cells results in the assembly and secretion of rubella virus-like particles (VLPs).[108,222] The VLPs, which resemble native virions in terms of morphology and antigenicity, have served as a useful tool for studying virus assembly, and as a consequence, the roles of RUBV structural proteins and their domains in the assembly process are relatively well understood. The fact that rubella VLPs are efficiently assembled and secreted in the absence of genomic RNA indicates that virus budding is not tightly linked to *bona fide* nucleocapsid assembly with viral genomic RNA. Whether RUBV capsid can form nucleocapsid-like structures with host RNAs or the viral subgenomic RNA has not been investigated.

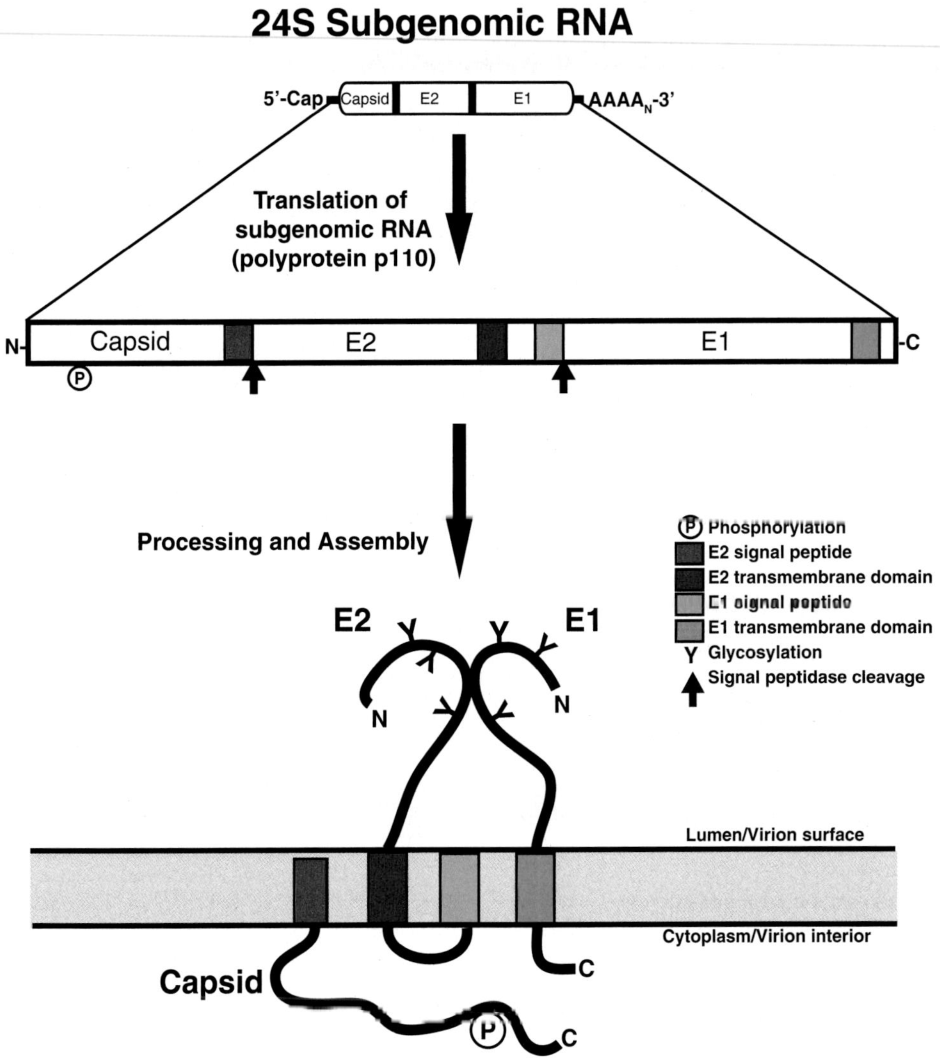

24S Subgenomic RNA

FIGURE 4.9 Processing of RUBV structural proteins. The 24S RNA serves as the mRNA for translation of a structural polyprotein precursor, which is then cleaved by host signal peptidase to produce capsid, E2 and E1. The relative membrane orientations of the structural proteins immediately following translocation into the ER are shown. The amino (N) and carboxyl (C) termini of the proteins are indicated.

Capsid

The capsid protein is a phosphoprotein with an apparent molecular mass of 33 to 35 kDa.[158] The protein contains 300 amino acid residues and is rich in arginine and proline residues, particularly at its amino terminus, which gives it a net positive charge[52] and facilitates its interaction with genomic RNA during nucleocapsid formation. The protein often migrates as a doublet on SDS-PAGE gels. The reason for this remains unknown, but it is not due to the use of an alternate translation start site.[53,158] Virion-associated capsid protein can be isolated as disulfide-linked dimers, but intermolecular disulfide bonding is not necessary for formation of virus particles.[14,141] X-ray crystallography was used to determine the structure of the carboxyl-terminal 150 amino acids residues (127 to 277) of RUBV capsid protein.[157] In addition to confirming that this protein homo-dimerizes via disulfide bonds between cysteine residues 153 and 197, it was discovered that RUBV capsid contains a

unique peptide fold not found in other proteins. There are five antiparallel β-strands and a short α-helix in each capsid monomer, and interactions between the two of the β-strands on one monomer and a flexible loop on the other monomer help stabilize capsid dimers. The dimers are further arranged into rows via lateral interactions between the dimers (Fig. 4.10).

Cleavage of the RUBV capsid from the polyprotein precursor differs from alphaviruses whose capsid proteins have autoprotease activity that separates them from the polyprotein.[170] As a consequence, alphavirus capsids are free in the cytoplasm of infected cells. RUBV capsid protein, in contrast, lacks autoprotease activity, and separation from E2 is carried out by host cell signal peptidase.[52] The E2 signal peptide is therefore retained as the carboxyl terminus of capsid protein (Fig. 4.9) where it confers membrane association of the protein.[105,158,253] The membrane association of RUBV capsid protein may account for some of the unusual morphogenetic features of

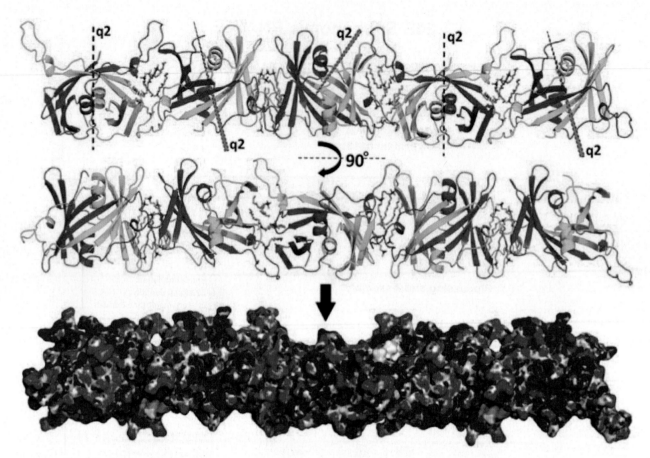

FIGURE 4.10 Capsid dimers are arranged into rows. A row of the C2 crystal form of capsid with its dimer axe parallel and perpendicular to the plane of the paper, respectively, is shown. The *dashed lines* correspond to quasi-twofold axes (q2). For each crystal form, the molecular surface that presumably faces the viral membrane is colored according to its electrostatic potential. The potentials at 300 K are in the range +125 mV (+5 kT/e) (*blue*) to −125 mV (−5 kT/e) (*red*) where k = Boltzmann constant, T = temperature, e = electronic charge, and mV = millivolts. The detergent molecules in the C2 space group are shown in *orange*. A *black arrow* indicates the site of the detergent binding region that possibly also binds the cytosolic part of E2. (Adapted with permission from Mangala Prasad V, Willows SD, Fokine A, et al. Rubella virus capsid protein structure and its role in virus assembly and infection. *Proc Natl Acad Sci U S A* 2013;110(50):20105–20110.)

the virus. Indeed, retention of the E2 signal peptide on capsid protein is necessary for assembly of VLPs and presumably infectious virions.[135]

Role of the capsid protein in virus assembly

The primary function of capsid protein during virus assembly is to homo-oligomerize and bind viral genomic RNA to form the nucleocapsid. The RNA-binding domain of capsid protein resides within amino acid residues 28 to 56 and binds to a packaging signal (nucleotides 347 to 375) in the genomic RNA.[149] Posttranslational modification of capsid protein may play an important role in regulating the formation of nucleocapsids because phosphorylation of serine 46 within the RNA-binding domain negatively regulates RNA binding.[136,137] This is believed to limit nonspecific binding of cellular RNAs to capsid protein and/or to delay binding of genomic RNA until the virion components are targeted to the budding site. *In vitro*, capsid protein is a substrate for protein phosphatase IA, an enzyme has been implicated in Golgi-associated functions.[136] Accordingly, targeting of capsid protein to the Golgi complex, followed by dephosphorylation at this site could explain how nucleocapsid

assembly is synchronized with virus assembly (Fig. 4.11). Supporting this scenario is the observation that virion-associated capsid protein has a higher affinity for viral RNA and contains significantly less phosphate than cell-associated capsid protein.[136,137] Similar to alphaviruses,[252] it is thought that capsid protein drives virus budding through interactions with the envelope glycoproteins. Direct binding between RUBV capsid protein and E2 and/or E1 has yet to be demonstrated, but structural analyses of the capsid revealed a potential binding site for the cytoplasmic tail of E2.[157]

Nonstructural roles of the capsid protein

In addition to nucleocapsid assembly, the RUBV capsid protein plays a role in regulating viral transcription and replication. The first indication of this nonstructural function came from the observation that expression of capsid protein rescues the replication of an RUBV replicon containing an in-frame deletion of p150.[269] Further analyses indicated that the capsid protein is involved in modulating viral genomic and subgenomic RNA synthesis.[270] In the absence of capsid protein expression, the ratio of genomic RNA to subgenomic RNA is

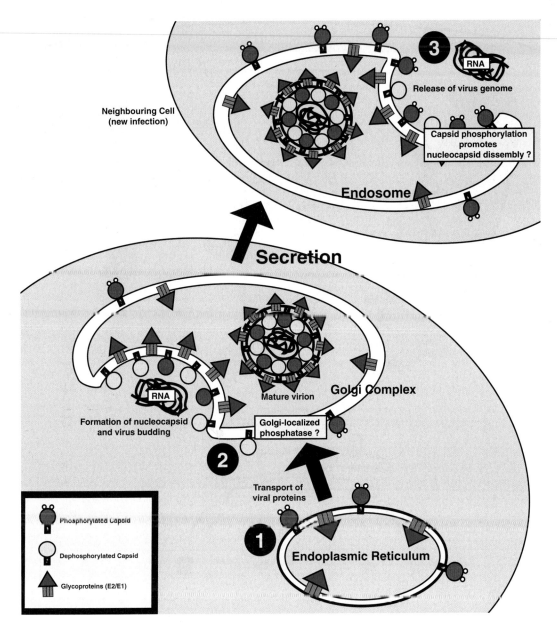

FIGURE 4.11 Model to illustrate the putative roles of dynamic phosphorylation of capsid protein in virus replication. (1) Phosphorylation of newly synthesized capsid protein prevents nonspecific binding of RNA and premature formation of nucleocapsid at the early stages of virus assembly. (2) Capsid protein is subsequently targeted to the Golgi complex, and dephosphorylation of the protein at this stage allows interaction with the genomic RNA, formation of the nucleocapsid and subsequent virus budding. (3) Timely rephosphorylation of capsid protein before or during virus entry promotes the disassembly of nucleocapsid.

substantially lower. The pool of capsid protein that associates with the replication complexes is thought to be responsible for regulating synthesis of viral RNAs. A self-dimerization motif in the amino-terminal region of capsid is required for interaction with p150 and infectivity of virions.[240] Some *Rubivirus* capsid proteins lack this motif,[66] and therefore, it is not clear whether capsid–p150 interactions are critical for replication of other viruses within this genus. Finally, it is interesting to note that the effects of capsid protein on viral transcription depend on the levels of RNA.[50] At low levels of viral RNA, capsid protein enhances replication of genomic RNA, but as the concentration of RNA increases, capsid protein becomes inhibitory for this process.

Given its multiple roles, it is not surprising that the RUBV capsid protein associates with multiple organelles. Consistent with its function in virus assembly, pools of capsid protein are localized to the Golgi.[13,108] Transport of capsid to the Golgi region from the site of its synthesis, the ER, depends upon E1 and E2.[86,135] Capsid also localizes to mitochondria and to virus replication complexes.[19,140] In contrast, the glycoproteins E1 and E2 are targeted mainly to the virus budding site (Golgi), which may indicate that they do not have significant nonstructural roles. Together with p150, replication complex-localized capsid protein[134] is thought to modulate replication of viral RNA, whereas the mitochondrial pool of capsid plays one or more critical roles in virus–host interactions (Fig. 4.12).

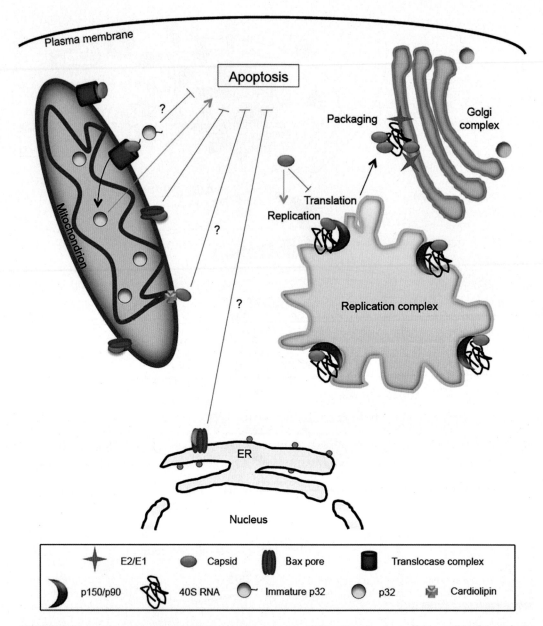

FIGURE 4.12 Integrated model of RUBV capsid nonstructural functions. At the replication complex, capsid associates with nonstructural proteins (p150 and p90) and regulates transcription and replication of viral RNA. Late in the infection cycle, local sequestration of translation initiation factors such as PABP may modulate the switch from translation to packaging of the genomic RNA; a mechanism that would leave the viral RNA available for packaging into nucleocapsids at the Golgi complex. Capsid prevents apoptosis by binding to Bax and inducing the formation of hetero-oligomers that are incompetent for pore formation at the mitochondria and potentially at the ER membranes. Capsid may also inhibit apoptosis by preventing translocation of proapoptotic proteins such as p32 into the mitochondria or by engaging in complexes with the mitochondrial lipid, cardiolipin. (Modified with permission of Future Medicine Ltd. from Ilkow CS, Willows SD, Hobman TC. Rubella virus capsid protein: a small protein with big functions. *Future Microbiol* 2010;5(4):571–584; permission conveyed through Copyright Clearance Center, Inc.)

Capsid potently blocks programmed cell death by sequestering the proapoptotic host protein Bax into nonfunctional complexes.[121] Membrane association and phosphorylation appear to be important for this function of capsid.[291] Intriguingly, hypophosphorylated capsid binds just as well to Bax, suggesting that interaction alone with this proapoptotic protein is not sufficient to block programmed cell death.

The RUBV capsid also interferes with mitochondrial import,[123] a critical process that is linked to apoptosis in mammalian cells.[205]

Capsid interacts with the mitochondrial matrix protein p32,[19] and several lines of evidence suggest that it is important for virus replication. First, ablation of the p32-binding site in capsid protein reduces the replication efficiency of RUBV by 1,000-fold.[18] Second, depletion of cellular p32 pools reduces virus replication.[55] Capsid protein–p32 interactions may also be important for synthesis of subgenomic RNA and/or translation of structural proteins. Finally, loss of stable binding between capsid protein and p32 is correlated with reduced mitochondrial clustering in the perinuclear region. Together, these results suggest that interactions between capsid protein and p32 are important for RUBV-induced rearrangement of mitochondria, a phenomenon that is associated with optimal replication. Finally, it was recently reported that RUBV capsid protein inhibits RNA interference by sequestering double-stranded RNA substrates from Dicer.[294] Whether this function of capsid is important for RUBV replication or interference with the innate immune response is not known.

Envelope glycoproteins E1 and E2

Both E1 and E2 are type I membrane proteins that dimerize to form the spike complexes on the surface of the virion (Fig. 4.9). The major functions of these spikes are to bind cell surface receptors and mediate fusion with cell membranes.[128] The envelope proteins, E1 in particular, are the major antigenic determinants against which neutralizing antibodies are directed.[283]

Receptor binding and membrane fusion of virions with host cell membranes are mediated by the E1 glycoprotein.[56,70 72] It is 481 amino acid residues in length and exhibits an apparent molecular mass of 58 kDa when analyzed by SDS-PAGE. The mature protein contains three asparagine-linked oligosaccharide moieties[109] and is further modified by palmitoylation.[107,284] An amino-terminal signal peptide facilitates translocation of E1 into the ER, and a 22 amino acid hydrophobic sequence at its carboxyl terminus mediates membrane association.[110] E1 also contains a carboxyl-terminal tail of 13 amino acid residues that is exposed to the cytoplasm.

The crystal structure of the E1 ectodomain has been solved at a resolution of **1.8 Å**. Similar to alphavirus E1 and flavivirus E proteins, which also mediate fusion of viral and host membranes, RUBV E1 is a class II membrane fusion protein and has a β-sheet structure. It is composed of three domains, DI, DII, and DIII, that are linked to the single transmembrane domain by a stem region (Fig. 4.13). In low pH environments such as endosomes, the DII domain inserts into the target host membrane and then forms a trimer with DI.[72,100,131] Whereas class II fusions proteins of alphaviruses and flaviviruses have companion proteins that protect them from the low pH environments of the late secretory and endocytic compartments, it is not clear how this occurs for RUBV E1. There are a number of other differences between E1 and the other class II viral fusion proteins,[232] but most are beyond the scope of this chapter. However, it is important to point out that unlike other class II viral fusion proteins, RUBV E1 has two fusion loops instead of one and requires calcium for fusion with early endosomal membranes during viral entry.[70-72] RUBV E1 shares more than 50% sequence similarity with E1 proteins of other rubiviruses (Ruhugu and Rustrela) including the amino acid residues that coordinate calcium binding.[21]

E2 glycoprotein (282 amino acids residues) is not as well characterized as E1, but it is critical for E1 function and virus assembly. It contains two stretches of hydrophobic amino acid residues near its carboxy terminus, an 18 amino acid residue transmembrane domain and the E1 signal peptide, which comprises the C-terminus.[13,52] These two hydrophobic domains are separated by a seven amino acid residue loop that is rich in basic amino acid residues. Similar to E1, translocation of E2 into ER membranes is mediated by an amino-terminal signal peptide.[105] E2 is heavily glycosylated and contains both asparagine-linked and O-linked carbohydrates,[110,153] and like E1, it is modified by the addition of palmitate prior to virus assembly.[107,283] The

role of this modification in spike protein function has not been investigated, but it is possible that acylation may serve to further stabilize and/or orientate E2 and E1 in the membrane. The membrane orientations of the RUBV structural proteins are shown in Figure 4.9.

Similar to binding partners for other viral class II fusion proteins, E2 is synthesized immediately before E1 in the RUBV structural polyprotein p110 and once released from the precursor, forms a heterodimer with the fusogenic protein E1.[130,232] However, unlike the companion proteins pE2 and prM, which protect alphavirus and flavivirus fusion proteins, respectively, from low pH in the secretory pathway, RUBV E2 is not known to be proteolytically processed by endoproteases such as furin.

Replication Strategy

The replication strategy of RUBV is similar to that of alphaviruses in many respects, but there are several quantitative and qualitative differences. As discussed previously, RUBV replication is less robust and kinetically much slower than that of alphaviruses.[101] In addition, it is not possible to obtain a uniformly infected population of cells within 24 hours, even at high MOIs.[243] The reason for this phenomenon is not clear, but given that eventually all cells within a permissive culture become infected, it is possible that a cell cycle–dependent factor is required for RUBV entry or early viral replication events. Another major difference from the alphaviruses is that a large pool of the nascent RUBV capsid protein remains membrane associated.[135,253] This may be one of the reasons that RUBV nucleocapsid assembly differs from that of alphaviruses, which are not membrane associated. Free nucleocapsids are rarely observed in RUBV-infected cells but rather assembly is coincident with virus budding at the Golgi complex, a process that is hypothesized to be regulated by reversible phosphorylation of the capsid protein.[136] A schematic diagram of how RUBV enters, replicates and exits from host cells is shown in Figure 4.14.[67]

Attachment and Internalization

The identity of host cell receptors for RUBV remained elusive until 10 years ago. Using an affinity purification approach, myelin oligodendrocyte glycoprotein was identified as an E1-binding protein by mass spectrometry.[56] Expression of this transmembrane host protein in HEK293T cells, which are not normally permissive for RUBV, resulted in the ability of this virus to infect these cells. The observation that RUBV can infect other cell types such as keratinocytes, which do not express myelin oligodendrocyte glycoprotein,[265] suggests that the virus employs multiple receptors. It has been known for many years that lipids are important for virus binding,[161] and more recently, it was reported that both cholesterol and sphingomyelin are required for entry of RUBV into host cells.[191] Following binding to the host cell, the virus is internalized by receptor-mediated endocytosis.[209] At low pH, the E1 glycoprotein becomes fusogenic, and capsid undergoes a conformational change and becomes hydrophobic,[128,165] indicating that the acidic environment within endosomes induces fusion of the viral envelope with cellular membranes and release of the nucleocapsid into the cytoplasm. While not required for binding to host cells or oligomerization of E1, calcium is critical for E1-dependent fusion of the viral envelope with endosomal membranes.[70,71]

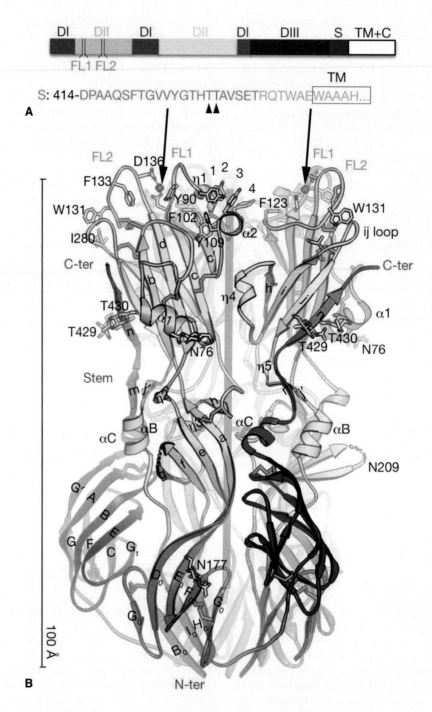

FIGURE 4.13 Domain and crystal structure of E1 protein. Linear **(A)** and three-dimensional **(B)** diagrams of E1 ectodomain color-coded by domain, with disulphide bonds in *green*. DI–DIII denote domains I to III, with the stem (S; sequence displayed in **A**) in *magenta* and the DI–DIII linker in *cyan*. FL1 and FL2 denote fusion loops 1 and 2. In **(A)**, the transmembrane (*TM*) and cytoplasmic (*C*) segments are indicated in *white*. *Gray* fonts in the stem sequence mark residues absent from the structure. Framed section denotes the beginning of the transmembrane segment. *Black triangles* denote *O*-linked glycan sites. *Arrows* point to the metal sites (*blue spheres*). Aromatic residues at the membrane-contact area are shown as ball-and-stick; the 1, 2, 3, 4 arc denotes tyrosine residues 95, 101, 112, and 108 in one subunit. The trimer axis is shown in *red* in **(B)** (side view). (Adapted by permission from Nature: DuBois RM, Vaney MC, Tortorici MA, et al. Functional and evolutionary insight from the crystal structure of rubella virus protein E1. *Nature* 2013;493(7433):552–556. Copyright © 2013 Springer Nature.)

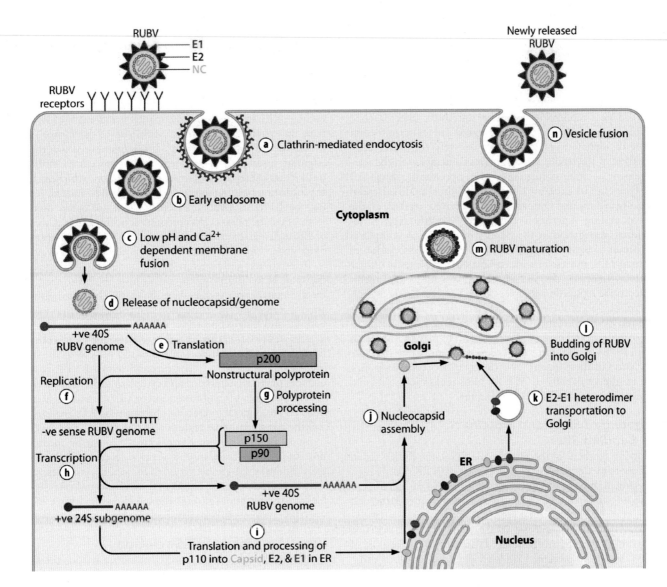

FIGURE 4.14 Life cycle of RUBV. In the upper left section, the three structural proteins E2 (*blue*), E1 (*red*), and nucleocapsid (NC; *cyan*) are indicated in the RUBV virion bound to host cell receptors on the plasma membrane. (*a*) RUBV enters host cells by clathrin-mediated endocytosis. (*b, c*) In the early endosome, low pH and Ca2+ activate virus membrane fusion. (*d*) Nucleocapsid or the genome is released into the cytoplasm. (*e, f*) The genomic RNA is translated to the nonstructural polyprotein p200, which synthesizes negative-strand RNAs. (*g, h*) p200 is processed to p150 and p90; transcription of positive polarity genomic and subgenomic RNAs then takes place. (*i*) The structural polyprotein precursor p110 is translated from subgenomic RNA and translocated into the endoplasmic reticulum (ER). Signal peptidase in the ER cleaves p110 to the capsid (*cyan*), E2 (*blue*), and E1 (*red*) proteins. (*j*) The capsid is suggested to assemble with genomic RNA into nucleocapsid on the rough ER and then to be transported to the Golgi by interactions with E2 and/or the E2–E1 dimer. (*k, l*) E2–E1 heterodimers are transported to the Golgi, where RUBV assembly and budding take place. (*m, n*) Transport vesicles deliver mature RUBV from the Golgi to the cell surface. During the process of maturation, immature particles with a uniformly dense core are believed to mature into particles with a defined internal core well separated from the virus membrane, while the smooth exterior adopts a spiky appearance. (Republished with permission of American Society for Microbiology from Das PK, Kielian M. Molecular and structural insights into the life cycle of rubella virus. *J Virol* 2021;95(10):e02349–20; permission conveyed through Copyright Clearance Center, Inc.)

Replication Complexes

Similar to all other RNA viruses that infect mammalian cells, replication of RUBV RNA occurs in association with cellular membranes. Cytoplasmic vacuoles (Fig. 4.6) with regularly shaped invaginations or spherules (60 nm in diameter) are present in RUBV-infected cells.[142] The spherules are connected to vacuolar membranes by thin membranous necks and can be stained with antibodies against p150 and double-stranded RNA, indicating that they are the sites of viral RNA synthesis.[134,143] These vacuoles are likely derived from endosomes and/or possibly lysosomes.[155]

Replication complexes in RUBV-infected cells have been analyzed using electron microscopy and freeze fracture techniques.[76] The replication of viral RNA occurs within protected membranous pockets of the cytopathic vacuoles. The vacuoles are surrounded by rough ER, an arrangement that may facilitate binding between RNA and the capsid protein (which is synthesized on the surface of the ER) to promote nucleocapsid formation. In a number of fundamental aspects, RUBV replication complexes are similar to those found in alphavirus-infected cells.[83] However, there are several important distinctions between them. First, assembled nucleocapsids are rarely observed near replication complexes in RUBV-infected cells. In contrast, nucleocapsids often surround the replication complexes of alphavirus-infected cells. In RUBV-infected cells, formation of the replication complexes coincides with the rearrangement of other cellular structures. Specifically, rough ER and Golgi are in close proximity to the virus-modified endocytic organelles, and mitochondria cluster to regions of the cell containing replication complexes.[140,142] Although mitochondrial aggregation in the vicinity of replication complexes also occurs in alphavirus-infected cells, the close association of the rough ER and Golgi with replication complexes is unique to RUBV-infected cells. Recruitment of ER and Golgi membranes to the replication complexes may be necessary to coordinate translation of the structural proteins and packaging of the genomic RNA. Mitochondria are also recruited to the replication complexes and have long been known to play an important role in RUBV replication.[9] This led to speculation that the close association of these organelles with replication complexes may increase the availability of ATP for virus replication, but solid evidence to support this theory is lacking.

Targeting of Structural Proteins to the Budding Site

Following synthesis of the subgenomic RNA, the RUBV structural proteins are translated in association with ER membranes. The structural polyprotein precursor is cleaved by signal peptidase at two sites (Fig. 4.9) to generate the three structural proteins.[105,110] The structural proteins are then posttranslationally modified and transported to the Golgi complex, which is the primary site of virus budding. Processing and transport of RUBV structural proteins have been extensively studied using transfection experiments. When coexpressed, E2 and E1 heterodimerize, form intramolecular disulfide bonds in the ER, and are transported to and retained in the Golgi.[13,112] Targeting of the virus glycoproteins to the Golgi complex is independent of capsid, indicating that accumulation of E2 and E1 in this organelle is the major factor in determining the budding site. In the absence of E2, E1 does not target to the Golgi but rather is retained in a smooth ER compartment.[111] The membrane proximal regions of the structural proteins have important roles in regulating the localization and transport of these proteins. For example, within the transmembrane and the cytoplasmic domains of E1 resides an ER retention signal that prevents or delays transport of nascent viral glycoproteins from the ER.[106] Coexpression of E2 appears to mask the ER retention signal in E1, thereby allowing transport of the E2–E1 heterocomplex from the ER to the Golgi after a maturation period. The transmembrane domain of E2, in turn, contains a retention signal that mediates retention of the E2–E1 heterodimer in the Golgi.[113]

The highly regulated transport of RUBV glycoproteins may serve as a quality control mechanism to ensure that only properly assembled subunits reach the virus-budding site. The half-life for transport of the RUBV glycoproteins to the Golgi is 60 to 90 minutes (whereas for alphavirus glycoproteins, it is ~25 minutes).[104] Dimerization of E1 and E2 in the ER is not rate limiting as evidenced by the fact that these two proteins associate rapidly following synthesis. E2 achieves its mature conformation shortly after synthesis and has been proposed to function as a scaffold for E1. Accordingly, the rate-limiting step for transport of the glycoproteins is the relatively slow maturation and folding of E1 in the ER.[112] The mature ectodomain of E1 contains 20 cysteine residues that participate in the formation of intramolecular disulfide bonds.[97] It is hypothesized that the ER retention signal in E1 is required to retain nascent E1 in the ER until it has achieved the proper conformation, which includes the formation of intramolecular disulfide bonds. Indeed, replacing the E1 transmembrane domain with analogous domains from other membrane glycoproteins actually increases the rate of ER to Golgi transport for E1 and E2.[86] The E2 transmembrane and cytoplasmic domains are required for assembly of E2–E1 heterodimers and therefore have an indirect role in regulating transport of the RUBV glycoproteins from the ER to the Golgi. Finally, mutagenesis studies have shown that N-linked glycosylation is important for maturation and intracellular transport of both E1 and E2 glycoproteins.[109,221]

As well as regulating targeting of E1 to the Golgi complex, E2 is required for transport of the capsid protein to the intracellular budding site.[13,108] The carboxyl terminus of E2, which includes the transmembrane and cytoplasmic domains, is essential for this process[86] and formation of VLPs[135] and likely infectious virions. Lateral interactions between the E2 signal peptide and the transmembrane regions of E2 and/or E1 may facilitate transport of capsid from the ER to the Golgi by incorporation into ER-derived transport vesicles. In contrast, the analogous regions of E1 are not required for localization of capsid to the juxtanuclear region. Together, these results indicate that the E2 carboxyl terminus governs the targeting of all three RUBV structural proteins to the virus-budding site.

Virus Assembly and Secretion

RUBV budding has been reported to occur at both the Golgi complex and the plasma membrane, depending on cell type and the time postinfection.[12,275] However, several lines of evidence suggest that the primary site for virus budding is the Golgi complex. First, the presence of a signal in E2 mediates retention of the structural proteins in the Golgi complex, and consequently, only a small fraction of the RUBV structural proteins reaches the plasma membrane.[112,113] Second, budding at the plasma membrane reportedly occurs late in infection, suggesting that this is not the principal budding site. Furthermore, virion membrane composition is more similar to that of intracellular membranes rather than the plasma membrane.[10]

Unlike alphavirus nucleocapsids, which are formed in the cytoplasm of infected cells prior to budding, RUBV nucleocapsids form in association with cellular membranes coincident with budding and are rarely observed in the cytoplasm of infected cells.[144] This suggests that RUBV employs a mechanism to prevent premature assembly of nucleocapsids (Fig. 4.11). Reversible phosphorylation of the RNA-binding region of capsid could regulate assembly and disassembly of RUBV nucleocapsids.[136,137] Subsequently, it was reported that a similar mechanism regulates binding of genomic RNA to alphavirus capsid proteins.[34,35]

The mechanisms that regulate interactions between the nucleocapsid and spike glycoproteins during virus budding are largely unknown. With respect to the budding reaction, it is tempting to speculate that electrostatic interactions between the cytoplasmic domain of E2, which is rich in basic amino acid residues, and clusters of acidic amino acid residues in the capsid are involved. Indeed, the manner in which RUBV capsid proteins are arranged in rows suggests that they can interact with the E2 cytoplasmic tail.[157] Moreover, nonconservative mutations in this segment of E2 drastically affect the assembly of VLPs.[86] It is also well established that the transmembrane domains of the structural proteins are important for targeting to the budding site. In this respect, lateral interactions between the transmembrane domains of E1, E2, and capsid protein may be important for the budding reaction. Finally, it is possible that interactions between RUBV structural proteins and host cell proteins contribute to efficient budding of virus particles.

Freeze-substitution electron microscopy revealed that rubella virions undergo a maturation process following budding into the Golgi.[233] At early time points, intra-Golgi virions exhibited homogenous interiors with fine contacts between the core and the particle membrane. Later, the virion cores appeared denser and were smaller in diameter such that they were clearly delineated from the virion membrane. These results indicate that the virion maturation process involves compaction of the nucleocapsid. Similar results were reported from tomographic studies of immature and mature RUBV virions, which also showed that E1 protrudes out more on mature particles giving them a more spiky appearance.[156] Several lines of evidence suggest that the E1 transmembrane and cytoplasmic domains also function in virion maturation and/or secretion. Replacement of the E1 transmembrane domain does not affect budding of VLPs in the Golgi, but secretion of the particles into the extracellular space is blocked.[85] Similarly, introduction of point mutations into the E1 transmembrane and/or cytoplasmic domains drastically reduces virus secretion without affecting the assembly process at the Golgi.[225,295] These rather surprising data indicate that virus assembly at the Golgi complex is not coupled to secretion and that E1 is involved in a late-stage maturation event that is necessary for virus secretion.

There is limited information regarding the interactions between RUBV virions and polarized cells. Because it causes a systemic infection, the virus must cross one or more epithelial layers, including the upper respiratory epithelium. Cultured epithelial cells can be infected from the apical and basal membranes, indicating that RUBV receptors are not confined to one surface.[85] The secretion of virus particles varies according to cell type. In two of the three polarized cell lines examined, virions were released primarily from the apical surface, but significant quantities were also secreted from the basolateral membrane. Presumably, secretion of rubella virions from the apical surface facilitates virus spread from person to person, whereas basolateral secretion could be important for establishing a systemic infection and/or crossing the placenta prior to fetal infection.

RUBV Persistence

RUBV can induce cell death by apoptosis in highly permissive cell lines that are infected at high MOI. However, infection of many cell types at low MOI often results in little cytopathology and viral persistence in vitro.[1,3,82,290] RUBV-infected cells are quite resistant to a variety of apoptotic stimuli as a result of interaction between the capsid protein and the host protein Bax.[121] These findings are consistent with earlier observations that while temperature-sensitive mutants and defective interfering (DI) particles develop in and may play a role in controlling replication in persistently infected cells, neither is required to establish persistent infection.[82,290] During long-term persistence in RUBV-infected Vero cells, DI RNAs become the dominant species of viral RNA with genomic RNA decreasing to low levels. Persistence in cultured cells is thus a chronic infection with the majority of cells expressing viral antigen and RNA, much of which is DI RNA. These cultures release low levels of temperature-sensitive progeny virus and DI particles. Finally, while it cannot be ruled out that interferons play a role in viral persistence, they are clearly not essential because persistent RUBV infections can be established in interferon-deficient cell lines such as Vero and BHK-/21 cells.[251] Moreover, exogenous interferon was not found to have an effect on RUBV persistence in these cell lines.

The virus can persist for many months in congenitally infected human fetuses, and multiple organ systems are affected (see "Mechanisms of Teratogenesis"). Following postnatal infection, PBMCs are an established reservoir for RUBV persistence in vivo, particularly in adults who develop rubella-associated arthritis following natural infection or immunization.[41] Viral persistence in vivo occurs in the presence of high levels of neutralizing antibody, which may not only limit viral spread but has even been suggested to promote viral persistence. To date, however, this theory has yet to be substantiated. Another site of persistence in vivo is joint tissue,[45,79] which has led to speculation that RUBV plays a role in development of degenerative joint disease (see "Complications").

In vitro, both wt+ and vaccine strains of RUBV can infect and persist in chondrocyte-derived cell lines[42] and in primary cultures of human joint tissue.[172] Except for the Cendehill vaccine strain, all other RUBV strains can replicate and persist in joint tissue for more than 3 months. Interestingly, virus derived from these chronically infected cultures was temperature sensitive, but no DI particles were detected.

Animal Models of Rubella Virus Infection

There are no reliable animal models for the study of clinically symptomatic rubella infection, even though a variety of laboratory animals (including nonhuman primates) can be asymptomatically infected with RUBV. Rhesus and African green monkeys develop viremia, shed virus in respiratory secretions, and produce humoral immune responses in a manner that is similar to acute rubella in humans.[115] However, attempts to model the teratogenic effects of rubella in various animals, including baboons, cynomolgus monkeys, marmosets, and rats, have produced inconsistent results with, at best, low incidence of defects such as cataracts or stillbirths.[281,285] Infection of the central nervous system (CNS) has been shown to occur in immunosuppressed BALB/c mice, and as such, it is possible that this system could work as a small animal model to understand the effects of RUBV on the brain.[160] Unfortunately, none of the animal systems has proven sufficiently reliable to study details of the pathogenesis of either acquired or congenital rubella.

Antigenic Composition and Determinants

Complement-Fixing and Hemagglutinating Antigens

Early serologic tests for rubella used crude complement fixation antigens extracted from virus-infected cells and purified on sucrose gradients. A more slowly sedimenting fraction from the gradients with a density of 1.08 to 1.10 in sucrose (as compared to a density of 1.18 to 1.20 for intact virions) was shown to have hemagglutinating (HA) activity.[267] HA activity is also associated with cell-free virus preparations[119] and can be extracted from infected cells or supernatant virus using Tween-80 and ether, resulting in a 26S particle that retains biological activity. By electron microscopy, it appears as a 15-nm rosette with a hollow core.[266]

B-Cell Epitopes

The E1 glycoprotein is the immunodominant surface molecule of the virus particle as evidenced by the fact that it is the major target for the host's humoral immune system.[292] Antibodies to both E2 and capsid are also found in humans, although at lower levels and of lower avidity. Mapping of antigenic domains on the viral proteins were first carried out using monoclonal antibodies.[292] Later, detailed studies on the fine antigenic structure of each viral protein were carried out using recombinant proteins, proteolytic peptide fragments, and synthetic peptides to deduce antigenic sites.[47,167,174] At least five distinct nonoverlapping immunoreactive regions were identified in the E1 protein ($E1_{11-39}$, $E1_{154-179}$, $E1_{199-239}$, $E1_{226-277}$, and $E1_{389-412}$). Cellular proliferative responses to these peptides were found in 29% to 83% of the subjects tested,[174] including one peptide ($E1_{208-239}$) that contained a previously identified neutralization domain.[293] When incorporated into a peptide-based enzyme-linked immunoassay (ELISA), reactivity with this peptide correlates well with results from conventional ELISAs that measure hemagglutination assay inhibition (HAI) and viral neutralization titers.[60,177] Four of the B-cell epitopes on RUBV E1 are conserved among E1 proteins of two other rubiviruses (Ruhugu and Rustrela viruses).[21] To date, two B-cell epitopes have been identified on the capsid protein, C_{1-30} and C_{96-123}, and one ($E2_{31-105}$) on the E2 glycoprotein.[47,167,195]

T-Cell Epitopes

There are at least 17 RUBV-specific T-cell epitopes, but the precise limit of each epitope is not known.[167,174,194] A minimum of four immunodominant sites are located on E1, and these display reactivity to T cells from several donors with different HLA haplotype backgrounds.[200] Subsequently, minimal T helper cell epitopes were identified at $E1_{280-287}$, $E1_{385-393}$, and $E1_{410-420}$ using T-cell lines from seropositive healthy donors, with variation in responsiveness found between individuals.[160] Interestingly, binding of the peptide $E1_{272-285}$ to HLA-DR and its recognition by RUBV-specific clones is influenced by DRβ polymorphisms.[199]

At least three T-cell epitopes have been found on the E2 protein.[174,194] One of these peptides ($E2_{54-65}$) is present in approximately 50% of T-cell lines derived from donors with the HLA-DR7 phenotype.[192] Epitopes on the capsid protein do not appear to be well conserved among rubiviruses with the exception of two potential T-cell epitopes shared between RUBV and Ruhugu virus.[21] A peptide ($C_{265-273}$) within the RUBV capsid is recognized by T-cell clones derived from donors expressing the DRB1*0403 and DRB1*0901 alleles.[193] However, this peptide is recognized promiscuously by HLA-DR molecules that have common residues in pocket 4 of the peptide-binding groove and therefore likely defines a DR supertype.[198]

EPIDEMIOLOGY

Incidence

Prior to the introduction of immunization programs, rubella was endemic worldwide, with regular seasonal peaks occurring in the spring months in temperate climates. In addition, epidemics of rubella occurred at intervals of 6 to 9 years as the pool of susceptible individuals reached a threshold. Epidemics still occur in developing and tropical countries, but the lack of effective monitoring programs, together with the absence of serious clinical symptoms in affected children, has made them difficult to assess.[236] Regional variation in the age of onset of rubella, the incidence of the disease, and the appearance and spread of epidemics are determined by population densities, socioeconomic factors, and levels of medical sophistication in a given community. When these rubella outbreaks occur, they are accompanied by birth defects associated with congenital rubella syndrome (CRS). The teratogenic effects of rubella were a significant factor that spurred vaccine development following the rubella pandemic between 1962 and 1965. In this epidemic alone, an estimated 12.5 million cases of rubella occurred in the United States alone, resulting in up to 20,000 children born with congenital abnormalities.[38] Today, fully documented and reported CRS cases have been reduced to a handful of cases in both Europe and North America. A declaration by the Centers for Disease Control and Prevention (CDC) in 2005 stated that endemic CRS had been eliminated from the United States,[2] and subsequently, as of the end of 2019, 81 countries have eliminated transmission of the virus.[206] Residual cases of rubella can still be associated with immigrants who may not have been immunized in their country of origin.[22] Indeed, multiple countries in Africa and Asia remain susceptible to rubella (Fig. 4.1) where hundreds of cases of CRS cases are still reported annually. The number of true cases of RUBV-linked teratogenesis is highly under reported, and by some estimates, there are still more than 100,000 infants born with CRS annually.

Age

Prior to introduction of universal rubella immunization, peak infection occurred in the 5- to 9-year-old age group.[116] After vaccine implementation, the disease shifted from children to young adults until its virtual elimination from Europe and North America in recent years.[39] In countries that have not implemented vaccination programs, infection at an early age is still the norm, with high seroconversion rates found in both preschool populations and in the 5- to 9-year-old age group.[91] A notable exception is Japan, a country in which rubella has not yet been eliminated and where 95% of infections occur in adults.[254] Finally, in some developing countries, women of childbearing age are susceptible to rubella and the incidence of CRS during rubella outbreaks can be 1 to 2 per 1,000 live births.[64]

Origin and Spread of Epidemics

There are no animal reservoirs for RUBV and therefore continued cycling of the virus within the human population is required for perpetuation of the disease between seasons of maximal endemic occurrence. In countries where rubella immunization is not carried out and congenital infection still occurs, the surviving infants shed high levels of virus for many months, forming a potential source for maintenance of the virus for relatively long periods. Enhanced vaccination programs have been very effective in disrupting virus circulation in much of the developed world. However, localized outbreaks of rubella still occur when vaccine refusal occurs on the basis of religious grounds[16,38] or when distribution of uptake of vaccine is interrupted by war.[120] Together, these studies demonstrate the importance of maintaining high levels of herd immunity in developed countries, because rubella can be reintroduced into the population by foreign travel or from recent immigrants travelling from endemic areas. To prevent outbreaks, it has been estimated that at least 85% of the population must be immune to RUBV,[4] whereas to maintain elimination, a 90% level of immunity among children is required.[102]

Molecular Epidemiology

Based on sequence comparison of the E1 gene, at least one genotypes of RUBV representing two clades (RG1 and 2) have been identified[300] (Fig. 4.3). The RG1 clade comprises viral isolates from North America, Europe, and Japan, whereas RG2 was identified using isolates from China and India. RG1 and RG2 differ by 8% to 10% at the nucleotide level, as opposed to less than 5% among genotypes within each clade. RG2 has more genetic diversity than RGI and may in fact consist of multiple clades. These genetic differences have been useful in tracking RUBV spread around the world and changes in endemic strains over time. Nevertheless, the differences in E1 genes result in only 1% to 3% substitutions at the amino acid, attesting to a high degree of genetic conservation between rubella strains. Finally, only one strain from clade 2 contained a mutation in one of the known epitopes defined by monoclonal antibodies, the first indication of a serotype variant.

CLINICAL FEATURES

Acute Rubella

Postnatal infection with RUBV is usually mild and frequently subclinical.[8,74] Typical symptoms, when present, include sore throat and low-grade fever, a maculopapular rash, lymphadenopathy, and, in some cases, conjunctivitis and/or arthralgia. The rash (Fig. 4.15) is first seen on the face and spreads in centripetal fashion. The lesions appear as distinct pink maculopapules that fade rapidly over several days. A pronounced posterior cervical and suboccipital adenopathy is often present. In the majority of cases, the clinical syndrome clears in days and is seldom attended by more significant symptoms, but arthropathy, thrombocytopenia, and encephalopathy can occur.[24] However, serious sequelae and death as a result of RUBV infection are rare. The course of the acquired infection and the accompanying immune response is shown in Figure 4.16.

The virus is transmitted through respiratory secretions and the mucosa of the upper respiratory tract and the nasopharyngeal lymphoid tissue serve as portals of virus entry as well as the initial sites for viral replication. Spread of virus via lymphatics

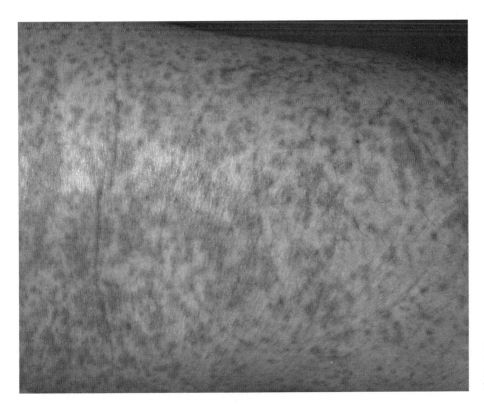

FIGURE 4.15 Characteristic skin rash on patient with acute rubella. (Reproduced with permission from VisualDx.)

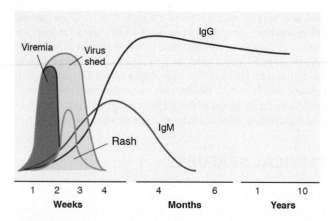

FIGURE 4.16 Time course showing viremic phase, rash, and IgM and IgG development during acute rubella from the time of infection initiation by droplet spray. Patients are infectious and shed virus from the time of infection until 1 to 2 weeks after the appearance of rash. IgM is present by day 10 and peaks around 4 weeks postinfection, by which time low-avidity IgG is also present.

or a transient viremia then seeds regional lymph nodes. Local replication of virus in these nodes accounts for the posterior cervical and occipital nodal enlargement that typically appears 5 to 9 days before the onset of the rash. The incubation period (~14 days) is followed by the appearance of virus in serum, and the onset of viral shedding into the nasopharynx and stool, providing a source of spread to susceptible individuals. High levels of virus can be found in nasopharyngeal secretions, exceeding 10^5 TCID$_{50}$ per 0.1 mL even in vaccinated individuals.[8] The viremic phase may be marked by mild prodromal symptoms and malaise. The maculopapular rash appears at 14 to 21 days after natural exposure, but somewhat earlier following experimental infection or vaccination. The presence of virus in serum ceases shortly after the rash appears, coincident with the onset of detectable circulating antibodies.

Immune Response

A serologic response can be detected at the onset of rash and continues to evolve over the next few weeks (Fig. 4.16). Generally, IgM antibody is first detected at 10 days postinfection after which peak levels occur at 4 weeks postinfection but can persist for more than 7 months after acute infection.[241,258] By 3 weeks, RUBV-specific antibodies are present in all immunoglobulin classes, including IgG, IgA, IgD, and IgE. At early stages of primary infection, IgG is of low avidity, maturing gradually during the next 3 months.[31]

When measured by immunoprecipitation or immunoblot techniques, the majority of the immunoglobulin response appears to be directed at the E1 glycoprotein, with proportionally lesser amounts of the response against E2 or capsid.[46] Interestingly, males have a more rapid and robust antibody response than females, although females have a higher anti-E2 response.[178] Whether there are pathological consequences of these differences is not known.

Transient depression of lymphocyte responsiveness to mitogenic stimulation follows natural or vaccine infections in children and adults.[32] Despite this generalized immune suppression, RUBV-specific cell-mediated immune responses develop and can be measured *in vitro* within 1 or 2 weeks of onset of

clinical illness. The cellular responses wane over the next few years but persist at low levels indefinitely after natural rubella. In contrast, they are difficult to detect following vaccination. More detailed studies have defined the epitope specificity of defined CD4+ and CD8+ T-cell clones[151,194,197] (see "Antigenic Composition and Determinants").

Complications

Joint symptoms

The most common complications of natural rubella are acute arthralgia and/or arthritis, particularly in adolescent and adult women.[248] Incidence rates for joint involvement range between 30% and 60% during outbreaks. For example, in one report, 52% of adult females and 9% of adult males developed arthropathy, with symptoms being more severe among women.[259] The joint symptoms usually begin within a week of the appearance of the rash and may involve any joint, with the fingers and knees being most commonly affected. Although these symptoms usually resolve within several weeks, they can persist for months or even years, in which case they are episodic. Rarely, chronic severe arthropathy that is significantly disabling has been reported.[41] A similar range of less severe symptoms occurs 9 to 27 days following vaccination but is less common than after natural rubella.[259] A report on rubella vaccine-associated arthritis, based on analysis of the Vaccine Adverse Events Reporting System (VAERS) database, has confirmed that rubella vaccine in adult women is associated with chronic arthritis that can persist for at least 1 year.[88]

Factors that affect the incidence of joint symptoms include age and gender,[259] as well as MHC type of the infected individual.[175] Hormonal influences also affect the incidence of joint symptoms with adult females being most susceptible. The underlying pathogenesis of rubella arthritis is unknown, but the mechanism may involve local viral replication. Several groups have reported the isolation of RUBV from synovial fluids of symptomatic joints for up to a month following acute infection.[79,183] Virus has also been isolated from PBMCs of symptomatic individuals[41] and can be detected in women with chronic arthropathy postvaccination by reverse transcriptase–polymerase chain reaction (RT-PCR) amplification of PBMC RNA using RUBV-specific primers.[176] Replication and persistence of virus in extra-articular sites and deposition of immune complexes on articular surfaces may therefore play a role in the acute stage.

RUBV can also infect and persist in joint tissue for prolonged periods *in vitro*, forming foci of infection that are positive for viral antigen.[172] Overall, the body of evidence indicates that RUBV is a highly arthrotropic virus and a plausible candidate as one of several viral triggers (including human parvovirus, hepatitis C, and HTLV-1) of chronic degenerative forms of arthritis.

Thrombocytopenia

A number of different viral infections result in reduced platelets either by inhibiting their production or causing their lysis.[225] For example, binding of viral immune complexes to Fc receptors on the platelet surface triggers immune-mediated clearing of both the complex and its associated platelet.[129] This causes a transient asymptomatic depression of thrombocyte counts and is quite common with rubella.[58] Thrombocytopenic purpura is seen following rubella infection; however, this condition is relatively rare (1 in 1,500 cases)[271] and is usually self-limiting. However, it may even occur in the absence of rash. Accordingly, undiagnosed RUBV infections are likely the cause of some cases of idiopathic thrombocytopenic purpura. Very rarely is epidemic rubella associated with hemolytic anemia.

Encephalopathy

The most serious complication of postnatal rubella is postinfectious encephalopathy or encephalomyelitis.[20] Estimated to occur in 1 in 6,000 cases of natural infection, rubella encephalitis is rarely reported in countries with comprehensive vaccination policies. However, occasionally, case reports indicate that this disorder can appear during rubella outbreaks. The symptoms of rubella encephalopathy appear abruptly 1 to 6 days following the onset of rash in an otherwise typical case of rubella. It has been reported that fatal rubella encephalitis can present without rash.[27] The most frequently encountered symptoms include headache, vomiting, stiff neck, lethargy, and generalized convulsions.[282] In rare cases, RUBV antigens have been detected within brain tissue,[57] and virus has been isolated from CSF, indicating that it has the capacity to invade the mature CNS.[249]

Postnatal rubella encephalopathy usually requires only supportive treatment, and the disease course is often concluded within a few days; the survival rate is approximating 80%. Among the 20% of patients who do not survive, the disease course typically includes coma, respiratory distress, apnea, and then death, usually within a few days of onset of symptoms.

Congenital Rubella Syndrome

Although postnatal rubella is rarely associated with severe complications, infection *in utero* following transplacental transmission of virus from the mother has dire consequences for the developing fetus. These are reflected in a constellation of symptoms collectively called congenital rubella syndrome.[58,285]

Pathogenesis of Congenital Rubella Syndrome

In general, maternal infection shortly before conception does not lead to intrauterine infection.[75] However, when infection occurs after conception, the virus is present in placental villi approximately 10 days after the onset of rash in the mother and can be detected in the fetus after 20 to 30 days.[127] Transplacental transmission occurs in up to 90% of cases during the first 8 weeks of gestation, falling to a low of 25% to 35% during the second trimester and rising again near term.[8,87,285] This fluctuating incidence of fetal infection is likely related to changes in the placenta during pregnancy. In early gestation, infection of the placenta causes scattered foci of necrotic syncytiotrophoblast and cytotrophoblast cells, as well as damage to the vascular endothelium, resulting in placental hypoplasia.[87] Infection at later stages is associated with multifocal mononuclear cell infiltrates in the placental membranes, cord, and decidua, along with vasculitis.[285] In cases where fetal infection occurs, the virus can spread widely and almost any organ may be infected. A chronic and generally nonlytic infection is then established in the fetus.[210]

Clinical Consequences

The effects of RUBV invasion of fetal tissue are quite varied, and early infection may result in resorption of the embryo. Whether placental infection alone can lead to spontaneous

TABLE 4.1	Manifestations of congenital rubella syndrome
Group A	**Group B**
Eye manifestations • Cataracts • Congenital glaucoma • Retinitis Congenital heart defects • Patent ductus arteriosus • Pulmonary artery stenosis Sensorineural hearing loss Pigmentary neuropathy	Purpura Hepatosplenomegaly Jaundice Microcephaly Meningoencephalitis Radiolucent bone disease Progressive or late-onset manifestations • Mental retardation • Diabetes mellitus • Progressive panencephalitis

abortion or abnormalities of fetal development is not established. In the majority of cases, the infected fetus will survive and the pregnancy continues to term, with premature delivery or stillbirths being rare outcomes.[173] In many countries, clinically recognized maternal rubella during the first 8 weeks of gestation is an indication for therapeutic abortion due to the high incidence of congenital defects. Although these are not universal, some degree of neurologic deficit including sensorineural deafness is found in most cases. The current rubella vaccine RA27/3 has extremely low teratogenicity, and inadvertent vaccination in early pregnancy is not considered an indication for therapeutic abortion, although immunization at this time should be avoided.[37,214]

The most common clinical manifestations of congenital rubella are listed in Table 4.1. In addition to the high incidence of sensorineural deafness (~80%), cataracts are detected in 50% to 60% of neonates infected in the first 8 weeks of pregnancy.[8] Congenital heart disease is also found in more than half of CRS babies, usually manifested as patent ductus arteriosus or pulmonary artery or valvular stenosis. Other common defects include glaucoma, retinopathy, psychomotor retardation, neonatal thrombocytopenia purpura, hepatomegaly and/or splenomegaly, and intrauterine growth retardation.[58] Less frequent features (present in 5% to 10%) include adenopathy, bony radiolucencies, hepatitis, and hemolytic anemia. Many of the clinical manifestations of congenital rubella are evident at birth or shortly thereafter. This includes a reddish-blue (purpuric) maculopapular rash termed the "blueberry muffin" rash (Fig. 4.17). Other clinical signs, including hepatosplenomegaly and jaundice, usually resolve within weeks. In addition, there are defects that are not recognized at birth but may be manifest in childhood (e.g., mental or physical retardation) or in adolescence (type 1 diabetes).

At birth, CRS is accompanied by clinical signs that include bulging anterior fontanel, microcephaly, lethargy, irritability, and motor tone abnormalities.[285] RUBV can be isolated from almost any organ at birth and from selected tissues for up to 1 year or more in surviving infants.[171] More than 80% of congenitally infected newborns contain substantial amounts of RUBV in their nasopharyngeal secretions and urine, and 3% will continue to shed virus for as long as 20 months. This chronic shedding of RUBV by neonates is an indicator of early

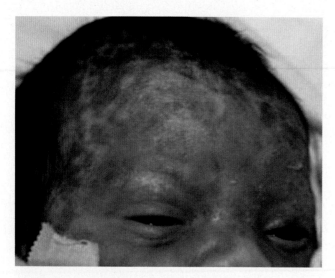

FIGURE 4.17 Infant with congenital rubella showing characteristic "blueberry muffin" maculopapular rash. (Reprinted with permission from Mehta V, Balachandran C, Lonikar V. Blueberry muffin baby: a pictoral differential diagnosis. *Dermatol Online J.* 2008;14(2):8. https://dx.doi.org/10.5070/D353q852nc. Retrieved from https://escholarship.org/uc/item/53q852nc.)

gestational infection[62] and a major source of virus for dissemination to others.

Mechanisms of Teratogenesis

Most of our information on rubella embryopathy comes from pathological analyses conducted following the major rubella pandemic of the 1960s. Together, these analyses supported the notion that the direct cytolytic effects of RUBV in cells of the retinal epithelium, myocardium, skeletal muscle, and neural tissue and inflammation associated vascular injury and systemic spread underlie much of the observed damage in CRS.[133,138,237,263] The widespread nature of the tissue damage indicates that RUBV infects most fetal organ systems. Infection of focal clones of cells and their progeny during critical stages of the ontogeny of fetal organs was believed to give rise to the wide range of abnormalities that together comprise CRS.

Because there are no animal models that recapitulate the teratogenic effects of RUBV infection, the direct effects of the on human fetal cells *in situ* can only be extrapolated from studies in cell culture. Multiple studies reporting that cultured cells infected with RUBV exhibited signs of apoptosis[73,114,139,169,217] and that human embryonic cells persistently infected with RUBV produce lower levels of collagen and are less responsive to epidermal growth factor[297] led to the hypothesis that altered cell physiology and induction of programmed cell death were integral to the teratogenic activity of the virus. However, a later study reported that RUBV infection does not induce apoptosis in human embryonic fibroblasts but rather induces expression of multiple of antiapoptotic genes.[3] These findings are consistent with a more recent report showing that the capsid protein blocks apoptosis in human embryonic and adult-cultured cell lines.[121] Morphological and transcriptomic analyses of RUBV-infected human-induced pluripotent stem cells that were differentiated into different embryonic lineages showed that viral infection induces chromatin remodeling and host gene expression changes that would be expected to affect human

development.[28] Accordingly, it seems likely that a predominantly noncytopathic RUBV infection of selected embryonic cell types *in utero* upsets the normal delicate balance of cellular growth and differentiation and has profound effects on organogenesis. These effects, alone or in concert, could explain the observation that the small but otherwise apparently normal organs of congenital rubella infants contain reduced numbers of cells.[181] Finally, demyelination associated with infection of oligodendrocytes, which express the known RUBV receptor myelin oligodendrocyte glycoprotein, may also play a role in the pathologies associated with CRS.[7] In addition to these direct effects of RUBV replication in host tissue, it is possible that immune-mediated damage occurs in CRS.

Fetal Immune Response in CRS

The persistence of RUBV in fetal tissue throughout gestation, and in infants with CRS for prolonged periods after birth, raises the question of how the virus avoids immune elimination. Clearly, neither transferred maternal IgG nor fetal IgM (detected at around 15 weeks' gestation[285]) can eliminate virus *in utero*, although both have neutralizing capacity *in vitro*.[59] It has been suggested that antibody may in fact promote persistence; however, this phenomenon has only been observed *in vitro*,[1,40] and it is not at all clear whether it can occur in the absence of the complement system and phagocytic cells. Multiple studies suggest that the ability of RUBV to block apoptosis may also play a role establishment and/or maintenance of persistence by thwarting innate antiviral defenses.[3,121] Moreover, because the thymus does not mature until 15 weeks, the fetus is highly vulnerable to viral infection prior to this time. Interferon-α is present early in gestation and therefore may limit viral spread; a scenario that could explain why only 0.1% to 0.001% of cells from fetal organs contained detectable virus.[227]

Postnatal infection induces IgG class antibodies against each of the three structural proteins of the virus; however, CRS infants often lack antibodies to the capsid protein and demonstrate weak humoral reactivity to the E2 protein.[68,220] Perhaps more telling, these children show selective tolerance to the E1 protein[166] and, more specifically, possess little or no antibody to the putative E1 neutralization domain.[177,220]

Infants with CRS also demonstrate prolonged impairment of RUBV-specific cell-mediated immune responses, including cytotoxicity, and lymphokine secretion *in vitro*.[32,68] T-cell lines derived from several congenital rubella children and adults failed to respond to RUBV peptides that stimulate lymphocyte proliferative responses in normal immune adult donor cells.[194] These data suggest that early fetal infection results in selective immune tolerance to a limited but critical number of RUBV epitopes that must be recognized to clear the virus.

Late-Onset Sequelae

Although many of the effects of fetal rubella that manifest at birth are transient, some defects such as retinopathy, mental retardation, hearing loss, and endocrine abnormalities may not become clinically apparent for several years.[168,244] Psychomotor retardation (62%), cardiac abnormalities (58%), and mental retardation (42%) are also associated with CRS, and multiorgan disease is found in 88% of patients.[90]

Delayed endocrine disease

Congenital rubella infection is also associated with a variety of delayed endocrine abnormalities, including type 1 diabetes, thyroid disease, and polyglandular autoimmunity.[224,244] Early reports suggested that type 1 diabetes occurs in as many as 10% to 40% of CRS patients. However, while more recent analyses from a diabetes-focused perspective confirmed that *in utero* RUBV infection undoubtedly predisposes to diabetes, the proportion is probably less than 10%.[84] Conversely, postnatal rubella does not have a clear association with type 1 diabetes.[29]

The mechanism by which RUBV causes diabetes is not understood, and certainly, the lack of a suitable animal model has limited progress in this area. However, a number of older studies in hamsters have provided some intriguing results. For example, Syrian hamster pups infected with an adapted rubella RA 27/3 vaccine virus exhibited hypoinsulinemia and hyperglycemia.[228] In these animals, cell-free RUBV was recoverable from pancreas, viral antigens were present in islet cells, and a mononuclear infiltration of the islets occurred over the first 3 weeks of the infection. Moreover, islet cell antibodies developed in 40% of the infected pups.

RUBV-induced damage to the pancreas may therefore be a combination of viral replication in islets, compounded by the triggering of an autoimmune reaction that perpetuates beta cell damage. Evidence in favor of this theory includes the identification of a monoclonal antibody to RUBV capsid protein that reacts with pancreatic islet cell Ia2 protein.[126] In addition, CD4 and CD8 T-cell clones isolated from CRS patients recognize peptides of the diabetes-associated autoantigen GAD65 in an HLA-restricted manner.[196,201] Also, 20% to 40% of sera from CRS patients in a selected series were found to contain antibodies that react with thyroid tissue.[54,89,245] Finally, CRS is also associated with growth hormone deficiency, and therefore, pituitary involvement is another complication. Relatedly, hamsters immunized with recombinant RUBV E1 or E2 were observed to develop pituitary autoantibodies.[298] In summary, these observations suggest that viral-induced autoimmune mechanisms may partially account for the late appearance of polyendocrine diseases that frequently complicate congenital rubella.

Delayed neurologic disease

A rare late-onset encephalitis following rubella has been described, referred to as progressive rubella panencephalitis (PRP).[264,286] Like other slow viral diseases of the CNS, PRP is characterized by a prolonged asymptomatic period, followed by the onset of symptoms of neural deterioration during the second decade of life. The pathogenesis of PRP is unclear; however, immune complexes are consistently identified, suggesting ongoing viral replication.[61] The near complete destruction of Purkinje cells indicates either some degree of selective tropism of RUBV for these cells within the CNS or a negative effect on their metabolism. This could also account for the selective loss of myelin and oligodendroglia, although immunopathological mechanisms could also be active.

DIAGNOSIS

Differential

The most common symptoms of rubella (lymphadenopathy, erythematous rash, and low-grade fever) can be readily confused with similar illnesses associated with maculopapular rash caused by other common viral and nonviral pathogens or even some drug treatments. The differential diagnosis includes parvovirus, measles, human herpesvirus 6 (roseola), and rash-associated enteroviruses, such as echovirus 9 and coxsackievirus A9.[8] In particular, parvovirus infections can be confused with rubella because their clinical presentations are so similar and both can be associated with arthritis or arthralgia.[246] Moreover, in endemic areas, dengue, West Nile, Sindbis, chikungunya, and Ross River virus infections should be considered.[8] Therefore, a definitive diagnosis of rubella can only be made using specific laboratory tests.

Similarly, confirmation of a diagnosis of CRS cannot be established solely on the basis of clinical findings. It requires either the direct isolation of RUBV or serologic evidence of acute infection in the infant. In the absence of confirmatory laboratory data, a clinical diagnosis compatible with CRS requires the presence of any two of the following: cataracts and/or congenital glaucoma, congenital heart disease, hearing loss, or pigmentary retinopathy. In the presence of only one of the preceding manifestations, the additional finding of purpura, hepatosplenomegaly, jaundice, microcephaly, mental retardation, meningoencephalitis, or radiolucent bone disease is indicative of CRS (Table 4.1).[36] In countries in which rubella vaccination is not carried out (or is in the process of being implemented), surveillance for CRS is important to monitor for prevalence or effectiveness of the vaccination policy. A combination of eye and congenital heart anomalies has been proposed as a sensitive and specific sentinel for CRS to identify infants for further laboratory investigation.[234]

Laboratory

Diagnosis of postnatal rubella and congenital infection (following birth) is normally carried out by detection of rubella-specific IgM by enzyme immunoassay (EIA) using commercial assays.[262] The capture assay is preferred over indirect assays, which have been shown to give false-positive results with other acute viral infections such as parvovirus, Epstein-Barr virus, or cytomegalovirus,[256] or when rheumatoid factor is present.[94] IgM is usually detectable for 6 to 8 weeks after acute rubella[8] but can be detected for longer in some patients and is present for up to a year in congenitally infected infants.[257]

Virus isolation may occasionally be warranted, particularly to confirm infection during pregnancy. In acute infection, RUBV is readily isolated from throat swabs or nasopharyngeal secretions for approximately 1 week before and up to 2 weeks after the appearance of rash.[301] Virus can also be isolated from circulating lymphocytes for up to 1 month postinfection,[44] but this is too expensive for routine clinical diagnostic purposes. Cord blood or placental tissue may be used to confirm congenital infection at time of birth. In addition, virus can readily be isolated from throat swabs or urine of the neonate.[62]

A variety of nucleic acid amplification–based techniques have been developed to detect RUBV genomic RNA in clinical samples. Reverse transcription of RNA isolated from patient tissue/cells or fluid is required prior to amplification of the cDNA by polymerase chain reaction (PCR) using primers specific for a selected region of the RUBV genome (usually the E1 gene). PCR-based detection of RUBV RNA has been used to detect virus in cases of suspected congenital infection using samples obtained by amniocentesis, cordocentesis, and chorionic villus sampling for *in utero* diagnosis.[30,230] A comparison of nested RT-PCR on amniotic fluid with measurement of rubella

IgM in fetal blood has confirmed both the specificity and the sensitivity of the genome amplification technique.[154] Finally, adaption of multiplexed real-time–based PCR assays allows molecular genotyping as well as exquisitely accurate and sensitive detection of as little as one plaque-forming unit of RUBV in clinical samples.[184,185]

PREVENTION AND CONTROL

Vaccines

Development

Following isolation of RUBV in cell culture in 1962,[204] attenuation of the virus was carried out by serial passage in a variety of cell lines, giving rise to several vaccine strains that came into use around 1970. These included the original vaccine used widely in North America, HPV77/DE5[33]; the Cendehill strain, used more extensively in Europe[208]; and several Japanese strains.[247] The HPV77/DE5 strain was the predominant strain used in North America until 1979, when it was replaced by the RA27/3 vaccine due to concerns of waning immunity in HPV77/DE5 vaccine recipients.[117] The RA27/3 strain was derived from an isolate from the kidney of an RUBV-infected fetus and was attenuated by passaging 4 times in human embryonic kidney followed by passaging 17 to 25 times in WI-38 fibroblasts.[211] This strain of virus induces a more vigorous immune response than HPV77/DE5 and has the added advantage that it was attenuated in human cells and is therefore not subject to possible side effects associated with vaccines grown in nonhuman cells. RA27/3 was licensed in 1979 and is now the only rubella vaccine available in North America. It is also widely used in other countries, including the majority of those in Europe, in Australia and New Zealand, and in South America. However, in parts of Asia, locally produced rubella vaccine strains are used. In Japan, five vaccine strains (KRT, TO-336, Matsuura, TCRB19, and Matsuba) have been developed,[190] whereas in China, BRD-2 has been compared in clinical studies to RA27/3.[280] As approximately 75% of the global population lives in countries where rubella has not been eliminated, there remains substantial risk for continuing rubella outbreaks in parts of Africa and Asia in particular (Fig. 4.1).

Vaccine Administration

Rubella vaccine is usually given in combination with measles and mumps as the measles–mumps–rubella (MMR) vaccine between 12 and 15 months of age, with a subsequent booster dose prior to school entry or in adolescence. Subcutaneous administration induces an antibody response in approximately 95% of recipients older than 12 months of age, detectable at 4 weeks postimmunization. The majority of vaccinated children report only mild symptoms, and transmission to susceptible bystanders seems not to occur. Although the antibody titers are lower than those following natural infection, protection is believed to endure for more than 21 years in the majority of those immunized.[189] However, in 10% of women tested in the United States, titers had dropped to low or undetectable levels in 5 years, although they responded rapidly to challenge with high-titer RA27/3.[188] In view of this, rubella vaccination should be given to all women of childbearing age found to have low or undetectable antibody titers, preferably 1 month before conception or postpartum. Immunization during pregnancy should be avoided (see "Risk in Pregnancy").

Adverse Reactions

The current RA27/3 vaccine is well tolerated but not problem free. Certainly, the incidence of acute adverse reactions is lower than after natural rubella[259] but still higher than that reported for some other vaccine strains.[25] Symptoms include fever, lymphadenopathy, arthralgia/arthritis, paresthesia, and carpal tunnel syndrome. Between 10% and 30% of adult rubella seronegative women vaccinated with the RA27/3 vaccine develop acute, usually transient, arthritis or arthralgia.[212,259,261] The joint reactions can be recurrent or persistent, similar to symptoms following natural rubella, and viral persistence may be associated with ongoing symptoms.[41] Subsequent studies have questioned the link between RUBV vaccination and joint manifestations, and it is probably prudent to conclude that the incidence of vaccine-induced chronic arthritis is lower than previously reported.[259] However, the finding of an association of certain HLA-DR haplotypes with a higher incidence of joint symptoms following RA27/3 rubella vaccination[175] suggests that the virus may cause joint symptoms in small numbers of genetically predisposed individuals. This factor should be taken into account in any future studies based on analysis of populations.

Vaccine side effects and complications are a serious challenge to maintaining herd immunity, and the higher incidence of arthralgia and arthritis particularly in female vaccines has most certainly had negative consequences. However, by far, the most damage to effective uptake of MMR vaccine stems from a report by Wakefield et al.[277] that ultimately led to the belief among a significant number of people that this vaccine was linked to autism. Numerous larger and much better controlled studies failed to confirm a causal relationship between the MMR vaccine and autism, but unfortunately the damage was done and the rate of vaccine uptake dropped dramatically. Predictably, this led to an increase in the number of cases of measles and to a lesser extent rubella. Fortunately, the journal that published the Wakefield et al. paper, the Lancet, retracted the paper from the published record in 2010. However, it will still be some time before we have fully recovered from the effects of this fraudulent report.

Risk in Pregnancy

A serious concern of rubella vaccination programs has been the potential risk to the developing fetus in mothers who are immunized during early pregnancy. In such instances, the placenta and fetus may become infected, although the isolation rate is only 3%.[235] Moreover, one survey of 515 children born of mothers inadvertently immunized within 3 months of conception showed that none had malformations compatible with CRS.[23] This included cases of vaccination with the earlier Cendehill and HPV-77 vaccines, as well as with the current RA27/3 vaccine. Vaccine strains of RUBV therefore appear to be far less teratogenic than wt+ RUBV and even in one case where the fetus was infected no signs of CRS were detected at birth. Because a potential risk to the fetus still exists (estimated at 1.3% when the mother is vaccinated 1 to 2 weeks before to 4 to 6 weeks after conception[231]), pregnancy remains a contraindication to rubella vaccination. However, inadvertent vaccination of a seronegative pregnant woman is not sufficient reason for termination of pregnancy.

New Vaccine Strategies

Because the current rubella vaccines are considered highly effective, there is limited interest in developing a subunit vaccine. Nevertheless, live attenuated vaccines are not recommended for children with immunodeficiency diseases or for women in the early stages of pregnancy who might be living or working in a situation where they risk exposure. For these situations, a subunit vaccine that provides some protection, even if only for a limited time, may be appropriate. Use of the E1 protein, which contains the major neutralizing epitopes, has been proposed[293] but such vaccine platforms have not been developed further. In addition, DNA vaccines incorporating genes for all three structural proteins, or just E1 and E2, have been constructed and have shown some promise in mice.[213] However, for general use, a live attenuated vaccine that promotes the strongest and most enduring immune response is still advisable. With current knowledge on the genetic determinants of virulence and joint tropism, the potential exists for development of a recombinant vaccine designed to be highly immunogenic but not associated with unwanted side effects. Nevertheless, the overall success of current vaccines likely precludes further development of next-generation recombinant vaccines.

PERSPECTIVE

With the availability of relatively inexpensive and safe vaccines, rubella is most certainly a preventable disease. Indeed, much of the industrialized world has adopted comprehensive immunization policies that have curtailed virus circulation and CRS; however, much of the global birth cohort is still susceptible to rubella.[206,229] The cost of medical care for children with CRS has been shown to easily justify implementation of comprehensive immunization programs on economic grounds alone.[103] Yet RUBV is still endemic in many developing countries, and sadly, these are the least well-equipped nations to deal with the very high costs of caring for CRS children.

To prevent RUBV transmission, herd immunity needs to exceed 85%[4] and the cost of proper surveillance for RUBV can be prohibitive. As a result of inadequate or absent surveillance, the actual numbers of rubella and CRS are vastly underreported according to modeling from seroprevalence and vaccine coverage. Of the more than 100,000 estimated cases of CRS that occurred in 2010, only 31 were reported to the WHO.[276,289] Accordingly, RUBV is still a significant human pathogen that impacts the health of the world's population through the widespread manifestations of CRS, most notably in relation to blindness and hearing defects.

On the positive side, significant progress has been made with respect to understanding virus–host interactions at the molecular level, and the complete sequences of multiple wild-type and vaccine strains of RUBV are known. By pooling the knowledge from these studies through further investigation, we will be in a better position to understand the underlying mechanisms of teratogenicity and virus-induced autoimmune diseases such as diabetes and arthritis.

REFERENCES

1. Abernathy ES, Wang CY, Frey TK. Effect of antiviral antibody on maintenance of long-term rubella virus persistent infection in Vero cells. *J Virol* 1990;64(10):5183–5187.
2. Achievements in public health: elimination of rubella and congenital rubella syndrome-US, 1969–2004. *Ann Pharmacother* 2005;39(6):1151–1152.
3. Adamo P, Asis L, Silveyra P, et al. Rubella virus does not induce apoptosis in primary human embryo fibroblast cultures: a possible way of viral persistence in congenital infection. *Viral Immunol* 2004;17(1):87–100.
4. Anderson RM, May RM. Immunisation and herd immunity. *Lancet* 1990;335(8690):641–645.
5. Atreya CD, Kulkarni S, Mohan KV. Rubella virus P90 associates with the cytokinesis regulatory protein Citron-K kinase and the viral infection and constitutive expression of P90 protein both induce cell cycle arrest following S phase in cell culture. *Arch Virol* 2004;149(4):779–789.
6. Auewarakul P. Composition bias and genome polarity of RNA viruses. *Virus Res* 2005;109(1):33–37.
7. Backovic M, Rey FA. Virus entry: old viruses, new receptors. *Curr Opin Virol* 2012;2(1):4–13.
8. Banatvala JE, Brown DW. Rubella. *Lancet* 2004;363(9415):1127–1137.
9. Bardeletti G. Respiration and ATP level in BHK21/13S cells during the earliest stages of rubella virus replication. *Intervirology* 1977;8(2):100–109.
10. Bardeletti G, Gautheron DC. Phospholipid and cholesterol composition of rubella virus and its host cell BHK 21 grown in suspension cultures. *Arch Virol* 1976;52(1–2):19–27.
11. Bardeletti G, Kessler N, Aymard-Henry M. Morphology, biochemical analysis and neuraminidase activity of rubella virus. *Arch Virol* 1975;49(2–3):175–186.
12. Bardeletti G, Tektoff J, Gautheron D. Rubella virus maturation and production in two host cell systems. *Intervirology* 1979;11(2):97–103.
13. Baron MD, Ebel T, Suomalainen M. Intracellular transport of rubella virus structural proteins expressed from cloned cDNA. *J Gen Virol* 1992;73(Pt 5):1073–1086.
14. Baron MD, Forsell K. Oligomerization of the structural proteins of rubella virus. *Virology* 1991;185(2):811–819.
15. Bart SW, Stetler HC, Preblud SR, et al. Fetal risk associated with rubella vaccine: an update. *Rev Infect Dis* 1985;7(Suppl 1):S95–S102.
16. Basrur S, Stewart A. *Information for Health Care Professionals: Rubella Outbreak in Southern Ontario.* Vol. 5, issue 5. Ontario Ministry of Health; 2005.
17. Battisti AJ, Yoder JD, Plevka P, et al. Cryo-electron tomography of rubella virus. *J Virol* 2012;86(20):11078–11085.
18. Beatch MD, Everitt JC, Law LJ, et al. Interactions between rubella virus capsid and host protein p32 are important for virus replication. *J Virol* 2005;79(16):10807–10820.
19. Beatch MD, Hobman TC. Rubella virus capsid associates with host cell protein p32 and localizes to mitochondria. *J Virol* 2000;74(12):5569–5576.
20. Bechar M, Davidovich S, Goldhammer G, et al. Neurological complications following rubella infection. *J Neurol* 1982;226(4):283–287.
21. Bennett AJ, Paskey AC, Ebinger A, et al. Relatives of rubella virus in diverse mammals. *Nature* 2020;586(7829):424–428.
22. Berger BE, Omer SB. Could the United States experience rubella outbreaks as a result of vaccine refusal and disease importation? *Hum Vaccin* 2010;6(12):1016–1020.
23. Best JM. Rubella vaccines: past, present and future. *Epidemiol Infect* 1991;107(1):17–30.
24. Best J, Banatvala J. Rubella. In: Zuckerman A, Banatvala J, Pattison J, et al., eds. *Principles and Practice of Clinical Virology.* New York: John Wiley & Sons; 2004:428–457.
25. Best JM, Banatvala JE, Bowen JM. New Japanese rubella vaccine: comparative trials. *Br Med J* 1974;3(5925):221–224.
26. Best JM, Thomson A, Nores JR, et al. Rubella virus strains show no major antigenic differences. *Intervirology* 1993;34:164–168.
27. Bharadwaj SD, Sahay RR, Yadav PD, et al. Acute encephalitis with atypical presentation of rubella in family cluster, India. *Emerg Infect Dis* 2018;24(10):1923–1925.
28. Bilz NC, Willscher E, Binder H, et al. Teratogenic rubella virus alters the endodermal differentiation capacity of human induced pluripotent stem cells. *Cells* 2019;8(8).
29. Bodansky HJ, Dean BM, Grant PJ, et al. Does exposure to rubella virus generate endocrine autoimmunity? *Diabet Med* 1990;7(7):611–614.
30. Bosma TJ, Corbett KM, O'Shea S, et al. PCR for detection of rubella virus RNA in clinical samples. *J Clin Microbiol* 1995;33(5):1075–1079.
31. Bottiger B, Jensen IP. Maturation of rubella IgG avidity over time after acute rubella infection. *Clin Diagn Virol* 1997;8(2):105–111.
32. Buimovici-Klein E, Cooper LZ. Cell-mediated immune response in rubella infections. *Rev Infect Dis* 1985;7(Suppl 1):S123–S128.
33. Buynak EB, Hilleman MR, Weibel RE, et al. Live attenuated rubella virus vaccines prepared in duck embryo cell culture. I. Development and clinical testing. *JAMA* 1968;204(3):195–200.
34. Carey BD, Akhrymuk I, Dahal B, et al. Protein Kinase C subtype delta interacts with Venezuelan equine encephalitis virus capsid protein and regulates viral RNA binding through modulation of capsid phosphorylation. *PLoS Pathog* 2020;16(3):e1008282.
35. Carey BD, Ammosova T, Pinkham C, et al. Protein Phosphatase 1alpha interacts with venezuelan equine encephalitis virus capsid protein and regulates viral replication through modulation of capsid phosphorylation. *J Virol* 2018;92(15).
36. Centers for Disease Control and Prevention (CDC). Rubella and congenital rubella—United States, 1984–1986. *MMWR Morb Mortal Wkly Rep* 1987;36(40):664–666, 671–665.
37. Centers for Disease Control and Prevention (CDC). Revised ACIP recommendation for avoiding pregnancy after receiving a rubella-containing vaccine. *MMWR Morb Mortal Wkly Rep* 2001;50(49):1117.
38. Centers for Disease Control and Prevention (CDC). Elimination of rubella and congenital rubella syndrome—United States, 1969–2004. *MMWR Morb Mortal Wkly Rep* 2005;54(11):279–282.
39. Centers for Disease Control and Prevention (CDC). Progress toward elimination of measles and prevention of congenital rubella infection—European region, 1990–2004. *MMWR Morb Mortal Wkly Rep* 2005;54(7):175–178.
40. Chantler JK, Davies MA. The effect of antibody on rubella virus infection in human lymphoid cells. *J Gen Virol* 1987;68(Pt 5):1277–1288.
41. Chantler JK, Ford DK, Tingle AJ. Persistent rubella infection and rubella-associated arthritis. *Lancet* 1982;1(8285):1323–1325.
42. Chantler JK, Lund KD, Miki NP, et al. Characterization of rubella virus strain differences associated with attenuation. *Intervirology* 1993;36(4):225–236.

43. Chantler JK, Tingle AJ. Replication and expression of rubella virus in human lymphocyte populations. *J Gen Virol* 1980;50(2):317–328.
44. Chantler JK, Tingle AJ. Isolation of rubella virus from human lymphocytes after acute natural infection. *J Infect Dis* 1982;145(5):673–677.
45. Chantler JK, Tingle AJ, Petty RE. Persistent rubella virus infection associated with chronic arthritis in children. *N Engl J Med* 1985;313(18):1117–1123.
46. Chaye HH, Mauracher CA, Tingle AJ, et al. Cellular and humoral immune responses to rubella virus structural proteins E1, E2, and C. *J Clin Microbiol* 1992;30(9):2323–2329.
47. Chaye H, Ou D, Chong P, et al. Human T- and B-cell epitopes of E1 glycoprotein of rubella virus. *J Clin Immunol* 1993;13(2):93–100.
48. Chen MH, Frey TK. Mutagenic analysis of the 3′ cis-acting elements of the rubella virus genome. *J Virol* 1999;73(4):3386–3403.
49. Chen MH, Frolov I, Icenogle J, et al. Analysis of the 3′ cis-acting elements of rubella virus by using replicons expressing a puromycin resistance gene. *J Virol* 2004;78(5):2553–2561.
50. Chen MH, Icenogle JP. Rubella virus capsid protein modulates viral genome replication and virus infectivity. *J Virol* 2004;78(8):4314–4322.
51. Chen JP, Strauss JH, Strauss EG, et al. Characterization of the rubella virus nonstructural protease domain and its cleavage site. *J Virol* 1996;70(7):4707–4713.
52. Clarke DM, Loo TW, Hui I, et al. Nucleotide sequence and in vitro expression of rubella virus 24S subgenomic messenger RNA encoding the structural proteins E1, E2 and C. *Nucleic Acids Res* 1987;15(7):3041–3057.
53. Clarke DM, Loo TW, McDonald H, et al. Expression of rubella virus cDNA coding for the structural proteins. *Gene* 1988;65(1):23–30.
54. Clarke WL, Shaver KA, Bright GM, et al. Autoimmunity in congenital rubella syndrome. *J Pediatr* 1984;104(3):370–373.
55. Claus C, Chey S, Heinrich S, et al. Involvement of p32 and microtubules in alteration of mitochondrial functions by rubella virus. *J Virol* 2011;85(8):3881–3892.
56. Cong H, Jiang Y, Tien P. Identification of the myelin oligodendrocyte glycoprotein as a cellular receptor for rubella virus. *J Virol* 2011;85(21):11038–11047.
57. Connolly JH, Hutchinson WM, Allen IV, et al. Carotid artery thrombosis, encephalitis, myelitis and optic neuritis associated with rubella virus infections. *Brain* 1975;98(4):583–594.
58. Cooper LZ. The history and medical consequences of rubella. *Rev Infect Dis* 1985;7 Suppl 1:S2–S10.
59. Cooper LZ, Ziring PR, Ockerse AB, et al. Rubella. Clinical manifestations and management. *Am J Dis Child* 1969;118(1):18–29.
60. Cordoba P, Lanoel A, Grutadauria S, et al. Evaluation of antibodies against a rubella virus neutralizing domain for determination of immune status. *Clin Diagn Lab Immunol* 2000;7(6):964–966.
61. Coyle PK, Wolinsky JS. Characterization of immune complexes in progressive rubella panencephalitis. *Ann Neurol* 1981;9(6):557–562.
62. Cradock-Watson JE, Miller E, Ridehalgh MK, et al. Detection of rubella virus in fetal and placental tissues and in the throats of neonates after serologically confirmed rubella in pregnancy. *Prenat Diagn* 1989;9(2):91–96.
63. Cui T, Porter AG. Localization of binding site for encephalomyocarditis virus RNA polymerase in the 3′-noncoding region of the viral RNA. *Nucleic Acids Res* 1995;23(3):377–382.
64. Cutts FT, Robertson SE, Diaz-Ortega JL, et al. Control of rubella and congenital rubella syndrome (CRS) in developing countries, Part 1: burden of disease from CRS. *Bull World Health Organ* 1997;75(1):55–68.
65. Das I, Basantray I, Mamidi P, et al. Heat shock protein 90 positively regulates Chikungunya virus replication by stabilizing viral non-structural protein nsP2 during infection. *PLoS One* 2014;9(6):e100531.
66. Das PK, Kielian M. The enigmatic capsid protein of an encephalitic Rubivirus. *J Virol* 2021;95(8).
67. Das PK, Kielian M. Molecular and structural insights into the life cycle of rubella virus. *J Virol* 2021;95(10).
68. de Mazancourt A, Waxham MN, Nicolas JC, et al. Antibody response to the rubella virus structural proteins in infants with the congenital rubella syndrome. *J Med Virol* 1986;19(2):111–122.
69. Dominguez G, Wang CY, Frey TK. Sequence of the genome RNA of rubella virus: evidence for genetic rearrangement during togavirus evolution. *Virology* 1990;177(1):225–238.
70. Dube M, Etienne L, Fels M, et al. Calcium-dependent rubella virus fusion occurs in early endosomes. *J Virol* 2016;90(14):6303–6313.
71. Dube M, Rey FA, Kielian M. Rubella virus: first calcium-requiring viral fusion protein. *PLoS Pathog* 2014;10(12):e1004530.
72. DuBois RM, Vaney MC, Tortorici MA, et al. Functional and evolutionary insight from the crystal structure of rubella virus protein E1. *Nature* 2013;493(7433):552–556.
73. Duncan R, Muller J, Lee N, et al. Rubella virus-induced apoptosis varies among cell lines and is modulated by Bcl-XL and caspase inhibitors. *Virology* 1999;255(1):117–128.
74. Dwyer DE, Robertson PW, Field PR. Broadsheet: clinical and laboratory features of rubella. *Pathology* 2001;33(3):322–328.
75. Enders G, Nickerl-Pacher U, Miller E, et al. Outcome of confirmed periconceptional maternal rubella. *Lancet* 1988;1(8600):1445–1447.
76. Fontana J, Lopez-Iglesias C, Tzeng WP, et al. Three-dimensional structure of Rubella virus factories. *Virology* 2010;405(2):579–591.
77. Forbes JA. Rubella: historical aspects. *Am J Dis Child.* 1969;118(1):5–11.
78. Ford D, Tingle A, Chantler J. Rubella arthritis. In: Espinoza L, Goldberg G, Arnett F, Alarcon G, eds. *Infections in the Rheumatic Diseases.* New York: Grune and Stratton; 1988:103–106.
79. Fraser JR, Cunningham AL, Hayes K, et al. Rubella arthritis in adults. Isolation of virus, cytology and other aspects of the synovial reaction. *Clin Exp Rheumatol* 1983;1(4):287–293.
80. Frey TK. Molecular biology of rubella virus. *Adv Virus Res* 1994;44:69–160.
81. Frey TK, Abernathy ES, Bosma TJ, et al. Molecular analysis of rubella virus epidemiology across three continents, North America, Europe, and Asia, 1961–1997. *J Infect Dis* 1998;178(3):642–650.
82. Frey TK, Hemphill ML. Generation of defective-interfering particles by Rubella virus in Vero cells. *Virology* 1988;164:22–29.
83. Froshauer S, Kartenbeck J, Helenius A. Alphavirus RNA replicase is located on the cytoplasmic surface of endosomes and lysosomes. *J Cell Biol* 1988;107(6 Pt 1):2075–2086.
84. Gale EA. Congenital rubella: citation virus or viral cause of type 1 diabetes? *Diabetologia* 2008;51(9):1559–1566.
85. Garbutt M, Chan H, Hobman TC. Secretion of rubella virions and virus-like particles in cultured epithelial cells. *Virology* 1999;261(2):340–346.
86. Garbutt M, Law LM, Chan H, et al. Role of rubella virus glycoprotein domains in assembly of virus-like particles. *J Virol* 1999;73(5):3524–3533.
87. Garcia AG, Marques RL, Lobato YY, et al. Placental pathology in congenital rubella. *Placenta* 1985;6(4):281–295.
88. Geier DA, Geier MR. Rubella vaccine and arthritic adverse reactions: an analysis of the Vaccine Adverse Events Reporting System (VAERS) database from 1991 through 1998. *Clin Exp Rheumatol* 2001;19(6):724–726.
89. Ginsberg-Fellner F, Witt ME, Fedun B, et al. Diabetes mellitus and autoimmunity in patients with the congenital rubella syndrome. *Rev Infect Dis* 1985;7(Suppl 1):S170–S176.
90. Givens KT, Lee DA, Jones T, et al. Congenital rubella syndrome: ophthalmic manifestations and associated systemic disorders. *Br J Ophthalmol* 1993;77(6):358–363.
91. Gomwalk NE, Ahmad AA. Prevalence of rubella antibodies on the African continent. *Rev Infect Dis* 1989;11(1):116–121.
92. Gorbalenya AE, Koonin EV, Lai MM. Putative papain-related thiol proteases of positive-strand RNA viruses. Identification of rubi- and aphthovirus proteases and delineation of a novel conserved domain associated with proteases of rubi-, alpha- and coronaviruses. *FEBS Lett* 1991;288(1–2):201–205.
93. Gould JJ, Butler M. Differentiation of rubella virus strains by neutralization kinetics. *J Gen Virol* 1980;49(2):423–426.
94. Grangeot-Keros L, Pustowoit B, Hobman T. Evaluation of Cobas Core Rubella IgG EIA recomb, a new enzyme immunoassay based on recombinant rubella-like particles. *J Clin Microbiol* 1995;33(9):2392–2394.
95. Gregg NM. Congenital cataract following German measles in the mother. *Trans Ophthalmol Soc Aust* 1941;(3):35–46.
96. Grimwood RM, Holmes EC, Geoghegan JL. A novel rubi-like virus in the pacific electric ray (*Tetronarce californica*) reveals the complex evolutionary history of the *Matonaviridae*. *Viruses* 2021;13(4):585.
97. Gros C, Linder M, Wengler G, et al. Analyses of disulfides present in the rubella virus E1 glycoprotein. *Virology* 1997;230:179–186.
98. Gros C, Wengler G. Identification of an RNA-stimulated NTPase in the predicted helicase sequence of the Rubella virus nonstructural polyprotein. *Virology* 1996;217(1):367–372.
99. Hahn YS, Grakoui A, Rice CM, et al. Mapping of RNA- temperature-sensitive mutants of Sindbis virus: complementation group F mutants have lesions in nsP4. *J Virol* 1989;63(3):1194–1202.
100. Harrison SC. Viral membrane fusion. *Virology* 2015;479–480:498–507.
101. Hemphill ML, Forng RY, Abernathy ES, et al. Time course of virus-specific macromolecular synthesis during rubella virus infection in Vero cells. *Virology* 1988;162(1):65–75.
102. Hethcote HW. Measles and rubella in the United States. *Am J Epidemiol* 1983;117(1):2–13.
103. Hinman AR, Irons B, Lewis M, et al. Economic analyses of rubella and rubella vaccines: a global review. *Bull World Health Organ* 2002;80(4):264–270.
104. Hobman TC. Targeting of viral glycoproteins to the Golgi complex. *Trends Microbiol* 1993;1(4):124–130.
105. Hobman TC, Gillam S. In vitro and in vivo expression of rubella virus glycoprotein E2: the signal peptide is contained in the C-terminal region of capsid protein. *Virology* 1989;173(1):241–250.
106. Hobman TC, Lemon HF, Jewell K. Characterization of an endoplasmic reticulum retention signal in the rubella virus E1 glycoprotein. *J Virol* 1997;71(10):7670–7680.
107. Hobman TC, Lundstrom ML, Gillam S. Processing and intracellular transport of rubella virus structural proteins in COS cells. *Virology* 1990;178(1):122–133.
108. Hobman TC, Lundstrom ML, Mauracher CA, et al. Assembly of rubella virus structural proteins into virus-like particles in transfected cells. *Virology* 1994;202(2):574–585.
109. Hobman TC, Qiu ZY, Chaye H, et al. Analysis of rubella virus E1 glycosylation mutants expressed in COS cells. *Virology* 1991;181(2):768–772.
110. Hobman TC, Shukin R, Gillam S. Translocation of rubella virus glycoprotein E1 into the endoplasmic reticulum. *J Virol* 1988;62(11):4259–4264.
111. Hobman TC, Woodward L, Farquhar MG. The rubella virus E1 glycoprotein is arrested in a novel post-ER, pre-Golgi compartment. *J Cell Biol* 1992;118(4):795–811.
112. Hobman TC, Woodward L, Farquhar MG. The rubella virus E2 and E1 spike glycoproteins are targeted to the Golgi complex. *J Cell Biol* 1993;121(2):269–281.
113. Hobman TC, Woodward L, Farquhar MG. Targeting of a heterodimeric membrane protein complex to the Golgi: rubella virus E2 glycoprotein contains a transmembrane Golgi retention signal. *Mol Biol Cell* 1995;6(1):7–20.
114. Hofmann J, Pletz MW, Liebert UG. Rubella virus-induced cytopathic effect in vitro is caused by apoptosis. *J Gen Virol* 1999;80(Pt 7):1657–1664.
115. Horstmann DM. Discussion paper: the use of primates in experimental viral infections—rubella and the rubella syndrome. *Ann N Y Acad Sci* 1969;162(1):594–597.
116. Horstmann DM. The rubella story, 1881–1985. *S Afr Med J* 1986;Suppl:60–63.
117. Horstmann DM, Schluederberg A, Emmons JE, et al. Persistence of vaccine-induced immune responses to rubella: comparison with natural infection. *Rev Infect Dis* 1985;7(Suppl 1):S80–S85.
118. Horzinek M. *Non-arthropod-born Togaviruses.* London: Academic Press; 1981.
119. Ho-Terry L, Londesborough P, Cohen A. Analysis of rubella virus complement-fixing antigens by polyacrylamide gel electrophoresis. *Arch Virol* 1986;87(3–4):219–228.
120. Hukic M, Hubschen JM, Seremet M, et al. An outbreak of rubella in the Federation of Bosnia and Herzegovina between December 2009 and May 2010 indicates failure to vaccinate during wartime (1992–1995). *Epidemiol Infect* 2012;140:447–453.
121. Ilkow CS, Goping IS, Hobman TC. The Rubella virus capsid is an anti-apoptotic protein that attenuates the pore-forming ability of Bax. *PLoS Pathog* 2011;7(2):e1001291.
122. Ilkow CS, Mancinelli V, Beatch MD, et al. Rubella virus capsid protein interacts with poly(a)-binding protein and inhibits translation. *J Virol* 2008;82(9):4284–4294.
123. Ilkow CS, Weckbecker D, Cho WJ, et al. The rubella virus capsid protein inhibits mitochondrial import. *J Virol* 2010;84(1):119–130.

124. Johnstone P, Whitby JE, Bosma T, et al. Sequence variation in 5′ termini of rubella virus genomes: changes affecting structure of the 5′ proximal stem-loop. *Arch Virol* 1996;141(12):2471–2477.
125. Kamer G, Argos P. Primary structural comparison of RNA-dependent polymerases from plant, animal and bacterial viruses. *Nucleic Acids Res* 1984;12(18):7269–7282.
126. Karounos DG, Wolinsky JS, Thomas JW. Monoclonal antibody to rubella virus capsid protein recognizes a beta-cell antigen. *J Immunol* 1993;150(7):3080–3085.
127. Katow S. Rubella virus genome diagnosis during pregnancy and mechanism of congenital rubella. *Intervirology* 1998;41(4–5):163–169.
128. Katow S, Sugiura A. Low pH-induced conformational change of rubella virus envelope proteins. *J Gen Virol* 1988;69(Pt 11):2797–2807.
129. Kelton JG, Smith JW, Santos AV, et al. Platelet IgG Fc receptor. *Am J Hematol* 1987;25(3):299–310.
130. Kielian M. Class II virus membrane fusion proteins. *Virology* 2006;344(1):38–47.
131. Kielian M. Mechanisms of virus membrane fusion proteins. *Annu Rev Virol* 2014;1(1):171–189.
132. Kouri G, Aguilera A, Rodriguez P, et al. A study of microfoci and inclusion bodies produced by rubella virus in the RK-13 cell line. *J Gen Virol* 1974;22(1):73–80.
133. Kresky B, Nauheim JS. Rubella retinitis. *Am J Dis Child* 1967;113(3):305–310.
134. Kujala P, Ahola T, Ehsani N, et al. Intracellular distribution of rubella virus nonstructural protein P150. *J Virol* 1999;73(9):7805–7811.
135. Law LM, Duncan R, Esmaili A, et al. Rubella virus E2 signal peptide is required for perinuclear localization of capsid protein and virus assembly. *J Virol* 2001;75(4):1978–1983.
136. Law LM, Everitt JC, Beatch MD, et al. Phosphorylation of rubella virus capsid regulates its RNA binding activity and virus replication. *J Virol* 2003;77(3):1764–1771.
137. Law LJ, Ilkow CS, Tzeng WP, et al. Analyses of phosphorylation events in the rubella virus capsid protein: role in early replication events. *J Virol* 2006;80(14):6917–6925.
138. Lazar M, Perelygina L, Martines R, et al. Immunolocalization and distribution of rubella antigen in fatal congenital rubella syndrome. *EBioMedicine* 2016;3:86–92.
139. Lee JY, Bowden DS. Rubella virus replication and links to teratogenicity. *Clin Microbiol Rev* 2000;13(4):571–587.
140. Lee JY, Bowden DS, Marshall JA. Membrane junctions associated with rubella virus infected cells. *J Submicrosc Cytol Pathol* 1996;28(1):101–108.
141. Lee JY, Hwang D, Gillam S. Dimerization of rubella capsid protein is not required for virus particle formation. *Virology* 1996;216:223–227.
142. Lee JY, Marshall JA, Bowden DS. Replication complexes associated with the morphogenesis of rubella virus. *Arch Virol* 1992;122(1–2):95–106.
143. Lee JY, Marshall JA, Bowden DS. Characterization of rubella virus replication complexes using antibodies to double-stranded RNA. *Virology* 1994;200(1):307–312.
144. Lee JY, Marshall JA, Bowden DS. Localization of rubella virus core particles in vero cells. *Virology* 1999;265(1):110–119.
145. Liang Y, Gillam S. Mutational analysis of the rubella virus nonstructural polyprotein and its cleavage products in virus replication and RNA synthesis. *J Virol* 2000;74(11):5133–5141.
146. Liang Y, Yao J, Gillam S. Rubella virus nonstructural protein protease domains involved in trans- and cis-cleavage activities. *J Virol* 2000;74(12):5412–5423.
147. Liu X, Ropp SL, Jackson RJ, et al. The rubella virus nonstructural protease requires divalent cations for activity and functions in trans. *J Virol* 1998;72(5):4463–4466.
148. Liu X, Yang J, Ghazi AM, et al. Characterization of the zinc binding activity of the rubella virus nonstructural protease. *J Virol* 2000;74(13):5949–5956.
149. Liu Z, Yang D, Qiu Z, et al. Identification of domains in rubella virus genomic RNA and capsid protein necessary for specific interaction. *J Virol* 1996;70:2184–2190.
150. Londesborough P, Ho-Terry L, Terry G. Sequence variation and biological activity of rubella virus isolates. *Arch Virol* 1995;140(3):563–570.
151. Lovett AE, McCarthy M, Wolinsky JS. Mapping cell-mediated immunodominant domains of the rubella virus structural proteins using recombinant proteins and synthetic peptides. *J Gen Virol* 1993;74(Pt 3):445–452.
152. Lund KD, Chantler JK. Mapping of genetic determinants of rubella virus associated with growth in joint tissue. *J Virol* 2000;74(2):796–804.
153. Lundstrom ML, Mauracher CA, Tingle AJ. Characterization of carbohydrates linked to rubella virus glycoprotein E2. *J Gen Virol* 1991;72(Pt 4):843–850.
154. Mace M, Cointe D, Six C, et al. Diagnostic value of reverse transcription-PCR of amniotic fluid for prenatal diagnosis of congenital rubella infection in pregnant women with confirmed primary rubella infection. *J Clin Microbiol* 2004;42(10):4818–4820.
155. Magliano D, Marshall J, Bowden DS, et al. Rubella virus replication complexes are virus-modified lysosomes. *Virology* 1998;240:57–63.
156. Mangala Prasad V, Klose T, Rossmann MG. Assembly, maturation and three-dimensional helical structure of the teratogenic rubella virus. *PLoS Pathog* 2017;13(6):e1006377.
157. Mangala Prasad V, Willows SD, Fokine A, et al. Rubella virus capsid protein structure and its role in virus assembly and infection. *Proc Natl Acad Sci U S A* 2013;110(50):20105–20110.
158. Marr LD, Sanchez A, Frey TK. Efficient in vitro translation and processing of the rubella virus structural proteins in the presence of microsomes. *Virology* 1991;180(1):400–405.
159. Marr LD, Wang CY, Frey TK. Expression of the rubella virus nonstructural protein ORF and demonstration of proteolytic processing. *Virology* 1994;198(2):586–592.
160. Marttila J, Ilonen J, Lehtinen M, et al. Definition of three minimal T helper cell epitopes of rubella virus E1 glycoprotein. *Clin Exp Immunol* 1996;104(3):394–397.
161. Mastromarino P, Cioe L, Rieti S, et al. Role of membrane phospholipids and glycolipids in the Vero cell surface receptor for rubella virus. *Med Microbiol Immunol* 1990;179(2):105–114.
162. Maton W. Some account of a rash liable to be mistaken for scarlatina. *Med Trans Coll Physicians* 1815;5:149–165.
163. Matsumoto A, Higashi M. Electron micrographic studies on the morphology and morphogenesis of togaviruses. *Ann Rep Inst Virus Res*, Kyoto Univ 1974;17:11–12.
164. Matthews JD, Tzeng WP, Frey TK. Determinants in the maturation of rubella virus p200 replicase polyprotein precursor. *J Virol* 2012;86(12):6457–6469.
165. Mauracher CA, Gillam S, Shukin R, et al. pH-dependent solubility shift of rubella virus capsid protein. *Virology* 1991;181(2):773–777.
166. Mauracher CA, Mitchell LA, Tingle AJ. Differential IgG avidity to rubella virus structural proteins. *J Med Virol* 1992;36(3):202–208.
167. McCarthy M, Lovett A, Kerman RH, et al. Immunodominant T-cell epitopes of rubella virus structural proteins defined by synthetic peptides. *J Virol* 1993;67(2):673–681.
168. McIntosh ED, Menser MA. A fifty-year follow-up of congenital rubella. *Lancet* 1992;340(8816):414–415.
169. Megyeri K, Berencsi K, Halazonetis TD, et al. Involvement of a p53-dependent pathway in rubella virus-induced apoptosis. *Virology* 1999;259(1):74–84.
170. Melancon P, Garoff H. Processing of the Semliki Forest virus structural polyprotein: role of the capsid protease. *J Virol* 1987;61(5):1301–1309.
171. Menser MA, Dods L, Harley JD. A twenty-five-year follow-up of congenital rubella. *Lancet* 1967;2(7530):1347–1350.
172. Miki NP, Chantler JK. Differential ability of wild-type and vaccine strains of rubella virus to replicate and persist in human joint tissue. *Clin Exp Rheumatol* 1992;10(1):3–12.
173. Miller E, Cradock-Watson JE, Pollock TM. Consequences of confirmed maternal rubella at successive stages of pregnancy. *Lancet* 1982;2(8302):781–784.
174. Mitchell LA, Decarie D, Tingle AJ, et al. Identification of immunoreactive regions of rubella virus E1 and E2 envelope proteins by using synthetic peptides. *Virus Res* 1993;29(1):33–57.
175. Mitchell LA, Tingle AJ, MacWilliam L, et al. HLA-DR class II associations with rubella vaccine-induced joint manifestations. *J Infect Dis* 1998;177(1):5–12.
176. Mitchell LA, Tingle AJ, Shukin R, et al. Chronic rubella vaccine-associated arthropathy. *Arch Intern Med* 1993;153(19):2268–2274.
177. Mitchell LA, Zhang T, Ho M, et al. Characterization of rubella virus-specific antibody responses by using a new synthetic peptide-based enzyme-linked immunosorbent assay. *J Clin Microbiol* 1992;30(7):1841–1847.
178. Mitchell LA, Zhang T, Tingle AJ. Differential antibody responses to rubella virus infection in males and females. *J Infect Dis* 1992;166(6):1258–1265.
179. Murphy F. Togavirus morphology and morphogenesis. In: Schlesinger RW, ed. *The Togaviruses*. New York: Academic Press; 1980:241–316.
180. Murphy FA, Halonen PE, Harrison AK. Electron microscopy of the development of rubella virus in BHK-21 cells. *J Virol* 1968;2(10):1223–1227.
181. Naeye RL, Blanc W. Pathogenesis of congenital rubella. *JAMA* 1965;194(12):1277–1283.
182. Nam S, Ga YJ, Lee JY, et al. Radicicol inhibits chikungunya virus replication by targeting nonstructural protein-2. *Antimicrob Agents Chemother* 2021;65:e0013521.
183. Ogra PL, Herd JK. Arthritis associated with induced rubella infection. *J Immunol* 1971;107(3):810–813.
184. Oka JA, Weigel PH. Microtubule-depolymerizing agents inhibit asialo-orosomucoid delivery to lysosomes but not its endocytosis or degradation in isolated rat hepatocytes. *Biochim Biophys Acta* 1983;763:368–376.
185. Okamoto K, Fujii K, Komase K. Development of a novel TaqMan real-time PCR assay for detecting rubella virus RNA. *J Virol Methods* 2010;168(1–2):267–271.
186. Oker-Blom C. The gene order for rubella virus structural proteins is NH_2-C-E2-E1-COOH. *J Virol* 1984;51:354–358.
187. Oker-Blom C, Ulmanen I, Kaariainen L, et al. Rubella virus 40S genome RNA specifies a 24S subgenomic mRNA that codes for a precursor to structural proteins. *J Virol* 1984;49(2):403–408.
188. O'Shea S, Best JM, Banatvala JE. Viremia, virus excretion, and antibody responses after challenge in volunteers with low levels of antibody to rubella virus. *J Infect Dis* 1983;148(4):639–647.
189. O'Shea S, Woodward S, Best JM, et al. Rubella vaccination: persistence of antibodies for 10–21 years. *Lancet* 1988;2(8616):909.
190. Otsuki N, Abo H, Kubota T, et al. Elucidation of the full genetic information of Japanese rubella vaccines and the genetic changes associated with in vitro and in vivo vaccine virus phenotypes. *Vaccine* 2011;29(10):1863–1873.
191. Otsuki N, Sakata M, Saito K, et al. Both sphingomyelin and cholesterol in the host cell membrane are essential for rubella virus entry. *J Virol* 2018;92(1).
192. Ou D, Chong P, Choi Y, et al. Identification of T-cell epitopes on E2 protein of rubella virus, as recognized by human T-cell lines and clones. *J Virol* 1992;66(11):6788–6793.
193. Ou D, Chong P, McVeish P, et al. Characterization of the specificity and genetic restriction of human CD4+ cytotoxic T cell clones reactive to capsid antigen of rubella virus. *Virology* 1992;191(2):680–686.
194. Ou D, Chong P, Tingle AJ, et al. Mapping T-cell epitopes of rubella virus structural proteins E1, E2, and C recognized by T-cell lines and clones derived from infected and immunized populations. *J Med Virol* 1993;40(3):175–183.
195. Ou D, Chong P, Tripet B, et al. Analysis of T- and B-cell epitopes of capsid protein of rubella virus by using synthetic peptides. *J Virol* 1992;66(3):1674–1681.
196. Ou D, Jonsen LA, Metzger DL, et al. CD4+ and CD8+ T-cell clones from congenital rubella syndrome patients with IDDM recognize overlapping GAD65 protein epitopes. Implications for HLA class I and II allelic linkage to disease susceptibility. *Hum Immunol* 1999;60(8):652–664.
197. Ou D, Mitchell LA, Decarie D, et al. Characterization of an overlapping CD8+ and CD4+ T-cell epitope on rubella capsid protein. *Virology* 1997;235(2):286–292.
198. Ou D, Mitchell LA, Decarie D, et al. Promiscuous T-cell recognition of a rubella capsid protein epitope restricted by DRB1*0403 and DRB1*0901 molecules sharing an HLA DR supertype. *Hum Immunol* 1998;59(3):149–157.
199. Ou D, Mitchell LA, Domeier ME, et al. Characterization of the HLA-restrictive elements of a rubella virus-specific cytotoxic T cell clone: influence of HLA-DR4 beta chain residue 74 polymorphism on antigenic peptide-T cell interaction. *Int Immunol* 1996;8(10):1577–1586.
200. Ou D, Mitchell LA, Ho M, et al. Analysis of overlapping T- and B-cell antigenic sites on rubella virus E1 envelope protein. Influence of HLA-DR4 polymorphism on T-cell clonal recognition. *Hum Immunol* 1994;39(3):177–187.
201. Ou D, Mitchell LA, Metzger DL, et al. Cross-reactive rubella virus and glutamic acid decarboxylase (65 and 67) protein determinants recognised by T cells of patients with type I diabetes mellitus. *Diabetologia* 2000;43(6):750–762.
202. Pappas CL, Tzeng WP, Frey TK. Evaluation of cis-acting elements in the rubella virus subgenomic RNA that play a role in its translation. *Arch Virol* 2006;151(2):327–346.
203. Parkman PD. Biological characteristics of rubella virus. *Arch Gesamte Virusforsch* 1965;16:401–411.

204. Parkman PD, Buescher EL, Artenstein MS. Recovery of rubella virus from army recruits. *Proc Soc Exp Biol Med* 1962;111:225–230.
205. Paschen SA, Weber A, Hacker G. Mitochondrial protein import: a matter of death? *Cell Cycle* 2007;6(20):2434–2439.
206. Patel MK, Antoni S, Danovaro-Holliday MC, et al. The epidemiology of rubella, 2007–18: an ecological analysis of surveillance data. *Lancet Glob Health* 2020;8(11):e1399–e1407.
207. Peetermans J. Factors affecting the stability of viral vaccines. *Dev Biol Stand* 1996;87:97–101.
208. Peetermans J, Huygelen C. Attenuation ob rubella virus by serial passage in primary rabbit kidney cell cultures. I. Growth characteristics in vitro and production of experimental vaccines at different passage levels. *Arch Gesamte Virusforsch* 1967;21(2):133–143.
209. Petruzziello R, Orsi N, Macchia S, et al. Pathway of rubella virus infectious entry into Vero cells. *J Gen Virol* 1996;77(Pt 2):303–308.
210. Plotkin SA. Routes of fetal infection and mechanisms of fetal damage. *Am J Dis Child* 1975;129(4):444–449.
211. Plotkin SA, Farquhar J, Katz M, et al. A new attenuated rubella virus grown in human fibroblasts: evidence for reduced nasopharyngeal excretion. *Am J Epidemiol* 1967;86(2):468–477.
212. Polk BF, Modlin JF, White JA, et al. A controlled comparison of joint reactions among women receiving one of two rubella vaccines. *Am J Epidemiol* 1982;115(1):19–25.
213. Pougatcheva SO, Abernathy ES, Vzorov AN, et al. Development of a rubella virus DNA vaccine. *Vaccine* 1999;17(15–16):2104–2112.
214. Preblud SR, Williams NM. Fetal risk associated with rubella vaccine: implications for vaccination of susceptible women. *Obstet Gynecol* 1985;66(1):121–123.
215. Pugachev KV, Abernathy ES, Frey TK. Improvement of the specific infectivity of the rubella virus (RUB) infectious clone: determinants of cytopathogenicity induced by RUB map to the nonstructural proteins. *J Virol* 1997;71(1):562–568.
216. Pugachev KV, Abernathy ES, Frey TK. Genomic sequence of the RA27/3 vaccine strain of rubella virus. *Arch Virol* 1997;142(6):1165–1180.
217. Pugachev KV, Frey TK. Rubella virus induces apoptosis in culture cells. *Virology* 1998;250(2):359–370.
218. Pugachev KV, Frey TK. Effects of defined mutations in the 5′ nontranslated region of rubella virus genomic RNA on virus viability and macromolecule synthesis. *J Virol* 1998;72(1):641–650.
219. Pugachev KV, Galinski MS, Frey TK. Infectious cDNA clone of the RA27/3 vaccine strain of Rubella virus. *Virology* 2000;273(1):189–197.
220. Pustowoit B, Liebert UG. Predictive value of serological tests in rubella virus infection during pregnancy. *Intervirology* 1998;41(4–5):170–177.
221. Qiu Z, Hobman TC, McDonald HL, et al. Role of N-linked oligosaccharides in processing and intracellular transport of E2 glycoprotein of rubella virus. *J Virol* 1992;66(6): 3514–3521.
222. Qiu Z, Ou D, Hobman TC, et al. Expression and characterization of virus-like particles containing rubella virus structural proteins. *J Virol* 1994;68(6):4086–4091.
223. Qiu Z, Yao J, Cao H, et al. Mutations in the E1 hydrophobic domain of rubella virus impair virus infectivity but not virus assembly. *J Virol* 2000;74(14):6637–6642.
224. Rabinowe SL, George KL, Loughlin R, et al. Congenital rubella. Monoclonal antibody-defined T cell abnormalities in young adults. *Am J Med* 1986;81(5):779–782.
225. Rand ML, Wright JF. Virus-associated idiopathic thrombocytopenic purpura. *Transfus Sci* 1998;19(3):253–259.
226. Rathore AP, Haystead T, Das PK, et al. Chikungunya virus nsP3 & nsP4 interacts with HSP-90 to promote virus replication: HSP-90 inhibitors reduce CHIKV infection and inflammation in vivo. *Antiviral Res* 2014;103:7–16.
227. Rawls WE. Congenital rubella: the significance of virus persistence. *Prog Med Virol* 1968;10:238–285.
228. Rayfield EJ, Kelly KJ, Yoon JW. Rubella virus-induced diabetes in the hamster. *Diabetes* 1986;35(11):1278–1281.
229. Reef SE, Strebel P, Dabbagh A. Progress toward control of rubella and prevention of congenital rubella syndrome—worldwide, 2009. *MMWR Morb Mortal Wkly Rep* 2010;59(40):1307–1310.
230. Revello MG, Baldanti F, Sarasini A, et al. Prenatal diagnosis of rubella virus infection by direct detection and semiquantitation of viral RNA in clinical samples by reverse transcription-PCR. *J Clin Microbiol* 1997;35(3):708–713.
231. Revised ACIP recommendations for avoiding pregnancy after receiving a Rubella-containing vaccine. *JAMA* 2002;287:311–312.
232. Rey FA, Lok SM. Common features of enveloped viruses and implications for immunogen design for next-generation vaccines. *Cell* 2018;172(6):1319–1334.
233. Risco C, Carrascosa JL, Frey TK. Structural maturation of rubella virus in the Golgi complex. *Virology* 2003;312(2):261–269.
234. Rittler M, Lopez-Camelo J, Castilla EE. Monitoring congenital rubella embryopathy. *Birth Defects Res A Clin Mol Teratol* 2004;70(12):939–943.
235. Robertson SE, Cutts FT, Samuel R, et al. Control of rubella and congenital rubella syndrome (CRS) in developing countries, Part 2: vaccination against rubella. *Bull World Health Organ* 1997;75(1):69–80.
236. Robertson SE, Featherstone DA, Gacic-Dobo M, et al. Rubella and congenital rubella syndrome: global update. *Rev Panam Salud Publica* 2003;14(5):306–315.
237. Rorke LB. Nervous system lesions in the congenital rubella syndrome. *Arch Otolaryngol* 1973;98(4):249–251.
238. Rozanov MN, Koonin EV, Gorbalenya AE. Conservation of the putative methyltransferase domain: a hallmark of the 'Sindbis-like' supergroup of positive-strand RNA viruses. *J Gen Virol* 1992;73(Pt 8):2129–2134.
239. Sakata M, Katoh H, Otsuki N, et al. Heat shock protein 90 ensures the integrity of rubella virus p150 protein and supports viral replication. *J Virol* 2019;93(22).
240. Sakata M, Otsuki N, Okamoto K, et al. Short self-interacting N-terminal region of rubella virus capsid protein is essential for cooperative actions of capsid and nonstructural p150 proteins. *J Virol* 2014;88(19):11187–11198.
241. Sarnesto A, Ranta S, Vaananen P, et al. Proportions of Ig classes and subclasses in rubella antibodies. *Scand J Immunol* 1985;21(3):275–282.
242. Schluter WW, Reef SE, Redd SC, et al. Changing epidemiology of congenital rubella syndrome in the United States. *J Infect Dis* 1998;178(3):636–641.
243. Sedwick WD, Sokol F. Nucleic acid of rubella virus and its replication in hamster kidney cells. *J Virol* 1970;5(4):478–489.
244. Sever JL, South MA, Shaver KA. Delayed manifestations of congenital rubella. *Rev Infect Dis* 1985;7(Suppl 1):S164–S169.
245. Shaver KA, Boughman JA, Nance WE. Congenital rubella syndrome and diabetes: a review of epidemiologic, genetic, and immunologic factors. *Am Ann Deaf* 1985;130(6):526–532.
246. Shirley JA, Revill S, Cohen BJ, et al. Serological study of rubella-like illnesses. *J Med Virol* 1987;21(4):369–379.
247. Shishido A, Ohtawara M. Development of attenuated rubella virus vaccines in Japan. *Jpn J Med Sci Biol* 1976;29(5):227–253.
248. Smith CA, Petty RE, Tingle AJ. Rubella virus and arthritis. *Rheum Dis Clin North Am* 1987;13(2):265–274.
249. Squadrini F, Taparelli F, De Rienzo B, et al. Rubella virus isolation from cerebrospinal fluid in postnatal rubella encephalitis. *Br Med J* 1977;2(6098):1329–1330.
250. Standardization of the nomenclature for genetic characteristics of wild-type rubella viruses. *Wkly Epidemiol Rec* 2005;80(14):126–132.
251. Stanwick TL, Hallum JV. Role of interferon in six cell lines persistently infected with rubella virus. *Infect Immun* 1974;10(4):810–815.
252. Strauss JH, Strauss EG, Kuhn RJ. Budding of alphaviruses. *Trends Microbiol* 1995;3(9):346–350.
253. Suomalainen M, Garoff H, Baron MD. The E2 signal sequence of rubella virus remains part of the capsid protein and confers membrane association in vitro. *J Virol* 1990;64(11):5500–5509.
254. Takeshita K, Takeuchi N, Ohkusu M, et al. Population-based study of a free rubella-specific antibody testing and immunization campaign in Chiba city in response to the 2018–2019 nationwide rubella outbreak in Japan. *Hum Vaccin Immunother* 2021;17:1779–1784.
255. Takkinen K, Vidgren G, Ekstrand J, et al. Nucleotide sequence of the rubella virus capsid protein gene reveals an unusually high G/C content. *J Gen Virol* 1988;69(Pt 3):603–612.
256. Thomas HI, Barrett E, Hesketh LM, et al. Simultaneous IgM reactivity by EIA against more than one virus in measles, parvovirus B19 and rubella infection. *J Clin Virol* 1999;14(2):107–118.
257. Thomas HI, Morgan-Capner P, Cradock-Watson JE, et al. Slow maturation of IgG1 avidity and persistence of specific IgM in congenital rubella: implications for diagnosis and immunopathology. *J Med Virol* 1993;41(3):196–200.
258. Thomas HI, Morgan-Capner P, Enders G, et al. Persistence of specific IgM and low avidity specific IgG1 following primary rubella. *J Virol Methods* 1992;39(1–2):149–155.
259. Tingle AJ, Allen M, Petty RE, et al. Rubella-associated arthritis. I. Comparative study of joint manifestations associated with natural rubella infection and RA 27/3 rubella immunisation. *Ann Rheum Dis* 1986;45(2):110–114.
260. Tingle AJ, Chantler JK, Kettyls GD, et al. Failed rubella immunization in adults: association with immunologic and virological abnormalities. *J Infect Dis* 1985;151(2):330–336.
261. Tingle AJ, Mitchell LA, Grace M, et al. Randomised double-blind placebo-controlled study on adverse effects of rubella immunisation in seronegative women. *Lancet* 1997;349(9061):1277–1281.
262. Tipples G, Hiebert J. Detection of measles, mumps, and rubella viruses. *Methods Mol Biol* 2011;665:183–193.
263. Tondury G, Smith DW. Fetal rubella pathology. *J Pediatr* 1966;68(6):867–879.
264. Townsend JJ, Baringer JR, Wolinsky JS, et al. Progressive rubella panencephalitis. Late onset after congenital rubella. *N Engl J Med* 1975;292(19):990–993.
265. Trinh QD, Pham NTK, Takada K, et al. Myelin oligodendrocyte glycoprotein-independent rubella infection of keratinocytes and resistance of first-trimester trophoblast cells to rubella virus in vitro. *Viruses* 2018;10(1).
266. Trudel M, Marchessault F, Payment P. Characterisation of rubella virus hemagglutinin rosettes. *J Virol Methods* 1981;2(4):195–201.
267. Trudel M, Ravaoarinoro M, Payment P. Reconstitution of rubella hemagglutinin on liposomes. *Can J Microbiol* 1980;26(8):899–904.
268. Tzeng WP, Chen MH, Derdeyn CA, et al. Rubella virus DI RNAs and replicons: requirement for nonstructural proteins acting in cis for amplification by helper virus. *Virology* 2001;289(1):63–73.
269. Tzeng WP, Frey TK. Complementation of a deletion in the rubella virus p150 nonstructural protein by the viral capsid protein. *J Virol* 2003;77(17):9502–9510.
270. Tzeng WP, Frey TK. Rubella virus capsid protein modulation of viral genomic and subgenomic RNA synthesis. *Virology* 2005;337(2):327–334.
271. Ueda K, Shingaki Y, Sato T, et al. Hemolytic anemia following postnatally acquired rubella during the 1975–1977 rubella epidemic in Japan. *Clin Pediatr (Phila)* 1985;24(3): 155–157.
272. Vaheri A, Sedwick WD, Plotkin SA. Growth of rubella virus in BHK21 cells. II. Enhancing effect of DEAE-dextran, semicarbazide and low doses of metabolic inhibitors. *Proc Soc Exp Biol Med* 1967;125(4):1092–1098.
273. Vaheri A, Sedwick WD, Plotkin SA, et al. Cytopathic effect of rubella virus in RHK21 cells and growth to high titers in suspension culture. *Virology* 1965;27(2):239–241.
274. Veale H. History of an epidemic of Rötheln with observations on its pathology. *Edinb Med J* 1866;12:404–414.
275. von Bonsdorff C-H, Vaheri A. Growth of rubella virus in BHK-21 cells: electron microscopy of morphogenesis. *J Gen Virol* 1969;5:47–51.
276. Vynnycky E, Adams EJ, Cutts FT, et al. Using seroprevalence and immunisation coverage data to estimate the global burden of congenital rubella syndrome, 1996–2010: a systematic review. *PLoS One* 2016;11(3):e0149160.
277. Wakefield AJ, Murch SH, Anthony A, et al. Ileal-lymphoid-nodular hyperplasia, non-specific colitis, and pervasive developmental disorder in children. *Lancet* 1998;351(9103):637–641.
278. Walker PJ, Siddell SG, Lefkowitz EJ, et al. Changes to virus taxonomy and the International Code of Virus Classification and Nomenclature ratified by the International Committee on Taxonomy of Viruses (2019). *Arch Virol* 2019;164(9):2417–2429.
279. Wang C-Y, Dominguez G, Frey TK. Construction of rubella virus genome-length cDNA clones and synthesis of infectious RNA transcripts. *J Virol* 1994;68:3550–3557.
280. Wang SS, Han YR, Su WN, et al. Studies on the reactogenicity and immunogenicity of the BRD-2 and RA27/3 live attenuated rubella vaccines. *Vaccine* 1984;2(4):277–280.

281. Wang Z, Yao P, Song Y, et al. Characteristics and mechanisms of isolated rubella virus, strain JR23: infection of the central nervous system of BALB/c mice. *Intervirology* 2003;46(2):79–85.

282. Waxham MN, Wolinsky JS. Rubella virus and its effects on the central nervous system. *Neurol Clin* 1984;2(2):367–385.

283. Waxham MN, Wolinsky JS. Detailed immunologic analysis of the structural polypeptides of rubella virus using monoclonal antibodies. *Virology* 1985;143(1):153–165.

284. Waxham MN, Wolinsky JS. A model of the structural organization of rubella virions. *Rev Infect Dis* 1985;7(Suppl 1):S133–S139.

285. Webster WS. Teratogen update: congenital rubella. *Teratology* 1998;58(1):13–23.

286. Weil ML, Itabashi H, Cremer NE, et al. Chronic progressive panencephalitis due to rubella virus simulating subacute sclerosing panencephalitis. *N Engl J Med* 1975;292(19):994–998.

287. Weller TH, Neva FA. Propagation in tissue culture of cytopathic agents from patients with rubella-like illness. *Proc Soc Exp Biol Med* 1962;111:215–225.

288. Wesselhoeft C. Rubella (German Measles). *N Engl J Med* 1947;236:943–950.

289. WHO. Reported cases of selected vaccine preventable diseases. 2019.

290. Williams MP, Brawner TA, Riggs HG Jr, et al. Characteristics of a persistent rubella infection in a human cell line. *J Gen Virol* 1981;52(Pt 2):321–328.

291. Willows S, Ilkow CS, Hobman TC. Phosphorylation and membrane association of the Rubella virus capsid protein is important for its anti-apoptotic function. *Cell Microbiol* 2014;16(8):1201–1210.

292. Wolinsky JS, McCarthy M, Allen-Cannady O, et al. Monoclonal antibody-defined epitope map of expressed rubella virus protein domains. *J Virol* 1991;65(8):3986–3994.

293. Wolinsky JS, Sukholutsky E, Moore WT, et al. An antibody- and synthetic peptide-defined rubella virus E1 glycoprotein neutralization domain. *J Virol* 1993;67(2):961–968.

294. Xu J, Kong J, Lyu B, et al. The capsid protein of rubella virus antagonizes RNA interference in mammalian cells. *Viruses* 2021;13(2).

295. Yao J, Gillam S. Mutational analysis, using a full-length rubella virus cDNA clone, of rubella virus E1 transmembrane and cytoplasmic domains required for virus release. *J Virol* 1999;73(6):4622–4630.

296. Yao J, Yang D, Chong P, et al. Proteolytic processing of rubella virus nonstructural proteins. *Virology* 1998;246(1):74–82.

297. Yoneda T, Urade M, Sakuda M, et al. Altered growth, differentiation, and responsiveness to epidermal growth factor of human embryonic mesenchymal cells of palate by persistent rubella virus infection. *J Clin Invest* 1986;77(5):1613–1621.

298. Yoon JW, Choi DS, Liang HC, et al. Induction of an organ-specific autoimmune disease, lymphocytic hypophysitis, in hamsters by recombinant rubella virus glycoprotein and prevention of disease by neonatal thymectomy. *J Virol* 1992;66(2):1210–1214.

299. Zheng DP, Frey TK, Icenogle J, et al. Global distribution of rubella virus genotypes. *Emerg Infect Dis* 2003;9(12):1523–1530.

300. Zhou Y, Ushijima H, Frey TK. Genomic analysis of diverse rubella virus genotypes. *J Gen Virol* 2007;88(Pt 3):932–941.

301. Zimmernman L, Reef S. Rubella. In: *VPD Surveillance Manual.* Atlanta: CDC; 2002:1–12.

Arteriviruses

Ying Fang • Eric J. Snijder • Udeni B. R. Balasuriya

History and Classification of Arteriviruses
Virion Structure
Genome Structure and Organization
The Arterivirus Replication Cycle
  Replication in Cultured Cells
  Attachment and Entry
  Genome Translation and Replication
  Synthesis and Translation of Subgenomic mRNAs
  Arterivirus Proteinases and Posttranslational Processing of the
    Replicase
  Replicase Proteins and the Replication Complex
  Assembly and Release
  Major Structural Proteins
  Minor Structural Proteins
  Arterivirus–Host Cell Interactions
Pathogenesis and Pathology of Arterivirus Infections
  Site of Primary Replication, Spread, and Cell and Tissue
    Tropism
  Immune Responses and Immune Evasion
  Release From the Host and Transmission
  Virulence
  Persistence
Epidemiology
  EAV
  PRRSV
  LDV
  SHFV
Clinical Features
  EAV
  PRRSV
  LDV
  SHFV
  WPDV
Prevention and Control
  Diagnosis
  Disease Control
  Vaccines
Perspectives

HISTORY AND CLASSIFICATION OF ARTERIVIRUSES

The family *Arteriviridae* was one of the four families within the order *Nidovirales* when it was established in 1996. It then included a single genus *Arterivirus*, which initially comprised four enveloped, positive-stranded RNA viruses: equine arteritis virus (EAV), lactate dehydrogenase-elevating virus (LDV), porcine reproductive and respiratory syndrome virus (PRRSV), and simian hemorrhagic fever virus (SHFV). EAV, LDV, SHFV, and PRRSV were first isolated and characterized in 1953, 1960, 1964, and 1991–1992, respectively.[32,57,223,264,311] Application of molecular biological techniques revealed an intriguing evolutionary relationship among arteriviruses, coronaviruses, and toroviruses (e-Fig. 5.1A). Despite striking differences in genome size and virion structure, the genome organization and expression strategy of these virus groups were found to be very similar, and their replicase genes were postulated to share common ancestry.[81] One of the most prominent features of their genome expression strategy is the generation of a nested set of subgenomic (sg) messenger RNAs (mRNAs), which provided the basis for the name *Nidovirales* (L. *nidus* = nest). Subsequently, the relationship between arteriviruses and coronaviruses was formalized by promoting the genus *Arterivirus* to a new family (named *Arteriviridae*),[29] and grouping it along with the family *Coronaviridae* in a new positive-stranded RNA virus order, *Nidovirales* (e-Fig. 5.1A). This group of viruses represents a distinct lineage among positive-stranded RNA viruses. The complex evolutionary relationship between arteriviruses and nidoviruses with larger genomes has been reviewed extensively elsewhere.[33,115,146,229] In this virus order, related replicase genes and replication strategies have been combined with seemingly unrelated sets of structural protein genes. RNA recombination likely was an important factor in nidovirus evolution and was also invoked to explain some internal rearrangements of arterivirus genomes.[79,114,148]

During the past decade, due to the advancement of next-generation sequencing and metagenomic analysis technologies, a range of previously unknown arterivirus species have been discovered. These include the wobbly possum disease virus (WPDV) in Australian brushtail possums (*Trichosurus vulpecula*),[48,93] the African pouched rat arterivirus (APRAV-1) in African pouched rats[144] (*Cricetomys emini*), Chinese rodent arteriviruses,[321] a novel arterivirus causing fatal encephalitis in European Hedgehogs[67] (*Erinaceus europaeus*), and Olivier's shrew virus (OSV) in African giant shrews (*Crocidura olivieri*).[299] Furthermore, a substantial number of additional simian arteriviruses have been identified in various species of African

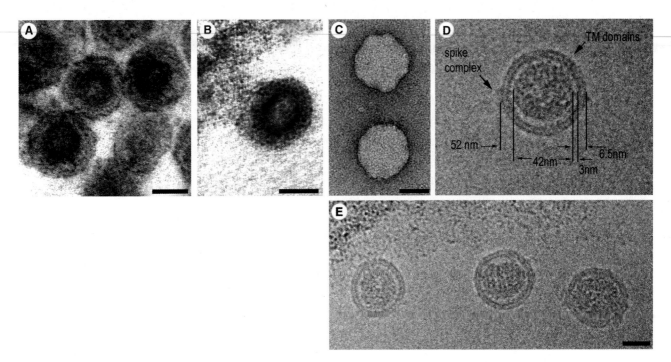

FIGURE 5.1 Electron micrographs of arterivirus particles. A: Transmission electron microscopic (EM) image of extracellular porcine reproductive and respiratory syndrome virus (PRRSV) particles. **B:** Transmission EM image of an equine arteritis virus (EAV) particle budding from smooth intracellular membranes. **C:** Negatively stained, purified PRRSV particles. **D–E:** Cryo-EM of PRRSV particles in vitreous ice. **Panel D** shows a typical PRRSV particle with dimensions indicated. A possible spike protein complex and the striated appearance that most likely corresponds to the transmembrane domains of envelope proteins are visible. All bars are 25 nm. (**A** and **B** adapted with permission of Microbiology Society from Snijder EJ, Meulenberg JJM. The molecular biology of arteriviruses. *J Gen Virol* 1998;79(Pt 5): 961–979; permission conveyed through Copyright Clearance Center, Inc; **C–E** reprinted from Dokland T. The structural biology of PRRSV. *Virus Res* 2010;154(1–2):86–97. Copyright © 2010 Elsevier. With permission.)

nonhuman primates.[144,149] The discovery of these additional arteriviruses, mostly documented in the form of only a genome sequence, warranted the reclassification of all members of the family *Arteriviridae*.[29,144,299] In the latest classification by the International Committee on Taxonomy of Viruses (ICTV), the family belongs to the suborder *Arnidovirineae* of the order *Nidovirales*. The members of the family *Arteriviridae* have been reclassified into six subfamilies currently containing 13 genera, 11 subgenera, and 23 species (e-Fig. 5.1B). The two PRRSV genotypes (previously known as type I and II) were promoted to separate species (PRRSV-1 and PRRSV-2). As virus isolates have not been obtained for most of these 23 species, our understanding of arterivirus (molecular) biology and pathogenesis, as summarized in this chapter, is still largely based on studies with the four viruses that were grouped together when the arterivirus family was first established. Compared to other families in the order *Nidovirales*, arterivirus genomes are the smallest, and the size, structure, and composition of their virions is unique.

VIRION STRUCTURE

Arterivirus particles are pleomorphic but roughly spherical, 50 to 74 nm in diameter (Fig. 5.1; see Refs.[88,247] and references therein). The buoyant density of arteriviruses is 1.13 to 1.17 g/cm³ in sucrose, and their sedimentation coefficient ranges from 214S to 230S. Virions are readily inactivated by lipid solvents, low concentration of nonionic detergents, commonly used disinfectants, and a pH other than 5 to 7; the virus quickly loses its infectivity when stored at temperatures higher than 4°C.[25,282]

The nucleocapsid structure of arteriviruses has long been assumed to be isometric, but cryoelectron tomography studies of PRRSV revealed a rather pleomorphic and "disorganized" core structure.[255] These findings are clearly incompatible with an icosahedral core and suggest a resemblance to the nucleocapsid structure proposed for coronaviruses, a helical coil, or an even more loosely organized filamentous structure. The arterivirus nucleocapsid (Fig. 5.2, e-Fig. 5.2) is composed of the positive-stranded RNA genome and the nucleocapsid protein (N). The crystal structure for the capsid-forming C-terminal domain of PRRSV N[85] (e-Fig. 5.2) suggests that it represents a new class of capsid–forming domains, a hypothesis further supported by cryo-EM studies.

Based on studies with EAV and PRRSV, the lipid bilayer that surrounds the nucleocapsid is now presumed to contain seven envelope proteins (Table 5.1; Fig. 5.2), an unusually large number compared to other positive-stranded RNA viruses. In simian arteriviruses, this number may even go up to eleven (see Table 5.1).[300] An overview of the current structural protein nomenclature for EAV, LDV, PRRSV-1 and PRRSV-2, and SHFV is presented in Table 5.1 and Figures 5.2 and 5.3.[29] Among arterivirus envelope proteins, two major (GP5 and M) and five minor (E, GP2, GP3, GP4, and the ORF5a protein) species have been identified. The two major envelope proteins, the nonglycosylated triple-spanning M protein and GP5, form a disulfide-linked heterodimer in the mature virus particle,[71,95]

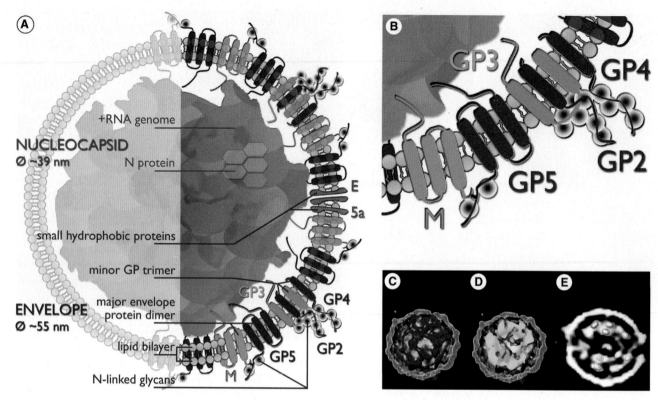

FIGURE 5.2 Arterivirus structure. A: The presumed location and topology of the envelope proteins GP2 to GP5, E, M, open reading frame (ORF) 5a protein, and N protein are shown (see also Table 5.1 and Fig. 5.3). The major envelope proteins GP5 and M form a disulfide-linked heterodimer. The minor glycoproteins GP2, GP3, and GP4 form a disulfide-linked heterotrimer. See **Panel B** for a close-up. In addition, also GP2–GP4 dimers (not depicted) have been identified in equine arteritis virus (EAV) particles. It should be noticed that not all proteins depicted here have been identified in all arterivirus particles and that member of the subfamily *Simarterivirinae* may contain up to four additional envelope proteins.[300] **C–E:** Cryo-electron microscopy–based tomographic reconstruction of a porcine reproductive and respiratory syndrome virus (PRRSV) particle,[255] revealing that the virion core is not solid, but consists of a two-layered shell that surrounds a hollow central cavity. **C:** Cutaway view of the internal core, obtained by peeling away the envelope (shown in mesh representation). The core, which is separated from the envelope by a 3-nm gap, appears to be disorganized and consist of density strands that are bundled together into a ball. The data suggest a model for the core in which two layers of N dimers form a linked chain (see also **Panel E**). The core is shown as an isosurface, colored by the radius from the center of the particle (from *red* to *blue*). **D:** The core has been cut open to show the internal structure, including the central density (*red-orange*) typically seen in the tomograms. **E:** A 6.3-nm thick slab through the center of one PRRSV particle tomogram, with several copies of the crystal structure of the dimeric C-terminal domain of N, rendered at a comparable resolution and superimposed on the oblong densities in the core. (See also e-Fig. 5.2.) (**C–E** reprinted with permission of Microbiology Society from Spilman MS, Welbon C, Nelson E, et al. Cryo-electron tomography of porcine reproductive and respiratory syndrome virus: organization of the nucleocapsid. *J Gen Virol* 2009;90(Pt 3):527–535; permission conveyed through Copyright Clearance Center, Inc.)

while the three minor envelop proteins (GP2, GP3, and GP4) form a heterotrimer in the virion[314,317] (Fig. 5.2). By separately knocking out the expression of each of the structural proteins, it was established that all major and minor structural proteins are required for the production of infectious progeny,[188,317] with the possible exception of the recently discovered ORF5a protein.[103,132] Knockout mutants for minor structural protein genes produced noninfectious subviral particles consisting of GP5, M, N, and the genome RNA.[315,317,332] When one of the components of the GP2-GP3-GP4 trimer or the small nonglycosylated envelope protein (E)[248] was lacking, the incorporation of the three minor GPs into virions was abolished.[315] Taken together, these data indicate that the protein scaffold of the arterivirus core is formed by the three major structural polypeptides, N, M, and GP5. Whether the incorporation of (genome) RNA is a prerequisite for the formation of the nucleocapsid structure,

and which RNA sequences/structures specifically interact with N, remains to be established.

GENOME STRUCTURE AND ORGANIZATION

The arterivirus genome is a positive-sense, 3′-polyadenylated single-stranded RNA molecule of 12.7 to 15.7 kb, with a 5′-terminal type I cap structure.[230] It contains untranslated regions (UTRs) of 157–245 nt and 59–152 nt at the 5′ and 3′ ends of the genome, respectively, and a 3′-terminal poly(A) tail of variable length. Full-length genomic sequences (see also Table 5.1) have been obtained for prototypic virus strains in each of the six subfamilies. Next-generation sequencing and metagenomic analysis have further expanded the number of species within

TABLE 5.1 Molecular properties of typical arteriviruses

			Replicase Proteins			Structural Proteins[a]		
Virus[b]	Host	Genome Size (kb)	ORF	Size (aa)	nsps[c]	ORF	Protein Name[d]	Size (aa)
EAV	Horse	12.7	1a	1,727	9	2a	E	67
	Donkey		1ab	3,175	13	2b	GP2 (GP2b/G$_S$)	227
	Mule					3	GP3	163
	Zebra					4	GP4	152
						5	GP5 (G$_L$)	255
						5a	ORF5a protein	59
						6	M	162
						7	N	110
LDV	Mouse	14.1	1a	2,206	12	2a	E	70
			1ab	3,616	16	2b	GP2 (VP3-M)	227
						3	GP3	191
						4	GP4	175
						5	GP5 (VP3-P)	199
						5a	ORF5a protein	47
						6	M (VP2)	171
						7	N (VP1)	115
PRRSV-1	Pig	15.1	1a	2,396	12	2a	GP2 (GP2a)	249
			1ab	3,854	16	2b	E	70
						3	GP3	265
						4	GP4	183
						5	GP5	201
						5a	ORF5a protein	43
						6	M	173
						7	N	128
PRRSV-2	Pig	15.4	1a	2,503	12	2a	GP2 (GP2a)	256
			1ab	3,960	16	2b	E	73
						3	GP3	254
						4	GP4	178
						5	GP5	200
						5a	ORF5a protein	51
						6	M	174
						7	N	123
SHFV	Monkey	15.7	1a	2,105	13	2a'	GP2' protein	281
			1ab	3,594	17	2b'	E' protein	94
						3'	GP3' protein	204
						4'	GP4' protein	182
						2a	E	80
						2b	GP2 (GP2b)	214
						3	GP3	179
						4	GP4	205
						5	GP5	278
						5a	ORF5a protein	64
						6	M	162
						7	N	111

ORF, open reading frame; EAV, equine arteritis virus; aa, amino acid; GP, glycoprotein; nsp, nonstructural protein; LDV, lactate dehydrogenase-elevating virus; PRRSV, porcine reproductive and respiratory syndrome virus; SHFV, simian hemorrhagic fever virus.

[a]Not all proteins listed here have been identified in all five arterivirus particles.

[b]Molecular characteristics were based on the GenBank sequences of the EAV-Bucyrus (accession #NC_002532), PRRSV-1 Lelystad (accession #M96262), PRRSV-2 VR2332 (accession #AY150564), LDV-P (accession #U15146), and the SHFV-LVR (accession #NC_003092).

[c]Numbers of nsps are based on the known (EAV/PRRSV) or predicted (LDV/SHFV) replicase processing schemes as depicted in Figure 5.3 and e-Figure 5.6; Two frameshifting products (nsp2TF and nsp2N) generated by −2/−1 PRF in nsp2 region (except EAV) are also included. Nsp8 is identical to the N-terminal domain of nsp9 due to −1 PRF.

[d]Alternative names used in other (older) publications are indicated in brackets.

several of the subfamilies and added a significant number of full-length genome sequences to the databases.

Arterivirus genomes are polycistronic and contain 10 to 16 recognized ORFs encoding nonstructural and structural proteins (Table 5.1). The two most 5'-proximal ORFs (1a and 1b) occupy approximately three-quarters of the genome (Fig. 5.3). These replicase ORFs are translated to produce polyproteins pp1a and pp1ab, with the latter being a C-terminally extended version of pp1a, which is derived from a −1 programmed ribosomal frameshift (PRF) occurring just before termination of ORF1a translation. In contrast to the more conserved ORF1b, the size of ORF1a is variable (encoding between 1,727 [EAV] and about 2,600 [PRRSV; RatAV] amino acids). This partially explains the genome size differences encountered among arteriviruses. Within the nsp2-coding region of ORF1a, a short transframe (TF) ORF was identified in the −2 reading frame, which is expressed by −2 PRF.[101] Remarkably, this TF ORF is conserved in the genomes of all currently known arteriviruses, except EAV and WPDV. The same frameshift site also induces −1 PRF, which generates nsp2N, a C-terminally truncated version of nsp2 or a variant carrying a short unique C-terminal

extension.[101,162] The region downstream of the replicase gene contains 8 to 12 relatively small ORFs, most of which have both 5'- and 3'-terminal sequences that overlap with neighboring genes. These genes encode mostly (or exclusively) structural proteins and are translated from sg mRNAs (see section of "Synthesis and Translation of Subgenomic mRNAs" below). Their organization is generally well conserved among arteriviruses. An exception is the region immediately downstream of the replicase gene of simarteriviruses, which contains three or four additional ORFs that likely have arisen from the duplication of ORFs 2a/b to 4.[114] These duplicated genes are identified with a "prime" annotation (ORFs 2b', 2a', 3', and 4'; encoding E', GP2', GP3', and GP4', respectively). A recent detailed analysis of the SHFV transcriptome, performed using next-generation sequencing technology, revealed a number of previously undetected viral transcripts that may be used to express additional short ORFs or truncated versions of previously identified ORFs.[84] These findings potentially expand the coding capacity of the arterivirus genome, although the biological relevance of most of these (predicted) additional viral protein products remains to be established.

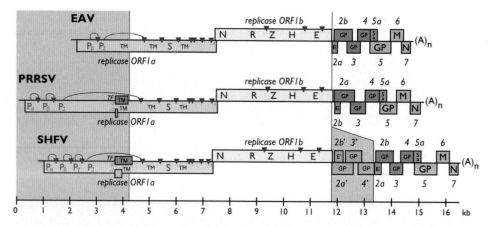

FIGURE 5.3 Arterivirus genome organization. The family prototype equine arteritis virus (EAV; subfamily *Equarterivirinae*) is shown at the **top**, followed by porcine reproductive and respiratory syndrome virus (PRRSV; subfamily *Variarterivirinae*) and simian hemorrhagic fever virus (SHFV; subfamily *Simarterivirinae*). Together, these viruses represent the major genomic variations encountered among the six subfamilies of the family *Arteriviridae*. These major variations involve (a) the number of (active) papain-like proteinase domains in the nsp1 region (between one and three), (b) the presence of a −1/−2 programmed ribosomal frameshift signal in the nsp2-coding region of ORF1a, resulting in the production of additional C-terminally truncated nsp2 proteins (nsp2TF/ nsp2N), (c) a large insertion downstream of ORF1b (highlighted in *grey*) containing four ORFs encoding additional virion proteins[300] (only in the subfamily *Simarterivirinae*). The replicase open reading frames (ORFs) 1a and 1b are followed by the genes encoding the minor envelope proteins and the genes for the three major structural proteins GP5, M, and N (*blue*). In the replicase ORFs, the positions corresponding to known or predicted cleavage sites in the encoded polyproteins are depicted. *Red arrowheads* represent sites cleaved by the nsp4 serine proteinase (S), the viral main protease. The various papain-like proteinase domains (P) in the variable nsp1-nsp2 region and their (predicted) cleavage sites (*blue*) are also shown. Putative transmembrane domains (TM) in the replicase polyproteins are indicated. In ORF1b, the domains encoding five highly conserved nidovirus replicase domains are depicted: the nsp9 nidovirus RdRp-associated nucleotidyltransferase (NiRAN; N), the nsp9 RNA-dependent RNA polymerase (RdRp; R), the nsp10 multinuclear zinc-binding domain (Z), the nsp10 RNA helicase (H), and the nsp11 nidovirus uridylate-specific endonuclease (NendoU; E). Programmed ribosomal frameshifts at the ORF1a/1b junction and in the nsp2-coding region of ORF1a are indicated with −1 and −2. Depending on the virus species/isolate, the −1 frameshift in the nsp2-coding region is immediately followed by a stop codon or results in a small C-terminal extension of nsp2 (as depicted here for PRRSV and SHFV).

THE ARTERIVIRUS REPLICATION CYCLE

Replication in Cultured Cells

Arteriviruses are highly species specific, and macrophages are known to be their primary target cells (for reviews, see Refs.[92,136,150,172,213,247] and references therein). However, EAV can infect and replicate in cells from a variety of hosts, including primary equine alveolar or blood-derived macrophages, equine pulmonary artery endothelial cells,[125] horse, rabbit, and hamster kidney cells, and a number of continuous cell lines, including baby hamster kidney (BHK-21),[130,177] rabbit kidney-13 (RK-13), African green monkey kidney (Vero),[141] rhesus monkey kidney (LLC-MK2), MARC-145, and hamster lung (HmLu) cells.[141] In contrast, other members in the family exhibit a limited cell tropism. LDV infects only a subset of primary peritoneal macrophages of mice. Attempts to infect other cells from mice, rats, guinea pigs, and rabbits with LDV have been unsuccessful. In addition to primary peritoneal macrophages from their respective hosts (i.e., African green monkeys, patas, and rhesus), SHFV (and possibly other simarteriviruses) also replicate in the MA-104 cell line and derivatives thereof, including the MARC-145 cell line.[213,228,264] Similarly, PRRSV can only replicate in a limited number of cell types, including porcine alveolar macrophages (PAMs), the African green monkey cell line MA-104, and its derivative MARC-145.[136] Recently, a PAM cell line derived from the lung lavages of porcine fetuses (ZMAC; ATCCC PTA-8764) has been developed, and this new cell line is highly susceptible to PRRSV infection.[39,329] The recently identified WPDV can only be propagated in primary brushtail possum macrophages.[109]

In general, arterivirus infection of macrophages and cell lines is highly cytocidal, resulting in rounding of the cells and detachment from the culture plate surface, although cell culture models for persistent noncytopathic infection with EAV and PRRSV were established.[119,335] One-step growth kinetic analysis of prototype arterivirus strains (EAV, PRRSV, LDV, SHFV) showed that maximal viral progeny titers in cell culture can be reached at 10^6 to 10^7 tissue culture infectious dose (TCID)$_{50}$/mL for PRRSV and 10^4 PFU/mL for SHFV but may exceed 10^8 PFU/mL for EAV.[213,247]

Attachment and Entry

The entry of EAV and PRRSV requires a low-pH step, suggesting that it occurs via the standard endocytic route[142,197] (Fig. 5.4). Clathrin heavy-chain knockdown suppressed EAV infection[197] and electron microscopy revealed arterivirus particles contained in relatively small vesicles that appeared to be clathrin coated.[142] For EAV and PRRSV, key attachment factors and host cell receptors have been identified. Recently, it has been demonstrated that the equine CXCL16 protein (EqCXCL16) acts as an EAV entry receptor in susceptible equine cells (e.g., monocytes).[231,232] PRRSV entry has been studied most extensively (e-Fig. 5.3; for a recent review, see Ref.[338]) and at least six host cell molecules have been described as putative attachment factors or receptors. These include heparan sulfate (linear polysaccharide), vimentin, CD151, CD163 (scavenger receptor cysteine-rich [SCRR]), CD169 (sialoadhesin or sialic acid–binding immunoglobulin-like lectin 1, also known as siglec-1), and CD209 (dendritic cell-specific intercellular adhesion molecule-3-grabbing nonintegrin; DC-SIGN). Heparan sulfate (a glycos-aminoglycan) was identified as one of the PRRSV attachment factors on its *in vivo* target cell, the PAM.[78] Unlike attachment factors, virus receptors actively promote entry into cells, and accordingly sialoadhesin (siglec-1) was identified as a PRRSV receptor that mediates both virus binding and internalization into PAMs.[75,297] The interaction between PRRSV and siglec-1 was shown to occur via sialic acids on the virion and the N-terminal sialic acid–binding immunoglobulin domain of sialoadhesin.[76,77]

CD163 was shown to be a cellular receptor capable of mediating infection of cell lines otherwise nonpermissive to PRRSV infection.[38] Expression of CD163 from various species rendered a variety of nonpermissive cell lines (e.g., BHK-21, PK0809 porcine kidney, and NLFK feline kidney cell lines) susceptible to PRRSV infection, in the absence of detectable CD169 expression. Siglec-1 and CD163 were postulated to join forces during PRRSV entry based on two findings[291]: (a) in PAMs, both siglec-1– and CD163-specific antibodies strongly reduce infection, and a combination of both completely blocks virus infectivity; (b) cells expressing both siglec-1 and CD163 are highly susceptible to PRRSV infection when compared with cells expressing only siglec-1 or CD163, which were not susceptible and partially susceptible, respectively, depending on the cell line used. These findings clearly showed that CD163 is essential for PRRSV entry. Furthermore, incubation of PAMs with CD163-specific antibodies at 37°C, but not at 4°C, reduced PRRSV infection of macrophages. However, CD163 probably does not serve as an attachment factor,[297] but rather as a mediator of PRRSV entry that is involved in virus uncoating (i.e., virion disassembly and release of the viral genome) (e-Fig. 5.3). The exact role of CD163 and the molecular events during PRRSV entry remain to be investigated in more detail.

Based on data from cell culture–based studies, siglec-1 (CD169) is thought to be responsible for PRRSV's specific cell tropism. However, in pigs, siglec-1 gene knockout (siglec-1$^{-/-}$) did not alter the course of PRRSV infection, including clinical disease and histopathology. This indicates that siglec-1 expression is not required for PRRSV infection of pigs,[216] which resembles the situation in MARC-145 cells, which do not express CD169 on their surface.[90] Recently, siglec-10, a member of the same family as siglec-1, was shown to be able to significantly improve PRRSV infection and production in a CD163-expressing cell line.[323] Siglec-10 was concluded to play a role in PRRSV endocytosis, suggesting that the virus may use multiple siglecs to enter PAMs, which may explain the PRRSV susceptibility of CD169-negative cells. It was postulated that in PAMs, CD169 (and/or other siglecs) and CD163 work together, with the former serving as receptor for internalization and the latter playing a key role in virus uncoating and genome release, which are thought to occur in association with the early endosome, following its acidification[291] (e-Fig. 5.3).

Several reports indicate that the depletion of full-length CD163 or its SRCR5 region (the interaction site for the virus) confers resistance to infection with several PRRSV isolates in pigs or cultured host cells (reviewed in Ref.[258]). Challenge experiments with various PRRSV strains, including highly pathogenic variants, showed that CD163-knockout pigs are completely resistant to viral infection. This was evident from the absence of viremia, antibody responses, high fever, and all other PRRS-associated clinical signs. In contrast, wild-type control animals displayed typical signs of PRRSV infection.

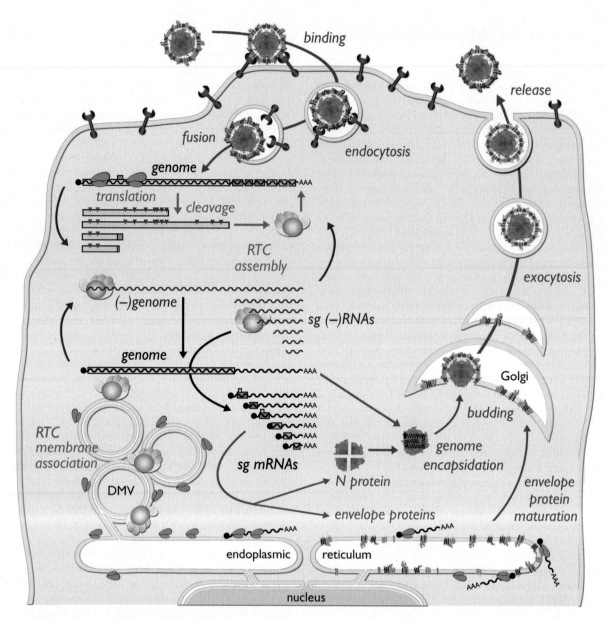

FIGURE 5.4 Overview of the arterivirus infection cycle. Following entry by receptor-mediated endocytosis and release of the genome into the cytosol, genome translation yields the pp1a and pp1ab replicase polyproteins (shown as *yellow bars*), as well as two truncated versions of nsp2 that derive from −2/−1 ribosomal frameshifting. Following polyprotein cleavage by multiple internal proteases, the viral nonstructural proteins assemble into a replication and transcription complex (RTC) that first engages in minus-strand RNA synthesis. Both full-length and subgenome-length minus strands are produced, with the latter templating the synthesis of subgenomic messenger RNAs (mRNAs) required to express the structural protein genes in the 3'-proximal quarter of the genome. Ultimately, novel genomes are packaged into nucleocapsids that become enveloped by budding from smooth intracellular membranes, after which the new virions leave the cell by following the exocytic pathway. (See text for more details.)

Thus, the results obtained with CD163-knockout pigs suggest that CD163 is the primary PRRSV entry mediator that determines the susceptibility of host cells to the virus.

Which arterivirus envelope protein(s) direct the fusion between the viral envelope and the endosomal membrane remains one of the key questions to be addressed for this virus family. A role for the minor glycoproteins in arterivirus receptor recognition and tropism has been demonstrated in previous studies.[65,268] PRRSV proteins GP2 and GP4 were shown to interact with CD163.[65] A chimeric PRRSV carrying E, GP2, GP3, and GP4 of EAV acquired the broad tropism for cultured cells that is typical of the latter virus.[268] These findings are in line with the previously observed phenotypes of recombinant viruses, in which replacing the GP5 or M ectodomain of EAV, did not alter the tropism in cell culture.[86,304] However, a more recent study showed that an M/GP5 ectodomain chimera was able to bind to heparan sulfate and block PRRSV infection in susceptible cells.[127] These studies, together with the identification of several other host factors as potential "PRRSV entry mediators", illustrate that several questions and controversies regarding arterivirus entry remain to be resolved.

Genome Translation and Replication

The arterivirus replication cycle (Fig. 5.4) is presumed to be entirely cytoplasmic, despite the fact that at least two viral proteins are (in part) targeted to the nucleus (see section of "Arterivirus-Host Cell Interactions" below). The incoming genome is translated into the two large replicase polyproteins pp1a (1,727 to 2,586 amino acids) and pp1ab (3,175 to 4,054 amino acids), which comprise all functions required for viral RNA synthesis.[188] Despite the relatively large 5′ UTR, translation presumably starts following "conventional" ribosomal scanning of the genomic 5′ end.[284] ORF1b translation requires a −1 PRF (estimated efficiency of 15% to 20%) just before ORF1a translation is terminated[81] (Fig. 5.3). The ORF1a/1b overlap region contains two signals that promote this event: a so-called "slippery" sequence, which is the actual ribosomal frameshift site, and a downstream RNA pseudoknot structure. In addition to the ORF1a/1b −1 PRF mechanism, a highly efficient −2 PRF element operates during translation of ORF1a in all currently known arteriviruses except EAV and WPDV.[101,162] Unlike the ORF1a/1b PRF site, this novel PRF signal lacks an RNA pseudoknot structure; instead, a downstream conserved RNA sequence (CCCANCUCC) is critically required for frameshifting. The −2 PRF expresses a conserved TF ORF that overlaps with the nsp2-coding region, while the same frameshift site also dictates an efficient −1 PRF. Consequently, two frameshift products (nsp2TF and nsp2N) are produced, which are N-terminally collinear with nsp2. The two PRF mechanisms extensively regulate the expression ratios of arteriviral ORF1a- and ORF1b-encoded replicase proteins. For PRRSV, of the ribosomes that produce nsp1α and nsp1β, approximately 20% and approximately 7% subsequently synthesize nsp2TF and nsp2N, respectively; the remaining approximately 73% synthesize nsp3–8 from the remainder of ORF1a, and only approximately 15% are thought to subsequently produce nsp9–12 from ORF1b.

Following proteolytic processing of the replicase polyproteins, an enzymatic complex for viral RNA synthesis is formed that generates a genome-length minus strand (or "antigenome"), the template for genome replication. In addition, a complex transcription mechanism operates to produce complementary nested sets of sg-length minus-strand RNAs and sg mRNAs[69,80] (see below and Fig. 5.5). The RNA signals involved in arterivirus genome replication remain to be studied in detail. The coding regions of the genomes are flanked by 5′ and 3′ UTRs of 157–245 and 59–152 nucleotides, respectively. However, natural and synthetic defective interfering RNAs of EAV invariably require at least 300 nucleotides from both genome termini for efficient replication, indicating that replication signals must extend into the coding sequences.[187,273] Likewise, in the case of PRRSV, a so-called "kissing interaction" between the loop sequences of RNA hairpin structures in 3′ UTR and N gene was found to be crucial for viral RNA synthesis.[303]

Using a combination of approaches, detailed RNA secondary structure models were developed for the EAV 5′ and 3′ UTRs. In the 5′ UTR, which is involved in translation, replication, and transcription,[283] (e-Fig. 5.4B), one domain in particular was found to be crucial for sg RNA production. This so-called "leader TRS [transcription-regulating sequence] hairpin" (LTH) is potentially conserved in the 5′ UTR of other arteriviruses (e-Fig 5.4C). The importance of other structural features of the EAV 5′ UTR and, for example, their involvement in RNA–protein interactions, remains to be investigated, because few of these elements are conserved in other arteriviruses.[283] A possible exception is EAV hairpin C (termed SL2 in PRRSV)[171] that was reported to be crucial for PRRSV replication and sg RNA synthesis in particular (e-Fig. 5.4C).

The 3′ UTR of the arterivirus genome does not contain obviously conserved primary sequences. For EAV, the 3′-terminal CC motif immediately upstream of the poly(A) tail plays a critical role in viral RNA synthesis.[23] A stem-loop structure near the 3′-terminus of the EAV genome is also required for RNA synthesis[24] (e-Fig. 5.5A), and its loop was implicated in an essential pseudoknot interaction with an upstream stem-loop structure residing in the N protein gene.[23] This conformation was predicted to be conserved in other arteriviruses and proposed to constitute a molecular switch that could regulate the specificity or timing of viral (minus strand) RNA synthesis (e-Fig. 5.5B).

Synthesis and Translation of Subgenomic mRNAs

One of the hallmarks of the replication cycle of arteriviruses (and other nidoviruses) is the synthesis of a 3′-coterminal nested set of sg mRNAs (Fig. 5.5) from which the genes in the 3′-proximal region of the genome are expressed. In the case of arteriviruses, all these genes encode structural proteins. Arterivirus sg mRNAs also have a common 5′-terminal sequence, the so-called "leader sequence," which is derived from the 5′-terminal region of the genome.[69] This property is shared with coronaviruses, but—remarkably—not with some other nidoviruses (like toroviruses and roniviruses; for reviews, see Refs.[115,204,234]). Supported by the presumed common ancestry of the arterivirus and coronavirus replicase genes, leader-to-body fusion during arterivirus sg RNA synthesis was proposed to rely on a mechanism of discontinuous RNA synthesis similar to that previously proposed for coronaviruses.[114,144] In both virus groups, short conserved TRSs are present at the 3′ end of the leader sequence ("leader TRS") and at the 5′ end of each of the transcription units specifying a sg mRNA "body" ("body TRS"; reviewed in Refs.[204,234,247]). The observation that arterivirus-infected cells contain a nested set of sg-length minus-strand RNAs, which are complementary to the sg mRNAs, is another important parallel with coronaviruses.[50,80] With the exception of the smallest species, the arterivirus sg mRNAs are structurally polycistronic, but most of them are presumed to be functionally monocistronic. Notable exceptions are EAV/PRRSV/LDV mRNAs 2 and 5 (Fig. 5.3), which are functionally bicistronic transcripts from which the partially overlapping gene sets E/GP2 and ORF5a/GP5 are expressed, presumably by leaky ribosomal scanning.[103,132,248] Arterivirus sg RNAs are produced in nonequimolar, but relatively constant amounts, thus providing a mechanism to regulate the relative expression of the various structural protein genes.

Different models for coronavirus and arterivirus sg mRNA synthesis have been proposed (Refs.[204,234,247], and references therein). The concept of discontinuous extension of minus-strand RNA synthesis was supported by data from biochemical and genetic studies with coronaviruses and arteriviruses and resulted in a model for the production of a set of sg-length minus-strand templates for sg mRNA synthesis (Fig. 5.5; e-Fig. 5.4).[234] Many details remain to be elucidated regarding the mechanism by which the transcriptase is translocated

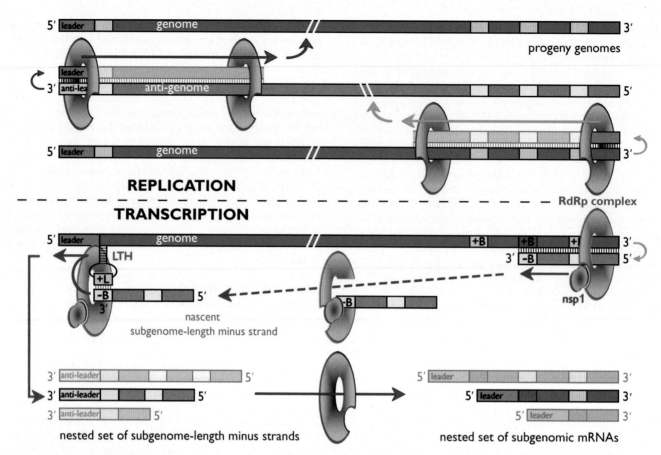

FIGURE 5.5 Arterivirus RNA synthesis. Model for arterivirus (and coronavirus) replication and transcription[204,233,234] using a hypothetical arterivirus genome encoding three subgenomic messenger RNAs (mRNAs). The top half of the scheme depicts the replication of the genome by the viral RNA-dependent RNA polymerase (RdRp) complex, which requires a full-length minus-strand intermediate (antigenome). The bottom half illustrates how minus-strand RNA synthesis can be interrupted at a body transcription-regulating sequence (TRS) (+B), after which the nascent minus strand, having a body TRS complement (−B) at its 3′-end, is redirected to the leader TRS (+L) near the 5′-end of the genome. This +L sequence is thought to be "presented" for base pairing by an RNA structure, the leader TRS hairpin (LTH), that is critical for subgenomic RNA synthesis. Guided by a base-pairing interaction between the complementary −B and +L sequences, RNA synthesis is resumed to add the complement of the genomic leader sequence (antileader) to each of the nascent subgenome-length minus strands. Subsequently, each of the latter serves as template to produce one of the subgenomic mRNAs. The RdRp complexes engaged in replication and transcription may be (partially) different. For example, in the equine arteritis virus (EAV) model, nsp1 has been identified as a regulatory factor that is dispensable for replication but required to regulate the accumulation levels of the different subgenomic RNAs, most likely by controlling a step during minus strand RNA synthesis. See text for more details.

between the body and leader TRS in the genomic template, a step that may resemble copy-choice RNA recombination.[205,295] EAV reverse genetics studies have rigorously demonstrated that discontinuous RNA synthesis depends on duplex formation between the leader TRS and one of the body TRS complements at the 3′ end of a nascent minus strand. In general, the relative amount of a sg mRNA correlates with the calculated stability of this duplex.[205,206,295] Sequences flanking the body TRS, the relative order and/or location of body TRSs in the genomic template, and possibly also higher order RNA structures were shown or postulated to also influence transcription efficiencies.[203] Structural studies on the 5′-proximal part of the EAV genome[283] placed the leader TRS in a single-stranded loop of the "leader TRS hairpin" (or LTH; e-Fig. 5.4B and C), which was characterized as a critical player in transcription.[284]

At the protein level, transcription-specific functions have been attributed to several replicase subunits, in particular nonstructural protein 1 (nsp1) and nsp10, for which introduction of certain mutations resulted in the (near-) complete inactivation

of sg mRNA synthesis, while genome replication was up-regulated 2.5- to 3-fold.[193,273,287] EAV nsp1 controls the accumulation levels of the viral genome and individual sg mRNAs in the infected cell by determining the levels at which the minus strand templates for each of these molecules are produced.[193] An N-terminal zinc finger (ZF) domain was implicated in this function, but also other nsp1 sequences appear to be important. Mutagenesis of nsp1 triggered the emergence of numerous nsp1 pseudorevertants with compensatory mutations that invariably rescued both balanced EAV mRNA accumulation and efficient virus production.[193] In the case of PRRSV, where nsp1 is internally cleaved into nsp1α and nsp1β, the ZF-containing nsp1α subunit is presumed to fulfill a similar role in transcriptional regulation.[143]

A recent next-generation sequencing-based analysis of viral RNA products in SHFV-infected cells revealed the presence of a large number of additional sg RNAs, in addition to the expected transcripts produced from the previously identified "canonical" body TRS sequences.[84] These additional RNA species were detected both in SHFV-infected MA-104 cells and in macrophages from infected macaques. Most of the newly identified TRSs were located in the 3'-proximal region of the genome, but some mapped to internal sites in the replicase gene. A total of 137 different sg mRNA species was reported, each with a unique leader-to-body junction, leading to the conclusion that multiple transcripts are used to express most of the SHFV ORFs, with some of these newly discovered transcripts being more abundant than those produced from "canonical" body TRSs. Furthermore, some of these RNAs may express short ORFs in alternative reading frames or 3'-terminal fragments of established genes. A proteomics analysis provided support for the expression of several of such SHFV polypeptides.[84] Taken together, these findings paint a much more complex picture of both transcription and translation in the arterivirus-infected cell, similar to recent reports for coronaviruses.[102,135] For both virus families, this potential expansion of their coding capacity warrants more detailed studies in order to establish the function and biological relevance of these (predicted) additional viral proteins in the replication cycle.

Arterivirus Proteinases and Posttranslational Processing of the Replicase

The proteolytic maturation of the arterivirus pp1a and pp1ab replicase polyproteins involves the rapid autoproteolytic release of two to four N-terminal nsps and the subsequent cleavage of the remaining part of both polyproteins by the viral nsp4 "main proteinase." The posttranslational processing of the replicase polyproteins has been studied most extensively for EAV (see Refs.[247,281,340], and references therein; e-Fig. 5.6A and B) in which pp1a and pp1ab are cleaved 8 and 11 times, respectively, by three ORF1a-encoded proteinases (see below). In combination with the ORF1a/1b PRF mechanism, this yields at least 13 processing end products (named nonstructural protein [nsp] 1 to 12, including nsp7α and nsp7β; Fig. 5.3; e-Fig. 5.6E). Of these, nsp1–8 are generated from ORF1a, whereas nsp10–12 are entirely ORF1b-encoded; and due to the ribosomal frameshift, nsp9 consists of a small, ORF1a-encoded N-terminal domain (identical to nsp8) and a large C-terminal part that is encoded by ORF1b, which includes the viral RNA-dependent RNA polymerase (RdRp) domain. EAV reverse genetics studies with cleavage site mutants underscored the critical importance of replicase polyprotein processing for virus replication.[281,288] The nsp3–8 region of pp1a (and likely also pp1ab) is subjected to two alternative processing cascades, with the "major pathway" requiring an interaction with nsp2 as a cofactor to trigger the cleavage of the nsp4/5 site[309] (e-Fig. 5.6D), a mechanism that was independently confirmed for PRRSV.[165]

The three EAV proteinase domains in nsp1, nsp2, and nsp4 (e-Fig. 5.6) and their corresponding cleavage sites are conserved across arteriviruses[100,247,340] (Fig. 5.3). EAV nsp1 and nsp2 both contain a papain-like proteinase domain (PLP; formerly referred to as PCP or CP for [papain-like] cysteine protease) that mediate their rapid release from the polyprotein,[250] whereas nsp4 includes a chymotrypsin-like serine proteinase (SP) domain, which is the arterivirus main proteinase.[252] PRRSV and LDV, in addition to having homologs of these three EAV proteinases, possess a fourth nonstructural proteinase,[79] which mediates the rapid release of an additional N-terminal cleavage product. This PLPα possibly is a duplication of the proteinase (PLPβ) present in the C-terminal domain of EAV nsp1 and appears to have

become inactivated in EAV.[79] The sequence analysis of the nsp1 region of SHFV and other members of the subfamily *Simarterivirinae* revealed an even more complex situation, with an array of three PLP domains (PLPα, PLPβ, PLPγ) present in the 480-residue region upstream of the nsp1/nsp2 junction. All of these were reported to be proteolytically active,[301] raising the number of nonstructural proteinases in the replicase polyproteins of *Simarterivirinae* to five. This further testifies to the complex evolutionary history of this part of the genome, in which functions appear to have been acquired, duplicated, and lost when different arterivirus lineages are compared.[118]

The nsp4 SP combines the His-Asp-Ser catalytic triad of classical chymotrypsin-like proteinases with the substrate specificity of the so-called 3C-like cysteine proteinases, a subgroup of chymotrypsin-like enzymes named after the picornavirus 3C proteinases. Specific residues in the substrate-binding region of the SP are assumed to determine its specificity for cleavage sites containing Glu (or sometimes Gln) as the P1 residue and mainly Gly, Ala, or Ser at the P1' position. Nine such sites were identified in pp1a/pp1ab, which are all conserved across the arterivirus family.[247,281,340]

Nsp4 structures have been obtained for EAV and PRRSV by x-ray crystallography[21,271] (e-Fig. 5.7). The protein consists of three domains, with domains I and II forming the typical chymotrypsin-like two-β-barrel fold of the SP. The C-terminal domain III is dispensable for proteolytic activity and may be involved in fine-tuning replicase polyprotein cleavage.[280] Also the structures of PRRSV nsp1α[259] and nsp1β[325] were elucidated, including their respective PLP domains (e-Fig. 5.7), which—in line with previous studies—were both confirmed to employ a Cys-His tandem as active site residues. Both PLPα and PLPβ appear to act exclusively *in cis* and the two crystal structures indeed revealed the presence of the C-terminal region of the two proteins in the PLP substrate-binding pocket, suggesting an intramolecular cleavage mechanism that would preclude further proteolytic activity toward other substrates. Both nsp1α and nsp1β of PRRSV have also been implicated in evasion of the host's immune response (see below), but this was most directly demonstrated for the PLP residing in the N-terminal domain of the highly variable nsp2 subunit. This PLP2 proteinase[251] is distantly related to the ovarian tumor domain (OTU) family of deubiquitinating enzymes (DUBs), which represents a unique subclass of zinc-dependent OTU DUBs.[104,179] It possesses both *cis* and *trans* cleavage activities[121,293] and not only directs the critical cleavage of the nsp2/3 site in pp1a and pp1ab, but is also able to remove ubiquitin (Ub) and Ub-like modifiers like ISG15 from yet-to-be-identified substrates in the infected cell.[260,261,293,294] A recent study showed that the PLP2 domain of PRRSV nsp2TF is able to deconjugate Ub from the major envelope proteins GP5 and M, thus counteracting the proteasomal degradation of these key viral structural proteins and promoting the production of viral progeny.[120]

Replicase Proteins and the Replication Complex

In arteriviruses, with the notable exception of the role of nsp1 in sg mRNA synthesis (see section of "Synthesis and Translation of Subgenomic mRNAs" above), the ORF1a-encoded functions mainly appear to be important for the regulation of replicase gene expression (by controlling proteolytic processing and nsp2TF/nsp2N expression) and the formation of a membrane-anchored "scaffold" for viral RNA synthesis. The ORF1b-encoded proteins, on the other hand, are more directly involved in replication and transcription. Except for the proteins from the nsp1 region and nsp2TF/nsp2N,[51,101,272] all arterivirus replicase subunits studied so far localize to the perinuclear region of the infected cell[164,286] (e-Fig. 5.8A–D), where they are associated with "replication organelles" that are derived from the endoplasmic reticulum (ER). Upon infection, these host cell membranes are modified into double-membrane structures and vesicles (DMVs). The latter have an average diameter of about 90 nm and presumably carry the viral RNA-synthesizing machinery (e-Fig. 5.9A–F).[208,249,292] Electron tomography of EAV-infected cells revealed that DMVs are interconnected and part of a network of modified ER[140] (e-Fig. 5.9E). Biochemical and electron microscopy studies have implicated ORF1a-encoded subunits that contain trans-membrane domains (in particular nsp2, nsp3, and nsp5; e-Fig. 5.6C) in the formation of these membrane structures.[208,215,249,285,286] Recent studies with coronaviruses, which induce DMVs that are about three times larger in diameter, have identified DMVs as the main viral RNA-synthesizing platform in the infected cell.[246] Furthermore, advanced cryo-EM methods revealed the existence of a molecular pore that spans the DMV membrane and may serve to export newly made viral RNA from the DMV interior to the cytosol, for translation and packaging.[318]

An analysis of interactions between PRRSV nsps identified a complex network that was centered around the ORF1b-encoded nsps, which were mainly connected by the nsp2, nsp3, and nsp5 transmembrane subunits.[254] Replicase ORF1b is the most conserved part of the arterivirus genome and encodes the core enzymes for viral RNA synthesis—RdRp (nsp9) and helicase (nsp10).[81,115,196] The predicted NTP binding and superfamily-1 helicase activities of arterivirus nsp10 were corroborated by in vitro assays with recombinant nsp10. These also revealed the 5′-to-3′ polarity of the unwinding reaction, a property shared with coronaviruses.[22,235] This property remains to be reconciled with the protein's presumed role in unwinding local double-stranded RNA structures that might hinder the RdRp during viral RNA synthesis, which proceeds in the opposite direction. As in all nidoviruses, the helicase is linked to an N-terminal zinc-binding domain (ZBD) that might assist the proper folding of nsp10 and/or mediate interactions of the protein with its RNA substrates. This domain was also implicated in a remarkable transcription-specific defect that abolished the synthesis of all EAV sg mRNAs, while allowing genome replication to proceed.[287,289] Crystal structures were obtained for both EAV[83] and PRRSV[240] nsp10 and revealed the presence of an uncharacterized domain 1B that connects the helicase domains 1A and 2A to a long linker of the ZBD, which consists of a novel RING-like module and treble-clef zinc finger, together coordinating three Zn atoms. Helicase activity was found to depend on the extensive relay of interactions between the ZBD and HEL1 domains.[154]

The bioinformatics and biochemical characterization of EAV nsp9 revealed a second enzymatic activity, in addition to the C-terminal RdRp domain. This nucleotidyl transferase (nucleoside monophosphate [NMP] transferase) domain is conserved among nidoviruses and was therefore coined nidovirus RdRp-associated nucleotidyltransferase (NiRAN).[153] The substrate(s) of NiRAN remains undetermined thus far. In the case of EAV nsp9, it was found to mediate (self-)UMPylation

and GMPylation in vitro, but recent coronavirus studies have revealed that the substrates may (also) include other replicase subunits or viral RNA, in the context of the initiation of RNA synthesis or mRNA capping.[242,326] Both the RdRp-associated NiRAN domain and the helicase-associated ZBD are unique for nidoviruses and considered genetic markers of this virus order.[229]

Bioinformatics studies provided the first evidence to suggest that nsp11, and its coronavirus homolog nsp15, contain a nidovirus-specific endoribonuclease activity (NendoU).[243] Subsequently, this prediction was experimentally verified in biochemical assays for recombinant coronavirus nsp15[131] and EAV nsp11.[194] The site-directed mutagenesis of key NendoU residues was found to exert pleiotropic effects on EAV RNA synthesis, including a complete block in some of the mutants and more moderate effects in others.[214] Recombinant NendoU-containing proteins exhibit broad substrate specificity in vitro, processing both single-stranded and double-stranded RNA substrates 3′ of pyrimidines.[194] However, in the context of the infected cell, NendoU activity or substrate specificity likely is controlled via specific protein–protein interactions or compartmentalization within replication organelles. The exact function of the NendoU domain, a genetic marker of vertebrate nidoviruses,[196] remains to be elucidated, but recent coronavirus studies have implicated the enzyme in mediating innate immune evasion by reducing the innate immune sensing of viral double-stranded RNA, thus preventing or delaying activation of the cell's antiviral responses.[82,139]

The final ORF1b-encoded replicase subunit of arteriviruses, nsp12, has not been studied in great detail, although sequence comparisons identified an arterivirus-specific domain (AsD) that is considered a genetic marker of the family.[29]

Assembly and Release

EAV N protein partially colocalizes with the viral replication organelles[272] (e-Fig. 5.8D). Although the N protein is not required for replication or transcription,[188,287,317] genome encapsidation may occur (or begin) at the site of viral RNA synthesis. Electron tomography studies of EAV-infected cells revealed a network of N-containing sheets and tubules in close vicinity of DMVs, but the functional significance of these N-containing structures remains to be studied in more detail.[140]

Arteriviruses acquire their envelope by the budding of preformed nucleocapsids into the lumen of the smooth endoplasmic reticulum and/or the Golgi complex (e-Figs. 5.8E and F and 5.9G and H). The role of the various envelope proteins (GP5-M heterodimer, GP2–GP3–GP4 complex, and the small E and ORF5a proteins) in virus assembly is only partially understood.[302] Most arterivirus envelope proteins are retained in intracellular membranes (e-Fig. 5.8E and F), and the formation of the GP5-M heterodimer is a primary determinant of virus budding.[315,317,332] The transport of GP5 and M to the Golgi complex depends on their heterodimerization and correlates with the production of infectious virus.[86,244,304] After budding, virions accumulate in intracellular vesicles, which merge with the plasma membrane to release the progeny virus. In PRRSV-infected cells, nsp2TF was recently detected in the exocytic pathway (ERGIC and Golgi complex), where it uses its PLP2 domain to deubiquitinate GP5 and M, thus reducing the proteasome-driven turnover of these viral proteins and promoting virus assembly.[120]

Major Structural Proteins

The three major structural proteins GP5, M, and N are encoded—in this order—by the three most 3′-proximal ORFs in the arterivirus genome (Fig. 5.3 and Table 5.1). N is a small protein and contains many basic residues, in particular in its presumably disordered N-terminal domain, which is thought to interact with the genomic RNA during nucleocapsid assembly.[85,88] The C-terminal "capsid-forming" half of N forms dimers and is the basis for a proposed "nidovirus nucleocapsid fold" that is also encountered in the much larger coronavirus N protein.[88] The EAV and PRRSV N proteins are phosphorylated.[70,320] In the case of PRRSV N, phosphoserines map to both the RNA-binding domain and the capsid-forming domain, where they may modulate nucleic acid–binding activity or protein–protein interactions.[320]

The nonglycosylated M protein is the most conserved envelope protein of arteriviruses.[70] The M protein has three internal membrane-spanning segments and a short amino-terminus exposed at the virion surface (aa 10 to 18), and its carboxy-terminus (approximately aa 72) is buried within the virus' interior.[70,247] The M protein resembles the coronavirus M protein in that its N-terminal half presumably traverses the membrane three times,[70,96,184] resulting in an N_{exo}-C_{endo} configuration with a short ectodomain exposed on the virion surface. One of the membrane-spanning fragments is thought to function as an internal signal sequence. The M protein forms disulfide-linked heterodimers with GP5 through a disulfide bridge between cysteine residues in their respective ectodomains (e.g., position 8 [Cys-8] of M and Cys-34 of GP5 of EAV). The mutagenesis of either cysteine residue completely inhibited heterodimerization of the two proteins.[71,95,244] GP5-M heterodimerization is thought to be essential for virus assembly, possibly by inducing the membrane curvature required for virus budding.[71,86,244] Furthermore, the covalent association of the GP5 and M proteins is indispensable for producing infectious arteriviruses.[244,304] Hetero dimerization of the GP5 and M proteins is also critical for the authentic posttranslational modification and conformational maturation of the major neutralization determinants in GP5 of EAV and PRRSV.[11,17]

Despite considerable differences in primary structure, the GP5 proteins of arteriviruses share common structural features. They contain an N-terminal signal sequence that is assumed to be cleaved from a short ectodomain. The central hydrophobic region probably spans the membrane three times and is followed by a cytoplasmic domain. EAV GP5 is predicted to have an ectodomain of 98 residues, while the GP5 proteins of LDV and PRRSV have ectodomains of approximately 30 amino acids, which all contain variable N-linked glycosylation sites.[96,184] The EAV GP5 ectodomain usually possesses a single N-linked polylactosamine side chain,[70] although in some strains one or two additional N-linked glycans are present. The short (21-aa) N-terminal ectodomain of SHFV GP5 contains only one putative glycosylation site, whereas glycosylation of LDV GP5 occurs by the addition of variable numbers of lactosamine repeats. The major neutralization epitopes of EAV, PRRSV, SHFV, and LDV have been mapped to the N-terminal ectodomain of GP5.[12]

Minor Structural Proteins

Arterivirus minor envelope proteins are encoded in ORFs 2a, 2b, 3, 4, and 5a. The small E protein is encoded by ORF2a in EAV (ORF2b in PRRSV). Its higher order structure is unknown, but the protein is essential for virus infectivity[248] and might be associated with the trimer of minor GPs.[315] The protein has been proposed to oligomerize and form an ion channel that could play a role during viral entry.[152] Furthermore, its N-terminus contains a myristoylation signal that is functional in EAV and PRRSV. A block of the fatty acid addition was not lethal, but knockout mutants were crippled and displayed a small-plaque phenotype.[265] A recent study showed that the E protein's C-terminal endodomain is essential to interact with tubulin-α, suggesting that during the early stages of infection, PRRSV requires the microtubule network, while the interaction of E and tubulin-α may contribute to microtubule depolymerization during the later stages of infection.[337]

The GP2 protein is expressed from ORF2a or ORF2b (Fig. 5.3). It is a conventional class I integral membrane protein with an N-terminal signal peptide, a C-terminal transmembrane segment, and 1 to 4 potential N-glycosylation sites in its ectodomain. The GP2 protein occurs in several distinct conformations—as four monomers resulting from different disulfide-bonded structures or as a disulfide-linked dimer (i.e., intramolecular and intermolecular cysteine bridges).[71] However, only the dimeric form of GP2 is further associated with GP3 and GP4 proteins as a heterotrimeric complex, which is incorporated into viral particles.[312,315,317]

The GP3 protein has two putative N-myristoylation sites and three casein kinase II phosphorylation motifs, but it is unclear whether they are used. EAV GP3 is a heavily glycosylated integral membrane protein with an uncleaved N-terminal signal sequence and a hydrophobic C-terminal domain, suggesting the protein is anchored in the membrane with both termini.[313] Like GP2 and GP4, EAV GP3 localizes to the endoplasmic reticulum.[313] Following virus release, GP3 becomes disulfide-linked to the GP2–GP4 heterodimers, and this post assembly maturation event yields a complex of three covalently bound minor GPs. As a result, EAV particles contain both GP2–GP4 heterodimers and GP2–GP3–GP4 heterotrimers.[314,315]

Like GP2, GP4 is a predicted class I membrane protein with a cleaved signal sequence and multiple N-glycosylation sites in its ectodomain.[186,296,313] Little is known about the properties or function of GP4, apart from the oligomerization described above and the finding that GP4 may be responsible for an interaction of the GP2–GP3–GP4 trimer with GP5.[65] Reverse genetics studies with PRRSV mutants lacking specific glycans in GP2, GP3, or GP4 showed that GP2 and GP3 mutants failed to produce progeny virus.[66] Although single-site mutants of GP4 produced infectious virus, mutation of any two sites in GP4 was lethal. Furthermore, only GP2 and GP4 glycosylation are critical for their interactions with CD163.

In SHFV and other simarteriviruses, a large insertion downstream of ORF1b contains four ORFs encoding additional four minor structural proteins (E′, GP2′, GP3′, and GP4′). These additional ORFs likely derive from an ancient duplication of the ORF 2 to 4 gene block. A recent study indicated that the duplicated set of SHFV minor structural proteins is not functionally redundant and that all eight minor structural proteins are required to produce infectious extracellular viruses.[300]

Bioinformatics analyses of the EAV genome revealed an additional ORF (ORF5a) that overlaps the 5′ end of ORF5 and is conserved in all arteriviruses.[103,132] The small hydrophobic ORF5a protein is thought to be expressed from the same subgenomic mRNA (sg mRNA5) as GP5, possibly involving a leaky ribosomal scanning mechanism, although (co)expression from a separate sg mRNA has been postulated for SHFV.[84] The ORF5a protein was identified in purified PRRSV virions.

It is predicted to be a type III membrane protein with a short (5 to 12 aa) amino-terminal domain in the lumen, a central signal transmembrane sequence, and its carboxy terminal domain in the cytosol.[132] The function of this protein remains to be characterized in detail. EAV reverse genetics revealed that the ORF5a protein is not essential, although knockout mutants showed a significant reduction of progeny virus titers.[103]

Arterivirus–Host Cell Interactions

Arteriviruses interact with a variety of host factors and pathways, for example to modulate innate immune responses, the unfolded protein response,[107] and apoptosis in cell lines and/or cultured macrophages.[5,60,343] PRRSV also induces apoptosis in germinal cells *in vivo*.[262] In both macrophages and MARC-145 cells, PRRSV stimulates antiapoptotic pathways during early infection, but late in infection, cells die from caspase-dependent apoptosis, culminating in secondary necrosis.[4,60]

Over the past decade, several additional (potential) host cell factors were reported to interact with specific arterivirus replicase subunits, which unfortunately cannot be discussed in detail due to space limitations.[72,89,167,218] For example, various proteins from MA-104 cells were reported to bind to SHFV-derived RNA sequences.[129,178] In EAV, the *in vitro* RNA-synthesizing activity of semipurified viral replication and transcription complexes depends on the presence of a soluble host protein of 59 to 70 kDa that remains to be identified.[292] Recent studies on PRRSV and SHFV showed that the $-2/-1$ PRF mechanism during ORF1a translation is in part controlled by an interaction of viral protein nsp1β with specific viral RNA sequences and host poly(C)-binding proteins.[162,192,207]

Despite the cytoplasmic replication cycle of arteriviruses, some viral proteins are directed (in part) to the nucleus of infected cells (e-Fig. 5.8), specifically the nsp1 (see above) and N protein. A nuclear localization signal (NLS) interacting with the nuclear transporters importin α and β was identified at positions 41 to 47 of PRRSV N,[227] which—like its EAV counterpart—accumulates in the nucleoli of infected cells.[227,272] Remarkably, a block of exportin1-mediated nuclear export with the drug leptomycin B resulted in the nuclear accumulation of EAV N, indicating that the protein apparently shuttles between cytoplasm and nucleus before playing its role in cytoplasmic virus assembly.[272] Various nuclear host proteins interacting with PRRSV N protein were identified (reviewed by Refs.[330]), including fibrillarin, nucleolin, and poly(A)-binding protein, but the functional implications of these findings remain to be unraveled. Using reverse genetics, a knockout mutation for the NLS of PRRSV N protein was engineered and yielded a viable, although seriously attenuated, mutant virus.[151] Compared to the wild-type control, pigs infected with this mutant virus showed reduced viremia; however, reversions occurred in the NLS region that were able to translocate the mutated N proteins to the nucleus, indicating an important role of N protein nuclear localization in viral pathogenesis *in vivo*.

PATHOGENESIS AND PATHOLOGY OF ARTERIVIRUS INFECTIONS

Site of Primary Replication, Spread, and Cell and Tissue Tropism

The natural host range of arteriviruses is restricted to members of the family *Equidae* (horses, donkeys, mules, and zebras;

EAV), pigs (PRRSV), rodents (LDV and rat arteriviruses), Australian brushtail possums (WPDV), Oliver's shrews (OSV),[299] and nonhuman primates (SHFV and other simarteriviruses). Based on the studies of prototypic arterivirus species, macrophages appear to be their primary target cell in the respective hosts. Disease outcome is highly variable and includes persistent asymptomatic infections, respiratory disease, reproductive failure (abortion), lethal hemorrhagic fever, neurological disorders, and fatal encephalitis.[7,67,93,213]

Following respiratory transmission, EAV initially replicates in alveolar macrophages, and bronchiolar epithelial cells, after which the virus spreads to regional lymph nodes (e.g., bronchial).[126] However, recent *ex vivo* (i.e., mucosal explants) and *in vitro* studies aimed at elucidating the early events in the pathogenesis of EAV infection demonstrated that the virus localizes in CD3+ T lymphocytes, CD172a+ myeloid cells, and a small population of IgM+ B lymphocytes found in the connective tissue.[279] Interestingly, the virus was not detected in epithelial cells from the upper respiratory tract during the early phase of infection.[278,279] These studies suggested that the nasopharynx and tubal nasopharyngeal tonsils play an important role as primary sites of EAV replication during early infection, and high viral titers were detected during the first 7 days post infection (dpi).[151] Previously, *in vivo* experimental infections of horses have shown cell-associated viremia within 3 dpi, which frequently extended to 3 to 19 dpi. The virus is distributed throughout the body, replicating in macrophages, vascular smooth muscle cells, and endothelial cells, which causes a systemic panvasculitis (reviewed in Ref.[7] and references therein). Thus, the clinical manifestations of equine viral arteritis (EVA) reflect endothelial cell injury and increased vascular permeability. EAV infection of pregnant mares can result in abortion, and aborted fetuses are usually (partially) autolyzed at the time of expulsion. With the exception of infected stallions, viral clearance usually occurs by 28 dpi and coincides with the appearance and rise of serum neutralizing antibodies. EAV exclusively persists in the reproductive tract of carrier stallions (mainly the ampullae of the vas deferens),[43,195] which leads to continuous virus shedding in semen.

The primary target cells for PRRSV replication *in vivo* are fully differentiated porcine pulmonary alveolar macrophages (PAM) in the lung, pulmonary intravascular macrophages (PIM) of the placenta and umbilical cord, and monocyte-derived macrophages (MDM) in lymph nodes and spleen.[91,266] PRRSV replicates to a lesser extent in dendritic cells and in MDM. PRRSV infection can be divided into three stages: acute infection, persistence, and extinction.[173] Acute infection follows exposure to PRRSV and virus replication in lung and lymphoid tissues. Viremia usually is detected 6 to 48 hpi, and viral loads peak by 4 to 14 dpi. After the peak of viremia, virus titers in serum drop rapidly, and most pigs are no longer viremic by 21 to 28 dpi. The persistence stage begins when viremia ends, and clinical signs subside. However, PRRSV replicates in tonsils and lymph nodes, and pigs continue to shed the virus. Boars can become persistently infected and shed virus in their semen. The extinction phase begins when the virus is cleared from lymphoid tissues and viral shedding ends, which may take as long as 250 days postexposure to the virus (reviewed in Refs.[173,267]).

LDV replicates in permissive macrophages in the spleen, lymph nodes, thymus, and liver of infected mice.[176] The virus attains extremely high titer in serum within 12 to 14 hours after experimental inoculation, due to rapid cytolysis of the targeting macrophages, which releases massive numbers of infectious virions into the circulation. The subpopulation of macrophages that is susceptible to LDV infection normally is responsible for the clearance of lactate dehydrogenase (LDH), explaining the elevated LDH levels in blood and the name of this arterivirus. Persistent infection is a characteristic of LDV infection in mice, which is maintained by virus replication in new permissive macrophages, which are continuously generated from apparently nonpermissive precursor cells.

Like the other arteriviruses, SHFV principally replicates in macrophages, although there is considerable variation in the cellular tropism, virulence, and immunogenicity of individual strains of SHFV in African monkeys. Long-term viremia in these monkey species (e.g., patas monkeys, African green monkeys, and baboons) can occur without disease and without detectable antibody responses. Detection of asymptomatic carriers through culture of peritoneal macrophages has been described. Asian monkeys (e.g., rhesus macaques) are highly susceptible to SHFV infection and develop fatal hemorrhagic disease.[176]

The experimental intraperitoneal inoculation of wild-caught brushtail possum with purified WPDV has been described.[108] The viral nucleic acid was detected in the serum, retropharyngeal lymph node, spleen, liver, salivary gland, kidney, bladder, forebrain, and urine of infected possums. The possums developed neurologic signs of wobbly possum disease.

Immune Responses and Immune Evasion

Several arteriviruses cause persistent infections despite the development of an adaptive immune response. Neither neutralizing antibodies nor effective helper and cytolytic T lymphocytes are able to control virus replication in these persistently infected animals. Therefore, arteriviruses must have developed strategies to evade immune responses, highlighting the importance of studying immunity in natural and experimental infections in order to enhance our knowledge of the underlying mechanisms. For a more detailed overview of arterivirus immune evasion and host responses to arterivirus infection, the reader is also referred to a variety of review articles (reviewed in Refs.[4,9,12,170,173,219,220] and references therein).

Innate Immune Response

It remains rather unclear which pattern recognition receptors (PRRs) of the innate immune system recognize arterivirus infection in different cell types. Several reports have suggested the involvement of toll-like receptors in lung cells and lymphoid tissues of PRRSV-infected pigs (reviewed in Ref.[170] and references therein). Retinoic acid–inducible gene 1 (RIG-I) and melanoma differentiation–associated gene (MDA5) expression were found to be increased in alveolar macrophages infected with PRRSV, but the level was rather weak compared to that induced by swine influenza virus.[87] PLP2 has deubiquitinase activity, which suppresses activated RIG-I to control innate immune signaling in arterivirus-infected cells. A study with EAV in knockout mouse embryonic fibroblasts suggested that of the cytosolic retinoic acid inducible I–like receptors (RLRs), MDA5 is predominantly involved in recognition of this virus.[294] Experimental LDV infection of TLR7[−/−] mice revealed the importance of this TLR expressed by plasmacytoid dendritic cells (pDCs) for the induction of type I interferon (IFN) and the activation of lymphocytes during LDV infection.[2]

The innate immune response to EAV infection has not been characterized comprehensively. *In vitro* studies using alveolar and blood-derived macrophages demonstrated that tumor necrosis factor (TNF)-α and other proinflammatory cytokines are induced following infection with virulent EAV strains.[189] In the case of PRRSV, the innate immune response, particularly the type 1 IFN response, is weakly induced or could even be actively suppressed following viral infection.[170,173] The induction level of TNF-α, IFN-α, and other innate cytokines appears to depend on the viral isolate, host age, and host immune status. Several PRRSV proteins have been identified as innate immune antagonists (see section "Immune Evasion" below). LDV infection induces natural killer (NK) cells in infected mice, and as a consequence, a large increase in serum IFN-γ was observed, but these responses were unable to control LDV replication.[180] LDV also elicits IFN-α through TLR7 activation in pDCs, but the virus is not sensitive to a systemic IFN-α response in mice.[2]

Humoral Immune Response

Following infection, both EAV-specific complement-fixing (CF) and virus-neutralizing (VN) antibodies develop between 7 and 14 dpi, which provide long-lasting immunity (3 years or more) and protection from reinfection with most (if not all) viral strains (reviewed in Ref.[7] and references therein) (e-Fig. 5.10). Sera from infected horses recognize N, M, GP5, and GP2.[175] In addition, antibodies against nsp2, nsp4, nsp5, and nsp12 were found in experimentally or persistently infected horses, whereas animals vaccinated with a modified live virus (MLV) vaccine against EAV produced antibodies against nsp2, nsp12, and nsp4 (weak response), but not against nsp5.[112] PRRSV-infected pigs produce antibodies directed against the structural proteins GP2 to GP5, M, and N, with the antibodies recognizing N being detected earliest and most abundantly.[168,185] The early humoral response against PRRSV also includes antibodies against nsp1α/β, nsp2, and nsp7, which develop to titers as high as those of the anti-N antibodies and can be detected as long as 202 dpi[31,133] (e-Fig. 5.11). It has been proposed that LDV- and PRRSV-specific antibodies contribute to antibody-dependent enhancement (ADE) of infection.[37,331] For PRRSV, certain nonneutralizing epitopes in the N and GP5 proteins induce antibodies that seem to be responsible for ADE through opsonization, leading to enhance internalization of the virus into macrophages.[41]

Neutralizing antibodies in arterivirus-infected animals are predominantly directed to the major glycoprotein GP5.[13,36,200,212] The neutralization site in EAV, PRRSV, and LDV GP5 was mapped to the ectodomain of the protein.[8,160,212] In EAV, four major neutralization sites were identified in the GP5 ectodomain, and some of these epitopes appear to be conformational.[8] The PRRSV GP5 epitope was initially thought to be linear, but more recent data show that it is conformational.[97,159] Consistent with that conclusion, no linear neutralization epitopes were identified in GP5 by peptide scanning analysis. As the M protein forms a heterodimer with GP5, it may contribute to the conformation of neutralization epitopes in GP5. The M protein itself was also reported to contain a neutralization epitope.[327] Recently, a single amino acid (Tyr-10) in the PRRSV M protein was identified as critical for swine antibodies to mediate broadly neutralizing activity.[277] Besides the major envelope proteins, earlier studies identified a neutralization epitope in the PRRSV minor glycoprotein GP4,[62,63,186,296] and subsequently peptide scanning identified linear neutralization epitopes in all three minor glycoproteins GP2, GP3, and GP4.[298]

The induction of a strong neutralizing antibody response in EAV-infected horses coincides with virus clearance, suggesting that the humoral immune response plays an important role in recovery (e-Fig. 5.10).[106] However, despite the presence of high levels of neutralizing antibodies, EAV persists in the reproductive tract of carrier stallions. In contrast, neutralizing antibodies against LDV and PRRSV are detected only very late, 1 to 2 months after infection, and are produced at relatively low levels.[36,168,331] One of the most common hypotheses for the delayed neutralizing antibody production in PRRSV infection, or after vaccination, is the presence of an immuno-dominant decoy epitope. This decoy epitope just upstream of the GP5 neutralization epitope and induces a strong nonneutralizing antibody response.[200] Insertion of another epitope between the neutralizing and decoy epitopes increased the neutralizing response, suggesting that the juxtapositioning of the two original epitopes indeed plays a role.[98] In addition, the glycosylation state of the GP5 ectodomain in the vicinity of the neutralizing epitope and GP3 glycosylation may influence the efficiency of neutralizing antibody production.[305] Similarly, in the case of nonneuropathogenic LDV strains, the GP5 ectodomain contains three polylactosaminoglycan chains, as opposed to a single polylactosaminoglycan in the ectodomain of neuropathogenic strains. It was postulated that the nonneuropathogenic strains can establish persistent infections because neutralizing antibodies bind less efficiently to the highly glycosylated ectodomain of their GP5. In contrast, neuropathogenic strains are not able to persist.[55,160,213] Yet another explanation for inefficient neutralization was inspired by the observation that PRRSV infection in piglets manipulates the development of the B-cell repertoire.[34] Together with the general idea that PRRSV suppresses (innate) immune responses, this may explain the delayed and aberrant antibody production that is observed (reviewed in Refs.[170,219]).

The humoral immune response against SHFV varies with the species of monkey and the virus isolate that is tested.[116,117] The rapid death of macaques after SHFV infection precludes an effective host immune response. Virulent SHFV strains, which cause acute disease in patas monkeys, induced neutralizing antibodies at 7 dpi. The production of neutralizing antibodies correlated with the complete clearance of the virus from the circulation by 21 dpi. On the other hand, SHFV strains that cause a persistent infection in these monkeys induce very low antibody titers.

Cell-Mediated Immune Response

Cell-mediated immunity (CMI) to arterivirus infection has not yet been characterized in much detail. Studies in ponies experimentally infected with EAV have shown that the cytotoxicity induced by EAV-stimulated peripheral blood mononuclear cells (PBMC) was virus-specific, genetically restricted, mediated by CD8+ T cells, and that the precursors persist for at least 1 year after infection.[9,46]

Cell-mediated responses in PRRSV-infected animals include CD4+, CD8+, and double-positive T cells, which appear transiently between 2 and 8 weeks after experimental infection (reviewed in Refs.[170,220,322]) or become more pronounced at later stages.[182] The abundance of PRRSV-specific T cells and IFN-γ–producing cells in both acute and persistently infected animals is highly variable and does not correlate

with virus levels in lymphoid tissue.[182,322] The cytotoxic effector function of CD8+ T cells (CTLs) has not been directly linked to the control of primary PRRSV infection, since the CTL activity was only detected after viremia was cleared[61] (e-Fig. 5.11). Several studies indicate that the strongest CMI inducers of PRRSV are M, N, GP4, and GP5 proteins.[170] In addition, nsp9 and nsp10 were reported to contain a number of potential T-cell epitopes.[202]

Cytotoxic and helper T-cell responses were detected in LDV-infected mice but did not reduce LDV replication.[94] Additional studies are required to determine whether there is a correlation between T-cell responses *in vitro* and protection *in vivo*, and the overall data suggest that the arteriviruses probably directly, or indirectly, manipulate CMI.

Immune Evasion

Not much is known about the mechanistic details of immune evasion by arteriviruses, but it is clear that modulation of the immune response occurs on different levels. An expanding body of data documents the suppression of innate immune responses (reviewed for PRRSV in Refs.[4,100,330]), as for example recently demonstrated for EAV.[111] Several reports suggest that arteriviruses also manipulate the CMI. Down-regulation of major histocompatibility complex class I and II (MHCI and MHC-II) molecules on the surface of antigen-presenting cells (APCs) was shown for PRRSV,[170] and coinfection with LDV causes a delay of the CD8+ T-cell–mediated immune response to Friend virus in mice, suggesting manipulation of the MHC-I presentation pathway.[225]

The molecular mechanisms underlying immune-suppressive activities of arteriviruses have been mostly studied for EAV and PRRSV. One of the critical features of EAV long-term persistent infection (LTPI) in the reproductive tract of the stallion is that the virus does not exploit immunologically privileged tissues, such as the testes. Instead, EAV primarily replicates in the ampulla of the vas deferens and accessory sex glands in the presence of active immune responses (humoral and CMI), as evidenced by the presence of inflammatory infiltrates.[42,43,45] At present, it is not known why these apparently active immune responses fail to eliminate the virus. Potential explanations include continuous EAV evolution leading to the emergence of antigenic variants,[191] a local immunosuppressive environment mediated by cytokines and hormones such as androgens, induction of peripheral tolerance via T-regulatory lymphocytes, or even immune exhaustion caused by continual antigenic stimulation that results in effector T cells becoming progressively dysfunctional and less responsive.[7] Such mechanisms are not mutually exclusive and could occur in combination, but further studies will be needed. Recent studies indicate that EAV may be hijacking the CXCL16/CXCR6 axis to subvert the local immune response to the virus at the site of persistent infection in the stallion.[42] Several reports suggested that PRRSV induces significant IL-10 production in pigs during the first 2 weeks of infection. This immunosuppressive cytokine interacts with a wide array of immune cells, including the PRRSV target cells from the monocyte/macrophage lineage, to down-regulate in particular cell-mediated innate and adaptive immunity. Recent experiments suggest that PRRSV N may be responsible for IL-10 up-regulation during infection and that this may be achieved through induction of specific regulatory T-cell populations.[170,241,319,330]

In addition to N, several nonstructural proteins have been implicated in arterivirus immune evasion: nsp1 (nsp1α and nsp1β in PRRSV), nsp2 (EAV and PRRSV), nsp2TF/nsp2N (PRRSV), nsp4 (PRRSV), and nsp11 (PRRSV).[4,163,330] Three of these proteins (nsp1, nsp2, and nsp11) were suggested to suppress innate immune signaling induced by the RLR- or TLR-innate sensors, or TNF-α, which lead to IFN-β and/or nuclear factor kappa B (NF-kB) expression. PRRSV nsp1α and nsp1β both inhibit the expression of IFN-β after induction of innate responses by Sendai virus or double-stranded DNA (dsRNA),[26] and nsp1β also inhibits signaling downstream of type 1 IFN by inhibiting nuclear translocation of STAT1.[51] Furthermore, both nsp1α and nsp1β suppress NF-kB activation.[26,253] Kim et al.[137] showed degradation of cAMP response element-binding (CREB) protein induced by PRRSV nsp1 during infection, causing inhibition of interferon regulatory transcription factor 3 (IRF3) activity in the nucleus. Besides localizing to the perinuclear region with other nsps, nsp1 is partially transported to the nucleus,[51,137,272] which may be connected to at least some of its immune evasive activities.

Arterivirus nsp2 contains a papain-like proteinase (PLP2) in its N-terminal domain. The enzyme not only cleaves the nsp2/nsp3 site in the replicase polyproteins but also is a deubiquitinating enzyme (DUB). Upon overexpression, EAV and PRRSV PLP2 show a general DUB activity toward cellular ubiquitin conjugates and also cleave the IFN-induced ubiquitin homolog ISG15, which is thought to have antiviral activity.[104] Indications that these DUB activities could be functional in the suppression of innate immune responses were obtained from experiments in which the EAV PLP2-DUB suppressed TNFα-induced NF-kB signaling in 293T cells. Also the PRRSV PLP2-DUB inhibits NF-kB signaling, as well as the IRF3-dependent IFN-β pathway induced by Sendai virus infection.[158,163,260] PRRSV PLP2-DUB appears to remove K48-linked polyubiquitin from IkBα to prevent its proteasomal degradation and thereby downstream signaling toward NF-kB activation. Further studies on PLP2 of four prototypic arteriviruses (EAV, PRRSV, SHFV, and LDV) showed that PLP2 suppresses RLR-mediated IFN-β induction by removing K63-linked polyubiquitin from RIG-I, which results in inhibition of downstream signaling.[294] Besides the PLP2 domain of PRRSV nsp2, also the variable regions in the central part of this large protein could influence antiviral responses.[56,100]

Recent studies showed that PRRSV nsp4 is able to antagonize IFN-β transcription in the nucleus.[54,263] This innate immune antagonist function depends on the serine proteinase (SP) encoded in nsp4, which can cleave multiple sites in NF-κB essential modulator (NEMO) and thus suppresses activation of the NF-κB pathway and downstream IFN-β production.[49,128]

Arterivirus nsp11 (containing the NendoU endoribonuclease) was proposed to be an IFN antagonist. The RNase activity of PRRSV NendoU was implicated in immune evasion,[239,330] and recent studies demonstrated that nsp11 may induce STAT2 degradation and inhibit ISG expression.[328] Another study showed that nsp11 interacts with IRF9 and impairs the formation of IFN-stimulated gene factor 3 (ISGF3).[307] As these data were mostly generated using nsp11 overexpression, it remains to be established that they reflect the natural situation in the infected cell, where NendoU activity may be controlled by interaction with other viral proteins and/or compartmentalization within replication organelles. Whether the RNase activity

of nsp11 specifically targets certain innate immune responses in the infected cell, or perhaps the overall mRNA population of the cell to induce a translational shut-off, should therefore be probed more rigorously in future studies.

The replication of LDV and SHFV in macrophages allows the virus to avoid host defense mechanisms.[176] In addition, LDV successfully evades host immune response in a number of ways, thereby establishing lifelong persistent infection in mice. LDV infection modulates a variety of immune responses through a number of direct and indirect effects, including depression of cellular immunity, cytokine perturbations, and macrophage function. However, the precise mechanisms of LDV and SHFV immune evasion and persistent infection are still unclear.

Release From the Host and Transmission

The two principal modes of EAV and PRRSV transmission are horizontal transmission by aerosolization of infectious respiratory tract secretions from acutely infected animals and venereal transmission during natural or artificial insemination with infective semen from persistently infected stallions or boars (reviewed in Refs.[7,174,310] and references therein). It has been demonstrated that EAV can be transmitted during embryo transfer from mares inseminated with infective semen. EAV can also be transmitted through indirect contact with fomites or personnel. Congenital infection results from transplacental transmission (vertical transmission) of the virus when pregnant mares are infected late in gestation.

PRRSV is shed in respiratory tract secretions, saliva, semen, mammary secretions (i.e., milk), urine, and feces of infected animals (reviewed in Refs.[59,126]). Susceptible pigs are naturally infected by inhalation of infectious aerosols or ingestion of PRRSV-contaminated food (horizontal transmission). Congenital infection results from transplacental transmission (vertical transmission) of the virus. Transmission of PRRSV to females has been demonstrated during breeding with semen from persistently infected carrier boars that harbor the virus in their tonsils long after the virus is cleared from other tissues. PRRSV was shown to replicate in testicular germ cells such as spermatids and spermatocytes.[262] PRRSV can also be transmitted through indirect contact with fomites or personnel, needles, contaminated boots, and coveralls.[59,201,210] There is evidence that flies and mosquitoes might serve as mechanical vectors of PRRSV.

LDV establishes lifelong viremia in infected mice, and the virus is shed in urine, feces, and saliva.[342] Feces contain high titers of virus, and thus, coprophagic behavior of mice probably plays an important role in the transmission of the virus. LDV transmission from mother to offspring through the placenta or via breast milk is highly efficient if the mother is immunologically naive.[213] However, transmission via these routes from persistently infected mothers is rare because anti-LDV antibodies block transplacental transmission of the virus and its release into milk. Also, horizontal transmission of LDV does occur among laboratory mice that fight and bite one another. The sexual transmission of LDV among mice has not been clearly demonstrated.[35]

Transmission of SHFV among African monkeys most likely occurs through wounds and biting, but sexual transmission has not been ruled out. SHFV is not transmitted transplacentally from persistently infected mothers to their offspring.[116] Several epizootics of SHF in captive macaque colonies originated from the accidental mechanical transmission of SHFV from asymptomatic, persistently infected African monkeys.

Once illness becomes apparent in the macaque colony, the SHFV spreads rapidly throughout the colony, most likely by direct contact and aerosols.

Virulence

Outbreaks of virulent field strains of EAV and PRRSV have been reported; however, molecular determinants of virulence have not been fully characterized. Several full-length infectious cDNA clones of EAV have been developed, and the virulence phenotypes of the derived recombinant chimeric viruses have been characterized in horses.[15,19,287] These sequences are derived from several well-characterized attenuated strains (i.e., the current modified vaccine strain, and several highly cell culture–adapted laboratory viruses) and the virulent EAV Bucyrus strain. The recombinant chimeric viruses were used to characterize neutralization and virulence determinants of EAV, clearly showing that multiple viral genes codetermine the viral phenotype (e.g., virulence/attenuation, viral persistence, cellular tropism, and neutralization). These studies confirmed that amino acid substitutions in both structural and nonstructural proteins may allow field strains of EAV to evade protective host immune responses to facilitate persistent infection of stallions. Specifically, reverse genetics experiments showed that substitutions in the structural proteins may lead to more severe attenuation than those in the nonstructural proteins.[333] Collectively, interactions of both major (GP5 and M) and minor (GP2, GP3, and GP4) envelope proteins seem to influence tropism, and thus, mutations in these proteins can affect virulence.[113] Furthermore, it has been also demonstrated that EAV CD3+ T lymphocyte tropism is primarily determined by specific amino acid residues in the GP2, GP4, GP5, and M envelope proteins but not the GP3 minor envelope protein. Unlike the virulence determinants of EAV, the E and GP3 minor envelope proteins appeared to play an important role in the establishment of persistent infection in mammalian cells *in vitro*.

Sequence comparisons revealed that the highly pathogenic PRRSV (HP-PRRSV) strain causing the "porcine high fever disease" in Asia since 2006 originated from Chinese domestic viruses (which are related to VR-2332, the prototype strain of PRRSV-2).[236] They share the same striking deletions of a conserved leucine and a 29 amino acid stretch in nsp2.[156,236,270] Similarly, several virulent isolates reported in the United States contain variable nsp2 deletions; for example, isolates MN184 and NADC30 contained three discontinuous deletions of 111, 1, and 19 amino acids when compared to the VR-2332 prototype.[30,122] However, these typical differences do not seem to be a primary determinant of the increased virulence.[30,339] Using chimeric infectious clones of a highly virulent PRRSV (FL12) and their counterparts of an attenuated vaccine strain (Prime Pac, Merck Animal Health), the major virulence determinants were mapped to the nsp3–8 and ORF5 region.[145] Recent studies on Chinese HP-PRRSV suggested that nsp9 and nsp10 are virulence factors, and residues 586 and 592 of nsp9 were identified as critical sites for fatal virulence.[166,324]

The virulence determinants of LDV and SHFV are not well characterized.[183,213] However, it has been reported that the LDV-P and LDV-vx strains readily establish persistent infections in mice, but are not neurovirulent. In contrast, two laboratory mutant strains of LDV (e.g., LDV-C and LDV-v) are highly susceptible to antibody neutralization and incapable of establishing persistent infection in mice.[52] Interestingly, the LDV-C and LDV-v strains are neurovirulent in immunosuppressed

C58 and AKR mice.[53] The GP5 ectodomain of these mutant viruses lacks the two N-terminal glycans (Asn-36 and Asn-45), flanking the major neutralization epitope of LDV and losing these two glycosylation sites makes the neutralization epitope both highly immunogenic and susceptible to *in vivo* neutralization by antibodies. Loss of these glycosylation sites also alters cellular tropism of LDV-C and LDV-v, leading to infection of spinal cord anterior horn neurons and subsequent paralysis of the infected mice (see below).[211]

Persistence

Persistent infection constitutes the main epidemiological challenge in the control and eradication of arterivirus infections. Persistently infected animals serve as a source of infection for susceptible individuals. Following natural EAV infection, the majority of the stallions (~70%) can become persistently infected and continuously shed virus in their semen for either a short (several weeks to 1 year; short-term carriers or short-term shedders [STS]) or a long period of time (1 year to lifelong; long-term carriers or long-term persistently infected [LTPI] shedders) without adverse effects on semen quality or reproductive capacity (e-Fig. 5.10).[40] The virus persists exclusively in the male reproductive tract, despite the presence of high levels of neutralizing and mucosal antibodies.[45] Moreover, maintenance of EAV LTPI is testosterone-dependent and, therefore, does not cause persistent infection in mares, foals, and sexually immature colts (reviewed in Ref.[9] and references therein). The analysis of multiple tissues from the reproductive tract of EAV carrier stallions unequivocally confirmed the ampullae of the vas deferens as the primary site of EAV persistence in the stallion's reproductive tract. In addition, using immunohistochemistry and dual immunofluorescence microscopy, it has been demonstrated that EAV has a specific tropism for vimentin-positive stromal cells (e.g., fibrocytes and tissue macrophages) and CD8+ T and CD21+ B lymphocytes but not for cytokeratin-positive glandular epithelial cells in the male reproductive tract. Recently, it has been demonstrated that establishment of EAV LTPI correlates with the *in vitro* susceptibility of a subpopulation of CD3+ T lymphocytes to EAV infection, and, consequently, stallions with the CD3+ T lymphocyte susceptibility phenotype are at higher risk of becoming LTPI carriers compared to those that lack this phenotype.[110,112,113] A genome-wide association study (GWAS) demonstrated that these phenotypes are associated with the *CXCL16* gene located in equine chromosome 11 (ECA11). Subsequent studies have identified two allelic variants of *CXCL16* (namely *CXCL16S* and *CXCL16R*) that differ by four nonsynonymous nucleotide substitutions in exon 2 and show a very strong association with the two CD3+ T lymphocyte phenotypes (susceptible and resistant) and with either the establishment of LTPI (*CXCL16S*) or the early viral clearance (STS) in stallions (*CXCL16R*).[42,231] The role of CXCL16 and its receptor CXCR6 (CXCL16–CXCR6 chemokine axis) in the pathogenesis of persistent EAV infection is under further investigation.

In contrast to EAV, PRRSV can establish a chronic, persistent infection in lymph nodes (e.g., inguinal, mandibular and sternal) and tonsils of infected animals without sex predilection, as well as in the reproductive tract of infected boars.[217,226,316] The virus has been isolated from tonsils and lymph nodes of infected pigs for up to 157 dpi and can be detectable by RT-PCR up to 251 dpi.[1,316] During the persistent infection stage, virus is no longer detected in blood and lungs, and pigs no longer exhibit significant clinical signs. At this asymptomatic stage, lymphoid organs, including tonsil and lymph nodes, are the primary sites of viral replication, and the virus can still transmit to sentinel pigs. The presence of PRRSV in semen of infected boars could be due to either local virus replication and shedding from reproductive tract tissues (testes, epididymis, and bulbourethral glands) or direct dissemination (via infected monocytes and macrophages) from tissues other than those of the reproductive tract (reviewed in Ref.[217] and references therein). Nevertheless, it is believed that this virus most likely reaches the tissues of the male reproductive tract and semen by migration of infected macrophages. Although the mechanisms underlying the failure to promptly clear PRRSV infection are poorly understood, it appears that a major reason is the inability of pigs to rapidly develop effective protective immune responses, which is likely due to the concerted immune evasion strategies exploited by the virus (reviewed in Refs.[4,170,173]).

LDV is able to establish a largely asymptomatic persistent infection in mice, which is maintained by virus replication in permissive macrophages that are continuously generated from apparently nonpermissive precursor cells.[213] SHFV appears to be endemic among several species of African monkeys, in which it causes asymptomatic or persistent infections.[169]

EPIDEMIOLOGY

EAV

EAV has a worldwide distribution primarily in domestic equine populations in North and South America, Europe, Australia, Africa, and various countries in Asia (reviewed in Ref.[16] and references therein). Other countries, such as Iceland, Japan, and New Zealand, are free of the disease.[181] Although the vast majority of EAV infections are subclinical, outbreaks of the disease do occur and are most importantly associated with abortion, neonatal mortality, and establishment of persistent infection in stallions. The first recognized and most severe epizootic occurred in 1953 in Bucyrus, Ohio, USA.[32] Subsequently, EVA outbreaks have been reported from elsewhere in the United States, Canada, and a number of European countries, with more significant outbreaks occurring in Normandy (France, 2006) and New Mexico (USA, 2007).[126,334,336] EAV seroprevalence varies between countries and horses of different breeds and age in the same country. Persistently infected stallions play a central role in the maintenance, perpetuation, and evolution of the virus in the horse population. An increase in the incidence of the disease has been observed in the past 20 years, associated *inter alia* with increased national and international movement of horses and shipment of frozen or chilled semen. A recent GWAS (see section "Persistence" above) pinpointed genetic differences within and among horse populations that are associated with susceptibility of CD3+ T lymphocytes to EAV infection *in vitro*.[110] EAV genetic variation, evolution during LTPI in the stallion reproductive tract, and the molecular epidemiology EVA have been previously described.[14,18,124,191,334,336] Phylogenetic analysis based on ORF5 segregates EAV strains into North American and European lineages, with the European lineage subdivided into two subgroups.[224] Further analysis of 101 EAV ORF5 sequences from horses divided the North American and European strains of EAV into seven clusters.[257] Recently, an analysis of 170 EAV ORF5 reference sequences from horses and donkeys demonstrated that donkey isolates from Chile and South Africa belong to a single monophyletic group.[224] This asinine cluster represents a new genotype that circulates in South America and South Africa, which is clearly distinct from the well-characterized EAV strains that are prevalent in horses.

PRRSV

PRRSV-2 was first detected in 1987 in the United States,[57] and the first outbreaks of PRRSV-1 in Europe were recognized in Germany in 1990.[311] Today, PRRSV infection is ubiquitous in most of swine-producing areas of the world, including North and South America, Europe, and Asia. Severe abortion storms had a resurgence in 1996–1998 in the United States. More recently, high-virulent PRRSV-2 variants have been reported in U.S. swine farms, where the emerging strains were characterized as 1-8-4, 1-7-4, and 1-4-4 (1c lineage) cutting pattern based on an ORF5 restriction fragment length polymorphism (RFLP) analysis.[122,275,290] In Eastern Europe, an enhanced pathogenic PRRSV-1 Lena strain was isolated from a Belarusian farm.[134] Sequence analysis on strains from Belarus, Lithuania, and Russia revealed a high degree of variability compared with other global PRRSV-1 strains.[20] In China, HP-PRRSV variants emerged in 2006, causing outbreaks of fatal disease that were unparalleled in severity.[270] In the following years, this highly pathogenic PRRSV spread to all Chinese swine-producing areas as well as surrounding Asian countries. About 60% of the pigs were infected with PRRSV in the 5 years after the virulent virus emerged.[156] In addition to HP-PRRSV, pathogenic NADC30-like strains have been emerged in China since 2014 (reviewed in Ref.[269]). Detailed analysis of PRRSV molecular epidemiology has been reported previously.[28,105,236–238,256] Globally, PRRSV presents as genetically diversified populations, with PRRSV-1 strains mainly distributed in Europe and PRRSV-2 stains mainly distributed in North America and Asia. The high genetic variation among the strains is primarily due to the natural characteristics of RNA viruses, which lack RdRp proofreading ability and exhibit genetic recombination among different strains. Besides the effect of local divergent evolution, the transboundary movement of infected animals and the use of MLV vaccines are important factors to influence the genetic diversity.

LDV

LDV was first discovered in laboratory mice.[213,223] The virus was also isolated from wild mice in several countries, although the worldwide incidence is not known.

SHFV

SHFV appears to be endemic among several species of African monkeys (*Erythrocebus patas*, *Cercopithecus aethiops*, *Papio anubis*, and *Papio cynocephalus*).[116,148,169] Nevertheless, the virus was first isolated from Asian macaques, during outbreaks of fatal hemorrhagic fever in research centers in the Soviet Union and the United States.[264] These epizootics were probably caused by inadvertent transmission by humans from African monkeys to the macaques. During these outbreaks, SHFV was readily transmitted from the initially infected rhesus monkeys (*Macaca mulatta*) to other macaque species (*Macaca fascicularis* and *Macaca arctoides*). Subsequently, similar epizootics among macaques occurred in various other primate centers.

Until recently, the etiological agent of SHF was thought to be a single virus, SHFV, which was isolated in cell culture from clinical samples during the 1964 outbreak in the United States.[306] However, in subsequent SHFV outbreaks, there were monkeys with severe neurologic signs, which suggested that different strains may cause SHF. Recently, a few preserved tissue samples from these past SHF outbreaks were sequenced. These studies demonstrated that at least the 1964 Sukhumi outbreak and an outbreak in Alamogordo, NM, in 1989 were caused by two previously uncharacterized SHFV-related viruses, which are now named simian hemorrhagic encephalitis virus (SHEV) and Pebjah virus (PBJV).[147] The natural reservoir(s) of these viruses remains to be identified, but African nonhuman primates are suspected of being natural reservoirs. Furthermore, using next-generation sequencing, eleven additional divergent simian arteriviruses have been detected recently in diverse and apparently healthy African cercopithecid monkeys.[306] The discovery of these novel viruses has expanded the simian arteriviruses, which require isolation and further molecular characterization.

CLINICAL FEATURES

EAV

Clinical signs of EVA vary considerably among individual horses and among outbreaks.[9,32,126] A substantial percentage of all infections are subclinical (i.e., asymptomatic), especially those that occur in mares bred to persistently infected stallions. Typically, clinical cases of EVA have an incubation period of 2 to 14 days (6 to 8 days following venereal exposure), with the most consistent clinical features of EAV being pyrexia, leukopenia, flu-like symptoms in adult animals, abortion in pregnant mares (e-Fig. 5.12A), persistent infection in stallions, and interstitial pneumonia in neonates. Typical cases of the disease can present with all or any combination of the following signs: fever up to 41°C (105.8°F) (2- to 9-day duration), anorexia, serous nasal discharge, conjunctivitis, urticaria, leukopenia, edema of the lower limbs, scrotum, prepuce, eyelids, ventral body wall, and udder, abortion in the mare (3 to 10 months gestation), (e-Fig. 5.12), fatal interstitial pneumonia, or pneumoenteritis in young foals. As with most infectious diseases, old, debilitated, or immunosuppressed horses and very young foals are predisposed to more severe disease.[9,126] Clinical features are characteristic vascular lesions, necrosis of small muscular arteries (from which the name of the family prototype EAV was derived). Virulence and clinical signs are strain dependent, but the genetic basis for these differences in EAV field strains has not been established.[274]

PRRSV

At 12 to 24 hours after exposure to PRRSV, young pigs, sows, and boars become viremic, a state that can last from 1 to 2 weeks in mature animals to 8 weeks in young pigs. Clinical manifestations of PRRSV include occasional discoloring and blotching of the skin, most often on the ears (which gave PRRS the name "blue ear disease") and vulva, and occasionally on the trunk. Further symptoms are fever, anorexia, breathing difficulties, lymphadenopathy, gross and microscopic lesions in the lung, and reproductive failure characterized by delivery of weak or stillborn piglets (e-Fig. 5.13A), or autolyzed fetuses.[341] The clinical features of the highly pathogenic PRRSV variants that emerged in China in 2006 are strikingly more severe than those reported

for the older isolates (e-Fig. 5.14). The new variant affected pigs of all ages and was characterized by high fever (40°C to 42°C [104.0°F to 107.6°F]), depression, anorexia, lethargy, and rubefaction of the skin and ears. Most diseased pigs showed obvious respiratory distress, such as sneezing, coughing, and asthma, as well as intestinal problems including diarrhea. At autopsy, the severe lesions in skin, lung, gastrointestinal tract, and brain were considered unique for this atypical form of PRRS[270] (e-Fig. 5.14F). Mortality rates ranged from 20% to 100%, depending on the age and health of the infected animals.

LDV

Infection of mice with LDV leads to a life-long viremia, but the infection is asymptomatic. It is maintained by continuous rounds of cytocidal virus replication in a renewable subpopulation of macrophages.[199] By 24 hours after infection, LDV titers of 10^{10} infectious dose $(ID)_{50}$/mL are present in the plasma, which then decrease to a level of 10^4 to 10^6 ID_{50}/mL. These titers remain present throughout the life of the mouse, together with elevated levels of LDH and other serum enzymes. LDV can be detected in the spleen, lymph nodes, thymus, and liver of persistently infected mice. Neurovirulent LDV variants can cause a fatal age-dependent poliomyelitis in certain inbred mouse strains that are of the Fv-$1^{n/n}$ genotype and carry N-tropic, ecotropic murine leukemia virus (MuLV) proviruses[58] (e-Fig. 5.15). The replication of these ecotropic MuLVs in the glial cells of the spinal cord was proposed to render the anterior horn neurons susceptible to cytocidal LDV infection. Consequently, the development of age-dependent poliomyelitis may result from a combination of increased expression of ecotropic MuLVs and a decreasing ability to mount a motor neuron-protective anti-LDV response. LDV can also induce severe thrombocytopenia in animals that have been treated with antiplatelet antibodies at a dose that in itself was insufficient to induce clinical disease.[190] The mechanism is unknown, but macrophage activation by virus-induced IFN-γ production is likely to play an important role.

SHFV

Depending on the virus strain, SHFV causes asymptomatic acute or persistent infections in several species of African monkeys,[116,169] whereas in captive macaques, fatal hemorrhagic fever was reported upon SHFV infection[264] (e-Fig. 5.16). Clinical signs in the latter animals consist of early fever, mild facial erythema, and edema, followed by anorexia, dehydration, and various hemorrhagic manifestations. The macaques usually die within 2 weeks, with mortality rates approaching 100%. Very little is known about SHFV pathogenesis in macaques. Macrophages are the primary target cells for SHFV, and a causal relationship exists between the cytocidal infection of these cells and the clinical symptoms of hemorrhagic fever.[117]

WPDV

Wobbly possum disease (WPD) was first recognized in an Australian brushtail possum (*T. vulpecula*) with fatal neurological disease in a research facility in 1995.[174] Subsequently, WPD has been observed among free-living possums in New Zealand, and the neurologic disease was experimentally reproduced by inoculating healthy possums with filtered materials prepared from spleen or liver homogenates of WPDV-infected animals.[198,209] The infected possum developed early clinical signs of inappetence, decreased responsiveness to environmental stimuli, and temperament changes. The disease progressed to head tremors, ataxia, apparent blindness, and cachexia. Histologically, perivascular mononuclear infiltrates were observed in a variety of tissues of WPDV-infected possums, including brain, liver, spleen, and kidney. Viral nucleic acid was detected by RT-PCR in some of these tissues.

PREVENTION AND CONTROL

Diagnosis

Diagnosis of EAV or PRRSV infections on the basis of clinical signs alone is generally difficult, and therefore not reliable. This is due to the often subclinical or mild symptoms that resemble the symptoms of other respiratory diseases of horses and swine. Differential diagnosis of EAV- or PRRSV-induced abortions are also not straightforward, although these are generally characterized by (partial) autolysis of the fetuses and a lack of pathognomonic lesions.

For laboratory diagnosis of EAV, nasopharyngeal swabs or washings, conjunctival swabs, semen, blood and tissue specimens can be used. Several standard and real-time reverse transcriptase polymerase chain reaction (RT-PCR) assays are available for detection of EAV RNA in such clinical samples. EAV can be also isolated in cell cultures using these specimens, and virus isolation in semen is currently the OIE prescribed test for international trade. In addition, immunohistochemistry using monoclonal antibodies to EAV proteins and chromogenic RNA in situ hybridization assays (conventional and RNAscope®) are reliable methods for EAV diagnosis in tissues.[44] Several laboratories have developed enzyme-linked immunosorbent assays (ELISAs) and microsphere immunoassay (Luminex®) for detecting antibody response against EAV; however, virus neutralization assay remains the gold standard for detection of serum antibodies against EAV (reviewed in Ref.[9]).

PRRSV can be detected by using virus isolation and fluorescent antibody (both direct FA and indirect [IFA]) tests in serum or using immunohistochemistry in tissue samples. For detecting swine antibody response against PRRSV, the IDEXX ELISA is the most widely used test, and microsphere immunoassay, IFA, and neutralization assays have also been used to detect antibodies in serum and oral fluid samples. In addition, real-time RT-PCR tests are routinely used to detect viral RNA in serum, oral fluid, semen, processing fluids, and tissue samples.[276] Sequence analysis of the ORF5 region has been used for identification and differentiation of PRRSV field strains.[341] In traditional tests for antibody detection, N protein is the antigen, but certain nonstructural proteins, including nsp1α/β, nsp2, and nsp7, have also been explored as an alternative or more accurate indicators of PRRSV infection.[31,133]

LDV can only be quantitated by an end-point dilution assay in mice, which is based on the increase in plasma LDH activity that accompanies LDV infection in mice. The presence of LDV in mice or in other materials is readily detected by injecting plasma, tissue homogenates, or other materials (e.g., transplantable mouse tumors) into groups of two to three mice and assaying their plasma LDH activity 4 to 5 days later.[161] LDV also can be detected by IFA and in situ hybridization with cDNA probes.[123]

Persistently infected monkeys can be identified by the presence of SHFV that replicates in primary cultures of peritoneal macrophages from rhesus and patas monkeys.[264] The most sensitive method for detection of persistent infection in monkeys is experimental inoculation of macaque monkeys, and there currently are no molecular diagnostic assays for detection of SHFV. Indirect immunofluorescent assay, ELISA, and neutralization assays are available for serological diagnosis of SHFV infection. However, these assays are not reliable because of the low level of anti-SHFV antibodies found in many persistently infected monkeys.

Disease Control

Currently, there are no means available for eliminating the carrier state in stallions persistently infected with EAV other than surgical castration. There is no specific treatment for horses infected with EAV. Current EVA control and prevention strategies are aimed at preventing EAV spread in susceptible equine populations, which is achieved with appropriate quarantine and laboratory testing procedures. The management and biosecurity practices used to mitigate the risk of spreading EAV include the identification of carrier stallions, the quarantine of new arrivals, the segregation of pregnant mares and foals from other horses, implementation of biosecurity measures, and enforcement of vaccination programs.[16]

Changes in swine management have proven effective in preventing PRRSV outbreaks and are presently thought to be the key to control the disease in the less intensive swine industry. The method of herd closure, for example, involves the uniform exposure of a confined herd to PRRSV, followed by a continued isolation of the herd for more than 200 days. This effectively eliminates PRRSV, as long as no new animals, and thereby possibly new PRRSV strains, are introduced from outside. In addition, strict biosecurity protocols, including air filtration, have been shown effective (reviewed in Refs.[59,73] and references therein). In areas with highly intensive pig farming, this type of relatively costly strategies is often difficult to implement, and the need for better PRRSV vaccines than those currently available is clear (see below).

LDV vaccines are not available, and there is no need for them, as control of LDV infection in laboratory mice is by exclusion. LDV can be eliminated from contaminated cell lines and tumors by in vitro culture or passage through athymic nude rats. By doing so, the requisite mouse macrophage subpopulation that is essential for virus replication is eliminated and subsequently cleared of virus.[64]

Currently, there are no vaccines to prevent SHFV infection in macaques. Repeated administration of an IFN-inducer (e.g., polyriboinosinic–polyribocytidylic acid containing poly-L-lysine and carboxymethylcellulose) prevented fatalities in rhesus macaques that were experimentally infected with SHFV.[155] Supportive care including administration of heparin to treat disseminated intravascular coagulation has been suggested, but euthanasia is more often elected to control disease outbreaks.

Because arteriviruses generally infect production or laboratory animals, low priority has been given to the development of antiviral treatments. Infected animals either die quickly from the disease or are culled as a way to prevent further spread of the virus.

Vaccines

For EAV, a MLV vaccine, ARVAC® (Zoetis Animal Health, Kalamazoo, MI), has been widely used in North America. In some European countries, an adjuvanted killed virus vaccine, Artervac® (Zoetis Animal Health, Kalamazoo, MI), has been approved for use in the field. Although the current MLV vaccine is believed to be safe and efficacious, it is not recommended by the manufacturer for use in pregnant mares. Several genetically engineered candidate vaccines have been developed and tested in experimental infections (reviewed in Ref.[9]). Some promising results were obtained with a vaccine based on Venezuelan equine encephalitis virus replicon particles expressing both EAV GP5 and M. Horses vaccinated with this recombinant vaccine produced neutralizing antibodies, shed little or no virus, and developed only mild symptoms after a challenge with virulent EAV.[10] An EAV candidate live marker vaccine was developed on the basis of the deletion of the immunodominant domain of GP5, for which a peptide-specific ELISA is available.[47] This recombinant virus caused an asymptomatic infection in ponies and induced neutralizing antibodies, albeit only against the recombinant and not against the wild-type virus. The vaccinated animals were fully protected against disease following a challenge with virulent EAV.[47] The ELISA for the deleted immunodominant domain can be used to distinguish between vaccinated and naturally infected animals.

For PRRSV, a variety of live-attenuated and killed vaccines are commercially available. The MLV vaccines induce long-lasting protection, but when derived from a single PRRSV vaccine strain, they do not fully protect against heterologous PRRSV infection.[138,222,267] Furthermore, MLV vaccines do not completely prevent reinfection with wild-type virus and virus transmission. Adverse effects of vaccination of Danish pig herds with a modified live PRRS vaccine have been described, which were probably caused by reversion of the vaccine virus to virulence.[27] Acute PRRS-like symptoms, including an increasing number of abortions and stillborn piglets, were experienced in vaccinated herds. Furthermore, vaccine virus was transmitted from vaccinated to nonvaccinated boars in several cases, resulting in viremia and shedding of vaccine virus in the semen. In addition, in Thai swine farms, vaccine-derived viruses were found to spread,[3] and homologous recombination with circulating virus was observed in China.[157] In some situations, it is impossible to discriminate between vaccinated and naturally infected animals. Either a subunit vaccine or a genetically modified live marker vaccine could overcome this problem, although the use of recombinant viruses in the field continues to be debated between vaccine developers, swine practitioners, and animal health authorities. Using reverse genetic systems, chimeric infectious cDNA clones have been engineered aimed at developing attenuated MLV (marker) vaccines.[68,99] Chimeric infectious clones in which sequences from virulent field strains were combined with attenuated vaccine strains gave some promising results.[308] Removal/reduce of viral activities that suppresses innate immune responses is a strategy that has been developed, in which the viral gene encoding for immune "evasion" protein was modified to produce a viable, attenuated vaccine virus (reviewed in Refs.[100,222,245]).

In contrast to MLV vaccines, the killed (autogenous vaccines) and subunit vaccines are safer, but vaccine efficacy needs to be improved. Since the discovery of PRRSV, a large amount of studies have been directed to develop effective PRRSV inactivated and subunit vaccines, including various virus inactivation methods, adjuvants, nanoparticle-based vaccine delivery systems, DNA vaccines, and recombinant subunit vaccines using baculovirus, plant, and different viral vector systems (reviewed in Refs.[138,221,267]). Considering the genetically diversified field strains of PRRSV, there remains a need to find innovative strategies to generate cross-protective and noninfectious vaccines.[173,221]

PERSPECTIVES

Arteriviruses are part of a unique group of positive-stranded RNA viruses united in the order *Nidovirales*, which is characterized by having the largest and most complicated replication machinery among currently known positive-stranded RNA viruses. The SARS-CoV-2 pandemic, and the enormous attention for the replicative enzymes of coronaviruses in the context of basic and antiviral drug research, have highlighted the value of studying distantly related nidoviruses, in particular arteriviruses. For several universal nidovirus features, like the ZBD-helicase, the NiRAN domain, discontinuous sg RNA synthesis, and replication organelle formation, prior studies on arteriviruses have helped to advance our understanding of the replication of other nidoviruses. In anticipation of systems allowing the complete *in vitro* reconstitution of arterivirus/nidovirus RNA synthesis, progress will continue to depend on successfully combining bioinformatics, biochemistry, and structural and molecular biology. This powerful approach has already provided detailed insights in some of the intricacies of arterivirus RNA synthesis, replication, and virus–host interactions. However, a variety of important issues remains to be addressed, including basic questions on the unresolved mRNA capping pathway, the composition of the RdRp complex and its relation to the DMVs, and functions of several undercharacterized nsps (e.g., nsp2N, nsp6-7-8, nsp12). The further characterization of the "arterivirus nsp interactome," especially inside the living infected cell, will undoubtedly provide more clues on the spatial and temporal organization of arterivirus replication and immune evasion.

The characterization of the eight to twelve arterivirus structural proteins and their functional interactions during particle assembly and disassembly promises to be a complex issue, which also links to the many unanswered questions regarding host cell functions relevant for arterivirus attachment and entry. Although progress has been made toward understanding host factors involved in PRRSV and EAV entry, the in-depth mechanisms of how these host proteins interact with the viral surface proteins remain to be addressed, for example, which arterivirus GP supplies membrane fusion activity and how does the virus enter into host cells. Most of the viral structural proteins have been defined in basic terms only, and understanding the molecular details of their role in the viral replication cycle is another major challenge for molecular arterivirus research. The −2 PRF noncanonical translation mechanism first discovered in PRRSV (and likely conserved in most other arteriviruses) adds another layer of complexity to arterivirus genome expression. The stabilizing role of the −2 PRF product (nsp2TF) toward the major envelope proteins GP5 and M provides a novel regulatory mechanism and possibly also new starting points for the development of vaccines and antivirals.

During the past two decades, prompted in particular by the enormous PRRSV problems in Asia, determinants of arterivirus pathogenesis and virulence have received more attention. Research tools and model systems to study the highly complex interplay between arterivirus and host have been established. Host genome studies have been added to better understand the host (immune) responses to PRRSV/EAV infection. Pig and horse whole-genome sequencing data are now available, and host genetic markers associated with PRRSV/EAV susceptibility are being sought. This knowledge can be applied in breeding programs to optimize viral resistance and in balance with other traits of economic importance in animal production. In addition, modern technologies, including meta-transcriptomic sequencing, single-cell sequencing, CRISPR/Cas-based genome editing, and genetically modified/engineered pigs, will be valuable tools to study the basic mechanisms of viral pathogenesis and host factors responding to viral infection. In combination with reverse genetics, these tools will help us to better understand arterivirus–host interactions and elucidate the immune mechanisms of antigen-specific protection, which will ultimately lead to the development of a new generation of vaccines and novel antiviral strategies.

Our understanding of arterivirus epidemiology and evolution must be improved to prevent problems like the Asian PRRS outbreak in the future. This field also connects to the interesting question of the potential for arterivirus cross-species transmission. Considering the inapparent and persistent infections frequently caused by currently known arteriviruses, clinical symptoms may not be the most direct indicator for arterivirus infections in other species. Modern virus hunting techniques have enormously increased our capability to identify such additional family members, as evidenced by the recent discovery of many previously unknown arteriviruses from African nonhuman primates. This group of simian viruses represent a rapidly expanding subfamily (simarteriviruses) of poorly characterized arteriviruses. Historically, wild nonhuman primates are important sources or reservoirs of human pathogens, generating serious concerns that some simian arteriviruses may have zoonotic potential.[6] Future studies are warranted to elucidate the nature of interspecies transmission and pathogenic significance of these simarteriviruses.

Although a human arterivirus is yet to be identified, there is significant concern about cross-species arterivirus transmission following xenotransplantation. There is no indication that humans can be infected with SHFV or any other arterivirus during disease outbreaks. However, transplantation to humans of organs or tissues from SHFV-infected baboons or PRRSV-infected pigs could result in the transfer of a considerable amount of these viruses, potentially leading to selection of a variant(s) that can replicate in humans. In this respect, PRRSV and SHFV should be considered as a serious threat upon xenotransplantation of organs and tissues from baboons and pigs.

REFERENCES

1. Allende R, Laegreid WW, Kutish GF, et al. Porcine reproductive and respiratory syndrome virus: description of persistence in individual pigs upon experimental infection. *J Virol* 2000;74:10834–10837.
2. Ammann CG, Messer RJ, Peterson KE, et al. Lactate dehydrogenase-elevating virus induces systemic lymphocyte activation via TLR7-dependent IFNalpha responses by plasmacytoid dendritic cells. *PLoS One* 2009;4:e6105.
3. Amonsin A, Kedkovid R, Puranaveja S, et al. Comparative analysis of complete nucleotide sequence of porcine reproductive and respiratory syndrome virus (PRRSV) isolates in Thailand (US and EU genotypes). *Virol J* 2009;6:143.
4. An TQ, Li JN, Su CM, et al. Molecular and cellular mechanisms for PRRSV pathogenesis and host response to infection. *Virus Res* 2020;286:197980.
5. Archambault D, St-Laurent G. Induction of apoptosis by equine arteritis virus infection. *Virus Genes* 2000;20:143–147.
6. Bailey AL, Lauck M, Sibley SD, et al. Zoonotic potential of simian arteriviruses. *J Virol* 2016;90:630–635.
7. Balasuriya UB, Carossino M. Reproductive effects of arteriviruses: equine arteritis virus and porcine reproductive and respiratory syndrome virus infections. *Curr Opin Virol* 2017;27:57–70.
8. Balasuriya UB, Dobbe JC, Heidner HW, et al. Characterization of the neutralization determinants of equine arteritis virus using recombinant chimeric viruses and site-specific mutagenesis of an infectious cDNA clone. *Virology* 2004;321:235–246.
9. Balasuriya UB, Go YY, MacLachlan NJ. Equine arteritis virus. *Vet Microbiol* 2013;167:93–122.
10. Balasuriya UB, Heidner HW, Davis NL, et al. Alphavirus replicon particles expressing the two major envelope proteins of equine arteritis virus induce high level protection against challenge with virulent virus in vaccinated horses. *Vaccine* 2002;20:1609–1617.
11. Balasuriya UB, Heidner HW, Hedges JF, et al. Expression of the two major envelope proteins of equine arteritis virus as a heterodimer is necessary for induction of neutralizing antibodies in mice immunized with recombinant Venezuelan equine encephalitis virus replicon particles. *J Virol* 2000;74:10623–10630.
12. Balasuriya UB, MacLachlan NJ. The immune response to equine arteritis virus: potential lessons for other arteriviruses. *Vet Immunol Immunopathol* 2004;102:107–129.
13. Balasuriya UB, Patton JF, Rossitto PV, et al. Neutralization determinants of laboratory strains and field isolates of equine arteritis virus: identification of four neutralization sites in the amino-terminal ectodomain of the G(L) envelope glycoprotein. *Virology* 1997;232:114–128.
14. Balasuriya UB, Timoney PJ, McCollum WH, et al. Phylogenetic analysis of open reading frame 5 of field isolates of equine arteritis virus and identification of conserved and nonconserved regions in the GL envelope glycoprotein. *Virology* 1995;214:690–697.
15. Balasuriya UB, Zhang J, Go YY, et al. Experiences with infectious cDNA clones of equine arteritis virus: lessons learned and insights gained. *Virology* 2014;462–463:388–403.
16. Balasuriya UBR, Carossino M, Timoney PJ. Equine viral arteritis: a respiratory and reproductive disease of significant economic importance to the equine industry. *Equine Vet Educ* 2018;30:497–512.
17. Balasuriya UBR, Dobbe JC, Heidner HW, et al. Characterization of the neutralization determinants of equine arteritis virus using recombinant chimeric viruses and site-specific mutagenesis of an infectious cDNA clone. *Virology* 2004;327:318–319.
18. Balasuriya UBR, Hedges JF, Smalley VL, et al. Genetic characterization of equine arteritis virus during persistent infection of stallions. *J Gen Virol* 2004;85:379–390.
19. Balasuriya UBR, Snijder EJ, Heidner HW, et al. Development and characterization of an infectious cDNA clone of the virulent Bucyrus strain of Equine arteritis virus. *J Gen Virol* 2007;88:918–924.
20. Balka G, Podgorska K, Brar MS, et al. Genetic diversity of PRRSV 1 in Central Eastern Europe in 1994–2014: origin and evolution of the virus in the region. *Sci Rep* 2018;8:7811.
21. Barrette-Ng IH, Ng KK, Mark BL, et al. Structure of arterivirus nsp4. The smallest chymotrypsin-like proteinase with an alpha/beta C-terminal extension and alternate conformations of the oxyanion hole. *J Biol Chem* 2002;277:39960–39966.
22. Bautista EM, Faaberg KS, Mickelson D, et al. Functional properties of the predicted helicase of porcine reproductive and respiratory syndrome virus. *Virology* 2002;298:258–270.
23. Beerens N, Snijder EJ. An RNA pseudoknot in the 3′ end of the arterivirus genome has a critical role in regulating viral RNA synthesis. *J Virol* 2007;81:9426–9436.
24. Beerens N, Snijder EJ. RNA signals in the 3′ terminus of the genome of Equine arteritis virus are required for viral RNA synthesis. *J Gen Virol* 2006;87:1977–1983.
25. Benfield DA, Nelson E, Collins JE, et al. Characterization of swine infertility and respiratory syndrome (SIRS) virus (isolate ATCC VR-2332). *J Vet Diagn Invest* 1992;4:127–133.
26. Beura LK, Sarkar SN, Kwon B, et al. Porcine reproductive and respiratory syndrome virus nonstructural protein 1beta modulates host innate immune response by antagonizing IRF3 activation. *J Virol* 2010;84:1574–1584.
27. Botner A, Strandbygaard B, Sorensen KJ, et al. Appearance of acute PRRS-like symptoms in sow herds after vaccination with a modified live PRRS vaccine. *Vet Rec* 1997;141:497–499.
28. Brar MS, Shi M, Murtaugh MP, et al. Evolutionary diversification of type 2 porcine reproductive and respiratory syndrome virus. *J Gen Virol* 2015;96:1570–1580.
29. Brinton MG, Gulyaeva AA, Balasuriya UBR, et al. ICTV Taxonomy Report: Arteriviridae. *J Gen Virol* 2021;102(8):001632.
30. Brockmeier SL, Loving CL, Vorwald AC, et al. Genomic sequence and virulence comparison of four Type 2 porcine reproductive and respiratory syndrome virus strains. *Virus Res* 2012;169:212–221.
31. Brown E, Lawson S, Welbon C, et al. Antibody response to porcine reproductive and respiratory syndrome virus (PRRSV) nonstructural proteins and implications for diagnostic detection and differentiation of PRRSV types I and II. *Clin Vaccine Immunol* 2009;16:628–635.
32. Bryans JT, Crowe ME, Doll ER, et al. Isolation of a filterable agent causing arteritis of horses and abortion by mares; its differentiation from the equine abortion (influenza) virus. *Cornell Vet* 1957;47:3–41.
33. Bukhari K, Mulley G, Gulyaeva AA, et al. Description and initial characterization of metatranscriptomic nidovirus-like genomes from the proposed new family Abyssoviridae, and from a sister group to the Coronavirinae, the proposed genus Alphaletovirus. *Virology* 2018;524:160–171.
34. Butler JE, Wertz N, Weber P, et al. Porcine reproductive and respiratory syndrome virus subverts repertoire development by proliferation of germline-encoded B cells of all isotypes bearing hydrophobic heavy chain CDR3. *J Immunol* 2008;180:2347–2356.
35. Cafruny WA, Bradley SE. Trojan Horse macrophages: studies with the murine lactate dehydrogenase-elevating virus and implications for sexually transmitted virus infection. *J Gen Virol* 1996;77(Pt 12):3005–3012.
36. Cafruny WA, Chan SP, Harty JT, et al. Antibody response of mice to lactate dehydrogenase-elevating virus during infection and immunization with inactivated virus. *Virus Res* 1986;5:357–375.
37. Cafruny WA, Plagemann PG. Immune response to lactate dehydrogenase-elevating virus: serologically specific rabbit neutralizing antibody to the virus. *Infect Immun* 1982;37:1007–1012.
38. Calvert JG, Slade DE, Shields SL, et al. CD163 expression confers susceptibility to porcine reproductive and respiratory syndrome viruses. *J Virol* 2007;81:7371–7379.
39. Calzada-Nova G, Husmann RJ, Schnitzlein WM, et al. Effect of the host cell line on the vaccine efficacy of an attenuated porcine reproductive and respiratory syndrome virus. *Vet Immunol Immunopathol* 2012;148:116–125.
40. Campos JR, Breheny P, Araujo RR, et al. Semen quality of stallions challenged with the Kentucky 84 strain of equine arteritis virus. *Theriogenology* 2014;82:1068–1079.
41. Cancel-Tirado SM, Evans RB, Yoon KJ. Monoclonal antibody analysis of porcine reproductive and respiratory syndrome virus epitopes associated with antibody-dependent enhancement and neutralization of virus infection. *Vet Immunol Immunopathol* 2004;102:249–262.

42. Carossino M, Dini P, Kalbfleisch TS, et al. Equine arteritis virus long-term persistence is orchestrated by CD8+ T lymphocyte transcription factors, inhibitory receptors, and the CXCL16/CXCR6 axis. *PLoS Pathog* 2019;15:e1007950.

43. Carossino M, Loynachan AT, Canisso IF, et al. Equine arteritis virus has specific tropism for stromal cells and CD8(+) T and CD21(+) B lymphocytes but not for glandular epithelium at the primary site of persistent infection in the stallion reproductive tract. *J Virol* 2017;91:e00418-17.

44. Carossino M, Loynachan AT, James MacLachlan N, et al. Detection of equine arteritis virus by two chromogenic RNA in situ hybridization assays (conventional and RNAscope((R))) and assessment of their performance in tissues from aborted equine fetuses. *Arch Virol* 2016;161:3125–3136.

45. Carossino M, Wagner B, Loynachan AT, et al. Equine arteritis virus elicits a mucosal antibody response in the reproductive tract of persistently infected stallions. *Clin Vaccine Immunol* 2017;24:e00215-17.

46. Castillo-Olivares J, Tearle JP, Montesso F, et al. Detection of equine arteritis virus (EAV)-specific cytotoxic CD8+ T lymphocyte precursors from EAV-infected ponies. *J Gen Virol* 2003;84:2745–2753.

47. Castillo-Olivares J, Wieringa R, Bakonyi T, et al. Generation of a candidate live marker vaccine for equine arteritis virus by deletion of the major virus neutralization domain. *J Virol* 2003;77:8470–8480.

48. Chang WS, Eden JS, Hartley WJ, et al. Metagenomic discovery and co-infection of diverse wobbly possum disease viruses and a novel hepacivirus in Australian brushtail possums. *One Health Outlook* 2019;1:5.

49. Chen J, Wang D, Sun Z, et al. Arterivirus nsp4 antagonizes interferon beta production by proteolytically cleaving NEMO at multiple sites. *J Virol* 2019;93:e00385-19.

50. Chen Z, Faaberg KS, Plagemann PG. Determination of the 5' end of the lactate dehydrogenase-elevating virus genome by two independent approaches. *J Gen Virol* 1994;75 (Pt 4):925–930.

51. Chen Z, Lawson S, Sun Z, et al. Identification of two auto-cleavage products of nonstructural protein 1 (nsp1) in porcine reproductive and respiratory syndrome virus infected cells: nsp1 function as interferon antagonist. *Virology* 2010;398:87–97.

52. Chen Z, Li K, Plagemann PG. Neuropathogenicity and sensitivity to antibody neutralization of lactate dehydrogenase-elevating virus are determined by polylactosaminoglycan chains on the primary envelope glycoprotein. *Virology* 2000;266:88–98.

53. Chen Z, Li K, Rowland RR, et al. Lactate dehydrogenase-elevating virus variants: cosegregation of neuropathogenicity and impaired capability for high viremic persistent infection. *J Neurovirol* 1998;4:560–568.

54. Chen Z, Li M, He Q, et al. The amino acid at residue 155 in nonstructural protein 4 of porcine reproductive and respiratory syndrome virus contributes to its inhibitory effect for interferon-beta transcription in vitro. *Virus Res* 2014;189:226–234.

55. Chen Z, Rowland RR, Anderson GW, et al. Coexistence in lactate dehydrogenase-elevating virus pools of variants that differ in neuropathogenicity and ability to establish a persistent infection. *J Virol* 1997;71:2913–2920.

56. Chen Z, Zhou X, Lunney JK, et al. Immunodominant epitopes in nsp2 of porcine reproductive and respiratory syndrome virus are dispensable for replication, but play an important role in modulation of the host immune response. *J Gen Virol* 2010;91:1047–1057.

57. Collins JE, Benfield DA, Christianson WT, et al. Isolation of swine infertility and respiratory syndrome virus (isolate ATCC VR-2332) in North America and experimental reproduction of the disease in gnotobiotic pigs. *J Vet Diagn Invest* 1992;4:117–126.

58. Contag CH, Plagemann PG. Age-dependent poliomyelitis of mice: expression of endogenous retrovirus correlates with cytocidal replication of lactate dehydrogenase-elevating virus in motor neurons. *J Virol* 1989;63:4362–4369.

59. Corzo CA, Mondaca E, Wayne S, et al. Control and elimination of porcine reproductive and respiratory syndrome virus. *Virus Res* 2010;154:185–192.

60. Costers S, Lefebvre DJ, Delputte PL, et al. Porcine reproductive and respiratory syndrome virus modulates apoptosis during replication in alveolar macrophages. *Arch Virol* 2008;153:1453–1465.

61. Costers S, Lefebvre DJ, Goddeeris B, et al. Functional impairment of PRRSV-specific peripheral CD3+CD8 high cells. *Vet Res* 2009;40:46.

62. Costers S, Lefebvre DJ, Van Doorsselaere J, et al. GP4 of porcine reproductive and respiratory syndrome virus contains a neutralizing epitope that is susceptible to immunoselection in vitro. *Arch Virol* 2010;155:371–378.

63. Costers S, Vanhee M, Van Breedam W, et al. GP4-specific neutralizing antibodies might be a driving force in PRRSV evolution. *Virus Res* 2010;154:104–113.

64. Coutelier J-P, Brinton MA. Lactate dehydrogenase-elevating virus. In: Fox JG, Davisson MT, Quimby FW, et al. (eds.), *The Mouse in Biomedical Research*. 2nd ed., Vol. II. Cambridge, MA: Academic Press; 2007:215–234.

65. Das PB, Dinh PX, Ansari IH, et al. The minor envelope glycoproteins GP2a and GP4 of porcine reproductive and respiratory syndrome virus interact with the receptor CD163. *J Virol* 2010;84:1731–1740.

66. Das PB, Vu HL, Dinh PX, et al. Glycosylation of minor envelope glycoproteins of porcine reproductive and respiratory syndrome virus in infectious virus recovery, receptor interaction, and immune response. *Virology* 2011;410:385–394.

67. Dastjerdi A, Inglese N, Partridge T, et al. Novel arterivirus associated with outbreak of fatal encephalitis in European Hedgehogs, England, 2019. *Emerg Infect Dis* 2021;27:578–581.

68. de Lima M, Kwon B, Ansari IH, et al. Development of a porcine reproductive and respiratory syndrome virus differentiable (DIVA) strain through deletion of specific immunodominant epitopes. *Vaccine* 2008;26:3594–3600.

69. de Vries AA, Chirnside ED, Bredenbeek PJ, et al. All subgenomic mRNAs of equine arteritis virus contain a common leader sequence. *Nucleic Acids Res* 1990;18:3241–3247.

70. de Vries AA, Chirnside ED, Horzinek MC, et al. Structural proteins of equine arteritis virus. *J Virol* 1992;66:6294–6303.

71. de Vries AA, Post SM, Raamsman MJ, et al. The two major envelope proteins of equine arteritis virus associate into disulfide-linked heterodimers. *J Virol* 1995;69:4668–4674.

72. de Wilde AH, Boomaars-van der Zanden AL, de Jong AWM, et al. Adaptive mutations in replicase transmembrane subunits can counteract inhibition of equine arteritis virus RNA synthesis by cyclophilin inhibitors. *J Virol* 2019;93:e00490-19.

73. Dee S, Otake S, Deen J. Use of a production region model to assess the efficacy of various air filtration systems for preventing airborne transmission of porcine reproductive and respiratory syndrome virus and Mycoplasma hyopneumoniae: results from a 2-year study. *Virus Res* 2010;154:177–184.

74. Delano WL. The PyMOL Molecular Graphics System. 2002. http://www.pymol.org

75. Delputte PL, Costers S, Nauwynck HJ. Analysis of porcine reproductive and respiratory syndrome virus attachment and internalization: distinctive roles for heparan sulphate and sialoadhesin. *J Gen Virol* 2005;86:1441–1445.

76. Delputte PL, Nauwynck HJ. Porcine arterivirus infection of alveolar macrophages is mediated by sialic acid on the virus. *J Virol* 2004;78:8094–8101.

77. Delputte PL, Van Breedam W, Delrue I, et al. Porcine arterivirus attachment to the macrophage-specific receptor sialoadhesin is dependent on the sialic acid-binding activity of the N-terminal immunoglobulin domain of sialoadhesin. *J Virol* 2007;81:9546–9550.

78. Delputte PL, Vanderheijden N, Nauwynck HJ, et al. Involvement of the matrix protein in attachment of porcine reproductive and respiratory syndrome virus to a heparinlike receptor on porcine alveolar macrophages. *J Virol* 2002;76:4312–4320.

79. den Boon JA, Faaberg KS, Meulenberg JJ, et al. Processing and evolution of the N-terminal region of the arterivirus replicase ORF1a protein: identification of two papainlike cysteine proteases. *J Virol* 1995;69:4500–4505.

80. den Boon JA, Kleijnen MF, Spaan WJ, et al. Equine arteritis virus subgenomic mRNA synthesis: analysis of leader-body junctions and replicative-form RNAs. *J Virol* 1996;70: 4291–4298.

81. den Boon JA, Snijder EJ, Chirnside ED, et al. Equine arteritis virus is not a togavirus but belongs to the coronaviruslike superfamily. *J Virol* 1991;65:2910–2920.

82. Deng X, Hackbart M, Mettelman RC, et al. Coronavirus nonstructural protein 15 mediates evasion of dsRNA sensors and limits apoptosis in macrophages. *Proc Natl Acad Sci U S A* 2017;114:E4251–E4260.

83. Deng Z, Lehmann KC, Li X, et al. Structural basis for the regulatory function of a complex zinc-binding domain in a replicative arterivirus helicase resembling a nonsense-mediated mRNA decay helicase. *Nucleic Acids Res* 2014;42:3464–3477.

84. Di H, Madden JC Jr, Morantz EK, et al. Expanded subgenomic mRNA transcriptome and coding capacity of a nidovirus. *Proc Natl Acad Sci U S A* 2017;114:E8895–E8904.

85. Doan DN, Dokland T. Structure of the nucleocapsid protein of porcine reproductive and respiratory syndrome virus. *Structure* 2003;11:1445–1451.

86. Dobbe JC, van der Meer Y, Spaan WJ, et al. Construction of chimeric arteriviruses reveals that the ectodomain of the major glycoprotein is not the main determinant of equine arteritis virus tropism in cell culture. *Virology* 2001;288:283–294.

87. Dobrescu I, Levast B, Lai K, et al. In vitro and ex vivo analyses of co-infections with swine influenza and porcine reproductive and respiratory syndrome viruses. *Vet Microbiol* 2014;169:18–32.

88. Dokland T. The structural biology of PRRSV. *Virus Res* 2010;154:86–97.

89. Dong J, Zhang N, Ge X, et al. The interaction of nonstructural protein 9 with retinoblastoma protein benefits the replication of genotype 2 porcine reproductive and respiratory syndrome virus in vitro. *Virology* 2014;464–465:432–440.

90. Duan X, Nauwynck HJ, Favoreel HW, et al. Identification of a putative receptor for porcine reproductive and respiratory syndrome virus on porcine alveolar macrophages. *J Virol* 1998;72:4520–4523.

91. Duan X, Nauwynck HJ, Pensaert MB. Effects of origin and state of differentiation and activation of monocytes/macrophages on their susceptibility to porcine reproductive and respiratory syndrome virus (PRRSV). *Arch Virol* 1997;142:2483–2497.

92. Duan X, Nauwynck HJ, Pensaert MB. Virus quantification and identification of cellular targets in the lungs and lymphoid tissues of pigs at different time intervals after inoculation with porcine reproductive and respiratory syndrome virus (PRRSV). *Vet Microbiol* 1997;56:9–19.

93. Dunowska M, Biggs PJ, Zheng T, et al. Identification of a novel nidovirus associated with a neurological disease of the Australian brushtail possum (*Trichosurus vulpecula*). *Vet Microbiol* 2012;156:418–424.

94. Even C, Rowland RR, Plagemann PG. Cytotoxic T cells are elicited during acute infection of mice with lactate dehydrogenase-elevating virus but disappear during the chronic phase of infection. *J Virol* 1995;69:5666–5676.

95. Faaberg KS, Even C, Palmer GA, et al. Disulfide bonds between two envelope proteins of lactate dehydrogenase-elevating virus are essential for viral infectivity. *J Virol* 1995;69: 613–617.

96. Faaberg KS, Plagemann PG. The envelope proteins of lactate dehydrogenase-elevating virus and their membrane topography. *Virology* 1995;212:512–525.

97. Fan B, Liu X, Bai J, et al. The amino acid residues at 102 and 104 in GP5 of porcine reproductive and respiratory syndrome virus regulate viral neutralization susceptibility to the porcine serum neutralizing antibody. *Virus Res* 2015;204:21–30.

98. Fang L, Jiang Y, Xiao S, et al. Enhanced immunogenicity of the modified GP5 of porcine reproductive and respiratory syndrome virus. *Virus Genes* 2006;32:5–11.

99. Fang Y, Christopher-Hennings J, Brown E, et al. Development of genetic markers in the non-structural protein 2 region of a US type 1 porcine reproductive and respiratory syndrome virus: implications for future recombinant marker vaccine development. *J Gen Virol* 2008;89:3086–3096.

100. Fang Y, Snijder EJ. The PRRSV replicase: exploring the multifunctionality of an intriguing set of nonstructural proteins. *Virus Res* 2010;154:61–76.

101. Fang Y, Treffers EE, Li Y, et al. Efficient −2 frameshifting by mammalian ribosomes to synthesize an additional arterivirus protein. *Proc Natl Acad Sci U S A* 2012;109: E2920-2928.

102. Finkel Y, Mizrahi O, Nachshon A, et al. The coding capacity of SARS-CoV-2. *Nature* 2021;589:125–130.

103. Firth AE, Zevenhoven-Dobbe JC, Wills NM, et al. Discovery of a small arterivirus gene that overlaps the GP5 coding sequence and is important for virus production. *J Gen Virol* 2011;92:1097–1106.

104. Frias-Staheli N, Giannakopoulos NV, Kikkert M, et al. Ovarian tumor domain-containing viral proteases evade ubiquitin- and ISG15-dependent innate immune responses. *Cell Host Microbe* 2007;2:404–416.

105. Frossard JP, Hughes GJ, Westcott DG, et al. Porcine reproductive and respiratory syndrome virus: genetic diversity of recent British isolates. *Vet Microbiol* 2013;162:507–518.
106. Fukunaga Y, Imagawa H, Tabuchi E, et al. Clinical and virological findings on experimental equine viral arteritis in horses. *B Equine Res Inst* 1981;1981:110–118.
107. Gao P, Chai Y, Song J, et al. Reprogramming the unfolded protein response for replication by porcine reproductive and respiratory syndrome virus. *PLoS Pathog* 2019;15:e1008169.
108. Giles J, Perrott M, Roe W, et al. Viral RNA load and histological changes in tissues following experimental infection with an arterivirus of possums (wobbly possum disease virus). *Virology* 2018;522:73–80.
109. Giles JC, Perrott MR, Dunowska M. Primary possum macrophage cultures support the growth of a nidovirus associated with wobbly possum disease. *J Virol Methods* 2015;222:66–71.
110. Go YY, Bailey E, Cook DG, et al. Genome-wide association study among four horse breeds identifies a common haplotype associated with in vitro CD3+ T cell susceptibility/resistance to equine arteritis virus infection. *J Virol* 2011;85:13174–13184.
111. Go YY, Li Y, Chen Z, et al. Equine arteritis virus does not induce interferon production in equine endothelial cells: identification of nonstructural protein 1 as a main interferon antagonist. *Biomed Res Int* 2014;2014:420658.
112. Go YY, Snijder EJ, Timoney PJ, et al. Characterization of equine humoral antibody response to the nonstructural proteins of equine arteritis virus. *Clin Vaccine Immunol* 2011;18:268–279.
113. Go YY, Zhang J, Timoney PJ, et al. Complex interactions between the major and minor envelope proteins of equine arteritis virus determine its tropism for equine CD3+ T lymphocytes and CD14+ monocytes. *J Virol* 2010;84:4898–4911.
114. Godeny EK, de Vries AA, Wang XC, et al. Identification of the leader-body junctions for the viral subgenomic mRNAs and organization of the simian hemorrhagic fever virus genome: evidence for gene duplication during arterivirus evolution. *J Virol* 1998;72:862–867.
115. Gorbalenya AE, Enjuanes L, Ziebuhr J, et al. Nidovirales: evolving the largest RNA virus genome. *Virus Res* 2006;117:17–37.
116. Gravell M, London WT, Leon M, et al. Elimination of persistent simian hemorrhagic fever (SHF) virus infection in patas monkeys. *Proc Soc Exp Biol Med* 1986;181:219–225.
117. Gravell M, London WT, Leon ME, et al. Differences among isolates of simian hemorrhagic fever (SHF) virus. *Proc Soc Exp Biol Med* 1986;181:112–119.
118. Gulyaeva A, Dunowska M, Hoogendoorn E, et al. Domain organization and evolution of the highly divergent 5′ coding region of genomes of arteriviruses, including the novel possum nidovirus. *J Virol* 2017;91.
119. Guo R, Shang P, Carrillo CA, et al. Double-stranded viral RNA persists in vitro and in vivo during prolonged infection of porcine reproductive and respiratory syndrome virus. *Virology* 2018;524:78–89.
120. Guo R, Yan X, Li Y, et al. A swine arterivirus deubiquitinase stabilizes two major envelope proteins and promotes production of viral progeny. *PLoS Pathog* 2021;17:e1009403.
121. Han J, Rutherford MS, Faaberg KS. The porcine reproductive and respiratory syndrome virus nsp2 cysteine protease domain possesses both trans- and cis-cleavage activities. *J Virol* 2009;83:9449–9463.
122. Han J, Wang Y, Faaberg KS. Complete genome analysis of RFLP 184 isolates of porcine reproductive and respiratory syndrome virus. *Virus Res* 2006;122:175–182.
123. Haven TR, Rowland RR, Plagemann PG, et al. Regulation of transplacental virus infection by developmental and immunological factors: studies with lactate dehydrogenase-elevating virus. *Virus Res* 1996;41:153–161.
124. Hedges JF, Balasuriya UB, Timoney PJ, et al. Genetic divergence with emergence of novel phenotypic variants of equine arteritis virus during persistent infection of stallions. *J Virol* 1999;73:3672–3681.
125. Hedges JF, DeMaula CD, Moore BD, et al. Characterization of equine E-selectin. *Immunology* 2001;103:498–504.
126. Holyoak GR, Balasuriya UB, Broaddus CC, et al. Equine viral arteritis: current status and prevention. *Theriogenology* 2008;70:403–414.
127. Hu J, Ni Y, Meng XJ, et al. Expression and purification of a chimeric protein consisting of the ectodomains of M and GP5 proteins of porcine reproductive and respiratory syndrome virus (PRRSV). *J Chromatogr B Analyt Technol Biomed Life Sci* 2012;911:43–48.
128. Huang C, Zhang Q, Guo XK, et al. Porcine reproductive and respiratory syndrome virus nonstructural protein 4 antagonizes beta interferon expression by targeting the NF-kappaB essential modulator. *J Virol* 2014;88:10934–10945.
129. Hwang YK, Brinton MA. A 68-nucleotide sequence within the 3′ noncoding region of simian hemorrhagic fever virus negative-strand RNA binds to four MA104 cell proteins. *J Virol* 1998;72:4341–4351.
130. Hyllseth B. A plaque assay of equine arteritis virus in BHK-21 cells. *Arch Gesamte Virusforsch* 1969;28:26–33.
131. Ivanov KA, Hertzig T, Rozanov M, et al. Major genetic marker of nidoviruses encodes a replicative endoribonuclease. *Proc Natl Acad Sci U S A* 2004;101:12694–12699.
132. Johnson CR, Griggs TF, Gnanandarajah J, et al. Novel structural protein in porcine reproductive and respiratory syndrome virus encoded by an alternative ORF5 present in all arteriviruses. *J Gen Virol* 2011;92:1107–1116.
133. Johnson CR, Yu W, Murtaugh MP. Cross-reactive antibody responses to nsp1 and nsp2 of Porcine reproductive and respiratory syndrome virus. *J Gen Virol* 2007;88:1184–1195.
134. Karniychuk UU, Geldhof M, Vanhee M, et al. Pathogenesis and antigenic characterization of a new East European subtype 3 porcine reproductive and respiratory syndrome virus isolate. *BMC Vet Res* 2010;6:30.
135. Kim D, Lee JY, Yang JS, et al. The architecture of SARS-CoV-2 transcriptome. *Cell* 2020;181:914–921.e910.
136. Kim HS, Kwang J, Yoon IJ, et al. Enhanced replication of porcine reproductive and respiratory syndrome (PRRS) virus in a homogeneous subpopulation of MA-104 cell line. *Arch Virol* 1993;133:477–483.
137. Kim O, Sun Y, Lai FW, et al. Modulation of type I interferon induction by porcine reproductive and respiratory syndrome virus and degradation of CREB-binding protein by nonstructural protein 1 in MARC-145 and HeLa cells. *Virology* 2010;402:315–326.
138. Kimman TG, Cornelissen LA, Moormann RJ, et al. Challenges for porcine reproductive and respiratory syndrome virus (PRRSV) vaccinology. *Vaccine* 2009;27:3704–3718.
139. Kindler E, Gil-Cruz C, Spanier J, et al. Early endonuclease-mediated evasion of RNA sensing ensures efficient coronavirus replication. *PLoS Pathog* 2017;13:e1006195.
140. Knoops K, Barcena M, Limpens RW, et al. Ultrastructural characterization of arterivirus replication structures: reshaping the endoplasmic reticulum to accommodate viral RNA synthesis. *J Virol* 2012;86:2474–2487.
141. Konishi S, Akashi H, Sentsui H, et al. Studies on equine viral arteritis. 1. Characterization of virus and trial survey on antibody with Vero cell-cultures. *Jpn J Vet Sci* 1975;37:259–267.
142. Kreutz LC, Ackermann MR. Porcine reproductive and respiratory syndrome virus enters cells through a low pH-dependent endocytic pathway. *Virus Res* 1996;42:137–147.
143. Kroese MV, Zevenhoven-Dobbe JC, Bos-de Ruijter JNA, et al. The nsp1alpha and nsp1 papain-like autoproteinases are essential for porcine reproductive and respiratory syndrome virus RNA synthesis. *J Gen Virol* 2008;89:494–499.
144. Kuhn JH, Lauck M, Bailey AL, et al. Reorganization and expansion of the nidoviral family Arteriviridae. *Arch Virol* 2016;161:755–768.
145. Kwon B, Ansari IH, Pattnaik AK, et al. Identification of virulence determinants of porcine reproductive and respiratory syndrome virus through construction of chimeric clones. *Virology* 2008;380:371–378.
146. Lauber C, Goeman JJ, Parquet Mdel C, et al. The footprint of genome architecture in the largest genome expansion in RNA viruses. *PLoS Pathog* 2013;9:e1003500.
147. Lauck M, Alkhovsky SV, Bao Y, et al. Historical outbreaks of simian hemorrhagic fever in captive macaques were caused by distinct arteriviruses. *J Virol* 2015;89:8082–8087.
148. Lauck M, Hyeroba D, Tumukunde A, et al. Novel, divergent simian hemorrhagic fever viruses in a wild Ugandan red colobus monkey discovered using direct pyrosequencing. *PLoS One* 2011;6:e19056.
149. Lauck M, Sibley SD, Hyeroba D, et al. Exceptional simian hemorrhagic fever virus diversity in a wild African primate community. *J Virol* 2013;87:688–691.
150. Lawson SR, Rossow KD, Collins JE, et al. Porcine reproductive and respiratory syndrome virus infection of gnotobiotic pigs: sites of virus replication and co-localization with MAC-387 staining at 21 days post-infection. *Virus Res* 1997;51:105–113.
151. Lee C, Hodgins D, Calvert JG, et al. Mutations within the nuclear localization signal of the porcine reproductive and respiratory syndrome virus nucleocapsid protein attenuate virus replication. *Virology* 2006;346:238–250.
152. Lee C, Yoo D. The small envelope protein of porcine reproductive and respiratory syndrome virus possesses ion channel protein-like properties. *Virology* 2006;355:30–43.
153. Lehmann KC, Gulyaeva A, Zevenhoven-Dobbe JC, et al. Discovery of an essential nucleotidylating activity associated with a newly delineated conserved domain in the RNA polymerase-containing protein of all nidoviruses. *Nucleic Acids Res* 2015;43:8416–8434.
154. Lehmann KC, Snijder EJ, Posthuma CC, et al. What we know but do not understand about nidovirus helicases. *Virus Res* 2015;202:12–32.
155. Levy HB, London W, Fuccillo DA, et al. Prophylactic control of simian hemorrhagic fever in monkeys by an interferon inducer, polyriboinosinic-polyribocytidylic acid-poly-L-lysine. *J Infect Dis* 1976;133 Suppl:A256–A259.
156. Li B, Fang L, Guo X, et al. Epidemiology and evolutionary characteristics of the porcine reproductive and respiratory syndrome virus in China between 2006 and 2010. *J Clin Microbiol* 2011;49:3175–3183.
157. Li B, Fang L, Xu Z, et al. Recombination in vaccine and circulating strains of porcine reproductive and respiratory syndrome viruses. *Emerg Infect Dis* 2009;15:2032–2035.
158. Li H, Zheng Z, Zhou P, et al. The cysteine protease domain of porcine reproductive and respiratory syndrome virus non-structural protein 2 antagonizes interferon regulatory factor 3 activation. *J Gen Virol* 2010;91:2947–2958.
159. Li J, Murtaugh MP. Dissociation of porcine reproductive and respiratory syndrome virus neutralization from antibodies specific to major envelope protein surface epitopes. *Virology* 2012;433:367–376.
160. Li K, Chen Z, Plagemann P. The neutralization epitope of lactate dehydrogenase-elevating virus is located on the short ectodomain of the primary envelope glycoprotein. *Virology* 1998;242:239–245.
161. Li K, Schuler T, Chen Z, et al. Isolation of lactate dehydrogenase-elevating viruses from wild house mice and their biological and molecular characterization. *Virus Res* 2000;67:153–162.
162. Li Y, Firth AE, Brierley I, et al. Programmed −2/−1 ribosomal frameshifting in simarteriviruses: an evolutionarily conserved mechanism. *J Virol* 2019;93:e00370-19.
163. Li Y, Shang P, Shyu D, et al. Nonstructural proteins nsp2TF and nsp2N of porcine reproductive and respiratory syndrome virus (PRRSV) play important roles in suppressing host innate immune responses. *Virology* 2018;517:164–176.
164. Li Y, Tas A, Snijder EJ, et al. Identification of porcine reproductive and respiratory syndrome virus ORF1a-encoded non-structural proteins in virus-infected cells. *J Gen Virol* 2012;93:829–839.
165. Li Y, Tas A, Sun Z, et al. Proteolytic processing of the porcine reproductive and respiratory syndrome virus replicase. *Virus Res* 2015;202:48–59.
166. Li Y, Zhou L, Zhang J, et al. Nsp9 and Nsp10 contribute to the fatal virulence of highly pathogenic porcine reproductive and respiratory syndrome virus emerging in China. *PLoS Pathog* 2014;10:e1004216.
167. Liu L, Tian J, Nan H, et al. Porcine reproductive and respiratory syndrome virus nucleocapsid protein interacts with Nsp9 and cellular DHX9 to regulate viral RNA synthesis. *J Virol* 2016;90:5384–5398.
168. Loemba HD, Mounir S, Mardassi H, et al. Kinetics of humoral immune response to the major structural proteins of the porcine reproductive and respiratory syndrome virus. *Arch Virol* 1996;141:751–761.
169. London WT. Epizootiology, transmission and approach to prevention of fatal simian haemorrhagic fever in rhesus monkeys. *Nature* 1977;268:344–345.
170. Loving CL, Osorio FA, Murtaugh MP, et al. Innate and adaptive immunity against porcine reproductive and respiratory syndrome virus. *Vet Immunol Immunopathol* 2015;167:1–14.

171. Lu J, Gao F, Wei Z, et al. A 5′-proximal stem-loop structure of 5′ untranslated region of porcine reproductive and respiratory syndrome virus genome is key for virus replication. *Virol J* 2011;8:172.
172. Lu Z, Zhang J, Huang CM, et al. Chimeric viruses containing the N-terminal ectodomains of GP5 and M proteins of porcine reproductive and respiratory syndrome virus do not change the cellular tropism of equine arteritis virus. *Virology* 2012;432:99–109.
173. Lunney JK, Fang Y, Ladinig A, et al. Porcine reproductive and respiratory syndrome virus (PRRSV): pathogenesis and interaction with the immune system. *Annu Rev Anim Biosci* 2016;4:129–154.
174. Mackintosh CG, Crawford JL, Thompson EG, et al. A newly discovered disease of the brushtail possum: wobbly possum syndrome. *N Z Vet J* 1995;43:126.
175. MacLachlan NJ, Balasuriya UB, Hedges JF, et al. Serologic response of horses to the structural proteins of equine arteritis virus. *J Vet Diagn Invest* 1998;10:229–236.
176. MacLachlan NJ, Balasuriya UB, Murtaugh MP, et al. Arterivirus pathogenesis and immune response. *Nidoviruses* 2008:325–337.
177. Maess J, Reczko E, Bohm HO. Equine arteritis virus—multiplication in Bhk 21-cells, buoyant density and electron microscopical demonstration. *Arch Ges Virusforsch* 1970; 30:47–58.
178. Maines TR, Young M, Dinh NN, et al. Two cellular proteins that interact with a stem loop in the simian hemorrhagic fever virus 3′(+)NCR RNA. *Virus Res* 2005;109:109–124.
179. Makarova KS, Aravind L, Koonin EV. A novel superfamily of predicted cysteine proteases from eukaryotes, viruses and *Chlamydia pneumoniae*. *Trends Biochem Sci* 2000;25:50–52.
180. Markine-Goriaynoff D, Hulhoven X, Cambiaso CL, et al. Natural killer cell activation after infection with lactate dehydrogenase-elevating virus. *J Gen Virol* 2002;83:2709–2716.
181. McFadden AM, Pearce PV, Orr D, et al. Evidence for absence of equine arteritis virus in the horse population of New Zealand. *N Z Vet J* 2013;61:300–304.
182. Meier WA, Galeota J, Osorio FA, et al. Gradual development of the interferon-gamma response of swine to porcine reproductive and respiratory syndrome virus infection or vaccination. *Virology* 2003;309:18–31.
183. Meulenberg JJ, Hulst MM, de Meijer EJ, et al. Lelystad virus belongs to a new virus family, comprising lactate dehydrogenase-elevating virus, equine arteritis virus, and simian hemorrhagic fever virus. *Arch Virol Suppl* 1994;9:441–448.
184. Meulenberg JJ, Hulst MM, de Meijer EJ, et al. Lelystad virus, the causative agent of porcine epidemic abortion and respiratory syndrome (PEARS), is related to LDV and EAV. *Virology* 1993;192:62–72.
185. Meulenberg JJ, Petersen-den Besten A, De Kluyver EP, et al. Characterization of proteins encoded by ORFs 2 to 7 of Lelystad virus. *Virology* 1995;206:155–163.
186. Meulenberg JJ, van Nieuwstadt AP, van Essen-Zandbergen A, et al. Posttranslational processing and identification of a neutralization domain of the GP4 protein encoded by ORF4 of Lelystad virus. *J Virol* 1997;71:6061–6067.
187. Molenkamp R, Rozier BC, Greve S, et al. Isolation and characterization of an arterivirus defective interfering RNA genome. *J Virol* 2000;74:3156–3165.
188. Molenkamp R, van Tol H, Rozier BCD, et al. The arterivirus replicase is the only viral protein required for genome replication and subgenomic mRNA transcription. *J Gen Virol* 2000;81:2491–2496.
189. Moore BD, Balasuriya UB, Watson JL, et al. Virulent and avirulent strains of equine arteritis virus induce different quantities of TNF-alpha and other proinflammatory cytokines in alveolar and blood-derived equine macrophages. *Virology* 2003;314:662–670.
190. Musaji A, Cormont F, Thirion G, et al. Exacerbation of autoantibody-mediated thrombocytopenic purpura by infection with mouse viruses. *Blood* 2004;104:2102–2106.
191. Nam B, Mekuria Z, Carossino M, et al. Intrahost selection pressure drives equine arteritis virus evolution during persistent infection in the stallion reproductive tract. *J Virol* 2019;93:e00045-19.
192. Napthine S, Treffers EE, Bell S, et al. A novel role for poly(C) binding proteins in programmed ribosomal frameshifting. *Nucleic Acids Res* 2016;44:5491–5503.
193. Nedialkova DD, Gorbalenya AE, Snijder EJ. Arterivirus Nsp1 modulates the accumulation of minus-strand templates to control the relative abundance of viral mRNAs. *PLoS Pathog* 2010;6:e1000772.
194. Nedialkova DD, Ulferts R, van den Born E, et al. Biochemical characterization of arterivirus nonstructural protein 11 reveals the nidovirus-wide conservation of a replicative endoribonuclease. *J Virol* 2009;83:5671–5682.
195. Neu S, Timoney P, McCollum W. Proceedings of the 5th International Conference on Equine Infectious Diseases. 1987.
196. Nga PT, Parquet Mdel C, Lauber C, et al. Discovery of the first insect nidovirus, a missing evolutionary link in the emergence of the largest RNA virus genomes. *PLoS Pathog* 2011;7:e1002215.
197. Nitschke M, Korte T, Tielesch C, et al. Equine arteritis virus is delivered to an acidic compartment of host cells via clathrin-dependent endocytosis. *Virology* 2008;377:248–254.
198. O'Keefe JS, Stanislawek WL, Heath DD. Pathological studies of wobbly possum disease in New Zealand brushtail possums (*Trichosurus vulpecula*). *Vet Rec* 1997;141:226–229.
199. Onyekaba CO, Harty JT, Plagemann PG. Extensive cytocidal replication of lactate dehydrogenase-elevating virus in cultured peritoneal macrophages from 1-2-week-old mice. *Virus Res* 1989;14:327–338.
200. Ostrowski M, Galeota JA, Jar AM, et al. Identification of neutralizing and nonneutralizing epitopes in the porcine reproductive and respiratory syndrome virus GP5 ectodomain. *J Virol* 2002;76:4241–4250.
201. Otake S, Dee S, Corzo C, et al. Long-distance airborne transport of infectious PRRSV and *Mycoplasma hyopneumoniae* from a swine population infected with multiple viral variants. *Vet Microbiol* 2010;145:198–208.
202. Parida R, Choi IS, Peterson DA, et al. Location of T-cell epitopes in nonstructural proteins 9 and 10 of type-II porcine reproductive and respiratory syndrome virus. *Virus Res* 2012;169:13–21.
203. Pasternak AO, Spaan WJ, Snijder EJ. Regulation of relative abundance of arterivirus subgenomic mRNAs. *J Virol* 2004;78:8102–8113.
204. Pasternak AO, Spaan WJM, Snijder EJ. Nidovirus transcription: how to make sense…? *J Gen Virol* 2006;87:1403–1421.
205. Pasternak AO, van den Born E, Spaan WJ, et al. Sequence requirements for RNA strand transfer during nidovirus discontinuous subgenomic RNA synthesis. *EMBO J* 2001;20:7220–7228.
206. Pasternak AO, van den Born E, Spaan WJ, et al. The stability of the duplex between sense and antisense transcription-regulating sequences is a crucial factor in arterivirus subgenomic mRNA synthesis. *J Virol* 2003;77:1175–1183.
207. Patel A, Treffers EE, Meier M, et al. Molecular characterization of the RNA-protein complex directing −2/-1 programmed ribosomal frameshifting during arterivirus replicase expression. *J Biol Chem* 2020;295:17904–17921.
208. Pedersen KW, van der Meer Y, Roos N, et al. Open reading frame 1a-encoded subunits of the arterivirus replicase induce endoplasmic reticulum-derived double-membrane vesicles which carry the viral replication complex. *J Virol* 1999;73:2016–2026.
209. Perrott MR, Wilks CR, Meers J. Routes of transmission of wobbly possum disease. *N Z Vet J* 2000;48:3–8.
210. Pitkin A, Deen J, Dee S. Use of a production region model to assess the airborne spread of porcine reproductive and respiratory syndrome virus. *Vet Microbiol* 2009;136:1–7.
211. Plagemann PG. Complexity of the single linear neutralization epitope of the mouse arterivirus lactate dehydrogenase-elevating virus. *Virology* 2001;290:11–20.
212. Plagemann PG. The primary GP5 neutralization epitope of North American isolates of porcine reproductive and respiratory syndrome virus. *Vet Immunol Immunopathol* 2004;102:263–275.
213. Plagemann PG, Moennig V. Lactate dehydrogenase-elevating virus, equine arteritis virus, and simian hemorrhagic fever virus: a new group of positive-strand RNA viruses. *Adv Virus Res* 1992;41:99–192.
214. Posthuma CC, Nedialkova DD, Zevenhoven-Dobbe JC, et al. Site-directed mutagenesis of the Nidovirus replicative endoribonuclease NendoU exerts pleiotropic effects on the arterivirus life cycle. *J Virol* 2006;80:1653–1661.
215. Posthuma CC, Pedersen KW, Lu Z, et al. Formation of the arterivirus replication/transcription complex: a key role for nonstructural protein 3 in the remodeling of intracellular membranes. *J Virol* 2008;82:4480–4491.
216. Prather RS, Rowland RR, Ewen C, et al. An intact sialoadhesin (Sn/SIGLEC1/CD169) is not required for attachment/internalization of the porcine reproductive and respiratory syndrome virus. *J Virol* 2013;87:9538–9546.
217. Prieto C, Castro JM. Porcine reproductive and respiratory syndrome virus infection in the boar: a review. *Theriogenology* 2005;63:1–16.
218. Qi P, Liu K, Wei J, et al. Nonstructural protein 4 of porcine reproductive and respiratory syndrome virus modulates cell surface swine leukocyte antigen class I expression by downregulating beta2-microglobulin transcription. *J Virol* 2017;91:e01755-16.
219. Rahe MC, Murtaugh MP. Effector mechanisms of humoral immunity to porcine reproductive and respiratory syndrome virus. *Vet Immunol Immunopathol* 2017;186:15–18.
220. Rahe MC, Murtaugh MP. Mechanisms of adaptive immunity to porcine reproductive and respiratory syndrome virus. *Viruses* 2017;9:148.
221. Renukaradhya GJ, Meng XJ, Calvert JG, et al. Inactivated and subunit vaccines against porcine reproductive and respiratory syndrome: current status and future direction. *Vaccine* 2015;33:3065–3072.
222. Renukaradhya GJ, Meng XJ, Calvert JG, et al. Live porcine reproductive and respiratory syndrome virus vaccines: current status and future direction. *Vaccine* 2015;33: 4069–4080.
223. Riley V, Lilly F, Huerto E, et al. Transmissible agent associated with 26 types of experimental mouse neoplasms. *Science* 1960;132:545–547.
224. Rivas J, Neira V, Mena J, et al. Identification of a divergent genotype of equine arteritis virus from South American donkeys. *Transbound Emerg Dis* 2017;64:1655–1660.
225. Robertson SJ, Ammann CG, Messer RJ, et al. Suppression of acute anti-friend virus CD8+ T-cell responses by coinfection with lactate dehydrogenase-elevating virus. *J Virol* 2008;82:408–418.
226. Rowland RR, Lawson S, Rossow K, et al. Lymphoid tissue tropism of porcine reproductive and respiratory syndrome virus replication during persistent infection of pigs originally exposed to virus in utero. *Vet Microbiol* 2003;96:219–235.
227. Rowland RR, Schneider P, Fang Y, et al. Peptide domains involved in the localization of the porcine reproductive and respiratory syndrome virus nucleocapsid protein to the nucleolus. *Virology* 2003;316:135–145.
228. Rowson KEK, Mahy BWJ. *Lactic dehydrogenase virus*. New York: Springer-Verlag; 1975.
229. Saberi A, Gulyaeva AA, Brubacher JL, et al. A planarian nidovirus expands the limits of RNA genome size. *PLoS Pathog* 2018;14:e1007314.
230. Sagripanti JL, Zandomeni RO, Weinmann R. The cap structure of simian hemorrhagic fever virion RNA. *Virology* 1986;151:146–150.
231. Sarkar S, Bailey E, Go YY, et al. Allelic variation in CXCL16 determines CD3+ T lymphocyte susceptibility to equine arteritis virus infection and establishment of long-term carrier state in the stallion. *PLoS Genet* 2016;12:e1006467.
232. Sarkar S, Chelvarajan L, Go YY, et al. Equine arteritis virus uses equine CXCL16 as an entry receptor. *J Virol* 2016;90:3366–3384.
233. Sawicki SG, Sawicki DL. Coronavirus transcription: a perspective. *Curr Top Microbiol* 2005;287:31–55.
234. Sawicki SG, Sawicki DL, Siddell SG. A contemporary view of coronavirus transcription. *J Virol* 2007;81:20–29.
235. Seybert A, van Dinten LC, Snijder EJ, et al. Biochemical characterization of the equine arteritis virus helicase suggests a close functional relationship between arterivirus and coronavirus helicases. *J Virol* 2000;74:9586–9593.
236. Shi M, Lam TT, Hon CC, et al. Molecular epidemiology of PRRSV: a phylogenetic perspective. *Virus Res* 2010;154:7–17.
237. Shi M, Lam TT, Hon CC, et al. Phylogeny-based evolutionary, demographical, and geographical dissection of North American type 2 porcine reproductive and respiratory syndrome viruses. *J Virol* 2010;84:8700–8711.
238. Shi M, Lemey P, Singh Brar M, et al. The spread of type 2 porcine reproductive and respiratory syndrome virus (PRRSV) in North America: a phylogeographic approach. *Virology* 2013;447:146–154.

239. Shi X, Wang L, Li X, et al. Endoribonuclease activities of porcine reproductive and respiratory syndrome virus nsp11 was essential for nsp11 to inhibit IFN-beta induction. *Mol Immunol* 2011;48:1568–1572.

240. Shi Y, Tong X, Ye G, et al. Structural characterization of the Helicase nsp10 encoded by porcine reproductive and respiratory syndrome virus. *J Virol* 2020;94:e02158-19.

241. Silva-Campa E, Flores-Mendoza L, Resendiz M, et al. Induction of T helper 3 regulatory cells by dendritic cells infected with porcine reproductive and respiratory syndrome virus. *Virology* 2009;387:373–379.

242. Slanina H, Madhugiri R, Bylapudi G, et al. Coronavirus replication-transcription complex: vital and selective NMPylation of a conserved site in nsp9 by the NiRAN-RdRp subunit. *Proc Natl Acad Sci U S A* 2021;118.

243. Snijder EJ, Bredenbeek PJ, Dobbe JC, et al. Unique and conserved features of genome and proteome of SARS-coronavirus, an early split-off from the coronavirus group 2 lineage. *J Mol Biol* 2003;331:991–1004.

244. Snijder EJ, Dobbe JC, Spaan WJ. Heterodimerization of the two major envelope proteins is essential for arterivirus infectivity. *J Virol* 2003;77:97–104.

245. Snijder EJ, Kikkert M, Fang Y. Arterivirus molecular biology and pathogenesis. *J Gen Virol* 2013;94:2141–2163.

246. Snijder EJ, Limpens R, de Wilde AH, et al. A unifying structural and functional model of the coronavirus replication organelle: tracking down RNA synthesis. *PLoS Biol* 2020;18: e3000715.

247. Snijder EJ, Meulenberg JJ. The molecular biology of arteriviruses. *J Gen Virol* 1998;79 (Pt 5):961–979.

248. Snijder EJ, van Tol H, Pedersen KW, et al. Identification of a novel structural protein of arteriviruses. *J Virol* 1999;73:6335–6345.

249. Snijder EJ, van Tol H, Roos N, et al. Non-structural proteins 2 and 3 interact to modify host cell membranes during the formation of the arterivirus replication complex. *J Gen Virol* 2001;82:985–994.

250. Snijder EJ, Wassenaar AL, Spaan WJ. Proteolytic processing of the replicase ORF1a protein of equine arteritis virus. *J Virol* 1994;68:5755–5764.

251. Snijder EJ, Wassenaar AL, Spaan WJ, et al. The arterivirus Nsp2 protease. An unusual cysteine protease with primary structure similarities to both papain-like and chymotrypsin-like proteases. *J Biol Chem* 1995;270:16671–16676.

252. Snijder EJ, Wassenaar AL, van Dinten LC, et al. The arterivirus nsp4 protease is the prototype of a novel group of chymotrypsin-like enzymes, the 3C-like serine proteases. *J Biol Chem* 1996;271:4864–4871.

253. Song C, Krell P, Yoo D. Nonstructural protein 1alpha subunit-based inhibition of NF-kappaB activation and suppression of interferon-beta production by porcine reproductive and respiratory syndrome virus. *Virology* 2010;407:268–280.

254. Song J, Liu Y, Gao P, et al. Mapping the nonstructural protein interaction network of porcine reproductive and respiratory syndrome virus. *J Virol* 2018;92:e01112-18.

255. Spilman MS, Welbon C, Nelson E, et al. Cryo-electron tomography of porcine reproductive and respiratory syndrome virus: organization of the nucleocapsid. *J Gen Virol* 2009;90:527–535.

256. Stadejek T, Stankevicius A, Murtaugh MP, et al. Molecular evolution of PRRSV in Europe: current state of play. *Vet Microbiol* 2013;165:21–28.

257. Steinbach F, Westcott DG, McGowan SL, et al. Re-emergence of a genetic outlier strain of equine arteritis virus: impact on phylogeny. *Virus Res* 2015;202:144–150.

258. Su CM, Rowland RRR, Yoo D. Recent advances in PRRS virus receptors and the targeting of receptor-ligand for control. *Vaccines (Basel)* 2021;9:354.

259. Sun Y, Xue F, Guo Y, et al. Crystal structure of porcine reproductive and respiratory syndrome virus leader protease Nsp1alpha. *J Virol* 2009;83:10931–10940.

260. Sun Z, Chen Z, Lawson SR, et al. The cysteine protease domain of porcine reproductive and respiratory syndrome virus nonstructural protein 2 possesses deubiquitinating and interferon antagonism functions. *J Virol* 2010;84:7832–7846.

261. Sun Z, Li Y, Ransburgh R, et al. Nonstructural protein 2 of porcine reproductive and respiratory syndrome virus inhibits the antiviral function of interferon-stimulated gene 15. *J Virol* 2012;86:3839–3850.

262. Sur JH, Doster AR, Christian JS, et al. Porcine reproductive and respiratory syndrome virus replicates in testicular germ cells, alters spermatogenesis, and induces germ cell death by apoptosis. *J Virol* 1997;71:9170–9179.

263. Tao R, Fang L, Bai D, et al. Porcine reproductive and respiratory syndrome virus nonstructural protein 4 cleaves porcine DCP1a to attenuate its antiviral activity. *J Immunol* 2018;201:2345–2353.

264. Tauraso NM, Shelokov A, Palmer AE, et al. Simian hemorrhagic fever. 3. Isolation and characterization of a viral agent. *Am J Trop Med Hyg* 1968;17:422–431.

265. Thaa B, Kabatek A, Zevenhoven-Dobbe JC, et al. Myristoylation of the arterivirus E protein: the fatty acid modification is not essential for membrane association but contributes significantly to virus infectivity. *J Gen Virol* 2009;90:2704–2712.

266. Thanawongnuwech R, Halbur PG, Thacker EL. The role of pulmonary intravascular macrophages in porcine reproductive and respiratory syndrome virus infection. *Anim Health Res Rev* 2000;1:95–102.

267. Thanawongnuwech R, Suradhat S. Taming PRRSV: revisiting the control strategies and vaccine design. *Virus Res* 2010;154:133–140.

268. Tian D, Wei Z, Zevenhoven-Dobbe JC, et al. Arterivirus minor envelope proteins are a major determinant of viral tropism in cell culture. *J Virol* 2012;86:3701–3712.

269. Tian K. NADC30-like porcine reproductive and respiratory syndrome in China. *Open Virol J* 2017;11:59–65.

270. Tian K, Yu X, Zhao T, et al. Emergence of fatal PRRSV variants: unparalleled outbreaks of atypical PRRS in China and molecular dissection of the unique hallmark. *PLoS One* 2007;2:e526.

271. Tian X, Lu G, Gao F, et al. Structure and cleavage specificity of the chymotrypsin-like serine protease (3CLSP/nsp4) of porcine reproductive and respiratory syndrome virus (PRRSV). *J Mol Biol* 2009;392:977–993.

272. Tijms MA, van der Meer Y, Snijder EJ. Nuclear localization of non-structural protein 1 and nucleocapsid protein of equine arteritis virus. *J Gen Virol* 2002;83:795–800.

273. Tijms MA, van Dinten LC, Gorbalenya AE, et al. A zinc finger-containing papain-like protease couples subgenomic mRNA synthesis to genome translation in a positive-stranded RNA virus. *Proc Natl Acad Sci U S A* 2001;98:1889–1894.

274. Timoney PJ, McCollum WH. Equine viral arteritis. *Vet Clin North Am Equine Pract* 1993;9:295–309.

275. Trevisan G, Li G, Moura CAA, et al. Complete coding genome sequence of a novel porcine reproductive and respiratory syndrome virus 2 restriction fragment length polymorphism 1-4-4 lineage 1C variant identified in Iowa, USA. *Microbiol Resour Announc* 2021;10:e0044821.

276. Trevisan G, Linhares LCM, Crim B, et al. Macroepidemiological aspects of porcine reproductive and respiratory syndrome virus detection by major United States veterinary diagnostic laboratories over time, age group, and specimen. *PLoS One* 2019;14:e0223544.

277. Trible BR, Popescu LN, Monday N, et al. A single amino acid deletion in the matrix protein of porcine reproductive and respiratory syndrome virus confers resistance to a polyclonal swine antibody with broadly neutralizing activity. *J Virol* 2015;89:6515–6520.

278. Vairo S, Favoreel H, Scagliarini A, et al. Identification of target cells of a European equine arteritis virus strain in experimentally infected ponies. *Vet Microbiol* 2013;167:235–241.

279. Vairo S, Van den Broeck W, Favoreel H, et al. Development and use of a polarized equine upper respiratory tract mucosal explant system to study the early phase of pathogenesis of a European strain of equine arteritis virus. *Vet Res* 2013;44:22.

280. van Aken D, Snijder EJ, Gorbalenya AE. Mutagenesis analysis of the nsp4 main proteinase reveals determinants of arterivirus replicase polyprotein autoprocessing. *J Virol* 2006;80:3428–3437.

281. van Aken D, Zevenhoven-Dobbe J, Gorbalenya AE, et al. Proteolytic maturation of replicase polyprotein pp1a by the nsp4 main proteinase is essential for equine arteritis virus replication and includes internal cleavage of nsp7. *J Gen Virol* 2006;87:3473–3482.

282. Van Alstine WG, Kanitz CL, Stevenson GW. Time and temperature survivability of PRRS virus in serum and tissues. *J Vet Diagn Invest* 1993;5:621–622.

283. Van Den Born E, Gultyaev AP, Snijder EJ. Secondary structure and function of the 5'-proximal region of the equine arteritis virus RNA genome. *RNA* 2004;10:424–437.

284. van den Born E, Posthuma CC, Gultyaev AP, et al. Discontinuous subgenomic RNA synthesis in arteriviruses is guided by an RNA hairpin structure located in the genomic leader region. *J Virol* 2005;79:6312–6324.

285. van der Hoeven B, Oudshoorn D, Koster AJ, et al. Biogenesis and architecture of arterivirus replication organelles. *Virus Res* 2016;220:70–90.

286. van der Meer Y, van Tol H, Locker JK, et al. ORF1a-encoded replicase subunits are involved in the membrane association of the arterivirus replication complex. *J Virol* 1998;72: 6689–6698.

287. van Dinten LC, den Boon JA, Wassenaar AL, et al. An infectious arterivirus cDNA clone: identification of a replicase point mutation that abolishes discontinuous mRNA transcription. *Proc Natl Acad Sci U S A* 1997;94:991–996.

288. van Dinten LC, Rensen S, Gorbalenya AE, et al. Proteolytic processing of the open reading frame 1b-encoded part of arterivirus replicase is mediated by nsp4 serine protease and Is essential for virus replication. *J Virol* 1999;73:2027–2037.

289. van Dinten LC, van Tol H, Gorbalenya AE, et al. The predicted metal-binding region of the arterivirus helicase protein is involved in subgenomic mRNA synthesis, genome replication, and virion biogenesis. *J Virol* 2000;74:5213–5223.

290. van Geelen AGM, Anderson TK, Lager KM, et al. Porcine reproductive and respiratory disease virus: evolution and recombination yields distinct ORF5 RFLP 1 7 4 viruses with individual pathogenicity. *Virology* 2018;513:168–179.

291. Van Gorp H, Van Breedam W, Delputte PL, et al. Sialoadhesin and CD163 join forces during entry of the porcine reproductive and respiratory syndrome virus. *J Gen Virol* 2008;89:2943–2953.

292. van Hemert MJ, de Wilde AH, Gorbalenya AE, et al. The in vitro RNA synthesizing activity of the isolated arterivirus replication/transcription complex is dependent on a host factor. *J Biol Chem* 2008;283:16525–16536.

293. van Kasteren PB, Bailey-Elkin BA, James TW, et al. Deubiquitinase function of arterivirus papain-like protease 2 suppresses the innate immune response in infected host cells. *Proc Natl Acad Sci U S A* 2013;110:E838–E847.

294. van Kasteren PB, Beugeling C, Ninaber DK, et al. Arterivirus and nairovirus ovarian tumor domain-containing Deubiquitinases target activated RIG-I to control innate immune signaling. *J Virol* 2012;86:773–785.

295. van Marle G, Dobbe JC, Gultyaev AP, et al. Arterivirus discontinuous mRNA transcription is guided by base pairing between sense and antisense transcription-regulating sequences. *Proc Natl Acad Sci U S A* 1999;96:12056–12061.

296. van Nieuwstadt AP, Meulenberg JJ, van Essen-Zanbergen A, et al. Proteins encoded by open reading frames 3 and 4 of the genome of Lelystad virus (Arteriviridae) are structural proteins of the virion. *J Virol* 1996;70:4767–4772.

297. Vanderheijden N, Delputte PL, Favoreel HW, et al. Involvement of sialoadhesin in entry of porcine reproductive and respiratory syndrome virus into porcine alveolar macrophages. *J Virol* 2003;77:8207–8215.

298. Vanhee M, Van Breedam W, Costers S, et al. Characterization of antigenic regions in the porcine reproductive and respiratory syndrome virus by the use of peptide-specific serum antibodies. *Vaccine* 2011;29:4794–4804.

299. Vanmechelen B, Vergote V, Laenen L, et al. Expanding the arterivirus host spectrum: Olivier's Shrew virus 1, A novel arterivirus discovered in African Giant Shrews. *Sci Rep* 2018;8:11171.

300. Vatter HA, Di H, Donaldson EF, et al. Each of the eight simian hemorrhagic fever virus minor structural proteins is functionally important. *Virology* 2014;462–463:351–362.

301. Vatter HA, Di H, Donaldson EF, et al. Functional analyses of the three simian hemorrhagic fever virus nonstructural protein 1 papain-like proteases. *J Virol* 2014;88:9129–9140.

302. Veit M, Matczuk AK, Sinhadri BC, et al. Membrane proteins of arterivirus particles: structure, topology, processing and function. *Virus Res* 2014;194:16–36.

303. Verheije MH, Olsthoorn RC, Kroese MV, et al. Kissing interaction between 3' noncoding and coding sequences is essential for porcine arterivirus RNA replication. *J Virol* 2002;76:1521–1526.

304. Verheije MH, Welting TJ, Jansen HT, et al. Chimeric arteriviruses generated by swapping of the M protein ectodomain rule out a role of this domain in viral targeting. *Virology* 2002;303:364–373.

305. Vu HL, Kwon B, Yoon KJ, et al. Immune evasion of porcine reproductive and respiratory syndrome virus through glycan shielding involves both glycoprotein 5 as well as glycoprotein 3. *J Virol* 2011;85:5555–5564.

306. Wahl-Jensen V, Johnson JC, Lauck M, et al. Divergent simian arteriviruses cause simian hemorrhagic fever of differing severities in macaques. *mBio* 2016;7:e02009–e02015.

307. Wang D, Chen J, Yu C, et al. Porcine reproductive and respiratory syndrome virus nsp11 antagonizes type I interferon signaling by targeting IRF9. *J Virol* 2019;93:e00623-19.

308. Wang Y, Liang Y, Han J, et al. Attenuation of porcine reproductive and respiratory syndrome virus strain MN184 using chimeric construction with vaccine sequence. *Virology* 2008;371:418–429.

309. Wassenaar AL, Spaan WJ, Gorbalenya AE, et al. Alternative proteolytic processing of the arterivirus replicase ORF1a polyprotein: evidence that NSP2 acts as a cofactor for the NSP4 serine protease. *J Virol* 1997;71:9313–9322.

310. Wensvoort G, de Kluyver EP, Pol JM, et al. Lelystad virus, the cause of porcine epidemic abortion and respiratory syndrome: a review of mystery swine disease research at Lelystad. *Vet Microbiol* 1992;33:185–193.

311. Wensvoort G, Terpstra C, Pol JM, et al. Mystery swine disease in The Netherlands: the isolation of Lelystad virus. *Vet Q* 1991;13:121–130.

312. Wieringa R, De Vries AA, Post SM, et al. Intra- and intermolecular disulfide bonds of the GP2b glycoprotein of equine arteritis virus: relevance for virus assembly and infectivity. *J Virol* 2003;77:12996–13004.

313. Wieringa R, de Vries AA, Raamsman MJ, et al. Characterization of two new structural glycoproteins, GP(3) and GP(4), of equine arteritis virus. *J Virol* 2002;76:10829–10840.

314. Wieringa R, de Vries AA, Rottier PJ. Formation of disulfide-linked complexes between the three minor envelope glycoproteins (GP2b, GP3, and GP4) of equine arteritis virus. *J Virol* 2003;77:6216–6226.

315. Wieringa R, de Vries AA, van der Meulen J, et al. Structural protein requirements in equine arteritis virus assembly. *J Virol* 2004;78:13019–13027.

316. Wills RW, Doster AR, Galeota JA, et al. Duration of infection and proportion of pigs persistently infected with porcine reproductive and respiratory syndrome virus. *J Clin Microbiol* 2003;41:58–62.

317. Wissink EH, Kroese MV, van Wijk HA, et al. Envelope protein requirements for the assembly of infectious virions of porcine reproductive and respiratory syndrome virus. *J Virol* 2005;79:12495–12506.

318. Wolff G, Limpens R, Zevenhoven-Dobbe JC, et al. A molecular pore spans the double membrane of the coronavirus replication organelle. *Science* 2020;369:1395–1398.

319. Wongyanin P, Buranapraditkun S, Chokeshai-Usaha K, et al. Induction of inducible CD4+CD25+Foxp3+ regulatory T lymphocytes by porcine reproductive and respiratory syndrome virus (PRRSV). *Vet Immunol Immunopathol* 2010;133:170–182.

320. Wootton SK, Rowland RR, Yoo D. Phosphorylation of the porcine reproductive and respiratory syndrome virus nucleocapsid protein. *J Virol* 2002;76:10569–10576.

321. Wu Z, Lu L, Du J, et al. Comparative analysis of rodent and small mammal viromes to better understand the wildlife origin of emerging infectious diseases. *Microbiome* 2018; 6:178.

322. Xiao Z, Batista L, Dee S, et al. The level of virus-specific T-cell and macrophage recruitment in porcine reproductive and respiratory syndrome virus infection in pigs is independent of virus load. *J Virol* 2004;78:5923–5933.

323. Xie J, Christiaens I, Yang B, et al. Molecular cloning of porcine Siglec-3, Siglec-5 and Siglec-10, and identification of Siglec-10 as an alternative receptor for porcine reproductive and respiratory syndrome virus (PRRSV). *J Gen Virol* 2017;98:2030–2042.

324. Xu L, Zhou L, Sun W, et al. Nonstructural protein 9 residues 586 and 592 are critical sites in determining the replication efficiency and fatal virulence of the Chinese highly pathogenic porcine reproductive and respiratory syndrome virus. *Virology* 2018;517:135–147.

325. Xue F, Sun Y, Yan L, et al. The crystal structure of porcine reproductive and respiratory syndrome virus nonstructural protein Nsp1beta reveals a novel metal-dependent nuclease. *J Virol* 2010;84:6461–6471.

326. Yan L, Ge J, Zheng L, et al. Cryo-EM structure of an extended SARS-CoV-2 replication and transcription complex reveals an intermediate state in cap synthesis. *Cell* 2021;184:184–193.e110.

327. Yang L, Frey ML, Yoon KJ, et al. Categorization of North American porcine reproductive and respiratory syndrome viruses: epitopic profiles of the N, M, GP5 and GP3 proteins and susceptibility to neutralization. *Arch Virol* 2000;145:1599–1619.

328. Yang L, He J, Wang R, et al. Nonstructural protein 11 of porcine reproductive and respiratory syndrome virus induces STAT2 degradation to inhibit interferon signaling. *J Virol* 2019;93:e01352-19.

329. Yim-Im W, Huang H, Park J, et al. Comparison of ZMAC and MARC-145 cell lines for improving porcine reproductive and respiratory syndrome virus isolation from clinical samples. *J Clin Microbiol* 2021;59:e01757-20.

330. Yoo D, Song C, Sun Y, et al. Modulation of host cell responses and evasion strategies for porcine reproductive and respiratory syndrome virus. *Virus Res* 2010;154:48–60.

331. Yoon KJ, Wu LL, Zimmerman JJ, et al. Antibody-dependent enhancement (ADE) of porcine reproductive and respiratory syndrome virus (PRRSV) infection in pigs. *Viral Immunol* 1996;9:51–63.

332. Zevenhoven-Dobbe JC, Greve S, van Tol H, et al. Rescue of disabled infectious single-cycle (DISC) equine arteritis virus by using complementing cell lines that express minor structural glycoproteins. *J Gen Virol* 2004;85:3709–3714.

333. Zhang J, Go YY, MacLachlan NJ, et al. Amino acid substitutions in the structural or nonstructural proteins of a vaccine strain of equine arteritis virus are associated with its attenuation. *Virology* 2008;378:355–362.

334. Zhang J, Miszczak F, Pronost S, et al. Genetic variation and phylogenetic analysis of 22 French isolates of equine arteritis virus. *Arch Virol* 2007;152:1977–1994.

335. Zhang J, Timoney PJ, MacLachlan NJ, et al. Persistent equine arteritis virus infection in HeLa cells. *J Virol* 2008;82:8456–8464.

336. Zhang J, Timoney PJ, Shuck KM, et al. Molecular epidemiology and genetic characterization of equine arteritis virus isolates associated with the 2006–2007 multi-state disease occurrence in the USA. *J Gen Virol* 2010;91:2286–2301.

337. Zhang M, Zakhartchouk A. Porcine reproductive and respiratory syndrome virus envelope (E) protein interacts with tubulin. *Vet Microbiol* 2017;211:51–57.

338. Zhang Q, Yoo D. PRRS virus receptors and their role for pathogenesis. *Vet Microbiol* 2015;177:229–241.

339. Zhou L, Zhang J, Zeng J, et al. The 30-amino-acid deletion in the Nsp2 of highly pathogenic porcine reproductive and respiratory syndrome virus emerging in China is not related to its virulence. *J Virol* 2009;83:5156–5167.

340. Ziebuhr J, Snijder EJ, Gorbalenya AE. Virus-encoded proteinases and proteolytic processing in the Nidovirales. *J Gen Virol* 2000;81:853–879.

341. Zimmerman JJ. *Diseases of Swine*. 11th ed. Hoboken, NJ: Wiley-Blackwell; 2019.

342. Zitterkopf NL, Haven TR, Huela M, et al. Transplacental lactate dehydrogenase-elevating virus (LDV) transmission: immune inhibition of umbilical cord infection, and correlation of fetal virus susceptibility with development of F4/80 antigen expression. *Placenta* 2002;23:438–446.

343. Zitterkopf NL, McNeal DW, Eyster KM, et al. Lactate dehydrogenase-elevating virus induces apoptosis in cultured macrophages and in spinal cords of C58 mice coincident with onset of murine amyotrophic lateral sclerosis. *Virus Res* 2004;106:35–42.

W. Ian Lipkin • Christiane Herden • Jürgen A. Richt • Thomas Briese

History
Taxonomy
The virion
  Morphology and physical characteristics
  Genome and coding strategy
  Proteins
Cycle of infection
  Attachment and entry
  Transcription, replication, and gene expression
  Assembly and release
Bornavirus infection in mammals
  Borna disease
  Human infections
Bornavirus infection in avians
  Epidemiology, geographic distribution, and host range
  Clinical signs and seroprevalence
  Route of infection and transmission
  Pathogenesis
  Gross findings and histopathology
Models of bornavirus infection
  Cell culture models
  Infection in mammals
Diagnosis of bornavirus infection
  Differential diagnoses
  Intra vitam diagnosis
  Postmortem diagnosis
Therapy and control
  Vaccination
  Therapeutics
Perspectives and public health considerations

HISTORY

The syndrome we know as Borna disease (BD) was first described in European veterinary textbooks in the 1700s[408,440] as a disease of farm horses using various names like "Hitzige Kopfkrankheit" (German; "hot-headed disease") or "Seuchenhafte Gehirn-Rückenmarksentzündung" (German; "epidemic encephalomyelitis"). The contemporary name Borna disease was coined after the occurrence of major outbreaks in the years 1894–1896 in the district around the town of Borna in Saxony, Germany.[440] The name contains the "classifying" letters "RNA," a classification that was only justified at the end of the 20th century, when the etiologic agent Borna disease

virus (BoDV, formerly BDV) was identified as an RNA virus. BD predominantly affects horses and sheep, but also other Equidae, certain farm and zoo animals, and companion animals are occasionally diagnosed with natural BD (reviewed in Refs.[73,133,305,315,377]).

During the first decades of the 20th century, studies of BD focused primarily on defining the etiology, pathology, and pathophysiology of the disease. Initial evidence for a viral etiology was presented by Zwick[440] by reproducing the disease with bacteria-free filtrates of brain homogenates from affected horses. Histopathologic studies demonstrated a nonpurulent encephalomyelitis characterized by massive lymphohistiocytic infiltrates affecting the gray, and to a lesser extent, the white matter of the central nervous system, reactive astrogliosis, and intranuclear eosinophilic, so-called "Joest-Degen," inclusion bodies.[101,147,168,169,228,359] Pathologic changes were preferentially localized in the limbic system, most likely resulting in the observed behavioral disturbances.[162,315] Detailed studies have been performed on the spectrum of susceptible host species and on the clinical manifestations of the infection. Transmission experiments between naturally infected horses and sheep as well as other host species—including rabbits, guinea pigs, rats, chickens, and monkeys—established the infectious nature of the BD agent and confirmed that the same agent afflicted horses and sheep.[133,219,248,269,315,440,441]

Interest in BD and its causative agent was rather limited until the late 1970s/early 1980s, when the optimization of tissue and cell culture techniques for propagating the agent paved the way for work on the identification of the agent and on mechanisms of its pathogenesis in rabbit, rat, and tree shrew models.[215,231,245,374] Milestones in pathogenesis included the adaptation to Lewis and Wistar rats, the demonstration of an age-dependent outcome in experimentally infected rats,[148,245,251] and the recognition of its T-cell–dependent immunopathology.[148,245,246,309,310,381,386] Narayan's observations of a biphasic disease in adult-infected rats characterized by initial hyperactivity and followed by hypoactivity prompted efforts to determine whether humans were infected with a related agent. Serologic findings suggestive of a potential role for BoDV in affective disorders[316] intrigued many investigators (including the authors of this chapter), resulting in new efforts to identify the causative agent and explore in more detail the pathobiology and epidemiology/epizootiology of the infection. However, the causative agent remained elusive until the late 1990s, when BoDV was isolated and classified as a negative, single-stranded, nonsegmented RNA virus, the first member of the new family *Bornaviridae* in the order *Mononegavirales*.[29,48,55,214,310,341,345,403] With the advent of reverse genetics systems to produce infectious cDNA clones, detailed molecular analyses of the genome and its gene products, regulation of their expression, and detailed pathogenicity studies using constructs stably expressing fluorescent proteins became possible.[1,56,266,346,350,434]

In the first decade of the 21st century, a novel bornavirus, designated avian bornavirus, was identified in parrots with proventricular dilatation disease (PDD).[153,181] PDD is a progressive, variably contagious and often fatal disease of domesticated and wild psittacine birds worldwide. Typical clinical signs such as gastrointestinal (GI) dysfunction and associated wasting with or without neurologic symptoms are caused by nonpurulent inflammation of the enteric, autonomic, and central nervous system. A viral etiology for PDD has been assumed for over 40 years; recent work provides evidence for the etiologic role of ABV in the development of clinically manifest PDD. Avian bornaviruses have been detected worldwide not only in many captive parrots but also in other nonpsittacine species.[59,130,154,262,421] More recently, additional members of the family were discovered by molecular means that include bornaviruses found in snakes and fish but virus isolates to assess their biology are missing.[165,360,379]

Studies during the last decade are also beginning to solve the enigma of human bornavirus infections. During 2011–2014, cases of classical and fatal encephalitis in three breeders of variegated squirrels were shown to be caused by a bornavirus transmitted from the squirrels to their handlers.[151] Due to targeted studies triggered by this finding, BoDV was shortly thereafter also identified as the cause of fatal encephalitis in three patients that had received solid organ transplants from a common donor and in an additional case of unexplained fatal encephalitis not associated with transplantation.[194,336]

Until recently, it has been believed that no endogenous nonretroviral viruses exist in animal genomes. Surprisingly, endogenous elements homologous to BoDV genes were detected in the genomes of a large variety of vertebrates that, among others, reach from reptiles to bats and primates, including humans.[12,158] Phylogenetic analyses of such endogenous bornavirus-like elements (EBLs) indicate an evolutionary history of bornaviruses for at least 100 million years.[177]

TAXONOMY

Although the syndrome known as BD has been described since the 1700s, its causative agent, BoDV, eluded characterization until the late 1980s, when the application of a novel technique, subtractive cDNA cloning, yielded the first cDNA clones of the agent.[214,403] Thereafter, analysis of concentrated, partially purified virus preparations[26,303] led to the identification of BoDV as a nonsegmented, negative-strand RNA virus, distantly related to rhabdo-, paramyxo-, and filoviruses.[29,48] Identification of distinctive features including nuclear replication and transcription,[26,45,310] differential use of transcription initiation and termination signals,[29,340] and the use of alternative mRNA splicing[29,49,345] resulted in the creation of a new family *Bornaviridae* within the order *Mononegavirales* in 1996.[293] BoDV is the prototype of the family and was its sole member until avian bornaviruses were recognized in 2008.[153,181] Since then, the detection of additional family members[165,360,379] let to the establishment of several genera. The 2020 taxonomy of the family *Bornaviridae* encompasses three genera, *Orthobornavirus*, *Carbovirus*, and *Cultervirus*, of which the genus *Cultervirus* includes only one member species, *Sharpbelly cultervirus*, and the genus *Carbovirus* two species, *Queensland carbovirus* and *Southwest carbovirus* (https://talk.ictvonline.org/ictv-reports/ictv_online_report/negative-sense-rna-viruses/w/bornaviridae).[317] The majority of known bornaviruses are assigned to the genus *Orthobornavirus* that includes eight species: *Mammalian 1 orthobornavirus*, represented by BoDV; *Mammalian 2 orthobornavirus*, represented by variegated squirrel bornavirus (VSBV); the five avian orthobornavirus (ABV) species *Passeriform 1 orthobornavirus*, *Passeriform 2 orthobornavirus*, *Psittaciform 1 orthobornavirus*, *Psittaciform 2 orthobornavirus*, and *Waterbird 1 orthobornavirus*; and *Elapid 1 orthobornavirus*, represented by Loveridge's garter snake virus-1 (LGSV-1), a virus sequenced from an African snake.

THE VIRION

Most of what we know about the basic features of bornaviral virions is derived from studies of BoDV. The biology of many other bornaviruses is largely unknown since no virus isolate exists for members of the genera *Cultervirus* and *Carbovirus* or the Loveridge's garter snake virus-1, that are only known by sequence. Therefore, unless explicitly stated, features described below are based on experimental evidence obtained with representatives of the genus *Orthobornavirus*.

Morphology and Physical Characteristics

Spherical, enveloped particles of 80 to 100 nm with an electron dense core have been visualized by electron microscopy (EM) in extracts of BoDV-infected cultured cells.[189,438] Smaller structures also identified in these extracts presumably represent defective particles. No similar structures have been reported in tissues or fluids from infected mammals.[4,43,330] ABV viral particles of 83 to 104 nm in diameter have been detected in the brain, eye, or small intestine of ABV-infected birds, and detection of comparable particles more than 30 years ago led to the conclusion that PDD is caused by a virus infection.[154,224,432] The virion M_r and the S_{20},ω are not known; partially purified virus has a buoyant density of 1.15 to 1.22 g/cm^3 in CsCl, 1.18 to 1.22 g/cm^3 in sucrose, and 1.13 g/cm^3 in renografin.[51,97,261,303,438] Virus infectivity is only marginally affected after 24 hours in serum or by incubation at 37°C. In tissues and cell-free virus preparations, the virus can be more stable than in culture extracts, and depending on the mode of desiccation, dried preparations can remain infectious for months (tissue at ambient temperature) to years (brain suspension under vacuum).[51,215,216,248,440,442] At 4°C, BoDV infectivity is stable for more than 3 months. BoDV can withstand both alkaline and acidic environments but is most stable at neutral pH.[51,77,132] Heating to 56°C for more than 3 hours inactivates the virus, and common disinfection methods are appropriate as BoDV is sensitive to organic solvents, detergents, pH below 4, and to UV light.[51,68,132,133,245,248,261,440]

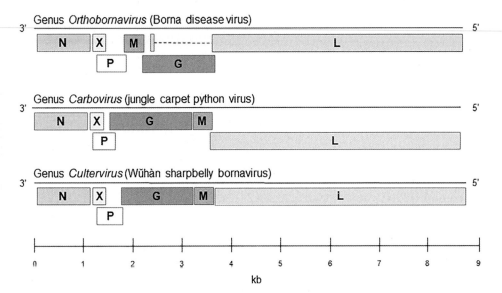

FIGURE 6.1 Variation of genome organization in representative viruses of the genera *Orthobornavirus*, *Carbovirus*, and *Cultervirus*. Schematic illustrating different organization of open reading frames for viral proteins N (nucleocapsid protein), X (X protein), P (phosphoprotein), M (matrix protein), G (glycoprotein), and L (RNA-dependent RNA polymerase) along bornaviral genomes.

Genome and Coding Strategy

The bornaviral genome is a negative-sense, single-stranded, nonsegmented RNA comprising approximately 8,900 nucleotides (nt) that includes six major open reading frames (ORF) with structural proteins in a 3′ and the viral polymerase in a 5′ position.[29,153,181,253,280] Short noncoding complementary sequences are found at the termini (Fig. 6.1). Unlike other nonsegmented negative-strand (NNS) RNA viruses, bornaviruses lack specific intergenic regions and instead have mostly overlapping ORFs. The first transcription unit of BoDV encodes the nucleocapsid protein (N) (Fig. 6.2). N exists in two isoforms, p40 (40 kDa) and p38 (38 kDa), that differ in the presence or absence of an amino terminal basic sequence that mediates nuclear localization.[186,295] Although nucleocytoplasmic shuttling can be deduced from immunohistochemical and *in situ* hybridization results for ABV,[418,419] there is no proof for the existence of N isoforms in ABV.[105,404,405] The viral phosphoprotein (P, p23) and the regulatory X protein (X, p10) are encoded by the second transcription unit.[416] The 5′ end of the P ORF overlaps with the 3′ portion of the X ORF in the +1 reading frame, an organization that resembles the P/C/C′ organization of the second gene of vesiculoviruses.[199,373] However, X is the first ORF in the RNA transcript, and there is no evidence of cotranscriptional mRNA editing, a mechanism used by some paramyxoviruses to regulate expression of multiple reading frames from their second transcription unit.[191,395] The first and second transcription units of bornaviruses overlap, because the transcription start S2 is located upstream of the termination/polyadenylation signal T1 (Fig. 6.2).[340] The start S3 of the third transcription unit is located 2 nt downstream of T2 and generates multiple transcripts for the matrix protein (M, p16), the type I surface glycoprotein (G, p57), and the L-polymerase (L, p190). The G ORF overlaps the M ORF in the +1 reading frame. The L gene initiates with a short ORF of 6 amino acids (aa) that is spliced to the large 5′ ORF (Fig. 6.2).[345,411]

BoDV isolates and strains reveal a remarkably high degree of genetic stability and homology. Among wild-type and experimentally host-adapted viruses, sequence identity is about 95% or greater at the nucleotide level and 1.5% to 3% at the predicted amino acid level.[18,29,48,143,192,253,280,342,377] Phylogenetic analyses of wild-type isolates and laboratory strains indicate distinct clusters, which correspond to the different endemic areas in Central Europe.[192] Geographical virus clusters exhibited a higher degree of identity to each other than isolates from distant regions, independent of host species or year of isolation. There is only one more divergent strain, No/98, that originated from Styria in Austria where BD is not endemic.[253] In contrast to this high genome conservation, ABV strains and isolates display remarkable genetic variability. Multiple genotypes have been described within the psittacine bornaviruses that share less than 70% sequence identity to any described BoDV.[153,181,262,418,421] These ABV genotypes vary considerably in their gene sequences with a homology range of 50% to 90% without clustering according to country of origin or avian species.[153,154,181,182,311,376,418,421]

Bornaviruses are phylogenetically distinct from other taxa. The region where bornaviruses have significant sequence similarity to other known viruses is in the conserved signature motifs of RNA-dependent RNA polymerases (RdRp).[284,285] When compared to the other members of the order *Mononegavirales*, some sequence relationship exists to rhabdo- and paramyxoviruses,[29,48] with the N-terminal part of the L sequence appearing closer to rhabdoviruses, whereas the C-terminal part more closely related to paramyxoviruses. However, the closest phylogenetic relations appear to exist to members of the families *Nyamiviridae* and *Xinmoviridae* and *Mymonaviridae*.

Sequences distantly related to BoDV L, M, N, P, and G sequences were identified in the genomes of several animal species, including bats, elephants, fish, lemurs, rodents, squirrels, primates, and man.[12,158,159,177] Detailed phylogenetic analyses

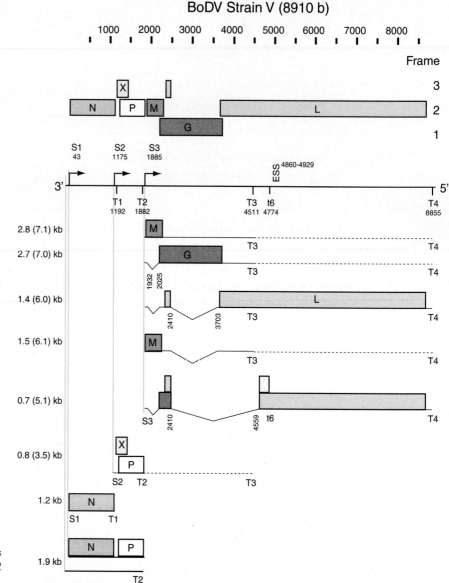

FIGURE 6.2 Genome and subgenomic transcript map of BoDV. S1 through S3, transcriptional initiation sites; T1 through T4, and t6, transcriptional termination sites; ESS, exon-splicing suppressor. *Dashed lines* indicate readthrough at termination sites T2 and T3. See text for details.

suggest multiple ancient independent integration events. An intriguing example is a BoDV N-related sequence that likely integrated before the separation of marmosets and macaques 40 million years ago.[12,158] In few instances, the endogenous bornavirus-like (EBL) element comprises a complete ORF that includes BoDV-like transcription initiation and termination signals. The finding of mRNA transcripts of such EBL elements suggests potential functional roles that may include protection from BoDV infection.[12,94,184] Recent findings indicate also the existence of EBL elements with similarity to carbo- and culter-virus sequences, and the overall history of bornaviruses may extend to almost 100 million years.[177]

Proteins

Nucleocapsid Protein (N)

In BoDV, N exists as a 40- and 38-kDa isoform.[28,186,295] Additionally, minority isoforms of N can be generated from

alternative splice sites in the N mRNA of BoDV, generating three truncated products with distinct subcellular distributions that may participate in the regulation of mRNA transcription and genomic RNA replication.[190] However, these splice sites are only conserved in BoDV and VSBV, not in other orthobornaviruses. The 38-kDa isoform of N has also not yet been observed in ABV.[105,404,405] The 40-kDa variant (p40) is derived from the full-length ORF, while the 38-kDa variant (p38) initiates at a second in-frame AUG, resulting in the lack of 13 aa at the amino terminus (Fig. 6.3). Although an RNA with coding information for p38 has been found that starts downstream of S1,[295] it is unknown whether p40 and p38 can both be translated from mRNA transcripts starting at the S1 transcriptional initiation site. The 13 aa amino terminal sequence present in p40 contains a nuclear localization signal (NLS; $P_3KRRLVDDA_{11}$) compatible with the differential cellular distribution of the two isoforms seen in cells transfected with

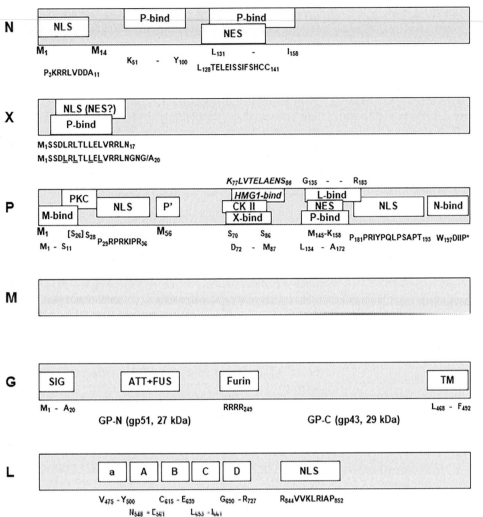

FIGURE 6.3 Map of motifs identified in BoDV proteins. M1 and M14 in N and M1 and M56 in P indicate start sites of p40 and p38, or P and P', respectively; NLS, nuclear localization signal; NES, nuclear export signal; P-bind, site of interaction with P; M-bind, site of interaction with M; X-bind, site of interaction with X; L-bind, site of interaction with L; N-bind, site of interaction with N; HMG1-bind, site of interaction with host-cell protein amphoterin; PKCε, protein kinase Cε phosphorylation; CK II, casein kinase II phosphorylation; SIG, signal peptide; TM, transmembrane domain; ATT+FUS, attachment and fusion domain; Furin, Furin cleavage site; a, A, B, C, D, conserved L-polymerase motifs. See text for further details.

constructs expressing only one of the isoforms, while p40 is primarily nuclear, p38 is primarily cytoplasmic.[186,295] However, both p38 and p40 bind to P. As P contains potent NLS (Fig. 6.3), the *in vivo* significance of the two N isoforms is unknown; p38 may enter the nucleus through interaction with P. Experimental evidence with expression constructs indicates that p38 can accumulate in the nucleus to levels similar to those of p40; however, p38 alone cannot support transcription/replication of BoDV (mini-)genomes.[266] Thus, the amino terminal sequence of p40 may have functions in addition to N protein translocation to the nucleus. Both p40 and p38 bind to P through two motifs (K_{51}–Y_{100} and L_{131}–I_{158}; Fig. 6.3).[13,185] and p38 appears to regulate cellular levels of free p40 by blocking the respective binding site on P, thus modulating cellular ratios of free p40 to P.[348] In addition, p38 and p40 contain a nuclear export signal (NES; L_{128}TELEISSIFSHCC$_{141}$)[185] that overlaps the binding motif for P (Fig. 6.3). It is therefore hypothesized that p38, which lacks the NLS motif, may redistribute to the cytosol after dissociation from bound P, possibly once assembled in ribonucleoprotein (RNP) complexes.[185] As indicated by purification experiments and colocalization studies, both p38 and

p40, as well as P and M, are included with genomic RNA in the nuclear RNP.[38,230] Association of genomic RNA with N relies on basic amino acid residues located in a cleft formed between the amino- and carboxy-terminal helical domains of N.[149,325] However, binding to N in the multimeric RNP appears not to shield the genomic RNA from enzymatic attack.

Together with P, N constitutes the BoDV s-antigen, a complex found in the noninfectious supernatant fluid obtained after high-speed centrifugation of sonicated infected brain tissue or cultured cells. Characterization of the s-antigen provided the first evidence of protein–protein interactions[9,112,215] and until the development of molecular assays, served as the critical diagnostic marker for infection.[256,409,410]

X Protein (X)

BoDV X or p10[416] is a nonstructural protein[230,353] that, together with P, modulates BoDV polymerase activity as a function of the relative abundance of the two proteins.[287,353] X effects appear to be differently pronounced in different cell types.[434] Although X is not essential for the formation of infectious particles,[265] it does perform crucial functions during the BoDV life cycle because recombinant BoDV constructs carrying a non-functional X ORF are not viable.[289] Mammalian two-hybrid and coimmunoprecipitation experiments indicate an interaction between X and P,[358] and recombinant BoDV systems showed that X inhibited BoDV RNA replication and transcription through binding to P[266,288,349] in the absence of viral M and G.[265] The site of X interaction with P has been mapped to the N-terminal motif $S_3DLRLTLLELVRRL_{16}$, with aa 8 through 15 being probably most essential.[223,288,429] X is small (10 kDa) and can be found in the nucleus and cytoplasm. A leucine-rich amino-terminal motif with primary sequence similarity to the NES of cellular and viral export proteins like HIV-1 Rev or PKI (Fig. 6.3, underlined leucines) led to the speculation that X may mediate nucleocytoplasmic shuttling through its interaction with the RNP via P. However, X has been shown in association with BoDV nuclear proteins,[38] and other data suggest that this motif functions as an NLS rather than an NES ($R_6LTL-LELVRRNGN_{19}$).[430] These experiments also showed that transport of X through the nuclear pore complex is mediated by direct binding to importin-alpha. The cytoplasmic fraction of X colocalizes with mitochondria also through this N-terminal, alpha-helical sequence since alanine mutagenesis showed that R_6A/L_7A and $R_{14}A/R_{15}A$ mutants lose the mitochondrial localization.[286] Mitochondrial localization of X is necessary for antiapoptotic and neuroprotective effects of X in cell culture and animal models, and neuroprotection has been shown to be mediated by a peptide encompassing the 29 C-terminal aa of the X protein.[286,387] Antiapoptotic effects of X may relate to its interference with type I interferon signaling.[423]

Phosphoprotein (P)

P, a cofactor of the viral polymerase L, is phosphorylated at multiple serine residues by two different cellular kinases.[354,394] P is phosphorylated predominantly by protein kinase Cε (PKCε) at Ser28 (and Ser26, which is not present in all BoDV strains) and to a lesser extent by casein kinase II (CK II) at Ser 70 and Ser 86 (Fig. 6.3). As in other NNS virus phosphoproteins, phosphorylation status may regulate P's ability to form homomultimers, bind to other viral proteins, and serve as a transcriptional activator. P interacts with itself, X, N, M, and L as shown by mammalian two-hybrid and co-immunoprecipitation analyses. Regions of interaction of P with P (aa 135–172), with N (aa 197–201),[358] with M (aa 1–11),[38] and with X (aa 72–87)[188] were mapped through analysis of truncation mutants of P. The region of interaction with L (aa 135–183) overlaps that identified for homooligomerization; however, the sites are functionally separated as shown by analyses of P mutants that bound to L but had lost the ability to oligomerize.[347] These analyses also demonstrated that P-oligomerization is essential for polymerase activity. Furthermore, the oligomerization motif in P overlaps with the NES and the L-binding motif adjacent to the aminoterminal NLS of P; two NLS have been mapped at the amino- and carboxyl-terminus of P (Fig. 6.3).[357,361] The NES (M_{145}-K_{158}) includes four methionine residues that were shown to be essential to the export function of that sequence but not to P binding or for functioning as polymerase cofactor.[435] Overlap also exists between the CK II phosphorylation sites and the region of interaction with X. Although it is conceivable that phosphorylation of P (or X at S_{34}) may be involved in differentially regulating protein function, nucleocytoplasmic

trafficking of P or its interaction with X appear not affected.[188] In this context, it is intriguing that PKCε is highly concentrated in limbic circuitry,[328] as it suggests that PKCε phosphorylation may be important to the limbic distribution of BoDV. BoDV infection of neurons interferes with synaptic vesicle recycling through blockade of PKC phosphorylation of myristoylated alanine-rich C kinase substrate (MARCKS) and mammalian uncoordinated-18 (Munc-18). There is speculation that P may contribute to BoDV pathogenesis by competing with neuronal substrates for phosphorylation by PKC.[172,291,429]

Matrix Protein (M)

Like the BoDV s-antigen, a 14.5-kDa protein purified from infected brain homogenate had been linked to the unidentified BD agent prior to molecular characterization of BoDV.[334] Once genome sequence data became available, microsequencing indicated that this protein is the product of the 16-kDa ORF of BoDV (p16).[183] Subsequent analyses showed that p16 forms noncovalently linked tetramers and constitutes a nonglycosylated viral matrix protein.[197,198] M is a component of the viral RNP, can bind to P and to RNA, and has features compatible with membrane association.[38,230,247] However, in contrast to M proteins of other NNS RNA viruses, BoDV M appears to have no inhibitory effect on polymerase activity.[38]

Glycoprotein (G)

The BoDV glycoprotein is a classical type I membrane protein that is generated from the 57-kDa ORF and posttranslationally modified by N-glycosylation to yield a 94-kDa primary product (gp94).[304,343] The primary product is processed by cellular furin protease into an amino-terminal GP-N (27 kDa, gp51) and a carboxy-terminal GP-C (29 kDa, gp43) through cleavage after arginine$_{249}$ (Fig. 6.3).[180,304] Whereas the gp94 precursor contains only high-mannose glycans, analysis of the cleaved fragments indicated glycan maturation by showing mixtures of high-mannose and complex-type glycans on both GP-N and GP-C.[180] Anchored by its transmembrane domain, GP-C is transferred to the cell membrane, while the gp94 precursor predominantly accumulates in the endoplasmic reticulum. The final composition of mature virions is not clear; gp94 as well as GP-C and GP-N have been found in infectious particles,[96,97,267] but GP-N and GP-C were also demonstrated in infectious particles that lacked the gp94 precursor after virus purification.[74,180] Computational analyses indicate an arrangement of structural features of BoDV G that is colinear to that of rhabdoviral G, suggesting that BoDV G also belongs to the class III viral fusion proteins.[92]

RNA-Dependent RNA Polymerase (L)

The large polymerase protein (L) of BoDV is the product of alternative splicing, a mechanism unique among NNS RNA viruses.[29,345] The generated continuous ORF translates a 190-kDa protein[332,411] that displays motifs characteristic of RNA-dependent RNA polymerases (RdRp). L interacts with P and, analogous to other NNS L-polymerases, is phosphorylated by cellular kinases (Fig. 6.3).[411] Plasmid constructs directing expression of the continuous 190-kDa protein that supported replication of recombinant BoDV genomes confirmed the RNA polymerase activity of the protein.[226,266,349,350,434] Translocation of L to the nucleus of the infected cell may be promoted by an NLS motif (R_{844}VVKLRIAP$_{852}$; Fig. 6.3) located toward the center of L,[412] or in association with BoDV P.[349]

CYCLE OF INFECTION

Attachment and Entry

BoDV attachment and entry appear to be analogous to the pH-dependent entry via intracellular vesicles described for rhabdo- and filoviruses, as opposed to the pH-independent surface fusion mechanism used by paramyxoviruses.[279,312,329] BoDV G binds to one or more still unidentified cellular surface receptor(s).[68,74,97,152,343] Receptor interaction of G triggers BoDV internalization through energy-dependent, clathrin-mediated endocytosis and subsequent pH-dependent membrane fusion leads to release of the RNP from intracellular vesicles into the cytosol.[41,96] Protease inhibitor studies indicate that cleavage of the precursor gp94 is essential for infectivity.[304] Whereas the amino-terminal 244 aa of GP-N and/or gp94 are involved in receptor binding, the hydrophobic amino-terminus of GP-C is hypothesized to initiate membrane fusion upon a conformational change induced by acidification in the early to intermediate endosome.[41,74,96,267,343]

Despite its predilection for neuronal cell types *in vivo*, BoDV has the capacity to infect a wide variety of cultured neuronal as well as nonneuronal cell types from many species. Only hematopoietic cells[323] and mouse cell lines[85] have been reported as resistant to infection *in vitro*. This may indicate potential exploitation of secondary receptors and has also led to hypotheses about a nonreceptor–mediated cell-to-cell spread of BoDV that is supported by *in vitro* as well as *in vivo* observations.[45,99,218] Subsequent studies with a CHO cell line that apparently was resistant to infection by BoDV virions, and with furin protease-deficient CHO cells, indicated that BoDV may disseminate by G receptor–independent pathways.[40] However, correct G maturation enhanced the proposed receptor independent cell-to-cell spread and is mandatory for the formation of infectious progeny virions.[6] More recent analyses support the view that cleaved G is necessary for efficient virus spread, although predominantly to directly neighboring cells without excluding a contribution of direct cell-to-cell transfer of RNPs in certain cell types.[37,207]

Transcription, Replication, and Gene Expression

Recombinant virus systems confirm that BoDV N, P, and L are essential and sufficient for transcription and replication of the viral genome.[226,265,266,349,350,434] As with other negative-strand RNA viruses, genomic RNA packaged by N constitutes the RNP that serves as a template for the associated polymerase complex components L and P.[149,230] The BoDV X protein, although not part of the incoming ribonucleocapsid complex released after membrane fusion,[230,353] appears to modulate the formation and activity of functional polymerase complexes later in the infection cycle by buffering the crucial N-to-P ratio and likely attenuating the enzymatic activity of the polymerase through association with the nuclear RNP.[38,127,265,287,415] Furthermore, BoDV is unique among known animal NNS RNA viruses in its nuclear

location for transcription and replication.[26,45] To generate its proteins, BoDV uses predominantly polycistronic mRNAs that are transcribed from three transcriptional initiation sites characterized by a CUU consensus sequence and terminate at four AU$_6$ termination/polyadenylation sites (Fig. 6.2).[29,340]

The first and second transcription units overlap such that the initiation signal S2 lies upstream of the termination signal T1.[29,48,290,340] A similar organization was postulated to serve as an attenuation signal for the control of polymerase expression in respiratory syncytial virus.[42] However, attenuation appears not to take place in BoDV as the two transcription units are found at similar levels,[29] in contrast to the usual transcriptional gradient observed in other viruses of the order *Mononegavirales*. Other factors may modify mRNA levels beyond effects attributable to the typical 3′-to-5′ transcriptional gradient, including the incorporation of regulatory sequences in spliced introns.[362]

Read-through at termination/polyadenylation signals is a vital feature of BoDV transcription, leading to primary, subgenomic RNA transcripts of 0.8, 1.2, 1.9, 2.8, 3.5, and 7.1 kb. The 1.2-kb transcript is the only monocistronic product. It is colinear with the p40 ORF and directs translation of the p40 and p38 isoforms of BoDV N from alternative in-frame AUG codons.[186,295] The second transcription unit generates the 0.8-kb transcript that codes for the X and the P protein in overlapping ORFs. There is no evidence of splicing to eliminate the AUG initiating translation of X.[29,340,416] Thus, it is likely that P is expressed through a leaky scanning mechanism, possibly analogous to the termination-mediated reinitiation of X translation from the small upstream ORF included in the 0.8-kb transcript. The expression of X may be further modulated by cellular protein interactions with the long 5′-untranslated region (UTR) of this BoDV transcript.[414] The long 5′-UTR region also includes poorly defined regulatory elements controlling RNA polymerase read-through at the T1 signal.[287,290] Interestingly, the region containing the AUG of the upstream small ORF has been found deleted in sequenced psittacine ABV genomes but not in ABV genomes from geese.[262,311] In BoDV, a truncated 16-kDa P′ product of undefined function may result from initiation at a downstream in-frame AUG.[187]

Read-through at T2 produces an elongated 0.8-kb derivative of 3.5 kb. Two primary transcripts of 2.8 and 7.1 kb are generated from the third transcription unit through differential read-through at T3. The 2.8- and 7.1-kb transcripts include the p16 and p57, or the p16, p57, and pol ORF, respectively; in addition, several secondary transcripts are derived from these RNAs through alternative splicing (Fig. 6.2).

Transcripts of the third transcription unit include two intron sequences, intron-1 and intron-2, that are subject to alternative splicing.[345] Whereas the 2.8- and 7.1-kb transcripts direct translation of M, the expression of G likely requires removal of intron-1. Although G may also be expressed *in vitro* from unspliced transcripts by leaky ribosomal scanning, splicing of intron-1 creates a stop-codon after the 13th aa of the p16 ORF that facilitates translational initiation at the AUG of G.[344] Splicing of intron-2 removes almost the complete p57 ORF and fuses a small 17 nt ORF located upstream of the splice donor site to the large downstream ORF that, in the case of the 2.8-kb RNA transcript, terminates at T3, generating a truncated L protein of unknown function (Fig. 6.2). Expression of L is, analogous to G, likely facilitated by splicing of intron-1. In addition, an alternative splice acceptor site, controlled by a downstream exon-splicing suppressor, has been identified at nt 4559.[399] Splicing of this potential intron-3 (nt 2410–4559), and transcriptional read-through at t6,[29] may result in expression of two additional BoDV coded proteins.[47,399] However, the splice acceptor side at nt 4559 is not strictly conserved among sequenced BoDV isolates. The lack of conservation in BoDV No/98[280] as well as in ABV isolates indicates that the potential gene products are unlikely to fulfill essential functions in the life cycle of most orthobornaviruses.

There have been reports of multiple types of BoDV 1.9-kb RNA transcripts with unspecified function. Analyses based on RNA circularization and sequencing over the junction indicated the presence of a noncapped RNA complementary to position 1 to 1882 of the BoDV genome that interacted with oligo(dT)-beads, but was not fully polyadenylylated.[340] Such transcripts may represent abortive replication intermediates or subgenomic RNAs analogous to leader RNAs found in other mononegaviruses. On the other hand, studies employing precipitation with a cap-specific antibody characterized a capped 1.9-kb mRNA with a long poly(A)-tail, extending from S1 to T2[290] (Fig. 6.2).

Initiation of transcription and replication in negative-strand RNA viruses is commonly mediated by sequences located in the UTR. A single transcriptional promoter located in the 3′-UTR of the genome generates the usual transcriptional gradient, and promoter sequences driving genome replication are located in both the complementary 3′- and 5′-genomic termini. However, BoDV analyses indicated remarkable terminal heterogeneity.[280] Kinetic analyses comparing the genomic termini in acute and persistent BoDV infection showed an accumulation of terminal truncations in the course of infection, which in several cases resulted in strongly attenuated replicational and transcriptional promoter activity, possibly contributing to BoDV's persistent lifestyle.[313] In addition, rescue of infectious recombinant BoDV constructs demonstrated trimmed 5′ genomic termini generated from originally perfectly complementary constructs.[350] In this system, when recessed 5′ ends aligned to the 3′ terminus were generated, there was strong attenuation of replication while transcriptional activity appeared to be unaffected. This finding is compatible with the high antigen levels in conjunction with low levels of infectious virus that are observed during persistent BoDV infection. The four 5′ terminal bases of the genome and antigenome appear to be copied from internal template motifs through backfolding of the termini followed by specific elongation and termination on the template motifs.[225] This allows later cleavage of these terminal bases to generate monophosphorylated 5′ termini of progeny strands without the loss of genetic information. Trimming of the termini in BoDV may support its persistent infection by escape from innate immune responses through RIG-I–mediated recognition of triphosphorylated genomic termini.[113] It is not known whether viral and/or host functions are responsible for the terminal trimming. Further characterization of these unique BoDV transcriptional and replicational promoter sequences may help to resolve results obtained in various recombinant test systems.

Assembly and Release

As with other negative-strand RNA viruses, a first step in the production of BoDV progeny is packaging of the replicated nascent genomic RNA by N. The 5′-trailer RNA specifically promotes its association with N via basic residues in the cleft between the amino- and carboxy-terminal domains of the protein.[149,325] Formation of progeny RNP complexes includes

association of P via its carboxy-terminal aa residues and the inclusion of L via P's binding motif for L (see Fig. 6.3). The viral RNP assembles in the nucleus to larger structures that have been termed vSPOTs (viral speckles of transcripts).[228] These correspond in location to the pathognomonic nuclear inclusion bodies described by Joest and Degen[168,169] that also elicit the characteristic staining pattern in the diagnostic IFA test.[140] The structures appear as porous cage-like assemblies where N is condensed to the rims, like an exoskeleton, P as the central protein-binding hub with interaction to all viral proteins except G distributed in a web-like fashion throughout the interior, but X and M also present in a more random distribution.[147] Due to the additional presence of negative-sense (genomic) as well as positive-sense (antigenomic and messenger) viral RNA, they are considered "viral factories" where replication and transcription take place.[147,228] The factories are linked to the host chromosome mediated by the HMGB1 binding site on P (see Fig. 6.3). Synchronized with the breakdown of nuclear structure during mitosis, the factories dissemble and relocate to mitotic chromosomes to ensure segregation to the daughter cells and persistent infection.[228] Due to the overlap of the HMGB1 with the X binding site on P (see Fig. 6.3) and the known relocation of nuclear P upon X expression,[188,435] this may also provide pathways for virus maturation and nucleocytoplasmic shuttling of individual RNP for packaging into mature virions. Based on NLS motifs located in N, P, L, and X, and NES motifs in the two N isotypes and in P upon activation through X-binding,[188,435] various hypotheses concerning nucleocytoplasmic shuttling of BoDV RNP have been proposed and are conceivable but experimental support for each remains fragmentary. No distinct packaging signals have been defined for BoDV.

BORNAVIRUS INFECTION IN MAMMALS

Borna Disease

Epidemiology, Geographic Distribution, and Host Range

In general, seroepidemiological studies point to a widespread, possibly worldwide distribution of orthobornaviruses. Natural BD is endemic in areas of central Europe such as southern and eastern Germany, Switzerland, Liechtenstein, and Austria.[32,50,71,133,140,233,417,422,440] Reports of natural BD outside these endemic areas suggest a potentially wider distribution.[90,114,115,171,174,436] Virus-specific serum antibodies and/or nucleic acids in the absence of disease or in association with unusual clinical signs have been reported in animals from different geographic areas, including European countries, such as France, Sweden, Finland, and Italy, as well as Turkey, Israel, Japan, Iran, China, Australia, and the United States.[71,90,114,115,171,174,217,305,315,436] However, as some of these data are debated and require more confirmation, further epidemiologic studies are warranted, especially to clarify whether these data might point to novel bornaviruses or possibly the expression of EBLs.

A seasonal accumulation of BD cases in April, May, and June—with a significant decrease in late fall and winter—is quite characteristic and argues, in combination with the geographically limited occurrence, for a natural reservoir.[71,73,102,133,219,402] Clinically apparent BD infection is restricted to endemic areas of Germany, Switzerland, and Austria that correspond to the distribution of the bicolored white-toothed shrew (*Crocidura leucodon*). This shrew species has been confirmed to serve as a natural reservoir for BoDV,[24,72,146,417] and phylogenetic analyses indicate the presence of stable geographic virus clusters.[18,192,402] Typical for reservoir hosts, shrews show a widespread viral organ distribution and virus shedding but do not develop clinical signs and neuroinflammation is absent. In incidental dead-end host species, such as horses or humans, a nonpurulent meningoencephalitis is the typical clinical outcome.

BD is reported most commonly in horses and sheep, but disease has also been reported in other *Equidae*, farm animals (cattle and goats), rabbits, lynx, zoo animals (alpacas, sloths, various monkeys, hippopotamuses), and rarely in companion animals (dogs and cats).[21,33,50,58,73,133,166,167,220,232,315,377,422,440] Recently, BoDV infections have been confirmed in llama and alpaca herds in endemic areas in Switzerland and Germany.[167,222] Susceptibility to infection depends on host species and viral strains.[50,315,431]

Clinical Signs and Seroprevalence

Animal accidental dead-end hosts, such as horses and sheep, typically suffer from a severe neurological disorder after BoDV infection with a mortality of about 80% to 90%; in horses death occurs within 1 to 4 weeks after onset of clinical signs.[73,102,104,305] In 72% of stables with equine BD cases, only individual animals develop clinically manifested BD. In cattle and sheep, death was noted in more than 50% of animals after 1 to 6 weeks or 1 to 3 weeks after onset of clinical signs, respectively.[21,307]

Seroepidemiological studies point to frequent inapparent infections in horses and sheep (reviewed in Ref.[135]). Clinical signs of BD are composed of various neurologic symptoms affecting psyche, sensorium, sensibility, motility, and autonomous nervous system, depending on the stage of infection and the respective brain area affected by neuroinflammation (reviewed in Ref.[135]). In other host species, clinical signs are mainly similar to the symptoms in horses.[21,32,33,219,232,257,315] In contrast, in the shrew reservoir species, no inflammatory infiltrate or degenerative lesions can be found in the central nervous system despite high viral loads.[24,72,294]

In contrast to the epidemic course of BD at the end of the 19th century, the incidence of BD decreased significantly during recent decades; usually less than 100 horses or sheep are diagnosed with BD per year.[71,140,240] However, BoDV infections in horses and sheep can be inapparent as indicated by seroepidemiologic surveys in Germany. The average seroprevalence of BoDV-specific antibodies in clinically healthy horses in Germany is approximately 11.5%[140] and increases in endemic areas up to 22.5%, reaching 50% in stables with a history of clinical BD.[104] There is a higher frequency of BD on farms with mixed stock of horses, sheep, and cattle, operating under lower hygiene standards.[71] Repeated outbreaks of BD within the same premises have been noted but usually are spaced several months or years apart.[104,305] Recurring outbreaks have recently also been observed in llama and alpaca herds.[222,352] The reason for the discrepancy between the high BoDV seroprevalence and the low BD incidence in horses remains unknown but may relate to age, immune status, genetic background, virus strain, and/or dose and route of infection.

Route of Infection and Transmission

There is evidence that nerve endings in the nasal and pharyngeal mucosa represent the most likely natural route of entry.[169,229,238] Experimental BDV infection of neonatal rats results in virus

persistence and disseminated virus distribution with presence of viral gene products and infectious virus in saliva, urine, and feces.[229,238] Such secreta or excreta are important in transmission of other pathogenic viruses (e.g., lymphocytic choriomeningitis virus and hantaviruses). This finding further supports the concept of a natural reservoir of BDV, which is substantiated by stable geographic virus clusters,[18,192,402] despite substantial horse movement and trade. This was recently confirmed by a case of natural BD in Great Britain that was traced back to a likely origin of infection in Germany.[292] It seems that widespread horse-to-horse or sheep-to-sheep transmissions do not occur.[16,71,306,377] The infectious dose for natural infections is unknown.

Pathogenesis

Manifestations of mammalian orthobornavirus infections vary. Whereas reservoir hosts such as shrews and squirrels do not develop inflammation or disease, dead-end host species, such as horses or humans, typically suffer from a strictly neurotropic and lethal infection associated with neurological signs and a severe nonpurulent meningoencephalitis. The disease in these end hosts is based on immunopathological mechanisms; for BoDV, it is known that a T-cell–mediated delayed-type hypersensitivity reaction with a key role of immunopathogenic CD8+ and CD4+ T cells trigger the disease[375,381] (reviewed in Ref.[135]).

Gross Findings and Histopathology

In animals, the pattern and type of inflammatory lesions in the central nervous system have been described in detail[101,168] (reviewed in Ref.[135]). In BoDV-1–infected horses, gross findings may include leptomeningeal hyperemia, edema, or hydrocephalus internus in later disease stages.[133,176,440,443] Histopathological changes after BoDV infection are similar in all mammalian species and mainly restricted to gray matter areas of the central nervous system, spinal cord, and retina. A severe nonpurulent poliomeningoencephalomyelitis with severe perivascular and parenchymal immune cell infiltrates accompanied by activation of astrocytes and microglia is characteristic, and diagnosis can be confirmed if pathognomonic intranuclear "Joest-Degen" inclusion bodies are present in neurons. Some cases have loss of pyramidal cells of the hippocampus. In BoDV-infected horses, the brain regions most impacted are the olfactory bulb, basal cortex, caudate nucleus, thalamus, hippocampus, and periventricular areas of the medulla oblongata.

Although viral antigen is commonly found in the retina, blindness is commonly central.[15,137] However, degeneration of retinal neurons resulting in blindness has been reported.[65] In contrast, BDV-infected rats and rabbits typically develop blindness caused by a nonpurulent chorioretinitis with degeneration of rods and cones.[200,245,246] No inflammation of neuropathology is seen in the reservoir host species *C. leucodon*.

Human Infections

Much of the impetus for characterization of BoDV came from concerns that it could infect humans and might be implicated in major depressive disorder, bipolar disorder, schizophrenia, autism, chronic fatigue syndrome, AIDS encephalopathy, multiple sclerosis, motor neuron disease, and brain tumors (glioblastoma multiforme) (Tables 6.1 and 6.2). Over a period of three decades, investigators reported findings of human infection using mostly PCR and serologic assays, including the

TABLE 6.1 Serum immunoreactivity to borna disease virus in subjects with various diseases (1985–2010)

Disease	Prevalence Disease (%)	Control (%)	Assay	Reference
Psychiatric (various)	0.6 (4/694)	0 (0/200)	IFA	Rott et al. (1985) *Science* 228:755
	2 (13/642)	2 (11/540)	IFA	Bode et al. (1988) *Lancet* 2:689
	4–7 (200–350/5,000)	1 (10/1,000)	WB/IFA	Rott et al. (1991) *Arch Virol* 118:143
	12 (6/49)		IFA	Bode et al. (1993) *Arch Virol* S7:159
	30 (18/60)		WB	Kishi et al. (1995) *FEBS Lett* 364:293
	14 (18/132)	1.5 (3/203)	WB	Sauder et al. (1996) *J Virol* 70:7713
	24 (13/55)	11 (4/36)	IFA	Igata-Yi et al. (1996) *Nat Med* 2:948
	0 (0/44)	0 (0/70)	IFA/WB	Kubo et al. (1997) *Clin Diagn Lab Immunol* 4:189
	2.8 (35/126)	1.1 (10/917)	ECLIA	Yamaguchi et al. (1999) *Clin Diagn Lab Immunol* 6:696
	9.8 (4/41)		IFA	Bachmann et al. (1999) *J Neurovirol* 5:190
	15 (4/27)	0 (0/13)	IFA	Vahlenkamp et al. (2000) *Vet Microbiol* 76:229
	0 (0/89)	0 (0/210)	IFA/WB	Tsuji et al. (2000) *J Med Virol* 61:336
	5.5 (5/90)	0 (0/45)	WB (N[a])	Fukuda et al. (2001) *J Clin Microbiol* 39:419
	2.1 (17/816)		ECLIA	Rybakowski et al. (2001) *Eur Psychiatry* 16:191
	2.4 (23/946)	1.0 (4/412)	ECLIA	Rybakowski et al. (2002) *Med Sci Monit* 8:CR642
				Rybakowski et al. (2001) *Psychiatr Pol* 35:819
	13 (11/87)	16 (45/290)	IFA	Lebain et al. (2002) *Schizophr Res* 57:303
	15 (26/171)	2 (1/50)	RLA	Matsunaga et al. (2005) *Clin Diagn Lab Immunol* 12:671
	23 (39/171)	0 (0/9)	WB	Matsunaga et al. (2005) *Clin Diagn Lab Immunol* 12:671
	29 (24/84)	20 (77/378)	RLA	Matsunaga et al. (2008) *J Clin Virol* 43:317
	67 (26/39)	22 (28/126)	CIC	Rackova et al. (2009) *Neuro Endocrinol Lett* 30:414
	4.5 (12/265)	0 (0/105)	IFA	Amsterdam et al. (1995) *Arch Gen Psych* 42:1093
Affective disorders	4.2 (12/285)	0 (0/200)	IFA	Rott et al. (1985) *Science* 228:755
	38 (53/138)	16 (19/117)	WB (P[a])	Fu et al. (1993) *J Affect Disord* 27:61
	37 (10/27)		IFA	Bode et al. (1993) *Arch Virol* S7:159
	12 (6/52)	1.5 (3/203)	WB	Sauder et al. (1996) *Virol* 70:7713
	0–0.8 (0–1/122)	0 (0/70)	IFA/WB	Kubo et al. (1997) *Clin Diagn Lab Immunol* 4:189
	2.2 (1/45)	0 (0/45)	WB	Fukuda et al. (2001) *J Clin Microbiol* 39:419
	93 (26/28)	32 (21/65)	CIC	Bode et al. (2001) *Mol Psychiatry* 6:481
	27 (9/33)	4 (1/25)	WB	Terayama et al. (2003) *Psychiatry Res* 120:201
	19 (25/129)	20 (77/378)	RLA	Matsunaga et al. (2008) *J Clin Virol* 43:317
	4.8 (5/104)	0 (0/42)	ELISA	Flower et al. (2008) *APMIS Suppl* (124):89
	0 (0/138)	0 (0/60)	IFA	Na et al. (2009) *Psychiatry Investig* 6:306
Schizophrenia	25 (1/4)		IFA	Bode et al. (1993) *Arch Virol* S7:159
	32 (29/90)	20 (4/20)	WB	Waltrip et al. (1995) *Psychiat Res* 56:33
	17 (15/90)	15 (3/20)	IFA	Waltrip et al. (1995) *Psychiat Res* 56:33
	14 (16/114)	1.5 (3/203)	WB	Sauder et al. (1996) *J Virol* 70:7713
	20 (2/10)		WB	Richt et al. (1997) *J Neurovirol* 3:174
	0–1 (0–2/167)	0 (0/70)	IFA/WB	Kubo et al. (1997) *Clin Diagn Lab Immunol* 4:189
	14 (964)	0 (0/20)	WB	Waltrip et al. (1997) *Schizoph Res* 23:253
	36 (24/67)	0 (0/26)	WB (P[a])	Iwahashi et al. (1997) *Acta Psych Scand* 96:412
	12 (38/276)		WB	Chen et al. (1999) *Mol Psychiatry* 4:33

TABLE 6.1 Serum immunoreactivity to borna disease virus in subjects with various diseases (1985–2010) (*Continued*)

Disease	Prevalence		Assay	Reference
	Disease (%)	Control (%)		
	10 (3/29)	23 (6/26)	IFA	Selten et al. (2000) *Med Microbiol Immunol* 189:55
	8.9 (4/45)	0 (0/45)	WB	Fukuda et al. (2001) *J Clin Microbiol* 39:419
	13 (11/87)	16 (45/290)	IFA	Lebain et al. (2002) *Schizoph Res* 57:303
	8.6 (10/116)	0 (0/54)	WB	Yang et al. (2003) *Zhanghua Shi Yan He Lin Chuang Bing Du Xue Za Zhi* 1:85
	22 (7/32)	4 (1/25)	WB	Terayama et al. (2003) *Psychiatry Res* 120:201
	23 (21/91)	20 (77/378)	RLA	Matsunaga et al. (2008) *J Clin Virol* 43:317
	0 (0/60)	0 (0/60)	IFA	Na et al. (2009) *Psychiatry Investig* 6:306
Childhood neuropsychiatric disorder	56 (93/166)	51 (50/98)	CIC	Donfrancesco et al. (2008) *APMIS Suppl* (124):80
CFS	24 (6/25)		WB	Nakaya et al. (1996) *FEBS Lett* 378:145
	34 (30/89)		WB	Kitani et al. (1996) *Microbiol Immunol* 40:459
				Nakaya et al. (1997) *Nippon Rinsho* 55:3064
	0 (0/69)	0 (0/62)	WB	Evengard et al. (1999) *J Neurovirol* 5:495
	100 (7/7)	33 (1/3)	WB	Nakaya et al. (1999) *Microbiol Immunol* 43:679
	11 (7/61)	0 (0/73)	WB	Li et al. (2003) *Zhonghua Shi Yan He Lin Chuang Bing Du Xue Za Zhi* 17:330
	21 (17/82)	0 (0/73)	WB	Li et al. (2005) *Zhonghua Yi Xue Za Zhi* 85:701
MS	13 (15/114)	2.3 (11/483)	IP/IFA	Bode et al. (1992) *J Med Virol* 36:309
	0 (0/50)		IFA	Kitze et al. (1996) *J Neurol* 243:660
HIV-positive	7.8 (36/460)	2.0 (11/540)	IFA	Bode et al. (1988) *Lancet* ii:689
HIV-early	8.1 (61/751)	2.3 (11/483)	IP/IFA	Bode et al. (1992) *J Med Virol* 36:309
HIV-LAP	14 (34/244)	2.3 (11/483)	IP/IFA	Bode et al. (1992) *J Med Virol* 36:309
Schisto/malaria	9.8 (19/193)	2.3 (11/483)	IP/IFA	Bode et al. (1992) *J Med Virol* 36:309
SSPE-associated BDV antibody	22 (39/174)	23 (39/173[b])	ELISA	Güngör et al. (2005) *Pediatr Infect Dis J* 24:833
Mental healthcare workers	9.8 (8/82)	2.9 (8/277)	WB	Chen et al. (1999) *Mol Psychiatry* 4:33
Family of schizophrenic patients	12 (16/132)	2.9 (8/277)	WB	Chen et al. (1999) *Mol Psychiatry* 4:33
Living near horse farms	15 (16/108)	1 (1/100)	ELISA	Takahashi et al. (1997) *J Med Virol* 52:330
Ostrich exposure	46 (19/41)	10 (4/41)	ELISA	Weisman et al. (1994) *Lancet* 344:1732
Veterinarians	0.7 (1/138)		IFA	Kinnunen et al. (2007) *J Clin Virol* 38:64
Suspected hanta virus infection	0.2 (1/361)		IFA	Kinnunen et al. (2007) *J Clin Virol* 38:64
Alcohol and drug addiction	37 (15/41)	37 (47/126)	CIC	Rackova et al. (2010) *BMC Psychiatry* 10:70
Multitransfused	8.3 (14/168)	0 (0/42)	ELISA	Flower et al. (2008) *APMIS Suppl* (124):89
Pregnant women	0.9 (2/214)		ELISA	Flower et al. (2008) *APMIS Suppl* (124):89
Blood donors	2.3 (5/219)		ELISA	Flower et al. (2008) *APMIS Suppl* (124):89
Normal population	59 (1,204/2,101)		TELISA	Patti et al. (2008) *APMIS Suppl* (124):70
	37 (591/1,588)		TELISA	Patti et al. (2008) *APMIS Suppl* (124):74
	50 (130/258)		TELISA	Patti et al. (2008) *APMIS Suppl* (124):77

[a]Immunoreactivity to BDV N and P was measured, and the higher prevalence is given.
[b]Epilepsy, headache, and cerebral palsy.
CFS, chronic fatigue syndrome; CIC, circulating immune complexes; ECLIA, enhanced chemiluminescence immunoassay, ELISA, enzyme-linked immunosorbent assay; HIV, human immunodeficiency virus; IFA, immunofluorescence assay; IP, immunoprecipitation; LAP, lymphadenopathy; MS, multiple sclerosis; RLA, radioligand assay; Schisto/malaria, schistosomiasis and malaria; SSPE, subacute sclerosing panencephalitis; TELISA, triple ELISA–CIC, Ab, Ag; WB, western immunoblot.

TABLE 6.2 Borna disease virus nucleic acid in subjects with various diseases (1995–2009)

Disease	Tissue	Prevalence Disease (%)	Prevalence Control (%)	Divergence[a]	Reference
Psychiatric (various)	PBMC	67 (4/6)	0 (0/10)	0–3.6	Bode et al. (1995) *Nat Med* 1:232
	PBMC	37 (22/60)	6.5 (5/77)	4.2–9.3	Kishi et al. (1995) *FEBS Lett* 364:293
					Kishi et al. (1996) *J Virol* 70:635
	PBMC-coculture	9.1 (3/33)	0 (0/5)	0.07–0.83	Bode et al. (1996) *Mol Psych* 1:200
					de la Torre et al. (1996) *Virus Res* 44:33
	PBMC	1.9 (2/106)	0 (0/12)		Kubo et al. (1997) *Clin Diagn Lab Immunol* 4:189
	PBMC	0 (0/24)	0 (0/4)		Richt et al. (1997) *J Neurovirol* 3:174
	PB	0 (0/159)			Lieb et al. (1997) *Lancet* 350:1002
	Blood	(1/1)			Planz et al. (1998) *Lancet* 352:623
	PBMC	4 (5/126)	2.4 (2/84)		Iwata et al. (1998) *J Virol* 72:10044
	PBMC	20 (3/15)	0 (0/3)		Planz et al. (1999) *J Virol* 73:6251
	PBMC	0 (0/81)			Kim et al. (1999) *J Neurovirol* 5:196
	PBMC	0 (0/27)			Bachmann et al. (1999) *J Neurovirol* 5:190
	CSF	0 (0/27)			Bachmann et al. (1999) *J Neurovirol* 5:190
	PBMC	1.8 (1/56)	0.6 (1/173)		Tsuji et al. (2000) *J Med Virol* 61:336
	PBMC	37 (10/27)	15 (2/13)		Vahlenkamp et al. (2000) *Vet Microbiol* 76:229
	PBMC	1.1 (1/90)	0 (0/45)		Fukuda et al. (2001) *J Clin Microbiol* 39:419
	PBMC	33 (10/30)	13 (4/30)		Miranda et al. (2006) *J Affect Disord* 90:43
Affective disorders	PBMC	33 (1/3)	0 (0/23)		Sauder et al. (1996) *J Virol* 70:7713
	PBMC	17 (1/6)	0 (0/36)		Igata-Yi et al. (1996) *Nat Med* 2:948
	PBMC	0 (0/9)			Richt et al. (1997) *J Neurovirol* 3:174
	Brain	40 (2/5)	0 (0/10)		Salvatore et al. (1997) *Lancet* 349:1813
	PBMC	4.1 (2/49)	2.4 (2/84)	0–5.1	Iwata et al. (1998) *J Virol* 72:10044
	CSF	4.6 (3/65)	0 (0/69)	[Protein]	Deuschle et al. (1988) *Lancet* 352:1828
	PBMC	2.2 (1/45)	0 (0/45)		Fukuda et al. (2001) *J Clin Microbiol* 39:419
	PBMC	11 (6/53)	0 (0/32)		Wang et al. (2006). *Zhonghua Liu Xing Bing Xue Za Zhi* 27(6):479
PBMC	0 (0/138)	0 (0/38)	0 (0/60)		Na et al. (2009) *Psychiatry Investig* 6:306
Schizophrenia	Brain	0 (0/3)	0 (0/3)		Sierra-Honigman et al. (1995) *Br J Psych* 166:55
	CSF	0 (0/48)	0 (0/9)		Sierra-Honigman et al. (1995) *Br J Psych* 166:55
	PBMC	0 (0/9)	0 (0/9)		Sierra-Honigman et al. (1995) *Br J Psych* 166:55
	PBMC	64 (7/11)	0 (0/23)		Sauder et al. (1996) *J Virol* 70:7713
	PBMC	10 (5/49)	0 (0/36)		Igata-Yi et al. (1996) *Nat Med* 2:948
	PBMC	0 (0/26)	0 (0/14)		Richt et al. (1997) *J Neurovirol* 3:174
	Brain	53 (9/17)	0 (0/10)		Salvatore et al. (1997) *Lancet* 349:1813
	PBMC	9.8 (6/61)	0 (0/26)		Iwahashi et al. (1997) *Acta Psych Scand* 96:412
	PBMC	3.9 (3/77)	2.4 (2/84)	0–5.1	Iwata et al. (1998) *J Virol* 72:10044
	PBMC	14 (10/74)	1.4 (1/69)		Chen et al. (1999) *Mol Psychiatry* 4:566
	Brain	24 (1/4)		[RNA, virus, and protein]	Nakamura et al. (2000) *J Virol* 74:4601
	PBMC	14 (4/29)	35 (9/26)		Selten et al. (2000) *Med Microbiol Immunol* 189:55

TABLE 6.2 **Borna disease virus nucleic acid in subjects with various diseases (1995–2009)** (*Continued*)

Disease	Tissue	Prevalence Disease (%)	Prevalence Control (%)	Divergence[a]	Reference
	PBMC	0 (0/45)	0 (0/45)		Fukuda et al. (2001) *J Clin Microbiol* 39:419
	PBMC	12 (3/25)		6.0–14	Nakaya et al. (1996) *FEBS Lett* 378:145
					Kitani et al. (1996) *Microbiol Immunol* 40:459
	PBMC	12 (7/57)	4.9 (8/172)		Nakaya et al. (1997) *Nippon Rinsho* 55:3064
	PBMC	0 (0/18)			Evengard et al. (1999) *J Neurovirol* 5:495
	PBMC	0 (0/60)	0 (0/60)		Na et al. (2009) *Psychiatry Investig* 6:306
Schizoaffective	PBMC	44 (12/27)	15 (4/27)		Nunes et al. (2008) *J Clin Lab Analysis* 22:314
Viral encephalitis	CSFMC	12 (6/52)	0 (0/32)		Wang et al. (2006) *Zhonghua Liu Xing Bing Xue Za Zhi* 27(6):479
	PBMC	14 (6/43)	0 (0/98)	2.3–4.5	Wang et al. (2008) *Zhonghua Liu Xing Bing Xue Za Zhi* 29:1213
	PBMC	15 (6/40)	0 (0/46)		Li et al. (2009) *Eur J Neurol* 16:399
	PBMC	10 (6/59)	0 (0/60)	4.7	Ma et al. (2009) *Zhonghua Liu Xing Bing Xue Za Zhi* 30:1284
FMS	CSF	0 (0/18)	0 (0/6)		Wittrup et al. (2000) *Scand J Rheumatol* 29:387
CFS	PBMC	12 (3/25)		6.0–14	Nakaya et al. (1996) *FEBS Lett* 378:145
	Brain	80 (4/5)			de la Torre et al. (1996) *Virus Res* 44:33
Hippocampal sclerosis	Brain	15 (3/20)	0 (0/85)		Czygan et al. (1999) *J Infect Dis* 180:1695
Epilepsy	Brain	0 (0/106)			Hofer et al. (2006) *J Clin Virol* 36:84
MS	CSF	11 (2/19)	0 (0/69)	[Protein]	Deuschle et al. (1998) *Lancet* 352:1828
	PBMC	0 (0/34)	0 (0/40)		Hasse et al. (2001) *Ann Neurol* 50:423
	PBMC	22 (2/9)	0 (0/98)	2.3–4.5	Wang et al. (2008) *Zhonghua Liu Xing Bing Xue Za Zhi* 29:1213
	PBMC	0 (0/9)	0 (0/46)		Li et al. (2009) *Eur J Neurol* 16:399
Peripheral neuropathy	PBMC	0 (0/7)	0 (0/98)		Wang et al. (2008) *Zhonghua Liu Xing Bing Xue Za Zhi* 29:1213
	PBMC	0 (0/16)	0 (0/46)		Li et al. (2009) *Eur J Neurol* 16:399
Parkinson disease	PBMC	0 (0/5)	0 (0/98)		Wang et al. (2008) *Zhonghua Liu Xing Bing Xue Za Zhi* 29:1213
HIV infection	PBMC	13 (11/82)			Cotto et al. (2003) *J Clin Microbiol* 41:5577
Immunosuppressive treatment	PBMC	1.3 (1/80)			Cotto et al. (2003) *J Clin Microbiol* 41:5577
Multiple transfusions	PBMC	0.8 (1/127)	2 (2/200)		Lefrere et al. (2004) *Transfusion* 44:1396
Mental healthcare workers	PBMC	15 (7/45)	1.4 (1/69)		Chen et al. (1999) *Mol Psychiatry* 4:566
Normal controls	PBMC		4.7 (8/172)		Kishi et al. (1995) *Med Microbiol Immunol* 184:135
	Brain		6.7 (2/30)		Haga et al. (1997) *Brain Res* 770:307
	PBMC		0 (0/100)		Davidson et al. (2004) *Vax Sang* 86:148
	Plasma		0 (0/275[b]		Davidson et al. (2004) *Vox Sang* 86:148

[a]Divergence of P gene nucleotide sequence from Borna disease virus strain V and He/80.
[b]Plasma minipools of 91 individual samples.
CFS, Chronic fatigue syndrome; CSF, cerebrospinal fluid; PBMC, peripheral blood mononuclear cells; PB, peripheral blood; FMS, fibromyalgia syndrome; MS, multiple sclerosis.

detection of circulating immune complexes,[20,22,428] but there were also occasional reports of infectious virus isolated from humans or viral gene products detected in human brain by *in situ* hybridization and immunohistochemistry.[57,244] Failure to independently replicate positive results in the majority of laboratories undermined confidence in the association of BoDV with human psychiatric disease.[213,428] Another concern was the possibility of cross-contamination suggested by sequence similarity of putative human BoDV sequences with those of the laboratory strains and field isolates handled in the laboratories reporting the human sequences.[70,161,302,356,377,428] A blinded multicenter analysis failed to find either molecular or serologic evidence for BoDV infection in psychiatric illness.[161] Thus, although the potential for human infection has not been excluded, it is exceedingly unlikely that a bornavirus similar to those identified to date is responsible for a significant burden of psychiatric disease. However, bornaviruses have recently been unequivocally implicated as zoonotic pathogens in human encephalitis.

Infection With Variegated Squirrel Bornavirus

A cluster of unexplained encephalitis cases in Germany among breeders of exotic squirrels native to Central America let to the discovery of variegated squirrel bornavirus (VSBV) by unbiased viral high-throughput nucleic acid sequencing.[151] These and other clusters provided the first solid evidence for human bornavirus infections. Extended screening of captive squirrels in private holdings and zoological gardens indicated the presence of VSBV in species of two subfamilies, Central American *Sciurinae* (*Sciurinae variegatoides* and *Sciurinae granatensis*) and Southeast Asian *Callosciurinae* (*Callosciurinae prevostii*, *Callosciurinae finlaysonii*, and *Tamiops swinhoei*).[3,337,338] Human VSBV infection manifests as an acute, commonly fatal encephalitis with immunopathology analogous to that known from classical BD in animals.[392,393] The VSBV found in Germany was presumably imported through Prevost's squirrels.[30,389] However, this origin has not been confirmed. The public health risk of VSBV appears to be limited, at least in Europe from where sufficient data are available, and restricted to specific risk populations of breeders and handlers that constitute dead-end hosts. Bites and scratches have been proposed as potential routes of cutaneous entry.[151]

Virus isolates of VSBV have been obtained through cocultivation of infected squirrel cells with permanent C6 or Vero lines.[339] Intracranial infection of neonate Lewis rats with cultured VSBV induces meningoencephalitis.

Infection With Borna Disease Virus

Although the original reports linking BoDV to psychiatric syndromes have been refuted, BoDV has been confirmed as a rare cause of human encephalitis. BoDV infection was first unequivocally demonstrated in four cases of nonsuppurative encephalopathy: three recipients of a solid organ transplant from a nonsymptomatic donor[336] and one unrelated case of acute idiopathic viral encephalitis in a previously healthy 25-year-old man.[194] A total of 30 cases have been identified through analyses of mainly banked samples from encephalitis cases in endemic regions of Germany collected over a period of two decades (1999 to 2020).[44,76,81,194,211,250,336] Ten of the cases were analyzed by multiple investigators, using various approaches

including RT-PCR, serology, histology, immunohistochemistry, *in situ* hybridization, and/or brain imaging. In summary, these human cases closely match the picture known from natural BoDV infections of horse and sheep. Each of these patients had a rapidly progressing encephalitis with fatal outcome in all but two patients. One survivor remained in an unresponsive state.[44] The other liver transplant recipient of the initial case cluster survived with neurologic damage and progressing optic nerve atrophy during ribavirin and intravenous immunoglobulin treatment.[336] The organ donor did not have any neurologic symptoms or signs of infection; no samples from the time of donation are available, and the nature and source of the BoDV infection remain unknown. All patients had a high viral load in brain tissue. Identical virus isolates were obtained in parallel by three laboratories from brain samples of one confirmed case.[250] All but one of these cases originated from the endemic areas in Southern Germany, and the virus sequence of the patient matched those determined for the respective regional BoDV genotype known from animal BD cases or white-toothed shrews.[250,319] Most recently, another fatal human case originating from a nonendemic area in Northeast Germany has been reported that was related to an outbreak in alpacas.[391] Epidemiologic surveys in areas endemic for BD indicated a low seroprevalence among veterinarians (0.001%) and blood donors (0%),[390] which together with the observed high clinical case fatality rate and the limited overall case number identified over a period of 20 years suggest that human BoDV infections are rare events.

BORNAVIRUS INFECTION IN AVIANS

Epidemiology, Geographic Distribution, and Host Range

Avian orthobornaviruses were identified in 2008 as etiological cause of proventricular dilatation disease (PDD) in birds.[153,181] PDD was known since the 1970 in macaws exported from Bolivia.[14,108,224] Avian orthobornaviruses comprise a heterogeneous group of virus species within the genus *Orthobornavirus*; within the 5 virus species, at least 15 different viruses have been identified.[317] These avian bornaviruses have been detected in not only more than 80 captive and free-ranging psittacine and nonpsittacine species worldwide, including pet and wild birds, but also critically endangered species such as the Spix's macaw (*Cyanopsitta spixii*).[52,59,108,154,179,227,249,268,270,271,327,418] Infection with avian bornaviruses has also been reported in nonpsittacine species such as songbirds (canaries, finches) and free-ranging waterfowl such as swans (*Cygnus buccinators*, *Cygnus olor*, *Cygnus buccinator*), geese (*Branta canadensis*, *Chen rossii*, *Chen caerulescens*) and wild ducks.[59,62,109–111,130,154,249,262,264,318,320,421] Aquatic bird bornavirus 1 and 2 are found mainly in wild aquatic bird species in North America and Europe, and it cannot be excluded that some of them might represent natural reservoirs.[60,110,262,396] All other avian bornaviruses are detected in captive and wild birds with a worldwide distribution for parrot bornaviruses 1 to 8.[25,67,78,130,153,179,181,202,227,241,271,274,296,311,327] Passeriformes serve as natural hosts of canary bornaviruses 1 to 3, munia bornavirus 1, and estrildid finch bornavirus 1.[318,320,421] Among the different avian bornaviruses, parrot bornavirus 2 and 4 (PaBV-2 and 4; Psittacine 1 orthobornaviruses) are the most frequently detected viruses.[321,418] Cockatiels and canaries have been established as experimental models of avian orthobornavirus infections. Whereas clinical signs can be consistently be reproduced in cockatiels, canaries usually do not develop clinical signs.

Clinical Signs and Seroprevalence

Typical clinical signs of PPD are progressive GI dysfunction and wasting.[14,108,154,224,376] Avian bornaviruses can be detected in about 60% to 100% of birds with PDD[91,105,130,153,154,181,258,263,296,311,314] (reviewed in Refs.[19,377]). Affected animals have a progressive decrease in GI motility resulting in anorexia, lethargy, weight loss leading to cachexia, and vomiting. Neurological signs include lethargy, ataxia, tremor, seizures, and motor deficits. Blindness has been described in a few cases.[378] The mortality rate approaches 100%.[108] Besides the typical clinical course, clinically silent infections have been reported, with antibody-positive animals shedding viral RNA continuously or intermittently.[54,131,139,134,209,264,404,432] Sudden death is occasionally reported, which might be associated with cardiac disease.[203] Some studies report that 15% to 40% healthy animals are positive for avian bornavirus infection[130,156,314] (reviewed in Ref.[135]). Feather-damaging behavior in seropositive psittacines has also recently been described.[82,160] In a follow-up study in an aviary with naturally infected cockatiels over 5 years, a decline of viral shedding and lack of detection of viral RNA in various tissues was found in birds previously found to be RT-PCR positive in cloacal swabs.[241]

A wide variation in the pathological lesions of infected animals has been noted and also healthy animals that show typical histologic lesions at necropsy, clinically inconspicuous birds with widespread virus distribution or restriction of viral RNA to the nervous tissue, and any variation thereof.[54,60,209,264,272,296,404,432] Asymptomatic carriers may contribute to virus maintenance. Some animals do not become infected despite being in close contact to infected birds.[131,182,296,320] Virus-specific antibodies can be detected in clinically healthy or diseased birds[53,54,82,111,130,131,139] (reviewed in Ref.[157]). Recently, it was shown that chicks infected with PaBV-4 on the first day of life did not develop clinically manifest PDD despite virus persistence.[93] Surveillance studies in naturally infected animal found that birds with high viral RNA loads and high virus-specific antibody titers are at higher risk to develop clinically manifest PDD.[131] Importantly, virus-specific antibodies do not show a protective effect[131] (reviewed in Ref.[135]).

Route of Infection and Transmission

Field observations favor horizontal transmission since viral RNA is present in feces, cloacal, and crop swabs in naturally infected animals including free ranging waterfowl.[60,321] Virus transmission may also occur via wounds or skin lesions with subsequent infection of adjacent nerve fibers and retrograde viral spread to the central nervous system.[128,203,204] Experimental transmission is possible via the intramuscular and subcutaneous route even with low virus doses.[326] In contrast to mammalian orthobornaviruses, the oronasal route is ineffective.[129,326] Vertical transmission has been proposed based on the demonstration of avian orthobornaviral RNA and specific antibodies in embryos, but no infectious virus has been described.[61,178,210,237,433] The incubation period typically ranges from 20 to 60 days but may be as long as 200 days.[91,105,182,204,205,264,272,273] Virus-specific serum

antibodies are detected between 7 and 60 days after experimental infection.

Pathogenesis

Avian orthobornaviruses are neurotropic and distribute through the central, peripheral and autonomic nervous systems. Viral RNA and/or antigen can be found most frequently in the brain, spinal cord and gastrointestinal tract (crop, proventriculus, gizzard, small intestine), as well as in peripheral organs such as adrenal gland, eye, heart, liver, kidney, spleen, pancreas, lungs, gonads, thyroid, and skin[139,182,272,296] (reviewed in Refs.[156,263]). It has been suggested that the vagus nerve might be involved in viral dissemination due to direct vagal innervation of major visceral organs[272,273,296] (reviewed in Ref.[314]).

Gross Findings and Histopathology

Typical gross pathology findings in clinical PDD comprise emaciation with atrophy of pectoral, proventricular and ventricular muscles, dilatation or rupture of the proventriculus, and duodenal distension.[14,91] Characteristic mononuclear infiltrates can be present in ganglia and nerves of the enteric autonomic nervous system (ENS) of proventriculus and ventriculus, esophagus, crop and duodenum. It has been proposed that inflammation within the ENS is responsible for gastrointestinal dysfunction and paralytic dilatation of the esophagus and proventriculus.

Our knowledge of the pathogenesis of avian orthobornavirus infections is less advanced than for mammalian bornavirus infection. Nonetheless, given the common features of viral persistence and inflammatory lesion, one can anticipate mechanistic similarities. This concept is substantiated by a comparable correlation of onset of clinical signs with the appearance of CD3[+] T cells in the brain[264] and a similar composition of the inflammatory infiltrates (lymphocytes; further characterized as CD4[+] and CD8[+] T cells), macrophages, and variable numbers of plasma cells,[272,273] which points to a role of the adaptive cellular immune response for pathogenesis (reviewed in Ref.[397]).

MODELS OF BORNAVIRUS INFECTION

Cell Culture Models

Studies in cell culture systems are providing further insights into the mechanisms by which BoDV interferes with cellular functions and induces neuropathology. Interference with basic cellular signaling pathways and modulation of cellular protein functions through direct binding by, or indirect interaction with, individual viral proteins has been recognized. The N-terminal portion (aa 13–171) of BoDV N binds to the Cdc2-cyclin B1 complex and delays cell cycle progression in primary rat and mouse fibroblasts.[278] Direct protein–protein interaction was also shown between BoDV P and the neurite outgrowth factor amphoterin (also designated HMG1).[173] Complex formation between amphoterin's A-box and BoDV P (aa 77–86; see Fig. 6.3) leads to competitive inhibition of p53 binding to amphoterin, resulting in down-regulation of cyclin G promoter activity.[437] Through interference with the transcriptional activity of p53, BoDV may affect cell cycle regulation as well as apoptosis. BoDV P interaction with amphoterin also causes altered intracellular distribution of amphoterin in infected cells, leading to an inhibition of neurite outgrowth and migration that has been ascribed to interference with the normal interaction between amphoterin and its receptor RAGE (Receptor for Advanced Glycation End-products).[173] Studies of neuronal differentiation of PC12 cells indicate an interaction of BoDV with cellular MAPK signaling pathways.[119] Persistently infected PC12 cells demonstrate constitutive phosphorylation of MAPK/ERK kinase (MEK), extracellular signal-regulated kinase (ERK), and the E 26 (ETS)–like transcription factor 1 (Elk-1); however, nuclear translocation of ERK is impaired, contributing to the failure of the cells to differentiate with nerve growth factor (NGF) treatment. Activation of MAPK signaling is evident within 1 hour after acute infection, suggesting that gene expression is not required for BoDV activation of the MAPK cascade, whereas sustained MAPK activation appears essential to virus transmission. Chemical blockade of MEK inhibited virus spread to neighboring cells.[277] BoDV impairment of ERK-mediated neurotrophin signaling also modulates synaptic functioning by interfering with synaptogenesis and synaptic protein synthesis.[118] Analogous to findings in the neonatal rat,[98] BoDV infection of neuronal cells specifically down-regulates the expression of proteins related to synaptic plasticity, such as synaptophysin and growth-associated protein 43 (GAP-43).[119] In addition, infection interfered with synaptic activity by inhibiting synaptic vesicle recycling in response to stimulus-induced potentiation in hippocampal neuronal cultures.[407] Several cellular kinases participate in the phosphorylation events involved in synaptic vesicle recycling, including protein kinase C (PKC), the epsilon isoform of which phosphorylates BoDV P.[354] Thus, it is conceivable that the high levels of BoDV P that are expressed in the cytoplasm as well as in the nucleus of BoDV-infected cells may act as a decoy substrate for PKC, analogous to the BoDV P phosphorylation by Traf family member–associated NF-κB (TANK)–binding kinase 1 (TBK-1) that results in the suppression of TBK-1–dependent interferon (IFN) expression in non-neuronal cells.[401] However, species-specific differences appear to exist in the susceptibility of BoDV to the antiviral action of IFNγ. Human IFNγ efficiently prevented BoDV infection of human and monkey cell lines, whereas rat IFN only ineffectively inhibited the infection of rat cell lines or rat hippocampal slice cultures.[333] Moreover, experiments in mouse brain slice cultures indicated a tissue-specific action of IFNγ, with a more pronounced effect of IFNγ on BoDV proliferation in cerebellar than in hippocampal cultures.[85]

Infection in Mammals

Early virus detection and isolation experiments by Zwick and colleagues were performed in rabbits.[440] Rabbits are highly susceptible and after early weight loss develop neurologic disease 3 weeks after infection with BoDV-infected brain homogenates. Symptoms include slow movement, depression, and somnolence followed by flaccid back musculature, paresis starting from the hind limbs, and spasm of the jaw muscle.[216] Rats have been become the most common model for BoDV infection in mammals.[148,245,246,251] Susceptibility to disease in rats is genetically determined. Wistar rats and black-hooded rats show less severe disease than Lewis rats, a strain with deficiencies in the hypothalamic–pituitary–adrenal axis associated with enhanced susceptibility to immune-mediated disorders.[39,148,380] Resistance to BD is inherited as a dominant trait independent

of MHC genes in black-hooded and Lewis hybrids.[141,148] Serial passage in rat brain may enhance the virulence of BoDV strains for rats.[251] BoDV infection of susceptible adult rats results in a biphasic disorder that manifests approximately 10 to 20 days after intracerebral infection as an acute immunopathologic disease, presenting clinically as hyperactivity and exaggerated startle responses.[245,246] The onset of acute disease coincides with infiltration of mononuclear cells into the brain, particularly in areas of high viral burden such as the hippocampus, amygdala, and other limbic structures.[34] After the initial acute phase, the animals enter a chronic disease phase characterized by somnolence, apathy, paralysis, dystonia, dyskinesia, stereotyped and self-mutilation behaviors, and blindness.[245,246,365,366] Chronic disease is paralleled by widespread distribution of virus in the limbic system and prefrontal cortex, and 5% to 10% of animals become obese, developing up to 3 times the weight of normal rats.[216] BoDV variant strains have been described that cause a higher percentage of obesity. The obese phenotype is correlated with inflammation and viral antigen expression in the septum, hippocampus, amygdala, and ventromedian tuberal hypothalamus.[136]

Infection of adult rats is associated with behavioral changes, disturbances in monoamine neurotransmitter systems and limbic circuitry, marked central nervous system inflammation, loss of brain mass, and gliosis. In contrast, neonatally infected rats have hippocampal and cerebellar dysgenesis and display behavioral changes without inflammation. Rats inoculated as neonates with low passage virus during the first day of life become persistently infected, are smaller than uninfected littermates, and display only mild behavioral disturbances manifest as cognitive, emotional, or social deficits.[11,35,66,162,201,281,282,324]

BoDV has been experimentally transmitted to a variety of other animal species. Susceptibility to infection varies according to species and virus strain. Compared to the highly susceptible rabbits, guinea pigs, gerbils, and rats, other species, such as mice, cattle, chickens, monkeys, and tree shrews, appear to be less susceptible to disease.[5,50,100,175,216,229,243,307,315,322,374,382] Ferrets, pigeons, dogs, and hamsters develop no disease symptoms although they become persistently infected.[50,315]

BoDV Infection of the Adult Rat

Intracranial, intraocular, or intranasal inoculation routes have all been used to infect adult rats. The onset of disease correlates with distance from the inoculation site to the central nervous system,[34] indicating that BoDV spreads primarily through neural networks. This is supported by the finding that sciatic nerve transection after footpad infection prevents central nervous system infection.[34] Further, after olfactory, ophthalmic, or intraperitoneal inoculation, viral proteins or nucleic acids move centripetally via synaptic connections.[34] Analogous to rabies virus, spread of viral RNPs instead of mature virus within neural networks has been hypothesized for BoDV,[99] and the possibility of G-receptor–independent dissemination of BoDV has been described in vitro.[40,218] Although viral RNA can be found in peripheral blood mononuclear cells (PBMC) of infected animals, viremia is currently not considered to play a significant role in the pathogenesis and dissemination of BoDV.

BoDV infection of adult Lewis rats results in severe central nervous system immunopathology and pronounced behavioral disturbances.[245,246,309,381] Monocyte infiltration, glial activation, and Th₁-type cytokines in limbic structures coincide with the onset of hyperactivity and exaggerated startle responses 2 to 3 weeks after infection and persist until the animals enter the chronic phase approximately 12 weeks later. This is associated with a switch of the Th1 to a Th2 response.[120] Microglial activation precedes astroglial reaction but seems to depend on persistent infection of neurons and activation of astrocytes.[138,259] In many other viral central nervous system infections, the presence of an intact immune response results in viral clearance or death of the host. However, in BoDV infection, the virus persists at high titer in the presence of a robust cellular immune response during the acute phase and also during the chronic phase when Th₂-type cytokines increase while immune cell infiltrates decline in the presence of almost unchanged viral load in the central nervous system and continued glial activation.[120] While lymphocytes isolated from the brains of acutely infected rats had potent cytolytic activity *in vitro* and can recreate BD-specific pathology after adoptive transfer into healthy, immunosuppressed BoDV-infected rats, the lymphocytes isolated from brains of chronically infected rats do not lyse BoDV-infected target cells *in vitro* or to induce pathology after adoptive transfer.[363] Furthermore, levels of IgG antibodies produced intrathecally increase during the chronic disease phase, accompanied by high titer neutralizing antibodies in peripheral blood,[121,122] in addition to the nonneutralizing anti-N and anti-P serum antibodies generated during the acute phase.[27,88] Although the increasing titer of neutralizing antibodies does not result in viral clearance, it may nonetheless restrict the virus to the nervous system. Passive immunization of rats immunocompromised by cyclosporine treatment restricts viral replication to cells of the central, peripheral, and autonomic nervous system, whereas rats not passively immunized showed viral replication outside of the nervous system.[383]

The observation that infection of immunocompromised animals does not result in overt disease and combined with the fact that BoDV does not show cytopathic effects in cultured cells suggested a primarily immune-mediated pathology in immunocompetent adult rats.[145,245,246,386] This model is supported by the finding that adoptive transfer of spleen cells from diseased rats, or of BoDV-specific CD4⁺ T-cell lines, triggered classical disease in such animals.[245,276,301,308,309,363] Infiltrating cells in infected animals include CD4⁺ and CD8⁺ T cells, macrophages and B cells, with CD4⁺ cells accumulating primarily in perivascular cuffs and CD8⁺ cells distributing in the parenchyma.[17,64,275] A crucial role for CD8⁺ cells has been deduced from the effects of antibody treatment against CD4⁺ and CD8⁺ cells, which led in both cases to neuroprotection and abrogation of severe immunopathology.[17,276,385] However, the ultimate mechanisms of immune-mediated pathologic cell death remain undefined. Both CD4⁺cell lines possessing or lacking cytotoxic capacity have been established, and although current evidence is compatible with an involvement of classical cytotoxic T-cell action,[252] a role of indirect mechanisms elaborated through proinflammatory cytokines and their potentially cytotoxic effects, particularly in neuronal cell death, is also possible.[260] The immunopathology in adult-infected rats represents a delayed-type hypersensitivity response with contribution of both CD8+ and CD4+ T cells in the immunopathologic events.

Behavioral and movement disturbances in adult infected rats have been linked to dysfunction of the dopamine (DA)

neurotransmitter system.[365–368,370] Both pre- and postsynaptic sites appear to be damaged. DA reuptake sites are reduced in the caudate–putamen and nucleus accumbens.[368,370] DA receptor losses vary by receptor subtype and brain region. D2 receptor binding is markedly reduced in the caudate–putamen. Both D2 and D3 receptor binding are reduced in nucleus accumbens.[366–368] In contrast, postsynaptic DA receptors (D1, D2, D3) are intact in the prefrontal cortex.[367] Selective losses of D2 receptors and resultant D1 receptor hypersensitivity may be implicated in behavioral disturbances. Whereas treatment with D1 receptor antagonists such as SCH23390, or clozapine—an atypical antipsychotic with mixed D1, D2, D3, and D4 antagonist activity—reduces repetitive and self-injurious behaviors, D2-selective antagonists such as raclopride do not.[366] Neurochemical studies indicate a lesion in DA transmission consistent with partial DA deafferentation and compensatory metabolic hyperactivity in nigrostriatal and mesolimbic DA systems.

In addition to disturbances in the DA system, decreased mRNA levels for somatostatin, cholecystokinin, and glutamic acid decarboxylase have been recorded in adult infected rats during the acute phase of disease, while recovery to normal levels was observed during the chronic phase.[212] Decreases are also evident in choline acetyltransferase-positive fibers of the cholinergic system involved in learning and memory. Losses in cholinergic fibers become evident by 6 days postinfection (dpi), and almost complete absence of choline acetyltransferase-positive fibers is reported in the hippocampus and neocortex by 15 dpi.[95] Infected animals also respond abnormally to the opiate antagonist naloxone with hyperkinesis and seizures.[369] Normal rats show increased levels of the endogenous cannabinoid anandamide in hippocampus and amygdala after naloxone treatment and develop no seizures. In virus-infected rats, seizures develop after naloxone treatment, while anandamide levels remain comparable to baseline levels recorded in the same structures of mock-treated BoDV-infected or normal rats.[364] Blockade of anandamide transport in infected rats prevented naloxone-induced seizures. Furthermore, levels of mRNA encoding the opioid precursor preproenkephalin were elevated in striatum of infected rats 14, 21, and 45 dpi, and virus and met-enkephalin colocalized in a high percentage of cells.[86,371] Induction of enkephalin expression in infected cells may relate to increased levels of phosphorylated cyclic AMP response element binding (phosphoCREB) protein due to activation of the mitogen-activated protein kinase (MAPK) pathway.[193] Indeed, interaction of BoDV with MAPK signaling has been demonstrated in cell culture systems.[119,277] The marked central nervous system inflammation in adult infected rats makes it difficult to determine to what extent monoamine, cholinergic, and opiatergic dysfunction results from direct effects of the virus, indirect effects on resident cells of the central nervous system, or cellular immune responses to viral gene products.

BoDV Infection of the Neonatal Rat

The neonatal rat model is characterized by lifelong persistence of high virus load in the brain and mild behavioral disturbances that are compatible with cerebellar and hippocampal dysgenesis.[35,163,246] Infected animals exhibit learning deficits, increased motor activity, decreased anxiety responses, stereotypic behaviors, reduced initiation of and response to play interactions, and a preference for salt solutions.[11,66,163,283,324] Compared to normal littermates, rats neonatally infected with BoDV show an altered circadian rhythm and have a smaller size, although food ingestion and levels of glucose, growth hormone, and insulin-like growth factor 1 appear to remain at normal levels.[10,11,35] Neuropathologic, physiologic, and neurobehavioral features of the neonatal BoDV infection are therefore suitable for exploring the mechanisms by which viral and immune factors may damage developing neurocircuitry.

Despite significant astrocytosis and microgliosis, the overall brain architecture of neonatally infected rats appears maintained, although there are losses in granule cells of the dentate gyrus, Purkinje cell subsets of the cerebellum, and pyramidal neurons in the cortex.[75,163,324,355,420,425,426] Consistent with Purkinje cell loss in the cerebellum, testing of cerebellar function demonstrated deficits in motor coordination and postural stability.[163] Neuronal loss in the dentate gyrus correlates with the severity of the spatial learning and memory deficiencies also observed.[281,324]

BoDV infection in neonates results in more modest immune responses than those observed in adult infected rats. Serum antibody titers measured in an immunofluorescence assay are low in comparison to adult infected rats, but persist for more than 10 months.[35] A brief surge of T-cell infiltration is observed starting at 4 weeks and resolving by 6 weeks postinfection, paralleled by elevated expression of proinflammatory cytokine, chemokine, and chemokine receptor transcripts,[163,299,331,332,439] whereas the observed neuropathology parallels regions and time course of microglial proliferation and expression of MHC class I and class II, ICAM, CD4, and CD8 molecules.[420]

Abnormal regulation of apoptosis also contributes to the disturbance of brain architecture in neonatal BoDV infection. Excitotoxic stimulation, including activation of glutamatergic circuitry, may trigger neuronal apoptosis. There are complex alterations in mRNAs for apoptosis mediators in the hippocampus, amygdala, prefrontal cortex, nucleus accumbens, and cerebellum consistent with prolonged promotion of apoptosis throughout the brains of rats neonatally infected with BoDV.[163] Levels of mRNAs for FAS and ICE (caspase-1), two promoters of apoptosis, are increased. Levels of mRNA for bcl-x, a factor that inhibits apoptosis, are decreased. Terminal deoxynucleotidyl transferase dUTP-biotin nick end labeling (TUNEL) can be seen in cerebral cortex and dentate gyrus and in the granule cell layer of the cerebellum.[163,420] Degeneration of cells in the hippocampal formation is related to activation of caspase 3, PARP-1, and deregulation of zinc homeostasis.[425] Although apoptosis is described in the normally developing rat hippocampus as late as days 7 to 10 of postnatal life, it is normally not found at later time points.[400]

Brain dysfunction in neonatally infected animals may be linked to direct viral effects on morphogenesis of the hippocampus and cerebellum, two structures that continue to mature postnatally in rodents. BoDV-induced down-regulation of the neuronal gap junction protein connexin 36 occurs first throughout the hippocampal formation and at 8 weeks postinfection in the cerebellum. These findings are anticipated to correlate with impaired neuronal functioning in these structures.[195]

BoDV Infection of Tree Shrews
Nonacute infection in the prosimian tree shrew (*Tupaia glis*) establishes a persistent infection and transient mild encephalitis,

resulting in a disorder characterized primarily by hyperactivity and alterations in sociosexual behavior rather than motor dysfunction.[374] Housing of animals as mating pairs revealed pronounced disturbances in social and breeding behavior.[374] Females, not males, initiated mating and despite increased sexual activity, the infected animals failed to reproduce. The behavioral changes were attributed to dysfunction of the limbic system, although neuroanatomic analyses were not performed.

BoDV Infection of Nonhuman Primates
The only reported studies of experimentally infected primates employed adult immunocompetent rhesus macaques (*Macaca mulatta*). Following intracerebral infection, an acute neurologic syndrome ensued, during which animals were initially hyperactive and subsequently became apathetic and hypokinetic, similar to BoDV-infected adult rats. Pathologic changes were remarkable and severe meningoencephalitis and retinopathy were observed.[36,248,269,382,440]

BoDV Infection of Mice
Adult mice develop high virus titers in the brain after BoDV inoculation, but most strains do not develop encephalitis.[175] However, disease may be induced by infection of certain mouse strains during the neonatal period[116] or by adaptation of virus through multiple passages in mice.[322] Serial passage results in adaptive mutations in the viral polymerase that may contribute to pathogenicity.[2] The reason for the different course of experimental BoDV infection in adult vs. newborn mice, and in rats, remains unclear but may reflect the time point of antigen presentation in the periphery.[123]

The incidence and severity of BoDV-induced clinical manifestations varies considerably between different mouse strains. Similar to the adult rat model, the occurrence of clinical signs is associated with immune cell infiltration in the brain and glial activation, mainly in the cerebral cortex and hippocampus. An immunopathologic syndrome mediated by MHC class I–restricted CD8+ T cells in a CD4+ T-cell–dependent manner is most pronounced in mouse strains such as MRL with the MHC H-2k allele.[116,124] This MHC I haplotype is associated with severity of clinical disease, but the incidence of disease is most likely associated with other, to date unknown, genetic factors.[116] The BoDV N peptide T_{129}ELEISSI was the dominant epitope shown to sensitize cytotoxic T cells.[335] Transgenic expression of BoDV-N in neurons or astrocytes in B10.BR mice did not result in clinical disease and prevented induction of BoDV-N-specific CD8+ T cells.[298] Moreover, down-regulation of the functional avidity of virus-specific CD8+ T cells in experimentally infected mice seemed to be involved in controlling the inflammatory reaction and facilitating viral persistence.[79] Overexpression of cytokines such as IL-12 or TNF in mice less susceptible to BoDV-induced disease sensitize the mice to develop an immune-mediated disorder and clinical disease, for example, epileptic seizures in the case of TNF overexpression.[84,116,150,196] The IL-12 effect seems to be mediated via IFN-γ, which also exerts neuroprotective effects in the mouse model.[125,150]

A behavioral syndrome similar to that of neonatally infected rats has been described after expression of an individual BoDV gene product in transgenic mice. High glial expression of BoDV-P decreases synaptic density, serotonin receptors, and levels of brain-derived neurotropic factor (BDNF), resulting in behavioral disturbances.[172] Thus, at least one viral product interferes with neural function, but in natural disease, replication of the virus itself and other viral components are also likely to contribute.[286]

DIAGNOSIS OF BORNAVIRUS INFECTION

Differential Diagnoses

Neurologic signs of BD are characteristic of encephalitis due to a wide range of viral pathogens. Thus, laboratory tests are needed for diagnosis. The differential diagnosis includes other neurotropic virus infections such as equine herpesviruses,[427] rabies,[106] tick-borne encephalitis,[239] as well as bacterial diseases such as botulism[343,424] and bacterial meningitis,[83] and parasitic infections such as verminous myeloencephalitis[69] and equine protozoal myeloencephalitis (EPM).[221] In certain geographic regions, arthropod-borne flaviviruses (e.g., West Nile virus) and alphaviruses (e.g., western, eastern, Venezuelan equine encephalitis viruses) must also be considered. The differential diagnosis of human bornavirus infection also includes bacterial, fungal, autoimmune, and prion diseases.[81]

The differential diagnosis of PDD and ABV infection includes bacterial, parasitic, or mycotic infections of the GI tract, ingestion of foreign bodies, intoxications, or neoplasia. An additional challenge is that repeated laboratory testing may be required to detect ABV.[108,130,154,264]

Intra Vitam Diagnosis

BD can be confirmed by the demonstration of BoDV-specific antibodies in the serum and cerebrospinal fluid,[102,104] or BoDV-specific antigens, RNA, or virus in blood or cerebrospinal fluid specimens. As serologic test systems, Western blot (WB) analysis, enzyme-linked immunosorbent assay (ELISA) and an indirect immunofluorescence assay (IFA) have been established (Fig. 6.4).[22,104,140,142,144] IFA with BoDV-infected and control cells is considered to be the most reliable method for the detection of BoDV-specific antibodies with high sensitivity and specificity.[142] Titers of BoDV-specific antibodies vary widely from 1:2 to 1:1280 in serum and cerebrospinal fluid and do not correlate with the clinical course of the infection.[104,140] In very early stages of acute BD, or after treatment with corticosteroids, BoDV-specific antibodies may not be detectable. Clinically healthy horses can have BoDV-specific antibodies in the serum but not in the cerebrospinal fluid.[104,140] In acute BD, the quantity of cerebrospinal fluid protein content can be elevated, and a mononuclear pleocytosis is regularly present.[104]

The same test methods as established for BD in animals have been used to diagnose human bornavirus infection. A clinical presentation of encephalitis or encephalopathy combined with the detection of viral RNA in cerebrospinal fluid is sufficient even without demonstration of virus-specific antigen or RNA in brain tissues. Clinical signs of encephalitis or encephalopathy in the absence of other evidence and detection of bornavirus-reactive IgG in serum or cerebrospinal fluid with full virus (e.g., IFA) combined with a confirmatory assay for individual antigens (e.g., WB or ELISA) constitutes a probable diagnosis.[76]

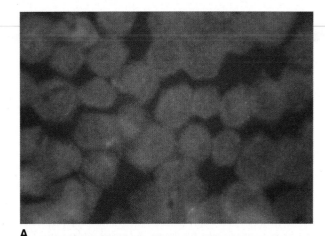

A

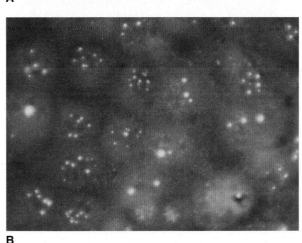

B

FIGURE 6.4 Indirect immunofluorescence assay (IFA) for the demonstration of BoDV-specific antibodies in horse sera employing Madin-Darby canine kidney (MDCK) cells. A: BoDV-positive serum incubated with uninfected MDCK cells. **B:** BoDV-positive serum incubated with BoDV-infected MDCK cells. (From Richt JA, Grabner A, Herzog S, et al. Borna disease in Equines. In: Sellon DC, Long M, eds. *Equine Infectious Diseases.* St Louis: Saunders Elsevier; 2007:201–216, with permission.)

Reliable *antemortem* diagnosis of PDD and ABV infection is challenging because clinical signs are not pathognomonic. Dilatation of the proventriculus and possibly other parts of the upper GI tract can be visualized by radiography/imaging techniques.[63] A definite diagnosis of PDD has to be substantiated by histopathologic examination of upper GI tract biopsies and the demonstration of mononuclear infiltrates of ganglia. In one study, crop biopsies revealed false-negative results in approximately 24% of cases.[107] ABV-specific serum antibodies can be demonstrated by WB assay,[54,209,404] ELISA,[54] and IFA (Fig. 6.5).[105,139] ABV infection has also been diagnosed by detection of ABV RNA in feces, swabs of crop and cloaca, blood, and feather calami using RT-PCR.[53,105,183,209,311] The diversity of known ABV may require several RT-PCR assays. Parrot bornavirus genotypes 4 and 2 have been detected most frequently in PDD.[91,105,183,234,272]

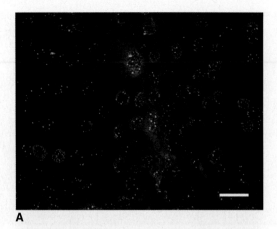

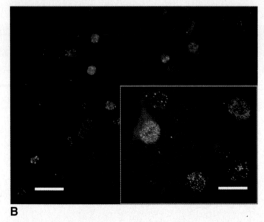

FIGURE 6.5 Indirect immunofluorescence assay for the demonstration of ABV-specific antibodies. A: IFA for demonstration of ABV-specific antibodies employing BDV-infected MDCK cells. Note the brilliant granular fluorescence in the nucleus. **Bar:** 50 μm. **B:** IFA for demonstration of ABV-specific antibodies employing ABV-infected CEC cells. Note the brilliant granular fluorescence in the nucleus. **Bar:** 100 μm; **Insert:** 50 μm. (From Herzog S, Enderlein D, Heffels-Redmann U, et al. Indirect immunofluorescence assay for intra vitam diagnosis of avian bornavirus infection in psittacine birds. *J Clin Microbiol* 2010;48:2282–2284, with permission.)

Postmortem Diagnosis

For the postmortem diagnosis of natural BD, typical histopathologic lesions (Fig. 6.6), viral proteins, and/or RNA in the central nervous system are usually demonstrated. Monoclonal or polyclonal antibodies recognizing N, P, M, X, or G proteins have been used in immunohistochemical (IHC) (Fig. 6.7) or WB analyses.[15,104] Histopathology, IHC, WB, and nested RT-PCR gave identical diagnostic results in a comparative study of over 150 horses with or without BD.[136] Furthermore, isolation of infectious BoDV and demonstration of BoDV RNA by *in situ* hybridization (ISH) (Fig. 6.7) can be used with adequately preserved tissue specimens. The same approaches have been used in the diagnosis of human infection.[44,194,211,250,336]

Postmortem investigations in PDD show typical histopathologic lesions predominantly in the GI tract and central nervous system (Fig. 6.8). ABV RNA can be demonstrated not only in the nervous system and GI tract but often in many other tissues.[105,130,153,182,183,209,296,311,404,432] ABV RNA may be visualized by ISH[419] and ABV antigens by IHC, applying either cross-reactive anti-BoDV antibodies against the N, P, or X protein, or ABV-specific antibodies against the N protein (Fig. 6.9).[139,258,272,296,311,418,432]

THERAPY AND CONTROL

Vaccination

Although there is only limited experience with vaccines in BD, better success has been reported with live attenuated than with killed virus vaccines.[50,255] A lapinized live vaccine[444] was used for many years in the eastern federal states of Germany. Because efficacy was questionable, and there were concerns regarding the possible postvaccination shedding of infectious virus as well as potential establishment of a persistent virus reservoir, the vaccine was abandoned in 1992.[236,351] High virus titer may be important for the successful implementation of live vaccines.[236,351] Cell culture–attenuated BoDV-protected rats against intracerebral challenge with a virulent inoculum only when administered at high titer (10^5–10^6 vs. 10^2–10^4).[255]

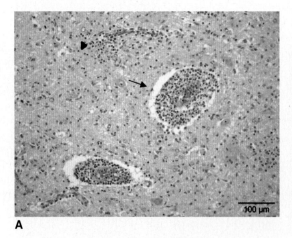

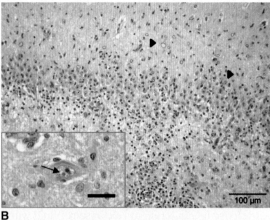

FIGURE 6.6 Characteristic histopathologic lesions in a horse suffering from BD. A: Severe perivascular (*arrow*) and moderate parenchymal (*arrowhead*) mononuclear immune cell infiltrates in the CNS. **B:** Moderate to severe parenchymal immune cell infiltrates with astroglial and microglial activation (*arrowhead*) in a more advanced stage of BD. **Insert:** Intranuclear Joest-Degen inclusion body (*arrow*). **Bar:** a, b: 100 μm, **Insert:** 25 μm. (From Herden C, Richt JA. Equine Borna disease. *Equine Vet Educ Manual* 2009;8:113–127, with permission.)

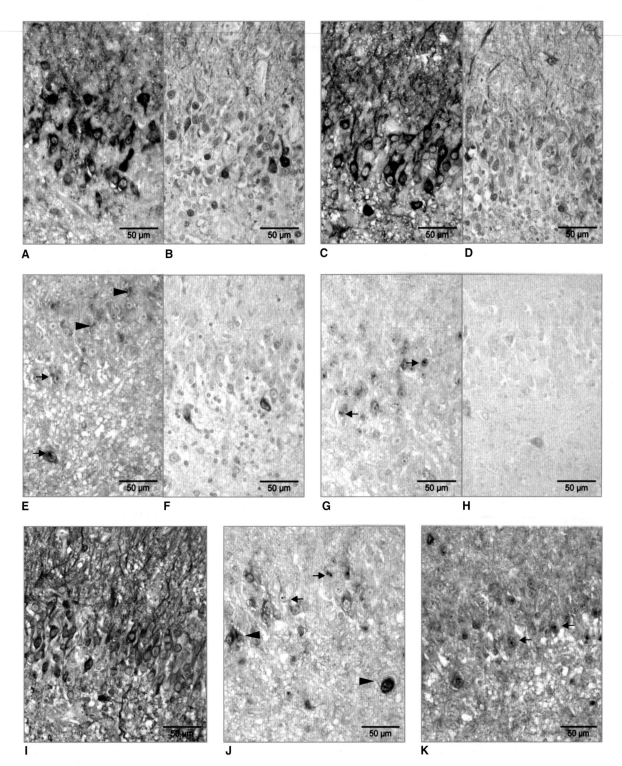

FIGURE 6.7 Demonstration of BoDV RNAs and proteins in a horse with typical BD by *in situ* hybridization and immunohistochemistry.
A, C, E, G, J, K: Demonstration of BoDV-specific RNAs by *in-situ* hybridization (ISH). **B, D, F, H, I:** Demonstration of BoDV-specific proteins by immunohistochemistry (IHC). **A:** Widespread BoDV N mRNA mainly in the cytoplasm and processes of neurons. **B:** Widespread BoDV N (monoclonal antibody Bo 18) in the cytoplasm and nuclei of infected neurons and in the neuropil. **C:** Widespread BoDV P mRNA mainly in the cytoplasm and processes of neurons. **D:** Widespread BoDV-P (polyclonal monospecific anti-BoDV P antibody) in the cytoplasm and a few nuclei of neurons and in the neuropil. **E:** Demonstration of BoDV M mRNA in the cytoplasm (*arrowhead*) and few nuclei as dot-like signal (*arrow*) in some neurons. **F:** Detection of the BoDV M (polyclonal anti-BoDV M antibody) mainly in the cytoplasm of some neurons. **G:** Demonstration of BoDV G mRNA mainly in the nuclei as dot-like signal (*arrow*) in some neurons. **H:** Detection of the BoDV G (monospecific polyclonal anti-BoDV G antibody) only in the cytoplasm of a few neurons. **I:** Detection of BoDV X (polyclonal anti-BoDV X antibody) mainly in the cytoplasm of neurons and the neuropil. **J:** Demonstration of BoDV L mRNA in the cytoplasm (*arrowhead*) and nuclei as dot-like signal (*arrow*) in some neurons. **K:** Demonstration of genomic BoDV RNA mainly in the nuclei as dot-like signal (*arrow*) in some neurons. N, nucleoprotein; P, phosphoprotein; X, X protein; M, matrix protein; G, glycoprotein; L, polymerase; **Bar:** 50 μm. (From Herden C, Richt JA. Equine Borna disease. *Equine Vet Educ Manual* 2009;8:113–127, with permission.)

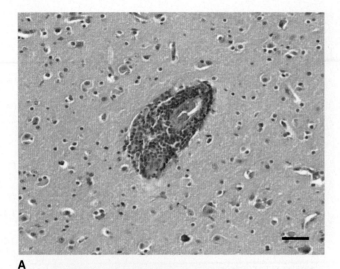

A

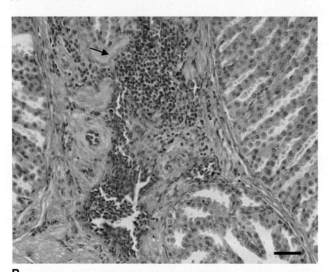

B

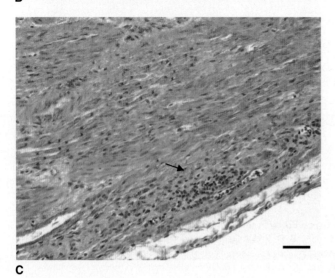

C

FIGURE 6.8 Typical histopathologic lesions in PDD. A: Perivascular lymphohistiocytic infiltrate in the brain. **B:** Severe lymphohistiocytic infiltrate in the proventriculus (*arrow*). **C:** Lymphohistiocytic infiltrate in and around ganglia of the gizzard (*arrow*). **Bar:** 50 μm.

Similarly, a high dose of another extensively passaged virus resulted in strong humoral and cellular immunity. A lower dose inoculum did not provide this protection.[87] Neither of these studies investigated virus shedding by the vaccinated animals or the biology of progeny virus.

There have been several efforts to develop recombinant BoDV vaccines. A vaccinia virus recombinant expressing BoDV N primed rats not only for enhanced viral clearance after challenge but also for aggravated disease due to increased immunopathology.[208] Expression of BoDV N by a parapoxvirus vector system was reported to protect rats from challenge.[134] No data are available on vaccines based on BoDV G; however, the observation that a monoclonal anti-G antibody was protective in rats suggests that such an approach could be successful.[88]

A number of different vector vaccines against avian orthobornavirus infection have been designed and tested in various prime boost strategies.[254,297,326] Recombinant Newcastle disease virus (NDV) and modified vaccinia virus (MVA) vectors expressing N and P of PaBV-4 or CnBv-2 in either cockatiels and canaries led to decreased viral shedding and viral tissue loads when applied in a homologous challenge but protection against PDD and sterile immunity were not achieved.[254]

Using a heterologous challenge regime in cockatiels after vaccination with both vectors, an enhanced protection against a lower dose of heterologous PaBV-2 was observed.[326] Evaluation of each vaccine individually showed that the MVA vaccine was able to protect cockatiels from PDD after heterologous PaBV-2 challenge.[297] Immunization of persistently PaBV-4–infected birds showed that neither the MVA nor the NDV vaccine led to exacerbated immunopathology or disease severity and did not lower viral load.[297]

Therapeutics

Amantadine sulfate, a drug with antiviral activity against influenza A,[126] has been proposed as antiviral treatment for BoDV infection.[23] However, the efficacy of the drug for treatment of persistently BoDV-infected cell cultures and animals is controversial.[46,117,384] In a small clinical study of horses with acute BD, 2 mg/kg orally had no effect in 8 out of 9 animals.[103] This lack of efficacy was corroborated by disease progression in a confirmed human patient despite high-dose therapy with amantadine-hemisulfate (200 mg/500 mL qd for 12 days).[44]

Ribavirin inhibits transcription and replication of both He/80 and strain V BoDV in a variety of cell lines.[170,235] In addition to its antiviral effects through depletion of cellular GTP pools, interference with mRNA capping, and direct interaction with viral polymerases, ribavirin can promote a Th₁-type immune response.[164,388] This led to concerns that enhancement of cellular immunity might aggravate immunopathology of BD.[120,208,363] In one study, the efficacy of ribavirin administered directly to the brain by intraventricular injection was assessed in the rat model. Although ribavirin had no effect on viral load, treated animals had less inflammation and milder disease presumably due to antimitotic effects on microglia.[372] In another animal model, the Mongolian gerbil, in which BoDV can cause direct neuronal damage independent of immunopathology,[413] ribavirin at a higher dosage than tolerated in the rat model reduced virus load in the brain.[206]

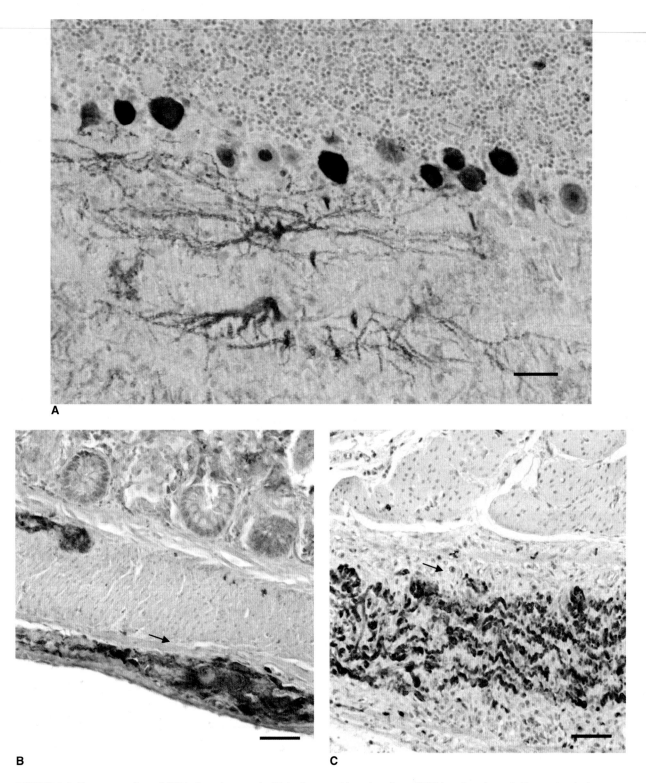

A

B

C

FIGURE 6.9 Demonstration of ABV phosphoprotein (P) by immunohistochemistry (IHC) in psittacines. A: Expression in the nucleus, cytoplasm, and processes of numerous Purkinje cells and a few granule cells in the cerebellum. **B:** Expression in ganglia (*arrow*) of the small intestine. **C:** Expression in nerve fibers (*arrow*) of the gizzard. **Bar:** 50 μm.

1-β-D-arabinofuranosylcytosine (Ara-C) inhibits BoDV replication in cultured cells and inhibits viral replication, improving clinical outcome in infected rats.[7,51] Ara-C is a DNA polymerase inhibitor and has no effect on polymerases of influenza or measles viruses but has antiviral activity against rabies virus.[31] In BoDV, Ara-C appears to act as a competitive inhibitor of cytidine.[406] A related cytosine nucleoside, 2′-fluoro-2′-deoxycytidine, shows similar antiviral activity *in vitro* and may be preferable due to its reduced cytotoxicity.[8]

Another potent RdRp inhibitor with broad anti-RNA virus activity is favipiravir (T-705; 6-fluoro-3-hydroxy-2-pyrazinecarboxamide; [Avigan]) acting as a purine analogue.[89] The oral drug is approved in Japan for treatment of infections with emerging influenza strains and drug resistant mutants, and received clearance for investigational new drug application against COVID-19 from the US Food and Drug Administration (FDA). Against bornavirus infection, favipiravir showed improved efficacy compared to ribavirin since no recurrence of virus replication was detected after removal of the drug, whereas virus replication resumes after cessation of ribavirin treatment.[398] Favipiravir was active against both BoDV and an isolate of avian orthobornavirus (PaBV-4),[398] as had also been shown for ribavirin,[242,300] suggesting that these drugs are likely active against a broader range of orthobornaviruses.

In naturally ABV-infected birds with end-stage PDD, cyclosporine A treatment has been used successfully along with a COX-2 inhibitor to ameliorate clinical signs and prolong life.[156] In a recent study, no effect of nonsteroidal anti-inflammatory drugs (NSAIDs) was found in cockatiels infected experimentally with PaBV-2.[80] Thus, the value of NSAIDs remains controversial[155] (reviewed in Refs.[19,314]).

PERSPECTIVES AND PUBLIC HEALTH CONSIDERATIONS

In the past 30 years since the recognition of BoDV as a negative-strand RNA virus, substantial progress has been achieved regarding the molecular characterization of the agent, its natural distribution, mechanisms of viral persistence, and the underlying immunopathogenesis of BD. Nonetheless, we still have only an incomplete understanding of the ecology and epidemiology, mechanisms for natural transmission, and the underpinnings of its capacity for persistence and neurotropism. The pathogenesis and clinical manifestations of infection reflect not only viral factors but also the genetic predisposition of the host. Although the genomic fossil record indicates infection of primates, including human ancestors for over 40 million years, there is no current evidence of widespread human infection and linkages to neuropsychiatric disease have been rigorously refuted. The family has grown to include 11 species in three genera, comprising viruses with host ranges that expand beyond mammals to birds, reptiles, and possibly fish.

REFERENCES

1. Ackermann A, Guelzow T, Staeheli P, et al. Visualizing viral dissemination in the mouse nervous system, using a green fluorescent protein-expressing Borna disease virus vector. *J Virol* 2010;84(10):5438–5442.
2. Ackermann A, Staeheli P, Schneider U. Adaptation of Borna disease virus to new host species attributed to altered regulation of viral polymerase activity. *J Virol* 2007;81(15):7933–7940.
3. Allendorf V, Rubbenstroth D, Schlottau K, et al. Assessing the occurrence of the novel zoonotic variegated squirrel bornavirus 1 in captive squirrels in Germany -A prevalence study. *Zoonoses Public Health* 2021;68(2):110–120.
4. Anzil AP, Blinzinger K. Electron microscopic studies of rabbit central and peripheral nervous system in experimental Borna disease. *Acta Neuropathol* 1972;22(4):305–318.
5. Anzil AP, Blinzinger K, Mayr A. Persistent Borna virus infection in adult hamsters. *Arch Gesamte Virusforsch* 1973;40(1):52–57.
6. Bajramovic JJ, Munter S, Syan S, et al. Borna disease virus glycoprotein is required for viral dissemination in neurons. *J Virol* 2003;77(22):12222–12231.
7. Bajramovic JJ, Syan S, Brahic M, et al. 1-beta-D-arabinofuranosylcytosine inhibits borna disease virus replication and spread. *J Virol* 2002;76(12):6268–6276.
8. Bajramovic JJ, Volmer R, Syan S, et al. 2'-fluoro-2'-deoxycytidine inhibits Borna disease virus replication and spread. *Antimicrob Agents Chemother* 2004;48(4):1422–1425.
9. Bause-Niedrig I, Jackson M, Schein E, et al. Borna disease virus-specific antigens. II. The soluble antigen is a protein complex. *Vet Immunol Immunopathol* 1992;31(3–4):361–369.
10. Bautista JR, Rubin SA, Moran TH, et al. Developmental injury to the cerebellum following perinatal Borna disease virus infection. *Brain Res Dev Brain Res* 1995;90(1–2):45–53.
11. Bautista JR, Schwartz GJ, De La Torre JC, et al. Early and persistent abnormalities in rats with neonatally acquired Borna disease virus infection. *Brain Res Bull* 1994;34(1):31–40.
12. Belyi VA, Levine AJ, Skalka AM. Unexpected inheritance: multiple integrations of ancient bornavirus and ebolavirus/marburgvirus sequences in vertebrate genomes. *PLoS Pathog* 2010;6:e1001030.
13. Berg M, Ehrenborg C, Blomberg J, et al. Two domains of the Borna disease virus p40 protein are required for interaction with the p23 protein. *J Gen Virol* 1998;79(Pt 12):2957–2963.
14. Berhane Y, Smith DA, Newman S, et al. Peripheral neuritis in psittacine birds with proventricular dilatation disease. *Avian Pathol* 2001;30(5):563–570.
15. Bilzer T, Grabner A, Stitz L. [Immunopathology of Borna disease in the horse: clinical, virological and neuropathologic findings]. *Tierarztl Prax* 1996;24(6):567–576.
16. Bilzer T, Planz O, Lipkin WI, et al. Presence of CD4+ and CD8+ T cells and expression of MHC class I and MHC class II antigen in horses with Borna disease virus-induced encephalitis. *Brain Pathol* 1995;5(3):223–230.
17. Bilzer T, Stitz L. Immune-mediated brain atrophy. CD8+ T cells contribute to tissue destruction during borna disease. *J Immunol* 1994;153(2):818–823.
18. Binz T, Lebelt J, Niemann H, et al. Sequence analyses of the p24 gene of Borna disease virus in naturally infected horse, donkey and sheep. *Virus Res* 1994;34(3):281–289.
19. Boatright-Horowitz SL. Avian bornaviral ganglioneuritis: current debates and unanswered questions. *Vet Med Int* 2020;2020:6563723.
20. Bode L. Human bornavirus infection—towards a valid diagnostic system. *APMIS Suppl* 2008;(124):21–39.
21. Bode L, Durrwald R, Ludwig H. Borna virus infections in cattle associated with fatal neurological disease. *Vet Rec* 1994;135(12):283–284.
22. Bode L, Reckwald P, Severus WE, et al. Borna disease virus-specific circulating immune complexes, antigenemia, and free antibodies—the key marker triplet determining infection and prevailing in severe mood disorders. *Mol Psychiatry* 2001;6(4):481–491.
23. Bode L, Dietrich DE, Stoyloff R, et al. Amantadine and human Borna disease virus in vitro and in vivo in an infected patient with bipolar depression. *Lancet* 1997;349(9046):178–179.
24. Bourg M, Herzog S, Encarnação JA, et al. Bicolored white-toothed shrews as reservoir for borna disease virus, Bavaria, Germany. *Emerg Infect Dis* 2013;19(12):2064–2066.
25. Bourque L, Laniesse D, Beaufrere H, et al. Identification of avian bornavirus in a Himalayan monal (Lophophorus impejanus) with neurological disease. *Avian Pathol* 2015;44(4):323–327.
26. Briese T, de la Torre JC, Lewis A, et al. Borna disease virus, a negative-strand RNA virus, transcribes in the nucleus of infected cells. *Proc Natl Acad Sci U S A* 1992;89(23):11486–11489.
27. Briese T, Hatalski CG, Kliche S, et al. Enzyme-linked immunosorbent assay for detecting antibodies to Borna disease virus-specific proteins. *J Clin Microbiol* 1995;33(2):348–351.
28. Briese T, Lipkin WI, de la Torre JC. Molecular biology of Borna disease virus. *Curr Top Microbiol Immunol* 1995;190:1–16.
29. Briese T, Schneemann A, Lewis AJ, et al. Genomic organization of Borna disease virus. *Proc Natl Acad Sci U S A* 1994;91(10):4362–4366.
30. Cadar D, Allendorf V, Schulze V, et al. Introduction and spread of variegated squirrel bornavirus 1 (VSBV-1) between exotic squirrels and spill-over infections to humans in Germany. *Emerg Microbes Infect* 2021;10(1):602–611.
31. Campbell JB, Maes RF, Wiktor TJ, et al. The inhibition of rabies virus by arabinosyl cytosine. Studies on the mechanism and specificity of action. *Virology* 1968;34:701–708.
32. Caplazi P, Melzer K, Goetzmann R, et al. [Borna disease in Switzerland and in the principality of Liechtenstein]. *Schweiz Arch Tierheilkd* 1999;141(11):521–527.
33. Caplazi P, Waldvogel A, Stitz L, et al. Borna disease in naturally infected cattle. *J Comp Pathol* 1994;111(1):65–72.
34. Carbone KM, Duchala CS, Griffin JW, et al. Pathogenesis of Borna disease in rats: evidence that intra-axonal spread is the major route for virus dissemination and the determinant for disease incubation. *J Virol* 1987;61(11):3431–3440.
35. Carbone KM, Park SW, Rubin SA, et al. Borna disease: association with a maturation defect in the cellular immune response. *J Virol* 1991;65(11):6154–6164.
36. Cervos-Navarro J, Roggendorf W, Ludwig H, et al. Die BORNA-Krankheit beim Affen unter besonderer Berücksichtigung der encephalitischen Reaktion. *Verh Dtsch Ges Pathol* 1981;65:208–212.
37. Charlier CM, Wu YJ, Allart S, et al. Analysis of borna disease virus trafficking in live infected cells by using a virus encoding a tetracysteine-tagged p protein. *J Virol* 2013;87(22):12339–12348.
38. Chase G, Mayer D, Hildebrand A, et al. Borna disease virus matrix protein is an integral component of the viral ribonucleoprotein complex that does not interfere with polymerase activity. *J Virol* 2007;81(2):743–749.
39. Cizza G, Sternberg EM. The role of the hypothalamic-pituitary-adrenal axis in susceptibility to autoimmune/inflammatory disease. *Immunomethods* 1994;5:73–78.
40. Clemente R, de la Torre JC. Cell-to-cell spread of Borna disease virus proceeds in the absence of the virus primary receptor and furin-mediated processing of the virus surface glycoprotein. *J Virol* 2007;81(11):5968–5977.
41. Clemente R, de la Torre JC. Cell entry of Borna disease virus follows a clathrin-mediated endocytosis pathway that requires Rab5 and microtubules. *J Virol* 2009;83(20):10406–10416.
42. Collins PL, Olmsted RA, Spriggs MK, et al. Gene overlap and site-specific attenuation of transcription of the viral polymerase L gene of human respiratory syncytial virus. *Proc Natl Acad Sci U S A* 1987;84:5134–5138.
43. Compans RW, Melsen LR, de la Torre JC. Virus-like particles in MDCK cells persistently infected with Borna disease virus. *Virus Res* 1994;33(3):261–268.

44. Coras R, Korn K, Kuerten S, et al. Severe bornavirus-encephalitis presenting as Guillain-Barre-syndrome. *Acta Neuropathol* 2019;137(6):1017–1019.
45. Cubitt B, de la Torre JC. Borna disease virus (BDV), a nonsegmented RNA virus, replicates in the nuclei of infected cells where infectious BDV ribonucleoproteins are present. *J Virol* 1994;68(3):1371–1381.
46. Cubitt B, de la Torre JC. Amantadine does not have antiviral activity against Borna disease virus. *Arch Virol* 1997;142(10):2035–2042.
47. Cubitt B, Ly C, de la Torre JC. Identification and characterization of a new intron in Borna disease virus. *J Gen Virol* 2001;82(Pt 3):641–646.
48. Cubitt B, Oldstone C, de la Torre JC. Sequence and genome organization of Borna disease virus. *J Virol* 1994;68(3):1382–1396.
49. Cubitt B, Oldstone C, Valcarcel J, et al. RNA splicing contributes to the generation of mature mRNAs of Borna disease virus, a non-segmented negative strand RNA virus. *Virus Res* 1994;34(1):69–79.
50. Danner K. *Borna-Virus und Borna-Infektionen*. Stuttgart, Germany: Enke Copythek; 1982.
51. Danner K, Mayr A. In vitro studies on Borna virus. II. Properties of the virus. *Arch Virol* 1979;61(4):261–271.
52. Daoust PY, Julian RJ, Yason CV, et al. Proventricular impaction associated with nonsuppurative encephalomyelitis and ganglioneuritis in two Canada geese. *J Wildl Dis* 1991;27(3):513–517.
53. De Kloet AH, Kerski A, de Kloet SR. Diagnosis of Avian bornavirus infection in psittaciformes by serum antibody detection and reverse transcription polymerase chain reaction assay using feather calami. *J Vet Diagn Invest* 2011;23(3):421–429.
54. De Kloet SR, Dorrestein GM. Presence of avian bornavirus RNA and anti-avian bornavirus antibodies in apparently healthy macaws. *Avian Dis* 2009;53(4):568–573.
55. De la Torre JC. Molecular biology of borna disease virus: prototype of a new group of animal viruses. *J Virol* 1994;68(12):7669–7675.
56. De la Torre JC. Reverse-genetic approaches to the study of Borna disease virus. *Nat Rev Microbiol* 2006;4(10):777–783.
57. De La Torre JC, Gonzalez-Dunia D, Cubitt B, et al. Detection of borna disease virus antigen and RNA in human autopsy brain samples from neuropsychiatric patients. *Virology* 1996;223(2):272–282.
58. Degiorgis MP, Berg AL, Hard Af Segerstad C, et al. Borna disease in a free-ranging lynx (Lynx lynx). *J Clin Microbiol* 2000;38(8):3087–3091.
59. Delnatte P, Berkvens C, Kummrow M, et al. New genotype of avian bornavirus in wild geese and trumpeter swans in Canada. *Vet Rec* 2011;169(4):108.
60. Delnatte P, Nagy É, Ojkic D, et al. Avian bornavirus in free-ranging waterfowl: prevalence of antibodies and cloacal shedding of viral RNA. *J Wildl Dis* 2014;50(3):512–523.
61. Delnatte P, Nagy E, Ojkic D, et al. Investigation into the possibility of vertical transmission of avian bornavirus in free-ranging Canada geese (Branta canadensis). *Avian Pathol* 2014;43(4):301–304.
62. Delnatte P, Ojkic D, DeLay J, et al. Pathology and diagnosis of avian bornavirus infection in wild Canada geese (Branta canadensis), trumpeter swans (Cygnus buccinator) and mute swans (Cygnus olor) in Canada: a retrospective study. *Avian Pathol* 2013;42(2):114–128.
63. Dennison SE, Paul-Murphy JR, Adams WM. Radiographic determination of proventricular diameter in psittacine birds. *J Am Vet Med Assoc* 2008;232:709–714.
64. Deschl U, Stitz L, Herzog S, et al. Determination of immune cells and expression of major histocompatibility complex class II antigen in encephalitic lesions of experimental Borna disease. *Acta Neuropathol* 1990;81(1):41–50.
65. Dietzel J, Kuhrt H, Stahl T, et al. Morphometric analysis of the retina from horses infected with the Borna disease virus. *Vet Pathol* 2007;44(1):57–63.
66. Dittrich W, Bode L, Ludwig H, et al. Learning deficiencies in Borna disease virus-infected but clinically healthy rats. *Biol Psychiatry* 1989;26(8):818–828.
67. Donatti RV, Resende M, Ferreira FC, et al. Fatal proventricular dilatation disease in captive native psittacines in Brazil. *Avian Dis* 2014;58(1):187–193.
68. Duchala CS, Carbone KM, Narayan O. Preliminary studies on the biology of Borna disease virus. *J Gen Virol* 1989;70(Pt 12):3507–3511.
69. Duckett WM. *Verminous Myelitis*. Vol 3. Philadelphia, PA: Saunders; 1992.
70. Durrwald R, Kolodziejek J, Herzog S, et al. Meta-analysis of putative human bornavirus sequences fails to provide evidence implicating Borna disease virus in mental illness. *Rev Med Virol* 2007;17(3):181–203.
71. Durrwald R, Kolodziejek J, Muluneh A, et al. Epidemiological pattern of classical Borna disease and regional genetic clustering of Borna disease viruses point towards the existence of to-date unknown endemic reservoir host populations. *Microbes Infect* 2006;8(3): 917–929.
72. Dürrwald R, Kolodziejek J, Weissenböck H, et al. The bicolored white-toothed shrew Crocidura leucodon (HERMANN 1780) is an indigenous host of mammalian Borna disease virus. *PLoS One* 2014;9(4):e93659.
73. Durrwald R, Ludwig H. Borna disease virus (BDV), a (zoonotic?) worldwide pathogen. A review of the history of the disease and the virus infection with comprehensive bibliography. *Zentralbl Veterinarmed B* 1997;44(3):147–184.
74. Eickmann M, Kiermayer S, Kraus I, et al. Maturation of Borna disease virus glycoprotein. *FEBS Lett* 2005;579(21):4751–4756.
75. Eisenman LM, Brother R, Tran MH, et al. Neonatal Borna disease virus infection in the rat causes a loss of Purkinje cells in the cerebellum. *J Neurovirol* 1999;5:181–189.
76. Eisermann P, Rubbenstroth D, Cadar D, et al. Active case finding of current bornavirus infections in human encephalitis cases of unknown etiology, Germany, 2018–2020. *Emerg Infect Dis* 2021;27(5):1371–1379.
77. Elford WJ, Galloway IA. Filtration of the virus of Borna disease through graded collodion membranes. *Br J Exp Pathol* 1933;14(No. 3):196–205.
78. Encinas-Nagel N, Enderlein D, Piepenbring A, et al. Avian bornavirus in free-ranging psittacine birds, Brazil. *Emerg Infect Dis* 2014;20(12):2103–2106.
79. Engelhardt KR, Richter K, Baur K, et al. The functional avidity of virus-specific CD8+ T cells is down-modulated in Borna disease virus-induced immunopathology of the central nervous system. *Eur J Immunol* 2005;35(2):487–497.
80. Escandon P, Heatley JJ, Tizard I, et al. Treatment with nonsteroidal anti-inflammatory drugs fails to ameliorate pathology in cockatiels experimentally infected with parrot bornavirus-2. *Vet Med (Auckl)* 2019;10:185–195.
81. Finck T, Liesche-Starnecker F, Probst M, et al. Bornavirus encephalitis shows a characteristic magnetic resonance phenotype in humans. *Ann Neurol* 2020;88(4):723–735.
82. Fluck A, Enderlein D, Piepenbring A, et al. Correlation of avian bornavirus-specific antibodies and viral ribonucleic acid shedding with neurological signs and feather-damaging behaviour in psittacine birds. *Vet Rec* 2019;184(15):476.
83. Foreman JH. *Bacterial Meningitis and Cerebral Abscesses*. Vol 3. Philadelphia, PA: Saunders; 1992.
84. Freude S, Hausmann J, Hofer M, et al. Borna disease virus accelerates inflammation and disease associated with transgenic expression of interleukin-12 in the central nervous system. *J Virol* 2002;76(23):12223–12232.
85. Friedl G, Hofer M, Auber B, et al. Borna disease virus multiplication in mouse organotypic slice cultures is site-specifically inhibited by gamma interferon but not by interleukin-12. *J Virol* 2004;78(3):1212–1218.
86. Fu ZF, Weihe E, Zheng YM, et al. Differential effects of rabies and borna disease viruses on immediate-early- and late-response gene expression in brain tissues. *J Virol* 1993;67(11):6674–6681.
87. Furrer E, Bilzer T, Stitz L, et al. High-dose Borna disease virus infection induces a nucleoprotein-specific cytotoxic T-lymphocyte response and prevention of immunopathology. *J Virol* 2001;75(23):11700–11708.
88. Furrer E, Bilzer T, Stitz L, et al. Neutralizing antibodies in persistent borna disease virus infection: prophylactic effect of gp94-specific monoclonal antibodies in preventing encephalitis. *J Virol* 2001;75(2):943–951.
89. Furuta Y, Komeno T, Nakamura T. Favipiravir (T-705), a broad spectrum inhibitor of viral RNA polymerase. *Proc Jpn Acad Ser B Phys Biol Sci* 2017;93(7):449–463.
90. Galabru J, Saron MF, Berg M, et al. Borna disease virus antibodies in French horses. *Vet Rec* 2000;147(25):721–722.
91. Gancz AY, Kistler AL, Greninger AL, et al. Experimental induction of proventricular dilatation disease in cockatiels (Nymphicus hollandicus) inoculated with brain homogenates containing avian bornavirus 4. *Virol J* 2009;6:100.
92. Garry CE, Garry RF. Proteomics computational analyses suggest that the bornavirus glycoprotein is a class III viral fusion protein (gamma penetrene). *Virol J* 2009;6:145.
93. Gartner AM, Enderlein D, Link J, et al. Age dependent development and clinical characteristics of parrot bornavirus-4 (PaBV-4) infection in cockatiels (Nymphicus hollandicus). In: *Proceedings of the 4th International Conference on Avian, Herpetological and Exotic Mammal Medicine 2019*. 2019.
94. Geib T, Sauder C, Venturelli S, et al. Selective virus resistance conferred by expression of Borna disease virus nucleocapsid components. *J Virol* 2003;77(7):4283–4290.
95. Gies U, Bilzer T, Stitz L, et al. Disturbance of the cortical cholinergic innervation in Borna disease prior to encephalitis. *Brain Pathol* 1998;8(1):39–48.
96. Gonzalez-Dunia D, Cubitt B, de la Torre JC. Mechanism of Borna disease virus entry into cells. *J Virol* 1998;72(1):783–788.
97. Gonzalez-Dunia D, Cubitt B, Grasser FA, et al. Characterization of Borna disease virus p56 protein, a surface glycoprotein involved in virus entry. *J Virol* 1997;71(4):3208–3218.
98. Gonzalez-Dunia D, Watanabe M, Syan S, et al. Synaptic pathology in Borna disease virus persistent infection. *J Virol* 2000;74(8):3441–3448.
99. Gosztonyi G, Dietzschold B, Kao M, et al. Rabies and borna disease. A comparative pathogenetic study of two neurovirulent agents. *Lab Invest* 1993;68(3):285–295.
100. Gosztonyi G, Leiskau T, Ludwig H. The significance of the Borna disease virus infection for the non-mammal, the chicken. *Zentralbl Bakt Mikrobiol Hyg [A]* 1983;255:170.
101. Gosztonyi G, Ludwig H. Borna disease of horses. An immunohistological and virological study of naturally infected animals. *Acta Neuropathol* 1984;64(3):213–221.
102. Grabner A, Fischer A. [Symptomatology and diagnosis of Borna encephalitis of horses. A case analysis of the last 13 years]. *Tierarztl Prax* 1991;19(1):68–73.
103. Grabner A, Herzog S, Kailer S, et al. BDV infections and BD in horses in Germany: clinical and epidemiological aspects. *In Abstracts of the International Bornavirus Meeting, Freiburg, 1998*. 1998.
104. Grabner A, Herzog S, Lange-Herbst H, et al. Die intra-vitam-Diagnose der Bornaschen Krankheit (BD) bei Equiden. *Pferdeheilkunde* 2002;18:579–586.
105. Gray P, Hoppes S, Suchodolski P, et al. Use of avian bornavirus isolates to induce proventricular dilatation disease in conures. *Emerg Infect Dis* 2010;16(3):473–479.
106. Green SL. Rabies. *Vet Clin North Am Equine Pract* 1997;13:1–11.
107. Gregory CR, Latimer K, Campagnoli R, et al. Histologic evaluation of the crop for diagnosis of proventricular dilatation syndrome in psittacine birds. *J Vet Diagn Invest* 1996;8: 76–80.
108. Gregory CR, Latimer KS, Niagro FD, et al. Review of proventricular dilatation syndrome. *J Assoc Avian Vet* 1994;8:68–75.
109. Guo J, Baroch J, Randall A, et al. Complete genome sequence of an avian bornavirus isolated from a healthy Canadian Goose (Branta canadensis). *Genome Announc* 2013;1(5):e00839-13.
110. Guo J, Covaleda L, Heatley JJ, et al. Widespread avian bornavirus infection in mute swans in the Northeast United States. *Vet Med (Auckl)* 2012;3:49–52.
111. Guo J, Payne S, Zhang S, et al. Avian bornaviruses: diagnosis, isolation, and genotyping. *Curr Protoc Microbiol* 2014;34:15I.11.11-33.
112. Haas B, Becht H, Rott R. Purification and properties of an intranuclear virus-specific antigen from tissue infected with Borna disease virus. *J Gen Virol* 1986;67(Pt 2):235–241.
113. Habjan M, Andersson I, Klingstrom J, et al. Processing of genome 5' termini as a strategy of negative-strand RNA viruses to avoid RIG-I-dependent interferon induction. *PLoS One* 2008;3(4):e2032.
114. Hagiwara K, Asakawa M, Liao L, et al. Seroprevalence of Borna disease virus in domestic animals in Xinjiang, China. *Vet Microbiol* 2001;80(4):383–389.
115. Hagiwara K, Momiyama N, Taniyama H, et al. Demonstration of Borna disease virus (BDV) in specific regions of the brain from horses positive for serum antibodies to BDV

but negative for BDV RNA in the blood and internal organs. *Med Microbiol Immunol* 1997;186(1):19–24.
116. Hallensleben W, Schwemmle M, Hausmann J, et al. Borna disease virus-induced neurological disorder in mice: infection of neonates results in immunopathology. *J Virol* 1998;72(5):4379–4386.
117. Hallensleben W, Zocher M, Staeheli P. Borna disease virus is not sensitive to amantadine. *Arch Virol* 1997;142(10):2043–2048.
118. Hans A, Bajramovic JJ, Syan S, et al. Persistent, noncytolytic infection of neurons by Borna disease virus interferes with ERK 1/2 signaling and abrogates BDNF-induced synaptogenesis. *FASEB J* 2004;18(7):863–865.
119. Hans A, Syan S, Crosio C, et al. Borna disease virus persistent infection activates mitogen-activated protein kinase and blocks neuronal differentiation of PC12 cells. *J Biol Chem* 2001;276(10):7258–7265.
120. Hatalski CG, Hickey WF, Lipkin WI. Evolution of the immune response in the central nervous system following infection with Borna disease virus. *J Neuroimmunol* 1998;90(2):137–142.
121. Hatalski CG, Hickey WF, Lipkin WI. Humoral immunity in the central nervous system of Lewis rats infected with Borna disease virus. *J Neuroimmunol* 1998;90(2):128–136.
122. Hatalski CG, Kliche S, Stitz L, et al. Neutralizing antibodies in Borna disease virus-infected rats. *J Virol* 1995;69(2):741–747.
123. Hausmann J, Baur K, Engelhardt KR, et al. Vaccine-induced protection against Borna disease in wild-type and perforin-deficient mice. *J Gen Virol* 2005;86(Pt 2):399–403.
124. Hausmann J, Hallensleben W, de la Torre JC, et al. T cell ignorance in mice to Borna disease virus can be overcome by peripheral expression of the viral nucleoprotein. *Proc Natl Acad Sci U S A* 1999;96(17):9769–9774.
125. Hausmann J, Pagenstecher A, Baur K, et al. CD8 T cells require gamma interferon to clear borna disease virus from the brain and prevent immune system-mediated neuronal damage. *J Virol* 2005;79(21):13509–13518.
126. Hay A. The action of amantadines against influenza A viruses: inhibition of the M2 ion channel protein. *Semin Virol* 1992;3:21.
127. Hayashi Y, Horie M, Daito T, et al. Heat shock cognate protein 70 controls Borna disease virus replication via interaction with the viral non-structural protein X. *Microbes Infect* 2009;11(3):394–402.
128. Heckmann J, Enderlein D, Gartner AM, et al. Wounds as the Portal of Entrance for Parrot Bornavirus 4 (PaBV-4) and Retrograde Axonal Transport in Experimentally Infected Cockatiels (Nymphicus hollandicus). *Avian Dis* 2020;64(3):247–253.
129. Heckmann J, Enderlein D, Piepenbring AK, et al. Investigation of Different Infection Routes of Parrot Bornavirus in Cockatiels. *Avian Dis* 2017;61(1):90–95.
130. Heffels-Redmann U, Enderlein D, Herzog S, et al. Occurrence of avian bornavirus infection in captive psittacines in various European countries and its association with proventricular dilatation disease. *Avian Pathol* 2011;40(4):419–426.
131. Heffels-Redmann U, Enderlein D, Herzog S, et al. Follow-up investigations on different courses of natural avian bornavirus infections in psittacines. *Avian Dis* 2012;56(1): 153–159.
132. Heinig A. Die pH-Resistenz des Virus der Borna'schen Krankheit der Pferde. *Arch Exp Veterinarmed* 1955;9:517–521.
133. Heinig A. Die Bornasche Krankheit der Pferde und Schafe. In: Röhrer H, ed. *Handbuch der Virusinfektionen bei Tieren*. Vol Band 4. Jena, Germany: VEB G. Fischer; 1969:83–148.
134. Henkel M, Planz O, Fischer T, et al. Prevention of virus persistence and protection against immunopathology after Borna disease virus infection of the brain by a novel Orf virus recombinant. *J Virol* 2005;79(1):314–325.
135. Herden C, Briese T, Lipkin WI, et al. Bornaviridae. In: Knipe DM, Howley PM, eds. *Fields Virology*. 6th ed. Philadelphia, PA: Wolters Kluver Health/Lippincott Williams & Wilkins; 2013:1124.
136. Herden C, Herzog S, Richt JA, et al. Distribution of Borna disease virus in the brain of rats infected with an obesity-inducing virus strain. *Brain Pathol* 2000;10(1):39–48.
137. Herden C, Herzog S, Wehner T, et al. Comparison of different methods of diagnosing Borna disease in horses post mortem. In: Wernery U, Wade J, Mumford JA, Kaaden OR, eds. *Equine Infectious Diseases VIII*. Newmarket: R&W Publications; 1999:286–290.
138. Herden C, Schluesener HJ, Richt JA. Expression of allograft inflammatory factor-1 and haeme oxygenase-1 in brains of rats infected with the neurotropic Borna disease virus. *Neuropathol Appl Neurobiol* 2005;31(5):512–521.
139. Herzog S, Enderlein D, Heffels-Redmann U, et al. Indirect immunofluorescence assay for intra vitam diagnosis of avian bornavirus infection in psittacine birds. *J Clin Microbiol* 2010;48(6):2282–2284.
140. Herzog S, Frese K, Richt JA, et al. Ein Beitrag zur Epizootiologie der Bornaschen Krankheit der Pferde. *Wien Tierarztl Monschr* 1994;81:374–379.
141. Herzog S, Frese K, Rott R. Studies on the genetic control of resistance of black hooded rats to Borna disease. *J Gen Virol* 1991;72 (Pt 3):535–540.
142. Herzog S, Herden C, Frese K, et al. Borna disease of horses: contradictory results between antemortem and postmortem investigations. *Pferdeheilkunde* 2008;24:766–774.
143. Herzog S, Pfeuffer I, Haberzettl K, et al. Molecular characterization of Borna disease virus from naturally infected animals and possible links to human disorders. *Arch Virol Suppl* 1997;13:183–190.
144. Herzog S, Rott R. Replication of Borna disease virus in cell cultures. *Med Microbiol Immunol* 1980;168(3):153–158.
145. Herzog S, Wonigeit K, Frese K, et al. Effect of Borna disease virus infection on athymic rats. *J Gen Virol* 1985;66 (Pt 3):503–508.
146. Hilbe M, Herrsche R, Kolodziejek J, et al. Shrews as reservoir hosts of borna disease virus. *Emerg Infect Dis* 2006;12(4):675–677.
147. Hirai Y, Hirano Y, Matsuda A, et al. Borna disease virus assembles porous cage-like viral factories in the nucleus. *J Biol Chem* 2016;291(50):25789–25798.
148. Hirano N, Kao M, Ludwig H. Persistent, tolerant or subacute infection in Borna disease virus-infected rats. *J Gen Virol* 1983;64 (Pt 7):1521–1530.
149. Hock M, Kraus I, Schoehn G, et al. RNA induced polymerization of the Borna disease virus nucleoprotein. *Virology* 2010;397(1):64–72.
150. Hofer M, Hausmann J, Staeheli P, et al. Cerebral expression of interleukin-12 induces neurological disease via differential pathways and recruits antigen-specific T cells in virus-infected mice. *Am J Pathol* 2004;165(3):949–958.
151. Hoffmann B, Tappe D, Hoper D, et al. A Variegated Squirrel Bornavirus Associated with Fatal Human Encephalitis. *N Engl J Med* 2015;373(2):154–162.
152. Honda T, Horie M, Daito T, et al. Molecular chaperone BiP interacts with Borna disease virus glycoprotein at the cell surface. *J Virol* 2009;83(23):12622–12625.
153. Honkavuori KS, Shivaprasad HL, Williams BL, et al. Novel borna virus in psittacine birds with proventricular dilatation disease. *Emerg Infect Dis* 2008;14(12):1883–1886.
154. Hoppes S, Gray PL, Payne S, et al. The isolation, pathogenesis, diagnosis, transmission, and control of avian bornavirus and proventricular dilatation disease. *Vet Clin North Am Exot Anim Pract* 2010;13(3):495–508.
155. Hoppes S, Heatley JJ, Guo J, et al. Meloxicam treatment in cockatiels (Nymphicus hollandicus) infected with avian bornavirus Nymphicus hol- landicus) infected with avian bornaviruses. *J Exot Pet Med* 2013;22(3):275–279.
156. Hoppes SM, Shivaprasad HL. Update on avian bornavirus and proventricular dilatation disease: diagnostics, pathology, prevalence, and control. *Vet Clin North Am Exot Anim Pract* 2020;23(2):337–351.
157. Hoppes SM, Tizard I, Shivaprasad HL. Avian bornavirus and proventricular dilatation disease: diagnostics, pathology, prevalence, and control. *Vet Clin North Am Exot Anim Pract* 2013;16(2):339–355.
158. Horie M, Honda T, Suzuki Y, et al. Endogenous non-retroviral RNA virus elements in mammalian genomes. *Nature* 2010;463(7277):84–87.
159. Horie M, Kobayashi Y, Suzuki Y, et al. Comprehensive analysis of endogenous bornavirus-like elements in eukaryote genomes. *Philos Trans R Soc Lond B Biol Sci* 2013;368(1626):20120499.
160. Horie M, Ueda K, Ueda A, et al. Detection of Avian bornavirus 5 RNA in Eclectus roratus with feather picking disorder. *Microbiol Immunol* 2012;56(5):346–349.
161. Hornig M, Briese T, Licinio J, et al. Absence of evidence for bornavirus infection in schizophrenia, bipolar disorder and major depressive disorder. *Mol Psychiatry* 2012;17(5): 486–493.
162. Hornig M, Briese T, Lipkin WI. Bornavirus tropism and targeted pathogenesis: virus-host interactions in a neurodevelopmental model. *Adv Virus Res* 2001;56:557–582.
163. Hornig M, Weissenböck H, Horscroft N, et al. An infection-based model of neurodevelopmental damage. *Proc Natl Acad Sci U S A* 1999;96:12102–12107.
164. Hultgren C, Milich DR, Weiland O, et al. The antiviral compound ribavirin modulates the T helper (Th) 1/Th2 subset balance in hepatitis B and C virus-specific immune responses. *J Gen Virol* 1998;79:2381–2391.
165. Hyndman TH, Shilton CM, Stenglein MD, et al. Divergent bornaviruses from Australian carpet pythons with neurological disease date the origin of extant Bornaviridae prior to the end-Cretaceous extinction. *PLoS Pathog* 2018;14(2):e1006881.
166. Ihlenburg H. [Experimental tests of the susceptibility of cats to the virus of Borna disease]. *Arch Exp Veterinarmed* 1966;20(4):859–864.
167. Jacobsen B, Algermissen D, Schaudien D, et al. Borna disease in an adult alpaca stallion (Lama pacos). *J Comp Pathol* 2010;143(2–3):203–208.
168. Joest E, Degen K. Über eigentümliche Kerneinschlüsse der Ganglienzellen bei der enzootischen Gehirn-Rückenmarksentzündung der Pferde. *Z Infkrankh Haustiere* 1909;6: 348–356.
169. Joest E, Degen K. Untersuchungen über die pathologische Histologie, Pathogenese und postmortale Diagnose der seuchenhaften Gehirn-Rückenmarksentzündung (Bornasche Krankheit) des Pferdes. *Z Infkrankh Haustiere* 1911;9(1/2):1–98.
170. Jordan I, Briese T, Averett DR, et al. Inhibition of Borna disease virus replication by ribavirin. *J Virol* 1999;73(9):7903–7906.
171. Kamhieh S, Hodgson J, Bode L, et al. No evidence of endemic Borna disease virus infection in Australian horses in contrast with endemic infection in other continents. *Arch Virol* 2006;151(4):709–719.
172. Kamitani W, Ono E, Yoshino S, et al. Glial expression of Borna disease virus phosphoprotein induces behavioral and neurological abnormalities in transgenic mice. *Proc Natl Acad Sci U S A* 2003;100(15):8969–8974.
173. Kamitani W, Shoya Y, Kobayashi T, et al. Borna disease virus phosphoprotein binds a neurite outgrowth factor, amphoterin/HMG-1. *J Virol* 2001;75(18):8742–8751.
174. Kao M, Hamir AN, Rupprecht CE, et al. Detection of antibodies against Borna disease virus in sera and cerebrospinal fluid of horses in the USA. *Vet Rec* 1993;132(10):241–244.
175. Kao M, Ludwig H, Gosztonyi G. Adaptation of Borna disease virus to the mouse. *J Gen Virol* 1984;65(Pt 10):1845–1849.
176. Katz JB, Alstad D, Jenny AL, et al. Clinical, serologic, and histopathologic characterization of experimental Borna disease in ponies. *J Vet Diagn Invest* 1998;10(4):338–343.
177. Kawasaki J, Kojima S, Mukai Y, et al. 100-My history of bornavirus infections hidden in vertebrate genomes. *Proc Natl Acad Sci U S A* 2021;118(20):e2026235118.
178. Kerski A, de Kloet AH, de Kloet SR. Vertical transmission of avian bornavirus in Psittaciformes: avian bornavirus RNA and anti-avian bornavirus antibodies in eggs, embryos, and hatchlings obtained from infected sun conures (Aratinga solstitialis). *Avian Dis* 2012;56(3):471–478.
179. Kessler S, Heenemann K, Krause T, et al. Monitoring of free-ranging and captive Psittacula populations in Western Europe for avian bornaviruses, circoviruses and polyomaviruses. *Avian Pathol* 2020;49(2):119–130.
180. Kiermayer S, Kraus I, Richt JA, et al. Identification of the amino terminal subunit of the glycoprotein of Borna disease virus. *FEBS Lett* 2002;531(2):255–258.
181. Kistler AL, Gancz A, Clubb S, et al. Recovery of divergent avian bornaviruses from cases of proventricular dilatation disease: identification of a candidate etiologic agent. *Virol J* 2008;5:88.
182. Kistler AL, Smith JM, Greninger AL, et al. Analysis of naturally occurring avian bornavirus infection and transmission during an outbreak of proventricular dilatation disease among captive psittacine birds. *J Virol* 2010;84(4):2176–2179.
183. Kliche S, Briese T, Henschen AH, et al. Characterization of a Borna disease virus glycoprotein, gp18. *J Virol* 1994;68(11):6918–6923.

184. Kobayashi Y, Horie M, Nakano A, et al. Exaptation of bornavirus-like nucleoprotein elements in Afrotherians. *PLoS Pathog* 2016;12(8):e1005785.

185. Kobayashi T, Kamitani W, Zhang G, et al. Borna disease virus nucleoprotein requires both nuclear localization and export activities for viral nucleocytoplasmic shuttling. *J Virol* 2001;75(7):3404–3412.

186. Kobayashi T, Shoya Y, Koda T, et al. Nuclear targeting activity associated with the amino terminal region of the Borna disease virus nucleoprotein. *Virology* 1998;243(1):188–197.

187. Kobayashi T, Watanabe M, Kamitani W, et al. Translation initiation of a bicistronic mRNA of Borna disease virus: a 16-kDa phosphoprotein is initiated at an internal start codon. *Virology* 2000;277(2):296–305.

188. Kobayashi T, Zhang G, Lee BJ, et al. Modulation of Borna disease virus phosphoprotein nuclear localization by the viral protein X encoded in the overlapping open reading frame. *J Virol* 2003;77(14):8099–8107.

189. Kohno T, Goto T, Takasaki T, et al. Fine structure and morphogenesis of Borna disease virus. *J Virol* 1999;73(1):760–766.

190. Kojima S, Sato R, Yanai M, et al. Splicing-dependent subcellular targeting of borna disease virus nucleoprotein isoforms. *J Virol* 2019;93(5):e01621-18.

191. Kolakofsky D, Roux L, Garcin D, et al. Paramyxovirus mRNA editing, the 'rule of six' and error catastrophe: a hypothesis. *J Gen Virol* 2005;86:1869–1877.

192. Kolodziejek J, Durrwald R, Herzog S, et al. Genetic clustering of Borna disease virus natural animal isolates, laboratory and vaccine strains strongly reflects their regional geographical origin. *J Gen Virol* 2005;86(Pt 2):385–398.

193. Konradi C, Kobierski LA, Nguyen TV, et al. The cAMP-response-element-binding protein interacts, but Fos protein does not interact, with the proenkephalin enhancer in rat striatum. *Proc Natl Acad Sci U S A* 1993;90.7005–7009.

194. Korn K, Coras R, Bobinger T, et al. Fatal encephalitis associated with borna disease virus 1. *N Engl J Med* 2018;379(14):1375–1377.

195. Koster-Patzlaff C, Hosseini SM, Reuss B. Loss of connexin36 in rat hippocampus and cerebellar cortex in persistent Borna disease virus infection. *J Chem Neuroanat* 2009;37(2):118–127.

196. Kramer K, Schaudien D, Eisel U, et al. Epileptic seizures in TNF-transgenic mice infected with the neurotropic Borna disease virus are associated with altered prodynorphin mRNA levels in the brain. *Acta Neuropathol* 2008;116:349.

197. Kraus I, Bogner E, Lilie H, et al. Oligomerization and assembly of the matrix protein of Borna disease virus. *FEBS Lett* 2005;579(12):2686–2692.

198. Kraus I, Eickmann M, Kiermayer S, et al. Open reading frame III of borna disease virus encodes a nonglycosylated matrix protein. *J Virol* 2001;75(24):12098–12104.

199. Kretzschmar E, Peluso R, Schnell M, et al. Normal replication of vesicular stomatitis virus without C proteins. *Virology* 1996;216:309–316.

200. Krey HF, Ludwig H, Boschek CB. Multifocal retinopathy in Borna disease virus infected rabbits. *Am J Ophthalmol* 1979;87(2):157–164.

201. Lancaster K, Dietz DM, Moran TH, et al. Abnormal social behaviors in young and adult rats neonatally infected with Borna disease virus. *Behav Brain Res* 2007;176(1):141–148.

202. Last RD, Weissenbock H, Nedorost N, et al. Avian bornavirus genotype 4 recovered from naturally infected psittacine birds with proventricular dilatation disease in South Africa. *J S Afr Vet Assoc* 2012;83(1):938.

203. Leal de Araujo J, Hameed SS, Tizard I, et al. Cardiac lesions of natural and experimental infection by parrot bornaviruses. *J Comp Pathol* 2020;174:104–112.

204. Leal de Araujo J, Rech RR, Heatley JJ, et al. From nerves to brain to gastrointestinal tract: a time-based study of parrot bornavirus 2 (PaBV-2) pathogenesis in cockatiels (Nymphicus hollandicus). *PLoS One* 2017;12(11):e0187797.

205. Leal de Araujo J, Rodrigues-Hoffmann A, Giaretta PR, et al. Distribution of viral antigen and inflammatory lesions in the central nervous system of cockatiels (Nymphicus hollandicus) experimentally infected with parrot bornavirus 2. *Vet Pathol* 2019;56(1):106–117.

206. Lee BJ, Matsunaga H, Ikuta K, et al. Ribavirin inhibits Borna disease virus proliferation and fatal neurological diseases in neonatally infected gerbils. *Antiviral Res* 2008;80(3):380–384.

207. Lennartz F, Bayer K, Czerwonka N, et al. Surface glycoprotein of Borna disease virus mediates virus spread from cell to cell. *Cell Microbiol* 2016;18(3):340–354.

208. Lewis AJ, Whitton JL, Hatalski CG, et al. Effect of immune priming on Borna disease. *J Virol* 1999;73(3):2541–2546.

209. Lierz M, Hafez HM, Honkavuori KS, et al. Anatomical distribution of avian bornavirus in parrots, its occurrence in clinically healthy birds and ABV-antibody detection. *Avian Pathol* 2009;38(6):491–496.

210. Lierz M, Piepenbring A, Herden C, et al. Vertical transmission of avian bornavirus in psittacines. *Emerg Infect Dis* 2011;17(12):2390–2391.

211. Liesche F, Ruf V, Zoubaa S, et al. The neuropathology of fatal encephalomyelitis in human Borna virus infection. *Acta Neuropathol* 2019;138(4):653–665.

212. Lipkin WI, Carbone KM, Wilson MC, et al. Neurotransmitter abnormalities in Borna disease. *Brain Res* 1988;475(2):366–370.

213. Lipkin WI, Hornig M, Briese T. Borna disease virus and neuropsychiatric disease--a reappraisal. *Trends Microbiol* 2001;9(7):295–298.

214. Lipkin WI, Travis GH, Carbone KM, et al. Isolation and characterization of Borna disease agent cDNA clones. *Proc Natl Acad Sci U S A* 1990;87(11):4184–4188.

215. Ludwig H, Becht H, Groh L. Borna disease (BD), a slow virus infection. *Med Microbiol Immunol* 1973;158:275–289.

216. Ludwig H, Bode L, Gosztonyi G. Borna disease: a persistent virus infection of the central nervous system. *Prog Med Virol* 1988;35:107–151.

217. Ludwig H, Bode L. Borna disease virus: new aspects on infection, disease, diagnosis and epidemiology. *Rev Sci Tech* 2000;19(1):259–288.

218. Ludwig H, Furuya K, Bode L, et al. Biology and neurobiology of Borna disease viruses (BDV), defined by antibodies, neutralizability and their pathogenic potential. *Arch Virol Suppl* 1993;7:111–133.

219. Ludwig H, Kraft W, Kao M, et al. [Borna virus infection (Borna disease) in naturally and experimentally infected animals: its significance for research and practice]. *Tierarztl Prax* 1985;13(4):421–453.

220. Lundgren AL, Lindberg R, Ludwig H, et al. Immunoreactivity of the central nervous system in cats with a Borna disease-like meningoencephalomyelitis (staggering disease). *Acta Neuropathol* 1995;90(2):184–193.

221. MacKay RJ. Equine protozoal myeloencephalitis. *Vet Clin North Am Equine Pract* 1997;13:79–96.

222. Malbon AJ, Durrwald R, Kolodziejek J, et al. New World camelids are sentinels for the presence of Borna disease virus. *Transbound Emerg Dis* 2022;69(2):451–464.

223. Malik TH, Kishi M, Lai PK. Characterization of the P protein-binding domain on the 10-kilodalton protein of Borna disease virus. *J Virol* 2000;74(7):3413–3417.

224. Mannl A, Gerlach H, Leipold R. Neuropathic gastric dilatation in psittaciformes. *Avian Dis* 1987;31(1):214–221.

225. Martin A, Hoefs N, Tadewaldt J, et al. Genomic RNAs of Borna disease virus are elongated on internal template motifs after realignment of the 3' termini. *Proc Natl Acad Sci U S A* 2011;108(17):7206–7211.

226. Martin A, Staeheli P, Schneider U. RNA polymerase II-controlled expression of antigenomic RNA enhances the rescue efficacies of two different members of the Mononegavirales independently of the site of viral genome replication. *J Virol* 2006;80(12):5708–5715.

227. Marton S, Bányai K, Gál J, et al. Coding-complete sequencing classifies parrot bornavirus 5 into a novel virus species. *Arch Virol* 2015;160(11):2763–2768.

228. Matsumoto Y, Hayashi Y, Omori H, et al. Bornavirus closely associates and segregates with host chromosomes to ensure persistent intranuclear infection. *Cell Host Microbe* 2012;11(5):492–503.

229. Matthias D. Der Nachweis von latent infizierten Pferden, Schafen und Rindern und deren Bedeutung als Virusreservoir bei der Bornaschen Krankheit. *Arch Exp Veterinarmed* 1954;8:506–511.

230. Mayer D, Baginsky S, Schwemmle M. Isolation of viral ribonucleoprotein complexes from infected cells by tandem affinity purification. *Proteomics* 2005;5(17):4483–4487.

231. Mayr A, Danner K. Production of Borna virus in tissue culture. *Proc Soc Exp Biol Med* 1972;140(2):511–515.

232. Metzler A, Ehrensperger F, Wyler R. [Natural borna virus infection in rabbits]. *Zentralbl Veterinarmed B* 1978;25(2):161–164.

233. Metzler A, Minder HP, Wegmann C, et al. [Borna disease, a veterinary problem of regional significance]. *Schweiz Arch Tierheilkd* 1979;121(4):207–213.

234. Mirhosseini N, Gray PL, Hoppes S, et al. Proventricular dilatation disease in cockatiels (Nymphicus hollandicus) after infection with a genotype 2 avian bornavirus. *J Avian Med Surg* 2011;25(3):199–204.

235. Mizutani T, Inagaki H, Araki K, et al. Inhibition of Borna disease virus replication by ribavirin in persistently infected cells. *Arch Virol* 1998;143(10):2039–2044.

236. Möhlmann H. 10 Jahre Forschungsinstitut für Impfstoffe Dessau. *Arch Exp Veterinarmed* 1965;19:253–260.

237. Monaco E, Hoppes S, Guo J, et al. The detection of avian bornavirus within psittacine eggs. *J Avian Med Surg* 2012;26(3):144–148.

238. Morales JA, Herzog S, Kompter C, et al. Axonal transport of Borna disease virus along olfactory pathways in spontaneously and experimentally infected rats. *Med Microbiol Immunol* 1988;177(2):51–68.

239. Müller K, König M, Thiel HJ. [Tick-borne encephalitis (TBE) with special emphasis on infection in horses]. *Dtsch Tierarztl Wochenschr* 2006;113(4):147–151.

240. Muller-Doblies D, Baumann S, Grob P, et al. The humoral and cellular immune response of sheep against Borna disease virus in endemic and non-endemic areas. *Schweiz Arch Tierheilkd* 2004;146(4):159–172.

241. Murray M, Guo J, Tizard I, et al. Aquatic bird bornavirus-associated disease in free-living Canada Geese (Branta canadensis) in the Northeastern USA. *J Wildl Dis* 2017;53(3):607–611.

242. Musser JM, Heatley JJ, Koinis AV, et al. Ribavirin inhibits parrot bornavirus 4 replication in cell culture. *PLoS One* 2015;10(7):e0134080.

243. Nakamura Y, Nakaya T, Hagiwara K, et al. High susceptibility of Mongolian gerbil (Meriones unguiculatus) to Borna disease virus. *Vaccine* 1999;17(5):480–489.

244. Nakamura Y, Takahashi H, Shoya Y, et al. Isolation of Borna disease virus from human brain tissue. *J Virol* 2000;74(10):4601–4611.

245. Narayan O, Herzog S, Frese K, et al. Behavioral disease in rats caused by immunopathological responses to persistent borna virus in the brain. *Science* 1983;220(4604):1401–1403.

246. Narayan O, Herzog S, Frese K, et al. Pathogenesis of Borna disease in rats: immune-mediated viral ophthalmoencephalopathy causing blindness and behavioral abnormalities. *J Infect Dis* 1983;148(2):305–315.

247. Neumann P, Lieber D, Meyer S, et al. Crystal structure of the Borna disease virus matrix protein (BDV-M) reveals ssRNA binding properties. *Proc Natl Acad Sci U S A* 2009;106(10):3710–3715.

248. Nicolau S, Galloway IA. *Borna Disease and Enzootic Encephalo-myelitis of Sheep and Cattle*. London: H M Stat Office; 1928:1–115.

249. Nielsen AMW, Ojkic D, Dutton CJ, et al. Aquatic bird bornavirus 1 infection in a captive Emu (Dromaius novaehollandiae): presumed natural transmission from free-ranging wild waterfowl. *Avian Pathol* 2018;47(1):58–62.

250. Niller HH, Angstwurm K, Rubbenstroth D, et al. Zoonotic spillover infections with Borna disease virus 1 leading to fatal human encephalitis, 1999–2019: an epidemiological investigation. *Lancet Infect Dis* 2020;20(4):467–477.

251. Nitzschke E. Untersuchungen über die experimentelle Bornavirus-Infektion bei der Ratte. *Zentralbl Veterinarmed B* 1963;10:470–527.

252. Noske K, Bilzer T, Planz O, et al. Virus-specific CD4+ T cells eliminate borna disease virus from the brain via induction of cytotoxic CD8+ T cells. *J Virol* 1998;72(5):4387–4395.

253. Nowotny N, Kolodziejek J, Jehle CO, et al. Isolation and characterization of a new subtype of Borna disease virus. *J Virol* 2000;74(12):5655–5658.

254. Olbert M, Römer-Oberdörfer A, Herden C, et al. Viral vector vaccines expressing nucleoprotein and phosphoprotein genes of avian bornaviruses ameliorate homologous challenge infections in cockatiels and common canaries. *Sci Rep* 2016;6:36840.

255. Oldach D, Zink MC, Pyper JM, et al. Induction of protection against Borna disease by inoculation with high-dose-attenuated Borna disease virus. *Virology* 1995;206(1):426–434.

256. Otta J. Die Komplementbindungsreaktion bei der Meningo-Encephlomyelitis enzootica equorum (Bornasche Krankheit). *Arch Exp Veterinarmed* 1957;11:235–252.

257. Otta J, Jentzsch KD. Spontane Infektion mit dem Virus der Bornaschen Krankheit bei Kaninchen. *Monatsh Vet Med* 1960;15:127.

258. Ouyang N, Storts R, Tian Y, et al. Histopathology and the detection of avian bornavirus in the nervous system of birds diagnosed with proventricular dilatation disease. *Avian Pathol* 2009;38(5):393–401.

259. Ovanesov MV, Moldovan K, Smith K, et al. Persistent Borna Disease Virus (BDV) infection activates microglia prior to a detectable loss of granule cells in the hippocampus. *J Neuroinflammation* 2008;5:16.

260. Ovanesov MV, Sauder C, Rubin SA, et al. Activation of microglia by borna disease virus infection: in vitro study. *J Virol* 2006;80(24):12141–12148.

261. Pauli G, Ludwig H. Increase of virus yields and releases of Borna disease virus from persistently infected cells. *Virus Res* 1985;2(1):29–33.

262. Payne S, Covaleda L, Jianhua G, et al. Detection and characterization of a distinct bornavirus lineage from healthy Canada geese (Branta canadensis). *J Virol* 2011;85(22):12053–12056.

263. Payne SL, Delnatte P, Guo J, et al. Birds and bornaviruses. *Anim Health Res Rev* 2012;13(2):145–156.

264. Payne S, Shivaprasad HL, Mirhosseini N, et al. Unusual and severe lesions of proventricular dilatation disease in cockatiels (Nymphicus hollandicus) acting as healthy carriers of avian bornavirus (ABV) and subsequently infected with a virulent strain of ABV. *Avian Pathol* 2011;40(1):15–22.

265. Perez M, de la Torre JC. Identification of the Borna disease virus (BDV) proteins required for the formation of BDV-like particles. *J Gen Virol* 2005;86(Pt 7):1891–1895.

266. Perez M, Sanchez A, Cubitt B, et al. A reverse genetics system for Borna disease virus. *J Gen Virol* 2003;84(Pt 11):3099–3104.

267. Perez M, Watanabe M, Whitt MA, et al. N-terminal domain of Borna disease virus G (p56) protein is sufficient for virus receptor recognition and cell entry. *J Virol* 2001;75(15):7078–7085.

268. Perpinan D, Fernandez-Bellon H, Lopez C, et al. Lymphoplasmacytic myenteric, subepicardial, and pulmonary ganglioneuritis in four nonpsittacine birds. *J Avian Med Surg* 2007;21(3):210–214.

269. Pette H, Környey S. Über die Pathogenese und die Histologie der Bornaschen Krankheit im Tierexperiment. *Dtsch Z Nervenheilkd* 1935;136:20–63.

270. Philadelpho NA, Davies YM, Guimaraes MB, et al. Detection of avian bornavirus in wild and captive passeriformes in Brazil. *Avian Dis* 2019;63(2):294–297.

271. Philadelpho NA, Rubbenstroth D, Guimaraes MB, et al. Survey of bornaviruses in pet psittacines in Brazil reveals a novel parrot bornavirus. *Vet Microbiol* 2014;174(3–4):584–590.

272. Piepenbring AK, Enderlein D, Herzog S, et al. Pathogenesis of avian bornavirus in experimentally infected cockatiels. *Emerg Infect Dis* 2012;18(2):234–241.

273. Piepenbring AK, Enderlein D, Herzog S, et al. Parrot bornavirus (PaBV)-2 isolate causes different disease patterns in cockatiels than PaBV-4. *Avian Pathol* 2016;45(2):156–168.

274. Pinto MC, Rondahl V, Berg M, et al. Detection and phylogenetic analysis of parrot bornavirus 4 identified from a Swedish Blue-winged macaw (Primolius maracana) with unusual nonsuppurative myositis. *Infect Ecol Epidemiol* 2019;9(1):1547097.

275. Planz O, Bilzer T, Sobbe M, et al. Lysis of major histocompatibility complex class I-bearing cells in Borna disease virus-induced degenerative encephalopathy. *J Exp Med* 1993;178(1):163–174.

276. Planz O, Bilzer T, Stitz L. Immunopathogenic role of T-cell subsets in Borna disease virus-induced progressive encephalitis. *J Virol* 1995;69(2):896–903.

277. Planz O, Pleschka S, Ludwig S. MEK-specific inhibitor U0126 blocks spread of Borna disease virus in cultured cells. *J Virol* 2001;75(10):4871–4877.

278. Planz O, Pleschka S, Oesterle K, et al. Borna disease virus nucleoprotein interacts with the CDC2-cyclin B1 complex. *J Virol* 2003;77(20):11186–11192.

279. Plemper RK, Brindley MA, Iorio RM. Structural and mechanistic studies of measles virus illuminate paramyxovirus entry. *PLoS Pathog* 2011;7(6):e1002058.

280. Pleschka S, Staeheli P, Kolodziejek J, et al. Conservation of coding potential and terminal sequences in four different isolates of Borna disease virus. *J Gen Virol* 2001;82(Pt 11):2681–2690.

281. Pletnikov MV, Rubin SA, Carbone KM, et al. Neonatal Borna disease virus infection (BDV)-induced damage to the cerebellum is associated with sensorimotor deficits in developing Lewis rats. *Brain Res Dev Brain Res* 2001;126(1):1–12.

282. Pletnikov MV, Rubin SA, Schwartz GJ, et al. Persistent neonatal Borna disease virus (BDV) infection of the brain causes chronic emotional abnormalities in adult rats. *Physiol Behav* 1999;66(5):823–831.

283. Pletnikov MV, Rubin SA, Vasudevan K, et al. Developmental brain injury associated with abnormal play behavior in neonatally Borna disease virus-infected Lewis rats: a model of autism. *Behav Brain Res* 1999;100(1–2):43–50.

284. Poch O, Blumberg BM, Bougueleret L, et al. Sequence comparison of five polymerase (L proteins) of unsegmented negative-strand RNA viruses: theoretical assignment of functional domains. *J Gen Virol* 1990;71:1153–1162.

285. Poch O, Sauvaget I, Delarue M, et al. Identification of four conserved motifs among the RNA-dependent polymerase encoding elements. *EMBO J* 1989;8:3867–3874.

286. Poenisch M, Burger N, Staeheli P, et al. Protein X of Borna disease virus inhibits apoptosis and promotes viral persistence in the central nervous systems of newborn-infected rats. *J Virol* 2009;83(9):4297–4307.

287. Poenisch M, Staeheli P, Schneider U. Viral accessory protein X stimulates the assembly of functional Borna disease virus polymerase complexes. *J Gen Virol* 2008;89(Pt 6):1442–1445.

288. Poenisch M, Unterstab G, Wolff T, et al. The X protein of Borna disease virus regulates viral polymerase activity through interaction with the P protein. *J Gen Virol* 2004;85(Pt 7):1895–1898.

289. Poenisch M, Wille S, Ackermann A, et al. The X protein of borna disease virus serves essential functions in the viral multiplication cycle. *J Virol* 2007;81(13):7297–7299.

290. Poenisch M, Wille S, Staeheli P, et al. Polymerase read-through at the first transcription termination site contributes to regulation of borna disease virus gene expression. *J Virol* 2008;82(19):9537–9545.

291. Prat CM, Schmid S, Farrugia F, et al. Mutation of the protein kinase C site in borna disease virus phosphoprotein abrogates viral interference with neuronal signaling and restores normal synaptic activity. *PLoS Pathog* 2009;5(5):e1000425.

292. Priestnall SL, Schoniger S, Ivens PA, et al. Borna disease virus infection of a horse in Great Britain. *Vet Rec* 2011;168(14):380b.

293. Pringle CR. Virus taxonomy 1996—a bulletin from the Xth International Congress of Virology in Jerusalem. *Arch Virol* 1996;141(11):2251–2256.

294. Puorger ME, Hilbe M, Müller J-P, et al. Distribution of Borna disease virus antigen and RNA in tissues of naturally infected bicolored white-toothed shrews, Crocidura leucodon, supporting their role as reservoir host species. *Vet Pathol* 2010;47(2):236–244.

295. Pyper JM, Gartner AE. Molecular basis for the differential subcellular localization of the 38- and 39-kilodalton structural proteins of Borna disease virus. *J Virol* 1997;71(7):5133–5139.

296. Raghav R, Taylor M, Delay J, et al. Avian bornavirus is present in many tissues of psittacine birds with histopathologic evidence of proventricular dilatation disease. *J Vet Diagn Invest* 2010;22(4):495–508.

297. Rall I, Amann R, Malberg S, et al. Recombinant modified Vaccinia Virus Ankara (MVA) vaccines efficiently protect cockatiels against parrot bornavirus infection and proventricular dilatation disease. *Viruses* 2019;11(12):1130.

298. Rauer M, Gotz J, Schuppli D, et al. Transgenic mice expressing the nucleoprotein of Borna disease virus in either neurons or astrocytes: decreased susceptibility to homotypic infection and disease. *J Virol* 2004;78(7):3621–3632.

299. Rauer M, Pagenstecher A, Schulte-Monting J, et al. Upregulation of chemokine receptor gene expression in brains of Borna disease virus (BDV)-infected rats in the absence and presence of inflammation. *J Neurovirol* 2002;8(3):168–179.

300. Reuter A, Horie M, Hoper D, et al. Synergistic antiviral activity of ribavirin and interferon-alpha against parrot bornaviruses in avian cells. *J Gen Virol* 2016;97(9):2096–2103.

301. Richt J, Stitz L, Deschl U, et al. Borna disease virus-induced meningoencephalomyelitis caused by a virus-specific CD4+ T cell-mediated immune reaction. *J Gen Virol* 1990;71 (Pt 11):2565–2573.

302. Richt JA, Alexander RC, Herzog S, et al. Failure to detect Borna disease virus infection in peripheral blood leukocytes from humans with psychiatric disorders. *J Neurovirol* 1997;3(2):174–178.

303. Richt JA, Clements JE, Herzog S, et al. Analysis of virus-specific RNA species and proteins in Freon-113 preparations of the Borna disease virus. *Med Microbiol Immunol* 1993;182(5):271–280.

304. Richt JA, Furbringer T, Koch A, et al. Processing of the Borna disease virus glycoprotein gp94 by the subtilisin-like endoprotease furin. *J Virol* 1998;72(5):4528–4533.

305. Richt JA, Grabner A, Herzog S, et al. *Borna Disease*. St. Louis, MO: Saunders Elsevier; 2007.

306. Richt JA, Herzog S, Pyper J, et al. Borna disease virus: nature of the etiologic agent and significance of infection in man. *Arch Virol Suppl* 1993;7:101–109.

307. Richt JA, Pfeuffer I, Christ M, et al. Borna disease virus infection in animals and humans. *Emerg Infect Dis* 1997;3(3):343–352.

308. Richt JA, Schmeel A, Frese K, et al. Borna disease virus-specific T cells protect against or cause immunopathological Borna disease. *J Exp Med* 1994;179(5):1467–1473.

309. Richt JA, Stitz L, Wekerle H, et al. Borna disease, a progressive meningoencephalomyelitis as a model for CD4+ T cell-mediated immunopathology in the brain. *J Exp Med* 1989;170(3):1045–1050.

310. Richt JA, VandeWoude S, Zink MC, et al. Infection with Borna disease virus: molecular and immunobiological characterization of the agent. *Clin Infect Dis* 1992;14(6):1240–1250.

311. Rinder M, Ackermann A, Kempf H, et al. Broad tissue and cell tropism of avian bornavirus in parrots with proventricular dilatation disease. *J Virol* 2009;83(11):5401–5407.

312. Roche S, Albertini AA, Lepault J, et al. Structures of vesicular stomatitis virus glycoprotein: membrane fusion revisited. *Cell Mol Life Sci* 2008;65(11):1716–1728.

313. Rosario D, Perez M, de la Torre JC. Functional characterization of the genomic promoter of borna disease virus (BDV): implications of 3′-terminal sequence heterogeneity for BDV persistence. *J Virol* 2005;79(10):6544–6550.

314. Rossi G, Dahlhausen RD, Galosi L, et al. Avian Ganglioneuritis in clinical practice. *Vet Clin North Am Exot Anim Pract* 2018;21(1):33–67.

315. Rott R, Becht H. Natural and experimental Borna disease in animals. *Curr Top Microbiol Immunol* 1995;190:17–30.

316. Rott R, Herzog S, Fleischer B, et al. Detection of serum antibodies to Borna disease virus in patients with psychiatric disorders. *Science* 1985;228(4700):755–756.

317. Rubbenstroth D, Briese T, Durrwald R, et al. ICTV virus taxonomy profile: bornaviridae. *J Gen Virol* 2021;102(7):001613.

318. Rubbenstroth D, Rinder M, Stein M, et al. Avian bornaviruses are widely distributed in canary birds (Serinus canaria f. domestica). *Vet Microbiol* 2013;165(3–4):287–295.

319. Rubbenstroth D, Schlottau K, Schwemmle M, et al. Human bornavirus research: Back on track! *PLoS Pathog* 2019;15(8):e1007873.

320. Rubbenstroth D, Schmidt V, Rinder M, et al. Discovery of a new avian bornavirus genotype in estrildid finches (Estrildidae) in Germany. *Vet Microbiol* 2014;168(2–4):318–323.

321. Rubbenstroth D, Schmidt V, Rinder M, et al. Phylogenetic analysis supports horizontal transmission as a driving force of the spread of avian bornaviruses. *PLoS One* 2016;11(8):e0160936.

322. Rubin SA, Waltrip RW II, Bautista JR, et al. Borna disease virus in mice: host-specific differences in disease expression. *J Virol* 1993;67(1):548–552.

323. Rubin SA, Sierra-Honigmann AM, Lederman HM, et al. Hematologic consequences of Borna disease virus infection of rat bone marrow and thymus stromal cells. *Blood* 1995;85(10):2762–2769.

324. Rubin SA, Sylves P, Vogel M, et al. Borna disease virus-induced hippocampal dentate gyrus damage is associated with spatial learning and memory deficits. *Brain Res Bull* 1999;48(1):23–30.

325. Rudolph MG, Kraus I, Dickmanns A, et al. Crystal structure of the borna disease virus nucleoprotein. *Structure* 2003;11(10):1219–1226.
326. Runge S, Olbert M, Herden C, et al. Viral vector vaccines protect cockatiels from inflammatory lesions after heterologous parrot bornavirus 2 challenge infection. *Vaccine* 2017;35(4):557–563.
327. Sa-Ardta P, Rinder M, Sanyathitiseree P, et al. First detection and characterization of Psittaciform bornaviruses in naturally infected and diseased birds in Thailand. *Vet Microbiol* 2019;230:62–71.
328. Saito N, Itouji A, Totani Y, et al. Cellular and intracellular localization of e-subspecies of protein kinase C in the rat brain; presynaptic localization of the e-subspecies. *Brain Res* 1993;607:241–248.
329. Sanchez A. Analysis of filovirus entry into vero e6 cells, using inhibitors of endocytosis, endosomal acidification, structural integrity, and cathepsin (B and L) activity. *J Infect Dis* 2007;196 (Suppl 2):S251–S258.
330. Sasaki S, Ludwig H. In borna disease virus infected rabbit neurons 100 nm particle structures accumulate at areas of Joest-Degen inclusion bodies. *Zentralbl Veterinarmed B* 1993;40(4):291–297.
331. Sauder C, de la Torre JC. Cytokine expression in the rat central nervous system following perinatal Borna disease virus infection. *J Neuroimmunol* 1999;96(1):29–45.
332. Sauder C, Hallensleben W, Pagenstecher A, et al. Chemokine gene expression in astrocytes of Borna disease virus-infected rats and mice in the absence of inflammation. *J Virol* 2000;74(19):9267–9280.
333. Sauder C, Herpfer I, Hassler C, et al. Susceptibility of Borna disease virus to the antiviral action of gamma-interferon: evidence for species-specific differences. *Arch Virol* 2004;149(11):2171–2186.
334. Schadler R, Diringer H, Ludwig H. Isolation and characterization of a 14500 molecular weight protein from brains and tissue cultures persistently infected with borna disease virus. *J Gen Virol* 1985;66(Pt 11):2479–2484.
335. Schamel K, Staeheli P, Hausmann J. Identification of the immunodominant H-2K(k) restricted cytotoxic T-cell epitope in the Borna disease virus nucleoprotein. *J Virol* 2001;75(18):8579–8588.
336. Schlottau K, Forth L, Angstwurm K, et al. Fatal encephalitic borna disease virus 1 in solid-organ transplant recipients. *N Engl J Med* 2018;379(14):1377–1379.
337. Schlottau K, Hoffmann B, Homeier-Bachmann T, et al. Multiple detection of zoonotic variegated squirrel bornavirus 1 RNA in different squirrel species suggests a possible unknown origin for the virus. *Arch Virol* 2017;162(9):2747–2754.
338. Schlottau K, Jenckel M, van den Brand J, et al. Variegated squirrel bornavirus 1 in squirrels, Germany and the Netherlands. *Emerg Infect Dis* 2017;23(3):477–481.
339. Schlottau K, Nobach D, Herden C, et al. First isolation, in-vivo and genomic characterization of zoonotic variegated squirrel Bornavirus 1 (VSBV-1) isolates. *Emerg Microbes Infect* 2020;9(1):2474–2484.
340. Schneemann A, Schneider PA, Kim S, et al. Identification of signal sequences that control transcription of borna disease virus, a nonsegmented, negative-strand RNA virus. *J Virol* 1994;68(10):6514–6522.
341. Schneemann A, Schneider PA, Lamb RA, et al. The remarkable coding strategy of borna disease virus: a new member of the nonsegmented negative strand RNA viruses. *Virology* 1995;210(1):1–8.
342. Schneider PA, Briese T, Zimmermann W, et al. Sequence conservation in field and experimental isolates of Borna disease virus. *J Virol* 1994;68(1):63–68.
343. Schneider PA, Hatalski CG, Lewis AJ, et al. Biochemical and functional analysis of the Borna disease virus G protein. *J Virol* 1997;71(1):331–336.
344. Schneider PA, Kim R, Lipkin WI. Evidence for translation of the Borna disease virus G protein by leaky ribosomal scanning and ribosomal reinitiation. *J Virol* 1997;71(7): 5614–5619.
345. Schneider PA, Schneemann A, Lipkin WI. RNA splicing in Borna disease virus, a nonsegmented, negative-strand RNA virus. *J Virol* 1994;68(8):5007–5012.
346. Schneider U. Novel insights into the regulation of the viral polymerase complex of neurotropic Borna disease virus. *Virus Res* 2005;111(2):148–160.
347. Schneider U, Blechschmidt K, Schwemmle M, et al. Overlap of interaction domains indicates a central role of the P protein in assembly and regulation of the Borna disease virus polymerase complex. *J Biol Chem* 2004;279(53):55290–55296.
348. Schneider U, Naegele M, Staeheli P. Regulation of the Borna disease virus polymerase complex by the viral nucleoprotein p38 isoform. Brief Report. *Arch Virol* 2004;149(7): 1409–1414.
349. Schneider U, Naegele M, Staeheli P, et al. Active borna disease virus polymerase complex requires a distinct nucleoprotein-to-phosphoprotein ratio but no viral X protein. *J Virol* 2003;77(21):11781–11789.
350. Schneider U, Schwemmle M, Staeheli P. Genome trimming: a unique strategy for replication control employed by Borna disease virus. *Proc Natl Acad Sci U S A* 2005;102(9): 3441–3446.
351. Schulz JA, Müller H, Lippmann R. Untersuchungen zur Prophylaxe der Bornaschen Krankheit bei Schafen mittels aktiver Immunisierung. *Arch Exp Veterinarmed* 1968;22(3):571–583.
352. Schulze V, Grosse R, Furstenau J, et al. Borna disease outbreak with high mortality in an alpaca herd in a previously unreported endemic area in Germany. *Transbound Emerg Dis* 2020;67:2093–2107.
353. Schwardt M, Mayer D, Frank R, et al. The negative regulator of Borna disease virus polymerase is a non-structural protein. *J Gen Virol* 2005;86(Pt 11):3163–3169.
354. Schwemmle M, De B, Shi L, et al. Borna disease virus P-protein is phosphorylated by protein kinase Cepsilon and casein kinase II. *J Biol Chem* 1997;272(35):21818–21823.
355. Schwemmle M, Heimrich B. Viral interference with neuronal integrity: what can we learn from the Borna disease virus? *Cell Tissue Res* 2011;344(1):13–16.
356. Schwemmle M, Jehle C, Formella S, et al. Sequence similarities between human bornavirus isolates and laboratory strains question human origin. *Lancet* 1999;354(9194):1973–1974.
357. Schwemmle M, Jehle C, Shoemaker T, et al. Characterization of the major nuclear localization signal of the Borna disease virus phosphoprotein. *J Gen Virol* 1999;80(Pt 1): 97–100.
358. Schwemmle M, Salvatore M, Shi L, et al. Interactions of the borna disease virus P, N, and X proteins and their functional implications. *J Biol Chem* 1998;273(15):9007–9012.
359. Seifried O, Spatz H. Die Ausbreitung der encephalitischen Reaktion bei der Bornaschen Krankheit der Pferde und deren Beziehungen zu der Encephalitis epidemica, der Heine-Medinschen Krankheit und der Lyssa des Menschen. Eine vergleichend-pathologische Studie. *Z Gesamte Neurol Psychiatr* 1930;124:317–382.
360. Shi M, Lin XD, Chen X, et al. The evolutionary history of vertebrate RNA viruses. *Nature* 2018;556(7700):197–202.
361. Shoya Y, Kobayashi T, Koda T, et al. Two proline-rich nuclear localization signals in the amino- and carboxyl-terminal regions of the Borna disease virus phosphoprotein. *J Virol* 1998;72(12):9755–9762.
362. Siemetzki U, Ashok MS, Briese T, et al. Identification of RNA instability elements in Borna disease virus. *Virus Res* 2009;144(1–2):27–34.
363. Sobbe M, Bilzer T, Gommel S, et al. Induction of degenerative brain lesions after adoptive transfer of brain lymphocytes from Borna disease virus-infected rats: presence of CD8+ T cells and perforin mRNA. *J Virol* 1997;71(3):2400–2407.
364. Solbrig MV, Adrian R, Baratta J, et al. A role for endocannabinoids in viral-induced dyskinetic and convulsive phenomena. *Exp Neurol* 2005;194(2):355–362.
365. Solbrig MV, Fallon JH, Lipkin WI. Behavioral disturbances and pharmacology of Borna disease. *Curr Top Microbiol Immunol* 1995;190:93–101.
366. Solbrig MV, Koob GF, Fallon JH, et al. Tardive dyskinetic syndrome in rats infected with Borna disease virus. *Neurobiol Dis* 1994;1(3):111–119.
367. Solbrig MV, Koob GF, Fallon JH, et al. Prefrontal cortex dysfunction in Borna disease virus (BDV)—infected rats. *Biol Psychiatry* 1996;40(7):629–636.
368. Solbrig MV, Koob GF, Joyce JN, et al. A neural substrate of hyperactivity in borna disease; changes in brain dopamine receptors. *Virology* 1996;222(2):332–338.
369. Solbrig MV, Koob GF, Lipkin WI. Naloxone-induced seizures in rats infected with Borna disease virus. *Neurology* 1996;46(4):1170–1171.
370. Solbrig MV, Koob GF, Lipkin WI. Cocaine sensitivity in Borna disease virus-infected rats. *Pharmacol Biochem Behav* 1998;59(4):1047–1052.
371. Solbrig MV, Koob GF, Lipkin WI. Key role for enkephalinergic tone in cortico-striatal-thalamic function. *Eur J Neurosci* 2002;16(9):1819–1822.
372. Solbrig MV, Schlaberg R, Briese T, et al. Neuroprotection and reduced proliferation of microglia in ribavirin-treated bornavirus-infected rats. *Antimicrob Agents Chemother* 2002;46(7):2287–2291.
373. Spiropoulou C, Nichol S. A small highly basic protein Is encoded in overlapping frame within the P gene of vesicular Stomatitis virus. *J Virol* 1993;67:3103–3110.
374. Sprankel H, Richarz K, Ludwig H, et al. Behavior alterations in tree shrews (Tupaia glis, Diard 1820) induced by Borna disease virus. *Med Microbiol Immunol* 1978;165(1):1–18.
375. Staeheli P. Bornaviruses. *Virus Res* 2002;82(1–2):55–59.
376. Staeheli P, Rinder M, Kaspers B. Avian bornavirus associated with fatal disease in psittacine birds. *J Virol* 2010;84(13):6269–6275.
377. Staeheli P, Sauder C, Hausmann J, et al. Epidemiology of Borna disease virus. *J Gen Virol* 2000;81(Pt 9):2123–2135.
378. Steinmetz A, Pees M, Schmidt V, et al. Blindness as a sign of proventricular dilatation disease in a grey parrot (Psittacus Erithacus Erithacus). *J Small Anim Pract* 2008;49:660–662.
379. Stenglein MD, Leavitt EB, Abramovitch MA, et al. Genome sequence of a bornavirus recovered from an African Garter Snake (Elapsoidea loveridgei). *Genome Announc* 2014;2(5):e00779-14.
380. Sternberg EM, Wilder RL, Gold PW, et al. A defect in the central component of the immune system—hypothalamic-pituitary-adrenal axis feedback loop is associated with susceptibility to experimental arthritis and other inflammatory diseases. *Ann N Y Acad Sci* 1990;594:289–292.
381. Stitz L, Bilzer T, Planz O. The immunopathogenesis of Borna disease virus infection. *Front Biosci* 2002;7:d541–d555.
382. Stitz L, Krey H, Ludwig H. Borna disease in rhesus monkeys as a models for uveo-cerebral symptoms. *J Med Virol* 1981;6(4):333–340.
383. Stitz L, Noske K, Planz O, et al. A functional role for neutralizing antibodies in Borna disease: influence on virus tropism outside the central nervous system. *J Virol* 1998;72(11):8884–8892.
384. Stitz L, Planz O, Bilzer T. Lack of antiviral effect of amantadine in Borna disease virus infection. *Med Microbiol Immunol* 1998;186(4):195–200.
385. Stitz L, Sobbe M, Bilzer T. Preventive effects of early anti-CD4 or anti-CD8 treatment on Borna disease in rats. *J Virol* 1992;66(6):3316–3323.
386. Stitz L, Soeder D, Deschl U, et al. Inhibition of immune-mediated meningoencephalitis in persistently Borna disease virus-infected rats by cyclosporine A. *J Immunol* 1989;143(12):4250–4256.
387. Szelechowski M, Betourne A, Monnet Y, et al. A viral peptide that targets mitochondria protects against neuronal degeneration in models of Parkinson's disease. *Nat Commun* 2014;5:5181.
388. Tam RC, Pai B, Bard J, et al. Ribavirin polarizes human T cell responses towards a Type 1 cytokine profile. *J Hepatol* 1999;30(3):376–382.
389. Tappe D, Frank C, Homeier-Bachmann T, et al. Analysis of exotic squirrel trade and detection of human infections with variegated squirrel bornavirus 1, Germany, 2005 to 2018. *Euro Surveill* 2019;24(8):1800483.
390. Tappe D, Frank C, Offergeld R, et al. Low prevalence of Borna disease virus 1 (BoDV-1) IgG antibodies in humans from areas endemic for animal Borna disease of Southern Germany. *Sci Rep* 2019;9(1):20154.
391. Tappe D, Portner K, Frank C, et al. Investigation of fatal human Borna disease virus 1 encephalitis outside the previously known area for human cases, Brandenburg, Germany—a case report. *BMC Infect Dis* 2021;21(1):787.
392. Tappe D, Schlottau K, Cadar D, et al. Occupation-associated fatal limbic encephalitis caused by variegated squirrel bornavirus 1, Germany, 2013. *Emerg Infect Dis* 2018;24(6):978–987.
393. Tappe D, Schmidt-Chanasit J, Rauch J, et al. Immunopathology of fatal human variegated squirrel bornavirus 1 encephalitis, Germany, 2011–2013. *Emerg Infect Dis* 2019; 25(6):1058–1065.

394. Thiedemann N, Presek P, Rott R, et al. Antigenic relationship and further characterization of two major Borna disease virus-specific proteins. *J Gen Virol* 1992;73(Pt 5):1057–1064.

395. Thomas SM, Lamb RA, Paterson RG. Two mRNA's that differ by two nontemplated nucleotides encode the amino coterminal proteins P and V of the paramyxovirus SV5. *Cell* 1988;54:891–902.

396. Thomsen AF, Nielsen JB, Hjulsager CK, et al. Aquatic bird bornavirus 1 in wild geese, Denmark. *Emerg Infect Dis* 2015;21(12):2201–2203.

397. Tizard I, Shivaprasad HL, Guo J, et al. The pathogenesis of proventricular dilatation disease. *Anim Health Res Rev* 2016;17(2):110–126.

398. Tokunaga T, Yamamoto Y, Sakai M, et al. Antiviral activity of favipiravir (T-705) against mammalian and avian bornaviruses. *Antiviral Res* 2017;143:237–245.

399. Tomonaga K, Kobayashi T, Lee BJ, et al. Identification of alternative splicing and negative splicing activity of a nonsegmented negative-strand RNA virus, Borna disease virus. *Proc Natl Acad Sci U S A* 2000;97(23):12788–12793.

400. Toth Z, Yan XX, Haftoglou S, et al. Seizure-induced neuronal injury: vulnerability to febrile seizures in an immature rat model. *J Neurosci* 1998;18(11):4285–4294.

401. Unterstab G, Ludwig S, Anton A, et al. Viral targeting of the interferon-{beta}-inducing Traf family member-associated NF-{kappa}B activator (TANK)-binding kinase-1. *Proc Natl Acad Sci U S A* 2005;102(38):13640–13645.

402. Vahlenkamp TW, Konrath A, Weber M, et al. Persistence of Borna disease virus in naturally infected sheep. *J Virol* 2002;76(19):9735–9743.

403. VandeWoude S, Richt JA, Zink MC, et al. A borna virus cDNA encoding a protein recognized by antibodies in humans with behavioral diseases. *Science* 1990;250(4985):1278–1281.

404. Villanueva I, Gray P, Mirhosseini N, et al. The diagnosis of proventricular dilatation disease: use of a Western blot assay to detect antibodies against avian Borna virus. *Vet Microbiol* 2010;143(2–4):196–201.

405. Villanueva I, Gray P, Tizard I. Detection of an antigen specific for proventricular dilation disease in psitticine birds. *Vet Rec* 2008;163(14):426.

406. Volmer R, Bajramovic JJ, Schneider U, et al. Mechanism of the antiviral action of 1-beta-D-arabinofuranosylcytosine on Borna disease virus. *J Virol* 2005;79(7):4514–4518.

407. Volmer R, Monnet C, Gonzalez-Dunia D. Borna disease virus blocks potentiation of presynaptic activity through inhibition of protein kinase C signaling. *PLoS Pathog* 2006;2(3):e19.

408. von Sind JB. *Der im Feld und auf der Reise geschwind heilende Pferdearzt, welcher einen gründlichen Unterricht von den gewöhnlichsten Krankheiten der Pferde im Feld und auf der Reise wie auch einen auserlesenen Vorrath der nützlichsten und durch die Erfahrung bewährtesten Heilungsmitteln eröffnet.* Frankfurt und Leipzig: Heinrich Ludwig Brönner; 1767.

409. von Sprockhoff H. Untersuchungen über die Komplementbindungsreaktion bei der Borna'schen Krankheit. *Zentralbl Veterinarmed B* 1954;1:494–503.

410. von Sprockhoff H, Nitzschke E. Untersuchungen über das komplementbindende Antigen in Gehirnen bornavirus-infizierter Kaninchen. 1. Mitteilung: Nachweis eines löslichen Antigens. *Zentralbl Veterinarmed B* 1955;2(Heft 2):185–192.

411. Walker MP, Jordan I, Briese T, et al. Expression and characterization of the Borna disease virus polymerase. *J Virol* 2000;74(9):4425–4428.

412. Walker MP, Lipkin WI. Characterization of the nuclear localization signal of the borna disease virus polymerase. *J Virol* 2002;76(16):8460–8467.

413. Watanabe M, Lee BJ, Yamashita M, et al. Borna disease virus induces acute fatal neurological disorders in neonatal gerbils without virus- and immune-mediated cell destructions. *Virology* 2003;310(2):245–253.

414. Watanabe Y, Ohtaki N, Hayashi Y, et al. Autogenous translational regulation of the Borna disease virus negative control factor X from polycistronic mRNA using host RNA helicases. *PLoS Pathog* 2009;5(11):e1000654.

415. Watanabe M, Zhong Q, Kobayashi T, et al. Molecular ratio between borna disease viral-p40 and -p24 proteins in infected cells determined by quantitative antigen capture ELISA. *Microbiol Immunol* 2000;44(9):765–772.

416. Wehner T, Ruppert A, Herden C, et al. Detection of a novel Borna disease virus-encoded 10 kDa protein in infected cells and tissues. *J Gen Virol* 1997;78(Pt 10):2459–2466.

417. Weissenbock H, Bago Z, Kolodziejek J, et al. Infections of horses and shrews with Bornaviruses in Upper Austria: a novel endemic area of Borna disease. *Emerg Microbes Infect* 2017;6(6):e52.

418. Weissenbock H, Bakonyi T, Sekulin K, et al. Avian bornaviruses in psittacine birds from Europe and Australia with proventricular dilatation disease. *Emerg Infect Dis* 2009;15(9):1453–1459.

419. Weissenbock H, Fragner K, Nedorost N, et al. Localization of avian bornavirus RNA by in situ hybridization in tissues of psittacine birds with proventricular dilatation disease. *Vet Microbiol* 2010;145(1–2):9–16.

420. Weissenbock H, Hornig M, Hickey WF, et al. Microglial activation and neuronal apoptosis in Bornavirus infected neonatal Lewis rats. *Brain Pathol* 2000;10(2):260–272.

421. Weissenbock H, Sekulin K, Bakonyi T, et al. Novel avian bornavirus in a nonpsittacine species (Canary; Serinus canaria) with enteric ganglioneuritis and encephalitis. *J Virol* 2009;83(21):11367–11371.

422. Weissenbock H, Suchy A, Caplazi P, et al. Borna disease in Austrian horses. *Vet Rec* 1998;143(1):21–22.

423. Wensman JJ, Munir M, Thaduri S, et al. The X proteins of bornaviruses interfere with type I interferon signalling. *J Gen Virol* 2013;94(Pt 2):263–269.

424. Whitlock RH, Buckley, C. Botulism. *Vet Clin North Am Equine Pract* 1997;13:107–128.

425. Williams BL, Hornig M, Yaddanapudi K, et al. Hippocampal poly(ADP-Ribose) polymerase 1 and caspase 3 activation in neonatal bornavirus infection. *J Virol* 2008;82(4):1748–1758.

426. Williams BL, Yaddanapudi K, Hornig M, et al. Spatiotemporal analysis of purkinje cell degeneration relative to parasagittal expression domains in a model of neonatal viral infection. *J Virol* 2007;81(6):2675–2687.

427. Wilson WD. Equine herpesvirus 1 myeloencephalopathy. *Vet Clin North Am Equine Pract* 1997;13:53–72.

428. Wolff T, Heins G, Pauli G, et al. Failure to detect Borna disease virus antigen and RNA in human blood. *J Clin Virol* 2006;36(4):309–311.

429. Wolff T, Pfleger R, Wehner T, et al. A short leucine-rich sequence in the Borna disease virus p10 protein mediates association with the viral phospho- and nucleoproteins. *J Gen Virol* 2000;81(Pt 4):939–947.

430. Wolff T, Unterstab G, Heins G, et al. Characterization of an unusual importin alpha binding motif in the borna disease virus p10 protein that directs nuclear import. *J Biol Chem* 2002;277(14):12151–12157.

431. Wu Y-J, Schulz H, Lin C-C, et al. Borna disease virus-induced neuronal degeneration dependent on host genetic background and prevented by soluble factors. *Proc Natl Acad Sci U S A* 2013;110(5):1899–1904.

432. Wunschmann A, Honkavuori K, Briese T, et al. Antigen tissue distribution of Avian bornavirus (ABV) in psittacine birds with natural spontaneous proventricular dilatation disease and ABV genotype 1 infection. *J Vet Diagn Invest* 2011;23(4):716–726.

433. Wüst E. *Untersuchungen zur vertikalen Übertragung des Parrot Bornavirus bei Psittaziden [Dissertation].* Justus-Liebig-Universität Gießen; 2017.

434. Yanai H, Hayashi Y, Watanabe Y, et al. Development of a novel Borna disease virus reverse genetics system using RNA polymerase II promoter and SV40 nuclear import signal. *Microbes Infect* 2006;8(6):1522–1529.

435. Yanai H, Kobayashi T, Hayashi Y, et al. A methionine-rich domain mediates CRM1-dependent nuclear export activity of Borna disease virus phosphoprotein. *J Virol* 2006;80(3):1121–1129.

436. Yilmaz H, Helps CR, Turan N, et al. Detection of antibodies to Borna disease virus (BDV) in Turkish horse sera using recombinant p40. Brief report. *Arch Virol* 2002;147(2):429–435.

437. Zhang G, Kobayashi T, Kamitani W, et al. Borna disease virus phosphoprotein represses p53-mediated transcriptional activity by interference with HMGB1. *J Virol* 2003;77(22):12243–12251.

438. Zimmermann W, Breter H, Rudolph M, et al. The Borna disease virus: immunoelectron microscopic characterization of cell-free virus and further information on the genome. *J Virol* 1994;68:6755–6758.

439. Zocher M, Czub S, Schulte-Monting J, et al. Alterations in neurotrophin and neurotrophin receptor gene expression patterns in the rat central nervous system following perinatal Borna disease virus infection. *J Neurovirol* 2000;6(6):462–477.

440. Zwick W. Bornasche Krankheit und Enzephalomyelitis der Tiere. In: Gildemeister E, Haagen E, Waldmann O, eds. *Handbuch der Viruskrankheiten, 2. Band.* Jena, Germany: G. Fischer; 1939:254–354.

441. Zwick W, Seifried O. Uebertragbarkeit der seuchenhaften Gehirn- und Rückenmarksentzündung des Pferdes (Borna'schen Krankheit) auf kleine Versuchstiere (Kaninchen). *Berl Tierarztl Wochenschr* 1925;41(Nr. 9):129–132.

442. Zwick W, Seifried O, Witte J. Experimentelle Untersuchungen über die seuchenhafte Gehirn- und Rückenmarksentzündung der Pferde (Bornasche Krankheit). *Z Infkrankh Haustiere* 1926;30:42–136.

443. Zwick W, Seifried O, Witte J. Weitere Untersuchungen über die seuchenhafte Gehirn- und Rückenmarksentzündung der Pferde (Bornasche Krankheit). *Z Infkrankh Haustiere* 1927;32:150–179.

444. Zwick W, Witte J. Zur Frage der Schutzimpfung und der Inkubations frist bei der Bornaschen Krankheit. *Arch Wiss Prakt Tierheilkd* 1931;64:116–124.

Rhabdoviridae

Sean P. J. Whelan • Louis-Marie Bloyet

Introduction
History
   Lyssaviruses
   Vesiculoviruses
   Ephemeroviruses
   Novirhabdoviruses
   Sigma virus
Taxonomy
Virion structure
Genome organization and encoded proteins
   The nucleoprotein
   The phosphoprotein
   The matrix protein
   The glycoprotein
   The large polymerase protein
Stages of replication
   Mechanism of attachment
   Mechanism of penetration
   Uncoating and primary transcription
   Genome replication
   Secondary transcription
   Viral replication compartment
   Assembly of progeny virions
Molecular genetics of rhabdoviruses
   Defective interfering particles
   Genetic engineering of rhabdoviruses
Molecular and cellular basis of pathogenesis
   Induction and suppression of host antiviral responses
   Induction of cytopathic effects
Mouse models of rhabdovirus infection
   Entry and site of initial replication
   Virus spread and tissue tropism
   Immune responses involved in recovery from rhabdovirus
     infection
   Immune response to vesiculovirus infection
   Immune response to lyssavirus infection
   Determinants of viral virulence
Epidemiology of rhabdovirus infections
   Epidemiology of lyssavirus infections
   Epidemiology of vesiculovirus infections
   Epidemiology of ephemerovirus infections
   Epidemiology of novirhabdovirus infections
Clinical features of rhabdovirus infections
   Lyssavirus infections
   Vesiculovirus infections
   Ephemerovirus infections
   Novirhabdovirus infections

Diagnosis of rhabdovirus infections
   Lyssavirus infections
   Vesiculovirus infections
   Ephemerovirus infections
   Novirhabdovirus infections
Prevention and control of rhabdovirus infections
   Lyssavirus infections in humans
   Control of rabies in animals
   Control of vesiculovirus infections
   Control of ephemerovirus infections
   Control of novirhabdovirus infections
Perspectives
Acknowledgments

INTRODUCTION

The family *Rhabdoviridae* comprises viruses with single-stranded, nonsegmented, negative-sense RNA genomes with an elongated rod-like or bullet-like shape. This distinctive morphology gave its name to the rhabdoviruses (*rhabdos* means "rod" in ancient Greek and separates them from other families in the order *Mononegavirales*. Rhabdoviruses can replicate in plants, invertebrates, or vertebrates and many are transmitted to their animal or plant hosts by arthropods. Significant medical, veterinary, and agricultural pathogens include rabies virus, bovine ephemeral fever virus, and maize mosaic virus.

HISTORY

Lyssaviruses

Rabies is one of the oldest recognized infectious diseases. The dangers of dog bites are described in the pre-Mosaic Eshnunna Code of Mesopotamia, circa the 23rd century BC. In The Iliad (700 BC), Hector is compared to a rabid dog. Chinese scholars warned of rabid dogs in 500 BC, and Aristotle (4th century BC) associated the disease with contracting it from a mad dog's bite. In Rome, Cordamus guessed that a poison (i.e., a "virus") was present in saliva, and Celsus described clinical aspects of human infection: "The patient is tortured at the same time by thirst and by invincible repulsion toward water." For prevention, he recommended immediate excision of the bitten tissue, cauterization of the wound by a hot iron, and dunking the victim into a pool. The Hebrew Talmud also makes several references to the disease.[36]

In 1546, the Italian physician Fracastoro described human infection by rabies: Its incubation [following a bite by a rabid animal] is so stealthy, slow, and gradual that the infection is very rarely manifest before the 20th day, in most cases after the 30th, and in many cases not until 4 or 6 months have elapsed. There are cases recorded in which it became manifest a year after the bite. [Once the disease takes hold] the patient can neither stand nor lie down; like a madman he flings himself hither and thither, tears his flesh with his hands, and feels intolerable thirst. This is the most distressing symptom, for he so shrinks from water and all liquids that he would rather die than drink or be brought near to water; it is then that they bite other persons, foam at the mouth, their eyes look twisted, and finally they are exhausted and painfully breathe their last.[272] This portrayal of human rabies is accurate in that the incubation periods can extend from months to years after initial exposure, but a biting attack on others by a rabid patient with resultant disease is uncommon.[159] In 1804, Zinke used dog saliva to transmit infection, and in 1879, Galtier reported rabies transmission and serial passage in rabbits. Clinical descriptions formed the basis for diagnosis until the advent of light microscopy. In 1903, Negri, a student of Golgi, reported detection of cytoplasmic inclusions (Negri bodies) in neurons of rabid animals.[296] Although the diagnostic value of Negri bodies was established by 1913, their viral composition had to wait until the later development of electron microscopy, and their importance in viral replication until the 21st century.

Pasteur's research on rabies included adaptation of "street" (wild-type) virus to laboratory animals, and the development of the first vaccine against rabies. Desiccated spinal cords from rabies virus–infected rabbits were supposedly safe, although now it is known that the fixed viruses from which these vaccines were derived were not apathogenic but could actually cause disease. On July 6, 1885, 9-year-old Joseph Meister was bitten at multiple sites by a rabid dog and received the first postexposure prophylaxis with Pasteur's vaccine and survived. Pasteur's vaccine became the accepted rabies prophylactic throughout the world in the early 20th century. However, improperly inactivated virus caused rabies, and animal brain tissue induced allergic reactions leading to neuroparalytic accidents. Moreover, the vaccine was not very effective in cases of severe bites, such as those inflicted on the face and neck.

Postexposure prophylaxis against rabies through simultaneous administration of antirabies serum and vaccine was introduced in 1889[27]; ultimately, the combined use of serum and vaccine was found to be more protective than vaccine alone.[213] The combination of immune globulin and vaccine is the recommended standard for prophylaxis in human rabies exposure. In the 1960s, rabies virus (RABV) grown in human diploid cells was used to produce an inactivated vaccine eliminating many of the problems connected with vaccines produced in brain tissue. This vaccine and others derived from cell culture are used widely throughout the world.

Vesiculoviruses

Vesicular stomatitis virus (VSV) is a widely studied prototype of the nonsegmented, negative-strand RNA viruses. VSV produces an acute disease in cattle, horses, and pigs characterized by fever and vesicles in the mucosa of the oral cavity and in the skin of the coronary band and teat. The symptoms are similar to livestock infection by foot-and-mouth disease (FMD). VSV can also cause an acute febrile disease in humans but laboratory-adapted strains are rarely pathogenic in humans. The disease was first reported in the United States in 1916 during an epidemic in cattle and horses.[521] The disease could be transmitted from horse to horse by rubbing the saliva of a sick animal on the tongue of a healthy one, establishing its infectious nature.[219] In 1925, cattle transported from Kansas City, Missouri, to Richmond, Indiana, initiated an outbreak of VS. The disease was experimentally transmitted to horses and the infectious agent was maintained by serial passage in animals to eventually become the VS-Indiana virus (VSIV) strain. An outbreak in cattle in New Jersey in 1926 similarly resulted in the VS-New Jersey virus (VSNJV) strain.[113] VSIV and VSNJV viruses represent the two serotypes most commonly isolated in the Americas. Most laboratory-adapted strains of VSV (e.g., Glasgow, Orsay, San Juan, Mudd-Summers) belong to the VSIV serotype. In the United States, the last reported outbreak of the VSIV serotype occurred in 2020.[19] The VSNJV serotype was responsible for outbreaks in the United States in 1944, 1949, 1957, 1959, 1963, 1982–1983, 1985, and 1995.[65] VSV is endemic in many Latin American countries and is responsible for important economic losses in the livestock industry.

Other vesiculoviruses are endemic in the Americas, Asia, and Africa. Piry virus was isolated from an opossum (Philander opossum) in Brazil in 1960[527] and caused a febrile disease in humans. Cocal virus (COCV) was isolated from mites of the genus *Gigantolaelaps* from rice rats (*Oryzomys laticeps velutinus*) trapped during 1961, on Bush Bush Island in the Nariva swamp in eastern Trinidad.[269] The VS Alagoas virus (VSAV) was isolated from domestic animals in the state of Alagoas, Brazil, during a VS outbreak, and subsequently from sand flies and seropositive livestock in Colombia.[525] Maraba virus (MARAV) was isolated from sand flies (*Lutzomyia* sp.) collected in the state of Pará, Brazil.[533]

Chandipura virus (CHPV) and Isfahan virus (ISFV). ISFV was isolated from sand flies (*Phlebotomus papatasii*) collected in Dormian, Isfahan Province, Iran, in 1975.[524] From serologic analyses, the presence of ISFV has been detected in India, Iran, Turkmenistan, and other Asian countries. CHPV was obtained from the sera of two patients with a febrile illness in Nagpur City, Maharashtra State, India, in 1965 during an epidemic of chikungunya and dengue.[51] This virus was also isolated from phlebotomine sand flies in West Africa in 1991.[176] CHPV can cause fatal viral encephalitis in children.[443]

Several vesiculoviruses infect fish. Infectious dropsy of the common carp, *Cyprinus carpio*, in central and eastern European pond culture led to the identification of the causative virus spring viremia of carp virus (SVCV).[164] SVCV infections in Europe, Russia, and the Middle East are associated with significant economic losses and mortality of up to 70% of young carps.[10] In the United States, SVCV was first identified in a North Carolina koi hatchery, but not before koi had been distributed to most of the 48 contiguous states. The first common carp die-off of wild fish that tested positive for SVC occurred in 2002 at Cedar Lake, Wisconsin.[135] The virus has rapidly disseminated to other states and spread to infect centrarchid fish such as bluegill and largemouth bass. In 2015, the virus was isolated from a salamander underscoring how this exotic virus is not only a threat to native fish but also amphibian species in North America.

Ephemeroviruses

In the 20th century, bovine ephemeral fever was described in ruminants throughout the tropical and subtropical regions of Africa, Asia, Australia, and the Middle East. Bovine ephemeral fever virus (BEFV) was grown in mice[543] and characterized genetically and biochemically.[550] Ephemeroviruses have also been isolated from mosquitoes.

Novirhabdoviruses

Infectious hematopoietic necrosis virus (IHNV) was discovered in sockeye salmon (*Oncorhynchus nerka*) dying at hatcheries in Washington in 1953.[465] Similar outbreaks among hatchery-reared salmonid fish in California were reported in the following decades. The virus spread during the 1970s to the eastern United States, Europe, Japan, Korea, Taiwan, and China by shipment of infected fish and eggs.[64] Electron microscopy of IHNV particles along with physicochemical and serologic analysis placed it in the family *Rhabdoviridae*.[360] In addition to the structural genes common to all rhabdoviruses, IHNV encodes a nonstructural, nonvirion (NV) gene between G and L.[301] Hirame rhabdovirus, snakehead virus, and viral hemorrhagic septicemia (VHS) virus also have a similar arrangement. These viruses were identified not only in North America but also in eastern and southern Asia, where they appear to be endemic.[274]

Sigma Virus

Sigma virus was first described in Drosophila in 1937. The virus has an unusual mode of transmission: it is only transmitted vertically through both eggs and sperm and does not move horizontally between hosts.[406] Sigma virus was initially placed in the *Rhabdoviridae* based on its bullet shape and confirmed using sequence data.[55]

TAXONOMY

The rhabdoviruses share a variety of gross morphologic and functional attributes with other members of the order *Mononegavirales*. Indeed, (a) the virions are large structures decorated with membrane-bound spikes and contain a helical nucleocapsid; (b) their genome is carried by a single-stranded, nonsegmented, negative-sense RNA; and (c) they share common strategies for genome expression and replication. The assignment to the *Rhabdoviridae* family is mainly based on the virion's morphology, which generates a heterogeneous group with relatively low sequence conservation and a great diversity in terms of genome composition (from five to more than ten genes) or site of replication (cytoplasmic or nuclear) (Fig. 7.1, see Fig. 7.4, Table 7.1).[131] Two exceptions are the

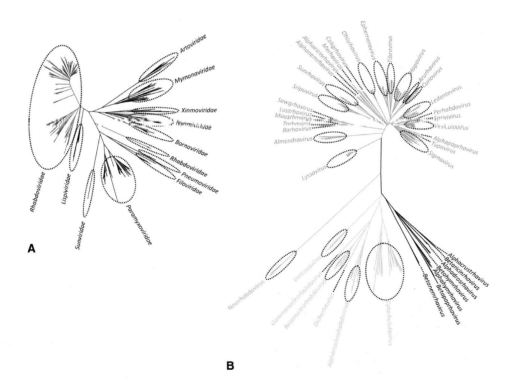

FIGURE 7.1 Phylogenetic tree of the *Mononegavirales* order and the *Rhabdoviridae* family.
A: Phylogenetic tree of the *Mononegavirales* order generated from an alignment of the RNA-dependent RNA polymerase domains of the L protein. Members of the *Rhabdoviridae* family are colored in *red*. **B:** Phylogenetic tree of the *Rhabdoviridae* family generated from an alignment of the full-length L proteins. The *Alpharhabdovirinae*, *Betarhabdovirinae*, and *Gammarhabdovirinae* subfamilies are colored in *teal*, *olive green*, and *yellow*, respectively. For both trees, one sequence per species was used (when available and complete). The sequences were selected based on the GenBank accession numbers given by the 2020 taxonomy of the International Committee on Taxonomy of Viruses.

TABLE 7.1   Organization of the *Rhabdoviridae* family

Genera	Hosts	Example Viruses	Genera	Hosts	Example Viruses
Subfamily *Alpharhabdovirinae*			**Subfamily *Betarhabdovirinae***		
Almendravirus	I	Puerto Almendras virus	Alphanucleorhabdovirus	P	Potato yellow dwarf virus
Alphanemrhavirus	I	Xinzhou nematode virus 4	Betanucleorhabdovirus	P	Datura yellow vein virus
Alphapaprhavirus	I	Hubei lepidoptera virus 2	Cytorhabdovirus	P, I	Lettuce necrotic yellows virus
Alpharicinrhavirus	I	Wuhan tick virus 1	Dichorhavirus*	P, I	Orchid fleck virus
Arurhavirus	I	Xiburema virus	Gammanucleorhabdovirus	P	Maize fine streak virus
Barhavirus	I	Bahia Grande virus	Varicosavirus*	P	Lettuce big vein-associated virus
Caligrhavirus	I	Caligus rogercresseyi rhabdovirus			
Curiovirus	I	Curionopolis virus	**Subfamily**		
Ephemerovirus	I, V	Bovine ephemeral fever virus	***Gammarhabdovirinae***		
Hapavirus	I, V	Flanders virus	Novirhabdovirus	V	Infectious hematopoietic necrosis virus
Ledantevirus	I, V	Le Dantec virus			
Lostrhavirus	I	Lone star tick rhabdovirus	**Other genera**		
Lyssavirus	V	Rabies virus	Alphacrustrhavirus	I	Wenling crustacean virus 11
Merhavirus	I	Merida virus	Alphadrosrhavirus	I	Wuhan house fly virus 2
Mousrhavirus	I	Moussa virus	Alphahymrhavirus	I	Hymenopteran rhabdo-related virus 38
Ohlsrhavirus	I	Ohlsdorf virus	Betahymrhavirus	I	Hymenopteran rhabdo-related virus 24
Perhabdovirus	V	Perch rhabdovirus	Betanemrhavirus	I	Hubei rhabdo-like virus 9
Sawgrhavirus	I	Long Island tick rhabdovirus	Betapaprhavirus	I	Spodoptera frugiperda rhabdovirus
Sigmavirus	I	Drosophila melanogaster sigmavirus	Betaricinrhavirus	I	Chimay rhabdovirus
Sprivivirus	V	Spring viremia of carp virus			
Sripuvirus	I, V	Niakha virus			
Sunrhavirus	I, V	Sunguru virus			
Tibrovirus	I, V	Tibrogargan virus			
Tupavirus	I, V	Durham virus			
Vesiculovirus	I, V	Vesicular stomatitis Indiana virus			
Zarhavirus	I	Zahedan rhabdovirus			

*Genera with bipartite genomes are marked with an asterisk.

members of the *Varicosavirus* and the *Dichorhavirus* genera, which have bipartite genomes and mostly produce nonenveloped virions.[291,471] The 2020 taxonomy of the International Committee on Taxonomy of Viruses recognizes a total of 3 subfamilies, 40 genera, and 246 species (Table 7.1).[297]

VIRION STRUCTURE

Rhabdoviruses are enveloped, rod- or cone-shaped particles (Fig. 7.2), approximately 100 to 430 nm long and 45 to 100 nm in diameter. Animal rhabdoviruses are usually approximately 180 nm long and 80 nm wide, but those isolated from plants can be longer. The length of the virion is dictated by the length of the RNA genome, so that incorporation of additional genes into the viral genome results in correspondingly longer virions. Typically, mature virions appear either as bullet-shaped particles with one rounded and one flattened end or as bacilliform particles that appear hemispheric at both ends.

The virions contain a single copy of the viral genome and at least five proteins. The genome is enwrapped into a homopolymer of nucleoprotein (N), thus forming a helical

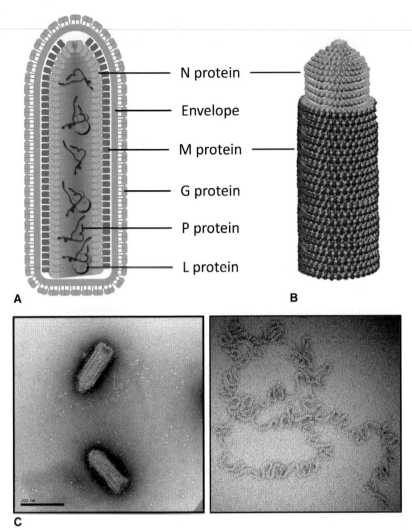

A

B

FIGURE 7.2 The viral particle. A: Representation of the viral particle of VSIV. The nucleocapsid, made of the viral genome enwrapped in a homopolymer of N proteins, is in a condensed helical conformation (*green*). A layer of matrix proteins (*violet*) coats the nucleocapsid and interacts with the lipid bilayer (*gray*). The exterior of the particle is decorated with trimeric transmembrane glycoproteins (*yellow*). Some L and P proteins are present in the particle. **B:** Model of the VSV nucleocapsid–M protein complex derived from cryoelectron microscopy data of Ge et al. (ref #194). **C:** Negative stain electron micrographs. VSIV virions (*left*), nucleocapsid (*right*).

C

ribonucleoprotein complex termed nucleocapsid. In the particles, the nucleocapsid is condensed into a bullet-shaped structure forming the core of the virions and is responsible for the particle's morphology (Fig. 7.2). This core is surrounded by matrix protein (M), which link the nucleocapsid to the membrane. Outside, the particles are decorated by transmembrane glycoproteins (G) required for entry of the virus into the host cell. The genome is negative sense and is delivered into cells as a ribonucleocapsid together with the viral polymerase complex, which comprises the catalytic large polymerase protein (L) and an essential phosphoprotein (P) cofactor. Biochemical estimates of the composition of VSIV virions indicated that they contain approximately 1,258 copies of N, 1826 of M, 1205 of G, 466 of P, and 50 copies of L.[528]

The structure of the nucleocapsid within the virions has been determined by cryo-electron microscopy to 10.6 Å and 15 Å resolution for VSIV[194] and RABV.[447] The orientation of N protein subunits of VSIV indicate that the 3′ end of the genome RNA is at the tip of the bullet, and the 5′ end is at the base. The conical tip of the VSIV bullet is formed by approximately seven successive turns of the N protein helix expanding gradually from 10 subunits per turn to 37.5 subunits per turn,

with two turns forming a helical repeat. This pattern continues for approximately 29 turns to form the cylindrical trunk of the bullet. For both VSV and RABV, the cryo-EM structures at the resolutions reported do not reveal details of the contacts, nor account for the full extent of M in the virion.

The lipids of the envelope are derived from the host cell membrane during virus assembly by budding. The lipid composition of the envelope generally reflects that of the host membrane from which the virus buds, consisting primarily of phospholipids and cholesterol, although virus envelopes appear to be enriched in cholesterol and sphingomyelin compared with the host membranes from which they were derived.[340]

GENOME ORGANIZATION AND ENCODED PROTEINS

Genomes of rhabdoviruses are single-stranded, nonsegmented RNA of negative polarity ranging from 10 to 16 kb. They lack a 5′ cap and a 3′ poly(A) tail and are fully encased by a nucleocapsid protein sheath and cannot function as templates for translation. The genome comprises a 3′ leader region, that functions as a promoter for transcription and replication, followed by adjacent genes separated by short nontranscribed intergenic regions and concludes with a trailer region, the complement of which functions as the promoter for genome synthesis (Fig. 7.3A). Rhabdoviruses possess at least five genes, always found in the same 3′-5′ order encoding the N, P, M, G, and L proteins. Each gene contains a gene start signal (GS) and a gene end signal (GE) required for the initiation and termination of transcription, respectively. The GE includes a homopolymeric U tract element that is reiteratively transcribed to generate the mRNA poly(A) tail. In some cases, the GS precedes the GE and the polymerase must scan the genome backward to reach the GS.[46] These signals are essential and show some degree of conservation (Fig. 7.3B). The length of the IR varies from one to about a hundred nucleotides but always starts and ends with a purine residue. The GS begins with two pyrimidine residues and have a U at position +4. In general, the 5′ and 3′ untranslated regions of the viral mRNA are short (10 to 50 nt).

Genomes from different genera differ in the number of additional open reading frames (ORFs, from five to more than ten ORFs) (Fig. 7.4). Additional ORFs can be found within the five essential genes as overlapping, alternative, or successive ORFs, and within additional genes. Sequence conservation suggests that some additional genes were generated by gene duplication.[551] The second ORF of a bicistronic mRNA can be translated by translational coupling.[551] Splicing of the mRNA has been reported for a member of *Culex tritaeniorhynchus* rhabdovirus (*Merhavirus*), which replicates in the cell nucleus.[302]

The Nucleoprotein

The N protein is an essential component of the RNA synthesis machinery since the viral polymerase can only use an encapsidated genome as a template.[54,153] Each N molecule covers nine nucleotides[12,207] although unlike the paramyxoviruses and the *rule of six*, there is no requirement that genomes of rhabdoviruses conform to a similar integer rule.[417]

In an infected cell, before its addition into a growing nucleocapsid, N is kept soluble by P. When expressed alone, N binds to and self-assembles on cellular RNAs, generat-

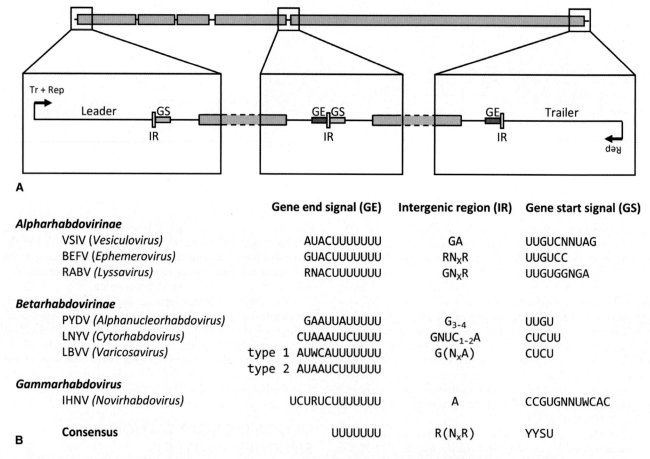

	Gene end signal (GE)	Intergenic region (IR)	Gene start signal (GS)
Alpharhabdovirinae			
VSIV (*Vesiculovirus*)	AUACUUUUUUU	GA	UUGUCNNUAG
BEFV (*Ephemerovirus*)	GUACUUUUUUU	RN_xR	UUGUCC
RABV (*Lyssavirus*)	RNACUUUUUUU	GN_xR	UUGUGGNGA
Betarhabdovirinae			
PYDV (*Alphanucleorhabdovirus*)	GAAUUAUUUUU	G_{3-4}	UUGU
LNYV (*Cytorhabdovirus*)	CUAAAUUCUUUU	$GNUC_{1-2}A$	CUCUU
LBVV (*Varicosavirus*)	type 1 AUWCAUUUUUUU	$G(N_xA)$	CUCU
	type 2 AUAAUCUUUUUU		
Gammarhabdovirus			
IHNV (*Novirhabdovirus*)	UCURUCUUUUUUU	A	CCGUGNNUWCAC
Consensus	UUUUUUU	$R(N_xR)$	YYSU

B

FIGURE 7.3 Transcription signals. A: Representation of a genome of rhabdoviruses. The five essential open reading frames are shown as *gray rectangles*. On the genome, the leader region contains a promoter for both transcription and replication. On the antigenome, the trailer region contains a replication promoter. Each gene starts with a gene start signal (GS) and ends with a gene end signal (GE). The genes are interspaced with nontranscribed intergenic regions (IR). **B:** Sequences of the transcription signals. For each subfamily, the consensus sequences of the GE, IR, and GS of representative members are shown. LBVV has two types of GE. The consensus sequences of the three subfamilies are shown on the last lane. PYDV: potato yellow dwarf virus, LNYV: lettuce necrotic yellows virus, LBVV: lettuce big-vein virus.

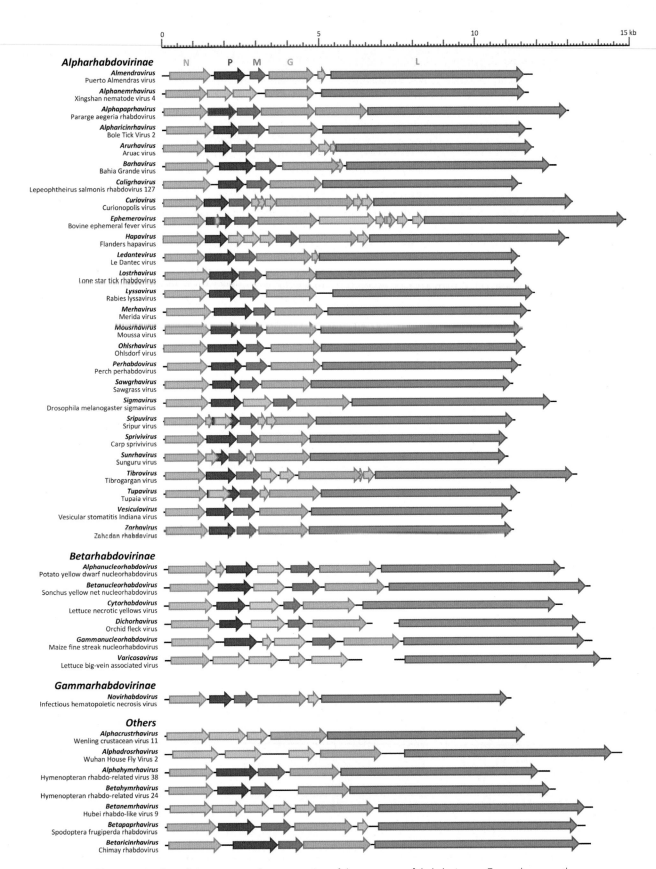

FIGURE 7.4 The organization of the genome. Representation of the genomes of rhabdoviruses. For each genus, the genome of one species is represented. Genes were drawn according to the GenBank files (GenBank accession numbers given by the 2020 taxonomy of the International Committee on Taxonomy of Viruses). The five common genes encoding for the N, P, M, G, and L proteins are colored in *green*, *red*, *violet*, *yellow*, and *blue*, respectively. For few genomes, the position of the N, P, M, or G genes has not yet been determined.

ing nucleocapsid-like structures.[252] These complexes can form closed rings, the atomic structures of which were determined for VSIV[207] and RABV.[12] The N protein comprises two globular domains (N-terminal (N_{NTD}) and C-terminal (N_{CTD}) domains) forming a groove that accommodates the RNA (Fig. 7.5A–D). An N-terminal arm (N_{arm}) and a loop (N_{loop}) protrude from the N_{NTD} and N_{CTD}, respectively. These extensions bind the adjacent N monomers and participate in oligomerization. Contacts between the N_{CTD} also contribute to the stability of the nucleocapsid. On one side of one N_i monomer, its N_{arm} interacts with both the N_{CTD} of the preceding N_{i-1}, and the N_{loop} of the N_{i-2}. On the other side, its N_{loop} interacts with both the N_{CTD} of the following N_{i+1}, and the N_{arm} of the N_{i+2} monomer. Thus, in the nucleocapsid, each N molecule interacts with four monomers (Fig. 7.5E). The structures are very stable and persist even after the removal of the RNA.[206,252]

The N protein interacts with both the backbone and some bases of the RNA. Depending on the register, the base can face the interior or exterior of the cavity.[12,207] For nucleocapsid-like rings and the condensed nucleocapsids in virions, the RNA molecule is found on the inside of the helix[194] (Fig. 7.5F). The nucleocapsid can adopt different conformations depending on the ionic strength, pH, or presence of M protein. When released from virions by treatment with detergents at high ionic strength, the nucleocapsid is loosely coiled and flexible (Fig. 7.2C), with a total length of 3.6 μm.[528] Upon diminution of the ionic strength and/or the pH, the nucleocapsid forms dense helical structures similar to the structures found in viral particles[129](Fig. 7.5F). Similarly, upon the addition of M, the nucleocapsid condenses into bullet-shaped structures.

The Phosphoprotein

The P protein interacts with both N and L and plays several key roles in the viral life cycle: it keeps N monomeric and soluble,[356] stabilizes and increases the processivity of the polymerase,[78,379] and recruits L on the nucleocapsid.[369] The P proteins of some rhabdoviruses also interact with cellular proteins to counteract innate immune responses.

The P protein is a modular protein composed of three main domains linked together with long intrinsically disordered regions (Fig. 7.6A and B).[197] The N-terminal domain (P_{NTD}) binds the monomeric RNA-free N protein (N^0).[91,359] Binding of the P_{NTD} to N prevents self-assembly of nucleocapsid-like structures and the binding to cellular RNA.[356] The N^0–P complexes are used as substrates for the encapsidation of nascent viral genomes during RNA replication.[242,424] The P_{NTD} is intrinsically disordered but a upon binding to N a short stretch of P adopts an alpha-helical conformation[325] (Fig. 7.6B and C).

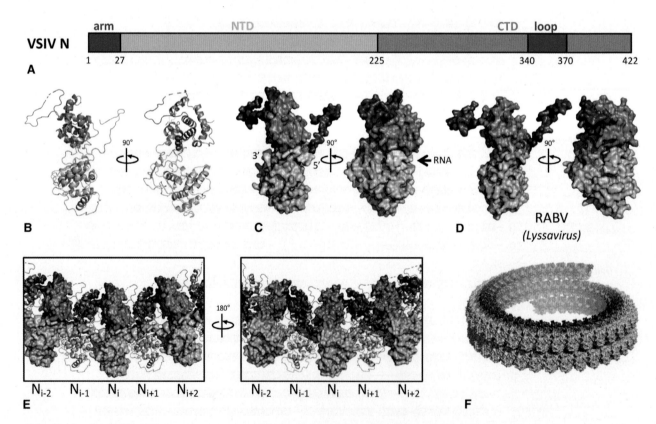

FIGURE 7.5 The nucleoprotein. A: Organization of the nucleoprotein of VSIV (NTD: N-terminal domain, CTD: C-terminal domain). **B:** Cartoon representation of the atomic structure of the VSIV nucleoprotein in the nucleocapsid conformation (PDB: 2WYY). **C:** Same as **(B)** in surface representation with the RNA in *gray*. **D:** Surface representation of the atomic structure of the nucleocapsid of RABV bound to RNA (PDB: 2GTT). **E:** Representation of the atomic structure of VSIV nucleocapsid with the RNA in *gray* and the N protomers in surface or cartoon representation. **F:** Surface representation of the structure of several turns of the condensed helical nucleocapsid of VSIV.

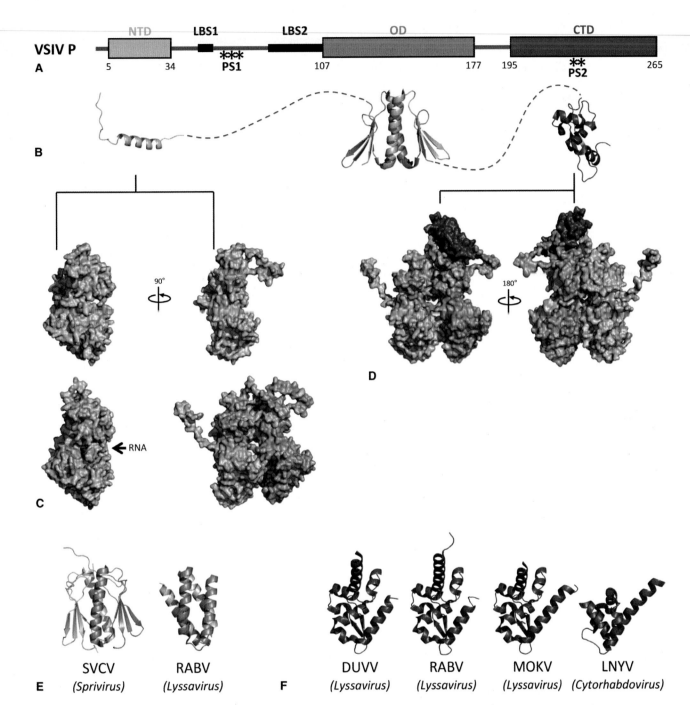

FIGURE 7.6 The phosphoprotein A: Organization of the phosphoprotein of VSIV (NTD: N-terminal domain, LBS1: L-binding site 1, LBS2: L-binding site 2, OD: oligomerization domain, CTD: C-terminal domain, PS1: phosphorylation site 1, PS2: phosphorylation site 2). **B:** Cartoon representation of the atomic structure of the VSIV P_{NTD} (PDB: 3PMK), P_{OD} (PDB: 2FQM), and P_{CTD} (PDB: 3HHZ). For the P_{OD}, one protomer is in *orange* and the other in *gray*. **C:** Surface representation of the atomic structure of the nucleoprotein (in *olive green*) in complex with the P_{NTD} (PDB: 3PMK) (*top*), the nucleoprotein in the nucleocapsid conformation with the RNA in the groove (*bottom left*), and two adjacent N protomers of the nucleocapsid (PDB: 2WYY) (*bottom right*). **D:** Surface representation of the atomic structure of the P_{CTD} in complex with two N protomers of the nucleocapsid (PDB: 3HHZ). **E:** Cartoon representation of the atomic structure of the P_{OD} of SVCV (PDB: 7C5Z) and RABV (PDB: 3L32). One protomer is in *orange* and the other in *gray*. **F:** Cartoon representation of the atomic structure of the P_{CTD} of DuvV (PDB: 7C21), RABV (PDB: 1VYI), MokV (PDB: 2WZL), and LNYV (PDB: 3T4R).

The N-terminus interacts with the N_{CTD} on the binding site of the N_{arm} of the adjacent N molecule in the nucleocapsid structure, thus preventing the oligomerization of N. The C-terminus of the P_{NTD} reaches the RNA-binding groove and blocks the binding to RNA (Fig. 7.6C).

The central domain, or oligomerization domain (P_{OD}), is responsible for the multimerization of the P. The P proteins of VSIV (*Vesiculovirus*), SVCV (*Sprivirus*), and RABV (*Lyssavirus*), all form dimers, but their respective P_{OD} adopt different structures[136,196,255,324] (Fig. 7.6B and E). In solution, each protomer of the P dimer can bind an N protein via their P_{NTD}.[587] For VSIV, the P_{OD} is not essential but may enhance viral replication, possibly by increasing the concentration of N^0 proteins at the site of encapsidation.[61,198] The C-terminal domain (P_{CTD}) binds the nucleocapsid, thus allowing the recruitment of the polymerase to its template. The structures of isolated P_{CTD} of RABV, MOKV, DUVV, LNYV, and VSIV have been determined by x-ray crystallography and NMR spectroscopy[23,205,354,358] (Fig. 7.6B and F). Although the sequence conservation is low, the structures are similar. The P_{CTD} of VSIV binds the N_{CTD} of two adjacent N proteins, thus explaining why P_{CTD} only binds N in the oligomerized form present on the template[205] (Fig. 7.6D).

The P protein also interacts and stabilizes L[78,369] and is essential for polymerase activity on the nucleocapsid. The L protein can synthesize short RNA products from a naked RNA template but P stimulates polymerase activity and processivity, with the template N required for full processivity.[379] For VSIV and RABV, the structure of L in complex with a fragment of the N-terminus of P was solved by cryo-electron microscopy.[241,263,331] Two fragments of P, located in the disordered region between the P_{NTD} and the P_{OD}, bind the polymerase (P_{LBS1} and P_{LBS2}) (Fig. 7.6A). A short peptide binds the C-terminal domain of L, and a second longer fragment meanders between different domains of L.

Phosphorylation of P by cellular kinases regulates polymerase activity.[45,89,285,502,516] VSIV P has two main phosphorylation sites (P_{PS}): residues S60, T62, S64 (P_{PS1}), phosphorylated by the casein kinase II, and S226, S227 (P_{PS2}), phosphorylated by an unidentified kinase[187] (Fig. 7.6A). Several studies show that phosphorylation of P_{PS1} enhances transcription but may be dispensable for replication.[419,516] VSIV P_{PS1} is located between the two L-binding sites and phosphorylation may affect the binding of P to L.[202] The P_{PS2}, located in the P_{CTD}, goes through cycles of phosphorylation/dephosphorylation and may play a role in genome replication.[248,419] RABV P is phosphorylated on S63 and S64 by an unknown kinase, and on S162, S210, and S271 by protein kinase C isomers.[210] Like VSIV P_{PS2}, S210 and S271 are also located in the P_{CTD} and their phosphorylation may affect the domain structure.[358] The tyrosine Y14 of VSIV P, which is essential for transcription and replication in a cell-based assay, can also be phosphorylated.[375]

The Matrix Protein

The matrix protein is one of the most abundant proteins in the virion[528] and binds to the nucleocapsid and lipid membranes.[24,143] At the right ionic strength, M condenses the nucleocapsid into a tightly coiled helical nucleocapsid–M protein complex sometimes referred to as the virus *skeleton*, which gives the virion its bullet-like shape.[368,389] When expressed alone, M causes invagination of the plasma membrane and release of vesicles.[330] Evidence also suggests that M interacts with the glycoprotein.[143,344,368]

The matrix protein is composed of a globular domain (M_{core}) preceded by a 40 to 60 amino acid-long N-terminal disordered region (M_{NTR}) (Fig. 7.7A).[190,203] Residues of the M_{NTR} participate in the M–N, M–M, and M–membrane interactions.[123,322,401] The atomic structure of M has been solved for VSIV, VSNJV, and LBV[191,203] (Fig. 7.7B and C). In the crystals of VSNJV and LBV M, a peptide of the M_{NTR} (M_{clip}) binds to the M_{core} of an adjacent M protein, which may mediate the self-association of M on the nucleocapsid.[203]

The structures of the core of the virions of VSIV and RABV have also been solved by cryo-electron microscopy.[194,447] For both viruses, the matrix proteins form a layer between the helical nucleocapsid and the envelope (Fig. 7.7D and E). The M interacts with N from two adjacent turns of the helix, thus stabilizing the helical conformation. Matrix proteins also interact with their neighboring M proteins from the same turn for RABV, and from both the same turn and the upstream and downstream turns for VSIV. The initial cryo-EM structure for VSV particles accounted for 1,200 of the 1,800 copies of M estimated to be present in the virion. The remaining 600 M protein subunits may be present in a nonhelical arrangement, thus rendering them undetectable in the analysis, or were not resolved clearly by the low resolution structure. One likely location is in association with the envelope lipid bilayer. M protein interacts with the lipid bilayer of the virus envelope, which was shown using lipophilic photoreactive probes.[322] The M protein sequences involved in the interaction are present in the N-terminal region, partially overlapping the sequences involved in interaction with the nucleocapsid.[123,322] This supports the idea that there are two populations of M protein in the virion, one involved in the nucleocapsid–M protein complex and the other involved in interaction with the envelope lipid bilayer.

A "late domain" in the form of a PPxY motif in their M_{NTR} (PPPY, aa 24 to 27, for VSIV and VSNJV, and PPEY, aa 35 to 38, for RABV). This motif plays a role in the release of the viral particles through engagement of host machinery.[222] The M protein also inhibits viral RNA synthesis[102] and as discussed later interacts with cellular proteins to inhibit host gene expression.

The Glycoprotein

The virus envelope contains approximately 300 to 400 spike-like projections composed of a single species of viral glycoprotein (G protein). The individual spikes are trimers of G,[192,572] which function in attachment and fusion of the virus envelope with endosome membranes. VSIV G protein is anchored in the envelope lipid bilayer by a 20–amino acid hydrophobic transmembrane domain near the C-terminus, which is followed by a 29–amino acid cytoplasmic domain, which is inside the virus envelope.[460] The structure of the 446–amino acid external domain (ectodomain) of VSV G has been determined by x-ray crystallography in both prefusion and postfusion conformations (Fig. 7.8).[453,454] Like other viral fusion proteins, the two conformations are dramatically different, indicating that major structural rearrangements must occur during the fusion process. Unlike the class I and class II fusion proteins exemplified by influenza A virus and flaviviruses, respectively, the conformational rearrangements in the glycoprotein are reversible in the absence of a target membrane. The two states exist in a dynamic equilibrium that is controlled by pH. The structure of the VSV G is homologous to that of GP64 of baculoviruses, the gB glycoprotein of herpesviruses, and the GP of thogotoviruses.

The Large Polymerase Protein

The L protein contains all the catalytic activities required for the transcription and replication of the viral genome: RNA synthesis,[154] addition of the cap to the mRNA,[3,327,404] methylation of the cap and the first nucleotide,[204,231,326,328,526] and polyadenylation.[246] Inhibitors of host cell chaperones including heat shock protein of 90 kDa (HSP90) suppress viral replication likely by impeding the correct folding of L.[110]

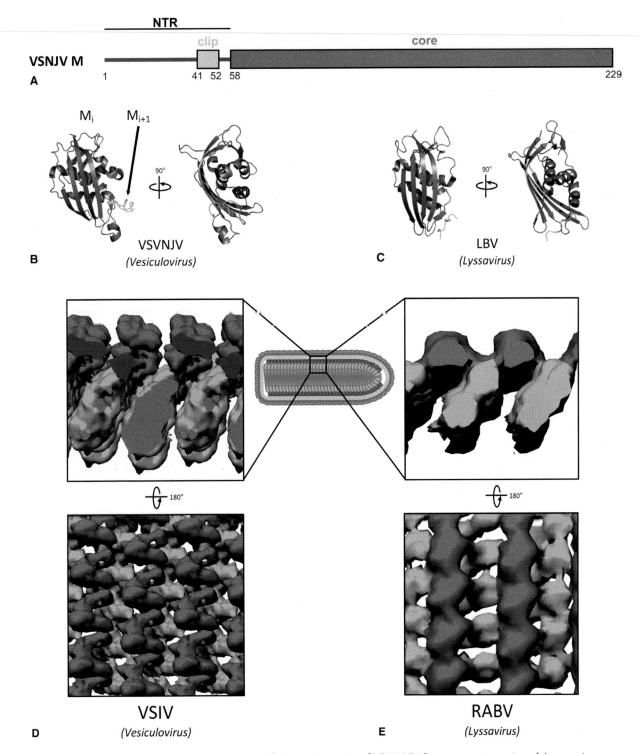

FIGURE 7.7 The matrix protein. A: Organization of the matrix protein of VSNJV. **B:** Cartoon representation of the atomic structure of the matrix protein of VSNJV with the M_{core} of one matrix protein (in *violet*) and the M_{clip} of an adjacent protein (in *yellow*) (PDB: 2W2R). **C:** Same as **(B)** for LBV (PDB: 2W2S). **D:** Density map of a portion of the VSIV particle (EMDB: EMD-1663). **E:** Same as **(D)** for RABV (EMDB: EMD-4995).

The first structure of L for any virus in the order *Mononega-virales* was provided by negative stain electron microscopy.[441] The L protein adopts a complex architecture with several globular domains linked together by flexible linkers, which adopt a preferred conformation when in complex with the P protein.[440] Subsequent use of electron cryo-microscopy provided atomic structural models of L in complex with a fragment of P for both VSIV and RABV.[241,263,331] The L protein comprises five structural domains: the RNA-dependent RNA polymerase (L_{RdRp}), capping (L_{Cap}), connector (L_{CD}), methyltransferase (L_{MT}), and C-terminal (L_{CTD}) domains (Fig. 7.9A). The overall structure is highly conserved between VSIV and RABV (Fig. 7.9B and C). The core of

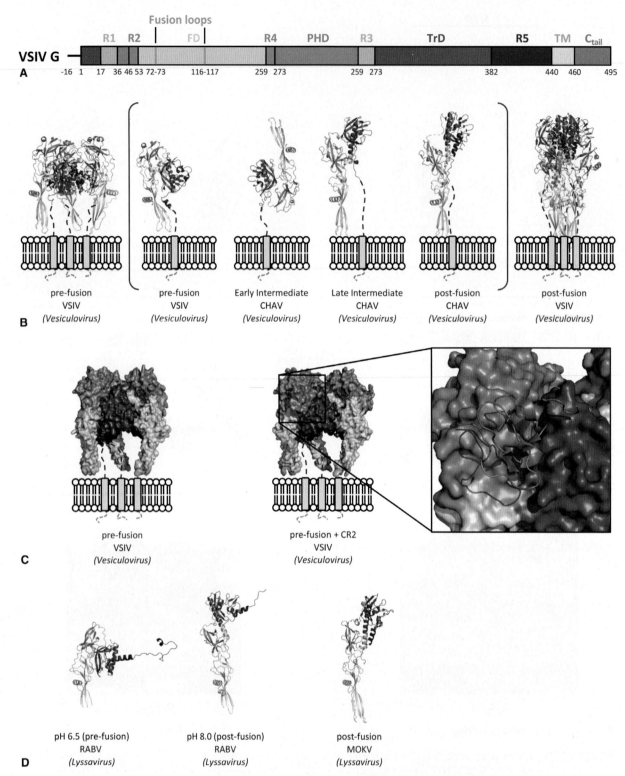

FIGURE 7.8 The glycoprotein protein. A: Organization of the glycoprotein of VSIV (TrD: trimerization domain, PHD: pleckstrin homology domain, FD: fusion domain, TM: transmembrane segment, C$_{tail}$: cytoplasmic tail). **B:** Cartoon representation of the atomic structure of the glycoprotein of vesiculoviruses in different conformations. *Left:* trimer of VSIV glycoprotein in the prefusion conformation (PDB: 5I2S). *Right:* trimer of VSIV glycoprotein in the postfusion conformation (PDB: 5I2M). A model of the glycoprotein conformation changes is shown in brackets. From left to right in the brackets: a protomer of the prefusion trimer of VSIV (PDB: 5I2S), a monomer of the glycoprotein of CHAV in an early intermediate conformation (PDB: 5MDM), in a late intermediate conformation (PDB: 5MDM), and a protomer of the postfusion trimer of CHAV (PDB: 4D6W). Blue and gray dotted lines represent the missing residues of the R5 segments and the C$_{tail}$, respectively. **C:** Surface representations of the prefusion trimer of VSIV alone (*left*, PDB: 5I2S) or in complex with the CR2 domain (*violet*) of the LDL-R (center, PDB: 5OYL). *Right:* enlargement with the CR2 domain in cartoon representation. **D:** Cartoon representations of a monomer of RABV glycoprotein crystallized at pH 6.5 (*left*, PDB: 6LGX) or at pH 8.0 (*center*, PDB: 6LGW). A monomer of the glycoprotein of MOKV in the postfusion conformation (*right*, PDB: 6TMR).

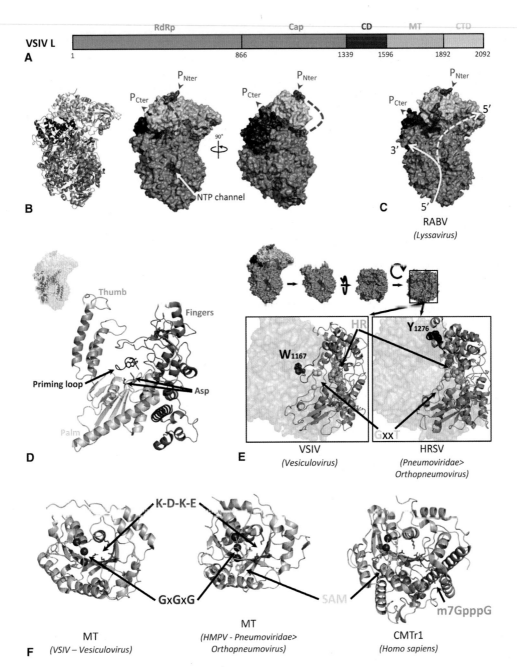

FIGURE 7.9 The polymerase protein. A: Organization of the polymerase of VSIV (RdRp: RNA-dependent RNA polymerase domain, Cap: capping domain, CD: connector domain, MT: methyltransferase domain, CTD: C-terminal domain). **B:** Cartoon and surface representations of the atomic structure of the polymerase of VSIV (PDB: 6U1X). Densities attributed to P are colored in *red*. The missing part between the two L-binding sites of P is shown as a *dotted line*. The orientation of P is shown with *arrows*. **C:** Same as **(B)** or the polymerase of RABV (PDB: 6UEB). The proposed internal paths of the template and the product are shown with *white solid* and *dotted arrows*, respectively. **D:** Cartoon representations of the right-hand structure forming the catalytic core of the RNA polymerase. The priming loop protrudes from the Cap domain into the catalytic cavity. The aspartic residues essential to the catalysis are shown with *red sticks*. **E:** Atomic structures of the VSIV (PDB: 6U1X) and HRSV polymerases (PDB: 6PZK). Top view of the RdRp and Cap domains with the RdRp represented with a transparent surface and the Cap domain with a cartoon. The priming loop is colored in *black*. The conserved aromatic residue of each priming loops, and the conserved residues of the "GxxT" and "HR" motifs, are shown with *spheres*. The "GxxT" and "HR" motifs are colored in *yellow* and *olive green*, respectively. **F:** Atomic structures of MT domain of VSIV (PDB: 6U1X) and HPMV (PDB: 4UCI) and the cellular methyltransferase CMTr1 (PDB: 4N49). The conserved "GxGxG" and "K-D-K-E" motifs are shown with *green spheres* and *red sticks*, respectively. On the HMPV MT and the CMTr1, the methyl group donor S-adenosylmethionine (SAM) is shown with *yellow sticks*. For CMTr1, the substrate is shown with *blue sticks*.

the molecule comprises the L_{RdRp} and L_{Cap} domains to which the three other globular domains are connected by flexible linkers. For VSIV, the L_{CD}, L_{MT}, and L_{CTD} domains can adopt different conformations and are stabilized onto the core by P.[440]

The L_{RdRp} domain contains a standard right-hand structure with the catalytic activity formed by the thumb, palm, and fingers subdomains (Fig. 7.9D). A priming loop protrudes from the L_{Cap} domain and enters the catalytic cavity to facilitate initiation of RNA synthesis.[331] Consistent with this an aromatic residue at the tip of the priming loop (W1180 for RABV and W1167 for VSIV) is required for efficient initiation from the 3'-terminus of the genome.[402]

Unlike the guanylyl transferase activity used by eukaryotic cells to cap their mRNA, L employs a unique polyribonucleotide transferase activity (PRNTase).[327,403,404] During transcription, the nascent 5' triphosphate RNA is covalently linked to the histidine residue of a conserved "HR" motif in the L_{Cap} domain.[327,405] The polyribonucleotide is then transferred onto GDP, possibly bound at the conserved "GxxT" motif. For VSIV, addition of the cap-structure requires a nascent mRNA chain length of 31-nucleotides.[522] Failure to cap the nascent RNA results in premature termination of transcription,[327,509] underscoring the intimate connection between these two functional domains of L. The structure of L of parainfluenza virus 5 (*Paramyxoviridae* family),[1] human metapneumovirus,[415] and human respiratory syncytial virus (both from the *Pneumoviridae* family)[79,200] shows the priming loop is retracted from the L_{RdRp} cavity. In this conformation, the conserved "GxxT" motif located at the base of the priming loop is brought closer to the "HR" motif, thus potentially creating the catalytic site of the capping enzyme (Fig. 7.9E). Mutational analysis of residues in the priming loop of VSV L support a role in both RNA synthesis initiation and mRNA capping.[327,402]

The L protein catalyzes the addition of methyl groups onto the N-7 position of the guanine of the cap and the 2'-O of the ribose of the first nucleotide, yielding a m^5GpppN_m structure.[526] The L_{MT} domain shares a similar fold with cellular and viral 2'-O methyltransferases[331,411] (Fig. 7.9F). A "GxGxG" motif implicated in the binding to the S-adenosylmethionine (SAM), the methyl group donor, and the "K-D-K-E" catalytic tetrad are conserved. However, the mechanism of methylation of the viral mRNA cap is unusual. Instead of having separate enzymes that catalyze either ribose 2'-O methylation or guanine-N-7 methylation, both activities reside in a single domain of L.[204,326,328] This domain has a single SAM-binding site and transfers the methyl groups in an unconventional order, in which 2'-O methylation precedes and facilitates guanine-N-7 methylation.[439] Abolition of cap methylation by treatment with S-adenosylhomocysteine or mutation of key residues in the L_{MT} domain is also accompanied by the hyperpolyadenylation of mRNAs, thus further highlighting the interconnection between the different catalytic activities of L.[439,459]

The L_{CD} and L_{CTD} are thought to participate in the structural organization of the domains and the conformation changes occurring during transcription and replication.[1,331] Two fragments of P bind the L protein: a first short peptide binds to the top of the L_{CTD} (P_{LBS1}) and a second longer segment meanders between the L_{RdRp}, L_{CD}, and L_{CTD} domains (P_{LBS2}) (Fig. 7.9B and C). For VSIV, the tyrosine 53 of the P_{LBS1} binds to a cavity in the L_{CTD} and is essential for viral growth but dispensable for transcription, thus suggesting the P_{LBS1}–L_{CTD} interaction may play a role in the replication of the genome.[263]

STAGES OF REPLICATION

The replication cycle of rhabdoviruses is typical of that of most nonsegmented, negative-strand RNA viruses (Fig. 7.10). The initial events of attachment, endocytosis, endosome acidification, and fusion of the viral and cellular membranes result in the release of the viral nucleocapsid into the cytoplasm of the host cell. The encapsidated parental genome RNA serves as a template for primary transcription by the virion polymerase, resulting in the synthesis of all viral mRNAs. These mRNAs are translated by the host translation machinery and newly made polymerases participate in primary transcription. The accumulation of viral proteins leads to replication of the genome, which involves synthesis and encapsidation of full-length positive-strand RNA, or antigenomes. The antigenomes, in turn, serve as templates for the synthesis of progeny negative-strand genomes. Progeny nucleocapsids are used for three different purposes: as templates for further rounds of replication; as templates for secondary transcription, which is the major amplification step for viral gene expression; and for assembly into progeny virions, which occurs by budding from host membranes. In single-cycle growth of virus in cells in culture, the early events including attachment, endocytosis, membrane fusion, and primary transcription occur within the first few hours postinfection. The processes of genome replication, secondary transcription, and virus assembly occur continuously throughout the remainder of the infectious cycle, which lasts for an additional 12 to 18 hours for VSIV or several days for RABV.

Mechanism of Attachment

Rhabdoviruses appear to use a variety of different receptors for attachment to different types of host cells. The RABV G protein binds most effectively to cells of neuronal origin[537] reflecting the neurotropism of RABV *in vivo*. Several different surface molecules expressed at high levels on neurons have been identified as potential receptors, including the nicotinic acetyl choline receptor[189] the neural cell adhesion molecule (CD56),[530] low-affinity nerve-growth factor receptor p75NTR,[538] integrin-β1,[492] and metabotropic glutamate receptor 2.[553] Expression of CD56 and p75NTR confer susceptibility to RABV on cells that are normally resistant to infection. Transgenic mice that lack CD56 show a delay in RABV spread through the central nervous system (CNS) and in RABV-induced mortality, but the mice still die following virus infection[530] indicating that other receptors are involved. RABV infection of transgenic mice that lack p75NTR was found to be similar to that of wild-type mice of the same strain indicating that p75NTR was not an important receptor for RABV pathogenesis. However, RABV G protein binds to a region of p75NTR that is present on a splice variant of p75NTR that is still expressed in the transgenic mice.[311] RABV can also use receptors that are widely distributed among many cell types.[514,585] The importance of the identified molecules in rabies infection and pathogenesis remains to be resolved.

VSV also binds to many different cell types in culture by interactions that appear to be of low affinity and often are not easily saturable. Negatively charged lipids were proposed to be cellular receptors for virus attachment including phosphatidyl serine.[476] The mammalian cell receptor for VSV was identified as low-density lipoprotein receptor (LDLR),[168] and the structure

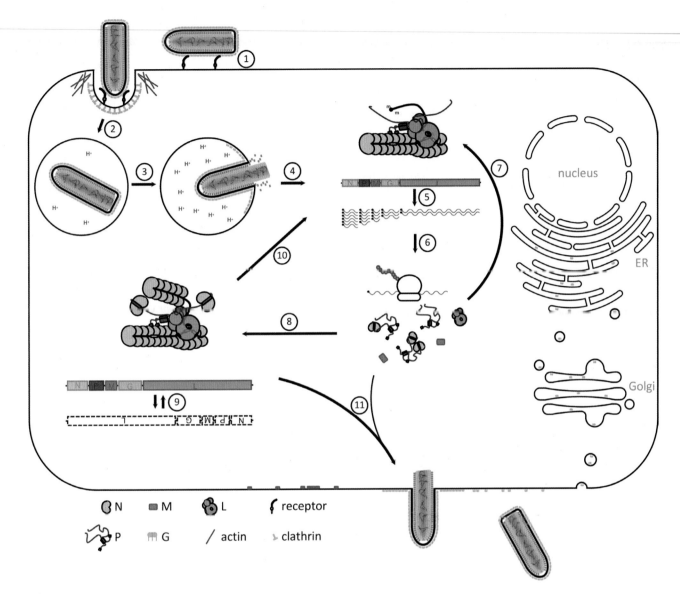

FIGURE 7.10 The viral life cycle. (*1*) The virion comes into contact with a host cell and the glycoproteins bind to their receptors. (*2*) The virion enters the cell through endocytosis using a clathrin- and actin-depend mechanism. (*3*) The pH decreases inside the endosome which triggers conformation changes of the glycoproteins and fusion of the viral and cellular membranes. (*4*) The content of the virion is released in the cytoplasm and matrix proteins dissociate from the nucleocapsid. (*5*) Primary transcription: the encapsidated genome is transcribed by the polymerase complexes present in the virion. (*6*) Viral mRNAs are translated by the host cell machinery. (*7*) Newly made polymerases transcribe the genome and increase primary transcription. (*8*) Once the N protein concentration reaches a certain threshold, the polymerase replicates the genome and uses N^0–P complexes to encapsidate the nascent RNA. (*9*) The antigenomes are used as a template to generate viral genomes. (*10*) Secondary transcription: newly made genomes are used as a template for transcription. (*11*) Nucleocapsids are transported to the cytoplasmic membrane where they assemble with M and G proteins into viral particles.

of the glycoprotein in complex with domains of LDLR receptor resolved.[393]

Attachment of VSV and RABV to cells is markedly enhanced at lower pH in the range from pH 6.5 to 5.6.[182,585] The pH dependence of attachment is similar to that of envelope fusion with cellular membranes, although fusion occurs most efficiently at slightly lower pH than attachment. Furthermore, G protein mutations that shift the pH dependence of fusion also shift the pH dependence of attachment.[182] This suggests that attachment to many cell types is mediated by G protein in a conformation that is similar to the fusion-active form of the

viral G protein. Imaging single virion attachment and hemifusion by TIRF microscopy on supported planar bilayers identifies that particles undergo an initial reversible engagement with the target membrane at pH 6.8 that depends on the hydrophobic fusion loops.[282] Earlier work had identified the hydrophobic loops of G are inserted into target membranes under the optimal conditions for both attachment and fusion.[148,413] This would also account for the affinity of the VSV G protein for phosphatidyl serine and other negatively charged phospholipids, because the presence of negatively charged lipids in the target membrane appears to be necessary for virus envelope fusion.[151]

Mechanism of Penetration

VSV and RABV are internalized into cells by clathrin-dependent endocytosis.[357,427] Following attachment to host cell surfaces, virions are internalized through clathrin-coated pits[120,264] where they undergo endocytosis into coated vesicles (Fig. 7.10, steps 1 and 2). Rhabdovirus particles are longer than the typical diameter of a coated vesicle, the final closure of the endocytic vesicle requires participation of the actin cytoskeleton.[120,121] The contents of early endosomes are transported to late endosomes and lysosomes for degradation. During this process, the endosomal vesicles often invaginate to form multiple intraluminal vesicles or multivesicular bodies (MVBs). As virions progress through the endocytic pathway, they are exposed to progressively lower pH. At a pH threshold of 6.2, the G protein mediates fusion of the viral envelope with the endosome membrane. This fusion event releases the internal virion components into the cytoplasm (Fig. 7.10, steps 3 and 4). Most of the available evidence indicates that VSV virions fuse primarily with the membranes of early endosomes.[264,373] Other evidence, however, suggests that many fusion events occur within MVBs, releasing the internal virion contents into the cytoplasmic contents trapped within the MVBs and requiring back-fusion of internal vesicles with the limiting membrane of the MVBs to release the viral nucleocapsid into the cytoplasm of the cell.[315] Viral proteins that fail to be released into the cytoplasm are degraded by proteases and other enzymes in lysosomes.[357] During infection of neuronal cells by RABV, evidence suggests that fusion and content release requires endocytic transport to the cell body.[428]

The mechanism by which rhabdovirus G proteins induce fusion of the virus envelope with cellular membranes shares many features with other viral envelope fusion proteins but is distinct. The VSV G protein and the structurally similar fusion proteins of herpesviruses, baculoviruses, and thogotoviruses are referred to as class III fusion proteins to distinguish them from class I proteins, which are structurally similar to the influenza virus hemagglutinin, and class II proteins, which include the envelope glycoproteins of the alphaviruses, flaviviruses, and some bunyaviruses.[30] As with class I fusion proteins, rhabdovirus G proteins exist as a trimer of subunits held together by noncovalent bonds (Fig. 7.8, B and C).[138,192,572] Unlike most viral envelope proteins, however, the subunits of G protein are in a dynamic equilibrium between monomers and trimers because of the rapid dissociation and reassociation of subunits.[347] As with most low pH-dependent fusion proteins, the effects of low pH are mediated by conformational changes in G. Unlike other viral fusion proteins, the conformational changes in G protein are reversible upon returning the pH to neutrality, whereas those of class I and II viral fusion proteins are not reversible.[138,193]

A general principle by which viral envelope proteins promote fusion is that they must insert into the target membrane through a region of their sequence referred to as the fusion peptide. In the class I fusion proteins, such as the influenza virus hemagglutinin (HA) and the paramyxovirus F proteins, the fusion peptide resides at the N-terminus of one of the subunits (HA2 or F1, respectively) generated by proteolysis of an inactive precursor. In contrast, proteolysis of rhabdovirus G proteins is not involved in activating fusion. This is similar to the case of the class II fusion proteins, in which the fusion peptide appears to be an internal region of the protein sequence. The regions of G protein that insert into target membranes at low pH were first mapped using photoactivatable

lipid probes and mutagenesis studies in both the RABV and VSV G proteins.[148,181,513] These sequences form two loops containing hydrophobic amino acids that extend from the protein structure ("fusion loops," Fig. 7.8A and B). In the neutral pH "prefusion" state, the fusion loops are oriented toward the viral membrane. Upon lowering the pH, there is a proposed intermediate, in which the domain containing the fusion loops is reoriented to insert into the target membrane (Fig. 7.8B). Fusion of the viral and target membrane involves another domain rearrangement that brings the two membranes together in the "postfusion" state.

A second region of the G protein sequence functionally involved in fusion is the membrane-proximal ectodomain sequence immediately N-terminal to the membrane anchor sequence. Most of this sequence is not visible in the x-ray structures, because it was cleaved to solubilize the G protein. Mutations in this region dramatically inhibit fusion.[262] G protein truncations containing part of this region (amino acids 421 to 461) together with the membrane anchor sequence and the cytoplasmic domain (G stems) enhance the fusion activity of other membrane fusion proteins and are able to cause hemifusion (mixing of the outer phospholipid leaflets of the two membranes).[262]

Uncoating and Primary Transcription

Following fusion of the virus envelope with endosome membranes, which releases the internal virion components into the cytoplasm of the host cell, the viral M protein dissociates from the nucleocapsid[123,373] (Fig. 7.10 step 4). This step is necessary for viral RNA synthesis to occur because M protein inhibits viral transcription.[102] The binding of most of the M protein to nucleocapsids is readily reversible,[345] and dissociation following envelope fusion is believed to occur spontaneously, although acidification of the virion interior appears to promote M protein dissociation from the nucleocapsid, similar to the M1 protein of influenza virus.[372] Rhabdoviruses do not encode a separate ion channel protein analogous to the M2 protein of influenza viruses. Instead, the G protein is responsible for the permeability of the envelope to protons.[372] Following dissociation of M, the ribonucleoproteins complex of the N-RNA template associated with the L-P polymerase is competent for transcription.

The first biosynthetic step in the viral replicative cycle is primary transcription (Fig. 7.10, step 5). The mechanism of primary transcription, defined as transcription from the parental template, appears to be identical to that of secondary transcription, or transcription from progeny templates following genome replication. The viral RNA polymerase is fully competent to synthesize all of the viral mRNAs without new synthesis of viral proteins, as shown by the transcriptase activity of virion cores following solubilization of the envelope.[41] This cell-free transcriptase system led to the dissociation of the virion into components that established the requirement for both the L and P proteins for RNA polymerase activity[154] and the requirement that the template RNA be encapsidated.[153]

Using this detergent activated transcription system, the gene-order of VSV was deduced by measuring the effect of ultra-violet irradiation on the accumulation of viral transcripts. Surprisingly, the only gene that showed inactivation kinetics similar to its physical size was that of the N gene with the P, M, and G genes having a target size of 2 to 4 times their physical size. This led to the conclusion that a single entry point exists for the viral RNA polymerase at the 3' end of the genome, and the viral mRNAs are transcribed in sequence N-P-M-G-L, which corresponds to the order they appear in the viral genome.[2,40] Two possible models could account for this finding, either nucleolytic processing of a precursor to yield individual viral mRNAs or sequential transcription where polymerase stops transcribing the upstream gene before starting transcription of the downstream gene. The stop–start model for sequential transcription became widely accepted and identification of specific cis-acting signals in the template RNA sequence that govern the activities of the transcriptase complex at each gene junction strongly support the model (Figs. 7.3 and 7.11A). Those signals and their functions are described below.

During transcription, the polymerase recognizes a 3' promoter within the 50-nt leader region.[497] Initiation at the 3' terminus of the genome yields a 47-nucleotide leader RNA that contains an uncapped 5' triphosphate and lacks a poly(A) tail (Fig. 7.11A).[104] Initiation at the 3' end of the genome requires a conserved tryptophan residue within a priming loop of the L_{Cap} that projects into the active site of the L_{RdRP}.[402] The priming loop likely stabilizes the initiation complex and facilitates the first catalytic event of formation of the 5' pppApC. Following termination of synthesis of the leader RNA, the stop–start model of sequential transcription posits that the polymerase can then initiate at the N gene-start to generate the N mRNA. Accordingly, the obligatorily sequential transcription would require that leader is always synthesized in excess of N, which is inconsistent with findings for a VSIV mutant (polR1) that synthesizes N mRNA in excess over leader RNA.[97] This discrepancy led to an examination of the requirement for the synthesis of the leader RNA prior to sequential transcription of the viral

genes. By insertion of a short 60-nt synthetic gene between the 50-nt leader promoter and the 1.3 kb N gene, it was possible to apply the technique of UV mapping to determine whether transcription of the first gene required prior transcription of the leader. In the cell-free system, synthesis of leader RNA was required for transcription of the short gene, but in cells, the UV target size of the short gene was independent of the leader.[569]

Each viral gene starts with a GS, which functions as a signal for initiation of the mRNA, and in the corresponding sequence of the nascent mRNA strand functions as key cis-acting sequences for mRNA capping.[481,509,554] The tryptophan of the L priming loop that is required for the initiation at the 3' end of the genome is not required for initiation at internal GS sites.[402] One possible interpretation of this findings is that during initiation at a gene-start sequence, the priming loop is retracted, as seen in the structures of the paramyxovirus polymerases. In contrast to initiation at the 3' end of the genome, the nascent mRNA is modified by the L mRNA capping machinery and this process is intimately coupled to subsequent transcriptional elongation. Sequence differences in the first 5-nt of the leader RNA versus an mRNA serve as a cis-acting signal for mRNA cap addition in the latter. For VSV, addition of the mRNA cap requires a nascent mRNA chain length of 31-nucleotides[522] (Fig. 7.11A, step iii) but does not require further elongation for subsequent cap methylation by the L_{MT} (Fig. 7.11A, step iv).

Termination of transcription is coupled with polyadenylation and is governed by a conserved GE sequence. That sequence fails to be recognized unless it is positioned a minimum of 60-nt from the gene-start sequence. During transcriptional termination, an element of the GE sequence signals the polymerase to "stutter" on the U track, which provides

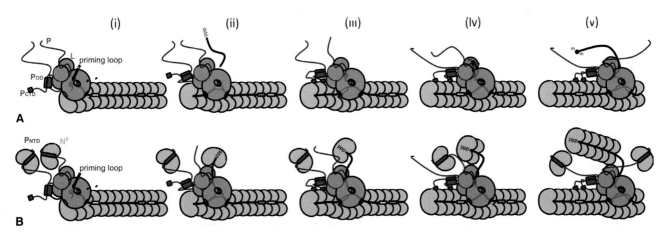

FIGURE 7.11 Models of the transcription and replication. A: Models of the transcription. (i) The polymerase, in complex with a dimer of phosphoproteins, engages the encapsidated genome at its 3' end. The priming loop is inserted in the RdRp cavity to facilitate RNA synthesis initiation. (ii) The polymerase synthesizes the leader RNA with a 5' triphosphate and releases it upon recognition of the first gene start sequence (GS, in *yellow*). (iii) The polymerase re-initiates RNA synthesis on the GS. The priming loop is no longer required for the internal RNA synthesis initiation. The 5' end of the nascent RNA reaches the catalytic site of the Cap domain where a cap is added. (iv) The nascent RNA reaches the methyltransferase domain where the cap and the first nucleotide are methylated. (v) The polymerase recognizes the gene end signal (GE, in *violet*), adds a poly(A) tail, and releases the mRNA. The polymerase then scans the genome to find the next GS. **B:** Model of the replication. (i) The replication complex is made of a polymerase in complex with a dimer of phosphoproteins bound to N⁰ proteins via their P_{NTD}. The polymerase engages the encapsidated genome at its 3' end. The priming loop is inserted in the RdRp cavity to facilitate RNA synthesis initiation. (ii, iii) The polymerase synthesizes the leader RNA with a 5' triphosphate and adds N proteins to the nascent RNA. (iv, v) In this context, the polymerase does not recognize the GS and GE sequences and generates a full-length encapsidated copy of the genome.

the mRNA a poly(A) tail[47,48] of roughly 50 to 200 residues[150] (Fig. 7.11A, step v). Precisely how the polymerase transitions from reiterative copying of the U tract to termination is unclear. Occasionally, the termination signal is ignored, resulting in read-through by the polymerase to give a polycistronic transcript.[48,232] The fate of the polymerase that terminates at a gene-end sequence is uncertain, but in most cases, the polymerase traverses the IR and resumes transcription at the GS of the downstream gene. Approximately 20% to 30% of transcriptase complexes fail to resume transcription of the downstream gene, however, and presumably dissociate from the template, leading to a 20% to 30% attenuation of expression of the downstream gene at each gene junction.[256] This transcription attenuation results in a gradient of mRNA and protein expression, such that the abundance of each gene product depends on its distance from the 3' end of the genome (Fig. 7.10, step 5).

Transcription attenuation is a hallmark of nonsegmented, negative-strand RNA viruses and is the major mechanism regulating the abundance of the individual mRNA. The importance of the gene order in regulating the relative levels of viral proteins was dramatically illustrated by genetic engineering experiments to change the order of the genes of VSIV. The resulting changes in the relative abundance of the viral proteins resulted in substantial reductions in viral replication and pathogenesis.[39,564] The similarity of the basic mechanisms in virus replication among nonsegmented, negative-strand RNA viruses and their dependence on the relative levels of each viral protein presumably accounts for the conservation of the basic gene order among these viruses.

For VSIV, by 6 hours postinfection, the viral mRNAs represent more than 60% of the total mRNA in the host cell.[335,388] Although the viral mRNAs are chemically identical to cellular mRNAs (i.e., capped and polyadenylated), the mechanism of their translation is different. Indeed, the dephosphorylation of the translation factor eIF4E and the activation of its repressor 4E-BP during VSIV infection reduce the translation of cellular mRNAs but not viral mRNAs.[107] Similarly, silencing of eIF4GI and eIF4GII decreases cellular translation while the translation of VSIV mRNAs is not affected.[561] Inversely, silencing of the large ribosomal subunit protein rpL40 only inhibits translation of the viral mRNAs.[316] However, like cellular mRNAs, viral mRNAs translation still depends on some cellular eIF factors since phosphorylation of eIF2α inhibits VSIV translation.[108] The insensitivity of viral mRNA to translation inhibition does not depend on cis-acting sequences on the mRNA but depends on their transcription by the viral polymerase.[570] The M protein of RABV also inhibits canonical translation through its interaction with eIF3h.[289]

Genome Replication

A fundamental principle in replication of nonsegmented, negative-strand RNA viruses is that the ability of the polymerase to replicate the viral genome depends on new viral protein synthesis to encapsidate the newly synthesized RNA (Fig. 7.10, steps 8 and 9). For example, treating infected cells with inhibitors of protein synthesis (e.g., cycloheximide) allows the synthesis of viral mRNA but inhibits replication of genome RNA.[243,563] The critical viral protein required for replication is the N protein, as shown by its ability to support the synthesis of genome RNA in the cell-free system.[420] In infected cells, however, both P and N are required since P interacts with N to maintain the nucleoprotein in a monomeric and soluble conformation so that the nascent genomes and antigenomes can be encapsidated.[356,423]

During replication, the polymerase initiates RNA synthesis at the 3' end of the genome, ignores the GEs, IRs, and GSs, and synthesizes a full-length copy of the genome (Fig. 7.11B). Using the same strategy, the antigenome is used as a template to synthesize new encapsidated genomes from the replication promoter at its 3' terminus. In addition to serving as a template for progeny genomes, the antigenome can be used as a template to generate a short, uncapped, nonpolyadenylated RNA complementary to the 3' end of the antigenome that is analogous to the leader RNA. Variously called the *minus strand leader* or *trailer* RNA, this RNA is found in small amounts in infected cells and is the primary product produced in the cell-free system when antigenomes are used as templates in the absence of a source of new viral proteins.[323,562]

The critical cis-acting RNA sequences that govern replication are located in the leader and trailer regions of the genome and antigenome, respectively (Fig. 7.3A). These sequences in the templates serve as promoters to initiate RNA synthesis, and their complementary sequences at the 5' end of the product RNA serve as encapsidation signals, with the resulting encapsidation permitting elongation of the RNA into full-length products. The sequences required for encapsidation have been mapped using cell-based replication assays and synthetic RNA in cell-free encapsidation assays.[382,417,568] The sequences in the templates that serve as promoters for replication and transcription have been defined by mutagenesis studies.[417,565,568] The 3' termini of the genome and antigenome of VSIV are identical at 15 of 18 positions. These 18 nucleotides are essential elements of both the genomic and antigenomic promoters. The extensive similarity between the 3' termini of the genome and antigenome led to the suggestion that complementarity between the termini may serve an important role in viral gene expression. In cell-based reconstitution assays conducted with VSV, enhanced complementarity between the termini correlated with an increased in the abundance of replication products.[565] Although it was concluded that base pairing of the termini is an important element of promoter recognition by the VSIV RNA polymerase, there is no direct evidence to show that the genomic termini are involved in an interaction that drives replication.

The genomic and antigenomic promoters of VSIV differ substantially at positions 19 to 29 and 34 to 46. These sequences in the genomic promoter are required for mRNA synthesis, but not for replication.[329,565,568] The different promoters help ensure that replication is asymmetric such that an excess of genomes are synthesized in virus-infected cells. The functional differences between the genomic and antigenomic promoters were exploited to engineer an *ambisense* RABV that contained the sequence of the genomic promoter at the 3' ends of both the genome and antigenome.[166] The promoter in the antigenome of this virus was engineered to drive the transcription of a foreign gene. As a result, both the genome and antigenome of this virus were used as templates for mRNA synthesis—the genome as a template for the five viral mRNAs and the antigenome as a template for the foreign mRNA. Furthermore, the normal asymmetry of replication was abolished, so that genomes and antigenomes were synthesized in approximately equal amounts.

The mechanism underlying the transition between transcription and replication is not yet clearly established.

The encapsidation of the nascent genomes and antigenomes suggests the concentration of N^0–P could regulate the transition. In agreement with this idea, diminution of the level of monomeric N^0 proteins in the host cell inhibits genome replication.[22] In the early stages of the viral life cycle, when the concentration of N^0–P complexes is low, the nascent leader RNA is not encapsidated, which triggers its release and the re-initiation of transcription on the next GS. Later in the cycle, with the increasing concentration of N^0–P, the leader RNA is fully encapsidated, which suppresses termination of RNA synthesis until the polymerase reaches the 5′ end of the genome[22,62] (Fig. 7.11B).

However, other factors modulate the transition between transcription and replication. The matrix protein of RABV has been shown to inhibit transcription in favor of genome replication.[167] The composition of the "transcriptase" and "replicase" complexes may be distinct. Indeed, as discussed earlier, the phosphorylation status of P differently affects transcription and replication. Moreover, different complexes involving L and P have been identified. An L–P–N complex was detected in insect cells and proposed to be the replicase.[211] The structures of the polymerase complex of VSIV compared to PIV5 highlight the conformational differences in L.[1] It will be of significant interest to determine whether there are conformational rearrangements in the polymerase complex during the different modes of RNA synthesis.

Secondary Transcription

Once nucleocapsids containing progeny genomes begin to accumulate in infected cells, they are used as templates for secondary transcription, and they are assembled into progeny virions (Fig. 7.10, steps 10 and 11). In the case of VSIV, most of the viral nucleocapsids that are made during the infectious cycle remain associated with infected cells and are not released in the form of progeny virions,[501] suggesting that use of these nucleocapsids as templates predominates over their use for virion assembly. Although conceptually it is the last step in the virus replication cycle, for VSIV assembly begins at approximately the same time as secondary transcription, around 2 to 3 hours postinfection, reaches a maximum rate around 8 to 10 hours postinfection when viral protein synthesis is at its maximum and declines concomitantly with a decline in viral protein synthesis toward the end of the infectious cycle around 16 to 20 hours postinfection.

Viral Replication Compartment

Studies of the subcellular localization of the viral proteins in infected cells have defined that the N, P, and L proteins of VSV and RABV are present within a fluid-like compartment that is not associated with membranes.[223,310,484] These compartments resemble Negri bodies, first observed in neurons of postmortem samples of patients with rabies. For both VSV and RABV, these inclusions have been shown to be sites of RNA synthesis, with subsequent transport of the mRNA for translation.[223,310] The compartments share properties with phase-separated structures in that they undergo fission and fusion.[224,394] Similar organized replication sites have been reported for many other mononegaviruses. A promising avenue of further investigation is exemplified by work with respiratory syncytial virus demonstrates that molecules that inhibit the fluidity of these compartments are antiviral.[449] The transport of viral components within cells for the replication and assembly of virions is a central and incompletely understood aspect of the viral replicative cycle. Work with VSV demonstrates that the viral nucleocapsids are rapidly transported within the cells on microtubular networks[223,224,588] and undergo "hopping" from one location to another.[238] How such processes relate to gene expression and virus assembly remains uncertain.

Assembly of Progeny Virions

As with most viruses, the individual components of rhabdoviruses are assembled in separate cellular compartments and only come together in the final steps of virus assembly: the nucleocapsid is assembled during the process of RNA replication as described in the previous section, the G protein is assembled in the secretory pathway, and the M protein is synthesized as a soluble protein that then associates with the cytoplasmic surface of the host plasma membrane.[286]

Assembly of G Protein

The assembly of the VSV G protein in the secretory pathway of host cells has been studied for many years by both virologists and cell biologists, not only for its importance for virus assembly but also as a prototype for the assembly of other host and viral integral membrane proteins. G protein is synthesized by ribosomes bound to the rough endoplasmic reticulum (ER) and is inserted into the ER membrane in the typical *type I* orientation.[460] An N-terminal signal sequence of 16 amino acids targets the protein for insertion and is cleaved from the nascent polypeptide.[333] The new N-terminus and most of the protein sequence (446 amino acids) are transferred to the luminal side of the ER membrane to form the protein's ectodomain.[278] A hydrophobic sequence of 20 amino acids near the C-terminus serves as a stop–transfer sequence and becomes the membrane anchor.[460] The 29 C-terminal amino acids remain on the cytoplasmic side of the ER membrane and form the protein's cytoplasmic domain.[278] Two asparagine residues in G protein are glycosylated during translation.[279] The initial oligosaccharides added to G protein are of the high mannose type, which are later modified by enzymes in Golgi membranes to the complex type of oligosaccharides.

Following insertion into the ER, G protein associates with two molecular chaperones, BiP (GRP78) and calnexin,[215] which assist in the formation of the proper disulfide bonds and correct folding of the ectodomain. Mutations that prevent correct folding of the ectodomain or that prevent glycosylation, which is required for calnexin binding, result in the formation of aggregates of misfolded G protein together with BiP, which are not transported from the ER.[350] Therefore, the ability of a mutant protein to be transported from the ER is a minimal criterion by which it can be said to be properly folded. Shortly after release of the properly folded G protein from the chaperones, G protein monomers associate into trimers and are transported to Golgi membranes by vesicles that bud from the ER and subsequently fuse with Golgi membranes.[531] G protein is one of the most rapidly transported integral membrane proteins, requiring approximately 15 minutes to be transported from ER to Golgi membranes and then appears at the plasma membrane within 30 minutes.[50] This rapid transport is dependent on a six–amino acid sequence in the cytoplasmic domain, which can function to concentrate G protein at the sites of vesicle budding.[487]

Once G protein is transported to Golgi membranes, it undergoes further posttranslational modifications, including conversion of its oligosaccharides from the high-mannose type to the complex type, containing additional N-acetyl glucosamine, galactose, and sialic acid. Although these modifications are not required for G protein function, they provide a convenient and widely used marker for transport of G protein through successive Golgi membranes.[485] Another G protein modification that occurs in Golgi membranes is the addition of the fatty acid palmitate to a cysteine residue in the cytoplasmic domain.[477] This modification does not appear to be critical, because some strains of VSV lack this modification, and mutation of the target cysteine residue, which abolishes palmitoylation, does not affect G protein function.[573]

In polarized epithelial cells, G protein is preferentially transported to the basolateral surface.[455] The same amino acid sequence in the cytoplasmic domain that promotes the rapid transport of G protein from ER to Golgi membranes is also necessary for the preferential transport to the basolateral surface of polarized epithelial cells.[529] Sorting of G and other basolaterally targeted proteins from those destined for the apical surface occurs first in Golgi membranes, and from Golgi membranes G protein is transported to the recycling endosome compartment prior to transport to the basolateral plasma membrane.[77] This intermediate step presumably reflects additional sorting steps by which cells regulate the protein composition of their plasma membranes.

At the plasma membrane of infected cells, G protein is organized into clusters or *microdomains* that are approximately 100 to 150 nm in diameter.[69] These G protein–containing microdomains are formed independently of other viral components[69] and appear to be similar to cholesterol- and sphingolipid-rich *lipid rafts* that serve as sites of assembly for other viruses, such as influenza viruses.[429] Lipid rafts have been defined in part by their resistance to solubilization with detergents at low temperatures.[68] In contrast to envelope glycoproteins of influenza virus and other viruses that assemble at lipid rafts, G protein in host plasma membranes and in virion envelopes is detergent soluble.[474] Nonetheless, the plasma membrane microdomains (and virus envelopes) that contain G protein resemble lipid rafts in that they are enriched in cholesterol and sphingolipids,[429] but these lipids must not be in sufficiently high amounts to confer detergent resistance.[474]

The G protein–containing microdomains at sites of virus budding are somewhat larger (300 to 400 nm) than the microdomains in the plasma membrane outside of virus budding sites (100 to 150 nm), implying that formation of virus budding sites involves clustering of membrane microdomains.[70] Remarkably, envelope glycoproteins from many unrelated viruses, as well as some host integral membrane proteins, can be incorporated into the envelopes of VSV or RABV in a process referred to as *pseudotype formation* or *phenotypic mixing*. Pseudotype formation was originally demonstrated by coinfection of cells with two different viruses.[596] With the development of reverse genetic approaches to manipulate the viral genome, multiple chimeric viruses in which the native glycoprotein gene (G) is replaced by one or more heterologous glycoproteins have been generated.[480,517] The resulting chimeric viruses contain only the heterologous envelope protein and it remains unclear whether clustering of microdomains containing the heterologous glycoprotein facilitates virus assembly.[70] It is not known what causes microdomains containing G protein or other glycoproteins to cluster at the sites of virus budding, but a model has been proposed in which clustering is driven by formation of the viral nucleocapsid–M protein complex.[70]

The efficiency with which heterologous glycoproteins are incorporated into the virus envelope varies over a considerable range. In the case of RABV, interaction of the G protein cytoplasmic domain with the internal virion components may promote incorporation into the virus budding site, because appending the G protein cytoplasmic domain to foreign glycoproteins enhances their incorporation into RABV virions.[365] In the case of VSV, the cytoplasmic tail can enhance incorporation of glycoproteins into the envelope but it is not required as substituting foreign sequences for the cytoplasmic domain of G protein or deleting the cytoplasmic domain does not appear to alter the efficiency of G protein incorporation.[479] Replacement of the cytoplasmic tail of the human immunodeficiency virus (HIV) envelope glycoprotein and that of human endogenous retrovirus K[451] promotes their incorporation into the virus envelope.[480] Thus, the ability of a foreign glycoprotein to be incorporated into the VSV envelope can be influenced by its cytoplasmic tail, and the composition or physical properties of the microdomains containing the foreign glycoprotein.

The presence of G in the plasma membrane is not essential for virus budding, as shown by studies with recombinant VSV and RABV in which the G gene has been mutated or deleted[366,517] In the absence of a complementing source of G protein, these viruses produce noninfectious or "bald" particles that lack G protein but are otherwise indistinguishable from wild-type viruses. The efficiency of virus budding, however, is reduced by at least an order of magnitude in the absence of G protein, indicating that G protein plays a role in virus assembly to enhance the budding process. Thus, not only is it likely that internal virion components promote incorporation of G protein into the envelope as described earlier but also it appears that G protein promotes assembly of internal virion components. As with the ability to be incorporated into the envelope, the ability of the VSV G protein to promote assembly is independent of the sequence of the cytoplasmic domain, although a minimal length of eight amino acids in the cytoplasmic domain does appear to be required.[479] Other evidence that the length of the cytoplasmic tail influences incorporation comes from studies of incorporation of the S protein of coronaviruses, where truncation of the S tail enhances the incorporation into virions.[82] Sequences in the membrane-proximal region of the ectodomain may promote membrane curvature and help drive virus budding.[452]

Role of M Protein in Virus Assembly

Unlike G protein, the M protein is synthesized as a soluble protein[286,362] and associates with membranes in the manner of peripheral membrane proteins (i.e., through a combination of ionic and hydrophobic interactions and without spanning the membrane lipid bilayer).[322,339,340,401,589,592,593] In virus-infected cells, most of M protein is usually localized in the cytoplasm and is found in the soluble cytosolic fraction in subcellular fractionation experiments, with smaller amounts being membrane associated.[174,286,407,409] This distribution is also observed in transfected cells that express M protein in the absence of other VSV components,[93,94,589] indicating that association of M protein with membranes does not depend on other viral components. In addition, membrane association does not appear to require posttranslational modification, such as phosphorylation or covalent modification with lipids.[273,322] Instead, M protein appears to spontaneously associate with membranes containing negatively charged phospholipids,[339,340,401,589,592] which are enriched on the cytoplasmic surface of host plasma membranes. The N-terminal 20 amino acids of M protein, which are enriched in positively charged residues, appear to be responsible for membrane association, as shown using photoactivatable membrane probes.[322] Mutational analysis has also implicated the N-terminal region of M protein in membrane binding.[94,123,589] The membrane-bound M protein in infected cells is organized into membrane microdomains whose size is similar to G protein microdomains.[515] However, M protein and G protein reside in separate microdomains except at the sites of virus budding.[515]

Both the cytosolic and membrane-bound M protein are recruited into nucleocapsid–M protein complexes at the site of virus budding from host plasma membranes.[173,399] Nucleocapsids clearly get selected for assembly with M protein, because most of the intracellular nucleocapsids, which are being used as templates for viral RNA synthesis, are not able to bind M protein.[173,407,409] The only place in infected cells where colocalization of nucleocapsids and M protein is observed is in the nucleocapsid–M protein complexes in the process of budding from the plasma membrane.[361,399,407,409] In the case of VSV, nucleocapsids containing genome RNA are incorporated into virus particles much more efficiently than those containing antigenomes.[464,493,501,563] An RNA sequence near the 5′ end of the genome has been identified that is required for nucleocapsids containing this RNA to be incorporated into virus particles.[567] If such a sequence is present in the RABV genome, it must also be present in the antigenome, because the recombinant ambisense RABV described earlier, which contains the genomic promoter in both the genome and antigenome, incorporates both genome and antigenome RNA into virions with equal efficiency.[166] One of the important questions about virus assembly that needs to be addressed is how this RNA sequence promotes incorporation into virions, because selection of nucleocapsids for virion assembly is a critical step.

Once assembly of nucleocapsid–M protein complexes has begun, the recruitment of M protein into the complex appears to occur spontaneously. This process can be recreated in a cell-free system using purified M protein and virion nucleocapsids that have been stripped of most of their M protein by treatment with high ionic strength buffers.[44,345,389,390] Nucleocapsids, from which M protein has been completely removed, however, cannot rebind M protein with the same high affinity observed in virion nucleocapsid–M protein complexes.[173,345] This suggests that addition of the initial one or a few molecules of M protein to nucleocapsids (and, therefore, their removal) is fundamentally different from that of most M protein molecules in the nucleocapsid–M protein complex. Although the basis for this difference has yet to be discovered, it is tempting to think that it may be connected to the process of selection of intracellular nucleocapsids for virus assembly described in the previous paragraph.

Release of Assembled Virions

Following assembly of the nucleocapsid–M protein complex, the final step in virus assembly is release of the budding virion. This process is mediated by interaction of M protein with host proteins involved in MVB formation.[221,222,250,251,260] The MVB machinery is also involved in release of retroviruses and filoviruses mediated by "late budding domains" in their Gag proteins or matrix proteins (VP40), respectively.[432] In the formation of MVBs, vesicles derived from endosome membranes bud into the lumen of the endosome, carrying elements of the cytoplasm as their internal contents. Modification of proteins on the cytoplasmic surface of the endosome membrane by covalent attachment of ubiquitin appears to be an important signal for incorporation of such cargo molecules into MVBs. The process of virus budding has the same membrane topology (cytoplasmic contents are internal), except that the process occurs at the plasma membrane rather than at the endosome membrane. A short sequence in M protein (PPPY in VSV, PPEY in RABV) appears to be responsible for redirecting this cellular machinery to the plasma membrane.[221,222,250,251,260,581] No other viral components appear to be required, because expression of M protein in transfected cells in the absence of other viral components results in budding of membrane vesicles containing M protein.[118,270,330] The PPPY sequence interacts with an E3 ubiquitin ligase called Nedd4, which is able to ubiquitinate M protein, in a cell-free assay.[221] It has yet to be established whether Nedd4 itself, or one of its numerous family members, ubiquitinate M protein in infected cells, because this is likely to involve only a small proportion of the total M protein. Nonetheless, it is likely that ubiquitination of M protein is critical for release of budding virions, because mutation of the PPPY motif in M protein, or depletion of free ubiquitin in infected cells, dramatically reduces the release of virions and causes the accumulation of budding particles at the plasma membrane because of inhibition of their release.[221,260] One of the questions that needs to be resolved is which cellular factors involved in MVB formation are involved in virus budding? Tsg101, a protein involved in recognizing ubiquitinated cargo proteins, and Vps4a, an adenosine triphosphatase (ATPase) involved in recycling the membrane trafficking machinery, have been implicated in budding of HIV but were reported not to be involved in budding of VSV or RABV.[250,251] However, a more recent report indicated that Vps4a is involved in VSV budding.[520]

MOLECULAR GENETICS OF RHABDOVIRUSES

Rhabdoviruses are classic examples of RNA viruses capable of undergoing rapid evolution. This is because of the high error rates of their RNA polymerases and their lack of proofreading activity. As a result, the rate of base substitutions during replication of genome RNA is approximately 1 in 10^4.[139] Because their genomes are only slightly larger than 10^4 bases, this implies that nearly every genome contains at least one base substitution. Thus, even clonal populations of these viruses are actually collections of viruses with closely related sequences (i.e., they are quasispecies). Because of their diversity of genome sequences, these viruses are capable of rapid genetic adaptation when placed under selective pressure of replication under different conditions. These viruses are genetically reasonably stable, however, when replication is maintained under a constant set of conditions.[456] This is because the collection of genome sequences quickly reaches a consensus sequence representing the sequence with the highest level of fitness within a few replication cycles in a new host. This rapid adaptability may be advantageous in nature for viruses that alternate replication among different hosts. For example, VSV replicates both in arthropod hosts, where it establishes persistent infection, and in mammalian hosts, where it causes an acute infection. Transfer from one type of host to the other requires substantial increases in viral fitness to maintain optimal replication in the new host.[595] In principle, this adaptation can occur through random mutation of the consensus sequence from the original host to one with greater fitness in the new host. However, in a virus population undergoing periodic cycling between insect and mammalian hosts, rapid adaptation to the mammalian host likely involves maintenance of a minority population of genomes in the insect host that quickly became dominant during mammalian infection.[397]

The high rate of spontaneous mutation makes it feasible to isolate a variety of different types of viral mutants in the laboratory. For example, several large collections of temperature-sensitive mutants of VSV were isolated, which fall into five or more complementation groups, corresponding to mutants with defects in each of the five viral genes.[169,237,437] Similarly, antigenic variants that escape neutralization with monoclonal antibodies are readily isolated in the laboratory.[309,319,343] Unlike influenza viruses and HIV, however, relatively little antigenic drift is found in rhabdoviruses during outbreaks in nature. This may reflect the harmful effects on G protein function of accumulating the multiple mutations necessary to escape neutralization by a polyclonal antibody response in intact animal hosts.[398]

Despite the advantages for rapid adaptation, the high rate of mutation makes these viruses susceptible to the harmful effects of genetic bottlenecks, in which only one or a few genomes are selected for further replication. In a process known as Muller's ratchet, successive passage under conditions of limited genetic diversity, such as sequential passage by isolation of individual virus plaques, leads to progressive accumulation of base substitutions, most of which decrease virus replication, thus leading to progressively lower viral fitness.[142]

Defective Interfering Particles

Another major mechanism of genetic alteration of rhabdoviruses is the generation of defective interfering (DI) particles. DI particles are generated when the viral RNA polymerase switches from copying one region of the template to copying an alternate template or an alternate region of the same template during replication. Because this inevitably results in generation of defective genomes, DI particles can replicate only in cells coinfected with standard virus to provide a source of viral proteins. If the polymerase switches to copying a distant region of the same template, this generates large deletions of the viral genome, referred to as internal deletion DI particles.[105] In other cases, the polymerase will switch to copying the terminal sequences of the nascent product RNA strand, generating RNA products with terminal complementarity, referred to as panhandle or snap-back DI particles.[425] Panhandle DI particles derived during synthesis of progeny negative-strand RNA thus have the sequence of the 5′ end of the viral genome, but the 3′ region of terminal complementarity has the sequence of the antigenome, including the antigenomic promoter. The minus-strand promoter drives more genomic replication than the plus-strand promoter—which needs to also promote transcription—DI genomes that have such "minus-strand" promoters for both genome and antigenome synthesis have a substantial

replicative advantage over standard viral genomes and interfere with the replication of standard virus, resulting in reductions in virus titer.[105] Although they have the same genomic promoter as standard virus, internal deletion DI particles also have a replicative advantage over standard virus, presumably because of their smaller size, and they also interfere with replication of standard virus.

Defective interfering particles are readily generated during virus replication in culture, so that repeated passage at high multiplicity leads to substantial reductions in virus titer because of accumulation of DI particles.[105] Because of the smaller size of their genomes, virions containing DI genomes are shorter than standard virions and can be separated from standard virus by centrifugation on density gradients. This ability to physically separate virions containing DI genomes from those containing standard genomes has proved to be useful in studies of the generation and replication of DI particles.

In contrast to the facile production of DI genomes in cell culture, recombination between viral genomes has not been reported experimentally. As recombination and DI particle formation depend upon a similar copy-choice mechanism principle, rhabdoviruses should be able to generate recombinants between genetically distinct viruses in coinfected cells. Despite many years of the genetic study of these viruses, no convincing evidence indicates that this type of RNA recombination occurs, although the possibility of rare occurrences in nature has been proposed.[87]

Genetic Engineering of Rhabdoviruses

The methods for genetically engineering viral genomes developed with rhabdoviruses have become the standard methods used for genetic modification of many nonsegmented, negative-strand RNA viruses. A major hurdle is that RNA transcribed from complementary DNA (cDNA) needs to be encapsidated to function as a viral genome. This process, which occurs so efficiently when RNA is replicated by the viral RNA polymerase, occurs inefficiently when RNA is transcribed from cDNA. Shorter RNAs expressed from cDNA appear to be encapsidated more efficiently than longer RNA. Thus, the first viral genomes to be recovered from cDNA were a VSV DI genome[418] and an RABV minigenome containing the terminal sequences of the viral genome required for transcription and replication flanking a foreign gene.[111] These genomes were expressed from plasmid cDNA in transfected cells together with plasmids encoding the N, P, and L proteins required for encapsidation and replication. Another hurdle to the recovery of viral genomes from cDNA was the requirement for the 3′ end of the RNA to reflect precisely the sequence of the viral genome (or antigenome) without additional nucleotides, in order to be recognized and replicated by the viral RNA polymerase. This was addressed by incorporating into the cDNA the sequence of the hepatitis delta virus ribozyme engineered to cleave the RNA transcript to generate a precise 3′ end.[418] Apparently, the sequence requirements at the 5′ end of the viral RNA are not as critical, because additional nucleotides derived from cDNA are removed during replication.

The experimental approach used to generate minigenomes from cDNA led to recovery of complete viral genomes from cDNA for RABV[483] and VSV.[313,566] A key insight was that the RNA transcribed from cDNA needed to be the antigenome rather than the genome. Otherwise, the mRNA derived from the helper plasmids encoding N, P, and L proteins would interfere with recovery by hybridization to the genomic RNA transcribed from cDNA. In most recovery experiments, high levels of expression of the antigenome RNA and the mRNA from the helper plasmids have been achieved by infecting cells with a recombinant vaccinia virus encoding T7 RNA polymerase and transfecting them with plasmids driven by T7 promoters.[313,483,566] Because this requires isolation of the recovered virus from contaminating vaccinia virus, methods for isolating recombinant rhabdoviruses without the use of vaccinia virus have been developed.[220,254]

The ability to engineer specific mutations into viral genomes has become an important tool for studying the mechanistic aspects of virus replication. In addition, it has made possible the use of rhabdoviruses as vectors for expression of foreign genes for potential use as vaccines and therapeutic agents. Several reviews have appeared on the use of rhabdoviruses as potential recombinant vaccines and as oncolytic agents.[12,332,364] The basic methodology to express foreign genes is to introduce a new transcription unit containing the gene stop–start signals and the foreign gene between two of the native viral genes, such as between the G and L genes.[367,481] The foreign gene is subject to the same transcriptional attenuation as the other viral genes. Thus, incorporation of a new gene reduces the expression of downstream genes by approximately 20% to 30%. Although this attenuation has the potential to reduce the efficiency of virus replication, incorporation of a single foreign gene usually does not notably reduce virus yields unless the foreign gene product itself has the potential to interfere with virus replication.[480] The processes of genome encapsidation and envelopment are sufficiently flexible that incorporation of new genes into rhabdovirus genomes simply leads to longer nucleocapsids and, therefore, longer virions.[481] In principle, no limit exists for packaging new genetic information, so that multiple foreign genes can be incorporated into genomes of recombinant viruses. Reductions in virus yield owing to multiple new transcription attenuation sites, as well as the difficulty of recovering longer genomes, however, probably places practical limits on the amount of new genetic information that can be incorporated into rhabdovirus genomes.

Use of this approach led to the development of a licensed human vaccine to combat Ebola virus infection. The G gene of VSV was replaced with that of Ebola virus and a single dose of the resulting virus was shown to protect hamsters and nonhuman primates against a lethal challenge with Ebola virus. Induction of neutralizing antibodies appears to be one correlate of protection against Ebola.

MOLECULAR AND CELLULAR BASIS OF PATHOGENESIS

Induction and Suppression of Host Antiviral Responses

Two of the major determinants of viral pathogenesis are the nature of the antiviral response mounted by the infected host and the mechanisms used by viruses to suppress or evade this response. In order for cells to mount an antiviral response, viral products have to be recognized by sensors known as pattern recognition receptors (PRRs). For most cell types, the major PRR that initiates the response to many negative-strand RNA viruses appears to be a cytoplasmic RNA helicase, RIG-I (retinoic acid–inducible gene I).[276,277] The other major PRRs that have been implicated in the host response to these viruses are toll-like receptors (TLRs). TLRs act either at the plasma membrane or in the endocytic compartment to recognize molecules that may be associated with infection by bacteria, fungi, and protozoa as well as viruses. Activation of RIG-I or TLRs results in formation of signaling complexes through a variety of adapter proteins, which activate protein kinases that turn on the expression of antiviral genes.[387,518] Most of the recent research in this area has focused on the production of type I (α and β) interferons (IFNs) and IFN-stimulated gene products, although other cytokines produced by virus-infected cells also play a major role in innate antiviral responses.

One of the principal ligands for RIG-I is 5′ phosphorylated RNA that is part of a short double-stranded RNA (dsRNA).[240,475] In the normal replication cycle of nonsegmented negative-strand RNA viruses, 5′ phosphorylated RNAs are produced during the process of transcription in the form of leader and trailer RNAs and during genome replication as either genomic or antigenomic RNAs (see earlier). However, the 5′ ends of these RNAs are shielded by the nucleocapsid protein. Thus, removal of the nucleocapsid protein would appear to be necessary to expose free 5′ ends of viral RNA and formation of dsRNA for recognition by RIG-I.[444] Another potential source of such RNAs would be aberrant transcription products that are not capped by the viral polymerase. Thus, the origin of the signals that activate RIG-I is not clear, but to a large extent these signals are coupled to the production of viral RNAs.

Unlike RIG-I–dependent signaling, which is widely distributed among many cell types, the distribution of TLRs and the relative importance of their signaling pathways is often cell type dependent. For example, TLR7 is a major PRR in the response to VSV in plasmacytoid dendritic cells,[342] while TLR13 and perhaps TLR4 are major PRRs in the response to VSV of splenic conventional dendritic cells and macrophages.[195,491] The signal that activates TLR7 appears to be the presence of single-stranded RNA in the endocytic compartment.[130] Such single-stranded RNA can arise during virus penetration by degradation of virions or can be generated from viral RNA in the cytoplasm, which enters the endocytic compartment by autophagy.[317] The signal that activates TLR4 in macrophages appears to be the VSV G protein, which interacts with TLR4 during virus attachment and penetration.[195] The signal that activates TLR13 is not known but does not appear to be related to viral RNA.[491]

The only TLR that has been implicated thus far in the innate response to RABV is TLR3.[259,435] TLR3 responds to the presence of dsRNA in the endocytic compartment.[13] As pointed out earlier, dsRNAs are not part of the normal replication cycle but may arise from abnormal replication products. TLR3 may play a role in the antiviral response to RABV, but surprisingly TLR3−/− mice are less susceptible to RABV than their wild-type controls.[370] This appears to be due to a role for TLR3 in the formation of Negri bodies, which are sites of virus replication.[310,370]

Nearly all viruses have mechanisms to evade or suppress host antiviral responses. Mutations in viruses that either increase the induction or decrease the suppression of antiviral responses almost inevitably decrease virus replication in susceptible hosts. VSV and RABV use different approaches. VSV uses a rapid and potent means of inhibiting these responses, involving the general inhibition of nearly all host gene expression. By contrast, RABV exploits a more subtle means of inhibiting host responses that do not involve the general inhibition of host gene expression.

Suppression of Interferon Signaling by RABV

The P protein of RABV functions both as a subunit of the viral RNA-dependent RNA polymerase and as a suppressor of IFN production and IFN signaling. P protein inhibits IFN production by preventing the phosphorylation of the transcription factor IRF-3 by two cellular protein kinases, TBK1 and IKK-ε (Fig. 7.12A).[74] Mutations in P protein that inactivate its IFN inhibitory function without affecting its RNA synthesis function have been identified.[448] Recombinant viruses that express either mutant P protein or lower levels of P protein than their wild-type controls[74,165] are less effective in suppressing IFN production. These viruses are able to replicate in cell types that are defective in their IFN responses but are rapidly eliminated from IFN-competent cell types and are less virulent in mice.[74,165,448]

In addition to inhibiting IFN production, RABV P protein inhibits signal transduction in response to IFN (Fig. 7.12B). RABV P is expressed not only as full-length P protein but also as four truncated forms (P2 through P5) that are synthesized from internal start codons.[416] P3, P4, and P5 proteins are found only in the nucleus. The ability of P protein and its truncated derivatives to inhibit IFN signaling is due to their ability to interfere with the transcription factors that activate interferon-stimulated genes (ISGs). Type I IFNs bind to a common receptor that is coupled to two tyrosine kinases, Jak1 and Tyk2.[442] Receptor activation leads to activation of these kinases, which in turn phosphorylate two cytoplasmic proteins, STAT1 and STAT2. Phospho-STAT1 and -STAT2 are transported to the nucleus, where they associate with IRF9 to form the ISGF-3 transcription factor that activates expression of ISGs. RABV P protein does not interfere with STAT phosphorylation. Instead, it binds to phosphorylated STAT1 and STAT2 and inhibits their translocation to the nucleus and binding to target DNAs (Fig. 7.12B).[75,90,380,546,547] This appears to be due to association of the P protein–STAT complex with microtubules in the cytoplasm, which prevents transport to the nucleus.[380] STAT1–STAT2 complexes that do get transported to the nucleus associate with P protein or its truncated derivatives, which interferes with DNA-binding activity.[547]

Inhibition of Host Gene Expression by VSV

VSV inhibits host gene expression at three different levels: (a) transcription of host mRNA, (b) transport of host mRNA from the nucleus to the cytoplasm, and (c) translation of host mRNA into proteins (Fig. 7.12A). The inhibition of all three processes presumably reflects the fact that no single inhibitory mechanism is completely effective in suppressing host antiviral responses. The inhibition of both host transcription and translation generally occurs in parallel and is usually 80% to 90% complete by 4 to 6 hours postinfection.[8,144] Some evidence indicates that the inhibition of nuclear-cytoplasmic RNA transport may occur earlier after infection, although a direct comparison with the inhibition at other levels has not been made.[510,548]

The VSV gene product that is primarily responsible for inhibiting host gene expression is M protein. Expression of VSV M protein in transfected cells in the absence of other viral components inhibits expression of cotransfected genes driven by a wide variety of different promoters.[6,56,162,346,412] This inhibitory activity of M protein is very potent and is evident even when M protein is expressed at 100 to 1,000 times lower levels than those in VSV-infected cells.[346] Viruses containing a variety of M protein mutations are defective in their ability to inhibit host gene expression.[5,8,57,115,128,162,178,261,510] Most of these mutations that render M protein defective in its ability to inhibit host gene expression do not affect its functions in virus assembly. Conversely, M protein mutations such as truncation of the N-terminal sequences that are important for virus assembly do not affect the ability of M protein to inhibit host gene expression.[57,261] Thus, the functions of M protein in the inhibition of host gene expression are genetically separable from its virus assembly functions. Although no separate M protein domains appear to mediate these two classes of functions, the point mutations that affect inhibition of host gene expression do map to one face of the M protein three-dimensional structure. Presumably, this face of M protein is involved in interaction with host components involved in the inhibition.

Because M protein lacks any enzymatic activity, it probably interferes with host gene expression by interacting with cellular proteins to alter their function. Thus far, the only host protein whose binding to M protein is correlated with the inhibition of host gene expression is Rae1.[158] Rae1 was originally implicated in mRNA transport, but more recent experiments suggest its principal function is in mitotic spindle assembly and mitotic checkpoint regulation.[28,60,494,582] M protein and Rae1 form complexes with multiple proteins involved in mRNA transport and other cellular functions, such as Nup98, hnRNP-U, and E1B-AP5.[86,158,548] However, deleting the Rae1 gene in cultured mouse embryo cells or silencing its expression in Drosophila does not lead to mRNA transport inhibition.[28,494] Given the observation that Rae1 is not essential for nuclear-cytoplasmic RNA transport, it is unlikely that the VSV M protein inhibits host gene expression simply by interfering with Rae1 function. Instead, it is more likely that the complex of M protein and Rae1 interferes with the function of other factors that are essential for host gene expression.

Because Rae1 is distributed throughout the cytoplasm and the nucleus of the cell, M protein–Rae1 complexes may be involved in inhibition of multiple steps in host gene expression. In support of this idea, the inhibition of transcription by host RNA polymerase II involves inactivation of the general transcription factor TFIID,[86] which binds to the TATA box upstream of most RNA polymerase II–dependent promoters and recruits other general transcription factors to these promoters. M protein, however, does not appear to interact directly with TFIID,[591] suggesting that the inactivation is indirect. The mechanisms involved in such an indirect effect have yet to be discovered.

The inhibition of host translation in VSV-infected cells does not result from depletion of cellular mRNA secondary to the inhibition of mRNA transcription and transport. As described earlier, the inhibition of host translation occurs early in the infectious cycle on a time scale too rapid to be caused by turnover of cellular mRNA. Instead, the translation apparatus is reprogrammed such that only new mRNAs are translated.[571]

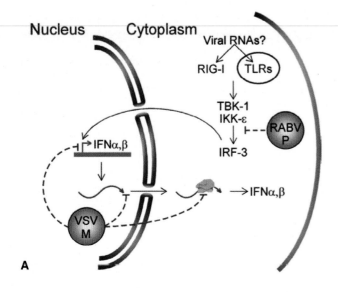

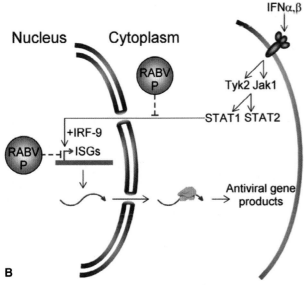

FIGURE 7.12 Induction and suppression of host interferon (IFN) responses by rabies virus (RABV) and vesicular stomatitis virus (VSV). A: Induction of synthesis of type I (a and b) IFN and its suppression by RABV P protein and VSV M protein. **B:** Response to IFN and its suppression by RABV P protein.

Preexisting host mRNAs are incorporated into translationally inactive messenger ribonucleoproteins (mRNPs), where they are stably maintained in infected cells.[462,570] Thus, the inhibition of host translation reflects the inhibition of translation of preexisting mRNAs together with the lack of production of new host mRNAs due to the inhibition of transcription and transport by M protein. The reprogramming of the translation apparatus appears to be due at least in part to alterations in the cap-binding translation factor eIF4F.[107,108,140] How the changes in the eIF4F complex result in the altered translation in VSV-infected cells is a major question that remains to be addressed.

Viral transcription provides a continuous supply of newly synthesized viral mRNAs, which are efficiently translated by the reprogrammed translation apparatus. Translation of viral mRNAs continues until late in the infectious cycle, when translation is inhibited because of phosphorylation of eIF2α by the antiviral kinase PKR, as well as other mechanisms.[107,108,570] Viral mRNAs do not appear to have cis-acting sequences that promote their translation analogous to the internal ribosome entry sites in picornavirus mRNAs.[570] Regardless of their sequences, new mRNAs are translated more efficiently in VSV-infected cells than in uninfected cells.[571] This enhancement of translation of new mRNAs appears to involve M protein, because M protein mutant viruses have been identified that inhibit host translation as effectively as their wild-type controls but are defective in promoting translation of viral mRNAs.[109,374]

Induction of Cytopathic Effects

As in the case of suppression of host antiviral responses, lyssaviruses and vesiculoviruses present strikingly different abilities to induce cytopathic effects in infected cells. In the case of most RABV strains, usually few, if any, morphologic changes occur in infected cells that would be interpreted as cytopathic effects until several days after infection. Indeed, some cell types infected with RABV continue to divide and establish persistent infections.[161] In contrast, many strains of VSV are among the most cytocidal of animal viruses, at least in mammalian and avian cells. In many insect cells, however, VSV replication is attenuated and a persistent infection is established with little, if any, cytopathic effect. In most cases, cytopathic effects are a result of host responses to virus infection involving activation of programmed cell death or apoptosis.

Induction of Apoptosis by Vesicular Stomatitis Virus

It is widely appreciated that many viruses induce apoptosis in infected cells, and, in general, apoptosis is a form of antiviral response in which death of the host cell should reduce the number of progeny resulting from the infectious cycle. VSV was one of the early viruses shown to induce apoptosis in infected cells.[295] In fact, most, if not all, of the cytopathic effects of VSV infection are caused by the induction of apoptosis. These effects include nearly all of the morphologic and biochemical changes typical of apoptosis in cell culture.[293,295] One of the earliest effects is cell rounding, followed by membrane blebbing, nuclear condensation and DNA fragmentation, cytoplasmic shrinkage, and cell lysis. Despite the general opinion that apoptosis of infected cells reduces virus yield, little, if any, difference exists in yield of VSV if apoptosis is delayed by overexpression of the antiapoptotic host protein Bcl-2,[292] indicating that the VSV replication cycle is largely complete before the infected cell has a chance to die.

At least two distinct mechanisms exist by which VSV infection can induce apoptosis in infected cells.[81,185,293,421] One appears to be a direct result of the inhibition of host gene expression by M protein, and thus is only activated by viruses with wild-type M protein. The other mechanism appears to be a cellular response to virus replication and is induced by both wild-type and M protein mutant viruses. The relative importance of these two mechanisms varies widely among different cell types, depending on the nature of the proteins that regulate apoptosis preexisting in the cell before infection and the contribution of newly synthesized proapoptotic protein induced after infection.[81,185,186,292,421,469] Such newly synthesized proapoptotic proteins can contribute to apoptosis induced by M protein mutant viruses but are suppressed by viruses with wild-type M protein.

Wild-type M protein induces apoptosis when expressed in transfected cells in the absence of other viral components.[293] In contrast, mutant M proteins that are defective in their ability to inhibit host gene expression cannot induce apoptosis in the absence of other viral components.[292,293] Induction of apoptosis by M protein appears to be similar to that induced by pharmacologic inhibitors of host gene expression (e.g., actinomycin D). As with most forms of intracellular damage, both M protein and pharmacologic inhibitors of host RNA synthesis activate the mitochondrial pathway, involving the release of cytochrome c and other proapoptotic proteins from mitochondria, which activate the upstream caspase, caspase-9.[38,292] As a result, induction of apoptosis by M protein can be inhibited by overexpression of antiapoptotic proteins like Bcl-2 and Bcl-XL, which prevent release of proapoptotic factors from mitochondria.

Despite the inability of mutant M proteins to induce apoptosis in the absence of other viral components, M protein mutant viruses, which are defective in their ability to inhibit host gene expression, are still very effective inducers of apoptosis in infected cells.[81,185,186,292,293,490] The induction of apoptosis by M protein mutant viruses appears to be part of the antiviral response induced by virus replication. In contrast to apoptosis induced by M protein alone, the death receptor pathway is the major mechanism of cell death, in which caspase-8 is the major upstream caspase, rather than caspase-9.[81,186] The Fas death receptor appears to be the major death receptor involved. In contrast to viruses such as influenza virus, in which Fas signaling is mediated through the adaptor protein FADD,[38] VSV infection appears to activate an alternative adapter protein Daxx, which is involved in the induction of apoptosis.[186] In some cell types, cross-talk between the death receptor and mitochondrial apoptotic pathways is required for efficient induction of cell death. This cross-talk is mediated through caspase-8 cleavage of the proapoptotic BH3-only protein Bid. Cleaved Bid (tBid) then promotes destabilization of the mitochondria through activation of proapoptotic mitochondrial proteins. Death receptor signaling has been classified as type I or type II depending on whether signaling is independent of the mitochondrial pathway (type I) or depends on amplification by the mitochondrial pathway (type II).[472,473] Cells that respond to death receptor ligands by a type II pathway also respond to VSV infection by a similar pathway.[81]

Induction of Apoptosis by Lyssaviruses

As pointed out earlier, there are cell types in which RABV induces little, if any, cytopathic effect and establishes persistent infections.[161] In other cell types, the infected cells eventually die as a result of induction of apoptosis.[258,539] Furthermore, RABV induces apoptosis in infected neurons *in vivo* during experimentally induced encephalitis in mice.[258] Inhibition of host gene expression does not play a role in the induction of apoptosis by RABV as it does in the case of VSV. Indeed, RABV infection induces the expression of host proapoptotic proteins, such as Bax,[539] and in this regard, resembles the induction of apoptosis by M protein mutants of VSV that do not inhibit host gene expression. Also analogous to VSV M protein mutants, the induction of apoptosis depends on activation of the death receptor pathway involving caspase-8, in the case of two other lyssaviruses, MOKV and LBV.[275] In contrast to the activation of the Fas death receptor by VSV M protein mutants, however, MOKV and LBV activate apoptosis through interaction of the death ligand tumor necrosis factor (TNF)-related apoptosis-inducing ligand (TRAIL) with its receptor.[275] Transfection

of cells with plasmids encoding lyssavirus M proteins induced apoptosis by the same caspase-8–dependent and TRAIL-dependent mechanism and also through mitochondrial disruption.[199,275] It is unlikely, however, that the lyssavirus M proteins induce apoptosis by a mechanism similar to VSV M protein, because they do not inhibit host gene expression. In addition to M protein, G proteins of some RABV strains also induce apoptosis.[434,436] Thus, it is likely that multiple viral components are involved in the induction of apoptosis in cells infected with lyssaviruses.

MOUSE MODELS OF RHABDOVIRUS INFECTION

Both RABV and VSV are highly neurotropic in mice, and virulence is largely due to virus-induced encephalomyelitis. Laboratory rodents (e.g., mice) have been extensively used for rabies diagnosis, vaccine potency testing, and pathogenic studies, although these taxa are epidemiologically insignificant as lyssavirus vectors or reservoirs,[92,299] compared with the families Carnivora and Chiroptera. Similarly, rodents are not known to be natural hosts for vesiculoviruses. In fact, the disease induced by VSV in rodents bears little resemblance to the disease in natural hosts, such as horses and cattle (described later). Nonetheless, much of what we know about the mechanisms of pathogenesis and immunity for these viruses is derived from experimental infection of mice.

Entry and Site of Initial Replication

Infection of mice with RABV is usually fatal regardless of the route of inoculation. Intramuscular inoculation is often used as a model for virus transmission by animal bites, and intranasal inoculation is used as a model for the occasional transmission of RABV by inhalation. In contrast to RABV, the ability of VSV to invade the CNS is highly dependent on the age of the mice and route of inoculation,[468] as well as the strain of mice infected.[147,177] In general, adult mice are relatively resistant to VSV inoculated intravenously or intraperitoneally, although systemic virus infection clearly occurs in these mice, as shown by the potent induction of immune responses (described later). In contrast to intravenous or intraperitoneal inoculation, mice are very sensitive to VSV introduced by intranasal or intracerebral inoculation. As an example of strain differences, mice of the 129 strain, which are often used in the generation of transgenic mice, were found to be five orders of magnitude more resistant than strains such as BALB/c, which are often used in studies of immunology and pathogenesis.[147]

Virus entry into the host is accompanied by initial virus replication at the site of entry. In the case of RABV infection of mice, initial replication following intramuscular inoculation can occur in either sensory or motor neurons without apparent replication in muscle,[114,488] although in natural hosts, virus can replicate in muscle tissue before progressing to the peripheral nervous tissue via neuromuscular connections.[88,160,386] In the case of either RABV or VSV infection following intranasal inoculation (Fig. 7.13), the primary site of virus replication is in olfactory receptor neurons and other cells of the olfactory epithelium.[308,431] In addition to olfactory epithelium, VSV can also infect cells of the respiratory epithelium and spread

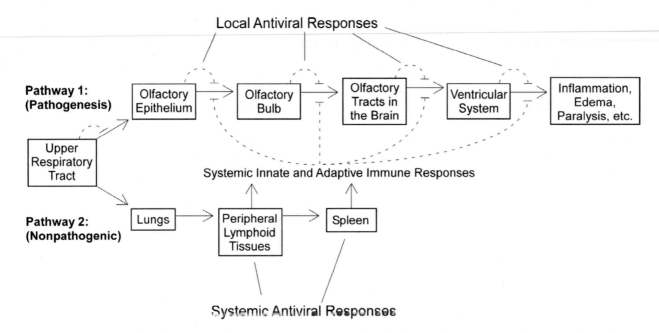

FIGURE 7.13 Diagram of pathogenesis and immune response in mice infected with vesicular stomatitis virus by intranasal inoculation. *Pathway 1* is the route of virus spread through the central nervous system by neuronal transmission leading to encephalitis. *Pathway 2* is a hypothetical route of spread from the respiratory tract to peripheral and central lymphoid organs. Also shown are sites at which local and systemic antiviral responses exert an inhibitory effect on spread of virus to the next stage. The outcome of infection depends on the relative ability of the virus to replicate and spread versus the ability of the host to inhibit virus replication at each step.

through the respiratory tract to the lungs, although little, if any, pathology is associated with virus replication in the lungs.[177]

Virus Spread and Tissue Tropism

Both RABV and VSV are transmitted to the CNS primarily by neural spread along the tracts served by the initially infected neurons. For example, following intramuscular inoculation, RABV spreads from the initially infected sensory and motor neurons to the spinal cord and sensory ganglia in subsequent rounds of replication.[114] Similarly, following intranasal inoculation (Fig. 7.13), both VSV and RABV quickly spread to the glomerular cells of the olfactory bulb as well as the anterior olfactory nuclei.[245,308] From these sites, the viruses spread to other parts of the CNS that are served by the neurons that innervate the olfactory bulb. These viruses have a clear preference for some classes of neurons over others. For example, RABV can also enter the CNS through neurons of the trigeminal ganglia,[308,488] whereas VSV cannot.[431] Similarly, RABV infects mitral cells of the olfactory bulb and spreads along tracts served by these cells,[308] whereas VSV does not.[245] In addition to neural spread, VSV infects cells lining the ventricular system, where it can be released into the cerebrospinal fluid (CSF) and can spread to other parts of the brain and spinal cord, leading to paralysis.[177,245,431]

The pathology associated with infection of mice by either RABV or VSV is typical of viral encephalomyelitis, involving both death of infected cells and inflammation at the infection sites. The inflammatory changes include activation of resident inflammatory cells (e.g., microglia) and infiltration of inflammatory cells (e.g., monocytes, natural killer [NK] cells, and T cells).[52,96,177,239] The morbidity and mortality associated with virus infection is usually attributed to virus-induced death

of infected cells that are critical for the host, rather than to immunopathologic mechanisms, because nearly all experimental manipulations that reduce the immune response to virus infection either enhance mortality by allowing more virus replication or have little effect. For example, virus infection of T-cell–deficient mice results in more extensive spread of virus throughout the brain and higher mortality than in immunocompetent mice.[239,244]

Immune Responses Involved in Recovery From Rhabdovirus Infection

The immune response to VSV infection in mice has been studied for many years by viral immunologists as a prototype immune response to virus infection. In addition, the development of recombinant VSV as a potential vaccine vector[450] has stimulated additional research into the anti-VSV immune response. In most cases, the infection resulting from intraperitoneal or intravenous inoculation has been studied, which often is asymptomatic and results in complete recovery in immunocompetent mice. Less frequently studied is the infection resulting from intranasal inoculation. In this case, nearly all mice develop clinical signs, and only about half of the mice survive. Clearly, differences in the immune responses resulting in resistance or recovery must exist between these two situations. In the case of RABV, there is little incidence of recovery from a productive CNS infection. The immune response to attenuated virus strains is often studied as a model for the immune response to potential live virus vaccine strains.

Immune Response to Vesiculovirus Infection

In the case of VSV infection, elements of both the innate and adaptive immune response are critical for survival (Fig. 7.13).

One of the most striking effects on VSV pathogenesis occurs in the absence of a response to type I (α and β) IFN. Mice that lack the type I IFN receptor, or the STAT1 transcription factor that mediates many of the effects of type I IFN, are extremely susceptible to the lethal effects of VSV infection.[146,385] In contrast to immunocompetent mice, in which virus replication occurs primarily in the CNS, in IFN receptor– or STAT1-deficient mice VSV replicates to high titer in all of the tissues tested.[146,385] In fact, the brains of these mice had the lowest titers of any of the organs examined.[385] This result implies that the pronounced neurotropism of VSV in immunocompetent mice is not caused by the inherent ability of different tissues to support virus replication, but rather differences in their ability to produce or respond to type I IFN.

As in the case of most viruses, no single IFN-inducible gene product is responsible for the effect of IFN in protecting nonneural tissues from VSV infection. No deletion of a single IFN-inducible gene has as profound an effect as deficiency of IFN receptor or STAT1. The antiviral protein kinase PKR is notable, however, in that its deletion leads to enhanced virus replication in the lung following intranasal inoculation, leading to enhanced morbidity and mortality caused by respiratory infection.[147]

The major source of type I IFN in mice following systemic inoculation appears to be a subclass of plasmacytoid dendritic cells residing in the marginal zone of the spleen.[43] This would be consistent with the ability of VSV to suppress IFN production by most other cell types, as described in the previous section. Dendritic cells containing TLR7, such as plasmacytoid dendritic cells, appear to be resistant to the inhibition of IFN production following VSV infection.[9,342,549] Other cell types involved in innate immunity also appear to be involved in protecting neural and nonneural tissues from VSV infection. Following systemic inoculation, chemokine-secreting marginal zone macrophages in the spleen are particularly important,[100,400] and following subcutaneous inoculation, subcapsular macrophages in draining lymph nodes are critical for preventing VSV neuroinvasion through peripheral nerves in the lymph nodes.[249]

Whereas the host IFN response and other innate immune mechanisms can protect most nonneural tissues from VSV infection, they do not fully protect the CNS, particularly following intranasal or intracerebral inoculation. This inability to protect the CNS is not because of a failure of neurons to respond to IFN.[534] Instead, the problem appears to reside in the amount of IFN produced in the CNS and the timing of the peripheral IFN response relative to virus invasion.[535] Indeed, treating mice with exogenous IFN can increase their resistance to CNS infection by VSV.[125,209,532] In addition to the IFN response, other innate immune mechanisms affect the susceptibility of the CNS to VSV infection. For example, deficiency in the production of nitric oxide by neuronal nitric oxide synthase-1 (NOS-1) enhances the susceptibility of the CNS to infection.[290] In contrast, deficiency of the inducible NOS (NOS-2) or NOS-3 has little effect on VSV infection of the CNS.

In addition to innate immune responses, adaptive immune responses are critical for recovery from VSV infection. Particularly important is the production of neutralizing antibodies. As with most viruses, the envelope glycoprotein of VSV (G protein) is the viral antigen that elicits neutralizing antibodies.[80,271,318] Induction of antibodies by G protein expressed on the surface of infected cells requires T cells.[29] The high density of G protein in virions is able to induce a T-cell–independent IgM response, however, which is consistent with the induction of T-cell–independent responses by antigens with highly repetitive epitopes.[29] T cells are required for isotype switching to produce immunoglobulin G (IgG) and other isotypes.[320,352] VSV-infected dendritic cells appear to be responsible for transporting the virus to secondary lymphoid organs, such as the spleen (Fig. 7.13), where they present viral antigens to virus-specific T cells and B cells.[99,100,341] The CD4+ T-helper cell (Th) response to VSV infection includes elicitation of both Th1 and Th2 cells. The response is predominantly of the Th1 type, resulting in secretion of IFN-γ and isotype switching in B cells to produce predominantly IgG2a antibodies. Isotype switching to IgG2a is also mediated by IFN-γ–producing γ-D T cells.[352] This polarization of the T-cell response presumably reflects secretion of IL-12 by dendritic cells and other antigen-presenting cells. Depletion of phagocytic cells, including marginal zone dendritic cells and macrophages, largely eliminates the Th1 response, although the Th2 response is left largely intact, suggesting that a different class of antigen-presenting cells is responsible for activation of Th2 cells.[100]

VSV infection also effectively elicits CD8+ cytolytic T cells (Tc). In contrast to neutralizing antibodies, which are serotype specific, many of the Tc cells are cross-reactive between Indiana and New Jersey serotypes of VSV.[463] These cells recognize peptides containing conserved sequences derived from G protein or N protein (and perhaps other viral proteins) presented in the context of class I major histocompatibility complex (MHC) molecules on virus-infected cells.[438,542,590] In addition to CD8+ Tc, VSV also elicits CD4+ cytotoxic T cells, which recognize epitopes derived from G protein presented in the context of class II MHC molecules.[71]

The importance of the antibody response in recovery from VSV infection is demonstrated by the observation that mice containing disruptions of the immunoglobulin μ gene are highly susceptible to VSV infection.[72] These mice die from CNS infection, even when infected by intraperitoneal inoculation. In contrast, depletion of either CD4+ or CD8+ T cells has little effect on susceptibility to VSV infection by this route.[320] Depletion of either T-cell subset or both subsets, however, enhances the susceptibility of mice to infection with VSV by intranasal inoculation,[244] indicating that T cells are important for reducing virus replication once infection is established in the CNS.

Immune Response to Lyssavirus Infection

Antibodies induced by vaccination, particularly those with neutralizing activity, play a prominent role in immune defense against RABV infection.[239] On rare occasions, immunity can also be naturally acquired after multiple exposures to virus.[175] The G protein represents the only antigen that induces neutralizing antibodies and is able to confer immunity against a lethal challenge.[117] Antibodies can mediate viral clearance from the CNS without other immune effectors.[133] The presence of other immune mechanisms, including IFN responses, and both CD4+ and CD8+ T-cell responses, however, hastens the clearance of virus from the CNS.[239] Although G protein is the only antigen that elicits neutralizing antibodies, the RNP is a major antigenic complex that induces a virus-specific antibody response, and antibodies directed against RNP can contribute to protection against infection.[134,155,336] Animals treated with anti-N sera can be protected against a subsequent challenge with RABV, and anti-N sera can exhibit an antiviral activity *in vitro*.[336] The mechanism by which anti-RNP antibodies inhibit viral replication, however, remains unclear.

Infection with RABV results in the generation of virus-specific CD8+ and CD4+ T cells. The G protein is one of the antigens that induces Tc responses.[348,349] Some mouse strains infected with virus also develop strong Tc responses to the P protein.[312] The role of CD8+ T cells in immune defense is unclear, however. Some investigators report clearance of rabies virus after transfer of RABV-specific T cells and protection against rabies by a Tc clone, whereas other investigators showed that Tc are insufficient to protect against challenge, and *in vivo* depletion of CD8+ T cells had no effect on host resistance to street virus infection.[280,312,426,433] In contrast, Tc may actually be involved in the immunopathology and have been implicated in neuritic paralysis.[512,560] By comparison, the induction of CD4+ T cells is an integral part of the protective immune response against rabies.[132] Elimination of CD4+ cells abrogates the production of IgG neutralizing antibody in response to virus infection.[476] The RNP contains major epitopes that induce CD4+ T-cell responses, and most of these T cells cross-react with other lyssaviruses.[155] The RNP-specific T cells, which can augment the production of neutralizing antibody, are believed to be the major factor that mediates the protective immune response induced by internal viral antigens.[134,184]

Determinants of Viral Virulence

In general, determinants of viral virulence among rhabdoviruses can be classified into those that enhance virus replication and those that enhance the suppression or evasion of host antiviral responses. Mutations in such virulence determinants are of considerable interest, because of their potential to generate live virus vaccines. In the case of RABV, much attention has focused on mutations in G protein that attenuate viral pathogenicity. For example, antigenic variants selected with neutralizing monoclonal antibodies against G protein often display reduced neurovirulence in mice. These variants contain mutations that change R/K333 in G protein to other amino acids. These changes reduce the ability of G protein to attach to neuron-specific receptors,[116,537] although virus replication in non-neuronal cells is not affected. Similarly, mutations in VSV that compromise its ability to replicate often result in attenuated virus strains. For example, truncation of the G protein cytoplasmic domain reduces the efficiency of virus budding, as described earlier. Such mutants are attenuated in their pathogenicity and form the basis for candidate recombinant viral vaccines.[450,461] Likewise, recombinant viruses in which the order of the VSV genes has been altered usually display reduced pathogenicity as a result of reduced virus replication and are candidate recombinant vaccines.[112,172]

An example of the second class of virulence determinants—those that lead to suppression of host antiviral responses—would be the VSV M protein. Mutations in M protein that render it defective in its ability to inhibit host gene expression attenuate viral virulence in mice without compromising the ability of the virus to replicate in cell culture.[4,7,510] In this case, the attenuation is caused by the enhanced innate immune responses elicited in infected cells because of the failure of the virus to suppress host gene expression.[535]

Similar to VSV M protein mutants, RABV P protein mutants have been generated that are defective in their ability

to block IRF-3 phosphorylation[448] or STAT1 nuclear translocation.[253] These viruses are also attenuated in their pathogenicity in mice, emphasizing the importance of P protein–mediated suppression of IFN responses as a virulence factor for RABV. However, equally important virulence factors for RABV are viral mechanisms that suppress production of the activators of innate antiviral responses. The difference in pathogenicity of attenuated viruses compared to field strains (i.e., street viruses) is correlated with lower levels of viral gene expression by the more virulent strains.[377,555] This leads to correspondingly lower induction of antiviral responses by the more virulent viruses. Similarly, strain differences in the N protein have been linked to differences in RIG-I signaling and corresponding differences in virulence.[355] Thus, the key to the pathogenicity of RABV is the combination of having a potent suppressive mechanism to inhibit IFN responses in susceptible cells together with a sufficiently low level of viral gene expression to reduce the responses generated in the cells of the innate immune system. In other words, RABV is said to "[use] stealth to reach the brain".[482]

EPIDEMIOLOGY OF RHABDOVIRUS INFECTIONS

Epidemiology of Lyssavirus Infections

Lyssavirus epidemiology is partially influenced by host species distribution, abundance, demographics, behavioral ecology, dispersal, and interactions with humans.[467] Rabies is a reportable disease in many countries, although surveillance is inadequate, particularly in sylvatic hosts. Biased epidemiologic information usually derives from clinical reports or the examination of suitable brain material submitted to public health or veterinary diagnostic laboratories only after infectious contact with animals is suspected. Exposure is generally defined as transdermal contact, typically by a bite, or mucosal contamination with potentially infectious material (e.g., saliva or CNS tissue).[583] The relative risk associated with other scenarios is difficult to define.

The domestic dog is the principal host and major vector of rabies throughout the world.[552] International reporting of both human and animal rabies cases grossly underestimates the magnitude of the problem.[371] Predominant wild reservoirs and maintenance hosts belong to the family Carnivora and include foxes in the Arctic (*Vulpes lagopus*), Canada, central and western Europe, and moderate latitudes of Asia (*V. vulpes, V. corsac*), and scattered foci elsewhere throughout North America (e.g., *Urocyon cinereoargenteus*); the raccoon dog (*Nyctereutes procyonoides*) in eastern Europe, Scandinavia, and portions of Asia[298]; coyotes, jackals (*Canis* species), and other wild canids in North America, Asia, and Africa[188]; skunks (*Mephitis mephitis, Spilogale putorius*) in North America[208]; procyonids, such as the raccoon (*Procyon lotor*), in eastern North America[53]; and herpestids (e.g., the yellow mongoose, *Cynictis penicillata*; the small Asian mongoose, *Herpestes javanicus*) and their relatives throughout Africa, Asia, and the Middle East.[545] Additionally, the ferret badger (*Melogale moschata*) was documented as a rabies reservoir in several regions of China.[334] Rabies detection in rodents is rare.[92]

Bat rabies predominates in the New World, described primarily among insectivorous bats of the United States and Canada (over 40 species) and the three hematophagous vampire species (principally, *Desmodus rotundus*) ranging from northern Mexico to Argentina.[34] Many bat species may also be important throughout Latin America.[126] Other lyssaviruses are transmitted by bats in Africa, Europe, Asia, and Australia.[17,305]

Surveillance efforts in the United States follow changes in indigenous and translocated cases in space and over time. For example, in 2009, 49 states and Puerto Rico reported 6,690 rabid animals and 4 human rabies cases to the Centers for Disease Control and Prevention (CDC). Approximately 92% of reported rabid animals were wildlife. Relative contributions by the major animal groups were 34.8% raccoons, 24.3% bats, 24.0% skunks, 7.5% foxes, 4.5% cats, 1.2% dogs, and 1.1% cattle. Compared with 2008, reported numbers of rabid raccoons and bats decreased, whereas reported numbers of rabid skunks, foxes, cats, cattle, dogs, and horses increased.[58] Historically, Hawaii has remained the only rabies-free state, never having reported a case of indigenously acquired rabies.[470]

Combined with historical, temporal, and spatial disease surveillance data, antigenic characterization with monoclonal antibodies (MAbs) and nucleotide sequence analysis can assist in the assignment of isolates to different animal reservoirs.[500] Arctic RABV circulates circumpolarly, although local variability was documented in several areas, such as Alaska and Ontario. Although *V. lagopus* historically has been recognized as the major reservoir of Arctic RABV, *V. vulpes* increasingly participates in circulation of this virus variant due to climate changes. Skunk rabies isolates appear to be distinct variants defining separate outbreaks in the north-central and south-central parts of North America and California. Additionally, smaller independent foci involve foxes, dogs, and coyotes in Texas, as well as foxes in Arizona and portions of the southwestern United States.[58]

Analysis of human rabies cases from the United States implicated viruses associated with insectivorous bats as the most frequent source of infection after elimination of canine rabies[58] and some bat isolates appear to possess unique pathogenic properties compared with isolates from the family Carnivora.[378] During 2003, a first reported occurrence of rabies in a human infected with the raccoon rabies virus variant was documented in Virginia; however, the exposure history was unknown. During 2004, transplantation from an infected donor resulted in four human cases in the United States[504] and three in Germany,[227] demonstrating the devastating consequences when rabies is not suspected.

Host switching from bats to terrestrial mammals during the history of lyssavirus evolution has been inferred from RABV phylogeny.[32] Based on the relatedness of carnivore RABV variants to bat RABV variants, the switch is proposed to have occurred approximately 1,000 to 1,500 years ago. Moreover, relatively frequent spill-over cases and host shifts of bat RABV variants to terrestrial mammals have been documented repeatedly during recent years.[20] More controversial is a proposed cross-species shift in lyssaviruses, given that a variety of non-RABV lyssaviruses, but not RABV, have been detected in bats in the Eastern Hemisphere, and only RABV detected in all reservoir hosts, including bats, in the Western Hemisphere.

In western and central Europe, where fox rabies has been largely eliminated via oral vaccination, bat rabies still poses public health concerns. The EBLV-1, first isolated in 1954 in Germany, was later identified across Europe, from Spain to the Ukraine.[304] About 95% of EBLV-1 cases have been observed in

E. serotinus bats.[17] However, it has also been reported in numerous other bat species.[486] Spill-over infections of EBLV-1 were documented in sheep in Denmark,[458] in stone marten in Germany,[384] and in domestic cats in France.[122] In contrast to EBLV-1, distribution of EBLV-2 is limited to northwestern Europe. This virus circulates primarily among bats of the *Myotis* genus. Five human rabies cases of bat origin have been documented in Europe. In one case, the virus was identified as EBLV-1, in two others EBLV-2 was identified, and in two cases the virus was not characterized.

Bat lyssavirus surveillance in southeastern Europe and Asia is extremely limited. Nevertheless, such viruses as ARAV and KHUV were isolated from *Myotis* bats in Central Asia.[307] IRKV was isolated from *Murina leucogaster* in Eastern Siberia[63] and later caused a human rabies case in the Far East,[49] and WCBV was isolated in the Caucasus region from *Miniopterus schreibersii*.[303] Historical records indicate isolation of lyssaviruses from bats in India and Thailand,[414] and serologic surveys demonstrated the presence of lyssavirus antibodies in bats from the Philippines, Cambodia, Thailand, and Bangladesh.[446] Presumed human rabies of bat origin was reported from China, although no virological examination was performed.[519] Indeed, significant surveillance efforts are needed in this large part of the world to elucidate ecology and epidemiology of lyssaviruses.

In Africa, several divergent lyssavirus species have been documented. Dog rabies is widely distributed and represents the major burden for humans and domestic animals. At least three phylogenetic lineages of dog RABV were described, along with a separate lineage associated with mongooses.[545] Epizootics in dogs frequently spread to wildlife.[321] Several outbreaks have been described that significantly reduced populations of such endangered species as African wild dog (*Lycaon pictus*)[236] and Ethiopian wolf (*Canis simensis*).[266] Another African lyssavirus, MOKV, has been sporadically isolated from shrews, domestic cats and dogs, and a rodent in various localities of sub-Saharan Africa.[353] MOKV is the only lyssavirus species never documented in bats. However, the principal reservoir host of this virus is still unknown. Two human cases of MOKV infection were documented via active surveillance efforts, both with unknown exposure history.[157] In contrast to MOKV, LBV is clearly associated with bats from the *Pteropodidae* family, such as *Eidolon helvum*, *Rousettus aegyptiacus*, *Micropteropus pussilus*, *Epomophorus wahlbergi*, and likely others, with only infrequent spill-over infections into terrestrial mammals, such as cats, dogs, and a mongoose.[306] LBV is broadly distributed in sub-Saharan Africa and at least once was translocated to France with *R. aegyptiacus* fruit bats, imported from Togo or Egypt.[26] The other two African bat lyssaviruses are less studied. Of the four known isolates of DUVV, three came from humans, who died of rabies after bites of insectivorous bats in South Africa and Kenya, and only one was obtained from a bat, presumably of the *Miniopterus* genus, in Zimbabwe.[544] The last member of the genus, SHIBV, is known by a single isolate, obtained from an insectivorous bat *Hipposideros commersonii* in Kenya.[305] Indeed, more studies are needed to understand ecology and epidemiology of African non-RABV lyssaviruses.

Prior to 1996, Australia had been considered free of rabies and rabies-like viruses. An outbreak of rabies involving several dogs occurred in the island state of Tasmania in 1867 but was quickly eradicated. Since then, only a few imported rabies cases were registered. Following the discovery that flying foxes were a reservoir of Hendra virus, surveillance of these animals was increased, which resulted in the discovery of ABLV in 1996.[180] ABLV has been identified in all four flying fox species in continental Australia: *P. alecto, P. poliocephalus, P. scapulatus,* and *P. conspicillatus,* in locations along the eastern coastal territory of the continent, where the surveillance was enhanced.[212] A distinct ABLV variant was identified in insectivorous bats *Saccolaimus albiventris.*[201] Human cases of ABLV infection from insectivorous bats were first documented in 1996,[15] and infection by a pteropid ABLV variant in 2002.[558] Both cases were fatal, and clinical symptoms were compatible with rabies. The distribution range of *P. alecto* bats extends into Papua, New Guinea, and the eastern islands of Indonesia.[180] The presence of antibodies to ABLV in 9.5% bat serum samples collected in the Philippines emphasizes that the geographic distribution of the virus is not restricted to Australia.[21]

Epidemiology of Vesiculovirus Infections

The mechanisms of VSV transmission are not completely understood. Ecologic factors and special conditions regarding the host and the etiologic agent have been implicated in the clinical presentation of the disease.[218] Experimental transmission from animal to animal by direct contact has produced irregular results. The virus is unable to penetrate intact skin or mucosa; for a successful transmission, it needs to be introduced beneath the skin and mucous membranes via wounds and abrasions. The virus can also be transmitted by the bite of insect vectors such as mosquitoes (*Aedes* spp.),[527] sand flies (*Lutzomyia* spp.),[106] blackflies (*Simulium* spp.),[119] and other Diptera.[163] Virus isolations from nonbiting insects (e.g., *Musca domestica*) have been reported.[179] Many potential biological vectors of VSV have been suggested, but the phlebotomine sand fly, *Lutzomyia shannoni,* is the only one confirmed in the United States.

The disease is present only in the Western Hemisphere, and it is enzootic in southern Mexico, in Central America, in some regions of South America,[559] and on Ossabaw Island, off the coast of Georgia.[507] In temperate zones, VSV outbreaks begin in late summer and end with the arrival of frost. In the United States, the outbreak during 1982–1983 was unusual because it continued throughout the winter months until the following spring.[65] In tropical areas, the disease appears at the end of the rainy season and disappears with the advent of the dry season. Typically, the disease affects only horses, cattle, and swine. During outbreaks, morbidity rates in a herd usually range from 10% to 15%.[559] Cattle generally recover in a few days, but horses and pigs can develop lameness.[559] A broad spectrum of wild mammals can also be affected.[559] Factors that influence the disease spread in dairy cattle include coarse roughage, hard pelleted concentrates, poor general and milking hygiene, and insufficient teat sanitation.[218] In the southeastern United States, feral swine had 10% to 100% antibody prevalence from 1979 to 1985 and on Ossabaw Island showed 12% and 60% seroconversion between June and September in 1982 and 1983.[508] In some enzootic areas of Central America, over 80% of the cattle have antibodies against VSV, but only 9% of the animals may present clinical signs in a particular year. In the same regions, wildlife also have a high VSV seroprevalence. In tropical areas where the disease is enzootic, VSV seroprevalence in the human population can be as high as 48%.[267] Serologic studies during outbreaks in Panama demonstrated a seroprevalence of 71% and 34% in personnel working with infected and

noninfected cattle.[67] A similar situation has been observed during VSV outbreaks in Colorado, where personnel (veterinarians, researchers, and regulatory staff) handling sick livestock showed an antibody prevalence of 13%, whereas unexposed humans had a 6% seroprevalence.[445]

The mechanism by which VSV is maintained in enzootic regions is not fully understood. Sand flies may transmit the virus from a reservoir (e.g., plants, wildlife, cattle) to livestock. Alternatively, VSV may be maintained in the sand fly population by transovarial transmission, and the insects infect susceptible animals during feeding.[106] In enzootic areas, feral swine have been suggested as a potential amplifying host.[507] Molecular epidemiologic studies indicate that enzootic areas may be the origin of the virus responsible for outbreaks in epizootic zones.[391] VSV may be introduced in a particular area by the movement of infected animals, wildlife, or insects, but the actual mechanism is unknown. Viruses circulating in enzootic areas present a high genetic diversity, with several lineages coexisting in the same region.[392] Within enzootic areas, the viruses seem to adapt under selective pressures exerted by ecologic factors. Viruses from different ecologic areas within enzootic regions belong to different genotypes. Viral adaptation to different insect vectors or mammalian reservoirs might be determinant factors for this divergent evolution.[456] Viruses obtained from a particular outbreak are genetically homogeneous.[391]

Epidemiology of Ephemerovirus Infections

Bovine ephemeral fever is distributed throughout Africa, the Middle East, Southeast Asia, and northern Australia.[505] It has never been reported in the Americas. The disease occurs during summer and autumn and disappears with the arrival of the first frosts in subtropical areas. In the tropics, yearly occurrence is associated with the rainy season.[505,550] Although transmission of the virus occurs via insect vectors, the difficulty of isolating the virus from insects hampers the recognition of the vector species involved in its transmission. BEFV was isolated from *Culicoides* spp. and from mosquitoes. In Australia, the geographic range of the disease is greater than that of the *Culicoides* species from which the virus was isolated. Two species of mosquitoes, *Culex annulirostris* and *Anopheles annulipes,* may be implicated in transmission in these areas.[505] In general, morbidity is low, but in some outbreaks, all of the animals in a herd may be affected. In other instances, only 2% or 3% of the animals show clinical signs.[505,550] Natural disease occurs only in cattle and water buffalo. Although seroprevalences of 13% to 38% were reported in cattle in enzootic areas, a higher prevalence of 64% has been observed during outbreaks.[124] The role of wild ruminants in the maintenance of BEFV in nature is not understood. Seroprevalences between 28% and 54% are found in wild ruminants in Kenya, Zimbabwe, and Tanzania.

Epidemiology of Novirhabdovirus Infections

Novirhabdoviruses cause severe economic losses to the salmonid farming industries.[235] IHNV is endemic to western North America, and dispersal of the virus outside North America has occurred by inadvertent transport of infected eggs and juvenile fish.[234] Within North America, dispersal of IHNV is thought to have involved the historical use of unpasteurized salmon viscera in feed for salmon hatcheries, and possibly the historically common practice of salmon transplantations.[76] Following the introduction to the Eastern Hemisphere, European and Asian

IHNV isolates demonstrate relatedness to specific phylogenetic lineages within the endemic area from which they were derived.[283,395,410]

VHSV was first discovered in Western Europe and has been isolated from over 60 fish species from both marine and freshwater habitats in North America, Asia, and Europe.[496] VHSV is endemic to numerous marine species in both the Atlantic and Pacific Oceans of the northern hemisphere and could have been introduced into freshwater habitats by marine fish species (e.g., herring, sprat, sand eel) that are used as fresh feed for commercial farming in some countries.[496] The freshwater isolates of VHSV appear to be evolving approximately 2.5 times faster than the marine isolates.[152] The successful recent viral adaptation in new hosts is one of the possible explanations for such higher evolutionary rates of VHSV in freshwater fish.[381] Alternative explanations for the increased substitution rates in freshwater VHSV are the intensive aquaculture practices and the higher water temperature in culture ponds, which could cause an increase in virus replication rates.[152] A similar pattern has also been observed for IHNV in North America, where the evolutionary rate was found to be three to four times higher in regions with intensive aquaculture, as compared with other regions.[536]

HIRRV was first isolated in Japan from Japanese flounder[284] and subsequently was also reported in Korea.[281] The virus infects several fish species endemic to Japan.[284] SHRV that causes epizootic ulcerative syndrome was first isolated from snakehead fish in Thailand[274] and infects warm water wild and cultured species in South East Asia.

CLINICAL FEATURES OF RHABDOVIRUS INFECTIONS

Lyssavirus Infections

Rabies cases are almost always attributable to the bite of a rabid animal. For example, animal bites were the cause of 99.8% of 3,920 human rabies cases examined at various Pasteur Institutes between 1927 and 1946.[363] Nonbite exposures, which rarely cause rabies, include inhalation of aerosols,[579] licks,[314] transdermal scratches, or other unusual events that lead to contamination of an open wound or mucous membrane, such as tissue or organ transplantation.[504] Bat RABV-associated human deaths in the United States may not have a reported exposure source,[84] but these cases are most likely caused by bat bites in which either the risk was not appreciated or the bites were not immediately recognized by the patient. Disease development after exposure depends on the location and severity of a bite, the species of animal responsible for the exposure, and the virus variant.[27,35] In the absence of vaccination, the highest mortality tends to occur in persons bitten on the head and face (40% to 80%), with intermediate mortality in those bitten on the hands or arms (15% to 40%), and least in those bitten on the trunk or legs (5% to 10%) or through clothing (<5%).[27]

The incubation period (the length of time between exposure to virus and development of clinical signs) is usually 1 to 2 months.[556] Because it can vary from less than a week[228] to several years,[11] rabies is one of the most variable infectious diseases. The length of the incubation period may depend on the bite site and relative proximity to the CNS,[11,265] severity of the bite,

type and quantity of virus introduced, host age, and immune status.[11,226,363]

Development of clinical rabies in humans can be divided into three general phases: a prodromal period, the acute neurologic phase, and coma preceding death.[228] During the prodromal period, lasting 2 to 10 days, symptoms are usually mild and almost entirely nonspecific; they include general malaise, chills, fever, headache, photophobia, anorexia, nausea, vomiting, diarrhea, sore throat, cough, and musculoskeletal pain. One specific early symptom is abnormal sensation around the bite site, such as itching, burning, numbness, or paresthesia.[145]

During the acute neurologic phase, patients exhibit signs of nervous system dysfunction such as anxiety, agitation, dysphagia, hypersalivation, paralysis, and episodes of delirium. Occasionally, priapism or increased libido may be observed.[149] Cases in which hyperactivity is predominant are classified as furious rabies. When paralysis dominates, it is classified as paralytic or dumb rabies.[95,287] From 17% to 80% of patients exhibit hydrophobia, a pathognomonic sign of rabies believed to be caused by an exaggerated respiratory tract protective reflex.[11,18] Hydrophobic episodes, initially triggered by attempts to drink[228] can last from 1 to 5 minutes. In furious rabies, the neurologic period ends after 2 to 7 days with coma or sudden death from respiratory or cardiac arrest.[59]

Paralytic rabies occurs in about 20% of patients and may be more frequent in persons exposed to certain strains, such as vampire bat RABV.[247] In marked contrast to furious rabies, the sensorium is largely spared[229,247] Patients initially develop paresthesia and weakness, and finally flaccid paralysis, usually in the bitten extremity.[95] Paralysis progresses to paraplegia and quadriplegia. In paralytic rabies, the course is usually less rapidly progressive, with some patients living up to 30 days without intensive care. The final stage of the disease is coma, which lasts 3 to 7 days and results in death.[59] In patients receiving respiratory assistance, survival may be prolonged for weeks[59,396] with death caused by other complications.

A handful of cases of human recovery from clinical rabies have been documented following exposure from an animal bites,[16,577] or after suspected inhalation of rabies virus in the laboratory.[83] Only one of these occurred in a patient who had never been vaccinated,[577] whereas the other cases were attributed as exposures and vaccination failures. In the nonvaccinated patient, an experimental treatment included induction of ketamine coma in conjunction with antiviral compounds and intensive care.[577] Attempts to repeat such experimental treatment (although with deviations and modifications) have largely failed,[257] except in a vaccination failure case (immunoglobulin was not administered, although all five doses of vaccine were administered on time). This is also the first documented survival case where the virus variant was identified (vampire bat RABV). In all other survivors neither antigen detection nor virus isolation nor RNA amplification was successful, and rabies diagnosis was based on the history of exposure, compatible incubation period and clinical signs, and serologic tests. Another case of presumptive abortive rabies infection in a human, who never required intensive care, and only once received rabies biologics after establishment of the diagnosis, has also been reported.[85] Most recently, a case of abortive rabies in a child in South Africa that was bitten by rabid dogs on two separate occasions and received incomplete propylaxis.[565a]

Clinical disease in animals is not unlike that of humans, except for the absence of hydrophobia. Signs are variable but can include altered phonation, pica, cranial nerve deficits, altered activity patterns, and loss of fear of humans.[33]

Vesiculovirus Infections

In natural infection, the incubation period of vesiculovirus varies from 2 to 9 days, but usually lesions develop between 2 and 5 days after exposure.[225] The lesions of vesiculovirus are indistinguishable from those of FMD. In cattle, the initial lesions are characterized by pink to white papules in the mouth that progress in 1 to 2 days to vesicles. The vesicles can coalesce and rupture, leaving a denuded area that heals in 1 or 2 weeks if no secondary infections occur. These lesions can also occur in the dental pad, lips, gums, muzzle, nose, teats, and feet. In experimental inoculation of horses, vesicles appeared in the mouth 42 hours after inoculation, and 2 days later, part of the dorsal epithelial covering of the tongue sloughed off. Vesicles also appeared on the feet. At necropsy, the spleen was enlarged, but no other lesions were observed in the internal organs.[113] In natural infection of horses, lesions are found in the lips, corners of the mouth, muzzle, nostrils, ears, belly, prepuce, and udder.[225] The lesions in pigs are similar to those described for cattle. Affected animals have increased salivation and a sharp reduction in milk production. Eating is difficult because of the sore mouth, with a consequent decline in physical condition. Lameness develops with foot lesions.

Although development of secondary lesions in places other than the point of inoculation is suggestive of viremia, the virus has not been isolated from blood even at 6 hours after the experimental inoculation of pigs.[101,506] The virus is present at its highest titer in the vesicular fluid, which represents a transient but very efficient source of virus for contact transmission. The virus can be isolated from specimens taken from saliva, tonsils, vesicular fluids of feet, and, in some cases, feces.[101,306]

Ephemerovirus Infections

After an incubation period of 2 to 4 days, the first clinical sign is fever (40°C to 42°C), accompanied by malaise and a severe drop in milk production. In 12 to 24 hours, fever remits, followed by a second febrile phase. During this second phase, the animals are depressed, are anorexic, and show muscle stiffness and lameness. Ruminal stasis, nasal and ocular discharges, and swelling of one or more joints are present. Subcutaneous emphysema can develop in some animals.[505,550] The clinical signs persist for 1 or 2 days, followed by rapid recovery. Clinical signs are much more severe in adults than in calves. Calves under 6 months of age show no clinical signs.

Novirhabdovirus Infections

VHS generally occurs at temperatures between 4°C and 14°C. At water temperatures between 15°C and 18°C, the disease generally has a short course with a modest accumulated mortality. VHS rarely occurs at higher temperatures. Low water temperatures (1°C to 5°C) generally result in an extended disease course with low daily mortality but high accumulated mortality. For IHNV, the temperature optimum is slightly greater, 3°C to 18°C. VHS outbreaks occur during all seasons but are most common in spring when water temperatures are rising or fluctuating. VHS progresses in three stages. The acute stage includes

a rapid onset of high mortalities (up to 90%, particularly in young fish) often with severe clinical signs such as darkening of body color, exophthalmia (bulging eye), bleeding around eyes and fin bases, pale gills, and petechial (pinpoint) hemorrhaging on the surfaces of the gills and viscera and in the muscle. Virus multiplication in endothelial cells of blood capillaries, hematopoietic tissues, and cells of the kidney underlies the clinical signs. Gross pathology includes generalized petechial hemorrhaging in the skin, muscle tissue (especially in dorsal muscles), and internal organs.

During the second subacute, or chronic, stage, the body continues to darken and exophthalmia may become more pronounced, but hemorrhaging around the eyes and fin bases is often reduced. Fish are severely anemic and paleness is particularly evident in the abdomen. Fish may develop a spiraling swimming motion. The final, nervous stage involves reduced mortality and clinical signs are usually absent, but the corkscrew swimming motion becomes more pronounced. The disease is transmitted horizontally through contact with infected fish or water. Large amounts of virus are shed in the feces, urine, and sexual fluids. There is no vertical transmission of the VHSV. However, vertical transmission has been documented for IHNV. Virus is shed from infected fish via the urine and reproductive fluids and can also be transferred by piscivorous birds as external mechanical vectors.[408] Incubation time is dependent on temperature and dose; it is 5 to 12 days at higher temperatures. During and immediately following an outbreak, virus can be isolated readily from kidney, heart, and spleen tissues.

VHSV can also establish a carrier state in freshwater fish species.[268] The virological status of such carriers will be dependent on a range of parameters including the length of time following initial exposure and geographical proximity to fish-farm outlets. Based on virus isolation in cell culture, the prevalence of VHSV in marine fish species has been found to be in the range of 0.0% to 16.7%.[496]

DIAGNOSIS OF RHABDOVIRUS INFECTIONS

Lyssavirus Infections

Absent a documented exposure to a rabid animal, rabies should be considered in any acute, unexplained neurologic disease that rapidly progresses to coma and death. Routine diagnosis is established by standard laboratory tests for specific virus isolates, antigens, nucleic acids, or neutralizing antibodies.[217] Postmortem diagnosis should be performed on CNS specimens, especially the brainstem and cerebellum.[523] The fluorescent antibody and avidin-biotin immunohistochemical technique[214] are sensitive and specific methods for detecting virus antigen (Fig. 7.14).

Examination of skin biopsies from the face[73] or hair-covered occipital portions of the neck for virus antigen[396] is a rapid method to diagnose human rabies before death. Rabies virus can be isolated from saliva by direct intracerebral inoculation into mice[294] or by infection of neuroblastoma cells.[498] Fluorescent antibody examinations of corneal impressions may occasionally lead to the diagnosis of human rabies.[288] The reverse transcriptase-polymerase chain reaction (RT-PCR) assay has

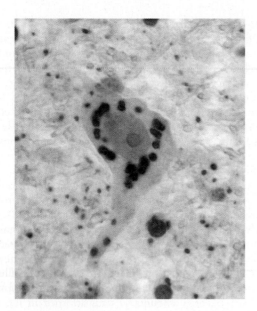

FIGURE 7.14 Immunohistochemical staining of intracytoplasmic viral inclusions in the neuron of a human rabies patient (630×). (Courtesy of M. Niezgoda, CDC/OID/NCEZID/DHPP/PRB.)

been used to amplify and sequence parts of the lyssavirus genome directly from brain, saliva, and other affected tissues.[103] This allows detection of rabies virus–specific RNA and also permits insights into the identity of the virus variant by genetic sequencing. Detection of specific antibodies in serum,[396] late in the clinical course can be diagnostic for rabies, if the patient has not been previously vaccinated. Except for certain cases of postvaccinal encephalomyelitis, CSF antibodies are produced only in rabies-infected, not in vaccinated, individuals.[557] Several diagnostic tests have been developed for detection of virus-neutralizing antibodies, such as the rapid fluorescent focus inhibition test (RFFIT) and the fluorescent antibody viral neutralization (FAVN) test, which are recommended by national and international authorities, such as the World Health Organization (WHO), Office International des Epizooties (OIE), and Advisory Commission on Immunization Practices (ACIP).[503] Lentiviral pseudotypes containing glycoproteins of different lyssaviruses have been developed for replacement of infectious RABV in such virus-neutralizing tests.[584] Several modifications of enzyme-linked immunosorbent assays (ELISAs) have been developed for capture and measure of antiglycoprotein antibodies of RABV but are not recommended for the cases where diagnostic accuracy is critical.[376] Other serologic methods have been developed that detect antibodies against other components of RABV, primarily the nucleocapsid, which is most abundant in the infected cells. Of these, the best established is the indirect fluorescent antibody test (IFA). Antibodies detected by IFA appear earlier than virus-neutralizing antibodies and sometimes are the only positive result obtained antemortem.[499]

Vesiculovirus Infections

Because vesiculovirus is clinically similar to FMD, differential diagnosis between the two diseases is critical in countries free of the latter disease. VSV can be isolated from vesicular fluid or epithelium of the lesions by inoculation in mice, embryonated eggs, or cell culture. The virus can be identified by virus

neutralization, complement fixation, or immunofluorescence. Complement fixation provides a rapid, sensitive, and accurate method for the differentiation of VSV and FMD virus.[219] A rise in virus neutralization or ELISA antibody titer in serum samples taken during the clinical and convalescent phases of the disease is evidence that the infection was caused by VSV.[14] RT-PCR is highly sensitive and specific, providing a rapid diagnosis and material for genetic characterization of the virus.[457]

Ephemerovirus Infections

Clinical diagnosis of BEF is based on its rapidity of spread and transient nature. For confirmation, virus isolation or the demonstration of an increase in virus neutralization or ELISA antibody in paired serum samples is needed.[137] A blocking ELISA compares favorably with neutralization and does not detect cross-reacting antibodies to Kimberly or Berrimah viruses.[594] Although impractical for routine diagnosis, cattle inoculation with blood from BEFV-affected animals is the most sensitive method for viral isolation. Isolation of BEFV in *Aedes albopictus* cells from the blood of infected animals, followed by direct immunofluorescence to detect the presence of viral antigens, has been used in experimental studies.[540]

Novirhabdovirus Infections

The occurrence of clinical signs of VHS described earlier should suggest the presence of IHNV and VHSV. Gross pathology includes generalized petechial hemorrhaging in the skin, muscle tissue (especially in dorsal muscles), and internal organs. Histopathologic findings reveal degenerative necrosis in the hematopoietic tissues, kidney, spleen, liver, pancreas, and digestive tract. Necrosis of eosinophilic granular cells in the intestinal wall is pathognomic of IHNV infection. The kidney, liver, and spleen show extensive focal necrosis and degeneration—cytoplasmic vacuoles, pyknosis, karyolysis, and lymphocytic invasion. In case of VHSV, diagnosis can involve immunohistochemistry analysis of VHSV-positive endothelial cells in the vascular system.[156] The standard surveillance method to detect carrier fish for IHNV and VHSV is based on direct isolation of the virus in cell culture followed by identification using antibody-based methods (IFA, ELISA) or nucleic acid–based methods (e.g., RT-PCR), followed by gene sequencing. PCR-based detection of viral genomes in fish tissue has also been described.[127]

PREVENTION AND CONTROL OF RHABDOVIRUS INFECTIONS

Lyssavirus Infections in Humans

Rabies has the highest case-to-fatality ratio of any infectious disease. With rare exceptions, comfort care, sedation, and life support measures may prolong life but do not prevent death. In most situations, use of the term treatment is a misnomer and refers to medical aid related to animal bite and disease prevention by postexposure prophylaxis.[574] However, the establishment of a protocol for experimental treatment of clinical rabies[577] has led to more attempts to combat the clinical disease. The majority of these have failed[257] although at least one positive result, with recovery of the patient, was reported. Indeed, more studies in suitable animal models are needed to investigate different components of the protocol, potential ways of their modifications, and improvements.[257] More than 12 million humans are exposed and may undergo antirabies prophylaxis annually, but in excess of an estimated 50,000 to 100,000 die, primarily from the bite of an infected dog.[371] Regional epidemiologic surveillance and knowledge of viral pathogenesis, development of vaccination algorithms, and communication of risk to different occupational groups can significantly reduce human morbidity from inappropriate prophylaxis and rabies mortality.[489] Eliminating primary exposure to rabid animals is a fundamental means of rabies prevention. Human rabies deaths are infrequent in regions with controlled canine rabies. Nevertheless, tens of thousands of potential exposure cases are treated annually in Europe and North America because of enzootic wildlife rabies.[217]

Postexposure prophylaxis in humans includes proper wound care and the administration of rabies vaccine and antirabies immune globulin. Although the inclusion of antirabies serum or immune globulin in the prophylaxis protocol is not new, it is infrequent. Most cases of human rabies prophylaxis in Africa, Asia, and Latin America are with vaccine only, often a nervous system tissue vaccine.[130] Cell culture–based rabies vaccines (e.g., human diploid cell rabies vaccine [HDCV]) are used in much of the developed world and form the standard for historical comparison with the Pasteurian neural vaccines from the 19th century. Inactivated cell culture–based vaccines[511] and antirabies immune globulin, which are major improvements over cruder biologicals, decrease the adverse events related to anaphylaxis or serum sickness.[575] Other major rabies vaccines are produced in avian embryo fibroblasts (e.g., purified chick embryo cell culture rabies vaccine [PCEC], Rabipur) or in rhesus monkey kidney cells (purified Vero cell rabies vaccine [PVRV], Verorab), with aluminum phosphate as an adjuvant. Production of HDCV is relatively difficult, with limited viral yields, resulting in high production costs. Primary hamster kidney cell vaccines are used in Russia, China, and other parts of Asia.[23] Efficacy trials using reduced doses, different immunization schedules, and alternative routes (e.g., intradermal administration) have been conducted and have demonstrated both high efficacy and safety.[98]

Vaccine failures are usually associated with inadequate wound care, omission of potent serum, failure to infiltrate the wound with immune globulin, delay, or failure to follow recommended procedures.[576] Future tactics for global human rabies prevention will continue to focus on the need for enhanced public health communications; continuing professional education; potent, inexpensive pre- and postexposure vaccines,[183] and new schedules; and viable alternatives to rabies immune globulin including monoclonal antibodies.[37] Based on the recognition that rabies at its source can be effectively controlled and sometimes eliminated, safer, more effective, and inexpensive veterinary vaccines are a necessity for animal reservoirs, vectors, or victims of the disease.[170]

Although available rabies biologics provide reliable protection against related lyssaviruses (RABV, DUVV, EBLV-1, EBLV-2, ABLV, ARAV, KHUV, DUVV), they do not protect against lyssaviruses LBV, MOKV, SHIBV, or WCBV, because of the significant antigenic differences.[31] Given broad distribution of the latter divergent lyssaviruses in Africa, in southeastern Europe, and perhaps more widely in the world,[305,353] there is a need to develop new biologicals, capable of providing reliable protection against them. Efforts to develop small molecule

inhibitors of RABV infection have led to the advancement of molecules that impede G's function during entry, and to the development of additional molecules that target polymerase functions.[141]

Control of Rabies in Animals

The numerous and diverse wild reservoirs for rabies pose significant challenges for control. The correlation between canine rabies and human fatalities, however, has led to the successful application of domestic animal vaccines, particularly in developed countries. A comprehensive domestic animal program also requires responsible pet ownership. Such a program entails stray animal management; leash law amendments; humane population curtailment (e.g., early spay and neuter programs); animal importation, translocation, and quarantine regulations; schedules for early preexposure vaccination of companion animals (in light of potential maternal immune inhibition); and rational postexposure management. Unlike postexposure prophylaxis of humans, euthanasia is usually recommended for the naïve animal exposed to rabies.

Current veterinary vaccines are more potent than earlier attenuated and inactivated vaccines.[25] Because no vaccine is 100% effective, given poor cross-reactivity with some viral species,[216] and because correct identification of the properly immunized animal may be confusing, the vaccinated dog or cat is not exempt from confinement and close observation. This strict period of observation of the biting animal applies to dogs, cats, and, in some countries, domestic ferrets. Human prophylaxis may be delayed during this time in areas that are not enzootic for canine rabies.[495] Pet vaccination status does not necessarily alter the need for euthanasia regardless of vaccine potency or efficacy, if rabies is suspected.

For wild mammals, population reduction has been practiced for centuries but is not regarded as a humane, long-term, cost-effective, or ecologically sound tool to control widespread lyssavirus infection. For more than five decades, efforts have been made to protect free-ranging wildlife against virulent street virus by oral consumption of vaccine contained within bait.[578] Millions of rabies virus vaccine–laden baits have been distributed over rural and urban areas in western Europe, eastern Canada, and the United States for wildlife rabies control. Historically, attenuated rabies virus strains (such as ERA, SAD) were broadly used for oral vaccination of wild carnivores in Western Europe and North America.[478] However, sporadically these vaccine strains caused rabies in wildlife.[383] A vaccinia-rabies glycoprotein (V-RG) vaccine was the first recombinant rabies vaccine to be constructed, field tested, and considered for regulation in Europe and North America for wildlife rabies control. This vaccine has been extensively reviewed to ensure safety (tested in more than 40 species of mammals and birds) and efficacy (proved against severe rabies challenge in target species). Thermostability of the vaccine has been demonstrated under laboratory and field conditions. Following the success of the V-RG vaccine against fox rabies in Belgium[66] and France, preliminary field trials suggest its potential utility for rabies control in raccoons, foxes, and coyotes in the United States. Other orthopoxviruses have been considered as vectors of lyssavirus antigens, but these have not yet been field tested.[337] A number of attenuated and recombinant rabies vaccines have been developed[466] including oral vaccines for red, Arctic, and gray foxes; coyotes; raccoon dogs; raccoons; skunks; and domestic dogs.[466]

If future recombinant, replication-incompetent, inactivated, or DNA-based vaccines[466,586] prove both efficacious and economical, they may render most previous biosafety concerns obsolete, paving the way for more widespread, free-ranging wildlife and dog rabies control, particularly in developing countries. Another promising approach is combination of rabies vaccination with immunocontraception, which can significantly reduce the population of the disease vectors, particularly stray dogs.

Control of Vesiculovirus Infections

Supportive veterinary care of affected animals helps to prevent complications that can delay recovery from VSV infection. Vaccination against VSV has been practiced to only a limited extent. A modified live vaccine, attenuated in cell culture or chicken embryos, has been used in parts of the United States, Central America, and Peru. This vaccine, administered intramuscularly in cattle, protects from disease for at least 1 year. A recombinant vaccinia virus expressing the VSV-I glycoprotein was developed and used experimentally to immunize cattle. Inoculated animals developed antibodies and resisted intradermal lingual challenge.[351] VSV-I with rearranged gene orders were also demonstrated to be effective in protecting mice and pigs against challenge with wild type virus.[171]

Control of Ephemerovirus Infections

Vector control of BEFV is very difficult. International efforts to prevent the introduction of disease and vaccination may be the only practical methods for prevention of BEF.[550] Several attenuated vaccines, produced by serial passage in mouse or cell culture, provided protection against experimental challenge when mixed with adjuvants and given in several doses. Inactivated vaccines were developed in Japan and Australia, but they induced poor and unreliable immunity. Vaccinia virus expressing the G protein elicited neutralizing antibodies in cattle, which were resistant to a subsequent viral challenge.[233] Additionally, an experimental subunit vaccine consisting of purified G protein mixed with Quil adjuvant conferred protection against viral challenge.[541]

Control of Novirhabdovirus Infections

Control methods for IHNV currently rely on avoidance of exposure to the virus through the implementation of strict control policies and sound hygiene practices.[580] The thorough disinfection of fertilized eggs, the use of virus-free water supplies for incubation and rearing, and the operation of facilities under established biosecurity measures are all critical for preventing infectious hematopoietic necrosis at a fish production site.

Vaccination of salmonids against IHNV is at an early stage of development; however, a range of vaccine preparations have shown promise in both laboratory and field trials.[300] Both autogenous, killed vaccines and a DNA vaccine have been licensed for commercial use in Atlantic salmon net-pen aquaculture on the West Coast of North America, where such vaccines can be delivered economically by injection. Vaccines against IHNV have not yet been licensed in other countries, where the application of vaccines to millions of small fish will require additional research on novel mass delivery methods. Although research on vaccine development against VHSV has been ongoing for more than three decades, a commercial vaccine is not yet available. DNA-based vaccines have proven to be very promising, inducing good protection from VHS.[338]

Several immunostimulants, such as yeast-derived β-glucans, IL-1β–derived peptides, and probiotics, have been assessed for enhancing protection against VHS.[422] Disinfection of eggs is a highly effective method to block egg-associated transmission of novirhabdoviruses in aquaculture settings.[580] The method is widely practiced in areas where the virus is endemic. Other experimental approaches include resistance breeding and restocking with a resistant fish species.[230]

PERSPECTIVES

VSV remains an important prototype for understanding nonsegmented, negative-strand RNA viruses. We now have complete structures of the viral proteins and the virion and are beginning to understand how those proteins function in each step of viral replication and pathogenesis. Ongoing studies of important pathogens in the family *Rhabdoviridae* will continue to be important as we do not understand RABV as a dreaded cause of disease in animals and humans, and the ephemeroviruses and novirhabdoviruses as important animal pathogens. Study of these viruses should continue to provide fundamental insights into the basis for virus–host interactions, neurotropism, and neuropathogenesis.

In terms of the basic molecular biology of negative-strand RNA viruses, a number of important questions that have yet to be fully addressed have been pointed out through the course of this chapter. For example, the question of how the large, multifunctional L protein is able to respond to the many different cis-acting sequences that regulate its activity, and the issue of how different intracellular nucleocapsids are selected for envelopment during the process of virus assembly are fundamental questions. Understanding how the polymerase navigates the nucleocapsid template and how the various activities of L are coordinated during mRNA synthesis, and how genome replication is coupled to encapsidation remain enduring puzzles. Understanding the cellular compartments in which viral replication occurs presents a fascinating story of host–viral interactions that we are just beginning to understand and may provide new approaches for antiviral development. The atomic structures of the viral proteins and the now straightforward genetic manipulation of the viral genomes provide important components of the tool kit for advancing new countermeasures against rhabdovirus infections. The questions of viral virulence determinants and how rhabdoviruses suppress host responses among the different cell types involved in viral pathogenesis and immunity remain key questions for understanding the basis for viral pathogenesis in intact animals. In terms of the control of rabies, advances will come from the enhanced ability to control the spread of RABV among wild animal populations as well as the development of newer, more effective vaccine strategies.

One of the exciting areas of development with rhabdoviruses is the use of genetically engineered viruses as vaccine vectors or therapeutic agents. The use of recombinant VSV, ISFV, and RABV as vectors has been mentioned several times throughout the chapter, as vaccines, oncolytic agents, and tracers. The successful deployment of VSV-Ebola as a licensed human vaccine paves the way for the advancement of additional VSV vectored vaccines and therapeutics. The use of VSV and RABV as neuronal tracers continues to provide new insights into neuronal circuits. Despite this success, our understanding of rhabdovirus biology remains incomplete. Understanding fundamental aspects of the replication of this family of viruses is likely to continue to be at least as exciting in the future as it has in the past.

ACKNOWLEDGMENTS

The authors acknowledge Douglas S. Lyles, Ivan V. Kuzmin, and Charles E. Rupprecht for the previous edition of this chapter that we updated and edited.

REFERENCES

1. Abdella R, Aggarwal M, Okura T, et al. Structure of a paramyxovirus polymerase complex reveals a unique methyltransferase-CTD conformation. *Proc Natl Acad Sci U S A* 2020;117(9):4931–4941.
2. Abraham G, Banerjee AK. Sequential transcription of the genes of vesicular stomatitis virus. *Proc Natl Acad Sci U S A* 1976;73(5):1504–1508.
3. Abraham G, Rhodes DP, Banerjee AK. The 5′ terminal structure of the methylated mRNA synthesized in vitro by vesicular stomatitis virus. *Cell* 1975;5(1):51–58.
4. Ahmed M, Cramer SD, Lyles DS. Sensitivity of prostate tumors to wild type and M protein mutant vesicular stomatitis viruses. *Virology* 2004;330(1):34–49.
5. Ahmed M, Lyles DS. Identification of a consensus mutation in M protein of vesicular stomatitis virus from persistently infected cells that affects inhibition of host-directed gene expression. *Virology* 1997;237(2):378–388.
6. Ahmed M, Lyles DS. Effect of vesicular stomatitis virus matrix protein on transcription directed by host RNA polymerases I, II, and III. *J Virol* 1998;72(10):8413–8419.
7. Ahmed M, Marino TR, Puckett S, et al. Immune response in the absence of neurovirulence in mice infected with m protein mutant vesicular stomatitis virus. *J Virol* 2008;82(18):9273–9277.
8. Ahmed M, McKenzie MO, Puckett S, et al. Ability of the matrix protein of vesicular stomatitis virus to suppress beta interferon gene expression is genetically correlated with the inhibition of host RNA and protein synthesis. *J Virol* 2003;77(8):4646–4657.
9. Ahmed M, Mitchell LM, Puckett S, et al. Vesicular stomatitis virus M protein mutant stimulates maturation of Toll-like receptor 7 (TLR7)-positive dendritic cells through TLR-dependent and -independent mechanisms. *J Virol* 2009;83(7):2962–2975.
10. Ahne W, Bjorklund HV, Essbauer S, et al. Spring viremia of carp (SVC). *Dis Aquat Organ* 2002;52(3):261–272.
11. Ahuja ML, Brooks AG. Hydrophobia in India. *Ind Med Gaz* 1950;85(10):449–453.
12. Albertini AA, Wernimont AK, Muziol T, et al. Crystal structure of the rabies virus nucleoprotein-RNA complex. *Science* 2006;313(5785):360–363.
13. Alexopoulou L, Holt AC, Medzhitov R, et al. Recognition of double-stranded RNA and activation of NF-kappaB by Toll-like receptor 3. *Nature* 2001;413(6857):732–738.
14. Allende R, Germano PM. Comparison of virus neutralisation and enzyme-linked immunosorbent assay for the identification of antibodies against vesicular stomatitis (Indiana 3) virus. *Rev Sci Tech* 1993;12(3):849–855.
15. Allworth A, Murray K, Morgan J. A human case of encephalitis due to a lyssavirus, recently identified in fruit bats. *Communicable Dis Intell* 1996;20:504.
16. Alvarez L, Fajardo R, Lopez E, et al. Partial recovery from rabies in a nine-year-old boy. *Pediatr Infect Dis J* 1994;13(12):1154–1155.
17. Amengual B, Whitby JE, King A, et al. Evolution of European bat lyssaviruses. *J Gen Virol* 1997;78(Pt 9):2319–2328.
18. Anderson LJ, Nicholson KG, Tauxe RV, et al. Human rabies in the United States, 1960 to 1979: epidemiology, diagnosis, and prevention. *Ann Intern Med* 1984;100(5):728–735.
19. APHIS. Published 2020. https://www.aphis.usda.gov/animal_health/downloads/animal_diseases/vsv/sitrep-11-13-20.pdf. Accessed May 5, 2022.
20. Aréchiga-Ceballos N, Velasco-Villa A, Shi M, et al. New rabies virus variant found during an epizootic in white-nosed coatis from the Yucatan Peninsula. *Epidemiol Infect* 2010;138(11):1586–1589.
21. Arguin PM, Murray-Lillibridge K, Miranda ME, et al. Serologic evidence of Lyssavirus infections among bats, the Philippines. *Emerg Infect Dis* 2002;8(3):258–262.
22. Arnheiter H, Davis NL, Wertz G, et al. Role of the nucleocapsid protein in regulating vesicular stomatitis virus RNA synthesis. *Cell* 1985;41(1):259–267.
23. Assenberg R, Delmas O, Ren J, et al. Structure of the nucleoprotein binding domain of Mokola virus phosphoprotein. *J Virol* 2010;84(2):1089–1096.
24. Atkinson PH, Moyer SA, Summers DF. Assembly of vesicular stomatitis virus glycoprotein and matrix protein into HeLa cell plasma membranes. *J Mol Biol* 1976;102(3):613–631.
25. Aubert M. Rabies vaccines for veterinary use: difficulties in establishing potency acceptability thresholds. *Dev Biol Stand* 1992;79:113–120.
26. Aubert M. Rabies in individual countries, France. *Rabies Bull Europe* 1999;23(2):6.
27. Babes V. *Traité de la rage*. Paris: J.-B. Baillière, et fils; 1912.
28. Babu JR, Jeganathan KB, Baker DJ, et al. Rae1 is an essential mitotic checkpoint regulator that cooperates with Bub3 to prevent chromosome missegregation. *J Cell Biol* 2003;160(3):341–353.
29. Bachmann MF, Hengartner H, Zinkernagel RM. T helper cell-independent neutralizing B cell response against vesicular stomatitis virus: role of antigen patterns in B cell induction? *Eur J Immunol* 1995;25(12):3445–3451.
30. Backovic M, Jardetzky TS. Class III viral membrane fusion proteins. *Curr Opin Struct Biol* 2009;19(2):189–196.
31. Badrane H, Bahloul C, Perrin P, et al. Evidence of two Lyssavirus phylogroups with distinct pathogenicity and immunogenicity. *J Virol* 2001;75(7):3268–3276.
32. Badrane H, Tordo N. Host switching in Lyssavirus history from the Chiroptera to the Carnivora orders. *J Virol* 2001;75(17):8096–8104.
33. Baer GM. Pathogenesis to the central nervous system. In: Baer GM, ed. *The Natural History of Rabies*. New York: Academic Press; 1975:181–198.
34. Baer GM. Vampire bat and bovine paralytic rabies. In: Baer GM, ed. *The Natural History of Rabies*. Boca Raton, FL: CRC Press; 1991:389–403.
35. Baer GM, Cleary WF, Díaz AM, et al. Characteristics of 11 rabies virus isolates in mice: titers and relative invasiveness of virus, incubation period of infection, and survival of mice with sequelae. *J Infect Dis* 1977;136(3):336–345.
36. Baer GM, Neville J, Turner GS. *Rabbis and Rabies: A Pictorial History Through the Ages*. Mexico City: Laboratorios Baer; 1996.
37. Bakker AB, Marissen WE, Kramer RA, et al. Novel human monoclonal antibody combination effectively neutralizing natural rabies virus variants and individual in vitro escape mutants. *J Virol* 2005;79(14):9062–9068.
38. Balachandran S, Roberts PC, Kipperman T, et al. Alpha/beta interferons potentiate virus-induced apoptosis through activation of the FADD/Caspase-8 death signaling pathway. *J Virol* 2000;74(3):1513–1523.
39. Ball LA, Pringle CR, Flanagan B, et al. Phenotypic consequences of rearranging the P, M, and G genes of vesicular stomatitis virus. *J Virol* 1999;73(6):4705–4712.
40. Ball LA, White CN. Order of transcription of genes of vesicular stomatitis virus. *Proc Natl Acad Sci U S A* 1976;73(2):442–446.
41. Baltimore D, Huang AS, Stampfer M. Ribonucleic acid synthesis of vesicular stomatitis virus, II. An RNA polymerase in the virion. *Proc Natl Acad Sci U S A* 1970;66(2):572–576.
42. Barber GN. Vesicular stomatitis virus as an oncolytic vector. *Viral Immunol* 2004;17(4):516–527.
43. Barchet W, Cella M, Odermatt B, et al. Virus-induced interferon alpha production by a dendritic cell subset in the absence of feedback signaling in vivo. *J Exp Med* 2002;195(4):507–516.
44. Barge A, Gaudin Y, Coulon P, et al. Vesicular stomatitis virus M protein may be inside the ribonucleocapsid coil. *J Virol* 1993;67(12):7246–7253.
45. Barik S, Banerjee AK. Phosphorylation by cellular casein kinase II is essential for transcriptional activity of vesicular stomatitis virus phosphoprotein P. *Proc Natl Acad Sci U S A* 1992;89(14):6570–6574.
46. Barr JN, Tang X, Hinzman E, et al. The VSV polymerase can initiate at mRNA start sites located either up or downstream of a transcription termination signal but size of the intervening intergenic region affects efficiency of initiation. *Virology* 2008;374(2):361–370.
47. Barr JN, Wertz GW. Polymerase slippage at vesicular stomatitis virus gene junctions to generate poly(A) is regulated by the upstream 3′-AUAC-5′ tetranucleotide: implications for the mechanism of transcription termination. *J Virol* 2001;75(15):6901–6913.
48. Barr JN, Whelan SP, Wertz GW. cis-Acting signals involved in termination of vesicular stomatitis virus mRNA synthesis include the conserved AUAC and the U7 signal for polyadenylation. *J Virol* 1997;71(11):8718–8725.
49. Belikov SI, Leonova GN, Kondratov IG, et al. Isolation and genetic characterisation of a new lyssavirus strain in the Primorskiy kray. *East Siberian J Infect Pathol* 2009;16:68–69.
50. Bergmann JE, Tokuyasu KT, Singer SJ. Passage of an integral membrane protein, the vesicular stomatitis virus glycoprotein, through the Golgi apparatus en route to the plasma membrane. *Proc Natl Acad Sci U S A* 1981;78(3):1746–1750.
51. Bhatt PN, Rodrigues FM. Chandipura: a new Arbovirus isolated in India from patients with febrile illness. *Indian J Med Res* 1967;55(12):1295–1305.
52. Bi Z, Barna M, Komatsu T, et al. Vesicular stomatitis virus infection of the central nervous system activates both innate and acquired immunity. *J Virol* 1995;69(10):6466–6472.
53. Biek R, Henderson JC, Waller LA, et al. A high-resolution genetic signature of demographic and spatial expansion in epizootic rabies virus. *Proc Natl Acad Sci U S A* 2007;104(19):7993–7998.
54. Bishop DH, Roy P. Kinetics of RNA synthesis by vesicular stomatitis virus particles. *J Mol Biol* 1971;57(3):513–527.
55. Björklund HV, Higman KH, Kurath G. The glycoprotein genes and gene junctions of the fish rhabdoviruses spring viremia of carp virus and hirame rhabdovirus: analysis of relationships with other rhabdoviruses. *Virus Res* 1996;42(1-2):65–80.
56. Black BL, Lyles DS. Vesicular stomatitis virus matrix protein inhibits host cell-directed transcription of target genes in vivo. *J Virol* 1992;66(7):4058–4064.
57. Black BL, Rhodes RB, McKenzie M, et al. The role of vesicular stomatitis virus matrix protein in inhibition of host-directed gene expression is genetically separable from its function in virus assembly. *J Virol* 1993;67(8):4814–4821.
58. Blanton JD, Palmer D, Rupprecht CE. Rabies surveillance in the United States during 2009. *J Am Vet Med Assoc* 2010;237(6):646–657.
59. Blatt ML, Hoffman SJ, Schneider M. Rabies: Report of twelve cases with a discussion of prophylaxis. *J Am Med Assoc* 1938;11:688–691.
60. Blower MD, Nachury M, Heald R, et al. A Rae1-containing ribonucleoprotein complex is required for mitotic spindle assembly. *Cell* 2005;121(2):223–234.
61. Bloyet LM, Morin B, Brusic V, et al. Oligomerization of the vesicular stomatitis virus phosphoprotein is dispensable for mRNA synthesis but facilitates RNA replication. *J Virol* 2020;94(13).
62. Blumberg BM, Leppert M, Kolakofsky D. Interaction of VSV leader RNA and nucleocapsid protein may control VSV genome replication. *Cell* 1981;23(3):837–845.
63. Botvinkin AD, Poleschuk EM, Kuzmin IV, et al. Novel lyssaviruses isolated from bats in Russia. *Emerg Infect Dis* 2003;9(12):1623–1625.
64. Bovo G, Giorgetti G, Jorgensen PEV, et al. Infectious haematopoietic necrosis: first detection in Italy. *Bull Eur Ass Fish Path* 1987;7:124.
65. Bridges VE, McCluskey BJ, Salman MD, et al. Review of the 1995 vesicular stomatitis outbreak in the western United States. *J Am Vet Med Assoc* 1997;211(5):556–560.
66. Brochier B, Kieny MP, Costy F, et al. Large-scale eradication of rabies using recombinant vaccinia-rabies vaccine. *Nature* 1991;354(6354):520–522.

67. Brody JA, Fischer GF, Peralta PH. Vesicular stomatitis virus in Panama. Human serologic patterns in a cattle raising area. *Am J Epidemiol* 1967;86(1):158–161.
68. Brown DA, Rose JK. Sorting of GPI-anchored proteins to glycolipid-enriched membrane subdomains during transport to the apical cell surface. *Cell* 1992;68(3):533–544.
69. Brown EL, Lyles DS. Organization of the vesicular stomatitis virus glycoprotein into membrane microdomains occurs independently of intracellular viral components. *J Virol* 2003;77(7):3985–3992.
70. Brown EL, Lyles DS. Pseudotypes of vesicular stomatitis virus with CD4 formed by clustering of membrane microdomains during budding. *J Virol* 2005;79(11):7077–7086.
71. Browning MJ, Huang AS, Reiss CS. Cytolytic T lymphocytes from the BALB/c-H-2dm2 mouse recognize the vesicular stomatitis virus glycoprotein and are restricted by class II MHC antigens. *J Immunol* 1990;145(3):985–994.
72. Bründler MA, Aichele P, Bachmann M, et al. Immunity to viruses in B cell-deficient mice: influence of antibodies on virus persistence and on T cell memory. *Eur J Immunol* 1996;26(9):2257–2262.
73. Bryceson AD, Greenwood BM, Warrell DA, et al. Demonstration during life of rabies antigen in humans. *J Infect Dis* 1975;131(1):71–74.
74. Brzózka K, Finke S, Conzelmann KK. Identification of the rabies virus alpha/beta interferon antagonist: phosphoprotein P interferes with phosphorylation of interferon regulatory factor 3. *J Virol* 2005;79(12):7673–7681.
75. Brzózka K, Finke S, Conzelmann KK. Inhibition of interferon signaling by rabies virus phosphoprotein P: activation-dependent binding of STAT1 and STAT2. *J Virol* 2006;80(6):2675–2683.
76. Burgner RL. Life history of sockeye salmon (Oncorhynchus nerka). In: Groot C, Margolis L, eds. *Pacific Salmon Life Histories.* Vancouver, BC: UBC Press; 1991:1–118.
77. Cancino J, Torrealba C, Soza A, et al. Antibody to AP1B adaptor blocks biosynthetic and recycling routes of basolateral proteins at recycling endosomes. *Mol Biol Cell* 2007;18(12):4872–4884.
78. Canter DM, Perrault J. Stabilization of vesicular stomatitis virus L polymerase protein by P protein binding: a small deletion in the C-terminal domain of L abrogates binding. *Virology* 1996;219(2):376–386.
79. Cao D, Gao Y, Roesler C, et al. Cryo-EM structure of the respiratory syncytial virus RNA polymerase. *Nat Commun* 2020;11(1):368.
80. Cartwright B, Brown F. Serological relationships between different strains of vesicular stomatis virus. *J Gen Virol* 1972;16(3):391–398.
81. Cary ZD, Willingham MC, Lyles DS. Oncolytic vesicular stomatitis virus induces apoptosis in U87 glioblastoma cells by a type II death receptor mechanism and induces cell death and tumor clearance in vivo. *J Virol* 2011;85(12):5708–5717.
82. Case JB, Rothlauf PW, Chen RE, et al. Neutralizing antibody and soluble ACE2 inhibition of a replication-competent VSV-SARS-CoV-2 and a clinical isolate of SARS-CoV-2. *Cell Host Microbe* 2020;28(3):475–485.e5.
83. Centers for Disease Control. Rabies in a laboratory worker—New York. *MMWR Morb Mortal Wkly Rep* 1977;26:183–184.
84. Centers for Disease Control and Prevention (CDC). Human rabies—Virginia, 1998. *MMWR Morb Mortal Wkly Rep* 1999;48(5):95–97.
85. Centers for Disease Control and Prevention (CDC). Presumptive abortive human rabies—Texas, 2009. *MMWR Morb Mortal Wkly Rep* 2010;59(7):185–190.
86. Chakraborty P, Seemann J, Mishra RK, et al. Vesicular stomatitis virus inhibits mitotic progression and triggers cell death. *EMBO Rep* 2009;10(10):1154–1160.
87. Chare ER, Gould EA, Holmes EC. Phylogenetic analysis reveals a low rate of homologous recombination in negative-sense RNA viruses. *J Gen Virol* 2003;84(Pt 10):2691–2703.
88. Charlton KM, Casey GA. Experimental rabies in skunks: immunofluorescence light and electron microscopic studies. *Lab Invest* 1979;41(1):36–44.
89. Chattopadhyay D, Banerjee AK. Phosphorylation within a specific domain of the phosphoprotein of vesicular stomatitis virus regulates transcription in vitro. *Cell* 1987;49(3):407–414.
90. Chelbi-Alix MK, Vidy A, El Bougrini J, et al. Rabies viral mechanisms to escape the IFN system: the viral protein P interferes with IRF-3, Stat1, and PML nuclear bodies. *J Interferon Cytokine Res* 2006;26(5):271–280.
91. Chen M, Ogino T, Banerjee AK. Interaction of vesicular stomatitis virus P and N proteins: identification of two overlapping domains at the N terminus of P that are involved in N0-P complex formation and encapsidation of viral genome RNA. *J Virol* 2007;81(24):13478–13485.
92. Childs JE, Colby L, Krebs JW, et al. Surveillance and spatiotemporal associations of rabies in rodents and lagomorphs in the United States, 1985–1994. *J Wildl Dis* 1997;33(1):20–27.
93. Chong LD, Rose JK. Membrane association of functional vesicular stomatitis virus matrix protein in vivo. *J Virol* 1993;67(1):407–414.
94. Chong LD, Rose JK. Interactions of normal and mutant vesicular stomatitis virus matrix proteins with the plasma membrane and nucleocapsids. *J Virol* 1994;68(1):441–447.
95. Chopra JS, Banerjee AK, Murthy JM, et al. Paralytic rabies: a clinico-pathological study. *Brain* 1980;103(4):789–802.
96. Christian AY, Barna M, Bi Z, et al. Host immune response to vesicular stomatitis virus infection of the central nervous system in C57BL/6 mice. *Viral Immunol* 1996;9(3):195–205.
97. Chuang JL, Perrault J. Initiation of vesicular stomatitis virus mutant polR1 transcription internally at the N gene in vitro. *J Virol* 1997;71(2):1466–1475.
98. Chutivongse S, Wilde H, Benjavongkulchai M, et al. Postexposure rabies vaccination during pregnancy: effect on 202 women and their infants. *Clin Infect Dis* 1995;20(4):818–820.
99. Ciavarra RP, Greene AR, Horeth DR, et al. Antigen processing of vesicular stomatitis virus in situ. Interdigitating dendritic cells present viral antigens independent of marginal dendritic cells but fail to prime CD4(+) and CD8(+) T cells. *Immunology* 2000;101(4):512–520.
100. Ciavarra RP, Taylor L, Greene AR, et al. Impact of macrophage and dendritic cell subset elimination on antiviral immunity, viral clearance and production of type 1 interferon. *Virology* 2005;2:2.
101. Clarke GR, Stallknecht DE, Howerth EW. Experimental infection of swine with a sandfly (Lutzomyia shannoni) isolate of vesicular stomatitis virus, New Jersey serotype. *J Vet Diagn Invest* 1996;8(1):105–108.
102. Clinton GM, Little SP, Hagen FS, et al. The matrix (M) protein of vesicular stomatitis virus regulates transcription. *Cell* 1978;15(4):1455–1462.
103. Coertse J, Weyer J, Nel LH, et al. Improved PCR methods for detection of African rabies and rabies-related lyssaviruses. *J Clin Microbiol* 2010;48(11):3949–3955.
104. Colonno RJ, Banerjee AK. A unique RNA species involved in initiation of vesicular stomatitis virus RNA transcription in vitro. *Cell* 1976;8(2):197–204.
105. Colonno RJ, Lazzarini RA, Keene JD, et al. In vitro synthesis of messenger RNA by a defective interfering particle of vesicular stomatitis virus. *Proc Natl Acad Sci U S A* 1977;74(5):1884–1888.
106. Comer JA, Tesh RB, Modi GB, et al. Vesicular stomatitis virus, New Jersey serotype: replication in and transmission by Lutzomyia shannoni (Diptera: Psychodidae). *Am J Trop Med Hyg* 1990;42(5):483–490.
107. Connor JH, Lyles DS. Vesicular stomatitis virus infection alters the eIF4F translation initiation complex and causes dephosphorylation of the eIF4E binding protein 4E-BP1. *J Virol* 2002;76(20):10177–10187.
108. Connor JH, Lyles DS. Inhibition of host and viral translation during vesicular stomatitis virus infection. eIF2 is responsible for the inhibition of viral but not host translation. *J Biol Chem* 2005;280(14):13512–13519.
109. Connor JH, McKenzie MO, Lyles DS. Role of residues 121 to 124 of vesicular stomatitis virus matrix protein in virus assembly and virus-host interaction. *J Virol* 2006;80(8):3701–3711.
110. Connor JH, McKenzie MO, Parks GD, et al. Antiviral activity and RNA polymerase degradation following Hsp90 inhibition in a range of negative strand viruses. *Virology* 2007;362(1):109–119.
111. Conzelmann KK, Schnell M. Rescue of synthetic genomic RNA analogs of rabies virus by plasmid-encoded proteins. *J Virol* 1994;68(2):713–719.
112. Cooper D, Wright KJ, Calderon PC, et al. Attenuation of recombinant vesicular stomatitis virus-human immunodeficiency virus type 1 vaccine vectors by gene translocations and g gene truncation reduces neurovirulence and enhances immunogenicity in mice. *J Virol* 2008;82(1):207–219.
113. Cotton WE. The causal agent of vesicular stomatitis proved to be a filter-passing virus. *J Am Vet Med Assoc* 1926;23:168–179.
114. Coulon P, Derbin C, Kucera P, et al. Invasion of the peripheral nervous systems of adult mice by the CVS strain of rabies virus and its avirulent derivative AvO1. *J Virol* 1989;63(8):3550–3554.
115. Coulon P, Deutsch V, Lafay F, et al. Genetic evidence for multiple functions of the matrix protein of vesicular stomatitis virus. *J Gen Virol* 1990;71(Pt 4):991–996.
116. Coulon P, Ternaux JP, Flamand A, et al. An avirulent mutant of rabies virus is unable to infect motoneurons in vivo and in vitro. *J Virol* 1998;72(1):273–278.
117. Cox JH, Dietzschold B, Schneider LG. Rabies virus glycoprotein. II. Biological and serological characterization. *Infect Immun* 1977;16(3):754–759.
118. Craven RC, Harty RN, Paragas J, et al. Late domain function identified in the vesicular stomatitis virus M protein by use of rhabdovirus-retrovirus chimeras. *J Virol* 1999;73(4):3359–3365.
119. Cupp EW, Maré CJ, Cupp MS, et al. Biological transmission of vesicular stomatitis virus (New Jersey) by Simulium vittatum (Diptera: Simuliidae). *J Med Entomol* 1992;29(2):137–140.
120. Cureton DK, Massol RH, Saffarian S, et al. Vesicular stomatitis virus enters cells through vesicles incompletely coated with clathrin that depend upon actin for internalization. *PLoS Pathog* 2009;5(4):e1000394.
121. Cureton DK, Massol RH, Whelan SP, et al. The length of vesicular stomatitis virus particles dictates a need for actin assembly during clathrin-dependent endocytosis. *PLoS Pathog* 2010;6(9):e1001127.
122. Dacheux L, Larrous F, Mailles A, et al. European bat Lyssavirus transmission among cats, Europe. *Emerg Infect Dis* 2009;15(2):280–284.
123. Dancho B, McKenzie MO, Connor JH, et al. Vesicular stomatitis virus matrix protein mutations that affect association with host membranes and viral nucleocapsids. *J Biol Chem* 2009;284(7):4500–4509.
124. Daniels PW, Sendow I, Soleha E, Sukarsih, Hunt NT, Bahri S. Australian-Indonesian collaboration in veterinary arbovirology—a review. *Vet Microbiol* 1995;46(1-3):151–174.
125. De Clercq E, De Somer P. Comparative study of the efficacy of different forms of interferon therapy in the treatment of mice challenged intranassaly with vesicular stomatitis virus (VSV). *Proc Soc Exp Biol Med* 1971;138(1):301–307.
126. de Mattos CA, de Mattos CC, Smith JS, et al. Genetic characterization of rabies field isolates from Venezuela. *J Clin Microbiol* 1996;34(6):1553–1558.
127. Deering RE, Arakawa CK, Oshima KH, et al. Development of a biotinylated DNA probe for detection and identification of infectious hematopoietic necrosis virus. *Dis Aquat Org* 1991;11:57–65.
128. Desforges M, Charron J, Bérard S, et al. Different host-cell shutoff strategies related to the matrix protein lead to persistence of vesicular stomatitis virus mutants on fibroblast cells. *Virus Res* 2001;76(1):87–102.
129. Desfosses A, Ribeiro EA Jr, Schoehn G, et al. Self-organization of the vesicular stomatitis virus nucleocapsid into a bullet shape. *Nat Commun* 2013;4:1429.
130. Diebold SS, Kaisho T, Hemmi H, et al. Innate antiviral responses by means of TLR7-mediated recognition of single-stranded RNA. *Science* 2004;303(5663):1529–1531.
131. Dietzgen RG, Kondo H, Goodin MM, et al. The family Rhabdoviridae: mono- and bipartite negative-sense RNA viruses with diverse genome organization and common evolutionary origins. *Virus Res* 2017;227:158–170.
132. Dietzschold B, Ertl HC. New developments in the pre- and post-exposure treatment of rabies. *Crit Rev Immunol* 1991;10(5):427–439.
133. Dietzschold B, Kao M, Zheng YM, et al. Delineation of putative mechanisms involved in antibody-mediated clearance of rabies virus from the central nervous system. *Proc Natl Acad Sci U S A* 1992;89(15):7252–7256.
134. Dietzschold B, Wang HH, Rupprecht CE, et al. Induction of protective immunity against rabies by immunization with rabies virus ribonucleoprotein. *Proc Natl Acad Sci U S A* 1987;84(24):9165–9169.
135. Dikkeboom AL, Radi C, Toohey-Kurth K, et al. First report of spring viremia of carp virus (SVCV) in wild common carp in North America. *J Aquat Anim Health* 2004;16:169–178.
136. Ding H, Green TJ, Lu S, et al. Crystal structure of the oligomerization domain of the phosphoprotein of vesicular stomatitis virus. *J Virol* 2006;80(6):2808–2814.

137. Doherty RL, George TD, Carley JG. Arbovirus infections of sentinel cattle in Australia and New Guinea. *Aust Vet J* 1973;49(12):574–579.
138. Doms RW, Keller DS, Helenius A, et al. Role for adenosine triphosphate in regulating the assembly and transport of vesicular stomatitis virus G protein trimers. *J Cell Biol* 1987;105(5):1957–1969.
139. Drake JW, Holland JJ. Mutation rates among RNA viruses. *Proc Natl Acad Sci U S A* 1999;96(24):13910–13913.
140. Dratewka-Kos E, Kiss I, Lucas-Lenard J, et al. Catalytic utilization of eIF-2 and mRNA binding proteins are limiting in lysates from vesicular stomatitis virus infected L cells. *Biochemistry* 1984;23(25):6184–6190.
141. Du Pont V, Wirblich C, Yoon JJ, et al. Identification and characterization of a small-molecule rabies virus entry inhibitor. *J Virol* 2020;94(13).
142. Duarte E, Clarke D, Moya A, et al. Rapid fitness losses in mammalian RNA virus clones due to Muller's ratchet. *Proc Natl Acad Sci U S A* 1992;89(13):6015–6019.
143. Dubovi EJ, Wagner RR. Spatial relationships of the proteins of vesicular stomatitis virus: induction of reversible oligomers by cleavable protein cross-linkers and oxidation. *J Virol* 1977;22(2):500–509.
144. Dunigan DD, Baird S, Lucas-Lenard J. Lack of correlation between the accumulation of plus-strand leader RNA and the inhibition of protein and RNA synthesis in vesicular stomatitis virus infected mouse L cells. *Virology* 1986;150(1):231–246.
145. Dupont JR, Earle KM. Human rabies encephalitis. A study of forty-nine fatal cases with a review of the literature. *Neurology* 1965;15(11):1023–1034.
146. Durbin JE, Hackenmiller R, Simon MC, et al. Targeted disruption of the mouse Stat1 gene results in compromised innate immunity to viral disease. *Cell* 1996;84(3):443–450.
147. Durbin RK, Mertz SE, Koromilas AE, et al. PKR protection against intranasal vesicular stomatitis virus infection is mouse strain dependent. *Viral Immunol* 2002;15(1):41–51.
148. Durrer P, Gaudin Y, Ruigrok RW, et al. Photolabeling identifies a putative fusion domain in the envelope glycoprotein of rabies and vesicular stomatitis viruses. *J Biol Chem* 1995;270(29):17575–17581.
149. Dutta JK. Excessive libido in a woman with rabies. *Postgrad Med J* 1996;72(851):554.
150. Ehrenfeld E, Summers DF. Adenylate-rich sequences in vesicular stomatitis virus messenger ribonucleic acid. *J Virol* 1972;10(4):683–688.
151. Eidelman O, Schlegel R, Tralka TS, et al. pH-dependent fusion induced by vesicular stomatitis virus glycoprotein reconstituted into phospholipid vesicles. *J Biol Chem* 1984;259(7):4622–4628.
152. Einer-Jensen K, Ahrens P, Forsberg R, et al. Evolution of the fish rhabdovirus viral haemorrhagic septicaemia virus. *J Gen Virol* 2004;85(Pt 5):1167–1179.
153. Emerson SU, Wagner RR. Dissociation and reconstitution of the transcriptase and template activities of vesicular stomatitis B and T virions. *J Virol* 1972;10(2):297–309.
154. Emerson SU, Yu Y. Both NS and L proteins are required for in vitro RNA synthesis by vesicular stomatitis virus. *J Virol* 1975;15(6):1348–1356.
155. Ertl HC, Dietzschold B, Gore M, et al. Induction of rabies virus-specific T-helper cells by synthetic peptides that carry dominant T-helper cell epitopes of the viral ribonucleoprotein. *J Virol* 1989;63(7):2885–2892.
156. Evensen Ø, Meier W, Wahli T, et al. Comparison of immunohistochemistry and virus cultivation for detection of viral haemorrhagic septicaemia virus in experimentally infected rainbow trout Oncorhynchus mykiss. *Dis Aquat Org* 1994;20:101–109.
157. Familusi JB, Osunkoya BO, Moore DL, et al. A fatal human infection with Mokola virus. *Am J Trop Med Hyg* 1972;21(6):959–963.
158. Faria PA, Chakraborty P, Levay A, et al. VSV disrupts the Rae1/mrnp41 mRNA nuclear export pathway. *Mol Cell* 2005;17(1):93–102.
159. Fekadu M, Endeshaw T, Alemu W, et al. Possible human-to-human transmission of rabies in Ethiopia. *Ethiop Med J* 1996;34(2):123–127.
160. Fekadu M, Shaddock JH. Peripheral distribution of virus in dogs inoculated with two strains of rabies virus. *Am J Vet Res* 1984;45(4):724–729.
161. Fernandes MV, Wiktor TJ, Koprowski H. Mechanism of the cytopathic effect of rabies virus in tissue culture. *Virology* 1963;21:128–131.
162. Ferran MC, Lucas-Lenard JM. The vesicular stomatitis virus matrix protein inhibits transcription from the human beta interferon promoter. *J Virol* 1997;71(1):371–377.
163. Ferris DH, Hanson RP, Dicke RJ, et al. Experimental transmission of vesicular stomatitis virus by Diptera. *J Infect Dis* 1955;96(2):184–192.
164. Fijan N, Petrinec Z, Sulimanovic D, et al. Isolation of the viral causative agent from the acute form of infectious dropsy of carp. *Vet Arh* 1971;41:125–138.
165. Finke S, Brzózka K, Conzelmann KK. Tracking fluorescence-labeled rabies virus: enhanced green fluorescent protein-tagged phosphoprotein P supports virus gene expression and formation of infectious particles. *J Virol* 2004;78(22):12333–12343.
166. Finke S, Conzelmann KK. Ambisense gene expression from recombinant rabies virus: random packaging of positive- and negative-strand ribonucleoprotein complexes into rabies virions. *J Virol* 1997;71(10):7281–7288.
167. Finke S, Mueller-Waldeck R, Conzelmann KK. Rabies virus matrix protein regulates the balance of virus transcription and replication. *J Gen Virol* 2003;84(Pt 6):1613–1621.
168. Finkelshtein D, Werman A, Novick D, et al. LDL receptor and its family members serve as the cellular receptors for vesicular stomatitis virus. *Proc Natl Acad Sci U S A* 2013;110(18):7306–7311.
169. Flamand A. [Genetic study of vesicular stomatitis virus: classification of spontaneous thermosensitive mutants into complementation groups]. *J Gen Virol* 1970;8(3):187–195.
170. Flamand A, Coulon P, Lafay F, et al. Eradication of rabies in Europe. *Nature* 1992;360(6400):115–116.
171. Flanagan EB, Schoeb TR, Wertz GW. Vesicular stomatitis viruses with rearranged genomes have altered invasiveness and neuropathogenesis in mice. *J Virol* 2003;77(10):5740–5748.
172. Flanagan EB, Zamparo JM, Ball LA, et al. Rearrangement of the genes of vesicular stomatitis virus eliminates clinical disease in the natural host: new strategy for vaccine development. *J Virol* 2001;75(13):6107–6114.
173. Flood EA, Lyles DS. Assembly of nucleocapsids with cytosolic and membrane-derived matrix proteins of vesicular stomatitis virus. *Virology* 1999;261(2):295–308.
174. Flood EA, McKenzie MO, Lyles DS. Role of M protein aggregation in defective assembly of temperature-sensitive M protein mutants of vesicular stomatitis virus. *Virology* 2000;278(2):520–533.
175. Follmann EH, Ritter DG, Beller M. Survey of fox trappers in northern Alaska for rabies antibody. *Epidemiol Infect* 1994;113(1):137–141.
176. Fontenille D, Traore-Lamizana M, Trouillet J, et al. First isolations of arboviruses from phlebotomine sand flies in West Africa. *Am J Trop Med Hyg* 1994;50(5):570–574.
177. Forger JM III, Bronson RT, Huang AS, et al. Murine infection by vesicular stomatitis virus: initial characterization of the H-2d system. *J Virol* 1991;65(9):4950–4958.
178. Francoeur AM, Poliquin L, Stanners CP. The isolation of interferon-inducing mutants of vesicular stomatitis virus with altered viral P function for the inhibition of total protein synthesis. *Virology* 1987;160(1):236–245.
179. Francy DB, Moore CG, Smith GC, et al. Epizoötic vesicular stomatitis in Colorado, 1982: isolation of virus from insects collected along the northern Colorado Rocky Mountain Front Range. *J Med Entomol* 1988;25(5):343–347.
180. Fraser GC, Hooper PT, Lunt RA, et al. Encephalitis caused by a Lyssavirus in fruit bats in Australia. *Emerg Infect Dis* 1996;2(4):327–331.
181. Fredericksen BL, Whitt MA. Vesicular stomatitis virus glycoprotein mutations that affect membrane fusion activity and abolish virus infectivity. *J Virol* 1995;69(3):1435–1443.
182. Fredericksen BL, Whitt MA. Attenuation of recombinant vesicular stomatitis viruses encoding mutant glycoproteins demonstrate a critical role for maintaining a high pH threshold for membrane fusion in viral fitness. *Virology* 1998;240(2):349–358.
183. Fries LF, Tartaglia J, Taylor J, et al. Human safety and immunogenicity of a canarypox-rabies glycoprotein recombinant vaccine: an alternative poxvirus vector system. *Vaccine* 1996;14(5):428–434.
184. Fu ZF, Dietzschold B, Schumacher CL, et al. Rabies virus nucleoprotein expressed in and purified from insect cells is efficacious as a vaccine. *Proc Natl Acad Sci U S A* 1991;88(5):2001–2005.
185. Gaddy DF, Lyles DS. Vesicular stomatitis viruses expressing wild-type or mutant M proteins activate apoptosis through distinct pathways. *J Virol* 2005;79(7):4170–4179.
186. Gaddy DF, Lyles DS. Oncolytic vesicular stomatitis virus induces apoptosis via signaling through PKR, Fas, and Daxx. *J Virol* 2007;81(6):2792–2804.
187. Gao Y, Lenard J. Multimerization and transcriptional activation of the phosphoprotein (P) of vesicular stomatitis virus by casein kinase-II. *EMBO J* 1995;14(6):1240–1247.
188. Gascoyne SC, Laurenson MK, Lelo S, et al. Rabies in African wild dogs (Lycaon pictus) in the Serengeti region, Tanzania. *J Wildl Dis* 1993;29(3):396–402.
189. Gastka M, Horvath J, Lentz TL. Rabies virus binding to the nicotinic acetylcholine receptor alpha subunit demonstrated by virus overlay protein binding assay. *J Gen Virol* 1996;77(Pt 10):2437–2440.
190. Gaudier M, Gaudin Y, Knossow M. Cleavage of vesicular stomatitis virus matrix protein prevents self-association and leads to crystallization. *Virology* 2001;288(2):308–314.
191. Gaudier M, Gaudin Y, Knossow M. Crystal structure of vesicular stomatitis virus matrix protein. *EMBO J* 2002;21(12):2886–2892.
192. Gaudin Y, Ruigrok RW, Tuffereau C, et al. Rabies virus glycoprotein is a trimer. *Virology* 1992;187(2):627–632.
193. Gaudin Y, Tuffereau C, Segretain D, et al. Reversible conformational changes and fusion activity of rabies virus glycoprotein. *J Virol* 1991;65(9):4853–4859.
194. Ge P, Tsao J, Schein S, et al. Cryo-EM model of the bullet-shaped vesicular stomatitis virus. *Science* 2010;327(5966):689–693.
195. Georgel P, Jiang Z, Kunz S, et al. Vesicular stomatitis virus glycoprotein G activates a specific antiviral Toll-like receptor 4-dependent pathway. *Virology* 2007;362(2):304–313.
196. Gerard FC, Ribeiro Ede A Jr, Albertini AA, et al. Unphosphorylated rhabdoviridae phosphoproteins form elongated dimers in solution. *Biochemistry* 2007;46(36):10328–10338.
197. Gerard FC, Ribeiro Ede A Jr, Leyrat C, et al. Modular organization of rabies virus phosphoprotein. *J Mol Biol* 2009;388(5):978–996.
198. Gerard FCA, Jamin M, Blackledge M, et al. Vesicular stomatitis virus phosphoprotein dimerization domain is dispensable for virus growth. *J Virol* 2020;94(6).
199. Gholami A, Kassis R, Real E, et al. Mitochondrial dysfunction in lyssavirus-induced apoptosis. *J Virol* 2008;82(10):4774–4784.
200. Gilman MSA, Liu C, Fung A, et al. Structure of the respiratory syncytial virus polymerase complex. *Cell* 2019;179(1):193–204.e14.
201. Gould AR, Kattenbelt JA, Gumley SG, et al. Characterisation of an Australian bat lyssavirus variant isolated from an insectivorous bat. *Virus Res* 2002;89(1):1–28.
202. Gould JR, Qiu S, Shang Q, et al. Consequences of phosphorylation in a mononegavirales polymerase-cofactor system. *J Virol* 2021;95.
203. Graham SC, Assenberg R, Delmas O, et al. Rhabdovirus matrix protein structures reveal a novel mode of self-association. *PLoS Pathog* 2008;4(12):e1000251.
204. Grdzelishvili VZ, Smallwood S, Tower D, et al. A single amino acid change in the L-polymerase protein of vesicular stomatitis virus completely abolishes viral mRNA cap methylation. *J Virol* 2005;79(12):7327–7337.
205. Green TJ, Luo M. Structure of the vesicular stomatitis virus nucleocapsid in complex with the nucleocapsid-binding domain of the small polymerase cofactor, P. *Proc Natl Acad Sci U S A* 2009;106(28):11713–11718.
206. Green TJ, Rowse M, Tsao J, et al. Access to RNA encapsidated in the nucleocapsid of vesicular stomatitis virus. *J Virol* 2011;85(6):2714–2722.
207. Green TJ, Zhang X, Wertz GW, et al. Structure of the vesicular stomatitis virus nucleoprotein-RNA complex. *Science* 2006;313(5785):357–360.
208. Greenwood RJ, Newton WE, Pearson GL, et al. Population and movement characteristics of radio-collared striped skunks in North Dakota during an epizootic of rabies. *J Wildl Dis* 1997;33(2):226–241.
209. Gresser I, Tovey MG, Bourali-Maury C. Efficacy of exogenous interferon treatment initiated after onset of multiplication of vesicular stomatitis virus in the brains of mice. *J Gen Virol* 1975;27(3):395–398.
210. Gupta AK, Blondel D, Choudhary S, et al. The phosphoprotein of rabies virus is phosphorylated by a unique cellular protein kinase and specific isomers of protein kinase C. *J Virol* 2000;74(1):91–98.
211. Gupta AK, Shaji D, Banerjee AK. Identification of a novel tripartite complex involved in replication of vesicular stomatitis virus genome RNA. *J Virol* 2003;77(1):732–738.
212. Guyatt KJ, Twin J, Davis P, et al. A molecular epidemiological study of Australian bat lyssavirus. *J Gen Virol* 2003;84(Pt 2):485–496.

213. Habel K, Koprowski H. Laboratory data supporting the clinical trial of anti-rabies serum in persons bitten by a rabid wolf. *Bull World Health Organ* 1955;13(5):773–779.

214. Hamir AN, Moser G, Wampler T, et al. Use of a single anti-nucleocapsid monoclonal antibody to detect rabies antigen in formalin-fixed, paraffin-embedded tissues. *Vet Rec* 1996;138(5):114–115.

215. Hammond C, Helenius A. Folding of VSV G protein: sequential interaction with BiP and calnexin. *Science* 1994;266(5184):456–458.

216. Hanlon CA, Kuzmin IV, Blanton JD, et al. Efficacy of rabies biologics against new lyssaviruses from Eurasia. *Virus Res* 2005;111(1):44–54.

217. Hanlon CA, Smith JS, Anderson GR. Recommendations of a national working group on prevention and control of rabies in the United States. Article II: laboratory diagnosis of rabies. The National Working Group on Rabies Prevention and Control. *J Am Vet Med Assoc* 1999;215(10):1444–1446.

218. Hansen DE, Thurmond MC, Thorburn M. Factors associated with the spread of clinical vesicular stomatitis in California dairy cattle. *Am J Vet Res* 1985;46(4):789–795.

219. Hanson RP. The natural history of vesicular stomatitis. *Bact Rev* 1952;16:179–204.

220. Harty RN, Brown ME, Hayes FP, et al. Vaccinia virus-free recovery of vesicular stomatitis virus. *J Mol Microbiol Biotechnol* 2001;3(4):513–517.

221. Harty RN, Brown ME, McGettigan JP, et al. Rhabdoviruses and the cellular ubiquitin-proteasome system: a budding interaction. *J Virol* 2001;75(22):10623–10629.

222. Harty RN, Paragas J, Sudol M, et al. A proline-rich motif within the matrix protein of vesicular stomatitis virus and rabies virus interacts with WW domains of cellular proteins: implications for viral budding. *J Virol* 1999;73(4):2921–2929.

223. Heinrich BS, Cureton DK, Rahmeh AA, et al. Protein expression redirects vesicular stomatitis virus RNA synthesis to cytoplasmic inclusions. *PLoS Pathog* 2010;6(6):e1000958.

224. Heinrich BS, Maliga Z, Stein DA, et al. Phase transitions drive the formation of vesicular stomatitis virus replication compartments. *MBio* 2018;9(5).

225. Heiny E. Vesicular stomatitis in cattle and horses in Colorado. *North Am Vet* 1945;26:726–730.

226. Held JR, Tierkel ES, Steele JH. Rabies in man and animals in the United States, 1946-65. *Public Health Rep* 1967;82(11):1009–1018.

227. Hellenbrand W, Meyer C, Rasch G, et al. Cases of rabies in Germany following organ transplantation. *Euro Surveill* 2005;10(2):E050224.6.

228. Hemachudha T. Human rabies: clinical aspects, pathogenesis, and potential therapy. *Curr Top Microbiol Immunol* 1994;187:121–143.

229. Hemachudha T, Phanuphak P, Sriwanthana B, et al. Immunologic study of human encephalitic and paralytic rabies. Preliminary report of 16 patients. *Am J Med* 1988;84(4):673–677.

230. Henryon M, Berg P, Olesen NJ, et al. Selective breeding provides an approach to increase resistance of rainbow trout to the diseases, enteric redmouth disease, rainbow trout fry syndrome, and viral haemorrhagic septicaemia. *Aquaculture* 2005;250:621–636.

231. Hercyk N, Horikami SM, Moyer SA. The vesicular stomatitis virus L protein possesses the mRNA methyltransferase activities. *Virology* 1988;163(1):222–225.

232. Herman RC, Schubert M, Keene JD, et al. Polycistronic vesicular stomatitis virus RNA transcripts. *Proc Natl Acad Sci U S A* 1980;77(8):4662–4665.

233. Hertig C, Pye AD, Hyatt AD, et al. Vaccinia virus-expressed bovine ephemeral fever virus G but not G(NS) glycoprotein induces neutralizing antibodies and protects against experimental infection. *J Gen Virol* 1996;77(Pt 4):631–640.

234. Hill BJ. Impact of viral diseases of salmonid fish in the European community. In: Kimura T, ed. *Proceedings of the OJI International Symposium on Salmonid Diseases.* Sapporo: Hokkaido Univ Press; 1992:48–59.

235. Hoffmann B, Beer M, Schütze H, et al. Fish rhabdoviruses: molecular epidemiology and evolution. *Curr Top Microbiol Immunol* 2005;292:81–117.

236. Hofmeyr M, Bingham J, Lane EP, et al. Rabies in African wild dogs (Lycaon pictus) in the Madikwe Game Reserve, South Africa. *Vet Rec* 2000;146(2):50–52.

237. Holloway AF, Wong PK, Cormack DV. Isolation and characterization of temperature-sensitive mutants of vesicular stomatitis virus. *Virology* 1970;42(4):917–926.

238. Holzwarth G, Bhandari A, Tommervik L, et al. Vesicular stomatitis virus nucleocapsids diffuse through cytoplasm by hopping from trap to trap in random directions. *Sci Rep* 2020;10(1):10643.

239. Hooper DC, Morimoto K, Bette M, et al. Collaboration of antibody and inflammation in clearance of rabies virus from the central nervous system. *J Virol* 1998;72(5):3711–3719.

240. Hornung V, Ellegast J, Kim S, et al. 5′-Triphosphate RNA is the ligand for RIG-I. *Science* 2006;314(5801):994–997.

241. Horwitz JA, Jenni S, Harrison SC, et al. Structure of a rabies virus polymerase complex from electron cryo-microscopy. *Proc Natl Acad Sci U S A* 2020;117(4):2099–2107.

242. Howard M, Wertz G. Vesicular stomatitis virus RNA replication: a role for the NS protein. *J Gen Virol* 1989;70(Pt 10):2683–2694.

243. Huang AS, Manders EK. Ribonucleic acid synthesis of vesicular stomatitis virus. IV. Transcription by standard virus in the presence of defective interfering particles. *J Virol* 1972;9(6):909–916.

244. Huneycutt BS, Bi Z, Aoki CJ, et al. Central neuropathogenesis of vesicular stomatitis virus infection of immunodeficient mice. *J Virol* 1993;67(11):6698–6706.

245. Huneycutt BS, Plakhov IV, Shusterman Z, et al. Distribution of vesicular stomatitis virus proteins in the brains of BALB/c mice following intranasal inoculation: an immunohistochemical analysis. *Brain Res* 1994;635(1-2):81–95.

246. Hunt DM, Mehta R, Hutchinson KL. The L protein of vesicular stomatitis virus modulates the response of the polyadenylic acid polymerase to S-adenosylhomocysteine. *J Gen Virol* 1988;69(Pt 10):2555–2561.

247. Hurst EW, Pawan JL. An outbreak of rabies in Trinidad without history of bites, and with the symptoms of acute ascending myelitis. *Caribb Med J* 1959;21:11–24.

248. Hwang LN, Englund N, Das T, et al. Optimal replication activity of vesicular stomatitis virus RNA polymerase requires phosphorylation of a residue(s) at carboxy-terminal domain II of its accessory subunit, phosphoprotein P. *J Virol* 1999;73(7):5613–5620.

249. Iannacone M, Moseman EA, Tonti E, et al. Subcapsular sinus macrophages prevent CNS invasion on peripheral infection with a neurotropic virus. *Nature* 2010;465(7301):1079–1083.

250. Irie T, Licata JM, Jayakar HR, et al. Functional analysis of late-budding domain activity associated with the PSAP motif within the vesicular stomatitis virus M protein. *J Virol* 2004;78(14):7823–7827.

251. Irie T, Licata JM, McGettigan JP, et al. Budding of PPxY-containing rhabdoviruses is not dependent on host proteins TGS101 and VPS4A. *J Virol* 2004;78(6):2657–2665.

252. Iseni F, Barge A, Baudin F, et al. Characterization of rabies virus nucleocapsids and recombinant nucleocapsid-like structures. *J Gen Virol* 1998;79(Pt 12):2909–2919.

253. Ito N, Moseley GW, Blondel D, et al. Role of interferon antagonist activity of rabies virus phosphoprotein in viral pathogenicity. *J Virol* 2010;84(13):6699–6710.

254. Ito N, Takayama-Ito M, Yamada K, et al. Improved recovery of rabies virus from cloned cDNA using a vaccinia virus-free reverse genetics system. *Microbiol Immunol* 2003;47(8):613–617.

255. Ivanov I, Crepin T, Jamin M, et al. Structure of the dimerization domain of the rabies virus phosphoprotein. *J Virol* 2010;84(7):3707–3710.

256. Iverson LE, Rose JK. Localized attenuation and discontinuous synthesis during vesicular stomatitis virus transcription. *Cell* 1981;23(2):477–484.

257. Jackson AC. Why does the prognosis remain so poor in human rabies? *Expert Rev Anti Infect Ther* 2010;8(6):623–625.

258. Jackson AC, Rossiter JP. Apoptosis plays an important role in experimental rabies virus infection. *J Virol* 1997;71(7):5603–5607.

259. Jackson AC, Rossiter JP, Lafon M. Expression of Toll-like receptor 3 in the human cerebellar cortex in rabies, herpes simplex encephalitis, and other neurological diseases. *J Neurovirol* 2006;12(3):229–234.

260. Jayakar HR, Murti KG, Whitt MA. Mutations in the PPPY motif of vesicular stomatitis virus matrix protein reduce virus budding by inhibiting a late step in virion release. *J Virol* 2000;74(21):9818–9827.

261. Jayakar HR, Whitt MA. Identification of two additional translation products from the matrix (M) gene that contribute to vesicular stomatitis virus cytopathology. *J Virol* 2002;76(16):8011–8018.

262. Jeetendra E, Ghosh K, Odell D, et al. The membrane-proximal region of vesicular stomatitis virus glycoprotein G ectodomain is critical for fusion and virus infectivity. *J Virol* 2003;77(23):12807–12818.

263. Jenni S, Bloyet LM, Diaz-Avalos R, et al. Structure of the vesicular stomatitis virus L protein in complex with its phosphoprotein cofactor. *Cell Rep* 2020;30(1):53–60.e5.

264. Johannsdottir HK, Mancini R, Kartenbeck J, et al. Host cell factors and functions involved in vesicular stomatitis virus entry. *J Virol* 2009;83(1):440–453.

265. Johnson HN. Rabies virus. In: Horsfall F, Tamm I, eds. *Viral and Rickettsial Infections of Man.* Philadelphia, PA: JB Lippincott; 1965:814–840.

266. Johnson N, Mansfield KL, Marston DA, et al. A new outbreak of rabies in rare Ethiopian wolves (Canis simensis). *Arch Virol* 2010;155(7):1175–1177.

267. Johnson KM, Tesh RB, Peralta PH. Epidemiology of vesicular stomatitis virus: some new data and a hypothesis for transmission of the Indian serotype. *J Am Vet Med Assoc* 1969;155(12):2133–2140.

268. Jorgensen PEV. Egtved virus: occurrence of inapparent infections with virulent virus in free-living rainbow trout, Salmo gairdneri Richardson, at low temperature. *J Fish Dis* 1982;5:251–255.

269. Jonkers AH, Shope RE, Aitken TH, et al. Cocal virus, a new agent in trinidad related to vesicular stomatitis virus, type Indiana. *Am J Vet Res* 1964;25:236–242.

270. Justice PA, Sun W, Li Y, et al. Membrane vesiculation function and exocytosis of wild-type and mutant matrix proteins of vesicular stomatitis virus. *J Virol* 1995;69(5):3156–3160.

271. Kang CY, Prevec L. Proteins of vesicular stomatitis virus. II. Immunological comparisons of viral antigens. *J Virol* 1970;6(1):20–27.

272. Kaplan MM, Koprowski H. Rabies. *Sci Am* 1980;242(1):120–134.

273. Kaptur PE, McKenzie MO, Wertz GW, et al. Assembly functions of vesicular stomatitis virus matrix protein are not disrupted by mutations at major sites of phosphorylation. *Virology* 1995;206(2):894–903.

274. Kasornchandra J, Engelking HM, Lannan CJ, et al. Characteristics of three rhabdoviruses from snakehead fish (Ophicephalus striatus). *Dis Aquat Organ* 1992;13:89–94.

275. Kassis R, Larrous F, Estaquier J, et al. Lyssavirus matrix protein induces apoptosis by a TRAIL-dependent mechanism involving caspase-8 activation. *J Virol* 2004;78(12):6543–6555.

276. Kato H, Sato S, Yoneyama M, et al. Cell type-specific involvement of RIG-I in antiviral response. *Immunity* 2005;23(1):19–28.

277. Kato H, Takeuchi O, Sato S, et al. Differential roles of MDA5 and RIG-I helicases in the recognition of RNA viruses. *Nature* 2006;441(7089):101–105.

278. Katz FN, Lodish HF. Transmembrane biogenesis of the vesicular stomatitis virus glycoprotein. *J Cell Biol* 1979;80(2):416–426.

279. Katz FN, Rothman JE, Lingappa VR, et al. Membrane assembly in vitro: synthesis, glycosylation, and asymmetric insertion of a transmembrane protein. *Proc Natl Acad Sci U S A* 1977;74(8):3278–3282.

280. Kawano H, Mifune K, Ohuchi M, et al. Protection against rabies in mice by a cytotoxic T cell clone recognizing the glycoprotein of rabies virus. *J Gen Virol* 1990;71(Pt 2):281–287.

281. Kim DH, Oh HK, Eou JI, et al. Complete nucleotide sequence of the hirame rhabdovirus, a pathogen of marine fish. *Virus Res* 2005;107(1):1–9.

282. Kim IS, Jenni S, Stanifer ML, et al. Mechanism of membrane fusion induced by vesicular stomatitis virus G protein. *Proc Natl Acad Sci U S A* 2017;114(1):E28–E36.

283. Kim WS, Oh MJ, Nishizawa T, et al. Genotyping of Korean isolates of infectious hematopoietic necrosis virus (IHNV) based on the glycoprotein gene. *Arch Virol* 2007;152(11):2119–2124.

284. Kimura T, Yoshimizu M, Gorie S. A new rhabdovirus isolated in Japan from cultured hirame (Japanese flounder) Paralichthys olivaceus and ayu Plecoglossus altivelis. *Dis Aquat Organ* 1986;1:209–217.

285. Kingsford L, Emerson SU. Transcriptional activities of different phosphorylated species of NS protein purified from vesicular stomatitis virions and cytoplasm of infected cells. *J Virol* 1980;33(3):1097–1105.

286. Knipe DM, Baltimore D, Lodish HF. Separate pathways of maturation of the major structural proteins of vesicular stomatitis virus. *J Virol* 1977;21(3):1128–1139.

287. Knutti RE. Acute ascending paralysis and myelitis due to the virus of rabies. *J Am Vet Med Assoc* 1929;93:754–758.

288. Koch FJ, Sagartz JW, Davidson DE, et al. Diagnosis of human rabies by the cornea test. *Am J Clin Pathol* 1975;63(4):509–515.

289. Komarova AV, Real E, Borman AM, et al. Rabies virus matrix protein interplay with eIF3, new insights into rabies virus pathogenesis. *Nucleic Acids Res* 2007;35(5):1522–1532.

290. Komatsu T, Ireland DD, Chen N, et al. Neuronal expression of NOS-1 is required for host recovery from viral encephalitis. *Virology* 1999;258(2):389–395.

291. Kondo H, Maeda T, Shirako Y, et al. Orchid fleck virus is a rhabdovirus with an unusual bipartite genome. *J Gen Virol* 2006;87(Pt 8):2413–2421.

292. Kopecky SA, Lyles DS. Contrasting effects of matrix protein on apoptosis in HeLa and BHK cells infected with vesicular stomatitis virus are due to inhibition of host gene expression. *J Virol* 2003;77(8):4658–4669.

293. Kopecky SA, Willingham MC, Lyles DS. Matrix protein and another viral component contribute to induction of apoptosis in cells infected with vesicular stomatitis virus. *J Virol* 2001;75(24):12169–12181.

294. Koprowski H. The mouse inoculation test. In: Meslin F-X, Kaplan MM, Koprowski H, eds. *Laboratory Techniques in Rabies.* 4th ed. Geneva, Switzerland: World Health Organization; 1996:80–87.

295. Koyama AH. Induction of apoptotic DNA fragmentation by the infection of vesicular stomatitis virus. *Virus Res* 1995;37(3):285–290.

296. Kristensson K, Dastur DK, Manghani DK, et al. Rabies: interactions between neurons and viruses. A review of the history of Negri inclusion bodies. *Neuropathol Appl Neurobiol* 1996;22(3):179–187.

297. Kuhn JH, Adkins S, Agwanda BR, et al. 2021 Taxonomic update of phylum Negarnaviricota (Riboviria: Orthornavirae), including the large orders Bunyavirales and Mononegavirales. *Arch Virol* 2021;166(12):3513–3566.

298. Kulonen K, Boldina I. Differentiation of two rabies strains in Estonia with reference to recent Finnish isolates. *J Wildl Dis* 1993;29(2):209–213.

299. Kulonen K, Boldina I. No rabies detected in voles and field mice in a rabies-endemic area. *Zentralbl Veterinarmed B* 1996;43:445–447.

300. Kurath G. Biotechnology and DNA vaccines for aquatic animals. *Rev Sci Tech* 2008;27(1):175–196.

301. Kurath G, Leong JC. Characterization of infectious hematopoietic necrosis virus mRNA species reveals a nonvirion rhabdovirus protein. *J Virol* 1985;53(2):462–468.

302. Kuwata R, Isawa H, Hoshino K, et al. RNA splicing in a new rhabdovirus from Culex mosquitoes. *J Virol* 2011;85(13):6185–6196.

303. Kuzmin IV, Hughes GJ, Botvinkin AD, et al. Phylogenetic relationships of Irkut and West Caucasian bat viruses within the Lyssavirus genus and suggested quantitative criteria based on the N gene sequence for lyssavirus genotype definition. *Virus Res* 2005;111(1):28–43.

304. Kuzmin IV, Hughes GJ, Rupprecht CE. Phylogenetic relationships of seven previously unclassified viruses within the family Rhabdoviridae using partial nucleoprotein gene sequences. *J Gen Virol* 2006;87(Pt 8):2323–2331.

305. Kuzmin IV, Mayer AE, Niezgoda M, et al. Shimoni bat virus, a new representative of the Lyssavirus genus. *Virus Res* 2010;149(2):197–210.

306. Kuzmin IV, Niezgoda M, Franka R, et al. Lagos bat virus in Kenya. *J Clin Microbiol* 2008;46(4):1451–1461.

307. Kuzmin IV, Orciari LA, Arai YT, et al. Bat lyssaviruses (Aravan and Khujand) from Central Asia: phylogenetic relationships according to N, P and G gene sequences. *Virus Res* 2003;97(2):65–79.

308. Lafay F, Coulon P, Astic L, et al. Spread of the CVS strain of rabies virus and of the avirulent mutant AvO1 along the olfactory pathways of the mouse after intranasal inoculation. *Virology* 1991;183(1):320–330.

309. Lafon M, Wiktor TJ, Macfarlan RI. Antigenic sites on the CVS rabies virus glycoprotein: analysis with monoclonal antibodies. *J Gen Virol* 1983;64(Pt 4):843–851.

310. Lahaye X, Vidy A, Pomier C, et al. Functional characterization of Negri bodies (NBs) in rabies virus-infected cells: evidence that NBs are sites of viral transcription and replication. *J Virol* 2009;83(16):7948–7958.

311. Langevin C, Jaaro H, Bressanelli S, et al. Rabies virus glycoprotein (RVG) is a trimeric ligand for the N-terminal cysteine-rich domain of the mammalian p75 neurotrophin receptor. *J Biol Chem* 2002;277(40):37655–37662.

312. Larson JK, Wunner WH, Ertl HC. Immune response to the nominal phosphoprotein of rabies virus. *Virus Res* 1992;23(1-2):73–88.

313. Lawson ND, Stillman EA, Whitt MA, et al. Recombinant vesicular stomatitis viruses from DNA. *Proc Natl Acad Sci U S A* 1995;92(10):4477–4481.

314. Leach CN, Johnson HN. Human rabies, with a special reference to virus distribution and titer. *Am J Trop Med* 1940;20:335–340.

315. Le Blanc I, Luyet PP, Pons V, et al. Endosome-to-cytosol transport of viral nucleocapsids. *Nat Cell Biol* 2005;7(7):653–664.

316. Lee AS, Burdeinick-Kerr R, Whelan SP. A ribosome-specialized translation initiation pathway is required for cap-dependent translation of vesicular stomatitis virus mRNAs. *Proc Natl Acad Sci U S A* 2013;110(1):324–329.

317. Lee HK, Lund JM, Ramanathan B, et al. Autophagy-dependent viral recognition by plasmacytoid dendritic cells. *Science* 2007;315(5817):1398–1401.

318. Lefrancois L, Lyles DS. The interaction of antibody with the major surface glycoprotein of vesicular stomatitis virus. I. Analysis of neutralizing epitopes with monoclonal antibodies. *Virology* 1982;121(1):157–167.

319. Lefrancois L, Lyles DS. Antigenic determinants of vesicular stomatitis virus: analysis with antigenic variants. *J Immunol* 1983;130(1):394–398.

320. Leist TP, Cobbold SP, Waldmann H, et al. Functional analysis of T lymphocyte subsets in antiviral host defense. *J Immunol* 1987;138(7):2278–2281.

321. Lembo T, Haydon DT, Velasco-Villa A, et al. Molecular epidemiology identifies only a single rabies virus variant circulating in complex carnivore communities of the Serengeti. *Proc Biol Sci* 2007;274(1622):2123–2130.

322. Lenard J, Vanderoef R. Localization of the membrane-associated region of vesicular stomatitis virus M protein at the N terminus, using the hydrophobic, photoreactive probe 125I-TID. *J Virol* 1990;64(7):3486–3491.

323. Leppert M, Rittenhouse L, Perrault J, et al. Plus and minus strand leader RNAs in negative strand virus-infected cells. *Cell* 1979;18(3):735–747.

324. Leyrat C, Schneider R, Ribeiro EA Jr, et al. Ensemble structure of the modular and flexible full-length vesicular stomatitis virus phosphoprotein. *J Mol Biol* 2012;423(2):182–197.

325. Leyrat C, Yabukarski F, Tarbouriech N, et al. Structure of the vesicular stomatitis virus N(0)-P complex. *PLoS Pathog* 2011;7(9):e1002248.

326. Li J, Fontaine-Rodriguez EC, Whelan SP. Amino acid residues within conserved domain VI of the vesicular stomatitis virus large polymerase protein essential for mRNA cap methyltransferase activity. *J Virol* 2005;79(21):13373–13384.

327. Li J, Rahmeh A, Morelli M, et al. A conserved motif in region v of the large polymerase proteins of nonsegmented negative-sense RNA viruses that is essential for mRNA capping. *J Virol* 2008;82(2):775–784.

328. Li J, Wang JT, Whelan SP. A unique strategy for mRNA cap methylation used by vesicular stomatitis virus. *Proc Natl Acad Sci U S A* 2006;103(22):8493–8498.

329. Li T, Pattnaik AK. Overlapping signals for transcription and replication at the 3′ terminus of the vesicular stomatitis virus genome. *J Virol* 1999;73(1):444–452.

330. Li Y, Luo L, Schubert M, et al. Viral liposomes released from insect cells infected with recombinant baculovirus expressing the matrix protein of vesicular stomatitis virus. *J Virol* 1993;67(7):4415–4420.

331. Liang B, Li Z, Jenni S, et al. Structure of the L protein of vesicular stomatitis virus from electron cryomicroscopy. *Cell* 2015;162(2):314–327.

332. Lichty BD, Power AT, Stojdl DF, et al. Vesicular stomatitis virus: re-inventing the bullet. *Trends Mol Med* 2004;10(5):210–216.

333. Lingappa VR, Katz FN, Lodish HF, et al. A signal sequence for the insertion of a transmembrane glycoprotein. Similarities to the signals of secretory proteins in primary structure and function. *J Biol Chem* 1978;253(24):8667–8670.

334. Liu Y, Zhang S, Wu X, et al. Ferret badger rabies origin and its revisited importance as potential source of rabies transmission in Southeast China. *BMC Infect Dis* 2010;10:234.

335. Lodish HF, Porter M. Translational control of protein synthesis after infection by vesicular stomatitis virus. *J Virol* 1980;36(3):719–733.

336. Lodmell DL, Esposito JJ, Ewalt LC. Rabies virus antinucleoprotein antibody protects against rabies virus challenge in vivo and inhibits rabies virus replication in vitro. *J Virol* 1993;67(10):6080–6086.

337. Lodmell DL, Sumner JW, Esposito JJ, et al. Raccoon poxvirus recombinants expressing the rabies virus nucleoprotein protect mice against lethal rabies virus infection. *J Virol* 1991;65(6):3400–3405.

338. Lorenzen N, LaPatra SE. DNA vaccines for aquacultured fish. *Rev Sci Tech* 2005;24(1):201–213.

339. Luan P, Glaser M. Formation of membrane domains by the envelope proteins of vesicular stomatitis virus. *Biochemistry* 1994;33(15):4483–4489.

340. Luan P, Yang L, Glaser M. Formation of membrane domains created during the budding of vesicular stomatitis virus. A model for selective lipid and protein sorting in biological membranes. *Biochemistry* 1995;34(31):9874–9883.

341. Ludewig B, Maloy KJ, López-Macías C, et al. Induction of optimal anti-viral neutralizing B cell responses by dendritic cells requires transport and release of virus particles in secondary lymphoid organs. *Eur J Immunol* 2000;30(1):185–196.

342. Lund JM, Alexopoulou L, Sato A, et al. Recognition of single-stranded RNA viruses by Toll-like receptor 7. *Proc Natl Acad Sci U S A* 2004;101(15):5598–5603.

343. Luo LH, Li Y, Snyder RM, et al. Point mutations in glycoprotein gene of vesicular stomatitis virus (New Jersey serotype) selected by resistance to neutralization by epitope-specific monoclonal antibodies. *Virology* 1988;163(2):341–348.

344. Lyles DS, McKenzie M, Parce JW. Subunit interactions of vesicular stomatitis virus envelope glycoprotein stabilized by binding to viral matrix protein. *J Virol* 1992;66(1):349–358.

345. Lyles DS, McKenzie MO. Reversible and irreversible steps in assembly and disassembly of vesicular stomatitis virus: equilibria and kinetics of dissociation of nucleocapsid-M protein complexes assembled in vivo. *Biochemistry* 1998;37(2):439–450.

346. Lyles DS, McKenzie MO, Ahmed M, et al. Potency of wild-type and temperature-sensitive vesicular stomatitis virus matrix protein in the inhibition of host-directed gene expression. *Virology* 1996;225(1):172–180.

347. Lyles DS, Varela VA, Parce JW. Dynamic nature of the quaternary structure of the vesicular stomatitis virus envelope glycoprotein. *Biochemistry* 1990;29(10):2442–2449.

348. Macfarlan RI, Dietzschold B, Koprowski H. Stimulation of cytotoxic T-lymphocyte responses by rabies virus glycoprotein and identification of an immunodominant domain. *Mol Immunol* 1986;23(7):733–741.

349. Macfarlan RI, Dietzschold B, Wiktor TJ, et al. T cell responses to cleaved rabies virus glycoprotein and to synthetic peptides. *J Immunol* 1984;133(5):2748–2752.

350. Machamer CE, Doms RW, Bole DG, et al. Heavy chain binding protein recognizes incompletely disulfide-bonded forms of vesicular stomatitis virus G protein. *J Biol Chem* 1990;265(12):6879–6883.

351. Mackett M, Yilma T, Rose JK, et al. Vaccinia virus recombinants: expression of VSV genes and protective immunization of mice and cattle. *Science* 1985;227(4685):433–435.

352. Maloy KJ, Odermatt B, Hengartner H, et al. Interferon gamma-producing gammadelta T cell-dependent antibody isotype switching in the absence of germinal center formation during virus infection. *Proc Natl Acad Sci U S A* 1998;95(3):1160–1165.

353. Markotter W, Van Eeden C, Kuzmin IV, et al. Epidemiology and pathogenicity of African bat lyssaviruses. *Dev Biol* 2008;131:317–325.

354. Martinez N, Ribeiro EA Jr, Leyrat C, et al. Structure of the C-terminal domain of lettuce necrotic yellows virus phosphoprotein. *J Virol* 2013;87(17):9569–9578.

355. Masatani T, Ito N, Shimizu K, et al. Amino acids at positions 273 and 394 in rabies virus nucleoprotein are important for both evasion of host RIG-I-mediated antiviral response and pathogenicity. *Virus Res* 2011;155(1):168–174.

356. Masters PS, Banerjee AK. Complex formation with vesicular stomatitis virus phosphoprotein NS prevents binding of nucleocapsid protein N to nonspecific RNA. *J Virol* 1988;62(8):2658–2664.

357. Matlin KS, Reggio H, Helenius A, et al. Pathway of vesicular stomatitis virus entry leading to infection. *J Mol Biol* 1982;156(3):609–631.

358. Mavrakis M, McCarthy AA, Roche S, et al. Structure and function of the C-terminal domain of the polymerase cofactor of rabies virus. *J Mol Biol* 2004;343(4):819–831.

359. Mavrakis M, Mehouas S, Real E, et al. Rabies virus chaperone: identification of the phosphoprotein peptide that keeps nucleoprotein soluble and free from non-specific RNA. *Virology* 2006;349(2):422–429.

360. McAllister PE, Wagner RR. Structural proteins of two salmonid rhabdoviruses. *J Virol* 1975;15(4):733–738.
361. McCreedy BJ Jr, Lyles DS. Distribution of M protein and nucleocapsid protein of vesicular stomatitis virus in infected cell plasma membranes. *Virus Res* 1989;14(3):189–205.
362. McCreedy BJ Jr, McKinnon KP, Lyles DS. Solubility of vesicular stomatitis virus M protein in the cytosol of infected cells or isolated from virions. *J Virol* 1990;64(2):902–906.
363. McKendrick AG. A ninth analytical review of reports from Pasteur Institutes. *Bull World Health Organ* 1941;9:31–78.
364. McKenna PM, McGettigan JP, Pomerantz RJ, et al. Recombinant rhabdoviruses as potential vaccines for HIV-1 and other diseases. *Curr HIV Res* 2003;1(2):229–237.
365. Mebatsion T, Conzelmann KK. Specific infection of CD4+ target cells by recombinant rabies virus pseudotypes carrying the HIV-1 envelope spike protein. *Proc Natl Acad Sci U S A* 1996;93(21):11366–11370.
366. Mebatsion T, Konig M, Conzelmann KK. Budding of rabies virus particles in the absence of the spike glycoprotein. *Cell* 1996;84(6):941–951.
367. Mebatsion T, Schnell MJ, Cox JH, et al. Highly stable expression of a foreign gene from rabies virus vectors. *Proc Natl Acad Sci U S A* 1996;93(14):7310–7314.
368. Mebatsion T, Weiland F, Conzelmann KK. Matrix protein of rabies virus is responsible for the assembly and budding of bullet-shaped particles and interacts with the transmembrane spike glycoprotein G. *J Virol* 1999;73(1):242–250.
369. Mellon MG, Emerson SU. Rebinding of transcriptase components (L and NS proteins) to the nucleocapsid template of vesicular stomatitis virus. *J Virol* 1978;27(3):560–567.
370. Ménager P, Roux P, Mégret F, et al. Toll-like receptor 3 (TLR3) plays a major role in the formation of rabies virus Negri Bodies. *PLoS Pathog* 2009;5(2):e1000315.
371. Meslin FX, Fishbein DB, Matter HC. Rationale and prospects for rabies elimination in developing countries. *Curr Top Microbiol Immunol* 1994;187:1–26.
372. Mire CE, Dube D, Delos SE, et al. Glycoprotein-dependent acidification of vesicular stomatitis virus enhances release of matrix protein. *J Virol* 2009;83(23):12139–12150.
373. Mire CE, White JM, Whitt MA. A spatio-temporal analysis of matrix protein and nucleocapsid trafficking during vesicular stomatitis virus uncoating. *PLoS Pathog* 2010;6(7):e1000994.
374. Mire CE, Whitt MA. The protease-sensitive loop of the vesicular stomatitis virus matrix protein is involved in virus assembly and protein translation. *Virology* 2011;416(1-2):16–25.
375. Mondal A, Victor KG, Pudupakam RS, et al. Newly identified phosphorylation site in the vesicular stomatitis virus P protein is required for viral RNA synthesis. *J Virol* 2014;88(3):1461–1472.
376. Moore SM, Hanlon CA. Rabies-specific antibodies: measuring surrogates of protection against a fatal disease. *PLoS Negl Trop Dis* 2010;4(3):e595.
377. Morimoto K, Foley HD, McGettigan JP, et al. Reinvestigation of the role of the rabies virus glycoprotein in viral pathogenesis using a reverse genetics approach. *J Neurovirol* 2000;6(5):373–381.
378. Morimoto K, Patel M, Corisdeo S, et al. Characterization of a unique variant of bat rabies virus responsible for newly emerging human cases in North America. *Proc Natl Acad Sci U S A* 1996;93(11):5653–5658.
379. Morin B, Rahmeh AA, Whelan SP. Mechanism of RNA synthesis initiation by the vesicular stomatitis virus polymerase. *EMBO J* 2012;31(5):1320–1329.
380. Moseley GW, Filmer RP, DeJesus MA, et al. Nucleocytoplasmic distribution of rabies virus P-protein is regulated by phosphorylation adjacent to C-terminal nuclear import and export signals. *Biochemistry* 2007;46(43):12053–12061.
381. Moya A, Elena SF, Bracho A, et al. The evolution of RNA viruses: a population genetics view. *Proc Natl Acad Sci U S A* 2000;97(13):6967–6973.
382. Moyer SA, Smallwood-Kentro S, Haddad A, et al. Assembly and transcription of synthetic vesicular stomatitis virus nucleocapsids. *J Virol* 1991;65(5):2170–2178.
383. Müller T, Bätza HJ, Beckert A, et al. Analysis of vaccine-virus-associated rabies cases in red foxes (Vulpes vulpes) after oral rabies vaccination campaigns in Germany and Austria. *Arch Virol* 2009;154(7):1081–1091.
384. Müller T, Cox J, Peter W, et al. Spill-over of European bat lyssavirus type 1 into a stone marten (Martes foina) in Germany. *J Vet Med B Infect Dis Vet Public Health* 2004;51(2):49–54.
385. Müller U, Steinhoff U, Reis LF, et al. Functional role of type I and type II interferons in antiviral defense. *Science* 1994;264(5167):1918–1921.
386. Murphy FA, Harrison AK, Winn WC, et al. Comparative pathogenesis of rabies and rabies-like viruses: infection of the central nervous system and centrifugal spread of virus to peripheral tissues. *Lab Investig* 1973;29(1):1–16.
387. Nakhaei P, Genin P, Civas A, et al. RIG-I-like receptors: sensing and responding to RNA virus infection. *Semin Immunol* 2009;21(4):215–222.
388. Neidermyer WJ Jr, Whelan SPJ. Global analysis of polysome-associated mRNA in vesicular stomatitis virus infected cells. *PLoS Pathog* 2019;15(6):e1007875.
389. Newcomb WW, Brown JC. Role of the vesicular stomatitis virus matrix protein in maintaining the viral nucleocapsid in the condensed form found in native virions. *J Virol* 1981;39(1):295–299.
390. Newcomb WW, Tobin GJ, McGowan JJ, et al. In vitro reassembly of vesicular stomatitis virus skeletons. *J Virol* 1982;41(3):1055–1062.
391. Nichol ST. Molecular epizootiology and evolution of vesicular stomatitis virus New Jersey. *J Virol* 1987;61(4):1029–1036.
392. Nichol ST. Genetic diversity of enzootic isolates of vesicular stomatitis virus New Jersey. *J Virol* 1988;62(2):572–579.
393. Nikolic J, Belot L, Raux H, et al. Structural basis for the recognition of LDL-receptor family members by VSV glycoprotein. *Nat Commun* 2018;9(1):1029.
394. Nikolic J, Le Bars R, Lama Z, et al. Negri bodies are viral factories with properties of liquid organelles. *Nat Commun* 2017;8(1):58.
395. Nishizawa T, Kinoshita S, Kim WS, et al. Nucleotide diversity of Japanese isolates of infectious hematopoietic necrosis virus (IHNV) based on the glycoprotein gene. *Dis Aquat Organ* 2006;71(3):267–272.
396. Noah DL, Drenzek CL, Smith JS, et al. Epidemiology of human rabies in the United States, 1980 to 1996. *Ann Intern Med* 1998;128(11):922–930.
397. Novella IS, Ebendick-Corpus BE, Zárate S, et al. Emergence of mammalian cell-adapted vesicular stomatitis virus from persistent infections of insect vector cells. *J Virol* 2007;81(12):6664–6668.
398. Novella IS, Gilbertson DL, Borrego B, et al. Adaptability costs in immune escape variants of vesicular stomatitis virus. *Virus Res* 2005;107(1):27–34.
399. Odenwald WF, Arnheiter H, Dubois-Dalcq M, et al. Stereo images of vesicular stomatitis virus assembly. *J Virol* 1986;57(3):922–932.
400. Oehen S, Odermatt B, Karrer U, et al. Marginal zone macrophages and immune responses against viruses. *J Immunol* 2002;169(3):1453–1458.
401. Ogden JR, Pal R, Wagner RR. Mapping regions of the matrix protein of vesicular stomatitis virus which bind to ribonucleocapsids, liposomes, and monoclonal antibodies. *J Virol* 1986;58(3):860–868.
402. Ogino M, Gupta N, Green TJ, et al. A dual-functional priming-capping loop of rhabdoviral RNA polymerases directs terminal de novo initiation and capping intermediate formation. *Nucleic Acids Res* 2019;47(1):299–309.
403. Ogino M, Ito N, Sugiyama M, et al. The rabies virus L protein catalyzes mRNA capping with GDP polyribonucleotidyltransferase activity. *Viruses* 2016;8(5).
404. Ogino T, Banerjee AK. Unconventional mechanism of mRNA capping by the RNA-dependent RNA polymerase of vesicular stomatitis virus. *Mol Cell* 2007;25(1):85–97.
405. Ogino T, Yadav SP, Banerjee AK. Histidine-mediated RNA transfer to GDP for unique mRNA capping by vesicular stomatitis virus RNA polymerase. *Proc Natl Acad Sci U S A* 2010;107(8):3463–3468.
406. Ohanessian A. Vertical transmission of the Piry rhabdovirus by sigma virus-infected Drosophila melanogaster females. *J Gen Virol* 1989;70(Pt 1):209–212.
407. Ohno S, Ohtake N. Immunocytochemical study of the intracellular localization of M protein of vesicular stomatitis virus. *Histochem J* 1987;19(5):297–306.
408. Olesen NJ, Vestergard-Jorgrnsen PE. Can and do herons serve as vectors for Egtved virus? *Bull Eur Assoc Fish Pathol* 1982;2:48.
409. Ono K, Dubois-Dalcq ME, Schubert M, et al. A mutated membrane protein of vesicular stomatitis virus has an abnormal distribution within the infected cell and causes defective budding. *J Virol* 1987;61(5):1332–1341.
410. Padhi A, Verghese B. Detecting molecular adaptation at individual codons in the glycoprotein gene of the geographically diversified infectious hematopoietic necrosis virus, a fish rhabdovirus. *Virus Res* 2008;132(1-2):229–236.
411. Paesen GC, Collet A, Sallamand C, et al. X-ray structure and activities of an essential Mononegavirales L-protein domain. *Nat Commun* 2015;6:8749.
412. Paik SY, Banerjea AC, Harmison GG, et al. Inducible and conditional inhibition of human immunodeficiency virus proviral expression by vesicular stomatitis virus matrix protein. *J Virol* 1995;69(6):3529–3537.
413. Pak CC, Puri A, Blumenthal R. Conformational changes and fusion activity of vesicular stomatitis virus glycoprotein: [125I]iodonaphthyl azide photolabeling studies in biological membranes. *Biochemistry* 1997;36(29):8890–8896.
414. Pal SR, Arora B, Chhuttani PN, et al. Rabies virus infection of a flying fox bat, Pteropus policephalus in Chandigarh, Northern India. *Trop Geogr Med* 1980;32(3):265–267.
415. Pan J, Qian X, Lattmann S, et al. Structure of the human metapneumovirus polymerase phosphoprotein complex. *Nature* 2020;577(7789):275–279.
416. Pasdeloup D, Poisson N, Raux H, et al. Nucleocytoplasmic shuttling of the rabies virus P protein requires a nuclear localization signal and a CRM1-dependent nuclear export signal. *Virology* 2005;334(2):284–293.
417. Pattnaik AK, Ball LA, LeGrone A, et al. The termini of VSV DI particle RNAs are sufficient to signal RNA encapsidation, replication, and budding to generate infectious particles. *Virology* 1995;206(1):760–764.
418. Pattnaik AK, Ball LA, LeGrone AW, et al. Infectious defective interfering particles of VSV from transcripts of a cDNA clone. *Cell* 1992;69(6):1011–1020.
419. Pattnaik AK, Hwang L, Li T, et al. Phosphorylation within the amino-terminal acidic domain I of the phosphoprotein of vesicular stomatitis virus is required for transcription but not for replication. *J Virol* 1997;71(11):8167–8175.
420. Patton JT, Davis NL, Wertz GW. N protein alone satisfies the requirement for protein synthesis during RNA replication of vesicular stomatitis virus. *J Virol* 1984;49(2):303–309.
421. Pearce AF, Lyles DS. Vesicular stomatitis virus induces apoptosis primarily through Bak rather than Bax by inactivating Mcl-1 and Bcl-XL. *J Virol* 2009;83(18):9102–9112.
422. Peddie S, McLauchlan PE, Ellis AE, et al. Effect of intraperitoneally administered IL-1beta-derived peptides on resistance to viral haemorrhagic septicaemia in rainbow trout Oncorhynchus mykiss. *Dis Aquat Organ* 2003;56(3):195–200.
423. Peluso RW. Kinetic, quantitative, and functional analysis of multiple forms of the vesicular stomatitis virus nucleocapsid protein in infected cells. *J Virol* 1988;62(8):2799–2807.
424. Peluso RW, Moyer SA. Viral proteins required for the in vitro replication of vesicular stomatitis virus defective interfering particle genome RNA. *Virology* 1988;162(2):369–376.
425. Perrault J, Leavitt RW. Inverted complementary terminal sequences in single-stranded RNAs and snap-back RNAs from vesicular stomatitis defective interfering particles. *J Gen Virol* 1978;38(1):35–50.
426. Perry LL, Lodmell DL. Role of CD4+ and CD8+ T cells in murine resistance to street rabies virus. *J Virol* 1991;65(7):3429–3434.
427. Piccinotti S, Kirchhausen T, Whelan SP. Uptake of rabies virus into epithelial cells by clathrin-mediated endocytosis depends upon actin. *J Virol* 2013;87(21):11637–11647.
428. Piccinotti S, Whelan SP. Rabies internalizes into primary peripheral neurons via clathrin coated pits and requires fusion at the cell body. *PLoS Pathog* 2016;12(7):e1005753.
429. Pickl WF, Pimentel-Muiños FX, Seed B. Lipid rafts and pseudotyping. *J Virol* 2001;75(15):7175–7183.
430. Piyasirisilp S, Schmeckpeper BJ, Chandanayingyong D, et al. Association of HLA and T-cell receptor gene polymorphisms with Semple rabies vaccine-induced autoimmune encephalomyelitis. *Ann Neurol* 1999;45(5):595–600.
431. Plakhov IV, Arlund EE, Aoki C, et al. The earliest events in vesicular stomatitis virus infection of the murine olfactory neuroepithelium and entry of the central nervous system. *Virology* 1995;209(1):257–262.

432. Pornillos O, Garrus JE, Sundquist WI. Mechanisms of enveloped RNA virus budding. *Trends Cell Biol* 2002;12(12):569–579.
433. Prabhakar BS, Fischman HR, Nathanson N. Recovery from experimental rabies by adoptive transfer of immune cells. *J Gen Virol* 1981;56(Pt 1):25–31.
434. Préhaud C, Lay S, Dietzschold B, et al. Glycoprotein of nonpathogenic rabies viruses is a key determinant of human cell apoptosis. *J Virol* 2003;77(19):10537–10547.
435. Préhaud C, Mégret F, Lafage M, et al. Virus infection switches TLR-3-positive human neurons to become strong producers of beta interferon. *J Virol* 2005;79(20):12893–12904.
436. Préhaud C, Wolff N, Terrien E, et al. Attenuation of rabies virulence: takeover by the cytoplasmic domain of its envelope protein. *Sci Signal* 2010;3(105):ra5.
437. Pringle CR. Genetic characteristics of conditional lethal mutants of vesicular stomatitis virus induced by 5-fluorouracil, 5-azacytidine, and ethyl methane sulfonate. *J Virol* 1970;5(5):559–567.
438. Puddington L, Bevan MJ, Rose JK, et al. N protein is the predominant antigen recognized by vesicular stomatitis virus-specific cytotoxic T cells. *J Virol* 1986;60(2):708–717.
439. Rahmeh AA, Li J, Kranzusch PJ, et al. Ribose 2′-O methylation of the vesicular stomatitis virus mRNA cap precedes and facilitates subsequent guanine-N-7 methylation by the large polymerase protein. *J Virol* 2009;83(21):11043–11050.
440. Rahmeh AA, Morin B, Schenk AD, et al. Critical phosphoprotein elements that regulate polymerase architecture and function in vesicular stomatitis virus. *Proc Natl Acad Sci U S A* 2012;109(36):14628–14633.
441. Rahmeh AA, Schenk AD, Danek EI, et al. Molecular architecture of the vesicular stomatitis virus RNA polymerase. *Proc Natl Acad Sci U S A* 2010;107(46):20075–20080.
442. Randall RE, Goodbourn S. Interferons and viruses: an interplay between induction, signalling, antiviral responses and virus countermeasures. *J Gen Virol* 2008;89(Pt 1):1–47.
443. Rao BL, Basu A, Wairagkar NS, et al. A large outbreak of acute encephalitis with high fatality rate in children in Andhra Pradesh, India, in 2003, associated with Chandipura virus. *Lancet* 2004;364(9437):869–874.
444. Rehwinkel J, Tan CP, Goubau D, et al. RIG-I detects viral genomic RNA during negative-strand RNA virus infection. *Cell* 2010;140(3):397–408.
445. Reif JS, Webb PA, Monath TP, et al. Epizootic vesicular stomatitis in Colorado, 1982: infection in occupational risk groups. *Am J Trop Med Hyg* 1987;36(1):177–182.
446. Reynes JM, Molia S, Audry L, et al. Serologic evidence of lyssavirus infection in bats, Cambodia. *Emerg Infect Dis* 2004;10(12):2231–2234.
447. Riedel C, Vasishtan D, Prazak V, et al. Cryo EM structure of the rabies virus ribonucleoprotein complex. *Sci Rep* 2019;9(1):9639.
448. Rieder M, Brzózka K, Pfaller CK, et al. Genetic dissection of interferon-antagonistic functions of rabies virus phosphoprotein: inhibition of interferon regulatory factor 3 activation is important for pathogenicity. *J Virol* 2011;85(2):842–852.
449. Risso-Ballester J, Galloux M, Cao J, et al. A condensate-hardening drug blocks RSV replication in vivo. *Nature* 2021;595(7868):596–599.
450. Roberts A, Buonocore L, Price R, et al. Attenuated vesicular stomatitis viruses as vaccine vectors. *J Virol* 1999;73(5):3723–3732.
451. Robinson LR, Whelan SP. Infectious entry pathway mediated by the human endogenous retrovirus K envelope protein. *J Virol* 2016;90(7):3640–3649.
452. Robison CS, Whitt MA. The membrane-proximal stem region of vesicular stomatitis virus G protein confers efficient virus assembly. *J Virol* 2000;74(5):2239–2246.
453. Roche S, Bressanelli S, Rey FA, et al. Crystal structure of the low-pH form of the vesicular stomatitis virus glycoprotein G. *Science* 2006;313(5784):187–191.
454. Roche S, Rey FA, Gaudin Y, et al. Structure of the prefusion form of the vesicular stomatitis virus glycoprotein G. *Science* 2007;315(5813):843–848.
455. Rodriguez Boulan E, Sabatini DD. Asymmetric budding of viruses in epithelial monlayers: a model system for study of epithelial polarity. *Proc Natl Acad Sci U S A* 1978;75(10):5071–5075.
456. Rodríguez LL, Fitch WM, Nichol ST. Ecological factors rather than temporal factors dominate the evolution of vesicular stomatitis virus. *Proc Natl Acad Sci U S A* 1996;93(23):13030–13035.
457. Rodriguez LL, Letchworth GJ, Spiropoulou CF, et al. Rapid detection of vesicular stomatitis virus New Jersey serotype in clinical samples by using polymerase chain reaction. *J Clin Microbiol* 1993;31(8):2016–2020.
458. Ronsholt LA. New case of European bat lyssavirus (EBL) infection in Danish sheep. *Rabies Bull Europe* 2002;26:15.
459. Rose JK, Lodish HF, Brock ML. Giant heterogeneous polyadenylic acid on vesicular stomatitis virus mRNA synthesized in vitro in the presence of S-adenosylhomocysteine. *J Virol* 1977;21(2):683–693.
460. Rose JK, Welch WJ, Sefton BM, et al. Vesicular stomatitis virus glycoprotein is anchored in the viral membrane by a hydrophobic domain near the COOH terminus. *Proc Natl Acad Sci U S A* 1980;77(7):3884–3888.
461. Rose NF, Marx PA, Luckay A, et al. An effective AIDS vaccine based on live attenuated vesicular stomatitis virus recombinants. *Cell* 2001;106(5):539–549.
462. Rosen CA, Ennis HL, Cohen PS. Translational control of vesicular stomatitis virus protein synthesis: isolation of an mRNA-sequestering particle. *J Virol* 1982;44(3):932–938.
463. Rosenthal KL, Zinkernagel RM. Cross-reactive cytotoxic T cells to serologically distinct vesicular stomatitis virus. *J Immunol* 1980;124(5):2301–2308.
464. Roy P, Repik P, Hefti E, et al. Complementary RNA species isolated from vesicular stomatitis (HR strain) defective virions. *J Virol* 1973;11(6):915–925.
465. Rucker RR, Whipple WJ, Parvin JR, et al. A contagious disease of sockeye salmon possibly of virus origin. *US Fish Wildl Serv Fish Bull* 1953;54:35–46.
466. Rupprecht CE, Dietzschold B, Campbell JB, et al. Consideration of inactivated rabies vaccines as oral immunogens of wild carnivores. *J Wildl Dis* 1992;28(4):629–635.
467. Rupprecht CE, Smith JS, Fekadu M, et al. The ascension of wildlife rabies: a cause for public health concern or intervention? *Emerg Infect Dis* 1995;1(4):107–114.
468. Sabin AB, Olitsky PK. Influence of host factors on neuroinvasiveness of vesicular stomatitis virus. III. Effect of age and pathway of infection on the character and localization of lesions in the central nervous system. *J Exp Med* 1938;67:201–227.
469. Samuel S, Tumilasci VF, Oliere S, et al. VSV oncolysis in combination with the BCL-2 inhibitor obatoclax overcomes apoptosis resistance in chronic lymphocytic leukemia. *Mol Ther* 2010;18(12):2094–2103.
470. Sasaki DM, Middleton CR, Sawa TR, et al. Rabid bat diagnosed in Hawaii. *Hawaii Med J* 1992;51(7):181–185.
471. Sasaya T, Ishikawa K, Koganezawa H. The nucleotide sequence of RNA1 of Lettuce big-vein virus, genus Varicosavirus, reveals its relation to nonsegmented negative-strand RNA viruses. *Virology* 2002;297(2):289–297.
472. Scaffidi C, Fulda S, Srinivasan A, et al. Two CD95 (APO-1/Fas) signaling pathways. *EMBO J* 1998;17(6):1675–1687.
473. Scaffidi C, Schmitz I, Zha J, et al. Differential modulation of apoptosis sensitivity in CD95 type I and type II cells. *J Biol Chem* 1999;274(32):22532–22538.
474. Scheiffele P, Rietveld A, Wilk T, et al. Influenza viruses select ordered lipid domains during budding from the plasma membrane. *J Biol Chem* 1999;274(4):2038–2044.
475. Schlee M, Roth A, Hornung V, et al. Recognition of 5′ triphosphate by RIG-I helicase requires short blunt double-stranded RNA as contained in panhandle of negative-strand virus. *Immunity* 2009;31(1):25–34.
476. Schlegel R, Tralka TS, Willingham MC, et al. Inhibition of VSV binding and infectivity by phosphatidylserine: is phosphatidylserine a VSV-binding site? *Cell* 1983;32(2):639–646.
477. Schmidt MF, Schlesinger MJ. Fatty acid binding to vesicular stomatitis virus glycoprotein: a new type of post-translational modification of the viral glycoprotein. *Cell* 1979;17(4):813–819.
478. Schneider LG. Rabies virus vaccines. *Dev Biol Stand* 1995;84:49–54.
479. Schnell MJ, Buonocore L, Boritz E, et al. Requirement for a non-specific glycoprotein cytoplasmic domain sequence to drive efficient budding of vesicular stomatitis virus. *EMBO J* 1998;17(5):1289–1296.
480. Schnell MJ, Buonocore L, Kretzschmar E, et al. Foreign glycoproteins expressed from recombinant vesicular stomatitis viruses are incorporated efficiently into virus particles. *Proc Natl Acad Sci U S A* 1996;93(21):11359–11365.
481. Schnell MJ, Buonocore L, Whitt MA, et al. The minimal conserved transcription stop-start signal promotes stable expression of a foreign gene in vesicular stomatitis virus. *J Virol* 1996;70(4):2318–2323.
482. Schnell MJ, McGettigan JP, Wirblich C, et al. The cell biology of rabies virus: using stealth to reach the brain. *Nat Rev* 2010;8(1):51–61.
483. Schnell MJ, Mebatsion T, Conzelmann KK. Infectious rabies viruses from cloned cDNA. *EMBO J* 1994;13(18):4195–4203.
484. Schott DH, Cureton DK, Whelan SP, et al. An antiviral role for the RNA interference machinery in Caenorhabditis elegans. *Proc Natl Acad Sci U S A* 2005;102(51):18420–18424.
485. Schwaninger R, Beckers CJ, Balch WE. Sequential transport of protein between the endoplasmic reticulum and successive Golgi compartments in semi-intact cells. *J Biol Chem* 1991;266(20):13055–13063.
486. Serra-Cobo J, Amengual B, Abellán C, et al. European bat lyssavirus infection in Spanish bat populations. *Emerg Infect Dis* 2002;8(4):413–420.
487. Sevier CS, Weisz OA, Davis M, et al. Efficient export of the vesicular stomatitis virus G protein from the endoplasmic reticulum requires a signal in the cytoplasmic tail that includes both tyrosine-based and di-acidic motifs. *Mol Biol Cell* 2000;11(1):13–22.
488. Shankar V, Dietzschold B, Koprowski H. Direct entry of rabies virus into the central nervous system without prior local replication. *J Virol* 1991;65(5):2736–2738.
489. Shannon LM, Poulton JL, Emmons RW, et al. Serological survey for rabies antibodies in raptors from California. *J Wildl Dis* 1988;24(2):264–267.
490. Sharif-Askari E, Nakhaei P, Oliere S, et al. Bax-dependent mitochondrial membrane permeabilization enhances IRF3-mediated innate immune response during VSV infection. *Virology* 2007;365(1):20–33.
491. Shi Z, Cai Z, Sanchez A, et al. A novel Toll-like receptor that recognizes vesicular stomatitis virus. *J Biol Chem* 2011;286(6):4517–4524.
492. Shuai L, Wang J, Zhao D, et al. Integrin beta1 promotes peripheral entry by rabies virus. *J Virol* 2020;94(2).
493. Simonsen CC, Batt-Humphries S, Summers DF. RNA synthesis of vesicular stomatitis virus-infected cells: in vivo regulation of replication. *J Virol* 1979;31(1):124–132.
494. Sitterlin D. Characterization of the Drosophila Rae1 protein as a G1 phase regulator of the cell cycle. *Gene* 2004;326:107–116.
495. Siwasontiwat D, Lumlertdacha B, Polsuwan C, et al. Rabies: is provocation of the biting dog relevant for risk assessment? *Trans R Soc Trop Med Hyg* 1992;86(4):443.
496. Skall HF, Olesen NJ, Mellergaard S. Prevalence of viral haemorrhagic septicaemia virus in Danish marine fishes and its occurrence in new host species. *Dis Aquat Organ* 2005;66(2):145–151.
497. Smallwood S, Moyer SA. Promoter analysis of the vesicular stomatitis virus RNA polymerase. *Virology* 1993;192(1):254–263.
498. Smith AL, Tignor GH, Emmons RW, et al. Isolation of field rabies virus strains in CER and murine neuroblastoma cell cultures. *Intervirology* 1978;9(6):359–361.
499. Smith JS, Fishbein DB, Rupprecht CE, et al. Unexplained rabies in three immigrants in the United States. A virologic investigation. *N Engl J Med* 1991;324(4):205–211.
500. Smith JS, Seidel HD. Rabies: a new look at an old disease. *Prog Med Virol* 1993;40:82–106.
501. Soria M, Little SP, Huang AS. Characterization of vesicular stomatitis virus nucleocapsids. I. Complementary 40 S RNA molecules in nucleocapsids. *Virology* 1974;61(1):270–280.
502. Spadafora D, Canter DM, Jackson RL, et al. Constitutive phosphorylation of the vesicular stomatitis virus P protein modulates polymerase complex formation but is not essential for transcription or replication. *J Virol* 1996;70(7):4538–4548.
503. Springfeld C, Darai G, Cattaneo R. Characterization of the Tupaia rhabdovirus genome reveals a long open reading frame overlapping with P and a novel gene encoding a small hydrophobic protein. *J Virol* 2005;79(11):6781–6790.
504. Srinivasan A, Burton EC, Kuehnert MJ, et al. Transmission of rabies virus from an organ donor to four transplant recipients. *N Engl J Med* 2005;352(11):1103–1111.
505. St. George TD, Standfast HA. Bovine ephemeral fever. In: Monath TP, ed. *The Arboviruses: Epidemiology and Ecology*. Vol. II. Boca Raton, FL: CRC Press; 1988:71–86.
506. Stallknecht DE, Howerth EW, Reeves CL, et al. Potential for contact and mechanical vector transmission of vesicular stomatitis virus New Jersey in pigs. *Am J Vet Res* 1999;60(1):43–48.

507. Stallknecht DE, Kavanaugh DM, Corn JL, et al. Feral swine as a potential amplifying host for vesicular stomatitis virus New Jersey serotype on Ossabaw Island, Georgia. *J Wildl Dis* 1993;29(3):377–383.
508. Stallknecht DE, Nettles VF, Fletcher WO, et al. Enzootic vesicular stomatitis New Jersey type in an insular feral swine population. *Am J Epidemiol* 1985;122(5):876–883.
509. Stillman EA, Whitt MA. Transcript initiation and 5′-end modifications are separable events during vesicular stomatitis virus transcription. *J Virol* 1999;73(9):7199–7209.
510. Stojdl DF, Lichty BD, tenOever BR, et al. VSV strains with defects in their ability to shutdown innate immunity are potent systemic anti-cancer agents. *Cancer Cell* 2003;4(4): 263–275.
511. Strady A, Lang J, Lienard M, et al. Antibody persistence following preexposure regimens of cell-culture rabies vaccines: 10-year follow-up and proposal for a new booster policy. *J Infect Dis* 1998;177(5):1290–1295.
512. Sugamata M, Miyazawa M, Mori S, et al. Paralysis of street rabies virus-infected mice is dependent on T lymphocytes. *J Virol* 1992;66(2):1252–1260.
513. Sun X, Belouzard S, Whittaker GR. Molecular architecture of the bipartite fusion loops of vesicular stomatitis virus glycoprotein G, a class III viral fusion protein. *J Biol Chem* 2008;283(10):6418–6427.
514. Superti F, Hauttecoeur B, Morelec MJ, et al. Involvement of gangliosides in rabies virus infection. *J Gen Virol* 1986;67(Pt 1):47–56.
515. Swinteck BD, Lyles DS. Plasma membrane microdomains containing vesicular stomatitis virus M protein are separate from microdomains containing G protein and nucleocapsids. *J Virol* 2008;82(11):5536–5547.
516. Takacs AM, Barik S, Das T, et al. Phosphorylation of specific serine residues within the acidic domain of the phosphoprotein of vesicular stomatitis virus regulates transcription in vitro. *J Virol* 1992;66(10):5842–5848.
517. Takada A, Robison C, Goto H, et al. A system for functional analysis of Ebola virus glycoprotein. *Proc Natl Acad Sci U S A* 1997;94(26):14764–14769.
518. Takeuchi O, Akira S. Pattern recognition receptors and inflammation. *Cell* 2010;140(6):805–820.
519. Tang X, Luo M, Zhang S, et al. Pivotal role of dogs in rabies transmission, China. *Emerg Infect Dis* 2005;11(12):1970–1972.
520. Taylor GM, Hanson PI, Kielian M. Ubiquitin depletion and dominant-negative VPS4 inhibit rhabdovirus budding without affecting alphavirus budding. *J Virol* 2007;81(24):13631–13639.
521. Teidebold TC, Mather CS, Merrillat LA. *Gangrenous Glossitis of Horses.* Report of the 20th Annual Meeting of the United States Livestock Sanitary Association. 1916:29–42.
522. Tekes G, Rahmeh AA, Whelan SP. A freeze frame view of vesicular stomatitis virus transcription defines a minimal length of RNA for 5′ processing. *PLoS Pathog* 2011;7(6):e1002073.
523. Tepsumethanon V, Lumlertdacha B, Mitmoonpitak C, et al. Fluorescent antibody test for rabies: prospective study of 8,987 brains. *Clin Infect Dis* 1997;25(6):1459–1461.
524. Tesh R, Saidi S, Javadian E, et al. Isfahan virus, a new vesiculovirus infecting humans, gerbils, and sandflies in Iran. *Am J Trop Med Hyg* 1977;26(2):299–306.
525. Tesh RB, Boshell J, Modi GB, et al. Natural infection of humans, animals, and phlebotomine sand flies with the Alagoas serotype of vesicular stomatitis virus in Colombia. *Am J Trop Med Hyg* 1987;36(3):653–661.
526. Testa D, Banerjee AK. Two methyltransferase activities in the purified virions of vesicular stomatitis virus. *J Virol* 1977;24(3):786–793.
527. Theiler M, Downs WG. Minor groups of arboviruses. In: Theiler M, Downs WG, eds. *The Arthropod-Borne Viruses of Vertebrates: An Account of the Rockefeller Foundation Virus Program 1951—1970.* New Haven, CT: Yale University Press; 1973:263–280.
528. Thomas D, Newcomb WW, Brown JC, et al. Mass and molecular composition of vesicular stomatitis virus: a scanning transmission electron microscopy analysis. *J Virol* 1985;54(2):598–607.
529. Thomas DC, Brewer CB, Roth MG. Vesicular stomatitis virus glycoprotein contains a dominant cytoplasmic basolateral sorting signal critically dependent upon a tyrosine. *J Biol Chem* 1993;268(5):3313–3320.
530. Thoulouze MI, Lafage M, Schachner M, et al. The neural cell adhesion molecule is a receptor for rabies virus. *J Virol* 1998;72(9):7181–7190.
531. Tisdale EJ, Bourne JR, Khosravi-Far R, et al. GTP-binding mutants of rab1 and rab2 are potent inhibitors of vesicular transport from the endoplasmic reticulum to the Golgi complex. *J Cell Biol* 1992;119(4):749–761.
532. Tovey MG, Maury C. Oromucosal interferon therapy: marked antiviral and antitumor activity. *J Interferon Cytokine Res* 1999;19(2):145–155.
533. Travassos da Rosa AP, Tesh RB, Travassos da Rosa JF, et al. Carajas and Maraba viruses, two new vesiculoviruses isolated from phlebotomine sand flies in Brazil. *Am J Trop Med Hyg* 1984;33(5):999–1006.
534. Trottier MD Jr, Palian BM, Reiss CS. VSV replication in neurons is inhibited by type I IFN at multiple stages of infection. *Virology* 2005;333(2):215–225.
535. Trottier MD, Lyles DS, Reiss CS. Peripheral, but not central nervous system, type I interferon expression in mice in response to intranasal vesicular stomatitis virus infection. *J Neurovirol* 2007;13(5):433–445.
536. Troyer RM, Kurath G. Molecular epidemiology of infectious hematopoietic necrosis virus reveals complex virus traffic and evolution within southern Idaho aquaculture. *Dis Aquat Organ* 2003;55(3):175–185.
537. Tuffereau C, Benejean J, Alfonso AM, et al. Neuronal cell surface molecules mediate specific binding to rabies virus glycoprotein expressed by a recombinant baculovirus on the surfaces of lepidopteran cells. *J Virol* 1998;72(2):1085–1091.
538. Tuffereau C, Bénéjean J, Blondel D, et al. Low-affinity nerve-growth factor receptor (P75NTR) can serve as a receptor for rabies virus. *EMBO J* 1998;17(24):7250–7259.
539. Ubol S, Sukwattanapan C, Utaisincharoen P. Rabies virus replication induces Bax-related, caspase dependent apoptosis in mouse neuroblastoma cells. *Virus Res* 1998;56(2):207–215.
540. Uren MF, St George TD, Murphy GM. Studies on the pathogenesis of bovine ephemeral fever in experimental cattle. III. Virological and biochemical data. *Vet Microbiol* 1992;30(4):297–307.
541. Uren MF, Walker PJ, Zakrzewski H, et al. Effective vaccination of cattle using the virion G protein of bovine ephemeral fever virus as an antigen. *Vaccine* 1994;12(9):845–850.
542. Van Bleek GM, Nathenson SG. Isolation of an endogenously processed immunodominant viral peptide from the class I H-2Kb molecule. *Nature* 1990;348(6298):213–216.
543. van der Westhuizen B. Studies on bovine ephemeral fever. I. Isolation and preliminary characterization of a virus from natural and experimentally produced cases of bovine ephemeral fever. *Onderstepoort J Vet Res* 1967;34(1):29–40.
544. van Thiel PP, van den Hoek JA, Eftimov F, et al. Fatal case of human rabies (Duvenhage virus) from a bat in Kenya: The Netherlands, December 2007. *Euro Surveill* 2008;13(2).
545. Van Zyl N, Markotter W, Nel LH. Evolutionary history of African mongoose rabies. *Virus Res* 2010;150(1-2):93–102.
546. Vidy A, Chelbi-Alix M, Blondel D. Rabies virus P protein interacts with STAT1 and inhibits interferon signal transduction pathways. *J Virol* 2005;79(22):14411–14420.
547. Vidy A, El Bougrini J, Chelbi-Alix MK, et al. The nucleocytoplasmic rabies virus P protein counteracts interferon signaling by inhibiting both nuclear accumulation and DNA binding of STAT1. *J Virol* 2007;81(8):4255–4263.
548. von Kobbe C, van Deursen JM, Rodrigues JP, et al. Vesicular stomatitis virus matrix protein inhibits host cell gene expression by targeting the nucleoporin Nup98. *Mol Cell* 2000;6(5):1243–1252.
549. Waibler Z, Detje CN, Bell JC, et al. Matrix protein mediated shutdown of host cell metabolism limits vesicular stomatitis virus-induced interferon-alpha responses to plasmacytoid dendritic cells. *Immunobiology* 2007;212(9-10):887–894.
550. Walker PJ. Bovine ephemeral fever in Australia and the world. *Curr Top Microbiol Immunol* 2005;292:57–80.
551. Walker PJ, Firth C, Widen SG, et al. Evolution of genome size and complexity in the rhabdoviridae. *PLoS Pathog* 2015;11(2):e1004664.
552. Wandeler AI, Matter HC, Kappeler A, et al. The ecology of dogs and canine rabies: a selective review. *Rev Sci Tech* 1993;12(1):51–71.
553. Wang J, Wang Z, Liu R, et al. Metabotropic glutamate receptor subtype 2 is a cellular receptor for rabies virus. *PLoS Pathog* 2018;14(7):e1007189.
554. Wang JT, McElvain LE, Whelan SP. Vesicular stomatitis virus mRNA capping machinery requires specific cis-acting signals in the RNA. *J Virol* 2007;81(20):11499–11506.
555. Wang ZW, Sarmento L, Wang Y, et al. Attenuated rabies virus activates, while pathogenic rabies virus evades, the host innate immune responses in the central nervous system. *J Virol* 2005;79(19):12554–12565.
556. Warner CK, Whitfield SG, Fekadu M, et al. Procedures for reproducible detection of rabies virus antigen mRNA and genome in situ in formalin-fixed tissues. *J Virol Methods* 1997;67(1):5–12.
557. Warrell DA, Warrell MJ. Human rabies and its prevention: an overview. *Rev Infect Dis* 1988;10(Suppl 4):S726–S731.
558. Warrilow D, Smith IL, Harrower B, et al. Sequence analysis of an isolate from a fatal human infection of Australian bat lyssavirus. *Virology* 2002;297(1):109–119.
559. Watson WA. Vesicular diseases: recent advances and concepts of control. *Can Vet J* 1981;22(10):311–320.
560. Weiland F, Cox JH, Meyer S, et al. Rabies virus neuritic paralysis: immunopathogenesis of nonfatal paralytic rabies. *J Virol* 1992;66(8):5096–5099.
561. Welnowska E, Castello A, Moral P, et al. Translation of mRNAs from vesicular stomatitis virus and vaccinia virus is differentially blocked in cells with depletion of eIF4GI and/or eIF4GII. *J Mol Biol* 2009;394(3):506–521.
562. Wertz GW. Replication of vesicular stomatitis virus defective interfering particle RNA in vitro: transition from synthesis of defective interfering leader RNA to synthesis of full-length defective interfering RNA. *J Virol* 1983;46(2):513–522.
563. Wertz GW, Levine M. RNA synthesis by vesicular stomatitis virus and a small plaque mutant: effects of cycloheximide. *J Virol* 1973;12(2):253–264.
564. Wertz GW, Perepelitsa VP, Ball LA. Gene rearrangement attenuates expression and lethality of a nonsegmented negative strand RNA virus. *Proc Natl Acad Sci U S A* 1998;95(7): 3501–3506.
565. Wertz GW, Whelan S, LeGrone A, et al. Extent of terminal complementarity modulates the balance between transcription and replication of vesicular stomatitis virus RNA. *Proc Natl Acad Sci U S A* 1994;91(18):8587–8591.
565a. Weyer J, Msimang-Dermaux V, Paweska J, et al. A case of human survival of rabies, South Africa. *S Afr J Infect Dis* 2016;31(2):66–68. https://doi.org/10.4102/sajid.v31i2.93
566. Whelan SP, Ball LA, Barr JN, et al. Efficient recovery of infectious vesicular stomatitis virus entirely from cDNA clones. *Proc Natl Acad Sci U S A* 1995;92(18):8388–8392.
567. Whelan SP, Wertz GW. The 5′ terminal trailer region of vesicular stomatitis virus contains a position-dependent cis-acting signal for assembly of RNA into infectious particles. *J Virol* 1999;73(1):307–315.
568. Whelan SP, Wertz GW. Regulation of RNA synthesis by the genomic termini of vesicular stomatitis virus: identification of distinct sequences essential for transcription but not replication. *J Virol* 1999;73(1):297–306.
569. Whelan SP, Wertz GW. Transcription and replication initiate at separate sites on the vesicular stomatitis virus genome. *Proc Natl Acad Sci U S A* 2002;99(14):9178–9183.
570. Whitlow ZW, Connor JH, Lyles DS. Preferential translation of vesicular stomatitis virus mRNAs is conferred by transcription from the viral genome. *J Virol* 2006;80(23):11733–11742.
571. Whitlow ZW, Connor JH, Lyles DS. New mRNAs are preferentially translated during vesicular stomatitis virus infection. *J Virol* 2008;82(5):2286–2294.
572. Whitt MA, Buonocore L, Prehaud C, et al. Membrane fusion activity, oligomerization, and assembly of the rabies virus glycoprotein. *Virology* 1991;185(2):681–688.
573. Whitt MA, Rose JK. Fatty acid acylation is not required for membrane fusion activity or glycoprotein assembly into VSV virions. *Virology* 1991;185(2):875–878.
574. Wiktor TJ. Historical aspects of rabies treatment. In: Koprowski H, Plotkin S, eds. *World's Debt to Pasteur.* New York: Alan Liss Press; 1985.
575. Wilde H, Chutivongse S. Equine rabies immune globulin: a product with an undeserved poor reputation. *Am J Trop Med Hyg* 1990;42(2):175–178.

576. Wilde H, Sirikawin S, Sabcharoen A, et al. Failure of postexposure treatment of rabies in children. *Clin Infect Dis* 1996;22(2):228–232.

577. Willoughby RE Jr, Tieves KS, Hoffman GM, et al. Survival after treatment of rabies with induction of coma. *N Engl J Med* 2005;352(24):2508–2514.

578. Winkler WG, Bögel K. Control of rabies in wildlife. *Sci Am* 1992;266(6):86–92.

579. Winkler WG, Fashinell TR, Leffingwell L, et al. Airborne rabies transmission in a laboratory worker. *JAMA* 1973;226(10):1219–1221.

580. Winton JR. Recent advances in the detection and control of infectious hematopoietic necrosis virus (IHNV) in aquaculture. *Ann Rev Fish Dis* 1991;1:83–93.

581. Wirblich C, Tan GS, Papaneri A, et al. PPEY motif within the rabies virus (RV) matrix protein is essential for efficient virion release and RV pathogenicity. *J Virol* 2008;82(19):9730–9738.

582. Wong RW, Blobel G, Coutavas E. Rae1 interaction with NuMA is required for bipolar spindle formation. *Proc Natl Acad Sci U S A* 2006;103(52):19783–19787.

583. World Health Organization. *WHO Expert Committee on Rabies, 8th Report.* Geneva, Switzerland: World Health Organization; 1992.

584. Wright E, McNabb S, Goddard T, et al. A robust lentiviral pseudotype neutralisation assay for in-field serosurveillance of rabies and lyssaviruses in Africa. *Vaccine* 2009;27(51):7178–7186.

585. Wunner WH, Reagan KJ, Koprowski H. Characterization of saturable binding sites for rabies virus. *J Virol* 1984;50(3):691–697.

586. Xuan X, Tuchiya K, Sato I, et al. Biological and immunogenic properties of rabies virus glycoprotein expressed by canine herpesvirus vector. *Vaccine* 1998;16(9-10):969–976.

587. Yabukarski F, Leyrat C, Martinez N, et al. Ensemble structure of the highly flexible complex formed between vesicular stomatitis virus unassembled nucleoprotein and its phosphoprotein chaperone. *J Mol Biol* 2016;428(13):2671–2694.

588. Yacovone SK, Smelser AM, Macosko JC, et al. Migration of nucleocapsids in vesicular stomatitis virus-infected cells is dependent on both microtubules and actin filaments. *J Virol* 2016;90(13):6159–6170.

589. Ye Z, Sun W, Suryanarayana K, et al. Membrane-binding domains and cytopathogenesis of the matrix protein of vesicular stomatitis virus. *J Virol* 1994;68(11):7386–7396.

590. Yewdell JW, Bennink JR, Mackett M, et al. Recognition of cloned vesicular stomatitis virus internal and external gene products by cytotoxic T lymphocytes. *J Exp Med* 1986;163(6):1529–1538.

591. Yuan H, Puckett S, Lyles DS. Inhibition of host transcription by vesicular stomatitis virus involves a novel mechanism that is independent of phosphorylation of TATA-binding protein (TBP) or association of TBP with TBP-associated factor subunits. *J Virol* 2001;75(9):4453–4458.

592. Zakowski JJ, Petri WA Jr, Wagner RR. Role of matrix protein in assembling the membrane of vesicular stomatitis virus: reconstitution of matrix protein with negatively charged phospholipid vesicles. *Biochemistry* 1981;20(13):3902–3907.

593. Zakowski JJ, Wagner RR. Localization of membrane-associated proteins in vesicular stomatitis virus by use of hydrophobic membrane probes and cross-linking reagents. *J Virol* 1980;36(1):93–102.

594. Zakrzewski H, Cybinski DH, Walker PJ. A blocking ELISA for the detection of specific antibodies to bovine ephemeral fever virus. *J Immunol Methods* 1992;151(1-2):289–297.

595. Zárate S, Novella IS. Vesicular stomatitis virus evolution during alternation between persistent infection in insect cells and acute infection in mammalian cells is dominated by the persistence phase. *J Virol* 2004;78(22):12236–12242.

596. Závada J. The pseudotypic paradox. *J Gen Virol* 1982;63(Pt 1):15–24.

Mumps Virus

Steven A. Rubin • Linda J. Rennick • W. Paul Duprex

History
Infectious agent
  Classification
  Virion morphology and structure
  Genomic organization
  Virus proteins and replication
  Virus infection of host cells
Pathology and pathogenesis
  Infection in experimental animals
  Infection in humans
  Molecular basis of virulence
Clinical features
Immune responses
  Humoral immunity
  Cell-mediated immunity
Epidemiology
  Age
  Morbidity and mortality
  Origin and spread of epidemics
  Prevalence and seroepidemiology
  New epidemiologic approaches
Diagnosis
  Clinical diagnosis
  Laboratory diagnosis
Differential diagnosis
Treatment
Prevention and control
  Vaccines and adverse events
  Vaccine use
Acknowledgments

HISTORY

In the 5th century BC, Hippocrates described a mild epidemic illness associated with nonsuppurative swelling near the ears and, variably, with painful swelling of one or both testes. These descriptions of parotitis and orchitis, respectively, are the hallmarks of mumps virus (MuV) infection. The name *mumps* may derive from an old English verb that means to grimace, grin, or mumble. In his description of the neuropathology of a fatal case, Hamilton, an 18th century physician, is credited as the first to associate central nervous system (CNS) involvement with mumps. Later studies would reveal MuV as a highly neurotropic agent and a leading cause of virus-induced aseptic meningitis and encephalitis.[21,50,199]

Laboratory investigations in the early 1900s suggested the disease had a viral etiology.[153,300,451] This was proven in 1935 by Johnson and Goodpasture who fulfilled Koch's postulates by inoculating children residing in one of the investigator's neighborhood with bacteria-free oral fluids from infected monkeys.[200,201]

The demonstration by Habel[157] and Enders[116] in 1945 that MuV could be isolated and propagated in embryonated eggs enabled the demonstration of the hemagglutinating, hemolytic,[285] and neuraminidase[195] activities of the virus and led to the development of an inactivated vaccine in 1946[158] and a live-attenuated vaccine in 1958.[381] The introduction of tissue culture as a practical alternative for the propagation and study of the virus in 1948[443] was pivotal for advancing studies of the epidemiology and pathogenesis of the disease as well as the molecular biology of the virus, permitting the development of cell-grown vaccines.

Historically seen as a benign childhood disease, mumps was viewed as a major concern for the military, particularly in times of mobilization. Mumps was a notable issue during the Civil War of the United States,[179] World War I,[149] and during World War II.[272,325] During World War I, mumps was a leading cause of days lost from active duty in the U.S. Army in France, exceeded only by losses due to influenza and gonorrhea infections. Mumps remained as a significant problem for the military until the generation of efficacious vaccines and their widespread use.

Live, attenuated mumps vaccines have nearly eliminated the disease from countries with high vaccine coverage rates of a two-dose regimen.[135,323] However, sporadic and sometimes large mumps outbreaks continue to occur even in highly vaccinated populations.[102]

INFECTIOUS AGENT

Classification

MuV is a nonsegmented, negative-strand RNA virus in the family *Paramyxoviridae*, subfamily *Rubulavirinae*, genus *Orthorubulavirus*. See *Fields Virology: Emerging Viruses*, 7th Edition, Chapter 12 for a detailed overview of the *Paramyxoviridae*.

Virion Morphology and Structure

Mumps virions are enveloped, pleomorphic particles ranging from 100 to 600 nm in size, consisting of a helical ribonucleoprotein (RNP) complex surrounded by a host cell–derived

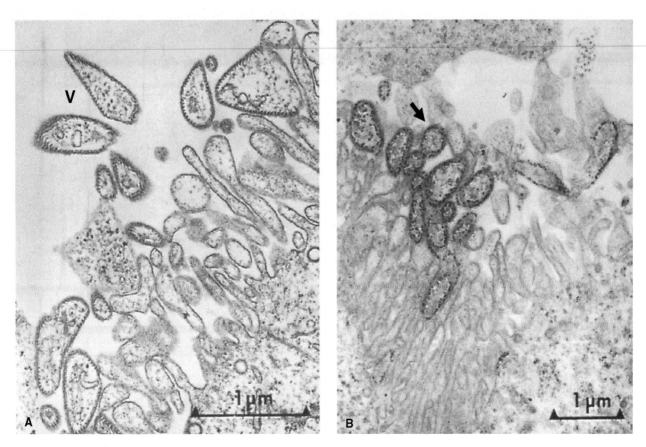

FIGURE 8.1 A: Pleomorphic mumps virions (V) budding from a choroid plexus epithelial cell. **B:** A subjacent section processed for postembedding localization of the major nucleocapsid-associated protein using monoclonal anti-N antibody. The N protein is localized by punctate, electron-dense reaction products below the surface membranes of the infected cell (arrow).

lipid bilayer (Fig. 8.1). The RNP complex consists of a single-stranded, negative sensed (−)RNA (ssRNA) molecule encapsidated with nucleocapsid (N) protein and associated with the phospho- (P) and large (L) proteins that function as the viral RNA-dependent RNA polymerase (RdRp).[88] The RNP appears to be a hollow tube with a unit length of approximately 1 μm, a diameter of 17 to 20 nm, and a central core of 5 to 6 nm.[182,183,270] The viral host cell–derived envelope contains the viral glycoproteins that project 12 to 15 nm from the virion surface.

Full-length genomic RNA (gRNA) is a nonsegmented, single-stranded macromolecule of negative polarity that consists of 15,384 nucleotides. The presence of multiple (−)RNPs in MuV virion preparations has been reported, but only one of the genomes is believed to be biologically active.[269]

Genomic Organization

The MuV genome contains seven tandemly linked transcription units (genes): the *N*, V/P-/I (*V/P/I*), matrix (*M*), fusion (*F*), small hydrophobic (*SH*), hemagglutinin-neuraminidase (*HN*), and large (*L*) (glyco)protein genes. The gene order is 3′-N-V/P/I-M-F-SH-HN-L-5′.[112,115] The MuV genome is flanked at the 3′ end by an extracistronic leader (Le) sequence of 55 nucleotides[399] and at the 5′ end by a trailer (Tr) sequence of 24 nucleotides.[308] The terminal 10 nucleotides share inverse complementarity. These regions are essential for vRdRp-mediated transcription and replication of the RNPs. Genes are

separated from each other by intergenic (Ig) sequences of 1 to 7 nucleotides. Unlike most paramyxoviruses, MuV does not have identical gene-start (GS) and gene-end (GE) sequences. The consensus GS sequence is 3′-U-U/C-C-G/U-G/U-N-C/U-U/C-U and the GE sequence is 3′-A-A/U-U/A-U-C/A-U6-7.[112]

Each gene encodes a single protein, with the exception of the *V/P/I* gene (conventionally referred to as the *P* gene), which gives rise to additional mRNA species as a result of the cotranscriptional insertion of nontemplated G nucleotides at the editing site located between positions 461 and 466.[115,319] Faithful transcription of the gene produces the V protein (formerly referred to as NS1 protein). Insertion of two G residues produces an mRNA encoding the P protein, and insertion of one or four G residues produces an mRNA encoding the I protein (formerly referred to as NS2 protein and analogous to the W protein reported in related paramyxoviruses). Thus, the V, P, and I proteins have identical amino-terminal sequence, different carboxyl-termini and have different lengths. The size of the monocistronic mRNAs as well as the number of amino acids and molecular weights of the MuV proteins are provided in Table 8.1.

Genome transcription occurs by a stop–start mechanism at GE/GS sequences in which the vRdRp expresses more monocistronic mRNAs from promoter proximal genes (*N*, *V/P/I* etc.) at the 3′-end of the genome compared to promoter distal genes (*HN* and *L*) at the 5′ end (See *Fields Virology: Emerging Viruses*, 7th Edition, Chapter 12). Due to the occasional failure of the vRdRp to recognize the GE and Ig signals, bi-,

TABLE 8.1   Mumps genes and gene products

| Gene | mRNA[a] | Amino Acids | MW in kD | | Biological Activity |
			Predicted	Observed[b]	
N	1,845	549	61.4	69–73[c]	• Encapsidates (−)RNA and (+)RNA • Protects RNA from nucleases • Confers helical structure of RNP • Binds to RdRp
P	1,314	391	41.6	45–47	• Part of the vRdRp • Tethers vRdRp to RNP
V	1,312	224	24.2	22–28	• Antagonizes IFN-β induction • Inhibits IFN-α/β and INF-γ signaling
I	1,313/1,315	170–171	18.3	16–19	Unknown
M	1,253	375	41.6	39–42	Virus assembly and budding
F₀	1,721	538	58.8	65–74	Fusion glycoprotein precursor
F₁		436	47.4	58–61	Viral attachment and entry
F₂		83[d]	9.4	10–16	Viral attachment and entry
SH	310	57	6.71	6	Antiapoptotic activity
HN	1,887	582	64	74–80	Viral attachment, entry, and release
L	6,925	2,261	256.6	160–200	Part of the vRdRp containing all the known catalytic activities

[a]Without polyA tail.
[b]Approximate molecular weight as observed by gel electrophoresis.
[c]Difference between calculated and observed weight likely due to phosphorylation.
[d]Without the cleaved 10 amino acid signal sequence.

tri-, tetra-, penta- and hexacistronic read-through transcripts can be detected in MuV-infected cells.[5,95,114] Only the first gene is translated from these transcripts.

Virus Proteins and Replication

N, P, and L Proteins

The promoter proximal *N* gene is expressed at the highest level. The N protein complexes with the gRNA to form the (−)RNP, which acts as a template for RNA transcription and replication. Unencapsidated (−)RNA cannot be transcribed. Much of what is known about MuV transcription and replication is inferred from other studies of highly homologous viruses.[150,160] Replication begins with the binding of the vRdRp to the genomic promoter (GP) in the 3′ Le region in the (−)RNP. The GE/Ig/GS sequences between the seven genes are ignored and concomitant encapsidation by the N protein generates an antigenomic, positive-sensed (+)RNP. Replication from the antigenomic promoter (AGP) in the 3′ end of the complementary RNA (cRNA) generates (−)RNPs, which are packaged into nascent virions. The AGP is a stronger promoter than the GP.[150,160]

The MuV N protein is a bipartite molecule consisting of a globular amino-terminal assembly domain (amino acids 1 to 398) mediating RNA binding and an unstructured hypervariable carboxyl-terminal tail believed, based on studies of related viruses, to interact with the MuV M protein during virion assembly.[42,94,368] The N protein is phosphorylated and this is important for regulating viral RNA synthesis.[470]

The MuV P protein forms homotrimers via a centrally located coiled-coil domain[93] and complexes with the L protein to form the vRdRp. The carboxyl-terminal 48 amino acids of the P protein is a nucleocapsid-binding domain (NBD), responsible for tethering of the vRdRp to RNPs by binding

to the assembly domain of the N protein (amino acids 1 to 398).[224] The three-dimensional structure of the NBD has been obtained using X-ray crystallography which revealed formation of a compact bundle of three α-helices, a feature that appears to be conserved among *Paramyxovirinae*.[225] Unlike the NBD of measles virus and Sendai virus, that of MuV lacks defined tertiary structure and is unstable.[224] Cryoelectron microscopy has been used to solve the structure of the nucleocapsid and suggests a role for the amino-terminal domain of P in uncoiling the nucleocapsid.[89] The carboxyl-terminal domain of P protein interacts with the L protein.[329] As indicated by its name, the MuV P protein is heavily phosphorylated,[297] an action believed to regulate vRdRp activity[132,390,391]; this has not been clearly demonstrated for MuV[132,390,391] although mutational analysis of the serine and threonine residues present in MuV P protein has identified amino acids that are phosphorylated and critical for viral RNA synthesis.[330] MuV P protein is phosphorylated by human kinase Polo-like kinase 1 and this phosphorylation is enhanced by the N protein.[332] MuV grows better in cells lacking the human kinase ribosomal protein S6 kinase beta-1 (RPS6KB1).[47] RPS6KB1 has been shown to bind to P protein, and in cells lacking RPS6KB1, there was a significant decrease in P protein phosphorylation indicating that RPS6KB1 may phosphorylate P by directly binding the protein.[47]

Six functional domains have been identified in the MuV L protein based on sequence similarity with L proteins from related viruses.[335,378] The L protein contains all the requisite catalytic functions such as execution of transcription and replication, as well as methylation, capping, and polyadenylation of mRNAs (See *Fields Virology: Emerging Viruses*, 7th Edition, Chapter 12). A detailed functional and structural analysis of the MuV L protein has not been carried out. However, heat shock protein 90 (Hsp90)[213] and the Hsp90 co-chaperone R2TP complex[215] are required for the formation and regulation of the polymerase complex, respectively, and recombinant viruses containing substitutions in the methyltransferase domain of L protein are attenuated in cotton rats.[163]

Matrix Protein

The MuV M protein orchestrates virion assembly and budding. Expression of the MuV M protein is sufficient to produce virus-like particles (VLP), although in the absence of coexpression with other viral proteins, efficiency is low.[249] The M protein binds to the cytoplasmic tails of assembled F and HN glycoproteins at distinct locations on cellular membranes, presumably lipid raft microdomains. There, the M protein functions as an adapter, physically linking the region of host cell membrane expressing the viral F and HN glycoproteins with the (−)RNP via its interaction with the N protein.[165,249] Budding appears to be mediated by an interaction between the MuV M protein and the cellular endosomal sorting complex required for transport (ESCRT) machinery.[249] The MuV M protein interacts with host proteins angiomotin like 1 (AmotL1) and 14-3-3.[320,321,346] Whereas the AmotL1–M protein interaction appears to promote MuV VLP production, based on studies of human paramyxovirus 5 (HPIV-5), M protein interaction with 14-3-3 decreases the efficiency of virus budding. Interestingly, the MuV M protein 14-3-3 binding site is adjacent to a sequence motif conserved among rubulaviruses, presumably functioning as a binding site for the host protein caveolin 1 (Cav-1), an essential structural component of caveolae that are considered a subset of lipid rafts. It is, therefore, likely that MuV budding, like that of HPIV-5, occurs from caveolae. The close proximity of the 14-3-3 and postulated Cav-1 binding sites raises the possibility that the MuV M protein switches between either binding to 14-3-3 or Cav-1, thereby regulating the amount of M protein that can participate in virus budding.[321] MuV M protein traffics between the nucleus and cytoplasm by ubiquitin-regulated active transport, and it has been suggested that some paramyxoviral M proteins have nonstructural functions.[324]

Surface Glycoproteins

The F and HN are type I and II transmembrane glycoproteins, respectively. The F glycoprotein is synthesized as an inactive precursor (F_0) that is targeted to the rough endoplasmic reticulum (RER) via a 19 amino acid signal peptide, which is subsequently cleaved.[438] Following N-linked glycosylation, the precursor is transported to the trans-Golgi network where it is proteolytically cleaved between amino acids 102 and 103 by the host cell protease furin at the R-R-H-K-R motif to produce two disulfide-linked heterodimers (F_1 and F_2).[176,276,297,413,439] Cleavage of F_0 is essential for virus-to-cell and cell-to-cell membrane fusion and for viral infectivity. The amino-terminus of the F_1 subunit possesses the fusion peptide, a conserved hydrophobic domain exposed following cleavage (See *Fields Virology: Emerging Viruses*, 7th Edition, Chapter 12). Evidence indicates that a second cleavage event occurs during which F_1 is processed into two subunits, F_{1a} and F_{1b}; this event may be important in mediating fusion activity.[429]

At least two heptad repeat (HR) domains are found in the F1 ectodomain: HR1 at the amino-terminus adjacent to the fusion peptide and HR2 at the carboxyl-terminus adjacent to the transmembrane domain.[254] The MuV F glycoprotein forms homotrimers and the HR1 and HR2 domains interact to form a stable six-helix bundle structure.[254,268] The HR2 domain is also involved in the binding of the F and HN glycoproteins, which form the fusion complex. Additional HR domains have been identified in related viruses, although this has not been confirmed for MuV.[141,287] The specific processes involved in MuV fusion have not been delineated. However, based on similarity with the six-helix bundle structure of the HPIV-5 F protein, the events that mediate MuV fusion are likely to be very similar (See *Fields Virology: Emerging Viruses*, 7th Edition, Chapter 12).

In its native state, the HN glycoprotein is a disulfide-bonded oligomer assembled as homotetramers. The glycoprotein is held in the lipid bilayer by a hydrophobic domain of 19 residues near the amino terminus, a domain that probably also serves as a signal sequence in a manner similar to other paramyxovirus HN glycoproteins. A membrane proximal stalk in monomers supports a globular head comprised of a six-blade β-propeller structure.[91,234] The globular head is responsible for both attachment to glycolipid and/or glycoprotein sialic acid containing receptors and neuraminidase activity.[195,312] The HN glycoprotein stalk in conjunction with the F glycoprotein mediates virus-to-cell and cell-to-cell fusion.[400,409] Based on inference from related viruses, a single site mediates both neuraminidase and receptor binding activities likely using a conformational switch mechanism to toggle between the two functions.[84,91,242] There may be a second sialic acid binding site within the globular head region, theorized to stabilize viral–cellular membrane interactions in addition to the large binding pocket that fluxes between neuraminidase and receptor binding activity.[45,340,469] A "stalk exposure" model has been proposed for the HN glycoprotein assisted activation of the F glycoprotein.[43] Briefly, this model proposes that a change in the structure of HN upon receptor binding exposes an F activation domain in the HN protein stalk. Upon interaction with this domain, F is destabilized resulting in membrane fusion.

V Protein

The MuV V protein is involved in inhibiting interferon (IFN) production and signaling (See *Fields Virology: Emerging Viruses*, 7th Edition, Chapter 12). The 69 amino acid carboxyl-terminal cysteine-rich domain of the MuV V protein appears to be the key player in these activities. This region directly interacts with melanoma differentiation–associated gene 5 (MDA5), a pattern recognition receptor that recognizes cytosolic, unencapsidated viral RNA, and with the TANK-binding kinase 1 (TBK-1)/inhibitor of kB kinase-ε (IKKε) kinases responsible for interferon regulatory factor-3 (IRF-3) phosphorylation. Interaction of the V protein with MDA5 inhibits its ability to induce transactivation of the IFN-β promoter[13,344] and, in the case of TBK-1/IKKε, leads to ubiquitination and subsequent proteasomal degradation.[258] This in turn prevents IRF-3 phosphorylation, which is required for transcription of IFN and IFN-stimulated genes. The carboxyl-terminus of the MuV V protein also interacts with the cellular signal transducer and activator of transcription (STAT) proteins, STAT-1, STAT-2, and STAT-3.[164,302,464,465] STAT-1 and STAT-2 play a central role in the IFN signal transduction pathway that lead to activation of IFN-stimulated genes. STAT-3 has also been implicated in cellular antiviral responses.[343,416] Inhibition of STAT-3 by the MuV V protein in a recombinant (r) virus led to accelerated clearance, and reduced neurovirulence, of the virus in animals.[262] Binding of MuV V protein leads to the ubiquitination and subsequent degradation through the proteasomal pathway of

STAT-1 and STAT-3, but not of STAT-2. However, the latter is required for targeting of STAT-1 for degradation.[232,415,416,465] The carboxyl-terminus of the MuV V protein is not the only region important in these interactions, as exemplified in a study demonstrating that a single point mutation at amino acid position 95 abrogates the ability of the MuV V protein to degrade STAT-3, while retaining the virus's ability to target STAT-1.[343] A recombinant (r)MuV based on a wild-type MuV strain associated with recent outbreaks, has been engineered to be unable to express the V protein.[458] This virus was used to confirm the role of V protein in blocking IFN induction and suggests an additional role in suppressing IL-6 production.[458]

The MuV V protein has also been shown to be a tetherin antagonist.[307]

The observation that the MuV V protein oligomerizes to form spherical particles suggests that the MuV protein provides a scaffold for coordinating the assembly of the cellular components (e.g., UV-damaged DNA binding protein 1 [DDB1], cullin 4A [Cul4A], and regulator of cullin 1 [Roc1]) involved in ubiquitination, collectively referred to as V-dependent degradation complexes (VDC).[415] For more details on VDC, See *Fields Virology: Emerging Viruses*, 7th Edition, Chapter 12.

SH Protein

The SH protein consists of 57 amino acids, 25 of which are highly hydrophobic and clustered at the amino-terminus serving as a membrane anchor region with its carboxyl-terminus facing the cytoplasm.[111,114,396] The predicted SH mRNA 5′ end contains two AUG start codons the second being used for translation of the protein. The first AUG, located at positions 4 to 6, gives rise to a minicistron with a stop codon at nucleotides 19 to 21.[114,396] Due to the proximity of this small minicistron to the 5′ mRNA cap, it is predicted that ribosomes will skip the first AUG and initiate at the second at a frequency of about 50%,[229] translating the SH protein, at reduced efficiency. The biological significance of this minicistron and its proposed role in reducing the amount of SH protein remains unknown. The protein can be tagged with enhanced green fluorescent protein and is trafficked through the ER (Fig. 8.2).

In certain MuV isolates, such as the Enders and Rubini strains, a point mutation exists in the putative *F* gene polyadenylation signal resulting in an F-SH bicistronic mRNA,[235,396,397] from which only the F glycoprotein is made. This demonstrates that the SH protein is not essential for virus replication and this has been confirmed for HPIV-5.[170] Similarly, routine molecular surveillance of circulating MuVs has detected viruses with mutations in the *SH* gene that result in the generation of premature stop codons in the protein.[386]

Deletion of the SH open reading frame from the wild-type MuV strain associated with recent outbreaks demonstrated that the SH protein facilitates evasion of the host antiviral response in L929 cells by decreasing NF-κB activation, TNF-α production, and apoptosis.[170,171,457] The virus was also attenuated in rats. The reduction of NF-κB activation was subsequently shown to be due to decreased IKKβ, IκBα, and p65 phosphorylation, and reduced translocation of p65 into the nucleus of infected cells.[128] In the same study, the SH protein coimmunoprecipitated with TNFR1, RIP1, and IRAK1. Yeast two-hybrid and coimmunoprecipitation studies identified ataxin-1 ubiquitin-like interacting protein (A1Up) as a cellular target of the MuV SH protein. This protein plays a role in proteasomal degradation, but the biological significance of its interaction with the MuV SH protein is not clear.[454]

I Protein

Expression of the I protein in infected cells was confirmed, but its role in the life cycle of the virus is unknown.[319]

Virus Infection of Host Cells

Sialic acid, an acyl derivative of neuraminic acid, is found on cellular glycoproteins and glycolipids and serves as a receptor for MuV. More recently, it has been shown that MuV preferentially uses a trisaccharide containing 2,3-linked sialic acid as a receptor.[231] Infection of murine Sertoli and Leydig cells, pretreated with α2,3-sialidase to remove sialic acid, demonstrated that the virus was internalized less efficiently but that binding was not affected,[435] suggesting a role for sialic acid in virus internalization rather than binding, at least in these testicular cells.

Following attachment of the virus to cell surface receptors, the viral and cellular membranes fuse and the (−)RNP is liberated into the cytoplasm. Primary transcription is mediated by the incoming vRdRp and both existing and nascent vRdRp replicates the genome via a (+)RNP intermediate. Secondary transcription from (−)RNPs increases the amount of viral mRNAs and proteins in the infected cell. These events occur in an analogous manner to most paramyxoviruses (See *Fields Virology: Emerging Viruses*, 7th Edition, Chapter 12 for a detailed description of these and other events such as viral assembly and release).

Since MuV receptor(s) are expressed ubiquitously on mammalian cells, the virus infects a wide range of cell types. After infection of differentiated human airway epithelial cells[113] or polarized epithelial cells[214] *in vitro*, the virus is predominantly released from the apical surface. In polarized epithelial cells, this release is Rab11 dependent.[214] The replication of MuV is typically detected *in vitro* by the induction of multinucleated syncytia and subsequent cell lysis. Reverse genetics approaches

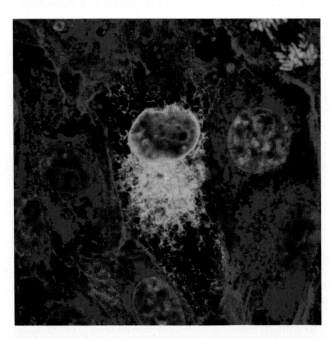

FIGURE 8.2 Localization of the SH protein in cells. EGFP-tagged SH protein (*green*) localizes in the endoplasmic reticulum (ER) of Vero cells. Actin (*red*), DNA (*yellow*), and protein disulfide isomerase (*blue*), a multifunctional redox chaperone of the ER.

permit the insertion of an additional transcription unit (ATU) expressing fluorescent proteins, for example EGFP, into the viral genome and this permits the study of cell-to-cell spread and cytopathic effect (CPE) over time *in vitro* (Fig. 8.3). CPE in MuV-infected monolayers varies considerably among isolates and substrates, and in some instances, there is little evident morphologic change.[4,154,269] The type of CPE produced *in vitro* does not correlate with the *in vivo* behavior of the virus.

PATHOLOGY AND PATHOGENESIS

Infection in Experimental Animals

Humans are the only natural host of MuV, although experimental infection has been induced in animal models of disease, including nonhuman primates,[246,354,362,456] hamsters,[203,316,447] mice,[221,316,331,456] and rats.[341,359] The use of rMuV expressing

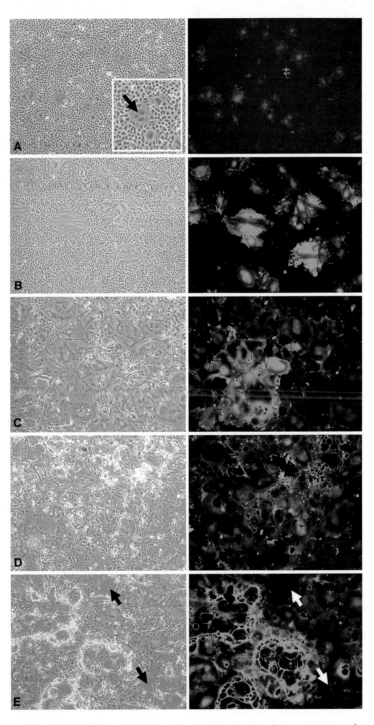

FIGURE 8.3 Phase contrast and fluorescent photomicrographs showing the progression of cytopathic effects of a recombinant mumps virus clinical isolate expressing enhanced green fluorescent protein after incubation on Vero cells for 24 (A), 50 (B), 69 (C), 79 (D), and 92 (E) hours. The classic cytopathic effect of cell-to-cell fusion and syncytium formation (**A**, *inset*) with nuclei clustering in the center (*arrow*) appear 1 day postinfection (d.p.i.). Cell lysis and disintegration of the cell monolayer occurs around 4 d.p.i. after which time the cells detach (E, *arrows*).

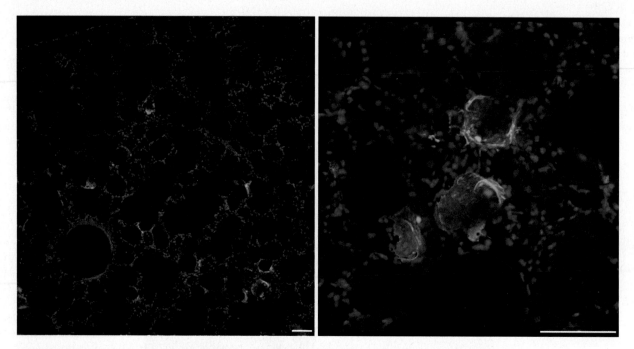

FIGURE 8.4 Fluorescent photomicrographs of a recombinant mumps virus based on a clinical isolate (genotype G) expressing enhanced green fluorescent protein (EGFP) replicating in the cotton rat lung following intranasal infection. Cell-to-cell spread in pneumocytes in the absence of overt CPE is observed in the lung parenchyma. Nuclei counterstained with Hoechst. Scale bars represent 100 µm (Rennick and Duprex, unpublished)

EGFP has permitted the examination of the primary sites of replication in the cotton rat lung (Fig. 8.4). These *in vivo* approaches permit cell-to-cell spread to be examined in the absence of overt CPE. Experimental infection of animals has mostly been used to study the pathogenesis of MuV neurotropism and neurovirulence. Intracerebral inoculation of MuV into the suckling hamster results in a massive inflammatory response, including meningitis, encephalitis, and ventriculitis. Intraperitoneal inoculation of virulent laboratory-adapted strains into suckling hamsters also leads to CNS infection.[448] Associated neuropathology includes hydrocephalus, Chiari type I cerebellar malformation, and neuronal necrosis.[220,316,395,398,449] Many of these are reported features of CNS infection in humans, suggesting the applicability of the hamster model for studying the pathogenesis of MuV infection in humans. Similar findings have also been reported in nonhuman primates.[78,256,353,362,468] Very little, if any, work has been accomplished in mice because MuV infection tends to be abortive, thereby limiting the value of this model system.[169,342,410] Early studies also indicated MuV infection to be abortive in rats, unless laboratory adapted by serial passage in brain.[341] Subsequent studies, however, determined that intracerebral inoculation of the virus into newborn rats resulted in inflammation of the ventricular system (choroiditis, ependymitis) and hydrocephalus, but not meningitis or encephalitis.[359] Interestingly, the severity of hydrocephalus in rats correlates with strain-specific neurovirulence potential for humans, suggesting the relevance of this model of disease in examining the pathogenesis and molecular basis of MuV neurovirulence.[360] The severity of virus-induced neuropathology in marmosets, but not other nonhuman primate species, was also found to correlate with virus neurovirulence potential for humans.[355]

Infection in Humans

Transmissibility after nasal or buccal mucosal inoculation of virus[201] suggests that natural infection is initiated by droplet spread. The incubation period is 16 to 18 days,[181,277] during which the virus multiplies in the upper respiratory mucosa before spreading to draining lymph nodes. Based on infection of hamsters, virus disseminates via a transient plasma viremia,[448] potentially infecting multiple tissues and organ systems.[186] The most common sites of virus dissemination are glandular tissues (parotid glands, testes, breasts, and pancreas) and the CNS. If viruria is used as an indication of kidney infection, then kidney involvement is common in mumps, although clinical nephritis is rarely diagnosed.[419,421] In rare cases, MuV can be transmitted transplacentally.

Virus is shed in saliva as early as 6 days before the onset of parotitis[173] and mostly cleared by day 4 of symptom onset based on virus isolation efforts.[336] This timing correlates with the local appearance of virus-specific secretory IgA and IgM.[75,327] However, in a study by Fanoy *et al.*, greater than 100 genome copies/100 µL saliva were detected by reverse transcription/polymerase chain reaction (RT/PCR) for up to 15 days after symptom onset in unvaccinated persons, and for up to 7 days in 2-dose vaccinated persons.[120] The proportion of these copies that represent replication competent virus is unknown. Overall, these studies indicate that mumps patients are capable of spreading virus by the respiratory route over a 10-day period and likely longer.

Plasma viremia disappears coincident with the development of MuV-specific antibody, which can be detected in serum as early as 11 days after infection of humans.[173] Animal models suggest that circulating infected lymphocytes facilitate the spread of virus in the face of mounting humoral immunity.[448] Despite the apparent high frequency of viremia during mumps, infectious virions have only rarely been isolated from blood,[196,217,315] possibly due to the presence of anti-mumps virus antibodies, which begin to appear at the time of symptoms.[49]

Parotid Gland

Initial clinical symptoms usually relate to infection of the parotid gland, but viral involvement of this gland is neither a primary nor obligate step in the infection.[218] Virus infects the ductal epithelium, resulting in desquamation of involved cells, periductal interstitial edema, and a local inflammatory reaction primarily involving lymphocytes. Swelling, inflammation, and tissue damage in the parotid gland can produce elevation of serum and urine amylase levels.[373]

Central Nervous System

MuV CNS invasion, as demonstrated by cerebrospinal fluid (CSF) pleocytosis, occurs in more than one third of patients presenting with clinical mumps.[21,50,53,119] Symptomatic CNS infection (i.e., meningitis) is less common, occurring in approximately 10% of cases.[21,161,211] Encephalitis occurs in less than 0.5% of cases. In the prevaccine era, MuV was a leading cause of viral meningitis and encephalitis in most developed countries and continues to be a leading cause in unvaccinated populations worldwide.[19,134,174,278] Neurologic manifestations appear with a 3:1 or greater male–female ratio[37,227,244] and are generally preceded by parotitis 4 to 5 days earlier but can occur before or in complete absence of detectable salivary gland swelling.

Lymphocytes are the predominant cell type found in the CSF, with white blood cell (WBC) counts averaging 250/mm³.[218,452] Cells counts peak around the third day of neurologic symptoms and then gradually decline over a period of several weeks.[130,446] In some instances, CSF pleocytosis can persist for as long as a year.[426] The CSF is usually under normal pressure[53] and the protein content in the CSF is elevated in 60% to 70% of all cases.[130,218] Protein levels up to 100 mg/dL can be seen; on occasion, they exceed 700 mg/dL. This appears to reflect damage to the blood–brain barrier, as indicated by elevated albumin indices that do not normalize for several weeks to months after the onset of CNS symptoms.[252] The CSF glucose content is modestly depressed to 17% to 41% of the serum value in 6% to 29% of all cases.[107,206,446] About one third of patients have evidence of intrathecal IgG synthesis and demonstrable oligoclonal immunoglobulins during the first week of CNS symptoms; this oligoclonal antibody can persist for more than 2 years.[130] More than one half show increased IgG indices by the 3rd month following mumps meningitis.[130,252,427] Up to 90% of patients with acute mumps meningitis produce virus-specific IgG within the CNS compartment,[252,414,427] and one half show MuV-specific IgM.[125] Since mumps antibodies are uncommon in the CSF during other CNS infections,[105] in many instances of mumps meningitis, a diagnosis can be confirmed by elevated CSF-to-serum antibody ratios using samples taken during illness.[286,414]

As inferred from animal infection studies, viral invasion of the CNS occurs across the choroid plexus.[448] Blood-borne infected mononuclear cells, and possibly cell-free virus, can cross the fenestrated endothelium of the choroid plexus stroma and serve as a source for subsequent infection of the choroidal

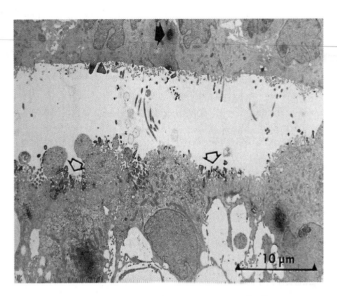

FIGURE 8.5 Postembedding electron micrograph of immunocytochemical staining of a region of the lateral ventricle of a hamster 5 days after intraperitoneal infection with the Kilham strain of MuV. Anti-N monoclonal antibody was used as the primary reagent. The reaction product defines nucleocapsids located below the cytoplasmic membranes at sites of virion budding along both the ependymal and choroidal (*unfilled arrows*) surfaces. Intracytoplasmic nucleocapsid inclusions are also demarcated by the reaction product in both choroid plexus and individual ependymal (*filled arrow*) cells.

epithelium. Maturation of virus from the ventricular surfaces of choroidal cells releases virions that are distributed widely throughout ventricular pathways and the subarachnoid space in CSF (Fig. 8.5). Virus can penetrate brain parenchyma and infect neurons by cell-to-cell spread in ependymal cells that line the ventricular cavities of the brain. Once within neurons, virus most likely spreads along neuronal pathways, as reported in nonhuman primates.[246] Although primary encephalitis is typically the response to direct viral invasion of neural cells, cases of postinfectious encephalitis, an autoimmune attack on CNS myelin sheaths, also occurs. Symptoms of primary encephalitis appear before or during the development of parotitis; symptoms of postinfectious encephalitis and associated demyelination appear 1 to 3 weeks after the onset of parotitis.[253,401]

Typical CNS pathology of MuV encephalitis includes edema and congestion throughout the brain with hemorrhage, lymphocytic perivascular infiltration, perivascular gliosis, and demyelination. Findings in the spinal cord include early degenerative changes in the anterior horn cells and perineuronal edema.[108,142,401] When seen, the selective periventricular myelin loss with relative sparing of axons is typical of parainfectious autoimmune encephalitis.

Most cases of CNS infection resolve without sequelae. However, permanent neurologic damage such as obstructive hydrocephalus,[306] deafness,[251] and myelitis[304,423] can occur in some cases.

Hydrocephalus can develop days to years after initial MuV infection and can lead to progressively worsening headaches, mental status changes, and gait abnormalities.[79,148,306] The pathogenesis of hydrocephalus is inferred from animal studies that suggest desquamation of virus-infected ventricular ependymal cells blocks egress of CSF through the aqueduct of Sylvius.

Abnormally restricted flow of CSF to adsorptive sites over the cerebral convexities results in progressive enlargement of the lateral and third ventricles.[202,203] The presence of ependymal cell debris in the CSF of humans presenting with MuV CNS infection suggests a similar mechanism of hydrocephalus induction.[175,306,407] Hydrocephalus has also been observed before, or in the total absence of, aqueductal stenosis,[204,393,394,447] indicating this could be a secondary consequence of external compression by surrounding edematous tissue and not causally related to the pathogenesis of hydrocephalus.

Deafness

MuV is the most frequent cause of acquired sensorineural hearing loss in children. Transient, high-frequency deafness is the most common form, occurring in approximately 4% of mumps cases.[431] Permanent deafness occurs in less than 1 per 20,000 cases[34,166] and is usually unilateral. Deafness is believed to be the result of direct viral invasion of the cochlea, likely via the perilymph, which freely communicates with the CSF.[159,273,380,444] However, deafness does not occur more frequently in persons with CNS complications, suggesting an alternative or contributing etiology, such as via a hematogenous route.[283] Hearing loss caused by indirect effects of virus infection (e.g., immune-mediated damage) have also been suggested.[417] Pathology includes degeneration of the stria vascularis, tectorial membrane, and organ of Corti and collapse of Reissner membrane.[118]

Gonads

Orchitis, usually unilateral, occurs in approximately 20% of postpubertal men who develop mumps.[17,133,240] Orchitis rarely occurs in children, suggesting that certain hormonal factors, such as receptors for luteinizing hormone and follicle-stimulating hormone expressed during adolescence, might promote testicular tropism of the virus.[403] Virus has been isolated from testicular biopsies of the affected gland within the first 4 days of symptoms, and from semen,[36,192] strongly suggesting that symptomatic gonadal involvement reflects local virus replication. The seminiferous tubules may be the primary site of viral replication, with local lymphocytic infiltration and edema of interstitial tissues.

Infection of the ovaries is diagnosed in less than 5% of postpubertal women who develop mumps,[46,68,103,212,267,389] which may be an underestimate because unless a pelvic examination is performed, abdominal or pelvic pain from inflamed ovaries might be attributed to pancreatic infection.

Kidneys

Based on the frequency of viruria, virus frequently disseminates to the kidneys, where epithelial cells of the distal tubules, calyces, and ureters appear to be primary sites of virus replication.[442] Viruria can be detected in most patients, sometimes for as long as 14 days after the onset of clinical symptoms.[419,420] Mild abnormalities of renal function have been described, but they are usually of little clinical importance.[419] Although virus dissemination to, and replication in, the parotid gland and kidney can occur simultaneously, replication in renal tissue is more prolonged and continues well beyond the appearance of neutralizing antibody in serum.

Pancreas

Pancreatic involvement, diagnosed in 1% to 27% of cases,[46,54,68,247,317,372,384,403,445] is usually expressed as mild epigastric pain, but

severe hemorrhagic pancreatitis[122] and transient exocrine function abnormalities[97] have been reported. MuV infects human pancreatic beta cells *in vitro*,[432] and virus infection of the pancreas has been demonstrated in hamsters inoculated intraperitoneally.[448] Viral infections have been considered a possible precipitating event leading to the onset of about one third of all cases of juvenile-onset or type I insulin-dependent diabetes mellitus (IDDM). However, whether MuV causes IDDM is unclear,[90,136,147,371] and no association has been found between mumps and type II diabetes.[255] Serum amylase levels are elevated in cases of pancreatitis, which can be differentiated from parotitis by isoenzyme analysis or serum pancreatic lipase determinations.[253]

Heart

Myocardial invasion occurs frequently in mumps, as indicated by electrocardiographic abnormalities.[15] Although it is seldom symptomatic, interstitial lymphocytic myocarditis and mild pericarditis may occur following mumps replication in cells of the myocardium and pericardium.[51] MuV myocarditis can lead to the rare but serious sequelae of endocardial fibroelastosis.[298]

Of all cases of mumps with symptoms sufficiently severe to warrant hospitalization, less than 10% can be expected to show transient electrocardiograph abnormalities consistent with myocardial damage. These usually consist of ST-segment depression, but patients can show evidence of atrioventricular conduction defects, including complete heart block.[15] Seldom is the cardiac involvement acutely symptomatic.

Fetus and Newborn

MuV can be transmitted transplacentally as demonstrated in nonhuman primates[385] and by the isolation of the virus from the human fetus following spontaneous first-trimester abortion during maternal mumps.[236,463] The virus can produce a fetal wastage in humans, with or without subsequent spread of virus to involve fetal tissues directly.[463] MuV has also been isolated from fetal tissues following planned therapeutic abortion of seronegative women 1 week after vaccination with live, attenuated MuV, although it is unclear if the virus detected was vaccine virus, or wild-type virus coincidentally contracted at or shortly before the time of vaccination.[460] A proliferative necrotizing villitis with decidual cells containing intracytoplasmic inclusions has been described in the products of spontaneous and induced abortions.[139] Late-gestation intrauterine infection was reported in an infant born to a mother who developed mumps more than 4 weeks before delivery, diagnosed by RT-PCR testing of the cord blood cells from the infant.[392] This infant developed severe pulmonary symptoms, including hypertension and hemorrhage.

MuV is excreted in breast milk,[219] but few cases of perinatal mumps have been described[208,238] and it is not clear if breast milk was responsible for these cases. There appears to be a somewhat different mode of pathogenesis of mumps in newborns. In the first year or two of life, infants may have only pulmonary involvement without evidence of parotitis.[208,392] Split immunologic recognition in the infants can follow maternal parotitis, resulting in MuV-specific cell-mediated immune responses without a concomitant antibody response.[1,385,405]

Molecular Basis of Virulence

While comprehensive studies on the molecular basis of MuV virulence have yet to be performed, it is clear that the genetic basis of MuV virulence does not lie within any one gene[7,356,365,376,455] and no simple pattern of genomic mutations capable of discriminating virulent from attenuated MuV strains has been identified.[9,190,365]

CLINICAL FEATURES

The clinical features of mumps reflect the pathogenesis of the infection. Approximately one third of all MuV infections occur without recognized symptoms.[52,85,119,328,347] Moderate fever is often present at the onset of disease, with defervescence a few days later. The feature most characteristic of mumps is salivary gland swelling, particularly the parotid glands (Fig. 8.6),[328] which constitutes the basis of a clinical diagnosis. Submaxillary gland enlargement and involvement of the sublingual glands also occur. Enlargement of individual glands is painful, usually lasting 2 to 3 days, but may persist 10 days or longer.[172] Virus is present in the saliva for several days before the onset of clinical disease[173] and for up to 5 days later.[75] The virus can be detected in urine for several weeks after the onset of mumps.[420]

Various organs and tissues can be symptomatically involved during mumps, including the testes, CNS, mammary glands, ovary, pancreas, kidneys, and heart.[186] Parotitis usually precedes manifestations of involvement of other sites of virus infection, but the latter can be clinically evident before, during, or even in the absence of parotitis.

The most common complication of mumps (aside from parotitis) is epididymo-orchitis. Testicular pain and swelling has a time course similar to that of the parotid gland. Mumps orchitis often leads to testicular atrophy of the involved and,

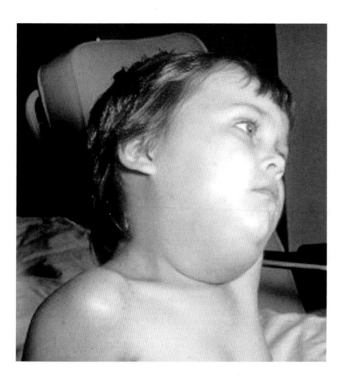

FIGURE 8.6 Mumps patient with parotitis. (Courtesy of Centers for Disease Control and Prevention, Atlanta, GA.)

occasionally, the clinically uninvolved gland.[29] Atrophy after mumps orchitis is rarely implicated as a cause of male sterility.[377] About 15% of females complain of breast swelling and tenderness. As with orchitis in men, the incidence of mastitis is significantly higher after puberty.[328]

Nausea and vomiting with or without epigastric or left upper-quadrant pain are frequent features of mumps, occurring in approximately half of all cases during the St. Lawrence Island epidemic.[328] It is unclear whether these symptoms reflect involvement of the pancreas or other viscera. Some of these generalized features of the illness may reflect the effects of circulating IFN, which can be found in serum early in the clinical course of mumps.[286,434]

More than one third of mumps cases develop CSF pleocytosis, but symptomatic CNS involvement is far less frequent.[21,50,328] Mumps meningitis may precede parotitis, but it typically develops 5 days following parotitis. However, as many as half of those with mumps meningitis may not have detectable salivary gland enlargement.[206,218]

IMMUNE RESPONSES

Humoral Immunity

Virus-specific salivary IgM and IgA and serum IgA, IgM, IgG and neutralizing antibody are all detectable at the time of symptom onset. During natural infection, salivary IgM appears to be the first detectable immunoglobulin class, followed by salivary IgA. The latter is capable of virus neutralization and is detectable for approximately 10 weeks after symptom onset.[76,127,129] Levels of serum IgA and IgM peak approximately 1 to 2 weeks after symptom onset and decline to undetectable levels by week 8 after symptom onset.[49,414] MuV-specific IgG has been detected as early as 4 days before symptom development,[299] peaking 4 to 8 weeks later and detectable for decades.[49,414] In naïve individuals, IgG is of low avidity[296] and IgG3 antibodies predominate early in the course of disease, whereas in later stages, isotypes IgG1 and IgG2 predominate. Upon a second exposure to MuV, serum IgM and IgA antibodies are typically absent or are produced at very low levels; the IgG1 subclass, typically of high avidity, predominates.[155]

Virus-neutralizing antibodies are detectable as early as day 2 after symptom onset, peaking 4 to 8 weeks later, and are detectable for decades. The role of antibody in arresting the infection cannot be underestimated. Seropositive patients challenged intravenously with up to 10^9 plaque-forming units of MuV showed only transient fever and no symptoms of reinfection developed, although an anamnestic rise in antibody titer was seen 4 to 5 days later.[309]

The evidence that virus-neutralizing antibodies confer protection is clear and seronegative individuals are highly susceptible to infection, maternal antibody confers protection in infants, and passive immunization with mumps virus-specific IgG is protective.[86,140,180,237,450] Studies conducted during the prevaccine era indicated that neutralizing antibody titers in the range of 1:4 to 1:8 confer protection.[27,52,117,279] However, multiple studies of mumps outbreaks in the postvaccine era found persons with very high levels of IgG and virus-neutralizing antibody to be susceptible to mumps and that no specific level of antibody could reliably predict protection.[151,152,301]

Only antibodies directed against the F and HN glycoproteins have been definitively shown to neutralize the virus and protect against infection.[184,250,257,382] Use of polyclonal antisera in virus neutralization assays demonstrates a broad cross-reactivity among different MuV genotypes.[189,312,314,361,461] However, neutralizing antibody titers can differ substantially against different MuV strains, suggesting significant antigenic differences between strains, and possibly the existence of virus strain–specific neutralizing epitopes. Despite such demonstrations in the laboratory, MuV appears serologically monotypic in clinical situations as suggested empirically by the dramatic reductions in mumps incidence in countries with high two-dose vaccine coverage.[135,322,379,437] However, as discussed later, such antigenic differences between the older vaccine viruses and contemporary wild-type circulating strains may lead to the occurrence of breakthrough cases in individuals whose immunity has waned.

Cell-Mediated Immunity

In vitro lymphocyte-proliferative responses to MuV antigens are readily measured in seropositive individuals.[187] CD8+ and γ/δ cytotoxic T lymphocytes have been demonstrated in blood and CSF following infection with wild-type or vaccine MuV strains.[32,77,124,230] Mononuclear cell inflammation in MuV-infected tissues is well developed at the time of onset of clinical disease, suggesting that specific cellular responses develop during the incubation period. The presence of major histocompatibility (MHC) antigen (e.g., MHC Ia)-restricted T lymphocytes and specifically sensitized cells in both the blood and the CSF of some patients with active mumps meningitis support this view.[130] After immunization, peak cell-mediated immune responses are found 2 to 4 weeks later and can last for decades.[77,162,207] Circulating cytotoxic T-cell responses restricted to autologous-infected target cells are found within the first few weeks of mumps meningitis.

Although the presence or absence of MuV-specific cell-mediated responses often correlates with the presence or absence of virus-specific antibody, the magnitude of the two types of immune responses do not correlate[74,350]; in some instances, cell-mediated immune responses have been detected in seronegative persons.[162,207] Immunologic studies of closely related viruses (e.g., measles) indicate the importance of the cellular response in the recovery and long-term protection from disease,[28,137,193,194,326,436] but this has not been established for MuV. For example, levels of interferon-γ induced by MuV infection do not correlate with illness severity[239,434] and patients with severely compromised T-cell responses experience a course of disease that does not differ from that seen in healthy individuals.[104] Similarly, neither severe symptoms of mumps nor a protracted course of illness has been reported in persons with acquired immunodeficiency syndrome (AIDS).

Considering data demonstrating that MuV targets MDA-5 and STAT proteins for degradation (discussed earlier), MuV may impede cytotoxic T lymphocyte (CTL) activation, by suppressing IFN production and signaling, which regulate MHC class-I expression.[57]

EPIDEMIOLOGY

Age

Before widespread vaccine use, mumps was most commonly seen in children between 5 and 9 years of age[83]; by 15 years of age, greater than 90% of most populations had serologic evidence of infection with MuV.[59,288] Despite a high seroprevalence in older individuals in the prevaccine era, large outbreaks were common, particularly in high-density, close-contact environments, such as military settings.[149,325]

In the years following mumps vaccine licensure in 1967, a gradual shift was seen in the typical age of infection in the general U.S. population from young children toward those 10 to 19 years of age, likely reflecting protection of younger children by vaccination, while older children and young adults not eligible for vaccination at the time remained susceptible.[61,422] By 1992, the highest age-specific incidence in the United States shifted back to the 5- to 9-year-old age group, where it remained until a large multistate mumps outbreak occurred in 2006, predominantly on university campuses.[274,275] In the years following the 2006 mumps outbreak, the age-specific incidence returned to the younger age group,[66,67] until the recent mumps outbreaks in New York and New Jersey in 2009–2010, where again most cases occurred in young adults.[68] A similar pattern has been observed in many other countries and the occurrence of mumps predominantly in young adults is now common.

Mumps is rarely seen in children younger than 1 year of age, most likely because of acquisition of immunity by placental transfer of maternal antibody. In premature infants born to seropositive mothers, little maternal antibody can be detected at birth; by 3 months of age, no antibody can be detected in these babies.[144] Thus, premature infants may be particularly susceptible to MuV infection.

Morbidity and Mortality

The major morbidity from mumps results from meningitis, encephalitis, and orchitis. These occur as age- and sex-specific hazards, with peak risk in postpubertal boys.[11] With the case fatality ratio for mumps between 1.6 and 3.8 per 10,000,[58] and with 0.5% to 2.3% of all mumps encephalitis cases being fatal,[284] it is apparent that most fatal mumps cases have CNS infection.

Origin and Spread of Epidemics

Humans are the only natural host for MuV infection; there is no known animal reservoir, although an immunologically cross-reactive virus with over 90% amino acid similarity to MuV was identified in bats in the Democratic Republic of Congo[109] and South Africa.[289] There is no evidence of transmission of MuV from bats to humans.

MuV requires a population of about 200,000 people to sustain endemic transmission. Such population densities were first achieved some four to five millennia ago,[38] so it follows that MuV could have first evolved about 5,000 years ago. Mumps is a geographically unrestricted disease, except for its absence among a few remote tribes or isolated small-island populations. In modern-day urban populations and in the absence of immunization, mumps is endemic, with peak incidence rates in the winter and spring months.[284] In the prevaccine era, preschool-aged children were an important source of virus introduced into families, given that inapparent infections are common in children of this age.[85,328]

In the present era of high vaccine coverage of children, most cases now occur among young adults, suggesting waning immunity.[56,82,87,131,372,425] Data from multiple studies showed that geometric mean titer of neutralizing antibody decline by approximately 50% over a 10-year period after vaccination.[90,243,361] More dramatic declines linked to time since vaccination have been reported by others, including seronegativity.[44,48,99,281] However, these were not longitudinal studies. Nonetheless, the evidence for waning of vaccine-induced immunity is clear. Numerous groups reported time since last vaccination as a susceptibility risk, with estimates of the odds of developing mumps after the first year postvaccination to increase by 7% to 27% annually.[425,433] This is reflected in a recent investigation of a university campus mumps outbreak during the 2015–2016 academic year, which found that students who had received the second dose of vaccine 13 to 15 years or 16 to 24 years before the outbreak had a ninefold and 14-fold, respectively, greater risk of contracting mumps than students who had received the second dose within the past 2 years.[55] Vaccine efficacy estimates also track accordingly. Cohen et al., reported a decline in vaccine effectiveness from 96% in the immediate postvaccination period to 66% 10 years later,[82] and Fu et al., reported a gradual decline in vaccine effectiveness from 98.5% 1 year postvaccination to 53.0% 12 years later.[131]

The less than desirable performance of mumps vaccines is highlighted by the global resurgence of the disease despite very high vaccine coverage. After many years of steadily declining disease incidence in the United States following the institution of mumps vaccination, the reported number of cases surged in 2006 and periodic large outbreaks have continued since (Fig. 8.7). Nearly all cases occurred in fully vaccinated individuals, including in populations with 98% to 100% vaccine coverage.[8,55,68,87,98,264,352] Similar occurrences were reported in other countries.[2,14,22,46,349,364] Despite the occurrence of these outbreaks, the effectiveness of the vaccine was still good, with attack rates ranging from 2% to 8%, while attack rates in unvaccinated persons ranged from 25% to 49%.[181,222,277]

In addition to waning immunity as a possible factor in the persistence of the disease and continued epidemics, there is also evidence of possible evolvement of strains under immune pressure. As described (see "New Epidemiologic Approaches") for molecular epidemiological purposes, mumps virus isolates are grouped by genotype based on the nucleotide sequence of the *SH* gene. Although historically many different MuV genotypes have been cocirculating, the resurgence of mumps experienced globally over the past 15 years is characterized by a single genotype, genotype G. While MuVs are serologically monotypic, there are antigenic differences between strains and it has been hypothesized that such differences between the contemporary circulating genotype G viruses and older vaccine genotypes could lead to vaccine escape in individuals with low levels of mumps antibody. In virus neutralization assays, sera from vaccinees have substantially lower potency against genotype G viruses as compared to the homologous vaccine virus.[152,345,357,424,428] While as yet there is no evidence that genotype G viruses can fully escape neutralization by sera possessing high levels of antibody, the relatively low potency of vaccine sera against genotype G viruses is a concern, particularly for persons whose immunity has waned (see "Origin and Spread of Epidemics").

Prevalence and Seroepidemiology

Data on the incidence of mumps are complicated by the fact that approximately 30% of all MuV infections are subclinical.[52,85,119,248,265,328,347] Furthermore, only 25% of all cases are seen by a clinician and fewer than 30% are reported to public health agencies.[119,248] Annual incidence rates vary, with an interepidemic period of approximately 3 years.[11,25,303]

The highest incidence of mumps reported in the United States since 1922 was almost 250 per 100,000 population in 1941. In 1968, when mumps vaccine was introduced, the yearly incidence was 76 per 100,000 population, steadily declining to less than 1 case per 100,000 population by 1993 and then to an all-time low of less than 0.1 per 100,000 population by 2003 (Fig. 8.7).[50,64] Mumps incidence remained low until 2006 when the United States experienced its largest mumps outbreak in 19 years, with 6,584 cases reported, representing a 20-fold increase in disease incidence from the prior year. Mumps incidence rapidly returned to baseline, a pattern that has repeated (Fig. 8.7). Despite averaging about 2,300 cases per year between 2006 (when the resurgence began in the United States) and 2020, which has reversed the previous trend that was approaching disease elimination, disease incidence is still greater than 96% lower than it was before widespread vaccine use. Similar success in mumps control through vaccination was achieved in other countries.[23,31,40,106,259,369]

In the prevaccine era, or in countries not incorporating mumps vaccine in national immunization programs, most persons become seropositive by adolescence. In the United States, where vaccination is required for school entry, by 1996, approximately 90% of 19- to 35-month-old children had received at least one dose of mumps-containing vaccine[62,65,69] and among adolescents aged 13 to 17 years, by 2006 coverage with two or more doses was 89%.[70] Based on the most up to date information, coverage with two doses of mumps-containing vaccine among kindergartners during the 2019–2020 school year in the United States was estimated to be 95.2%,[374] exceeding the herd immunity threshold, estimated to be 90% to 92% based on theoretical studies[12,333] and the 95% figure based on evidence from the experience in Finland where indigenous mumps has been eliminated.[100]

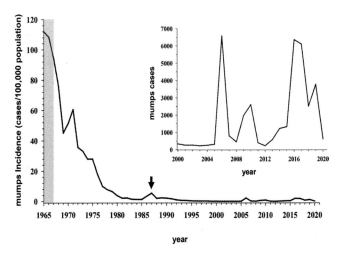

FIGURE 8.7 Mumps cases/100,000 population in the United States from 1965 to 2020. *Shaded box* indicated prevaccine era and vaccine introduction in 1967. *Inset*: Larger scale showing disease incidence between 2000 and 2020, with large outbreaks in 2006, 2009–2010, and 2016–2018 and previously 1987–1989 (*arrow*).

MuV was the most common cause of viral encephalitis in the United States until 1975, when high coverage rates of vaccination were attained.[63] In unvaccinated populations, mumps accounts for up to half of all encephalitis cases.[337] In an epidemic setting, 11% of clinical mumps cases have CNS disease, 90% with meningitis and 10% with encephalitis.[328] Severe mumps meningitis or encephalitis is most common between the ages of 5 and 9 years, with a clear male predominance in all age groups.[37]

New Epidemiologic Approaches

Routine nucleotide sequencing of virus isolates has become a key element in mumps surveillance and is a definitive means of identifying transmission pathways. MuV genotyping is conventionally performed based on the nucleotide sequence of the *SH* gene, the most variable sequence in the genome. Phylogenetic analyses of these sequences place the virus strains into distinct clusters that form the basis for genotype assignment.[462] Virus strains belonging to the same SH genotype vary at the nucleotide level within the *SH* gene by up to −11%, whereas intergenotype variation is typically on the order of 5% to 21%.[197,198,291] It has been suggested that establishment of new genotypes should not be based on variation from existing genotypes by a fixed minimal amount of sequence diversity, rather the new genotype should be phylogenetically distinct and represent ongoing transmission of MuV with epidemiological relevance.[291] Currently, 12 MuV genotypes have been described, designated A through N (genotype designations E and M have been merged with genotypes C and K, respectively) (Fig. 8.8).

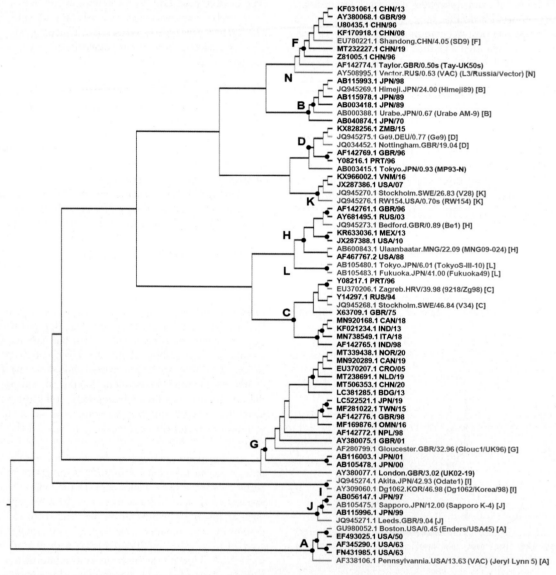

FIGURE 8.8 Phylogenetic tree showing the 12 MuV genotypes, A through N (omitting E and M), based on the *SH* gene nucleotide sequence. For clarity, sequence names have been condensed to accession number, country and year, except for reference sequences (shown in *red*) and three unclassified sequences (shown in *blue*). The tree was constructed based on comparison of complete sequences of *SH* gene using the neighbor-joining method of MEGA program. The robustness of the internal branches was determined by 1,000 bootstrap replications and the p-distance Model. The nodes denoted with a dot have support of at least 0.75. (Tree constructed courtesy of Ben Wulf and Felix Drexler, Charité—Universitätsmedizin Berlin.)

Genotypes A, C, D, G, and H were predominantly observed in the Western hemisphere, whereas genotypes B, F, I, K, and L were typically found in countries of the Asia-Pacific region.[290,291] Since 2005, genotype G has gained prominence and is now the predominant strain circulating globally. There is no established association between genotype designation and transmissibility or virulence.[9,190,365]

Relationships among MuV strains have also been inferred from nucleotide sequence analyses of the N,[191] P,[363,459] F,[126,402,411] and HN[245,358,461] genes. While these genes are more conserved in sequence and, thus, their use in discriminating among virus strains is not as powerful, phylogenetic analyses of these sequences may prove useful. For example, because the HN protein is the major cell surface target of neutralizing antibody,[312,313,375] it stands to reason that HN-based genotyping will provide valuable information on antigenic diversity and protective immunity.[96,228,314] Sequence analysis of this and other genes may also provide valuable information on the evolution of MuV.

RT/PCR and sequencing of viruses has proved particularly useful in investigation of possible vaccine-associated adverse events, such as aseptic meningitis. It was not until the availability of this technology that reports of this complication of vaccination could be confirmed.[18,209,292,294,366,404,430]

DIAGNOSIS

Clinical Diagnosis

A clinical diagnosis of mumps is made on the basis of fever and constitutional symptoms (e.g., parotitis) usually developing within 3 weeks after known exposure. Meningeal symptoms include headache, vomiting, fever, and nuchal rigidity, usually appearing 3 to 5 days after the onset of parotitis with a range of 1 week before to 2 weeks afterward.[21,348] Seizures occur in 20% to 30% of patients with CNS symptoms.[20,143] Meningeal involvement is also suggested by positive Brudzinski and Kernig signs and can be differentiated from encephalitis by a normal electroencephalogram (EEG), although the EEG findings can be normal in subjects with encephalitis, even when clinical seizures occur.[143] In many cases, the diagnosis can be confirmed by an elevated CSF-to-serum antibody ratio.[286,414] Mumps associated meningitis is generally a benign condition with complete recovery in 3 to 4 days. Frank delirium and focal neurologic deficits are uncommon. Patients with mumps meningitis and encephalitis without focal deficits, prolonged or recurrent focal seizures, or papilledema have marked clinical improvement of neurologic function within 2 to 4 days. Even with profound obtundation, patients recover with few sequelae.[20,50,53]

Laboratory confirmation is often required because a number of infectious agents, drugs, and conditions can cause mumps-like symptoms (see "Differential Diagnosis" below).

Laboratory Diagnosis

Typically, detection of virus-specific IgM in an acute serum sample or a significant rise in IgG between paired acute and convalescent samples has been the basis of a laboratory diagnosis of the disease. However, in the present era of widespread vaccine use, such markers are now unreliable given that the IgM response to "reinfection" may not be detectable and IgG levels may already be high.[351] RT/PCR testing of oral swabs is significantly more likely to confirm infection as compared to IgM or IgG testing.[26,35,72,167,168,352] Virus genome can also be detected by RT/PCR in CSF, and urine samples, but with much lower success. Despite the apparent high frequency of viremia (based on the clinical symptomatology), virus has rarely been detected in blood.

Virus detection rates are highest on samples collected within the first 2 days of illness and diminish rapidly thereafter. Rota *et al.*, reported a greater than threefold decrease in case confirmation by RT/PCR when comparing samples collected 3 or more days after symptom onset to samples collected within 2 days of symptom onset (21% vs. 68% positivity).[352] Similarly, Patel *et al.*, reported an RT/PCR-based case confirmation rate of 44% for samples collected 2 or more days after symptom onset compared to 83% for samples collected less than 2 days after symptom onset.[318]

DIFFERENTIAL DIAGNOSIS

For cases of parotitis reported during an outbreak or for cases epidemiologically linked, the clinical diagnosis of mumps is straightforward. However, in the absence of a mumps outbreak, other causes of parotitis should be considered. For example, Epstein-Barr virus has been identified in 20% of laboratory rejected cases of presumed mumps.[260] Other viruses that can cause parotitis include HPIV-1, -2, and -3, influenza A virus, coxsackieviruses, and adenovirus.[24,156,260] Nonviral causes of parotitis include suppurative infections, such as *Staphylococcus aureus* and atypical mycobacteria, starch ingestion, drugs (e.g., phenylbutazone, thiouracil, iodides, and phenothiazines), metabolic disorders (e.g., diabetes mellitus, cirrhosis, and uremia), and malnutrition. Rare conditions such as Mikulicz, Parinaud, and Sjogren syndromes can also be confused with mumps.[253] Other possible causes of parotid swelling include tumors, cysts, and salivary stones.

TREATMENT

Treatment of mumps and its various complications is generally symptomatic. In a controlled study, adult men presenting with parotitis were alternatively given either an intramuscular injection of 20 mL of gammaglobulin prepared from human convalescent serum or simply confined to a hospital for routine, nonspecific symptomatic therapy.[140] Orchitis developed in 4 of 51 antibody-treated and 14 of 51 symptomatically treated patients ($p < 0.01$). No protective effect was seen with gammaglobulin obtained from a normal donor serum pool.[140] This study suggests that immunotherapy with high-titer polyvalent or monoclonal antibody preparations could be useful in selected cases but should be used very early in the course of the illness. However, such treatment has been generally found to be of limited value for postexposure prophylaxis and immunoglobulin for the treatment of mumps is no longer available in most countries.

PREVENTION AND CONTROL

The apparent ineffectiveness of passive protection and the near impossibility of preventing virus spread by case isolation (considering that virus is shed before the appearance of clinical symptoms and a significant portion of infected individuals are asymptomatically infected) leaves vaccination as the only practical control measure.

Vaccines and Adverse Events

Two general types of MuV vaccines have been used, formalin-inactivated (killed) vaccines and live, attenuated vaccines. Use of formalin-inactivated MuV vaccines (used in the United States from 1950 to 1978) has been discontinued worldwide due to short-lived (<1 year) immunity and relatively poor efficacy.[188,334] All mumps vaccines currently in use are live, attenuated viruses (Table 8.2) and have been responsible for the remarkable decline in the incidence of mumps and related sequelae.

Live, attenuated virus mumps vaccines were developed through continuous serial passage of wild-type isolates. At present, no clear distinguishing marker exists for attenuation of MuV strains apart from the failure of a passaged isolate to produce clinical symptoms in vaccinees, although various animal tests of mumps vaccine virulence are under evaluation. In the United States, the only licensed mumps vaccine is the Jeryl Lynn (JL) strain which is currently only available in combination with MSD's measles and rubella vaccines (MMR-II) or measles, rubella, and varicella vaccines (ProQuad). Monovalent Jeryl Lynn vaccine is no longer manufactured.

Because of demonstrated and theoretical considerations about spread of virus to placenta and fetal tissues, administration of live viral vaccines (including mumps-containing vaccines) is generally contraindicated in women known to be pregnant or attempting to become pregnant.[334]

Prelicensure studies demonstrated that a single dose of the Jeryl Lynn vaccine strain induces virus neutralizing antibodies in greater than 95% of recipients.[178,388,440] Similar results have been found for most other mumps vaccine strains licensed for use elsewhere.[30,110,261,295,339]

The Jeryl Lynn vaccine is composed of two distinct but genetically related viruses, designated Jeryl Lynn-5 (JL-5) and Jeryl Lynn-2 (JL-2), existing in an approximate 5:1 ratio.[6] These two viruses differ from each other at 414 nucleotides (3%), leading to 87 amino acid substitutions.[10] Over 500 million doses of the Jeryl Lynn–based MuV vaccines have been distributed worldwide, with few serious adverse effects noted.[177] Most reported complications (e.g., rash, pruritus, and purpura) have been allergic in nature; these complications are both uncommon and usually mild and self-limited.[63] Approaches for the immunization of egg-allergic children have been detailed.[241] A comprehensive survey of the literature by the Vaccine Safety Committee of the Institute of Medicine failed to find adequate information to establish or reject a causal relationship between the administration of Jeryl Lynn MuV–containing vaccines and the development of encephalopathy, encephalitis, residual seizure disorders, optic neuritis, transverse myelitis, Guillain-Barré syndrome, IDDM, or sterility caused by orchitis, all of which have been extensively reviewed elsewhere.[39,387] Parotitis following Jeryl Lynn vaccination occurs in approximately 1% of vaccinees.[123,282,339]

Other widely distributed vaccine strains include the RIT 4385, Urabe AM9, Leningrad-Zagreb, and Rubini (discontinued). The RIT 4385 strain, produced by GlaxoSmithKline (Philadelphia, PA), was derived from the Jeryl Lynn strain by clonally isolating the JL-5 population.[406] The Jeryl Lynn and RIT 4385 strains of vaccine appear to have similar safety and efficacy profiles.[92,280,418]

In contrast to the Jeryl Lynn–based strains, most other strains have been linked to aseptic meningitis,[80,185,216,223,266,293,305,412] mostly 2 to 3 weeks after vaccination,

TABLE 8.2   Mumps virus vaccine strains in current use

Vaccine Strain	Genotype	Manufacturer	Vaccine Name	Main Area of Use
Hoshino	B	Kitasato Institute	Hokken, Hoshino	Japan, Korea
NK M-46		Chiba Serum Institute	NK M-46	Japan
Torii		Takeda Pharmaceutical	Torii	Japan
Urabe	B	Sanofi-Pasteur	Trimovax® (trivalent)	Worldwide
Leningrad-3	Classification pending	Moscow State Facility for Bacterial Preparations	Leningrad-3	Russia
Leningrad-Zagreb	Classification pending	Inst. of Immunol., Zagreb	Leningrad-Zagreb	Croatia, Slovenia
		Serum Institute of India	Tresivac® (trivalent)	Worldwide
Jeryl Lynn	A	Merck/Aventis Pasteur MSD	MMRII® (trivalent) MMR-Vaxpro® (trivalent) ProQuad® (quadrivalent)	Worldwide Europe Worldwide
		GlaxoSmithKline (RIT 4385 strain)	Priorix® (trivalent) PriorixTetra® (quadrivalent)	Worldwide Europe
		Netherlands Vaccine Inst.	BMR vaccine® (trivalent)	Netherlands
		Sevapharma Inc.	Pavivac® Trivivac® (trivalent)	Czech Republic Slovak Republic
		Dalian Jingang-Andi Bioproducts	S79	China
S-12	H	Razi State Serum and Vaccine Institute	S-12	Iran

with a male predominance. The reported rate of vaccine-associated aseptic meningitis ranges from more than 1 case per 400 doses to less than 1 case per 100,000 doses, a range influenced by vaccine manufacturer, stringency of adverse event reporting, method of surveillance, study size, clinical definition, and background rates of aseptic meningitis.[41] The course of illness is mild, with no sequelae noted. Other, less frequent adverse events following vaccination include orchitis[3,81,233] and pancreatitis.[121,408] Vaccine-associated sensorineural deafness has been reported but is exceedingly rare.[16] Symptomatic transmission of certain vaccine viruses, including the Leningrad-3, Leningrad-Zagreb, and Urabe strains, has been reported.[18,209,366] Although mumps and its complications are usually mild, most analyses of cost-to-benefit ratios favor an intensive vaccination program for developed nations.[135,212,226,383,471]

The Rubini vaccine strain, which was extensively passaged in embryonated chicken eggs and WI-38 and MRC-5 human diploid cells,[145] was found to offer little protection against mumps.[146,310,338,367] As of 2001, the World Health Organization (WHO) no longer recommended its use for national immunization programs.[453]

Vaccine Use

The Advisory Committee on Immunization Practices (ACIP) recommends administration of the first dose of MMR at 12 to 15 months of age and administration of a second dose at 4 to 6 years of age. The 1-dose schedule was instituted in 1977 and modified to a 2-dose schedule in 1989.[60] Quadrivalent measles, mumps, rubella, and varicella vaccine can be used in place of MMR for the second dose at any age, or for the first dose at 48 months of age or older.[263] Administration of mumps vaccine to infants younger than 9 months of age is associated with vaccine failure, both due to interference by maternal antibody and an underdeveloped humoral response at this age. Buynak et al., reported a seroconversion rate of only 50% in infants younger than 6 months compared to 95% in infants 6 to 11 months of age.[441] A similar finding was reported by Gans et al.[138] Overall, across many studies, seroconversion rates and geometric mean titers of antibody increased with increasing infant age at the time of vaccination.[63,205,210,243,370] Seroconversion rates among adults are similar to those observed among children[101,466] and there is no gender effect on the response to vaccination.[33]

Vaccination in the face of recent chemotherapy or radiation therapy is unlikely to induce adequate serologic responses and should be delayed for at least 3 months following such treatment.[334] Studies of MuV-containing vaccines in nonimmunocompromised HIV-1–infected patients, primarily in the form of trivalent mumps, measles, and rubella vaccines, have not documented serious or unusual adverse effects and, therefore, vaccination is recommended.[71,271]

Early studies of the Jeryl Lynn mumps vaccine demonstrated that a single dose was ≥95% effective.[178,440] However, in subsequent field studies, the effectiveness varied widely. The overall effectiveness of a single dose of the Jeryl Lynn strain is approximately 77% and that of two doses is approximately 85%.[334] These differences may be attributed to waning immunity. Whereas the initial clinical trials involved mostly young children followed over a relatively short time frame and during an era where opportunities for natural boosting were common, modern day field studies involve persons with long intervals

since vaccination during an era of virtually no circulating wild type virus. Under the latter conditions, antibody titers may decline and could result in diminished immunity (see "Origin and Spread of Epidemics").

It is important to point out that in cases of breakthrough infections, the course of disease, complications, and complication severity are substantially reduced as compared to outcomes of infection in unvaccinated individuals.[26,46,73,311,364,467] Thus, the term "vaccine failure" is misleading.

ACKNOWLEDGMENTS

This research was supported in part by the Center for Vaccine Research, University of Pittsburgh and funding from NIH (R01AI099100) to WPD.

REFERENCES

1. Aase JM, Noren GR, Reddy DV, et al. Mumps-virus infection in pregnant women and the immunologic response of their offspring. N Engl J Med 1972;286:1379–1382.
2. Aasheim ET, Inns T, Trindall A, et al. Outbreak of mumps in a school setting, United Kingdom, 2013. Hum Vaccin Immunother 2014;10:2446–2449.
3. Abdelbaky AM, Channappa DB, Islam S. Unilateral epididymo-orchitis: a rare complication of MMR vaccine. Ann R Coll Surg Engl 2008;90:336–337.
4. Afzal MA, Dussupt V, Minor PD, et al. Assessment of mumps virus growth on various continuous cell lines by virological, immunological, molecular and morphological investigations. J Virol Methods 2005;126:149–156.
5. Afzal MA, Elliott GD, Rima BK, et al. Virus and host cell-dependent variation in transcription of the mumps virus genome. J Gen Virol 1990;71:615–619.
6. Afzal MA, Pickford AR, Forsey T, et al. The Jeryl Lynn vaccine strain of mumps virus is a mixture of two distinct isolates. J Gen Virol 1993;74:917–920.
7. Afzal MA, Yates PJ, Minor PD. Nucleotide sequence at position 1081 of the hemagglutinin-neuraminidase gene in the mumps Urabe vaccine strain. J Infect Dis 1998;177:265–266.
8. Albertson JP, Clegg WJ, Reid HD, et al. Mumps outbreak at a university and recommendation for a third dose of measles-mumps-rubella vaccine—Illinois, 2015–2016. MMWR Morb Mortal Wkly Rep 2016;65:731–734.
9. Amexis G, Rubin S, Chatterjee N, et al. Identification of a new genotype H wild-type mumps virus strain and its molecular relatedness to other virulent and attenuated strains. J Med Virol 2003;70:284–286.
10. Amexis G, Rubin S, Chizhikov V, et al. Sequence diversity of Jeryl Lynn strain of mumps virus: quantitative mutant analysis for vaccine quality control. Virology 2002;300:171–179.
11. Anderson RM, Crombie JA, Grenfell BT. The epidemiology of mumps in the UK: a preliminary study of virus transmission, herd immunity and the potential impact of immunization. Epidemiol Infect 1987;99:65–84.
12. Anderson RM, May RM. Vaccination and herd immunity to infectious diseases. Nature 1985;318:323–329.
13. Andrejeva J, Childs KS, Young DF, et al. The V proteins of paramyxoviruses bind the IFN-inducible RNA helicase, mda-5, and inhibit its activation of the IFN-beta promoter. Proc Natl Acad Sci U S A 2004;101:17264–17269.
14. Anis E, Grotto I, Moerman L, et al. Mumps outbreak in Israel's highly vaccinated society: are two doses enough? Epidemiol Infect 2012;140:439–446.
15. Arita M, Ueno Y, Masuyama Y. Complete heart block in mumps myocarditis. Br Heart J 1981;46:342–344.
16. Asatryan A, Pool V, Chen RT, et al. Live attenuated measles and mumps viral strain-containing vaccines and hearing loss: Vaccine Adverse Event Reporting System (VAERS), United States, 1990–2003. Vaccine 2008;26:1166–1172.
17. Association for the Study of Infectious Disease. A retrospective survey of the complications of mumps. J R Coll Gen Pract 1974;24:552–556.
18. Atrasheuskaya A, Neverov A, Rubin S, et al. Horizontal transmission of the Leningrad-3 live attenuated mumps vaccine virus. Vaccine 2006;24:1530–1536.
19. Aygun AD, Kabakus N, Celik I, et al. Long-term neurological outcome of acute encephalitis. J Trop Pediatr 2001;47:243–247.
20. Azimi PH. Mumps meningoencephalitis. Prolonged abnormality of cerebrospinal fluid. JAMA 1975;234:1161–1162.
21. Bang HO, Bang J. Involvement of the central nervous system in mumps. Acta Med Scand 1943;113:487–505.
22. Bangor-Jones RD, Dowse GK, Giele CM, et al. A prolonged mumps outbreak among highly vaccinated Aboriginal people in the Kimberley region of Western Australia. Med J Aust 2009;191:398–401.
23. Barchitta M, Basile G, Lopalco PL, et al. Vaccine-preventable diseases and vaccination among Italian healthcare workers: a review of current literature. Future Microbiol 2019;14:15–19.
24. Barrabeig I, Costa J, Rovira A, et al. Viral etiology of mumps-like illnesses in suspected mumps cases reported in Catalonia, Spain. Hum Vaccin Immunother 2015;11:282–287.
25. Barskey AE, Glasser JW, LeBaron CW. Mumps resurgences in the United States: a historical perspective on unexpected elements. Vaccine 2009;27:6186–6195.

26. Barskey AE, Schulte C, Rosen JB, et al. Mumps outbreak in Orthodox Jewish communities in the United States. *N Engl J Med* 2012;367:1704–1713.
27. Bashe WJ Jr, Gotlieb T, Henle G, et al. Studies on the prevention of mumps. VI. The relationship of neutralizing antibodies to the determination of susceptibility and to the evaluation of immunization procedures. *J Immunol* 1953;71:76–85.
28. Bautista-López N, Ward BJ, Mills E, et al. Development and durability of measles antigen-specific lymphoproliferative response after MMR vaccination. *Vaccine* 2000;18:1393–1401.
29. Beard CM, Benson RC Jr, Kelalis PP, et al. The incidence and outcome of mumps orchitis in Rochester, Minnesota, 1935 to 1974. *Mayo Clin Proc* 1977;52:3–7.
30. Beck M, Welsz-Malecek R, Mesko-Prejac M, et al. Mumps vaccine L-Zagreb, prepared in chick fibroblasts. I. Production and field trials. *J Biol Stand* 1989;17:85–90.
31. Belmar-George S, Cassius-Frederick J, Leon P, et al. MMR2 vaccination coverage and timeliness among children born in 2004–2009: a national survey in Saint Lucia, 2015. *Rev Panam Salud Publica* 2018;42:e76.
32. Bertotto A, Spinozzi F, Gerli R, et al. CD8+ and γ/δ lymphocytes in mumps meningitis patients. *Acta Paediatr* 1995;84:1268–1270.
33. Bianchi FP, De Nitto S, Stefanizzi P, et al. Long time persistence of antibodies against mumps in fully MMR immunized young adults: an Italian retrospective cohort study. *Hum Vaccin Immunother* 2020;16:2649–2655.
34. Bitnun S, Rakover Y, Rosen G. Acute bilateral total deafness complicating mumps. *J Laryngol Otol* 1986;100:943–945.
35. Bitsko RH, Cortese MM, Dayan GH, et al. Detection of RNA of mumps virus during an outbreak in a population with a high level of measles, mumps, and rubella vaccine coverage. *J Clin Microbiol* 2008;46:1101–1103.
36. Bjorvatn B. Mumps virus recovered from testicles by fine-needle aspiration biopsy in cases of mumps orchitis. *Scand J Infect Dis* 1973;5:3–5.
37. Bjorvatn B, Wolontis S. Mumps meningoencephalitis in Stockholm November 1964—July 1971: I. Analysis of a hospitalized study group. Questions of selection and representativity. *Scand J Infect Dis* 1973;5:253–260.
38. Black FL, Hierholzer WJ, Pinheiro FD, et al. Evidence for persistence of infectious agents in isolated human populations. *Am J Epidemiol* 1974;100:230–250.
39. Black S, Shinefield H, Ray P, et al. Risk of hospitalization because of aseptic meningitis after measles-mumps-rubella vaccination in one- to two-year-old children: an analysis of the Vaccine Safety Datalink (VSD) Project. *Pediatr Infect Dis J* 1997;16:500–503.
40. Bogusz J, Paradowska-Stankiewicz I. Mumps in Poland in 2017. *Przegl Epidemiol* 2019;73:311–315.
41. Bonnet M-C, Dutta A, Weinberger C, et al. Mumps vaccine virus strains and aseptic meningitis. *Vaccine* 2006;24:7037–7045.
42. Boriskin YS, Booth JC, Yamada A. Sequence variation within the carboxyl terminus of the nucleoprotein gene of mumps virus strains. *Clin Diagn Virol* 1994;2:79–85.
43. Bose S, Song AS, Jardetzky TS, et al. Fusion activation through attachment protein stalk domains indicates a conserved core mechanism of paramyxovirus entry into cells. *J Virol* 2014;88:3925–3941.
44. Boulianne N, De Serres G, Ratnam S, et al. Measles, mumps, and rubella antibodies in children 5–6 years after immunization: effect of vaccine type and age at vaccination. *Vaccine* 1995;13:1611–1616.
45. Bousse TL, Taylor G, Krishnamurthy S, et al. Biological significance of the second receptor binding site of Newcastle disease virus hemagglutinin-neuraminidase protein. *J Virol* 2004;78:13351–13355.
46. Boxall N, Kubinyiova M, Prikazsky V, et al. An increase in the number of mumps cases in the Czech Republic, 2005–2006. *Euro Surveill* 2008;13:18842.
47. Briggs K, Wang L, Nagashima K, et al. Regulation of mumps virus replication and transcription by kinase RPS6KB1. *J Virol* 2020;94:e00387.
48. Broliden K, Abreu ER, Arneborn M, et al. Immunity to mumps before and after MMR vaccination at 12 years of age in the first generation offered the two-dose immunization programme. *Vaccine* 1998;16:323–327.
49. Brown GC, Baublis JV, O'Leary TP. Development and duration of mumps fluorescent antibodies in various immunoglobulin fractions of human serum. *J Immunol* 1970;104:86–94.
50. Brown JW, Kirkland HB, Hein GE. Central nervous system involvement during mumps. *Am J Med Sci* 1948;215:434–441.
51. Brown NJ, Richmond SJ. Fatal mumps myocarditis in an 8-month-old child. *Br Med J* 1980;281:356–357.
52. Brunell PA, Brickman A, O'Hare D, et al. Ineffectiveness of isolation of patients as a method of preventing the spread of mumps. *N Engl J Med* 1968;279:1357–1361.
53. Bruyn HB, Sexton HM, Brainerd HD. Mumps meningoencephalitis; a clinical review of 119 cases with one death. *Calif Med* 1957;86:153–160.
54. Buxton J, Craig C, Daly P, et al. An outbreak of mumps among young adults in Vancouver, British Columbia, associated with 'rave' parties. *Can J Public Health* 1999;90:160–163.
55. Cardemil CV, Dahl RM, James L, et al. Effectiveness of a third dose of MMR vaccine for mumps outbreak control. *N Engl J Med* 2017;377:947–956.
56. Castilla J, García Cenoz M, Arriazu M, et al. Effectiveness of Jeryl Lynn-containing vaccine in Spanish children. *Vaccine* 2009;27:2089–2093.
57. Cebulla CM, Miller DM, Sedmak DD. Viral inhibition of interferon signal transduction. *Intervirology* 1999;42:325–330.
58. Centers for Disease Control and Prevention. Mumps surveillance report. *MMWR Morb Mortal Wkly Rep* 1972;21:1–12.
59. Centers for Disease Control and Prevention. Current trends Mumps—United States, 1984–1985. *MMWR Morb Mortal Wkly Rep* 1986;35:216–219.
60. Centers for Disease Control and Prevention. Measles prevention. *MMWR Morb Mortal Wkly Rep* 1989;38:1–18.
61. Centers for Disease Control and Prevention. Summary of notifiable diseases, United States, 1996. *MMWR Morb Mortal Wkly Rep* 1996;45:1–88.
62. Centers for Disease Control and Prevention. Status report on the Childhood Immunization Initiative: national, state, and urban area vaccination coverage levels among children aged 19–35 months–United States, 1996. *MMWR Morb Mortal Wkly Rep* 1997;46:657–664.
63. Centers for Disease Control and Prevention. Measles, mumps, and rubella—Vaccine use and strategies for the elimination of measles, rubella, and congenital rubella syndrome and control of mumps: recommendations of the Advisory Committee on Immunization Practices (ACIP). *MMWR Morb Mortal Wkly Rep* 1998;47:1–48.
64. Centers for Disease Control and Prevention. Summary of notifiable diseases, 2003. *MMWR Morb Mortal Wkly Rep* 2005;52:17–71.
65. Centers for Disease Control and Prevention. National, state, and urban area vaccination coverage among children aged 19–35 months–United States, 2005. *MMWR Morb Mortal Wkly Rep* 2006;55:988–993.
66. Centers for Disease Control and Prevention. Summary of notifiable diseases—United States, 2007. *MMWR Morb Mortal Wkly Rep* 2009;56:1–94.
67. Centers for Disease Control and Prevention. Summary of notifiable diseases—United States, 2008. *MMWR Morb Mortal Wkly Rep* 2009;57:1–94.
68. Centers for Disease Control and Prevention. Update: mumps outbreak—New York and New Jersey, June 2009–January 2010. *MMWR Morb Mortal Wkly Rep* 2010;59:125–129.
69. Centers for Disease Control and Prevention. National, state, and local area vaccination coverage among children aged 19–35 months—United States, 2009. *MMWR Morb Mortal Wkly Rep* 2010;59:1171–1177.
70. Centers for Disease Control and Prevention. National, state, and local area vaccination coverage among adolescents aged 13–17 years—United States, 2009. *MMWR Morb Mortal Wkly Rep* 2010;59:1018–1023.
71. Centers for Disease Control and Prevention. Guide to vaccine contraindications and precautions [Internet]. March 15, 2022. [cited 2022 April 22]. https://www.cdc.gov/vaccines/hcp/acip-recs/general-recs/contraindications.html.
72. Centers for Disease Control and Prevention. Mumps outbreak on a university campus—California, 2011. *MMWR Morb Mortal Wkly Rep* 2012;61:986–989.
73. Chen CC, Lu CC, Su BH, et al. Epidemiologic features of mumps in Taiwan from 2006 to 2011: a new challenge for public health policy. *World J Pediatr* 2015;11:141–147.
74. Chiba Y, Dzierba JL, Morag A, et al. Cell-mediated immune response to mumps virus infection in man. *J Immunol* 1976;116:12–15.
75. Chiba Y, Horino K, Umetsu M, et al. Virus excretion and antibody response in saliva in natural mumps. *Tohoku J Exp Med* 1973;111:229–238.
76. Chiba Y, Nakao T. Mumps virus neutralizing antibody in saliva following natural infection. *Tohoku J Exp Med* 1972;106:75–81.
77. Chiba Y, Tsutsumi H, Nakao T, et al. Human leukocyte antigen-linked genetic controls for T-cell mediated cytotoxicity response to mumps virus in humans. *Infect Immun* 1982;35:600–604.
78. Chu TH, Cheever FS, Coons AH, et al. Distribution of mumps virus in the experimentally infected monkey. *Exp Biol Med* 1951;76:571–574.
79. Cinalli G, Spennato P, Ruggiero C, et al. Aqueductal stenosis 9 years after mumps meningoencephalitis: treatment by endoscopic third ventriculostomy. *Childs Nerv Syst* 2004;20:61–64.
80. Cizman M, Mozetic M, Radescek-Rakar R, et al. Aseptic meningitis after vaccination against measles and mumps. *Pediatr Infect Dis J* 1989;8:302–308.
81. Clifford V, Wadsley J, Jenner B, et al. Mumps vaccine associated orchitis: evidence supporting a potential immune-mediated mechanism. *Vaccine* 2010;28:2671–2673.
82. Cohen C, White JM, Savage EJ, et al. Vaccine effectiveness estimates, 2004–2005 mumps outbreak, England. *Emerg Infect Dis* 2007;13:12–17.
83. Collins SD. Age incidence of the common communicable diseases of children: a study of case rates among all children and among children not previously attacked and of death rates and the estimated case fatality. *Pub Health Rep (1896–1970)* 1929;44:763.
84. Connaris H, Takimoto T, Russell R, et al. Probing the sialic acid binding site of the hemagglutinin-neuraminidase of Newcastle disease virus: identification of key amino acids involved in cell binding, catalysis, and fusion. *J Virol* 2002;76:1816–1824.
85. Cooney MK, Fox JP, Hall CE. The Seattle Virus Watch. VI. Observations of infections with and illness due to parainfluenza, mumps and respiratory syncytial viruses and Mycoplasma pneumoniae. *Am J Epidemiol* 1975;101:532–551.
86. Copelovici Y, Strulovici D, Cristea AL, et al. Data on the efficiency of specific antimumps immunoglobulins in the prevention of mumps and of its complications. *Virologie* 1979;30:171–177.
87. Cortese MM, Jordan HT, Curns AT, et al. Mumps vaccine performance among university students during a mumps outbreak. *Clin Infect Dis* 2008;46:1172–1180.
88. Cox R, Green TJ, Qiu S, et al. Characterization of a mumps virus nucleocapsidlike particle. *J Virol* 2009;83:11402–11406.
89. Cox R, Pickar A, Qiu S, et al. Structural studies on the authentic mumps virus nucleocapsid showing uncoiling by the phosphoprotein. *Proc Natl Acad Sci U S A* 2014;111:15208–15213.
90. Craighead JE. The role of viruses in the pathogenesis of pancreatic disease and diabetes mellitus. *Prog Med Virol* 1975;19:161–214.
91. Crennell S, Takimoto T, Portner A, et al. Crystal structure of the multifunctional paramyxovirus hemagglutinin-neuraminidase. *Nat Struct Biol* 2000;7:1068–1074.
92. Crovari P, Gabutti G, Giammanco G, et al. Reactogenicity and immunogenicity of a new combined Measles–Mumps–Rubella vaccine: results of a multicentre trial. *Vaccine* 2000;18:2796–2803.
93. Curran J, Boeck R, Lin-Marq N, et al. Paramyxovirus phosphoproteins form homotrimers as determined by an epitope dilution assay, via predicted coiled coils. *Virology* 1995;214:139–149.
94. Curran J, Homann H, Buchholz C, et al. The hypervariable C-terminal tail of the Sendai paramyxovirus nucleocapsid protein is required for template function but not for RNA encapsidation. *J Virol* 1993;67:4358–4364.
95. Curran JA, Quinn JP, Hoey EM, et al. cDNA cloning of the nucleocapsid and nucleocapsid-associated protein genes of mumps virus. *J Gen Virol* 1985;66:977–985.
96. Cusi MG, Fischer S, Sedlmeier R, et al. Localization of a new neutralizing epitope on the mumps virus hemagglutinin–neuraminidase protein. *Virus Res* 2001;74:133–137.
97. Dacou-Voutetakis C. Diabetes mellitus following mumps. *Am J Dis Child* 1974;127:890.
98. Date AA, Kyaw MH, Rue AM, et al. Long-term persistence of mumps antibody after receipt of 2 measles-mumps-rubella (MMR) vaccinations and antibody response after a third MMR vaccination among a university population. *J Infect Dis* 2008;197:1662–1668.

99. Davidkin I, Jokinen S, Broman M, et al. Persistence of measles, mumps, and rubella antibodies in an MMR-vaccinated cohort: a 20-year follow-up. *J Infect Dis* 2008;197:950–956.
100. Davidkin I, Kontio M, Paunio M, et al. MMR vaccination and disease elimination: the Finnish experience. *Expert Rev Vaccines* 2010;9:1045–1053.
101. Davidson WL, Buynak EB, Leagus MB, et al. Vaccination of adults with live attenuated mumps virus vaccine. *JAMA* 1967;201:995–998.
102. Dayan GH, Rubin S. Mumps outbreaks in vaccinated populations: are available mumps vaccines effective enough to prevent outbreaks? *Clin Infect Dis* 2008;47:1458–1467.
103. Dayan GH, Quinlisk MP, Parker AA, et al. Recent resurgence of mumps in the United States. *N Engl J Med* 2008;358:1580–1589.
104. de Boer AW, de Vaan GAM. Mild course of mumps in patients with acute lymphoblastic leukaemia. *Eur J Pediatr* 1989;148:618–619.
105. Deibel R, Schryver GD. Viral antibody in the cerebrospinal fluid of patients with acute central nervous system infections. *J Clin Microbiol* 1976;3:397–401.
106. Di Pietro A, Visalli G, Antonuccio GM, et al. Today's vaccination policies in Italy: the National Plan for Vaccine Prevention 2017–2019 and the Law 119/2017 on the mandatory vaccinations. *Ann Ig* 2019;31:54–64.
107. Donald PR, Burger PJ, Becker WB. Mumps meningo-encephalitis. *S Afr Med J* 1987;71:283–285.
108. Donohue WL, Playfair FD, Whitaker L. Mumps encephalitis. *J Pediatr* 1955;47:395–412.
109. Drexler JF, Corman VM, Muller MA, et al. Bats host major mammalian paramyxoviruses. *Nat Commun* 2012;3:796.
110. Ehrengut W, Georges AM, André FE. The reactogenicity and immunogenicity of the Urabe Am 9 live mumps vaccine and persistence of vaccine induced antibodies in healthy young children. *J Biol Stand* 1983;11:105–113.
111. Elango N, Kövamees J, Varsanyi TM, et al. mRNA sequence and deduced amino acid sequence of the mumps virus small hydrophobic protein gene. *J Virol* 1989;63:1413–1415.
112. Elango N, Varsanyi TM, Kovamees J, et al. Molecular cloning and characterization of six genes, determination of gene order and intergenic sequences and leader sequence of mumps virus. *J Gen Virol* 1988;69:2893–2900.
113. Elderfield RA, Parker L, Stilwell P, et al. Ferret airway epithelial cell cultures support efficient replication of influenza B virus but not mumps virus. *J Gen Virol* 2015;96:2092–2098.
114. Elliott GD, Afzal MA, Martin SJ, et al. Nucleotide sequence of the matrix, fusion and putative SH protein genes of mumps virus and their deduced amino acid sequences. *Virus Res* 1989;12:61–75.
115. Elliott GD, Yeo RP, Afzal MA, et al. Strain-variable editing during transcription of the P gene of mumps virus may lead to the generation of non-structural proteins NS1 (V) and NS2. *J Gen Virol* 1990;71:1555–1560.
116. Enders JF. Mumps: techniques of laboratory diagnosis, tests for susceptibility, and experiments on specific prophylaxis. *J Pediatr* 1946;29:129–142.
117. Ennis FA. Immunity to mumps in an institutional epidemic. Correlation of insusceptibility to mumps with serum plaque neutralizing and hemagglutination-inhibiting antibodies. *J Infect Dis* 1969;119:654–657.
118. Everberg BG. Deafness following mumps. *Acta Otolaryngol* 1957;48:397–403.
119. Falk WA, Buchan K, Dow M, et al. The epidemiology of mumps in southern alberta, 1980–1982. *Am J Epidemiol* 1989;130:736–749.
120. Fanoy EB, Cremer J, Ferreira JA, et al. Transmission of mumps virus from mumps-vaccinated individuals to close contacts. *Vaccine* 2011;29:9551–9556.
121. Feldman G, Zer M. Infantile acute pancreatitis after mumps vaccination simulating an acute abdomen. *Pediatr Surg Int* 2000;16:488–489.
122. Feldstein JD, Johnson FR, Kallick CA, et al. Acute hemorrhagic pancreatitis and pseudocyst due to mumps. *Ann Surg* 1974;180:85–88.
123. Fescharek R, Quast U, Maass G, et al. Measles-mumps vaccination in the FRG: an empirical analysis after 14 years of use. II. Tolerability and analysis of spontaneously reported side effects. *Vaccine* 1990;8:446–456.
124. Fleischer B, Kreth HW. Clonal analysis of HLA-restricted virus-specific cytotoxic T lymphocytes from cerebrospinal fluid in mumps meningitis. *J Immunol* 1983;130:2187–2190.
125. Forsberg P, Frydén A, Link H, et al. Viral IgM and IgG antibody synthesis within the central nervous system in mumps meningitis. *Acta Neurol Scand* 1986;73:372–380.
126. Forsey T, Mawn JA, Yates PJ, et al. Differentiation of vaccine and wild mumps viruses using the polymerase chain reaction and dideoxynucleotide sequencing. *J Gen Virol* 1990;71:987–990.
127. Frankova V, Sixtova E. Specific IgM antibodies in the saliva of mumps patients. *Acta Virol* 1987;31:357–364.
128. Franz S, Rennert P, Woznik M, et al. Mumps virus SH protein inhibits NF-kappaB activation by interacting with tumor necrosis factor receptor 1, interleukin-1 receptor 1, and toll-like receptor 3 complexes. *J Virol* 2017;91:e01037.
129. Friedman MG. Salivary IgA antibodies to mumps virus during and after mumps. *J Infect Dis* 1981;143:617.
130. Fryden A, Link H, Moller E. Demonstration of cerebrospinal fluid lymphocytes sensitized against virus antigens in mumps meningitis. *Acta Neurol Scand* 1978;57:396–404.
131. Fu C, Liang J, Wang M. Matched case–control study of effectiveness of live, attenuated S79 mumps virus vaccine against clinical mumps. *Clin Vaccine Immunol* 2008;15:1425–1428.
132. Fuentes SM, Sun D, Schmitt AP, et al. Phosphorylation of paramyxovirus phosphoprotein and its role in viral gene expression. *Future Microbiol* 2010;5:9–13.
133. Fuller IC. Mumps and its complications: an example of the utilization of disease indices. *J R Coll Gen Pract* 1968;16:494–496.
134. Galazka A, Kraigher A, Robertson SE. Wide spread inflammation of the parotid glands (mumps): underestimated disease. I. Epidemiology of the mumps and its medical meaning in Poland. *Przegl Epidemiol* 1998;52:389–400.
135. Galazka AM, Robertson SE, Kraigher A. Mumps and mumps vaccine: a global review. *Bull World Health Organ* 1999;77:3–14.
136. Gamble DR. Relation of antecedent illness to development of diabetes in children. *Br Med J* 1980;281:99–101.
137. Gans HA, Maldonado Y, Yasukawa LL, et al. IL-12, IFN-gamma, and T cell proliferation to measles in immunized infants. *J Immunol* 1999;162:5569–5575.
138. Gans H, Yasukawa L, Rinki M, et al. Immune responses to measles and mumps vaccination of infants at 6, 9, and 12 months. *J Infect Dis* 2001;184:817–826.
139. Garcia AG, Pereira JM, Vidigal N, et al. Intrauterine infection with mumps virus. *Obstet Gynecol* 1980;56:756–759.
140. Gellis SS, McGuinness AC, Peters M. A study on the prevention of mumps orchitis by gamma globulin. *Am J Med Sci* 1945;210:661–664.
141. Ghosh JK, Ovadia M, Shai Y. A leucine zipper motif in the ectodomain of Sendai virus fusion protein assembles in solution and in membranes and specifically binds biologically-active peptides and the virus. *Biochemistry* 1997;36:15451–15462.
142. Gibbons JL, Miller HG, Stanton JB. Para-infectious encephalomyelitis and related syndromes; a critical review of the neurological complications of certain specific fevers. *Q J Med* 1956;25:427–505.
143. Gibbs FA. Common types of childhood encephalitis. *Arch Neurol* 1964;10:1.
144. Glick C, Feldman S, Norris MR, et al. Measles, mumps, and rubella serology in premature infants weighing less than 1,000 grams. *South Med J* 1998;91:159–160.
145. Gluck R, Hoskins JM, Wegmann A, et al. Rubini, a new live attenuated mumps vaccine virus strain for human diploid cells. *Dev Biol Stand* 1986;65:29–35.
146. Goh KT. Resurgence of mumps in Singapore caused by the Rubini mumps virus vaccine strain. *Lancet* 1999;354:1355–1356.
147. Goldacre MJ, Wotton CJ, Yeates D, et al. Hospital admission for selected single virus infections prior to diabetes mellitus. *Diabetes Res Clin Pract* 2005;69:256–261.
148. Gonzalez-Gil J, Zarrabeitia MT, Altuzarra E, et al. Hydrocephalus: a fatal late consequence of mumps encephalitis. *J Forensic Sci* 2000;45:204–207.
149. Gordon JE, Heeren RH. The epidemiology of mumps. *Am J Med Sci* 1940;200:338–359.
150. Gotoh H, Shioda T, Sakai Y, et al. Rescue of Sendai virus from viral ribonucleoprotein-transfected cells by infection with recombinant vaccinia viruses carrying Sendai virus L and P/C genes. *Virology* 1989;171:434–443.
151. Gouma S, Schurink-Van't Klooster TM, de Melker HE, et al. Mumps serum antibody levels before and after an outbreak to assess infection and immunity in vaccinated students. *Open Forum Infect Dis* 2014;1:ofu101.
152. Gouma S, Ten Hulscher HI, Schurink-van't Klooster TM, et al. Mumps-specific cross-neutralization by MMR vaccine-induced antibodies predicts protection against mumps virus infection. *Vaccine* 2016;34:4166–4171.
153. Granata S. Sulla etiologia degli orecchioni da virus filtrable. *Med Ital* 1908;6:647–649.
154. Gresser I, Enders JF. Cytopathogenicity of mumps virus in cultures of chick embryo and human amnion cells. *Proc Soc Exp Biol Med* 1961;107:804–807.
155. Gut J-P, Lablache C, Behr S, et al. Symptomatic mumps virus reinfections. *J Med Virol* 1995;45:17–23.
156. Guy RJ, Andrews RM, Kelly HA, et al. Mumps and rubella: a year of enhanced surveillance and laboratory testing. *Epidemiol Infect* 2004;132:391–398.
157. Habel K. Cultivation of mumps virus in the developing chick embryo and its application to studies of immunity to mumps in man. *Pub Health Rep (1896–1970)* 1945;60:201.
158. Habel K. Preparation of mumps vaccines and immunization of monkeys against experimental mumps infection. *Pub Health Rep (1896–1970)* 1946;61:1655.
159. Hall R, Richards H. Hearing loss due to mumps. *Arch Dis Child* 1987;62:189–191.
160. Hamaguchi M, Yoshida T, Nishikawa K, et al. Transcriptive complex of Newcastle disease virus. *Virology* 1983;128:105–117.
161. Hammer SM, Connolly KJ. Viral aseptic meningitis in the United States: clinical features, viral etiologies, and differential diagnosis. *Curr Clin Top Infect Dis* 1992;12:1–25.
162. Hanna-Wakim R, Yasukawa LL, Sung P, et al. Immune responses to mumps vaccine in adults who were vaccinated in childhood. *J Infect Dis* 2008;197:1669–1675.
163. Hao X, Wang Y, Zhu M, et al. Development of improved mumps vaccine candidates by mutating viral mRNA cap methyltransferase sites in the large polymerase protein. *Virol Sin* 2021;36:521–536.
164. Hariya Y, Yokosawa N, Yonekura N, et al. Mumps virus can suppress the effective augmentation of HPC-induced apoptosis by IFN-gamma through disruption of IFN signaling in U937 cells. *Microbiol Immunol* 2000;44:537–541.
165. Harrison MS, Sakaguchi T, Schmitt AP. Paramyxovirus assembly and budding: building particles that transmit infections. *Int J Biochem Cell Biol* 2010;42:1416–1429.
166. Hashimoto H, Fujioka M, Kinumaki H. An office-based prospective study of deafness in mumps. *Pediatr Infect Dis J* 2009;28:173–175.
167. Hassan J, Kelly J, De Gascun C. Presence of low mumps-specific IgG in oral fluids is associated with high mumps viral loads. *J Clin Virol* 2020;129:104517.
168. Hatchette T, Davidson R, Clay S, et al. Laboratory diagnosis of mumps in a partially immunized population: the Nova Scotia experience. *Can J Infect Dis Med Microbiol* 2009;20:e157–e162.
169. Hayashi K, Ross ME, Notkins AL. Persistence of mumps viral antigens in mouse brain. *Jpn J Exp Med* 1976;46:197–200.
170. He B, Leser GP, Paterson RG, et al. The paramyxovirus SV5 small hydrophobic (SH) protein is not essential for virus growth in tissue culture cells. *Virology* 1998;250:30–40.
171. He B, Lin GY, Durbin JE, et al. The SH integral membrane protein of the paramyxovirus simian virus 5 is required to block apoptosis in MDBK cells. *J Virol* 2001;75:4068–4079.
172. Henle G, Enders JF. *Mumps Virus*. Philadelphia, PA: Lippincott; 1965.
173. Henle G, Henle W, et al. Isolation of mumps virus from human beings with induced apparent or inapparent infections. *J Exp Med* 1948;88:223–232.
174. Hensel M, Gutjahr P, Kamin W, et al. Meningitis in 154 children of a pediatric clinic in Germany: clinical and epidemiologic aspects. *Klin Padiatr* 1992;204:163–170.
175. Herndon RM, Johnson RT, Davis LE, et al. Ependymitis in mumps virus meningitis. Electron microscopical studies of cerebrospinal fluid. *Arch Neurol* 1974;30:475–479.
176. Herrler G, Compans RW. Synthesis of mumps virus polypeptides in infected vero cells. *Virology* 1982;119:430–438.
177. Hilleman MR. Past, present, and future of measles, mumps, and rubella virus vaccines. *Pediatrics* 1992;90:149–153.

178. Hilleman MR, Weibel RE, Buynak EB, et al. Live, attenuated mumps-virus vaccine. *N Engl J Med* 1967;276:252–258.
179. Hirsch A. *Handbook of Geographical and Historical Pathology. Volume I: Acute Infective Diseases*. London: Sydenham Society; 1883.
180. Hodes D, Brunell PA. Mumps antibody: placental transfer and disappearance during the first year of life. *Pediatrics* 1970;45:99–101.
181. Hope-Simpson RE. Infectiousness of communicable diseases in the household (measles, chickenpox, and mumps). *Lancet* 1952;2:549–554.
182. Horne RW, Waterson AP, Wildy P, et al. The structure and composition of the myxoviruses. *Virology* 1960;11:79–98.
183. Hosaka Y, Shimizu K. Lengths of the nucleocapsids of Newcastle disease and mumps viruses. *J Mol Biol* 1968;35:369–373.
184. Houard S, Varsanyi TM, Milican F, et al. Protection of hamsters against experimental mumps virus (MuV) infection by antibodies raised against the MuV surface glycoproteins expressed from recombinant vaccinia virus vectors. *J Gen Virol* 1995;76:421–423.
185. Hrynash Y, Nadraga A, Dasho M. Effectiveness of a vaccination program against mumps in Ukraine. *Eur J Clin Microbiol Infect Dis* 2008;27:1171–1176.
186. Hyatt HW Sr. Complications of mumps. *GP* 1962;25:124–126.
187. Ilonen J. Lymphocyte blast transformation response of seropositive and seronegative subjects to herpes simplex, rubella, mumps and measles virus antigens. *Acta Pathol Microbiol Scand C* 1979;87C:151–157.
188. Ilonen J, Salmi A, Penttinen K, et al. Lymphocyte blast transformation and antibody responses after vaccination with inactivated mumps virus vaccine. *Acta Pathol Microbiol Scand C* 1981;89:303–309.
189. Inou Y, Nakayama T, Yoshida N, et al. Molecular epidemiology of mumps virus in Japan and proposal of two new genotypes. *J Med Virol* 2004;73:97–104.
190. Ivancic J, Gulija TK, Forcic D, et al. Genetic characterization of L-Zagreb mumps vaccine strain. *Virus Res* 2005;109:95–105.
191. Ivancic-Jelecki J, Santak M, Forcic D. Variability of hemagglutinin-neuraminidase and nucleocapsid protein of vaccine and wild-type mumps virus strains. *Infect Genet Evol* 2008;8:603–613.
192. Jalal H, Bahadur G, Knowles W, et al. Mumps epididymo-orchitis with prolonged detection of virus in semen and the development of anti-sperm antibodies. *J Med Virol* 2004;73:147–150.
193. Jaye A, Magnusen Albert F, Whittle Hilton C. Human leukocyte antigen class I- and class II-restricted cytotoxic T lymphocyte responses to measles antigens in immune adults. *J Infect Dis* 1998;177:1282–1289.
194. Jaye A, Magnusen AF, Sadiq AD, et al. Ex vivo analysis of cytotoxic T lymphocytes to measles antigens during infection and after vaccination in Gambian children. *J Clin Invest* 1998;102:1969–1977.
195. Jensik SC, Silver S. Polypeptides of mumps virus. *J Virol* 1976;17:363–373.
196. Jin L, Feng Y, Parry R, et al. Real-time PCR and its application to mumps rapid diagnosis. *J Med Virol* 2007;79:1761–1767.
197. Jin L, Rima B, Brown D, et al. Proposal for genetic characterisation of wild-type mumps strains: preliminary standardisation of the nomenclature. *Arch Virol* 2005;150:1903–1909.
198. Johansson B, Tecle T, Örvell C. Proposed criteria for classification of new genotypes of mumps virus. *Scand J Infect Dis* 2002;34:355–357.
199. Johnson RT. *Viral Infection of the Nervous System*. New York: Raven Press; 1982.
200. Johnson CD, Goodpasture EW. An investigation of the etiology of mumps. *J Exp Med* 1934;59:1–19.
201. Johnson CD, Goodpasture EW. The etiology of mumps. *Am J Epidemiol* 1935;21:46–57.
202. Johnson RT, Johnson KP. Hydrocephalus following viral infection: the pathology of aqueductal stenosis developing after experimental mumps virus infection. *J Neuropathol Exp Neurol* 1968;27:591–606.
203. Johnson RT, Johnson KP, Edmonds CJ. Virus-induced hydrocephalus: development of aqueductal stenosis in hamsters after mumps infection. *Science* 1967;157:1066–1067.
204. Johnson KP, Johnson RT. Granular ependymitis. Occurrence in myxovirus infected rodents and prevalence in man. *Am J Pathol* 1972;67:511–526.
205. Johnson CE, Kumar ML, Whitwell JK, et al. Antibody persistence after primary measles-mumps-rubella vaccine and response to a second dose given at four to six vs. eleven to thirteen years. *Pediatr Infect Dis J* 1996;15:687–692.
206. Johnstone JA, Ross CA, Dunn M. Meningitis and encephalitis associated with mumps infection. A 10-year survey. *Arch Dis Child* 1972;47:647–651.
207. Jokinen S, Österlund P, Julkunen I, et al. Cellular immunity to mumps virus in young adults 21 years after measles-mumps-rubella vaccination. *J Infect Dis* 2007;196:861–867.
208. Jones JF, Ray CG, Fulginiti VA. Perinatal mumps infection. *J Pediatr* 1980;96:912–914.
209. Kaic B, Gjenero-Margan I, Aleraj B, et al. Transmission of the L-Zagreb mumps vaccine virus, Croatia, 2005–2008. *Euro Surveill* 2008;13:18843.
210. Kakakios AM, Burgess MA, Bransby RD, et al. Optimal age for measles and mumps vaccination in Australia. *Med J Aust* 1990;152:472–474.
211. Kanra G, Isik P, Kara A, et al. Complementary findings in clinical and epidemiologic features of mumps and mumps meningoencephalitis in children without mumps vaccination. *Pediatr Int* 2004;46:663–668.
212. Kaplan KM, Marder DC, Cochi SL, et al. Mumps in the workplace. Further evidence of the changing epidemiology of a childhood vaccine-preventable disease. *JAMA* 1988;260:1434–1438.
213. Katoh H, Kubota T, Nakatsu Y, et al. Heat shock protein 90 ensures efficient mumps virus replication by assisting with viral polymerase complex formation. *J Virol* 2017;91:e02220.
214. Katoh H, Nakatsu Y, Kubota T, et al. Mumps virus is released from the apical surface of polarized epithelial cells, and the release is facilitated by a Rab11-mediated transport system. *J Virol* 2015;89:12026–12034.
215. Katoh H, Sekizuka T, Nakatsu Y, et al. The R2TP complex regulates paramyxovirus RNA synthesis. *PLoS Pathog* 2019;15:e1007749.
216. Ki M, Park T, Yi SG, et al. Risk analysis of aseptic meningitis after measles-mumps-rubella vaccination in Korean children by using a case-crossover design. *Am J Epidemiol* 2003;157:158–165.
217. Kilham L. Isolation of mumps virus from the blood of a patient. *Proc Soc Exp Biol Med* 1948;69:99.
218. Kilham L. Mumps meningoencephalitis with and without parotitis. *Am J Dis Child* 1949;78:324–333.
219. Kilham L. Mumps virus in human milk and in milk of infected monkey. *J Am Med Assoc* 1951;146:1231–1232.
220. Kilham L, Margolis G. Induction of congenital hydrocephalus in hamsters with attenuated and natural strains of mumps virus. *J Infect Dis* 1975;132:462–466.
221. Kilham L, Murphy HW. Propagation of mumps virus in suckling mice and in mouse embryo tissue cultures. *Exp Biol Med* 1952;80:495–498.
222. Kim-Farley R, Bart S, Stetler H, et al. Clinical mumps vaccine efficacy. *Am J Epidemiol* 1985;121:593–597.
223. Kimura M, Kuno-Sakai H, Yamazaki S, et al. Adverse events associated with MMR vaccines in Japan. *Pediatr Int* 1996;38:205–211.
224. Kingston RL, Baase WA, Gay LS. Characterization of nucleocapsid binding by the measles virus and mumps virus phosphoproteins. *J Virol* 2004;78:8630–8640.
225. Kingston RL, Gay LS, Baase WS, et al. Structure of the nucleocapsid-binding domain from the mumps virus polymerase; an example of protein folding induced by crystallization. *J Mol Biol* 2008;379:719–731.
226. Koplan JP, Preblud SR. A benefit-cost analysis of mumps vaccine. *Am J Dis Child* 1982;136:362–364.
227. Koskiniemi M, Donner M, Pettay O. Clinical appearance and outcome in mumps encephalitis in children. *Acta Paediatr Scand* 1983;72:603–609.
228. Kövamees J, Rydbeck R, Örvell C, et al. Hemagglutinin-neuraminidase (HN) amino acid alterations in neutralization escape mutants of Kilham mumps virus. *Virus Res* 1990;17:119–129.
229. Kozak M. A short leader sequence impairs the fidelity of initiation by eukaryotic ribosomes. *Gene Expr* 1991;1:111–115.
230. Kreth HW, Kress L, Kress HG, et al. Demonstration of primary cytotoxic T cells in venous blood and cerebrospinal fluid of children with mumps meningitis. *J Immunol* 1982;128:2411–2415.
231. Kubota M, Takeuchi K, Watanabe S, et al. Trisaccharide containing alpha2,3-linked sialic acid is a receptor for mumps virus. *Proc Natl Acad Sci U S A* 2016;113:11579–11584.
232. Kubota T, Yokosawa N, Yokota S, et al. C terminal CYS-RICH region of mumps virus structural V protein correlates with block of interferon alpha and gamma signal transduction pathway through decrease of STAT 1-alpha. *Biochem Biophys Res Commun* 2001;283:255–259.
233. Kuczyk MA, Denil J, Thon WF, et al. Orchitis following mumps vaccination in an adult. *Urol Int* 1994;53:179–180.
234. Kulkarni-Kale U, Ojha J, Manjari GS, et al. Mapping antigenic diversity and strain specificity of mumps virus: a bioinformatics approach. *Virology* 2007;359:436–446.
235. Kunkel U, Schreier E, Siegl G, et al. Molecular characterization of mumps virus strains circulating during an epidemic in eastern Switzerland 1992/93. *Arch Virol* 1994;136:433–438.
236. Kurtz JB, Tomlinson AH, Pearson J. Mumps virus isolated from a fetus. *Br Med J (Clin Res Ed)* 1982;284:471.
237. Kuske I, Karduck A, Bartholome W. Diagnostic value of nasopharyngeal endoscopy for the early recognition of tumours. *Endoscopy* 1977;9:199–202.
238. Lacour M, Maherzi M, Vienny H, et al. Thrombocytopenia in a case of neonatal mumps infection: evidence for further clinical presentations. *Eur J Pediatr* 1993;152:739–741.
239. Larke RP. Interferon in the cerebrospinal fluid of children with central nervous system disorders. *Can Med Assoc J* 1967;96:21–32.
240. Laurence D, McGavin D. The complications of mumps. *Br Med J* 1948;1:94–97.
241. Lavi S, Zimmerman B, Koren G, et al. Administration of measles, mumps, and rubella virus vaccine (live) to egg-allergic children. *JAMA* 1990;263:269–271.
242. Lawrence MC, Borg NA, Streltsov VA, et al. Structure of the haemagglutinin-neuraminidase from human parainfluenza virus type III. *J Mol Biol* 2004;335:1343–1357.
243. LeBaron CW, Forghani B, Beck C, et al. Persistence of mumps antibodies after 2 doses of measles-mumps-rubella vaccine. *J Infect Dis* 2009;199:552–560.
244. Leboreiro-Fernandez A, Moura-Ribeiro MVL, Leboreiro IEF, et al. Mumps meningoencephalitis: an epidemiological approach. *Arq Neuropsiquiatr* 1997;55:12–15.
245. Lee J-Y, Kim Y-Y, Shin G-C, et al. Molecular characterization of two genotypes of mumps virus circulated in Korea during 1998–2001. *Virus Res* 2003;97:111–116.
246. Levenbuk IS, Nikolayeva MA, Chigirinsky AE, et al. On the morphological evaluation of the neurovirulence safety of attenuated mumps virus strains in monkeys. *J Biol Stand* 1979;7:9–19.
247. Levine MI. A sponsored epidemic of mumps in a private school. *Am J Public Health Nations Health* 1944;34:1274–1276.
248. Levitt LP, Mahoney DH Jr, Casey HL, et al. Mumps in a general population. A sero-epidemiologic study. *Am J Dis Child* 1970;120:134–138.
249. Li M, Schmitt PT, Li Z, et al. Mumps virus matrix, fusion, and nucleocapsid proteins cooperate for efficient production of virus-like particles. *J Virol* 2009;83:7261–7272.
250. Liang Y, Ma S, Yang Z, et al. Immunogenicity and safety of a novel formalin-inactivated and alum-adjuvanted candidate subunit vaccine for mumps. *Vaccine* 2008;26:4276–4283.
251. Lindsay JR, Davey PR, Ward PH. LXVII inner ear pathology in deafness due to mumps. *Ann Otol Rhinol Laryngol* 1960;69:918–935.
252. Link H, Laurenzi MA, Frydén A. Viral antibodies in oligoclonal and polyclonal IgG synthesized within the central nervous system over the course of mumps meningitis. *J Neuroimmunol* 1981;1:287–298.
253. Litman N, Baum SG. Mumps virus. In: Mandell GL, Bennett JE, Donlin R, eds. *Principles and Practice of Infectious Diseases*. 7th ed. Philadelphia, PA: Churchill Livingstone: Elsevier; 2010:2201–2206.
254. Liu Y, Zhu J, Feng M-G, et al. Six-helix bundle assembly and analysis of the central core of mumps virus fusion protein. *Arch Biochem Biophys* 2004;421:143–148.
255. Lohr JM, Oldstone MBA. Detection of cytomegalovirus nucleic acid sequences in pancreas in type 2 diabetes. *Lancet* 1990;336:644–648.

256. London WT, Kent SG, Palmer AE, et al. Induction of congenital hydrocephalus with mumps virus in rhesus monkeys. *J Infect Dis* 1979;139:324–328.
257. Löve A, Rydbeck R, Utter G, et al. Monoclonal antibodies against the fusion protein are protective in necrotizing mumps meningoencephalitis. *J Virol* 1986;58:220–222.
258. Lu LL, Puri M, Horvath CM, et al. Select paramyxoviral V proteins inhibit IRF3 activation by acting as alternative substrates for inhibitor of kappaB kinase epsilon (IKKe)/TBK1. *J Biol Chem* 2008;283:14269–14276.
259. Ma R, Lu L, Zhou T, et al. Mumps disease in Beijing in the era of two-dose vaccination policy, 2005–2016. *Vaccine* 2018;36:2589–2595.
260. Magurano F, Baggieri M, Marchi A, et al. Mumps clinical diagnostic uncertainty. *Eur J Public Health* 2018;28:119–123.
261. Makino S, Sasaki K, Nakayama T, et al. A new combined trivalent live measles (AIK-C strain), mumps (Hoshino strain), and rubella (Takahashi strain) vaccine. Findings in clinical and laboratory studies. *Am J Dis Child* 1990;144:905–910.
262. Malik T, Ngo L, Bosma T, et al. A single point mutation in the mumps V protein alters targeting of the cellular STAT pathways resulting in virus attenuation. *Viruses* 2019;11:1016.
263. Marin M, Broder KR, Temte JL, et al.; Centers for Disease Control and Prevention. Use of combination measles, mumps, rubella, and varicella vaccine: recommendations of the Advisory Committee on Immunization Practices (ACIP). *MMWR Recomm Rep* 2010;59:1–12.
264. Marin M, Quinlisk P, Shimabukuro T, et al. Mumps vaccination coverage and vaccine effectiveness in a large outbreak among college students—Iowa, 2006. *Vaccine* 2008;26:3601–3607.
265. Maris EP, Enders JF, Stokes J, et al. Immunity in mumps: IV. The correlation of the presence of complement-fixing antibody and resistance to mumps in human beings. *J Exp Med* 1946;84:323–339.
266. Maruyama H. Reports on aseptic meningitis after MMR vaccination. *Clin Virol* 1994;22:77–82.
267. Maynard JE, Shramek G, Noble GR, et al. Use of attenuated live mumps virus vaccine during a "virgin soil" epidemic of mumps on St. Paul Island, Alaska. *Am J Epidemiol* 1970;92:301–306.
268. McAleer B, Rima B. Cloning and secreted expression of the extracellular domain of the mumps virus fusion protein in Pichia pastoris. *Virus Genes* 2000;20:127–133.
269. McCarthy M, Johnson RT. Morphological heterogeneity in relation to structural and functional properties of mumps virus. *J Gen Virol* 1980;48:395–399.
270. McCarthy M, Lazzarini RA. Intracellular nucleocapsid RNA of mumps virus. *J Gen Virol* 1982;58:205–209.
271. McFarland E. Immunizations for the immunocompromised child. *Pediatr Ann* 1999;28:487–496.
272. McGuiness AC, Gall EA. Mumps at army camps in 1943. *War Med* 1944;5:95–104.
273. McKenna MJ. Measles, mumps, and sensorineural hearing loss. *Ann N Y Acad Sci* 1997;830:291–298.
274. McNabb SJ, Jajosky RA, Hall-Baker PA, et al. Summary of notifiable diseases—United States, 2005. *MMWR Morb Mortal Wkly Rep* 2007;54:1–92.
275. McNabb SJ, Jajosky RA, Hall-Baker PA, et al. Summary of notifiable diseases–United States, 2006. *MMWR Morb Mortal Wkly Rep* 2008;55:1–92.
276. Merz DC, Server AC, Waxham MN, et al. Biosynthesis of mumps virus F glycoprotein: non-fusing strains efficiently cleave the F glycoprotein precursor. *J Gen Virol* 1983;64:1457–1467.
277. Meyer MB. An epidemiologic study of mumps, its spread in schools and families. *Am J Epidemiol* 1962;75:259–281.
278. Meyer HM, Johnson RT, Crawford IP, et al. Central nervous system syndromes of "viral" etiology. *Am J Med* 1960;29:334–347.
279. Meyer MB, Stifler WC, Joseph JM. Evaluation of mumps vaccine given after exposure to mumps, with special reference to the exposed adult. *Pediatrics* 1966;37:304–315.
280. Miller E, Andrews N, Stowe J, et al. Risks of convulsion and aseptic meningitis following measles-mumps-rubella vaccination in the United Kingdom. *Am J Epidemiol* 2007;165:704–709.
281. Miller E, Hill A, Morgan-Capner P, et al. Antibodies to measles, mumps and rubella in UK children 4 years after vaccination with different MMR vaccines. *Vaccine* 1995;13:799–802.
282. Miller C, Miller E, Rowe K, et al. Surveillance of symptoms following MMR vaccine in children. *Practitioner* 1989;233:69–73.
283. Mizushima N, Murakami Y. Deafness following mumps: the possible pathogenesis and incidence of deafness. *Auris Nasus Larynx* 1986;13:S55–S57.
284. Modlin JF, Orenstein WA, David Brandling-Bennett A. Current status of mumps in the United States. *J Infect Dis* 1975;132:106–109.
285. Morgan HR, Enders JF, Wagley PF. A hemolysin associated with the mumps virus. *J Exp Med* 1948;88:503–514.
286. Morishima T, Miyazu M, Ozaki T, et al. Local immunity in mumps meningitis. *Am J Dis Child* 1980;134:1060–1064.
287. Morrison TG. Structure and function of a paramyxovirus fusion protein. *Biochim Biophys Acta* 2003;1614:73–84.
288. Mortimer PP. Mumps prophylaxis in the light of a new test for antibody. *Br Med J* 1978;2:1523–1524.
289. Mortlock M, Dietrich M, Weyer J, et al. Co-circulation and excretion dynamics of diverse rubula- and related viruses in Egyptian rousette bats from South Africa. *Viruses* 2019;11.
290. Mühlemann K. The molecular epidemiology of mumps virus. *Infect Genet Evol* 2004;4:215–219.
291. Mumps virus nomenclature update: 2012. *Wkly Epidemiol Rec* 2012;87:217–224.
292. Nagai T, Nakayama T. Mumps vaccine virus genome is present in throat swabs obtained from uncomplicated healthy recipients. *Vaccine* 2001;19:1353–1355.
293. Nagai T, Okafuji T, Miyazaki C, et al. A comparative study of the incidence of aseptic meningitis in symptomatic natural mumps patients and monovalent mumps vaccine recipients in Japan. *Vaccine* 2007;25:2742–2747.
294. Nakayama T, Oka S, Komase K, et al. The relationship between the mumps vaccine strain and parotitis after vaccination. *J Infect Dis* 1992;165:186–187.
295. Nakayama T, Urano T, Osano M, et al. Evaluation of live trivalent vaccine of measles AIK-C strain, mumps Hoshino strain and rubella Takahashi strain, by virus-specific interferon-γ production and antibody response. *Microbiol Immunol* 1990;34:497–508.
296. Narita M, Matsuzono Y, Takekoshi Y, et al. Analysis of mumps vaccine failure by means of avidity testing for mumps virus-specific immunoglobulin G. *Clin Diagn Lab Immunol* 1998;5:799–803.
297. Naruse H, Nagai Y, Yoshida T, et al. The polypeptides of mumps virus and their synthesis in infected chick embryo cells. *Virology* 1981;112:119–130.
298. Ni J, Bowles NE, Kim Y-H, et al. Viral infection of the myocardium in endocardial fibroelastosis. *Circulation* 1997;95:133–139.
299. Nicolai-Scholten ME, Ziegelmaier R, Behrens F, et al. The enzyme-linked immunosorbent assay (ELISA) for determination of IgG and IgM antibodies after infection with mumps virus. *Med Microbiol Immunol* 1980;168:81–90.
300. Nicolle C, Conseil E. Essai de reproduction experimentale des oreillons chez le singe. *Compt Rend Soc de Biol* 1913;75:217.
301. Nielsen LE, Kelly DC, Gyorffy J, et al. Mumps outbreak and MMR IgG surveillance as a predictor for immunity in military trainees. *Vaccine* 2019;37:6139–6143.
302. Nishio M, Garcin D, Simonet V, et al. The carboxyl segment of the mumps virus V protein associates with STAT proteins in vitro via a tryptophan-rich motif. *Virology* 2002;300:92–99.
303. Nokes DJ, Wright J, Morgan-Capner P, et al. Serological study of the epidemiology of mumps virus infection in north-west England. *Epidemiol Infect* 1990;105:175–195.
304. Nussinovitch M, Brand N, Frydman M, et al. Transverse myelitis following mumps in children. *Acta Paediatr* 1992;81:183–184.
305. Odisseev H, Gacheva N. Vaccinoprophylaxis of mumps using mumps vaccine, strain Sofia 6, in Bulgaria. *Vaccine* 1994;12:1251–1254.
306. Ogata H, Oka K, Mitsudome A. Hydrocephalus due to acute aqueductal stenosis following mumps infection: report of a case and review of the literature. *Brain Dev* 1992;14:417–419.
307. Ohta K, Matsumoto Y, Ito M, et al. Tetherin antagonism by V proteins is a common trait among the genus Rubulavirus. *Med Microbiol Immunol* 2017;206:319–326.
308. Okazaki K, Tanabayashi K, Takeuchi K, et al. Molecular cloning and sequence analysis of the mumps virus gene encoding the L protein and the trailer sequence. *Virology* 1992;188:926–930.
309. Okuno Y, Asada T, Yamanishi K, et al. Studies on the use of mumps virus for treatment of human cancer. *Biken J* 1978;21:37–49.
310. Ong G, Goh KT, Ma S, et al. Comparative efficacy of Rubini, Jeryl–Lynn and Urabe mumps vaccine in an Asian population. *J Infect* 2005;51:294–298.
311. Orlikova H, Maly M, Lexova P, et al. Protective effect of vaccination against mumps complications, Czech Republic, 2007–2012. *BMC Public Health* 2016;16:293.
312. Orvell C. Immunological properties of purified mumps virus glycoproteins. *J Gen Virol* 1978;41:517–526.
313. Orvell C. The reactions of monoclonal antibodies with structural proteins of mumps virus. *J Immunol* 1984;132:2622–2629.
314. Orvell C, Alsheikhly AR, Johansson B, et al. Characterization of genotype-specific epitopes of the HN protein of mumps virus. *J Gen Virol* 1997;78:3187–3193.
315. Overman JR. Viremia in human mumps virus infections. *AMA Arch Intern Med* 1958;102:354–356.
316. Overman JR, Peers JH, Kilham L. Pathology of mumps virus meningoencephalitis in mice and hamsters. *AMA Arch Pathol* 1953;55:457–465.
317. Palihawadana P, Jayaratne IL, Wijemunige N. An outbreak of mumps in Dompe. *Ceylon Med J* 2007;52:35–36.
318. Patel LN, Arciuolo RJ, Fu J, et al. Mumps outbreak among a highly vaccinated university community-New York City, January-April 2014. *Clin Infect Dis* 2017;64:408–412.
319. Paterson RG, Lamb RA. RNA editing by G-nucleotide insertion in mumps virus P-gene mRNA transcripts. *J Virol* 1990;64:4137–4145.
320. Pei Z, Bai Y, Schmitt AP. PIV5 M protein interaction with host protein angiomotin-like 1. *Virology* 2010;397:155–166.
321. Pei Z, Harrison MS, Schmitt AP. Parainfluenza virus 5 M protein interaction with host protein 14-3-3 negatively affects virus particle formation. *J Virol* 2011;85:2050–2059.
322. Peltola H, Davidkin I, Paunio M, et al. Mumps and rubella eliminated from Finland. *JAMA* 2000;284:2643–2647.
323. Peltola H, Jokinen S, Paunio M, et al. Measles, mumps, and rubella in Finland: 25 years of a nationwide elimination programme. *Lancet Infect Dis* 2008;8:796–803.
324. Pentecost M, Vashisht AA, Lester T, et al. Evidence for ubiquitin-regulated nuclear and subnuclear trafficking among Paramyxovirinae matrix proteins. *PLoS Pathog* 2015;11:e1004739.
325. Penttinen K, Cantell K, Somer P, et al. Mumps vaccination in the Finnish defense forces. *Am J Epidemiol* 1968;88:234–244.
326. Permar SR, Klumpp SA, Mansfield KG, et al. Role of CD8(+) lymphocytes in control and clearance of measles virus infection of rhesus monkeys. *J Virol* 2003;77:4396–4400.
327. Perry KR, Brown DW, Parry JV, et al. Detection of measles, mumps, and rubella antibodies in saliva using antibody capture radioimmunoassay. *J Med Virol* 1993;40:235–240.
328. Philip RN, Reinhard KR, Lackman DB. Observations on a mumps epidemic in a virgin population. *Am J Hyg* 1959;69:91–111.
329. Pickar A, Elson A, Yang Y, et al. Oligomerization of mumps virus phosphoprotein. *J Virol* 2015;89:11002–11010.
330. Pickar A, Xu P, Elson A, et al. Roles of serine and threonine residues of mumps virus P protein in viral transcription and replication. *J Virol* 2014;88:4414–4422.
331. Pickar A, Xu P, Elson A, et al. Establishing a small animal model for evaluating protective immunity against mumps virus. *PLoS One* 2017;12:e0174444.
332. Pickar A, Zengel J, Xu P, et al. Mumps virus nucleoprotein enhances phosphorylation of the phosphoprotein by polo-like kinase 1. *J Virol* 2016;90:1588–1598.
333. Plans P. Prevalence of antibodies associated with herd immunity: a new indicator to evaluate the establishment of herd immunity and to decide immunization strategies. *Med Decis Making* 2010;30:438–443.

334. Plotkin SA, Rubin SA. *Mumps Vaccine*. 5th ed. Philadelphia, PA: Saunders Elsevier; 2008.
335. Poch O, Blumberg BM, Bougueleret L, et al. Sequence comparison of five polymerases (L proteins) of unsegmented negative-strand RNA viruses: theoretical assignment of functional domains. *J Gen Virol* 1990;71:1153–1162.
336. Polgreen PM, Bohnett LC, Cavanaugh JE, et al. The duration of mumps virus shedding after the onset of symptoms. *Clin Infect Dis* 2008;46:1447–1449.
337. Ponka A, Pettersson T. The incidence and aetiology of central nervous system infections in Helsinki in 1980. *Acta Neurol Scand* 1982;66:529–535.
338. Pons C, Pelayo T, Pachon I, et al. Two outbreaks of mumps in children vaccinated with the Rubini strain in Spain indicate low vaccine efficacy. *Euro Surveill* 2000;5:80–84.
339. Popow-Kraupp T, Kundi M, Ambrosch F, et al. A controlled trial for evaluating two live attenuated mumps-measles vaccines (Urabe Am 9-Schwarz and Jeryl Lynn-Moraten) in young children. *J Med Virol* 1986;18:69–79.
340. Porotto M, Murrell M, Greengard O, et al. Inhibition of parainfluenza virus type 3 and Newcastle disease virus hemagglutinin-neuraminidase receptor binding: effect of receptor avidity and steric hindrance at the inhibitor binding sites. *J Virol* 2004;78:13911–13919.
341. Pospisil L, Brycthova J. Adaptation of the mumps virus to the albino rat (Wistar). *Zentralbl Bakteriol Parasitenkd Infektionskr Hyg* 1956;165:1–8.
342. Powell HM, Culbertson CG. Detection of mumps virus in mice sacrificed at different periods of time after injection. *Proc Soc Exp Biol Med* 1949;72:145–147.
343. Puri M, Lemon K, Duprex WP, et al. A point mutation, E95D, in the mumps virus V protein disengages STAT3 targeting from STAT1 targeting. *J Virol* 2009;83:6347–6356.
344. Ramachandran A, Horvath CM. Dissociation of paramyxovirus interferon evasion activities: universal and virus-specific requirements for conserved V protein amino acids in MDA5 interference. *J Virol* 2010;84:11152–11163.
345. Rasheed MAU, Hickman CJ, McGrew M, et al. Decreased humoral immunity to mumps in young adults immunized with MMR vaccine in childhood. *Proc Natl Acad Sci U S A* 2019;116:19071–19076.
346. Ray G, Schmitt PT, Schmitt AP. Angiomotin-like 1 links paramyxovirus M proteins to NEDD4 family ubiquitin ligases. *Viruses* 2019;11:128.
347. Reed D, Brown G, Merrick R, et al. A mumps epidemic on St. George Island, Alaska. *JAMA* 1967;199:113–117.
348. Ritter BS. Mumps meningoencephalitis in children. *J Pediatr* 1958;52:424–433.
349. Roberts C, Porter-Jones G, Crocker J, et al. Mumps outbreak on the island of Anglesey, North Wales, December 2008-January 2009. *Euro Surveill* 2009;14:19109.
350. Rola-Pleszczynski M, Vincent MM, Hensen SA, et al. ^{51}Chromium-release microassay technique for cell-mediated immunity to mumps virus: correlation with humoral and delayed-type skin hypersensitivity responses. *J Infect Dis* 1976;134:546–551.
351. Rota JS, Rosen JB, Doll MK, et al. Comparison of the sensitivity of laboratory diagnostic methods from a well-characterized outbreak of mumps in New York city in 2009. *Clin Vaccine Immunol* 2013;20:391–396.
352. Rota JS, Turner JC, Yost-Daljev MK, et al. Investigation of a mumps outbreak among university students with two measles-mumps-rubella (MMR) vaccinations, Virginia, September-December 2006. *J Med Virol* 2009;81:1819–1825.
353. Rozina EE, Hilgenfeldt M. Comparative study on the neurovirulence of different vaccine strains of parotitis virus in monkeys. *Acta Virol* 1985;29:225–230.
354. Rozina EE, Kaptsova TI, Sharova OK, et al. Study of mumps virus invasiveness in monkeys. *Acta Virol* 1984;28:107–113.
355. Rubin SA, Afzal MA. Neurovirulence safety testing of mumps vaccines—Historical perspective and current status. *Vaccine* 2011;29:2850–2855.
356. Rubin SA, Amexis G, Pletnikov M, et al. Changes in mumps virus gene sequence associated with variability in neurovirulent phenotype. *J Virol* 2003;77:11616–11624.
357. Rubin SA, Link MA, Sauder CJ, et al. Recent mumps outbreaks in vaccinated populations: no evidence of immune escape. *J Virol* 2012;86:615–620.
358. Rubin S, Mauldin J, Chumakov K, et al. Serological and phylogenetic evidence of monotypic immune responses to different mumps virus strains. *Vaccine* 2006;24:2662–2668.
359. Rubin SA, Pletnikov M, Carbone KM. Comparison of the neurovirulence of a vaccine and a wild-type mumps virus strain in the developing rat brain. *J Virol* 1998;72:8037–8042.
360. Rubin SA, Pletnikov M, Taffs R, et al. Evaluation of a neonatal rat model for prediction of mumps virus neurovirulence in humans. *J Virol* 2000;74:5382–5384.
361. Rubin SA, Qi L, Audet SA, et al. Antibody induced by immunization with the Jeryl Lynn mumps vaccine strain effectively neutralizes a heterologous wild-type mumps virus associated with a large outbreak. *J Infect Dis* 2008;198:508–515.
362. Saika S, Kidokoro M, Ohkawa T, et al. Pathogenicity of mumps virus in the marmoset. *J Med Virol* 2001;66:115–122.
363. Saito H, Takahashi Y, Harata S, et al. Isolation and characterization of mumps virus strains in a mumps outbreak with a high incidence of aseptic meningitis. *Microbiol Immunol* 1996;40:271–275.
364. Sane J, Gouma S, Koopmans M, et al. Epidemic of mumps among vaccinated persons, The Netherlands, 2009–2012. *Emerg Infect Dis* 2014;20:643–648.
365. Sauder CJ, Zhang CX, Link MA, et al. Presence of lysine at aa 335 of the hemagglutinin-neuraminidase protein of mumps virus vaccine strain Urabe AM9 is not a requirement for neurovirulence. *Vaccine* 2009;27:5822–5829.
366. Sawada H, Yano S, Oka Y, et al. Transmission of Urabe mumps vaccine between siblings. *Lancet* 1993;342:371.
367. Schlegel M, Osterwalder JJ, Galeazzi RL, et al. Comparative efficacy of three mumps vaccines during disease outbreak in Eastern Switzerland: cohort study. *BMJ* 1999;319:352.
368. Schmitt PT, Ray G, Schmitt AP. The C-terminal end of parainfluenza virus 5 NP protein is important for virus-like particle production and M-NP protein interaction. *J Virol* 2010;84:12810–12823.
369. Schneider R, Reinau D, Schur N, et al. Coverage rates and timeliness of nationally recommended vaccinations in Swiss preschool children: a descriptive analysis using claims data. *Vaccine* 2020;38:1551–1558.
370. Schoub BD, Path MRC, Johnson S, et al. Measles, mumps and rubella immunization at nine months in a developing country. *Pediatr Infect Dis J* 1990;9:263–267.
371. Schulz B, Michaelis D, Hildmann W, et al. Islet cell surface antibodies (ICSA) in subjects with a previous mumps infection—a prospective study over a 4 year period. *Exp Clin Endocrinol* 1987;90:62–70.
372. Schwarz NG, Bernard H, Melnic A, et al. Mumps outbreak in the Republic of Moldova, 2007–2008. *Pediatr Infect Dis J* 2010;29:703–706.
373. Scully C, Eckersall PD, Emond RTD, et al. Serum α-amylase isozymes in mumps: estimation of salivary and pancreatic isozymes by isoelectric focusing. *Clin Chim Acta* 1981;113:281–291.
374. Seither R, McGill MT, Kriss JL, et al. Vaccination coverage with selected vaccines and exemption rates among children in kindergarten—United States, 2019–20 school year. *MMWR Morb Mortal Wkly Rep* 2021;70:75–82.
375. Server AC, Merz DC, Waxham MN, et al. Differentiation of mumps virus strains with monoclonal antibody to the HN glycoprotein. *Infect Immun* 1982;35:179–186.
376. Shah D, Vidal S, Link MA, et al. Identification of genetic mutations associated with attenuation and changes in tropism of Urabe mumps virus. *J Med Virol* 2008;81:130–138.
377. Shulman A, Shohat B, Gillis D, et al. Mumps orchitis among soldiers: frequency, effect on sperm quality, and sperm antibodies. *Fertil Steril* 1992;57:1344–1346.
378. Sidhu MS, Menonna JP, Cook SD, et al. Canine distemper virus L gene: sequence and comparison with related viruses. *Virology* 1993;193:50–65.
379. Slater PE, Anis E, Leventhal A. The control of mumps in Israel. *Eur J Epidemiol* 1999;15:765–767.
380. Smith GA, Gussen R. Inner ear pathologic features following mumps infection: report of a case in an adult. *Arch Otolaryngol Head Neck Surg* 1976;102:108–111.
381. Smorodintsev AA, Klyatchko NS. Live anti-mumps vaccine. I. Results of tests of the immunogenic properties of live vaccine when administered intradermally to susceptible children. *Acta Virol* 1958;2:137–144.
382. Somboonthum P, Yoshii H, Okamoto S, et al. Generation of a recombinant Oka varicella vaccine expressing mumps virus hemagglutinin-neuraminidase protein as a polyvalent live vaccine. *Vaccine* 2007;25:8741–8755.
383. Sosin DM, Cochi SL, Gunn RA, et al. Changing epidemiology of mumps and its impact on university campuses. *Pediatrics* 1989;84:779–784.
384. Spanaki A, Hajiioannou J, Varkarakis G, et al. Mumps epidemic among young british citizens on the island of Crete. *Infection* 2007;35:104–106.
385. St Geme JWS, Peralta H, Van Pelt LF. Intrauterine infection of the rhesus monkey with mumps virus: abbreviated viral replication in the immature fetus as an explanation for split immunologic recognition after birth. *J Infect Dis* 1972;126:249–256.
386. Stinnett RC, Beck AS, Lopareva EN, et al. Functional characterization of circulating mumps viruses with stop codon mutations in the small hydrophobic protein. *mSphere* 2020;5:e00840.
387. Stratton KR. Adverse events associated with childhood vaccines other than pertussis and rubella. *JAMA* 1994;271:1602.
388. Sugg WC, Finger JA, Levine RH, et al. Field evaluation of live virus mumps vaccine. *J Pediatr* 1968;72:461–466.
389. Sullivan KM, Halpin TJ, Kim-Farley R, et al. Mumps disease and its health impact: an outbreak-based report. *Pediatrics* 1985;76:533–536.
390. Sun M, Fuentes SM, Timani K, et al. Akt plays a critical role in replication of nonsegmented negative-stranded RNA viruses. *J Virol* 2008;82:105–114.
391. Sun D, Luthra P, Li Z, et al. PLK1 down-regulates parainfluenza virus 5 gene expression. *PLoS Pathog* 2009;5:e1000525.
392. Takahashi Y, Teranishi A, Yamada Y, et al. A case of congenital mumps infection complicated with persistent pulmonary hypertension. *Am J Perinatol* 1998;15:409–412.
393. Takano T, Mekata Y, Yamano T, et al. Early ependymal changes in experimental hydrocephalus after mumps virus inoculation in hamsters. *Acta Neuropathol* 1993;85:521–525.
394. Takano T, Takikita S, Shimada M. Experimental mumps virus-induced hydrocephalus. *NeuroReport* 1999;10:2215–2221.
395. Takano T, Uno M, Yamano T, et al. Pathogenesis of cerebellar deformity in experimental Chiari type I malformation caused by mumps virus. *Acta Neuropathol* 1994;87:168–173.
396. Takeuchi K, Tanabayashi K, Hishiyama M, et al. The mumps virus SH protein is a membrane protein and not essential for virus growth. *Virology* 1996;225:156–162.
397. Takeuchi K, Tanabayashi K, Hishiyama M, et al. Variations of nucleotide sequences and transcription of the SH gene among mumps virus strains. *Virology* 1991;181:364–366.
398. Takikita S, Takano T, Narita T, et al. Neuronal apoptosis mediated by IL-1 beta expression in viral encephalitis caused by a neuroadapted strain of the mumps virus (Kilham Strain) in hamsters. *Exp Neurol* 2001;172:47–59.
399. Tanabayashi K, Takeuchi K, Hishiyama M, et al. Nucleotide sequence of the leader and nucleocapsid protein gene of mumps virus and epitope mapping with the in vitro expressed nucleocapsid protein. *Virology* 1990;177:124–130.
400. Tanabayashi K, Takeuchi K, Okazaki K, et al. Expression of mumps virus glycoproteins in mammalian cells from cloned cDNAs: both F and HN proteins are required for cell fusion. *Virology* 1992;187:801–804.
401. Taylor FB. Primary mumps meningo-encephalitis. *Arch Intern Med* 1963;112:216.
402. Tecle T, Johansson B, Yun Z, et al. Antigenic and genetic characterization of the fusion (F) protein of mumps virus strains. *Arch Virol* 2000;145:1199–1210.
403. Ternavasio-de la Vega H-G, Boronat M, Ojeda A, et al. Mumps orchitis in the post-vaccine era (1967–2009). *Medicine* 2010;89:96–116.
404. Tešović G, Poljak M, Lunar MM, et al. Horizontal transmission of the Leningrad–Zagreb mumps vaccine strain: a report of three cases. *Vaccine* 2008;26:1922–1925.
405. Thompson JA, Glasgow LA. Intrauterine viral infection and the cell-mediated immune response. *Neurology* 1980;30:212–215.
406. Tillieux SL, Halsey WS, Sathe GM, et al. Comparative analysis of the complete nucleotide sequences of measles, mumps, and rubella strain genomes contained in Priorix-Tetra™ and ProQuad™ live attenuated combined vaccines. *Vaccine* 2009;27:2265–2273.
407. Timmons GD, Johnson KP. Aqueductal stenosis and hydrocephalus after mumps encephalitis. *N Engl J Med* 1970;283:1505–1507.

408. Toovey S, Jamieson A. Pancreatitis complicating adult immunisation with a combined mumps measles rubella vaccine. A case report and literature review. *Travel Med Infect Dis* 2003;1:189–192.

409. Tsurudome M, Yamada A, Hishiyama M, et al. Monoclonal antibodies against the glycoproteins of mumps virus: fusion inhibition by anti-HN monoclonal antibody. *J Gen Virol* 1986;67:2259–2265.

410. Tsurudome M, Yamada A, Hishiyama M, et al. Replication of mumps virus in mouse: transient replication in lung and potential of systemic infection. *Arch Virol* 1987;97:167–179.

411. Uchida K, Shinohara M, Shimada S-i, et al. Characterization of the F gene of contemporary mumps virus strains isolated in Japan. *Microbiol Immunol* 2003;47:167–172.

412. Ueda K, Miyazaki C, Hidaka Y, et al. Aseptic meningitis caused by measles-mumps-rubella vaccine in Japan. *Lancet* 1995;346:701–702.

413. Ueo A, Kubota M, Shirogane Y, et al. Lysosome-associated membrane proteins support the furin-mediated processing of the mumps virus fusion protein. *J Virol* 2020;94:e00050.

414. Ukkonen P, Penttinen K, Granström M-L. Mumps-specific immunoglobulin M and G antibodies in natural mumps infection as measured by enzyme-linked immunosorbent assay. *J Med Virol* 1981;8:131–142.

415. Ulane CM, Kentsis A, Cruz CD, et al. Composition and assembly of STAT-targeting ubiquitin ligase complexes: paramyxovirus V protein carboxyl terminus is an oligomerization domain. *J Virol* 2005;79:10180–10189.

416. Ulane CM, Rodriguez JJ, Parisien J-P, et al. STAT3 ubiquitylation and degradation by mumps virus suppress cytokine and oncogene signaling. *J Virol* 2003;77:6385–6393.

417. Unal M, Katircioglu S, Can Karatay M, et al. Sudden total bilateral deafness due to asymptomatic mumps infection. *Int J Pediatr Otorhinolaryngol* 1998;45:167–169.

418. Usonis V, Bakasenas V, Chitour K, et al. Comparative study of reactogenicity and immunogenicity of new and established measles, mumps and rubella vaccines in healthy children. *Infection* 1998;26:222–226.

419. Utz JP, Houk VN, Alling DW. Clinical and laboratory studies of mumps. IV. Viruria and abnormal renal function. *N Engl J Med* 1964;270:1283–1286.

420. Utz JP, Szwed CF. Mumps III. Comparison of methods for detection of viruria. *Exp Biol Med* 1962;110:841–844.

421. Utz JP, Szwed CF, Kasel JA. Clinical and laboratory studies of mumps II. Detection and duration of excretion of virus in urine. *Exp Biol Med* 1958;99:259–261.

422. van Loon FP, Holmes SJ, Sirotkin BI, et al. Mumps surveillance—United States, 1988–1993. *MMWR CDC Surveill Summ* 1995;44:1–14.

423. Vaheri A, Julkunen I, Koskiniemi ML. Chronic encephalomyelitis with specific increase in intrathecal mumps antibodies. *Lancet (London, England)* 1982;2:685–688.

424. Vaidya SR, Dvivedi GM, Jadhav SM. Cross-neutralization between three mumps viruses & mapping of haemagglutinin-neuraminidase (HN) epitopes. *Indian J Med Res* 2016;143:37–42.

425. Vandermeulen C, Roelants M, Vermoere M, et al. Outbreak of mumps in a vaccinated child population: a question of vaccine failure? *Vaccine* 2004;22:2713–2716.

426. Vandvik B, Nilsen RE, Vartdal F, et al. Mumps meningitis: Specific and non-specific antibody responses in the central nervous system. *Acta Neurol Scand* 1982;65:468–487.

427. Vandvik B, Norrby E, Steen-Johnsen J, et al. Mumps meningitis: Prolonged pleocytosis and occurrence of mumps virus-specific oligoclonal IgG in the cerebrospinal fluid. *Eur Neurol* 1978;17:13–22.

428. Vermeire T, Barbezange C, Francart A, et al. Sera from different age cohorts in Belgium show limited cross neutralization between the mumps vaccine and outbreak strains. *Clin Microbiol Infect* 2019;25:907.e1–907.e6.

429. von Messling V, Milosevic D, Devaux P, et al. Canine distemper virus and measles virus fusion glycoprotein trimers: partial membrane-proximal ectodomain cleavage enhances function. *J Virol* 2004;78:7894–7903.

430. Vukić BT, Pavić I, Milotić I, et al. Aseptic meningitis after transmission of the Leningrad–Zagreb mumps vaccine from vaccinee to susceptible contact. *Vaccine* 2008;26:4879.

431. Vuori M, Lahikainen EA, Peltonen T. Perceptive deafness in connection with mumps: a study of 298 servicemen suffering from mumps. *Acta Otolaryngol* 1962;55:231–236.

432. Vuorinen T, Nikolakaros G, Smell O, et al. Mumps and coxsackie B3 virus infection of human fetal pancreatic islet-like cell clusters. *Pancreas* 1992;7:460–464.

433. Vygen S, Fischer A, Meurice L, et al. Waning immunity against mumps in vaccinated young adults, France 2013. *Euro Surveill* 2016;21:30156.

434. Waddell DJ, Wilbur JR, Merigan TC. Interferon production in human mumps infections. *Exp Biol Med* 1968;127:320–324.

435. Wang F, Chen R, Jiang Q, et al. Roles of sialic acid, AXL, and MER receptor tyrosine kinases in mumps virus infection of mouse sertoli and leydig cells. *Front Microbiol* 2020;11:1292.

436. Ward BJ, Boulianne N, Ratnam S, et al. Cellular immunity in measles vaccine failure: demonstration of measles antigen-specific lymphoproliferative responses despite limited serum antibody production after revaccination. *J Infect Dis* 1995;172:1591–1595.

437. Watson JC, Hadler SC, Dykewicz CA, et al. Measles, mumps, and rubella—vaccine use and strategies for elimination of measles, rubella, and congenital rubella syndrome and control of mumps: recommendations of the Advisory Committee on Immunization Practices (ACIP). *MMWR Recomm Rep* 1998;47:1–57.

438. Waxham MN, Server AC, Goodman HM, et al. Cloning and sequencing of the mumps virus fusion protein gene. *Virology* 1987;159:381–388.

439. Waxham MN, Wolinsky JS. A fusing mumps virus variant selected from a nonfusing parent with the neuraminidase inhibitor 2-deoxy-2,3-dehydro-N-acetylneuraminic acid. *Virology* 1986;151:286–295.

440. Weibel RE, Stokes J, Buynak EB, et al. Live, attenuated mumps-virus vaccine. *N Engl J Med* 1967;276:245–251.

441. Weibel RE, Stokes J Jr, Buynak EB, et al. Jeryl Lynn strain live attenuated mumps virus vaccine. Durability of immunity following administration. *JAMA* 1968;203:14–18.

442. Weller TH, Craig JM. The isolation of mumps at autopsy. *Am J Pathol* 1949;25:1105–1115.

443. Weller TH, Enders JF. Production of hemagglutinin by mumps and influenza A viruses in suspended cell tissue cultures. *Exp Biol Med* 1948;69:124–128.

444. Westmore GA, Pickard BH, Stern H. Isolation of mumps virus from the inner ear after sudden deafness. *Br Med J* 1979;1:14–15.

445. Wharton M, Cochi SL, Hutcheson RH, et al. A large outbreak of mumps in the postvaccine era. *J Infect Dis* 1988;158:1253–1260.

446. Wilfert CM. Mumps meningoencephalitis with low cerebrospinal-fluid glucose, prolonged pleocytosis and elevation of protein. *N Engl J Med* 1969;280:855–859.

447. Wolinsky JS, Baringer JR, Margolis G, et al. Ultrastructure of mumps virus replication in newborn hamster central nervous system. *Lab Invest* 1974;31:403–412.

448. Wolinsky JS, Klassen T, Baringer JR. Persistence of neuroadapted mumps virus in brains of newborn hamsters after intraperitoneal inoculation. *J Infect Dis* 1976;133:260–267.

449. Wolinsky JS, Stroop WG. Virulence and persistence of three prototype strains of mumps virus in newborn hamsters. *Arch Virol* 1978;57:355–359.

450. Wolinsky JS, Waxham MN, Server AC. Protective effects of glycoprotein-specific monoclonal antibodies on the course of experimental mumps virus meningoencephalitis. *J Virol* 1985;53:727–734.

451. Wollstein M. An experimental study of parotitis (mumps). *J Exp Med* 1916;23:353–375.

452. Wolontis S, Bjorvatn B. Mumps meningoencephalitis in Stockholm November 1964—July 1971: II. Isolation attempts from the cerebrospinal fluid in a hospitalized study group. *Scand J Infect Dis* 1973;5:261–271.

453. World Health Organization. Mumps virus vaccines: WHO position paper. *Wkly Epidemiol Rec* 2001;76:346–355.

454. Woznik M, Rodner C, Lemon K, et al. Mumps virus small hydrophobic protein targets ataxin-1 ubiquitin-like interacting protein (ubiquilin 4). *J Gen Virol* 2010;91:2773–2781.

455. Wright KE, Dimock K, Brown EG. Biological characteristics of genetic variants of Urabe AM9 mumps vaccine virus. *Virus Res* 2000;67:49–57.

456. Xu P, Huang Z, Gao X, et al. Infection of mice, ferrets, and rhesus macaques with a clinical mumps virus isolate. *J Virol* 2013;87:8158–8168.

457. Xu P, Li Z, Sun D, et al. Rescue of wild-type mumps virus from a strain associated with recent outbreaks helps to define the role of the SH ORF in the pathogenesis of mumps virus. *Virology* 2011;417:126–136.

458. Xu P, Luthra P, Li Z, et al. The V protein of mumps virus plays a critical role in pathogenesis. *J Virol* 2012;86:1768–1776.

459. Yamada A, Takeuchi K, Tanabayashi K, et al. Sequence variation of the P gene among mumps virus strains. *Virology* 1989;172:374–376.

460. Yamauchi T, Wilson C, St. Geme JW. Transmission of live, attenuated mumps virus to the human placenta. *N Engl J Med* 1974;290:710–712.

461. Yates PJ, Afzal MA, Minor PD. Antigenic and genetic variation of the HN protein of mumps virus strains. *J Gen Virol* 1996;77:2491–2497.

462. Yeo RP, Afzal MA, Forsey T, et al. Identification of a new mumps virus lineage by nucleotide sequence analysis of the SH gene of ten different strains. *Arch Virol* 1993;128:371–377.

463. Ylinen O, Järvinen PA. Parotitis during pregnancy. *Acta Obstet Gynecol Scand* 1953;32:121–132.

464. Yokosawa N, Kubota T, Fujii N. Poor induction of interferon-induced 2′,5′-oligoadenylate synthetase (2–5 AS) in cells persistently infected with mumps virus is caused by decrease of STAT-1α. *Arch Virol* 1998;143:1985–1992.

465. Yokosawa N, Yokota S-I, Kubota T, et al. C-terminal region of STAT-1alpha is not necessary for its ubiquitination and degradation caused by mumps virus V protein. *J Virol* 2002;76:12683–12690.

466. Young ML, Dickstein B, Weibel RE, et al. Experiences with Jeryl Lynn strain live attenuated mumps virus vaccine in a pediatric outpatient clinic. *Pediatrics* 1967;40:798–803.

467. Yung CF, Andrews N, Bukasa A, et al. Mumps complications and effects of mumps vaccination, England and Wales, 2002–2006. *Emerg Infect Dis* 2011;17:661–667.

468. Yuzepchuk SA, Rozina EE, Kaptsova TI, et al. Morphological differences in the central nervous system and organs of monkeys inoculated intracerebrally with virulent and attenuated strains of mumps virus. *Acta Virol* 1975;19:305–310.

469. Zaitsev V, von Itzstein M, Groves D, et al. Second sialic acid binding site in Newcastle disease virus hemagglutinin-neuraminidase: implications for fusion. *J Virol* 2004;78:3733–3741.

470. Zengel J, Pickar A, Xu P, et al. Roles of phosphorylation of the nucleocapsid protein of mumps virus in regulating viral RNA transcription and replication. *J Virol* 2015;89:7338–7347.

471. Zhou F, Reef S, Massoudi M, et al. An economic analysis of the current universal 2-dose measles-mumps-rubella vaccination program in the United States. *J Infect Dis* 2004;189:S131–S145.

Measles Virus

Diane E. Griffin

History
Infectious agent
  Propagation and assay in cell culture
  Biological characteristics
  Evolution, antigenic composition, and strain variation
Pathogenesis and pathology
  Natural (wild type) measles
  Persistent infection
  Veterinary correlates
  Experimental infection in animals
Epidemiology
  Classic measles
  Subacute sclerosing panencephalitis
Clinical features
  Classic measles and its complications
  Atypical measles
  Measles in the immunocompromised host
  Subacute sclerosing panencephalitis
Diagnosis
  Isolation or detection of virus
  Detection of antibody
Prevention and control
  Treatment
  Prevention
  Prospects for eradication
Acknowledgments

Measles is a highly contagious disease characterized by a prodromal illness of fever, coryza, cough, and conjunctivitis followed by the appearance of a generalized maculopapular rash (Fig. 9.1). Introduction of measles into virgin populations and endemic transmission in populations with inadequate medical care is associated with high mortality. Despite the development of a successful live attenuated vaccine, measles remains a major cause of mortality in children, particularly in developing countries, and a cause of continuing outbreaks in industrialized nations.

HISTORY

Measles is a relatively new disease of humans and probably evolved from an animal morbillivirus. Phylogenetically, measles virus (MeV) is most closely related to rinderpest virus (RPV),

a pathogen of cattle (Fig. 9.2), and it is postulated that MeV evolved in an environment where cattle and humans lived in close proximity.[583] Phylogenetic analysis of the divergence of RPV and MeV is consistent with MeV emergence as early as the 6th century BCE in early centers of civilization where human populations attained sufficient densities to sustain continued transmission.[213]

Abu Becr, an Arab physician known as Rhazes of Baghdad, is generally credited with distinguishing smallpox from measles in the 9th century and dated its first description to the 6th century, but earlier "pestilence" descriptions likely include measles. Rhazes referred to measles as hasbah (eruption) and regarded it as a modification of smallpox with the distinction that "anxiety of mind, sick qualms and heaviness of heart oppress more in the measles than in the smallpox." Repeated epidemics of illnesses characterized by a rash are recorded in European and Far Eastern populations between 1 and 1,200, and it appears that measles spread across the Pyrenees into France with the Saracen invasion of the 8th century with epidemics identified as measles recorded in the 11th and 12th centuries and first mentioned as a childhood disease in 1224.

In the European literature, the name applied was "morbilli," derived from the Italian "little diseases" to distinguish it from plague, "il morbo," but morbilli included several exanthemata. Sanvages in 1763 defined morbilli as measles, but called it rubeola (derived from the Spanish), leading to a common confusion with rubella that persists to the present. Epidemics of rash illnesses were associated with episodes of depopulation in China, India, and the Mediterranean region, and introduction of measles into previously unexposed populations has been associated with high morbidity and mortality.[82,763,779] Approximately 56 million people died as a result of European exploration of the New World, largely due to the introduction into native Amerindian populations of Old World diseases, notably smallpox and measles. Decreases in population are likely to have facilitated the transfer of Spanish culture to South America.

Many of the basic principles of measles epidemiology were elucidated by Peter Panum, a Danish physician who worked in the Faroe Islands during a large measles epidemic in 1846.[628] Panum deduced the highly contagious nature of the disease, the 14-day incubation period, the lifelong immunity present in older residents, and postulated a respiratory route of transmission.

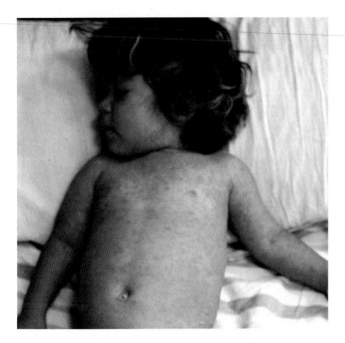

FIGURE 9.1 Typical maculopapular rash in a child with measles.

Complications of measles were first described in the 18th century. In 1790, James Lucas, an English surgeon, described post measles encephalomyelitis in a young woman who developed paraparesis as the rash was fading. Nineteenth century medical textbooks associated measles with the exacerbation of tuberculosis, and in 1908, while working at a tuberculosis hospital in Vienna, von Pirquet recorded the loss of delayed-type hypersensitivity skin test responses to tuberculin, the first experimental evidence of measles-induced immune suppression.

In 1933, Dawson described subacute sclerosing panencephalitis (SSPE) in a 16-year-old boy with progressive neurologic deterioration. Histologic examination of the brain showed

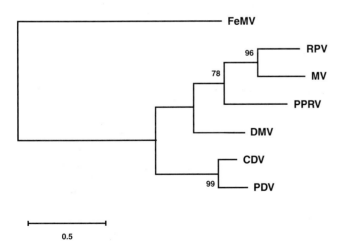

FIGURE 9.2 Maximum-likelihood phylogeny of the translated H gene of viruses in the genus Morbillivirus determined using MEGA-X software and applying the Whelan-and-Goldman substitution model and a complete deletion option. Numbers at nodes indicate support of grouping from 1,000 bootstrap replicates. Scale bar indicates substitutions per site. (Courtesy of Linda Murphy and Paul Duprex.)

eosinophilic intranuclear and intracytoplasmic inclusions in neurons and glial cells. After reports of paramyxovirus-like particles in the inclusions,[816] observations of elevated levels of MeV antibody in serum and cerebrospinal fluid (CSF) and the reactivity of the inclusions with antibody to MeV identified the paramyxovirus as MeV.[154]

INFECTIOUS AGENT

In 1757, an infectious agent was formally shown to be the cause of measles when the Scottish physician Francis Home, attempting immunization, transmitted the disease to naive individuals using blood taken from measles patients during the early stages of the rash. In 1905, Hektoen transmitted disease to volunteers with blood "free of bacteria" taken from measles cases in the acute stage and observed an incubation period of 13 days. In 1911, Goldberger and Anderson transmitted measles to rhesus macaques with filtered respiratory tract secretions from measles patients and successfully passaged disease from one monkey to another.

Propagation and Assay in Cell Culture
Primary Isolation
In 1954, Enders and Peebles first isolated MeV in tissue culture by inoculating primary human kidney cells with the blood of David Edmonston, a child with measles.[222] Isolates were also made using primary monkey kidney cells[222] and later continuous monkey kidney cell lines (e.g., Vero, CV-1).[790] However, isolation of wild-type strains of MeV is most often successful using an Epstein-Barr virus–transformed marmoset B lymphocyte line B95-8,[420] a human T-cell line from cord blood COBL-a,[419] or Vero cells engineered to express the human MeV receptor signaling lymphocyte activation molecule (SLAMF1).[618] Generally, the first observable sign of virus growth is cell–cell fusion and syncytia formation (Fig. 9.3).

Laboratory Propagation and Assay
Growth of MeV in cell culture enabled the development of live attenuated vaccine strains by adaptation of MeV to growth in cells from foreign hosts, such as the chick embryo and canine and bovine kidney cells.[402] Tissue culture–adapted strains are generally grown in Vero cells and wild-type strains in Vero/hSLAM cells using a low multiplicity of infection to avoid accumulation of defective interfering (DI) particles. Vero and Vero/hSLAM cells are also useful for virus titration by $TCID_{50}$ or plaque formation.[12] The virus replicates slowly, so 3 to 5 days of culture are usually needed for plaques to become visible. Wild-type strains can also be assayed by syncytia formation in B95-8 or human cord blood mononuclear cells.

Biological Characteristics
The morbilliviruses differ from other paramyxoviruses in formation of intranuclear inclusion bodies. Virions are pleomorphic, range in size from 120 to 500 nm, and may contain more than one genome.[162,682] Each genome encodes eight proteins of which six are found in the virion. The envelope carries surface projections composed of the viral transmembrane hemagglutinin (H) and fusion (F) glycoproteins. The matrix (M) protein lines the interior of the virion envelope and may coat the nucleocapsid.[464] The helical ribonucleocapsid (total length of

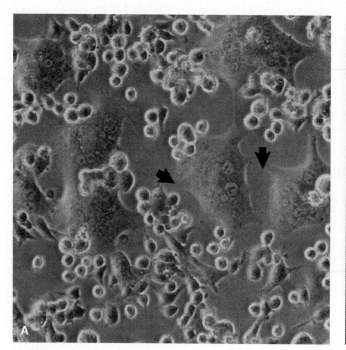 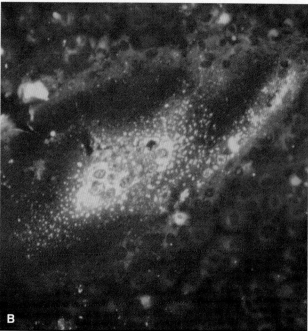

FIGURE 9.3 Typical cytopathic effects of syncytia formation and multinucleated giant cells associated with MeV replication in Vero cells. A: Unstained cells in culture. Arrows are next to syncytial cells. (Courtesy of William Bellini, CDC.) **B:** Cells stained with a fluorescently labeled antibody to MeV.

1.2 μm) formed from the 16-kb genomic RNA wrapped with the nucleocapsid (N) protein is packed within the envelope in the form of a symmetrical coil with the phosphoprotein (P) and large polymerase (L) proteins attached. Diagrams and detailed descriptions of the structures and functions of paramyxovirus virions, genomes, proteins, and replication are covered in Volume 1 Chapter 12. The following provides an overview and special features relevant to MeV and morbilliviruses.

Proteins

Nucleocapsid protein

As with other paramyxoviruses, the N protein mRNA is the first transcribed from the genome, and the N protein (525 residues) is the most abundant of the viral proteins. N appears as a 60-kDa band on polyacrylamide gels and can self-assemble but usually surrounds viral genomic or antigenomic RNAs to form flexible helical ribonucleocapsid structures that are the required template for both replication and transcription. N is organized into two functionally distinct regions. The folded N-terminal portion of the protein (residues 1 to 400, Ncore) is conserved and is required for RNA binding and assembly into nucleocapsids.[56,395] The C-terminal portion of the protein (residues 401 to 525, Ntail) is variable, intrinsically disordered, acidic, phosphorylated, and required for nucleocapsid flexibility.[54,74,319,476,677]

Ncore includes a nuclear localization signal,[732] and monomeric N (N⁰) can enter the nucleus but is usually retained in the cytoplasm by interaction with the disordered N-terminal residues of P to form N⁰P. The P chaperone shields the NLS, prevents N binding to cellular RNA, and maintains N as a monomer in the cytoplasm.[185,315,358] Interaction of N⁰P with viral RNA leads to assembly of a conformationally flexible nucleocapsid structure with 12.3 protomers per turn.[74,316,318] Serine/threonine phosphorylation of Ntail by PIM3 kinase regulates

oligomer formation and activation of transcription.[281,319,795] Each N monomer binds six nucleotides of genomic or antigenomic RNA with three bases pointing into the RNA-binding groove and three away from the groove consistent with the "rule of 6" for replication.[185,318,425] The open 3′ end of the RNA likely facilitates binding of L to initiate RNA synthesis.[185,316]

In the nucleocapsid structure, Ncore has two distinct globular domains, the N-terminal NTD (residues 37 to 265) and C-terminal CTD (residues 266 to 372), flanked before and after by short arms that link the protomers.[318] Viral RNA is stably bound in the groove between these domains. Ntail starts inside the helix before protruding to the outside[56,94,887] and has three short conserved motifs (Boxes 1 to 3) that serve as binding sites for cellular and viral proteins that regulate MeV replication. Box-2, alpha-helical molecular recognition element (α-MoRE, residues 489 to 506), interacts with the X domain in the C terminus of P (P-XD) to generate a four helix structure that likely positions the P-L polymerase complex near the encapsidated viral RNA to negotiate intergenic regions and prevent premature termination.[56,85,104,161,476,818] These interactions occur in liquid-like phase-separated cytoplasmic inclusions and residual disorder (fuzziness) in the Ntail-XD interaction modulates transcription and replication.[205,317,475] For instance, Box-2 and Box-3 (residues 517 to 525) bind heat shock protein (hsp) 70 in association with hsp40 to promote viral transcription, replication, and virulence.[160,894] Box-3 also binds the viral M protein to regulate viral RNA synthesis and virion assembly.[373] Ntail interacts with additional host proteins in virus strain- and cell type–specific ways. Documented interacting proteins include interferon (IFN) regulatory factor (IRF)-3, the cellular protein responsible for nuclear export of N, the p40 subunit of eIF3, FcγRII, and cyclophilins A and B.[151,436,731,817]

P, C, and V proteins

The P (phospho) protein (507 residues) is a polymerase cofactor regulated by phosphorylation that links L to N to form the replicase complex. While the 72-kDa P protein is abundant in the infected cell, only small amounts are present in the packaged virus. P is a multifunctional protein with a modular organization of ordered and disordered domains that functions as a tetramer. The N-terminus (P_{NT}, residues 1 to 303) is poorly conserved, intrinsically unstructured, acidic, phosphorylated, and required for replication. Residues 1 to 48 of P_{NT} bind to Ncore, which induces folding of P_{NT} and prevents N^0 binding to cellular RNAs, illegitimate N self-assembly and nuclear translocation.[315,396] In this complex, P_{NT} initiates encapsidation of genomic viral RNA by sequence-specific binding to the leader RNA.[315] Elongation of the nucleocapsid structure is independent of sequence. P_{NT} also interacts with cellular proteins to regulate the response to IFN (see discussion of V below).

The C-terminus (P_{CT}, residues 304 to 507) is conserved[58] and contains all domains required for transcription. The region between residues 304 and 321 contains the α-helical domain that binds to Ntail as part of the nucleocapsid structure and is responsible for tethering the polymerase L to its template.[412] P recruits hsp90 to chaperone the folding of L.[86] A coiled-coil domain between residues 344 and 411 is sufficient for P oligomerization. The unique P-XD (residues 459 to 507) has three α-helices arranged in antiparallel triple helix bundle that binds the Ntail α-MoRE and induces its folding.[78,269,476] Binding affinity is weak, consistent with a model in which P-XD is responsible for tethering L to the ribonucleocapsid in a way that allows it to progress during RNA synthesis.[93,412,887] P-XD also interacts with and stabilizes the ubiquitin ligase p53-induced RING-H2.[136]

The P gene of MeV, like other members of the *Paramyxoviridae* (see Chapter 12 in volume 1), also encodes proteins that regulate the innate response to infection. The C protein is a basic protein of 186 amino acids synthesized when an initiator methionine codon downstream from that for P is used to translate an overlapping reading frame.[72] The V protein shares the initiator methionine and the amino terminal 231 amino acids of the P protein, but RNA editing adds an extra non–template-directed guanosine (G) residue at position 751. This shifts the reading frame and results in a different 68 amino acid cysteine-rich C-terminus with zinc-binding properties that is highly conserved among paramyxoviruses.[128,472] Neither C nor V is necessary for MeV replication in Vero cells, but both regulate the cellular response to infection.[188,681,742,753]

C interacts with P_{CT} and is recruited into the replication complex where it modulates viral polymerase activity.[60,645] C improves the processivity of L for genome replication to decrease production of copyback DI RNAs that induce IFN and activate RNA-dependent protein kinase (PKR) to phosphorylate eIF-2α and inhibit translation.[582,647] In the absence of C, decreased L processivity results in a steepening of the mRNA transcription gradient.[648] C also interacts with immunity-related GTPase family M protein (IRGM) to induce autophagy and promote virus production.[696] Thus, C reduces induction of IFN and improves MeV replication in primary human cells and *in vivo*.[188,230,374,635,812]

The V protein interferes directly with IFN induction and signaling. The C-terminal zinc-binding domain of V (V_{CT}) prevents activation of melanoma differentiation–associated protein (MDA)-5 by inhibiting protein phosphatase 1–mediated dephosphorylation and the binding of dsRNA required for induction of IFN-β.[139,140,170,565] V also inhibits the response to IFN.[113,625,685] V_{CT} interacts with a number of IFN pathway proteins including STAT2 to disrupt formation of ISGF3 for induction of IFN-stimulated genes.[47,578] The intrinsically disordered N-terminal domains of both P and V interfere with IFN-induced JAK1 and STAT1 phosphorylation to prevent nuclear translocation and induction of IFN-stimulated genes.[113,114,190,886]

Matrix (M) protein

The envelope of the virion consists of the M protein (335 aa) and the two transmembrane glycoproteins F and H. M is a basic protein with several conserved hydrophobic domains that interacts with the surface glycoproteins and the ribonucleocapsid complex to regulate RNA synthesis and drive particle assembly and release.[71,217,373,403,463] The mRNAs for morbillivirus M proteins contain approximately 400 nucleotides of noncoding sequence at the 3′ end that increases M protein production.[71,807] M dimers form a lattice on the inner surface of the cell membrane in association with annexin A2 and interact with actin and the intracytoplasmic regions of the viral transmembrane glycoproteins to direct virus release from the apical surface of polarized epithelial cells and modulate the fusogenic capacity of the envelope glycoproteins.[198,373,403,422,464,579,666,853] Deletion of M increases cell-to-cell fusion and decreases production of infectious virus.[126] These properties are often defective in the mutated M proteins of viruses causing persistent infection.[3,347,633,797]

Fusion (F) protein

F is a highly conserved type I transmembrane glycoprotein synthesized as an inactive precursor (F_0) of about 60 kDa. The mRNAs for morbillivirus F_0 proteins contain unusually long (460 to 585 nucleotides) G-C–rich 5′-nontranslated regions that are predicted to have extensive secondary structure and are followed by clusters of 3 to 4 AUGs. The 5′ NTR influences the choice of AUG and regulates translation of F, virus production, and cytopathogenicity.[125,807] F_0 is glycosylated and trimerized in the ER[661] and cleaved by furin in the trans-Golgi at a multibasic site (108 to 112: Arg-Arg-His-Lys-Arg) to yield the 41-kDa (F_1) and 18-kDa (F_2) disulfide-linked fusion-competent mature class I fusion protein.[351] Mutation of Arg 112 results in a reduced rate of F transport to the cell surface, aberrant cleavage, and abolition of the fusogenic activity necessary for infection.[15] F_2 has all of the predicted N-linked glycosylation sites. Mutation of any of these asparagines decreases transport to the cell surface and impairs proteolytic cleavage, stability, and the fusion capacity.[16]

F_1 contains a highly conserved stretch of hydrophobic amino acid residues at the new N terminus (aa 113 to 145) that constitutes the fusion peptide. Insertion of the fusion peptide into the plasma membrane and formation of the six-helix bundle leads to fusion at the cell surface.[654,656] There are two heptad-repeat amphipathic α-helices in F_1: one adjacent to the fusion peptide and another N terminal to the transmembrane region. F_2 possesses a third heptad repeat region in a microdomain near residue 94.[657]

The structure of the prefusion F trimer is similar to other paramyxovirus fusion proteins with head and stalk domains (Fig. 9.4).[335] Fusion requires the expression of both H and cleaved F, interaction of the F trimer head with the H stalk, and binding of H to a cell surface receptor.[623,893] Fusogenicity

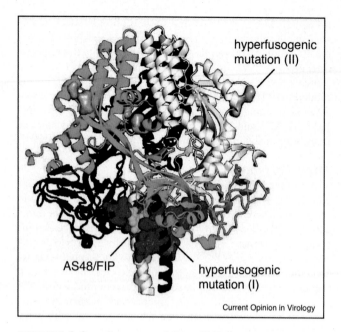

FIGURE 9.4 Crystal structure of the prefusion protein trimer.
Hyperfusogenic mutations (I) in the stalk region are colored *red*. The fusion inhibitors AS-48 and fusion inhibitor protein (FIP) target residues in this region. Other hyperfusogenic mutations (II) are distant from the stalk and colored *salmon*. (Reprinted from Fukuhara H, Mwaba MH, Maenaka K. Structural characteristics of measles virus entry. *Curr Opin Virol* 2020;41:52–58. Copyright © 2020 Elsevier. With permission. Ref.[256])

is determined by the stability of the prefusion structure and strength of the noncovalent interaction with H. These properties are regulated by sequences around the fusion peptide, the protomer interface, and a hydrophobic region of a neck domain between the head and stalk.[335,366] Mutations that decrease stability of the prefusion conformation result in hyperfusogenicity and are implicated in MeV-induced infection of the nervous system.[26,49,390,859,860] Inhibitors that bind to the neck domain increase stability and prevent the conformational change required for fusion (Fig. 9.4).[335,658,695,735]

The 33-residue cytoplasmic tail of F_1 possesses basolateral sorting and endocytosis signals[547] but can be redirected to the apical surface in polarized epithelial cells by interaction with M.[84,579] F tail mutations associated with persistent infection include premature stop codons, missense mutations, altered reading frames, and nonconservative amino acid substitutions that interfere with budding and increase cell-to-cell fusion and neurovirulence.[49,127,548,741] Progressive cell–cell fusion and post-fusion pore expansion to produce syncytia are regulated by interaction of M and F with actin and annexin A1.[144,581]

Hemagglutinin (H) protein

H (617 aa) is the receptor-binding and hemagglutinating (HA) protein and an important determinant of morbillivirus cellular tropism. H is a type II transmembrane glycoprotein with cysteine residues at 139 and 154 responsible for intermolecular disulfide bonding to form homodimers.[660] Homodimers then associate to form the H dimer of dimers present on the surfaces of infected cells and virions (Fig. 9.5).[97,336,660] The H protein has a cytoplasmic tail of 34 amino acids preceding a single hydrophobic transmembrane region and a large C-terminal ectodomain with 13 strongly conserved cysteines.

The cytoplasmic tail is essential for efficient transport to the cell surface and includes signals for basolateral sorting and endocytosis but can be redirected along with F by M to the apical surface of polarized epithelial cells for particle formation and virus release.[84,547,549] The ectodomain has 5 predicted N-linked glycosylation sites clustered between positions 168 and 238 of which 4 are used and necessary for proper folding, antigenicity, dimerization, and transport.[356] Presence of an additional glycosylation site at residue 416 in some isolates correlates with a loss of HA activity.[719]

The H ectodomain consists of an N-terminal α-helical stalk (aa 59 to 154), a connecting region (aa 155 to 187), and a large cubic-shaped six-blade β-propeller head domain (aa 188 to 617) (Fig. 9.5).[150,336] Three functionally distinct regions of the tetrameric stalk have been defined: a lower portion that interacts with and activates F, a spacer that facilitates H/F assembly, and a C-terminal linker important for H tetramer formation.[345,444,592,654] In the head domain, each of the blade modules contains four antiparallel β-strands connected sequentially through extended loops (Fig. 9.5). In the dimer, N-linked carbohydrates cover the top pocket and cause the two molecules to tilt away from each other optimizing exposure of neutralizing epitopes and the receptor-binding sites on the lateral surface away from the dimer interface[336] (see section on receptors). The H tetramer oligomerizes with the F trimer in the ER through interaction of the F head domain with the H stalk, and the two surface glycoproteins function together for budding and for fusion, entry, and syncytia formation.[96,623,661]

L protein

The L (large) protein (2183 aa) is a multidomain polymerase protein with several highly conserved regions that synthesize and cap viral RNAs. The N-terminus contains the Gly-Asp-Asn-Gln motif common to the RNA polymerases of negative-strand viruses adjacent to the capping domain with polyribonucleotidyl transferase activity.[163,208,815] A linker region connects these catalytic domains to the methyltransferase domain.[815] L is present in small quantities in the infected cell, interacts with and functions in association with P, and is part of the viral nucleocapsid both in the cell and in the virion. A domain in the N-terminal 408 amino acids binds to a trihelical binding domain in P_{CT} that links it to the nucleocapsid for transcription and replication.[354,413]

Cellular Receptors

MeV can infect several types of cells and uses multiple receptors in a virus strain and cell type–specific manner. Three cell surface receptors have been identified: membrane cofactor protein or CD46,[203,588] signaling lymphocytic activation molecule (SLAM) or CD150,[814] and poliovirus receptor–related 4 (PVRL4) or nectin 4.[570,602] The binding sites for these cellular receptors are all found on the lateral surface of the head structure of H[337,728] (Fig. 9.5).

SLAMF1/CD150

SLAMF1 is a 70-kDa glycoprotein that is the first member (F1) of the SLAM subfamily of CD2 immunomodulatory type 1 transmembrane proteins[117,186] and is the most important receptor for MeV replication in lymphoid tissue.[174] CD150 is expressed on the surface of cells of the immune system including immature thymocytes, invariant T cells, and activated T and B lymphocytes.[147,711] In dendritic cells (DCs) and macrophages,

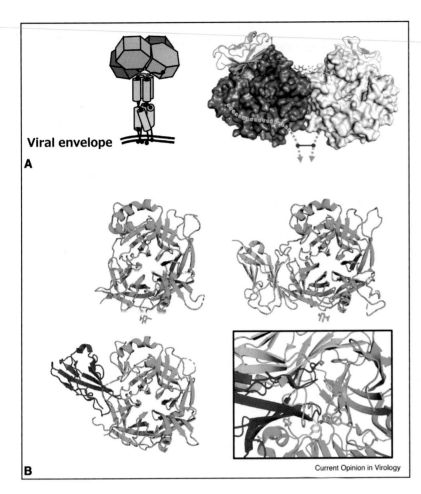

Viral envelope

A

B

Current Opinion in Virology

FIGURE 9.5 Structural features of the H protein.
(A) *Left*: Schematic image of the H protein dimer of dimers. The C-terminal head domains of the H protein homodimer (*cyan* and *blue*) linked to the tetrameric stalk domain. *Right*: Crystal structure of the H homodimer complexed with SLAM; MeV H (surface presentation, *grey* and *dark grey*), SLAM (cartoon presentation, *cyan*). Oligosaccharides are shown as a stick model. The connector regions are shown as *orange dotted lines* with the disulfide bond at Cys154 intimated in *red*. **(B)** Crystal structures of H (*green, left top*) and its receptor complexes SLAM (*cyan, right top*) and nectin 4 (*magenta, left bottom*). *Right bottom*: H (*green*) residues interacting with each receptor are shown in a stick model colored in *slate* (SLAM), *salmon* (nectin 4), and *yellow* (overlapped). (Reprinted from Fukuhara H, Mwaba MH, Maenaka K. Structural characteristics of measles virus entry. *Curr Opin Virol* 2020;41:52–58. Copyright © 2020 Elsevier. With permission.)

SLAMF1 is in endocytic recycling vesicles and trafficked to the surface with activation of acidic sphingomyelinase.[744,840] Most other morbilliviruses also use SLAM of the relevant species as a receptor suggesting that this is a common feature.[6,62,810,850] Only MeV uses human SLAMF1 efficiently.[755]

SLAMF1 is a dual function costimulatory molecule with two highly glycosylated immunoglobulin-like domains (V and C2).[781,884] The cytoplasmic domain has immunoreceptor tyrosine–based switch motifs that bind small SH2 domain adaptor proteins, such as SLAM-associated protein (SAP) and Ewing sarcoma–associated transcript-2 (EAT-2), important for cell signaling.[116,117,186,781] MeV H binds to the V domain of human, but not mouse, SLAM[610] leading to endocytosis and down-regulation of SLAMF1 expression on the surface of infected cells.[282,865] H residues comprising the critical four components for binding the V domain of SLAMF1 are located primarily on the side of H blade 5 contiguous to the binding site for CD46[337,505,593,851] (Fig. 9.5). Interactions with the extreme N-terminal region of SLAMF1 promote specificity for human SLAMF1.[757] Both vaccine and wild-type strains can use SLAMF1 as a receptor, but wild-type viruses with asparagine at H481 enter PBMCs more efficiently than vaccine viruses with tyrosine at this position.[228,743]

Nectin 4/poliovirus receptor–like 4
Poliovirus receptor–like 4/nectin 4, a transmembrane adherens junction protein of the immunoglobulin superfamily, is expressed on the basolateral surface of epithelial cells and serves as a MeV receptor.[570,602] Nectin 4 has two C2-type immunoglobulin domains and a V adhesive surface domain that interacts with the hydrophobic groove between H propellers 4 and 5[506,570,895] (Fig. 9.5). Nectin 4 is used by both vaccine and wild type strains, and a homologue serves as a receptor in chicken cells used for attenuation of the Edmonston vaccine strain of MeV.[756] Interaction of CDV with canine nectin 4 determines epithelial cell infection and its virulence.[675]

CD46/membrane cofactor protein
CD46 is a widely distributed human complement regulatory protein that acts as a cofactor in the proteolytic inactivation of C3b/C4b by factor I. CD46 is expressed on all nucleated cells and preferentially on the apical surface of polarized epithelial cells.[84,699] Monkeys have a CD46 homolog that is expressed on erythrocytes and is the basis for HA activity. All CD46 isoforms contain four short consensus repeats (SCRs), a serine/threonine/proline domain near the transmembrane segment and one of two alternative cytoplasmic tails.[699] The H protein β-propeller blades 4 and 5 bind to one planar face of SCR1, and SCR2 while SCRs 2, 3, and 4 bind C3b/C4b.[124,699] Most MeV vaccine strains use CD46 on cultured cells efficiently, while wild-type strains do not.[228,618] Tyrosine at position 481 and glycine at 546 are key determinants of the affinity of H for CD46.[598,721,728] However, there is little evidence of vaccine virus replication in CD46-expressing cells *in vivo* so the importance of this receptor is not clear.[173,177,811]

Other receptors and cell surface interactions
Several pieces of information suggest that MeV uses additional receptors and H-independent modes of entry. The currently

known H-interacting receptors do not account for the ability of MeV to infect endothelial cells,[233] epithelial cells through the apical surface,[471] or neurons.[521] Both endocytosis and macropinocytosis, in addition to fusion at the plasma membrane, can be important for MeV entry[164,183,248,642] and mutations that destabilize F enable infection and syncytia formation in the absence of known receptors (Fig. 9.4)[773,859,860] (see modes of entry below). Recently, synaptic cell adhesion molecules (CADM) 1 and 2 have been identified as neuronal receptors when expressed in the same cell as MeV H (*cis*) and trigger fusion with adjacent cells when combined with a hyperfusogenic mutant of F.[774]

Other cell surface molecules interact with MeV but do not serve as entry receptors. For instance, MeV H can bind Toll-like receptor (TLR) 2 and induce signaling,[76] and DC-specific ICAM-3 grabbing nonintegrin (DC-SIGN) is an attachment receptor that enhances infection and modulates function of DCs.[42,179,531]

Hemagglutination, Hemadsorption, and Hemolysis

Some strains of MeV bind to and agglutinate the erythrocytes of Old World monkeys, particularly African green, patas, and rhesus macaques. HA is indicative of binding to CD46 and dependent on the C-terminal 18 amino acids of H, amino acids 451 and 481, and absence of glycosylation at 416.[720,769] This is consistent with the distribution of the CD46 molecule, which is not present on human red blood cells, and with the molecular characteristics of primate CD46.[355] In baboons, lack of HA is due to an amino acid substitution in SCR2 and in New World monkeys to an absence of SCR1.[355] HA is followed within a few hours by lysis of the agglutinated erythrocytes. Hemolysis is a consequence of fusion that is dependent on F, as well as H.[16,872]

Entry

H attachment to a cellular receptor is followed by fusion of the virus envelope with the cellular plasma membrane and delivery of the viral ribonucleocapsid into the cytoplasm for initiation of infection. The H dimer of dimers associates with the prefusion F trimer in the secretory system of the host cell with interaction of the MeV H protein stalk and the MeV F protein head resulting in a staggered head domain arrangement on the virion surface.[96,444,623,656] Fusion at neutral pH is induced through cooperation of H and F oligomers from compatible virus species[611] and requires prior cleavage of F_0 into F_1 and F_2.[569] A series of structural rearrangements is initiated by the binding of H to a cellular receptor that induces a reorganization of the dimer–dimer head domains. Receptor binding is transmitted to the F protein head contact zone in the central segment of the H stalk. Signaling to the base of the F protein head triggers refolding of the F trimer followed by membrane fusion.[30,98,99,337,590,591,593] Separate regions in the H stalk are required for interaction with F and for triggering fusion suggesting that these are discrete functions.[444,623,656]

MeV fusogenicity correlates inversely with the strength of the interaction between F and H.[157,158,226,369,662] More avid binding decreases fusion, indicating the need for H and F dissociation during the process of entry and productive infection.[226] Likewise, mutations in F that decrease the stability of the prefusion trimer enhance fusogenicity and allow fusion and entry to occur even when H interactions with the cell surface are weak.[773]

Other modes of entry, such as endocytosis and macropinocytosis used by several paramyxoviruses, are likely to be important additional mechanisms for MeV entry, particularly into primary cells.[164,248,282,642] Macropinocytosis is used by several viruses for entry into epithelial cells,[528,706,824] facilitates nectin 4–dependent entry of MeV into colon and breast cancer cells,[183] and SLAMF1 entry into lymphocytes[282] and is suggested by the large membranous blebs and cytoplasmic vacuoles of the multinuclear giant cells formed by apically infected respiratory epithelial cells.[471]

Replication and Cytopathic Effects

After entry, sequential synthesis of viral mRNAs results in a transcriptional gradient of mRNAs for N through to L. mRNA translation is facilitated by the ATP-binding cassette transformer ABCE1, a cellular protein important for ribosomal recycling.[23] Replication is facilitated by activation of sphingosine kinase resulting in NF-κB signaling[846] and C protein interaction with IRGM to induce autophagy.[643,696] MeV-induced changes in cellular transcription are cell type–dependent and evolve over the course of infection with early up-regulation of antiviral genes and proteins in epithelial cells, but not lymphoid cells, followed by suppression of constitutively expressed genes.[77,729,733] Hsp 70 is induced and released from infected cells to interact with TLR2 and TLR4.[410]

MeV replication in cell culture results in cytopathic changes of three varieties: multinucleated giant cells (syncytia), altered cell shape, and inclusion bodies.[223] Cell-to-cell fusion occurs at neutral pH, and syncytia formation occurs *in vitro* (Fig. 9.3) and *in vivo*[222] using fusion mechanisms similar to those for virus entry. Syncytia formation is facilitated by basolateral expression of H and F, the actin filament–plasma membrane cross-linker moesin, and can be inhibited by cytochalasin B or expression of BST2/tetherin.[202,405] Fusion of infected cells with uninfected cells can produce syncytia with 50 or more nuclei. Nuclei in the center of the syncytia have marginated chromatin[222] and are often undergoing apoptotic cell death[232] leading to plaque formation *in vitro*. Infected cells may also change from a normal polygonal shape to a stellate, dendritic, or spindle shape with increased refractility to light. This type of "strand-forming" cytopathic effect appears after several passages and may be related to the production of DI particles.[520]

Both spindle-shaped cells and syncytial cells may contain intracytoplasmic and intranuclear inclusion bodies. Cytoplasmic inclusions are liquid-like phase-separated compartments formed in association with cofilin that are sites of viral transcription and replication with L- and N-encapsidated RNA decorated with P producing "fuzzy" or "granular" ribonucleocapsids.[88,317,424,898] Cellular proteins that facilitate virus replication such as WD repeat–containing protein 5 are selectively recruited to these cytoplasmic inclusion bodies.[484] Intranuclear Cowdry type A inclusion bodies are characteristic of morbillivirus infections, are generally smaller than cytoplasmic inclusions, contain N and hsp, and occur late in infection.[606,608] Because MeV N migrates to the nucleus[358] and assembles into nucleocapsids if not retained in the cytoplasm by P,[607] it has been postulated that late in infection amounts of P become limiting and allow formation of nuclear inclusions.[88,358]

Budding

M plays a central role in virus assembly and release.[403] Virion release is inefficient, dependent on M and independent of the cellular ESCRT system.[724] Expression of M alone can induce assembly and release of virus-like particles.[126,132,666,715] To initiate virus assembly, M interacts with N in the ribonucleocapsid and with the cytoplasmic domains of F oligomers and localizes with annexin A2 to the inner surface of plasma membrane detergent–resistant microdomains to form a 2D paracrystalline array that promotes virion assembly and release.[403,422,494,547,548,666] M association with F-actin regulates interaction with H and modulates choice between virion assembly and cell–cell fusion.[853] In polarized epithelial cells, particle release is directed to the apical surface by the M protein despite the intrinsic glycoprotein targeting to the basolateral surface.[489,579] Loss of apical targeting by M enhances cell–cell fusion at the expense of virus production.[126,127,715]

Cell-to-Cell Spread

MeV is highly cell associated and can spread cell-to-cell without releasing virus particles from the plasma membrane, a process that is regulated by relative fusogenicity of the membrane glycoproteins.[734] In addition to syncytia formation, cell–cell transfer of infection can occur by transfer of ribonucleocapsids to adjacent cells, a process most often observed in polarized epithelia and in the nervous system.[375,442,785,786] In epithelial cells, a nectin-dependent endocytic pathway has been identified,[271] and in neurons, there is cis-acting triggering of fusion by interaction of H with adhesion molecules CADM1 and CADM2.[774]

Evolution, Antigenic Composition, and Strain Variation

Antigenically, MeV is a monotypic virus.[66,798] Antisera from individuals infected decades ago as well as recipients of the live virus vaccine developed in the 1960s retain the ability to neutralize current wild-type strains of MeV, although with varying efficiency.[175,235,416] The observed rate of mutation of H in virus circulating in defined geographic locations is low, estimated at 4×10^{-4} per year for a given nucleotide.[701] The rate of mutation during growth under selective pressure *in vitro* is estimated at 9×10^{-5} per replication for a nucleotide[751] and 1.8×10^{-6} under nonselective conditions.[896] In addition to mutation, MeV may also evolve by cotransmission of multiple genomes to a single cell.[775]

Mutational analysis indicates that the H and F envelope proteins have little tolerance for change while other proteins and untranslated regions of the genome are less restricted.[260] The structure of H with carbohydrates masking the top surface and exposed receptor-binding sites on the side likely constrains acquisition of mutations (Fig. 9.5).[336,712] Nevertheless, evidence of vaccine-induced selective pressure on wild-type strains of MeV has been identified in the noose and receptor-binding regions of H, and this pressure may contribute to the decreasing diversity of MeV genotypes in circulation (see "Epidemiology").[103,244,798]

Strains separate into eight different clades (A to H) and at least 24 different genotypes based on sequencing of the C-terminal 450 nucleotides of the N gene or the entire coding region of H.[698,709] Live attenuated vaccines were all derived from genotype A wild-type strains and are quite similar.[59] New genotypes are designated if the nucleotide sequence differs from the closest reference sequence by more than 2.5% in N or 2.0% in H. Some genotypes are found in one geographic region, others are co-circulating, while an increasing number are probably extinct.[103] The main genotypes circulating currently are B3, D4, D8, and H1 (Fig. 9.6) with evidence that B3 may be both more transmissible and more likely to escape vaccine-induced immunity.[4,103,676]

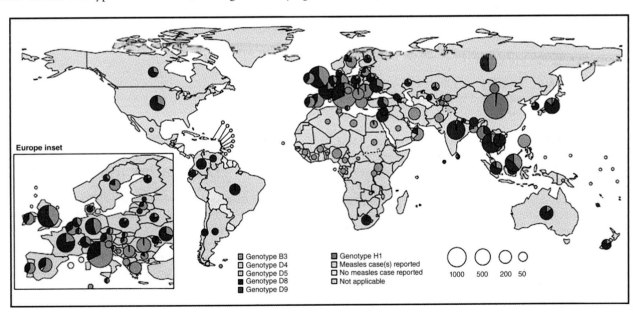

FIGURE 9.6 Geographic distribution of MeV genotypes 2016–2020. WHO currently recognizes 24 genotypes of wild-type MeV, but many are no longer in circulation. The map shows the global distribution of MeV genotypes and measles incidence in 2020. *Colored circles* indicate MeV genotypes reported to the WHO database, and the size of the circles is proportional to the number of genotypes reported for the indicated areas. Europe is also shown as an *inset* to provide more resolution. The boundaries and names shown and the designations used on this map do not imply the expression of any opinion whatsoever on the part of the WHO concerning the legal status of any country, territory, city or area or of its authorities, or concerning the delimitation of its frontiers of boundaries. *Dotted lines* on maps represent approximate borderlines for which there may not yet be full agreement. (From Brown KE, Rota PA, Goodson JL, et al. Genetic characterization of measles and rubella viruses detected through global measles and rubella elimination surveillance, 2016–2018. *MMWR Morb Mortal Wkly Rep* 2019;68(26):587–591.)

Nucleotide sequence variability has been a useful tool for the MeV genotyping required for molecular epidemiologic identification of transmission pathways. N genes differ by up to 7% in the C-terminal Ntail region that is used for strain identification.[277] However, for analysis of transmission, sequencing only this region has become less useful as the diversity of circulating strains has decreased. Alternatives include sequences of the P, H, or L genes, the noncoding region between M and F, or the entire genome.[87,334,408,637] The P gene is most variable in the shared PV$_{NTD}$.[58] The H gene nucleotide sequence is most variable between residues 167 and 241 where the N-linked glycosylation sites are located.[75,143] The M-F intergenic region tolerates insertions, deletions, and substitutions[57] and, aside from whole genome sequencing, is currently most useful for tracking chains of transmission.[275]

PATHOGENESIS AND PATHOLOGY

Natural (Wild Type) Measles

MeV is spread by the respiratory route and is typically a childhood infection in unvaccinated human populations with endemic transmission. Measles disease is characterized by a latent period of 10 to 14 days and a 2- to 3-day prodrome of fever, runny nose, cough, and conjunctivitis followed by the appearance of a characteristic maculopapular rash (Fig. 9.1).[417,452,631] The onset of the rash coincides with the appearance of the adaptive immune response and initiation of virus clearance (Fig. 9.7). Recovery is accompanied by lifelong immunity to reinfection.[628] Macaques exposed to infected humans or experimentally infected with wild-type strains of MeV develop a similar disease, and much of our more detailed understanding of pathogenesis, immune responses, and sites of virus replication come from studies of nonhuman primates, often facilitated by the use of engineered reporter viruses.[40,174,177,399,437,518]

Entry and Sites of Primary Replication

MeV is efficiently transmitted over short distances by respiratory droplets and over longer distances by small particle aerosols.[137] High MeV infectivity suggests that the cellular sites of initial virus replication are very susceptible to infection. However, the nature of these cells is unclear because it has been difficult to identify MeV-positive cells in the respiratory tract at early times after infection.[174,446] Although autopsy studies have shown abundant infection of respiratory epithelial cells,[546,722] studies of experimentally infected monkeys have identified alveolar macrophages and subepithelial DCs as most likely to be infected early.[174,177,446] In vitro studies of differentiated respiratory epithelial cells have shown that MeV infection from the basolateral surface through the nectin 4 receptor leads to epithelial spread and apical virus release,[483,787] while infection from the apical surface through an unidentified receptor leads to release of infectious virus and shedding of multinucleated giant cells without residual infection of or damage to the epithelial sheet.[471] MeV engineered to eliminate binding to nectin 4 can still initiate infection after intranasal inoculation, but shedding from the respiratory tract is reduced.[448] It is likely that pulmonary macrophages and DCs transport MeV to local lymphoid tissue where virus is amplified leading to viremia and subsequent systemic spread of infection to many tissues, including back to the lung.[805]

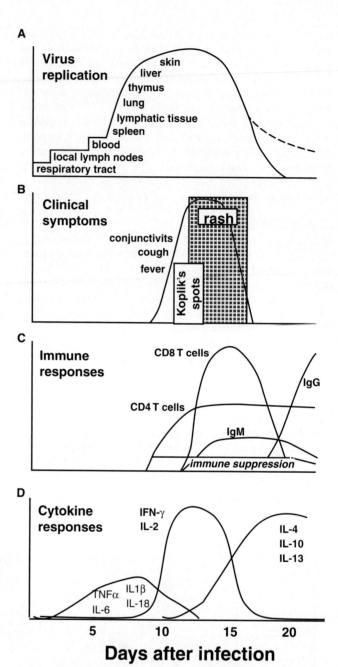

FIGURE 9.7 Diagrammatic representation of the pathogenesis of measles for the first 4 weeks after infection with wild-type MeV. Infection is initiated in the respiratory tract, and virus spreads to lymphocytes, monocyte/macrophages, endothelial cells, and epithelial cells in draining lymph nodes and then systemically through the blood to thymus, spleen, lymph nodes, liver, skin, and lung and to the conjunctivae and mucosal surfaces of the gastrointestinal, respiratory, and genitourinary tracts (A). The rash appears **(B)** at the time of the virus-specific adaptive immune response with activation of MeV-specific CD4+ and CD8+ T cells and synthesis of MeV-specific IgM and IgG antibody **(C)**. Clearance of infectious virus is approximately coincident with fading of the rash, but clearance of RNA (*dotted line*) is slower **(A)**. Cytokines produced are consistent with inflammasome and NF-κB activation followed by Th1 CD4+ and CD8+ T cells and then Th2 CD4+ T cells and regulatory cells **(D)**. Immune suppression is initiated during the rash and persists for months after its resolution **(C)**.

Spread

MeV interaction with DC-SIGN on DCs leads to up-regulation of SLAMF1, MeV entry, increased motility, and likely participation in transport of virus from the respiratory tract to draining lymph nodes[42,184,530,771] where they can transfer infection to susceptible lymphocytes.[44,174,180,421] Replication in local lymphatic tissue is efficient with virus production by SLAMF1-expressing monocytes, T cells, and B cells.[469] Infected mononuclear cells are detected in peripheral blood within 4 to 7 days after infection.[40,234,440] The viremia is cell-associated. and infectious virus has been only rarely isolated from plasma,[636] but viral RNA can sometimes be detected by RT-PCR. MeV-infected mononuclear cells increase expression of the integrins LFA-1 ($\alpha_L\beta_2$) and VLA-4 ($\alpha_4\beta_1$) that promote adherence to endothelial cells and cell-to-cell transmission of infection.[38,200,361,481] These properties likely facilitate virus dissemination by infected leukocytes to epithelial cells in the skin and respiratory tract.[251,482] The viremia is accompanied by lymphopenia due to viral or immune-mediated death of infected cells as well as changes in leukocyte trafficking (Fig. 9.8).[40,178,372,612,717,869]

Target Cells and Tissues

From the blood, infection is spread by infected leukocytes to distal lymphoid tissue and to epithelial cells, endothelial cells. and macrophages in nonlymphoid organs.[19,174,546] Transmigration across an endothelial barrier is impaired for MeV-infected lymphocytes,[200] so entry of MeV into tissues may occur primarily from endothelial cells infected by circulating leukocytes or by movement of other types of infected cells, such as monocytes, across blood vessel walls.[481] Once within tissue, spread is cell type– and virus strain–dependent and occurs by cell-to-cell transmission or by release of infectious virus.[145] Tyrosine residues in the cytoplasmic tails of F (aa 549) and H (aa 12) are important for basolateral glycoprotein sorting and determine the fusogenic spread of MeV in epithelial cells,[548,549] while only the H sorting signal determines wild-type MeV release versus cell–cell fusion in lymphocytes.[713,714]

Infection in lymphoid tissues (e.g., thymus, spleen, lymph nodes, appendix, and tonsils) is extensive[174] with formation of the giant cells first described by Warthin and Finkeldey. These cells can be 100 μm or more in diameter and contain up to 100 nuclei aggregated near the center and are most often located in or near germinal centers, in the thymus, and in submucosal lymphoid tissue.[603] There is extensive replication in both B and T cells with a higher percentage of MeV-positive B cells than T cells.[469] Replication occurs preferentially in SLAMF1-expressing double-positive thymocytes, naive and memory B cells, and memory T cells with acute depletion of these populations.[178,438,440,469] Decrease in the size of the thymic cortex is prolonged, but other lymphoid tissues recover cellularity promptly.[869]

MeV also spreads to the skin, conjunctivae, kidney, lung, gastrointestinal tract, respiratory mucosa, genital mucosa, and liver often through interaction with infected leukocytes.[251] In these nonlymphoid sites, the virus replicates in endothelial cells, epithelial cells, and tissue-resident myeloid and lymphoid cells.[233,439,546,801] Endothelial cell infection may be accompanied by vascular dilatation, increased permeability, mononuclear cell infiltration, and infection of surrounding tissue. The histopathology of the measles rash suggests that the initial event is infection of dermal myeloid and endothelial cells followed by spread of infection into the overlying epidermis with infection of keratinocytes in the stratum granulosum, focal keratosis, and multinucleated giant cells near hair follicles and sebaceous glands.[411,439,460,487,801] The hyperemic rash appears as immune cells accumulate at sites of virus replication (Fig. 9.9). Koplik spots found on the oral mucosa are pathologically similar and involve the submucous glands.

On rare occasions, there is spread to the nervous system. Infection of endothelial cells has been demonstrated in the brains of children dying of measles,[233,414] and *in vitro* studies have demonstrated infection of brain microvascular endothelial cells by cell-free virus and by adherent MeV-infected T lymphocytes.[200] Polarized endothelial cells can release virus from both the apical and basolateral cell surfaces, allowing access to the brain parenchyma, as well as the blood.[200] If neurons become infected, virus can spread through the CNS from neuron-to-neuron and to astrocytes without the release of infectious particles.[215,665]

Immune Responses

A vigorous MeV-specific cellular and humoral immune response associated with many of the clinical manifestations of measles is mounted to infection. This response results in virus clearance, clinical recovery, and establishment of lifelong protective immunity as well as a prolonged increase in susceptibility to other infections that accounts for most of the measles-associated mortality (Figs. 9.7–9.10). Although infectious

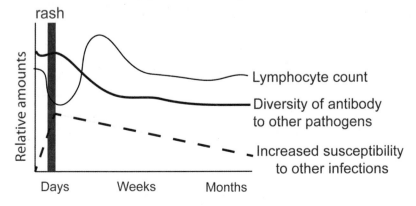

FIGURE 9.8 Diagrammatic representation of the immunosuppressive effects of MeV infection. Lymphopenia resolves within days after the rash has faded, while there is a long-term effect on the diversity of antibody in circulation and susceptibility to other infections. (Adapted from Griffin DE. Measles immunity and immunosuppression. *Curr Opin Virol* 2021;46:9–14. https://creativecommons.org/licenses/by/4.0/. Ref.[298])

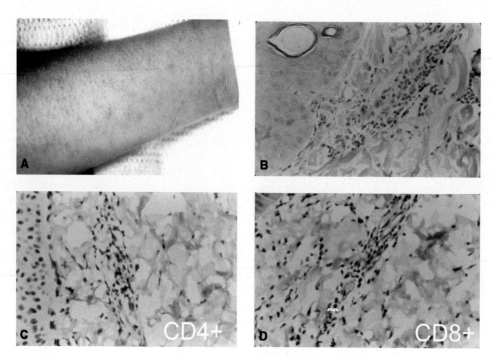

FIGURE 9.9 Histopathology of the measles rash. (A) Photograph of the maculopapular rash of measles. Skin biopsy stained with hematoxylin and eosin showing mononuclear inflammatory infiltrates **(B)** and stained for CD4+ T cells **(C)** and CD8+ T cells **(D)** indicative of the cellular immune response to MeV-infected keratinocytes in the skin. (Adapted by permission from Nature: Polack FP, Auwaerter PG, Lee SH, et al. Production of atypical measles in rhesus macaques: evidence for disease mediated by immune complex formation and eosinophils in the presence of fusion-inhibiting antibody. *Nat Med* 1999;5(6):629–634. Copyright © 1999 Springer Nature.)

virus cannot be isolated after the rash is cleared, viral RNA can be detected for many weeks in PBMCs and lymphoid tissue indicating that complete viral clearance is a prolonged process (Fig. 9.10).[466,595,596,641,697] The roles of various components of the immune response in recovery from infection have been

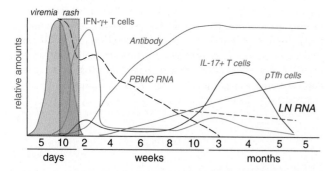

FIGURE 9.10 Diagram of the clearance of virus and prolonged evolution of the immune response after wild-type MeV infection of rhesus macaques. Ability to culture MeV from peripheral blood mononuclear cells (PBMCs) (viremia) ends soon after appearance of the rash and interferon (IFN)-γ–secreting T cells. However, clearance of MeV RNA from PBMCs is much slower, and RNA persists in lymph node (LN) tissues for months. IL-17–producing T cells are induced several weeks later and peripheral T follicular helper (pTfh) cells continuously increase. Amounts and avidity of antiviral antibody increase over weeks. (Reprinted from Griffin DE. Measles virus persistence and its consequences. *Curr Opin Virol* 2020;41:46–51. Copyright © 2020 Elsevier. With permission. Ref.[297])

deduced from the outcome of MeV infection in patients with deficiencies of immunological function, from the studies of monkeys depleted of specific immune components, and from mathematical modeling of in-host virus clearance.[283,555,638,639] In general, deficits in antibody production permit recovery, while deficits in cellular immune responses can lead to slowed clearance or progressive disease (see "Measles in Immunodeficiency"). In immunologically normal individuals, the onset of clinically apparent disease coincides with the appearance of the MeV-specific adaptive immune response (Fig. 9.7). Activation of the immune system as well as evidence of immune suppression continues for weeks to months after apparent recovery (Figs. 9.8 and 9.10).[305,308,504,541,595,596,813,856,857]

Early innate responses
Innate responses may contribute to eventual control of virus replication by the adaptive immune response but do not prevent systemic virus spread during the clinically silent 10- to 14-day incubation period. Type I IFN is an important component of the innate response to many virus infections, and MeV replication is sensitive to its inhibitory effects.[17,449] IFN-induced proteins that inhibit MeV replication include APOBEC3G, BST1/tetherin, RSAD2/Viperin, and Mx.[237,405,433,822,823] Mutations that affect IFN receptor or STAT2 signaling predispose to MeV vaccine complications[329,342] and a recombinant wild-type MeV that cannot interfere with STAT1 translocation is attenuated in macaques.[189] However, *in vitro* investigations related to IFN induction and its role in measles pathogenesis have been confounded by the frequent presence of 5' copyback DI RNAs in the stocks of the virus strains studied.[349,770,778] Vaccine strains

are more likely to induce IFN-α/β than wild-type strains,[589] but this may be related to the efficiency with which they generate DI RNAs that are potent inducers of IFN through activation of RIG-I.[407,726,803]

IFN responses that might be triggered by MeV replication in the absence of DIs through interaction with MDA5[726] are suppressed by the actions of the P, C, and V proteins that prevent production of and response to type I IFN.[47] In addition, interaction with DC-SIGN prevents the dephosphorylation required for activation of RNA sensors RIG-I and MDA5.[531,762] Likewise, during *in vivo* MeV infection, there is little evidence of type I or type III IFN production or activation of IFN-induced genes in humans or experimentally infected macaques.[188,306,772,777,843,899] However, during the incubation period in macaques, there is an increase in interleukin (IL)-1β, IL-12, IFN-γ, and chemokines CCL2/MCP1, CCL11/eotaxin, CCL22/MDC, CXCL9/MIG, and CXCL11/ITAC.[469] In naturally infected humans, inflammatory cytokines and chemokines that are increased in plasma at the time disease is recognized include inflammasome products IL-1β and IL-18 and NF-κB products IL-6 and TNF-α and chemokines CCL2, CCL4/MIP-1β, CCL11, CCL13/MCP-4, CCL22, CXCL8/IL-8, and CXCL10/IP10 (Fig. 9.7).[469,470,730,759,899] PBMCs cultured from patients after rash onset produce IL-1β,[857] and transcriptional analysis of PBMCs from children with measles has shown increases in mRNAs for cytokines IL-1β and TNF-α, and chemokines CCL4, CXCL2/MIP-2α and CXCL8, and CIAS-1/NALP3, a component of the inflammasome.[899] Induction of NF-κB signaling may occur through interaction of the viral H protein with TLR2,[76] but it is not clear how the inflammasome is activated.

Natural killer (NK) cells and complement activation constitute other potentially important early defense mechanisms. However, NK cell function is actually lower than normal during measles at the time of the rash.[407] MeV and MeV-infected cells can activate the factor B–dependent alternative complement pathway through F_1-mediated deposition of C3b rendering the cells susceptible to complement-mediated lysis because the CD46 and CD55 complement regulators are segregated into membrane microdomains that are separate from F.[187,272,788]

Antibody

Antibodies are first detectable when the rash appears (Figs. 9.7 and 9.10).[291] The isotype of MeV-specific antibody is initially IgM followed by a switch first to IgG2 and IgG3 and then, in the memory phase, to IgG1 and IgG4.[92] IgG is initially of low avidity, and this improves steadily over several months.[580,829] IgA, IgM, and IgG antibodies to MeV are found in secretions, and sampling of saliva has provided a noninvasive method for determining immune status.[102,365]

Antibodies are eventually produced to most viral proteins. The most abundant and most rapidly produced antibody is to N, and absence of this antibody is an indicator of seronegativity.[291] The smallest amount of antibody is to M, except in atypical measles.[291,485] The primary antibodies that neutralize virus infectivity are to H.[175,176,278] Neutralization is generally measured by reduction of plaque formation on CD46-expressing Vero cells by the Edmonston vaccine strain of MeV,[148] but this assay may not reflect neutralization of wild-type MeV infection of SLAM-expressing cells.[667] Neutralizing epitopes have been mapped by competitive binding of monoclonal antibodies and by analysis of different strains and escape mutants.[357,360,456,768] Human convalescent sera show reactivity to linear epitopes, as well as to epitopes dependent on conformation and glycosylation.[356,527,573] A highly conserved linear neutralizing epitope is in the H noose (aa 379 to 410).[678] Major conformational epitopes have been localized to regions between amino acids 368 to 396 and in the SLAM-binding region.[229,456] Essentially all of these epitopes are on exposed surfaces on the sides of the H head domain,[336,728] and mutations that alter head conformation decrease the neutralizing capacity of sera.[434] Although most neutralizing antibodies are specific for H, antibodies to F induced by regions encompassing amino acids 73 and 388 to 402 contribute to virus neutralization, probably by preventing fusion of the virus membrane with the cell membrane at the time of virus entry.[37,176,236,491,670] Human sera also recognize linear epitopes in six to seven regions spread over much of the F protein frequently close to T-cell epitopes.[572,871]

Antibody can protect from MeV infection, may contribute to recovery from infection, and may play a role in establishing persistent infection.[32,224,466,686] Antibody-dependent cellular cytotoxicity correlates temporally with cessation of cell-associated viremia,[247] and failure to mount an adequate antibody response carries a poor prognosis.[868] However, in primate studies, transient depletion of B cells did not affect clearance of infectious virus.[638] Antibody binding to the surface of infected cells as well as intracellular IgA inhibits virus replication and may contribute to control of infection *in vivo*.[255,279,746,897] The role of antibody in protection from infection is discussed under immunization, and the role in establishing persistence is discussed under persistent infection.

Cellular immunity

The ability to recover from measles was postulated by Burnet to be an indication of the adequacy of T lymphocyte–mediated immune responses,[107] and depletion of CD8$^+$ T cells in infected macaques impairs control of virus replication and slows clearance.[639] MeV-specific, proliferating, and clonally expanded CD8$^+$ T cells are present in blood at the time of the rash, in bronchoalveolar lavage fluid during pneumonitis and infiltrate sites of replication in the skin (Fig. 9.9).[383,551,576,837,856] IFN-γ, soluble CD8, and β2 microglobulin, a component of the MHC class I molecule, are increased in plasma (Fig. 9.7).[305,306,308,563] Culture of PBMCs with autologous MeV-infected or MeV peptide-pulsed cells after recovery expands CD8$^+$ T cells that produce IFN-γ and are cytotoxic demonstrating that effector CD8$^+$ T-cell memory is established by infection.[384,584,837] CD8$^+$ T- cell responses in humans show a broad pattern of reactivity with epitopes identified in all viral proteins.[346,382,383,620,739,839,841,842] Modeling of the data from macaques indicates that clearance of the acute viremia is dependent on T cells that deplete virus-infected lymphocytes, a process that also contributes to immune suppression.[24,555]

CD4$^+$ T cells are proliferating during the rash[856] and soluble CD4 becomes elevated in plasma and remains so for several weeks after recovery.[304] CD4$^+$ T-cell proliferation and cytokine production are induced in response to most MeV proteins.[502,563,571,839,891] Cytokines produced by CD4$^+$ T cells determine their function, and distinct populations of CD4$^+$ T cells are sequentially activated during measles (Fig. 9.10).

Type 1 CD4+ T (Th1) cells require IL-12 during differentiation and produce IFN-γ that activates macrophages and IL-2 that promotes T-cell proliferation. These are the primary mediators of classical delayed-type hypersensitivity. In measles, IL-12 is produced early, so that IFN-γ, neopterin (a product of IFN-γ–activated macrophages), and soluble IL-2 receptor rise during the prodrome with continued production of IFN-γ at the time of the rash followed by increases in IL-2 and soluble CD4.[304–307,469,470,563] Type 2 CD4+ T (Th2) cells require IL-4 during differentiation and produce IL-4, IL-5, IL-10, and IL-13 that are important for B-cell growth and differentiation and for macrophage deactivation. Later suppression of IL-12 production and induction of IL-10 likely contributes to development of the Th2 responses during recovery[120,304,651] as IL-12 supplementation decreases production of IL-4 and neutralizing antibody.[350] As the rash fades, IL-4, IL-10, and IL-13 increase (Fig. 9.7) and elevation of these cytokines persists in some individuals for weeks.[304,470,563,891] Th17 cells require IL-23 for differentiation, are associated with autoimmunity, and produce IL-17; T regulatory (Treg) cells produce IL-10 and TGF-β; and follicular helper (Tfh) cells promote germinal center formation and produce IL-21. At late times, after apparent recovery, numbers of MeV-specific IL-17–producing T cells and Tfh cells in circulation increase (Fig. 9.10).[470,595,596,766]

In addition to its regulatory properties, IFN-γ may have an important direct antiviral effect. IFN-γ suppresses MeV replication in epithelial and endothelial cells *in vitro* through induction of indoleamine 2,3 dioxygenase[604] and inhibits MeV replication in the brains of infected rodents.[243,632,862]

Durability of the immune response

Epidemiologic studies have documented long-term protection from reinfection without reexposure,[628] and high levels of antibody to MeV are sustained for decades.[21] After apparent recovery from the acute infection, there is continued development of lymph node germinal centers, production of antibody-secreting cells that traffic to the bone marrow, and progressive avidity maturation.[595] Extensive MeV replication in lymphoid tissue followed by persistence of MeV RNA may maximize and prolong the presentation of viral antigen by follicular DCs and stimulate long-term production of memory B cells and germinal center–matured plasma cells that become resident in the bone marrow (Fig. 9.10).[325,466,469] Immunologic memory to MeV also includes continued circulation of MeV-specific CD4+ and CD8+ T lymphocytes[584] and residence of memory CD4+ T cells in the bone marrow[615] so long-lasting cellular immunity may play an important supportive role in protection from reinfection and disease.

Immune suppression

MeV can suppress immune responses *in vivo* during measles, *in vitro* when immune cells are cultured with virus or viral proteins, and in some animal models.

During measles

Measles was the first disease recognized to increase susceptibility to other infections, and most measles deaths are caused by other infections.[67] Clemens von Pirquet first quantified the immunosuppressive effects of measles in his study of tuberculin delayed-type hypersensitivity skin test responses during

a measles outbreak in a Vienna tuberculosis sanitarium. This response is suppressed for weeks after the rash has cleared and recovery appears complete (Fig. 9.11).[813] In those who survive, the increase in susceptibility to infection and risk of hospitalization continues for 2 to 3 years (Fig. 9.8).[69,262,289,541]

Immune suppression is probably a multifactorial process and begins during a period of intense immune activation associated with the onset of the measles rash and generation of the immune response to MeV. Infection of immune cells likely plays an important role. Immune cells expressing SLAMF1 in lymphoid tissue are the main sites of virus amplification and fuel the viremia and systemic spread of MeV.[174] Both myeloid and lymphoid cells are infected and targets for immune elimination resulting in depletion due to cell death and functional abnormalities in surviving cells (Fig. 9.11).[24,178,232,234,372,469,555,869] Both B cells and T cells are infected with decreased numbers in circulation (Fig. 9.8) and reduced CD4:CD8 ratios during the acute phase of measles.[33,169,301,717,870] Lymphocytopenia is more marked in girls and in malnourished children and may be exacerbated by fever-induced changes in lymphocyte trafficking and bystander lymphocyte apoptosis.[5,39,612,717,852]

Ex vivo studies of virus replication in thymus organ cultures, tonsil explants, and PBMCs have shown preferential replication in double-positive thymocytes, B cells, and memory T cells consistent with SLAMF1 expression by these cells.[153,178,310,613] *In vivo*, there is extensive replication of MeV in B and T cells in blood and lymphoid tissues with a higher percentage of MeV-positive B cells than T cells. Replication occurs in both naive and memory B cells but primarily in memory T cells.[178,438,440,469] Leukopenia is followed by a rapid rebound in numbers of circulating cells with lymphocyte activation and proliferation and increased thymic output of naive CD4+ and CD8+ cells, while other immunologic abnormalities persist (Figs. 9.8 and 9.10).[40,640,717,856] In lymph nodes, the phase of B- and T-cell depletion is followed by lymph node enlargement due to repopulation with proliferating lymphocytes, B-cell follicle expansion, and formation of germinal centers as part of the adaptive immune response at the time of the rash.[178,595] The effects of cell depletion and subsequent proliferation change the relative representation of subtypes of immune cells in circulation over time.[438,717] In general, after recovery, naive T cells and memory B cells are decreased while activated and memory T cells and regulatory T cells are increased compared to before infection.[438]

PBMCs collected during both acute and convalescent phases of measles have suppressed lymphoproliferative responses to mitogens (Fig. 9.11) with inadequate production of IL-2 by lymphocytes and low levels of IL-12 and TNF-α production by monocytes.[36,40,300,348,669,857] During recovery, *in vitro* production of IFN-γ is low to normal and IL-4 is high compared to controls,[304,857] and the suppressive effects of Th2 production of IL-4 and IL-10 on Th1 cells and macrophages may contribute to suppression of delayed-type hypersensitivity. The role of persistent MeV RNA in these functional defects is not known. Th2 cytokine predominance produces an environment favoring B-cell maturation that facilitates the establishment of humoral memory important for lifelong protection from reinfection while depressing macrophage activation and induction of type 1 responses that may be required for combating new pathogens. Infection of monkeys with an IL-12–producing recombinant

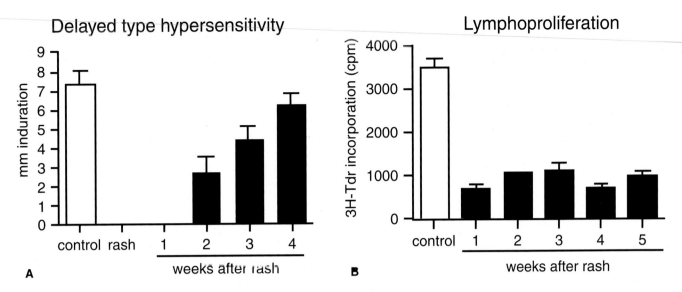

FIGURE 9.11 Immune suppression during measles. A; Changes during measles in tuberculin-induced delayed-type hypersensitivity (DTH) skin test responses in children with measles who had previously received immunization against tuberculosis. **B;** Changes in proliferation of peripheral blood mononuclear cells to the mitogen phytohemagglutinin. (Data from Tamashiro VG, Perez HH, Griffin DE. Prospective study of the magnitude and duration of changes in tuberculin reactivity during uncomplicated and complicated measles. *Pediatr Infect Dis J* 1987;6(5):451–454. Hirsch RL, Griffin DE, Johnson RT, et al. Cellular immune responses during complicated and uncomplicated measles virus infections of man. *Clin Immunol Immunopathol* 1984;31(1):1–12.)

MeV increased production of IFN-γ and suppressed production of MeV-specific antibody but did not improve lymphocyte proliferation.[350] Similarly, infection of cotton rats with an IL-4–producing recombinant MeV did not affect mitogen-induced lymphocyte proliferation.[120] These data suggest that the MeV-induced Th2 cytokine milieu may alter responses to other pathogens and thus contribute to increased susceptibility to infection but do not explain the characteristic measles-induced defect in lymphoproliferation.

Measles also increases long-term susceptibility to infection by altering the repertoire of pathogen-specific antibody responses and types of cells in circulation. Numbers of memory B cells are reduced, and there is an incomplete reconstitution of naive B cells.[438,644] In addition, diversity of antipathogen antibodies in plasma is decreased presumably due to MeV-induced loss of long-lived plasma cells that produce most of the antibody found in circulation, either due directly to MeV-induced or immune-mediated death or eviction from bone marrow niches during the response to MeV.[540]

In vitro infection of immune cells

In vitro infection of leukocytes and leukocyte cell lines with MeV induces abnormalities of DC, monocyte/macrophage, B-cell, T-cell, and epithelial cell function. T-cell proliferation to mitogens and soluble antigens,[514] cytotoxic function,[123] B-cell production of immunoglobulin,[123,515] and bone marrow stromal cell developmental support of hematopoietic stem cells[493] are suppressed by *in vitro* infection. These abnormalities may be relevant to immune suppression during measles, although some can be attributed to production of type I IFN in the MeV-infected cultures.

Infection of monocytes or macrophage lineage cells *in vitro* stimulates production of IFN-α/β, inhibits production of

TNF-α and IL-12, and may interfere with expression of peptide-loaded MHC class II complexes.[397,451,725,888] Virus production decreases as macrophages mature.[254,340] MeV infection of immature DCs induces maturation[749,761,778] but impairs CD40L signaling necessary for terminal differentiation.[761] Mannose receptor–mediated endocytosis is not affected.[311] Monocytes and DCs exposed to MeV or N protein have impaired production of IL-12 but preserved or increased production of the regulatory cytokine IL-10.[254,321,397,496,761] Suppression of IL-12 production in response to TLR4 ligation is facilitated by H interaction with SLAMF1,[321] and MeV interaction with DC-SIGN increases IL-10 transcription by inducing acetylation of NF-κB subunit p65.[309] Ncore interacts with FcγRII on B cells to inhibit antibody production *in vitro*, and Ntail binds to thymic epithelial cells and activated T cells through an unidentified receptor to induce cell cycle arrest.[689]

Analysis of antigen-presenting function has shown that MeV-infected monocytes can present MeV, but not an unrelated antigen, to T-cell clones.[450] Interaction with DC-SIGN increases MeV uptake, DC maturation, and mobilization, but MeV-infected DCs cannot support immune synapse formation with T cells and become apoptotic.[44,159,254,311] Likewise, MeV-exposed T cells are recruited into conjugates with DCs *in vitro* but have impaired clustering and maintenance of immune synapse proteins needed for sustained T-cell activation,[776] in part due to sphingomyelinase activation and accumulation of ceramide.[267,574]

Lymphocytes infected with MeV *in vitro* can be activated by mitogen but proliferate poorly because entry into S phase and progression through the cell cycle is impaired.[265,514,517,587,748,883] T-cell proliferation can also be suppressed by direct inhibitory signaling of the H and F₁–F₂ viral glycoprotein complex present on virions or infected cells.[206,740,749,864] Blocking the interaction of H with SLAMF1 or CD46 does not interfere with suppression of lymphocyte proliferation,[227] but antibody to H or F reverses the inhibition.[206] This contact-dependent inhibitory signal affects association of signaling molecules and their regulators with lipid rafts by inhibiting degradation of the cytoplasmic inhibitory protein Cbl-b and recruitment of Akt kinase and Vav.[45] This interference with T-cell activation of PI3 kinase/Akt prevents S phase entry and cell cycle progression in response to ligation of the T-cell receptor or the IL-2 receptor[41,45,740] and is not dependent on cell death, membrane fusion, production of soluble inhibitors, or T-cell infection.[206,225,748,863] In addition, induction of SIP110 phosphatase decreases availability of PIP_3 needed for phospholipid signaling.[43] Determination of the relevance of this process to *in vivo* suppression of lymphoproliferation requires further study, but ongoing interaction of T cells in lymphatic tissue or in circulation with MeV-infected cells could induce this refractory state and result in suppressed proliferation in response to stimulation *ex vivo*.

Animal models

Small animal models, primarily cotton rats and CD46 and SLAMF1 transgenic mice, have also been used to study immunosuppression *in vivo* after MeV infection. Respiratory infection of cotton rats results in decreased proliferation of cultured T cells.[599] Infected CD46 transgenic mice have impaired T-cell cytotoxicity and antibody production associated with increased susceptibility to bacterial infection.[616,789] MeV infection of SLAMF1 transgenic mice inhibits differentiation of DCs from bone marrow precursors through STAT1-independent, STAT2-dependent actions of type I IFN.[120,322] In IFN receptor-deficient SLAMF1-expressing mice, MeV infection leads to lymphopenia and Th2-mediated immunosuppression.[423] The relevance of these observations to the immune suppression that occurs during human infection is unclear.

Autoimmunity

An autoimmune demyelinating disease, postinfectious or acute disseminated encephalomyelitis (ADEM), is an important complication of measles[538] (Table 9.1; Fig. 9.12) and is associated with an immune response to myelin basic protein[388] similar to that seen in animals with experimental autoimmune encephalomyelitis. The similarity of these diseases and lack of MeV in the brain have led to the current understanding that ADEM is an autoimmune disease induced during measles.[388]

The mechanism of induction of autoimmune disease is not clear. Hypotheses have included altered presentation of myelin antigens due to MeV infection of oligodendrocytes, "molecular mimicry" of myelin antigens by MeV, and dysregulation of immune responses.[348,379] There is little evidence for MeV infection of cells in the nervous system.[270,388,546] Neither cross-reactive antibodies nor cross-reactive T-cell clones have been identified in humans or rats with demyelinating disease induced in conjunction with MeV infection.[457] Genetic susceptibility to ADEM has been postulated, but the numbers of patients studied have been insufficient to clearly identify a link between MHC antigens or other genetic factors and disease.[443]

Studies of immune regulation have shown that patients with encephalomyelitis differ from patients with uncomplicated disease by having a distinct pattern of immunologic abnormalities. IgE is more persistently elevated, and soluble IL-2 receptor is lower.[299,305] The timing of autoimmune disease suggests that immune dysregulation during measles may play a role in allowing activation and expansion of autoreactive lymphocytes.

Release and Transmission

Epidemiologic data suggest that infected individuals become infectious for nonimmune contacts a few days before the onset of the rash.[417] At this time, virus can be cultured from the nasopharynx, conjunctivae, and mouth[219] consistent with the respiratory tract as the site of virus release. Multinucleated epithelial giant cells are readily demonstrated in nasal secretions and conjunctivae during the prodrome and first days of the rash and are also shed into the urine.[462,738] A recombinant virus that cannot interact with nectin 4 to infect epithelial cells is not shed from the respiratory tract of infected macaques further suggesting that epithelial cells are the source of virus that is transmitted.[448] Strains of MeV may differ in the efficiency with which they are transmitted either due to decreased susceptibility to vaccine-induced protection or increased infectiousness.[4,676]

Virulence

There is increasing evidence that wild-type strains may differ both in transmissibility and virulence as evidenced by increased hospitalization rate and complications associated with the currently circulating B3 genotype compared to the D8 genotype.[4,676] More obvious and amenable to analysis are differences between the live attenuated virus vaccine that rarely causes disease and wild-type MeV that causes measles. Differences in the sites of replication have not been clearly identified, but vaccine strains induce little viremia and show limited replication in lymphoid tissue compared to wild-type strains.[40,173,177,469] Virulence has been assessed by the study of replication of MeV in human tissues explanted into culture or implanted into immunodeficient mice and in primary cells of different types. In general, vaccine strains replicate similarly to wild-type strains in primary endothelial cells and respiratory epithelial cells and tissues but not in lymphoid cells and tissues where vaccine virus entry into primary lymphocytes is similar but virus production is restricted.[153,469,471] In thymic explants and implants, wild-type viruses grow more rapidly, to higher titer, and cause more extensive thymocyte apoptosis than attenuated strains.[39,613] In tonsil explants, vaccine virus infects more naive T cells, but fewer B cells, macrophages, and NK cells than wild-type virus.[153]

Sequences have been compared and many changes that may contribute to attenuation have been identified,[809] but *in vivo* testing of virulence is difficult because of the lack of a good small animal model. Because adaptation of wild-type MeV to growth in Vero cells selects for a virus that no longer causes a rash in monkeys,[55] many studies of virulence have focused on the sequence changes required for wild-type viruses to grow in Vero cells. Changes in multiple protein genes (P/C/V, M, F, H, and L) are selected and associated with improved growth in Vero cells or chicken embryo fibroblasts.[58,204,373,542,764,799,800,806,808,826,882] The H protein of vaccine strains can use the CD46 receptor efficiently, while wild-type strains do not, but this alone does not determine virulence.[799] Construction of recombinant viruses using the Japanese IC-B wild-type and CAM-70 vaccine

TABLE 9.1 Summary of the neurologic complications of measles

Disease	Host	Age of Measles	Incidence	Pathology	Time Course
Acute disseminated encephalomyelitis (ADEM)	Normal	>2 y	1:1,000	Inflammation, demyelination	Monophasic, weeks
Measles inclusion body encephalitis (MIBE)	Immunocompromised	Any	1:10	Inclusion bodies	Progressive, months
Subacute sclerosing panencephalitis (SSPE)	Normal	<2 y	1:2,000	Inclusion bodies, inflammation	Progressive, years

strains has shown that changes in M, F, H, and L all contribute to efficient growth of CAM-70 in chicken fibroblasts,[398,764] but which one or combination of changes alters *in vivo* virulence has not been identified.

Persistent Infection

MeV can establish persistent infection *in vitro* and *in vivo*. A number of cell lines persistently infected with MeV have been established, and neurologic disease can be caused by persistent infection of neurons and glial cells.

Persistently Infected Cells in Culture

Replication of MeV usually causes death of cultured cells, but this is not necessarily the case *in vivo* or with primary cells. The elements determining persistent noncytopathic versus lytic infection are not completely understood, but properties of both the infected cell and the infecting virus contribute. Methods historically used to establish persistently infected cell lines include (a) passage of virus at high multiplicity with generation of DI particles[700]; (b) passage of infected cells in the presence of antibody[716]; (c) cultivation of cells surviving lytic infection[201,240,716]; and (d) cocultivation of cells with brain cells from persistently infected animals or humans.[526]

Persistent noncytopathic infection is most easily established in neuronal cells but has also been established in lymphoid, epithelial, and glial cell lines.[201,703,747,802] Persistent infection is usually accompanied by a marked decrease in the amount of infectious virus released. After persistence has been established, accumulation of N can suppress replication and form nuclear inclusion bodies.[201] Cellular factors that influence persistence include expression of heat shock proteins, cAMP, IFN-inducible proteins, miRNAs, and altered regulation of lipid metabolism.[537,577,700] Cellular protein synthesis is relatively unaffected by MeV infection, but specific cellular proteins (e.g., cell surface receptors) and functional responses (e.g., signal transduction, expression of transcription factors) may be altered, particularly in neural cells.[65,245] Some cell lines produce

no infectious virus, and infection is maintained by passage of encapsidated viral RNA to daughter cells during cell division.[108]

Defects in glycoprotein expression may be due in part to limited mRNA production associated with steep transcriptional gradients and an increase in bicistronic messages.[130] However, mutations in these genes also lead to proteins with altered expression or function. For instance, defects in the M protein facilitate persistence and hinder association of N with the viral glycoproteins.[639]

Persistence of Viral RNA After Clearance of Infectious Virus In Vivo

Clearance of infectious virus occurs during the rash, and within a few days after the rash has faded, virus cannot be recovered from any site. However, MeV RNA can be detected by RT-PCR in urine, PBMCs, and respiratory secretions for weeks to months after apparent recovery.[134,466,469,641,697] In experimentally infected macaques, lymph node biopsies demonstrate persistence of viral RNA in cells of the immune system for months after it is no longer detected in PBMCs (Fig. 9.10).[466,595,596] The nature and intracellular location of the RNA has not been defined, but studies of mice with CNS infection suggest that renewed virus replication occurs if immune control is eliminated.[539] Persistence of viral RNA with production of viral antigens may be important both for maturation of a durable immune response and development of late disease.

Subacute Sclerosing Panencephalitis

SSPE is a slowly progressive uniformly fatal CNS disease that develops years after the original MeV infection (Fig. 9.12).[543] The pathogenesis of SSPE remains poorly understood but occurs in approximately 1 in 10,000 cases overall and approximately 1 in 1,000 children infected under 2 years of age when the immune system is immature and maternal antibody may still be present (Table 9.1).[73,327,409,536,710,750,804,867] There may be a genetic predisposition to developing SSPE, but specific genetic risk factors have not been clearly identified.[370,371,394,652,653] At the

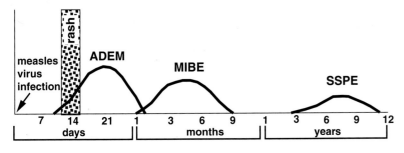

FIGURE 9.12 Time after infection of the occurrence of the three main neurologic complications of measles: postinfectious or acute disseminated encephalomyelitis (ADEM), measles inclusion body encephalitis (MIBE), and subacute sclerosing panencephalitis (SSPE).

time of disease onset, both white matter and gray matter are affected with nuclear and cytoplasmic viral inclusion bodies in neurons and glia.

Virus replication and spread

The route of virus entry into the CNS is unknown but may have occurred during acute infection through replication in brain endothelial cells[233,414] or trafficking of activated infected mononuclear cells from the blood into the CNS. Extensive sequence analysis of viral RNA from various parts of the brain in SSPE suggests that the virus in the CNS is clonal,[51] implying that virus entered the brain at one time (presumably during the original acute infection). Once in the CNS, CADM 1 and 2 can act as neuronal receptors and trigger fusion with adjacent cells.[774] No virus is seen being released from the surface of infected cells, and the cytoplasm contains "fuzzy" nucleocapsids that extend into neuronal processes consistent with virus spread through the CNS from neuron-to-neuron and to astrocytes by transmission of the ribonucleoprotein without the release of infectious particles.[209,215,442,511,665,736] Interaction with neurokinin-1, substance P, and glutamate transporters may facilitate transfer.[490,665]

There is no clustering of cases to suggest that the wild-type virus causing the initial infection is different from the virus causing uncomplicated disease. Analysis of viral RNA sequences has shown that SSPE viruses are related to wild-type strains circulating at the time of the primary infection but have accumulated mutations either before or after entry into the CNS that alters the M, F, or H envelope proteins to interfere with assembly and budding of infectious virus.[52,131,133,386,741]

In general, expression of M is low[455] due to lack of synthesis, instability, or mislocalization of the protein.[385,767,791] A variety of defects have been encountered in the mRNAs encoding M extracted from SSPE brain with mutations throughout the gene that include frequent U to C changes indicative of double-stranded RNA mutation by adenosine deaminase (biased or A/I hypermutation).[133,876] M transcripts often lack initiator AUGs necessary for expression, and when expressed, the proteins have defects in binding to viral nucleocapsids and in down-regulating transcription.[347,797] P gene mRNAs are edited less frequently to express V than in acute infection.[535] H proteins are often defective in intracellular transport and protein–protein interactions important for cell–cell fusion.[131] Neuropathogenicity and spread within the CNS is dependent on mutations in F that render it hyperfusogenic (Fig. 9.4)[366,390,508,859] so that truncations, mutations, and deletions in the cytoplasmic domain of F that interfere with virus budding and enhance fusion are almost universal.[48,50,131,741]

Immune responses

At the time of symptom onset, there are vigorous antiviral antibody responses in both serum and CSF and an extensive mononuclear inflammatory reaction in the CNS.[101,344] MeV-specific antibody is produced by plasma cells residing in the CNS,[106,622] and MeV-specific immunoglobulin in CSF is high and of restricted heterogeneity leading to the appearance of oligoclonal immunoglobulin bands on electrophoretic analysis.[231,825] Antibodies against the N and P ribonucleoprotein complex proteins are particularly abundant, and M protein antibody is particularly deficient.[324]

Antibody to MeV has been postulated to play a role in establishing persistent CNS infection either through alteration of the induction of the primary immune response at the time of infection[686] or through modulation of infection once virus is in the nervous system.[255] Treatment with antibody after intracerebral infection of small mammals with neuroadapted strains of MeV attenuates acute disease but increases the incidence of subacute or chronic encephalitis.[687] Cases of SSPE have been associated with passive transfer of immune globulin, and persistent infection has been induced experimentally by passive transfer of antibody.[686]

Studies of cellular immunity have been less extensive. MeV-specific lymphoproliferation is not impaired, but MeV-specific cytotoxic T-cell activity is decreased,[192,331] while production of IL-12, IL-23, IL-17, IL-22, and IFN-γ is increased compared with healthy seropositive individuals.[833] General measures of cellular immunity, such as skin test responses to various recall antigens and proliferative responses to mitogens, are normal. The mononuclear inflammatory response in the brain includes CD4$^+$ and CD8$^+$ T cells, as well as monocytes and Ig-secreting B cells.[27,231] Class I and class II MHC expression is increased in brain, and β2 microglobulin, soluble IL-2 receptor, and soluble CD8 are increased in CSF.[523] Thus, there is no evidence for a global defect in immune responses, but these immune responses are ineffective in clearing virus from the CNS.

Other Chronic Diseases

In addition to a clear role in SSPE, MeV in combination with genetic factors has also been implicated in the pathogenesis of Paget disease,[252,432,784] otosclerosis,[519,752] chronic active hepatitis,[702] and multiple sclerosis.[18] For most of these diseases, an etiologic link to measles is controversial[510,532,533,684] and for none has a definitive role for MeV been identified.

Veterinary Correlates

Canine Distemper

Canine distemper was described by Antonio de Ulloa in 1746 as a disease of dogs in Quito and is postulated to have arisen through adaptation of MeV to canines in South America.[680,830] The disease was subsequently imported into Spain and then spread through Europe.[83] Experimental transmission with secretions from a sick dog by Karle in 1844 demonstrated that the disease was infectious. It was shown to be of viral etiology in 1905 by Henri Carre, and the virus was isolated in primary canine kidney cells in 1959. Several effective live attenuated vaccines have been developed with the Onderstepoort strain most widely used.[500]

CDV is spread by aerosol, and the disease is characterized by fever, coryza, conjunctivitis, gastroenteritis, and pneumonitis. Through adaptive mutation in the H gene for interaction with SLAM and nectin 4 from different species, CDV has acquired a broader host range than many morbilliviruses and can cause fatal disease characterized by giant cell pneumonia, lymphocyte depletion, and immune suppression in all families of terrestrial carnivores and in macaques.[20,181,210,285,513,552,679,723] Canine distemper has many similarities to measles in humans, but infection of the CNS and neurologic disease are more common with glial cells as a primary target.[844] Using ferrets as a model system, it can be shown that CDV appears first in bronchial lymph nodes followed by a cell-associated viremia with spread to multiple lymphoid organs and epithelial tissues.[849] CDV enters the brain through infection of endothelial cells or CNS infiltration of infected monocytes.[46,737] Like measles, canine distemper is associated with profound short- and long-term immune suppression, and much of the mortality is due to secondary infections.

Neurologic disease is characterized by gait abnormalities and seizures, is most common in young animals, and can occur either early after infection or associated with demyelination 3 to 4 weeks later.[428,844] Persistence of virus in neural cells and in epithelial cells of the feet leads to chronic diseases known as old dog encephalitis and hard pad disease.[29,427] Some cases of old dog encephalitis have defective virus with intranuclear inclusions in the CNS coexisting with high levels of antiviral antibody, features in common with SSPE.

Rinderpest

Rinderpest was first recognized as a distinct clinical entity causing severe gastroenteritis in cattle during a 4th century European epizootic and produced a devastating pandemic when introduced into East Africa in 1889.[663] The causal agent of this disease was reported to be filterable in 1902 and was isolated in bovine embryonic kidney cells in 1957.[604] RPV causes a highly contagious disease of ruminants and swine characterized by inflammation, hemorrhage, necrosis, and erosion of the gastrointestinal tract.[63] RPV replicates in lymphocytes and macrophages leading to lymphoid necrosis, and in epithelial cells of the gastrointestinal, respiratory, and urinary tracts, and endocrine and exocrine glands, but not in the brain or spinal cord.[793,873] The success of vaccination campaigns in eradicating this disease from its last sites in Africa was declared in 2011.[497]

Peste des Petits Ruminants

Peste des petits ruminants virus (PPRV) causes an economically important disease of sheep, goats, buffalo, and camels in Africa, the Middle East, and Asia.[191,435] The disease was first discovered in West Africa in 1942 and is characterized by fever, erosive stomatitis, pneumonitis, diarrhea, and lymphoid cell depletion. PPRV replicates in epithelial cells, pneumocytes, macrophages, and lymphocytes.[68] PPRV is most closely related to RPV (Fig. 9.2), and four lineages are recognized.[207] Eradication efforts are underway with a target date of 2030[600] but have been complicated by the introduction of the more virulent lineage IV Asian strain into northern and eastern Africa.[207,435]

Morbillivirus Infections of Aquatic Mammals

In 1987, an epizootic of respiratory disease with high mortality due to secondary infections occurred in seals in the Baltic and North Seas.[848] Serology suggested infection with a morbillivirus related to CDV, and the causal agent, phocine distemper virus (PDV), was isolated in 1988 (Fig. 9.2).[406] Infection has since spread to otters in the Pacific Ocean and seals along the East Coast of the United States potentially associated with Arctic sea ice reduction.[280,387,650,845] Infection causes fever, nasal and ocular discharge, and signs of severe respiratory, gastrointestinal, and neurological disease. In the CNS, there is neuronal infection with inflammation.[792] Disease is complicated by a variety of secondary viral, bacterial, and parasitic infections suggesting the type of immune suppression seen in measles and canine distemper.[619]

Similar epizootics of severe respiratory disease were subsequently recognized in porpoises and dolphins, and morbilliviruses (PMV and DMV, now grouped together as cetacean morbillivirus, CeMV) distinct from PDV were isolated from these animals[64,387] and recognized subsequently in whales.[512] CeMV spreads along migration routes to cause strandings associated with giant cell pneumonia, encephalitis, and lymphoid depletion and virus demonstrable in the lung, brain, spleen, and bladder.[197,556]

Other Morbilliviruses

Feline morbillivirus (FeMV) was first isolated in 2012 in Hong Kong from stray domestic cats and associated with tubular interstitial nephritis.[877] Viral RNA is most often detected in urine with continued shedding over many months.[765] FeMV is distinct from other morbilliviruses and most closely related to bat morbillivirus sequences (Fig. 9.2). FeMV has now been identified worldwide with two main genotypes, but its role in the pathogenesis of chronic kidney disease in cats is unclear.[171]

Porcine morbillivirus, most closely related to CDV, was recently identified as a probable cause of fetal death, encephalitis, and placentitis in swine.[34] More viruses are likely to be discovered as morbillivirus sequences have been detected in specimens from many animals including bats.

Experimental Infection in Animals

Nonhuman primates can be infected naturally or experimentally with MeV and provide the only experimental model for the pathogenesis of human disease. Small laboratory mammals generally are not susceptible to systemic infection with wild-type strains of MeV, although replication has been reported in the respiratory tract of cotton rats[879] and in transgenic mice expressing the human receptor CD46[492] and/or SLAMF1.[771] Several neurotropic strains of MeV have been developed by repeated intracerebral passage in hamsters, mice, and rats. These strains do not produce acute disease like that seen in humans but rather serve as models for neurologic diseases such as SSPE.

Nonhuman Primates

Natural measles occurs only in humans. However, a number of species of nonhuman primates are susceptible to infection with wild-type MeV and can contract the disease through contact with humans.[692] Experimentally, monkeys can be infected by intranasal, intratracheal, or subcutaneous inoculation.[40,838] Disease in macaques is generally similar to that seen in humans, and when deaths occur, they are often caused by secondary infections.[692] Rhesus (*Macaca mulatta*) and cynomolgus (*Macaca fascicularis*) macaques have served as animal models for studies of measles pathogenesis, immune suppression, virus virulence, response to vaccines, and protective immunity.[40,216,447,465,466,469,516,518,627,838] Squirrel monkeys (*Saimiri sciureus*) are susceptible to infection and provide another potential experimental system.[182]

Marmosets and tamarins are also susceptible to MeV infection by the respiratory route but develop a fulminant disease with high mortality characterized by interstitial pneumonitis, gastroenterocolitis, and bacteremia.[477] Infection with vaccine strains produces little disease.[477] Intracerebral inoculation with the most virulent strains of MeV produces encephalitis, while attenuated strains do not.[13]

Cotton Rats

The respiratory tract of cotton rats (*Sigmodon hispidus*) can be infected with vaccine and wild-type strains of MeV, although SLAM is used inefficiently.[121,292,649,879] Virus replicates in the lungs and wild-type strains can spread to mediastinal lymph nodes and induce immunosuppression as measured by decreased proliferation of spleen cells to mitogen stimulation.[649] Cotton rats have been used for studies of pathogenesis, immune suppression, vaccine-induced immune responses, and protection from infection.[120,415,509,549,649,879,880]

Rats

The hamster neurotropic strain of MeV can infect laboratory rats after intracerebral inoculation. The CAM strain of MeV was adapted by serial passage to replicate in rat brain and causes fatal encephalitis in newborn rats.[459] The type of disease produced in older rats is determined by the strain of rat. In Brown Norway rats, 10% to 20% develop acute encephalitis, and there is no late disease in survivors. In Lewis rats, 80% to 90% develop acute fatal encephalitis, and the rest develop subacute disease. Infectious, cell-free virus can be recovered during acute, but not subacute, disease.[458] Rats have been used to identify determinants of neurovirulence and the role of the immune response in MeV-associated neurologic disease and persistent infection.[486,545] Acute encephalitis in newborn rats can be modulated by passive transfer of antibody to the H protein that results in persistent infection and a late onset of disease.[456] Features of subacute disease that are similar to SSPE include an inability to recover virus by routine methods, restricted expression of MeV envelope protein mRNAs in the brain, and intrathecal synthesis of oligoclonal MeV-specific antibody.[458,745]

Hamsters

Newborn hamsters are susceptible to CNS infection with wild-type vaccine and SSPE strains of MeV, develop hyperirritability leading to death within a few days, and have been used to assess determinants of neurovirulence.[49,50,380] Brains from young animals show giant cell encephalitis with intranuclear and intracytoplasmic inclusion bodies and a polymorphonuclear inflammatory response.[854] Older animals develop myoclonus with infection of cortical, thalamic, and hippocampal neurons without giant cell formation.[796,854] Ependymal infection may lead to hydrocephalus.[380] Cell-free virus can be easily recovered from the brains of newborn but not older hamsters.[111] Demyelination is uncommon,[854] but some hamsters inoculated as newborns with the LEC SSPE strain develop myelitis weeks later.[119]

Mice

Several strains of MeV have been adapted to grow in the brains of newborn mice and cause fatal disease after intracerebral, but not peripheral, inoculation.[31,368,594] Histopathology and immunocytochemical staining show neuronal and glial infection and giant cell encephalitis.[302,479,594] These viruses have mutations in H and P and are defective for replication in weanling mice where MeV antigen–positive neurons have only smooth nucleocapsid structures and no detectable H, F, or M proteins.[302,343,479] Disease consists of hyperexcitation and seizures associated with production of excitotoxic amino acids and destruction of pyramidal cells in the hippocampus that can be prevented by administration of glutamate receptor antagonists.[302,479] The genetic background of the mouse influences susceptibility with C3H/He mice most susceptible and SJL mice most resistant.[594,861] Deficiencies in cellular immunity increase susceptibility.[243,831]

A number of investigators have produced mice engineered, either by grafting human cells or by transgenic expression of human genes, to provide better murine systems for studying measles pathogenesis. Severely immunodeficient mice have been grafted with human PBMCs or hematopoietic stem cells or implanted with human fetal thymus and liver to provide lymphoid tissue sites for virus replication.[367] In thymic implants, MeV shows strain-specific differences in virus growth and thymocyte apoptosis that have been useful for assessing virulence and determinants of replication *in vivo*.[39,835,836] Immunologically normal mice with transplanted human leukocytes develop graft versus host disease and can also be infected with MeV.[363]

Transgenic mice expressing human CD46 or SLAM have been produced using genomic DNA or cDNAs with promoters designed to provide generalized or cell type–specific expression of the receptor transgene.[322,492,634,771,866] In general, little infectious virus can be recovered, and this is age-dependent with neonatal mice more permissive than older mice.[634] Blocks to MeV replication in mice are at multiple levels[847] so infection in transgenic mice is enhanced by the absence of components of the innate or adaptive immune system.[492,609,771] These mice and cells from these mice have been used for studies of pathogenesis, virulence, immunosuppression, CNS infection, and virus clearance.[241,320,322,423,539,758,808]

Ferrets

Intracerebral inoculation of ferrets with cells infected with certain SSPE strains of MeV causes acute encephalitis.[400] Subacute or chronic encephalitis is established if animals are immunized prior to intracerebral injection with infected cells.[820] Pathologic and clinical features in animals with chronic disease resemble SSPE with cerebral inflammation, gliosis and intranuclear inclusion bodies, electroencephalographic changes, bound immunoglobulin in brain, and high titers of antibody to MeV in serum and CSF.[400,820]

EPIDEMIOLOGY

Classic Measles

In the Absence of Vaccination

The study of island populations was important in establishing many of the principles of measles epidemiology. Pioneering observations on the transmissibility, incubation period, and lifelong immunity of measles were made by Panum during the 1846 epidemic in the Faroe Islands.[628] Measles is one of the most infectious of communicable diseases. It is estimated that 76% of household exposures of susceptible persons lead to measles and that the reproductive number (R_o), or average number of secondary cases produced by an infectious individual in a totally susceptible population, is approximately 12 to 18.[313,553] Transmission is most efficient through direct exposure to an infected symptomatic individual, but aerosolized MeV can survive for hours so direct contact is not required for infection to occur.[137] Individuals are most infectious from 4 to 5 days before through 4 days after the appearance of the rash with MeV RNA detectable in the environment of a patient with measles for up to 8 days after rash onset.[79,141]

There is no animal reservoir or evidence of latent or epidemiologically significant persistent infection. Therefore, maintenance of MeV in the human population requires a continuous supply of susceptible individuals. Because older members of a community are immune through previous infection with the virus, endemic measles is primarily a disease of childhood. If the population is too small to establish endemic transmission, the virus cannot be maintained.[81] Mathematical calculations and studies of islands and cities with populations of different sizes have shown a requirement for a population of 250,000 to 500,000 to establish measles as an endemic disease.[82,404] This is approximately the population size of the earliest urban civilizations in ancient Sumeria where MeV is postulated to have emerged.[213]

In large population centers, measles is endemic with occasional epidemics as the numbers of susceptible individuals increase. These epidemics spread in waves from large cities to smaller cities and then to rural areas over time.[295] In temperate climates, measles is more frequent in the winter and early spring. The frequency of epidemics is determined by numbers of susceptible individuals, the duration of infectiousness, and patterns of population mixing.[404] The size of the population is also a primary determinant of the age of seroconversion. In countries with high birth rates, infection occurs at an early age and is earlier in urban than in rural areas in both developed and developing countries.[167] In small isolated populations, measles epidemics are controlled by extinction and chance reintroduction of the virus and this leads on average to infection at older ages.[141,694]

Very young infants are protected from measles (and from response to vaccine) by maternal antibody.[11] The source of maternal immunity (vaccination vs. natural measles), gestational age, and presence of maternal infection (e.g., human immunodeficiency virus type 1 [HIV-1], malaria) are determinants of the amount of antibody passively transferred and therefore, the length of time required for initial levels of antibody to decay to the point that an infant will become susceptible to measles.[112]

Effect of Vaccination

Immunization alters the epidemiology of measles by reducing the numbers and proportion of susceptible individuals in the population. In countries with high rates of vaccination, the average age for measles is increased because herd immunity reduces transmission and indirectly protects children from infection. Vaccination also lengthens the interepidemic period.[167] When outbreaks occur in areas of sustained high vaccine coverage, an increasingly large portion of the cases will be in older individuals who are susceptible due to lack of prior vaccination or natural infection or to primary or secondary vaccine failure. In contrast to prevaccination populations, outbreaks are increasingly likely to be local and dependent on social networks.[855] Because of the infectiousness of MeV and the high R_0, it is estimated that ≥95% of the population needs to be immune to interrupt endemic transmission.[268] However, even highly immunized populations are vulnerable to localized outbreaks associated with importation from areas where measles remains endemic.[268] These risks are increased in communities that include individuals who refuse vaccination for philosophical or religious reasons.[238]

Molecular Epidemiology

Lineages of MeV include 24 genotypes within 8 distinct clades identified by the variable 450 nucleotides of the C terminus of N (see "Evolution, Antigenic Composition, and Strain Variation").[708] Sequence comparisons of Ntail; portions of the P, H, or L genes; the M-F intergenic region; and whole genomes have been useful for analysis of the molecular epidemiology of measles.[87,408,709] Identification of the source of the MeV causing disease and chains of transmission in a particular location has become increasingly important as control programs are improved and identification of cases as imported or indigenous is necessary. Assembly of a large database of MeV genotypes has aided in the identification of global measles transmission pathways and led to recognition of decreasing diversity of the genotypes in circulation worldwide (B3, D4, D8, H1) (Fig. 9.6). Strain dominance may be driven by vaccine escape and/or more efficient transmission.[4,103,381,676,885] As elimination is approached and diversity of wild-type viruses in circulation decreases, regional analysis of importations and chains of transmission becomes more complex and more reliant on targeted whole genome sequencing.[87,676]

Subacute Sclerosing Panencephalitis

SSPE occurs preferentially in boys from rural areas with a history of measles at an early age.[327,377,543] In developing countries with high birth rates, measles often occurs in young infants,[289,327,559,562] and these countries have a high burden of SSPE.[495,718,804] This is further exacerbated when there is a high prevalence of HIV-1 infection because children of HIV-1–infected mothers are more likely to acquire measles at an early age.[218,562] Several studies have identified exposure to birds as a risk factor, but this relationship has not yet been explained.[327] The incidence has decreased dramatically with the introduction of measles vaccination.[73,115,624] There is no evidence that the vaccine virus can cause SSPE.[543]

CLINICAL FEATURES

Classic Measles and Its Complications

Measles has an incubation period of 10 to 14 days spanning the time from exposure to the appearance of clinical disease (Fig. 9.7). The first prodromal symptoms of measles are fever, malaise, and anorexia followed by cough, coryza, and conjunctivitis. The prodrome lasts 2 to 3 days, and during this time, small bright red spots with a bluish-white speck at the center, Koplik spots, may become visible on the buccal mucosa, providing early diagnostic evidence of measles.[821,892] The maculopapular rash appears first on the face and behind the ears and then spreads to the trunk and extremities (Figs. 9.1 and 9.8) and lasts 3 to 5 days accompanied by lymphadenopathy. In malnourished children ,the rash may desquamate.[554] In uncomplicated measles, clinical recovery begins soon after the rash fades.

Respiratory Disease

The prominent respiratory symptoms are manifestations of diffuse mucosal inflammation in response to widespread infection of epithelial cells. Interstitial pneumonitis and bronchiolitis due to MeV replication and inflammation in the lower respiratory tract are common, but frequently detectable only by imaging studies or measuring the alveolar–arterial oxygen gradient.[9,294,341,392] Pneumonitis is more likely to be clinically severe during pregnancy.[14,605] Symptomatic giant cell pneumonia is seen primarily in immunocompromised individuals.[221,499] Most of the severe pneumonia that complicates measles and leads to chronic pulmonary disease is caused by secondary bacterial and viral infections.[67,294,323] Other common respiratory complications caused by secondary infections are otitis media and laryngotracheobronchitis.[67,141] In addition to increasing susceptibility to new infections, previously latent viral and bacterial infections may be reactivated.[141,794]

Gastrointestinal Disease

MeV replication in the liver, particularly bile duct epithelium, is common in all ages, but clinically evident hepatitis is most frequent in adults.[276,392,445] Diarrhea is a common complication of measles, particularly in children requiring hospitalization.[293] Many epithelial surfaces are infected with MeV, and this may lead directly to gastrointestinal symptoms. However, diarrhea is frequently associated with secondary bacterial and protozoal infections[293] that compound the borderline nutritional status of young children in developing countries.

Myocardial Disease

Electrocardiographic abnormalities, including prolongation of the PR interval, ST segment and T-wave changes, can be detected in 20% to 30% of children with uncomplicated measles. However, symptomatic cardiac disease is uncommon and is most often related to transient conduction abnormalities. In autopsy studies, myocardial and pericardial lesions are usually attributable to systemic bacterial infections.

Neurological Disease

There is little evidence that the brain parenchyma is an important target tissue for MeV replication during acute disease in immunologically normal individuals.[522,546] However, apparently uncomplicated measles is frequently accompanied by a CSF pleocytosis and changes in the electroencephalogram[273,330] suggesting the possibility of CNS infection. The occasional appearance of slowly progressive neurological disease (measles inclusion body encephalitis, MIBE) in immunosuppressed individuals[10,249,575] and the occurrence of late neurological disease (SSPE) in immunologically normal individuals infected at a young age (Table 9.1; Fig. 9.12) attests to the ability of MeV occasionally to enter the CNS and replicate in neurons and glial cells.

ADEM complicates 1 in 1,000 cases of measles, with the highest attack rate in children over the age of 5 years and usually occurs within 2 weeks after the onset of the rash[538] (Fig. 9.12). The disease is characterized by an abrupt onset of fever and obtundation, accompanied by seizures and multifocal neurological signs. Neurologic damage can be severe with approximately 30% mortality and neurologic sequelae in most survivors.[388] Pathologic studies show that this is a perivenular inflammatory demyelinating disease, not inclusion body encephalitis like MIBE and SSPE, suggesting immunologically mediated disease.[270,890] There is little evidence for virus in the brain either as assessed directly by virus isolation or by detection of viral antigen or RNA[270,546] or indirectly by the appearance of MeV-specific antibody in the CSF.[388] There is, however, the induction of an autoimmune response to myelin protein similar to that seen in animals with experimental autoimmune encephalomyelitis and humans with Semple rabies vaccine–induced encephalomyelitis.[95,195,388,441]

Eye Disease

In addition to conjunctivitis, measles can cause keratitis and be an important cause of childhood blindness.[617] In areas of vitamin A deficiency, the two problems are synergistic and corneal ulceration resembling keratomalacia is a frequent complication of measles.[727]

Risk Factors for Morbidity and Mortality

Measles remains one of the most important causes of child morbidity and mortality worldwide.[557,561,874] Predictors of poor outcome are severe lymphopenia, elevated C-reactive protein, desquamating rash, and poor antibody response.[155,474,559,868] Mortality is highest at the extremes of age, in girls, in those with low socioeconomic status, and in those without access to medical care.[141,196,266,704] Mortality is also increased in pregnant women,[605] malnourished individuals,[61,488] HIV-1 infection,[559] and secondary cases in a household.[1,426] Malnutrition affects the immune responses to MeV, impairs virus clearance, and may lead to lower rates of diagnosis.[169,673] Vitamin A is a particularly important nutrient influencing outcome.[61] Low serum retinol is common in severe measles due either to prior dietary deficiency or to impaired mobilization from hepatic stores.[61,110] Case fatality rates range from 0.1% in places with good access to medical care to 6% in developing countries and up to 25% in refugee camps and virgin populations.[167,289,559,585,763,874]

Atypical Measles

A severe form of measles with unusual clinical features was seen in individuals who had previously received a poorly protective inactivated MeV vaccine used in the mid-1960s. Atypical measles differs from typical measles by having higher and more prolonged fever, unusual skin lesions, and severe pneumonitis.[258] The rash often is accompanied by evidence of hemorrhage or vesiculation and begins on the extremities and spreads to the trunk. Pneumonitis is associated with distinct nodular parenchymal lesions and hilar adenopathy.[294,889] Abdominal pain, hepatic dysfunction, headache, eosinophilia, pleural effusions, and edema are also described. Cases of atypical measles were reported up to 16 years after receipt of the inactivated vaccine. Administration of live virus vaccine after two to three doses of killed vaccine did not eliminate subsequent susceptibility to atypical measles and was often associated with severe local reactions.[109,135,257]

Hypotheses about the pathogenesis of atypical measles included an abnormally intense cellular immune response,[257] an inability of the inactivated vaccine to induce local respiratory tract immunity,[70] and a lack of production of antibody to F, which allowed virus to spread from cell to cell despite the development of antibody to H.[529,601] In rhesus macaques, the formalin-inactivated vaccine induces transient neutralizing and fusion-inhibiting antibodies, but there is a poor T-cell response, and antibodies induced do not undergo avidity maturation. Subsequent infection with MeV induces an anamnestic response of low avidity antibody that cannot neutralize wild-type virus. This leads to immune complex deposition, vasculitis, pneumonitis, and atypical measles.[667]

Measles in the Immunocompromised Host

Children with hypogammaglobulinemia appear to recover uneventfully from MeV infection while those with deficiencies in cellular immune responses may not.[283] Virus clearance is compromised, and progressive pulmonary, myocardial, or neurologic disease may result from infection, often in the absence of the typical rash or other characteristic features of measles.[105,221,253,499,614]

Giant cell pneumonia is characterized by increasing respiratory insufficiency beginning 2 to 3 weeks after exposure to MeV. Virus can be isolated from lung tissue and bronchial and nasopharyngeal washings. Pathology shows multinucleated epithelial, alveolar, and bronchiolar giant cells with intranuclear and intracytoplasmic inclusion bodies.[221,881] There is often evidence of systemic disease with giant cells visualized in multiple organs.[221]

MIBE occasionally accompanies giant cell pneumonia[393] but is more often present as an isolated primary manifestation of progressive MeV infection in immunocompromised adults and children.[10,249,359,575,875] Neurologic disease usually becomes evident within 6 to 12 months after exposure (Fig. 9.12). Initial signs and symptoms include altered mental status, focal seizures or epilepsia partialis continua, and occasionally blindness or hearing loss.[7,10,328] The course is typically rapid with progression to coma and death within weeks to months.[575] Pathology shows gliosis with inclusions in glial cells and neurons.[287] Giant cell formation is unusual, and little inflammation is present.[7,575] MeV protein and RNA are abundant and detectable by immunocytochemical staining or in situ hybridization. Viral nucleocapsids without budding particles are seen intracellularly by electron microscopy.[7,705] The mRNAs for genes encoding the H, M, and F envelope proteins are reduced, and these proteins are often undetectable.[53,129] MeV is usually mutated, but infectious virus can occasionally be recovered from the brain.[7,53,333,509,705] MIBE may be fundamentally similar to SSPE, but clinical symptoms are manifested earlier after infection and are more rapidly progressive in the absence of an immune response.[705]

Subacute Sclerosing Panencephalitis

SSPE most commonly occurs in individuals under the age of 20 who present many years after measles with neurologic disease and is uniformly fatal. The average time to onset of SSPE is 6 to 10 years (Fig. 9.12), but ranges from 1 to 24 years.[115,543] The onset is insidious, and the diagnosis is often not suspected early in disease.[353,674] The typical presentation of SSPE is with mental deterioration and personality changes (stage I). Subsequently, there is myoclonus, and often seizures (stage II) followed by progressive neurologic deterioration marked by rigidity (stage III), optic atrophy, akinetic mutism, and coma (stage IV).[378] Death occurs within months to years after onset.[250] Antibody to MeV is elevated in both serum and CSF, and inclusions are present in glial cells and neurons.[344] Perinatal infection can lead to SSPE with an accelerated onset and a fulminant course.[115,783]

DIAGNOSIS

The classical clinical features of measles—Koplik spots, fever, erythematous maculopapular rash, coryza, cough, and conjunctivitis—are generally sufficient to make the diagnosis, especially in the setting of a community outbreak, but laboratory confirmation should be obtained. The clinical case definition for measles includes (a) a generalized maculopapular rash of 3 days or more; (b) fever of 38.3°C (101°F), and (c) one of the following: cough, coryza, or conjunctivitis. However, not all of these signs and symptoms may be present and many are shared with other diseases. The differential diagnosis includes all causes of rash and fever, such as scarlet fever, rubella, chikungunya and other alphaviruses, dengue and other flaviviruses, parvovirus B19, human herpesvirus-6, human herpesvirus-7, meningococcemia, Kawasaki disease, and toxic shock syndrome.[102,284,672] Fever and/or rash may be absent during measles in very young infants, immunocompromised patients, malnourished children, and previously immunized individuals.[214,673]

Laboratory diagnostic procedures consist of isolation of virus; direct detection of the virus, viral RNA, or viral antigens; detection of IgM or low avidity IgG antibody by enzyme immunoassay (EIA); or documentation of seroconversion using HI, complement fixation (CF), virus neutralization, or IgG-specific EIA on serum taken during the acute and convalescent phases of disease. In immune compromised patients and SSPE, the diagnosis can be difficult, often not suspected and is usually dependent on biopsy to detect MeV in tissue.[10,511,575,671]

Isolation or Detection of Virus

Virus can be cultured from PBMCs, respiratory secretions, conjunctival swabs, and urine, but culture is rarely used as the means of diagnosing acute disease. Cell lines vary in their susceptibility to infection by wild-type strains with human cord blood leukocytes, the COBLa cord blood T-cell line, marmoset B95-8 or B95a cells, and Vero cells expressing SLAMF1 being most sensitive.[246,419,420,618] Epithelial cells from the nasopharynx, buccal mucosa, conjunctivae, or urine can be used for direct cytologic examination for giant cells and inclusions and for antigen detection.[462,790] Generally, the most useful antibody for staining is one directed to N because this protein is most abundant in the infected cell and N antigen reactivity is retained using a wide variety of fixation methods.[790] Direct examination for virus is of particular importance for diagnosis in immunocompromised individuals where antibody responses may not be present. The detection of MeV RNA by RT-PCR using primers targeted to highly conserved regions of the N, M, or F genes has been successfully applied to a variety of clinical samples[8,365,641,819] and to most other morbilliviruses.[290,453,780]

Detection of Antibody

The clinical diagnosis of measles is most often confirmed by serology. Samples ideally consist of acute and convalescent serum pairs, but detection of MeV-specific IgM in serum or saliva or low avidity IgG in serum is diagnostic and may require only a single sample.[102,172,365,829] IgM antibody appears at the time of the rash and can be detected by 3 days and for up to 4 weeks after the onset of the rash in most individuals.[339] MeV-specific IgG peaks approximately 2 weeks later and gradually increases in avidity. EIA allows for differential detection of IgM and IgG and is widely used because of its convenience. Plates may be coated with lysates of MeV-infected cells or with recombinant MeV protein.[91,362]

The HI test detects antibody to H and correlates well with the neutralization test. Major limitations of the HI test include the requirement for fresh sensitive monkey erythrocytes and sufficient antigen for large numbers of tests, as well as the possible presence of nonspecific HA inhibitors in serum. The CF test has also been used to determine measles immunity, but titers are less stable over time. Neither of these tests is in common use. The virus plaque reduction neutralization assay remains the standard against which other tests are measured. It is more sensitive than HI or EIA tests[12,149] and provides the best correlate for protection from infection[138] and therefore remains the preferred measure of response to vaccination.[11]

PREVENTION AND CONTROL

Treatment

The only recommended treatment for measles, other than supportive care, is vitamin A. Administration of high doses of vitamin A during acute measles decreases morbidity and mortality by an unknown mechanism even in the absence of clinical evidence of vitamin A deficiency.[61,364] In areas of vitamin A deficiency and xerophthalmia, supplementation prevents blindness due to measles-induced corneal destruction. The World Health Organization recommends two doses of vitamin A for all children with measles.

No direct-acting antiviral treatment is currently available, but several drugs are in development that might aid in measles control and case management.[655] These drugs include polymerase inhibitors and fusion inhibitors in addition to drugs that affect cellular functions important for virus replication.[90,286,659] Most advanced are nucleoside analog GS-5734/Remdesivir[473] and ERDRP-0519, an orally available small molecule polymerase inhibitor.[163,431] These drugs may deserve further *in vivo* evaluation for treatment of measles.

Numerous therapeutic agents, including amantadine, IFN, isoprinosine, ribavirin, transfer factor, and neurokinin receptor antagonists, have been used for the treatment of SSPE. Evaluation of the efficacy of any of these regimens is difficult because the disease is rare, the course is variable, reports are anecdotal, and the benefits at best short term.[338]

Prevention

History of Vaccine Development

The earliest attempts at vaccination against measles by Home in 1749 were based on the principles of variolation with the reasoning that introduction of disease through the skin would lessen the effects on the lung, but "mobilization" was in general, unsuccessful. Subsequent approaches between 1920 and 1940 designed to inactivate or attenuate the virus by culture in chick embryos also met with limited success.[498] The isolation of MeV in tissue culture opened the way for a more concerted approach to vaccine development using the Edmonston strain of virus.[222] Killed virus vaccines were developed using formalin and Tween-ether for inactivation.[858] Simultaneously, attenuated vaccines based on adaptation of MeV to growth in chick cells were developed and are now widely used (Fig. 9.13).[401] The attenuated live virus vaccine has dramatically decreased the incidence of measles in all countries in which it has been effectively delivered and has saved millions of lives, estimated at more than 20 million from 2000 to 2017 (Fig. 9.14).[168,454,558]

The live attenuated MeV vaccine induces both neutralizing antibody and cellular immune responses that are long-lasting, but the immune responses necessary for protection from infection or disease have not been completely defined. Antibody is sufficient for protection because infants are protected by maternal antibody,[11] and passive transfer of immune serum can modify or interfere with measles vaccination and partially protect children from measles after exposure.[691] Amounts of neutralizing antibody in plasma at the time of exposure correlate with protection,[89,138,878] but the independent importance of memory B cells that can respond with antibody production after infection is not known.[391] Cellular immune responses are induced more readily than antibody in young infants and in the presence of maternal antibody,[263] but alone do not protect against measles.[467]

Inactivated Vaccines

The alum-precipitated inactivated vaccine was used in a three-dose regimen.[122,858] Recipients developed moderate levels of

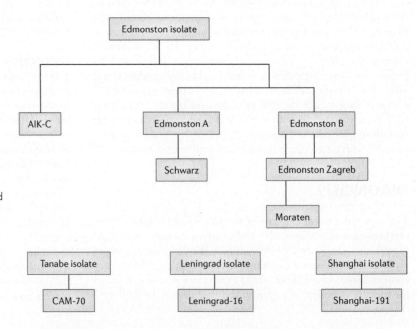

FIGURE 9.13 Measles virus vaccines. All attenuated measles vaccines in current use were developed from genotype A viruses and the most widely used vaccines (Moraten, Schwarz, and Edmonston-Zagreb) were developed from the Edmonston strain of MeV. (Reprinted by permission from Nature: Moss WJ, Griffin DE. Global measles elimination. *Nat Rev Microbiol* 2006;4(12):900–908. Copyright © 2006 Springer Nature.)

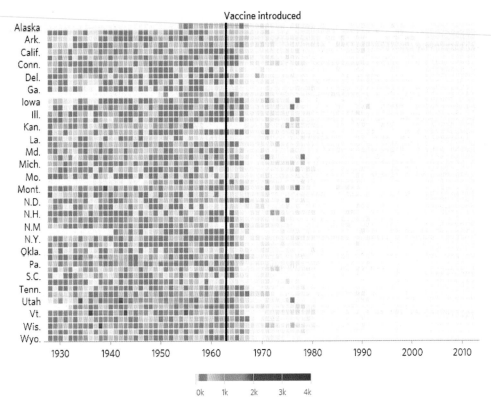

FIGURE 9.14 Reduction in numbers of cases of measles in the United States after introduction of measles vaccination.

neutralizing and HI antibodies and low levels of CF antibody.[122,239,601] Studies in rhesus macaques have shown that the inactivated vaccine induces no CD8+ T-cell response and that the avidity of MeV antibody does not mature.[667,668] The vaccine was protective when exposure to measles occurred soon after immunization.[239,259] However, antibody titers declined rapidly, and recipients again became susceptible to measles and, when infected, had a tendency to develop the more severe disease, atypical measles[259,667] discussed previously, and the vaccine was withdrawn.

Attenuated Live Virus Vaccines

The first attenuated live measles vaccine was developed by adaptation of the Edmonston strain of MeV to chick embryos and subsequently to chick embryo fibroblasts after passage in primary renal and amnion cells to produce the Edmonston B virus (Fig. 9.13).[220] Inoculation of this virus produced no detectable viremia, no spread to the respiratory tract. or disease in monkeys but did induce antibody and protected from subsequent challenge with wild-type MeV. This vaccine was efficacious[430] and licensed in 1963, but it produced fever and rash in a large proportion of immunized children.[401] Reactions were reduced when MeV antibody was given at the same time as the vaccine. Further passage of the Edmonston B virus in chick embryo fibroblasts produced a more attenuated vaccine virus[754] that was licensed in 1965. The Moraten/Attenuvax strain used in the United States was licensed in 1968 and is closely related to Schwarz.[707] Other Edmonston-derived vaccine strains (e.g., Zagreb, AIK-C) and attenuated strains developed independently (e.g., CAM, Leningard-16, Shanghai-191)

are also successful vaccines. Few differences have been described among MeV vaccine strains (all genotype A) regardless of the geographic origin of the parent virus, although differences in seroconversion rates in children less than 12 months of age have been identified.[376,707] The lyophilized vaccine is relatively stable but rapidly loses infectivity at room temperature after reconstitution.[525]

As with natural infection, antibody is induced to most viral proteins,[332] and neutralizing antibody to H correlates best with protection. Measles vaccine has a remarkable record of safety[461] and in many industrialized countries, it is given in combination with live virus vaccines for mumps and rubella (MMR) and sometimes varicella (MMRV). In resource-poor countries, MeV vaccine is often given alone, but there is an effort to transition to delivery of combined measles and rubella (MR) vaccine.[429,564]

The recommended age of initial vaccination varies from 6 to 15 months. The probability of seroconversion and the levels of antibody induced are determined by the level of persisting MeV-specific maternal antibody and by the age of the infant.[118,166,263,264,690] Age of immunization is determined by a region-specific balance between the optimum age for seroconversion and probability of acquiring measles before that age.[166] In areas where measles remains prevalent, measles vaccination is routinely performed at 9 months (85% response), whereas in areas with little measles, vaccination is often at 12 to 15 months of age (95% response).[167] Immunization as early as 6 months is recommended for protection during outbreaks but results in neutralizing antibody responses that are lower in titer and avidity.[100,501,597] Overall, the efficacy of a single dose of measles vaccine in infancy is estimated at 77% to 84% when administered at 9 to 11 months, 92% when administered at ≥12 months, and 94% after two doses.[263,834]

A second dose of vaccine is necessary to immunize persons who did not respond to the first dose[268] and can be delivered as a part of a routine vaccination program or in supplementary immunization campaigns. The two-dose strategy has been credited with elimination of indigenous measles in several countries.[558] However, low vaccine coverage in many regions due to weak health care systems or complacency, concerns about safety, and philosophical and religious objections to vaccination have resulted in gaps in coverage and a worldwide resurgence of measles.[35,165,212,630,832] Because an increasing proportion of susceptibles are unvaccinated adults, it has been suggested that coverage could be improved by immunization of parents at the same time as their children.[503]

The standard route of administration is either subcutaneous or intramuscular, but alternative routes that would avoid the need for needles and syringes have been explored. Transcutaneous delivery is being developed.[389] Intranasal administration of reconstituted liquid vaccine elicits a local, but not a systemic immune response, so is not an option.[782] Pulmonary delivery of aerosolized liquid vaccine can be effective, and inhalation of a small particle dry powder vaccine is safe in humans and induces protective immunity in macaques.[173,296,312]

Host factors including genetic differences affect the likelihood of seroconversion and level of antibody produced[199,683] with several polymorphisms identified that may affect responses.[146,193,194,621] The effect of common childhood illnesses on seroconversion is unclear,[326,534] and any potential decrease in seroconversion must be balanced against loss of the opportunity for vaccination and consequent risk of the child acquiring measles. Compromises must also be considered with respect to immunizing HIV-1–infected and other moderately immunocompromised individuals. In general, measles vaccine has been well tolerated in HIV-1–seropositive children, although the MeV seroconversion rate is lower, antibody is of lower avidity, and titers wane more quickly than in HIV-1–uninfected children.[524,580] Because of the potential severity of measles in these individuals, the vaccine is recommended for routine administration to infants without respect to HIV-1 serostatus in most countries, unless the CD4[+] T-cell count is known to be low. Progressive fatal measles vaccine virus infection can occur in severely immunocompromised children and adults[25,80,314,550] so immunization of these individuals is contraindicated.

The dose of MeV routinely used for immunization is between 10^3 and 10^4 plaque-forming units. Ten- to 100-fold higher doses improved seroconversion in younger infants, but subsequent follow-up of children receiving high titered vaccines in countries with high childhood mortality showed an increased mortality in girls over the subsequent 2 to 3 years.[352,418] Mortality was not due to measles, but rather to a relative increase in the deaths due to other infections.[2] The pathogenesis of delayed increased mortality after high titered vaccine is not understood but occurred primarily in those who developed a rash after vaccination and may be related to long-term suppression of immune responses similar to that induced by measles.[760]

The immune response to the live attenuated vaccine is similar to that induced by natural disease but levels of antibody induced are lower.[469] This results in lower levels of passively transferred maternal antibody and earlier susceptibility of infants to infection.[314] Also, the duration of vaccine-induced

immunity is more variable. Although antibody decays slowly,[28] both antibody titers and CD4[+] T-cell numbers decline with time.[142,156,274,586] Secondary vaccine failure rates 10 to 15 years after immunization have been estimated at approximately 5% but are probably lower when vaccine is administered after 12 months of age.[22,100,507] Failure rates may also depend on the circulating strain of wild-type MeV and was recently observed to be higher with exposure to the B3 genotype than the D8 genotype.[676] Attempts to boost immunity with repeated immunization have generally led to only transient improvements in either levels of neutralizing antibody or MeV-specific T-cell responses[242,544] and raise the possibility that new approaches to boosting immunity in adults may be required for measles control in the future.[303]

Postexposure Prophylaxis

Disease can be prevented after exposure either by vaccination or by passive transfer of immune globulin.[828] Currently, it is recommended that susceptible immunocompetent individuals 6 months or older be given measles vaccine within 72 hours of exposure. Alternatively, intramuscular or, if necessary, intravenous administration of human immunoglobulin should be used. However, levels of MeV antibody in these products are declining due to the increasing prevalence in donors of immunity induced by vaccination rather than natural infection.[544]

Experimental Vaccines

Development of new vaccines has been hampered by an incomplete understanding of protective immunity[89] and of the priming for enhanced disease by the inactivated vaccine. The primary motivations for development of a new vaccine are to increase thermostability, to provide a vaccine that can be given to young infants or boost immunity in adults, and to avoid the hazards associated with the use of needles and syringes. Vaccination with the H, F, and/or N protein expressed in bacterial, poxvirus, adenovirus, or bacille Calmette-Guerin vectors or as variously formulated DNAs, peptides, or proteins can induce cellular and humoral immunity in mice and cotton rats.[303] Macaques are the most relevant model system, and studies have shown different degrees of protection from infection and disease after vaccination with many of these experimental vaccines, but none has proven to be as protective as the current live attenuated virus vaccine.[303,468,626]

Measles Virus Vaccine Vectors and Oncolytics

Efficient systems have been developed for production of recombinant MeVs,[152,646,693] and these techniques are being applied to develop MeV vaccine as a vector for immunization against a variety of other virus infections (e.g., flavivirus, alphavirus, retrovirus, coronavirus).[478,480,567] For instance, a phase 1 trial of the MeV recombinant chikungunya virus vaccine showed that it was safe and induced antibody in adults with preexisting MeV immunity.[688] In addition, MeV vaccine virus is cytolytic for many tumor cells *in vitro*, and recombinant MeVs have been retargeted as oncolytic agents for cancer therapy.[566] These approaches have shown promise in animal models, and clinical trials, using doses orders of magnitude higher than those used for vaccination, have been initiated for treatment of multiple myeloma, ovarian and breast cancer, T-cell lymphoma, and glioblastoma.[566,568]

Prospects for Eradication

Theoretically, measles is an ideal virus for eradication through vaccination: there is only one serotype; most cases are clinically identifiable; there is no animal reservoir; and an effective vaccine is available.[560] However, measles remains a leading cause of vaccine-preventable childhood mortality with more than 100,000 deaths each year.[168] All WHO regions have established elimination goals, and in 2016, the region of the Americas was verified to have eliminated measles only to have this status reversed in 2018 when endemic transmission was reestablished.[564] The highly communicable nature of the virus requires continued maintenance of high vaccine coverage to prevent outbreaks, with 95% to 98% seropositivity needed to interrupt endemic transmission.[261,268,313] Global programs, such as the Expanded Program for Immunization, the Global Vaccine Action Plan, and the Measles and Rubella Initiative, have increased vaccine coverage worldwide and have resulted in significant decreases in measles and measles mortality.[564] However, coverage has plateaued at 84% to 85%, and delivery remains difficult in many areas due to civil strife, the COVID-19 pandemic, the need to maintain a cold chain, decreasing donor support, and religious or philosophical resistance to vaccination.[35,630,832] As elimination is approached, the average age of infection and year-to-year variability in numbers of cases increases while spatial clustering of unvaccinated individuals becomes more important in maintaining transmission.[288,629,827] Eradication remains a worthy but difficult goal.[211,564]

ACKNOWLEDGMENTS

Work from the author's laboratory has been supported by the National Institutes of Health (R01 AI131228, R01 AI153140, R21 AI095981) and the Bill and Melinda Gates Foundation. The contributions of many colleagues and members of the laboratory who have participated in these studies are gratefully acknowledged.

REFERENCES

1. Aaby P, Leeuwenburg J. Patterns of transmission and severity of measles infection: a reanalysis of data from the Machakos area, Kenya. *J Infect Dis* 1990;161(2):171–174.
2. Aaby P, Samb B, Simondon F, et al. A comparison of vaccine efficacy and mortality during routine use of high-titre Edmonston-Zagreb and Schwarz standard measles vaccines in rural Senegal. *Trans R Soc Trop Med Hyg* 1996;90(3):326–330.
3. Abe Y, Hashimoto K, Watanabe M, et al. Characteristics of viruses derived from nude mice with persistent measles virus infection. *J Virol* 2013;87(8):4170–4175.
4. Ackley SF, Hacker JK, Enanoria WTA, et al. Genotype-specific measles transmissibility: a branching process analysis. *Clin Infect Dis* 2018;66(8):1270–1275.
5. Addae MM, Komada Y, Zhang XL, et al. Immunological unresponsiveness and apoptotic cell death of T cells in measles virus infection. *Acta Paediatr Jpn* 1995;37(3):308–314.
6. Adombi CM, Lelenta M, Lamien CE, et al. Monkey CV1 cell line expressing the sheep-goat SLAM receptor a highly sensitive cell line for the isolation of peste des petits ruminants virus from pathological specimens. *J Virol Methods* 2011;173(2):306–313.
7. Aicardi J, Goutieres F, Arsenio-Nunes ML, et al. Acute measles encephalitis in children with immunosuppression. *Pediatrics* 1977;59(2):232–239.
8. Akiyama M, Kimura H, Tsukagoshi H, et al. Development of an assay for the detection and quantification of the measles virus nucleoprotein (N) gene using real-time reverse transcriptase PCR. *J Med Microbiol* 2009;58(Pt 5):638–643.
9. Albarello F, Cristofaro M, Busi Rizzi E, et al. Pulmonary measles disease: old and new imaging tools. *Radiol Med* 2018;123(12):935–943.
10. Albertyn C, van der Plas H, Hardie D, et al. Silent casualties from the measles outbreak in South Africa. *S Afr Med J* 2011;101(5):313–314, 316–317.
11. Albrecht P, Ennis FA, Saltzman EJ, et al. Persistence of maternal antibody in infants beyond 12 months: mechanism of measles vaccine failure. *J Pediatr* 1977;91(5):715–718.
12. Albrecht P, Herrmann K, Burns GR. Role of virus strain in conventional and enhanced measles plaque neutralization test. *J Virol Methods* 1981;3(5):251–260.
13. Albrecht P, Lorenz D, Klutch MJ. Encephalitogenicity of measles virus in marmosets. *Infect Immun* 1981;34(2):581–587.
14. Ali ME, Albar HM. Measles in pregnancy: maternal morbidity and perinatal outcome. *Int J Gynecol Obstet* 1997;59(2):109–113.
15. Alkhatib G, Roder J, Richardson C, et al. Characterization of a cleavage mutant of the measles virus fusion protein defective in syncytium formation. *J Virol* 1994;68(10):6770–6774.
16. Alkhatib G, Shen SH, Briedis D, et al. Functional analysis of N-linked glycosylation mutants of the measles virus fusion protein synthesized by recombinant vaccinia virus vectors. *J Virol* 1994;68(3):1522–1531.
17. Allagui F, Achard C, Panterne C, et al. Modulation of the type I interferon response defines the sensitivity of human melanoma cells to oncolytic measles virus. *Curr Gene Ther* 2017;16(6):419–428.
18. Allen I, Brankin B. Pathogenesis of multiple sclerosis—the immune diathesis and the role of viruses. *J Neuropathol Exp Neurol* 1993;52(2):95–105.
19. Allen IV, McQuaid S, Penalva R, et al. Macrophages and dendritic cells are the predominant cells infected in measles in humans. *mSphere* 2018;3(3).
20. Almberg ES, Cross PC, Smith DW. Persistence of canine distemper virus in the Greater Yellowstone ecosystem's carnivore community. *Ecol Appl* 2010;20(7):2058–2074.
21. Amanna IJ, Carlson NE, Slifka MK. Duration of humoral immunity to common viral and vaccine antigens. *N Engl J Med* 2007;357(19):1903–1915.
22. Anders JF, Jacobson RM, Poland GA, et al. Secondary failure rates of measles vaccines: a metaanalysis of published studies. *Pediatr Infect Dis J* 1996;15(1):62–66.
23. Anderson DE, Pfeffermann K, Kim SY, et al. Comparative loss-of-function screens reveal ABCE1 as an essential cellular host factor for efficient translation of *Paramyxoviridae* and *Pneumoviridae*. *mBio* 2019;10(3).
24. Anelone AJN, Hancock EJ, Klein N, et al. Control theory helps to resolve the measles paradox. *R Soc Open Sci* 2021;8(4):201891.
25. Angel JB, Walpita P, Lerch RA, et al. Vaccine-associated measles pneumonitis in an adult with AIDS. *Ann Intern Med* 1998;129(2):104–106.
26. Angius F, Smuts H, Rybkina K, et al. Analysis of a subacute sclerosing panencephalitis genotype B3 virus from the 2009–2010 South African measles epidemic shows that hyperfusogenic F proteins contribute to measles virus infection in the brain. *J Virol* 2019;93(4).
27. Anlar B, Soylemezoglu F, Aysun S, et al. Tissue inflammatory response in subacute sclerosing panencephalitis (SSPE). *J Child Neurol* 2001;16(12):895–900.
28. Antia A, Ahmed H, Handel A, et al. Heterogeneity and longevity of antibody memory to viruses and vaccines. *PLoS Biol* 2018;16(8):e2006601.
29. Appel MJ. Pathogenesis of canine distemper. *Am J Vet Res* 1969;30(7):1167–1182.
30. Apte-Sengupta S, Navaratnarajah CK, Cattaneo R. Hydrophobic and charged residues in the central segment of the measles virus hemagglutinin stalk mediate transmission of the fusion-triggering signal. *J Virol* 2013;87(18):10401–10404.
31. Arai T, Terao-Muto Y, Uchida S, et al. The P gene of rodent brain-adapted measles virus plays a critical role in neurovirulence. *J Gen Virol* 2017;98(7):1620–1629.
32. Arciuolo RJ, Jablonski RR, Zucker JR, et al. Effectiveness of measles vaccination and immune globulin post-exposure prophylaxis in an outbreak setting—New York City, 2013. *Clin Infect Dis* 2017;65(11):1843–1847.
33. Arneborn P, Biberfeld G. T-lymphocyte subpopulations in relation to immunosuppression in measles and varicella. *Infect Immun* 1983;39(1):29–37.
34. Arruda B, Shen H, Zheng Y, et al. Novel Morbillivirus as putative cause of fetal death and encephalitis among swine. *Emerg Infect Dis* 2021;27(7):1858–1866.
35. Arvin AM. Will measles virus or humanity win the international "fitness" challenge? *Annu Rev Virol* 2019;6(1):iii–vii.
36. Atabani SF, Byrnes AA, Jaye A, et al. Natural measles causes prolonged suppression of interleukin-12 production. *J Infect Dis* 2001;184(1):1–9.
37. Atabani SF, Obeid OE, Chargelegue D, et al. Identification of an immunodominant neutralizing and protective epitope from measles virus fusion protein by using human sera from acute infection. *J Virol* 1997;71(10):7240–7245.
38. Attibele N, Wyde PR, Trial J, et al. Measles virus-induced changes in leukocyte function antigen 1 expression and leukocyte aggregation: possible role in measles virus pathogenesis. *J Virol* 1993;67(2):1075–1079.
39. Auwaerter PG, Kaneshima H, McCune JM, et al. Measles virus infection of thymic epithelium in the SCID-hu mouse leads to thymocyte apoptosis. *J Virol* 1996;70(6):3734–3740.
40. Auwaerter PG, Rota PA, Elkins WR, et al. Measles virus infection in rhesus macaques: altered immune responses and comparison of the virulence of six different virus strains. *J Infect Dis* 1999;180(4):950–958.
41. Avota E, Avots A, Niewiesk S, et al. Disruption of Akt kinase activation is important for immunosuppression induced by measles virus. *Nat Med* 2001;7(6):725–731.
42. Avota E, Gulbins E, Schneider-Schaulies S. DC-SIGN mediated sphingomyelinase-activation and ceramide generation is essential for enhancement of viral uptake in dendritic cells. *PLoS Pathog* 2011;7(2):e1001290.
43. Avota E, Harms H, Schneider-Schaulies S. Measles virus induces expression of SIP110, a constitutively membrane clustered lipid phosphatase, which inhibits T cell proliferation. *Cell Microbiol* 2006;8(11):1826–1839.
44. Avota E, Koethe S, Schneider-Schaulies S. Membrane dynamics and interactions in measles virus dendritic cell infections. *Cell Microbiol* 2013;15(2):161–169.
45. Avota E, Muller N, Klett M, et al. Measles virus interacts with and alters signal transduction in T-cell lipid rafts. *J Virol* 2004;78(17):9552–9559.
46. Axthelm MK, Krakowka S. Canine distemper virus: the early blood-brain barrier lesion. *Acta Neuropathol* 1987;75(1):27–33.
47. Ayasoufi K, Pfaller CK. Seek and hide: the manipulating interplay of measles virus with the innate immune system. *Curr Opin Virol* 2020;41:18–30.
48. Ayata M, Shingai M, Ning X, et al. Effect of the alterations in the fusion protein of measles virus isolated from brains of patients with subacute sclerosing panencephalitis on syncytium formation. *Virus Res* 2007;130(1–2):260–268.
49. Ayata M, Takeuchi K, Takeda M, et al. The F gene of the Osaka-2 strain of measles virus derived from a case of subacute sclerosing panencephalitis is a major determinant of neurovirulence. *J Virol* 2010;84(21):11189–11199.

50. Ayata M, Tanaka M, Kameoka K, et al. Amino acid substitutions in the heptad repeat A and C regions of the F protein responsible for neurovirulence of measles virus Osaka-1 strain from a patient with subacute sclerosing panencephalitis. *Virology* 2016;487:141–149.

51. Baczko K, Lampe J, Liebert UG, et al. Clonal expansion of hypermutated measles virus in a SSPE brain. *Virology* 1993;197(1):188–195.

52. Baczko K, Liebert UG, Billeter M, et al. Expression of defective measles virus genes in brain tissues of patients with subacute sclerosing panencephalitis. *J Virol* 1986;59(2):472–478.

53. Baczko K, Liebert UG, Cattaneo R, et al. Restriction of measles virus gene expression in measles inclusion body encephalitis. *J Infect Dis* 1988;158(1):144–150.

54. Baczko K, Pardowitz I, Rima BK, et al. Constant and variable regions of measles virus proteins encoded by the nucleocapsid and phosphoprotein genes derived from lytic and persistent viruses. *Virology* 1992;190(1):469–474.

55. Bankamp B, Hodge G, McChesney MB, et al. Genetic changes that affect the virulence of measles virus in a rhesus macaque model. *Virology* 2008;373(1):39–50.

56. Bankamp B, Horikami SM, Thompson PD, et al. Domains of the measles virus N protein required for binding to P protein and self-assembly. *Virology* 1996;216(1):272–277.

57. Bankamp B, Liu C, Rivailler P, et al. Wild-type measles viruses with non-standard genome lengths. *PLoS One* 2014;9(4):e95470.

58. Bankamp B, Lopareva EN, Kremer JR, et al. Genetic variability and mRNA editing frequencies of the phosphoprotein genes of wild-type measles viruses. *Virus Res* 2008;135(2):298–306.

59. Bankamp B, Takeda M, Zhang Y, et al. Genetic characterization of measles vaccine strains. *J Infect Dis* 2011;204(Suppl 1):S533–S548.

60. Bankamp B, Wilson J, Bellini WJ, et al. Identification of naturally occurring amino acid variations that affect the ability of the measles virus C protein to regulate genome replication and transcription. *Virology* 2005;336(1):120–129.

61. Barclay AJ, Foster A, Sommer A. Vitamin A supplements and mortality related to measles: a randomised clinical trial. *Br Med J (Clin Res Ed)* 1987;294(6567):294–296.

62. Baron MD. Wild-type Rinderpest virus uses SLAM (CD150) as its receptor. *J Gen Virol* 2005;86(Pt 6):1753–1757.

63. Barrett T, Rossiter PB. Rinderpest: the disease and its impact on humans and animals. *Adv Virus Res* 1999;53:89–110.

64. Barrett T, Visser IK, Mamaev L, et al. Dolphin and porpoise morbilliviruses are genetically distinct from phocine distemper virus. *Virology* 1993;193(2):1010–1012.

65. Bazarsky E, Wolfson M, Galron D, et al. Persistent measles virus infection of murine neuroblastoma cells differentially affects the expression of PKC individual isoenzymes. *Virus Genes* 1997;15(3):227–234.

66. Beaty SM, Lee B. Constraints on the genetic and antigenic variability of measles virus. *Viruses* 2016;8(4):109.

67. Beckford AP, Kaschula RO, Stephen C. Factors associated with fatal cases of measles. A retrospective autopsy study. *S Afr Med J* 1985;68(12):858–863.

68. Begum S, Nooruzzaman M, Islam MR, et al. A sequential study on the pathology of peste des petits ruminants and tissue distribution of the virus following experimental infection of Black Bengal goats. *Front Vet Sci* 2021;8:635671.

69. Behrens L, Cherry JD, Heininger U; Swiss Measles Immune Amnesia Study Group. The susceptibility to other infectious diseases following measles during a three year observation period in Switzerland. *Pediatr Infect Dis J* 2020;39(6):478–482.

70. Bellanti JA, Sanga RL, Klutinis B, et al. Antibody responses in serum and nasal secretions of children immunized with inactivated and attenuated measles-virus vaccines. *N Engl J Med* 1969;280(12):628–633.

71. Bellini WJ, Englund G, Richardson CD, et al. Matrix genes of measles virus and canine distemper virus: cloning, nucleotide sequences, and deduced amino acid sequences. *J Virol* 1986;58(2):408–416.

72. Bellini WJ, Englund G, Rozenblatt S, et al. Measles virus P gene codes for two proteins. *J Virol* 1985;53(3):908–919.

73. Bellini WJ, Rota JS, Lowe LE, et al. Subacute sclerosing panencephalitis: more cases of this fatal disease are prevented by measles immunization than was previously recognized. *J Infect Dis* 2005;192(10):1686–1693.

74. Bhella D, Ralph A, Yeo RP. Conformational flexibility in recombinant measles virus nucleocapsids visualised by cryo-negative stain electron microscopy and real-space helical reconstruction. *J Mol Biol* 2004;340(2):319–331.

75. Bianchi S, Canuti M, Ciceri G, et al. Molecular epidemiology of B3 and D8 measles viruses through hemagglutinin phylogenetic history. *Int J Mol Sci* 2020;21(12).

76. Bieback K, Lien E, Klagge IM, et al. Hemagglutinin protein of wild-type measles virus activates toll-like receptor 2 signaling. *J Virol* 2002;76(17):8729–8736.

77. Billing AM, Kessler JR, Revets D, et al. Proteome profiling of virus-host interactions of wild type and attenuated measles virus strains. *J Proteomics* 2014;108:325–336.

78. Bischak CG, Longhi S, Snead DM, et al. Probing structural transitions in the intrinsically disordered C-terminal domain of the measles virus nucleoprotein by vibrational spectroscopy of cyanylated cysteines. *Biophys J* 2010;99(5):1676–1683.

79. Bischoff WE, McNall RJ, Blevins MW, et al. Detection of measles virus RNA in air and surface specimens in a hospital setting. *J Infect Dis* 2016;213(4):600–603.

80. Bitnun A, Shannon P, Durward A, et al. Measles inclusion-body encephalitis caused by the vaccine strain of measles virus. *Clin Infect Dis* 1999;29(4):855–861.

81. Black FL. Measles endemicity in insular populations: critical community size and its evolutionary implication. *J Theor Biol* 1966;11(2):207–211.

82. Black FL. Infectious diseases in primitive societies. *Science* 1975;187(4176):515–518.

83. Blancou J. Dog distemper: imported into Europe from South America? *Hist Med Vet* 2004;29(2):35–41.

84. Blau DM, Compans RW. Entry and release of measles virus are polarized in epithelial cells. *Virology* 1995;210(1):91–99.

85. Bloyet LM, Brunel J, Dosnon M, et al. Modulation of re-initiation of measles virus transcription at intergenic regions by PXD to NTAIL binding strength. *PLoS Pathog* 2016;12(12):e1006058.

86. Bloyet LM, Welsch J, Enchery F, et al. HSP90 Chaperoning in addition to phosphoprotein required for folding but not for supporting enzymatic activities of measles and Nipah virus L polymerases. *J Virol* 2016;90(15):6642–6656.

87. Bodewes R, Reijnen L, Zwagemaker F, et al. An efficient molecular approach to distinguish chains of measles virus transmission in the elimination phase. *Infect Genet Evol* 2021;91:104794.

88. Bohn W, Ciampor F, Rutter R, et al. Localization of nucleocapsid associated polypeptides in measles virus-infected cells by immunogold labelling after resin embedding. *Arch Virol* 1990;114(1–2):53–64.

89. Bolotin S, Hughes SL, Gul N, et al. What is the evidence to support a correlate of protection for measles? A systematic review. *J Infect Dis* 2020;221(10):1576–1583.

90. Booth L, Roberts JL, Ecroyd H, et al. AR-12 inhibits multiple chaperones concomitant with stimulating autophagosome formation collectively preventing virus replication. *J Cell Physiol* 2016;231(10):2286–2302.

91. Bouche F, Ammerlaan W, Berthet F, et al. Immunosorbent assay based on recombinant hemagglutinin protein produced in a high-efficiency mammalian expression system for surveillance of measles immunity. *J Clin Microbiol* 1998;36(3):721–726.

92. Bouche FB, Ertl OT, Muller CP. Neutralizing B cell response in measles. *Viral Immunol* 2002;15(3):451–471.

93. Bourhis JM, Canard B, Longhi S. Structural disorder within the replicative complex of measles virus: functional implications. *Virology* 2006;344(1):94–110.

94. Bourhis JM, Receveur-Brechot V, Oglesbee M, et al. The intrinsically disordered C-terminal domain of the measles virus nucleoprotein interacts with the C-terminal domain of the phosphoprotein via two distinct sites and remains predominantly unfolded. *Protein Sci* 2005;14(8):1975–1992.

95. Brilot F, Dale RC, Selter RC, et al. Antibodies to native myelin oligodendrocyte glycoprotein in children with inflammatory demyelinating central nervous system disease. *Ann Neurol* 2009;66(6):833–842.

96. Brindley MA, Chaudhury S, Plemper RK. Measles virus glycoprotein complexes preassemble intracellularly and relax during transport to the cell surface in preparation for fusion. *J Virol* 2015;89(2):1230–1241.

97. Brindley MA, Plemper RK. Blue native PAGE and biomolecular complementation reveal a tetrameric or higher-order oligomer organization of the physiological measles virus attachment protein H. *J Virol* 2010;84(23):12174–12184.

98. Brindley MA, Suter R, Schestak I, et al. A stabilized headless measles virus attachment protein stalk efficiently triggers membrane fusion. *J Virol* 2013;87(21):11693–11703.

99. Brindley MA, Takeda M, Plattet P, et al. Triggering the measles virus membrane fusion machinery. *Proc Natl Acad Sci U S A* 2012;109(44):E3018–E3027.

100. Brinkman ID, de Wit J, Smits GP, et al. Early measles vaccination during an outbreak in the Netherlands: short-term and long-term decreases in antibody responses among children vaccinated before 12 months of age. *J Infect Dis* 2019;220(4):594–602.

101. Brody JA, Detels R, Sever JL. Measles-antibody titres in sibships of patients with subacute sclerosing panencephalitis and controls. *Lancet* 1972;1(7743):177–178.

102. Brown DW, Ramsay ME, Richards AF, et al. Salivary diagnosis of measles: a study of notified cases in the United Kingdom, 1991–3. *BMJ* 1994;308(6935):1015–1017.

103. Brown KE, Rota PA, Goodson JL, et al. Genetic characterization of measles and rubella viruses detected through global measles and rubella elimination surveillance, 2016–2018. *MMWR Morb Mortal Wkly Rep* 2019;68(26):587–591.

104. Brunel J, Chopy D, Dosnon M, et al. Sequence of events in measles virus replication: role of phosphoprotein-nucleocapsid interactions. *J Virol* 2014;88(18):10851–10863.

105. Budka H, Urbanits S, Liberski PP, et al. Subacute measles virus encephalitis: a new and fatal opportunistic infection in a patient with AIDS. *Neurology* 1996;46(2):586–587.

106. Burgoon MP, Keays KM, Owens GP, et al. Laser-capture microdissection of plasma cells from subacute sclerosing panencephalitis brain reveals intrathecal disease-relevant antibodies. *Proc Natl Acad Sci U S A* 2005;102(20):7245–7250.

107. Burnet FM. Measles as an index of immunological function. *Lancet* 1968;2(7568):610–613.

108. Burnstein T, Jacobsen LB, Zeman W, et al. Persistent infection of BSC-1 cells by defective measles virus derived from subacute sclerosing panencephalitis. *Infect Immun* 1974;10(6):1378–1382.

109. Buser F. Side reaction to measles vaccination suggesting the Arthus phenomenon. *N Engl J Med* 1967;277(5):250–251.

110. Butler JC, Havens PL, Sowell AL, et al. Measles severity and serum retinol (vitamin A) concentration among children in the United States. *Pediatrics* 1993;91(6):1176–1181.

111. Byington DP, Johnson KP. Experimental subacute sclerosing panencephalitis in the hamster: correlation of age with chronic inclusion-cell encephalitis. *J Infect Dis* 1972;126(1):18–26.

112. Caceres VM, Strebel PM, Sutter RW. Factors determining prevalence of maternal antibody to measles virus throughout infancy: a review. *Clin Infect Dis* 2000;31(1):110–119.

113. Caignard G, Bourai M, Jacob Y, et al. Inhibition of IFN-alpha/beta signaling by two discrete peptides within measles virus V protein that specifically bind STAT1 and STAT2. *Virology* 2009;383(1):112–120.

114. Caignard G, Guerbois M, Labernardiere JL, et al. Measles virus V protein blocks Jak1-mediated phosphorylation of STAT1 to escape IFN-alpha/beta signaling. *Virology* 2007;368(2):351–362.

115. Campbell H, Andrews N, Brown KE, et al. Review of the effect of measles vaccination on the epidemiology of SSPE. *Int J Epidemiol* 2007;36(6):1334–1348.

116. Cannons JL, Schwartzberg PL. SAP and lessons learned from a primary immunodeficiency. *J Immunol* 2017;199(5):1531–1533.

117. Cannons JL, Tangye SG, Schwartzberg PL. SLAM family receptors and SAP adaptors in immunity. *Annu Rev Immunol* 2011;29:665–705.

118. Carazo Perez S, De Serres G, Bureau A, et al. Reduced antibody response to infant measles vaccination: effects based on type and timing of the first vaccine dose persist after the second dose. *Clin Infect Dis* 2017;65(7):1094–1102.

119. Carrigan DR, Johnson KP. Chronic, relapsing myelitis in hamsters associated with experimental measles virus infection. *Proc Natl Acad Sci U S A* 1980;77(7):4297–4300.

120. Carsillo M, Klapproth K, Niewiesk S. Cytokine imbalance after measles virus infection has no correlation with immune suppression. *J Virol* 2009;83(14):7244–7251.

121. Carsillo T, Huey D, Levinsky A, et al. Cotton rat (*Sigmodon hispidus*) signaling lymphocyte activation molecule (CD150) is an entry receptor for measles virus. *PLoS One* 2014;9(10):e110120.

122. Carter CH, Conway TJ, Cornfeld D, et al. Serologic response of children to in-activated measles vaccine. *JAMA* 1962;179:848–853.

123. Casali P, Rice GP, Oldstone MB. Viruses disrupt functions of human lymphocytes. Effects of measles virus and influenza virus on lymphocyte-mediated killing and antibody production. *J Exp Med* 1984;159(5):1322–1337.

124. Casasnovas JM, Larvie M, Stehle T. Crystal structure of two CD46 domains reveals an extended measles virus-binding surface. *EMBO J* 1999;18(11):2911–2922.

125. Cathomen T, Buchholz CJ, Spielhofer P, et al. Preferential initiation at the second AUG of the measles virus F mRNA: a role for the long untranslated region. *Virology* 1995;214(2):628–632.

126. Cathomen T, Mrkic B, Spehner D, et al. A matrix-less measles virus is infectious and elicits extensive cell fusion: consequences for propagation in the brain. *EMBO J* 1998;17(14):3899–3908.

127. Cathomen T, Naim HY, Cattaneo R. Measles viruses with altered envelope protein cytoplasmic tails gain cell fusion competence. *J Virol* 1998;72(2):1224–1234.

128. Cattaneo R, Kaelin K, Baczko K, et al. Measles virus editing provides an additional cysteine-rich protein. *Cell* 1989;56(5):759–764.

129. Cattaneo R, Rebmann G, Baczko K, et al. Altered ratios of measles virus transcripts in diseased human brains. *Virology* 1987;160(2):523–526.

130. Cattaneo R, Rebmann G, Schmid A, et al. Altered transcription of a defective measles virus genome derived from a diseased human brain. *EMBO J* 1987;6(3):681–688.

131. Cattaneo R, Rose JK. Cell fusion by the envelope glycoproteins of persistent measles viruses which caused lethal human brain disease. *J Virol* 1993;67(3):1493–1502.

132. Cattaneo R, Schmid A, Rebmann G, et al. Accumulated measles virus mutations in a case of subacute sclerosing panencephalitis: interrupted matrix protein reading frame and transcription alteration. *Virology* 1986;154(1):97–107.

133. Cattaneo R, Schmid A, Spielhofer P, et al. Mutated and hypermutated genes of persistent measles viruses which caused lethal human brain diseases. *Virology* 1989;173(2):415–425.

134. Charlier C, Dina J, Freymuth F, et al. Prolonged maternal shedding and maternal-fetal transmission of measles virus. *Clin Infect Dis* 2021;72(9):1631–1634.

135. Chatterji M, Mankad V. Failure of attenuated viral vaccine in prevention of atypical measles. *JAMA* 1977;238(24):2635.

136. Chen M, Cortay JC, Logan IR, et al. Inhibition of ubiquitination and stabilization of human ubiquitin E3 ligase PIRH2 by measles virus phosphoprotein. *J Virol* 2005;79(18):11824–11836.

137. Chen RT, Goldbaum GM, Wassilak SG, et al. An explosive point-source measles outbreak in a highly vaccinated population. Modes of transmission and risk factors for disease. *Am J Epidemiol* 1989;129(1):173–182.

138. Chen RT, Markowitz LE, Albrecht P, et al. Measles antibody: reevaluation of protective titers. *J Infect Dis* 1990;162(5):1036–1042.

139. Childs K, Stock N, Ross C, et al. mda-5, but not RIG-I, is a common target for paramyxovirus V proteins. *Virology* 2007;359(1):190–200.

140. Childs KS, Andrejeva J, Randall RE, et al. Mechanism of mda-5 Inhibition by paramyxovirus V proteins. *J Virol* 2009;83(3):1465–1473.

141. Christensen PE, Schmidt H, Bang HO, et al. An epidemic of measles in southern Greenland, 1951; measles in virgin soil. II. The epidemic proper. *Acta Med Scand* 1953;144(6):430–449.

142. Christenson B, Bottiger M. Measles antibody: comparison of long-term vaccination titres, early vaccination titres and naturally acquired immunity to and booster effects on the measles virus. *Vaccine* 1994;12(2):129–133.

143. Ciceri G, Canuti M, Bianchi S, et al. Genetic variability of the measles virus hemagglutinin gene in B3 genotype strains circulating in Northern Italy. *Infect Genet Evol* 2019;75:103943.

144. Ciechonska M, Key T, Duncan R. Efficient reovirus- and measles virus-mediated pore expansion during syncytium formation is dependent on annexin A1 and intracellular calcium. *J Virol* 2014;88(11):6137–6147.

145. Cifuentes-Munoz N, Dutch RE, Cattaneo R. Direct cell-to-cell transmission of respiratory viruses: the fast lanes. *PLoS Pathog* 2018;14(6):e1007015.

146. Clifford HD, Richmond P, Khoo SK, et al. SLAM and DC-SIGN measles receptor polymorphisms and their impact on antibody and cytokine responses to measles vaccine. *Vaccine* 2011;29(33):5407–5413.

147. Cocks BG, Chang CC, Carballido JM, et al. A novel receptor involved in T-cell activation. *Nature* 1995;376(6537):260–263.

148. Cohen BJ, Audet S, Andrews N, et al.; WHO working group on measles plaque reduction neutralization test. Plaque reduction neutralization test for measles antibodies: description of a standardised laboratory method for use in immunogenicity studies of aerosol vaccination. *Vaccine* 2007;26(1):59–66.

149. Cohen BJ, Doblas D, Andrews N. Comparison of plaque reduction neutralisation test (PRNT) and measles virus-specific IgG ELISA for assessing immunogenicity of measles vaccination. *Vaccine* 2008;26(50):6392–6397.

150. Colf LA, Juo ZS, Garcia KC. Structure of the measles virus hemagglutinin. *Nat Struct Mol Biol* 2007;14(12):1227–1228.

151. Colombo M, Bourhis JM, Chamontin C, et al. The interaction between the measles virus nucleoprotein and the Interferon Regulator Factor 3 relies on a specific cellular environment. *Virol J* 2009;6:59.

152. Combredet C, Labrousse V, Mollet L, et al. A molecularly cloned Schwarz strain of measles virus vaccine induces strong immune responses in macaques and transgenic mice. *J Virol* 2003;77(21):11546–11554.

153. Condack C, Grivel JC, Devaux P, et al. Measles virus vaccine attenuation: suboptimal infection of lymphatic tissue and tropism alteration. *J Infect Dis* 2007;196(4):541–549.

154. Connolly JH, Allen IV, Hurwitz LJ, et al. Measles-virus antibody and antigen in subacute sclerosing panencephalitis. *Lancet* 1967;1(7489):542–544.

155. Coovadia HM, Wesley A, Brain P. Immunological events in acute measles influencing outcome. *Arch Dis Child* 1978;53(11):861–867.

156. Coppeta L, Somma G, Di Giampaolo L, et al. Persistence of antibodies for measles among vaccinated medical students in Italy. *Infect Dis (Lond)* 2020;52(8):593–595.

157. Corey EA, Iorio RM. Mutations in the stalk of the measles virus hemagglutinin protein decrease fusion but do not interfere with virus-specific interaction with the homologous fusion protein. *J Virol* 2007;81(18):9900–9910.

158. Corey EA, Iorio RM. Measles virus attachment proteins with impaired ability to bind CD46 interact more efficiently with the homologous fusion protein. *Virology* 2009;383(1):1–5.

159. Coughlin MM, Bellini WJ, Rota PA. Contribution of dendritic cells to measles virus induced immunosuppression. *Rev Med Virol* 2013;23(2):126–138.

160. Couturier M, Buccellato M, Costanzo S, et al. High affinity binding between Hsp70 and the C-terminal domain of the measles virus nucleoprotein requires an Hsp40 co-chaperone. *J Mol Recognit* 2010;23(3):301–315.

161. Cox RM, Krumm SA, Thakkar VD, et al. The structurally disordered paramyxovirus nucleocapsid protein tail domain is a regulator of the mRNA transcription gradient. *Sci Adv* 2017;3(2):e1602350.

162. Cox RM, Plemper RK. Structure and organization of paramyxovirus particles. *Curr Opin Virol* 2017;24:105–114.

163. Cox RM, Sourimant J, Govindarajan M, et al. Therapeutic targeting of measles virus polymerase with ERDRP-0519 suppresses all RNA synthesis activity. *PLoS Pathog* 2021;17(2):e1009371.

164. Crimeen-Irwin B, Ellis S, Christiansen D, et al. Ligand binding determines whether CD46 is internalized by clathrin-coated pits or macropinocytosis. *J Biol Chem* 2003;278(47):46927–46937.

165. Cutts FT, Ferrari MJ, Krause LK, et al. Vaccination strategies for measles control and elimination: time to strengthen local initiatives. *BMC Med* 2021;19(1):2.

166. Cutts FT, Grabowsky M, Markowitz LE. The effect of dose and strain of live attenuated measles vaccines on serological responses in young infants. *Biologicals* 1995;23(1):95–106.

167. Cutts FT, Markowitz LE. Successes and failures in measles control. *J Infect Dis* 1994;170(Suppl 1):S32–S41.

168. Dabbagh A, Laws RL, Steulet C, et al. Progress toward regional measles elimination—worldwide, 2000–2017. *MMWR Morb Mortal Wkly Rep* 2018;67(47):1323–1329.

169. Dagan R, Phillip M, Sarov I, et al. Cellular immunity and T-lymphocyte subsets in young children with acute measles. *J Med Virol* 1987;22(2):175–182.

170. Davis ME, Wang MK, Rennick LJ, et al. Antagonism of the phosphatase PP1 by the measles virus V protein is required for innate immune escape of MDA5. *Cell Host Microbe* 2014;16(1):19–30.

171. De Luca E, Sautto GA, Crisi PE, et al. Feline morbillivirus infection in domestic cats: what have we learned so far? *Viruses* 2021;13(4).

172. de Souza VA, Pannuti CS, Sumita LM, et al. Enzyme-linked immunosorbent assay-IgG antibody avidity test for single sample serologic evaluation of measles vaccines. *J Med Virol* 1997;52(3):275–279.

173. de Swart RL, de Vries RD, Rennick LJ, et al. Needle-free delivery of measles virus vaccine to the lower respiratory tract of non-human primates elicits optimal immunity and protection. *NPJ Vaccines* 2017;2:22.

174. de Swart RL, Ludlow M, de Witte L, et al. Predominant infection of CD150+ lymphocytes and dendritic cells during measles virus infection of macaques. *PLoS Pathog* 2007;3(11):e178.

175. de Swart RL, Yuksel S, Langerijs CN, et al. Depletion of measles virus glycoprotein-specific antibodies from human sera reveals genotype-specific neutralizing antibodies. *J Gen Virol* 2009;90(Pt 12):2982–2989.

176. de Swart RL, Yuksel S, Osterhaus AD. Relative contributions of measles virus hemagglutinin- and fusion protein-specific serum antibodies to virus neutralization. *J Virol* 2005;79(17):11547–11551.

177. de Vries RD, Lemon K, Ludlow M, et al. In vivo tropism of attenuated and pathogenic measles virus expressing green fluorescent protein in macaques. *J Virol* 2010;84(9):4714–4724.

178. de Vries RD, McQuaid S, van Amerongen G, et al. Measles immune suppression: lessons from the macaque model. *PLoS Pathog* 2012;8(8):e1002885.

179. de Witte L, Abt M, Schneider-Schaulies S, et al. Measles virus targets DC-SIGN to enhance dendritic cell infection. *J Virol* 2006;80(7):3477–3486.

180. de Witte L, de Vries RD, van der Vlist M, et al. DC-SIGN and CD150 have distinct roles in transmission of measles virus from dendritic cells to T-lymphocytes. *PLoS Pathog* 2008;4(4):e1000049.

181. Deem SL, Spelman LH, Yates RA, et al. Canine distemper in terrestrial carnivores: a review. *J Zoo Wildl Med* 2000;31(4):441–451.

182. Delpeut S, Sawatsky B, Wong XX, et al. Nectin-4 interactions govern measles virus virulence in a new model of pathogenesis, the squirrel monkey (*Saimiri sciureus*). *J Virol* 2017;91(11).

183. Delpeut S, Sisson G, Black KM, et al. Measles virus enters breast and colon cancer cell lines through a PVRL4-mediated macropinocytosis pathway. *J Virol* 2017;91(10).

184. Derakhshani S, Kurz A, Japtok L, et al. Measles virus infection fosters dendritic cell motility in a 3D environment to enhance transmission to target cells in the respiratory epithelium. *Front Immunol* 2019;10:1294.

185. Desfosses A, Milles S, Jensen MR, et al. Assembly and cryo-EM structures of RNA-specific measles virus nucleocapsids provide mechanistic insight into paramyxoviral replication. *Proc Natl Acad Sci U S A* 2019;116(10):4256–4264.

186. Detre C, Keszei M, Romero X, et al. SLAM family receptors and the SLAM-associated protein (SAP) modulate T cell functions. *Semin Immunopathol* 2010;32(2):157–171.

187. Devaux P, Christiansen D, Plumet S, et al. Cell surface activation of the alternative complement pathway by the fusion protein of measles virus. *J Gen Virol* 2004;85(Pt 6):1665–1673.

188. Devaux P, Hodge G, McChesney MB, et al. Attenuation of V- or C-defective measles viruses: infection control by the inflammatory and interferon responses of rhesus monkeys. *J Virol* 2008;82(11):5359–5367.

189. Devaux P, Hudacek AW, Hodge G, et al. A recombinant measles virus unable to antagonize STAT1 function cannot control inflammation and is attenuated in rhesus monkeys. *J Virol* 2011;85(1):348–356.

190. Devaux P, Priniski L, Cattaneo R. The measles virus phosphoprotein interacts with the linker domain of STAT1. *Virology* 2013;444(1–2):250–256.

191. Dhar P, Sreenivasa BP, Barrett T, et al. Recent epidemiology of peste des petits ruminants virus (PPRV). *Vet Microbiol* 2002;88(2):153–159.

192. Dhib-Jalbut S, Jacobson S, McFarlin DE, et al. Impaired human leukocyte antigen-restricted measles virus-specific cytotoxic T-cell response in subacute sclerosing panencephalitis. *Ann Neurol* 1989;25(3):272–280.

193. Dhiman N, Ovsyannikova IG, Cunningham JM, et al. Associations between measles vaccine immunity and single-nucleotide polymorphisms in cytokine and cytokine receptor genes. *J Infect Dis* 2007;195(1):21–29.

194. Dhiman N, Poland GA, Cunningham JM, et al. Variations in measles vaccine-specific humoral immunity by polymorphisms in SLAM and CD46 measles virus receptors. *J Allergy Clin Immunol* 2007;120(3):666–672.

195. Di Pauli F, Mader S, Rostasy K, et al. Temporal dynamics of anti-MOG antibodies in CNS demyelinating diseases. *Clin Immunol* 2011;138(3):247–254.

196. Diaz T, Nunez JC, Rullan JV, et al. Risk factors associated with severe measles in Puerto Rico. *Pediatr Infect Dis J* 1992;11(10):836–840.

197. Diaz-Delgado J, Groch KR, Sierra E, et al. Comparative histopathologic and viral immunohistochemical studies on CeMV infection among Western Mediterranean, Northeast-Central, and Southwestern Atlantic cetaceans. *PLoS One* 2019;14(3):e0213363.

198. Dietzel E, Kolesnikova L, Maisner A. Actin filaments disruption and stabilization affect measles virus maturation by different mechanisms. *Virol J* 2013;10:249.

199. Dilraj A, Cutts FT, de Castro JF, et al. Response to different measles vaccine strains given by aerosol and subcutaneous routes to schoolchildren: a randomised trial. *Lancet* 2000;355(9206):798–803.

200. Dittmar S, Harms H, Runkler N, et al. Measles virus-induced block of transendothelial migration of T lymphocytes and infection-mediated virus spread across endothelial cell barriers. *J Virol* 2008;82(22):11273–11282.

201. Doi T, Kwon HJ, Honda T, et al. Measles virus induces persistent infection by autoregulation of viral replication. *Sci Rep* 2016;6:37163.

202. Doi Y, Kurita M, Matsumoto M, et al. Moesin is not a receptor for measles virus entry into mouse embryonic stem cells. *J Virol* 1998;72(2):1586–1592.

203. Dorig RE, Marcil A, Chopra A, et al. The human CD46 molecule is a receptor for measles virus (Edmonston strain). *Cell* 1993;75(2):295–305.

204. Druelle J, Sellin CI, Waku-Kouomou D, et al. Wild type measles virus attenuation independent of type I IFN. *Virol J* 2008;5:22.

205. Du Pont V, Jiang Y, Plemper RK. Bipartite interface of the measles virus phosphoprotein X domain with the large polymerase protein regulates viral polymerase dynamics. *PLoS Pathog* 2019;15(8):e1007995.

206. Dubois B, Lamy PJ, Chemin K, et al. Measles virus exploits dendritic cells to suppress CD4+ T-cell proliferation via expression of surface viral glycoproteins independently of T-cell trans-infection. *Cell Immunol* 2001;214(2):173–183.

207. Dundon WG, Diallo A, Cattoli G. Peste des petits ruminants in Africa: a review of currently available molecular epidemiological data, 2020. *Arch Virol* 2020;165(10):2147–2163.

208. Duprex WP, Collins FM, Rima BK. Modulating the function of the measles virus RNA-dependent RNA polymerase by insertion of green fluorescent protein into the open reading frame. *J Virol* 2002;76(14):7322–7328.

209. Duprex WP, McQuaid S, Roscic-Mrkic B, et al. In vitro and in vivo infection of neural cells by a recombinant measles virus expressing enhanced green fluorescent protein. *J Virol* 2000;74(17):7972–7979.

210. Duque-Valencia J, Sarute N, Olarte-Castillo XA, et al. Evolution and interspecies transmission of canine distemper virus—an outlook of the diverse evolutionary landscapes of a multi-host virus. *Viruses* 2019;11(7).

211. Durrheim DN. Measles eradication-retreating is not an option. *Lancet Infect Dis* 2020;20(6):e138–e141.

212. Durrheim DN, Crowcroft NS, Blumberg LH. Is the global measles resurgence a "public health emergency of international concern"? *Int J Infect Dis* 2019;83:95–97.

213. Dux A, Lequime S, Patrono LV, et al. Measles virus and rinderpest virus divergence dated to the sixth century BCE. *Science* 2020;368(6497):1367–1370.

214. Edmonson MB, Addiss DG, McPherson JT, et al. Mild measles and secondary vaccine failure during a sustained outbreak in a highly vaccinated population. *JAMA* 1990;263(18):2467–2471.

215. Ehrengruber MU, Ehler E, Billeter MA, et al. Measles virus spreads in rat hippocampal neurons by cell-to-cell contact and in a polarized fashion. *J Virol* 2002;76(11):5720–5728.

216. El Mubarak HS, Yuksel S, van Amerongen G, et al. Infection of cynomolgus macaques (*Macaca fascicularis*) and rhesus macaques (*Macaca mulatta*) with different wild-type measles viruses. *J Gen Virol* 2007;88(Pt 7):2028–2034.

217. El Najjar F, Schmitt AP, Dutch RE. Paramyxovirus glycoprotein incorporation, assembly and budding: a three way dance for infectious particle production. *Viruses* 2014;6(8):3019–3054.

218. Embree JE, Datta P, Stackiw W, et al. Increased risk of early measles in infants of human immunodeficiency virus type 1-seropositive mothers. *J Infect Dis* 1992;165(2):262–267.

219. Enders JF. Measles virus. Historical review, isolation, and behavior in various systems. *Am J Dis Child* 1962;103:282–287.

220. Enders JF, Katz SL, Holloway A. Development of attenuated measles-virus vaccines. A summary of recent investigation. *Am J Dis Child* 1962;103:335–340.

221. Enders JF, Mc CK, Mitus A, et al. Isolation of measles virus at autopsy in cases of giant-cell pneumonia without rash *N Engl J Med* 1959;261:875–881.

222. Enders JF, Peebles TC. Propagation in tissue cultures of cytopathogenic agents from patients with measles. *Proc Soc Exp Biol Med* 1954;86(2):277–286.

223. Enders JF, Peebles TC, McCarthy K, et al. Measles virus: a summary of experiments concerned with isolation, properties, and behavior. *Am J Public Health Nations Health* 1957;47(3):275–282.

224. Endo A, Izumi H, Miyashita M, et al. Current efficacy of postexposure prophylaxis against measles with immunoglobulin. *J Pediatr* 2001;138(6):926–928.

225. Engelking O, Fedorov LM, Lilischkis R, et al. Measles virus-induced immunosuppression in vitro is associated with deregulation of G1 cell cycle control proteins. *J Gen Virol* 1999;80(Pt 7):1599–1608.

226. Ennis MK, Hu C, Naik SK, et al. Mutations in the stalk region of the measles virus hemagglutinin inhibit syncytium formation but not virus entry. *J Virol* 2010;84(20):10913–10917.

227. Erlenhoefer C, Wurzer WJ, Loffler S, et al. CD150 (SLAM) is a receptor for measles virus but is not involved in viral contact-mediated proliferation inhibition. *J Virol* 2001;75(10):4499–4505.

228. Erlenhofer C, Duprex WP, Rima BK, et al. Analysis of receptor (CD46, CD150) usage by measles virus. *J Gen Virol* 2002;83(Pt 6):1431–1436.

229. Ertl OT, Wenz DC, Bouche FB, et al. Immunodominant domains of the Measles virus hemagglutinin protein eliciting a neutralizing human B cell response. *Arch Virol* 2003;148(11):2195–2206.

230. Escoffier C, Manie S, Vincent S, et al. Nonstructural C protein is required for efficient measles virus replication in human peripheral blood cells. *J Virol* 1999;73(2):1695–1698.

231. Esiri MM, Oppenheimer DR, Brownell B, et al. Distribution of measles antigen and immunoglobulin-containing cells in the CNS in subacute sclerosing panencephalitis (SSPE) and atypical measles encephalitis. *J Neurol Sci* 1982;53(1):29–43.

232. Esolen LM, Park SW, Hardwick JM, et al. Apoptosis as a cause of death in measles virus-infected cells. *J Virol* 1995;69(6):3955–3958.

233. Esolen LM, Takahashi K, Johnson RT, et al. Brain endothelial cell infection in children with acute fatal measles. *J Clin Invest* 1995;96(5):2478–2481.

234. Esolen LM, Ward BJ, Moench TR, et al. Infection of monocytes during measles. *J Infect Dis* 1993;168(1):47–52.

235. Fatemi Nasab GS, Salimi V, Abbasi S, et al. Comparison of neutralizing antibody titers against outbreak-associated measles genotypes (D4, H1 and B3) in Iran. *Pathog Dis* 2016;74(8).

236. Fayolle J, Verrier B, Buckland R, et al. Characterization of a natural mutation in an antigenic site on the fusion protein of measles virus that is involved in neutralization. *J Virol* 1999;73(1):787–790.

237. Fehrholz M, Kendl S, Prifert C, et al. The innate antiviral factor APOBEC3G targets replication of measles, mumps and respiratory syncytial viruses. *J Gen Virol* 2012;93(Pt 3):565–576.

238. Feikin DR, Lezotte DC, Hamman RF, et al. Individual and community risks of measles and pertussis associated with personal exemptions to immunization. *JAMA* 2000;284(24):3145–3150.

239. Feldman HA, Novack A, Warren J. Inactivated measles virus vaccine. II Prevention of natural and experimental measles with the vaccine. *JAMA* 1962;179:391–397.

240. Fernandez-Munoz R, Celma ML. Measles virus from a long-term persistently infected human T lymphoblastoid cell line, in contrast to the cytocidal parental virus, establishes an immediate persistence in the original cell line. *J Gen Virol* 1992;73(Pt 9):2195–2202.

241. Ferreira CS, Frenzke M, Leonard VH, et al. Measles virus infection of alveolar macrophages and dendritic cells precedes spread to lymphatic organs in transgenic mice expressing human signaling lymphocytic activation molecule (SLAM, CD150). *J Virol* 2010;84(6):3033–3042.

242. Fiebelkorn AP, Coleman LA, Belongia EA, et al. Measles virus neutralizing antibody response, cell-mediated immunity, and immunoglobulin G antibody avidity before and after receipt of a third dose of measles, mumps, and rubella vaccine in young adults. *J Infect Dis* 2016;213(7):1115–1123.

243. Finke D, Brinckmann UG, ter Meulen V, et al. Gamma interferon is a major mediator of antiviral defense in experimental measles virus-induced encephalitis. *J Virol* 1995;69(9):5469–5474.

244. Finsterbusch T, Wolbert A, Deitemeier I, et al. Measles viruses of genotype H1 evade recognition by vaccine-induced neutralizing antibodies targeting the linear haemagglutinin noose epitope. *J Gen Virol* 2009;90(Pt 11):2739–2745.

245. Fishman D, Wolfson M, Bazarski E, et al. The effects of measles virus persistent infection on AP-1 transcription factor binding in neuroblastoma cells. *FEBS Lett* 1997;410(2–3):191–194.

246. Forthal DN, Aarnaes S, Blanding J, et al. Degree and length of viremia in adults with measles. *J Infect Dis* 1992;166(2):421–424.

247. Forthal DN, Landucci G, Habis A, et al. Measles virus-specific functional antibody responses and viremia during acute measles. *J Infect Dis* 1994;169(6):1377–1380.

248. Frecha C, Levy C, Costa C, et al. Measles virus glycoprotein-pseudotyped lentiviral vector-mediated gene transfer into quiescent lymphocytes requires binding to both SLAM and CD46 entry receptors. *J Virol* 2011;85(12):5975–5985.

249. Freeman AF, Jacobsohn DA, Shulman ST, et al. A new complication of stem cell transplantation: measles inclusion body encephalitis. *Pediatrics* 2004;114(5):e657–e660.

250. Freeman JM. The clinical spectrum and early diagnosis of Dawson's encephalitis, with preliminary notes on treatment. *J Pediatr* 1969;75(4):590–603.

251. Frenzke M, Sawatsky B, Wong XX, et al. Nectin-4-dependent measles virus spread to the cynomolgus monkey tracheal epithelium: role of infected immune cells infiltrating the lamina propria. *J Virol* 2013;87(5):2526–2534.

252. Friedrichs WE, Reddy SV, Bruder JM, et al. Sequence analysis of measles virus nucleocapsid transcripts in patients with Paget's disease. *J Bone Miner Res* 2002;17(1):145–151.

253. Frustaci A, Abdulla AK, Caldarulo M, et al. Fatal measles myocarditis. *Cardiologia* 1990;35(4):347–349.

254. Fugier-Vivier I, Servet-Delprat C, Rivailler P, et al. Measles virus suppresses cell-mediated immunity by interfering with the survival and functions of dendritic and T cells. *J Exp Med* 1997;186(6):813–823.

255. Fujinami RS, Oldstone MB. Antiviral antibody reacting on the plasma membrane alters measles virus expression inside the cell. *Nature* 1979;279(5713):529–530.

256. Fukuhara H, Mwaba MH, Maenaka K. Structural characteristics of measles virus entry. *Curr Opin Virol* 2020;41:52–58.

257. Fulginiti VA, Arthur JH, Pearlman DS, et al. Altered reactivity to measles virus: local reactions following attenuated measles virus immunization in children who previously received a combination of inactivated and attenuated vaccines. *Am J Dis Child* 1968;115(6):671–676.

258. Fulginiti VA, Eller JJ, Downie AW, et al. Altered reactivity to measles virus. Atypical measles in children previously immunized with inactivated measles virus vaccines. *JAMA* 1967;202(12):1075–1080.

259. Fulginiti VA, Kempe CH. Measles exposure among vaccine recipients: response to measles exposure and antibody persistence among recipients of measles vaccines. *Am J Dis Child* 1963;106:450–461.

260. Fulton BO, Sachs D, Beaty SM, et al. Mutational analysis of measles virus suggests constraints on antigenic variation of the glycoproteins. *Cell Rep* 2015;11(9):1331–1338.

261. Funk S, Knapp JK, Lebo E, et al. Combining serological and contact data to derive target immunity levels for achieving and maintaining measles elimination. *BMC Med* 2019;17(1):180.

262. Gadroen K, Dodd CN, Masclee GMC, et al. Impact and longevity of measles-associated immune suppression: a matched cohort study using data from the THIN general practice database in the UK. *BMJ Open* 2018;8(11):e021465.

263. Gans HA, Yasukawa LL, Alderson A, et al. Humoral and cell-mediated immune responses to an early 2-dose measles vaccination regimen in the United States. *J Infect Dis* 2004;190(1):83–90.

264. Gans HA, Yasukawa LL, Sung P, et al. Measles humoral and cell-mediated immunity in children aged 5–10 years after primary measles immunization administered at 6 or 9 months of age. *J Infect Dis* 2013;207(4):574–582.

265. Garcia M, Yu XF, Griffin DE, et al. Measles virus inhibits human immunodeficiency virus type 1 reverse transcription and replication by blocking cell-cycle progression of CD4+ T lymphocytes. *J Gen Virol* 2008;89(Pt 4):984–993.

266. Garenne M. Sex differences in measles mortality: a world review. *Int J Epidemiol* 1994;23(3):632–642.

267. Gassert E, Avota E, Harms H, et al. Induction of membrane ceramides: a novel strategy to interfere with T lymphocyte cytoskeletal reorganisation in viral immunosuppression. *PLoS Pathog* 2009;5(10):e1000623.

268. Gay NJ. The theory of measles elimination: implications for the design of elimination strategies. *J Infect Dis* 2004;189(Suppl 1):S27–S35.

269. Gely S, Lowry DF, Bernard C, et al. Solution structure of the C-terminal X domain of the measles virus phosphoprotein and interaction with the intrinsically disordered C-terminal domain of the nucleoprotein. *J Mol Recognit* 2010;23(5):435–447.

270. Gendelman HE, Wolinsky JS, Johnson RT, et al. Measles encephalomyelitis: lack of evidence of viral invasion of the central nervous system and quantitative study of the nature of demyelination. *Ann Neurol* 1984;15(4):353–360.

271. Generous AR, Harrison OJ, Troyanovsky RB, et al. Trans-endocytosis elicited by nectins transfers cytoplasmic cargo, including infectious material, between cells. *J Cell Sci* 2019;132(16).

272. Ghannam A, Hammache D, Matias C, et al. High-density rafts preferentially host the complement activator measles virus F glycoprotein but not the regulators of complement activation. *Mol Immunol* 2008;45(11):3036–3044.

273. Gibbs FA, Gibbs EL, Carpenter PR, et al. Electroencephalographic abnormality in "uncomplicated" childhood diseases. *J Am Med Assoc* 1959;171:1050–1055.

274. Gidding HF, Quinn HE, Hueston L, et al. Declining measles antibodies in the era of elimination: Australia's experience. *Vaccine* 2018;36(4):507–513.

275. Gil H, Fernandez-Garcia A, Mosquera MM, et al. Measles virus genotype D4 strains with non-standard length M-F non-coding region circulated during the major outbreaks of 2011–2012 in Spain. *PLoS One* 2018;13(7):e0199975.

276. Giladi M, Schulman A, Kedem R, et al. Measles in adults: a prospective study of 291 consecutive cases. *Br Med J (Clin Res Ed)* 1987;295(6609):1314.

277. Giraudon P, Jacquier MF, Wild TF. Antigenic analysis of African measles virus field isolates: identification and localisation of one conserved and two variable epitope sites on the NP protein. *Virus Res* 1988;10(2–3):137–152.

278. Giraudon P, Wild TF. Monoclonal antibodies against measles virus. *J Gen Virol* 1981;54(Pt 2):325–332.

279. Goldman MB, O'Bryan TA, Buckthal DJ, et al. Suppression of measles virus expression by noncytolytic antibody in an immortalized macrophage cell line. *J Virol* 1995;69(2):734–740.

280. Goldstein T, Mazet JA, Gill VA, et al. Phocine distemper virus in northern sea otters in the Pacific Ocean, Alaska, USA. *Emerg Infect Dis* 2009;15(6):925–927.

281. Gombart AF, Hirano A, Wong TC. Nucleoprotein phosphorylated on both serine and threonine is preferentially assembled into the nucleocapsids of measles virus. *Virus Res* 1995;37(1):63–73.

282. Goncalves-Carneiro D, McKeating JA, Bailey D. The measles virus receptor SLAMF1 can mediate particle endocytosis. *J Virol* 2017;91(7).

283. Good RA, Zak SJ. Disturbances in gamma globulin synthesis as experiments of nature. *Pediatrics* 1956;18(1):109–149.

284. Gourinat AC, Cazorla C, Pfannstiel A, et al. Measles during arbovirus outbreak: a diagnostic challenge. *JMM Case Rep* 2018;5(8):e005156.

285. Gowtage-Sequeira S, Banyard AC, Barrett T, et al. Epidemiology, pathology, and genetic analysis of a canine distemper epidemic in Namibia. *J Wildl Dis* 2009;45(4):1008–1020.

286. Grafen A, Schumacher F, Chithelen J, et al. Use of acid ceramidase and sphingosine kinase inhibitors as antiviral compounds against measles virus infection of lymphocytes in vitro. *Front Cell Dev Biol* 2019;7:218.

287. Graham DG, Gordon A, Ashworth B, et al. Immunodeficiency measles encephalitis. *J Clin Lab Immunol* 1983;10(2):117–120.

288. Graham M, Winter AK, Ferrari M, et al. Measles and the canonical path to elimination. *Science* 2019;364(6440):584–587.

289. Grais RF, Dubray C, Gerstl S, et al. Unacceptably high mortality related to measles epidemics in Niger, Nigeria, and Chad. *PLoS Med* 2007;4(1):e16.

290. Grant RJ, Banyard AC, Barrett T, et al. Real-time RT-PCR assays for the rapid and differential detection of dolphin and porpoise morbilliviruses. *J Virol Methods* 2009;156(1–2):117–123.

291. Graves M, Griffin DE, Johnson RT, et al. Development of antibody to measles virus polypeptides during complicated and uncomplicated measles virus infections. *J Virol* 1984;49(2):409–412.

292. Green MG, Huey D, Niewiesk S. The cotton rat (*Sigmodon hispidus*) as an animal model for respiratory tract infections with human pathogens. *Lab Anim (NY)* 2013;42(5):170–176.

293. Greenberg BL, Sack RB, Salazar-Lindo E, et al. Measles-associated diarrhea in hospitalized children in Lima, Peru: pathogenic agents and impact on growth. *J Infect Dis* 1991;163(3):495–502.

294. Gremillion DH, Crawford GE. Measles pneumonia in young adults. An analysis of 106 cases. *Am J Med* 1981;71(4):539–542.

295. Grenfell BT, Bjornstad ON, Kappey J. Travelling waves and spatial hierarchies in measles epidemics. *Nature* 2001;414(6865):716–723.

296. Griffin DE. Current progress in pulmonary delivery of measles vaccine. *Expert Rev Vaccines* 2014;13(6):751–759.

297. Griffin DE. Measles virus persistence and its consequences. *Curr Opin Virol* 2020;41:46–51.

298. Griffin DE. Measles immunity and immunosuppression. *Curr Opin Virol* 2021;46:9–14.

299. Griffin DE, Cooper SJ, Hirsch RL, et al. Changes in plasma IgE levels during complicated and uncomplicated measles virus infections. *J Allergy Clin Immunol* 1985;76(2 Pt 1):206–213.

300. Griffin DE, Johnson RT, Tamashiro VG, et al. In vitro studies of the role of monocytes in the immunosuppression associated with natural measles virus infections. *Clin Immunol Immunopathol* 1987;45(3):375–383.

301. Griffin DE, Moench TR, Johnson RT, et al. Peripheral blood mononuclear cells during natural measles virus infection: cell surface phenotypes and evidence for activation. *Clin Immunol Immunopathol* 1986;40(2):305–312.

302. Griffin DE, Mullinix J, Narayan O, et al. Age dependence of viral expression: comparative pathogenesis of two rodent-adapted strains of measles virus in mice. *Infect Immun* 1974;9(4):690–695.

303. Griffin DE, Pan CH. Measles: old vaccines, new vaccines. *Curr Top Microbiol Immunol* 2009;330:191–212.

304. Griffin DE, Ward BJ. Differential CD4 T cell activation in measles. *J Infect Dis* 1993;168(2):275–281.

305. Griffin DE, Ward BJ, Jauregui E, et al. Immune activation in measles. *N Engl J Med* 1989;320(25):1667–1672.

306. Griffin DE, Ward BJ, Jauregui E, et al. Immune activation during measles: interferon-gamma and neopterin in plasma and cerebrospinal fluid in complicated and uncomplicated disease. *J Infect Dis* 1990;161(3):449–453.

307. Griffin DE, Ward BJ, Jauregui E, et al. Natural killer cell activity during measles. *Clin Exp Immunol* 1990;81(2):218–224.

308. Griffin DE, Ward BJ, Juaregui E, et al. Immune activation during measles: beta 2-microglobulin in plasma and cerebrospinal fluid in complicated and uncomplicated disease. *J Infect Dis* 1992;166(5):1170–1173.

309. Gringhuis SI, den Dunnen J, Litjens M, et al. C-type lectin DC-SIGN modulates Toll-like receptor signaling via Raf-1 kinase-dependent acetylation of transcription factor NF-kappaB. *Immunity* 2007;26(5):605–616.

310. Grivel JC, Garcia M, Moss WJ, et al. Inhibition of HIV-1 replication in human lymphoid tissues ex vivo by measles virus. *J Infect Dis* 2005;192(1):71–78.

311. Grosjean I, Caux C, Bella C, et al. Measles virus infects human dendritic cells and blocks their allostimulatory properties for CD4+ T cells. *J Exp Med* 1997;186(6):801–812.

312. MVDP author group, Cape S, Chaudhari A, et al. Safety and immunogenicity of dry powder measles vaccine administered by inhalation: a randomized controlled Phase I clinical trial. *Vaccine* 2014;32(50):6791–6797.

313. Guerra FM, Bolotin S, Lim G, et al. The basic reproduction number (R0) of measles: a systematic review. *Lancet Infect Dis* 2017;17(12):e420–e428.

314. Guerra FM, Crowcroft NS, Friedman L, et al. Waning of measles maternal antibody in infants in measles elimination settings—a systematic literature review. *Vaccine* 2018;36(10):1248–1255.

315. Guryanov SG, Liljeroos L, Kasaragod P, et al. Crystal Structure of the measles virus nucleoprotein core in complex with an N-terminal region of phosphoprotein. *J Virol* 2015;90(6):2849–2857.

316. Guseva S, Milles S, Blackledge M, et al. The nucleoprotein and phosphoprotein of measles virus. *Front Microbiol* 2019;10:1832.

317. Guseva S, Milles S, Jensen MR, et al. Measles virus nucleo- and phosphoproteins form liquid-like phase-separated compartments that promote nucleocapsid assembly. *Sci Adv* 2020;6(14):eaaz7095.

318. Gutsche I, Desfosses A, Effantin G, et al. Structural virology. Near-atomic cryo-EM structure of the helical measles virus nucleocapsid. *Science* 2015;348(6235):704–707.

319. Hagiwara K, Sato H, Inoue Y, et al. Phosphorylation of measles virus nucleoprotein upregulates the transcriptional activity of minigenomic RNA. *Proteomics* 2008;8(9):1871–1879.

320. Hahm B, Arbour N, Naniche D, et al. Measles virus infects and suppresses proliferation of T lymphocytes from transgenic mice bearing human signaling lymphocytic activation molecule. *J Virol* 2003;77(6):3505–3515.

321. Hahm B, Cho JH, Oldstone MB. Measles virus-dendritic cell interaction via SLAM inhibits innate immunity: selective signaling through TLR4 but not other TLRs mediates suppression of IL-12 synthesis. *Virology* 2007;358(2):251–257.

322. Hahm B, Trifilo MJ, Zuniga EI, et al. Viruses evade the immune system through type I interferon-mediated STAT2-dependent, but STAT1-independent, signaling. *Immunity* 2005;22(2):247–257.

323. Hai le T, Thach HN, Tuan TA, et al. Adenovirus type 7 pneumonia in children who died from measles-associated pneumonia, Hanoi, Vietnam, 2014. *Emerg Infect Dis* 2016;22(4):687–690.

324. Hall WW, Lamb RA, Choppin PW. Measles and subacute sclerosing panencephalitis virus proteins: lack of antibodies to the M protein in patients with subacute sclerosing panencephalitis. *Proc Natl Acad Sci U S A* 1979;76(4):2047–2051.

325. Halliley JL, Tipton CM, Liesveld J, et al. Long-lived plasma cells are contained within the CD19(−)CD38(hi)CD138(+) subset in human bone marrow. *Immunity* 2015;43(1):132–145.

326. Halsey NA, Boulos R, Mode F, et al. Response to measles vaccine in Haitian infants 6 to 12 months old. Influence of maternal antibodies, malnutrition, and concurrent illnesses. *N Engl J Med* 1985;313(9):544–549.

327. Halsey NA, Modlin JF, Jabbour JT, et al. Risk factors in subacute sclerosing panencephalitis: a case-control study. *Am J Epidemiol* 1980;111(4):415–424.

328. Haltia M, Paetau A, Vaheri A, et al. Fatal measles encephalopathy with retinopathy during cytotoxic chemotherapy. *J Neurol Sci* 1977;32(3):323–330.

329. Hambleton S, Goodbourn S, Young DF, et al. STAT2 deficiency and susceptibility to viral illness in humans. *Proc Natl Acad Sci U S A* 2013;110(8):3053–3058.

330. Hanninen P, Arstila P, Lang H, et al. Involvement of the central nervous system in acute, uncomplicated measles virus infection. *J Clin Microbiol* 1980;11(6):610–613.

331. Hara T, Yamashita S, Aiba H, et al. Measles virus-specific T helper 1/T helper 2-cytokine production in subacute sclerosing panencephalitis. *J Neurovirol* 2000;6(2):121–126.

332. Haralambieva IH, Simon WL, Kennedy RB, et al. Profiling of measles-specific humoral immunity in individuals following two doses of MMR vaccine using proteome microarrays. *Viruses* 2015;7(3):1113–1133.

333. Hardie DR, Albertyn C, Heckmann JM, et al. Molecular characterisation of virus in the brains of patients with measles inclusion body encephalitis (MIBE). *Virol J* 2013;10:283.

334. Harvala H, Wiman A, Wallensten A, et al. Role of sequencing the measles virus hemagglutinin gene and hypervariable region in the measles outbreak investigations in Sweden during 2013–2014. *J Infect Dis* 2016;213(4):592–599.

335. Hashiguchi T, Fukuda Y, Matsuoka R, et al. Structures of the prefusion form of measles virus fusion protein in complex with inhibitors. *Proc Natl Acad Sci U S A* 2018;115(10):2496–2501.

336. Hashiguchi T, Kajikawa M, Maita N, et al. Crystal structure of measles virus hemagglutinin provides insight into effective vaccines. *Proc Natl Acad Sci U S A* 2007;104(49):19535–19540.

337. Hashiguchi T, Ose T, Kubota M, et al. Structure of the measles virus hemagglutinin bound to its cellular receptor SLAM. *Nat Struct Mol Biol* 2011;18(2):135–141.

338. Hashimoto K, Hosoya M. Advances in antiviral therapy for subacute sclerosing panencephalitis. *Molecules* 2021;26(2).

339. Helfand RF, Heath JL, Anderson LJ, et al. Diagnosis of measles with an IgM capture EIA: the optimal timing of specimen collection after rash onset. *J Infect Dis* 1997;175(1):195–199.

340. Helin E, Salmi AA, Vanharanta R, et al. Measles virus replication in cells of myelomonocytic lineage is dependent on cellular differentiation stage. *Virology* 1999;253(1):35–42.

341. Henneman PL, Birnbaumer DM, Cairns CB. Measles pneumonitis. *Ann Emerg Med* 1995;26(3):278–282.

342. Hernandez N, Bucciol G, Moens L, et al. Inherited IFNAR1 deficiency in otherwise healthy patients with adverse reaction to measles and yellow fever live vaccines. *J Exp Med* 2019;216(9):2057–2070.

343. Herndon RM, Rena-Descalzi L, Griffin DE, et al. Age dependence of viral expression. Electron microscopic and immunoperoxidase studies of Measles virus replication in mice. *Lab Invest* 1975;33(5):544–553.

344. Herndon RM, Rubinstein LJ. Light and electron microscopy observations on the development of viral particles in the inclusions of Dawson's encephalitis (subacute sclerosing panencephalitis). *Neurology* 1968;18(1 Pt 2):8–20.

345. Herren M, Shrestha N, Wyss M, et al. Regulatory role of the morbillivirus attachment protein head-to-stalk linker module in membrane fusion triggering. *J Virol* 2018;92(18).

346. Hickman CJ, Khan AS, Rota PA, et al. Use of synthetic peptides to identify measles nucleoprotein T-cell epitopes in vaccinated and naturally infected humans. *Virology* 1997;235(2):386–397.

347. Hirano A, Ayata M, Wang AH, et al. Functional analysis of matrix proteins expressed from cloned genes of measles virus variants that cause subacute sclerosing panencephalitis reveals a common defect in nucleocapsid binding. *J Virol* 1993;67(4):1848–1853.

348. Hirsch RL, Griffin DE, Johnson RT, et al. Cellular immune responses during complicated and uncomplicated measles virus infections of man. *Clin Immunol Immunopathol* 1984;31(1):1–12.

349. Ho TH, Kew C, Lui PY, et al. PACT- and RIG-I-dependent activation of type I interferon production by a defective interfering RNA derived from measles virus vaccine. *J Virol* 2016;90(3):1557–1568.

350. Hoffman SJ, Polack FP, Hauer DA, et al. Vaccination of rhesus macaques with a recombinant measles virus expressing interleukin-12 alters humoral and cellular immune responses. *J Infect Dis* 2003;188(10):1553–1561.

351. Hoffmann HH, Schneider WM, Blomen VA, et al. Diverse viruses require the calcium transporter SPCA1 for maturation and spread. *Cell Host Microbe* 2017;22(4):460–470 e5.

352. Holt EA, Moulton LH, Siberry GK, et al. Differential mortality by measles vaccine titer and sex. *J Infect Dis* 1993;168(5):1087–1096.

353. Honarmand S, Glaser CA, Chow E, et al. Subacute sclerosing panencephalitis in the differential diagnosis of encephalitis. *Neurology* 2004;63(8):1489–1493.

354. Horikami SM, Smallwood S, Bankamp B, et al. An amino-proximal domain of the L protein binds to the P protein in the measles virus RNA polymerase complex. *Virology* 1994;205(2):540–545.

355. Hsu EC, Dorig RE, Sarangi F, et al. Artificial mutations and natural variations in the CD46 molecules from human and monkey cells define regions important for measles virus binding. *J Virol* 1997;71(8):6144–6154.

356. Hu A, Cattaneo R, Schwartz S, et al. Role of N-linked oligosaccharide chains in the processing and antigenicity of measles virus haemagglutinin protein. *J Gen Virol* 1994;75(Pt 5):1043–1052.

357. Hu A, Sheshberadaran H, Norrby E, et al. Molecular characterization of epitopes on the measles virus hemagglutinin protein. *Virology* 1993;192(1):351–354.

358. Huber M, Cattaneo R, Spielhofer P, et al. Measles virus phosphoprotein retains the nucleocapsid protein in the cytoplasm. *Virology* 1991;185(1):299–308.

359. Hughes I, Jenney ME, Newton RW, et al. Measles encephalitis during immunosuppressive treatment for acute lymphoblastic leukaemia. *Arch Dis Child* 1993;68(6):775–778.

360. Hummel KB, Bellini WJ. Localization of monoclonal antibody epitopes and functional domains in the hemagglutinin protein of measles virus. *J Virol* 1995;69(3):1913–1916.

361. Hummel KB, Bellini WJ, Offermann MK. Strain-specific differences in LFA-1 induction on measles virus-infected monocytes and adhesion and viral transmission to endothelial cells. *J Virol* 1998;72(10):8403–8407.

362. Hummel KB, Erdman DD, Heath J, et al. Baculovirus expression of the nucleoprotein gene of measles virus and utility of the recombinant protein in diagnostic enzyme immunoassays. *J Clin Microbiol* 1992;30(11):2874–2880.

363. Huppes W, Smit V. Efficient replication of human immunodeficiency virus type 1 and measles virus in a human-to-mouse graft versus host disease model permits immunization research. *J Gen Virol* 1995;76(Pt 11):2707–2715.

364. Hussey GD, Klein M. Routine high-dose vitamin A therapy for children hospitalized with measles. *J Trop Pediatr* 1993;39(6):342–345.

365. Hutse V, Van Hecke K, De Bruyn R, et al. Oral fluid for the serological and molecular diagnosis of measles. *Int J Infect Dis* 2010;14(11):e991–e997.

366. Ikegame S, Hashiguchi T, Hung CT, et al. Fitness selection of hyperfusogenic measles virus F proteins associated with neuropathogenic phenotypes. *Proc Natl Acad Sci USA* 2021;118(18).

367. Ikeno S, Suzuki MO, Muhsen M, et al. Sensitive detection of measles virus infection in the blood and tissues of humanized mouse by one-step quantitative RT-PCR. *Front Microbiol* 2013;4:298.

368. Imagawa DT, Adams JM. Propagation of measles virus in suckling mice. *Proc Soc Exp Biol Med* 1958;98(3):567–569.

369. Iorio RM, Mahon PJ. Paramyxoviruses: different receptors—different mechanisms of fusion. *Trends Microbiol* 2008;16(4):135–137.

370. Ishizaki Y, Takemoto M, Kira R, et al. Association of toll-like receptor 3 gene polymorphism with subacute sclerosing panencephalitis. *J Neurovirol* 2008;14(6):486–491.

371. Ishizaki Y, Yukaya N, Kusuhara K, et al. PD1 as a common candidate susceptibility gene of subacute sclerosing panencephalitis. *Hum Genet* 2010;127(4):411–419.

372. Iwasa T, Suga S, Qi L, et al. Apoptosis of human peripheral blood mononuclear cells by wild-type measles virus infection is induced by interaction of hemagglutinin protein and cellular receptor, SLAM via caspase-dependent pathway. *Microbiol Immunol* 2010;54(7):405–416.

373. Iwasaki M, Takeda M, Shirogane Y, et al. The matrix protein of measles virus regulates viral RNA synthesis and assembly by interacting with the nucleocapsid protein. *J Virol* 2009;83(20):10374–10383.

374. Iwasaki M, Yanagi Y. Expression of the Sendai (murine parainfluenza) virus C protein alleviates restriction of measles virus growth in mouse cells. *Proc Natl Acad Sci U S A* 2011;108(37):15384–15389.

375. Iwasaki Y, Koprowski H. Cell to cell transmission of virus in the central nervous system. I. Subacute sclerosing panencephalitis. *Lab Invest* 1974;31(2):187–196.

376. Izadi S, Zahraei SM, Salehi M, et al. Head-to-head immunogenicity comparison of Edmonston-Zagreb vs. AIK-C measles vaccine strains in infants aged 8–12 months: a randomized clinical trial. *Vaccine* 2018;36(5):631–636.

377. Jabbour JT, Duenas DA, Sever JL, et al. Epidemiology of subacute sclerosing panencephalitis (SSPE). A report of the SSPE registry. *JAMA* 1972;220(7):959–962.

378. Jabbour JT, Garcia JH, Lemmi H, et al. Subacute sclerosing panencephalitis. A multidisciplinary study of eight cases. *JAMA* 1969;207(12):2248–2254.

379. Jahnke U, Fischer EH, Alvord EC Jr. Sequence homology between certain viral proteins and proteins related to encephalomyelitis and neuritis. *Science* 1985;229(4710):282–284.

380. Janda Z, Norrby E, Marusyk H. Neurotropism of measles virus variants in hamsters. *J Infect Dis* 1971;124(6):553–564.

381. Javelle E, Colson P, Parola P, et al. Measles, the need for a paradigm shift. *Eur J Epidemiol* 2019;34(10):897–915.

382. Jaye A, Herberts CA, Jallow S, et al. Vigorous but short-term gamma interferon T-cell responses against a dominant HLA-A*02-restricted measles virus epitope in patients with measles. *J Virol* 2003;77(8):5014–5016.

383. Jaye A, Magnusen AF, Sadiq AD, et al. Ex vivo analysis of cytotoxic T lymphocytes to measles antigens during infection and after vaccination in Gambian children. *J Clin Invest* 1998;102(11):1969–1977.

384. Jaye A, Magnusen AF, Whittle HC. Human leukocyte antigen class I- and class II-restricted cytotoxic T lymphocyte responses to measles antigens in immune adults. *J Infect Dis* 1998;177(5):1282–1289.

385. Jiang DP, Ide YH, Nagano-Fujii M, et al. Single-point mutations of the M protein of a measles virus variant obtained from a patient with subacute sclerosing panencephalitis critically affect solubility and subcellular localization of the M protein and cell-free virus production. *Microbes Infect* 2009;11(4):467–475.

386. Jin L, Beard S, Hunjan R, et al. Characterization of measles virus strains causing SSPE: a study of 11 cases. *J Neurovirol* 2002;8(4):335–344.

387. Jo WK, Osterhaus AD, Ludlow M. Transmission of morbilliviruses within and among marine mammal species. *Curr Opin Virol* 2018;28:133–141.

388. Johnson RT, Griffin DE, Hirsch RL, et al. Measles encephalomyelitis—clinical and immunologic studies. *N Engl J Med* 1984;310(3):137–141.

389. Joyce JC, Carroll TD, Collins ML, et al. A microneedle patch for measles and rubella vaccination is immunogenic and protective in infant rhesus macaques. *J Infect Dis* 2018;218(1):124–132.

390. Jurgens EM, Mathieu C, Palermo LM, et al. Measles fusion machinery is dysregulated in neuropathogenic variants. *mBio* 2015;6(1).

391. Kakoulidou M, Ingelman-Sundberg H, Johansson E, et al. Kinetics of antibody and memory B cell responses after MMR immunization in children and young adults. *Vaccine* 2013;31(4):711–717.

392. Kakoullis L, Sampsonas F, Giannopoulou E, et al. Measles-associated pneumonia and hepatitis during the measles outbreak of 2018. *Int J Clin Pract* 2020;74(2):e13430.

393. Kaplan LJ, Daum RS, Smaron M, et al. Severe measles in immunocompromised patients. *JAMA* 1992;267(9):1237–1241.

394. Karakas-Celik S, Piskin IE, Keni MF, et al. May TLR4 Asp299Gly and IL17 His161Arg polymorphism be associated with progression of primary measles infection to subacute sclerosing panencephalitis? *Gene* 2014;547(2):186–190.

395. Karlin D, Longhi S, Canard B. Substitution of two residues in the measles virus nucleoprotein results in an impaired self-association. *Virology* 2002;302(2):420–432.

396. Karlin D, Longhi S, Receveur V, et al. The N-terminal domain of the phosphoprotein of Morbilliviruses belongs to the natively unfolded class of proteins. *Virology* 2002;296(2):251–262.

397. Karp CL, Wysocka M, Wahl LM, et al. Mechanism of suppression of cell-mediated immunity by measles virus. *Science* 1996;273(5272):228–231.

398. Kato S, Ohgimoto S, Sharma LB, et al. Reduced ability of hemagglutinin of the CAM-70 measles virus vaccine strain to use receptors CD46 and SLAM. *Vaccine* 2009;27(29):3838–3848.

399. Kato SI, Nagata K, Takeuchi K. Cell tropism and pathogenesis of measles virus in monkeys. *Front Microbiol* 2012;3:14.

400. Katz M, Rorke LB, Masland WS, et al. Subacute sclerosing panencephalitis: isolation of a virus encephalitogenic for ferrets. *J Infect Dis* 1970;121(2):188–195.

401. Katz SL, Enders JF, Holloway A. Studies on an attenuated measles-virus vaccine. II. Clinical, virologic and immunologic effects of vaccine in institutionalized children. *N Engl J Med* 1960;263:159–161.

402. Katz SL, Enders JF, Holloway A. The development and evaluation of an attenuated measles virus vaccine. *Am J Public Health Nations Health* 1962;52(2 Suppl):5–10.

403. Ke Z, Strauss JD, Hampton CM, et al. Promotion of virus assembly and organization by the measles virus matrix protein. *Nat Commun* 2018;9(1):1736.

404. Keeling MJ, Grenfell BT. Disease extinction and community size: modeling the persistence of measles. *Science* 1997;275(5296):65–67.

405. Kelly JT, Human S, Alderman J, et al. BST2/tetherin overexpression modulates morbillivirus glycoprotein production to inhibit cell-cell fusion. *Viruses* 2019;11(8).

406. Kennedy S, Smyth JA, McCullough SJ, et al. Confirmation of cause of recent seal deaths. *Nature* 1988;335(6189):404.

407. Kessler JR, Kremer JR, Muller CP. Interplay of measles virus with early induced cytokines reveals different wild type phenotypes. *Virus Res* 2011;155(1):195–202.

408. Kessler JR, Kremer JR, Shulga SV, et al. Revealing new measles virus transmission routes by use of sequence analysis of phosphoprotein and hemagglutinin genes. *J Clin Microbiol* 2011;49(2):677–683.

409. Khetsuriani N, Sanadze K, Abuladze M, et al. High risk of subacute sclerosing panencephalitis following measles outbreaks in Georgia. *Clin Microbiol Infect* 2020;26(6):737–742.

410. Kim MY, Shu Y, Carsillo T, et al. hsp70 and a novel axis of type I interferon-dependent antiviral immunity in the measles virus-infected brain. *J Virol* 2013;87(2):998–1009.

411. Kimura A, Tosaka K, Nakao T. Measles rash. I. Light and electron microscopic study of skin eruptions. *Arch Virol* 1975;47(4):295–307.

412. Kingston RL, Baase WA, Gay LS. Characterization of nucleocapsid binding by the measles virus and mumps virus phosphoproteins. *J Virol* 2004;78(16):8630–8640.

413. Kingston RL, Hamel DJ, Gay LS, et al. Structural basis for the attachment of a paramyxoviral polymerase to its template. *Proc Natl Acad Sci U S A* 2004;101(22):8301–8306.

414. Kirk J, Zhou AL, McQuaid S, et al. Cerebral endothelial cell infection by measles virus in subacute sclerosing panencephalitis: ultrastructural and in situ hybridization evidence. *Neuropathol Appl Neurobiol* 1991;17(4):289–297.

415. Kisich KO, Higgins MP, Park I, et al. Dry powder measles vaccine: particle deposition, virus replication, and immune response in cotton rats following inhalation. *Vaccine* 2011;29(5):905–912.

416. Klingele M, Hartter HK, Adu F, et al. Resistance of recent measles virus wild-type isolates to antibody-mediated neutralization by vaccinees with antibody. *J Med Virol* 2000;62(1):91–98.

417. Klinkenberg D, Nishiura H. The correlation between infectivity and incubation period of measles, estimated from households with two cases. *J Theor Biol* 2011;284(1):52–60.

418. Knudsen KM, Aaby P, Whittle H, et al. Child mortality following standard, medium or high titre measles immunization in West Africa. *Int J Epidemiol* 1996;25(3):665–673.

419. Kobune F, Ami Y, Katayama M, et al. A novel monolayer cell line derived from human umbilical cord blood cells shows high sensitivity to measles virus. *J Gen Virol* 2007;88(Pt 5):1565–1567.

420. Kobune F, Sakata H, Sugiura A. Marmoset lymphoblastoid cells as a sensitive host for isolation of measles virus. *J Virol* 1990;64(2):700–705.

421. Koethe S, Avota E, Schneider-Schaulies S. Measles virus transmission from dendritic cells to T cells: formation of synapse-like interfaces concentrating viral and cellular components. *J Virol* 2012;86(18):9773–9781.

422. Koga R, Kubota M, Hashiguchi T, et al. Annexin A2 mediates the localization of measles virus matrix protein at the plasma membrane. *J Virol* 2018;92(10).

423. Koga R, Ohno S, Ikegame S, et al. Measles virus-induced immunosuppression in SLAM knock-in mice. *J Virol* 2010;84(10):5360–5367.

424. Koga R, Sugita Y, Noda T, et al. Actin-modulating protein cofilin is involved in the formation of measles virus ribonucleoprotein complex at the perinuclear region. *J Virol* 2015;89(20):10524–10531.

425. Kolakofsky D, Pelet T, Garcin D, et al. Paramyxovirus RNA synthesis and the requirement for hexamer genome length: the rule of six revisited. *J Virol* 1998;72(2):891–899.

426. Koster FT. Mortality among primary and secondary cases of measles in Bangladesh. *Rev Infect Dis* 1988;10(2):471–473.

427. Koutinas AF, Baumgartner W, Tontis D, et al. Histopathology and immunohistochemistry of canine distemper virus-induced footpad hyperkeratosis (hard Pad disease) in dogs with natural canine distemper. *Vet Pathol* 2004;41(1):2–9.

428. Krakowka S, Koestner A. Age-related susceptibility to infection with canine distemper virus in gnotobiotic dogs. *J Infect Dis* 1976;134(6):629–632.

429. Kretsinger K, Strebel P, Kezaala R, et al. Transitioning lessons learned and assets of the global polio eradication initiative to global and regional measles and rubella elimination. *J Infect Dis* 2017;216(Suppl_1):S308–S315.

430. Krugman S. Present status of measles and rubella immunization in the United States: a medical progress report. *J Pediatr* 1971;78(1):1–16.

431. Krumm SA, Yan D, Hovingh ES, et al. An orally available, small-molecule polymerase inhibitor shows efficacy against a lethal morbillivirus infection in a large animal model. *Sci Transl Med* 2014;6(232):232ra52.

432. Kurihara N, Hiruma Y, Yamana K, et al. Contributions of the measles virus nucleocapsid gene and the SQSTM1/p62(P392L) mutation to Paget's disease. *Cell Metab* 2011;13(1):23–34.

433. Kurokawa C, Iankov ID, Galanis E. A key anti-viral protein, RSAD2/VIPERIN, restricts the release of measles virus from infected cells. *Virus Res* 2019;263:145–150.

434. Kweder H, Ainouze M, Cosby SL, et al. Mutations in the H, F, or M proteins can facilitate resistance of measles virus to neutralizing human anti-MV sera. *Adv Virol* 2014;2014:205617.

435. Kwiatek O, Ali YH, Saeed IK, et al. Asian lineage of peste des petits ruminants virus, Africa. *Emerg Infect Dis* 2011;17(7):1223–1231.

436. Laine D, Trescol-Biemont MC, Longhi S, et al. Measles virus (MV) nucleoprotein binds to a novel cell surface receptor distinct from FcgammaRII via its C-terminal domain: role in MV-induced immunosuppression. *J Virol* 2003;77(21):11332–11346.

437. Laksono BM, de Vries RD, Duprex WP, et al. Measles pathogenesis, immune suppression and animal models. *Curr Opin Virol* 2020;41:31–37.

438. Laksono BM, de Vries RD, Verburgh RJ, et al. Studies into the mechanism of measles-associated immune suppression during a measles outbreak in the Netherlands. *Nat Commun* 2018;9(1):4944.

439. Laksono BM, Fortugno P, Nijmeijer BM, et al. Measles skin rash: infection of lymphoid and myeloid cells in the dermis precedes viral dissemination to the epidermis. *PLoS Pathog* 2020;16(10):e1008253.

440. Laksono BM, Grosserichter-Wagener C, de Vries RD, et al. In vitro measles virus infection of human lymphocyte subsets demonstrates high susceptibility and permissiveness of both naive and memory B cells. *J Virol* 2018;92(8).

441. Lalive PH, Hausler MG, Maurey H, et al. Highly reactive anti-myelin oligodendrocyte glycoprotein antibodies differentiate demyelinating diseases from viral encephalitis in children. *Mult Scler* 2011;17(3):297–302.

442. Lawrence DM, Patterson CE, Gales TL, et al. Measles virus spread between neurons requires cell contact but not CD46 expression, syncytium formation, or extracellular virus production. *J Virol* 2000;74(4):1908–1918.

443. Lebon P, Ponsot G, Gony J, et al. HLA antigens in acute measles encephalitis. *Tissue Antigens* 1986;27(2):75–77.

444. Lee JK, Prussia A, Paal T, et al. Functional interaction between paramyxovirus fusion and attachment proteins. *J Biol Chem* 2008;283(24):16561–16572.

445. Lee KY, Lee HS, Hur JK, et al. Clinical features of measles according to age in a measles epidemic. *Scand J Infect Dis* 2005;37(6–7):471–475.

446. Lemon K, de Vries RD, Mesman AW, et al. Early target cells of measles virus after aerosol infection of non-human primates. *PLoS Pathog* 2011;7(1):e1001263.

447. Leonard VH, Hodge G, Reyes-Del Valle J, et al. Measles virus selectively blind to signaling lymphocytic activation molecule (SLAM; CD150) is attenuated and induces strong adaptive immune responses in rhesus monkeys. *J Virol* 2010;84(7):3413–3420.

448. Leonard VH, Sinn PL, Hodge G, et al. Measles virus blind to its epithelial cell receptor remains virulent in rhesus monkeys but cannot cross the airway epithelium and is not shed. *J Clin Invest* 2008;118(7):2448–2458.

449. Leopardi R, Hyypia T, Vainionpaa R. Effect of interferon-alpha on measles virus replication in human peripheral blood mononuclear cells. *APMIS* 1992;100(2):125–131.

450. Leopardi R, Ilonen J, Mattila L, et al. Effect of measles virus infection on MHC class II expression and antigen presentation in human monocytes. *Cell Immunol* 1993;147(2):388–396.

451. Leopardi R, Vainionpaa R, Hurme M, et al. Measles virus infection enhances IL-1 beta but reduces tumor necrosis factor-alpha expression in human monocytes. *J Immunol* 1992;149(7):2397–2401.

452. Lessler J, Reich NG, Brookmeyer R, et al. Incubation periods of acute respiratory viral infections: a systematic review. *Lancet Infect Dis* 2009;9(5):291–300.

453. Li L, Bao J, Wu X, et al. Rapid detection of peste des petits ruminants virus by a reverse transcription loop-mediated isothermal amplification assay. *J Virol Methods* 2010;170(1–2):37–41.

454. Li X, Mukandavire C, Cucunuba ZM, et al. Estimating the health impact of vaccination against ten pathogens in 98 low-income and middle-income countries from 2000 to 2030: a modelling study. *Lancet* 2021;397(10272):398–408.

455. Liebert UG, Baczko K, Budka H, et al. Restricted expression of measles virus proteins in brains from cases of subacute sclerosing panencephalitis. *J Gen Virol* 1986;67(Pt 11):2435–2444.

456. Liebert UG, Flanagan SG, Loffler S, et al. Antigenic determinants of measles virus hemagglutinin associated with neurovirulence. *J Virol* 1994;68(3):1486–1493.

457. Liebert UG, Hashim GA, ter Meulen V. Characterization of measles virus-induced cellular autoimmune reactions against myelin basic protein in Lewis rats. *J Neuroimmunol* 1990;29(1–3):139–147.

458. Liebert UG, ter Meulen V. Virological aspects of measles virus-induced encephalomyelitis in Lewis and BN rats. *J Gen Virol* 1987;68(Pt 6):1715–1722.

459. Liebert UG, ter Meulen V. Synergistic interaction between measles virus infection and myelin basic protein peptide-specific T cells in the induction of experimental allergic encephalomyelitis in Lewis rats. *J Neuroimmunol* 1993;46(1–2):217–223.

460. Liersch J, Omaj R, Schaller J. Histopathological and immunohistochemical characteristics of measles exanthema: a study of a series of 13 adult cases and review of the literature. *Am J Dermatopathol* 2019;41(12):914–923.

461. Lievano F, Galea SA, Thornton M, et al. Measles, mumps, and rubella virus vaccine (M-M-RII): a review of 32 years of clinical and postmarketing experience. *Vaccine* 2012;30(48):6918–6926.

462. Lightwood R, Nolan R. Epithelial giant cells in measles as an acid in diagnosis. *J Pediatr* 1970;77(1):59–64.

463. Liljeroos L, Butcher SJ. Matrix proteins as centralized organizers of negative-sense RNA virions. *Front Biosci (Landmark Ed)* 2013;18:696–715.

464. Liljeroos L, Huiskonen JT, Ora A, et al. Electron cryotomography of measles virus reveals how matrix protein coats the ribonucleocapsid within intact virions. *Proc Natl Acad Sci U S A* 2011;108(44):18085–18090.

465. Lin WH, Griffin DE, Rota PA, et al. Successful respiratory immunization with dry powder live-attenuated measles virus vaccine in rhesus macaques. *Proc Natl Acad Sci U S A* 2011;108(7):2987–2992.

466. Lin WH, Kouyos RD, Adams RJ, et al. Prolonged persistence of measles virus RNA is characteristic of primary infection dynamics. *Proc Natl Acad Sci U S A* 2012;109(37):14989–14994.

467. Lin WH, Pan CH, Adams RJ, et al. Vaccine-induced measles virus-specific T cells do not prevent infection or disease but facilitate subsequent clearance of viral RNA. *mBio* 2014;5(2):e01047.

468. Lin WH, Vilalta A, Adams RJ, et al. Vaxfectin adjuvant improves antibody responses of juvenile rhesus macaques to a DNA vaccine encoding the measles virus hemagglutinin and fusion proteins. *J Virol* 2013;87(12):6560–6568.

469. Lin WW, Moran E, Adams RJ, et al. A durable protective immune response to wild-type measles virus infection of macaques is due to viral replication and spread in lymphoid tissues. *Sci Transl Med* 2020;12(537):eaax7799.

470. Lin WW, Nelson AN, Ryon JJ, et al. Plasma cytokines and chemokines in Zambian children with measles: innate responses and association with HIV-1 coinfection and in-hospital mortality. *J Infect Dis* 2017;215(5):830–839.

471. Lin WW, Tsay AJ, Lalime EN, et al. Primary differentiated respiratory epithelial cells respond to apical measles virus infection by shedding multinucleated giant cells. *Proc Natl Acad Sci U S A* 2021;118(11).

472. Liston P, Briedis DJ. Measles virus V protein binds zinc. *Virology* 1994;198(1):399–404.

473. Lo MK, Jordan R, Arvey A, et al. GS-5734 and its parent nucleoside analog inhibit Filo-, Pneumo-, and Paramyxoviruses. *Sci Rep* 2017;7:43395.

474. Lo Vecchio A, Krzysztofiak A, Montagnani C, et al. Complications and risk factors for severe outcome in children with measles. *Arch Dis Child* 2020;105(9):896–899.

475. Longhi S, Bloyet LM, Gianni S, et al. How order and disorder within paramyxoviral nucleoproteins and phosphoproteins orchestrate the molecular interplay of transcription and replication. *Cell Mol Life Sci* 2017;74(17):3091–3118.

476. Longhi S, Receveur-Brechot V, Karlin D, et al. The C-terminal domain of the measles virus nucleoprotein is intrinsically disordered and folds upon binding to the C-terminal moiety of the phosphoprotein. *J Biol Chem* 2003;278(20):18638–18648.

477. Lorenz D, Albrecht P. Susceptibility of tamarins (Saguinus) to measles virus. *Lab Anim Sci* 1980;30(4 Pt 1):661–665.

478. Lorin C, Combredet C, Labrousse V, et al. A paediatric vaccination vector based on live attenuated measles vaccine. *Therapie* 2005;60(3):227–233.

479. Love A, Norrby E, Kristensson K. Measles encephalitis in rodents: defective expression of viral proteins. *J Neuropathol Exp Neurol* 1986;45(3):258–267.

480. Lu M, Dravid P, Zhang Y, et al. A safe and highly efficacious measles virus-based vaccine expressing SARS-CoV-2 stabilized prefusion spike. *Proc Natl Acad Sci U S A* 2021;118(12).

481. Ludlow M, Allen I, Schneider-Schaulies J. Systemic spread of measles virus: overcoming the epithelial and endothelial barriers. *Thromb Haemost* 2009;102(6):1050–1056.

482. Ludlow M, Lemon K, de Vries RD, et al. Measles virus infection of epithelial cells in the macaque upper respiratory tract is mediated by subepithelial immune cells. *J Virol* 2013;87(7):4033–4042.

483. Ludlow M, Rennick LJ, Sarlang S, et al. Wild-type measles virus infection of primary epithelial cells occurs via the basolateral surface without syncytium formation or release of infectious virus. *J Gen Virol* 2010;91(Pt 4):971–979.

484. Ma D, George CX, Nomburg JL, et al. Upon infection, cellular WD repeat-containing protein 5 (WDR5) localizes to cytoplasmic inclusion bodies and enhances measles virus replication. *J Virol* 2018;92(5).

485. Machamer CE, Hayes EC, Gollobin SD, et al. Antibodies against the measles matrix polypeptide after clinical infection and vaccination. *Infect Immun* 1980;27(3):817–825.

486. Maehlen J, Olsson T, Love A, et al. Persistence of measles virus in rat brain neurons is promoted by depletion of CD8+ T cells. *J Neuroimmunol* 1989;21(2–3):149–155.

487. Magdaleno-Tapial J, Valenzuela-Onate C, Giacaman-von der Weth M, et al. Follicle and sebaceous gland multinucleated cells in measles. *Am J Dermatopathol* 2019;41(4):289–292.

488. Mahamud A, Burton A, Hassan M, et al. Risk factors for measles mortality among hospitalized Somali refugees displaced by famine, Kenya, 2011. *Clin Infect Dis* 2013;57(8):e160–e166.

489. Maisner A, Klenk H, Herrler G. Polarized budding of measles virus is not determined by viral surface glycoproteins. *J Virol* 1998;72(6):5276–5278.

490. Makhortova NR, Askovich P, Patterson CE, et al. Neurokinin-1 enables measles virus trans-synaptic spread in neurons. *Virology* 2007;362(1):235–244.

491. Malvoisin E, Wild F. Contribution of measles virus fusion protein in protective immunity: anti-F monoclonal antibodies neutralize virus infectivity and protect mice against challenge. *J Virol* 1990;64(10):5160–5162.

492. Manchester M, Rall GF. Model systems: transgenic mouse models for measles pathogenesis. *Trends Microbiol* 2001;9(1):19–23.

493. Manchester M, Smith KA, Eto DS, et al. Targeting and hematopoietic suppression of human CD34+ cells by measles virus. *J Virol* 2002;76(13):6636–6642.

494. Manie SN, de Breyne S, Vincent S, et al. Measles virus structural components are enriched into lipid raft microdomains: a potential cellular location for virus assembly. *J Virol* 2000;74(1):305–311.

495. Manning L, Laman M, Edoni H, et al. Subacute sclerosing panencephalitis in Papua New Guinean children: the cost of continuing inadequate measles vaccine coverage. *PLoS Negl Trop Dis* 2011;5(1):e932.

496. Marie JC, Kehren J, Trescol-Biemont MC, et al. Mechanism of measles virus-induced suppression of inflammatory immune responses. *Immunity* 2001;14(1):69–79.

497. Mariner JC, House JA, Mebus CA, et al. Rinderpest eradication: appropriate technology and social innovations. *Science* 2012;337(6100):1309–1312.

498. Maris EP, Gellis SS, et al. Vaccination of children with various chorioallantoic passages of measles virus; a follow-up study. *Pediatrics* 1949;4(1):1–8.

499. Markowitz LE, Chandler FW, Roldan EO, et al. Fatal measles pneumonia without rash in a child with AIDS. *J Infect Dis* 1988;158(2):480–483.

500. Martella V, Blixenkrone-Moller M, Elia G, et al. Lights and shades on an historical vaccine canine distemper virus, the Rockborn strain. *Vaccine* 2011;29(6):1222–1227.

501. Martins C, Garly ML, Bale C, et al. Measles virus antibody responses in children randomly assigned to receive standard-titer Edmonston-Zagreb measles vaccine at 4.5 and 9 months of age, 9 months of age, or 9 and 18 months of age. *J Infect Dis* 2014;210(5):693–700.

502. Marttila J, Ilonen J, Norrby E, et al. Characterization of T cell epitopes in measles virus nucleoprotein. *J Gen Virol* 1999;80(Pt 7):1609–1615.

503. Marziano V, Poletti P, Trentini F, et al. Parental vaccination to reduce measles immunity gaps in Italy. *Elife* 2019;8.

504. Mascia C, Pozzetto I, Kertusha B, et al. Persistent high plasma levels of sCD163 and sCD14 in adult patients with measles virus infection. *PLoS One* 2018;13(5):e0198174.

505. Masse N, Ainouze M, Neel B, et al. Measles virus (MV) hemagglutinin: evidence that attachment sites for MV receptors SLAM and CD46 overlap on the globular head. *J Virol* 2004;78(17):9051–9063.

506. Mateo M, Navaratnarajah CK, Willenbring RC, et al. Different roles of the three loops forming the adhesive interface of nectin-4 in measles virus binding and cell entry, nectin-4 homodimerization, and heterodimerization with nectin-1. *J Virol* 2014;88(24):14161–14171.

507. Mathias RG, Meekison WG, Arcand TA, et al. The role of secondary vaccine failures in measles outbreaks. *Am J Public Health* 1989;79(4):475–478.

508. Mathieu C, Bovier FT, Ferren M, et al. Molecular features of the measles virus viral fusion complex that favor infection and spread in the brain. *mBio* 2021;12(3):e0079921.

509. Mathieu C, Ferren M, Jurgens E, et al. Measles virus bearing measles inclusion body encephalitis-derived fusion protein is pathogenic after infection via the respiratory route. *J Virol* 2019;93(8).

510. Matthews BG, Afzal MA, Minor PD, et al. Failure to detect measles virus ribonucleic acid in bone cells from patients with Paget's disease. *J Clin Endocrinol Metab* 2008;93(4):1398–1401.

511. Mawrin C, Lins H, Koenig B, et al. Spatial and temporal disease progression of adult-onset subacute sclerosing panencephalitis. *Neurology* 2002;58(10):1568–1571.

512. Mazzariol S, Centelleghe C, Beffagna G, et al. Mediterranean fin whales (*Balaenoptera physalus*) threatened by dolphin morbillivirus. *Emerg Infect Dis* 2016;22(2):302–305.

513. McCarthy AJ, Shaw MA, Goodman SJ. Pathogen evolution and disease emergence in carnivores. *Proc Biol Sci* 2007;274(1629):3165–3174.

514. McChesney MB, Altman A, Oldstone MB. Suppression of T lymphocyte function by measles virus is due to cell cycle arrest in G1. *J Immunol* 1988;140(4):1269–1273.

515. McChesney MB, Fujinami RS, Lampert PW, et al. Viruses disrupt functions of human lymphocytes. II. Measles virus suppresses antibody production by acting on B lymphocytes. *J Exp Med* 1986;163(5):1331–1336.

516. McChesney MB, Fujinami RS, Lerche NW, et al. Virus-induced immunosuppression: infection of peripheral blood mononuclear cells and suppression of immunoglobulin synthesis during natural measles virus infection of rhesus monkeys. *J Infect Dis* 1989;159(4):757–760.

517. McChesney MB, Kehrl JH, Valsamakis A, et al. Measles virus infection of B lymphocytes permits cellular activation but blocks progression through the cell cycle. *J Virol* 1987;61(11):3441–3447.

518. McChesney MB, Miller CJ, Rota PA, et al. Experimental measles. I. Pathogenesis in the normal and the immunized host. *Virology* 1997;233(1):74–84.

519. McKenna MJ, Kristiansen AG, Haines J. Polymerase chain reaction amplification of a measles virus sequence from human temporal bone sections with active otosclerosis. *Am J Otol* 1996;17(6):827–830.

520. McKimm-Breschkin JL, Breschkin AM, Rapp F. Characterization of the Halle SSPE measles virus isolate. *J Gen Virol* 1982;59(Pt 1):57–64.

521. McQuaid S, Cosby SL. An immunohistochemical study of the distribution of the measles virus receptors, CD46 and SLAM, in normal human tissues and subacute sclerosing panencephalitis. *Lab Invest* 2002;82(4):403–409.

522. McQuaid S, Cosby SL, Koffi K, et al. Distribution of measles virus in the central nervous system of HIV-seropositive children. *Acta Neuropathol* 1998;96(6):637–642.

523. Mehta PD, Kulczycki J, Mehta SP, et al. Increased levels of beta 2-microglobulin, soluble interleukin-2 receptor, and soluble CD8 in patients with subacute sclerosing panencephalitis. *Clin Immunol Immunopathol* 1992;65(1):53–59.

524. Mehtani NJ, Rosman L, Moss WJ. Immunogenicity and safety of the measles vaccine in HIV-infected children: an updated systematic review. *Am J Epidemiol* 2019;188(12):2240–2251.

525. Melnick JL. Thermostability of poliovirus and measles vaccines. *Dev Biol Stand* 1996;87:155–160.

526. Menna JH, Collins AR, Flanagan TD. Characterization of an in vitro persistent-state measles virus infection: establishment and virological characterization of the BGM/MV cell line. *Infect Immun* 1975;11(1):152–158.

527. Meqdam M, Mostratos A. Characterization of immune response to synthetic peptides derived from the hemagglutinin of measles virus. *New Microbiol* 2000;23(2):113–118.

528. Mercer J, Helenius A. Virus entry by macropinocytosis. *Nat Cell Biol* 2009;11(5):510–520.

529. Merz DC, Scheid A, Choppin PW. Importance of antibodies to the fusion glycoprotein of paramyxoviruses in the prevention of spread of infection. *J Exp Med* 1980;151(2):275–288.

530. Mesman AW, de Vries RD, McQuaid S, et al. A prominent role for DC-SIGN+ dendritic cells in initiation and dissemination of measles virus infection in non-human primates. *PLoS One* 2012;7(12):e49573.

531. Mesman AW, Zijlstra-Willems EM, Kaptein TM, et al. Measles virus suppresses RIG-I-like receptor activation in dendritic cells via DC-SIGN-mediated inhibition of PP1 phosphatases. *Cell Host Microbe* 2014;16(1):31–42.

532. Michou L, Orcel P. The changing countenance of Paget's Disease of bone. *Joint Bone Spine* 2016;83(6):650–655.

533. Mieli-Vergani G, Sutherland S, Mowat AP. Measles and autoimmune chronic active hepatitis. *Lancet* 1989;2(8664):688.

534. Migasena S, Simasathien S, Samakoses R, et al. Adverse impact of infections on antibody responses to measles vaccination. *Vaccine* 1998;16(6):647–652.

535. Millar EL, Rennick LJ, Weissbrich B, et al. The phosphoprotein genes of measles viruses from subacute sclerosing panencephalitis cases encode functional as well as non-functional proteins and display reduced editing. *Virus Res* 2016;211:29–37.
536. Miller C, Farrington CP, Harbert K. The epidemiology of subacute sclerosing panencephalitis in England and Wales 1970–1989. *Int J Epidemiol* 1992;21(5):998–1006.
537. Miller CA, Carrigan DR. Reversible repression and activation of measles virus infection in neural cells. *Proc Natl Acad Sci U S A* 1982;79(5):1629–1633.
538. Miller DL. Frequency of Complications of Measles, 1963. Report on a National Inquiry by the Public Health Laboratory Service in Collaboration with the Society of Medical Officers of Health. *Br Med J* 1964;2(5401):75–78.
539. Miller KD, Matullo CM, Milora KA, et al. Immune-mediated control of a dormant neurotropic RNA virus infection. *J Virol* 2019;93(18).
540. Mina MJ, Kula T, Leng Y, et al. Measles virus infection diminishes preexisting antibodies that offer protection from other pathogens. *Science* 2019;366(6465):599–606.
541. Mina MJ, Metcalf CJ, de Swart RL, et al. Vaccines. Long-term measles-induced immunomodulation increases overall childhood infectious disease mortality. *Science* 2015;348(6235):694–699.
542. Miyajima N, Takeda M, Tashiro M, et al. Cell tropism of wild-type measles virus is affected by amino acid substitutions in the P, V and M proteins, or by a truncation in the C protein. *J Gen Virol* 2004;85(Pt 10):3001–3006.
543. Modlin JF, Jabbour JT, Witte JJ, et al. Epidemiologic studies of measles, measles vaccine, and subacute sclerosing panencephalitis. *Pediatrics* 1977;59(4):505–512.
544. Modrof J, Tille B, Farcet MR, et al. Measles virus neutralizing antibodies in intravenous immunoglobulins: is an increase by revaccination of plasma donors possible? *J Infect Dis* 2017;216(8):977–980.
545. Moeller-Ehrlich K, Ludlow M, Beschorner R, et al. Two functionally linked amino acids in the stem 2 region of measles virus haemagglutinin determine infectivity and virulence in the rodent central nervous system. *J Gen Virol* 2007;88(Pt 11):3112–3120.
546. Moench TR, Griffin DE, Obriecht CR, et al. Acute measles in patients with and without neurological involvement: distribution of measles virus antigen and RNA. *J Infect Dis* 1988;158(2):433–442.
547. Moll M, Klenk HD, Herrler G, et al. A single amino acid change in the cytoplasmic domains of measles virus glycoproteins H and F alters targeting, endocytosis, and cell fusion in polarized Madin-Darby canine kidney cells. *J Biol Chem* 2001;276(21):17887–17894.
548. Moll M, Klenk HD, Maisner A. Importance of the cytoplasmic tails of the measles virus glycoproteins for fusogenic activity and the generation of recombinant measles viruses. *J Virol* 2002;76(14):7174–7186.
549. Moll M, Pfeuffer J, Klenk HD, et al. Polarized glycoprotein targeting affects the spread of measles virus in vitro and in vivo. *J Gen Virol* 2004;85(Pt 4):1019–1027.
550. Monafo WJ, Haslam DB, Roberts RL, et al. Disseminated measles infection after vaccination in a child with a congenital immunodeficiency. *J Pediatr* 1994;124(2):273–276.
551. Mongkolsapaya J, Jaye A, Callan MF, et al. Antigen-specific expansion of cytotoxic T lymphocytes in acute measles virus infection. *J Virol* 1999;73(1):67–71.
552. Monne I, Fusaro A, Valastro V, et al. A distinct CDV genotype causing a major epidemic in Alpine wildlife. *Vet Microbiol* 2011;150(1–2):63–69.
553. Monto AS. Interrupting the transmission of respiratory tract infections: theory and practice. *Clin Infect Dis* 1999;28(2):200–204.
554. Morley D. Severe measles in the tropics. I. *Br Med J* 1969;1(5639):297–300.
555. Morris SE, Yates AJ, de Swart RL, et al. Modeling the measles paradox reveals the importance of cellular immunity in regulating viral clearance. *PLoS Pathog* 2018;14(12):e1007493.
556. Morris SE, Zelner JL, Fauquier DA, et al. Partially observed epidemics in wildlife hosts: modelling an outbreak of dolphin morbillivirus in the northwestern Atlantic, June 2013–2014. *J R Soc Interface* 2015;12(112).
557. Moss WJ. Measles still has a devastating impact in unvaccinated populations. *PLoS Med* 2007;4(1):e24.
558. Moss WJ. Measles. *Lancet* 2017;390(10111):2490–2502.
559. Moss WJ, Fisher C, Scott S, et al. HIV type 1 infection is a risk factor for mortality in hospitalized Zambian children with measles. *Clin Infect Dis* 2008;46(4):523–527.
560. Moss WJ, Griffin DE. Global measles elimination. *Nat Rev Microbiol* 2006;4(12):900–908.
561. Moss WJ, Griffin DE. Measles. *Lancet* 2012;379(9811):153–164.
562. Moss WJ, Monze M, Ryon JJ, et al. Prospective study of measles in hospitalized, human immunodeficiency virus (HIV)-infected and HIV-uninfected children in Zambia. *Clin Infect Dis* 2002;35(2):189–196.
563. Moss WJ, Ryon JJ, Monze M, et al. Differential regulation of interleukin (IL)-4, IL-5, and IL-10 during measles in Zambian children. *J Infect Dis* 2002;186(7):879–887.
564. Moss WJ, Shendale S, Lindstrand A, et al. Feasibility assessment of measles and rubella eradication. *Vaccine* 2021;39(27):3544–3559.
565. Motz C, Schuhmann KM, Kirchhofer A, et al. Paramyxovirus V proteins disrupt the fold of the RNA sensor MDA5 to inhibit antiviral signaling. *Science* 2013;339(6120):690–693.
566. Msaouel P, Opyrchal M, Dispenzieri A, et al. Clinical trials with oncolytic measles virus: current status and future prospects. *Curr Cancer Drug Targets* 2018;18(2):177–187.
567. Muhlebach MD. Vaccine platform recombinant measles virus. *Virus Genes* 2017;53(5):733–740.
568. Muhlebach MD. Measles virus in cancer therapy. *Curr Opin Virol* 2020;41:85–97.
569. Muhlebach MD, Leonard VH, Cattaneo R. The measles virus fusion protein transmembrane region modulates availability of an active glycoprotein complex and fusion efficiency. *J Virol* 2008;82(22):11437–11445.
570. Muhlebach MD, Mateo M, Sinn PL, et al. Adherens junction protein nectin-4 is the epithelial receptor for measles virus. *Nature* 2011;480(7378):530–533.
571. Muller CP, Ammerlaan W, Fleckenstein B, et al. Activation of T cells by the ragged tail of MHC class II-presented peptides of the measles virus fusion protein. *Int Immunol* 1996;8(4):445–456.
572. Muller CP, Handtmann D, Brons NH, et al. Analysis of antibody response to the measles virus using synthetic peptides of the fusion protein. Evidence of non-random pairing of T and B cell epitopes. *Virus Res* 1993;30(3):271–280.
573. Muller CP, Schroeder T, Tu R, et al. Analysis of the neutralizing antibody response to the measles virus using synthetic peptides of the haemagglutinin protein. *Scand J Immunol* 1993;38(5):463–471.
574. Muller N, Avota E, Schneider-Schaulies J, et al. Measles virus contact with T cells impedes cytoskeletal remodeling associated with spreading, polarization, and CD3 clustering. *Traffic* 2006;7(7):849–858.
575. Mustafa MM, Weitman SD, Winick NJ, et al. Subacute measles encephalitis in the young immunocompromised host: report of two cases diagnosed by polymerase chain reaction and treated with ribavirin and review of the literature. *Clin Infect Dis* 1993;16(5):654–660.
576. Myou S, Fujimura M, Yasui M, et al. Bronchoalveolar lavage cell analysis in measles viral pneumonia. *Eur Respir J* 1993;6(10):1437–1442.
577. Naaman H, Rall G, Matullo C, et al. MiRNA-124 is a link between measles virus persistent infection and cell division of human neuroblastoma cells. *PLoS One* 2017;12(10):e0187077.
578. Nagano Y, Sugiyama A, Kimoto M, et al. The measles virus V protein binding site to STAT2 overlaps that of IRF9. *J Virol* 2020;94(17).
579. Naim HY, Ehler E, Billeter MA. Measles virus matrix protein specifies apical virus release and glycoprotein sorting in epithelial cells. *EMBO J* 2000;19(14):3576–3585.
580. Nair N, Moss WJ, Scott S, et al. HIV-1 infection in Zambian children impairs the development and avidity maturation of measles virus-specific immunoglobulin G after vaccination and infection. *J Infect Dis* 2009;200(7):1031–1038.
581. Nakatsu Y, Ma X, Seki F, et al. Intracellular transport of the measles virus ribonucleoprotein complex is mediated by Rab11A-positive recycling endosomes and drives virus release from the apical membrane of polarized epithelial cells. *J Virol* 2013;87(8):4683–4693.
582. Nakatsu Y, Takeda M, Ohno S, et al. Translational inhibition and increased interferon induction in cells infected with C protein-deficient measles virus. *J Virol* 2006;80(23):11861–11867.
583. Nambulli S, Sharp CR, Acciardo AS, et al. Mapping the evolutionary trajectories of morbilliviruses: what, where and whither. *Curr Opin Virol* 2016;16:95–105.
584. Nanan R, Carstens C, Kreth HW. Demonstration of virus-specific CD8+ memory T cells in measles-seropositive individuals by in vitro peptide stimulation. *Clin Exp Immunol* 1995;102(1):40–45.
585. Nandy R, Handzel T, Zaneidou M, et al. Case-fatality rate during a measles outbreak in eastern Niger in 2003. *Clin Infect Dis* 2006;42(3):322–328.
586. Naniche D, Garenne M, Rae C, et al. Decrease in measles virus-specific CD4 T cell memory in vaccinated subjects. *J Infect Dis* 2004;190(8):1387–1395.
587. Naniche D, Reed SI, Oldstone MB. Cell cycle arrest during measles virus infection: a G0-like block leads to suppression of retinoblastoma protein expression. *J Virol* 1999;73(3):1894–1901.
588. Naniche D, Varior-Krishnan G, Cervoni F, et al. Human membrane cofactor protein (CD46) acts as a cellular receptor for measles virus. *J Virol* 1993;67(10):6025–6032.
589. Naniche D, Yeh A, Eto D, et al. Evasion of host defenses by measles virus: wild-type measles virus infection interferes with induction of Alpha/Beta interferon production. *J Virol* 2000;74(16):7478–7484.
590. Navaratnarajah CK, Generous AR, Yousaf I, et al. Receptor-mediated cell entry of paramyxoviruses: mechanisms, and consequences for tropism and pathogenesis. *J Biol Chem* 2020;295(9):2771–2786.
591. Navaratnarajah CK, Oezguen N, Rupp L, et al. The heads of the measles virus attachment protein move to transmit the fusion-triggering signal. *Nat Struct Mol Biol* 2011;18(2):128–134.
592. Navaratnarajah CK, Rosemarie Q, Cattaneo R. A structurally unresolved head segment of defined length favors proper measles virus hemagglutinin tetramerization and efficient membrane fusion triggering. *J Virol* 2016;90(1):68–75.
593. Navaratnarajah CK, Vongpunsawad S, Oezguen N, et al. Dynamic interaction of the measles virus hemagglutinin with its receptor signaling lymphocytic activation molecule (SLAM, CD150). *J Biol Chem* 2008;283(17):11763–11771.
594. Neighbour PA, Rager-Zisman B, Bloom BR. Susceptibility of mice to acute and persistent measles infection. *Infect Immun* 1978;21(3):764–770.
595. Nelson AN, Lin WW, Shivakoti R, et al. Association of persistent wild-type measles virus RNA with long-term humoral immunity in rhesus macaques. *JCI Insight* 2020;5(3):e134992.
596. Nelson AN, Putnam N, Hauer D, et al. Evolution of T cell responses during measles virus infection and RNA clearance. *Sci Rep* 2017;7(1):11474.
597. Nic Lochlainn LM, de Gier B, van der Maas N, et al. Immunogenicity, effectiveness, and safety of measles vaccination in infants younger than 9 months: a systematic review and meta-analysis. *Lancet Infect Dis* 2019;19(11):1235–1245.
598. Nielsen L, Blixenkrone-Moller M, Thylstrup M, et al. Adaptation of wild-type measles virus to CD46 receptor usage. *Arch Virol* 2001;146(2):197–208.
599. Niewiesk S, Gotzelmann M, ter Meulen V. Selective in vivo suppression of T lymphocyte responses in experimental measles virus infection. *Proc Natl Acad Sci U S A* 2000;97(8):4251–4255.
600. Njeumi F, Bailey D, Soula JJ, et al. Eradicating the scourge of peste des petits ruminants from the world. *Viruses* 2020;12(3).
601. Norrby E, Enders-Ruckle G, Meulen V. Differences in the appearance of antibodies to structural components of measles virus after immunization with inactivated and live virus. *J Infect Dis* 1975;132(3):262–269.
602. Noyce RS, Bondre DG, Ha MN, et al. Tumor cell marker PVRL4 (nectin 4) is an epithelial cell receptor for measles virus. *PLoS Pathog* 2011;7(8):e1002240.
603. Nozawa Y, Ono N, Abe M, et al. An immunohistochemical study of Warthin-Finkeldey cells in measles. *Pathol Int* 1994;44(6):442–447.
604. Obojes K, Andres O, Kim KS, et al. Indoleamine 2,3-dioxygenase mediates cell type-specific anti-measles virus activity of gamma interferon. *J Virol* 2005;79(12):7768–7776.
605. Ogbuanu IU, Zeko S, Chu SY, et al. Maternal, fetal, and neonatal outcomes associated with measles during pregnancy: Namibia, 2009–2010. *Clin Infect Dis* 2014;58(8):1086–1092.
606. Oglesbee M. Intranuclear inclusions in paramyxovirus-induced encephalitis: evidence for altered nuclear body differentiation. *Acta Neuropathol* 1992;84(4):407–415.

607. Oglesbee M, Jackwood D, Perrine K, et al. In vitro detection of canine distemper virus nucleic acid with a virus-specific cDNA probe by dot-blot and in situ hybridization. *J Virol Methods* 1986;14(3–4):195–211.

608. Oglesbee M, Krakowka S. Cellular stress response induces selective intranuclear trafficking and accumulation of morbillivirus major core protein. *Lab Invest* 1993;68(1):109–117.

609. Ohno S, Ono N, Seki F, et al. Measles virus infection of SLAM (CD150) knockIn mice reproduces tropism and immunosuppression in human infection. *J Virol* 2007;81(4):1650–1659.

610. Ohno S, Seki F, Ono N, et al. Histidine at position 61 and its adjacent amino acid residues are critical for the ability of SLAM (CD150) to act as a cellular receptor for measles virus. *J Gen Virol* 2003;84(Pt 9):2381–2388.

611. Okada H, Itoh M, Nagata K, et al. Previously unrecognized amino acid substitutions in the hemagglutinin and fusion proteins of measles virus modulate cell-cell fusion, hemadsorption, virus growth, and penetration rate. *J Virol* 2009;83(17):8713–8721.

612. Okada H, Kobune F, Sato TA, et al. Extensive lymphopenia due to apoptosis of uninfected lymphocytes in acute measles patients. *Arch Virol* 2000;145(5):905–920.

613. Okamoto Y, Vricella LA, Moss WJ, et al. Immature CD4+CD8+ thymocytes are preferentially infected by measles virus in human thymic organ cultures. *PLoS One* 2012;7(9):e45999.

614. Okamura A, Itakura O, Yoshioka M, et al. Unusual presentation of measles giant cell pneumonia in a patient with acquired immunodeficiency syndrome. *Clin Infect Dis* 2001;32(3):E57–E58.

615. Okhrimenko A, Grun JR, Westendorf K, et al. Human memory T cells from the bone marrow are resting and maintain long-lasting systemic memory. *Proc Natl Acad Sci U S A* 2014;111(25):9229–9234.

616. Oldstone MB, Lewicki H, Thomas D, et al. Measles virus infection in a transgenic model: virus-induced immunosuppression and central nervous system disease. *Cell* 1999;98(5):629–640.

617. Ong APC, Watson A, Subbiah S. Rubeola keratitis emergence during a recent measles outbreak in New Zealand. *J Prim Health Care* 2020;12(3):289–292.

618. Ono N, Tatsuo H, Hidaka Y, et al. Measles viruses on throat swabs from measles patients use signaling lymphocytic activation molecule (CDw150) but not CD46 as a cellular receptor. *J Virol* 2001;75(9):4399–4401.

619. Osterhaus A. A morbillivirus causing mass mortality in seals. *Vaccine* 1989;7(6):483–484.

620. Ota MO, Ndhlovu Z, Oh S, et al. Hemagglutinin protein is a primary target of the measles virus-specific HLA-A2-restricted CD8+ T cell response during measles and after vaccination. *J Infect Dis* 2007;195(12):1799–1807.

621. Ovsyannikova IG, Haralambieva IH, Vierkant RA, et al. The role of polymorphisms in Toll-like receptors and their associated intracellular signaling genes in measles vaccine immunity. *Hum Genet* 2011;130(4):547–561.

622. Owens GP, Ritchie AM, Gilden DH, et al. Measles virus-specific plasma cells are prominent in subacute sclerosing panencephalitis CSF. *Neurology* 2007;68(21):1815–1819.

623. Paal T, Brindley MA, St Clair C, et al. Probing the spatial organization of measles virus fusion complexes. *J Virol* 2009;83(20):10480–10493.

624. Pallivathucal LB, Noymer A. Subacute sclerosing panencephalitis mortality, United States, 1979–2016: vaccine-induced declines in SSPE deaths. *Vaccine* 2018;36(35):5222–5225.

625. Palosaari H, Parisien JP, Rodriguez JJ, et al. STAT protein interference and suppression of cytokine signal transduction by measles virus V protein. *J Virol* 2003;77(13):7635–7644.

626. Pan CH, Greer CE, Hauer D, et al. A chimeric alphavirus replicon particle vaccine expressing the hemagglutinin and fusion proteins protects juvenile and infant rhesus macaques from measles. *J Virol* 2010;84(8):3798–3807.

627. Pan CH, Valsamakis A, Colella T, et al. Modulation of disease, T cell responses, and measles virus clearance in monkeys vaccinated with H-encoding alphavirus replicon particles. *Proc Natl Acad Sci U S A* 2005;102(33):11581–11588.

628. Panum P. Observations made during the epidemic of measles on the Faroe Islands in the year 1846. *Med Classics* 1938;3:829–886.

629. Patel MK, Antoni S, Nedelec Y, et al. The changing global epidemiology of measles, 2013–2018. *J Infect Dis* 2020;222(7):1117–1128.

630. Patel MK, Goodson JL, Alexander JP Jr, et al. Progress toward regional measles elimination—worldwide, 2000–2019. *MMWR Morb Mortal Wkly Rep* 2020;69(45):1700–1705.

631. Paterson BJ, Kirk MD, Cameron AS, et al. Historical data and modern methods reveal insights in measles epidemiology: a retrospective closed cohort study. *BMJ Open* 2013;3(1).

632. Patterson CE, Lawrence DM, Echols LA, et al. Immune-mediated protection from measles virus-induced central nervous system disease is noncytolytic and gamma interferon dependent. *J Virol* 2002;76(9):4497–4506.

633. Patterson JB, Cornu TI, Redwine J, et al. Evidence that the hypermutated M protein of a subacute sclerosing panencephalitis measles virus actively contributes to the chronic progressive CNS disease. *Virology* 2001;291(2):215–225.

634. Patterson JB, Manchester M, Oldstone MB. Disease model: dissecting the pathogenesis of the measles virus. *Trends Mol Med* 2001;7(2):85–88.

635. Patterson JB, Thomas D, Lewicki H, et al. V and C proteins of measles virus function as virulence factors in vivo. *Virology* 2000;267(1):80–89.

636. Peebles TC. Distribution of virus in blood components during the viremia of measles. *Arch Gesamte Virusforsch* 1967;22(1):43–47.

637. Penedos AR, Myers R, Hadef B, et al. Assessment of the utility of whole genome sequencing of measles virus in the characterisation of outbreaks. *PLoS One* 2015;10(11):e0143081.

638. Permar SR, Klumpp SA, Mansfield KG, et al. Limited contribution of humoral immunity to the clearance of measles viremia in rhesus monkeys. *J Infect Dis* 2004;190(5):998–1005.

639. Permar SR, Klumpp SA, Mansfield KG, et al. Role of CD8(+) lymphocytes in control and clearance of measles virus infection of rhesus monkeys. *J Virol* 2003;77(7):4396–4400.

640. Permar SR, Moss WJ, Ryon JJ, et al. Increased thymic output during acute measles virus infection. *J Virol* 2003;77(14):7872–7879.

641. Permar SR, Moss WJ, Ryon JJ, et al. Prolonged measles virus shedding in human immunodeficiency virus-infected children, detected by reverse transcriptase-polymerase chain reaction. *J Infect Dis* 2001;183(4):532–538.

642. Pernet O, Pohl C, Ainouze M, et al. Nipah virus entry can occur by macropinocytosis. *Virology* 2009;395(2):298–311.

643. Petkova DS, Verlhac P, Rozieres A, et al. Distinct contributions of autophagy receptors in measles virus replication. *Viruses* 2017;9(5).

644. Petrova VN, Sawatsky B, Han AX, et al. Incomplete genetic reconstitution of B cell pools contributes to prolonged immunosuppression after measles. *Sci Immunol* 2019;4(41).

645. Pfaller CK, Bloyet LM, Donohue RC, et al. The C protein is recruited to measles virus ribonucleocapsids by the phosphoprotein. *J Virol* 2020;94(4).

646. Pfaller CK, Cattaneo R, Schnell MJ. Reverse genetics of Mononegavirales: how they work, new vaccines, and new cancer therapeutics. *Virology* 2015;479–480:331–344.

647. Pfaller CK, Mastorakos GM, Matchett WE, et al. Measles virus defective interfering RNAs are generated frequently and early in the absence of C protein and can be destabilized by adenosine deaminase acting on RNA-1-like hypermutations. *J Virol* 2015;89(15):7735–7747.

648. Pfaller CK, Radeke MJ, Cattaneo R, et al. Measles virus C protein impairs production of defective copyback double-stranded viral RNA and activation of protein kinase R. *J Virol* 2014;88(1):456–468.

649. Pfeuffer J, Puschel K, Meulen V, et al. Extent of measles virus spread and immune suppression differentiates between wild-type and vaccine strains in the cotton rat model (*Sigmodon hispidus*). *J Virol* 2003;77(1):150–158.

650. Philip Earle JA, Melia MM, Doherty NV, et al. Phocine distemper virus in seals, east coast, United States, 2006. *Emerg Infect Dis* 2011;17(2):215–220.

651. Phillips RS, Enwonwu CO, Okolo S, et al. Metabolic effects of acute measles in chronically malnourished Nigerian children. *J Nutr Biochem* 2004;15(5):281–288.

652. Piskin IE, Calik M, Abuhandan M, et al. PD-1 gene polymorphism in children with subacute sclerosing panencephalitis. *Neuropediatrics* 2013;44(4):187–190.

653. Piskin IE, Karakas-Celik S, Calik M, et al. Association of interleukin 18, interleukin 2, and tumor necrosis factor polymorphisms with subacute sclerosing panencephalitis. *DNA Cell Biol* 2013;32(6):336–340.

654. Plattet P, Alves L, Herren M, et al. Measles virus fusion protein: structure, function and inhibition. *Viruses* 2016;8(4):112.

655. Plemper RK. Measles resurgence and drug development. *Curr Opin Virol* 2020;41:8–17.

656. Plemper RK, Brindley MA, Iorio RM. Structural and mechanistic studies of measles virus illuminate paramyxovirus entry. *PLoS Pathog* 2011;7(6):e1002058.

657. Plemper RK, Compans RW. Mutations in the putative HR-C region of the measles virus F2 glycoprotein modulate syncytium formation. *J Virol* 2003;77(7):4181–4190.

658. Plemper RK, Doyle J, Sun A, et al. Design of a small-molecule entry inhibitor with activity against primary measles virus strains. *Antimicrob Agents Chemother* 2005;49(9):3755–3761.

659. Plemper RK, Hammond AL. Synergizing vaccinations with therapeutics for measles eradication. *Expert Opin Drug Discov* 2014;9(2):201–214.

660. Plemper RK, Hammond AL, Cattaneo R. Characterization of a region of the measles virus hemagglutinin sufficient for its dimerization. *J Virol* 2000;74(14):6485–6493.

661. Plemper RK, Hammond AL, Cattaneo R. Measles virus envelope glycoproteins heterooligomerize in the endoplasmic reticulum. *J Biol Chem* 2001;276(47):44239–44246.

662. Plemper RK, Hammond AL, Gerlier D, et al. Strength of envelope protein interaction modulates cytopathicity of measles virus. *J Virol* 2002;76(10):5051–5061.

663. Plowright W. Rinderpest virus. *Ann N Y Acad Sci* 1962;101:548–563.

664. Plowright W, Ferris RD. Cytopathogenicity of rinderpest virus in tissue culture. *Nature* 1957;179(4554):316.

665. Poelaert KCK, Williams RM, Matullo CM, et al. Noncanonical transmission of a measles virus vaccine strain from neurons to astrocytes. *mBio* 2021;12(2).

666. Pohl C, Duprex WP, Krohne G, et al. Measles virus M and F proteins associate with detergent-resistant membrane fractions and promote formation of virus-like particles. *J Gen Virol* 2007;88(Pt 4):1243–1250.

667. Polack FP, Auwaerter PG, Lee SH, et al. Production of atypical measles in rhesus macaques: evidence for disease mediated by immune complex formation and eosinophils in the presence of fusion-inhibiting antibody. *Nat Med* 1999;5(6):629–634.

668. Polack FP, Hoffman SJ, Crujeiras G, et al. A role for nonprotective complement-fixing antibodies with low avidity for measles virus in atypical measles. *Nat Med* 2003;9(9):1209–1213.

669. Polack FP, Hoffman SJ, Moss WJ, et al. Altered synthesis of interleukin-12 and type 1 and type 2 cytokinesin rhesus macaques during measles and atypical measles. *J Infect Dis* 2002;185(1):13–19.

670. Polack FP, Lee SH, Permar S, et al. Successful DNA immunization against measles: neutralizing antibody against either the hemagglutinin or fusion glycoprotein protects rhesus macaques without evidence of atypical measles. *Nat Med* 2000;6(7):776–781.

671. Poon TP, Tchertkoff V, Win H. Subacute measles encephalitis with AIDS diagnosed by fine needle aspiration biopsy. A case report. *Acta Cytol* 1998;42(3):729–733.

672. Posey DL, O'Rourke T, Roehrig JT, et al. O'nyong-nyong fever in West Africa. *Am J Trop Med Hyg* 2005;73(1):32.

673. Prasad SR, Shaikh NJ, Verma S, et al. IgG & IgM antibodies against measles virus in unvaccinated infants from Pune: evidence for subclinical infections. *Indian J Med Res* 1995;101:1–5.

674. Prashanth LK, Taly AB, Sinha S, et al. Subacute sclerosing panencephalitis (SSPE): an insight into the diagnostic errors from a tertiary care university hospital. *J Child Neurol* 2007;22(6):683–688.

675. Pratakpiriya W, Seki F, Otsuki N, et al. Nectin4 is an epithelial cell receptor for canine distemper virus and involved in neurovirulence. *J Virol* 2012;86(18):10207–10210.

676. Probert WS, Glenn-Finer R, Espinosa A, et al. Molecular epidemiology of measles in California, USA—2019. *J Infect Dis* 2021;224(6):1015–1023.

677. Prodhomme EJ, Fack F, Revets D, et al. Extensive phosphorylation flanking the C-terminal functional domains of the measles virus nucleoprotein. *J Proteome Res* 2010;9(11):5598–5609.

678. Putz MM, Hoebeke J, Ammerlaan W, et al. Functional fine-mapping and molecular modeling of a conserved loop epitope of the measles virus hemagglutinin protein. *Eur J Biochem* 2003;270(7):1515–1527.

679. Qiu W, Zheng Y, Zhang S, et al. Canine distemper outbreak in rhesus monkeys, China. *Emerg Infect Dis* 2011;17(8):1541–1543.
680. Quintero-Gil C, Rendon-Marin S, Martinez-Gutierrez M, et al. Origin of canine distemper virus: consolidating evidence to understand potential zoonoses. *Front Microbiol* 2019;10:1982.
681. Radecke F, Billeter MA. The nonstructural C protein is not essential for multiplication of Edmonston B strain measles virus in cultured cells. *Virology* 1996;217(1):418–421.
682. Rager M, Vongpunsawad S, Duprex WP, et al. Polyploid measles virus with hexameric genome length. *EMBO J* 2002;21(10):2364–2372.
683. Rager-Zisman B, Bazarsky E, Skibin A, et al. Differential immune responses to primary measles-mumps-rubella vaccination in Israeli children. *Clin Diagn Lab Immunol* 2004;11(5):913–918.
684. Ralston SH, Afzal MA, Helfrich MH, et al. Multicenter blinded analysis of RT-PCR detection methods for paramyxoviruses in relation to Paget's disease of bone. *J Bone Miner Res* 2007;22(4):569–577.
685. Ramachandran A, Parisien JP, Horvath CM. STAT2 is a primary target for measles virus V protein-mediated alpha/beta interferon signaling inhibition. *J Virol* 2008;82(17):8330–8338.
686. Rammohan KW, McFarland HF, McFarlin DE. Induction of subacute murine measles encephalitis by monoclonal antibody to virus haemagglutinin. *Nature* 1981;290(5807):588–589.
687. Rammohan KW, McFarland HF, McFarlin DE. Subacute sclerosing panencephalitis after passive immunization and natural measles infection: role of antibody in persistence of measles virus. *Neurology* 1982;32(4):390–394.
688. Ramsauer K, Schwameis M, Firbas C, et al. Immunogenicity, safety, and tolerability of a recombinant measles-virus-based chikungunya vaccine: a randomised, double-blind, placebo-controlled, active-comparator, first-in-man trial. *Lancet Infect Dis* 2015;15(5):519–527
689. Ravanel K, Castelle C, Defrance T, et al. Measles virus nucleocapsid protein binds to FcgammaRII and inhibits human B cell antibody production. *J Exp Med* 1997;186(2):269–278.
690. Redd SC, King GE, Heath JL, et al. Comparison of vaccination with measles-mumps-rubella vaccine at 9, 12, and 15 months of age. *J Infect Dis* 2004;189(Suppl 1):S116–S122.
691. Reilly CM, Stokes J Jr, Buynak EB, et al. Living attenuated measles-virus vaccine in early infancy. Studies of the role of passive antibody in immunization. *N Engl J Med* 1961;265:165–169.
692. Remfry J. A measles epizootic with 5 deaths in newly-imported rhesus monkeys (Macaca mulatta). *Lab Anim* 1976;10(1):49–57.
693. Rennick LJ, de Vries RD, Carsillo TJ, et al. Live-attenuated measles virus vaccine targets dendritic cells and macrophages in muscle of nonhuman primates. *J Virol* 2015;89(4):2192–2200.
694. Rhodes CJ, Anderson RM. Power laws governing epidemics in isolated populations. *Nature* 1996;381(6583):600–602.
695. Richardson CD, Scheid A, Choppin PW. Specific inhibition of paramyxovirus and myxovirus replication by oligopeptides with amino acid sequences similar to those at the N-termini of the F1 or HA2 viral polypeptides. *Virology* 1980;105(1):205–222.
696. Richetta C, Gregoire IP, Verlhac P, et al. Sustained autophagy contributes to measles virus infectivity. *PLoS Pathog* 2013;9(9):e1003599.
697. Riddell MA, Moss WJ, Hauer D, et al. Slow clearance of measles virus RNA after acute infection. *J Clin Virol* 2007;39(4):312–317.
698. Riddell MA, Rota JS, Rota PA. Review of the temporal and geographical distribution of measles virus genotypes in the prevaccine and postvaccine eras. *Virol J* 2005;2:87.
699. Riley-Vargas RC, Gill DB, Kemper C, et al. CD46: expanding beyond complement regulation. *Trends Immunol* 2004;25(9):496–503.
700. Rima BK, Davidson WB, Martin SJ. The role of defective interfering particles in persistent infection of Vero cells by measles virus. *J Gen Virol* 1977;35(1):89–97.
701. Rima BK, Earle JA, Baczko K, et al. Sequence divergence of measles virus haemagglutinin during natural evolution and adaptation to cell culture. *J Gen Virol* 1997;78(Pt 1):97–106.
702. Robertson DA, Zhang SL, Guy EC, et al. Persistent measles virus genome in autoimmune chronic active hepatitis. *Lancet* 1987;2(8549):9–11.
703. Robinzon S, Dafa-Berger A, Dyer MD, et al. Impaired cholesterol biosynthesis in a neuronal cell line persistently infected with measles virus. *J Virol* 2009;83(11):5495–5504.
704. Rodgers DV, Gindler JS, Atkinson WL, et al. High attack rates and case fatality during a measles outbreak in groups with religious exemption to vaccination. *Pediatr Infect Dis J* 1993;12(4):288–292.
705. Roos RP, Graves MC, Wollmann RL, et al. Immunologic and virologic studies of measles inclusion body encephalitis in an immunosuppressed host: the relationship to subacute sclerosing panencephalitis. *Neurology* 1981;31(10):1263–1270.
706. Rossman JS, Leser GP, Lamb RA. Filamentous influenza virus enters cells via macropinocytosis. *J Virol* 2012;86(20):10950–10960.
707. Rota JS, Wang ZD, Rota PA, et al. Comparison of sequences of the H, F, and N coding genes of measles virus vaccine strains. *Virus Res* 1994;31(3):317–330.
708. Rota PA, Bellini WJ. Update on the global distribution of genotypes of wild type measles viruses. *J Infect Dis* 2003;187(Suppl 1):S270–S276.
709. Rota PA, Brown K, Mankertz A, et al. Global distribution of measles genotypes and measles molecular epidemiology. *J Infect Dis* 2011;204(Suppl 1):S514–S523.
710. Rota PA, Rota JS, Goodson JL. Subacute sclerosing panencephalitis. *Clin Infect Dis* 2017;65(2):233–234.
711. Rudak PT, Yao T, Richardson CD, et al. Measles virus infects and programs MAIT cells for apoptosis. *J Infect Dis* 2021;223(4):667–672.
712. Ruigrok RW, Gerlier D. Structure of the measles virus H glycoprotein sheds light on an efficient vaccine. *Proc Natl Acad Sci U S A* 2007;104(52):20639–20640.
713. Runkler N, Dietzel E, Carsillo M, et al. Sorting signals in the measles virus wild-type glycoproteins differently influence virus spread in polarized epithelia and lymphocytes. *J Gen Virol* 2009;90(Pt 10):2474–2482.
714. Runkler N, Dietzel E, Moll M, et al. Glycoprotein targeting signals influence the distribution of measles virus envelope proteins and virus spread in lymphocytes. *J Gen Virol* 2008;89(Pt 3):687–696.
715. Runkler N, Pohl C, Schneider-Schaulies S, et al. Measles virus nucleocapsid transport to the plasma membrane requires stable expression and surface accumulation of the viral matrix protein. *Cell Microbiol* 2007;9(5):1203–1214.
716. Rustigian R. Persistent infection of cells in culture by measles virus. I. Development and characteristics of HeLa sublines persistently infected with complete virus. *J Bacteriol* 1966;92(6):1792–1804.
717. Ryon JJ, Moss WJ, Monze M, et al. Functional and phenotypic changes in circulating lymphocytes from hospitalized Zambian children with measles. *Clin Diagn Lab Immunol* 2002;9(5):994–1003.
718. Saha V, John TJ, Mukundan P, et al. High incidence of subacute sclerosing panencephalitis in south India. *Epidemiol Infect* 1990;104(1):151–156.
719. Saito H, Nakagomi O, Morita M. Molecular identification of two distinct hemagglutinin types of measles virus by polymerase chain reaction and restriction fragment length polymorphism (PCR-RFLP). *Mol Cell Probes* 1995;9(1):1–8.
720. Saito H, Sato H, Abe M, et al. Cloning and characterization of the cDNA encoding the HA protein of a hemagglutination-defective measles virus strain. *Virus Genes* 1994;8(2):107–113.
721. Sajjadi S, Shirode A, Vaidya SR, et al. Molecular mechanism by which residues at position 481 and 546 of measles virus hemagglutinin protein define CD46 receptor binding using a molecular docking approach. *Comput Biol Chem* 2019;80:384–389.
722. Sakaguchi M, Yoshikawa Y, Yamanouchi K, et al. Growth of measles virus in epithelial and lymphoid tissues of cynomolgus monkeys. *Microbiol Immunol* 1986;30(10):1067–1073.
723. Sakai K, Nagata N, Ami Y, et al. Lethal canine distemper virus outbreak in cynomolgus monkeys in Japan in 2008. *J Virol* 2013;87(2):1105–1114.
724. Salditt A, Koethe S, Pohl C, et al. Measles virus M protein-driven particle production does not involve the endosomal sorting complex required for transport (ESCRT) system. *J Gen Virol* 2010;91(Pt 6):1464–1472.
725. Salonen R, Ilonen J, Salmi AA. Measles virus inhibits lymphocyte proliferation in vitro by two different mechanisms. *Clin Exp Immunol* 1989;75(3):376–380.
726. Sanchez David RY, Combredet C, Sismeiro O, et al. Comparative analysis of viral RNA signatures on different RIG-I-like receptors. *Elife* 2016;5:e11275.
727. Sandford-Smith JH, Whittle HC. Corneal ulceration following measles in Nigerian children. *Br J Ophthalmol* 1979;63(11):720–724.
728. Santiago C, Celma ML, Stehle T, et al. Structure of the measles virus hemagglutinin bound to the CD46 receptor. *Nat Struct Mol Biol* 2010;17(1):124–129.
729. Sato H, Honma R, Yoneda M, et al. Measles virus induces cell-type specific changes in gene expression. *Virology* 2008;375(2):321–330.
730. Sato H, Kobune F, Ami Y, et al. Immune responses against measles virus in cynomolgus monkeys. *Comp Immunol Microbiol Infect Dis* 2008;31(1):25–35.
731. Sato H, Masuda M, Kanai M, et al. Measles virus N protein inhibits host translation by binding to eIF3-p40. *J Virol* 2007;81(21):11569–11576.
732. Sato H, Masuda M, Miura R, et al. Morbillivirus nucleoprotein possesses a novel nuclear localization signal and a CRM1-independent nuclear export signal. *Virology* 2006;352(1):121–130.
733. Sato H, Yoneda M, Honma R, et al. Measles virus infection inactivates cellular protein phosphatase 5 with consequent suppression of Sp1 and c-Myc activities. *J Virol* 2015;89(19):9709–9718.
734. Sato Y, Watanabe S, Fukuda Y, et al. Cell-to-cell measles virus spread between human neurons is dependent on hemagglutinin and hyperfusogenic fusion protein. *J Virol* 2018;92(6).
735. Satoh Y, Yonemori S, Hirose M, et al. A residue located at the junction of the head and stalk regions of measles virus fusion protein regulates membrane fusion by controlling conformational stability. *J Gen Virol* 2017;98(2):143–154.
736. Sawaishi Y, Yano T, Watanabe Y, et al. Migratory basal ganglia lesions in subacute sclerosing panencephalitis (SSPE): clinical implications of axonal spread. *J Neurol Sci* 1999;168(2):137–140.
737. Sawatsky B, Wong XX, Hinkelmann S, et al. Canine distemper virus epithelial cell infection is required for clinical disease but not for immunosuppression. *J Virol* 2012;86(7):3658–3666.
738. Scheifele DW, Forbes CE. Prolonged giant cell excretion in severe African measles. *Pediatrics* 1972;50(6):867–873.
739. Schellens IM, Meiring HD, Hoof I, et al. Measles Virus epitope presentation by HLA: novel insights into epitope selection, dominance, and microvariation. *Front Immunol* 2015;6:546.
740. Schlender J, Schnorr JJ, Spielhoffer P, et al. Interaction of measles virus glycoproteins with the surface of uninfected peripheral blood lymphocytes induces immunosuppression in vitro. *Proc Natl Acad Sci U S A* 1996;93(23):13194–13199.
741. Schmid A, Spielhofer P, Cattaneo R, et al. Subacute sclerosing panencephalitis is typically characterized by alterations in the fusion protein cytoplasmic domain of the persisting measles virus. *Virology* 1992;188(2):910–915.
742. Schneider H, Kaelin K, Billeter MA. Recombinant measles viruses defective for RNA editing and V protein synthesis are viable in cultured cells. *Virology* 1997;227(2):314–322.
743. Schneider U, von Messling V, Devaux P, et al. Efficiency of measles virus entry and dissemination through different receptors. *J Virol* 2002;76(15):7460–7467.
744. Schneider-Schaulies J, Schneider-Schaulies S. Sphingolipids in viral infection. *Biol Chem* 2015;396(6–7):585–595.
745. Schneider-Schaulies S, Liebert UG, Baczko K, et al. Restriction of measles virus gene expression in acute and subacute encephalitis of Lewis rats. *Virology* 1989;171(2):525–534.
746. Schneider-Schaulies S, Liebert UG, Segev Y, et al. Antibody-dependent transcriptional regulation of measles virus in persistently infected neural cells. *J Virol* 1992;66(9):5534–5541.
747. Schnorr JJ, Schneider-Schaulies S, Simon-Jodicke A, et al. MxA-dependent inhibition of measles virus glycoprotein synthesis in a stably transfected human monocytic cell line. *J Virol* 1993;67(8):4760–4768.

748. Schnorr JJ, Seufert M, Schlender J, et al. Cell cycle arrest rather than apoptosis is associated with measles virus contact-mediated immunosuppression in vitro. *J Gen Virol* 1997;78(Pt 12):3217–3226.
749. Schnorr JJ, Xanthakos S, Keikavoussi P, et al. Induction of maturation of human blood dendritic cell precursors by measles virus is associated with immunosuppression. *Proc Natl Acad Sci U S A* 1997;94(10):5326–5331.
750. Schonberger K, Ludwig MS, Wildner M, et al. Epidemiology of subacute sclerosing panencephalitis (SSPE) in Germany from 2003 to 2009: a risk estimation. *PLoS One* 2013;8(7):e68909.
751. Schrag SJ, Rota PA, Bellini WJ. Spontaneous mutation rate of measles virus: direct estimation based on mutations conferring monoclonal antibody resistance. *J Virol* 1999;73(1):51–54.
752. Schrauwen I, Van Camp G. The etiology of otosclerosis: a combination of genes and environment. *Laryngoscope* 2010;120(6):1195–1202.
753. Schuhmann KM, Pfaller CK, Conzelmann KK. The measles virus V protein binds to p65 (RelA) to suppress NF-kappaB activity. *J Virol* 2011;85(7):3162–3171.
754. Schwarz AJ. Preliminary tests of a highly attenuated measles vaccine. *Am J Dis Child* 1962;103:386–389.
755. Seki F, Ohishi K, Maruyama T, et al. Phocine distemper virus uses phocine and other animal SLAMs as a receptor but not human SLAM. *Microbiol Immunol* 2020;64(8):578–583.
756. Seki F, Someya K, Komase K, et al. A chicken homologue of nectin-4 functions as a measles virus receptor. *Vaccine* 2016;34(1):7–12.
757. Seki F, Yamamoto Y, Fukuhara H, et al. Measles virus hemagglutinin protein establishes a specific interaction with the extreme N-terminal region of human signaling lymphocytic activation molecule to enhance infection. *Front Microbiol* 2020;11:1830.
758. Sellin CI, Horvat B. Current animal models: transgenic animal models for the study of measles pathogenesis. *Curr Top Microbiol Immunol* 2009;330:111–127.
759. Semmler G, Griebler H, Aberle SW, et al. Elevated CXCL10 serum levels in measles virus primary infection and reinfection correlate with the serological stage and hospitalization status. *J Infect Dis* 2020;222(12):2030–2034.
760. Seng R, Samb B, Simondon F, et al. Increased long term mortality associated with rash after early measles vaccination in rural Senegal. *Pediatr Infect Dis J* 1999;18(1):48–52.
761. Servet-Delprat C, Vidalain PO, Bausinger H, et al. Measles virus induces abnormal differentiation of CD40 ligand-activated human dendritic cells. *J Immunol* 2000;164(4):1753–1760.
762. Seya T. Measles virus takes a two-pronged attack on PP1. *Cell Host Microbe* 2014;16(1):1–2.
763. Shanks GD, Lee SE, Howard A, et al. Extreme mortality after first introduction of measles virus to the polynesian island of Rotuma, 1911. *Am J Epidemiol* 2011;173(10):1211–1222.
764. Sharma LB, Ohgimoto S, Kato S, et al. Contribution of matrix, fusion, hemagglutinin, and large protein genes of the CAM-70 measles virus vaccine strain to efficient growth in chicken embryonic fibroblasts. *J Virol* 2009;83(22):11645–11654.
765. Sharp CR, Nambulli S, Acciardo AS, et al. Chronic infection of domestic cats with feline morbillivirus, United States. *Emerg Infect Dis* 2016;22(4):760–762.
766. Shen W, Ye H, Zhang X, et al. Elevated expansion of follicular helper T cells in peripheral blood from children with acute measles infection. *BMC Immunol* 2020;21(1):49.
767. Sheppard RD, Raine CS, Bornstein MB, et al. Rapid degradation restricts measles virus matrix protein expression in a subacute sclerosing panencephalitis cell line. *Proc Natl Acad Sci U S A* 1986;83(20):7913–7917.
768. Sheshberadaran H, Norrby E. Characterization of epitopes on the measles virus hemagglutinin. *Virology* 1986;152(1):58–65.
769. Shibahara K, Hotta H, Katayama Y, et al. Increased binding activity of measles virus to monkey red blood cells after long-term passage in Vero cell cultures. *J Gen Virol* 1994;75(Pt 12):3511–3516.
770. Shingai M, Ebihara T, Begum NA, et al. Differential type I IFN-inducing abilities of wild-type versus vaccine strains of measles virus. *J Immunol* 2007;179(9):6123–6133.
771. Shingai M, Inoue N, Okuno T, et al. Wild-type measles virus infection in human CD46/CD150-transgenic mice: CD11c-positive dendritic cells establish systemic viral infection. *J Immunol* 2005;175(5):3252–3261.
772. Shiozawa S, Yoshikawa N, Iijima K, et al. A sensitive radioimmunoassay for circulating alpha-interferon in the plasma of healthy children and patients with measles virus infection. *Clin Exp Immunol* 1988;73(3):366–369.
773. Shirogane Y, Hashiguchi T, Yanagi Y. Weak cis and trans interactions of the hemagglutinin with receptors trigger fusion proteins of neuropathogenic measles virus isolates. *J Virol* 2020;94(2).
774. Shirogane Y, Takemoto R, Suzuki T, et al. CADM1 and CADM2 triggers neuropathogenic measles virus-mediated membrane fusion by acting in cis. *J Virol* 2021;95(14):e0052821.
775. Shirogane Y, Watanabe S, Yanagi Y. Cooperation between different variants: a unique potential for virus evolution. *Virus Res* 2019;264:68–73.
776. Shishkova Y, Harms H, Krohne G, et al. Immune synapses formed with measles virus-infected dendritic cells are unstable and fail to sustain T cell activation. *Cell Microbiol* 2007;9(8):1974–1986.
777. Shivakoti R, Hauer D, Adams RJ, et al. Limited in vivo production of type I or type III interferon after infection of macaques with vaccine or wild-type strains of measles virus. *J Interferon Cytokine Res* 2015;35(4):292–301.
778. Shivakoti R, Siwek M, Hauer D, et al. Induction of dendritic cell production of type I and type III interferons by wild-type and vaccine strains of measles virus: role of defective interfering RNAs. *J Virol* 2013;87(14):7816–7827.
779. Shulman ST, Shulman DL, Sims RH. The tragic 1824 journey of the Hawaiian king and queen to London: history of measles in Hawaii. *Pediatr Infect Dis J* 2009;28(8):728–733.
780. Si W, Zhou S, Wang Z, et al. A multiplex reverse transcription-nested polymerase chain reaction for detection and differentiation of wild-type and vaccine strains of canine distemper virus. *Virol J* 2010;7:86.
781. Sidorenko SP, Clark EA. The dual-function CD150 receptor subfamily: the viral attraction. *Nat Immunol* 2003;4(1):19–24.
782. Simon JK, Ramirez K, Cuberos L, et al. Mucosal IgA responses in healthy adult volunteers following intranasal spray delivery of a live attenuated measles vaccine. *Clin Vaccine Immunol* 2011;18(3):355–361.
783. Simsek E, Ozturk A, Yavuz C, et al. Subacute sclerosing panencephalitis (SSPE) associated with congenital measles infection. *Turk J Pediatr* 2005;47(1):58–62.
784. Singer FR. The etiology of Paget's disease of bone: viral and genetic interactions. *Cell Metab* 2011;13(1):5–6.
785. Singh BK, Li N, Mark AC, et al. Cell-to-cell contact and nectin-4 govern spread of measles virus from primary human myeloid cells to primary human airway epithelial cells. *J Virol* 2016;90(15):6808–6817.
786. Singh BK, Pfaller CK, Cattaneo R, et al. Measles Virus ribonucleoprotein complexes rapidly spread across well-differentiated primary human airway epithelial cells along F-actin rings. *mBio* 2019;10(6).
787. Sinn PL, Williams G, Vongpunsawad S, et al. Measles virus preferentially transduces the basolateral surface of well-differentiated human airway epithelia. *J Virol* 2002;76(5):2403–2409.
788. Sissons JG, Oldstone MB, Schreiber RD. Antibody-independent activation of the alternative complement pathway by measles virus-infected cells. *Proc Natl Acad Sci U S A* 1980;77(1):559–562.
789. Slifka MK, Homann D, Tishon A, et al. Measles virus infection results in suppression of both innate and adaptive immune responses to secondary bacterial infection. *J Clin Invest* 2003;111(6):805–810.
790. Smaron MF, Saxon E, Wood L, et al. Diagnosis of measles by fluorescent antibody and culture of nasopharyngeal secretions. *J Virol Methods* 1991;33(1–2):223–229.
791. Stephenson JR, Siddell SG, Meulen VT. Persistent and lytic infections with SSPE virus: a comparison of the synthesis of virus-specific polypeptides. *J Gen Virol* 1981;57(Pt 1):191–197.
792. Stimmer L, Siebert U, Wohlsein P, et al. Viral protein expression and phenotyping of inflammatory responses in the central nervous system of phocine distemper virus-infected harbor seals (*Phoca vitulina*). *Vet Microbiol* 2010;145(1–2):23–33.
793. Stolte M, Haas L, Wamwayi HM, et al. Induction of apoptotic cellular death in lymphatic tissues of cattle experimentally infected with different strains of rinderpest virus. *J Comp Pathol* 2002;127(1):14–21.
794. Suga S, Yoshikawa T, Asano Y, et al. Activation of human herpesvirus-6 in children with acute measles. *J Med Virol* 1992;38(4):278–282.
795. Sugai A, Sato H, Yoneda M, et al. PIM 3 kinase, a proto-oncogene product, regulates phosphorylation of the measles virus nucleoprotein tail domain at Ser 479 and Ser 510. *Biochem Biophys Res Commun* 2020;531(3):267–274.
796. Sugita T, Shiraki K, Ueda S, et al. Induction of acute myoclonic encephalopathy in hamsters by subacute sclerosing panencephalitis virus. *J Infect Dis* 1984;150(3):340–347.
797. Suryanarayana K, Baczko K, ter Meulen V, et al. Transcription inhibition and other properties of matrix proteins expressed by M genes cloned from measles viruses and diseased human brain tissue. *J Virol* 1994;68(3):1532–1543.
798. Tahara M, Burckert JP, Kanou K, et al. Measles virus hemagglutinin protein epitopes: the basis of antigenic stability. *Viruses* 2016;8(8).
799. Tahara M, Takeda M, Seki F, et al. Multiple amino acid substitutions in hemagglutinin are necessary for wild-type measles virus to acquire the ability to use receptor CD46 efficiently. *J Virol* 2007;81(6):2564–2572.
800. Tahara M, Takeda M, Yanagi Y. Contributions of matrix and large protein genes of the measles virus Edmonston strain to growth in cultured cells as revealed by recombinant viruses. *J Virol* 2005;79(24):15218–15225.
801. Takahashi H, Umino Y, Sato TA, et al. Detection and comparison of viral antigens in measles and rubella rashes. *Clin Infect Dis* 1996;22(1):36–39.
802. Takahashi M, Watari E, Shinya E, et al. Suppression of virus replication via down-modulation of mitochondrial short chain enoyl-CoA hydratase in human glioblastoma cells. *Antiviral Res* 2007;75(2):152–158.
803. Takaki H, Watanabe Y, Shingai M, et al. Strain-to-strain difference of V protein of measles virus affects MDA5-mediated IFN-beta-inducing potential. *Mol Immunol* 2011;48(4):497–504.
804. Takasu T, Mgone JM, Mgone CS, et al. A continuing high incidence of subacute sclerosing panencephalitis (SSPE) in the Eastern Highlands of Papua New Guinea. *Epidemiol Infect* 2003;131(2):887–898.
805. Takeda M. Measles virus breaks through epithelial cell barriers to achieve transmission. *J Clin Invest* 2008;118(7):2386–2389.
806. Takeda M, Kato A, Kobune F, et al. Measles virus attenuation associated with transcriptional impediment and a few amino acid changes in the polymerase and accessory proteins. *J Virol* 1998;72(11):8690–8696.
807. Takeda M, Ohno S, Seki F, et al. Long untranslated regions of the measles virus M and F genes control virus replication and cytopathogenicity. *J Virol* 2005;79(22):14346–14354.
808. Takeda M, Ohno S, Tahara M, et al. Measles viruses possessing the polymerase protein genes of the Edmonston vaccine strain exhibit attenuated gene expression and growth in cultured cells and SLAM knock-in mice. *J Virol* 2008;82(23):11979–11984.
809. Takeda M, Sakaguchi T, Li Y, et al. The genome nucleotide sequence of a contemporary wild strain of measles virus and its comparison with the classical Edmonston strain genome. *Virology* 1999;256(2):340–350.
810. Takeda M, Seki F, Yamamoto Y, et al. Animal morbilliviruses and their cross-species transmission potential. *Curr Opin Virol* 2020;41:38–45.
811. Takeuchi K, Nagata N, Kato SI, et al. Wild-type measles virus with the hemagglutinin protein of the Edmonston vaccine strain retains wild-type tropism in macaques. *J Virol* 2012;86(6):3027–3037.
812. Takeuchi K, Takeda M, Miyajima N, et al. Stringent requirement for the C protein of wild-type measles virus for growth both in vitro and in macaques. *J Virol* 2005;79(12):7838–7844.
813. Tamashiro VG, Perez HH, Griffin DE. Prospective study of the magnitude and duration of changes in tuberculin reactivity during uncomplicated and complicated measles. *Pediatr Infect Dis J* 1987;6(5):451–454.

814. Tatsuo H, Ono N, Tanaka K, et al. SLAM (CDw150) is a cellular receptor for measles virus. *Nature* 2000;406(6798):893–897.
815. Te Velthuis AJW, Grimes JM, Fodor E. Structural insights into RNA polymerases of negative-sense RNA viruses. *Nat Rev Microbiol* 2021;19(5):303–318.
816. Tellez-Negal I, Harter DH. Subacute sclerosing leukoencephalitis: ultrastructure of intranuclear and intracytoplasmic inclusions. *Science* 1966;154(3751):899–901.
817. tenOever BR, Servant MJ, Grandvaux N, et al. Recognition of the measles virus nucleocapsid as a mechanism of IRF-3 activation. *J Virol* 2002;76(8):3659–3669.
818. Thakkar VD, Cox RM, Sawatsky B, et al. The unstructured paramyxovirus nucleocapsid protein tail domain modulates viral pathogenesis through regulation of transcriptase activity. *J Virol* 2018;92(8).
819. Thomas B, Beard S, Jin L, et al. Development and evaluation of a real-time PCR assay for rapid identification and semi-quantitation of measles virus. *J Med Virol* 2007;79(10):1587–1592.
820. Thormar H, Mehta PD, Lin FH, et al. Presence of oligoclonal immunoglobulin G bands and lack of matrix protein antibodies in cerebrospinal fluids and sera of ferrets with measles virus encephalitis. *Infect Immun* 1983;41(3):1205–1211.
821. Tierney LM Jr, Wang KC. Images in clinical medicine. Koplik's spots. *N Engl J Med* 2006;354(7):740.
822. Tiwarekar V, Fehrholz M, Schneider-Schaulies J. KDELR2 competes with measles virus envelope proteins for cellular chaperones reducing their chaperone-mediated cell surface transport. *Viruses* 2019;11(1).
823. Tiwarekar V, Wohlfahrt J, Fehrholz M, et al. APOBEC3G-regulated host factors interfere with measles virus replication: role of REDD1 and mammalian TORC1 inhibition. *J Virol* 2018;92(17).
824. Torriani G, Mayor J, Zimmer G, et al. Macropinocytosis contributes to hantavirus entry into human airway epithelial cells. *Virology* 2019;531:57–68.
825. Tourtellotte WW, Ma BI, Brandes DB, et al. Quantification of de novo central nervous system IgG measles antibody synthesis in SSPE. *Ann Neurol* 1981;9(6):551–556.
826. Tran-Van H, Avota E, Börtlein C, et al. Measles virus modulates dendritic cell/T-cell communication at the level of plexinA1/neuropilin-1 recruitment and activity. *Eur J Immunol* 2011;41(1):151–163.
827. Truelove SA, Graham M, Moss WJ, et al. Characterizing the impact of spatial clustering of susceptibility for measles elimination. *Vaccine* 2019;37(5):732–741.
828. Tunis MC, Salvadori MI, Dubey V, et al.; National Advisory Committee on Immunization. Updated NACI recommendations for measles post-exposure prophylaxis. *Can Commun Dis Rep* 2018;44(9):226–230.
829. Tuokko H. Detection of acute measles infections by indirect and mu-capture enzyme immunoassays for immunoglobulin M antibodies and measles immunoglobulin G antibody avidity enzyme immunoassay. *J Med Virol* 1995;45(3):306–311.
830. Uhl EW, Kelderhouse C, Buikstra J, et al. New world origin of canine distemper: interdisciplinary insights. *Int J Paleopathol* 2019;24:266–278.
831. Urbanska EM, Chambers BJ, Ljunggren HG, et al. Spread of measles virus through axonal pathways into limbic structures in the brain of TAP1 −/− mice. *J Med Virol* 1997;52(4):362–369.
832. Utazi CE, Tatem AJ. Precise mapping reveals gaps in global measles vaccination coverage. *Nature* 2021;589(7842):354–355.
833. Uygun DFK, Uygun V, Burgucu D, et al. Role of the Th1 and Th17 pathway in subacute sclerosing panencephalitis. *J Child Neurol* 2019;34(13):815–819.
834. Uzicanin A, Zimmerman L. Field effectiveness of live attenuated measles-containing vaccines: a review of published literature. *J Infect Dis* 2011;204(Suppl 1):S133–S148.
835. Valsamakis A, Auwaerter PG, Rima BK, et al. Altered virulence of vaccine strains of measles virus after prolonged replication in human tissue. *J Virol* 1999;73(10):8791–8797.
836. Valsamakis A, Schneider H, Auwaerter PG, et al. Recombinant measles viruses with mutations in the C, V, or F gene have altered growth phenotypes in vivo. *J Virol* 1998;72(10):7754–7761.
837. van Binnendijk RS, Poelen MC, Kuijpers KC, et al. The predominance of CD8+ T cells after infection with measles virus suggests a role for CD8+ class I MHC-restricted cytotoxic T lymphocytes (CTL) in recovery from measles. Clonal analyses of human CD8+ class I MHC-restricted CTL. *J Immunol* 1990;144(6):2394–2399.
838. van Binnendijk RS, van der Heijden RW, Osterhaus AD. Monkeys in measles research. *Curr Top Microbiol Immunol* 1995;191:135–148.
839. van Binnendijk RS, Versteeg-van Oosten JP, Poelen MC, et al. Human HLA class I- and HLA class II-restricted cloned cytotoxic T lymphocytes identify a cluster of epitopes on the measles virus fusion protein. *J Virol* 1993;67(4):2276–2284.
840. van Driel BJ, Liao G, Engel P, et al. Responses to microbial challenges by SLAMF receptors. *Front Immunol* 2016;7:4.
841. van Els CA, Herberts CA, van der Heeft E, et al. A single naturally processed measles virus peptide fully dominates the HLA-A*0201-associated peptide display and is mutated at its anchor position in persistent viral strains. *Eur J Immunol* 2000;30(4):1172–1181.
842. van Els CA, Nanan R. T cell responses in acute measles. *Viral Immunol* 2002;15(3):435–450.
843. Van Nguyen N, Kato SI, Nagata K, et al. Differential induction of type I interferons in macaques by wild-type measles virus alone or with the hemagglutinin protein of the Edmonston vaccine strain. *Microbiol Immunol* 2016;60(7):501–505.
844. Vandevelde M, Zurbriggen A. Demyelination in canine distemper virus infection: a review. *Acta Neuropathol* 2005;109(1):56–68.
845. VanWormer E, Mazet JAK, Hall A, et al. Viral emergence in marine mammals in the North Pacific may be linked to Arctic sea ice reduction. *Sci Rep* 2019;9(1):15569.
846. Vijayan M, Seo YJ, Pritzl CJ, et al Sphingosine kinase 1 regulates measles virus replication. *Virology* 2014;450–451:55–63.
847. Vincent S, Tigaud I, Schneider H, et al. Restriction of measles virus RNA synthesis by a mouse host cell line: trans-complementation by polymerase components or a human cellular factor(s). *J Virol* 2002;76(12):6121–6130.
848. Visser IK, van Bressem MF, Barrett T, et al. Morbillivirus infections in aquatic mammals. *Vet Res* 1993;24(2):169–178.
849. von Messling V, Milosevic D, Cattaneo R. Tropism illuminated: lymphocyte-based pathways blazed by lethal morbillivirus through the host immune system. *Proc Natl Acad Sci U S A* 2004;101(39):14216–14221.
850. von Messling V, Oezguen N, Zheng Q, et al. Nearby clusters of hemagglutinin residues sustain SLAM-dependent canine distemper virus entry in peripheral blood mononuclear cells. *J Virol* 2005;79(9):5857–5862.
851. Vongpunsawad S, Oezgun N, Braun W, et al. Selectively receptor-blind measles viruses: identification of residues necessary for SLAM- or CD46-induced fusion and their localization on a new hemagglutinin structural model. *J Virol* 2004;78(1):302–313.
852. Vuorinen T, Peri P, Vainionpaa R. Measles virus induces apoptosis in uninfected bystander T cells and leads to granzyme B and caspase activation in peripheral blood mononuclear cell cultures. *Eur J Clin Invest* 2003;33(5):434–442.
853. Wakimoto H, Shimodo M, Satoh Y, et al. F-actin modulates measles virus cell-cell fusion and assembly by altering the interaction between the matrix protein and the cytoplasmic tail of hemagglutinin. *J Virol* 2013;87(4):1974–1984.
854. Waksman BH, Burnstein T, Adams RD. Histologic study of the encephalomyelitis produced in hamsters by a neurotropic strain of measles. *J Neuropathol Exp Neurol* 1962;21:25–49.
855. Wallinga J, Edmunds WJ, Kretzschmar M. Perspective: human contact patterns and the spread of airborne infectious diseases. *Trends Microbiol* 1999;7(9):372–377.
856. Ward BJ, Johnson RT, Vaisberg A, et al. Spontaneous proliferation of peripheral mononuclear cells in natural measles virus infection: identification of dividing cells and correlation with mitogen responsiveness. *Clin Immunol Immunopathol* 1990;55(2):315–326.
857. Ward BJ, Johnson RT, Vaisberg A, et al. Cytokine production in vitro and the lymphoproliferative defect of natural measles virus infection. *Clin Immunol Immunopathol* 1991;61(2 Pt 1):236–248.
858. Warren J, Crawford JG, Gallian MJ. Potency measurement of inactivated measles vaccines. *Am J Dis Child* 1962;103:452–457.
859. Watanabe S, Ohno S, Shirogane Y, et al. Measles virus mutants possessing the fusion protein with enhanced fusion activity spread effectively in neuronal cells, but not in other cells, without causing strong cytopathology. *J Virol* 2015;89(5):2710–2717.
860. Watanabe S, Shirogane Y, Suzuki SO, et al. Mutant fusion proteins with enhanced fusion activity promote measles virus spread in human neuronal cells and brains of suckling hamsters. *J Virol* 2013;87(5):2648–2659.
861. Weidinger G, Czub S, Neumeister C, et al. Role of CD4(+) and CD8(+) T cells in the prevention of measles virus-induced encephalitis in mice. *J Gen Virol* 2000;81(Pt 11):2707–2713.
862. Weidinger G, Henning G, ter Meulen V, et al. Inhibition of major histocompatibility complex class II-dependent antigen presentation by neutralization of gamma interferon leads to breakdown of resistance against measles virus-induced encephalitis. *J Virol* 2001;75(7):3059–3065.
863. Weidmann A, Fischer C, Ohgimoto S, et al. Measles virus-induced immunosuppression in vitro is independent of complex glycosylation of viral glycoproteins and of hemifusion. *J Virol* 2000;74(16):7548–7553.
864. Weidmann A, Maisner A, Garten W, et al. Proteolytic cleavage of the fusion protein but not membrane fusion is required for measles virus-induced immunosuppression in vitro. *J Virol* 2000;74(4):1985–1993.
865. Welstead GG, Hsu EC, Iorio C, et al. Mechanism of CD150 (SLAM) down regulation from the host cell surface by measles virus hemagglutinin protein. *J Virol* 2004;78(18):9666–9674.
866. Welstead GG, Iorio C, Draker R, et al. Measles virus replication in lymphatic cells and organs of CD150 (SLAM) transgenic mice. *Proc Natl Acad Sci U S A* 2005;102(45):16415–16420.
867. Wendorf KA, Winter K, Zipprich J, et al. Subacute sclerosing panencephalitis: the devastating measles complication that might be more common than previously estimated. *Clin Infect Dis* 2017;65(2):226–232.
868. Wesley AG, Coovadia HM, Kiepiela P. Further predictive indices of clinical severity of measles. *S Afr Med J* 1982;61(18):663–665.
869. White RG, Boyd JF. The effect of measles on the thymus and other lymphoid tissues. *Clin Exp Immunol* 1973;13(3):343–357.
870. Whittle HC, Dossetor J, Oduloju A, et al. Cell-mediated immunity during natural measles infection. *J Clin Invest* 1978;62(3):678–684.
871. Wiesmuller KH, Spahn G, Handtmann D, et al. Heterogeneity of linear B cell epitopes of the measles virus fusion protein reacting with late convalescent sera. *J Gen Virol* 1992;73 (Pt 9):2211–2216.
872. Wild TF, Malvoisin E, Buckland R. Measles virus: both the haemagglutinin and fusion glycoproteins are required for fusion. *J Gen Virol* 1991;72(Pt 2):439–442.
873. Wohlsein P, Trautwein G, Harder TC, et al. Viral antigen distribution in organs of cattle experimentally infected with rinderpest virus. *Vet Pathol* 1993;30(6):544–554.
874. Wolfson LJ, Grais RF, Luquero FJ, et al. Estimates of measles case fatality ratios: a comprehensive review of community-based studies. *Int J Epidemiol* 2009;38(1):192–205.
875. Wolinsky JS, Swoveland P, Johnson KP, et al. Subacute measles encephalitis complicating Hodgkin's disease in an adult. *Ann Neurol* 1977;1(5):452–457.
876. Wong TC, Ayata M, Ueda S, et al. Role of biased hypermutation in evolution of subacute sclerosing panencephalitis virus from progenitor acute measles virus. *J Virol* 1991;65(5):2191–2199.
877. Woo PC, Lau SK, Wong BH, et al. Feline morbillivirus, a previously undescribed paramyxovirus associated with tubulointerstitial nephritis in domestic cats. *Proc Natl Acad Sci U S A* 2012;109(14):5435–5440.
878. Woudenberg T, van Binnendijk R, Veldhuijzen I, et al. Additional evidence on serological correlates of protection against measles: an observational cohort study among once vaccinated children exposed to measles. *Vaccines (Basel)* 2019;7(4):158.
879. Wyde PR, Moore-Poveda DK, Daley NJ, et al. Replication of clinical measles virus strains in hispid cotton rats. *Proc Soc Exp Biol Med* 1999;221(1):53–62.
880. Wyde PR, Stittelaar KJ, Osterhaus AD, et al. Use of cotton rats for preclinical evaluation of measles vaccines. *Vaccine* 2000;19(1):42–53.
881. Wyplosz B, Lafarge M, Escaut L, et al. Fatal measles pneumonitis during Hodgkin's lymphoma. *BMJ Case Rep* 2013;2013.
882. Xin JY, Ihara T, Komase K, et al. Amino acid substitutions in matrix, fusion and hemagglutinin proteins of wild measles virus for adaptation to Vero cells. *Intervirology* 2011;54(4):217–228.

883. Yanagi Y, Cubitt BA, Oldstone MB. Measles virus inhibits mitogen-induced T cell proliferation but does not directly perturb the T cell activation process inside the cell. *Virology* 1992;187(1):280–289.

884. Yanagi Y, Ono N, Tatsuo H, et al. Measles virus receptor SLAM (CD150). *Virology* 2002;299(2):155–161.

885. Yang L, Grenfell BT, Mina MJ. Measles vaccine immune escape: should we be concerned? *Eur J Epidemiol* 2019;34(10):893–896.

886. Yang Y, Zhou D, Zhao B, et al. Immunoglobulin A targeting on the N-terminal moiety of viral phosphoprotein prevents measles virus from evading interferon-beta signaling. *ACS Infect Dis* 2020;6(5):844–856.

887. Yegambaram K, Kingston RL. The feet of the measles virus polymerase bind the viral nucleocapsid protein at a single site. *Protein Sci* 2010;19(4):893–899.

888. Yilla M, Hickman C, McGrew M, et al. Edmonston measles virus prevents increased cell surface expression of peptide-loaded major histocompatibility complex class II proteins in human peripheral monocytes. *J Virol* 2003;77(17):9412–9421.

889. Young LW, Smith DI, Glasgow LA. Pneumonia of atypical measles. Residual nodular lesions. *Am J Roentgenol Radium Ther Nucl Med* 1970;110(3):439–448.

890. Young NP, Weinshenker BG, Parisi JE, et al. Perivenous demyelination: association with clinically defined acute disseminated encephalomyelitis and comparison with pathologically confirmed multiple sclerosis. *Brain* 2010;133(Pt 2):333–348.

891. Yu XL, Cheng YM, Shi BS, et al. Measles virus infection in adults induces production of IL-10 and is associated with increased CD4+ CD25+ regulatory T cells. *J Immunol* 2008;181(10):7356–7366.

892. Zenner D, Nacul L. Predictive power of Koplik's spots for the diagnosis of measles. *J Infect Dev Ctries* 2012;6(3):271–275.

893. Zhang P, Li L, Hu C, et al. Interactions among measles virus hemagglutinin, fusion protein and cell receptor signaling lymphocyte activation molecule (SLAM) indicating a new fusion-trimer model. *J Biochem Mol Biol* 2005;38(4):373–380.

894. Zhang X, Bourhis JM, Longhi S, et al. Hsp72 recognizes a P binding motif in the measles virus N protein C-terminus. *Virology* 2005;337(1):162–174.

895. Zhang X, Lu G, Qi J, et al. Structure of measles virus hemagglutinin bound to its epithelial receptor nectin-4. *Nat Struct Mol Biol* 2013;20(1):67–72.

896. Zhang X, Rennick LJ, Duprex WP, et al. Determination of spontaneous mutation frequencies in measles virus under nonselective conditions. *J Virol* 2013;87(5):2686–2692.

897. Zhou D, Zhang Y, Li Q, et al. Matrix protein-specific IgA antibody inhibits measles virus replication by intracellular neutralization. *J Virol* 2011;85(21):11090–11097.

898. Zhou Y, Su JM, Samuel CE, et al. Measles virus forms inclusion bodies with properties of liquid organelles. *J Virol* 2019;93(21).

899. Zilliox MJ, Moss WJ, Griffin DE. Gene expression changes in peripheral blood mononuclear cells during measles virus infection. *Clin Vaccine Immunol* 2007;14(7):918–923.

Respiratory Syncytial Virus and Metapneumovirus

Ursula J. Buchholz • Larry J. Anderson • Peter L. Collins • Asuncion Mejias

History
Infectious agent
  Classification
  Virion
  RNA
  Proteins
  Replicative cycle
  Propagation *in vitro*
  Genetics and reverse genetics
  Infection of animals with HRSV and HMPV
  Antigenic subgroups and genotypes
  Animal viruses
Pathogenesis and pathology
Immune response
  Antigens
  Innate immunity and inflammation
  Antibodies
  T lymphocytes
  Viral evasion of host immunity
Epidemiology
  Infection of infants and young children
  Infection of adults
  Other high-risk populations
  The yearly HRSV pandemic
Clinical features
Diagnosis
  Differential diagnosis
  Laboratory diagnosis
Treatment and prevention
  Treatment
  Prevention
Perspective

HISTORY

Human respiratory syncytial virus (HRSV) was first isolated in 1955 from a laboratory chimpanzee with illness resembling the common cold, and transmission between chimpanzees and humans was recognized.[441] Shortly thereafter, the same virus was recovered from infants with respiratory illness, and serologic studies indicated that infection in infants and children was common, establishing HRSV as a common pathogen of humans.[92,93] HRSV is now recognized as the most important viral agent of pediatric lower respiratory tract illness (LRI) worldwide.[371,555] In many areas, it outranks other microbial pathogens as a cause of pneumonia and bronchiolitis in infants. HRSV also can infect and cause disease in individuals of all ages and severe disease in the elderly and in immunosuppressed individuals.[178,255] Worldwide, acute respiratory infection (ARI) is the leading cause of mortality due to infectious disease, and HRSV remains one of the pathogens deemed most important for vaccine development.[386] HRSV research is hampered by its poor growth *in vitro*, its physical instability, the heterogeneous and filamentous nature of its particles, and the difficulties of studies involving young children. HRSV has a single serotype with two antigenic subgroups A and B.

Human metapneumovirus (HMPV) was first described in 2001 following its isolation from infants and children experiencing HRSV-like disease of unknown etiology.[625] There is serologic evidence of extensive pediatric infection dating back more than 70 years, and thus HMPV was newly discovered rather than newly emerged.[625,662,663] The virus had been overlooked because it grows slowly *in vitro*, has a delayed cytopathic effect, and usually requires added trypsin for activation of the fusion F protein needed to initiate infection. HMPV is recognized as an important agent of respiratory tract disease worldwide, especially in the pediatric and elderly populations, although its impact is less than that of HRSV.[662] HMPV also has a single serotype with two subgroups A and B.[565]

INFECTIOUS AGENT

Classification

HRSV and HMPV are enveloped, cytoplasmic viruses with single-stranded nonsegmented negative-sense RNA genomes. They were reclassified in 2016 by the International Committee on Virus Taxonomy (ICTV) from the family *Paramyxoviridae* to create the new family *Pneumoviridae*, order *Mononegavirales*, because they represent a distinct phylogenetic clade within the negative-sense RNA viruses based on their L protein sequences and the presence of an M2 gene.[507] The *Pneumoviridae* family contains two genera, *Orthopneumovirus* and *Metapneumovirus* (e-Figs. 10.1 and 10.2). The genus *Orthopneumovirus* contains three species, HRSV, bovine RSV (BRSV), and murine pneumonia virus (MPV; formerly called pneumonia virus of mice [PVM]). The genus *Metapneumovirus* contains two species, HMPV, and avian metapneumovirus (AMPV, formerly called

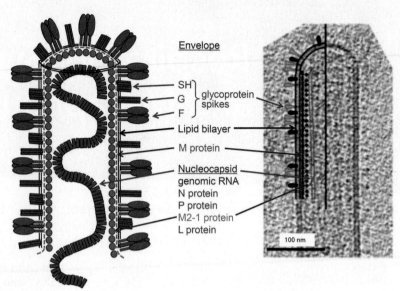

FIGURE 10.1 Diagrams of a filamentous HRSV particle: an idealized diagram of a budding filament is shown on the *left*, and a cryotomographic image of an HRSV particle is shown on the *right*, with a schematic drawing of the virion architecture superimposed over the left side of the tomogram. (Adapted with permission of American Society for Microbiology from Kiss G, Holl JM, Williams GM, et al. Structural analysis of respiratory syncytial virus reveals the position of M2-1 between the matrix protein and the ribonucleoprotein complex. *J Virol* 2014;88(13):7602-7617; permission conveyed through Copyright Clearance Center, Inc.) The G, SH, and F proteins are present in homo-oligomers that constitute the glycoprotein spikes. Separate layers composed of the M and M2-1 proteins underlie the lipid bilayer. The proteins of the nucleocapsid are not depicted individually. The HMPV particle architecture is thought to be similar.

turkey rhinotracheitis virus [TRTV] or avian pneumovirus [APV]). Comparisons of these viruses based on gene maps and nucleotide sequences are shown in e-Figures 10.1 and 10.2.

Virion

The HRSV virion consists of a nucleocapsid/polymerase complex that is packaged within two protein layers that underlie a lipid envelope derived from the host cell plasma membrane during budding (Figs. 10.1 and 10.2). Virus particles are heterogeneous in size and shape; when visualized by electron microscopy (Fig. 10.2C and D), virions appear primarily as long filamentous particles 0.5 to 12 μm in length (average: 1.5 μm) and 60 to 250 nm in diameter (average: 130 nm). Some irregular spherical particles of 100 to 350 nm in diameter are also present.[318,333] Structural studies suggest that long filamentous particles may contain more than one genome copy,[333] but UV inactivation kinetics of infectivity indicated that most particles do not contain more than a single functional genome.[154] During *in vitro* passage, approximately 90% of HRSV virions remain associated with the exterior face of the cell plasma membrane, suggestive of incomplete budding. Filaments can be visualized as projections from the surface of infected cells by fluorescence photomicroscopy[22,289] (Fig. 10.2B).

The nucleocapsid appears in electron micrographs as a herringbone structure that also is characteristic of *Paramyxoviridae*. However, the HRSV nucleocapsid is narrower than those of prototype members of *Paramyxoviridae* (12 to 16 nm compared to 17 to 20 nm) and has a steeper pitch.[22] The minimum components of the nucleocapsid—as isolated by centrifugation in CsCl gradients—are the viral RNA associated with the nucleoprotein N. This further associates with three additional proteins: the phosphoprotein P, the large polymerase subunit L, and the transcription processivity factor M2-1 (which also forms one of the protein layers underlying the envelope, see next paragraph) (Fig. 10.3A). This comprises the nucleocapsid/polymerase complex, also known as the ribonucleoprotein core (RNP). However, polymerase activity in purified virions, an activity found in prototypic members of *Mononegavirales*, has not been demonstrated for HRSV preparations.

The HRSV envelope contains three virally encoded transmembrane surface glycoproteins: the major attachment protein G, the fusion protein F, and the small hydrophobic SH protein (Figs. 10.3A and 10.4). The nonglycosylated matrix M protein forms a layer underneath the lipid envelope (Fig. 10.1). In between the M layer and the RNP, the M2-1 protein forms an additional layer.[318,333] The viral glycoproteins are present as transmembrane homo-oligomers that are visualized as short (11 to 20 nm), closely spaced (intervals of 6 to 10 nm) surface projections or "spikes." HRSV lacks a neuraminidase or a hemagglutinin; MPV is the only pneumovirus that agglutinates erythrocytes via its G protein.[379]

HRSV virions can readily lose infectivity during handling, especially during freeze–thawing. This is at least in part attributed to the metastable nature of the prefusion (pre-F) version of the F protein, which readily and irreversibly converts to the postfusion (post-F) conformation (see "Proteins" and "Antigens").[322,377] Loss of infectivity can be partly overcome by agents such as sugars that reduce aggregation and improve thermal stability.[19] The long filamentous shape of the particle may also contribute to fragility and loss of infectivity.

HMPV virions were visualized by electron microscopy as heterogeneous spheres and filaments that appear to have general similarity to those of HRSV[477,625] (Fig. 10.2E). The spherical particles had a reported diameter of 150 to 600 nm with envelope spikes of 13 to 17 nm. The nucleocapsid diameter was reported as 17 nm, suggesting a possible difference compared to HRSV.[477] HMPV has the same array of structural proteins as HRSV (Fig. 10.3B). The infectivity of HMPV particles is markedly more stable than that of HRSV.[611]

RNA

The HRSV genome (Fig. 10.3C) is a single negative-sense strand of RNA ranging in length from 15,191 to 15,226 nucleotides for the first six strains that were sequenced, namely the subgroup A strains A2 (15,222 nucleotides; GenBank accession number M74568), Long strain (15,226 nucleotides; AY911262), S2 (15,191 nucleotides; NC_001803), and line 19 (15,191 nucleotides; FJ614813), and the subgroup B strains B1 (15,225 nucleotides; NC_001781) and 9320 (15,225 nucleotides; AY353550). More recently, genetic lineages have emerged with duplications of 60 (subgroup B[615]) or 72 (subgroup A[169])

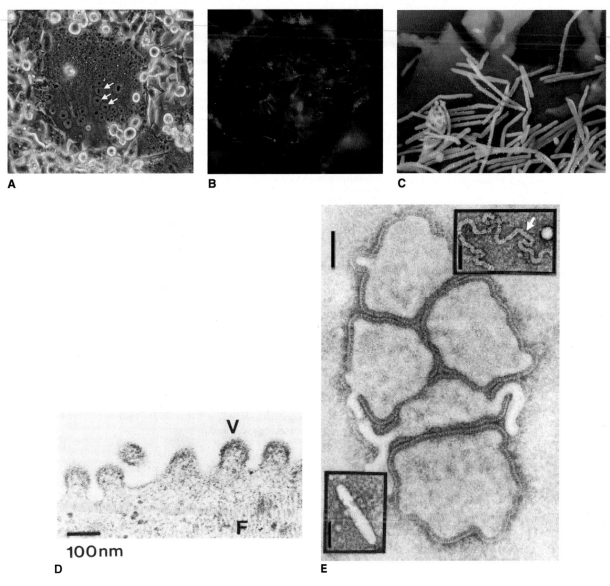

FIGURE 10.2 Photomicrographs (A and B) and electron micrographs (C–E) of HRSV-infected cells (A–D) and HMPV virions (E).
Panel **A** is a photomicrograph of an HRSV-infected HEp-2 cell monolayer showing a virus-induced syncytium (several nuclei are indicated with *arrows*; courtesy of Dr. Alexander Bukreyev). Panel **B** is a fluorescence photomicrograph of HRSV-infected human bronchial epithelial cell monolayers (cell line 16HBE14o) showing a syncytium stained with an antibody specific to the F protein, exhibiting filamentous viral projections. (Courtesy of Dr. Ursula J. Buchholz.) Panel **C** is a scanning electron micrograph of HRSV virions (pseudo-colored *blue*), labeled with immunogold-conjugated anti-HRSV F antibodies (pseudo-colored *yellow*, seen as *small dots*), shedding from the surface of human lung A549 cells. (Courtesy of Dr. Masfique Mehedi, University of North Dakota.) (NIAID stock photograph [NIAID Image Resources]). Panel **D** is a negatively strained electron micrograph of HRSV virions budding from a HeLa cell: V indicates a budding virion and F indicates filamentous cytoplasmic structures that likely are nucleocapsids. (Courtesy of Dr. Robert M. Chanock. Reprinted by permission from Springer: Kalica AR, Wright PF, Hetrick FM, et al. Electron microscopic studies of respiratory syncytial temperature-sensitive mutants. *Arch Gesamte Virusforsch* 1973;41(3):248-258. Copyright © 1973 Springer-Verlag.)[305] Panel **E** is a negatively stained electron micrograph of HMPV (bar markers represent 100 nm): the main panel shows spherical-type particles, the *upper insert* shows a free nucleocapsid (*arrow*), and the *lower insert* shows a filamentous or rod-like particle. (From Peret TC, Boivin G, Li Y, et al. Characterization of human metapneumoviruses isolated from patients in North America. *J Infect Dis* 2002;185(11):1660–1663. Reproduced by permission of the Infectious Diseases Society of America.)

nucleotides in hypervariable regions of the G ORF, increasing the genome length (see "Glycoprotein G").

The genome is neither capped nor polyadenylated. Both in virions and intracellularly, the genome is tightly and completely bound by N protein to create the RNAse-resistant nucleocapsid, as is typical of *Mononegavirales*. This tight encapsidation likely protects the genome, which lacks stabilizing features of capping and polyadenylation, from degradation. It also likely shields the genome from recognition by host cell pattern recognition receptors, in particular the cytoplasmic helicases

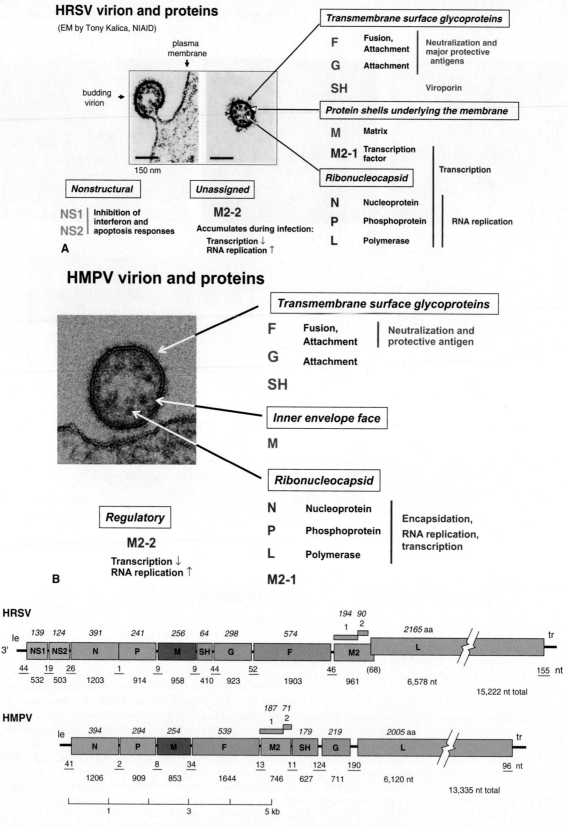

FIGURE 10.3 The proteins of HRSV (A) and HMPV (B), and maps of the viral genomic RNAs (C). Panels **A** and **B** indicate locations of the proteins in the virus particle and major functions when known. Panels **A–C** are color coded: proteins/genes that are part of the nucleocapsid and polymerase complex or that are involved in RNA synthesis are in *blue*, surface glycoproteins in *red*, matrix protein in *magenta*, and the two HRSV nonstructural proteins in *brown*. The electron micrographs of the HRSV virions are courtesy of Dr. Robert M. Chanock. Reprinted by permission from Springer: Kalica AR, Wright PF, Hetrick FM, et al. Electron microscopic studies of respiratory syncytial temperature-sensitive mutants. *Arch Gesamte Virusforsch* 1973;41(3):248–258. Copyright © 1973 Springer-Verlag. The electron micrograph of the HMPV virions is from Buchholz UJ, Nagashima K, Murphy BR, et al. Live vaccines for human metapneumovirus designed by reverse genetics. *Expert Rev Vaccines* 2006;5(5):695–706. Reprinted by permission of Taylor & Francis Ltd, https://www.tandfonline.com. The maps in Panel **C** are approximately to scale and show the 3′ to 5′ negative-sense genomes of HRSV strain A2 and HMPV strain CAN97-83. The overlapping ORFs of the M2 mRNAs are illustrated over the M2 genes. Numbers beneath each map indicate nucleotide (nt) lengths; those of the extragenic leader (le), trailer (tr) and intergenic regions are underlined, and that of the HRSV gene overlap is in parentheses. Italicized numbers above each map indicate amino acid (aa) lengths based on the complete ORFs.

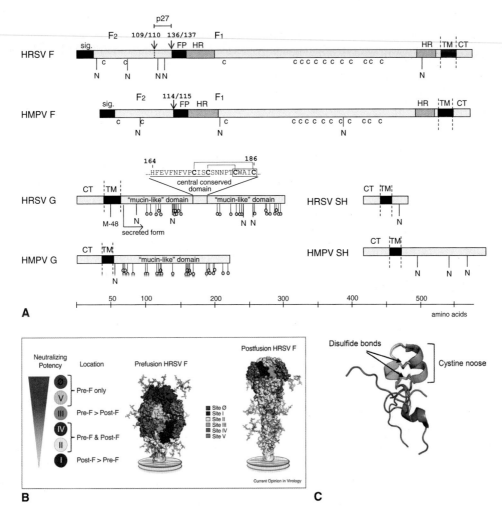

FIGURE 10.4 Glycoproteins of HRSV and HMPV. A: Primary structures (approximately to scale) of the F, G, and SH surface glycoproteins of HRSV strain A2 and HMPV strain CAN97-83. Hydrophobic domains are *black bars*: Sig., signal peptide; FP, fusion peptide representing the N-terminus of the F1 subunit; TM, transmembrane anchor; CT, cytoplasmic tail. Heptad repeats (HR) in the F protein are gray and cysteine residues conserved between the F proteins of HRSV and HMPV are indicated underneath (indicated as c). *Downward-facing arrows* identify the cleavage-activation site(s) in the F protein. Potential acceptor sites for N-linked carbohydrate are indicated as *downward facing stalks* with N. For each G protein, the 25 potential acceptor sites for O-linked sugars predicted by NetOGlyc 2.0 to be the most likely to be utilized are indicated as *downward facing stalks* with *small circles*. The sequence excerpt above the HRSV G protein shows the highly conserved 13-aa segment (underlined) and cystine noose; cysteine residues are bold; the disulfide bonding pattern is indicated by *dotted lines*[218]; and the fractalkine CX3C motif is *boxed*. M-48 in the HRSV G protein is the translational start site for the secreted form, and the N-terminus of the major mature secreted form is indicated.[511] **B:** Antigenic sites on the pre-F and post-F conformations of the HRSV F protein. RSV pre-F and post-F structures are shown as molecular surfaces, with N-linked glycans modeled as sticks and the viral membrane represented as a *gray disc*. There are two pre-F–specific antigenic sites (Ø and V) and four sites that are present on both conformations (I, II, III, IV). Antibodies against site III generally bind tighter to the pre-F conformation, whereas antibodies against site I bind tighter to the post-F conformation. The neutralization sensitivity of each antigenic site is directly related to exclusive or preferential binding to the pre-F conformation. The most potent MAbs bind to the apex of the pre-F trimer at sites Ø and V located at the apex of the pre-F trimer, and MAbs to those sites compete with antibodies that account for the large majority of neutralizing activity in human sera. (Images prepared by Morgan S. Gilman, PhD, Department of Biochemistry and Cell Biology, Giesel School of Medicine at Dartmouth. Reprinted from Graham BS. Vaccine development for respiratory syncytial virus. *Curr Opin Virol* 2017;23:107–112. Copyright © 2017 Elsevier. With permission.) **C:** Cystine noose of the HRSV G protein. A 36-amino acid region of the G protein of HRSV A2 (Asp162 to Lys196) encompassing the cystine noose and flanking regions is shown. The peptide is colored following the spectrum from *blue* (N-terminus) to *red* (C-terminus). The two disulfide bonds in the cystine noose are indicated. (Adapted by permission from Nature: Battles MB, McLellan JS. Respiratory syncytial virus entry and how to block it. *Nat Rev Microbiol* 2019;17(4):233–245. Copyright © 2019 Springer Nature.) This structure is derived from four crystal structures of the RSV G peptide in complex with four different antigen-binding fragments (Fabs). The Fabs are not shown. The four structures are superimposed, showing the invariant cystine noose and different alternative structures for the N-terminal and C-terminal ends.

retinoic acid–induced gene I (RIG-I) and melanoma differentiation–associated protein 5 (MDA-5), as well as RNA-inducible protein kinase R (PKR), which also activates NF-κB and phosphorylates eukaryotic translation initiation factor 2a (eIF-2a) to inhibit translational initiation as part of antiviral defense.

The HRSV genome contains 10 genes in the order 3′ NS1-NS2-N-P-M-SH-G-F-M2-L (Fig. 10.3C) that are transcribed sequentially into 10 separate mRNAs.[107,108,111,117,154,433] Each gene begins with a highly conserved 9-nucleotide gene-start (GS) transcription signal and ends with a moderately conserved 12- to 13-nucleotide gene-end (GE) signal[295,348] (e-Fig. 10.3A). The first nine genes are separated by intergenic regions that vary in length from 1 to 58 nucleotides.[107,295] These lack any conserved motifs, are poorly conserved between strains, and appear to be unimportant spacers. The last two HRSV genes, M2 and L, overlap by 68 nucleotides[116] (Fig. 10.3C and e-Fig. 10.3A). Specifically, the GS signal for the L gene is located upstream, rather than downstream, of the M2 GE signal. The same overlap occurs in BRSV; overlapping genes are not found in any other members of *Pneumoviridae* or *Paramyxoviridae*, but sometimes are found in *Rhabdoviridae* and *Filoviridae*. The 3′ and 5′ ends of the genome consist of short extragenic leader and trailer regions (44 and 155 nucleotides long, respectively, in strain A2).

The HRSV mRNAs contain a methylated 5′ cap structure m[7]G[5′]ppp[5′]Gp[27] and are polyadenylated at the 3′ end by reiterative copying on a U tract in each GE signal. Each HRSV mRNA encodes a single major protein except for M2, which has two separate ORFs encoding the M2-1 and M2-2 proteins. The M2-1 ORF is located in the upstream part of the mRNA, while the M2-2 ORF is located downstream and overlaps by 32 nucleotides in strain A2. Translation of the downstream M2-2 ORF depends on re-initiation by ribosomes exiting the upstream M2-1 ORF, a process that appears to be influenced by the structure of a region of RNA located approximately 150 nucleotides upstream of the M2-2 translational start site.[221] Whereas the P genes of *Paramyxoviridae* encode additional accessory proteins by overlapping ORFs, alternative translational start sites, and RNA editing, the P gene of HRSV (and HMPV) encodes only P (although MPV P contains a second ORF encoding a short protein; see "Animal Viruses").

HRSV transcription follows the general *Mononegavirales* model,[108,154] involving initiation at a single 3′ promoter and a start–stop–restart sequential mechanism guided by the GS and GE signals. RNA sequences important in the initiation of transcription and RNA replication are shown in e-Figure 10.4. Capping seems to be an essential step for efficient mRNA elongation: when capping was blocked using a novel HRSV-specific inhibitor, transcription produced uncapped abortive RNAs of approximately 45 to 50 nt.[382] Termination at the various GE signals typically is somewhat inefficient, resulting in readthrough transcription that creates mRNAs representing two or more adjacent genes and their intervening intergenic regions.[117] These readthrough mRNAs account for approximately 10% of total mRNA.

The M2/L gene overlap raised two questions for the model of sequential transcription: (a) how do polymerases that exit the M2 gene find the upstream L GS signal (or does polymerase enter independently at that site) and (b) how do polymerases that initiate at the L GS signal avoid premature termination when they cross the M2 GE signal? Studies with a mini-replicon system showed that when polymerase completes transcription of the M2 gene, it efficiently gains access to the L gene by retrograde scanning.[183] The polymerase appeared to scan in both directions. This led to the current proposal that scanning is a common function of the polymerase that occurs at each gene junction as well as during initiation of transcription and RNA replication at the viral promoter. The M2 GE signal within the L gene indeed causes premature termination for 90% of L gene transcripts, producing a 68-nucleotide polyadenylated RNA that does not appear to encode a protein and is not known to have any function.[116] The synthesis of full-length L mRNA depends on polymerase readthrough at the M2 GE signal. Thus, the "error" of reading through a GE signal is necessary for synthesis of this essential mRNA.[116] Premature termination of 90% of L gene transcripts might be expected to severely down-regulate the production of full-length mRNA, but the ability of the polymerase to recycle back to the L GS signal apparently relieves much of this effect, and the amount of L mRNA produced for HRSV relative to the other mRNAs appears to be about the same as for other members of *Pneumoviridae* and *Paramyxoviridae*. The gene overlap does not seem to be of any particular benefit to the virus and may be an accidental arrangement that can be tolerated due to the scanning function of the polymerase.

RNA replication by HRSV also follows the general *Mononegavirales* model. The replicating polymerase ignores the GS and GE signals and produces a complete positive-sense copy of the viral genome that is called the antigenome and also is tightly encapsidated. The antigenome serves in turn as the template for producing progeny genomes. Chain elongation of nascent genomes and antigenomes depends on concurrent encapsidation.[416] For viruses in the family *Paramyxoviridae*, the nucleotide length of the genome must be an even multiple of six in order for efficient RNA replication to occur ("rule of six"), reflecting a requirement for nucleocapsid organization, but there appears to be no comparable requirement for members of *Pneumoviridae*.[534]

The HMPV genome is approximately 13.2 kb—nearly 2 kb shorter than that of HRSV—and lacks the NS1 and NS2 genes (Fig. 10.3C). Also, the order of the SH, G, F, and M2 genes differs between HRSV (SH-G-F-M2) and HMPV (F-M2-SH-G). After correcting for the lack of NS1 and NS2 for HMPV and the difference in gene order, the genomes of HRSV and HMPV share 50% nucleotide sequence identity. HMPV strains for which the first complete genome sequences have been reported include CAN97-83 (13,335 nt, GenBank accession AY297749) and NL/00/1 (13,350, AF371337) of subgroup A, and CAN98-75 (13,280, AY297748) and NL/1/99 (13,293, AY525843) of subgroup B.[49,277] Duplications of 180 nucleotides and 111 nucleotides in the G ORF occur in some HMPV strains, increasing the genome length (see "Glycoprotein G").[454]

Features of the structure, encapsidation, transcription, and replication of the HMPV genome are generally similar to those described above for HRSV. The *cis*-acting signals of HMPV have considerable similarity to those of HRSV[49,624] (e-Fig. 10.3B). The HMPV intergenic regions can be longer than those of HRSV, up to 190 nt in the case of CAN97-83 (Fig. 10.3C and e-Fig. 10.3B). Unlike HRSV, the HMPV M2-2 protein appears to be translated independently of the upstream M2-1 ORF.[70]

Proteins

HRSV encodes 11 separate proteins (Fig. 10.3A). HMPV encodes nine proteins (Fig. 10.3B) that generally correspond to those of HRSV except for the lack of NS1 and NS2.[49,624] Table 10.1 shows amino acid sequence relatedness between members of the *Pneumoviridae* family.

Fusion F Glycoprotein

The HRSV F and L proteins are the ones that most closely resemble their counterparts in the *Paramyxoviridae* family. As is typical for *Paramyxoviridae* and *Pneumoviridae*, the HRSV F protein directs viral penetration by fusion between the virion envelope and the host cell plasma membrane or internal endosomal membranes (see "Replicative Cycle"). Later in infection, F protein expressed on the cell surface can mediate fusion with neighboring cells to form syncytia (Fig. 10.2A).

The HRSV F protein also appears to play a role in viral attachment. F binds to cellular glycosaminoglycans (GAGs), which are long unbranched chains of repeating disaccharide subunits that are part of the glycocalyx present on the outer surface of the cell.[188,189,599] GAGs are important for infection of cell lines *in vitro*, but not for infection of human airway epithelium (see "Replicative Cycle"). Interaction of F with the cellular protein nucleolin appears to be important in initiating infection.[597] HRSV attachment and entry are described in greater detail in "Glycoprotein G" and "Replicative Cycle" below.

F is a type I transmembrane surface protein that has a cleaved signal peptide at the N-terminus and a membrane anchor near the C-terminus[112] (Fig. 10.4A). Crystal structures of the pre- and post-F forms of the HRSV F protein have been resolved[419,591] (Fig. 10.4B).

As is typical for *Paramyxoviridae* and *Pneumoviridae*, F is synthesized as a fusion-inactive precursor F0 that assembles into a homotrimer. The F proteins of HRSV and BRSV are unique in *Paramyxoviridae* and *Pneumoviridae* in having two, rather than one, polybasic proteolytic cleavage sites, separated by 27 amino acids[216,688] (Fig. 10.4A). The site that

is immediately upstream of the fusion peptide (131-Lys-Lys-Arg-Lys-Arg-Arg↓, with cleavage between residues 136/137 in HRSV strain A2) is the one that corresponds to that of other pneumoviruses and paramyxoviruses. The second site is located 27 amino acids upstream (106-Arg-Ala-Arg-Arg↓, with cleavage between residues 109/110). Thus, both sites contain a furin cleavage motif (Arg-X-Arg/Lys-Arg↓). F is cleaved in the trans-Golgi complex by furin or a furin-like cellular endoprotease to yield two disulfide-linked subunits, NH2-F2–F1-COOH. One study indicated that F protein present in HRSV particles had been cleaved only at the upstream site, and that cleavage at the downstream site—necessary for activation—occurred only following endocytic uptake during the next round of infection.[343]

Newly synthesized, cleaved F protein is in the pre-F conformation, with the trimer forming a spheroidal shape that extends about 12 nm from the virus membrane[420] (Fig. 10.4B). The N-terminus of the F1 subunit that is created by cleavage contains a hydrophobic domain (the fusion peptide) that inserts directly into the target membrane to initiate fusion. The F1 subunit also contains two areas of heptad repeats that associate during fusion, driving a conformational shift that brings the viral and cellular membranes into close proximity.[31,112] HRSV F protein can direct efficient fusion independent of other viral proteins. This is characteristic of *Pneumoviridae* but differs from most members of *Paramyxoviridae*, for which efficient fusion requires interaction with the homologous attachment protein. As noted above, the 12 nm pre-F conformation of the F trimer is metastable and can be readily triggered to refold irreversibly into the post-F conformation, assuming an elongated shape of about 17 nm in length[591] (Fig. 10.4B). Both pre-F and post-F trimers are present on virus particles, and the proportion likely shifts toward post-F as trimers are triggered by environmental factors.[322,377]

Cleavage at the two sites in HRSV F0 releases a short peptide of 27 amino acids (p27) that has two N-linked sugar side chains; the remainder of F has two N-linked sugars in F2 and one in F1.[688] For BRSV, this peptide contains a tachykinin

TABLE 10.1   Percent amino acid sequence identity between the proteins of HRSV subgroup A (HRSV-A) or HMPV subgroup A (HMPV-A) and the indicated viruses[a]

Viruses Compared		% Amino Acid Sequence Identity for the Indicated Protein										
		NS1	NS2	N	P	M	SH	G	F	M2-1	M2-2	L
HRSV-A versus:	HRSV-B	87	92	96	91	91	76	53	89	92	72	93
	BRSV	69	84	93	81	89	38	30	81	80	42	84
	MPV	16	20	60	33	42	23	12	43	43	10	53
	HMPV-A	—[b]	—[b]	42	35	38	23	15	33	36	17	45
	AMPV-A	—[b]	—[b]	41	32	38	19	16	35	37	12	43
HMPV-A versus:	HMPV-B	—[b]	—[b]	96	85	97	59	37	95	96	89	94
	AMPV-C	—[b]	—[b]	88	68	87	24	23	81	83	56	80
	AMPV-A	—[b]	—[b]	70	58	77	20	12	68	73	25	64
	AMPV-B	—[b]	—[b]	69	53	76	20	13	67	71	27	ND[c]

[a]Viruses are listed in order of decreasing relatedness to HRSV-A or HMPV-A.
[b]Does not encode NS1 or NS2.
[c]ND, not done.

sequence motif and is processed and released from BRSV-infected cells to yield a virokinin that induces smooth muscle contraction *in vitro*, which is a property of tachykinins.[689] Tachykinins also have proinflammatory and immunomodulatory activities. Recombinant BRSV in which most of p27 was deleted, or in which the upstream cleavage site was mutated, replicated as efficiently as the wild-type parent in calves but induced less pulmonary inflammation and a somewhat lower titer of serum neutralizing antibody.[621,688] Thus, p27 of BRSV has the potential to augment viral disease by effects on smooth muscle contraction and pulmonary inflammation and might also stimulate the host immune response. In contrast, the sequence of p27 of HRSV does not resemble a tachykinin, and HRSV p27 does not have tachykinin-like properties *in vitro*.[689]

The HMPV F protein shares a moderate level of amino acid sequence identity with HRSV F (33%, Table 10.1)[49,624] and is similar in general organization and structure, except that it contains only a single cleavage activation site[30,412] (Fig. 10.4A). As with HRSV, HMPV F directs fusion involved in penetration and syncytium formation and does so efficiently without the need of the G and SH proteins.[47,51] HMPV F interacts with specific cellular integrins via an integrin-recognition motif 329-RGD-331, which is necessary for infection and might be involved in fusion activation[124] (see "Replicative Cycle").

The most common sequence at the HMPV cleavage site, Arg-Gln-Ser-Arg↓, does not conform to the consensus furin motif and, consistent with this, clinical isolates and most laboratory strains typically require exogenous trypsin for growth *in vitro*. *In vivo*, this cleavage depends on secreted protease present in the lumen of the respiratory tract. Several observations indicate that this is not a limiting factor in pathogenesis. For example, in some cases, serial passage of HMPV clinical isolates in cell culture resulted in the emergence of mutants that no longer required added trypsin, but these did not exhibit increased replication in hamsters.[540] Similarly, when the F cleavage site of recombinant HMPV was engineered so that it contained the furin motif and was cleaved intracellularly, this did not increase its replication or virulence in African green monkeys (AGMs).[48]

Glycoprotein G

The HRSV G protein is a type II membrane protein, with cytoplasmic (amino acids 1 to 37 in strain A2) and signal/transmembrane-anchor (amino acids 38 to 63) domains at the N-terminal end and the C-terminal two-thirds of the molecular oriented extracellularly (Fig. 10.4A). The extracellular domain consists mainly of two hypervariable domains that resemble mucin in having a high content of proline, serine, threonine, and alanine residues and O-linked sugars. These hypervariable mucin-like domains flank a central conserved domain (Fig. 10.4C).

The G protein was originally thought to be the sole viral attachment protein,[366] but recent evidence suggests that the F protein may also play a role, as noted above (see "Fusion F glycoprotein", also see "Replicative Cycle"). The HRSV G protein has no apparent relatedness by sequence or structure to the attachment HN, H, and G proteins of *Paramyxoviridae* and has only half the amino acid length.[297,652] A secreted version of G is produced by translational initiation at the second ATG in the ORF (codon 48), which lies within the signal/anchor sequence.[275,511] This truncated form is then trimmed by proteolysis, removing the remainder of the signal/anchor and creating a new N-terminus at Asn-66 for the final secreted form. The secreted form constituted approximately 20% of the total G protein expressed in HRSV-infected cells *in vitro*, but because of its rapid secretion, it accounted for 80% of the G protein released in cell culture by 24 hours postinfection, the remainder being virion associated.[275] The secreted form of G appears to be processed in a similar fashion to the membrane-anchored form, and no antigenic differences were detected when the secreted and membrane-bound forms were analyzed with an extensive panel of monoclonal antibodies (MAbs).[168]

The polypeptide backbone of full-length HRSV G has an Mr of approximately 32,000. In the case of strain A2, an estimated four N-linked sugar side chains (for strain A2) are added cotranslationally, increasing the Mr to 45,000.[653] The number of potential acceptor sites can vary considerably among strains. G assembles in the endoplasmic reticulum into oligomers that probably are trimers or tetramers, except that the secreted form of G remains a monomer. O-linked sugars are added subsequently in the trans-Golgi compartment or network.[653] Analysis of a chimeric F/G protein (created as a potential vaccine, see "Prevention") expressed in insect cells by a recombinant baculovirus indicated that G contains approximately 24 to 25 O-linked side chains.[646] Mature HRSV G grown in most immortalized cell lines such as HEp-2 migrates in gel electrophoresis as a broad, seemingly heterogeneous band of Mr up to about 95,000. In Vero cells, the G protein is cleaved by cathepsin L, resulting in an Mr of about 55,000.[121] This cleavage appears to be specific to Vero cells; it is not thought to occur *in vivo*, but it does reduce the infectivity of HRSV produced in Vero cells.

In vitro infection with HRSV also can be performed in differentiated polarized primary human airway epithelial (HAE) or human bronchial epithelial (HBE) cultures, which closely resemble authentic *in vivo* mucociliary pseudostratified airway epithelium (see "Propagation *In Vitro*" and Fig. 10.5).[330,682] When HRSV was grown in HBE, the Mr observed for the G protein was 170,000.[330] Since these cells are a more-authentic substrate than monolayer cultures of immortalized cell lines, this suggests that authentic G is either a covalently linked dimer or contains much more carbohydrate than previously thought.

Like mucins, the two hypervariable domains are thought to have an extended, nonglobular secondary structure. The significance of this mucin-like character remains unknown. One possibility is that it somehow helps the virus penetrate the protective mucus layer overlying the respiratory epithelium. The presence of a sheath of host-specified sugars might also shield the G protein from immune recognition and might interfere with antigen processing and presentation.

The central conserved domain of the G protein includes a 13-residue segment (positions 164 to 176 in strain A2) that is completely conserved among HRSV strains of subgroups A and B (Fig. 10.4A). This sequence partially overlaps a short downstream segment containing four closely spaced invariant cysteine residues (positions 173, 176, 182, and 186).[297] Disulfide linkages occur between Cys-173 and Cys-186, and between Cys-176 and Cys-182, to create a cystine noose.[218] The cysteine-rich segment contains a Cys-X$_3$-Cys (CX3C) motif involving the 3rd and 4th cysteine residues (Cys-182 and Cys-186) embedded in a region of limited sequence relatedness with the CX3C chemokine fractalkine.[618] Crystal structures of the central conserved domain bound to broadly neutralizing antibodies revealed the critical role of these disulfide linkages in

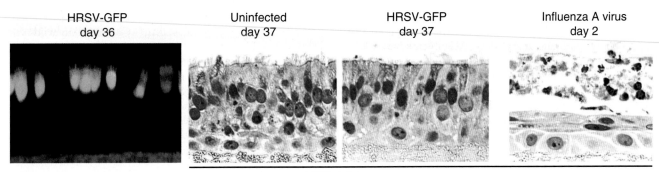

| HRSV-GFP day 36 | Uninfected day 37 | HRSV-GFP day 37 | Influenza A virus day 2 |

Fluorescence microscopy
Red: cilia marker

H&E staining

FIGURE 10.5 Infection of an *in vitro* model of human airway epithelium (HAE) with HRSV and influenza A virus, shown in cross-section. The cultures are primary HAE cells that have been seeded on filter supports and allowed to differentiate at an air–liquid interface into polarized pseudostratified mucociliary tissue that closely resembles authentic human airway epithelium. The *left-hand panel* is a fluorescence photomicrograph of cells 36 days following infection with HRSV expressing green fluorescent protein (GFP) and also stained with antibody specific to cilia (*red*; note that this antibody also nonspecifically stained the filter support underlying the cells). The *three panels to the right* show (from left to right) mock-infected, HRSV-GFP–infected, and influenza A virus–infected cultures visualized 37 (mock and HRSV-GFP) or 2 (influenza) days postinoculation. (Reprinted from Zhang L, Peeples ME, Boucher RC, et al. Respiratory syncytial virus infection of human airway epithelial cells is polarized, specific to ciliated cells, and without obvious cytopathology. *J Virol* 2002;76(11):5654–5666. Copyright © 2002 American Society for Microbiology.) In the *three right-hand panels*, the cells were stained with hematoxylin and eosin.

stabilizing the cystine noose and the conformational epitopes of the CX3C motif (Fig. 10.4C),[31,187,300] while the N-terminal flanking region seemed flexible and generally unstructured. A peptide containing the CX3C sequence mimicked the leukocyte chemoattractant activity of fractalkine in an *in vitro* assay. The G protein was shown to bind to the fractalkine receptor CX3CR1 by this CX3C motif, and antibodies specific to this region blocked interaction of the G protein with CX3CR1 and neutralized HRSV of both subgroups.[100] These findings strongly support a role for the central conserved domain of the G protein in mediating HRSV attachment to airway epithelial cells via the CX3CR1 receptor (see "Replicative Cycle").

Immortalized cell lines like HEp-2 and Vero cells are deficient in CX3CR1: in these cells, the G protein (and, to a lesser extent, F protein) participates in viral attachment by binding to specific GAGs on the cell surface. GAGs are important for infection in cell lines but not in human airway epithelium (see "Replicative Cycle"). The conserved central domain of G is not needed for infection of cell lines, since it can be deleted from recombinant HRSV with little effect on virus replication in HEp-2 cells (or in mice).[600] The exact region of G that is involved in binding to GAGs is not clear: one study implicated a region of positively charged amino acids located downstream from the central conserved domain,[189] but this region also could be deleted with little effect on HRSV infection and replication *in vitro* or in mice.[600]

Extensive passage of a subgroup B strain of HRSV in AGM Vero cells—in an attempt to attenuate the virus—resulted in mutants with various spontaneous deletions involving most of the G and SH genes.[310] This was the first evidence that, surprisingly, G is dispensable for replication in certain situations. One of these mutants was evaluated in humans as a potential live-attenuated intranasal vaccine and was highly attenuated, although it did appear to replicate at low levels.[310] Subsequently, HRSV strains that were isolated from immunocompromised children with LRI were found to have deletions of nearly the complete G ectodomain.[630] Recombinant HRSV strain A2 from which

the G gene was deleted by reverse genetics (ΔG) also replicated efficiently in Vero cells. However, the ΔG virus was restricted in HEp-2 cells, with defects at the levels of virus binding, fusion, and assembly and also was highly restricted in mice.[599,603] Thus, HRSV lacking all or most of the G protein can replicate efficiently in Vero cells and at low levels in the human host, suggestive of alternative attachment pathways, but G is needed for efficient replication in HEp-2 cells, mice, and humans.

In recent isolates, the C-terminal hypervariable domain of HRSV G contains a partial duplication (due to in-frame 60- and 72-nucleotide duplications, as noted above[169,616]). Other strains have a deletion of amino acids in this region, or an extension or shortening of the C-terminal end, which further illustrates the relative tolerance to change.[52] Some of these mutations appeared in recent years, which has allowed "real-time" monitoring of their subsequent worldwide spread.

The HMPV G protein (Fig. 10.4A) has a number of similarities with HRSV G, although it lacks significant sequence identity[49,624] (Table 10.1). HMPV G has a comparable N-terminal-proximal signal/anchor domain and a high content of serine/threonine/proline residues concentrated in the ectodomain.[49,624] It also is modified by the addition of N-linked and O-linked sugars to yield a mature form that migrates in gel electrophoresis as a diffuse band of Mr up to 97,000.[381] Its amino acid sequence also is highly divergent between the HMPV subgroups. As with HRSV G, HMPV strains containing partial internal duplications of G were recently found.[454] However, HMPV G differs from HRSV G in lacking the conserved central domain, cystine noose, and CX3C motif mentioned above and is correspondingly shorter in length. A secreted form of HMPV G has not been described, and the amino acid sequence gives no suggestion that such a species exists. As with HRSV, the HMPV G protein binds to cell surface GAGs, which likely reflects its role in attachment in cell lines.[604] Peptide binding studies suggested that two closely spaced clusters of basic amino acids at positions 149 to 155 and 159 to 166 may mediate binding to GAGs.[604]

Deletion of G from recombinant HMPV was less attenuating than for HRSV. Deletion of G had little effect on HMPV replication *in vitro*, and the HMPV ΔG mutant had a low-to-moderate level of replication in hamsters and AGMs.[47,51] Interestingly, infection of epithelial cells *in vitro* with the ΔG mutant resulted in increased activation of the transcription factors IFN regulatory factor 3 (IRF3) and nuclear factor kappa B (NF-κB) and increased expression of type I IFN and proinflammatory cytokines.[26] In explanation of this effect, the HMPV G protein was found to bind to RIG-I, and its deletion restored signaling from RIG-I.[25]

Small Hydrophobic SH Protein

The HRSV SH protein (Fig. 10.4A) is a short (64 amino acids for strain A2) transmembrane protein that is anchored by a hydrophobic signal–anchor sequence near the N-terminus, with the C-terminus oriented extracellularly.[114,200] Most of the SH protein remains nonglycosylated (Mr ~7,500), but there is a subpopulation containing a single N-linked side chain (resulting in Mr ~13,000 to 15,000), plus a subpopulation containing the further addition to the side chain of polylactosaminoglycan (resulting in Mr ~21,000 to 60,000 or more), as well as an N-terminally truncated subpopulation that arises from translational initiation at the second methionine codon in the ORF and has a pattern of glycosylation similar to that the full-length version.[11] However, the significance of these multiple forms is not known.

Chemical cross-linking and NMR-based modeling indicated that the HRSV SH protein associates into homopentamers[114,200] (e-Fig. 10.5A and B). Incorporation of SH into artificial membranes *in vitro* resulted in the formation of pore-like structures and the acquisition of cation-selective channel-like activity, activated at low pH.[200,372] Thus, the SH protein appears to be a viroporin, which typically are small proteins that modify membrane permeability and can have roles in budding and apoptosis. Interestingly, by increasing membrane permeability, the viroporin activity of HRSV SH also contributes to the activation of the Nod-like receptor (NLR) family pyrin domain–containing 3 (NLRP3) inflammasome.[617]

Recombinant HRSV from which SH was deleted replicates with wild-type efficiency *in vitro* and appears to be fully fusogenic.[76,598] The SH protein was reported to reduce apoptosis, but the effect was small.[198] SH also appeared to inhibit signaling from tumor necrosis factor (TNF)-α.[198] The ΔSH virus was slightly attenuated in mice and chimpanzees,[76,657] but deletion of the SH gene in an experimental live vaccine strain did not increase its level of attenuation in seronegative children.[315] Thus, the function(s) and impact of the HRSV SH protein seem unclear.

The SH protein of HMPV is nearly three times longer (177 to 183 amino acids) than its HRSV counterpart[49,624] (Fig. 10.4A). It has the same membrane orientation and a similar array of nonglycosylated and glycosylated forms. Passage of HMPV *in vitro* results in frequent mutations that ablate SH expression,[46] suggesting that there is a slight selective pressure against SH in cell culture. Infection of epithelial cells and mice with the ΔSH virus resulted in a modest increase in NF-κB activation and expression of proinflammatory proteins compared to wild-type virus, suggesting that the SH protein downregulates the innate response, but the effect may be small.[24]

In vivo, deletion of SH had little or no effect on HMPV replication in hamsters or in AGMs.[47] Compared to wild-type HMPV, HMPV with deletion of SH and G was internalized more efficiently by monocyte-derived dendritic cells (DCs) via macropinocytosis, indicating that SH and G may inhibit macropinocytosis. The presence of SH and G facilitated HMPV uptake by DCs via an alternative route, mediated by DC-SIGN. In addition, the presence of SH and G reduced T-cell activation by HMPV by reducing the number of immunological synapses between T cells and DCs.[355]

Matrix M Protein

The HRSV M protein is a nonglycosylated internal virion component that is smaller than its *Paramyxoviridae* counterparts (256 amino acids vs. 335 to 375 amino acids), with little apparent amino acid sequence relatedness. HRSV M appears to play two roles typical for *Mononegavirales*: it helps organize virion components at the plasma membrane for budding,[274] and it may silence viral RNA synthesis by nucleocapsids in preparation for packaging into the virus particle.[208] A crystal structure determined for the HRSV M protein revealed a monomer that is organized into compact N-terminal (residues 1 to 126) and C-terminal (residues 140 to 255) domains joined by a 13-residue linker.[438] The surface of M was found to contain a large positively charged area that extends across the two domains and the linker and may mediate association with the negatively charged membrane as well as with nucleocapsids[438]; this large positively charged domain also was a feature of a crystal structure of the HMPV M protein.[369]

Nucleocapsid/Polymerase Proteins N, P, L, and M2-1

The N, P, and L proteins of HRSV appear to be close functional analogs of their counterparts in members of the *Paramyxoviridae* family. The N protein binds tightly along the entire length of genomic and antigenomic RNA to form separate RNAse-resistant nucleocapsids that are templates for RNA synthesis. The P protein is a multifunctional adapter that helps mediate interactions between components of the nucleocapsid/polymerase complex. The L protein contains the polymerase catalytic domains. Studies with HRSV mini-replicons showed that N, P, and L are necessary and sufficient to direct RNA replication.[110] N, P, and L alone also have transcriptase activity, but fully processive transcription requires in addition the M2-1 protein.[110,184]

The 391-amino acid HRSV N protein is shorter than its counterparts in *Paramyxoviridae* (~490 to 555 amino acids), and sequence relatedness is limited to several conserved segments located toward the C-terminus.[595] HRSV N protein produced in bacteria was found to bind to bacterial RNA to form decamer rings, which are thought to mimic individual turns of the helical nucleocapsid, and a crystal structure was obtained[595] that is described in e-Figure 10.6A and B. The interaction of the N protein with viral RNA is shown in e-Figure 10.6C.

The HRSV P protein (241 amino acids) is shorter than its *Paramyxoviridae* counterparts (~390 to 605 amino acids) and lacks evident sequence relatedness. However, it is thought to have the same general array of functions. Like its counterparts in *Paramyxoviridae*, HRSV P forms a stable homotetramer through a multimerization domain in the middle of the molecule.[88,383] The C-terminal region of the P tetramer interacts with N protein in the nucleocapsid by binding to the C-terminal end of N that protrudes from the decamer ring[595] (e-Fig. 10.6B). In addition, low-resolution structural modeling indicated that the N-terminal domains of the P tetramer bind to the C-terminal domain of free monomeric N protein (called N_0).[170] In this way, P acts as a chaperone that prevents N_0 from self-aggregating or binding to nonviral RNA and delivers N_0 to nascent genomes/antigenomes during RNA replication.[88] P also binds to the L[212] (e-Fig. 10.7) and M2-1[16,613] proteins and helps mediate their interactions with the nucleocapsid. P may contribute to conformational changes that help the polymerase access the RNA template[88] and appears to be necessary for promoter clearance and chain elongation by the viral polymerase.[159] It also appears to have a role in dissociating the M protein from the nucleocapsid during uncoating to initiate infection.

P is the major phosphorylated HRSV protein and contains phosphate at more than 10 to 12 sites, with different sites exhibiting different rates of turnover: the C-terminal domain contains low-turnover phosphates and accounts for most of the total phosphate, the middle domain contains intermediate-turnover phosphates, and the N-terminal domain contains high-turnover phosphates.[17] Many of the activities of P described above appear to be affected by dynamic phosphorylation and dephosphorylation of P at a subset of these sites, usually involving a small percentage of the total phosphate content.[16,17] Most of the constitutive phosphorylation could be ablated in recombinant HRSV with only modest effects on virus growth.[387]

The 194-amino acid HRSV M2-1 protein is an essential transcription processivity factor; in its absence, the viral polymerase terminates prematurely and nonspecifically within several hundred nucleotides of the 3′ end of the genome, and downstream genes are not detectably transcribed.[109,110,184] M2-1 also decreases the efficiency of termination at the GE transcription signals—possibly a reflection of the same processivity activity—resulting in increased production of readthrough mRNAs.[267] HRSV M2-1 accumulates in phosphorylated and nonphosphorylated forms[266] and forms a homotetramer via an oligomerization domain at residues 32 to 63.[613] M2-1 contains a cysteine–histidine zinc finger motif ($C-X_7-C-X_5-C-X_3-H$) near its N-terminus (residues 7 to 25) that is essential for its activity[266]; this motif is conserved in *Pneumoviridae*.[624] The HRSV M2-1 protein binds positive-sense HRSV RNA, but not negative-sense RNA: M2-1 appears to transiently associate with nascent mRNA and is thought to help it extrude from the polymerase complex, likely indicating its role in transcription processivity.[64,202,613] M2-1 also binds discrete sites within specific cellular mRNAs, with a preference for A/U rich sequences.[64] Binding to specific cellular mRNAs may indicate a role for M2-1 in viral–host interactions. In the HRSV virion, M2-1 forms an additional protein layer between the M layer and the RNP, as already noted (Fig. 10.1). M2-1 is unique to *Pneumoviridae*, although VP30 of the family *Filoviridae* has some similarities, such as the presence of a conserved CCCH zinc finger motif.[266]

The 2,165-amino acid HRSV L protein is very similar in length to its *Paramyxoviridae* counterparts and has low but unambiguous sequence relatedness along nearly its entire length.[576] Specific segments of L are conserved within and beyond *Mononegavirales*.[576] The L protein contains an RNA-dependent RNA polymerase (RdRp) domain (amino acid residues 1 to 968), followed by a polyribonucleotidyl transferase (PRNTase) domain with mRNA capping function (residues 967 to 1,460), followed by a connector domain (residues 1,461 to 1,815), methyltransferase (MTase) domain (predicted: residues 1,816 to 1,890), and a C-terminal region enriched in basic amino acids (residues 1,891 to 2,165) (e-Fig. 10.7). A cryoelectron microscopy reconstruction of the N-terminal part of the L protein (residues 11 to 1,460; for details, see e-Fig. 10.7) in complex with the P protein at a resolution of 3.2 Å revealed the structure of the RdRp and capping domains[84,212] (e-Fig. 10.7). A nucleotide-binding domain involved in capping mRNA had previously been identified in the central region of the L protein based on sequence analysis of HRSV mutants selected for resistance to novel capping inhibitors, in which resistance was associated with an amino acid substitution at position 1381, 1269, or 1421.[382] The cap-dependent MTase activity of a fragment of the L protein spanning residues 1,755 to 2,165 has been confirmed experimentally.[590] In separate work, an amino acid substitution at position 1049 or 1169 in the L protein was associated with reduced efficiency of termination at the GE signals, resulting in increased synthesis of polycistronic mRNAs and reduced growth efficiency.[87,303]

The HMPV N, P, L, and M2-1 proteins are similar in size to their HRSV counterparts and share significant amino acid sequence identity[49,624] (Table 10.1). Crystal structures were determined for the HMPV N_0 protein bound to an N-terminal peptide of P, and for N protein complexed with RNA in nucleocapsid rings: these provided visualization of the role of the HMPV P protein in controlling nucleocapsid assembly and interaction with RNA, as noted above for HRSV.[504] A cryoelectron microscopy structure of the polymerase and capping domains of HMPV L bound to a tetramer of P revealed similarity to the structure described for HRSV.[470] One notable difference between HRSV and HMPV is that, whereas M2-1 appears to be essential for HRSV, recombinant HMPV in which the M2-1 ORF has been silenced was viable and replicated *in vitro* with an efficiency that was only marginally reduced.[70] However, in the hamster model, replication of HMPV lacking M2-1 could not be detected, indicating that M2-1 is important for replication *in vivo*. HMPV lacking M2-1 appeared to execute processive transcription efficiently, although the level of RNA accumulation was somewhat reduced. Thus, in contrast to HRSV, HMPV M2-1 is not completely essential, and its functions are less well understood.[70]

M2-2 Protein

HRSV M2-2 is a small (83-90 amino acids for strain A2, depending on the translational initiation site) protein that is expressed at a low level that may reflect inefficiency of the stop–restart mechanism of translation noted previously.[5] It is not known whether M2-2 is packaged in the virion. Recombinant HRSV in which the M2-2 ORF has been silenced grows more slowly *in vitro* than wild-type HRSV, although it eventually achieves a similar titer.[44,291] In ΔM2-2 virus-infected cells, there was a global increase in the accumulation of viral mRNAs (and viral proteins) and a decrease in the accumulation of genome and antigenome compared to wild-type virus. This implies that M2-2 plays a role in shifting RNA synthesis from transcription to RNA replication during the course of infection. When M2-2 was artificially overexpressed during HRSV infection—using a cotransfected plasmid or a recombinant HRSV in which expression of M2-2 was up-regulated by engineering it to be a separate gene—HRSV replication was inhibited, which is consistent with a regulatory role.[55,98] The ΔM2-2 virus retained the ability to replicate in mice and chimpanzees, but it was restricted approximately 500- to 1,000-fold compared to wild-type HRSV.[44,291,602] The features of up-regulation of antigen synthesis combined with attenuation make the ΔM2-2 deletion of interest for developing live-attenuated HRSV vaccines (see "Prevention").

HMPV encodes a 67-71-amino acid M2-2 protein from a comparable overlapping internal ORF in its M2 mRNA[49,624] (Fig. 10.3C). The HMPV M2-2 protein coimmunoprecipitated with the L protein and inhibited RNA synthesis by a mini-replicon, an activity that was lost by short deletions at the N- or C-terminus of M2-2.[334] As with HRSV, deletion of HMPV M2-2 from recombinant virus resulted in an attenuated virus in which transcription is increased and RNA replication decreased.[70] The HMPV M2-2 protein also has roles in interdicting host innate responses: it has been reported to inhibit mitochondrial antiviral–signaling protein (MAVS) activity and phosphorylation of IRF7 (e-Fig. 10.8).[569]

Nonstructural Proteins NS1 and NS2

The NS1 and NS2 proteins (139 and 124 amino acids, respectively) are unique to the genus *Orthopneumovirus*. Monomeric NS2 was unstable with a half-life of 30 minutes.[171] NS1 and NS2 can be coimmunoprecipitated[592] and may occur in mixed complexes of various stoichiometries.[171] The majority of NS1 and NS2 was found in a heterogeneous complex—called an "NS degradasome"—that had an apparent size of 300 to 750 kDa and was associated with mitochondria and stabilized in the presence of MAVS.[219] The NS degradasome has been speculated to function like a proteasome that degrades host cell proteins that perhaps have been marked by ubiquitination.[548] Crystal structures of NS1 and NS2 have been resolved separately.[95,476] Among other findings, the NS1 structure revealed similarities to the N-terminal region of the HRSV M protein that raised the possibility that NS1 arose from duplication of part of M followed by divergent evolution. The NS2 structure revealed details about the binding between its N-terminus and RIG-I to block IFN induction.

NS1 and NS2 strongly interfere with the induction and signaling of type I and type III IFN in human epithelial cells, macrophages, and DCs. This suppresses major components of host innate defense.[354] NS1 generally has a greater inhibitory effect than NS2. NS1 reduces levels of IRF3 and IRF7 and interferes with their nuclear translocation. The steps at which NS1 and NS2 subvert IFN induction and signaling are summarized in e-Figure 10.8 and have been described in detail elsewhere.[548]

Deletion of NS2 from recombinant HRSV decreased its ability to induce activation of NF-κB,[573] and siRNA-mediated knockdown of the expression of either NS1 or NS2 in HRSV-infected cells reduced activation of NF-κB and serine–threonine protein kinase (AKT) signaling.[54] This resulted in more rapid induction of apoptosis compared to wild-type HRSV-infected cells.[54] Thus, the two NS proteins appear to activate prosurvival pathways, thereby prolonging the life of the cell and increasing the viral yield.[54]

In addition, in HAE cultures and hamsters, NS2 promoted shedding of airway epithelial cells. This may contribute to obstruction of the distal airways leading to HRSV bronchiolitis.[375]

In a mini-replicon system, coexpression of NS1—and, to a lesser extent, NS2—inhibited transcription and RNA replication, affecting both the genomic and antigenomic promoters.[18] These effects remain unexplained but might resemble activities of the V and C accessory proteins of some members of *Paramyxoviridae*, which down-regulate viral RNA synthesis to prevent excessive RNA accumulation that otherwise activates the RIG-I/MDA5/PKR pattern recognition molecules.

As might be expected from the results described above, HRSV lacking NS1 and/or NS2 replicates to reduced titer in cultured cells competent for type I IFN, as well as in experimental animals, with the level of attenuation increasing in the order ΔNS2<ΔNS1≤ΔNS1+NS2.[292,572,602,657] These deletions are of interest for developing live-attenuated vaccines (see "Prevention").

Replicative Cycle

Efficient infection of immortalized monolayer cell lines *in vitro* by HRSV involves binding to cellular GAGs, especially heparan sulfate and chondroitin sulfate B.[259] The G and F proteins are each able to bind to GAGs, although binding by G appears to be more important.[188,189,599] However, the use of GAGs in attachment appears to be specific to cell lines and probably is not relevant to replication in the human respiratory tract. Heparan sulfate was not detected on surface epithelium cells of HAE and HBE cultures nor on the surface of human airway epithelium.[680] The ability of HRSV to utilize GAGs may be an adaptation to growth in cell lines, since HRSV that was grown in HBE cultures exhibited greatly reduced ability to bind GAGs and infect cell lines.[330]

Other potential receptor molecules for HRSV have been suggested, including intracellular adhesion molecule (ICAM)-1,[34] RhoA,[473] and annexin II.[399] The significance of these remains unclear. In primary differentiated HAE and HBE cultures, which closely resemble authentic human airway epithelium[330,682] (see "Propagation *In Vitro*" and Fig. 10.5), the CX3CR1 fractalkine receptor is now recognized as a major HRSV receptor and is bound by the G protein.[233,290,298] Thus, CX3CR1 plays the major role in viral attachment in HAE and HBE cultures and, by extrapolation, in the human airway, whereas GAGs play the major role in cultured cell lines. Interestingly, a hamster cell line that was engineered to stably express CX3CR1 remained unable to support CX3XR1-mediated HRSV infection, implying the involvement of additional factors in HAE cells.[332]

HRSV infection in several cell lines, in HAE cultures, and in mice also has been shown to involve the cellular protein nucleolin, which is bound by the F protein[597]; nucleolin also appears to play a role in attachment and entry by a variety of other viruses.[414] Interaction of HRSV F with nucleolin seems to be preceded by binding of pre-F to the insulin-like growth factor-1 receptor (IGF1R) on the surface of target cells, which triggers activation of protein kinase C zeta (PKCζ). This cellular signaling cascade then recruits nucleolin from the nuclei of cells to the plasma membrane, where it also binds to HRSV F on virions.[235] It may be that, at least in cell culture, efficient attachment and entry by HRSV depends on different binding events mediated by G and F.

HRSV entry occurs by fusion of the viral envelope with the cell plasma membrane or by macropinocytosis[343] or clathrin-mediated endocytosis[337] followed by fusion with internal endosomal membranes. When infection was monitored by video microscopy, the initiation of surface fusion by attached virions appeared to be a slow step, but once started the process was rapid.[21] HRSV entry does not require endosomal acidification, suggesting that there is no mechanistic difference between entry at the plasma membrane versus the endosomal membrane.[337] As already noted (see *Fusion F protein*) one report found that the F protein present in HRSV virions had mostly been cleaved only upstream of the two cleavage sites and thus presumably was not activated, and that endocytic uptake was required for the second cleavage—which was acid independent—downstream of the two sites, which was necessary for activation.[343]

Genome transcription and replication occur in the cytoplasm and the virus can grow in enucleated cells and in the presence of actinomycin D, indicating a lack of essential nuclear involvement. In cell lines such as HEp-2 cells, HRSV mRNAs and proteins can be detected intracellularly at 4 to 6 hours postinfection and reach a peak accumulation by 15 to 20 hours. The release of progeny virus in HEp-2 cells begins by 10 to 12 hours postinfection, reaches a peak after 24 hours, and continues until the cells deteriorate by 30 to 48 hours. The low-abundance M2-2 protein accumulates during infection and shifts the balance of RNA synthesis from transcription to RNA replication.[44] In mini-replicon experiments, increasing the level of accumulation of the N and P proteins did not shift the balance between RNA replication and transcription, indicating that the availability of protein to encapsidate replicative RNA does not affect this balance.[185] Analyses of the spatiotemporal relationships between the polymerase and other RNP components showed that the HRSV RNPs undergo a structural reorganization at 6 to 8 hours postinfection, concomitant with the onset of genome replication and secondary transcription (i.e., transcription from new genomes made by RNA replication). This RNP reorganization could be elicited by expression of the M2-2 protein.[55]

By 12 hours postinfection, the HRSV L, N, P, and M2-1 proteins are localized within dense cytoplasmic structures called inclusion bodies (e-Fig. 10.9). Inclusion bodies appear to be free of any enclosing membrane. During the course of infection, they increase in size and typically consolidate into a single large body. Inclusion bodies are the sites of viral transcription, RNA replication, and nucleocapsid assembly and thus might be regarded as viral factories. Nucleocapsids are then exported into the cytoplasm and transported to the plasma membrane for incorporation into virions. Inclusion bodies also sequester a number of cellular proteins including ones involved in host responses to infection and thereby reduce those responses.[55,194,199,293,376,508]

Several factors influence the relative levels of expression of the various HRSV genes. Like other *Mononegavirales*, sequential transcription has a polar gradient due to polymerase fall-off, and thus promoter-proximal genes are expressed more efficiently. The gradient of expression is not very steep for HRSV, with the exception of the low-abundance L mRNA.[117,338] However, the low abundance of the L mRNA compared to the other mRNAs appears to be due to a posttranscriptional effect rather than polymerase fall-off, with one possibility being mRNA stability.[350] Differences in the termination efficiency of the various HRSV GE signals also affect the relative levels of gene expression, whereas the intergenic regions generally do not have a major effect, although certain intergenic sequence assignments close to the GE signals may affect their efficiency.[265,442] When a GE signal is inefficient, a subpopulation of polymerases fail to terminate and instead continue transcription across the intergenic region and into the next downstream gene to produce a readthrough transcript, rather than re-initiating at the downstream gene to produce a separate transcript of that downstream gene. Because ORFs in internal positions in eukaryotic mRNAs generally are not efficiently translated, the downstream ORF(s) in a readthrough transcript would be poorly translated, effectively down-regulating protein expression from that gene. HMPV in particular has considerable variation in the efficiency of its GE signals, and readthrough transcription appears to sharply down-regulate the production of monocistronic SH mRNA. In particular, this appears to be responsible for the observed low level of expression of SH protein. For HRSV and HMPV, the relative abundance of the various mRNAs does not appear to change during infection.

HRSV assembly and budding occur at the plasma membrane. In polarized cells, this occurs at the apical surface.[510,682] Video microscopy showed that budding occurs within circumscribed regions on the cell surface.[21] These regions contain localized virus-modified lipid rafts involving all three viral surface proteins and the M protein.[274,673] The minimum viral protein requirements for the formation of virus-like particles capable of delivering the viral genome to target cells are the F, M, N, and P proteins,[601] and expression of F, M, and P is sufficient to induce formation of filaments.[430]

As has been observed for members of *Paramyxoviridae*, HRSV utilizes the host cytoskeleton in its replicative cycle. Viral substructures are associated with polymerized actin throughout the infectious cycle.[288] Both HRSV and HMPV induce actin rearrangement and stimulate the formation of extracellular extensions or filopodia in infected cells. HRSV-induced filopodia formation was dependent on the cellular actin nucleation factor actin-related protein 2 (ARP2). High-resolution microscopy revealed that newly formed HRSV and HMPV virions associate with filopodia. Filopodia seem to shuttle virions to neighboring cells: this may facilitate virus spread in the mucosal environment and also may shield cell-to-cell virus spread from virus-neutralizing antibodies.[165,328,424]

Efficient infection by HMPV *in vitro* in immortalized cell lines depends on binding to cell surface GAGs and specific cellular integrins.[124] DC-SIGN also has been identified as having a role in HMPV infection.[90,210] HMPV is thought to enter by fusion at the plasma membrane and also has been shown to internalize via clathrin-mediated endocytosis followed by fusion, which in that study did not require activation by low pH.[125] Activation of F appeared to depend on interaction with cellular integrins.[124] However, the F proteins of a small proportion (6%) of HMPV strains do depend on acidification for activation, indicating a dependence on endosomal uptake rather than fusion at the plasma membrane: this requirement mapped to the presence of glycine at position 294.[279,545] Another difference between HRSV and HMPV is that the kinetics of infection of the latter in cell culture are slower, with the peak of intracellular protein expression occurring at 48 to 72 hours postinfection.

Propagation *In Vitro*

In vitro replication by HRSV occurs most efficiently in immortalized cell lines derived from human epithelial cells, but HRSV can infect and replicate to a significant extent in a wide variety of cell lines representing various tissues from various hosts, including humans, monkeys, bovines, hamsters, and mice. The most commonly used cell line is human HEp-2, now thought to have been contaminated historically with, and outgrown by, the HeLa cell line.[413] Vero cells, an AGM kidney cell line, also are frequently used, and qualified Vero cells are used to produce HRSV for human administration.

HRSV is usually quantified by plaque titration or limiting dilution assay; immunostaining is often used to enhance visualization of plaques or infected wells. Fresh clinical isolates of HRSV may undergo adaptation for growth in cell lines[405]; this is poorly understood but might include adaptation to the use of GAGs for infection (see "Replicative Cycle"). However, passaged laboratory strains retain their virulence for chimpanzees and humans.[316,660]

As noted, cultures of primary differentiated HAE and HBE also are used and are recognized as a more authentic *in vitro* substrate than immortalized cell lines[330,682] (Fig. 10.5). HAE and HBE cultures are primary polarized pseudostratified mucociliary tissue that are grown on filter supports at an air–liquid interface and require weeks of differentiation following seeding. They closely resemble authentic human airway epithelium. HAE and HBE cultures are not to be confused with cultures such as A549 and BEAS-2B: although these latter two cell types are epithelial-like cells of human origin, they are immortalized cell lines grown in monolayers.

As noted above, most of the progeny HRSV virions remain cell associated, and virions can be visualized attached to the cell plasma membrane in a manner suggestive of incomplete budding. To make virus stocks, cell-associated virus is dislodged by freeze–thawing, sonication, or vortexing. The yield is low, typically 10 plaque-forming units (PFU) per cell. Virion preparations have substantial contamination by cellular debris. Particles are heterogeneous in shape and size. A large fraction of released virions appeared to be empty and presumably noninfectious.[22] Less than 5% of the infectivity of a preparation of HRSV could be passed through a 0.45-μm filter, while more than 85% passed through a 3-μm filter, consistent with the infectious particles being large filaments[510]; similar findings had been reported for BRSV.[468]

HMPV is more restricted in its *in vitro* host range than HRSV but is readily propagated in rhesus LLC-MK2 or Vero cell lines.[146,611] HMPV typically requires added trypsin to support cleavage of the F protein, although some strains mutated during passage to become trypsin independent, as noted above.[540] HMPV replicates more slowly than HRSV, its cytopathic effect is less prominent, and the yield of infectious virus is similarly low. Like HRSV, HMPV tends to remain cell associated but is more stable.

Genetics and Reverse Genetics

HRSV has a high mutation rate, as is typical for RNA viruses. The rate of nucleotide substitution in the G gene was estimated in natural isolates collected over 45 years to be $10^{-2.7}$ per position per year.[690] HRSV, like other *Mononegavirales*, also engages in nonhomologous recombination caused when the polymerase jumps from one template to another during RNA replication. This can create genomes that contain large deletions and, therefore, depend on complementation from standard virus for replication. These are called defective-interfering (DI) genomes or defective viral genomes (DVG).[190] Polymerase jumping also

can result in deletion of parts of genes[310] or sequence duplications.[615] Foreign sequence also can be acquired, as evidenced by a 1,015-nucleotide insert of unknown origin in the G gene of certain AMPV-C isolates.[42] Recombination between coinfecting viruses to create replication-competent mosaic genomes appears to be rare, although potential mosaic genomes are identified occasionally by sequence analysis.[683] One study designed to detect recombination between two coinfecting HRSV mutants in cell culture identified a single mosaic virus, which appeared to involve both homologous (i.e., guided by sequence relatedness) and nonhomologous recombination.[571] The difference in the order of the SH-G-F-M2 genes of HRSV versus HMPV, and the presence of NS1 and NS2 in HRSV but not HMPV, may be evidence of past recombination.

As with other *Mononegavirales*, HRSV and HMPV can be produced entirely from cloned cDNA by reverse genetics, involving cotransfection of plasmids encoding a copy of the genome or antigenome as well as the proteins of the nucleocapsid/polymerase complex. The viral protein requirements for recovering HRSV are N, P, L, and M2-1, whereas M2-1 is not required for HMPV.[50,70,109,277] A second type of reverse genetics system that has been used extensively for HRSV is based on cDNA-encoded mini-replicons in which the viral genes have been replaced by one or more foreign marker genes, with complementation by viral proteins supplied entirely from cotransfecting plasmids. Depending on the supplied proteins, this system can recreate genome encapsidation, transcription, RNA replication, and particle morphogenesis.[110,183,416,459,601] Because the complementing proteins are supplied from plasmids and do not depend on replication or transcription of the mini-replicon, this system allows analysis of mutations that might be lethal in complete virus.

Infection of Animals With HRSV and HMPV

A number of animal species can be infected in the respiratory tract by intranasal administration of HRSV, including cotton rats, mice, ferrets, guinea pigs, hamsters, marmosets, lambs, and various nonhuman primates.[38,79,230,492,570,660] Among experimental animals, only the chimpanzee approached the human in being highly susceptible to infection by contact, in supporting moderate to high levels of virus replication, and in exhibiting rhinorrhea and cough resembling that of humans. However, chimpanzees are no longer permitted to be used in HRSV studies. The most widely used experimental animals, cotton rats and mice, support a low to moderate level of virus replication that peaks on day 4 and is cleared quickly. *In situ* hybridization of lung tissue from cotton rats at the peak of virus replication showed that only scattered cells were infected.[451] Inbred strains of mice can vary 100-fold in permissiveness for replication.[492] The BALB/c mouse is one of the more permissive strains but is approximately 10-fold less permissive than cotton rats. Rodents do not exhibit overt HRSV respiratory tract disease, although pulmonary histopathologic changes are evident and illness can be monitored by weight loss and changes in pulmonary function. Newborn lambs have been used as models of neonatal HRSV disease.[570]

Intranasal administration of HMPV has been reported to infect guinea pigs, ferrets, mice, cotton rats, and hamsters, and several species of nonhuman primates.[6,261,391] BALB/c mice and hamsters may be more permissive for HMPV than for HRSV. Cynomolgus macaques and AGMs support moderate levels of HMPV replication.[344,565]

Unintentional transmission of HRSV and HMPV readily occurs to nonhuman primates in captivity and in the wild. The initial recovery of HRSV from captive chimpanzees presumably was preceded by a human-to-chimpanzee transmission.[441] Captive cynomolgus macaques, AGMs, chimpanzees, gorillas, and orangutans frequently have serum antibodies for HRSV and HMPV due to infection from their handlers and from other animals; in one report, seroprevalence for HRSV and HMPV was 79% and 47% in gorillas, 72% and 10% in orangutans, and 96% and 43% in chimpanzees, respectively.[75] Outbreaks of HMPV and human parainfluenza virus type 3 (HPIV3) were reported in wild chimpanzees, with HMPV causing 12% mortality and HPIV3 causing no direct mortality.[455]

Antigenic Subgroups and Genotypes

HRSV has a single serotype with two antigenic subgroups, A and B. These exhibited a three- to fourfold reciprocal difference in neutralization by polyclonal convalescent serum.[105] This was based on a neutralization assay performed in HEp-2 cells in the absence of complement, and since cell lines are deficient in the major HRSV receptor CX3CR1 (see "Replicative Cycle"), this analysis would not capture the contribution of those G-specific antibodies that neutralize by blocking binding to this receptor (see "Antigens"). The level of cross-neutralization by convalescent sera between the subgroups in HAE or HBE cells is unclear. Studies with MAbs demonstrated extensive antigenic differences in the G protein, with substantially fewer differences in the other viral proteins.[12,444] Analysis of glycoprotein-specific responses in cotton rats or human infants by enzyme-linked immunosorbent assay (ELISA) with purified F and G glycoproteins showed that F has 50% antigenic relatedness between subgroups compared to 1% to 7% relatedness for G.[276] Consistent with this, F protein expressed from a recombinant vaccinia virus was equally protective in cotton rats against infection with either subgroup, whereas the G protein was 13-fold less effective against the heterologous subgroup virus.[296] Thus, the F protein is responsible for most of the observed HRSV cross-subgroup protection. G has been reported to be less efficient than F in inducing cross-neutralizing antibodies, although this was based on neutralization assays in cell lines that, as noted above, typically do not capture the contribution of G-specific antibodies to the conserved CX3C domain.

The genomes of the two HRSV subgroups share 81% nucleotide identity. The various proteins vary considerably in their level of subgroup divergence, with M2-2, SH, and G being the most divergent (Table 10.1). The divergence is greatest for the ectodomains of SH and G, which exhibit only 50% and 44% sequence identity between subgroups, respectively.[115,297] The most recent common ancestor for the two HRSV subgroups was estimated to have occurred approximately 350 years ago.[690] There also is considerable variation within each subgroup: for example, the G glycoprotein can have 20% amino acid sequence difference between strains from the same subgroup.

The HRSV F protein is relatively stable antigenically, consistent with its high level of sequence conservation between the two HRSV subgroups. For example, analysis of 18 subgroup A strains and five subgroup B strains recovered from geographically diverse regions over 30 years using F-specific murine MAbs representing 16 separate neutralization epitopes in four antigenic sites showed that seven epitopes were conserved in all but one of the strains.[33] Similarly, a major epitope in the N

protein for CD8+ cytotoxic T lymphocytes (CTL) was highly conserved in field strains.[629]

The extensive diversity in the G protein has occurred incrementally over many years rather than through extensive change in a short time frame. The conservation of the central domain containing the CX3C domain involved in binding to CX3CR1 presumably represents a functional constraint on divergence of that major antigenic site. Sequence changes resulting in antigenic changes are evident in the hypervariable domains, presumably selected by immune pressure. These do not provide major antigenic change, but their occurrence implies that they provide sufficient advantage to be selected. Analysis of isolates collected over 38 years provided evidence of selection of progressive amino acid changes in G at an average rate of 0.25% per year that were paralleled by changes in reactivity with MAbs.[83] A study of strains collected over 11 years identified 18 sites, nine each in subgroups A and B strains, that appeared to change in response to selective immune pressure, and these changes frequently involved reversion back to a previous assignment ("flip-flop").[59]

The hypervariable domains are unusual in that they are more divergent at the amino acid level than at the nucleotide level,[297] suggestive of a selective pressure for amino acid change that would be consistent with selective immune pressure. These domains may be relatively tolerant of amino acid change because of their proposed extended, nonglobular structure. As noted above, G genes of both HRSV subgroups recently developed 72-nucleotide (subgroup A) or 60-nucleotide (subgroup B) in-frame duplications in sequence encoding the C-terminal mucin-like region,[169,616] changes that have become widespread worldwide. In contrast, while F presumably also would be subject to selective immune pressure, it likely is less tolerant of amino acid substitutions due to constraints from its folded structure and functional requirements. Analysis of BRSV isolates, including those from countries in which vaccination was in wide use, provided evidence of modest progressive changes not only in G but also in N and F.[622]

The HRSV antigenic subgroups can be further categorized into genotypes (also called clades or lineages). This has been based on the sequence of the G gene or, more usually, the downstream 270 nucleotides of the G ORF encoding the C-terminal hypervariable domain and identified as many as 13 and 20 genotypes for subgroups A and B, respectively.[225,498] More recently, whole-genome comparisons have been employed, identifying 23 and 6 proposed genotypes for subgroup A and B, respectively.[498] A consensus has recently been proposed for the naming of HRSV isolates (HRSV/subgroup identifier/geographic identifier/unique sequence identifier/year of sampling[533]), and efforts are underway to develop a consensus on HRSV genotype definitions.

HMPV also has a single serotype with two antigenic subgroups, A and B, that have extensive cross-reactivity and cross-protection.[277,565,625] The level of genome nucleotide sequence identity (80%) and the relatedness between the subgroups for the various proteins is somewhat similar to that described for HRSV (Table 10.1). The HMPV F protein is somewhat more conserved than that of HRSV and plays a major role in the high level of cross-neutralization and protection between the two subgroups.[565] The divergence of the HMPV G protein between the subgroups is even greater than for HRSV (Table 10.1). In-frame duplications in the sequence encoding the ectodomain of HMPV G have recently occurred and become predominant locally.[454] At least three and two genotypes have been described for HMPV subgroups A and B, respectively.[454]

Vaccination of poultry against AMPV appears to drive antigenic drift in the field, especially in the G and SH genes, resulting in virus that is sufficiently divergent from the vaccine strain that it is less restricted by vaccination.[89]

Animal Viruses

The animal virus members of the genus *Orthopneumovirus* are BRSV and MPV. BRSV, first reported in 1970, is a worldwide cause of respiratory disease in cattle, and can predispose animals to secondary infection by other pathogens leading to bovine respiratory disease complex.[527] The BRSV gene map is very similar to that of HRSV.[71] The genome of BRSV strain A51908 (NC_001989 and AF295543) contains 15,140 nucleotides and has 73% nucleotide identity with HRSV. Amino acid sequence identity with HRSV ranges from 30% (G protein) to 93% (N protein) (Table 10.1), and there is moderate antigenic cross-reactivity. BRSV and HRSV have broadly overlapping host ranges in cell culture; however, *in vivo*, BRSV is highly restricted in nonhuman primates.[72] Ovine and caprine RSV also have been described. Sequence analysis suggests that ovine RSV and BRSV represent two branches of ruminant RSV with a degree of divergence similar to that between the HRSV antigenic subgroups. Caprine RSV appears to be more closely related to BRSV than to ovine RSV.[127]

MPV was the first member of the current family *Pneumoviridae* to be identified. It was discovered during experiments in 1938 in which clinical material from patients with respiratory tract illness was passaged in mice in an effort to identify new human pathogens, and an apparent endogenous mouse respiratory virus became evident.[283] MPV is a respiratory pathogen that readily infects mice and other rodents and can be highly virulent. However, the natural host of MPV is unclear: the virus occasionally appears in colonies of laboratory mice, but serologic studies usually find little evidence of MPV-specific antibodies in wild rodents under conditions where there is extensive seropositivity for other common rodent viruses.[32,566] MPV became more virulent to mice during serial passage in mice.[283] There have been no reports of isolation of MPV from humans, and a low level of apparent MPV-seropositivity in adults appeared to be due to low-affinity polyreactive natural antibodies rather than to antibodies induced by MPV infection.[68] A virus that was recently isolated from dogs with acute respiratory disease appears to be a strain of MPV (e.g., the percent amino acid sequence identity between the isolate and MPV strain 15 ranged from a low of 90.2% [SH] to a high of 98.1% [M]).[505] Whether MPV commonly infects and causes respiratory tract disease in dogs remains unknown. The MPV gene map[339] is essentially the same as that of HRSV and BRSV except that (a) the M2 and L genes of MPV do not overlap and (b) expression of the MPV P mRNA is more complex. Specifically, the 295-codon P ORF is expressed intracellularly as full-length P protein and at least two shorter forms that initiate at internal in-frame start codons; in addition, the MPV P mRNA contains a second, overlapping, 137-codon ORF that encodes a protein that is detected intracellularly and represents a twelfth distinct MPV protein.[28] The complete nucleotide sequence of MPV strain 15 (AY729016) is 14,886 nucleotides in length and has 52% identity with that of HRSV.[339] The level of amino acid sequence identity between MPV and HRSV ranges from 10% (M2-2 protein) to 60% (N protein) (Table 10.1). There was no cross-neutralization between MPV and HRSV with convalescent antisera from experimental animals, and no cross-protection in mice.[68] MPV replicates at very low levels in non-human primates and is being developed as a vaccine vector.[69]

BRSV and MPV in their respective hosts are used as models for HRSV infection and disease,[207,517] although a review of these studies is beyond the scope of this chapter. The BRSV model is limited by the inconvenient nature of the large host. MPV differs from HRSV in that lethal infections are typical rather than an infrequent outcome, at least with the available MPV strains and in inbred mouse strains. Therefore, MPV can serve as a model for severe pneumovirus disease and has the advantage of the many available murine immunologic reagents and inbred mouse strains.

AMPV is the only animal virus member of the genus *Metapneumovirus*. It was first identified in 1978 as a virus associated with rhinotracheitis in turkeys. This disease is of economic importance, and AMPV also infects chickens and other birds.[458] Four AMPV antigenic subgroups have been described: subgroups A and B have been found in South Africa, Europe, Israel, and Asia; subgroup C in North America; and subgroup D in France.[458] Examples of complete prototype genomic sequences include subgroup A (AY640317) and subgroup C (AY590688 and AY579780). These range in length from 13,134 to 14,150 nucleotides, have the same general gene map as HMPV, and share 61% to 68% nucleotide sequence identity with HMPV subgroup A. Subgroups A, B, and D are more closely related to each other than to C[223,556] (e-Fig. 10.2B). Surprisingly, AMPV-C is more closely related to HMPV than to the other AMPV subgroups[624,625] (e-Fig. 10.2B). Sequence analysis of isolates collected over a 25-year period suggested that the most recent common ancestor for AMPV-C and HMPV existed approximately 200 years ago, implying a cross-species jump.[139] There is substantial host range restriction between human and avian MPV. AMPV-C (the subgroup most closely related to HMPV) is highly restricted in nonhuman primates.[480] HMPV has been reported to be unable to infect chickens and turkeys[625] or may transiently infect turkeys.[628]

PATHOGENESIS AND PATHOLOGY

HRSV disease involves contributions from viral factors—which may variously cause direct damage and illness, increase viral load and spread, and subvert host protective responses—and host factors—which may cause damage and illness even in the process of restricting viral infection. Some of these factors are depicted in Figure 10.6 and discussed throughout this chapter. These general themes also apply to HMPV.

In monolayer cultures of immortalized cell lines, infection with HRSV or HMPV results in long surface filaments that bear viral antigen and probably give rise to filamentous virus particles (Fig. 10.2B and C). The formation of HRSV filaments and filamentous virus depends on activation of RhoA and actin rearrangement: when activation was blocked, the production of infectious virus shifted to the nonfilamentous form.[224] HRSV-infected cells develop large electron-dense cytoplasmic inclusion bodies that are up to several microns in diameter and are not contained within a membrane (e-Fig. 10.9). As noted above ("Replicative Cycle"), the inclusion bodies are the sites of viral transcription and RNA replication[55,194,199,293,376,508] and also sequester specific cellular proteins involved in the host response to infection, thereby suppressing those responses.[194,293] HMPV

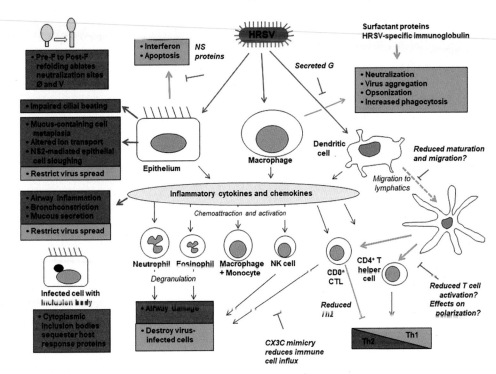

FIGURE 10.6 Selected factors in HRSV infection, disease, restriction, and immune evasion. In the respiratory tract, the virus (top) infects epithelial cells (the major site of virus replication), macrophages, and dendritic cells (DCs). Effects that increase virus replication and pathogenesis and/or decrease immune protection are in *red*; factors favoring protection are in *green*. *Top right*: surfactant proteins, virus-specific antibodies, and macrophages help restrict infection and spread; antibody-mediated clearance is countered by secreted G protein acting as a decoy. *Top left*: triggering of pre-F to refold irreversibly to post-F results in the loss of neutralization sites Ø and V, which may reduce virus neutralization and induction of antibodies specific to these sites. In infected cells, the viral NS proteins inhibit IFN induction and signaling and delay apoptosis. *Center left*: virus infection in epithelial cells impairs ciliary beating, increases mucus and airway fluid, and induces cell sloughing: these effects contribute to illness, but the latter two also may help restrict viral spread. *Center*: infected epithelial cells, macrophages, and DCs produce inflammatory cytokines and chemokines that promote airway reactivity and mucus production and attract and activate immune cells. These factors contribute to disease but also likely restrict virus spread (e.g., mucus, immune cells). *Bottom left*: cytoplasmic inclusion bodies sequester a number of specific cellular proteins involved in host responses, reducing those responses. *Bottom center*: immune cell influx is reduced by viral CX3C fractalkine mimicry. Degranulation by neutrophils and eosinophils, and cell killing by NK cells and CD8+ T cells, help restrict infection but also may contribute to disease. *Right*: antigen encounter by DCs leads to their maturation and migration to secondary lymphatic tissue: infection of DCs by HRSV is inefficient and subsequent maturation and migration is suboptimal. *Bottom right*: DCs induce CD4+ and CD8+ T-cell activation, polarization, and proliferation: these steps may be reduced due to HRSV exposure. Th2 responses may be suppressed by CD8+ T cells and NK cells. (Adapted from Brearey SP, Symth RL. Pathogenesis of RSV in children. In: Cane P, ed. *Respiratory Syncytial Virus*. Amsterdam, The Netherlands: Elsevier; 2007:143. Copyright © 2007 Elsevier. With permission.)

forms similar inclusions,[148] as also has been reported for some members of *Paramyxoviridae*. HRSV infection has slight inhibitory effects on cellular DNA and RNA synthesis and little effect on gross protein synthesis.[367] As one factor in the lack of inhibition of protein synthesis, the HRSV N protein binds to PKR and prevents it from phosphorylating eukaryotic translation initiation factor 2A (eIF-2A) and inhibiting protein synthesis.[239] Apoptosis of HRSV-infected cells occurs slowly and is inhibited by the NS1, NS2, and SH proteins. HRSV blocks the formation of stress granules, which can otherwise restrict HRSV replication, via expression of RNA derived from the trailer region.[263]

The formation of syncytia (Fig. 10.2A) is a major factor in cell death in nonpolarized monolayer cultures but usually is not a prominent histopathologic finding *in vivo* (below).

HRSV and HMPV are highly infectious viruses. Humans are their only natural host, although HRSV and HMPV can readily spread to nonhuman primates, as already noted. The major mode of spread by HRSV is by large droplets or through contaminated objects (i.e., fomites) and depends on close contact with infected individuals or contact of contaminated hands to nasal or conjunctival mucosa (self-inoculation). It was thought that small-particle aerosols (which can remain airborne

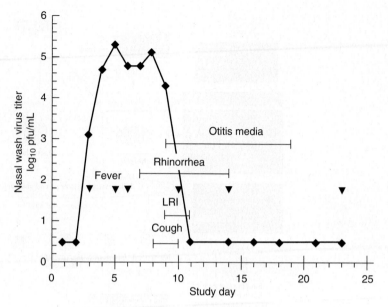

FIGURE 10.7 Time course of viral shedding and disease signs following experimental infection of a seronegative young vaccinee with 10^4 PFU of an investigational live-attenuated HRSV vaccine called *cpts*248/955. Fever (*filled triangles*) was intermittent. (Adapted from Karron RA, Wright PF, Crowe JE Jr, et al. Evaluation of two live, cold-passaged, temperature-sensitive respiratory syncytial virus vaccines in chimpanzees and in human adults, infants, and children. *J Infect Dis* 1997;176(6):1428–1436. Reproduced by permission of Oxford University Press.)

for extended periods and also can be inhaled deeply into the respiratory tract) are not an important mode of HRSV transmission,[249] although there are contrary data.[231] A recent study showed that infants hospitalized with HRSV produced large numbers of aerosol particles that were able to infect primary epithelial cell cultures.[346] The incubation period in humans from time of infection to onset of illness for HRSV is about 3 to 5 days[306,316] (Fig. 10.7). The incubation period for HMPV is not well defined but is thought to be longer than for HRSV and ranges from 4 to 7 days.[243]

HRSV replicates initially in the nasopharynx. Signs of LRI usually appear 1 to 3 days following the onset of rhinorrhea (Fig. 10.7). Viral spread to the lower respiratory tract likely involves aspiration of secretions. Infants hospitalized for HRSV disease shed infectious virus in nasal secretions with peak titers of 10^4 to 10^6 PFU per mL.[150,250,666] Shedding of infectious virus typically lasts from 7 to 10 days, although viral RNA can be detected by PCR for up to 3 to 4 weeks in infants following clinical recovery.[401] Limited data suggest that the titer of virus in the lower respiratory tract, sampled in bronchoalveolar lavage fluids of ventilated patients, is similar to that in the upper respiratory tract.[553] Infectious virus has been difficult to recover from adults during symptomatic infection despite positive serologic or RT-PCR tests, probably due to the presence of both preexisting and rapidly-induced neutralizing antibodies.

HRSV exhibits tropism for the superficial epithelial cells of the airways and lungs. *In vitro* studies in human adenoid or HAE cell cultures showed that HRSV nearly exclusively infected ciliated cells (Fig. 10.5).[682] Infection is limited to the superficial cells; it does not appear to spread to basal cells, and virus is released from the apical surface.[682] In HAE cultures, the infection continues through multiple rounds over several weeks, and infected cells are shed and replaced with little visible alteration of the microscopic appearance of the tissue, although ciliary beating usually is impaired.[682] Syncytia are not observed, probably because the F glycoprotein is expressed on the apical surface and does not contact adjacent cells. HRSV contrasts sharply with influenza A virus, which is rapidly destructive and quickly spreads to underlying cells (Fig. 10.5).[682] HRSV infection of epithelial cells induces a rapid inhibition of Na⁺ trans-

port, resulting in apical fluid accumulation. This might be a host mechanism to dilute and remove irritants but also might contribute to excess fluid and virus spread. This effect is not unique to HRSV and has been observed with HPIV and influenza viruses as well as with bacterial pathogens.

Histopathology of fatal HRSV infections also indicates that infection is limited to the superficial layer of the airway epithelium, although additional cells such as type I and II pneumonocytes also are infected[206,294,651] (Fig. 10.8). There is necrosis and destruction of ciliated cells and occasional proliferation of the bronchiolar epithelium, but basal cells are spared. Ciliated epithelial cells rarely reappear before 2 weeks postinfection, and complete restoration requires 4 to 8 weeks,[248] similar to the duration of postinfection altered lung function and airway reactivity in adults. There is an early influx of polymorphonuclear cells, and a peribronchiolar infiltrate of lymphocytes, CD69+ monocytes, plasma cells, and macrophages develops, with migration of the lymphocytes among the mucosal epithelial cells. Submucosal and adventitial tissues become edematous, and secretion of mucus is excessive, which combined with cell debris and inflammatory cells obstruct the bronchioles and alveoli, causing either collapse or air trapping of distal portions of the airway that is reflected in hyperinflation. When alveolar type I and II pneumocytes are infected, pneumonia can occur. In those instances, the interalveolar walls thicken as a result of mononuclear cell infiltration, and the alveolar spaces may fill with fluid. There is usually a patchy appearance of these pathologic changes, even though disease may be widespread.

Immunostaining identified virus-infected cells in the bronchial, bronchiolar, and alveolar epithelium[294,456] (Fig. 10.8). Syncytia are sometimes observed but are not prominent. However, syncytium formation and giant cell pneumonia are hallmarks of infection in individuals with extreme T-cell deficiency. HRSV antigen can be relatively abundant in lower respiratory tract infection, although the staining is usually focal, and in cases of fatal HRSV bronchiolitis, antigen may be present only in small amounts.[206,456]

The histopathology of HMPV infection is not well known, but HMPV also infects the upper and lower respiratory tract and has been reported to involve a characteristic enlarged,

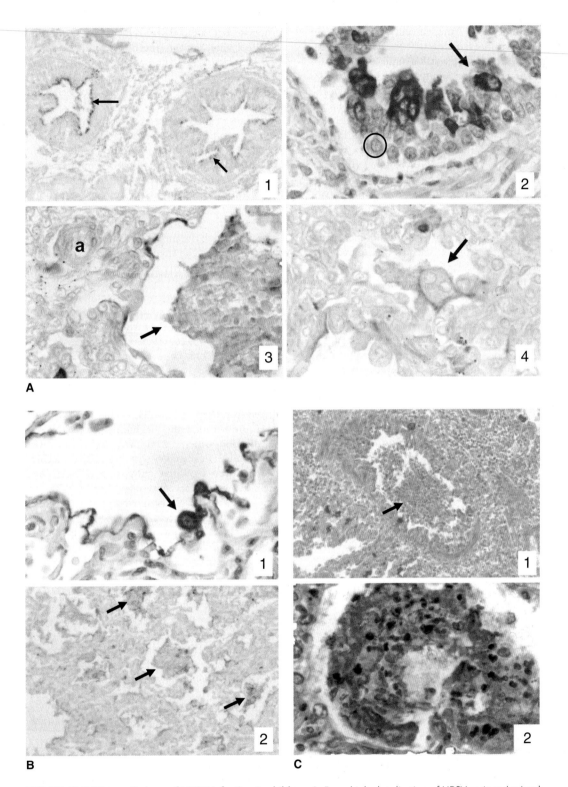

FIGURE 10.8 Histopathology of HRSV infection in children. A: Bronchiolar localization of HRSV antigen (stained *brown*) detected by immunohistochemistry. (*1*) HRSV antigen localized in the luminal epithelium of two bronchioles (*arrows* indicate examples of staining). (*2*) Higher magnification of infected ciliated cells of the luminal surface of the bronchiole (an example is indicated with the *arrow*), also showing that the basal progenitor cells (an example is *circled*) are not infected. (*3*) Intraluminal debris (the *arrow* indicates a large debris plug) in a small airway, staining positively for HRSV antigen (an arteriole is marked with "*a*"). (*4*) A small syncytium (*arrow*). **B:** Alveolar localization of HRSV antigen (*brown*) detected by immunohistochemistry. (*1*) HRSV-infected alveolar cells (the *arrow* indicates an infected cell). (*2*) Alveolar lumens and small airways clogged with debris (examples are indicated with the *arrows*) that stains positively for HRSV antigen. **C:** Histopathologic features of bronchiolar inflammation, with periodic acid–Schiff (PAS) staining of carbohydrate macromolecules. (*1*) Bronchiole occluded with an intraluminal plug of debris and inflammatory cells (*arrow*). (*2*) Higher magnification image of intraluminal debris. (Reprinted by permission from Nature: Johnson JE, Gonzales RA, Olson SJ, et al. The histopathology of fatal untreated human respiratory syncytial virus infection. *Mod Pathol* 2007;20(1):108–119. Copyright © 2006 United States and Canadian Academy of Pathology, Inc.)

darkly staining pneumocyte or "smudge cell" that is not seen with other respiratory paramyxoviruses.[586] Studies in nonhuman primates indicate that HMPV has a similar tropism for the bronchiolar respiratory epithelium type II alveolar cells.[344]

Infection by HRSV and HMPV is largely limited to the respiratory tract. Infectious virus is not recovered from the blood of HRSV- or HMPV-infected humans, and viral nucleic acid is infrequently detected in blood immune cells of HRSV-immunocompetent infected infants.[247,677] There are isolated reports of HRSV RNA detected in cerebrospinal fluid and myocardium.[536,584] HRSV, HMPV, and influenza viral RNA have been detected in sera of immunosuppressed individuals, and this was associated with worse clinical outcomes including mortality.[82] HRSV has been cultured from the myocardium of an infected infant with combined immunodeficiency as well as from a liver biopsy from an infected immunocompetent infant.[164] This suggests that HRSV has some potential to spread beyond the respiratory tract but usually is restricted by host immunity.

HRSV is not thought to cause latent or long-term infections in otherwise healthy individuals. However, there are some reports to the contrary suggesting the prolonged persistence of virus or viral RNA in otherwise healthy hosts. Infectious virus has been recovered from guinea pigs 60 to 100 days postinfection,[137] and BRSV RNA and proteins have been detected in bovine pulmonary lymph nodes 71 days following infection, and there was indirect evidence for in vitro infectivity from isolated bovine B lymphocytes.[619] There is conflicting evidence as to whether HRSV might persist in some individuals with stable chronic obstructive pulmonary disease (COPD).[177] HRSV shedding can be very prolonged in some cases of immunosuppression. For example, HRSV was shed for 199 days, largely without disease, in a child infected with human immunodeficiency virus (HIV),[329] and persistent shedding of HMPV has been described in asymptomatic hematopoietic stem cell transplant (HSCT) recipients.

There have not been clear, consistent differences in replication or clinical severity associated with any particular HRSV strain or genetic group. This also is the case with HMPV. However, evaluation of possible strain differences continues. A recent report describes a new genetic lineage of HRSV B that was associated with severe disease during an HRSV outbreak outside the regular respiratory season.[605] In another study, the subgroup A clade A/GA5 was associated with more severe disease.[515] An HRSV strain called line 19 was shown to induce increased lung IL-13 expression and mucus secretion in BALB/c mice, an effect that mapped to the F gene.[439] Thus, clinically relevant heterogeneity in strain virulence may be uncovered by further investigation. In addition, recent data suggest that defective HRSV genomes (DVG) might be associated with worse clinical outcomes.[190] With HMPV, there presently is no data suggesting that specific genotypes are associated with increased disease severity.[2]

Primary HRSV infection is usually symptomatic, but disease manifestations can vary greatly and may include upper respiratory tract illness (URI), fever, otitis media, or LRI ranging from mild disease to bronchiolitis and/or pneumonia with or without subsequent long-term abnormalities in pulmonary function (see "Clinical Features"). In high-income countries, death rarely occurs.[66] Infection in immunosuppressed individuals ranges from asymptomatic to highly lethal. A number of factors are thought to contribute to HRSV (and HMPV)

pathogenesis and the observed heterogeneity of disease, including direct viral damage, the host immune response, age, and other host factors including immune status, underlying disease, secondhand smoke exposure, or genetic polymorphisms affecting host defense.[108,271] These are discussed below and in subsequent sections.

Because HRSV can readily infect and cause disease during the first months of life, young age is a critical factor in disease pathogenesis (e-Fig. 10.10). Maternal antibodies and immunologic immaturity result in reduced immune responses during infancy (see "Immune Response"), and thus reduced ability to control the infection. Immune responses in the neonate and young infant have a reduced Th1 component, a situation that is protective for the fetus prior to birth but can contribute to a Th2 bias in early infancy[134] and may be associated with more severe disease.[402] The small diameter of bronchioles in infants makes them particularly susceptible to obstruction by edema, secretions, and immune and exfoliated cells. Infancy is a time of considerable lung growth and development. Developing lungs may be more susceptible to disease and to long-term respiratory morbidity. Studies in a rodent model suggest HRSV infection can lead to remodeling of neural networks that innervate the respiratory mucosa, contributing to recurrent airway inflammation and hyperreactivity.[612] There also is evidence from the mouse model that HRSV infection early in life can result in skewed primary and recall immune responses.[134] Other host risk factors are described in "Epidemiology".

A number of studies, including prospective studies of natural infection, experimental infection of adults with wild-type HRSV, and clinical studies with live HRSV vaccine candidates, have indicated a positive correlation between virus load and disease severity,[150,268,316] although there also are contradictory studies.[41,250,515,666] High nasopharyngeal viral load also has been associated with disease severity for HMPV.[519] Recent data, however, suggest that infants with mild HRSV infection have higher HRSV loads than those with more severe disease.[205,482,609] It is not clear whether correlations reflect pathogenesis due to direct viral damage or a heightened immune response. As noted, studies with HAE and HBE cultures indicate that HRSV is not very cytopathic or invasive, compared to other respiratory viruses such as influenza virus (Fig. 10.5). However, impaired ciliary function and increased cell shedding, possibly promoted by the HRSV NS2 protein,[375] would facilitate clogging of bronchioles and alveoli. In experimental infections in adults, the timing of HRSV disease coincided with the timing of viral shedding, suggesting that direct viral damage contributes to disease. HRSV and HMPV epidemics are associated with increased risk of S. pneumoniae infections in children.[9,648] In addition, the influence of the nasal microbiota, specifically of S. pneumoniae and H. influenzae, on clinical manifestations and the host immune response to HRSV has been appreciated in different studies.[142,153,568,582]

It is widely thought that host immunity plays a major role in HRSV (and presumably HMPV) disease. In HRSV-infected cotton rats or mice, treatment with HRSV-neutralizing antibodies rapidly reduced pulmonary viral titers but had little effect on lung histopathology.[425,495] In contrast, treatment with anti-inflammatory glucocorticoids reduced lung histopathology even though clearance of the virus was slowed, suggesting that in this model the host immune response played the major role in pathogenesis.[495] However, the situation is less clear in humans, where treatment with corticosteroids does not significantly reduce disease[74] (see "Treatment"). Immune factors that have been suggested to contribute to HRSV disease include (a) an unbalanced inflammatory response; (b) an overly robust CD8+ CTL response, resulting in excessive tissue damage; (c) impaired IFN responses; and (d) a Th2-biased CD4+ T-cell response that is not optimally effective against intracellular pathogens and results in excessive mucus production, and/or airway reactivity (see "Immune Response"). There are supporting and contrary data in each case, as will be shown, and it may be that the contributions of various factors vary in different individuals.

IMMUNE RESPONSE

In otherwise-healthy hosts, HRSV and HMPV cause acute infections that are restricted and resolved by host immunity. Cellular immunity is particularly important in resolving infection. Secretory and serum antibodies play the primary role in protection against reinfection. Many other aspects of innate and adaptive immunity are associated with HRSV infection, but their contributions to protection and disease often remain unclear. Figure 10.6 illustrates selected immune factors, among other factors, that may restrict HRSV infection but may also contribute to HRSV disease.

Antigens

Postinfection sera from experimental animals or humans contain antibodies that recognize a number of HRSV proteins. However, the F and G proteins are the only virus neutralization antigens and are the major, independent protective antigens.[118] For example, when cotton rats or mice were immunized with vaccinia virus recombinants expressing individual HRSV proteins and subsequently challenged with HRSV, F and G were the only proteins that induced neutralizing antibody responses and conferred long-lasting protection.[118,462] F was more protective than G.[118,462]

F generally has been reported to induce higher titers of serum HRSV-neutralizing antibodies than G based on traditional neutralization assays using monolayer cell lines. However, as noted above, cell lines are deficient in CX3CR1 and do not provide detection of antibodies that neutralize infectivity by blocking binding to this receptor. However, neutralization assays can be broadened to detect these antibodies by the use of HAE and HBE cells, which express CX3CR1.[85,123,332] Alternatively, the inclusion of complement in the traditional assays with cell lines broadens detection, but not all G-specific antibodies to the central conserved domain were detected.[123] More recently, neutralization studies of a limited number of sera using HAE cultures indicated that between 0% and 50% of the postinfection serum neutralizing titer from individual young children was G specific and thus was quite variable in that population.[85,332]

A large fraction of MAbs raised against the HRSV F protein neutralize infectivity efficiently, and many inhibit fusion.[33] Most epitopes of the F protein are conformation dependent. Structural biology studies have identified six major antigenic sites of the F protein (Ø to V, Fig. 10.4B).[226] Antigenic sites Ø and V are exclusively present on the pre-F conformation, and sites I to IV are shared between the pre-F and post-F conformation. Studies with mAbs showed that all known neutralizing epitopes are present on the pre-F conformation; some of these neutralizing epitopes are maintained after the F protein refolds to the post-F conformation, but to date, no neutralizing sites have been identified that are exclusively present on the post-F conformation. Sites eliciting the most potent neutralizing antibodies (antigenic sites Ø and V) are lost after refolding.[520] Interestingly, in young infants, site III is recognized by germline antibodies, which have HRSV-neutralizing activity.[217] Even though site III is shared between pre- and post-F, site III-specific antibodies recognize pre-F more efficiently.[217] The propensity of pre-F to be readily triggered to irreversibly refold into post-F, with the loss of sites Ø and V and reduced recognition of site III, may reduce the susceptibility of virions (containing both pre-F and post-F) to neutralization and reduce the induction of antibodies to these sites.

In contrast, HRSV G has a very different antigenic nature. Most G-specific MAbs bind efficiently to denatured G, such as in Western blots, and many bind efficiently to synthetic peptides, suggesting that reactivity does not depend on a complex folded structure. Most MAbs against the G protein are inefficient in neutralizing HRSV infectivity *in vitro* when tested individually in absence of complement, although neutralization can be achieved with mixtures of MAbs.[123,407,409] Most G-specific MAbs react with some HRSV strains but not others within an antigenic subgroup and thus are "strain specific": these MAbs often react only with glycosylated G, and their epitopes mostly are in the hypervariable domain in the C-terminal third of the molecule. Other MAbs react broadly within a subgroup, and a small number react with viruses from both subgroups: these MAbs typically do not depend on glycosylation of G for binding, and their epitopes usually are located in the central conserved region of G that contains the CX3C motif important for binding to CX3CR1.[123,407] A synthetic peptide representing this central region was protective in mice and calves,[29] confirming its importance in immunogenicity and antigenicity. Postinfection human serum antibodies to the G protein were found to be enriched for the IgG2 subclass, consistent with G being recognized in part as a polysaccharide antigen.[634]

Most of the HRSV proteins stimulate memory CD8+ and airway-resident CD4+ T cells in seropositive humans.[99,242,302] However, in both mice and humans, the G protein is a poor CTL antigen, possibly due to its skewed amino acid content and extensive glycosylation. In the commonly used BALB/c mouse model, the F, N, and M2-1 proteins have been shown to induce CD8+ CTL responses: the dominant CTL epitope recognized by this mouse strain is contained in amino acids 82 to 90 of the M2-1 protein, accounting for approximately 40% of the primary CTL response.[345] Immunization of BALB/c mice with vaccinia virus recombinants expressing the N or M2-1 proteins provided protective immunity that was not mediated by neutralizing antibodies and, in the case of M2-1, was confirmed to be mediated by CD8+ CTL.[118,345] However, protection waned within weeks, suggesting that pulmonary protection by CTL is short lived.

For HMPV, the F protein is a major neutralization and protective antigen, as shown in studies in which F was expressed by a HPIV1 vector and evaluated in rodents and nonhuman primates[565] or by an alphavirus replicon and evaluated in mice and cotton rats.[437] Surprisingly, vectors that individually expressed the G and SH proteins did not induce detectable neutralizing antibodies or protection in rodents.[437,564] Similarly, purified HMPV G protein administered to cotton rats did not induce neutralizing antibodies or protection.[526] Thus, HMPV appears to differ from members of *Orthopneumovirus* and *Paramyxoviridae* in having only a single surface glycoprotein as a major neutralization and protective antigen.

Innate Immunity and Inflammation

The first line of host defense includes the physical barriers of the glycocalyx of the superficial epithelial cells, the secreted mucus layer, and ciliary sweeping. A number of studies have highlighted the role of pulmonary surfactant proteins (SP), specifically SP-A, SP-C, and SP-D, in restricting HRSV while modulating the inflammatory response. SP are lipoprotein complexes produced by type II alveolar cells. SP-A and SP-D have been shown to bind to HRSV F or G glycoproteins, neutralize infectivity, and promote phagocytosis.[365] Mice with targeted disruption of SP-A, SP-C, or SP-D exhibited increased pulmonary HRSV titers and disease, which was ameliorated by topical administration of the missing surfactant.[365] Genetic polymorphisms in SP-A, SP-B, and SP-D have been associated with severe pediatric HRSV disease.[434] Infants with severe HRSV disease were found to have reduced surfactant concentration and function, although it is not known whether this was a cause or a result of severe disease.[319]

Toll-like receptors (TLRs) present on the plasma membrane and endosomes play a significant role in the host immune response to HRSV. The HRSV F protein stimulates TLR4 on leukocytes independent of viral replication, leading to activation of the NF-κB pathway to produce cytokines such as IL-6 and IL-8 and activation of IRF3 to induce type I IFN.[349] TLR4-deficient mice are less efficient than normal mice in resolving HRSV infection.[349] Studies have linked severe pediatric HRSV disease with genetic polymorphisms in TLR4, although other studies and a recent meta-analysis did not confirm this association.[81,685] Other TLRs have also been involved in the immune response to HRSV including TLR2, TLR3, TLR7, and TLR8.[384] HRSV has been shown to activate signaling from the TLR2/TLR6 heterodimer complex on the surface of leukocytes, resulting in the expression of proinflammatory cytokines, neutrophil influx, and DC activation in mice.[447] Mice lacking TLR2 or TLR6 were less able to restrict HRSV challenge compared to normal mice. HRSV also activates TLR3 in epithelial cells, resulting in the production of inflammatory cytokine and chemokines.[522] Studies in TLR3 knockout mice indicated that TLR3 did not make a significant contribution to restricting HRSV replication but helped prevent both IL-13 up-regulation and increased mucus production.[523] Also in mice, studies showed that TLR7 and RIG-I worked collaboratively to recruit and activate plasmacytoid DCs (pDCs) conferring protection against acute infection.[562] In addition, in infants hospitalized with HRSV LRI, TLR7, and TLR8 expression in mucosal samples was increased, while expression of TLR8 was decreased in blood monocytes.[40,538] Nevertheless, excessive stimulation of TLRs can potentially contribute to HRSV pathogenesis by promoting sensitivity both to HRSV and to possible coinfecting viruses or bacteria. In addition to TLRs, RIG-I plays a major role in innate responses.[404,675] As noted above, HRSV and HMPV have mechanisms that suppress activation of these signaling pathways (e-Fig. 10.8).

Infection of epithelial cells by HRSV (or HMPV) alters the cell transcriptional profile markedly, resulting in changes in expression (mostly up-regulation) of hundreds of genes.[408] This was mostly dependent on viral replication. These genes represented multiple biological pathways, showing a broad effect of viral infection. In infants with HRSV infection, mucosal transcriptional profiles corroborated those findings and showed a robust overexpression of genes of IFN and other innate immunity signaling pathways that correlated with clinical disease severity.[157,642] In human lung A549 epithelial cell cultures *in vitro*, in the mouse model and in children infected with HRSV, proteomic profiling identified changes in the expression of different proteins following HRSV infection, indicating a complex cellular response to infection.[643] Comparison of the responses in A549 cells infected with HRSV, HMPV, HPIV3, and measles virus identified a common core response that mainly involved defense against endoplasmic reticulum stress and induction of apoptosis.[627]

Airway epithelial cells and macrophages exposed to HRSV *in vitro* produce a broad array of proinflammatory cytokines, including IL-1, IL-8/CXCL8, RANTES/CCL5, IL-10, MIP-1α/CCL3, MCP-1/CCL2, IP-10/CXCL10, IL-6, TNF-α, and type I and type III IFNs.[431,572] Many of these cytokines have been found in upper and lower respiratory tract samples of infants and adults with HRSV LRI.[203,482,553,676] Bronchoalveolar washes from infants with severe HRSV disease had increased IL-9 mRNA expression, which is a T helper type-2 cell-derived pleiotropic cytokine that promotes inflammation and increased mucus production.[422]

Expression of cytokines described above promotes recruitment of immune cells to the infected lung. Furthermore, during HRSV infection, endothelial cells become activated and up-regulate endothelial intercellular adhesion molecule-1 (ICAM-1), which increases the adhesion of immature and mature neutrophils, thought to facilitate their migration into alveolar spaces.[304] Incoming immune cells become activated to express cytokines and other proinflammatory molecules such as cysteinyl leukotrienes that can heighten the inflammatory response. Activated granulocytes (neutrophils and eosinophils) also release degradative enzymes and other factors that may contribute to both protection and pathogenesis (see below). The total number of immune cells recovered in washes from the upper and lower respiratory tract of infants was several-fold higher in cases of severe HRSV disease compared with uninfected controls.[269,423,553] Neutrophils were by far the most abundant immune cells present in the airway, comprising 76% to 93% of recovered cells from the upper and lower respiratory tract, with lymphocytes and mononuclear cells being present at ≤10% each and eosinophils at less than 1%.[245,423]

Activated neutrophils release factors such as neutrophil elastase and extracellular traps (NETs) that potentially can restrict infection but also can cause tissue damage and airway obstruction.[122] What occurs during HRSV infection is not completely understood. In infants with severe HRSV disease, the appearance of neutrophil precursors in peripheral blood—which precedes their influx into the airways—closely followed the peak of viral load and clinical disease severity, whereas CD8+ T cells appeared later and seem less likely to have been a major contributor to disease when it was most severe[388] (e-Fig. 10.11). Levels of mRNA for IL-8—a cytokine that promotes neutrophil chemotaxis and survival—measured in nasal aspirates of children with bronchiolitis correlated with the severity of disease,[567] and an IL-8 haplotype characterized by increased IL-8 gene transcription was associated with increased susceptibility to HRSV disease.[246] A recent study conducted in the HRSV controlled-infection model in adults showed that greater mucosal neutrophil activation along with suppressed IL-17 responses before HRSV infection was predictive of the development of symptomatic HRSV disease.[245] These findings suggest that neutrophils have the potential to contribute to both viral clearance and disease.

Similarly, activated eosinophils release factors such as eosinophil-associated ribonucleases and cationic protein that have the potential to restrict infection as well as to cause tissue damage. The role of eosinophils in HRSV infection and pathogenesis is not completely understood.[481] On the one hand, the recruitment of these cells to the respiratory tract of HRSV-infected infants appears to be negligible, as noted above. On the other hand, studies suggest that blood eosinophils are activated during acute HRSV infection in humans and may contribute to clinical recovery.[378] Mice with eosinophilia due to increased IL-5 expression had increased viral clearance, indicating that eosinophils can be protective.[481]

Studies in mice showed that NK cells are prominent in the early response to infection, are an important source of IFN-γ, and have cytotoxic activity against infected cells.[284,614] In children with severe HRSV infection, numbers of NK cells are reduced in the blood, but increased in the lower respiratory tract, suggesting that these cells are activated and recruited to the site of the infection.[320]

Monocyte recruitment and activation is critical for effective control and clearance of HRSV infection.[209] Inadequate activation of monocytes in peripheral blood, assessed by HLA-DR expression or TNF-α production capacity, have been associated with more severe HRSV disease and increased risk of hospitalization.[271,429] Mice that are genetically deficient in monocyte/macrophage function, or in which macrophages have been depleted, are less able to restrict HRSV infection and exhibit increased lung inflammation.[501] This illustrates a key role for these phagocytic cells in restricting viral replication as well as in clearing the lung of debris that can cause further damage and inflammation. Macrophages also play an important role in the early response to HRSV infection by producing an immediate release of proinflammatory and immunomodulatory cytokines.[489] Studies in mice suggest that alveolar macrophages are the primary source of type I IFN in response to viral respiratory infection in general, with myeloid DC (mDCs) also contributing, while pDCs can play a role later in infection if virus replication is not controlled.[347,398,501] mDCs and pDCs are mobilized to the respiratory mucosal during the acute HRSV infection, and higher numbers of both subsets remained in respiratory samples for weeks after symptoms of HRSV infection have resolved.[209]

Type I IFN has well-known antiviral effects mediated by signaling through its ubiquitous receptor IFNAR. Type I IFN also is considered to stimulate both innate and adaptive immunity, although these effects can be complex.[324,446] Studies in which bovines were immunized with NS-gene-deletion mutants of BRSV provided evidence of increased humoral and cellular immune responses associated with deletion of NS2, which is the major IFN antagonist of BRSV (whereas NS1 is the major antagonist in HRSV).[620] Type III IFNs (IFN-λ1 to λ4) are less well characterized but also have important antiviral effects.[354] The IFN-λ receptor (IFN-λR1/IL-10R2) is expressed mainly on the epithelial cells of the respiratory and gastrointestinal tracts, and thus its effects appear to be largely limited to those sites.[354] Studies in mice lacking the receptor for either or both type I and III IFN showed that each is involved in restricting replication of respiratory viruses including HRSV,[440] although a

study with MPV suggested that type I IFN has a greater antiviral role.[272] In children with HRSV infection, increased expression of IFN in the blood was associated with decreased disease severity.[271,426] Data regarding the protective role of type III IFN in mucosal samples are limited, as detection of these cytokines at the site of the infection has not been consistent.[549] However, HRSV is notable in that IFN-α/β were detected less frequently and at very low levels in nasal washes from infants, young children, and adults infected with HRSV, compared to influenza and HPIVs.[252,253,417] In addition, HRSV infection and replication are more resistant to prophylaxis and treatment with IFN-α compared to influenza and HPIVs.[201,588] Thus, HRSV, because of the NS1/NS2 proteins, appears to be particularly effective at inhibiting the host IFN response. HMPV induces higher levels of IFN-α/β in mice and is more sensitive to IFN-α than HRSV.[240]

In contrast to studies noted above linking inflammation to severe HRSV disease, there also is evidence that, while HRSV may indeed induce high levels of certain inflammatory cytokines in children hospitalized with HRSV disease, this may not be the dominant factor driving disease severity. In fact, different studies suggest that, in the more severe forms of HRSV disease, some components of the innate immune response are inadequately activated or even suppressed.[41,203,271,426,429,553] Furthermore, a prospective study of primary HRSV and HMPV infections in infants showed that, while infants infected with either virus had similar clinical disease severity, the levels of inflammatory cytokines induced by HMPV were significantly lower than with HRSV.[352] Thus, while these viruses exhibited similar patterns of disease, they do not share a common pattern of overly robust innate immune responses that might be expected if that is the major determinant of disease.

Antibodies

Young infants possess maternally derived serum IgG antibodies against HRSV, HMPV, and other common pathogens.[129] Maternal antibodies are transmitted to the fetus from the mother during gestation by active transport across the placenta beginning at approximately 26 weeks of gestation and continuing until birth (Fig. 10.9). Infants who are born prematurely have lower titers, increasing their susceptibility to infection and disease. The IgG1 subclass is preferentially transferred, but otherwise the titer and specificity of maternally derived IgG antibodies in the full-term neonate are similar to or slightly higher than those of the mother. Thereafter, these antibodies decay with a half-life of approximately 21 to 26 days and protection diminishes. Maternally acquired serum HRSV-specific antibodies are generally thought to reduce the risk of HRSV disease in young infants. Epidemiologic studies indicate that HRSV disease in infants born with higher levels of maternally acquired HRSV-neutralizing and/or IgG antibodies, for example, pre-F IgG antibodies, was milder and/or occurred at an older age than in infants with lower antibody levels, suggesting a protective effect.[85,335,641] Some studies have not found such an association.[287] Breast milk may also contribute protective antibodies, although this has not been clearly documented and likely is a minor effect.

RSV infection induces IgG, IgA, and IgM antibodies to structural and nonstructural HRSV proteins.[43,397] In hospitalized infants, HRSV-specific serum IgA and IgG responses were detected 10 days following the onset of illness, and peak titers were achieved at 3 to 4 weeks.[650] The magnitude of serum

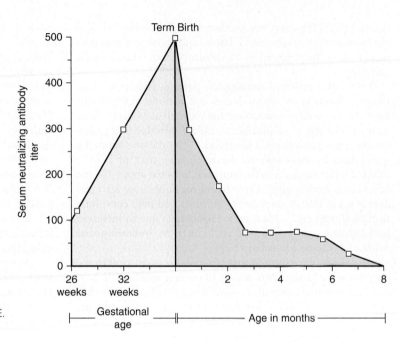

FIGURE 10.9 An idealized diagram, based on experimental data, illustrating the titer of HRSV-neutralizing maternal serum antibodies in the fetus[141] and newborn human infant[472] as a function of gestational and postnatal age. This illustration depicts the increase in serum antibody titer in the fetus during the transplacental transfer and the subsequent decrease in titer due to degradation following birth; this diagram shows only the HRSV-neutralizing component of the multivalent maternal antibodies. (Courtesy of Dr. James E. Crowe, Jr.)

and secretory antibody responses to HRSV in young infants (< ~6 months of age) typically is reduced compared to older individuals. For example, in a study of infants and young children undergoing a primary HRSV infection, the titers of serum antibodies that bound to the F or G glycoprotein or that neutralized HRSV were 8- to 10-fold lower in individuals of 4 to 8 months versus 9 to 21 months of age.[449] The frequency of a detectable secretory IgA response to HRSV in infected infants was also related to age, and these antibodies often were non-neutralizing *in vitro*.[317,418] The effect of age on the response of serum and nasal wash antibodies to an investigational live-attenuated HRSV vaccine is illustrated in e-Figure 10.12. In addition, antibody responses in the young infant are short lived compared to older individuals: the increases in HRSV-specific IgA and IgG antibodies observed shortly after infection in infants were absent or at very low titer 1 year later in one study.[650] This is particularly relevant to HRSV, since HRSV infection is very common in infancy (see "Epidemiology"). The antibody response to HMPV is less well studied but is assumed to be similar to HRSV except that seroprevalence increases with age more slowly than with HRSV.[403]

Reduced immune responses to HRSV (and HMPV) early in life are due to immunologic immaturity[368] and the immunosuppressive effects of maternal antibodies.[129,558] Immunologic immaturity has been characterized for a variety of antigens and has been shown to limit innate, antibody, and cellular responses during the first year of life, although these effects are not absolute and adult-like responses can be elicited under some circumstances.[368] Antibody responses of young infants to the HRSV F protein seem to be biased toward recognition of a limited number of antigenic sites that are distinct from those recognized by adults.[211,217] Examination of the human neonatal B-cell response to HRSV revealed a bias in the repertoire of antibody gene expression and a dramatically reduced frequency of somatic mutations compared to individuals older than 3 months, which likely contributes to the poorly neutralizing nature of the response in the young infant.[664] However, a subset of 450 antibodies isolated from very young infants exhibited

potent neutralizing activity despite lacking somatic hypermutations, indicating that it is possible to elicit protective antibodies in very young infants.[217] Interestingly, a large fraction of these antibodies was directed to antigenic site III and bound more efficiently to pre-F than to post-F. Immunosuppression by HRSV-specific maternal or administered passive serum antibodies has been documented in natural infection,[448] in experimental animals,[450] and in the setting of clinical evaluation of live HRSV vaccines in infants.[668] For example, in the case of live-attenuated vaccines, the titer of maternal antibody had little effect on virus replication in the upper respiratory tract but suppressed the serum and secretory antibody response.[668] In mice, passive HRSV-specific serum antibodies suppressed both serum and secretory antibody responses to infection with wild-type HRSV but did not suppress the cell-mediated response and priming for a secondary antibody response.[132] Surprisingly, in a cohort of infants of less than 6 months of age with very low titers of HRSV-specific maternal antibodies, natural wild-type HRSV infection induced neutralizing serum antibody titers that were indistinguishable from those of individuals aged 6 to 24 months.[557] This indicates that young infants are able to mount an effective neutralizing antibody response when maternal antibodies are low or no longer present to exert their suppressive role. Thus, maternal antibodies are beneficial in providing some disease sparing early in life but also suppress antibody responses.

Natural HRSV infection induces an anamnestic antibody response in adults that can be seen as early as 3 days after onset of illness.[640] In adults, reinfection has been associated with a higher antibody titer response in the elderly compared to young adults[636]: in one study, elderly adults had approximately an eightfold rise in serum HRSV-neutralizing antibodies, which subsequently declined greater than fourfold during the subsequent year, while younger adults had a less than fourfold rise in neutralizing antibody titers.[180] Titers in uninfected control subjects did not decline during this period, suggesting that, after an initial decrease, titers are relatively stable over time. Interestingly, elderly individuals had similar preinfection titers, but a greater increase in neutralizing antibodies postinfection with HRSV or HMPV, compared to younger adults.[179,636] This suggests that the age-associated increase in disease severity characteristic of HRSV is not due to lower preinfection antibody titers or an inability to mount a virus-neutralizing antibody response to infection. Although serum HRSV antibodies wane over time in children and adults, they persist throughout life, likely in part because of repeated infections.

In young infants, the appearance of secretory IgA antibodies usually corresponds with a decrease in HRSV shedding during infection, suggesting a contribution to resolving infection.[418] Secretory IgA antibodies are likely to be particularly efficient in restricting HRSV replication at mucosal surfaces. However, the secretory antibody response is not long lasting, though with increasing age and repeat infection it does last longer.[317] The potential role of IgA antibodies in protective immunity may be limited by its short duration.

F and G antibodies have been associated with decreased risk of human HRSV infection or disease in several studies. In a study of HRSV hospitalized children, higher titers of pre-F and G antibodies in acute-phase serum samples were associated with less severe disease.[85] In another study of HRSV disease in infants, F but not G antibody titers in acute-phase sera were associated with a decrease in a composite measure of illness severity.[641] In a challenge study, higher titers of neutralizing, anti-F and anti-G secretory or serum antibodies were associated with a decreased risk of reinfection,[257] and there are similar findings for natural infection.[637] In a study of HRSV-infected HSCT recipients, early recovery was associated with higher levels of antibodies against G but not against pre- or post-F.[197]

Studies of passive immunoprophylaxis in high-risk infants with either intravenous Ig containing high titers of HRSV-neutralizing antibodies (RSV-IGIV) or HRSV-neutralizing F MAbs (palivizumab, motavizumab; these products are described in "Prevention" below) support the protective effect of a high titer of serum HRSV-neutralizing antibodies against severe HRSV disease in young infants.[86,238,469] Studies of passively transferred antibodies in experimental animals also illustrate the protective effect of high titer serum HRSV-neutralizing antibodies (below). Serum IgG antibodies gain access to the respiratory tract primarily by the relatively inefficient process of passive transudation. Transfer is more effective into the lower than the upper respiratory tract. For example, in studies of passively transferred antibodies in the cotton rat model, serum titers of 1:390 and 1:3,500 were required to achieve a 99% reduction in HRSV replication in the lower and upper respiratory tract, respectively.[494] As another indication of the concentration gradient between the circulation and the lumen of the respiratory tract, the therapeutic effect of passive antibodies in reducing HRSV replication in cotton rats was 160-fold greater when administered directly to the respiratory tract versus systemically.[491] Studies in humans suggested an antibody concentration gradient of approximately 350:1 between sera and nasal washes.[633] The gradient between blood and the lower respiratory tract is thought to be lower (i.e., greater transfer), as shown in the cotton rat studies noted above. The consequence is that passive administration of HRSV-neutralizing antibodies is more effective at preventing LRI than URI.[86,238,469] Higher serum HMPV antibody titers were associated with lower rate of infection but not with less severe disease in one study.[179]

Development of stabilized pre-F protein and characterization of epitopes on pre-F and post-F have helped fine-tune our understanding of F-specific neutralizing antibodies.[31,419] Ngwuta et al. determined that most HRSV-neutralizing antibodies as measured in cell lines are readily absorbed out with pre-F protein, some with post-F protein, and some with G protein.[457] With epitope mutation and antibody competition studies, they also determined the relative binding at different epitopes. The antigenic site Ø was associated with binding of a substantial part of the neutralizing activity in many but not all serum specimens. A study of 364 F-specific MAbs developed from memory B cells from three adults also demonstrated variability in the proportion of antibodies against antigenic sites on F with another site, site V, being most common. In this study, some antibodies were 100-fold more potent than palivizumab, and some cross-reacted with HMPV.[211] Two other studies of MAbs derived from human memory B cells showed diversity in site-specific reactivity patterns, with most MAbs binding both pre-F and post-F, but usually with greater binding to pre-F[14]; potent neutralizing pre-F MAbs reacted at a variety of epitopes and some reacted against and neutralized both HRSV and HMPV.[671] The specificity of the HRSV–HMPV cross-reacting MAbs varied, including some that bound at antigenic site IV and others at site V.

Animal studies show that the G protein also induces HRSV-neutralizing antibodies and protective immunity.[118] G MAbs that bind to the relatively conserved central region of the G protein and block binding to CX3CR1, a major HRSV receptor, have direct HRSV neutralizing activity. As noted above (see "Replicative Cycle" and "Propagation In Vitro"), these antibodies are not detected by traditional neutralization assays that employ immortalized cell lines such as HEp-2 and Vero that are deficient in CX3CR1; detection requires the use of HAE or HBE cultures that express functional CX3CR1. Alternatively, detection of G-specific antibodies can be broadened by adding complement to the traditional assay, but this does not detect all antibodies to the central conserved domain.[123] Thus, the potential contribution of G-protein–specific antibodies to the neutralization of HRSV is likely underappreciated with the neutralization assays commonly used.

G MAbs that bind to the conserved central region of the G protein also have anti-inflammatory and Fc-dependent antiviral activity in animal studies.[61] In animal studies, Fc-mediated antiviral activity has also been associated with anti-F antibodies and F and SH vaccination and can be cell mediated through antibody-dependent cellular cytotoxicity (ADCC) or complement activation.[280,539] In animals, this combination of an antiviral and anti-inflammatory activity of G was highly effective at promptly decreasing HRSV replication and disease when given 3 days postinfection, while an anti-F neutralizing MAb was effective at promptly decreasing replication, but much less effective at decreasing disease.[62] The anti-inflammatory effects associated with G MAbs to the conserved central domain may be due to blocking G from inducing host responses that contribute to disease, such as host responses triggered by G binding to CX3CR1.

T Lymphocytes

Experience with patients with deficiencies in cell-mediated immunity has demonstrated its importance in restricting HRSV and other enveloped respiratory viruses.[255,329,655] Immunodeficient children fail to clear HRSV and can shed virus for months rather than the typical interval of 1 to 3 weeks. Severely immunocompromised adults, such as HSCT recipients or individuals with leukemia, are readily infected with HRSV and have a high incidence of serious disease and death. HMPV also can cause severe disease in HSCT recipients,[82] although there also can be prolonged shedding without disease.[145]

In the mouse model for HRSV, depletion of the CD4+ and CD8+ T-lymphocyte subsets individually or together showed that both are important in clearing a primary infection.[229] Both subsets also contributed to disease in that model, with CD8+ cells having the greater effect.[229] In contrast, depletion of B lymphocytes indicated that HRSV-specific antibodies are not required for clearance of a primary infection in mice, although they reduced disease and were important for restricting reinfection.[227] While treatment with HRSV-neutralizing antibodies can greatly reduce viral replication in HRSV-infected mice, it was inefficient in eliminating the virus, illustrating the importance of cellular immunity for viral clearance.[467]

In humans, robust CD8+ T-cell responses have been documented in the peripheral blood of infants and children during primary and secondary HRSV infections (e-Fig. 10.11B), which precedes the migration of these cells to the respiratory tract.[269,270] Infants with severe HRSV disease have increased numbers of T lymphocytes in the airways, with a greater abundance of the CD8+ versus CD4+ subset, and a greater proportion of airway CD8+ T cells compared with rhinovirus-infected children.[172,270,423] However, although the number of CD8+ T cells was increased by infection, they did not constitute a particularly abundant cell population either in fluid recovered from the airways of infants with severe HRSV disease[172,270,423] or in pulmonary tissue from infants that experienced severe or fatal HRSV infection.[294,651] In another study, increased disease was observed in a severely immunocompromised child with a long-term HRSV infection following transfer of donor lymphocytes.[166] However, in infants and children with HRSV LRI, the timing of the CD8+ T-cell response did not correlate with disease: specifically, the appearance of virus-specific CD8+ T cells in peripheral blood peaked during recovery 9 to 15 days following the onset of symptoms[269,388] (e-Fig. 10.11B). In addition, the magnitude of the systemic virus-specific CD8+ T-cell response did not correlate with disease severity.[269] In a controlled human infection model in adults, tissue resident memory CD4+ and CD8+ T cells specific for a broad spectrum of HRSV epitopes were detected in bronchial biopsies, and high frequencies of HRSV specific CD8+ T cells, but not CD4+ T cells, were associated with reduced symptoms and viral load.[242,302] Thus, while studies in mice suggest that CD8+ T cells make an important contribution to HRSV disease severity, this is less evident from observations in humans.

An increased response of Th2 versus Th1 CD4+ lymphocytes (defined by the signature cytokines IL-4 and IFN-γ, respectively) may contribute to pathogenic responses to HRSV infection and reinfection. The clinical picture of severe HRSV disease, including airway plugging, wheezing, and long-lasting effects on lung function, has some similarity with asthma, which involves a Th2 bias. As noted above, young infants can have a Th2 bias lingering from the prenatal period. Also, studies in rodents indicate that a Th2-biased response was involved in the enhanced HRSV disease that was associated with a formalin-inactivated HRSV vaccine evaluated in the 1960s (see "Prevention"). However, analogies to asthma and the formalin-inactivated vaccine are inexact because disease in those examples depends on prior sensitization, whereas HRSV disease during

natural infection is most severe during the initial exposure and is less severe with repeat exposures.

The evidence for Th2-biased responses in HRSV disease is mixed. In some studies, peripheral blood mononuclear cells from infants hospitalized with HRSV disease exhibited a Th2-biased HRSV-specific recall response when stimulated *in vitro*.[39,516] However, other studies documented Th1-biased responses[63] or heterogeneity in responses, with some infants having Th1-biased responses and others Th2.[360,435] Th2-biased cytokine responses detected in respiratory washes from infants infected with HRSV were significantly higher than from influenza virus–infected infants.[587] A positive association was found between HRSV disease and a genetic polymorphism in the IL-4 gene that increases gene expression.[434] Other studies detected Th2-biased responses predominantly in individuals with a history of asthma or allergy, suggesting that Th2 involvement is linked to those with this predisposition.[323,363] In another study, Th2-biased responses were observed with influenza and HPIV in addition to HRSV and were greater in individuals ≤3 months of age compared to those greater than 3 months of age, suggesting that this reflects a Th2 bias during the first few months of life but is not specific to HRSV.[341]

Studies in mice suggest that NK cells and HRSV-specific CD8+ CTLs play an important role in enhancing Th1 and limiting Th2 responses to HRSV antigens during infection, an effect mediated by secretion of IFN-γ and probably other regulatory molecules.[284,463,574] IFN-α/β also appeared to enhance Th1 and suppress Th2 responses.[160,446] In addition, HRSV-specific CD8+ T cells may reduce virus-induced inflammation through the secretion of IL-10.[579]

Viral Evasion of Host Immunity

HRSV readily reinfects symptomatically (but usually with reduced disease) throughout life without need for significant antigenic change, and symptomatic reinfection by HMPV also appears to be common (see "Epidemiology"). This contrasts with, for example, influenza A virus, for which symptomatic reinfection usually depends on significant antigenic change, or measles virus, for which infection typically confers lifelong protection. The ability of HRSV to reinfect throughout life is often taken as evidence of viral inhibition of host immune responses. HRSV (and HMPV) indeed has mechanisms that directly inhibit or interfere with host innate and adaptive immunity (e-Fig. 10.8).[548,569] Conversely, some features of HRSV (and HMPV) biology provide for avoidance of host immunity rather than direct inhibition.

Examples of direct inhibition of host responses have already been noted for HRSV, including very effective inhibition of type I and type III IFN production and signaling, inhibition of apoptosis, inhibition of TNF-α and NF-κB signaling, and inhibition of PKR activation and stress granule formation. HRSV also inhibits signaling from type II IFN (IFN-γ) in macrophages.[550]

In addition, studies in the mouse model with HRSV mutants showed that the presence of the fractalkine motif in the G protein reduces the pulmonary influx of CX3CR1-bearing leukocytes, including subsets of NK cells and CD4+ and CD8+ T cells.[264] In a separate effect, the central conserved domain of G was shown to reduce activation of TLR2, TLR4, and TLR9 in human monocytes, thus suppressing innate immune responses.[486] Maturation of mDC in response to HRSV infection was partly suppressed by the NS proteins.[446] In addition, expression of NS1 was associated with a shift toward Th2 polarization, reduced Th17 polarization, and reduced activation of CD8+ T cells bearing CD103, a homing integrin that directs CD8+ T cells to mucosal epithelial cells.[446]

Experimental viral infection studies in adults showed that peripheral IgA memory B cells were undetectable following HRSV infection, whereas they were detected following natural influenza virus infection, and levels of IgA against HRSV appeared to be reduced and transient compared to IgA against influenza virus.[244] The mechanism of this effect remains to be identified.

Some studies demonstrated reduced activation and altered polarization of CD4+ T lymphocytes *in vitro* in response to HRSV-exposed human mDCs,[140,241,518] although other results suggest that HRSV does not differ significantly from HMPV, HPIV3, and influenza A virus in this regard.[356,359] HRSV also can suppress T-cell proliferative responses *in vitro* by direct contact mediated by the F protein.[541] Some reports indicated that CD8+ CTL are functionally down-regulated in the HRSV-infected lung. This was originally suggested to reflect immune inhibition by HRSV,[91] but further studies showed that this effect does not appear to be specific to HRSV but rather is a property of the tissue.[155,623] This may be a mechanism to reduce lung injury, although it would also reduce immune protection.

Some features of HRSV biology provide for evasion rather than direct inhibition of host immunity. HRSV is highly infectious, which likely promotes infection and spread in a partly-immune population. The tropism of HRSV (and HMPV) for the superficial layer of the epithelium together with apical budding and low invasiveness and low cytopathogenicity (e.g., Fig. 10.5) likely reduce the display of viral antigen to the host immune system.[682] In addition, the effectiveness of host immune protection is reduced at the superficial airway epithelium, as has already been noted in regard to the gradient of antibody titer between the blood and respiratory surface (see "Antibodies" above).

As already noted, young infants mount weak and short-lived immune responses, which is due to host factors (immunologic immaturity and suppression by maternal antibodies) rather than viral factors. This is particularly relevant for HRSV because of its ability to infect in the first months of life, a time when maternal antibodies are protective against many other pathogens including other common respiratory viruses. Why HRSV is more efficient in infecting early in life despite maternal antibodies is not known. One factor may be its high infectivity as already noted. Another may be that HRSV expresses a secreted form of the G protein that acts as an antigen decoy to spare virus from neutralizing antibodies and reduce antibody-mediated clearance by immune cells.[77]

As noted above, another factor contributing to evasion of host immunity is that the HRSV G protein is less efficient than F as a protective antigen and generally is a poor inducer of CD8+ CTLs. The HMPV G protein also does not appear to be a significant protective antigen, at least in experimental animals. The unusual amino acid content, nonglobular structure, and high content of host-specified sugars for these G proteins may reduce their immunogenicity.

In the case of the F protein, the metastable nature of the pre-F protein and its propensity to be triggered to refold irreversibly into the post-F form limits the exposure of the most potent neutralizing epitopes to the host immune system. Consistent with this, analysis of the F-specific antibody response in humans by phage cloning identified heterogeneity in the ability of individual antibodies to react with F protein present in virions and infected cells.[531]

As noted, exposure of mDCs *in vitro* to HRSV and HMPV induced only a low-to-moderate level of mDC maturation.[140] In addition, in mDCs infected with HRSV or HMPV, up-regulation of the CCR7 receptor that is necessary for mDC migration to lymphatic tissue was inefficient.[357] As noted above, the HRSV NS proteins had a suppressive effect on maturation. However, weak maturation also was due to poor infection and insufficient stimulation, rather than strong inhibition.[357,359]

Newly formed HRSV and HMPV virions associate with filopodia on the surface of infected epithelial cells, which appear to deliver virions directly to neighboring epithelial cells in a manner that shields them from mucins and neutralizing antibodies.[165,328,424]

The sequestration of cellular response proteins into cytoplasmic viral inclusion bodies is another potentially potent means of interfering with host responses to infection but probably is not unique to HRSV (and HMPV) since a number of related viruses also form inclusion bodies that seem to be similar.

While these various mechanisms of immune evasion have been described for HRSV, their aggregate impact is not clear. Indeed, it is not clear that, beyond young infancy, protective responses to HRSV and HMPV are inherently weak. Primary infection of seronegative mice and cotton rats with HRSV induces robust antibody and cellular immune responses and long-lived protective immunity.[228,493] Infection of seronegative chimpanzees with wild-type HRSV or with strongly attenuated live vaccine candidates induced very robust serum antibody titers and protection.[130,602,657,660] With HMPV, infection of mice or cotton rats results in a strong neutralizing serum antibody response and clearance of the virus, although there was one report of prolonged virus replication for 60 days.[6,261] In one report, infection of cynomolgus macaques with HMPV resulted in neutralizing serum antibody responses that waned substantially over the course of several months and provided poor protection against challenge 8 months later,[626] but other studies in AGMs documented strong immune responses to live-attenuated HMPV vaccine candidates.[47] In young children ≥6 months of age, a single dose of live-attenuated HRSV candidates induced substantial levels of serum HRSV-neutralizing antibodies that appeared to be associated with protective immunity and were stable over the winter season.[308] Young children with low levels of maternal antibodies have very strong responses of serum virus-neutralizing antibodies in response to HRSV infection.[557] In human adults, titers of neutralizing antibodies to HMPV and HRSV are quite high.[179,180] Importantly, reinfection with either virus usually causes substantially reduced disease (see "Epidemiology"), indicating that prior infections induce substantial protection against clinically significant disease.

Thus, the ability of HRSV (and HMPV) to readily reinfect without significant antigenic change appears to be due to the ability to subvert some aspects of host protective mechanisms and to avoid other aspects, combined with its ability to infect early in life when immune responses are reduced. Most viruses possess multiple mechanisms to subvert host responses. Whether HRSV is particularly immunosuppressive remains unclear.

EPIDEMIOLOGY

The burden of HRSV (and HMPV) infection, morbidity, and mortality is greatest at both ends of life—in infancy and old age—and in individuals with certain underlying conditions, as discussed below. Older children and non-elderly adults who are otherwise healthy typically have substantially reduced HRSV (and HMPV) infection and disease.

Infection of Infants and Young Children

HRSV is the most important global cause of severe acute viral LRI in infants and young children. In a benchmark surveillance study from 1957 to 1976 in Washington, DC, HRSV was detected in 23.3% of hospitalizations for respiratory tract disease in infants and young children, compared with 11.5%, 6%, 3.2%, and 5.2% of hospitalizations with HPIV3, HPIV1, HPIV2, and influenza A virus, respectively.[325] Similar relative proportions of ARI hospitalizations have been attributed to HRSV and the other respiratory viruses in children less than 5 years of age in multiple subsequent studies in the United States and other countries.[258,286,485] HRSV infection is found in a high percentage of young children hospitalized with bronchiolitis (40% to 75%), commonly in those hospitalized with pneumonia, and less commonly in those hospitalized with bronchitis (around 10%) or croup (10% to 30%).[325,432] It has been estimated that there are between 57,527 and 126,306 hospitalizations for HRSV disease in children under 5 years of age annually in the United States.[258,361,552] The burden of HRSV disease is not confined to hospitalization. In the United States, an estimated 2.1 to 4.2 million children under the age of 5 years (representing 10% to 20% of that age group) receive medical care each year for HRSV-related illness.[258,361] Hall et al.[258] estimated that this involves 517,747 (1 of 38) visits to the emergency room and 1,534,064 (1 of 13) primary care office visits, in addition to the hospitalizations already noted. Pediatric deaths in high-income countries are uncommon as illustrated for the United States in one study, estimating approximately 300 deaths per year, mostly in children less than 1 year of age.[607] Similar estimated yearly deaths are reported in other studies.[78]

Less is known about the burden of HMPV disease in children, but it is usually detected in one-third to one-half of the numbers of hospitalizations for ARI due to HRSV.[286,661,662] Its clinical presentation is similar to HRSV, with upper respiratory tract symptoms with or without lower respiratory tract symptoms of bronchitis, bronchiolitis, or pneumonia. It can also present with fever without localizing symptoms.

Worldwide, HRSV is estimated to cause from 21.6 to 50.3 million episodes of acute LRI, 2.7 to 3.8 million hospital admissions, and 94,600 to 149,400 deaths each year in children under 5 years of age.[555] Since most HRSV deaths in developing countries likely occur outside the hospital where the cause of death is usually not determined, estimating HRSV deaths in these settings is difficult. However, studies are beginning to provide data on HRSV-associated deaths outside the hospital in low-income communities in a variety of settings. The results of these studies should improve the accuracy of these estimates. In preliminary results from postmortem diagnostics of deceased children in sub-Saharan Africa and South Asia, HRSV was associated with 6% of 304 deaths in children 1 to 60 months of age.[596] In a study in a low-income community in Argentina, HRSV was estimated to result in 0.26 in home deaths in children less than 1 year of age per 100 live births.[80] In a study of suspected bacterial infection in infants 1 to 59 days old in Southeast Asia, HRSV was the single most commonly identified pathogen at 5.4% of those suspected of having an infection and also was linked to about 2% of the deaths.[529]

HRSV infection is common in the first year of life, with around 50% to 70% of children having serologic evidence of infection by 1 year of age and most by 2 years of age.[13,214,273,325] Primary infection is usually symptomatic with 25% to 40% having symptoms of LRI.[214] Reinfections can occur throughout life without significant antigenic change: there can be variability in circulating strains due to the two antigenic subgroups and changes at a few antigenic sites, most commonly in G (see "Antigenic Subgroups and Genotypes" and "The Yearly HRSV Pandemic"), but reinfection does not require this variability. Reinfections usually are associated with a decrease in disease severity (see "Infection of Adults").[273] In one prospective study,[214] 47% and 45% of the children infected in their first year were reinfected during their 2nd and 3rd years of life, respectively.

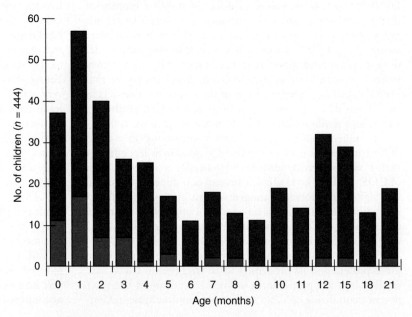

FIGURE 10.10 Age at time of hospitalization for HRSV disease at the Johns Hopkins Hospital during 1993–1996. The *red bars* indicate more severe disease. (Courtesy of Dr. Ruth A. Karron. Adapted from Karron RA, Singleton RJ, Bulkow L, et al. Severe respiratory syncytial virus disease in Alaska native children. RSV Alaska Study Group. *J Infect Dis* 1999;180(1):41–49.)

In a longitudinal day care center study, among young children infected during one HRSV outbreak, 74% and 65% were reinfected in outbreaks during the following 2 years, respectively.[273] Severe HRSV disease is most frequent between 1 and 6 months of life, with a peak incidence at 1 to 3 months of life (Fig. 10.10). However, infections and reinfections later in childhood are associated with a substantial disease burden as illustrated in one study where 61% of all HRSV-associated health care visits in the first 5 years of life occurred in children 2 to 5 years of age.[258]

Primary infections with HMPV typically occur slightly later in life than HRSV infections, with the peak of hospitalization occurring at about 6 months of life.[286] Acquisition of HMPV antibodies has usually been reported to occur later than acquisition of HRSV antibodies, with most children becoming positive by age 5.[625] As with HRSV, reinfection with HMPV is frequent during the first few years of life without significant antigenic change. In infants, the second HMPV infection can present with upper or lower respiratory tract disease, as with HRSV.[663]

Prematurity (birth at <36 weeks gestation, and especially <28 weeks of gestation), young age, underlying lung, cardiac disease, and immune deficiency are major risk factors for serious complications with HRSV infection.[236,421] Other factors associated with increased hospitalization include increased exposure (day care attendance, siblings under 5 years of age, and admission to the hospital during HRSV season) and other risk factors (low titers of maternal antibodies, lack of previous HRSV infection, young age at infection, asthma or a family history of asthma, poverty, exposure to smoke from tobacco or other sources in the household, and male gender).[128,585] In one study, the estimated number of HRSV hospitalizations per 1,000 during the first year of life was 388 for infants with chronic lung disease, 92 for those with congenital heart disease, 66 for those born at 29 to less than 33 weeks, and 30 for term infants with no underlying disease.[60] Very high rates of hospitalization can occur in certain populations. In American Indian and Alaska Native children, the risk of hospitalization for HRSV is three to five times greater than that of the general U.S. pediatric population,[57,314] and high rates of severe HRSV disease have been observed in other aboriginal populations. Recipients of HSCTs are at high risk for serious complications of HRSV infection.[192] Overall, however, the majority (50% to 70%) of HRSV hospitalizations occur in previously healthy full-term infants.[60,488] Children born prematurely or having comorbidities including underlying pulmonary, cardiac, neurologic, or immunodeficient conditions are at increased risk of HRSV-associated death.[649] Infection at a young age has been associated with a subsequent increased risk of respiratory disease including asthma.[427,465,559]

Host genetic factors likely also play a role in susceptibility to pediatric HRSV disease. One study found an increased concordance of severe pediatric HRSV infection in identical versus fraternal twins.[608] A number of studies have described positive or negative associations of severe pediatric HRSV disease with polymorphisms in a variety of host genes, notably ones involved in innate immunity and the Th2 subclass of CD4+ T lymphocytes. These include genes for surfactant proteins, TLR4, IL-4, IL-8, IL-9, IL-10, IL-13, IL-18, RANTES (CCL5), CX3CR1, vitamin D receptor, nitric oxide synthetase, transcription factor Jun, IFN-α5, and other innate immunity genes.[532] These gene-association studies remain preliminary and are sometimes contradictory, often because the study sizes were too small to validate associations, but they suggest that a number of genes likely contribute to resistance or susceptibility to severe HRSV disease but determining which

ones will require validation.[532] Biomarker and epigenetic changes have also been associated with severity of HRSV[464,672] but, as with the genetic associations, need to be validated.

Infection of Adults

All adults have been infected with HRSV in childhood, but the virus reinfects 2% to 10% each year.[175,178] Reinfection is more frequent in adults with increased exposure to the virus. For example, during a typical HRSV season, 25% to 50% of health care workers are reinfected, and family members of sick children are readily reinfected. It is likely that adults become susceptible to reinfection as titers of secretory and serum HRSV-neutralizing antibodies from previous exposure decline with time.[181,257] HRSV is considered to be second to influenza as a cause of medically significant respiratory tract disease in adults worldwide[610] and, like influenza, HRSV is associated with and can be misdiagnosed as an exacerbation of underlying chronic lung or heart disease or asthma. In one study, HRSV infection was associated with 10.6% of hospitalizations in the elderly for pneumonia, 11.4% for COPD, 5.4% for congestive heart failure, and 7.2% for asthma.[178] In a study in the United Kingdom using RT-PCR to identify pathogens in various age groups with medically attended respiratory disease, in individuals ≥15 years of age HRSV was identified in 11% to 22% (depending on the year) of cases compared to 16% to 43% with influenza virus.[678] Hospitalization of healthy, nonelderly adults for HRSV disease is rare. However, severe disease and even death due to HRSV can rarely occur in young, previously healthy adults.[551] HMPV reinfection occurs in 1% to 9% of adults each year, with a wide disease spectrum ranging from asymptomatic to severe respiratory disease.[174,638] HRSV is estimated to cause between 10,000 and 20,000 deaths annually in the United States, with 78% of these deaths in adults over age 65.[178,607] Thus, in more affluent countries, there are more deaths due to HRSV in the elderly than in the pediatric population, whereas in less affluent countries, the pediatric burden is likely to be greater. HMPV also afflicts the elderly with hospitalization rates similar to those for HRSV. In one study of adult patients hospitalized for cardiopulmonary conditions, 11% had evidence of HMPV infection, and the frail elderly appeared to be at increased risk of severe disease.[176] In another study of elderly adults hospitalized for respiratory tract disease, HMPV was identified in 8% of cases (ranging from 4.4% to 13.2%, depending on the year), compared to 10.5% for influenza A and 9.6% for HRSV.[174]

Risk of serious complications from HRSV infection is increased with increasing age, comorbidities such as chronic lung and cardiac disease, obesity, and immune suppression.[178,362,543] Though the risk of serious complications is greater with these risk factors, most infections do not require hospitalization. Increased risk of hospitalization with HRSV in adults has also been associated with living in census tracks with high levels of individuals living below the poverty level and high levels of household crowding.[282] Low serum neutralizing antibody titer is associated with increased risk of hospitalization.[639] Immune senescence,[475,577] resulting in a reduced ability to control infection, presumably is an important factor in the increased severity of HRSV and HMPV disease in the elderly.

Other High-Risk Populations

As noted above, HRSV infection is of higher risk in adults and older children with underlying pulmonary or cardiac disease or who are severely immunocompromised, especially with T-cell deficiencies.[655] Immune suppression from a variety of causes is associated with increased HRSV and HMPV disease severity, including congenital immunodeficiencies, HIV infection, immune suppressive treatment for cancer or hematologic malignancies, and solid organ or HSCT.[285,443,655] Mortality associated with HRSV infection in transplant patients is reported as high as 80% to 100%, but rates were lower in more recent studies.[192] The variation in severity of disease likely depends on the type and magnitude of immunosuppression, patient population, diagnostic testing, etc. For HSCT recipients, HRSV infection that occurs pre-engraftment is associated with the highest risk of pneumonia and death, but mortality also is high in those who develop pneumonia postengraftment. HMPV also can cause severe disease in individuals with hematologic malignancies and in HSCT recipients, although mild or asymptomatic infections also can occur. Both HRSV and HMPV can cause severe LRI in lung transplant recipients. HRSV infection also has been associated with chronic rejection and the development of bronchiolitis obliterans in some but not all studies.[396] HRSV is the leading viral cause of hospitalization and reduction in pulmonary function for children with cystic fibrosis.[321] The effect of HIV infection on the severity of HRSV appears to vary by setting. In the United States, prior infection with HIV does not appear to increase the morbidity and mortality associated with HRSV infections in children, though prolonged viral shedding has been reported.[329] In other settings such as South Africa, the severity of HRSV disease was higher in HIV-infected than in HIV-uninfected children and adults.[421]

The Yearly HRSV Pandemic

Community HRSV outbreaks occur each year worldwide with variability in timing in different locations.[461] In temperate climates, HRSV primarily occurs in yearly epidemics of 4 to 5 months duration in the winter and early spring (Fig. 10.11) with substantial variation in the timing and duration of outbreaks between years in the same community and between communities in the same region in the same year.[445,575] Within local variability, there are also regional differences in timing of HRSV outbreaks as illustrated by surveillance data from the United States.[471] In tropical settings, HRSV is often detected throughout the year without well-defined outbreak periods but with peak activity mostly during rainy seasons.[561] In temperate climates, HRSV can also be detected at low levels outside of outbreak periods throughout the year.[67] The seasonal patterns of HRSV outbreaks result, in part, from environmental factors including temperature, humidity, and precipitation.[23] Other factors that may contribute to outbreak timing include population immunity (possibly strain-specific immunity), travelers introducing HRSV from other communities, and superspreading events. HMPV also

occurs primarily in annual epidemics during the late winter and early spring in temperate climates, often overlapping in part or in whole with the annual HRSV epidemic.[2,663] Sporadic HMPV infections can be detected year-round in temperate climates.[163,662]

HRSV is highly infectious and easily spread by contact, especially in settings of close interaction such as day care facilities, hospitals, and families. HRSV is introduced into families primarily by a young school-age child, after which infection spreads to siblings and adults with high frequency.[4] In one prospective study, approximately 40% of all family members older than 1 year were infected after the introduction of HRSV.[254] HRSV can be a serious nosocomial pathogen. The rate of hospital-acquired infection for infants and children during an HRSV season was reported to range from 26% to 47% in newborn units and from 20% to 40% for older children. Hospital staff members appear to play a major role in nosocomial spread of HRSV infection. The likelihood that an individual infant or child will acquire nosocomial HRSV infection increases with the duration of stay and the number of individuals housed in his or her room.[251] Outbreaks in units caring for immunocompromised patients can be devastating.[285] Outbreaks with serious disease can also occur in facilities providing care for institutionalized adults.[191]

An evaluation of the HRSV strains circulating in distinct geographic regions during the same years found that five to seven distinct genotypes representing both antigenic subgroups circulated during the same season in a given location.[478] In a given year, the pattern of genotypes frequently is different in different locations. The pattern of local strains gradually changes in successive years. There typically are one or two dominant local genotypes that are replaced in dominance in successive years. In addition, there can be shifts in the predominance of subgroup A versus B occurring in 1- or 2-year cycles.[644] This presumably reflects an advantage of the heterologous strain in evading previously induced immunity,[656] but reinfection by the same subgroup also frequently occurs. Thus, HRSV outbreaks do not necessarily involve spread of a predominant new strain, as is the case with influenza A virus. Rather, epidemics appear to involve local endemic strains as well new genotypes introduced from other regions. The introduction, spread, and replacement by new strains is nicely illustrated by the subgroup B strain designated BA with a 60-nucleotide duplication in the G gene first detected in 1999[616] and by a subgroup A strain designated ON1 with a 72-nucleotide duplication in the G gene first detected in 2010.[169] Variants of these two strains have become the most common strains globally.[161,615] Similar to HRSV, different strains of HMPV cocirculate during the same season in the same community with the predominant strain and subgroup of that strain varying from year to year.[2,327] In-frame duplications of 180 and 111 nucleotides in the HMPV G ORF were detected in 2014 and 2017, respectively, and quickly became predominant locally.[454]

FIGURE 10.11 Variation in HRSV epidemics during six consecutive years (2014–2020) based on number of HRSV tests performed at Nationwide Children's Hospital in Columbus, Ohio. Each bar represents the number of HRSV cases per month. Numbers above bars indicate the total number of HRSV cases diagnosed each season that typically lasts from October to November until April to May (Courtesy of Dr. Asuncion Mejias.)

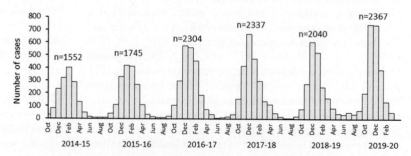

During the first year of the COVID-19 pandemic, the usually seasonal pattern of circulation of HRSV and other respiratory viruses was interrupted in many locations. This is attributed to COVID-19 mitigation measures, such as social distancing, masking, business and school closures, etc.[162] With reopening of businesses, children returning to schools, decreases in social distancing, and masking, HRSV circulation returned, but during times that usually have low levels of circulation and with more disease in older children.[193] Studies of the effect of this unprecedented interruption of respiratory virus circulation will likely provide new information on the epidemiology and disease of HRSV, HMPV, and other respiratory viruses.

CLINICAL FEATURES

HRSV infections are almost always symptomatic in previously healthy infants who encounter the virus for the first time. The clinical presentation is broad, ranging from URI, with or without fever, to LRI in 25% to 40% of children.[214] Bronchiolitis and pneumonia are the primary manifestations of severe HRSV and HMPV LRI, with laryngotracheobronchitis (croup) occurring less frequently. In those infants in whom LRI develops, there is a prodromal phase of rhinorrhea often accompanied by decrease in appetite. Dry cough may appear simultaneously but occurs more often after an interval of 1 to 3 days and can last up to 2 or 3 weeks (Fig. 10.7). At that time, there also may be sneezing and a low-grade fever. Soon after the cough has developed, the child may develop wheezing[66]; if the disease is mild, the symptoms may not progress beyond this stage. Examination in infants with LRI usually shows moderate tachypnea, subcostal and/or intercostal retractions, diffuse inspiratory crackles, and expiratory wheezes. Development of otitis media is common and occurs in up to 75% of infants during or after the acute episode.[606] In most instances, uneventful recovery occurs after an illness of 7 to 12 days (Fig. 10.7). Among infants who require hospitalization with HRSV or HMPV, the most common diagnoses include bronchiolitis and pneumonia. In toddlers and children less than 5 years of age, pneumonia and asthma exacerbations triggered by HRSV and HMPV are also common.[427] Cough is present in most infants, fever in 52% to 86%, and wheezing in about one half of cases.[662] The frequency of fever and wheezing appears to increase with age in infants and young children with HRSV infection.[66] In more severe cases, the child becomes tachypneic, with intercostal and subcostal retractions and/or nasal flaring. There is also evident hyperexpansion of the chest because of air trapping. Infants often feed poorly, because of the increased work of breathing; infants less than 6 months of age are obligate nose breathers, and nasal obstruction prevents adequate respiration during feedings. In advanced disease, the child tires and respiratory failure may occur.

Severe bacterial infections are unusual complications of HRSV[256] or HMPV infections, and clinical guidelines do not recommend routine use of antibiotics.[204] Nevertheless, in clinical trials conducted in infants, a pneumococcal vaccine significantly reduced the incidence of severe HRSV LRI[393] and HMPV LRI,[394] suggesting that there are bacterial–viral interactions that may not be appreciated clinically.[142,582] In contrast, bacterial otitis media is a common complication of HRSV and HMPV URI. HRSV and HMPV are two of the most common precipitating viruses associated with otitis media.[101] HRSV and

HMPV antigens and nucleic acids have been identified in middle ear fluids.[484]

Most infants who require hospitalization for HRSV or HMPV infection are hypoxemic on admission, and a reading on pulse oximeters of less than 90% is a criterion for admission. The hypoxemia is probably due to an abnormally low ventilation/perfusion ratio. In infants with underlying diseases, the progression of symptoms may be rapid, especially in those with cyanotic congenital heart disease or chronic lung disease in whom rates of intensive care unit admission and mechanical ventilation are higher compared to otherwise-healthy term infants.[204,236] Other groups of children at increased risk for severe HRSV and HMPV infection and subsequent respiratory morbidity include those with cystic fibrosis or neuromuscular disorders.[340]

The peak of severe HRSV infection in infants is 2 to 3 months of age, while that for severe HMPV infection tends to be later.[10] Newborn infants with HRSV infection may present with lethargy, irritability, and fever or temperature instability rather than classic bronchiolitis. Symptomatic HMPV infection is rare in newborns. In addition, infants who are born prematurely, and full-term infants younger than 4 to 6 weeks of age, can develop apnea as the first clinical manifestation of HRSV. Apnea often is seen even in the presence of minimal respiratory signs and may be the predominant symptom bringing the infant to medical attention.[496]

HRSV has been detected more frequently than HMPV in the lungs of children that died of sudden infant death syndrome (SIDS). However, the association between these viruses and SIDS is unclear, and the detection of HRSV in some SIDS cases likely reflects its prevalence as well as the concurrence of the peak incidence of both HRSV infection and SIDS in winter months.[385]

Recurrent wheezing and abnormalities in pulmonary function are common after HRSV bronchiolitis or pneumonia and have been reported in 10% to 60% of children for up to 12 years after HRSV infection and might persist even into adulthood.[406,427,559] Postexercise or pharmacologically induced bronchial lability also is increased, despite an absence of symptoms.[563] Evidence suggests that prevention of severe HRSV infections early in life reduces the incidence of recurrent wheezing, suggesting that HRSV can play a causal role,[56,425,560] whereas other evidence is inconclusive.[158] Most of the studies did not observe a link between these lingering respiratory abnormalities and allergic sensitization and the development of persistent asthma, but other studies have suggested such a link,[20,559] and this remains an area of controversy. To date, no such epidemiologic links have been reported for HMPV.

Thus, it remains unclear whether infection with HRSV (and possibly HMPV) causes subsequent abnormal pulmonary function, or whether the abnormalities observed preceded the infection and indeed may have contributed to disease. Martinez et al. measured pulmonary function in infants shortly after birth and found a strong association between reduced pulmonary function in infants at baseline and subsequent development of post-HRSV wheezing.[406] This correlation persisted in children in whom at least one additional lower respiratory infection developed during the first 3 years of life.[406] It is likely that respiratory disease and recurrent abnormalities in children are multifactorial. These factors may include genetic factors that have already been discussed (see "Infection of Infants and Young Children"). They may also include prior underlying anatomic (small airways) and functional abnormalities, as well as an immature immune response that might predispose to initial bronchiolitis and subsequent development of recurrent wheezing. Environmental factors such as secondhand smoke exposure may trigger episodes of lower respiratory dysfunction and aggravate long-term or recurrent airway pathology.

Symptomatic HRSV infections are common in adults, particularly in medical personnel or in individuals caring for small children.[251,254] Those infections are usually characterized by rhinorrhea, pharyngitis, cough, bronchitis, constitutional symptoms including headache, fatigue, and low-grade fever. Disease usually lasts about 5 days but may be more prolonged. In contrast, HMPV infection in adults is often asymptomatic, though the spectrum of clinical illness in symptomatic individuals is similar to HRSV, with hoarseness being particularly prominent in young adults.[638] In older people, particularly those with underlying cardiac or pulmonary diseases such as COPD, severe LRI may occur with HRSV or HMPV, requiring hospitalization and intensive care.[176,178,554] HRSV infection in severely immunocompromised individuals may not present with the classic symptoms identified in a noncompromised host and may evolve quickly into LRI that is associated with high morbidity and mortality.

DIAGNOSIS

Differential Diagnosis

The differential diagnosis of HRSV and HMPV infection in young infants must include all other causes of acute LRI. This includes HPIVs, particularly HPIV3, adenoviruses, influenza viruses, rhinoviruses, endemic coronaviruses, and enteroviruses. In infants younger than 3 months of age, *Chlamydia pneumoniae* should be considered, which causes afebrile interstitial pneumonia with cough and, in some cases, wheezing. *Mycoplasma pneumoniae* and *Bordetella pertussis* also are in the differential. In HIV-infected or immunocompromised infants, infection with *Pneumocystis jirovecii* should be considered. Differentiation from bacterial pneumonia may occasionally be difficult, although wheezing is rarely present in children with classic pyogenic bacterial pneumonia, and infants with bacterial pneumonia typically have lobar infiltrates. In older infants, infections with HRSV or HMPV must be differentiated from other causes of mild respiratory tract infection as well as causes of acute bronchospastic disease, including environmental allergens and aspiration of a foreign body.

In the elderly, HRSV or HMPV infection should be suspected in any patient (with or without underlying cardiopulmonary disease) who has acute bronchitis, pneumonia, or wheezing, with or without a low-grade fever, particularly when such an event occurs as part of a cluster of cases in the winter season.

Presumptive diagnosis of HRSV bronchiolitis in infants can often be made on the basis of the clinical syndrome combined with the time of year and other epidemiologic features. It is common to observe that other members of the family have respiratory illness at the time of, or just preceding, an episode of HRSV bronchiolitis or pneumonia in an infant. Usually, the infant has far more serious illness than other members of the family, as primary HRSV infections are more severe.[254]

Radiographic findings for HRSV and HMPV are common but relatively nonspecific. The classic chest radiographic findings of HRSV and HMPV bronchiolitis include hyperaeration, a flattened diaphragm because of the air trapping, diffuse prominent lung markings due to bronchial wall thickening, and focal areas of atelectasis.

Laboratory Diagnosis

Definitive diagnosis of HRSV and HMPV depends on laboratory tests. Rapid detection of HRSV or HMPV is desirable to guide the use of appropriate infection-control measures and to limit unnecessary antibiotic use. In practice, however, while diagnostic testing is typically performed in academic centers, it may be used less frequently in community hospitals or primary care settings.

Although the gold standard is isolation of virus in cell culture from nasal swabs, nasal washes, or nasopharyngeal aspirates, the lability of HRSV, the slow growth characteristics of HMPV, the expense of the technique, the duration of 4 to 7 days needed for results, and the increasing availability of rapid assays based on detection of viral antigen or—more frequently—nucleic acid have made cell culture an increasingly infrequent choice, and most diagnostic virology laboratories in academic centers have abandoned this technique.

More rapid diagnosis can be made by the detection of viral antigen in nasal swabs or washes using direct immunofluorescence assay (DFA), antigen-capture enzyme-linked immunoassay (EIA), or by lateral flow immunochromatography.[213] Both DFA and EIA for HRSV are commercially available (with the former being more sensitive than the latter), and DFA is commercially available for HMPV. The sensitivity of the EIA rapid commercial tests, which produce results in less than 30 minutes, generally is lower than that of DFA, and negative results should be confirmed by PCR. In addition, antigen-based tests in general often have reduced sensitivity in adults due to low levels of viral shedding.[175]

RT-PCR of viral RNA for detection of HRSV or HMPV in respiratory samples is an especially useful method of diagnosis for both pediatric and adult populations, because the sensitivity of these assays allows detection of small quantities of virus. RT-PCR can be used in multiplex formats capable of detecting multiple pathogens with a fast turn-around time (<1 hour) and no need for technical expertise.[205] RT-PCR is more sensitive than virus culture or antigen assay.

Serologic methods are used infrequently (apart from clinical studies) and provide only retrospective information, since serum antibody rises are detected by analysis of sera collected at least 2 to 4 weeks postinfection. Typically, serum antibodies are detected by ELISA or microneutralization assay, with fourfold or greater increases considered indicative of infection.

TREATMENT AND PREVENTION

Treatment

Most infants and children with mild HRSV LRI can be managed as outpatients. Treatment of more severe LRI can be guided by measurement of oxygenation, monitoring respiratory rate, and evaluation of dehydration. Severe respiratory distress, hypoxia, and dehydration are among the indications for hospitalization.

The American Academy of Pediatrics (AAP) has issued evidence-based recommendations for the diagnosis and management of bronchiolitis,[497] most cases of which can likely be attributed to HRSV, human rhinovirus, or HMPV. Where appropriate, AAP recommendations are cited below.

Symptomatic Interventions and Supportive Care

Inpatient treatment of HRSV infection requires supportive care: frequent suction of the airway to remove secretions is one of the most important aspects along with administration of humidified oxygen, administration of nasogastric or intravenous fluids if there are signs of dehydration or severe tachypnea, and, in the most severe cases, respiratory assistance with noninvasive or invasive mechanical ventilation. Current AAP guidelines suggest the use of supplemental oxygen if the percent oxygen saturation (SpO_2) falls below 90%. Antibiotic therapy should not be used unless there are indications that a bacterial coinfection is present, such as acute otitis media. The youngest premature and full-term infants infected with HRSV may require monitoring for apnea. Improvements in supportive care clearly have made a major impact on mortality from severe HRSV disease, resulting in the current low mortality rate in high-resource settings.

Corticosteroids are not recommended for the management of acute bronchiolitis as indicated by the current AAP guidance.[497] Systemic corticosteroids have been used for the treatment of HRSV bronchiolitis since the 1960s, based in part on their effectiveness in the treatment of acute asthma and on the premise that much of HRSV disease is immune mediated. However, observational studies, randomized clinical trials, and meta-analysis of placebo-controlled studies indicated that systemic glucocorticoids provided no improvement in oxygenation, respiratory rate, or length of hospitalization, but its use was associated with increased viral shedding.[74,205,474] In addition, a large controlled study indicated that inhaled glucocorticoids provided no improvement in wheezing following HRSV bronchiolitis.[167]

Other anti-inflammatory approaches for the treatment of HRSV have also been considered. Acute HRSV bronchiolitis is associated with elevations of cysteinyl leukotrienes in respiratory secretions[136]; however, the leukotriene receptor antagonist montelukast was not effective in ameliorating acute bronchiolitis.[8] Assessment of the utility of montelukast for prevention of post-HRSV wheezing episodes has yielded conflicting results[53] and further studies may be warranted.

Drugs used to treat reversible bronchospasm in asthma have also been used to treat HRSV infection. However, systematic reviews indicate that they provide only modest short term to no improvement and the current AAP guidance does not recommend the administration of bronchodilators to infants and children with bronchiolitis.[497] Nebulized hypertonic saline increases mucociliary clearance, and its use has been associated with modest reductions in length of stay and improved clinical disease severity scores. Current AAP guidance suggests that nebulized 3% hypertonic saline can be used for the management of infants and children hospitalized for bronchiolitis.[681]

Antiviral Interventions

Ribavirin, a nucleoside analog, is a broad-spectrum antiviral whose mode of action remains unclear, but which exhibits potent activity against HRSV and HMPV in cell culture and animal models.[670] Ribavirin was approved in 1986 in the United States for use in the treatment of severe HRSV infection.[631] A review showed that some improvement in a subjectively or objectively measured outcome was observed in 7 of 11 published randomized clinical trials of ribavirin, although the size and quality of the trials were highly variable.[331] Ribavirin is difficult to administer via aerosol, can cause anemia, and concerns have been raised about its teratogenic effect and health risks for caregivers.[513] Currently, the AAP does not recommend the routine use of ribavirin for the management of bronchiolitis, although it could be considered in immunocompromised children who are at increased risk for severe disease. Aerosolized and oral ribavirin have been used empirically for the management of HRSV LRI in HSCT or lung transplant patients[58,479] and retrospectively this has been reported to reduce mortality. Ribavirian also has been used anecdotally in immunocompromised children and adults with HMPV LRI.[500]

The incidence and severity of HRSV disease requiring hospitalization in high-risk infants can be reduced by prophylaxis with HRSV-neutralizing MAbs (see "Prevention"). MAbs (i.e., palivizumab and motavizumab) also have been evaluated for therapy of established HRSV infection.[400,499] In those studies, intravenous administration of mAbs reduced viral shedding by 10-fold, but a clear effect on clinical outcome was not demonstrated. It is possible that much of the LRI observed by the time infants reach the hospital (usually several days into their illnesses) is caused by existing viral damage or immune responses and will not be ameliorated by subsequent antiviral treatment. However, antibody preparations sometimes are used empirically for treating severely immunocompromised individuals, in whom viral shedding and infection can be prolonged,[96] although definite evidence of efficacy is lacking.[535]

Small-molecule antiviral drugs specific for HRSV targeting different viral proteins have undergone or are under evaluation in clinical trials.[382,583] There are three main categories depending on the viral target and the mechanisms of action: F protein inhibitors, N protein inhibitors, and RNA-dependent RNA polymerase (L protein) inhibitors. Of those, compounds that bind to the F protein (i.e., fusion inhibitors) have undergone the most extensive testing.

- N protein inhibitors: A drug specific to the N protein (RSV604)[94] was evaluated in 2006 in a phase 2 clinical trial in HRSV-infected adult HSCT recipients (ClinicalTrials. gov NCT00232635) and appeared to benefit a small subgroup of patients; however, it was discontinued because of its suboptimal potency and the challenge to achieve sufficient drug exposure. RSV604 has been replaced by EDP-938 that also targets the N protein and has a similar mechanism of action. Oral administration of EDP-938 demonstrated antiviral activity *in vitro*, in nonhuman primates, and in adult volunteers experimentally infected with HRSV.[506] EDP-938 is currently undergoing phase 2 clinical trials (ClinicalTrials. gov NCT04633187). A small interfering siRNA that targets the N gene (ALN-RSV01) was evaluated in two phase 2 trials of lung transplant patients with HRSV infection. In those studies, nebulized treatment with ALN-RSV01 for 3 to 5 days was associated with a reduction in the incidence of bronchiolitis obliterans syndrome.[220,679] However, its development has been abandoned.

- Fusion and polymerase inhibitors: Within the past years, orally administered inhibitors specific to the F protein (presatovir [GS-5806], JNJ-53718678, sisunatovir [RV521]) or L protein (lumicitabine [ALS-008176]) have shown antiviral and clinical efficacy in the adult HRSV challenge model.[149,151,152,578] Several other inhibitors targeting the F protein (enzaplatovir [BTA-C585], BTA988, MDT-637) and L protein (PC786 [ClinicalTrials.gov NCT03382431, JNJ-64417184]) have undergone or are undergoing proof of concept studies in the human challenge model. Unfortunately, despite the positive findings in experimentally infected adults, the development of some of these compounds have been abandoned for lack of clinical efficacy or antiviral effect in the main target populations. Presatovir was evaluated in clinical trials in hospitalized adults infected with HRSV and in lung transplant and HCT recipients but failed to improve virologic or clinical outcomes.[97,262,411] The development of lumicitabine was terminated because of toxicity concerns in infants with HRSV infection.[35] Ziresovir [AK0529] is another orally administered fusion inhibitor[684] that was recently shown to have antiviral and clinical effect in hospitalized infants with HRSV infection[35] and is currently being evaluated in adults (ClinicalTrials.gov NCT03699202). Phase 1 studies have evaluated JNJ-53718678 in infants hospitalized with HRSV infection with promising results. Randomized phase 2 trials in infants and young children hospitalized or evaluated in the outpatient setting with HRSV infection (ClinicalTrials.gov NCT03656510; NCT04068792), as well as in adults (ClinicalTrials.gov NCT03379675) are ongoing.[410] Sisunatovir[106] is also undergoing phase 2 clinical trials in hospitalized infants (ClinicalTrials.gov NCT04225897), and in adult HCT patients (ClinicalTrials.gov NCT04267822). Recently ALX-0171, an inhaled anti-F nanobody, was evaluated in two separate clinical trials in HRSV-infected children (ClinicalTrials.gov NCT02979431; NCT03418571) but did not show consistent differences in clinical outcomes and its development has been abandoned.[135]

Small molecule inhibitors are in preclinical development for HMPV. Lumicitabine was evaluated in phase 2 trials in adults with HPMV infection, but the study was terminated (ClinicalTrials.gov NCT03502694).

Because of concerns for development of antiviral resistance, as shown with the administration of presatovir,[581] and to achieve optimal clinical and virologic efficacy, combination therapies are being developed. These strategies involve either the combination of two different antiviral drugs to achieve a higher level of inhibition of viral replication or the combination of one or more antiviral drugs with an anti-inflammatory drug to restrict replication and reduce immune-mediated disease. This latter combination strategy effectively resolved viral replication and disease in the cotton rat model.[495] Similarly, early and aggressive combined therapy involving ribavirin and monoclonal or polyclonal antibody preparations has been used for severely immunocompromised patients. In the more-usual setting of acute HRSV infection of otherwise healthy individuals, antiviral therapy of a rapidly progressing infection such as HRSV is challenging because, by the time the viral agent is identified, it may be too late to control disease and its associated inflammation solely by inhibiting virus replication.

Prevention

Infection Control

Infection by HRSV is reduced by hand washing, limiting exposure to infected individuals, and avoiding self-inoculation of nasal and conjunctival mucosa. Nosocomial spread of HRSV is reduced by the use of gloves and gowns by care givers, strict observance of hand washing, active surveillance for HRSV infection, limiting visitors during the HRSV season, and cohorting infected patients and care givers.[392] As illustration of the effectiveness of infection-control measures to reduce HRSV infection, enhanced infection control using masks and social distancing during the recent SARS-CoV-2 pandemic was associated with a large decrease in infections by HRSV, among other viruses, followed by a resurgence in HRSV when restrictions were relaxed.[162,193] All of these preventive measures would also apply to HMPV.

Passive Immunoprophylaxis Against HRSV

Antibody products

Based on experimental data in animals[493,494] and epidemiologic data in humans[214] indicating that HRSV-neutralizing serum antibodies protected against HRSV LRI, products containing high titers of HRSV-neutralizing antibodies were developed for clinical administration.[512,514] Several of these antibody products proved to be effective for passive immunoprophylaxis (antibodies also have been evaluated for treatment of established infections, but definitive evidence of efficacy is lacking; see "Antiviral Interventions" above). Antibody immunoprophylaxis does not necessarily prevent HRSV infection completely but can restrict replication sufficiently to reduce disease. Serum antibodies are more effective in accessing and protecting the lower respiratory tract than the upper respiratory tract, as noted in "Antibodies".[633] Protection disappears as these passive serum antibodies degrade over the course of several months.

The first product, RSV Immune Globulin Intravenous (RSV-IGIV; RespiGam™, MedImmune), consisted of Ig purified from human donor sera prescreened for high HRSV-neutralizing titers. It was licensed in 1996 for use in infants and young children at high risk for severe HRSV disease due to prematurity or certain underlying conditions.[512] Administered in monthly intravenous infusions during the HRSV season, RSV-IGIV reduced the frequency of hospitalization for HRSV disease by 55% or more and reduced days spent in intensive care by 97%.[238,502] However, it had the disadvantages of a large intravenous infusion, the theoretical risk of adventitious agents, and potential interference with other pediatric vaccines due to the presence of antibodies against common pathogens. MedImmune RSV-IGIV has been superseded by the development of the MAb palivizumab (see below) and has not been available commercially since 2004.

Palivizumab (Synagis™, MedImmune) is an HRSV-neutralizing MAb directed against the F glycoprotein that was licensed in 1998. Palivizumab is based on a murine MAb called 1129[33] that was "humanized" by recombinantly transferring its complementarity-determining regions (~5% of the molecule) onto a human IgG1 backbone (95% of the molecule). Palivizumab recognizes antigenic site II present in both pre- and post-F (Fig.10.4). Palivizumab is 50- to 100-fold more effective on a weight basis than RSV-IGIV and, therefore, can be administered in a much smaller volume by monthly intramuscular injection given up to five times during the HRSV season.

Its clinical efficacy is similar to that of RSV-IGIV.[469] It is recommended for infants and children at high risk of HRSV disease due to prematurity (born <29 weeks gestational age) or certain underlying conditions including chronic lung and heart disease and immunosuppression.[7,512] The theoretical concern of emergence of antibody-resistant mutants has not been a significant problem: resistant mutants are detected in approximately 5% of treated individuals from whom HRSV was recovered but appear to have a modest reduction in growth fitness *in vitro*.[686]

The palivizumab MAb subsequently was modified by *in vitro* affinity maturation to create a better-binding derivative called motavizumab (MEDI-524 or Numax, MedImmune).[512] Motavizumab differs from palivizumab by 13 amino acid substitutions. It exhibited a 70-fold increase in antigen binding and a 20-fold increase in neutralization activity *in vitro*, was substantially more protective in cotton rats, and also protected the upper respiratory tract.[669] In term infants, motavizumab reduced HRSV hospitalizations by 87% and outpatient HRSV MALRIs by 71%,[460] and in preterm infants, it was 26% and 55% more effective than palivizumab in reducing HRSV hospitalization and MALRI, respectively.[86] However, motavizumab was associated with an increase in the incidence of hypersensitivity skin reactions and antidrug antibodies as well as a lack of clear superiority to palivizumab, and the FDA did not support commercialization.

Prior to the problematic clinical data, motavizumab was engineered by three amino acid substitutions (M252Y, S254T, and TD256E, called YTE) to increase its serum half-life by increasing its affinity for a receptor involved in recycling and sparing antibodies that have been taken up intracellularly for degradation.[138] Compared to motavizumab, motavizumab-YTE exhibited a two- to fourfold increase in serum half-life in adults, with serum HRSV-neutralizing activity persisting for 240 days versus 90 days for motavizumab.[509] Motavizumab-YTE has not been developed further due to the issues with motavizumab.

Screening of memory B cells from human donors resulted in the identification of an HRSV-neutralizing MAb called D25 that had more than fivefold greater neutralizing activity than motavizumab.[687] D25 was subjected to mutagenesis to enhance neutralizing activity and reduce its immunogenicity (to minimize the induction of antidrug antibodies). The lead molecule, called MEDI18897*, was 4-, 20-, and 150-fold more potent for *in vitro* neutralization than D25, motavizumab, and palivizumab, respectively. It contained five and four amino acid substitutions, respectively, in the complementarity-determining regions and the heavy chain framework.[687] MEDI18897* was found to bind to the highly conserved antigenic site Ø of the HRSV pre-F protein, which is the most potent neutralization site.[687] MEDI18897* was further modified by the YTE substitutions to create MEDI118897 (nirsevimab, MedImmune/AstraZeneca), which had a serum half-life in humans of 63 to 73 days compared to 19 to 27 days for palivizumab.[234] A single injection of MEDI18897 administered to 969 infants, who were ≤1 year of age and had been preterm, during the 2 months prior to the HRSV season reduced the incidence of HRSV hospitalization by 78% and outpatient HRSV-MALRI by 70% during the 150 days following administration compared to 484 placebo recipients, with no notable adverse or hypersensitivity events.[234] Nirsevimab is being developed for use as a single injection early in life, for both preterm and term infants, with the goal of providing protection that lasts through the first RSV season in life, when vulnerability to severe HRSV disease is greatest.

Not every antibody product has been successful: several other anti-F IgG and IgA MAbs evaluated in clinical trials were not sufficiently effective.[512] Some MAbs to HRSV G also can neutralize infectivity efficiently and in some cases (when directed against the central conserved domain) can reduce inflammatory responses (see "Antibodies") but are not presently in clinical studies.

Maternal immunization

Another strategy for passive HRSV immunoprophylaxis is maternal immunization,[102] whereby pregnant women are given an HRSV vaccine to increase their titers of serum HRSV-neutralizing antibodies. This results in higher transplacental transfer and higher titers in the newborn infants. Maternal serum antibodies degrade with a half-life of approximately 21 to 26 days, and higher titers at birth will prolong their protective effects. Date of birth relative to the local HRSV season is an important factor in maternal immunization; for example, in a location where the HRSV season begins in the fall/early winter, the passive antibody titer at the start of the HRSV season due to maternal immunization will be much higher for an infant born in October than in the preceding March. The mothers also would have the benefit of increased protection against HRSV illness.

A baculovirus-expressed HRSV F subunit nanoparticle vaccine developed by Novavax[342] was evaluated as a single dose vaccine in 4,636 pregnant women for safety and protective efficacy in infants born to immunized mothers.[395] This maternal vaccine had 39% and 44% efficacy against HRSV-MALRI and HRSV hospitalization, respectively, which did not meet the success criterion, but suggested a potential benefit of maternal immunization for protection against severe HRSV disease in infants.[395] Subunit vaccines based on F protein stabilized in the pre-F conformation, the most immunogenic form,[420,521] are under development as maternal vaccines. Pfizer and GlaxoSmithKline are separately evaluating pre-F subunit vaccines in up to 10,000 (NCT04424316) and 20,000 (NCT04605159) pregnant women, respectively, for safety and protection in infants born to immunized mothers. With the use of pre-F in maternal immunization, there is the theoretical concern that increasing the content of maternal antibodies specific to sites Ø and V on pre-F may suppress the induction of antibodies to these important neutralization sites in infants that become infected with HRSV.

Updated information on MAbs and maternal immunization for HRSV immunoprophylaxis is summarized on the PATH RSV Vaccine and mAB Snapshot (https://www.path.org/resources/rsv-vaccine-and-mab-snapshot/) and Trial Tracker (https://www.path.org/resources/rsv-and-mab-trial-tracker/).

In the case of HMPV, the development of products for passive immunoprophylaxis remains at the preclinical stage.[260,512,546] Several MAbs neutralize both HRSV and HMPV.[512,546]

Vaccines
General considerations

HRSV vaccines under development include pediatric vaccines for infants and young children and adult vaccines for the elderly and, as noted above, for maternal immunization. HRSV vaccine development poses challenges, but in recent years, substantial progress has been made. Given the high incidence of RSV disease in infancy and early childhood, a pediatric HRSV vaccine should be administered during infancy, but the optimal time with regard to safety, immunogenicity, and possible coordination with potential products such as nirsevimab remains to be established. Vaccines for infants and young children must satisfy stringent safety expectations. For example, to ensure early detection and assessment of possible reactogenicity, pediatric HRSV vaccine candidates typically must pass stepwise evaluation in the following groups: adults, seropositive older children, seronegative infants and younger children, and in some cases young infants of less than 6 months of age. As noted (see "Antibodies" and e-Fig. 10.12), immune responses in infancy are reduced due to immunologic immaturity and suppression of antibody responses by HRSV-specific maternal antibodies. These inhibitory effects decline substantially by 4 to 6 months of age, suggesting that this might be a suitable lower-age benchmark for HRSV vaccination. In adults, every vaccine recipient will already possess HRSV-specific immunity from prior HRSV infections during life. Preexisting HRSV immunity has been shown to highly restrict live-attenuated RSV vaccines resulting in poor immunogenicity.[215] Also, the immunogenicity of purified HRSV F and G proteins in rodents was reduced by passive transfer of serum HRSV-neutralizing antibodies, although this could be mostly overcome by increased dose of the vaccine.[450] Immune responses in the elderly can have age-related defects.[577] Another challenge to HRSV vaccine development in general is that available experimental animals are only semipermissive for HRSV infection, greatly limiting their usefulness in assessing attenuation, reactogenicity, immunogenicity, protection, and vaccine-enhanced HRSV disease (described below).

While various aspects of innate and adaptive immunity contribute to restricting HRSV infection (see "Immune Response"), serum virus-neutralizing antibodies remain the most reliable measure of protective immunity: higher titers typically correlate with reduced HRSV replication and disease (see "Antibodies"). Evaluating serum antibody responses to vaccines in adults is complicated in that they typically have variable preexisting reciprocal titers of upto approximately 2,000, and HRSV infection results in increases of approximately 3- to 14-fold (larger fold-increases tend to be associated with lower initial titers), followed by a mean decay of 4-fold over the next year.[180,637]

It is not anticipated that an HRSV vaccine will completely prevent HRSV infection and replication. Immune protection in the respiratory tract—especially the upper respiratory tract—is less efficient than protection of the lower respiratory tract. An example of this is the gradient of antibody titer between circulation and the lumen of the respiratory tract (see "Antibodies"). The ability of wild-type HRSV to reinfect without substantial antigenic change is another illustration of the difficulty in completely restricting HRSV infection. However, a successful HRSV vaccine will restrict replication sufficiently to reduce HRSV LRI and hospitalization and also should reduce HRSV illness of lesser severity.

The development of HRSV vaccines is aided by the presence of major neutralization sites that are highly conserved, by the existence of a single serotype, and by a slow rate of antigenic drift. HRSV vaccine development has largely focused on subgroup A strains. A vaccine based on subgroup A would be expected to induce substantial cross-protection against subgroup B strains, but it is not yet known whether this will be sufficient or whether a subgroup B component will be needed.

Vaccine-Enhanced HRSV Disease (ERD)

Development of HRSV vaccines—especially pediatric vaccines—is further complicated by the extraordinary phenomenon of ERD.[3] ERD was first observed in association with a formalin-inactivated pediatric HRSV vaccine (FI-RSV), given by IM injection to infants and children in the 1960s.[307,490] The vaccine was well tolerated but proved to be poorly protective. Unexpectedly, upon subsequent natural infection, vaccinees experienced much greater frequency and severity of HRSV disease: 80% of FI-RSV vaccinees required hospitalization for HRSV disease compared to 5% in the control group, and two toddlers (ages 14 and 16 months) died of what eventually became recognized as ERD. Their autopsies provided evidence of HRSV replication and pulmonary inflammation, the latter suggestive of immune-driven disease.[490]

Subsequent studies showed that the immune response to FI-RSV differed markedly from that to HRSV infection. The serum antibodies induced by FI-RSV in the original vaccinees and in experimental animals bound efficiently to HRSV antigen in ELISA but were inefficient in neutralizing infectivity, whereas those induced by natural infection neutralized efficiently.[453] The poor neutralizing activity of the FI-RSV–induced antibodies likely resulted from denaturation of neutralization epitopes in the vaccine as well as deficient antibody affinity maturation due to poor TLR stimulation by the nonreplicating vaccine.[147] Subsequent natural HRSV infection of the vaccinees induced even higher titers of these antibodies that bound antigen without neutralizing infectivity, resulting in excessive formation of antibody–antigen complexes and complement fixation, contributing to disease.[428] The cellular immune response also was aberrant. Peripheral blood lymphocytes from the original vaccinees exhibited an exaggerated proliferative response to HRSV antigen in vitro, suggestive of a heightened CD4+ T-cell response to FI-RSV compared to natural infection.[326] Consistent with this, subsequent studies in experimental animals showed that FI-RSV induced a disproportionately increased stimulation of the Th2 subset of CD4+ T cells compared with HRSV infection.[119,143] This Th2 bias was found to result from inefficient stimulation of CD8+ CTL and NK cells (presumably due to the lack of cytoplasmic expression of antigen and resulting poor MHC class I presentation), which normally down-regulate Th2 responses to HRSV antigens and likely have other immunomodulatory effects.[463,579] The Th2 bias may also have been enhanced by the presence in FI-RSV of carbonyl groups arising from the formalin treatment.[436] The importance of the Th2 biased response in ERD was confirmed by the finding that ERD did not occur when FI-RSV–immunized rodents were depleted of either CD4+ T cells or Th2 cytokines prior to HRSV challenge.[120,544] In summary, while our understanding of ERD remains incomplete, key factors include the induction of antibodies with low neutralizing activity and induction of a heightened Th2 response. Comparable vaccine enhancement of their respective diseases has been described with the clinical use of inactivated measles virus vaccines and in experimental animals receiving formalin-inactivated HPIV3[466] and HMPV[144,674] vaccines and thus occurs among several related viruses.

Further observations regarding ERD have important implications for HRSV (and HMPV) vaccine development. Markers for ERD were observed following HRSV challenge in experimental animals previously immunized with experimental HRSV F and G subunit vaccines.[452] This was the case even with the use of stabilized pre-F protein and Th1-biasing adjuvant.[544] In contrast, ERD does not occur with natural HRSV infection and reinfection; it also did not occur in pediatric clinical trials of a number of live-attenuated HRSV strains[308,309,667] or a live-attenuated chimeric bovine/human PIV3 vector expressing RSV F from an added gene (B/HPIV3-F).[45] This distinction between killed/subunit HRSV vaccines that prime for ERD versus live/vectored HRSV vaccines that do not likely reflects the greater efficiency of the latter in broadly stimulating innate and adaptive immunity, including stimulation of TLRs, NK cells, and CD8+ CTL important in regulating HRSV-specific immune responses. However, this distinction between killed/subunit and live/vectored is not fully defined,[351] and each new type of HRSV vaccine must be evaluated for ERD. This can be challenging because ERD is not reproduced exactly in available animal models and can be masked by strong protective immunity.[452] Another fundamental observation is that priming for ERD—in the original clinical trial and in experimental animals—occurred only during the first exposure to HRSV antigen in life and did not occur in recipients previously infected with HRSV.[645] (Incidentally, ERD did not reoccur in the original FI-RSV vaccinees during a second HRSV infection [Dr. Robert M. Chanock, personal communication]). Thus, a single natural infection with HRSV is sufficient to block or reverse priming for ERD.) Because of ERD, killed/subunit vaccines are contraindicated for pediatric use, but in contrast have been confirmed to be safe in adults, as expected since adults are HRSV seropositive. Pediatric HRSV vaccine development is focused on live/vector strategies.

Live-Attenuated HRSV Vaccines

Live-attenuated HRSV strains are being developed primarily for pediatric use. A live-attenuated vaccine provides all—or nearly all—of the viral antigens. It is administered intranasally and mimics a mild HRSV infection, broadly stimulating local and systemic innate, cellular, and antibody-mediated immunity. Local immunity is considered particularly effective for restricting respiratory viruses such as HRSV and reducing shedding and spread. Studies with influenza virus vaccines in infants and children suggest that live vaccines induced broader, more effective, and possibly more long-lasting immunity compared to protein vaccines.[37,281] The intranasal route for live HRSV vaccines partially avoids the replication-restricting and immunosuppressive effects of serum antibodies.[131] Beginning in the 1960s, a series of live-attenuated HRSV strains was developed by classic biological methods, notably multiple passages at increasingly low, suboptimal temperature[195] and by chemical mutagenesis and selection for temperature-sensitive mutants.[130] While some of these strains initially seemed promising, they fell short of satisfactory levels of attenuation and genetic stability in HRSV-naive infants and children.[668] All subsequent vaccine candidates have been made by reverse genetics.

Advantages of reverse genetics include (a) identification of attenuating mutations in existing viruses[658]; (b) new strategies for attenuation such as the deletion of genes,[44,602,632,657] deletion of one or more codons,[390] replacement of genes with counterparts from related animal viruses to obtain host-range restriction,[72,480,542] and large-scale genome recoding such as codon and

codon-pair deoptimization[358,580]; (c) moving the glycoprotein genes to promoter-proximal positions to increase the expression of protective antigens[338]; (d) increasing the stability of missense attenuating mutations by using codons whose sequences limit the possibilities for mutating to deattenuating assignments[389]; (e) introducing mutations in desired combinations to incrementally increase attenuation[390,659]; and (f) producing viruses with short, well-defined passage histories, important for safety.[589] Beyond the development of live-attenuated HRSV strains, molecular biology methods also have made possible other strategies including the development of vectored HRSV vaccines, large-scale synthesis of HRSV antigens and virus-like particles, and the engineering of viral antigen—particularly the HRSV F protein—for improved immunogenicity.

A number of attenuated HRSV strains produced by reverse genetics have been evaluated in clinical trials.[308,309] A lead candidate called ΔNS2/Δ1313/I1314L contains deletion of the NS2 gene combined with deletion of codon 1313 in the L gene, which confers attenuation and temperature-sensitivity phenotypes, combined with the missense mutation I1314L in the L gene, which confers phenotypic stability by preventing a second-site compensatory mutation at position 1314.[390] (In general, the temperature-sensitivity phenotype increases safety by restricting replication in the warmer lower respiratory tract to a greater extent compared to the cooler upper respiratory tract). In a phase 1 study in infants and young children, the ΔNS2/Δ1313/I1314L virus was genetically stable and had promising levels of attenuation and immunogenicity.[311] A potential advantage of deletion of the NS2 gene is that, as noted above (*Nonstructural Proteins NS1 and NS2*), this protein has been implicated in promoting the shedding of airway epithelial cells leading to airway obstruction, and thus its deletion may reduce virulence.[375] Other viruses were engineered by deletion of the M2-2 ORF on its own[312] or in combination with additional mutations such as a "stabilized" temperature sensitivity missense mutation in the L gene.[415] These ΔM2-2 viruses exhibited genetic stability and provided a promising range of attenuation and immunogenicity. As noted above (*M2-2 protein*), deletion of M2-2 shifts the balance of RNA synthesis from RNA replication towards transcription, resulting in restricted replication and a global increase in viral protein expression, which may provide for increased immunogenicity.[44] Examples of modifications in other candidates in clinical trials sponsored by several different laboratories include deletion of the G gene (International Clinical Trials Registry NTR7173)[632]; codon deoptimization of the NS1 and NS2 genes combined with deletion of secreted G and use of a heterologous F protein with greater stability (ClinicalTrials.gov NCT04444284)[580]; codon-pair deoptimization (NCT04919109); deletion of the NS2 gene combined with a stabilized missense mutation in L (NCT03387137); and deletion of the NS1 gene on its own or combined with shifting the F and G genes to the first two gene positions (NCT03596801). Recent analysis of five different regimens of immunization with live-attenuated HRSV strains in clinical studies in infants and young children showed that a single intranasal dose induced substantial serum neutralizing antibody responses in ≥80% of vaccinees; that these responses were relatively durable; and that upon natural exposure to wild-type HRSV, these vaccines in aggregate were 67% and 88% effective against RSV-MAARI and RSV-MAALRI, respectively, and primed for potent anamnestic responses.[308] Other candidate vaccine strains that were more attenuated were less immunogenic and protective, indicating the importance of identifying a suitable balance between restriction and immunogenicity.

Replication-Competent Vectors

Vectored HRSV vaccines also are in clinical trials for pediatric and/or adult use. The B/HPIV3 vector noted above comprises BPIV3 in which the F and HN surface glycoprotein genes were replaced with those of HPIV3, which combines the host range restriction of BPIV3 in primates with the major neutralization antigens of HPIV3.[542] B/HPIV3 expressing the wild-type HRSV F and/or G proteins from added genes was immunogenic in rodents and nonhuman primates.[542,594] B/HPIV3 expressing wild-type HRSV F protein was evaluated in infants and young children and found to be attenuated, but the expressed HRSV F protein had insufficient genetic stability and immunogenicity.[45] Promising new versions have been developed expressing stabilized HRSV pre-F protein as well as chimeric HRSV F protein containing the transmembrane and cytoplasmic domains of the vector HPIV3 F protein to direct efficient incorporation into the vector particles.[374] B/HPIV3 expressing HRSV protective antigen provides a bivalent intranasal vaccine against HPIV3 and HRSV. It has advantages over HRSV strains because the B/HPIV3 vector is more stable physically and is easier to manufacture and distribute than HRSV. Since the added HRSV F gene is not needed for B/HPIV3 replication, it can be expressed in the stabilized pre-F form, which is more immunogenic than wild-type F but is nonfunctional for fusion. Also, whereas attenuated HRSV strains are highly restricted and poorly immunogenic in hosts with preexisting HRSV immunity, B/HPIV3-vectored HRSV vaccines were not inhibited or suppressed in nonhuman primates possessing preexisting HRSV immunity.[373] Thus, these vectors would be effective in boosting immunity following a previous HRSV vaccine or for immunization of pediatric recipients who possess passive HRSV-neutralizing antibodies. The B/HPIV3 vector likely would be limited to pediatric use, since it likely would be overly restricted for replication in adults due to high HPIV3 seroprevalence.

An analogous approach employs Sendai virus (SeV) as a vector.[299,524] SeV is a murine relative of HPIV1 that is attenuated in primates by host-range restriction. SeV has sufficient antigenic cross-reactivity with HPIV1 that intranasal immunization protects AGMs against HPIV1 challenge. SeV was engineered to express HRSV wild-type F protein from an added gene (creating the virus SeVRSV) as a candidate bivalent vaccine against HPIV1 and HRSV. SeVRSV was attenuated and immunogenic in nonhuman primates.[299] In clinical trials, the empty SeV vector was well tolerated in adults and children of 3 to 6 years, and SeV/RSV was well tolerated in adults[537] and is a candidate for evaluation in younger individuals. High HPIV1 seroprevalence in adults would limit replication of SeV/RSV and likely reduce its immunogenicity in that population.

Replication-Incompetent Vectors

Replication-incompetent adenoviruses are another vectored strategy. To avoid neuralization by immunity to common adenovirus serotypes, these vaccines are based on nonhuman adenoviruses, namely chimpanzee adenovirus PanAd3 (Oxford Vaccine Group)[232] and chimpanzee adenovirus-155 (ChAd155, Oxford Vaccine Group and GlaxoSmithKline),[103] or low-seroprevalence human serotypes such as serotype 26 (Ad26, Janssen Vaccines and Prevention).[665] The PanAd3 and ChAd155 constructs express F protein lacking the transmembrane and cytoplasmic domains, plus the N and M2-1 proteins that were included to provide additional antigens for cellular immunity. The Ad26 construct expresses a stabilized pre-F protein. The Ad vectors usually are given parenterally and have been generally well tolerated and moderately immunogenic. The PanAd3-RSV construct was administered to adults 18 to 50 and 60 to 75 years of age by the intramuscular or intranasal routes in a single dose or a heterologous prime-boost with the host-range–restricted MVA (modified vaccinia Ankara) poxvirus vector (based on a strain that does not replicate in mammalian cells) expressing the same F, N, and M2-1 proteins. Of the different combinations, a single intramuscular dose of PanAd3-RSV induced the greatest increase in serum HRSV-neutralizing antibodies, less than 2.5-fold, whereas the intranasal route and boosting were poorly immunogenic.[232] Continued development has not been reported. ChAd155-RSV induced increases in serum HRSV-neutralizing antibodies of approximately 2.5-fold in adults of 18 to 45 years.[103] This vaccine also was evaluated in HRSV-seropositive children of 12 to 23 months (NCT02937873) and was being evaluated in HRSV-naïve infants of 6 to 7 months (NCT03636906) when development was suspended in 2021. Ad26.RSV.preF was evaluated in adults of ≥60 years as one dose or two doses at a 12-month interval and induced increases in serum HRSV-neutralizing antibodies of approximately three-fold[665] and presently is in an expanded study of 5,815 adults of ≥65 years with a single dose followed by a second dose at either 1, 2, or 4 years (NCT03982199). In a human infection model in adults, immunization with Ad26.RSV provided substantial protection against challenge 28 days later with the wild-type HRSV-A Memphis 37b strain.[528] Ad26.RSV.preF also has been evaluated in HRSV-seropositive children of 12 to 24 months (NCT03303625) and presently in HRSV-seronegative children aged 12 to 24 months (NCT03606512).

Another MVA-based construct, called MVA-BN-RSV, expresses the G protein from both HRSV subgroups, plus the F, N and M2-1 proteins from subgroup A.[301] In a study in adults aged ≥55 years, in which 337 individuals received vaccine versus 83 placebo recipients, a single intramuscular dose induced modest (<2-fold) increases in serum HRSV-neutralizing antibodies, and a second dose at 4 weeks had little effect.[301]

Moderna is developing a nonreplicating mRNA-based HRSV vaccine (mRNA-1345) expressing stabilized pre-F protein, using the same modified mRNA and lipid nanoparticle technologies that were used successfully with their recent COVID-19 vaccine. The HRSV vaccine presently is being evaluated in a study of up to 620 participants comprising four populations: healthy adults of 18 to 49 years, women of childbearing age of 18 to 40 years, healthy older adults of 65 to 79 years, and RSV-seropositive children of 12 to 59 months (NCT04528719). Preliminary data indicate that, in adults of 18 to 49 years, the HRSV vaccine was well tolerated and induced 20.5- and 11.7-fold increases in serum neutralizing antibodies against subgroups A and B, respectively (Moderna press release, April 14, 2021). This promising vaccine might be suitable for adults and potentially for pediatric use if free of ERD and suitably well tolerated.

HRSV Subunit Vaccines

In early pioneering work, wild-type F protein purified from HRSV-infected cells was evaluated in a number of studies in HRSV-seropositive older children and adults and was well tolerated but was poorly immunogenic and was discontinued.[36,182,237] Another approach involving a novel FG protein expressed from fused F and G ORFs in a recombinant baculovirus was similar in immunogenicity to the earlier subunits.[647] Another early experimental subunit vaccine, called BBG2Na, comprised a bacterially expressed fragment containing the central conserved domain of the HRSV G protein fused to the albumin-binding domain of the streptococcal G protein. This vaccine was poorly immunogenic in adults, with hypersensitivity observed in some recipients, and was discontinued.[487]

As already noted (*Maternal immunization*), Novavax developed an F subunit nanoparticle vaccine that proved to be insufficiently protective as a maternal vaccine.[395] This vaccine comprised baculovirus-expressed F protein that assembled into trimers that may represent multiple conformations on the pre-F to post-F continuum: these trimers aggregated into nanoparticles containing on average five trimers with a range of two to nine trimers.[342] In elderly adults, a single intramuscular dose of this vaccine induced less than twofold increases in serum HRSV-neutralizing antibodies, which probably is insufficient for further development.[196] A post-F subunit was developed by GlaxoSmithKline and evaluated in adults of 18 to 45 years of age: it induced up to a 4.5-fold increase in serum HRSV-neutralizing antibodies with no further increase from a boost at 28 days.[364] A post-F subunit vaccine developed by MedImmune was evaluated in elderly adults (mean age of 67 years): it induced increases in serum HRSV-neutralizing antibodies of less than 2.5-fold and did not protect from HRSV disease.[173]

Post-F subunits have largely been superseded by pre-F subunits, which in rhesus monkeys were 10-fold more immunogenic than post-F for serum HRSV-neutralizing antibodies[419] and were highly immunogenic in adults.[126,521] GlaxoSmithKline evaluated a pre-F subunit vaccine as a single intramuscular dose, with three dose levels, in women of 18 to 45 years of age. The vaccine induced increases of serum HRSV-neutralizing antibodies of 8- to 14-fold at day 8, which remained 5- to 6-fold increased at day 91, versus a 1-fold increase in placebo recipients.[547] As noted, this pre-F subunit is being evaluated as a single-dose maternal vaccine in up to 20,000 pregnant women (NCT04605159; GSK press release, November 23, 2020). This pre-F subunit also was evaluated in younger adults and elderly adults: it induced an almost 10-fold increase in serum HRSV-neutralizing antibodies (NCT03814590; GlaxoSmithKline press release February 16, 2021). This subunit presently is being evaluated in 1,717 participants ≥60 years of age, given as one dose alone or with up to two boosters at 12 and 36 months (NCT04732871), and also in four formulations in up to 25,000 participants of ≥60 years of age (NCT04886596). As noted, Pfizer is evaluating a pre-F maternal vaccine in up to 10,000 pregnant women (NCT04424316) and is evaluating a pre-F vaccine for the elderly in 304 subjects of 65 to 85 years of age, given as a single dose, or combined with an inactivated influenza vaccine, or boosted at 12 months (NCT03572062). This pre-F subunit also has been evaluated in a human-infection model in adults, in which participants were vaccinated and challenged with wild-type RSV (NCT04785612): the vaccine greatly reduced viral shedding, prevented the mild-to-moderate HRSV illness observed in the placebo recipients, and appeared to be more protective than the Ad26.RSV.preF vaccine described above (Pfizer Second Quarter 2021 Earnings Report).

A G-based subunit vaccine (BARS13) was made by expressing G protein, from which the transmembrane and cytoplasmic domains were deleted, in *E. coli* and combining the purified protein with cyclosporine A as an anti-inflammatory agent (Advaccine Biopharmaceuticals).[370] This vaccine candidate is being evaluated as a single intramuscular dose in a dose-ranging study in up to 120 elderly of 60 to 80 years of age (NCT04681833). A number of other F- or G-based subunit vaccines also are in early development (see PATH RSV Vaccine and mAB Snapshot; https://www.path.org/resources/rsv-vaccine-and-mab-snapshot/).

Other Approaches

Other varied approaches to an HRSV vaccine are being evaluated clinically, and there are many preclinical studies that mostly are not described here. A vaccine comprising pre-F linked to an immunostimulatory bacterium-like particle ("SynGEM") was administered intranasally to adults and was well tolerated but poorly immunogenic for serum HRSV-neutralizing antibodies (NCT02958540).[15] Another approach involves intramuscular immunization with the ectodomain of the SH protein in an oil emulsion (DPX-RSV(A); Immunovaccine).[353] In rodents, this experimental vaccine reduced viral load by the mechanism of antibody-mediated clearance of infected cells rather than direct neutralization of virus. In adults, this vaccine was safe and induced SH-specific antibodies detected by ELISA (NCT02472548).[353] Another approach involves a synthetic particle comprising a trimeric scaffold bearing a peptide representing the palivizumab epitope, plus a T-helper epitope: this vaccine (V-306 SVLP, Virometix) was immunogenic and protective in mice and is being evaluated in 60 women of child-bearing age (NCT04519073).[691] Mycobacterium bovis BCG, a live-attenuated vaccine in widespread use against tuberculosis, was engineered to express the HRSV N protein: in mice, this construct induced protective T-cell immunity, which provides a novel approach to HRSV immunoprophylaxis. When evaluated in adults of 18 to 50 years of age (NCT03213405, Pontificia Universidad Catolica de Chile), this construct was well tolerated and immunogenic against the N protein; in some subjects, it induced increases in serum HRSV-neutralizing antibodies, which remains unexplained since N-specific antibodies typically do not neutralize HRSV *in vitro*.[1] Several virus-like particles (VLPs) are in preclinical development as HRSV vaccines. In one approach, HRSV F and G proteins were engineered to contain the transmembrane and cytoplasmic domains of their Newcastle disease virus (NDV) counterparts in order to be assembled with the NDV nucleocapsid and matrix proteins into VLPs.[133] HRSV VLPs also have been assembled by coexpression of the HRSV F, G, and M proteins.[635] Another approach involved assembly of HRSV pre-F or post-F into particles with the HMPV M protein.[104]

Updated information on HRSV vaccines is summarized on the PATH RSV Vaccine and mAB Snapshot (https://www.path.org/resources/rsv-vaccine-and-mab-snapshot/) and Trial Tracker (https://www.path.org/resources/rsv-and-mab-trial-tracker/). In summary, substantial progress has been made for

HRSV vaccines. It seems likely that a live or vectored vaccine will be successfully developed for pediatric use and a subunit or vectored vaccine for adults.

HMPV Vaccines

The development of HMPV vaccines has received much less support compared to HRSV. The general properties needed for HMPV vaccines likely are very similar to those for HRSV vaccines. As noted, ERD has been described for HMPV in experimental animals; therefore, HMPV killed/subunit vaccines are contraindicated for pediatric use but are expected to be safe in adults.

With regard to live-attenuated HMPV vaccine candidates, deletion of the G and M2-2 genes by reverse genetics resulted in candidates with promising phenotypes of attenuation and immunogenicity in rodents and AGMs; these have not yet been evaluated in clinical studies.[47,70] Another approach has been to replace genes of HMPV with their AMPV counterparts to create chimeric viruses that are attenuated in primates due to host incompatibility effects of the AMPV genes. A chimera in which the HMPV P gene was replaced by its AMPV counterpart had promising phenotypes of attenuation and immunogenicity in AGMs.[480] When evaluated in a small phase 1 clinical study, this virus appeared to be satisfactorily attenuated in adults and HMPV-seropositive children but proved to be overattenuated and insufficiently immunogenic in HMPV-seronegative young children[313] and its development has been discontinued. Other HMPV vaccine candidates have been developed containing temperature-sensitivity and cold-passage point mutations, some of which had been described previously in HRSV; lead candidates were attenuated and immunogenic in hamsters, but further development has not been reported.[278] The B/HPIV3 vector described above was used to express the wild-type HMPV F protein from an added gene, resulting in a bivalent live-attenuated intranasal HPIV3-HMPV vaccine virus that had promising phenotypes of attenuation and bivalent immunogenicity in rodents and nonhuman primates.[564] SeV was modified to express a secreted form of the HMPV F protein; this construct was immunogenic and protective in cotton rats.[525]

HMPV vaccines focus on the F protein because it is by far the major neutralization and protective antigen and is highly conserved.[564] As noted, the structures for HMPV pre-F and post-F have general similarity with those of HRSV.[30,412] However, the apex of the HMPV pre-F trimer, which corresponds to the highly immunogenic antigenic site Ø of HRSV F, contains conserved N-linked glycans that appear to provide shielding from host immune recognition.[30] Perhaps due to this shielding, the pre-F form of HMPV F did not appear to be more efficient in inducing virus-neutralizing antibodies than the post-F form.[483] Further engineering, such as removal of *N*-glycans, might improve immunogenicity.

A bivalent mRNA-based vaccine against HMPV and HPIV3 (mRNA-1653, Moderna)—using the same technology as the recent Moderna COVID-19 vaccine—is being evaluated in adults followed by HPIV3- and HMPV-seropositive children 12 to 59 months of age (NCT04144348). Preliminary results from adults reported three- and sixfold increases in serum neutralizing antibodies against HPIV3 and HMPV, respectively, and a second dose 1 month later provided no boost (Moderna press release, February 12, 2019).

It is likely that successful HMPV vaccines for the pediatric and adult populations eventually will be developed, guided by experience with HRSV vaccines.

PERSPECTIVE

HRSV is one of the more complex members of *Mononegavirales* in terms of gene number. Differences between HRSV and HMPV compared to *Paramyxoviridae* led to their reclassification in 2016 to create the new family *Pneumoviridae*. A number of factors have impeded basic biochemical and molecular studies of HRSV, including its relatively poor replication *in vitro*, its physical instability, and the heterogeneous and filamentous nature of its particles. However, in recent years, there has been substantial progress in determining crystal structures of the HRSV proteins, as well as information on the activities of the viral proteins and RNAs in the viral replicative cycle and how they interact with and affect the host cell and host immune system. In particular, an exciting area of advance has been the identification of the pre-F and post-F conformations of the F protein, determination of their crystal structures, antigenic analysis including identification of the highly immunogenic site Ø, and structure-based stabilization of the pre-F conformation to obtain antigen with greatly increased immunogenicity for antibodies that efficiently neutralize infectivity. The identification and stabilization of the highly immunogenic HRSV pre-F structure guided similar advances with coronavirus spike proteins, resulting in improved immunogenicity of vaccines used during the COVID-19 pandemic.

HRSV is one of the most common, widespread, and infectious human viruses, appearing in yearly seasonal worldwide pandemics. It is notable for a historic and tragic vaccine failure, namely the FI-RSV pediatric vaccine in the 1960s. HRSV also is notable for the development of a successful strategy of passive antibody immunoprophylaxis, pioneering the use of MAbs in human medicine. Although the importance of HRSV in human disease has been known for more than 60 years, we still lack effective vaccines and antivirals. However, the last 10 years have seen a substantial increase in research and progress in modes of immunoprophylaxis and antiviral therapy. It seems likely that the next 5 to 10 years will see licensure of several products for immunoprophylaxis that might include a long half-life MAb for passive immunoprophylaxis and vaccines that might be based on live-attenuated HRSV strains, vectors, or subunits. This likely will include products for the pediatric and elderly populations as well as for maternal immunization. A substantial reduction in severe HRSV disease would be a major advance for human health.

HRSV is unusual in its ability to infect and cause disease in early infancy, partly due to inefficient restriction by maternal antibodies. The possible consequences of severe early HRSV infection in the context of the immature lung and immature immune system remain poorly understood. For example, severe HRSV disease early in life frequently is associated with lingering abnormalities in pulmonary function, but the extent to which these are due to preexisting deficiencies or were caused by infection remains controversial. It also has been speculated that early infection in life can have long-term effects on the immune response in some individuals. Further studies of infants who receive passive or (when available) active immuno-prophylaxis against HRSV may help to resolve these issues. The relative contributions of direct viral damage versus immune factors to HRSV disease remain unclear and likely will vary among individuals. HRSV also is notable for its ability to reinfect throughout life in the absence of significant antigenic change. The extent to which this reflects virus-mediated subversion of protective responses remains controversial.

HMPV is a close relative to HRSV that shares general features of tropism, epidemiology, and pathogenesis. However, the impact of HMPV on human health is less, and research on HMPV has received less attention. Many of the questions regarding disease mechanisms, immune response, and long-term consequences of HRSV infection early in life likely also apply to HMPV. Progress in HRSV vaccines and antivirals likely will guide progress with HMPV.

ACKNOWLEDGMENTS

UJB and PLC were funded by the Intramural Research Program of the National Institute of Allergy and Infectious Diseases, NIH.

Due to space limitations, references were limited to representative examples and emphasized more recent studies and classic pioneering studies. Many other relevant references could not be accommodated. We apologize to those authors. Additional references can be found in the previous edition.[113]

REFERENCES

1. Abarca K, Rey-Jurado E, Munoz-Durango N, et al. Safety and immunogenicity evaluation of recombinant BCG vaccine against respiratory syncytial virus in a randomized, double-blind, placebo-controlled phase I clinical trial. *EClinicalMedicine* 2020;27:100517.
2. Aberle JH, Aberle SW, Redlberger-Fritz M, et al. Human metapneumovirus subgroup changes and seasonality during epidemics. *Pediatr Infect Dis J* 2010;29:1016–1018.
3. Acosta PL, Caballero MT, Polack FP. Brief history and characterization of enhanced respiratory syncytial virus disease. *Clin Vaccine Immunol* 2015;23:189–195.
4. Agoti CN, Phan MVT, Munywoki PK, et al. Genomic analysis of respiratory syncytial virus infections in households and utility in inferring who infects the infant. *Sci Rep* 2019;9:10076.
5. Ahmadian G, Chambers P, Easton AJ. Detection and characterization of proteins encoded by the second ORF of the M2 gene of pneumoviruses. *J Gen Virol* 1999;80:2011–2016.
6. Alvarez R, Tripp RA. The immune response to human metapneumovirus is associated with aberrant immunity and impaired virus clearance in BALB/c mice. *J Virol* 2005;79:5971–5978.
7. American Academy of Pediatrics Committee on Infectious Diseases and American Academy of Pediatrics Bronchiolitis Guidelines Committee. Updated guidance for palivizumab prophylaxis among infants and young children at increased risk of hospitalization for respiratory syncytial virus infection. *Pediatrics* 2014;134:e620–e638.
8. Amirav I, Luder AS, Kruger N, et al. A double-blind, placebo-controlled, randomized trial of montelukast for acute bronchiolitis. *Pediatrics* 2008;122:e1249–e1255.
9. Ampofo K, Bender J, Sheng X, et al. Seasonal invasive pneumococcal disease in children: role of preceding respiratory viral infection. *Pediatrics* 2008;122:229–237.
10. Anderson EJ, Simoes EA, Buttery JP, et al. Prevalence and characteristics of human metapneumovirus infection among hospitalized children at high risk for severe lower respiratory tract infection. *J Pediatric Infect Dis Soc* 2012;1:212–222.
11. Anderson K, King AM, Lerch RA, et al. Polylactosaminoglycan modification of the respiratory syncytial virus small hydrophobic (SH) protein: a conserved feature among human and bovine respiratory syncytial viruses. *Virology* 1992;191:417–430.
12. Anderson LJ, Hierholzer JC, Tsou C, et al. Antigenic characterization of respiratory syncytial virus strains with monoclonal antibodies. *J Infect Dis* 1985;151:626–633.
13. Andeweg SP, Schepp RM, van de Kassteele J, et al. Population-based serology reveals risk factors for RSV infection in children younger than 5 years. *Sci Rep* 2021;11:8953.
14. Andreano E, Paciello I, Bardelli M, et al. The respiratory syncytial virus (RSV) prefusion F-protein functional antibody repertoire in adult healthy donors. *EMBO Mol Med* 2021;13:e14035.
15. Ascough S, Vlachantoni I, Kalyan M, et al. Local and systemic immunity against respiratory syncytial virus induced by a novel intranasal vaccine. A randomized, double-blind, placebo-controlled clinical trial. *Am J Respir Crit Care Med* 2019;200:481–492.
16. Asenjo A, Calvo E, Villanueva N. Phosphorylation of human respiratory syncytial virus P protein at threonine 108 controls its interaction with the M2-1 protein in the viral RNA polymerase complex. *J Gen Virol* 2006;87:3637–3642.
17. Asenjo A, Rodriguez L, Villanueva N. Determination of phosphorylated residues from human respiratory syncytial virus P protein that are dynamically dephosphorylated by cellular phosphatases: a possible role for serine 54. *J Gen Virol* 2005;86:1109–1120.
18. Atreya PL, Peeples ME, Collins PL. The NS1 protein of human respiratory syncytial virus is a potent inhibitor of minigenome transcription and RNA replication. *J Virol* 1998;72:1452–1461.
19. Ausar SF, Espina M, Brock J, et al. High-throughput screening of stabilizers for respiratory syncytial virus: identification of stabilizers and their effects on the conformational thermo-stability of viral particles. *Hum Vaccin* 2007;3:94–103.
20. Bacharier LB, Cohen R, Schweiger T, et al. Determinants of asthma after severe respiratory syncytial virus bronchiolitis. *J Allergy Clin Immunol* 2012;130:91–100.e103.
21. Bachi T. Direct observation of the budding and fusion of an enveloped virus by video microscopy of viable cells. *J Cell Biol* 1988;107:1689–1695.
22. Bachi T, Howe C. Morphogenesis and ultrastructure of respiratory syncytial virus. *J Virol* 1973;12:1173–1180.
23. Baker RE, Mahmud AS, Wagner CE, et al. Epidemic dynamics of respiratory syncytial virus in current and future climates. *Nat Commun* 2019;10:5512.
24. Bao X, Kolli D, Liu T, et al. Human metapneumovirus small hydrophobic protein inhibits NF-kappaB transcriptional activity. *J Virol* 2008;82:8224–8229.
25. Bao X, Kolli D, Ren J, et al. Human metapneumovirus glycoprotein G disrupts mitochondrial signaling in airway epithelial cells. *PLoS One* 2013;8:e62568.
26. Bao X, Liu T, Shan Y, et al. Human metapneumovirus glycoprotein G inhibits innate immune responses. *PLoS Pathog* 2008;4:e1000077.
27. Barik S. The structure of the 5′ terminal cap of the respiratory syncytial virus mRNA. *J Gen Virol* 1993;74:485–490.
28. Barr J, Chambers P, Harriott P, et al. Sequence of the phosphoprotein gene of pneumonia virus of mice: expression of multiple proteins from two overlapping reading frames. *J Virol* 1994;68:5330–5334.
29. Bastien N, Trudel M, Simard C. Complete protection of mice from respiratory syncytial virus infection following mucosal delivery of synthetic peptide vaccines. *Vaccine* 1999;17:832–836.
30. Battles MB, Mas V, Olmedillas E, et al. Structure and immunogenicity of pre-fusion-stabilized human metapneumovirus F glycoprotein. *Nat Commun* 2017;8:1528.
31. Battles MB, McLellan JS. Respiratory syncytial virus entry and how to block it. *Nat Rev Microbiol* 2019;17:233–245.
32. Becker SD, Bennett M, Stewart JP, et al. Serological survey of virus infection among wild house mice (Mus domesticus) in the UK. *Lab Anim* 2007;41:229–238.
33. Beeler JA, van Wyke Coelingh K. Neutralization epitopes of the F glycoprotein of respiratory syncytial virus: effect of mutation upon fusion function. *J Virol* 1989;63:2941–2950.
34. Behera AK, Matsuse H, Kumar M, et al. Blocking intercellular adhesion molecule-1 on human epithelial cells decreases respiratory syncytial virus infection. *Biochem Biophys Res Commun* 2001;280:188–195.
35. Beigel JH, Nam HH, Adams PL, et al. Advances in respiratory virus therapeutics—a meeting report from the 6th isirv Antiviral Group conference. *Antiviral Res* 2019;167:45–67.
36. Belshe RB, Anderson EL, Walsh EE. Immunogenicity of purified F glycoprotein of respiratory syncytial virus: clinical and immune responses to subsequent natural infection in children. *J Infect Dis* 1993;168:1024–1029.
37. Belshe RB, Edwards KM, Vesikari T, et al.; CAIV-T Comparative Efficacy Study Group. Live attenuated versus inactivated influenza vaccine in infants and young children. *N Engl J Med* 2007;356:685–696.
38. Belshe RB, Richardson LS, London WT, et al. Experimental respiratory syncytial virus infection of four species of primates. *J Med Virol* 1977;1:157–162.
39. Bendelja K, Gagro A, Bace A, et al. Predominant type-2 response in infants with respiratory syncytial virus (RSV) infection demonstrated by cytokine flow cytometry. *Clin Exp Immunol* 2000;121:332–338.
40. Bendelja K, Vojvoda V, Aberle N, et al. Decreased Toll-like receptor 8 expression and lower TNF-alpha synthesis in infants with acute RSV infection. *Respir Res* 2010;11:143.
41. Bennett BL, Garofalo RP, Cron SG, et al. Immunopathogenesis of respiratory syncytial virus bronchiolitis. *J Infect Dis* 2007;195:1532–1540.
42. Bennett RS, LaRue R, Shaw D, et al. A wild goose metapneumovirus containing a large attachment glycoprotein is avirulent but immunoprotective in domestic turkeys. *J Virol* 2005;79:14834–14842.
43. Berbers G, Mollema L, van der Klis F, et al. Antibody responses to respiratory syncytial virus: a cross-sectional serosurveillance study in the Dutch population focusing on infants younger than 2 years. *J Infect Dis* 2021;224:269–278.
44. Bermingham A, Collins PL. The M2-2 protein of human respiratory syncytial virus is a regulatory factor involved in the balance between RNA replication and transcription. *Proc Natl Acad Sci U S A* 1999;96:11259–11264.
45. Bernstein DI, Malkin E, Abughali N, et al. Phase 1 study of the safety and immunogenicity of a live, attenuated respiratory syncytial virus and parainfluenza virus type 3 vaccine in seronegative children. *Pediatr Infect Dis J* 2012;31:109–114.
46. Biacchesi S, Murphy BR, Collins PL, et al. Frequent frameshift and point mutations in the SH gene of human metapneumovirus passaged in vitro. *J Virol* 2007;81:6057–6067.
47. Biacchesi S, Pham QN, Skiadopoulos MH, et al. Infection of non-human primates with recombinant human metapneumovirus lacking the SH, G or M2-2 protein categorizes each as a nonessential accessory protein and identifies a vaccine candidate. *J Virol* 2005;79:12608–12613.
48. Biacchesi S, Pham QN, Skiadopoulos MH, et al. Modification of the trypsin-dependent cleavage activation site of the human metapneumovirus fusion protein to be trypsin independent does not increase replication or spread in rodents or nonhuman primates. *J Virol* 2006;80:5798–5806.
49. Biacchesi S, Skiadopoulos MH, Boivin G, et al. Genetic diversity between human metapneumovirus subgroups. *Virology* 2003;315:1–9.
50. Biacchesi S, Skiadopoulos MH, Tran KC, et al. Recovery of human metapneumovirus from cDNA: optimization of growth in vitro and expression of additional genes. *Virology* 2004;321:247–259.

51. Biacchesi S, Skiadopoulos MH, Yang L, et al. Recombinant human Metapneumovirus lacking the small hydrophobic SH and/or attachment G glycoprotein: deletion of G yields a promising vaccine candidate. *J Virol* 2004;78:12877–12887.
52. Bin L, Liu H, Tabor DE, et al. Emergence of new antigenic epitopes in the glycoproteins of human respiratory syncytial virus collected from a US surveillance study, 2015–17. *Sci Rep* 2019;9:3898.
53. Bisgaard H, Flores-Nunez A, Goh A, et al. Study of montelukast for the treatment of respiratory symptoms of post-respiratory syncytial virus bronchiolitis in children. *Am J Respir Crit Care Med* 2008;178:854–860.
54. Bitko V, Shulyayeva O, Mazumder B, et al. Nonstructural proteins of respiratory syncytial virus suppress premature apoptosis by an NF-kappaB-dependent, interferon-independent mechanism and facilitate virus growth. *J Virol* 2007;81:1786–1795.
55. Blanchard EL, Braun MR, Lifland AW, et al. Polymerase-tagged respiratory syncytial virus reveals a dynamic rearrangement of the ribonucleocapsid complex during infection. *PLoS Pathog* 2020;16:e1008987.
56. Blanken MO, Rovers MM, Molenaar JM, et al. Respiratory syncytial virus and recurrent wheeze in healthy preterm infants. *N Engl J Med* 2013;368:1791–1799.
57. Bockova J, O'Brien KL, Oski J, et al. Respiratory syncytial virus infection in Navajo and White Mountain Apache children. *Pediatrics* 2002;110:e20.
58. Boeckh M. The challenge of respiratory virus infections in hematopoietic cell transplant recipients. *Br J Haematol* 2008;143:455–467.
59. Botosso VF, Zanotto PM, Ueda M, et al. Positive selection results in frequent reversible amino acid replacements in the G protein gene of human respiratory syncytial virus. *PLoS Pathog* 2009;5:e1000254.
60. Boyce TG, Mellen BG, Mitchel EF Jr, et al. Rates of hospitalization for respiratory syncytial virus infection among children in medicaid. *J Pediatr* 2000;137:865–870.
61. Boyoglu-Barnum S, Gaston KA, Todd SO, et al. A respiratory syncytial virus (RSV) anti-G protein F(ab')2 monoclonal antibody suppresses mucous production and breathing effort in RSV rA2-line19F-infected BALB/c mice. *J Virol* 2013;87:10955–10967.
62. Boyoglu-Barnum S, Todd SO, Chirkova T, et al. An anti-G protein monoclonal antibody treats RSV disease more effectively than an anti-F monoclonal antibody in BALB/c mice. *Virology* 2015;483:117–125.
63. Brandenburg AH, Kleinjan A, van Het Land B, et al. Type 1-like immune response is found in children with respiratory syncytial virus infection regardless of clinical severity. *J Med Virol* 2000;62:267–277.
64. Braun MR, Noton SL, Blanchard EL, et al. Respiratory syncytial virus M2-1 protein associates non-specifically with viral messenger RNA and with specific cellular messenger RNA transcripts. *PLoS Pathog* 2021;17:e1009589.
65. Brearey SP, Symth RL. Pathogenesis of RSV in children. In: Cane P, ed. *Respiratory Syncytial Virus*. Amsterdam: Elsevier; 2007:141–162.
66. Brenes-Chacon H, Garcia-Maurino C, Moore-Clingenpeel M, et al. Age-dependent interactions among clinical characteristics, viral loads and disease severity in young children with respiratory syncytial virus infection. *Pediatr Infect Dis J* 2021;40:116–122.
67. Brittain-Long R, Andersson LM, Olofsson S, et al. Seasonal variations of 15 respiratory agents illustrated by the application of a multiplex polymerase chain reaction assay. *Scand J Infect Dis* 2012;44:9–17.
68. Brock LG, Karron RA, Krempl CD, et al. Evaluation of pneumonia virus of mice as a possible human pathogen. *J Virol* 2012;86:5829–5843.
69. Brock LG, Liu X, Liang B, et al. Murine pneumonia virus expressing the fusion glycoprotein of human respiratory syncytial virus from an added gene is highly attenuated and immunogenic in rhesus macaques. *J Virol* 2018;92.
70. Buchholz UJ, Biacchesi S, Pham QN, et al. Deletion of M2 gene open reading frames 1 and 2 of human metapneumovirus: effects on RNA synthesis, attenuation, and immunogenicity. *J Virol* 2005;79:6588–6597.
71. Buchholz UJ, Finke S, Conzelmann KK. Generation of bovine respiratory syncytial virus (BRSV) from cDNA: BRSV NS2 is not essential for virus replication in tissue culture, and the human RSV leader region acts as a functional BRSV genome promoter. *J Virol* 1999;73:251–259.
72. Buchholz UJ, Granzow H, Schuldt K, et al. Chimeric bovine respiratory syncytial virus with glycoprotein gene substitutions from human respiratory syncytial virus (HRSV): effects on host range and evaluation as a live-attenuated HRSV vaccine. *J Virol* 2000;74:1187–1199.
73. Buchholz UJ, Nagashima K, Murphy BR, et al. Live vaccines for human metapneumovirus designed by reverse genetics. *Expert Rev Vaccines* 2006;5:695–706.
74. Buckingham SC, Jafri HS, Bush AJ, et al. A randomized, double-blind, placebo-controlled trial of dexamethasone in severe respiratory syncytial virus (RSV) infection: effects on RSV quantity and clinical outcome. *J Infect Dis* 2002;185:1222–1228.
75. Buitendijk H, Fagrouch Z, Niphuis H, et al. Retrospective serology study of respiratory virus infections in captive great apes. *Viruses* 2014;6:1442–1453.
76. Bukreyev A, Whitehead SS, Murphy BR, et al. Recombinant respiratory syncytial virus from which the entire SH gene has been deleted grows efficiently in cell culture and exhibits site-specific attenuation in the respiratory tract of the mouse. *J Virol* 1997;71:8973–8982.
77. Bukreyev A, Yang L, Fricke J, et al. The secreted form of respiratory syncytial virus G glycoprotein helps the virus evade antibody-mediated restriction of replication by acting as an antigen decoy and through effects on Fc receptor-bearing leukocytes. *J Virol* 2008;82:12191–12204.
78. Byington CL, Wilkes J, Korgenski K, et al. Respiratory syncytial virus-associated mortality in hospitalized infants and young children. *Pediatrics* 2015;135:e24-e31.
79. Byrd LG, Prince GA. Animal models of respiratory syncytial virus infection. *Clin Infect Dis* 1997;25:1363–1368.
80. Caballero MT, Bianchi AM, Nuno A, et al. Mortality associated with acute respiratory infections among children at home. *J Infect Dis* 2019;219:358–364.
81. Caballero MT, Serra ME, Acosta PL, et al. TLR4 genotype and environmental LPS mediate RSV bronchiolitis through Th2 polarization. *J Clin Investig* 2015;125:571–582.
82. Campbell AP, Chien JW, Kuypers J, et al. Respiratory virus pneumonia after hematopoietic cell transplantation (HCT): associations between viral load in bronchoalveolar lavage samples, viral RNA detection in serum samples, and clinical outcomes of HCT. *J Infect Dis* 2010;201:1404–1413.
83. Cane PA, Pringle CR. Evolution of subgroup A respiratory syncytial virus: evidence for progressive accumulation of amino acid changes in the attachment protein. *J Virol* 1995;69:2918–2925.
84. Cao D, Gao Y, Roesler C, et al. Cryo-EM structure of the respiratory syncytial virus RNA polymerase. *Nat Commun* 2020;11:368.
85. Capella C, Chaiwatpongsakorn S, Gorrell E, et al. Prefusion F, postfusion F, G antibodies, and disease severity in infants and young children with acute respiratory syncytial virus infection. *J Infect Dis* 2017;216:1398–1406.
86. Carbonell-Estrany X, Simoes EA, Dagan R, et al. Motavizumab for prophylaxis of respiratory syncytial virus in high-risk children: a noninferiority trial. *Pediatrics* 2010;125:e35–e51.
87. Cartee TL, Megaw AG, Oomens AG, et al. Identification of a single amino acid change in the human respiratory syncytial virus L protein that affects transcriptional termination. *J Virol* 2003;77:7352–7360.
88. Castagne N, Barbier A, Bernard J, et al. Biochemical characterization of the respiratory syncytial virus P-P and P-N protein complexes and localization of the P protein oligomerization domain. *J Gen Virol* 2004;85:1643–1653.
89. Catelli E, Lupini C, Cecchinato M, et al. Field avian metapneumovirus evolution avoiding vaccine induced immunity. *Vaccine* 2010;28:916–921.
90. Chang A, Masante C, Buchholz UJ, et al. Human metapneumovirus (HMPV) binding and infection are mediated by interactions between the HMPV fusion protein and heparan sulfate. *J Virol* 2012;86:3230–3243.
91. Chang J, Braciale TJ. Respiratory syncytial virus infection suppresses lung CD8+ T-cell effector activity and peripheral CD8+ T-cell memory in the respiratory tract. *Nat Med* 2002;8:54–60.
92. Chanock RM, Finberg L. Recovery from infants with respiratory illness of a virus related to chimpanzee coryza agent (CCA). II Epidemiological aspects of infection in infants and young children. *Am J Hyg* 1957;66:291–300.
93. Chanock RM, Roizman B, Myers R. Recovery from infants with respiratory illness of a virus related to chimpanzee coryza agent. I. Isolation, properties and characterization. *Am J Hyg* 1957;66:281–290.
94. Chapman J, Abbott E, Alber DG, et al. RSV604, a novel inhibitor of respiratory syncytial virus replication. *Antimicrob Agents Chemother* 2007;51:3346–3353.
95. Chatterjee S, Luthra P, Esaulova E, et al. Structural basis for human respiratory syncytial virus NS1-mediated modulation of host responses. *Nat Microbiol* 2017;2:17101.
96. Chavez-Bueno S, Mejias A, Merryman RA, et al. Intravenous palivizumab and ribavirin combination for respiratory syncytial virus disease in high-risk pediatric patients. *Pediatr Infect Dis J* 2007;26:1089–1093.
97. Chemaly RF, Dadwal SS, Bergeron A, et al. A phase 2, randomized, double-blind, placebo-controlled trial of presatovir for the treatment of respiratory syncytial virus upper respiratory tract infection in hematopoietic-cell transplant recipients. *Clin Infect Dis* 2020;71:2777–2786.
98. Cheng X, Park H, Zhou H, et al. Overexpression of the M2-2 protein of respiratory syncytial virus inhibits viral replication. *J Virol* 2005;79:13943–13952.
99. Cherrie AH, Anderson K, Wertz GW, et al. Human cytotoxic T cells stimulated by antigen on dendritic cells recognize the N, SH, F, M, 22K, and 1b proteins of respiratory syncytial virus. *J Virol* 1992;66:2102–2110.
100. Choi Y, Mason CS, Jones LP, et al. Antibodies to the central conserved region of respiratory syncytial virus (RSV) G protein block RSV G protein CX3C-CX3CR1 binding and cross-neutralize RSV A and B strains. *Viral Immunol* 2012;25:193–203.
101. Chonmaitree T, Alvarez-Fernandez P, Jennings K, et al. Symptomatic and asymptomatic respiratory viral infections in the first year of life: association with acute otitis media development. *Clin Infect Dis* 2015;60:1–9.
102. Chu HY, Englund JA. Maternal immunization. *Birth Defects Res* 2017;109:379–386.
103. Cicconi P, Jones C, Sarkar E, et al. First-in-human randomized study to assess the safety and immunogenicity of an investigational respiratory syncytial virus (rsv) vaccine based on chimpanzee-adenovirus-155 viral vector-expressing rsv fusion, nucleocapsid, and antitermination viral proteins in healthy adults. *Clin Infect Dis* 2020;70:2073–2081.
104. Cimica V, Boigard H, Bhatia B, et al. Novel respiratory syncytial virus-like particle vaccine composed of the postfusion and prefusion conformations of the F glycoprotein. *Clin Vaccine Immunol* 2016;23:451–459.
105. Coates HV, Alling DW, Chanock RM. An antigenic analysis of respiratory syncytial virus isolates by a plaque reduction neutralization test. *Am J Epidemiol* 1966;83:299–313.
106. Cockerill GS, Angell RM, Bedernjak A, et al. Discovery of sisunatovir (RV521), an inhibitor of respiratory syncytial virus fusion. *J Med Chem* 2021;64:3658–3676.
107. Collins PL, Dickens LE, Buckler-White A, et al. Nucleotide sequences for the gene junctions of human respiratory syncytial virus reveal distinctive features of intergenic structure and gene order. *Proc Natl Acad Sci U S A* 1986;83:4594–4598.
108. Collins PL, Graham BS. Viral and host factors in human respiratory syncytial virus pathogenesis. *J Virol* 2008;82:2040–2055.
109. Collins PL, Hill MG, Camargo E, et al. Production of infectious human respiratory syncytial virus from cloned cDNA confirms an essential role for the transcription elongation factor from the 5′ proximal open reading frame of the M2 mRNA in gene expression and provides a capability for vaccine development. *Proc Natl Acad Sci U S A* 1995;92:11563–11567.
110. Collins PL, Hill MG, Cristina J, et al. Transcription elongation factor of respiratory syncytial virus, a nonsegmented negative-strand RNA virus. *Proc Natl Acad Sci U S A* 1996;93:81–85.
111. Collins PL, Huang YT, Wertz GW. Identification of a tenth mRNA of respiratory syncytial virus and assignment of polypeptides to the 10 viral genes. *J Virol* 1984;49:572–578.
112. Collins PL, Huang YT, Wertz GW. Nucleotide sequence of the gene encoding the fusion (F) glycoprotein of human respiratory syncytial virus. *Proc Natl Acad Sci U S A* 1984;81:7683–7687.
113. Collins PL, Karron RA. Respiratory syncytial virus and metapneumovirus. In: Knipe DM, Howley PM, Cohen JI, et al., eds. *Fields Virology*. Philadelphia, PA: Lippincott Williams & Wilkins; 2013:1086–1123.

114. Collins PL, Mottet G. Membrane orientation and oligomerization of the small hydrophobic protein of human respiratory syncytial virus. *J Gen Virol* 1993;74:1445–1450.
115. Collins PL, Olmsted RA, Johnson PR. The small hydrophobic protein of human respiratory syncytial virus: comparison between antigenic subgroups A and B. *J Gen Virol* 1990;71:1571–1576.
116. Collins PL, Olmsted RA, Spriggs MK, et al. Gene overlap and site-specific attenuation of transcription of the viral polymerase L gene of human respiratory syncytial virus. *Proc Natl Acad Sci U S A* 1987;84:5134–5138.
117. Collins PL, Wertz GW. cDNA cloning and transcriptional mapping of nine polyadenylylated RNAs encoded by the genome of human respiratory syncytial virus. *Proc Natl Acad Sci U S A* 1983;80:3208–3212.
118. Connors M, Collins PL, Firestone CY, et al. Respiratory syncytial virus (RSV) F, G, M2 (22K), and N proteins each induce resistance to RSV challenge, but resistance induced by M2 and N proteins is relatively short-lived. *J Virol* 1991;65:1634–1637.
119. Connors M, Giese NA, Kulkarni AB, et al. Enhanced pulmonary histopathology induced by respiratory syncytial virus (RSV) challenge of formalin-inactivated RSV-immunized BALB/c mice is abrogated by depletion of interleukin-4 (IL-4) and IL-10. *J Virol* 1994;68:5321–5325.
120. Connors M, Kulkarni AB, Firestone CY, et al. Pulmonary histopathology induced by respiratory syncytial virus (RSV) challenge of formalin-inactivated RSV-immunized BALB/c mice is abrogated by depletion of CD4+ T cells. *J Virol* 1992;66:7444–7451.
121. Corry J, Johnson SM, Cornwell J, et al. Preventing cleavage of the respiratory syncytial virus attachment protein in Vero cells rescues the infectivity of progeny virus for primary human airway cultures. *J Virol* 2016;90:1311–1320.
122. Cortjens B, de Boer OJ, de Jong R, et al. Neutrophil extracellular traps cause airway obstruction during respiratory syncytial virus disease. *J Pathol* 2016;238:401–411.
123. Cortjens B, Yasuda E, Yu X, et al. Broadly reactive anti-respiratory syncytial virus G antibodies from exposed individuals effectively inhibit infection of primary airway epithelial cells. *J Virol* 2017;91.
124. Cox RG, Livesay SB, Johnson M, et al. The human metapneumovirus fusion protein mediates entry via an interaction with RGD-binding integrins. *J Virol* 2012;86:12148–12160.
125. Cox RG, Mainou BA, Johnson M, et al. Human metapneumovirus is capable of entering cells by fusion with endosomal membranes. *PLoS Pathog* 2015;11:e1005303.
126. Crank MC, Ruckwardt TJ, Chen M, et al. A proof of concept for structure-based vaccine design targeting RSV in humans. *Science* 2019;365:505–509.
127. Cristina J, Yunus AS, Rockemann DD, et al. Genetic analysis of the G and P genes in ungulate respiratory syncytial viruses by RNase A mismatch cleavage method. *Vet Microbiol* 1998;62:185–192.
128. Crow R, Mutyara K, Agustian D, et al. Risk factors for respiratory syncytial virus lower respiratory tract infections: evidence from an Indonesian cohort. *Viruses* 2021;13.
129. Crowe JE Jr. Influence of maternal antibodies on neonatal immunization against respiratory viruses. *Clin Infect Dis* 2001;33:1720–1727.
130. Crowe JE Jr, Bui PT, Davis AR, et al. A further attenuated derivative of a cold-passaged temperature-sensitive mutant of human respiratory syncytial virus retains immunogenicity and protective efficacy against wild-type challenge in seronegative chimpanzees. *Vaccine* 1994;12:783–790.
131. Crowe JE Jr, Bui PT, Siber GR, et al. Cold-passaged, temperature-sensitive mutants of human respiratory syncytial virus (RSV) are highly attenuated, immunogenic, and protective in seronegative chimpanzees, even when RSV antibodies are infused shortly before immunization. *Vaccine* 1995;13:847–855.
132. Crowe JE Jr, Firestone CY, Murphy BR. Passively acquired antibodies suppress humoral but not cell-mediated immunity in mice immunized with live attenuated respiratory syncytial virus vaccines. *J Immunol* 2001;167:3910–3918.
133. Cullen LM, Schmidt MR, Torres GM, et al. Comparison of immune responses to different versions of VLP associated stabilized RSV pre-fusion F protein. *Vaccines (Basel)* 2019;7.
134. Culley FJ, Pollott J, Openshaw PJ. Age at first viral infection determines the pattern of T cell-mediated disease during reinfection in adulthood. *J Exp Med* 2002;196:1381–1386.
135. Cunningham S, Piedra PA, Martinon-Torres F, et al. Nebulised ALX-0171 for respiratory syncytial virus lower respiratory tract infection in hospitalised children: a double-blind, randomised, placebo-controlled, phase 2b trial. *Lancet Respir Med* 2021;9:21–32.
136. Da Dalt L, Callegaro S, Carraro S, et al. Nasal lavage leukotrienes in infants with RSV bronchiolitis. *Pediatr Allergy Immunol* 2007;18:100–104.
137. Dakhama A, Vitalis TZ, Hegele RG. Persistence of respiratory syncytial virus (RSV) infection and development of RSV-specific IgG1 response in a guinea-pig model of acute bronchiolitis. *Eur Respir J* 1997;10:20–26.
138. Dall'Acqua WF, Kiener PA, Wu H. Properties of human IgG1s engineered for enhanced binding to the neonatal Fc receptor (FcRn). *J Biol Chem* 2006;281:23514–23524.
139. de Graaf M, Osterhaus AD, Fouchier RA, et al. Evolutionary dynamics of human and avian metapneumoviruses. *J Gen Virol* 2008;89:2933–2942.
140. de Graaff PM, de Jong EC, van Capel TM, et al. Respiratory syncytial virus infection of monocyte-derived dendritic cells decreases their capacity to activate CD4 T cells. *J Immunol* 2005;175:5904–5911.
141. de Sierra TM, Kumar ML, Wasser TE, et al. Respiratory syncytial virus-specific immunoglobulins in preterm infants. *J Pediatr* 1993;122:787–791.
142. de Steenhuijsen Piters WA, Heinonen S, Hasrat R, et al. Nasopharyngeal microbiota, host transcriptome, and disease severity in children with respiratory syncytial virus infection. *Am J Respir Crit Care Med* 2016;194:1104–1115.
143. De Swart RL, Kuiken T, Timmerman HH, et al. Immunization of macaques with formalin-inactivated respiratory syncytial virus (RSV) induces interleukin-13-associated hypersensitivity to subsequent RSV infection. *J Virol* 2002;76:11561–11569.
144. de Swart RL, van den Hoogen BG, Kuiken T, et al. Immunization of macaques with formalin-inactivated human metapneumovirus induces hypersensitivity to hMPV infection. *Vaccine* 2007;25:8518–8528.
145. Debiaggi M, Canducci F, Terulla C, et al. Long-term study on symptomless human metapneumovirus infection in hematopoietic stem cell transplant recipients. *New Microbiol* 2007;30:255–258.
146. Deffrasnes C, Cote S, Boivin G. Analysis of replication kinetics of the human metapneumovirus in different cell lines by real-time PCR. *J Clin Microbiol* 2005;43:488–490.
147. Delgado MF, Coviello S, Monsalvo AC, et al. Lack of antibody affinity maturation due to poor Toll-like receptor stimulation leads to enhanced respiratory syncytial virus disease. *Nat Med* 2009;15:34–41.
148. Derdowski A, Peters TR, Glover N, et al. Human metapneumovirus nucleoprotein and phosphoprotein interact and provide the minimal requirements for inclusion body formation. *J Gen Virol* 2008;89:2698–2708.
149. DeVincenzo J, Tait D, Efthimiou J, et al. A randomized, placebo-controlled, respiratory syncytial virus human challenge study of the antiviral efficacy, safety, and pharmacokinetics of RV521, an inhibitor of the RSV-F protein. *Antimicrob Agents Chemother* 2020;64.
150. DeVincenzo JP, El Saleeby CM, Bush AJ. Respiratory syncytial virus load predicts disease severity in previously healthy infants. *J Infect Dis* 2005;191:1861–1868.
151. DeVincenzo JP, McClure MW, Symons JA, et al. Activity of oral ALS-008176 in a respiratory syncytial virus challenge study. *N Engl J Med* 2015;373:2048–2058.
152. DeVincenzo JP, Whitley RJ, Mackman RL, et al. Oral GS-5806 activity in a respiratory syncytial virus challenge study. *N Engl J Med* 2014;371:711–722.
153. Diaz-Diaz A, Bunsow E, Garcia-Maurino C, et al. Nasopharyngeal codetection of *H. influenzae* and *S. pneumoniae* and respiratory syncytial virus disease outcomes in children. *J Infect Dis* 2021. https://doi.org/10.1093/infdis/jiab481
154. Dickens LE, Collins PL, Wertz GW. Transcriptional mapping of human respiratory syncytial virus. *J Virol* 1984;52:364–369.
155. DiNapoli JM, Murphy BR, Collins PL, et al. Impairment of the CD8+ T cell response in lungs following infection with human respiratory syncytial virus is specific to the anatomical site rather than the virus, antigen, or route of infection. *Virol J* 2008;5:105.
156. Dinwiddie DL, Harrod KS. Human metapneumovirus inhibits IFN-alpha signaling through inhibition of STAT1 phosphorylation. *Am J Respir Cell Mol Biol* 2008;38:661–670.
157. Do LAH, Pellet J, van Doorn HR, et al. Host transcription profile in nasal epithelium and whole blood of hospitalized children under 2 years of age with respiratory syncytial virus infection. *J Infect Dis* 2017;217:134–146.
158. Driscoll AJ, Arshad SH, Bont L, et al. Does respiratory syncytial virus lower respiratory illness in early life cause recurrent wheeze of early childhood and asthma? Critical review of the evidence and guidance for future studies from a World Health Organization-sponsored meeting. *Vaccine* 2020;38:2435–2448.
159. Dupuy LC, Dobson S, Bitko V, et al. Casein kinase 2-mediated phosphorylation of respiratory syncytial virus phosphoprotein P is essential for the transcription elongation activity of the viral polymerase; phosphorylation by casein kinase 1 occurs mainly at Ser(215) and is without effect. *J Virol* 1999;73:8384–8392.
160. Durbin JE, Johnson TR, Durbin RK, et al. The role of IFN in respiratory syncytial virus pathogenesis. *J Immunol* 2002;168:2944–2952.
161. Duvvuri VR, Granados A, Rosenfeld P, et al. Genetic diversity and evolutionary insights of respiratory syncytial virus A ON1 genotype: global and local transmission dynamics. *Sci Rep* 2015;5:14268.
162. Edwards KM. The impact of social distancing for severe acute respiratory syndrome coronavirus 2 on respiratory syncytial virus and influenza burden. *Clin Infect Dis* 2021;72:2076–2078.
163. Edwards KM, Zhu Y, Griffin MR, et al. Burden of human metapneumovirus infection in young children. *N Engl J Med* 2013;368:633–643.
164. Eisenhut M. Extrapulmonary manifestations of severe respiratory syncytial virus infection—a systematic review. *Crit Care* 2006;10:R107.
165. El Najjar F, Cifuentes-Munoz N, Chen J, et al. Human metapneumovirus induces reorganization of the actin cytoskeleton for direct cell-to-cell spread. *PLoS Pathog* 2016;12:e1005922.
166. El Saleeby CM, Suzich J, Conley ME, et al. Quantitative effects of palivizumab and donor-derived T cells on chronic respiratory syncytial virus infection, lung disease, and fusion glycoprotein amino acid sequences in a patient before and after bone marrow transplantation. *Clin Infect Dis* 2004;39:e17–e20.
167. Ermers MJ, Rovers MM, van Woensel JB, et al. The effect of high dose inhaled corticosteroids on wheeze in infants after respiratory syncytial virus infection: randomised double blind placebo controlled trial. *BMJ* 2009;338:b897.
168. Escribano-Romero E, Rawling J, Garcia-Barreno B, et al. The soluble form of human respiratory syncytial virus attachment protein differs from the membrane-bound form in its oligomeric state but is still capable of binding to cell surface proteoglycans. *J Virol* 2004;78:3524–3532.
169. Eshaghi A, Duvvuri VR, Lai R, et al. Genetic variability of human respiratory syncytial virus A strains circulating in Ontario: a novel genotype with a 72 nucleotide G gene duplication. *PLoS One* 2012;7:e32807.
170. Esneau C, Raynal B, Roblin P, et al. Biochemical characterization of the respiratory syncytial virus N(0)-P complex in solution. *J Biol Chem* 2019;294:3647–3660.
171. Evans JE, Cane PA, Pringle CR. Expression and characterisation of the NS1 and NS2 proteins of respiratory syncytial virus. *Virus Res* 1996;43:155–161.
172. Everard ML, Swarbrick A, Wrightham M, et al. Analysis of cells obtained by bronchial lavage of infants with respiratory syncytial virus infection. *Arch Dis Child* 1994;71:428–432.
173. Falloon J, Yu J, Esser MT, et al. An adjuvanted, postfusion F protein-based vaccine did not prevent respiratory syncytial virus illness in older adults. *J Infect Dis* 2017;216:1362–1370.
174. Falsey AR. Human metapneumovirus infection in adults. *Pediatr Infect Dis J* 2008;27:S80–S83.
175. Falsey AR. Respiratory syncytial virus infection in adults. *Semin Respir Crit Care Med* 2007;28:171–181.
176. Falsey AR, Erdman D, Anderson LJ, et al. Human metapneumovirus infections in young and elderly adults. *J Infect Dis* 2003;187:785–790.
177. Falsey AR, Formica MA, Hennessey PA, et al. Detection of respiratory syncytial virus in adults with chronic obstructive pulmonary disease. *Am J Respir Crit Care Med* 2006;173:639–643.
178. Falsey AR, Hennessey PA, Formica MA, et al. Respiratory syncytial virus infection in elderly and high-risk adults. *N Engl J Med* 2005;352:1749–1759.

179. Falsey AR, Hennessey PA, Formica MA, et al. Humoral immunity to human metapneumovirus infection in adults. *Vaccine* 2010;28:1477–1480.

180. Falsey AR, Singh HK, Walsh EE. Serum antibody decay in adults following natural respiratory syncytial virus infection. *J Med Virol* 2006;78:1493–1497.

181. Falsey AR, Walsh EE. Relationship of serum antibody to risk of respiratory syncytial virus infection in elderly adults. *J Infect Dis* 1998;177:463–466.

182. Falsey AR, Walsh EE. Safety and immunogenicity of a respiratory syncytial virus subunit vaccine (PFP-2) in the institutionalized elderly. *Vaccine* 1997;15:1130–1132.

183. Fearns R, Collins PL. Model for polymerase access to the overlapped L gene of respiratory syncytial virus. *J Virol* 1999;73:388–397.

184. Fearns R, Collins PL. Role of the M2-1 transcription antitermination protein of respiratory syncytial virus in sequential transcription. *J Virol* 1999;73:5852–5864.

185. Fearns R, Peeples ME, Collins PL. Increased expression of the N protein of respiratory syncytial virus stimulates minigenome replication but does not alter the balance between the synthesis of mRNA and antigenome. *Virology* 1997;236:188–201.

186. Fearns R, Peeples ME, Collins PL. Mapping the transcription and replication promoters of respiratory syncytial virus. *J Virol* 2002;76:1663–1672.

187. Fedechkin SO, George NL, Nunez Castrejon AM, et al. Conformational flexibility in respiratory syncytial virus G neutralizing epitopes. *J Virol* 2020;94.

188. Feldman SA, Audet S, Beeler JA. The fusion glycoprotein of human respiratory syncytial virus facilitates virus attachment and infectivity via an interaction with cellular heparan sulfate. *J Virol* 2000;74:6442–6447.

189. Feldman SA, Hendry RM, Beeler JA. Identification of a linear heparin binding domain for human respiratory syncytial virus attachment glycoprotein G. *J Virol* 1999;73:6610–6617.

190. Felt SA, Sun Y, Jozwik A, et al. Detection of respiratory syncytial virus defective genomes in nasal secretions is associated with distinct clinical outcomes. *Nat Microbiol* 2021; 6:672–681.

191. Finger R, Anderson LJ, Dicker RC, et al. Epidemic infections caused by respiratory syncytial virus in institutionalized young adults. *J Infect Dis* 1987;155:1335–1339.

192. Fisher BT, Danziger-Isakov L, Sweet LR, et al. A multicenter consortium to define the epidemiology and outcomes of inpatient respiratory viral infections in pediatric hematopoietic stem cell transplant recipients. *J Pediatric Infect Dis Soc* 2018;7:275–282.

193. Foley DA, Yeoh DK, Minney-Smith CA, et al. The interseasonal resurgence of respiratory syncytial virus in Australian children following the reduction of coronavirus disease 2019-related public health measures. *Clin Infect Dis* 2021;73:e2829–e2830.

194. Fricke J, Koo LY, Brown CR, et al. p38 and OGT sequestration into viral inclusion bodies in cells infected with human respiratory syncytial virus suppresses MK2 activities and stress granule assembly. *J Virol* 2013;87:1333–1347.

195. Friedewald WT, Forsyth BR, Smith CB, et al. Low-temperature-grown RS virus in adult volunteers. *JAMA* 1968;203:690–694.

196. Fries L, Shinde V, Stoddard JJ, et al. Immunogenicity and safety of a respiratory syncytial virus fusion protein (RSV F) nanoparticle vaccine in older adults. *Immun Ageing* 2017;14:8.

197. Fuentes S, Hahn M, Chilcote K, et al. Antigenic fingerprinting of respiratory syncytial virus (RSV)-A-infected hematopoietic cell transplant recipients reveals importance of mucosal anti-RSV G antibodies in control of RSV infection in humans. *J Infect Dis* 2020;221:636–646.

198. Fuentes S, Tran KC, Luthra P, et al. Function of the respiratory syncytial virus small hydrophobic protein. *J Virol* 2007;81:8361–8366.

199. Galloux M, Risso-Ballester J, Richard CA, et al. Minimal elements required for the formation of respiratory syncytial virus cytoplasmic inclusion bodies in vivo and in vitro. *MBio* 2020;11.

200. Gan SW, Tan E, Lin X, et al. The small hydrophobic protein of the human respiratory syncytial virus forms pentameric ion channels. *J Biol Chem* 2012;287:24671–24689.

201. Gao L, Yu S, Chen Q, et al. A randomized controlled trial of low-dose recombinant human interferons alpha-2b nasal spray to prevent acute viral respiratory infections in military recruits. *Vaccine* 2010;28:4445–4451.

202. Gao Y, Cao D, Pawnikar S, et al. Structure of the human respiratory syncytial virus M2-1 protein in complex with a short positive-sense gene-end RNA. *Structure* 2020;28:979–990.e974.

203. Garcia C, Soriano-Fallas A, Lozano J, et al. Decreased innate immune cytokine responses correlate with disease severity in children with respiratory syncytial virus and human rhinovirus bronchiolitis. *Pediatr Infect Dis J* 2012;31:86–89.

204. Garcia CG, Bhore R, Soriano-Fallas A, et al. Risk factors in children hospitalized with RSV bronchiolitis versus non-RSV bronchiolitis. *Pediatrics* 2010;126:e1453–e1460.

205. Garcia-Maurino C, Moore-Clingenpeel M, Thomas J, et al. Viral load dynamics and clinical disease severity in infants with respiratory syncytial virus infection. *J Infect Dis* 2019;219:1207–1215.

206. Gardner PS, McQuillin J, Court SD. Speculation on pathogenesis in death from respiratory syncytial virus infection. *Br Med J* 1970;1:327–330.

207. Gershwin LJ. Bovine respiratory syncytial virus infection: immunopathogenic mechanisms. *Anim Health Res Rev* 2007;8:207–213.

208. Ghildyal R, Baulch-Brown C, Mills J, et al. The matrix protein of Human respiratory syncytial virus localises to the nucleus of infected cells and inhibits transcription. *Arch Virol* 2003;148:1419–1429.

209. Gill MA, Long K, Kwon T, et al. Differential recruitment of dendritic cells and monocytes to respiratory mucosal sites in children with influenza virus or respiratory syncytial virus infection. *J Infect Dis* 2008;198:1667–1676.

210. Gillespie L, Gerstenberg K, Ana-Sosa-Batiz F, et al. DC-SIGN and L-SIGN are attachment factors that promote infection of target cells by human metapneumovirus in the presence or absence of cellular glycosaminoglycans. *J Virol* 2016;90:7848–7863.

211. Gilman MS, Castellanos CA, Chen M, et al. Rapid profiling of RSV antibody repertoires from the memory B cells of naturally infected adult donors. *Sci Immunol* 2016;1.

212. Gilman MSA, Liu C, Fung A, et al. Structure of the respiratory syncytial virus polymerase complex. *Cell* 2019;179:193–204.e114.

213. Ginocchio CC, Swierkosz E, McAdam AJ, et al. Multicenter study of clinical performance of the 3M Rapid Detection RSV test. *J Clin Microbiol* 2010;48:2337–2343.

214. Glezen WP, Taber LH, Frank AL, et al. Risk of primary infection and reinfection with respiratory syncytial virus. *Am J Dis Child* 1986;140:543–546.

215. Gonzalez IM, Karron RA, Eichelberger M, et al. Evaluation of the live attenuated cpts 248/404 RSV vaccine in combination with a subunit RSV vaccine (PFP-2) in healthy young and older adults. *Vaccine* 2000;18:1763–1772.

216. Gonzalez-Reyes L, Ruiz-Arguello MB, Garcia-Barreno B, et al. Cleavage of the human respiratory syncytial virus fusion protein at two distinct sites is required for activation of membrane fusion. *Proc Natl Acad Sci U S A* 2001;98:9859–9864.

217. Goodwin E, Gilman MSA, Wrapp D, et al. Infants infected with respiratory syncytial virus generate potent neutralizing antibodies that lack somatic hypermutation. *Immunity* 2018;48:339–349.e335.

218. Gorman JJ, Ferguson BL, Speelman D, et al. Determination of the disulfide bond arrangement of human respiratory syncytial virus attachment (G) protein by matrix-assisted laser desorption/ionization time-of-flight mass spectrometry. *Protein Sci* 1997;6:1308–1315.

219. Goswami R, Majumdar T, Dhar J, et al. Viral degradasome hijacks mitochondria to suppress innate immunity. *Cell Res* 2013;23:1025–1042.

220. Gottlieb J, Zamora MR, Hodges T, et al. ALN-RSV01 for prevention of bronchiolitis obliterans syndrome after respiratory syncytial virus infection in lung transplant recipients. *J Heart Lung Transplant* 2016;35:213–221.

221. Gould PS, Easton AJ. Coupled translation of the second open reading frame of M2 mRNA is sequence dependent and differs significantly within the subfamily Pneumovirinae. *J Virol* 2007;81:8488–8496.

222. Goutagny N, Jiang Z, Tian J, et al. Cell type-specific recognition of human metapneumoviruses (HMPVs) by retinoic acid-inducible gene I (RIG-I) and TLR7 and viral interference of RIG-I ligand recognition by HMPV-B1 phosphoprotein. *J Immunol* 2010;184:1168–1179.

223. Govindarajan D, Samal SK. Analysis of the complete genome sequence of avian metapneumovirus subgroup C indicates that it possesses the longest genome among metapneumoviruses. *Virus Genes* 2005;30:331–333.

224. Gower TL, Pastey MK, Peeples ME, et al. RhoA signaling is required for respiratory syncytial virus-induced syncytium formation and filamentous virion morphology. *J Virol* 2005;79:5326–5336.

225. Goya S, Galiano M, Nauwelaers I, et al. Toward unified molecular surveillance of RSV: a proposal for genotype definition. *Influenza Other Respir Viruses* 2020;14:274–285.

226. Graham BS. Vaccine development for respiratory syncytial virus. *Curr Opin Virol* 2017;23:107–112.

227. Graham BS, Bunton LA, Rowland J, et al. Respiratory syncytial virus infection in anti-mu treated mice. *J Virol* 1991;65:4936–4942.

228. Graham BS, Bunton LA, Wright PF, et al. Reinfection of mice with respiratory syncytial virus [published erratum appears in J Med Virol 1991 Dec;35(4):307]. *J Med Virol* 1991;34:7–13.

229. Graham BS, Bunton LA, Wright PF, et al. Role of T lymphocyte subsets in the pathogenesis of primary infection and rechallenge with respiratory syncytial virus in mice. *J Clin Invest* 1991;88:1026–1033.

230. Graham BS, Perkins MD, Wright PF, et al. Primary respiratory syncytial virus infection in mice. *J Med Virol* 1988;26:153–162.

231. Grayson SA, Griffiths PS, Perez MK, et al. Detection of airborne respiratory syncytial virus in a pediatric acute care clinic. *Pediatr Pulmonol* 2017;52:684–688.

232. Green CA, Sande CJ, Scarselli E, et al. Novel genetically-modified chimpanzee adenovirus and MVA-vectored respiratory syncytial virus vaccine safely boosts humoral and cellular immunity in healthy older adults. *J Infect* 2019;78:382–392.

233. Green G, Johnson SM, Costello H, et al. CX3CR1 is a receptor for human respiratory syncytial virus in cotton rats. *J Virol* 2021;95:e0001021.

234. Griffin MP, Yuan Y, Takas T, et al. Single-dose nirsevimab for prevention of RSV in preterm infants. *N Engl J Med* 2020;383:415–425.

235. Griffiths CD, Bilawchuk LM, McDonough JE, et al. IGF1R is an entry receptor for respiratory syncytial virus. *Nature* 2020;583:615–619.

236. Groothuis JR, Gutierrez KM, Lauer BA. Respiratory syncytial virus infection in children with bronchopulmonary dysplasia. *Pediatrics* 1988;82:199–203.

237. Groothuis JR, King SJ, Hogerman DA, et al. Safety and immunogenicity of a purified F protein respiratory syncytial virus (PFP-2) vaccine in seropositive children with bronchopulmonary dysplasia. *J Infect Dis* 1998;177:467–469.

238. Groothuis JR, Simoes EA, Levin MJ, et al. Prophylactic administration of respiratory syncytial virus immune globulin to high-risk infants and young children. The Respiratory Syncytial Virus Immune Globulin Study Group. *N Engl J Med* 1993;329:1524–1530.

239. Groskreutz DJ, Babor EC, Monick MM, et al. Respiratory syncytial virus limits alpha subunit of eukaryotic translation initiation factor 2 (eIF2alpha) phosphorylation to maintain translation and viral replication. *J Biol Chem* 2010;285:24023–24031.

240. Guerrero-Plata A, Baron S, Poast JS, et al. Activity and regulation of alpha interferon in respiratory syncytial virus and human metapneumovirus experimental infections. *J Virol* 2005;79:10190–10199.

241. Guerrero-Plata A, Casola A, Suarez G, et al. Differential response of dendritic cells to human metapneumovirus and respiratory syncytial virus. *Am J Respir Cell Mol Biol* 2006;34:320–329.

242. Guvenel A, Jozwik A, Ascough S, et al. Epitope-specific airway-resident CD4+ T cell dynamics during experimental human RSV infection. *J Clin Invest* 2020;130:523–538.

243. Haas LE, Thijsen SF, van Elden L, et al. Human metapneumovirus in adults. *Viruses* 2013;5:87–110.

244. Habibi MS, Jozwik A, Makris S, et al. Impaired antibody-mediated protection and defective IgA B-cell memory in experimental infection of adults with respiratory syncytial virus. *Am J Respir Crit Care Med* 2015;191:1040–1049.

245. Habibi MS, Thwaites RS, Chang M, et al. Neutrophilic inflammation in the respiratory mucosa predisposes to RSV infection. *Science* 2020;370.

246. Hacking D, Knight JC, Rockett K, et al. Increased in vivo transcription of an IL-8 haplotype associated with respiratory syncytial virus disease-susceptibility. *Genes Immun* 2004;5:274–282.

247. Halfhide CP, Flanagan BF, Brearey SP, et al. Respiratory syncytial virus binds and undergoes transcription in neutrophils from the blood and airways of infants with severe bronchiolitis. *J Infect Dis* 2011;204:451–458.

248. Hall CB. Respiratory syncytial virus and parainfluenza virus. *N Engl J Med* 2001;344:1917–1928.

249. Hall CB, Douglas RG Jr, Geiman JM. Possible transmission by fomites of respiratory syncytial virus. *J Infect Dis* 1980;141:98–102.

250. Hall CB, Douglas RG Jr, Geiman JM. Quantitative shedding patterns of respiratory syncytial virus in infants. *J Infect Dis* 1975;132:151–156.

251. Hall CB, Douglas RG Jr, Geiman JM, et al. Nosocomial respiratory syncytial virus infections. *N Engl J Med* 1975;293:1343–1346.

252. Hall CB, Douglas RG Jr, Simons RL. Interferon production in adults with respiratory syncytial viral infection. *Ann Intern Med* 1981;94:53–55.

253. Hall CB, Douglas RG Jr, Simons RL, et al. Interferon production in children with respiratory syncytial, influenza, and parainfluenza virus infections. *J Pediatr* 1978;93:28–32.

254. Hall CB, Geiman JM, Biggar R, et al. Respiratory syncytial virus infections within families. *N Engl J Med* 1976;294:414–419.

255. Hall CB, Powell KR, MacDonald NE, et al. Respiratory syncytial viral infection in children with compromised immune function. *N Engl J Med* 1986;315:77–81.

256. Hall CB, Powell KR, Schnabel KC, et al. Risk of secondary bacterial infection in infants hospitalized with respiratory syncytial viral infection. *J Pediatr* 1988;113:266–271.

257. Hall CB, Walsh EE, Long CE, et al. Immunity to and frequency of reinfection with respiratory syncytial virus. *J Infect Dis* 1991;163:693–698.

258. Hall CB, Weinberg GA, Iwane MK, et al. The burden of respiratory syncytial virus infection in young children. *N Engl J Med* 2009;360:588–598.

259. Hallak LK, Collins PL, Knudson W, et al. Iduronic acid-containing glycosaminoglycans on target cells are required for efficient respiratory syncytial virus infection. *Virology* 2000;271:264–275.

260. Hamelin ME, Gagnon C, Prince GA, et al. Prophylactic and therapeutic benefits of a monoclonal antibody against the fusion protein of human metapneumovirus in a mouse model. *Antiviral Res* 2010;88:31–37.

261. Hamelin ME, Yim K, Kuhn KH, et al. Pathogenesis of human metapneumovirus lung infection in BALB/c mice and cotton rats. *J Virol* 2005;79:8894–8903.

262. Hanfelt-Goade D, Maimon N, Nimer A, et al. A phase 2b, randomized, double-blind, placebo-controlled trial of presatovir (GS-5806), a novel oral RSV fusion inhibitor, for the treatment of respiratory syncytial virus (RSV) in hospitalized adults. *Am J Respir Crit Care Med* 2018;197:A4457.

263. Hanley LL, McGivern DR, Teng MN, et al. Roles of the respiratory syncytial virus trailer region: effects of mutations on genome production and stress granule formation. *Virology* 2010;406:241–252.

264. Harcourt J, Alvarez R, Jones LP, et al. Respiratory syncytial virus G protein and G protein CX3C motif adversely affect CX3CR1+ T cell responses. *J Immunol* 2006;176:1600–1608.

265. Hardy RW, Harmon SB, Wertz GW. Diverse gene junctions of respiratory syncytial virus modulate the efficiency of transcription termination and respond differently to M2-mediated antitermination. *J Virol* 1999;73:170–176.

266. Hardy RW, Wertz GW. The Cys(3)-His(1) motif of the respiratory syncytial virus M2-1 protein is essential for protein function. *J Virol* 2000;74:5880–5885.

267. Hardy RW, Wertz GW. The product of the respiratory syncytial virus M2 gene ORF1 enhances readthrough of intergenic junctions during viral transcription. *J Virol* 1998;72:520–526.

268. Hasegawa K, Jartti T, Mansbach JM, et al. Respiratory syncytial virus genomic load and disease severity among children hospitalized with bronchiolitis: multicenter cohort studies in the United States and Finland. *J Infect Dis* 2015;211:1550–1559.

269. Heidema J, Lukens MV, van Maren WW, et al. CD8+ T cell responses in bronchoalveolar lavage fluid and peripheral blood mononuclear cells of infants with severe primary respiratory syncytial virus infections. *J Immunol* 2007;179:8410–8417.

270. Heidema J, Rossen JW, Lukens MV, et al. Dynamics of human respiratory virus-specific CD8+ T cell responses in blood and airways during episodes of common cold. *J Immunol* 2008;181:5551–5559.

271. Heinonen S, Velazquez VM, Ye F, et al. Immune profiles provide insights into respiratory syncytial virus disease severity in young children. *Sci Transl Med* 2020;12.

272. Heinze B, Frey S, Mordstein M, et al. Both nonstructural proteins 1 and 2 of pneumonia virus of mice are inhibitors of the interferon type I and III response in vivo. *J Virol* 2011;85:4071–4084.

273. Henderson FW, Collier AM, Clyde WA Jr, et al. Respiratory-syncytial-virus infections, reinfections and immunity. A prospective, longitudinal study in young children. *N Engl J Med* 1979;300:530–534.

274. Henderson G, Murray J, Yeo RP. Sorting of the respiratory syncytial virus matrix protein into detergent-resistant structures is dependent on cell-surface expression of the glycoproteins. *Virology* 2002;300:244–254.

275. Hendricks DA, McIntosh K, Patterson JL. Further characterization of the soluble form of the G glycoprotein of respiratory syncytial virus. *J Virol* 1988;62:2228–2233.

276. Hendry RM, Burns JC, Walsh EE, et al. Strain-specific serum antibody responses in infants undergoing primary infection with respiratory syncytial virus. *J Infect Dis* 1988;157:640–647.

277. Herfst S, de Graaf M, Schickli JH, et al. Recovery of human metapneumovirus genetic lineages a and B from cloned cDNA. *J Virol* 2004;78:8264–8270.

278. Herfst S, de Graaf M, Schrauwen EJA, et al. Generation of temperature-sensitive human metapneumovirus strains that provide protective immunity in hamsters. *J Gen Virol* 2008;89:1553–1562.

279. Herfst S, Mas V, Ver LS, et al. Low-pH-induced membrane fusion mediated by human metapneumovirus F protein is a rare, strain-dependent phenomenon. *J Virol* 2008;82:8891–8895.

280. Hiatt A, Bohorova N, Bohorov O, et al. Glycan variants of a respiratory syncytial virus antibody with enhanced effector function and in vivo efficacy. *Proc Natl Acad Sci U S A* 2014;111:5992–5997.

281. Hoft DF, Babusis E, Worku S, et al. Live and inactivated influenza vaccines induce similar humoral responses, but only live vaccines induce diverse T-cell responses in young children. *J Infect Dis* 2011;204:845–853.

282. Holmen JE, Kim L, Cikesh B, et al. Relationship between neighborhood census-tract level socioeconomic status and respiratory syncytial virus-associated hospitalizations in U.S. adults, 2015–2017. *BMC Infect Dis* 2021;21:293.

283. Horsfall FL, Hahn RG. A latent virus in normal mice capable of producing pneumonia in its natural host. *J Exp Med* 1940;71:391–408.

284. Hussell T, Openshaw PJ. Intracellular IFN-gamma expression in natural killer cells precedes lung CD8+ T cell recruitment during respiratory syncytial virus infection. *J Gen Virol* 1998;79:2593–2601.

285. Ison MG, Hirsch HH. Community-acquired respiratory viruses in transplant patients: diversity, impact, unmet clinical needs. *Clin Microbiol Rev* 2019;32.

286. Jain S, Williams DJ, Arnold SR, et al. Community-acquired pneumonia requiring hospitalization among U.S. children. *N Engl J Med* 2015;372:835–845.

287. Jans J, Wicht O, Widjaja I, et al. Characteristics of RSV-specific maternal antibodies in plasma of hospitalized, acute RSV patients under three months of age. *PLoS One* 2017;12:e0170877.

288. Jeffree CE, Brown G, Aitken J, et al. Ultrastructural analysis of the interaction between F-actin and respiratory syncytial virus during virus assembly. *Virology* 2007;369:309–323.

289. Jeffree CE, Rixon HW, Brown G, et al. Distribution of the attachment (G) glycoprotein and GM1 within the envelope of mature respiratory syncytial virus filaments revealed using field emission scanning electron microscopy. *Virology* 2003;306:254–267.

290. Jeong KI, Piepenhagen PA, Kishko M, et al. CX3CR1 is expressed in differentiated human ciliated airway cells and co-localizes with respiratory syncytial virus on cilia in a G protein-dependent manner. *PLoS One* 2015;10:e0130517.

291. Jin H, Cheng X, Zhou HZ, et al. Respiratory syncytial virus that lacks open reading frame 2 of the M2 gene (M2-2) has altered growth characteristics and is attenuated in rodents. *J Virol* 2000;74:74–82.

292. Jin H, Zhou H, Cheng X, et al. Recombinant respiratory syncytial viruses with deletions in the NS1, NS2, SH, and M2-2 genes are attenuated in vitro and in vivo. *Virology* 2000;273:210–218.

293. Jobe F, Simpson J, Hawes P, et al. Respiratory syncytial virus sequesters NF-kappaB subunit p65 to cytoplasmic inclusion bodies to inhibit innate immune signaling. *J Virol* 2020;94.

294. Johnson JE, Gonzales RA, Olson SJ, et al. The histopathology of fatal untreated human respiratory syncytial virus infection. *Mod Pathol* 2007;20:108–119.

295. Johnson PR, Collins PL. The A and B subgroups of human respiratory syncytial virus: comparison of intergenic and gene-overlap sequences. *J Gen Virol* 1988;69:2901–2906.

296. Johnson PR Jr, Olmsted RA, Prince GA, et al. Antigenic relatedness between glycoproteins of human respiratory syncytial virus subgroups A and B: evaluation of the contributions of F and G glycoproteins to immunity. *J Virol* 1987;61:3163–3166.

297. Johnson PR, Spriggs MK, Olmsted RA, et al. The G glycoprotein of human respiratory syncytial viruses of subgroups A and B: extensive sequence divergence between antigenically related proteins. *Proc Natl Acad Sci U S A* 1987;84:5625–5629.

298. Johnson SM, McNally BA, Ioannidis I, et al. Respiratory syncytial virus uses CX3CR1 as a receptor on primary human airway epithelial cultures. *PLoS Pathog* 2015;11:e1005318.

299. Jones BG, Sealy RE, Rudraraju R, et al. Sendai virus-based RSV vaccine protects African green monkeys from RSV infection. *Vaccine* 2012;30:959–968.

300. Jones HG, Ritschel T, Pascual G, et al. Structural basis for recognition of the central conserved region of RSV G by neutralizing human antibodies. *PLoS Pathog* 2018;14:e1006935.

301. Jordan E, Lawrence SJ, Meyer TPH, et al. Broad antibody and cellular immune response from a phase 2 clinical trial with a novel multivalent poxvirus-based respiratory syncytial virus vaccine. *J Infect Dis* 2021;223:1062–1072.

302. Jozwik A, Habibi MS, Paras A, et al. RSV-specific airway resident memory CD8+ T cells and differential disease severity after experimental human infection. *Nat Commun* 2015;6:10224.

303. Juhasz K, Murphy BR, Collins PL. The major attenuating mutations of the respiratory syncytial virus vaccine candidate cpts530/1009 specify temperature-sensitive defects in transcription and replication and a non-temperature-sensitive alteration in mRNA termination. *J Virol* 1999;73:5176–5180.

304. Juliana A, Zonneveld R, Plotz FB, et al. Neutrophil-endothelial interactions in respiratory syncytial virus bronchiolitis: an understudied aspect with a potential for prediction of severity of disease. *J Clin Virol* 2020;123:104258.

305. Kalica AR, Wright PF, Hetrick FM, et al. Electron microscopic studies of respiratory syncytial temperature-sensitive mutants. *Arch Gesamte Virusforsch* 1973;41:248–258.

306. Kapikian AZ, Bell JA, Mastrota FM, et al. An outbreak of febrile illness and pneumonia associated with respiratory syncytial virus infection. *Am J Hyg* 1961;74:234–248.

307. Kapikian AZ, Mitchell RH, Chanock RM, et al. An epidemiologic study of altered clinical reactivity to respiratory syncytial (RS) virus infection in children previously vaccinated with an inactivated RS virus vaccine. *Am J Epidemiol* 1969;89:405–421.

308. Karron RA, Atwell JE, McFarland EJ, et al. Live-attenuated vaccines prevent respiratory syncytial virus-associated illness in young children. *Am J Respir Crit Care Med* 2021;203:594–603.

309. Karron RA, Buchholz UJ, Collins PL. Live-attenuated respiratory syncytial virus vaccines. *Curr Top Microbiol Immunol* 2013;372:259–284.

310. Karron RA, Buonagurio DA, Georgiu AF, et al. Respiratory syncytial virus (RSV) SH and G proteins are not essential for viral replication in vitro: clinical evaluation and molecular characterization of a cold-passaged, attenuated RSV subgroup B mutant. *Proc Natl Acad Sci U S A* 1997;94:13961–13966.

311. Karron RA, Luongo C, Mateo JS, et al. Safety and immunogenicity of the respiratory syncytial virus vaccine RSV/DeltaNS2/Delta1313/I1314L in RSV-seronegative children. *J Infect Dis* 2020;222:82–91.

312. Karron RA, Luongo C, Thumar B, et al. A gene deletion that up-regulates viral gene expression yields an attenuated RSV vaccine with improved antibody responses in children. *Sci Transl Med* 2015;7:312ra175.

313. Karron RA, San Mateo J, Wanionek K, et al. Evaluation of a live attenuated human metapneumovirus vaccine in adults and children. *J Pediatric Infect Dis Soc* 2018;7:86–89.

314. Karron RA, Singleton RJ, Bulkow L, et al. Severe respiratory syncytial virus disease in Alaska native children. RSV Alaska Study Group. *J Infect Dis* 1999;180:41–49.

315. Karron RA, Wright PF, Belshe RB, et al. Identification of a recombinant live attenuated respiratory syncytial virus vaccine candidate that is highly attenuated in infants. *J Infect Dis* 2005;191:1093–1104.

316. Karron RA, Wright PF, Crowe JE Jr, et al. Evaluation of two live, cold-passaged, temperature-sensitive respiratory syncytial virus (RSV) vaccines in chimpanzees, adults, infants and children. *J Infect Dis* 1997;176:1428–1436.

317. Kaul TN, Welliver RC, Wong DT, et al. Secretory antibody response to respiratory syncytial virus infection. *Am J Dis Child* 1981;135:1013–1016.

318. Ke Z, Dillard RS, Chirkova T, et al. The morphology and assembly of respiratory syncytial virus revealed by cryo-electron tomography. *Viruses* 2018;10.

319. Kerr MH, Paton JY. Surfactant protein levels in severe respiratory syncytial virus infection. *Am J Respir Crit Care Med* 1999;159:1115–1118.

320. Kerrin A, Fitch P, Errington C, et al. Differential lower airway dendritic cell patterns may reveal distinct endotypes of RSV bronchiolitis. *Thorax* 2017;72:620–627.

321. Kiedrowski MR, Bomberger JM. Viral-bacterial co-infections in the cystic fibrosis respiratory tract. *Front Immunol* 2018;9:3067.

322. Killikelly AM, Kanekiyo M, Graham BS. Pre-fusion F is absent on the surface of formalin-inactivated respiratory syncytial virus. *Sci Rep* 2016;6:34108.

323. Kim CK, Kim SW, Park CS, et al. Bronchoalveolar lavage cytokine profiles in acute asthma and acute bronchiolitis. *J Allergy Clin Immunol* 2003;112:64–71.

324. Kim D, Niewiesk S. Synergistic induction of interferon alpha through TLR-3 and TLR-9 agonists identifies CD21 as interferon alpha receptor for the B cell response. *PLoS Pathog* 2013;9:e1003233.

325. Kim HW, Arrobio JO, Brandt CD, et al. Epidemiology of respiratory syncytial virus infection in Washington, D.C. I. Importance of the virus in different respiratory tract disease syndromes and temporal distribution of infection. *Am J Epidemiol* 1973;98: 216–225.

326. Kim HW, Leikin SL, Arrobio J, et al. Cell-mediated immunity to respiratory syncytial virus induced by inactivated vaccine or by infection. *Pediatr Res* 1976;10:75–78.

327. Kim JI, Park S, Lee I, et al. Genome-wide analysis of human metapneumovirus evolution. *PLoS One* 2016;11:e0152962.

328. Kinder JT, Moncman CL, Barrett C, et al. Respiratory syncytial virus and human metapneumovirus infections in three-dimensional human airway tissues expose an interesting dichotomy in viral replication, spread, and inhibition by neutralizing antibodies. *J Virol* 2020;94.

329. King JC Jr, Burke AR, Clemens JD, et al. Respiratory syncytial virus illnesses in human immunodeficiency virus- and noninfected children. *Pediatr Infect Dis J* 1993;12:733–739.

330. King T, Mejias A, Ramilo O, et al. The larger attachment glycoprotein of respiratory syncytial virus produced in primary human bronchial epithelial cultures reduces infectivity for cell lines. *PLoS Pathog* 2021;17:e1009469.

331. King VJ, Viswanathan M, Bordley WC, et al. Pharmacologic treatment of bronchiolitis in infants and children: a systematic review. *Arch Pediatr Adolesc Med* 2004;158: 127–137.

332. Kishko M, Catalan J, Swanson K, et al. Evaluation of the respiratory syncytial virus G-directed neutralizing antibody response in the human airway epithelial cell model. *Virology* 2020;550:21–26.

333. Kiss G, Holl JM, Williams GM, et al. Structural analysis of respiratory syncytial virus reveals the position of M2-1 between the matrix protein and the ribonucleoprotein complex. *J Virol* 2014;88:7602–7617.

334. Kitagawa Y, Zhou M, Yamaguchi M, et al. Human metapneumovirus M2-2 protein inhibits viral transcription and replication. *Microbes Infect* 2010;12:135–145.

335. Koivisto K, Nieminen T, Mejias A, et al. RSV specific antibodies in pregnant women and subsequent risk of RSV hospitalization in young infants. *J Infect Dis* 2021. https://doi.org/10.1093/infdis/jiab315

336. Kolli D, Bao X, Liu T, et al. Human metapneumovirus glycoprotein G inhibits TLR4-dependent signaling in monocyte-derived dendritic cells. *J Immunol* 2011;187:47–54.

337. Kolokoltsov AA, Deniger D, Fleming EH, et al. Small interfering RNA profiling reveals key role of clathrin-mediated endocytosis and early endosome formation for infection by respiratory syncytial virus. *J Virol* 2007;81:7786–7800.

338. Krempl C, Murphy BR, Collins PL. Recombinant respiratory syncytial virus with the G and F genes shifted to the promoter-proximal positions. *J Virol* 2002;76:11931–11942.

339. Krempl CD, Lamirande EW, Collins PL. Complete sequence of the RNA genome of pneumonia virus of mice (PVM). *Virus Genes* 2005;30:237–249.

340. Kristensen K, Hjuler T, Ravn H, et al. Chronic diseases, chromosomal abnormalities, and congenital malformations as risk factors for respiratory syncytial virus hospitalization: a population-based cohort study. *Clin Infect Dis* 2012;54:810–817.

341. Kristjansson S, Bjarnarson SP, Wennergren G, et al. Respiratory syncytial virus and other respiratory viruses during the first 3 months of life promote a local TH2-like response. *J Allergy Clin Immunol* 2005;116:805–811.

342. Krueger S, Curtis JE, Scott DR, et al. Structural characterization and modeling of a respiratory syncytial virus fusion glycoprotein nanoparticle vaccine in solution. *Mol Pharm* 2021;18:359–376.

343. Krzyzaniak MA, Zumstein MT, Gerez JA, et al. Host cell entry of respiratory syncytial virus involves macropinocytosis followed by proteolytic activation of the F protein. *PLoS Pathog* 2013;9:e1003309.

344. Kuiken T, van den Hoogen BG, van Riel DA, et al. Experimental human metapneumovirus infection of cynomolgus macaques (Macaca fascicularis) results in virus replication in ciliated epithelial cells and pneumocytes with associated lesions throughout the respiratory tract. *Am J Pathol* 2004;164:1893–1900.

345. Kulkarni AB, Collins PL, Bacik I, et al. Cytotoxic T cells specific for a single peptide on the M2 protein of respiratory syncytial virus are the sole mediators of resistance induced by immunization with M2 encoded by a recombinant vaccinia virus. *J Virol* 1995;69:1261–1264.

346. Kulkarni H, Smith CM, Lee Ddo H, et al. Evidence of respiratory syncytial virus spread by aerosol. Time to revisit infection control strategies? *Am J Respir Crit Care Med* 2016;194:308–316.

347. Kumagai Y, Takeuchi O, Kato H, et al. Alveolar macrophages are the primary interferon-alpha producer in pulmonary infection with RNA viruses. *Immunity* 2007;27:240–252.

348. Kuo L, Fearns R, Collins PL. Analysis of the gene start and gene end signals of human respiratory syncytial virus: quasi-templated initiation at position 1 of the encoded mRNA. *J Virol* 1997;71:4944–4953.

349. Kurt-Jones EA, Popova L, Kwinn L, et al. Pattern recognition receptors TLR4 and CD14 mediate response to respiratory syncytial virus. *Nat Immunol* 2000;1:398–401.

350. Kwilas AR, Yednak MA, Zhang L, et al. Respiratory syncytial virus engineered to express CFTR corrects the bioelectric phenotype of human cystic fibrosis airway epithelium in vitro. *J Virol* 2010;84:7770–7781.

351. Kwon YM, Hwang HS, Lee YT, et al. Respiratory syncytial virus fusion protein-encoding DNA vaccine is less effective in conferring protection against inflammatory disease than a virus-like particle platform. *Immune Netw* 2019;19:e18.

352. Laham FR, Israele V, Casellas JM, et al. Differential production of inflammatory cytokines in primary infection with human metapneumovirus and with other common respiratory viruses of infancy. *J Infect Dis* 2004;189:2047–2056.

353. Langley JM, MacDonald LD, Weir GM, et al. A respiratory syncytial virus vaccine based on the small hydrophobic protein ectodomain presented with a novel lipid-based formulation is highly immunogenic and safe in adults: a first-in-humans study. *J Infect Dis* 2018;218:378–387.

354. Lazear HM, Schoggins JW, Diamond MS. Shared and distinct functions of type I and type III interferons. *Immunity* 2019;50:907–923.

355. Le Nouen C, Hillyer P, Brock LG, et al. Human metapneumovirus SH and G glycoproteins inhibit macropinocytosis-mediated entry into human dendritic cells and reduce CD4+ T cell activation. *J Virol* 2014;88:6453–6469.

356. Le Nouen C, Hillyer P, Munir S, et al. Effects of human respiratory syncytial virus, metapneumovirus, parainfluenza virus 3 and influenza virus on CD4+ T cell activation by dendritic cells. *PLoS One* 2010;5:e15017.

357. Le Nouen C, Hillyer P, Winter CC, et al. Low CCR7-mediated migration of human monocyte derived dendritic cells in response to human respiratory syncytial virus (HRSV) and metapneumovirus (HMPV). *PLoS Pathog* 2011;17:e1002105.

358. Le Nouen C, McCarty T, Brown M, et al. Genetic stability of genome-scale deoptimized RNA virus vaccine candidates under selective pressure. *Proc Natl Acad Sci U S A* 2017;114:E386–E395.

359. Le Nouen C, Munir S, Losq S, et al. Infection and maturation of monocyte-derived human dendritic cells by human respiratory syncytial virus, human metapneumovirus, and human parainfluenza virus type 3. *Virology* 2009;385:169–182.

360. Lee FE, Walsh EE, Falsey AR, et al. Human infant respiratory syncytial virus (RSV)-specific type 1 and 2 cytokine responses ex vivo during primary RSV infection. *J Infect Dis* 2007;195:1779–1788.

361. Lee MS, Walker RE, Mendelman PM. Medical burden of respiratory syncytial virus and parainfluenza virus type 3 infection among US children. Implications for design of vaccine trials. *Hum Vaccin* 2005;1:6–11.

362. Lee N, Smith S, Zelyas N, et al. Burden of noninfluenza respiratory viral infections in adults admitted to hospital: analysis of a multiyear Canadian surveillance cohort from 2 centres. *CMAJ* 2021;193: E439–E446.

363. Legg JP, Hussain IR, Warner JA, et al. Type 1 and type 2 cytokine imbalance in acute respiratory syncytial virus bronchiolitis. *Am J Respir Crit Care Med* 2003;168:633–639.

364. Leroux-Roels G, De Boever F, Maes C, et al. Safety and immunogenicity of a respiratory syncytial virus fusion glycoprotein F subunit vaccine in healthy adults: results of a phase 1, randomized, observer-blind, controlled, dosage-escalation study. *Vaccine* 2019;37:2694–2703.

365. LeVine AM, Elliott J, Whitsett JA, et al. Surfactant protein-d enhances phagocytosis and pulmonary clearance of respiratory syncytial virus. *Am J Respir Cell Mol Biol* 2004;31: 193–199.

366. Levine S, Klaiber-Franco R, Paradiso PR. Demonstration that glycoprotein G is the attachment protein of respiratory syncytial virus. *J Gen Virol* 1987;68:2521–2524.

367. Levine S, Peeples M, Hamilton R. Effect of respiratory syncytial virus infection of HeLa-cell macromolecular synthesis. *J Gen Virol* 1977;37:53–63.

368. Levy O. Innate immunity of the newborn: basic mechanisms and clinical correlates. *Nat Rev Immunol* 2007;7:379–390.

369. Leyrat C, Renner M, Harlos K, et al. Structure and self-assembly of the calcium binding matrix protein of human metapneumovirus. *Structure* 2014;22:136–148.

370. Li C, Zhou X, Zhong Y, et al. A recombinant G protein plus cyclosporine a-based respiratory syncytial virus vaccine elicits humoral and regulatory T cell responses against infection without vaccine-enhanced disease. *J Immunol* 2016;196:1721–1731.

371. Li Y, Johnson EK, Shi T, et al. National burden estimates of hospitalisations for acute lower respiratory infections due to respiratory syncytial virus in young children in 2019 among 58 countries: a modelling study. *Lancet Respir Med* 2021;9:175–185.

372. Li Y, To J, Verdia-Baguena C, et al. Inhibition of the human respiratory syncytial virus small hydrophobic protein and structural variations in a bicelle environment. *J Virol* 2014;88:11899–11914.

373. Liang B, Matsuoka Y, Le Nouen C, et al. A parainfluenza virus vector expressing the respiratory syncytial virus (RSV) prefusion F protein is more effective than RSV for boosting a primary immunization with RSV. *J Virol* 2020;95.

374. Liang B, Ngwuta JO, Surman S, et al. Improved prefusion stability, optimized codon usage, and augmented virion packaging enhance the immunogenicity of respiratory syncytial virus fusion protein in a vectored-vaccine candidate. *J Virol* 2017;91.

375. Liesman RM, Buchholz UJ, Luongo CL, et al. RSV-encoded NS2 promotes epithelial cell shedding and distal airway obstruction. *J Clin Invest* 2014;124:2219–2233.

376. Lifland AW, Jung J, Alonas E, et al. Human respiratory syncytial virus nucleoprotein and inclusion bodies antagonize the innate immune response mediated by MDA5 and MAVS. *J Virol* 2012;86:8245–8258.

377. Liljeroos L, Krzyzaniak MA, Helenius A, et al. Architecture of respiratory syncytial virus revealed by electron cryotomography. *Proc Natl Acad Sci U S A* 2013;110:11133–11138.

378. Lindemans CA, Kimpen JL, Luijk B, et al. Systemic eosinophil response induced by respiratory syncytial virus. *Clin Exp Immunol* 2006;144:409–417.

379. Ling R, Pringle CR. Polypeptides of pneumonia virus of mice. II. Characterization of the glycoproteins. *J Gen Virol* 1989;70:1441–1452.
380. Ling Z, Tran KC, Teng MN. Human respiratory syncytial virus nonstructural protein NS2 antagonizes the activation of beta interferon transcription by interacting with RIG-I. *J Virol* 2009;83:3734–3742.
381. Liu L, Bastien N, Li Y. Intracellular processing, glycosylation, and cell surface expression of human metapneumovirus attachment glycoprotein. *J Virol* 2007;81:13435–13443.
382. Liuzzi M, Mason SW, Cartier M, et al. Inhibitors of respiratory syncytial virus replication target cotranscriptional mRNA guanylylation by viral RNA-dependent RNA polymerase. *J Virol* 2005;79:13105–13115.
383. Llorente MT, Garcia-Barreno B, Calero M, et al. Structural analysis of the human respiratory syncytial virus phosphoprotein: characterization of an alpha-helical domain involved in oligomerization. *J Gen Virol* 2006;87:159–169.
384. Lopez EL, Ferolla FM, Toledano A, et al. Genetic susceptibility to life-threatening respiratory syncytial virus infection in previously healthy infants. *Pediatr Infect Dis J* 2020;39:1057–1061.
385. Lormeau B, Foulongne V, Baccino E, et al. Epidemiological survey in a day care center following toddler sudden death due to human metapneumovirus infection. *Arch Pediatr* 2019;26:479–482.
386. Lozano R, Naghavi M, Foreman K, et al. Global and regional mortality from 235 causes of death for 20 age groups in 1990 and 2010: a systematic analysis for the Global Burden of Disease Study 2010. *Lancet* 2012;380:2095–2128.
387. Lu B, Ma CH, Brazas R, et al. The major phosphorylation sites of the respiratory syncytial virus phosphoprotein are dispensable for virus replication in vitro. *J Virol* 2002;76: 10776–10784.
388. Lukens MV, van de Pol AC, Coenjaerts FE, et al. A systemic neutrophil response precedes robust CD8(+) T-cell activation during natural respiratory syncytial virus infection in infants. *J Virol* 2010;84:2374–2383.
389. Luongo C, Winter CC, Collins PL, et al. Increased genetic and phenotypic stability of a promising live-attenuated respiratory syncytial virus vaccine candidate by reverse genetics. *J Virol* 2012;86:10792–10804.
390. Luongo C, Winter CC, Collins PL, et al. Respiratory syncytial virus modified by deletions of the NS2 gene and amino acid S1313 of the L polymerase protein is a temperature-sensitive, live-attenuated vaccine candidate that is phenotypically stable at physiological temperature. *J Virol* 2013;87:1985–1996.
391. MacPhail M, Schickli JH, Tang RS, et al. Identification of small-animal and primate models for evaluation of vaccine candidates for human metapneumovirus (hMPV) and implications for hMPV vaccine design. *J Gen Virol* 2004;85:1655–1663.
392. Madge P, Paton JY, McColl JH, et al. Prospective controlled study of four infection-control procedures to prevent nosocomial infection with respiratory syncytial virus. *Lancet* 1992;340:1079–1083.
393. Madhi SA, Klugman KP. A role for Streptococcus pneumoniae in virus-associated pneumonia. *Nat Med* 2004;10:811–813.
394. Madhi SA, Ludewick H, Kuwanda L, et al. Pneumococcal coinfection with human metapneumovirus. *J Infect Dis* 2006;193:1236–1243.
395. Madhi SA, Polack FP, Piedra PA, et al. Respiratory syncytial virus vaccination during pregnancy and effects in infants. *N Engl J Med* 2020;383:426–439.
396. Mahan LD, Points A, Mohanka MR, et al. Characteristics and outcomes among lung transplant patients with respiratory syncytial virus infection. *Transpl Infect Dis* 2021:e13661.
397. Maifeld SV, Ro B, Mok H, et al. Development of electrochemiluminescent serology assays to measure the humoral response to antigens of respiratory syncytial virus. *PLoS One* 2016;11:e0153019.
398. Makris S, Bajorek M, Culley FJ, et al. Alveolar macrophages can control respiratory syncytial virus infection in the absence of type I interferons. *J Innate Immun* 2016;8:452–463.
399. Malhotra R, Ward M, Bright H, et al. Isolation and characterisation of potential respiratory syncytial virus receptor(s) on epithelial cells. *Microbes Infect* 2003;5:123–133.
400. Malley R, DeVincenzo J, Ramilo O, et al. Reduction of respiratory syncytial virus (RSV) in tracheal aspirates in intubated infants by use of humanized monoclonal antibody to RSV F protein. *J Infect Dis* 1998;178:1555–1561.
401. Mansbach JM, Geller RJ, Hasegawa K, et al. Detection of respiratory syncytial virus or rhinovirus weeks after hospitalization for bronchiolitis and the risk of recurrent wheezing. *J Infect Dis* 2021;223:268–277.
402. Mariani TJ, Qiu X, Chu C, et al. Association of dynamic changes in the CD4 T-cell transcriptome with disease severity during primary respiratory syncytial virus infection in young infants. *J Infect Dis* 2017;216:1027–1037.
403. Marquez-Escobar VA. Current developments and prospects on human metapneumovirus vaccines. *Expert Rev Vaccines* 2017;16:419–431.
404. Marr N, Wang TI, Kam SH, et al. Attenuation of respiratory syncytial virus-induced and RIG-I-dependent type I IFN responses in human neonates and very young children. *J Immunol* 2014;192:948–957.
405. Marsh R, Connor A, Gias E, et al. Increased susceptibility of human respiratory syncytial virus to neutralization by anti-fusion protein antibodies on adaptation to replication in cell culture. *J Med Virol* 2007;79:829–837.
406. Martinez FD, Morgan WJ, Wright AL, et al. Initial airway function is a risk factor for recurrent wheezing respiratory illnesses during the first three years of life. Group Health Medical Associates. *Am Rev Respir Dis* 1991;143:312–316.
407. Martinez I, Dopazo J, Melero JA. Antigenic structure of the human respiratory syncytial virus G glycoprotein and relevance of hypermutation events for the generation of antigenic variants. *J Gen Virol* 1997;78:2419–2429.
408. Martinez I, Lombardia L, Garcia-Barreno B, et al. Distinct gene subsets are induced at different time points after human respiratory syncytial virus infection of A549 cells. *J Gen Virol* 2007;88:570–581.
409. Martinez I, Melero JA. Enhanced neutralization of human respiratory syncytial virus by mixtures of monoclonal antibodies to the attachment (G) glycoprotein. *J Gen Virol* 1998;79:2215–2220.
410. Martinon-Torres F, Rusch S, Huntjens D, et al. Pharmacokinetics, safety, and antiviral effects of multiple doses of the respiratory syncytial virus (RSV) fusion protein inhibitor, JNJ-53718678, in infants hospitalized with rsv infection: a randomized phase 1b study. *Clin Infect Dis* 2020;71:e594–e603.
411. Marty FM, Chemaly RF, Mullane KM, et al. A phase 2b, randomized, double-blind, placebo-controlled multicenter study evaluating antiviral effects, pharmacokinetics, safety, and tolerability of presatovir in hematopoietic cell transplant recipients with respiratory syncytial virus infection of the lower respiratory tract. *Clin Infect Dis* 2020;71:2787–2795.
412. Mas V, Rodriguez L, Olmedillas E, et al. Engineering, structure and immunogenicity of the human metapneumovirus F protein in the postfusion conformation. *PLoS Pathog* 2016;12:e1005859.
413. Masters JR. HeLa cells 50 years on: the good, the bad and the ugly. *Nat Rev Cancer* 2002;2:315–319.
414. Mastrangelo P, Chin AA, Tan S, et al. Identification of RSV fusion protein interaction domains on the virus receptor, nucleolin. *Viruses* 2021;13.
415. McFarland EJ, Karron RA, Muresan P, et al. Live respiratory syncytial virus attenuated by M2-2 deletion and stabilized temperature sensitivity mutation 1030s is a promising vaccine candidate in children. *J Infect Dis* 2020;221:534–543.
416. McGivern DR, Collins PL, Fearns R. Identification of internal sequences in the 3′ leader region of human respiratory syncytial virus that enhance transcription and confer replication processivity. *J Virol* 2005;79:2449–2460.
417. McIntosh K. Interferon in nasal secretions from infants with viral respiratory tract infections. *J Pediatr* 1978;93:33–36.
418. McIntosh K, Masters HB, Orr I, et al. The immunologic response to infection with respiratory syncytial virus in infants. *J Infect Dis* 1978;138:24–32.
419. McLellan JS, Chen M, Joyce MG, et al. Structure-based design of a fusion glycoprotein vaccine for respiratory syncytial virus. *Science* 2013;342:592–598.
420. McLellan JS, Chen M, Leung S, et al. Structure of RSV fusion glycoprotein trimer bound to a prefusion-specific neutralizing antibody. *Science* 2013;340:1113–1117.
421. McMorrow ML, Tempia S, Walaza S, et al. The role of human immunodeficiency virus in influenza- and respiratory syncytial virus-associated hospitalizations in South African children, 2011–2016. *Clin Infect Dis* 2019;68:773–780.
422. McNamara PS, Flanagan BF, Baldwin LM, et al. Interleukin 9 production in the lungs of infants with severe respiratory syncytial virus bronchiolitis. *Lancet* 2004;363:1031–1037.
423. McNamara PS, Ritson P, Selby A, et al. Bronchoalveolar lavage cellularity in infants with severe respiratory syncytial virus bronchiolitis. *Arch Dis Child* 2003;88:922–926.
424. Mehedi M, McCarty T, Martin SE, et al. Actin-related protein 2 (ARP2) and virus-induced filopodia facilitate human respiratory syncytial virus spread. *PLoS Pathog* 2016;12:e1006062.
425. Mejias A, Chavez-Bueno S, Rios AM, et al. Anti-respiratory syncytial virus (RSV) neutralizing antibody decreases lung inflammation, airway obstruction, and airway hyperresponsiveness in a murine RSV model. *Antimicrob Agents Chemother* 2004;48: 1811–1822.
426. Mejias A, Dimo B, Suarez NM, et al. Whole blood gene expression profiles to assess pathogenesis and disease severity in infants with respiratory syncytial virus infection. *PLoS Med* 2013;10:e1001549.
427. Mejias A, Wu B, Tandon N, et al. Risk of childhood wheeze and asthma after respiratory syncytial virus infection in full-term infants. *Pediatr Allergy Immunol* 2020;31:47–56.
428. Melendi GA, Hoffman SJ, Karron RA, et al. C5 modulates airway hyperreactivity and pulmonary eosinophilia during enhanced respiratory syncytial virus disease by decreasing C3a receptor expression. *J Virol* 2007;81:991–999.
429. Mella C, Suarez-Arrabal MC, Lopez S, et al. Innate immune dysfunction is associated with enhanced disease severity in infants with severe respiratory syncytial virus bronchiolitis. *J Infect Dis* 2013;207:564–573.
430. Meshram CD, Baviskar PS, Ognibene CM, et al. The respiratory syncytial virus phosphoprotein, matrix protein, and fusion protein carboxy-terminal domain drive efficient filamentous virus-like particle formation. *J Virol* 2016;90:10612–10628.
431. Miller AL, Bowlin TL, Lukacs NW. Respiratory syncytial virus-induced chemokine production: linking viral replication to chemokine production in vitro and in vivo. *J Infect Dis* 2004;189:1419–1430.
432. Miller EK, Gebretsadik T, Carroll KN, et al. Viral etiologies of infant bronchiolitis, croup and upper respiratory illness during 4 consecutive years. *Pediatr Infect Dis J* 2013;32:950–955.
433. Mink MA, Stec DS, Collins PL. Nucleotide sequences of the 3′ leader and 5′ trailer regions of human respiratory syncytial virus genomic RNA. *Virology* 1991;185:615–624.
434. Miyairi I, DeVincenzo JP. Human genetic factors and respiratory syncytial virus disease severity. *Clin Microbiol Rev* 2008;21:686–703.
435. Mobbs KJ, Smyth RL, O'Hea U, et al. Cytokines in severe respiratory syncytial virus bronchiolitis. *Pediatr Pulmonol* 2002;33:449–452.
436. Moghaddam A, Olszewska W, Wang B, et al. A potential molecular mechanism for hypersensitivity caused by formalin-inactivated vaccines. *Nat Med* 2006;12:905–907.
437. Mok H, Tollefson SJ, Podsiad AB, et al. An alphavirus replicon-based human metapneumovirus vaccine is immunogenic and protective in mice and cotton rats. *J Virol* 2008;82:11410–11418.
438. Money VA, McPhee HK, Mosely JA, et al. Surface features of a Mononegavirales matrix protein indicate sites of membrane interaction. *Proc Natl Acad Sci U S A* 2009;106: 4441–4446.
439. Moore ML, Chi MH, Luongo C, et al. A chimeric A2 strain of respiratory syncytial virus (RSV) with the fusion protein of RSV strain line 19 exhibits enhanced viral load, mucus, and airway dysfunction. *J Virol* 2009;83:4185–4194.
440. Mordstein M, Neugebauer E, Ditt V, et al. Lambda interferon renders epithelial cells of the respiratory and gastrointestinal tracts resistant to viral infections. *J Virol* 2010;84: 5670–5677.
441. Morris JA, Blount RE, Savage RE. Recovery of cytopathic agent from chimpanzees with coryza. *Proc Soc Exp Biol Med* 1956;92:544–550.
442. Moudy RM, Sullender WM, Wertz GW. Variations in intergenic region sequences of human respiratory syncytial virus clinical isolates: analysis of effects on transcriptional regulation. *Virology* 2004;327:121–133.
443. Moyes J, Walaza S, Pretorius M, et al. Respiratory syncytial virus in adults with severe acute respiratory illness in a high HIV prevalence setting. *J Infect* 2017;75:346–355.

444. Mufson MA, Orvell C, Rafnar B, et al. Two distinct subtypes of human respiratory syncytial virus. *J Gen Virol* 1985;66:2111–2124.
445. Mullins JA, LaMonte AC, Bresee JS, et al. Substantial variability in community RSV season timing: an analysis using the National Respiratory and Enteric Viruses Surveillance System (NREVSS). *Pediatric Infect Dis J* 2003;22:857–862.
446. Munir S, Hillyer P, Le Nouen C, et al. Respiratory syncytial virus interferon antagonist NS1 protein suppresses and skews the human T lymphocyte response. *PLoS Pathog* 2011;7:e1001336.
447. Murawski MR, Bowen GN, Cerny AM, et al. Respiratory syncytial virus activates innate immunity through Toll-like receptor 2. *J Virol* 2009;83:1492–1500.
448. Murphy BR, Alling DW, Snyder MH, et al. Effect of age and preexisting antibody on serum antibody response of infants and children to the F and G glycoproteins during respiratory syncytial virus infection. *J Clin Microbiol* 1986;24:894–898.
449. Murphy BR, Graham BS, Prince GA, et al. Serum and nasal-wash immunoglobulin G and A antibody response of infants and children to respiratory syncytial virus F and G glycoproteins following primary infection. *J Clin Microbiol* 1986;23:1009–1014.
450. Murphy BR, Prince GA, Collins PL, et al. Effect of passive antibody on the immune response of cotton rats to purified F and G glycoproteins of respiratory syncytial virus (RSV). *Vaccine* 1991;9:185–189.
451. Murphy BR, Prince GA, Lawrence LA, et al. Detection of respiratory syncytial virus (RSV) infected cells by in situ hybridization in the lungs of cotton rats immunized with formalin-inactivated virus or purified RSV F and G glycoprotein subunit vaccine and challenged with RSV. *Virus Res* 1990;16:153–162.
452. Murphy BR, Sotnikov AV, Lawrence LA, et al. Enhanced pulmonary histopathology is observed in cotton rats immunized with formalin-inactivated respiratory syncytial virus (RSV) or purified F glycoprotein and challenged with RSV 3–6 months after immunization. *Vaccine* 1990;8:497–502.
453. Murphy BR, Walsh EE. Formalin-inactivated respiratory syncytial virus vaccine induces antibodies to the fusion glycoprotein that are deficient in fusion-inhibiting activity. *J Clin Microbiol* 1988;26:1595–1597.
454. Nao N, Saikusa M, Sato K, et al. Recent molecular evolution of human metapneumovirus (HMPV): subdivision of HMPV A2b strains. *Microorganisms* 2020;8.
455. Negrey JD, Reddy RB, Scully EJ, et al. Simultaneous outbreaks of respiratory disease in wild chimpanzees caused by distinct viruses of human origin. *Emerg Microbes Infect* 2019;8:139–149.
456. Neilson KA, Yunis EJ. Demonstration of respiratory syncytial virus in an autopsy series. *Pediatr Pathol* 1990;10:491–502.
457. Ngwuta JO, Chen M, Modjarrad K, et al. Prefusion F-specific antibodies determine the magnitude of RSV neutralizing activity in human sera. *Sci Transl Med* 2015;7:309ra162.
458. Njenga MK, Lwamba HM, Seal BS. Metapneumoviruses in birds and humans. *Virus Res* 2003;91:163–169.
459. Noton SL, Cowton VM, Zack CR, et al. Evidence that the polymerase of respiratory syncytial virus initiates RNA replication in a nontemplated fashion. *Proc Natl Acad Sci U S A* 2010;107:10226–10231.
460. O'Brien KL, Chandran A, Weatherholtz R, et al. Efficacy of motavizumab for the prevention of respiratory syncytial virus disease in healthy Native American infants: a phase 3 randomised double-blind placebo-controlled trial. *Lancet Infect Dis* 2015;15:1398–1408.
461. Obando-Pacheco P, Justicia-Grande AJ, Rivero-Calle I, et al. Respiratory syncytial virus seasonality: a global overview. *J Infect Dis* 2018;217:1356–1364.
462. Olmsted RA, Elango N, Prince GA, et al. Expression of the F glycoprotein of respiratory syncytial virus by a recombinant vaccinia virus: comparison of the individual contributions of the F and G glycoproteins to host immunity. *Proc Natl Acad Sci U S A* 1986;83:7462–7466.
463. Olson MR, Varga SM. CD8 T cells inhibit respiratory syncytial virus (RSV) vaccine-enhanced disease. *J Immunol* 2007;179:5415–5424.
464. Oner D, Drysdale SB, McPherson C, et al. Biomarkers for disease severity in children infected with respiratory syncytial virus: a systematic literature review. *J Infect Dis* 2020;222:S648–S657.
465. Openshaw PJM, Chiu C, Culley FJ, et al. Protective and harmful immunity to RSV infection. *Annu Rev Immunol* 2017;35:501–532.
466. Ottolini MG, Porter DD, Hemming VG, et al. Enhanced pulmonary pathology in cotton rats upon challenge after immunization with inactivated parainfluenza virus 3 vaccines. *Viral Immunol* 2000;13:231–236.
467. Ottolini MG, Porter DD, Hemming VG, et al. Effectiveness of RSVIG prophylaxis and therapy of respiratory syncytial virus in an immunosuppressed animal model. *Bone Marrow Transplant* 1999;24:41–45.
468. Paccaud MF, Jacquier C. A respiratory syncytial virus of bovine origin. *Arch Gesamte Virusforsch* 1970;30:327–342.
469. Palivizumab, a humanized respiratory syncytial virus monoclonal antibody, reduces hospitalization from respiratory syncytial virus infection in high-risk infants. The IMpact-RSV Study Group. *Pediatrics* 1998;102:531–537.
470. Pan J, Qian X, Lattmann S, et al. Structure of the human metapneumovirus polymerase phosphoprotein complex. *Nature* 2020;577:275–279.
471. Panozzo CA, Fowlkes AL, Anderson LJ. Variation in timing of respiratory syncytial virus outbreaks: lessons from national surveillance. *Pediatr Infect Dis J* 2007;26: S41–S45.
472. Parrott RH, Kim HW, Arrobio JO, et al. Epidemiology of respiratory syncytial virus infection in Washington, D.C. II. Infection and disease with respect to age, immunologic status, race and sex. *Am J Epidemiol* 1973;98:289–300.
473. Pastey MK, Crowe JE Jr, Graham BS. RhoA interacts with the fusion glycoprotein of respiratory syncytial virus and facilitates virus-induced syncytium formation. *J Virol* 1999;73:7262–7270.
474. Patel H, Platt R, Lozano JM, et al. Glucocorticoids for acute viral bronchiolitis in infants and young children. *Cochrane Database Syst Rev* 2004;(4):CD004878.
475. Pawelec G, Larbi A, Derhovanessian E. Senescence of the human immune system. *J Comp Pathol* 2010;142(Suppl 1):S39–S44.
476. Pei J, Wagner ND, Zou AJ, et al. Structural basis for IFN antagonism by human respiratory syncytial virus nonstructural protein 2. *Proc Natl Acad Sci U S A* 2021:118.
477. Peret TC, Boivin G, Li Y, et al. Characterization of human metapneumoviruses isolated from patients in North America. *J Infect Dis* 2002;185:1660–1663.
478. Peret TC, Hall CB, Hammond GW, et al. Circulation patterns of group A and B human respiratory syncytial virus genotypes in 5 communities in North America. *J Infect Dis* 2000;181:1891–1896.
479. Permpalung N, Thaniyavarn T, Saullo JL, et al. Oral and inhaled ribavirin treatment for respiratory syncytial virus infection in lung transplant recipients. *Transplantation* 2020;104:1280–1286.
480. Pham QN, Biacchesi S, Skiadopoulos MH, et al. Chimeric recombinant human metapneumoviruses with the nucleoprotein or phosphoprotein open reading frame replaced by that of avian metapneumovirus exhibit improved growth in vitro and attenuation in vivo. *J Virol* 2005;79:15114–15122.
481. Phipps S, Lam CE, Mahalingam S, et al. Eosinophils contribute to innate antiviral immunity and promote clearance of respiratory syncytial virus. *Blood* 2007;110:1578–1586.
482. Piedra FA, Mei M, Avadhanula V, et al. The interdependencies of viral load, the innate immune response, and clinical outcome in children presenting to the emergency department with respiratory syncytial virus-associated bronchiolitis. *PLoS One* 2017;12:e0172953.
483. Pilaev M, Shen Y, Carbonneau J, et al. Evaluation of pre- and post-fusion Human metapneumovirus F proteins as subunit vaccine candidates in mice. *Vaccine* 2020;38:2122–2127.
484. Pitkaranta A, Jero J, Arruda E, et al. Polymerase chain reaction-based detection of rhinovirus, respiratory syncytial virus, and coronavirus in otitis media with effusion. *J Pediatr* 1998;133:390–394.
485. Pneumonia Etiology Research for Child Health Study Group. Causes of severe pneumonia requiring hospital admission in children without HIV infection from Africa and Asia: the PERCH multi-country case–control study. *Lancet* 2019;394:757–779.
486. Polack FP, Irusta PM, Hoffman SJ, et al. The cysteine-rich region of respiratory syncytial virus attachment protein inhibits innate immunity elicited by the virus and endotoxin. *Proc Natl Acad Sci U S A* 2005;102:8996–9001.
487. Power UF, Nguyen TN, Rietveld E, et al. Safety and immunogenicity of a novel recombinant subunit respiratory syncytial virus vaccine (BBG2Na) in healthy young adults. *J Infect Dis* 2001;184:1456–1460.
488. Prais D, Schonfeld T, Amir J. Admission to the intensive care unit for respiratory syncytial virus bronchiolitis: a national survey before palivizumab use. *Pediatrics* 2003;112:548–552.
489. Pribul PK, Harker J, Wang B, et al. Alveolar macrophages are a major determinant of early responses to viral lung infection but do not influence subsequent disease development. *J Virol* 2008;82:4441–4448.
490. Prince GA, Curtis SJ, Yim KC, et al. Vaccine-enhanced respiratory syncytial virus disease in cotton rats following immunization with Lot 100 or a newly prepared reference vaccine. *J Gen Virol* 2001;82:2881–2888.
491. Prince GA, Hemming VG, Horswood RL, et al. Effectiveness of topically administered neutralizing antibodies in experimental immunotherapy of respiratory syncytial virus infection in cotton rats. *J Virol* 1987;61:1851–1854.
492. Prince GA, Horswood RL, Berndt J, et al. Respiratory syncytial virus infection in inbred mice. *Infect Immun* 1979;26:764–766.
493. Prince GA, Horswood RL, Camargo E, et al. Mechanisms of immunity to respiratory syncytial virus in cotton rats. *Infect Immun* 1983;42:81–87.
494. Prince GA, Horswood RL, Chanock RM. Quantitative aspects of passive immunity to respiratory syncytial virus infection in infant cotton rats. *J Virol* 1985;55:517–520.
495. Prince GA, Mathews A, Curtis SJ, et al. Treatment of respiratory syncytial virus bronchiolitis and pneumonia in a cotton rat model with systemically administered monoclonal antibody (palivizumab) and glucocorticosteroid. *J Infect Dis* 2000;182:1326–1330.
496. Ralston S, Hill V. Incidence of apnea in infants hospitalized with respiratory syncytial virus bronchiolitis: a systematic review. *J Pediatr* 2009;155:728–733.
497. Ralston SL, Lieberthal AS, Meissner HC, et al. Clinical practice guideline: the diagnosis, management, and prevention of bronchiolitis. *Pediatrics* 2014;134:e1474–e1502.
498. Ramaekers K, Rector A, Cuypers L, et al. Towards a unified classification for human respiratory syncytial virus genotypes. *Virus Evol* 2020;6:veaa052.
499. Ramilo O, Lagos R, Saez-Llorens X, et al. Motavizumab treatment of infants hospitalized with respiratory syncytial virus infection does not decrease viral load or severity of illness. *Pediatr Infect Dis J* 2014;33:703–709.
500. Raza K, Ismailjee SB, Crespo M, et al. Successful outcome of human metapneumovirus (hMPV) pneumonia in a lung transplant recipient treated with intravenous ribavirin. *J Heart Lung Transplant* 2007;26:862–864.
501. Reed JL, Brewah YA, Delaney T, et al. Macrophage impairment underlies airway occlusion in primary respiratory syncytial virus bronchiolitis. *J Infect Dis* 2008;198:1783–1793.
502. Reduction of respiratory syncytial virus hospitalization among premature infants and infants with bronchopulmonary dysplasia using respiratory syncytial virus immune globulin prophylaxis. The PREVENT Study Group. *Pediatrics* 1997;99:93–99.
503. Ren J, Wang Q, Kolli D, et al. Human metapneumovirus M2-2 protein inhibits innate cellular signaling by targeting MAVS. *J Virol* 2012;86:13049–13061.
504. Renner M, Bertinelli M, Leyrat C, et al. Nucleocapsid assembly in pneumoviruses is regulated by conformational switching of the N protein. *Elife* 2016;5:e12627.
505. Renshaw R, Laverack M, Zylich N, et al. Genomic analysis of a pneumovirus isolated from dogs with acute respiratory disease. *Vet Microbiol* 2011;150:88–95.
506. Rhodin MHJ, McAllister NV, Castillo J, et al. EDP-938, a novel nucleoprotein inhibitor of respiratory syncytial virus, demonstrates potent antiviral activities in vitro and in a non-human primate model. *PLoS Pathog* 2021;17:e1009428.
507. Rima B, Collins P, Easton A, et al. ICTV virus taxonomy profile: Pneumoviridae. *J Gen Virol* 2017;98:2912–2913.
508. Rincheval V, Lelek M, Gault E, et al. Functional organization of cytoplasmic inclusion bodies in cells infected by respiratory syncytial virus. *Nat Commun* 2017;8:563.
509. Robbie GJ, Criste R, Dall'acqua WF, et al. A novel investigational Fc-modified humanized monoclonal antibody, motavizumab-YTE, has an extended half-life in healthy adults. *Antimicrob Agents Chemother* 2013;57:6147–6153.

510. Roberts SR, Compans RW, Wertz GW. Respiratory syncytial virus matures at the apical surfaces of polarized epithelial cells. *J Virol* 1995;69:2667–2673.
511. Roberts SR, Lichtenstein D, Ball LA, et al. The membrane-associated and secreted forms of the respiratory syncytial virus attachment glycoprotein G are synthesized from alternative initiation codons. *J Virol* 1994;68:4538–4546.
512. Rocca A, Biagi C, Scarpini S, et al. Passive immunoprophylaxis against respiratory syncytial virus in children: where are we now? *Int J Mol Sci* 2021:22.
513. Rodriguez WJ, Bui RH, Connor JD, et al. Environmental exposure of primary care personnel to ribavirin aerosol when supervising treatment of infants with respiratory syncytial virus infections. *Antimicrob Agents Chemother* 1987;31:1143–1146.
514. Rodriguez-Fernandez R, Mejias A, Ramilo O. Monoclonal antibodies for prevention of respiratory syncytial virus infection. *Pediatr Infect Dis J* 2021;40:S35–S39.
515. Rodriguez-Fernandez R, Tapia LI, Yang CF, et al. Respiratory syncytial virus genotypes, host immune profiles, and disease severity in young children hospitalized with bronchiolitis. *J Infect Dis* 2017;217:24–34.
516. Roman M, Calhoun WJ, Hinton KL, et al. Respiratory syncytial virus infection in infants is associated with predominant Th-2-like response. *Am J Respir Crit Care Med* 1997;156:190–195.
517. Rosenberg HF, Domachowske JB. Pneumonia virus of mice: severe respiratory infection in a natural host. *Immunol Lett* 2008;118:6–12.
518. Rothoeft T, Fischer K, Zawatzki S, et al. Differential response of human naive and memory/effector T cells to dendritic cells infected by respiratory syncytial virus. *Clin Exp Immunol* 2007;150:263–273.
519. Roussy JF, Carbonneau J, Ouakki M, et al. Human metapneumovirus viral load is an important risk factor for disease severity in young children. *J Clin Virol* 2014;60:133–140.
520. Ruckwardt TJ, Morabito KM, Graham BS. Immunological lessons from respiratory syncytial virus vaccine development. *Immunity* 2019;51:429–442.
521. Ruckwardt TJ, Morabito KM, Phung E, et al. Safety, tolerability, and immunogenicity of the respiratory syncytial virus prefusion F subunit vaccine DS-Cav1: a phase 1, randomised, open-label, dose-escalation clinical trial. *Lancet Respir Med* 2021;9:1111–1120.
522. Rudd BD, Burstein E, Duckett CS, et al. Differential role for TLR3 in respiratory syncytial virus-induced chemokine expression. *J Virol* 2005;79:3350–3357.
523. Rudd BD, Smit JJ, Flavell RA, et al. Deletion of TLR3 alters the pulmonary immune environment and mucus production during respiratory syncytial virus infection. *J Immunol* 2006;176:1937–1942.
524. Russell CJ, Hurwitz JL. Sendai virus-vectored vaccines that express envelope glycoproteins of respiratory viruses. *Viruses* 2021;13.
525. Russell CJ, Jones BG, Sealy RE, et al. A Sendai virus recombinant vaccine expressing a gene for truncated human metapneumovirus (hMPV) fusion protein protects cotton rats from hMPV challenge. *Virology* 2017;509:60–66.
526. Ryder AB, Tollefson SJ, Podsiad AB, et al. Soluble recombinant human metapneumovirus G protein is immunogenic but not protective. *Vaccine* 2010;28:4145–4152.
527. Sacco RE, McGill JL, Pillatzki AE, et al. Respiratory syncytial virus infection in cattle. *Vet Pathol* 2014;51:427–436.
528. Sadoff J, De Paepe E, DeVincenzo J, et al. Prevention of respiratory syncytial virus infection in healthy adults by a single immunization of Ad26.RSV.preF in a human challenge study. *J Infect Dis* 2021. https://doi.org/10.1093/infdis/jiab003
529. Saha SK, Schrag SJ, El Arifeen S, et al. Causes and incidence of community-acquired serious infections among young children in south Asia (ANISA): an observational cohort study. *Lancet* 2018;392:145–159.
530. Saitou N, Nei M. The neighbor-joining method: a new method for reconstructing phylogenetic trees. *Mol Biol Evol* 1987;4:406–425.
531. Sakurai H, Williamson RA, Crowe JE, et al. Human antibody responses to mature and immature forms of viral envelope in respiratory syncytial virus infection: significance for subunit vaccines. *J Virol* 1999;73:2956–2962.
532. Salas A, Pardo-Seco J, Cebey-Lopez M, et al. Whole exome sequencing reveals new candidate genes in host genomic susceptibility to respiratory syncytial virus disease. *Sci Rep* 2017;7:15888.
533. Salimi V, Viegas M, Trento A, et al. Proposal for human respiratory syncytial virus nomenclature below the species level. *Emerg Infect Dis* 2021;27:1–9.
534. Samal SK, Collins PL. RNA replication by a respiratory syncytial virus RNA analog does not obey the rule of six and retains a nonviral trinucleotide extension at the leader end. *J Virol* 1996;70:5075–5082.
535. Sanders SL, Agwan S, Hassan M, et al. Immunoglobulin treatment for hospitalised infants and young children with respiratory syncytial virus infection. *Cochrane Database Syst Rev* 2019;8:CD009417.
536. Saravanos GL, King CL, Deng L, et al. Respiratory syncytial virus-associated neurologic complications in children: a systematic review and aggregated case series. *J Pediatr* 2021;239:39–49.e9.
537. Scaggs Huang F, Bernstein DI, Slobod KS, et al. Safety and immunogenicity of an intranasal Sendai virus-based vaccine for human parainfluenza virus type I and respiratory syncytial virus (SeVRSV) in adults. *Hum Vaccin Immunother* 2021;17:554–559.
538. Scagnolari C, Midulla F, Pierangeli A, et al. Gene expression of nucleic acid-sensing pattern recognition receptors in children hospitalized for respiratory syncytial virus-associated acute bronchiolitis. *Clin Vaccine Immunol* 2009;16:816–823.
539. Schepens B, Sedeyn K, Vande Ginste L, et al. Protection and mechanism of action of a novel human respiratory syncytial virus vaccine candidate based on the extracellular domain of small hydrophobic protein. *EMBO Mol Med* 2014;6:1436–1454.
540. Schickli JH, Kaur J, Ulbrandt N, et al. An S101P substitution in the putative cleavage motif of the human metapneumovirus fusion protein is a major determinant for trypsin-independent growth in Vero cells and does not alter tissue tropism in hamsters. *J Virol* 2005;79:10678–10689.
541. Schlender J, Walliser G, Fricke J, et al. Respiratory syncytial virus fusion protein mediates inhibition of mitogen-induced T-cell proliferation by contact. *J Virol* 2002;76:1163–1170.
542. Schmidt AC, Wenzke DR, McAuliffe JM, et al. Mucosal immunization of rhesus monkeys against respiratory syncytial virus subgroups A and B and human parainfluenza virus type 3 using a live cDNA-derived vaccine based on a host range-attenuated bovine parainfluenza virus type 3 vector backbone. *J Virol* 2002;76:1089–1099.
543. Schmidt H, Das A, Nam H, et al. Epidemiology and outcomes of hospitalized adults with respiratory syncytial virus: a 6-year retrospective study. *Influenza Other Respir Viruses* 2019;13:331–338.
544. Schneider-Ohrum K, Snell Bennett A, Rajani GM, et al. CD4(+) T cells drive lung disease enhancement induced by immunization with suboptimal doses of respiratory syncytial virus fusion protein in the mouse model. *J Virol* 2019;93.
545. Schowalter RM, Chang A, Robach JG, et al. Low-pH triggering of human metapneumovirus fusion: essential residues and importance in entry. *J Virol* 2009;83:1511–1522.
546. Schuster JE, Cox RG, Hastings AK, et al. A broadly neutralizing human monoclonal antibody exhibits in vivo efficacy against both human metapneumovirus and respiratory syncytial virus. *J Infect Dis* 2015;211:216–225.
547. Schwarz TF, Johnson C, Grigat C, et al. Three dose levels of a maternal respiratory syncytial virus vaccine candidate are well tolerated and immunogenic in a randomized trial in non-pregnant women. *J Infect Dis* 2021. https://doi.org/10.1093/infdis/jiab317
548. Sedeyn K, Schepens B, Saelens X. Respiratory syncytial virus nonstructural proteins 1 and 2: exceptional disrupters of innate immune responses. *PLoS Pathog* 2019;15:e1007984.
549. Selvaggi C, Pierangeli A, Fabiani M, et al. Interferon lambda 1–3 expression in infants hospitalized for RSV or HRV associated bronchiolitis. *J Infect* 2014;68:467–477.
550. Senft AP, Taylor RH, Lei W, et al. Respiratory syncytial virus impairs macrophage IFN-alpha/beta- and IFN-gamma-stimulated transcription by distinct mechanisms. *Am J Respir Cell Mol Biol* 2010;42:404–414.
551. Shapiro JM, Jean RE. Respiratory syncytial virus. *N Engl J Med* 2001;345:1132–1133.
552. Shay DK, Holman RC, Newman RD, et al. Bronchiolitis-associated hospitalizations among US children, 1980–1996. *JAMA* 1999;282:1440–1446.
553. Sheeran P, Jafri H, Carubelli C, et al. Elevated cytokine concentrations in the nasopharyngeal and tracheal secretions of children with respiratory syncytial virus disease. *Pediatr Infect Dis J* 1999;18:115–122.
554. Shi T, Arnott A, Semogas I, et al. The etiological role of common respiratory viruses in acute respiratory infections in older adults: a systematic review and meta-analysis. *J Infect Dis* 2020;222:S563–S569.
555. Shi T, McAllister DA, O'Brien KL, et al. Global, regional, and national disease burden estimates of acute lower respiratory infections due to respiratory syncytial virus in young children in 2015: a systematic review and modelling study. *Lancet* 2017;390:946–958.
556. Shin HJ, Cameron KT, Jacobs JA, et al. Molecular epidemiology of subgroup C avian pneumoviruses isolated in the United States and comparison with subgroup a and B viruses. *J Clin Microbiol* 2002;40:1687–1693.
557. Shinoff JJ, O'Brien KL, Thumar B, et al. Young infants can develop protective levels of neutralizing antibody after infection with respiratory syncytial virus. *J Infect Dis* 2008;198:1007–1015.
558. Siegrist CA. Mechanisms by which maternal antibodies influence infant vaccine responses: review of hypotheses and definition of main determinants. *Vaccine* 2003;21:3406–3412.
559. Sigurs N, Aljassim F, Kjellman B, et al. Asthma and allergy patterns over 18 years after severe RSV bronchiolitis in the first year of life. *Thorax* 2010;65:1045–1052.
560. Simoes EA, Carbonell-Estrany X, Rieger CH, et al. The effect of respiratory syncytial virus on subsequent recurrent wheezing in atopic and nonatopic children. *J Allergy Clin Immunol* 2010;126:256–262.
561. Simoes EA, Mutyara K, Soh S, et al. The epidemiology of respiratory syncytial virus lower respiratory tract infections in children less than 5 years of age in Indonesia. *Pediatr Infect Dis J* 2011;30:778–784.
562. Simpson J, Lynch JP, Loh Z, et al. The absence of interferon-beta promotor stimulator-1 (IPS-1) predisposes to bronchiolitis and asthma-like pathology in response to pneumoviral infection in mice. *Sci Rep* 2017;7:2353.
563. Sims DG, Downham MA, Gardner PS, et al. Study of 8-year-old children with a history of respiratory syncytial virus bronchiolitis in infancy. *Br Med J* 1978;1:11–14.
564. Skiadopoulos MH, Biacchesi S, Buchholz UJ, et al. Individual contributions of the human metapneumovirus F, G, and SH surface glycoproteins to the induction of neutralizing antibodies and protective immunity. *Virology* 2006;345:492–501.
565. Skiadopoulos MH, Biacchesi S, Buchholz UJ, et al. The two major human metapneumovirus genetic lineages are highly related antigenically, and the fusion (F) protein is a major contributor to this antigenic relatedness. *J Virol* 2004;78:6927–6937.
566. Smith AL, Singleton GR, Hansen GM, et al. A serologic survey for viruses and Mycoplasma pulmonis among wild house mice (Mus domesticus) in southeastern Australia. *J Wildl Dis* 1993;29:219–229.
567. Smyth RL, Mobbs KJ, O'Hea U, et al. Respiratory syncytial virus bronchiolitis: disease severity, interleukin-8, and virus genotype. *Pediatr Pulmonol* 2002;33:339–346.
568. Sonawane AR, Tian L, Chu CY, et al. Microbiome-transcriptome interactions related to severity of respiratory syncytial virus infection. *Sci Rep* 2019;9:13824.
569. Soto JA, Galvez NMS, Benavente FM, et al. Human metapneumovirus: mechanisms and molecular targets used by the virus to avoid the immune system. *Front Immunol* 2018;9:2466.
570. Sow FB, Gallup JM, Olivier A, et al. Respiratory syncytial virus is associated with an inflammatory response in lungs and architectural remodeling of lung-draining lymph nodes of newborn lambs. *Am J Physiol Lung Cell Mol Physiol* 2011;300:L12–L24.
571. Spann KM, Collins PL, Teng MN. Genetic recombination during coinfection of two mutants of human respiratory syncytial virus. *J Virol* 2003;77:11201–11211.
572. Spann KM, Tran KC, Chi B, et al. Suppression of the induction of alpha, beta, and lambda interferons by the NS1 and NS2 proteins of human respiratory syncytial virus in human epithelial cells and macrophages *J Virol* 2004;78:4363–4369.
573. Spann KM, Tran KC, Collins PL. Effects of nonstructural proteins NS1 and NS2 of human respiratory syncytial virus on interferon regulatory factor 3, NF-kappaB, and proinflammatory cytokines. *J Virol* 2005;79:5353–5362.
574. Srikiatkhachorn A, Braciale TJ. Virus-specific CD8+ T lymphocytes downregulate T helper cell type 2 cytokine secretion and pulmonary eosinophilia during experimental murine respiratory syncytial virus infection. *J Exp Med* 1997;186:421–432.

575. Staadegaard L, Caini S, Wangchuk S, et al. Defining the seasonality of respiratory syncytial virus around the world: national and subnational surveillance data from 12 countries. *Influenza Other Respir Viruses* 2021;15:732–741.
576. Stec DS, Hill MG, Collins PL. Sequence analysis of the polymerase L gene of human respiratory syncytial virus and predicted phylogeny of nonsegmented negative-strand viruses. *Virology* 1991;183:273–287.
577. Stephens LM, Varga SM. Considerations for a respiratory syncytial virus vaccine targeting an elderly population. *Vaccines (Basel)* 2021;9.
578. Stevens M, Rusch S, DeVincenzo J, et al. Antiviral activity of oral JNJ-53718678 in healthy adult volunteers challenged with respiratory syncytial virus: a placebo-controlled study. *J Infect Dis* 2018;218:748–756.
579. Stevens WW, Sun J, Castillo JP, et al. Pulmonary eosinophilia is attenuated by early responding CD8(+) memory T cells in a murine model of RSV vaccine-enhanced disease. *Viral Immunol* 2009;22:243–251.
580. Stobart CC, Rostad CA, Ke Z, et al. A live RSV vaccine with engineered thermostability is immunogenic in cotton rats despite high attenuation. *Nat Commun* 2016;7:13916.
581. Stray K, Perron M, Porter DP, et al. Drug resistance assessment following administration of respiratory syncytial virus (RSV) fusion inhibitor presatovir to participants experimentally infected with RSV. *J Infect Dis* 2020;222:1468–1477.
582. Suarez-Arrabal MC, Mella C, Lopez SM, et al. Nasopharyngeal bacterial burden and antibiotics: influence on inflammatory markers and disease severity in infants with respiratory syncytial virus bronchiolitis. *J Infect* 2015;71:458–469.
583. Sudo K, Miyazaki Y, Kojima N, et al. YM-53403, a unique anti-respiratory syncytial virus agent with a novel mechanism of action. *Antiviral Res* 2005;65:125–131.
584. Sugimoto M, Morichi S, Kashiwagi Y, et al. A case of respiratory syncytial virus-associated encephalopathy in which the virus was detected in cerebrospinal fluid and intratracheal aspiration despite negative rapid test results. *J Infect Chemother* 2020;26:393–396.
585. Suleiman-Martos N, Caballero-Vazquez A, Gomez-Urquiza JL, et al. Prevalence and risk factors of respiratory syncytial virus in children under 5 years of age in the WHO European region: a systematic review and meta-analysis. *J Pers Med* 2021;11.
586. Sumino KC, Agapov E, Pierce RA, et al. Detection of severe human metapneumovirus infection by real-time polymerase chain reaction and histopathological assessment. *J Infect Dis* 2005;192:1052–1060.
587. Sung RY, Hui SH, Wong CK, et al. A comparison of cytokine responses in respiratory syncytial virus and influenza A infections in infants. *Eur J Pediatr* 2001;160:117–122.
588. Sung RY, Yin J, Oppenheimer SJ, et al. Treatment of respiratory syncytial virus infection with recombinant interferon alfa-2a. *Arch Dis Child* 1993;69:440–442.
589. Surman SR, Collins PL, Murphy BR, et al. An improved method for the recovery of recombinant paramyxovirus vaccine candidates suitable for use in human clinical trials. *J Virol Methods* 2007;141:30–33.
590. Sutto-Ortiz P, Tcherniuk S, Ysebaert N, et al. The methyltransferase domain of the Respiratory Syncytial Virus L protein catalyzes cap N7 and 2′-O-methylation. *PLoS Pathog* 2021;17:e1009562.
591. Swanson KA, Settembre EC, Shaw CA, et al. Structural basis for immunization with post-fusion RSV F to elicit high neutralizing antibody titers. *Proc Natl Acad Sci U S A* 2011;108:9619–9624.
592. Swedan S, Musiyenko A, Barik S. Respiratory syncytial virus nonstructural proteins decrease levels of multiple members of the cellular interferon pathways. *J Virol* 2009;83:9682–9693.
593. Tamura K, Dudley J, Nei M, et al. MEGA4: molecular evolutionary genetics analysis (MEGA) software version 4.0. *Mol Biol Evol* 2007;24:1596–1599.
594. Tang RS, Spaete RR, Thompson MW, et al. Development of a PIV-vectored RSV vaccine: preclinical evaluation of safety, toxicity, and enhanced disease and initial clinical testing in healthy adults. *Vaccine* 2008;26:6373–6382.
595. Tawar RG, Duquerroy S, Vonrhein C, et al. Crystal structure of a nucleocapsid-like nucleoprotein-RNA complex of respiratory syncytial virus. *Science* 2009;326:1279–1283.
596. Taylor AW, Blau DM, Bassat Q, et al. Initial findings from a novel population-based child mortality surveillance approach: a descriptive study. *Lancet Glob Health* 2020;8:e909–e919.
597. Tayyari F, Marchant D, Moraes TJ, et al. Identification of nucleolin as a cellular receptor for human respiratory syncytial virus. *Nat Med* 2011;17:1132–1135.
598. Techaarpornkul S, Barretto N, Peeples ME. Functional analysis of recombinant respiratory syncytial virus deletion mutants lacking the small hydrophobic and/or attachment glycoprotein gene. *J Virol* 2001;75:6825–6834.
599. Techaarpornkul S, Collins PL, Peeples ME. Respiratory syncytial virus with the fusion protein as its only viral glycoprotein is less dependent on cellular glycosaminoglycans for attachment than complete virus. *Virology* 2002;294:296–304.
600. Teng MN, Collins PL. The central conserved cystine noose of the attachment G protein of human respiratory syncytial virus is not required for efficient viral infection in vitro or in vivo. *J Virol* 2002;76:6164–6171.
601. Teng MN, Collins PL. Identification of the respiratory syncytial virus proteins required for formation and passage of helper-dependent infectious particles. *J Virol* 1998;72:5707–5716.
602. Teng MN, Whitehead SS, Bermingham A, et al. Recombinant respiratory syncytial virus that does not express the NS1 or M2-2 protein is highly attenuated and immunogenic in chimpanzees. *J Virol* 2000;74:9317–9321.
603. Teng MN, Whitehead SS, Collins PL. Contribution of the respiratory syncytial virus g glycoprotein and its secreted and membrane-bound forms to virus replication in vitro and in vivo. *Virology* 2001;289:283–296.
604. Thammawat S, Sadlon TA, Hallsworth PG, et al. Role of cellular glycosaminoglycans and charged regions of viral G protein in human metapneumovirus infection. *J Virol* 2008;82:11767–11774.
605. Thielen BK, Bye E, Wang X, et al. Summer outbreak of severe RSV-B disease, Minnesota, 2017 associated with emergence of a genetically distinct viral lineage. *J Infect Dis* 2020;222:288–297.
606. Thomas E, Mattila JM, Lehtinen P, et al. Burden of respiratory syncytial virus infection during the first year of life. *J Infect Dis* 2021;223:811–817.
607. Thompson WW, Shay DK, Weintraub E, et al. Mortality associated with influenza and respiratory syncytial virus in the United States. *JAMA* 2003;289:179–186.
608. Thomsen SF, Stensballe LG, Skytthe A, et al. Increased concordance of severe respiratory syncytial virus infection in identical twins. *Pediatrics* 2008;121:493–496.
609. Thwaites RS, Coates M, Ito K, et al. Reduced nasal viral load and IFN responses in infants with respiratory syncytial virus bronchiolitis and respiratory failure. *Am J Respir Crit Care Med* 2018;198:1074–1084.
610. Tin Tin Htar M, Yerramalla MS, Moisi JC, et al. The burden of respiratory syncytial virus in adults: a systematic review and meta-analysis. *Epidemiol Infect* 2020;148:e48.
611. Tollefson SJ, Cox RG, Williams JV. Studies of culture conditions and environmental stability of human metapneumovirus. *Virus Res* 2010;151:54–59.
612. Tortorolo L, Langer A, Polidori G, et al. Neurotrophin overexpression in lower airways of infants with respiratory syncytial virus infection. *Am J Respir Crit Care Med* 2005;172:233–237.
613. Tran TL, Castagne N, Dubosclard V, et al. The respiratory syncytial virus M2-1 protein forms tetramers and interacts with RNA and P in a competitive manner. *J Virol* 2009;83:6363–6374.
614. Tregoning JS, Wang BL, McDonald JU, et al. Neonatal antibody responses are attenuated by interferon-gamma produced by NK and T cells during RSV infection. *Proc Natl Acad Sci U S A* 2013;110:5576–5581.
615. Trento A, Casas I, Calderon A, et al. Ten years of global evolution of the human respiratory syncytial virus BA genotype with a 60-nucleotide duplication in the G protein gene. *J Virol* 2010;84:7500–7512.
616. Trento A, Galiano M, Videla C, et al. Major changes in the G protein of human respiratory syncytial virus isolates introduced by a duplication of 60 nucleotides. *J Gen Virol* 2003;84:3115–3120.
617. Triantafilou K, Kar S, Vakakis E, et al. Human respiratory syncytial virus viroporin SH: a viral recognition pathway used by the host to signal inflammasome activation. *Thorax* 2013;68:66–75.
618. Tripp RA, Jones LP, Haynes LM, et al. CX3C chemokine mimicry by respiratory syncytial virus G glycoprotein. *Nat Immunol* 2001;2:732–738.
619. Valarcher JF, Bourhy H, Lavenu A, et al. Persistent infection of B lymphocytes by bovine respiratory syncytial virus. *Virology* 2001;291:55–67.
620. Valarcher JF, Furze J, Wyld S, et al. Role of alpha/beta interferons in the attenuation and immunogenicity of recombinant bovine respiratory syncytial viruses lacking NS proteins. *J Virol* 2003;77:8426–8439.
621. Valarcher JF, Furze J, Wyld SG, et al. Bovine respiratory syncytial virus lacking the virokinin or with a mutation in furin cleavage site RA(R/K)R109 induces less pulmonary inflammation without impeding the induction of protective immunity in calves. *J Gen Virol* 2006;87:1659–1667.
622. Valarcher JF, Schelcher F, Bourhy H. Evolution of bovine respiratory syncytial virus. *J Virol* 2000;74:10714–10728.
623. Vallbracht S, Unsold H, Ehl S. Functional impairment of cytotoxic T cells in the lung airways following respiratory virus infections. *Eur J Immunol* 2006;36:1434–1442.
624. van den Hoogen BG, Bestebroer TM, Osterhaus AD, et al. Analysis of the genomic sequence of a human metapneumovirus. *Virology* 2002;295:119–132.
625. van den Hoogen BG, de Jong JC, Groen J, et al. A newly discovered human pneumovirus isolated from young children with respiratory tract disease. *Nat Med* 2001;7:719–724.
626. van den Hoogen BG, Herfst S, de Graaf M, et al. Experimental infection of macaques with human metapneumovirus induces transient protective immunity. *J Gen Virol* 2007;88:1251–1259.
627. van Diepen A, Brand HK, Sama I, et al. Quantitative proteome profiling of respiratory virus-infected lung epithelial cells. *J Proteomics* 2010;73:1680–1693.
628. Velayudhan BT, Nagaraja KV, Thachil AJ, et al. Human metapneumovirus in turkey poults. *Emerg Infect Dis* 2006;12:1853–1859.
629. Venter M, Rock M, Puren AJ, et al. Respiratory syncytial virus nucleoprotein-specific cytotoxic T-cell epitopes in a South African population of diverse HLA types are conserved in circulating field strains. *J Virol* 2003;77:7319–7329.
630. Venter M, van Niekerk S, Rakgantso A, et al. Identification of deletion mutant respiratory syncytial virus strains lacking most of the G protein in immunocompromised children with pneumonia in South Africa. *J Virol* 2011;85:8453–8457.
631. Ventre K, Randolph A. Ribavirin for respiratory syncytial virus infection of the lower respiratory tract in infants and young children. *Cochrane Database Syst Rev* 2004;(1):CD000181.
632. Verdijk P, van der Plas JL, van Brummelen EMJ, et al. First-in-human administration of a live-attenuated RSV vaccine lacking the G-protein assessing safety, tolerability, shedding and immunogenicity: a randomized controlled trial. *Vaccine* 2020;38:6088–6095.
633. Wagner DK, Clements ML, Reimer CB, et al. Analysis of immunoglobulin G antibody responses after administration of live and inactivated influenza A vaccine indicates that nasal wash immunoglobulin G is a transudate from serum. *J Clin Microbiol* 1987;25:559–562.
634. Wagner DK, Nelson DL, Walsh EE, et al. Differential immunoglobulin G subclass antibody titers to respiratory syncytial virus F and G glycoproteins in adults. *J Clin Microbiol* 1987;25:748–750.
635. Walpita P, Johns LM, Tandon R, et al. Mammalian cell-derived respiratory syncytial virus-like particles protect the lower as well as the upper respiratory tract. *PLoS One* 2015;10:e0130755.
636. Walsh EE, Falsey AR. Age related differences in humoral immune response to respiratory syncytial virus infection in adults. *J Med Virol* 2004;73:295–299.
637. Walsh EE, Falsey AR. Humoral and mucosal immunity in protection from natural respiratory syncytial virus infection in adults. *J Infect Dis* 2004;190:373–378.
638. Walsh EE, Peterson DR, Falsey AR. Human metapneumovirus infections in adults: another piece of the puzzle. *Arch Intern Med* 2008;168:2489–2496.
639. Walsh EE, Peterson DR, Falsey AR. Risk factors for severe respiratory syncytial virus infection in elderly persons. *J Infect Dis* 2004;189:233–238.
640. Walsh EE, Peterson DR, Kalkanoglu AE, et al. Viral shedding and immune responses to respiratory syncytial virus infection in older adults. *J Infect Dis* 2013;207:1424–1432.

641. Walsh EE, Wang L, Falsey AR, et al. Virus-specific antibody, viral load, and disease severity in respiratory syncytial virus infection. *J Infect Dis* 2018;218:208–217.

642. Wang L, Chu CY, McCall MN, et al. Airway gene-expression classifiers for respiratory syncytial virus (RSV) disease severity in infants. *BMC Med Genomics* 2021;14:57.

643. Wang XF, Zhang XY, Gao X, et al. Proteomic profiling of a respiratory syncytial virus-infected rat pneumonia model. *Jpn J Infect Dis* 2016;69:285–292.

644. Waris M. Pattern of respiratory syncytial virus epidemics in Finland: two-year cycles with alternating prevalence of groups A and B. *J Infect Dis* 1991;163:464–469.

645. Waris ME, Tsou C, Erdman DD, et al. Priming with live respiratory syncytial virus (RSV) prevents the enhanced pulmonary inflammatory response seen after RSV challenge in BALB/c mice immunized with formalin-inactivated RSV. *J Virol* 1997;71:6935–6939.

646. Wathen MW, Aeed PA, Elhammer AP. Characterization of oligosaccharide structures on a chimeric respiratory syncytial virus protein expressed in insect cell line Sf9. *Biochemistry* 1991;30:2863–2868.

647. Wathen MW, Brideau RJ, Thomsen DR, et al. Characterization of a novel human respiratory syncytial virus chimeric FG glycoprotein expressed using a baculovirus vector. *J Gen Virol* 1989;70:2625–2635.

648. Weinberger DM, Klugman KP, Steiner CA, et al. Association between respiratory syncytial virus activity and pneumococcal disease in infants: a time series analysis of US hospitalization data. *PLoS Med* 2015;12:e1001776.

649. Welliver RC, Checchia PA, Bauman JH, et al. Fatality rates in published reports of RSV hospitalizations among high-risk and otherwise healthy children. *Curr Med Res Opin* 2010;26:2175–2181.

650. Welliver RC, Kaul TN, Putnam TI, et al. The antibody response to primary and secondary infection with respiratory syncytial virus: kinetics of class-specific responses. *J Pediatr* 1980;96:808–813.

651. Welliver TP, Garofalo RP, Hosakote Y, et al. Severe human lower respiratory tract illness caused by respiratory syncytial virus and influenza virus is characterized by the absence of pulmonary cytotoxic lymphocyte responses. *J Infect Dis* 2007;195:1126–1136.

652. Wertz GW, Collins PL, Huang Y, et al. Nucleotide sequence of the G protein gene of human respiratory syncytial virus reveals an unusual type of viral membrane protein. *Proc Natl Acad Sci U S A* 1985;82:4075–4079.

653. Wertz GW, Krieger M, Ball LA. Structure and cell surface maturation of the attachment glycoprotein of human respiratory syncytial virus in a cell line deficient in O glycosylation. *J Virol* 1989;63:4767–4776.

654. Whelan JN, Tran KC, van Rossum DB, et al. Identification of respiratory syncytial virus nonstructural protein 2 residues essential for exploitation of the host ubiquitin system and inhibition of innate immune responses. *J Virol* 2016;90:6453–6463.

655. Whimbey E, Champlin RE, Couch RB, et al. Community respiratory virus infections among hospitalized adult bone marrow transplant recipients. *Clin Infect Dis* 1996;22:778–782.

656. White LJ, Waris M, Cane PA, et al. The transmission dynamics of groups A and B human respiratory syncytial virus (hRSV) in England & Wales and Finland: seasonality and cross-protection. *Epidemiol Infect* 2005;133:279–289.

657. Whitehead SS, Bukreyev A, Teng MN, et al. Recombinant respiratory syncytial virus bearing a deletion of either the NS2 or SH gene is attenuated in chimpanzees. *J Virol* 1999;73:3438–3442.

658. Whitehead SS, Firestone CY, Collins PL, et al. A single nucleotide substitution in the transcription start signal of the M2 gene of respiratory syncytial virus vaccine candidate cpts248/404 is the major determinant of the temperature-sensitive and attenuation phenotypes. *Virology* 1998;247:232–239.

659. Whitehead SS, Firestone CY, Karron RA, et al. Addition of a missense mutation present in the L gene of respiratory syncytial virus (RSV) cpts530/1030 to RSV vaccine candidate cpts248/404 increases its attenuation and temperature sensitivity. *J Virol* 1999;73:871–877.

660. Whitehead SS, Juhasz K, Firestone CY, et al. Recombinant respiratory syncytial virus (RSV) bearing a set of mutations from cold-passaged RSV is attenuated in chimpanzees. *J Virol* 1998;72:4467–4471.

661. Williams JV, Edwards KM, Weinberg GA, et al. Population-based incidence of human metapneumovirus infection among hospitalized children. *J Infect Dis* 2010;201:1890–1898.

662. Williams JV, Harris PA, Tollefson SJ, et al. Human metapneumovirus and lower respiratory tract disease in otherwise healthy infants and children. *N Engl J Med* 2004;350:443–450.

663. Williams JV, Wang CK, Yang CF, et al. The role of human metapneumovirus in upper respiratory tract infections in children: a 20-year experience. *J Infect Dis* 2006;193:387–395.

664. Williams JV, Weitkamp JH, Blum DL, et al. The human neonatal B cell response to respiratory syncytial virus uses a biased antibody variable gene repertoire that lacks somatic mutations. *Mol Immunol* 2009;47:407–414.

665. Williams K, Bastian AR, Feldman RA, et al. Phase 1 safety and immunogenicity study of a respiratory syncytial virus vaccine with an adenovirus 26 vector encoding prefusion F (Ad26.RSV.preF) in adults aged >/=60 Years. *J Infect Dis* 2020;222:979–988.

666. Wright PF, Gruber WC, Peters M, et al. Illness severity, viral shedding, and antibody responses in infants hospitalized with bronchiolitis caused by respiratory syncytial virus. *J Infect Dis* 2002;185:1011–1018.

667. Wright PF, Karron RA, Belshe RB, et al. The absence of enhanced disease with wild type respiratory syncytial virus infection occurring after receipt of live, attenuated, respiratory syncytial virus vaccines. *Vaccine* 2007;25:7372–7378.

668. Wright PF, Karron RA, Belshe RB, et al. Evaluation of a live, cold-passaged, temperature-sensitive, respiratory syncytial virus vaccine candidate in infancy. *J Infect Dis* 2000;182:1331–1342.

669. Wu H, Pfarr DS, Johnson S, et al. Development of motavizumab, an ultra-potent antibody for the prevention of respiratory syncytial virus infection in the upper and lower respiratory tract. *J Mol Biol* 2007;368:652–665.

670. Wyde PR, Chetty SN, Jewell AM, et al. Comparison of the inhibition of human metapneumovirus and respiratory syncytial virus by ribavirin and immune serum globulin in vitro. *Antiviral Res* 2003;60:51–59.

671. Xiao X, Tang A, Cox KS, et al. Characterization of potent RSV neutralizing antibodies isolated from human memory B cells and identification of diverse RSV/hMPV cross-neutralizing epitopes. *MAbs* 2019;11:1415–1427.

672. Xu X, Mann M, Qiao D, et al. Alternative mRNA processing of innate response pathways in respiratory syncytial virus (RSV) infection. *Viruses* 2021;13.

673. Yeo DS, Chan R, Brown G, et al. Evidence that selective changes in the lipid composition of raft-membranes occur during respiratory syncytial virus infection. *Virology* 2009;386:168–182.

674. Yim KC, Cragin RP, Boukhvalova MS, et al. Human metapneumovirus: enhanced pulmonary disease in cotton rats immunized with formalin-inactivated virus vaccine and challenged. *Vaccine* 2007;25:5034–5040.

675. Yoboua F, Martel A, Duval A, et al. Respiratory syncytial virus-mediated NF-kappa B p65 phosphorylation at serine 536 is dependent on RIG-I, TRAF6, and IKK beta. *J Virol* 2010;84:7267–7277.

676. Yu X, Lakerveld AJ, Imholz S, et al. Antibody and local cytokine response to respiratory syncytial virus infection in community-dwelling older adults. *mSphere* 2020;5.

677. Yui I, Hoshi A, Shigeta Y, et al. Detection of human respiratory syncytial virus sequences in peripheral blood mononuclear cells. *J Med Virol* 2003;70:481–489.

678. Zambon MC, Stockton JD, Clewley JP, et al. Contribution of influenza and respiratory syncytial virus to community cases of influenza-like illness: an observational study. *Lancet* 2001;358:1410–1416.

679. Zamora MR, Budev M, Rolfe M, et al. RNA interference therapy in lung transplant patients infected with respiratory syncytial virus. *Am J Respir Crit Care Med* 2011;183:531–538.

680. Zhang L, Bukreyev A, Thompson CI, et al. Infection of ciliated cells by human parainfluenza virus type 3 in an in vitro model of human airway epithelium. *J Virol* 2005;79:1113–1124.

681. Zhang L, Mendoza-Sassi RA, Wainwright C, et al. Nebulised hypertonic saline solution for acute bronchiolitis in infants. *Cochrane Database Syst Rev* 2017;12:CD006458.

682. Zhang L, Peeples ME, Boucher RC, et al. Respiratory syncytial virus infection of human airway epithelial cells is polarized, specific to ciliated cells, and without obvious cytopathology. *J Virol* 2002;76:5654–5666.

683. Zheng H, Storch GA, Zang C, et al. Genetic variability in envelope-associated protein genes of closely related group A strains of respiratory syncytial virus. *Virus Res* 1999;59:89–99.

684. Zheng X, Gao L, Wang L, et al. Discovery of ziresovir as a potent, selective, and orally bioavailable respiratory syncytial virus fusion protein inhibitor. *J Med Chem* 2019;62:6003–6014.

685. Zhou J, Zhang X, Liu S, et al. Genetic association of TLR4 Asp299Gly, TLR4 Thr399Ile, and CD14 C-159T polymorphisms with the risk of severe RSV infection: a meta-analysis. *Influenza Other Respir Viruses* 2016;10:224–233.

686. Zhu Q, McAuliffe JM, Patel NK, et al. Analysis of respiratory syncytial virus preclinical and clinical variants resistant to neutralization by monoclonal antibodies palivizumab and/or motavizumab. *J Infect Dis* 2011;203:674–682.

687. Zhu Q, McLellan JS, Kallewaard NL, et al. A highly potent extended half-life antibody as a potential RSV vaccine surrogate for all infants. *Sci Transl Med* 2017;9.

688. Zimmer G, Conzelmann KK, Herrler G. Cleavage at the furin consensus sequence RAR/KR(109) and presence of the intervening peptide of the respiratory syncytial virus fusion protein are dispensable for virus replication in cell culture. *J Virol* 2002;76:9218–9224.

689. Zimmer G, Rohn M, McGregor GP, et al. Virokinin, a bioactive peptide of the tachykinin family, is released from the fusion protein of bovine respiratory syncytial virus. *J Biol Chem* 2003;278:46854–46861.

690. Zlateva KT, Lemey P, Moes E, et al. Genetic variability and molecular evolution of the human respiratory syncytial virus subgroup B attachment G protein. *J Virol* 2005;79:9157–9167.

691. Zuniga A, Rassek O, Vrohlings M, et al. An epitope-specific chemically defined nanoparticle vaccine for respiratory syncytial virus. *NPJ Vaccines* 2021;6:85.

Terence S. Dermody • John S. L. Parker • Barbara Sherry

History
  Basic features of the *Reoviridae*
  Discovery of mammalian reoviruses
  Pathogenic *Reoviridae* viruses
  Reovirus as a model for studies of dsRNA virus replication and
    pathogenesis
Classification
  dsRNA viruses
  Family *Reoviridae*
  Genus *Orthoreovirus*
Virion structure
  Particle function
  Virions
  Infectious subvirion particles
  Core particles
  Recombinant particles
  Particles *in situ*
Genome structure and organization
  Physical characteristics
  Protein-coding strategies and nomenclature
  Terminal nontranslated regions
  Genetics
Stages of replication
  Aattachment
  Entry and intracellular trafficking
  Uncoating
  Membrane penetration
  Transcription
  Translation and viral factory formation
  Assortment and replication of genomic nucleic acid
  Assembly
  Release
Responses of the host cell to infection
  Induction of interferon and effects on viral replication
  Inhibition of cellular RNA and protein synthesis and induction
    of cellular stress responses
  Inhibition of cellular DNA synthesis and cell cycle progression
  Activation of NF-κB and induction of apoptosis or necroptosis
Pathogenesis and pathology
  Entry into the host
  Site of primary replication
  Spread of virus
  Cell and tissue tropism
  Innate immune responses
  Adaptive immune responses
Epidemiology
Clinical features
  Reovirus infections of humans

Diagnosis
Prevention and control
Reovirus oncolytics
Perspective
Acknowledgments

HISTORY

Basic Features of the *Reoviridae*

Members of the *Reoviridae* form nonenveloped virions composed of 1 to 3 concentric protein shells. The genomes of these viruses consist of 9 to 12 discrete segments of double-stranded RNA (dsRNA). Much of what is known about the *Reoviridae* comes from studies of orbiviruses, orthoreoviruses, and rotaviruses. Although these and other *Reoviridae* members display important structural and biological differences, there are several properties held in common across the family.

The dsRNA gene segments of the *Reoviridae* viruses are not thought to leave the inner capsid particle during the normal course of infection. Enzymes that catalyze RNA transcription, capping, and replication are contained within the inner capsid, which serves as the site for the RNA synthetic activities. The mRNA transcripts are capped but not polyadenylated. The infectious cycle is entirely cytoplasmic and occurs for the most part in structures that are termed viral factories, viral inclusions, or viroplasms. These viruses are sensed by the innate immune system and activate signaling cascades that induce an antiviral state or evoke cell death, often by apoptosis.

Discovery of Mammalian Reoviruses

Reoviruses were first isolated from stool specimens of children during the 1950s by Albert Sabin, Leon Rosen, and their colleagues.[379,381] Reovirus is an acronym for *r*espiratory *e*nteric *o*rphan virus; infections of humans by reovirus usually involve the respiratory and intestinal tracts with minimal or no associated disease symptoms. Therefore, the virus is referred to as an "orphan." In the early 1960s, Peter Gomatos and Igor Tamm noted that the inclusions in reovirus-infected cells fluoresce greenish-yellow when stained with acridine orange, whereas single-stranded RNA fluoresces orange.[177] Based on chemical and physical studies, the viral genome was demonstrated to consist of dsRNA. Reoviruses were the first dsRNA viruses to be described.

The *Reoviridae* now includes 15 genera of dsRNA viruses that infect a wide variety of animals, plants, algae, fungi, and protozoa (e-Table 11.1). The mammalian orthoreoviruses are the type species of the *Orthoreovirus* genus, which also contains viruses that infect birds and reptiles. The term "reovirus" refers to the mammalian orthoreoviruses and will be used as such in this chapter.

Pathogenic *Reoviridae* Viruses

Some members of the *Reoviridae* are pathogenic. Rotaviruses are responsible for gastroenteritis in animals and humans; they produce gastroenteritis in children and adults and are a major cause of infant illness and death in the developing world. Orbiviruses are transmitted by arthropod vectors and replicate in both mammalian and arthropod hosts. The best studied *Orbivirus* is bluetongue virus, an economically significant pathogen of sheep and cows named for a clinical sign sometimes seen in affected sheep. Coltiviruses also are transmitted by arthropod vectors, and the prototype member, Colorado tick fever virus, can cause neurologic disease in humans. Aquareoviruses infect fish and mollusks and are major pathogens in aquaculture. Fusogenic orthoreoviruses cause a variety of illnesses in birds, reptiles, and mammals and occasionally produce pneumonia in humans.

Reovirus as a Model for Studies of dsRNA Virus Replication and Pathogenesis

Reoviruses are useful experimental models for studies of viral replication and pathogenesis. Studies of reovirus RNA synthesis were the first to describe the methylated cap structure that modifies most eukaryotic mRNA molecules and is required for normal translation[164,165]; this work was done using RNAs synthesized *in vitro* from reovirus cores. Genetic approaches used to study the pathogenesis of reovirus infection in mice led to the discovery that phenotypic differences in specific steps in the virus–host encounter segregate with specific gene segments.[468] Reovirus was the first virus shown to traverse the intestinal mucosa by transcytosis across microfold (M) cells[478] and undergo proteolytic disassembly catalyzed by endosomal cathepsins.[143] Reovirus is being evaluated as an oncolytic agent in human clinical trials for a variety of cancers (see "Reovirus Oncolytics").

CLASSIFICATION

dsRNA Viruses

There are 11 taxonomic families of dsRNA viruses, the *Amalgaviridae, Birnaviridae, Chrysoviridae, Cystoviridae, Megabirnaviridae, Partitiviridae, Picobirnaviridae, Polymycoviridae, Quadriviridae, Reoviridae,* and *Totiviridae*[14] and https://talk.ictvonline.org/taxonomy/. The *Birnaviridae, Picobirnaviridae,* and *Reoviridae* infect vertebrates; the *Picobirnaviridae* and *Reoviridae* infect mammals including humans. The eleven families are distinguished by genome organization, coding strategy, particle structure, and host range, among other properties. Differences in RNA-dependent RNA polymerase sequences suggest independent evolutionary lineages of dsRNA viruses that arose from positive-sense RNA virus ancestors.[249] However, similarities beyond the existence of dsRNA genomes suggest common ancestry, most notably in the organization of the capsid components. Interestingly, not all dsRNA viruses encode capsids. Members of the *Hypoviridae* transfer their genomes vertically during propagation of their fungal hosts.[111]

Family *Reoviridae*

The *Reoviridae* is the largest and most diverse family of dsRNA viruses. The viral particles display icosahedral symmetry with a diameter of 60 to 95 nm. The protein capsid is organized as one, two, or three concentric capsid layers, which surround the dsRNA segments of the viral genome. Some genera have filamentous or rod-shaped attachment proteins, but most do not. The viral RNA species are usually monocistronic, although some segments have two or three in-frame initiation codons that lead to expression of additional open-reading frames (ORFs). Alternative out-of-frame ORFs, or nonoverlapping ORFs, are occasionally present. Proteins are encoded by only one strand of each duplex (the mRNA species).

The 15 genera of the *Reoviridae* are divided into two groups based on particle morphology[14] and https://talk.ictvonline.org/taxonomy/ (e-Table 11.1). The *Sedoreovirinae* subfamily includes genera-containing "smooth" viruses that are almost spherical in appearance, including *Cardoreovirus, Mimoreovirus, Orbivirus, Phytoreovirus, Rotavirus,* and *Seadornavirus*. The *Spinareovirinae* subfamily includes genera-containing viruses with large "spikes" or "turrets" at the 12 icosahedral vertices of either the virus or core particle, including *Aquareovirus, Coltivirus, Cypovirus, Dinovernavirus, Fijivirus, Idnoreovirus, Mycoreovirus, Orthoreovirus,* and *Oryzavirus*. The overall fold of several of the major inner and outer capsid proteins of *Reoviridae* members is similar, despite the absence of primary sequence identity.

The inner protein layer of the *Sedoreovirinae* (smooth) viruses has T = 1 symmetry (of homodimers) and is relatively fragile. This structure is surrounded by an additional protein layer, which has T = 13 symmetry, to form the transcriptionally active core particle. These double-layered particles are surrounded by an outer-capsid shell, giving rise to triple-layered particles. In contrast, the transcriptionally active core particle of the *Spinareovirinae* (turreted) viruses appears to contain only a single complete capsid layer, which has been interpreted as having T = 1 or T = 2 symmetry, to which the spikes are attached. Despite these different interpretations, the structure of the innermost complete capsid layer is almost identical for members of both the *Sedoreovirinae* and *Spinareovirinae*. In most cases, the core is surrounded by an additional protein layer with T = 13 symmetry that forms the outer capsid, which is penetrated by the spikes that arise from the core surface. These virus particles are therefore usually regarded as double-shelled (Fig. 11.1).

The innermost protein layer of *Reoviridae* viruses has an internal diameter of approximately 50 to 60 nm surrounding the 9 to 12 linear dsRNA gene segments. In the *Sedoreovirinae* viruses, the enzymatically active proteins of the virion (RNA-dependent RNA polymerase, NTPase, guanylyltransferase, and methyltransferase) also are situated within this central structure attached to the inner surface at the fivefold symmetry axes. In the *Spinareovirinae* viruses, some of these enzymes form the turrets on the surface of the core. These hollow projections also act as conduits for the exit of nascent mRNAs synthesized by the core-associated enzymes.

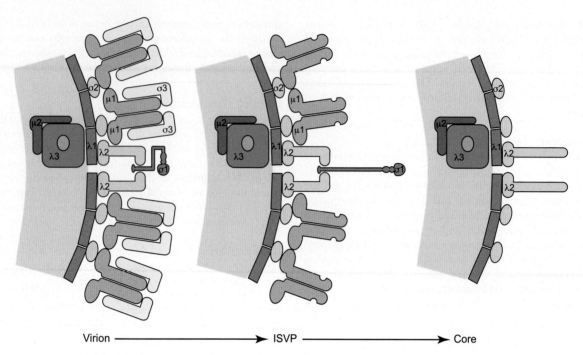

Virion ⟶ ISVP ⟶ Core

FIGURE 11.1 Schematic of reovirus particles with protein composition. Diagram of a cross-section from virions, infectious subvirion particles (ISVPs), and core particles showing the arrangement of the viral structural proteins in the double-layered shells of virions, the formation of ISVPs by removal of σ3, cleavage of μ1, and rearrangement of σ1, and the conversion to core particles by removal of the μ1 fragments, loss of σ1, and opening of the λ2 turret. See text for protein copy numbers in homo- and heteromeric complexes, simplified here for clarity.

Genus *Orthoreovirus*

The genus *Orthoreovirus* contains the nonfusogenic mammalian orthoreoviruses and the fusogenic orthoreoviruses, which infect a variety of vertebrate hosts. Common features of the members of the genus *Orthoreovirus* include (a) 2 protein shells with core spikes at the icosahedral fivefold vertices; (b) 10 dsRNA segments including three large (L), 3 medium (M), and 4 small (S) size class RNA gene segments; (c) 3 λ, 3 μ, and 4 σ primary translation products; (d) additional small gene products encoded by a polycistronic S1 gene segment; and (e) common serological characteristics. Related members of the genus *Orthoreovirus* can exchange gene segments following coinfection of host cells, producing viral progeny termed "reassortant viruses" containing mixtures of gene segments derived from both parents. The capacity of two strains to produce viable reassortant progeny can serve as the basis for designating species of virus within the genus. Nonfusogenic isolates can exchange gene segments with each other, as can fusogenic isolates, but reassortment between nonfusogenic and fusogenic viruses has not been reported.

Mammalian *Orthoreovirus* was the first species of the family *Reoviridae* to be isolated and identified.[381] The prefix "ortho-" was added to the name of the initial isolates (orthoreoviruses) and the corresponding genus (*Orthoreovirus*) to distinguish them from other members of the family, which also could be called "reoviruses." However, in common usage, the term "reovirus" refers to the mammalian orthoreoviruses.

Nonfusogenic Orthoreoviruses

Reoviruses have a wide geographic distribution, and virtually all mammals, including humans, serve as hosts for infection. Based on sequence analysis of reovirus strains isolated from a variety of mammalian hosts, there is no evidence that any of the gene segments confer host range restriction. Because of their near ubiquity, reoviruses are used as a marker for mammalian fecal contamination of water sources.[39] Human infections with reovirus are common, with most children demonstrating serological evidence of infection by the age of 5 years.[438] However, reovirus is rarely associated with disease, except in the very young. There is evidence suggesting an association between reovirus and infantile biliary atresia[355,455] and celiac disease,[56] but causal links have not been established. Newborn mice are exquisitely susceptible to reovirus infection and have been used as the preferred experimental system for studies of reovirus pathogenesis.

Three mammalian reovirus serotypes have been identified by classical neutralization and hemagglutination inhibition (HAI) tests. Four virus strains isolated from children in the 1950s, type 1 Lang (T1L), type 2 Jones (T2J), type 3 Abney (T3A), and type 3 Dearing (T3D), are used most frequently as prototype strains. A distinct reovirus strain (Ndelle) was isolated from a mouse in the Cameroon[13] and may represent a fourth mammalian reovirus serotype. Nucleotide sequences indicate that nonfusogenic mammalian isolates are a distinct phylogenetic group within the genus *Orthoreovirus*. General feature of the nonfusogenic mammalian orthoreoviruses are provided in Table 11.1.

TABLE 11.1 General features of nonfusogenic mammalian orthoreoviruses

Genome

Double-stranded RNA (dsRNA)

Ten gene segments in three size classes (L, M, S)

Total size ~23,500 base pairs

Gene segments each encode one or two proteins

Gene segments are transcribed into full-length mRNAs, which can have 5′ caps but are not polyadenylated

Plus strands of gene segments have 5′ caps

Nontranslated regions at segment termini are short

Gene segments can undergo reassortment if two or more strains infect a single cell

Particles

Nonenveloped

Spherical with icosahedral symmetry

Total diameter ~85 nm (excluding σ1 fibers)

Two concentric protein capsids: outer capsid subunits in T = 13 *laevo* lattice and arrangement of inner capsid subunits in T = 1 lattice

Eight structural proteins: four proteins in the outer capsid (λ2, μ1, σ1, and σ3) and five proteins in the core (λ1, λ2, λ3, μ2, and σ2)

Subvirion particles (ISVPs and cores) can be generated from fully intact particles (virions) by proteolysis

Protein λ2 forms pentamers that protrude from the core surface

Replication

Occurs in the cytoplasm of host cells

Viral attachment protein σ1 binds to two cell surface receptors, sialylated glycans and junctional adhesion molecule-A

Proteolysis of outer-capsid proteins σ3 and μ1 is required for infection and can occur either extracellularly or in the endocytic compartment

Transcription and capping of viral mRNAs occur within cores; both processes are catalyzed by particle-associated enzymes

Single-stranded, positive-sense RNAs are assorted into progeny cores

Minus-strand synthesis occurs within assembling particles

Mature virions are released from infected cells by lytic and nonlytic means

Many reovirus strains induce apoptosis of host cells; some strains also induce necroptosis

Fusogenic Orthoreoviruses

The fusogenic orthoreoviruses infect birds, mammals, and reptiles. In contrast to the nonfusogenic orthoreoviruses, fusogenic reoviruses induce the formation of large, multinucleated syncytia.[112] Fusion activity is mediated by virus-encoded fusion-associated small transmembrane (FAST) proteins, which are nonstructural proteins expressed on the surface of infected cells.[140] FAST proteins are small (<20 kDa), basic, acylated proteins that induce fusion of transfected cells in the absence of other viral proteins.[88] Fusogenic members of the related genus, *Aquareovirus*, also encode FAST proteins.[353] Extensive syncytium formation mediated by FAST proteins results in apoptosis and enhanced release of infectious virions.[384] Replication and virulence of a FAST-deficient fusogenic bat isolate are compromised relative to wild-type virus,[221] indicating that FAST proteins contribute to the pathogenicity of fusogenic orthoreoviruses. Other than this fusion activity, the replication strategies of fusogenic and nonfusogenic orthoreoviruses are similar.[32]

The fusogenic orthoreoviruses are divided into eight species: *Avian orthoreovirus, Neoavian orthoreovirus, Reptilian orthoreovirus, Testudine orthoreovirus, Mahlapitsi orthoreovirus, Nelson Bay orthoreovirus, Broome orthoreovirus,* and *Baboon orthoreovirus.* Colloquially, isolates in these species are referred to as avian reoviruses (ARV), neoavian reoviruses (NARV), reptilian reoviruses (RRV), chelonian reoviruses (ChRV), Mahlapitsi reovirus (MAHLV), Nelson Bay reoviruses (NBV), Broome reovirus (BrRV), and baboon reovirus (BRV), respectively[14] and https://talk.ictvonline.org/taxonomy/. ARVs and NARVs infect a variety of avian hosts, and ARVs are important pathogens in the poultry industry, causing gastroenteritis, hepatitis, malabsorption, myocarditis, and pneumonia. Birds that survive acute systemic infection can develop joint and tendon inflammation that resembles the pathology of human rheumatoid arthritis. RRVs and ChRVs have been isolated from numerous reptile species, and infected animals often develop pneumonia and neurologic symptoms.[469] MAHLV was isolated from a bat fly and is the only orthoreovirus isolated from arthropods.[215] Three fusogenic species have been isolated from mammals. BRV was isolated from baboons with meningoencephalomyelitis in a colony in Texas,[260] and NBV and BrRV were isolated from fruit bats with neurological symptoms.[444] Fusogenic reoviruses of bat origin have been isolated from humans with acute respiratory infections and may be capable of human-to-human transmission, raising concern that fusogenic bat reoviruses may be a potential source of emerging infections in humans.[85–87,465,484] BRV, BrRV, and MAHLV virions, like those of the aquareoviruses, lack the classical sigma-class fiber protein used for cell attachment by other reoviruses.[485]

VIRION STRUCTURE

Particle Function

Reovirus virions are spherical, nonenveloped particles approximately 85 nm in diameter[139] (Fig. 11.2), consisting of two concentric capsid protein shells that surround and protect the dsRNA genome. The inner-capsid shell or core particle encloses the genome, which is present in a condensed liquid crystalline form.[356] The outer-capsid shell surrounds the core particle, which protrudes radially into the outer-capsid layer at each of the fivefold axes of symmetry.[139]

Several different morphotypes of reovirus particles can be purified from infected cells or formed *in vitro* (Figs. 11.1 and 11.2). In addition, less well-defined particles have been purified from infected cells and are characterized by the capacity to transcribe the genome *in vitro* ("transcriptase" particles) or synthesize a negative-stranded RNA copy of particle-associated viral mRNA ("replicase" particles).[312,506] Physical properties of

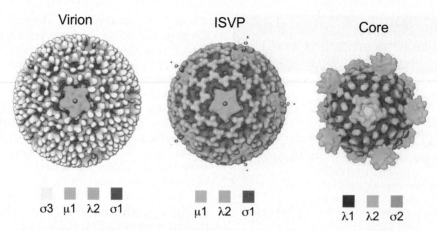

FIGURE 11.2 Cryo-EM image reconstructions of reovirus particles. Surface-shaded representations of cryo-EM image reconstructions of reovirus virions, infectious subvirion particles (ISVPs), and cores viewed along a fivefold axis of symmetry. The color coding is based on radial density and roughly approximates the individual capsid proteins as indicated. The *yellow color* corresponds to the interior of the particle. (Adapted with permission from Dryden KA, Wang G, Yeager M, et al. Early steps in reovirus infection are associated with dramatic changes in supramolecular structure and protein conformation: analysis of virions and subviral particles by cryoelectron microscopy and image reconstruction. *J Cell Biol* 1993;122(5):1023–1041. doi: https://doi.org/10.1083/jcb.122.5.1023. Copyright © 1993 Rockefeller University Press.)

virions, infectious subvirion particles (ISVPs), and cores are described in e-Table 11.2.

Virions

Reovirus virions are relatively stable in the environment and maintain infectivity for years when stored below 4°C. Large quantities of infectious virions can be purified from infected mouse L929 cells. A substantial proportion of particles that lack genomic dsRNA also are copurified. These empty particles have a lower buoyant density in CsCl gradients and band closer to the top of the gradient in comparison to genome-containing full particles and are called "top component." The ratio of full to empty particles purified from infected cells varies with viral strain and cell type. Protease treatment of empty particles can produce "empty" ISVPs and cores.

Virions are composed of a genome-containing inner T = 1 icosahedral core surrounded by a T = 13 *laevo* outer-capsid layer (Fig. 11.2). The outer capsid consists of 200 heterohexameric complexes of the M2-encoded μ1 (76 kDa, 708 aa) and S4-encoded σ3 (41 kDa, 365 aa) proteins. These complexes form a fenestrated shell that overlies the core. The outer-capsid shell is perforated at the icosahedral fivefold symmetry axes by turret-like structures formed by pentamers of the L2-encoded λ2 protein (144 kDa, 1288 to 1289 aa). The S1-encoded σ1 attachment protein (49 to 51 kDa, 455 to 470 aa) forms filamentous trimers that protrude from each of the λ2 turrets. In addition to encapsidating the 10 dsRNA gene segments, virions also contain short single-stranded RNA oligonucleotides (2 to 9 nucleotides) that can constitute up to 25% of the RNA. Most of these (70%) are abortive transcripts and terminate with 5'-GC(U)(A).[483] The remainder (~30%) are oligoadenylates that range in length from 2 to 20 residues.[405] Complete or partial atomic resolution structures are available for σ1 trimers,[130,358] σ3 dimers,[335] and μ1:σ3

heterohexamers.[266] Cryo-EM image reconstructions of reovirus virions, ISVPs, and cores[139,493,494] (Fig. 11.2) and an atomic resolution structure of the core[356] have been determined.

Infectious Subvirion Particles

Treatment of virions with chymotrypsin or trypsin using controlled conditions *in vitro*[320] or virion disassembly during infection of cells[434] or in the murine intestine[26] yields ISVPs (Figs. 11.1 and 11.2). These particles lack σ3 but retain σ1 and a proteolytically cleaved version of μ1 (see "Replication—Uncoating"). ISVPs of reovirus strain T1L are twofold more infectious than virions. In contrast, ISVPs from strain T3D are 10-fold less infectious than T3D virions as a consequence of a sequence polymorphism in σ1 that leads to its proteolytic cleavage,[78,320] which likely explains the decreased replication in the intestine and avirulence of T3D after peroral inoculation of newborn mice.[43] An additional intermediate particle, the ISVP*, is formed from ISVPs during infection of cells.[75] ISVP*s lack the σ1 attachment protein, have an altered conformer of μ1, and tend to aggregate. In contrast to virions and ISVPs, ISVP*s are transcriptionally active.[73] ISVP*s are formed following generation of ISVPs and interact with cell membranes leading to membrane penetration and release of the core particle into the cytosol (see "Replication—Membrane Penetration").

Core Particles

Like ISVPs, cores can be produced *in vitro* by treating virions with chymotrypsin or trypsin using specific conditions. Such treatment removes the outer-capsid proteins (μ1, σ3, and σ1) and exposes prominent turrets formed by pentamers of λ2. These turrets protrude from the capsid shell at each of the five-fold symmetry axes (Figs. 11.1 and 11.2) and form hollow cylinders that open to the interior of the particle. In virions and

TABLE 11.2 Functions of reovirus proteins

Gene Segment	Protein	Mass (Da)	Copy Number Per Virion	Functions[a]
L1	λ3	142,300	12	Minor inner-capsid protein; catalytic subunit of the viral RNA-dependent RNA polymerase; associates with nonstructural protein μNS. PDB: 1MUK
L2	λ2	144,000	60	Core spike protein; forms pentameric turret for insertion of attachment protein σ1; associates with nonstructural protein μNS; adds a 5′ methylated cap to mRNAs. PDB: 1EJ6
L3	λ1	142,000	120	Major inner-capsid protein; associates with nonstructural protein μNS; possible RNA helicase; may remove terminal phosphate from newly synthesized mRNA in preparation for capping. PDB: 1EJ6
M1	μ2	83,300	12–24[b]	Minor inner-capsid protein; probable RNA polymerase subunit; associates with nonstructural protein μNS; associates with and stabilizes microtubules; associates with cellular mRNA splicing complex in the nucleus; nonspecific RNA-binding protein; may remove terminal phosphate from newly synthesized [−] strand RNA after synthesis; interferon antagonist
M2	μ1	76,300	600	Major outer-capsid protein; required for penetration of endosomal membrane by the viral core; probably regulates late mRNA synthesis from secondary transcriptase particles; influences efficiency of reovirus-induced apoptosis. PDB: 1JMU
M3	μNS	80,000	NS[c]	Nonstructural replication protein; forms cytoplasmic inclusion structures; interacts with ER membranes; associates with nonstructural protein σNS and core proteins λ1, λ2, λ3, μ2, and σ2; first viral protein found in association with viral mRNA
M3	μNSC	75,000	NS	Nonstructural protein; function unknown; dispensable for replication in cell culture
S1	σ1	49,200 (T3D)–51,400 (T1L)	36	Attachment protein that binds to cell surface glycans and junctional adhesion molecule A (JAM-A); determines virus serotype; determines cell and tissue tropism and route of virus spread in the host. PDB: 1KKE, 6GA0
S1	σ1s	14,000	NS	Nonstructural protein; required for reovirus-induced cell cycle arrest and apoptosis; required for reovirus infection of endothelial cells and hematogenous dissemination
S2	σ2	47,200	150	Major inner-capsid protein; associates with nonstructural protein μNS; binds weakly to dsRNA. PDB: 1EJ6
S3	σNS	41,000	NS	Nonstructural protein found early in viral inclusions; interacts with ER membranes; associates with nonstructural protein μNS; nonspecific RNA-binding protein with high affinity for single-stranded RNA
S4	σ3	41,500	600	Major outer capsid protein; forms protective cap over μ1; nonspecific dsRNA-binding protein; influences efficiency of translation; associated with viral mRNA early in replication cycle; inhibits PKR activation. PDB: 1FN9, 1JMU

[a]Some functions are virus strain-specific. PDB accession numbers are provided when structural information is available.
[b]Stoichiometry not known with certainty.
[c]NS, nonstructural, not a component of viral particles.

ISVPs, the cavity within each turret is partially filled by a bulb-like structure that corresponds to a portion of the σ1 protein[139] (Fig. 11.2). The σ1 bulb is held in place by flap domains present on each of the five λ2 proteins. In cores, the flap domains of λ2 open outward. The interior surface of the pore formed by the λ2 turret possesses guanylyltransferase and methyltransferase activities, which allow the turrets to function as mRNA capping complexes[356] (see "Replication—Transcription"). Cores are approximately 1,000,000-fold less infectious than virions due to the loss of the outer-capsid proteins, which mediate virus attachment, entry, and membrane penetration. Cores can initiate an infectious cycle if introduced into cells by transfection.[216]

The T = 1 core shell is formed by 120 copies of the L3-encoded λ1 protein (142 kDa, 1275 aa) arranged in parallel asymmetric dimers. Five copies of λ1 (conformer λ1A) radiate from the fivefold axes of symmetry. These molecules interdigitate with a second set of five λ1 proteins (conformer λ1B) to form decamers; twelve decamers form the core shell.[356] The λ1 shell is stabilized by 150 copies of the S2-encoded σ2 protein (47 kDa, 418 aa), which clamps onto λ1 at three distinct sites within each icosahedral asymmetric unit of the shell.[356] Channels permeate the shell, with those at the fivefold symmetry axes allowing entry of nucleoside triphosphate (NTP) substrates and exit of newly synthesized viral mRNAs.

The reovirus core is described as a "molecular machine" owing to its capacity to synthesize capped viral mRNA transcripts *in vitro* when incubated with suitable substrates. During infection, particles thought to be similar to *in vitro*–generated cores initiate viral transcription after being deposited in the cytoplasm. Core particles contain approximately 12 copies of the L1-encoded λ3 polymerase (142 kDa, 1267 aa). Each λ3 protein is anchored to three λ1 proteins on the inner surface of the core and overlaps with, but is eccentric from, each of the icosahedral fivefold symmetry axes.[498] In addition, cores contain approximately 12 to 24 copies of the M1-encoded μ2 protein (83 kDa, 736 aa),[102] a polymerase cofactor. The precise location of μ2 within the core particle is not known, but one or two copies of μ2 are thought to associate with each copy of λ3. In the case of grass carp reovirus, an aquareovirus, a single copy of VP4 (μ2 equivalent) exists in complex with VP2 (λ3 equivalent).[466]

Recombinant Particles

Recombinant core-shell particles can be formed by coexpression of the λ1 and σ2 proteins or the λ1, λ2, and σ2 proteins.[482] Purified viral core particles prepared by *in vitro* digestion of virions with chymotrypsin or trypsin can be recoated with outer-capsid proteins μ1, σ3, and σ1 prepared using baculovirus expression systems.[77] Such recoated particles display infectivity similar to native virions and are useful tools for defining the consequences of lethal mutations in outer-capsid proteins on early steps in viral infection (see "Genome Structure and Organization—Genetic Complementation").

Particles *In Situ*

Icosahedral star-shaped single-layered particles (SLPs) within viral factories of reovirus serotype 3–infected MA104 cells can be detected using cryo-electron tomography.[436] A 5.4 Å structure obtained by subtomogram averaging revealed that SLPs have 120 copies of λ1 and 120 copies of σ2 (30 fewer than core particles). SLPs have a collapsed λ1 shell that is indented at the fivefold axes of symmetry giving rise to a star-like appearance. SLPs lack a genome and have no detectable density for the λ3 polymerase. Because of their similarity to φ8 cystovirus procapsids, SLPs have been suggested to be assembly intermediates on the pathway to assembly of core particles.[436]

GENOME STRUCTURE AND ORGANIZATION

Physical Characteristics

The reovirus genome consists of 10 discontiguous segments of dsRNA. The [+] and [−] strands of genomic dsRNA are collinear and complementary. The genomic dsRNA has an A-form structure with a right-handed double helix (10 base pairs per turn, 30 Å pitch, nucleotides oriented at 75 to 80 degrees to the long axis).

Gene Segments and Nomenclature

The 10 reovirus dsRNA gene segments are present in equimolar amounts in viral particles. The segments are grouped by size into large (L), medium (M), and small (S) classes according to their migration in polyacrylamide gels. There are three large (L1, L2, L3), three medium (M1, M2, M3), and four small (S1, S2, S3, S4) segments. Homologous gene segments from different reovirus isolates often migrate with different mobilities in polyacrylamide gels despite being of similar or identical length (e-Fig. 11.1). This property allows gene segments from different isolates to be unambiguously distinguished, which is essential for the assignment of gene segments in reassortant viruses to specific parental strains (see "Genome Structure and Organization—Reassortment"). The gene segments of prototype strain T3D are numbered according to their relative mobilities in Tris-acetate–buffered gels. Each gene segment encodes at least one protein product (Table 11.2).

Modifications to the Genomic RNA

The [+] strand RNA of each gene segment is capped. The [+] stranded RNA that is associated with the [−] strand RNA within core particles has a dimethylated cap-1 structure on its 5′ terminus,[165] which is added by viral guanylyltransferase and methyltransferase activities present in the λ2 protein. However, viral mRNAs that are present within infected cells can have a cap-1 or cap-2 structure with approximately 50% of viral mRNAs having a cap-2 structure in L929 cells.[125] The viral mRNA cap is recognized by translation initiation factor eIF4E[52] and protects the free 5′ ends of the viral mRNA from 5′ exonucleases.[163] The 5′ terminus of the [−] strand RNA of each gene segment has an unblocked diphosphate.[20] The terminal γ-phosphate of the [−] strand is removed by a phosphohydrolase activity (possibly mediated by the μ2 or λ1 protein) within reovirus particles.[234] The 3′ end of each gene segment has an unblocked hydroxyl group.[302] The viral [+] strand RNA does not contain a polyadenylate tract.

Sequence Features

Full-length sequences of the entire genomes of prototype mammalian orthoreovirus strains T1L, T2J, and T3D as well as those of several fusogenic orthoreovirus isolates have been determined (National Center for Biotechnology Information). The total length of the genome sequence is approximately 23,500 base pairs. The length of individual gene segments varies from 1,196 (T3D S4 gene segment) to 3,916 (T3D L2 gene segment) nucleotides. Apart from the S1 gene segment, homologous gene segments of different isolates display little (±4 base pairs) or no variation in segment length. The length of the S1 gene segment is 1,463, 1,440, and 1,416 base pairs for the T1L, T2J, and T3D S1 gene segments, respectively. Passage of the original isolate of the T3D strain in different laboratories has given rise to variants that have distinct phenotypic properties associated with numerous nonsynonymous changes in 8 of the 10 genome segments.[307] Whether serial passage of the T1L and T2J strains has led to similar changes is not known.

Protein-Coding Strategies and Nomenclature

Twelve proteins are translated from the 10 T3D reovirus gene segments (Table 11.2). Eight of these segments encode a single protein, and two encode two proteins each. Eight of the 12 proteins are structural components of virions (λ1, λ2, λ3, μ1, μ2, σ1, σ2, and σ3), and four are nonstructural (μNS, μNSC, σ1s, and σNS). The names of the proteins encoded by each of the gene segments are designated by a Greek symbol that corresponds to large (λ), medium (μ), and small (σ) sizes, which are encoded by gene segments of the L, M, and S classes, respectively. For historical reasons, the numbering of gene segments does not always correspond to the numbering of the proteins (Table 11.2).

During reovirus infection, the [−] strand of each dsRNA gene segment is transcribed to yield a full-length [+] strand RNA copy that is capped as it is released from the transcribing core particle. Viral mRNAs are not polyadenylated, but they are efficiently translated. ORFs of each gene segment are flanked by short nontranslated regions (NTRs). The AUG start codon for each gene segment is usually the first to be encountered by a scanning ribosome and, in most cases, it is found in an excellent context for translation initiation. The S1 gene segment encodes a second protein, σ1s, in an ORF overlapping that of the larger σ1 protein. The σ1s protein is translated from the first out-of-frame start codon within the σ1 ORF.[317] Like the S1 gene segment, the M3 gene segment encodes a second protein, which is called μNSC. Translation of μNSC is proposed to initiate from the second or third in-frame start codon of the m3 RNA, but this remains unconfirmed. There is no evidence that any reovirus protein is translated from a genomic [−] strand.

Terminal Nontranslated Regions

The reovirus gene segments contain short terminal NTRs (Fig. 11.3). The 5′ NTRs range in length from 12 to 32 nucleotides, and their relative sizes may affect their translation efficiency.[375] The 3′ NTRs are a little longer and vary in length from 35 to 83 nucleotides. In general, NTR length of homologous gene segments is conserved between different virus isolates.

The [+] strand of all reovirus gene segments contains the 5′ sequence GpCpUpA and the 3′ sequence UpCpApUpC.

Longer regions of sequence near the RNA termini and extending into the ORFs display less variability between isolates than sequences further from the ends[80,182,227] (Fig. 11.3). RNA-folding algorithms suggest that sequences near the ends of the reovirus [+] strands can form panhandle structures, which may be important for certain RNA functions. For example, the 5′ and 3′ NTRs include sequences and structural elements important for RNA packaging.[374,377,378]

Genetics

Reassortment

Gene segment exchange (or reassortment) among reovirus strains occurs during mixed infections of cultured cells or animal hosts. The progeny of such mixed infections are commonly referred to as reassortant viruses. Many reovirus strains are distinguishable by signature electrophoretic profiles of their dsRNA gene segments in polyacrylamide gels (e-Fig. 11.1A). Coinfection of cells with such strains produces a collection of reassortant viruses in which the parental origin of each gene segment can be determined following electrophoresis of viral genomic dsRNA (e-Fig. 11.1B). Studies of reassortant viruses have been used to assign biological polymorphisms displayed by different reovirus strains to specific viral gene segments. Thus, a phenotypic difference between two parental strains can be genetically mapped by screening the reassortant viruses in appropriate assays and correlating expression of the phenotype with a specific parental gene segment.

Reassortment of reovirus gene segments also occurs *in vivo*. Peroral inoculation of mice with strains T1L and T3D yields reassortant progeny in the stool and at sites of secondary replication.[470] In addition, topologies of phylogenetic trees constructed from protein-coding sequences of the L1,[257] M1,[487] S1,[121] S2,[80] S3,[182] and S4[227] gene segments derived from field isolate strains are distinct, providing evidence that these segments reassort in nature.

Reassortment is not entirely random. In a study of 83 reassortant viruses derived from strains T1L and T3D, statistically significant nonrandom associations of parental alleles were observed in the L1-L2, L1-M1, L1-S1, and L3-S1 gene segment pairs.[323] It is possible that these gene segments or their

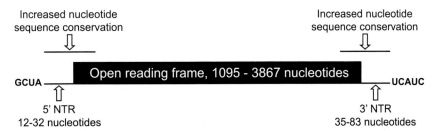

FIGURE 11.3 Reovirus gene segment coding strategies. The 10 reovirus gene segments demonstrate no significant sequence similarity except for the 5′-terminal four nucleotides [+] 5′-GCUA-3′) and 3′-terminal five nucleotides [+] 5′-UCAUC-3′), which are invariant among all 10 segments. However, sizable regions of subterminal sequence are conserved among homologous gene segments across individual strains. Each of the reovirus gene segments is monocistronic with the exception of the M3 gene segment, which encodes μNS and μNSC in the same reading frame (μNSC is an N-terminally truncated version of μNS), and the S1 gene segment, which encodes σ1 and σ1s in overlapping reading frames. Nucleotide sequence conservation extends inward from both nontranslated regions (NTRs) into the gene-segment open reading frames and is maintained even at synonymous positions. Only the plus strand is shown here. Sequence ranges are based on strain type 3 Dearing and include the larger of the two reading frames in the S1 gene segment.

protein products cannot accommodate exchange with gene segments from another strain without selection of fitness-compromising mutations. In particular, protein mismatches that occur as a consequence of reassortment can alter virus assembly and influence subsequent functions of the virus capsid including disassembly.[446] Additionally, the majority of progeny viruses resulting from mixed infections retain the genome constellation of the parental strains,[155] suggesting that viral replication is compartmentalized.

Selection of Mutants: "Forward Genetics"
Cell-adapted mutants
Although usually cytolytic, reoviruses are capable of establishing persistent infections in many types of cells in culture. These cultures are maintained by horizontal transmission of virus from cell to cell and can be cured of persistent infection by passage in the presence of reovirus-specific antibodies. During maintenance of L-cell cultures persistently infected with reovirus, mutations are selected in both cells and viruses.[4,122] Mutant cells selected during persistent infection have alterations in the expression of cathepsin L and do not support disassembly of wild-type virus.[18] These cells in turn select mutant viruses (termed persistent infection [PI] viruses) that have gained the capacity to bypass cellular blocks to infection by virtue of mutations in outer-capsid proteins σ1[476] and σ3,[473] which promote more efficient disassembly.

Non–sialic acid–binding reovirus strains have been adapted to replication in murine erythroleukemia (MEL) cells by serial passage.[81] These variants have single amino acid substitutions in the sialic acid–binding domain of σ1 protein and have gained the capacity to bind sialylated glycans.[81] Serial passage also has been used to select reovirus mutants for resistance to ammonium chloride,[89] which inhibits endosomal acidification, and E64,[144] which inhibits cysteine proteases. These mutants have alterations in σ3 protein that enhance kinetics of viral disassembly. Passage of strain T3D in murine L929 cells leads to selection of variants with enhanced replication capacity; these variants have mutations in the σ1 and λ2 proteins.[310,402] Other reovirus mutants have been selected during chronic infections of immunocompromised mice; these viruses are adapted to replicate more efficiently in the organs from which they were isolated.[190]

Mutants resistant to denaturants
Treatment of reovirus with harsh denaturants (e.g., heat, extremes of pH, ethanol, phenol, or SDS) results in substantial losses in infectivity.[138] Strain-specific differences in susceptibility to inactivation by heat and ethanol have been mapped using reassortant viruses to the σ3-encoding S4 gene and μ1-encoding M2 gene,[138] respectively. Concordantly, reovirus mutants selected for resistance to ethanol have mutations in the M2 gene.[202,471] These mutants display increased thermostability and a decreased capacity to penetrate host cell membranes.[202]

Deletion mutants
Some reovirus isolates lose portions of their genomes during serial high-MOI passage. Deletions in the L1 and L3 gene segments occur most commonly, but L2 and M1 deletions also occur. Analysis of a series of internally deleted M1 gene segments indicates that the minimum sizes for retained 5′- and 3′-terminal regions of message-sense RNA are 132 to 135 and

182 to 185 bases, respectively,[503] suggesting that these regions contain signals required for RNA synthesis or gene segment packaging. Some internal deletions appear to result from recombination within individual viral gene segments guided by direct sequence repeats.[411] Differences in the capacity of strains T1L and T3D to accumulate deletions segregates with the L2 gene segment, while the M3 gene segment is a determinant of which viral gene segments incur deletions.[63] Functions of the L2 and M3 gene products λ2 and μNS, respectively, in synthesis or packaging of reovirus RNA may influence the production or amplification of deletion mutations, but the underlying mechanism is unknown.

Directed Mutagenesis of the Genome: "Reverse Genetics"
Development of a plasmid-based reverse genetics system for members of the *Birnaviridae* family,[486] which contain two genomic dsRNA segments, suggested that delivery of viral positive-strand RNA alone could launch successful production of viral progeny for a dsRNA virus. This approach proved possible with the development of an entirely plasmid-based reverse genetics system for reovirus in which viable viruses are produced from a set of 10 cloned cDNAs representing the complete viral genome[239] (Fig. 11.4). Gene segment cDNAs corresponding to strains T1L[242] and T3D[239] were introduced into plasmids at

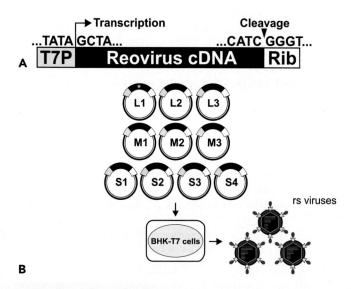

FIGURE 11.4 Recovery of reovirus from cDNA. A: Prototype reovirus gene segment cDNA in plasmid. Cloned cDNAs representing the 10 reovirus dsRNA gene segments are flanked by the bacteriophage T7 RNA polymerase promoter (T7P) and hepatitis delta virus ribozyme (Rib) sequences. **B:** The 10 plasmid constructs are transfected into baby hamster kidney (BHK) cells expressing T7 RNA polymerase. Transcription within the cells produces the 10 different viral mRNAs, each with its authentic 5′ end. Self-cleavage by the ribozyme produces authentic viral 3′ ends. These mRNAs are translated and yield all 12 reovirus proteins, which can then direct a productive infectious cycle. Following 1-to-2 days of incubation, transfected cells are lysed by freeze–thaw, and viable virus is isolated by a plaque assay using L929 cells. An engineered silent substitution in one of the cloned cDNAs (indicated by an *asterisk* in the L1 gene segment) produces a unique molecular signature to confirm the plasmid origin of the recombinant strain (rs) viruses.

sites flanked by the promoter sequence for T7 RNA polymerase and the hepatitis delta virus (HDV) ribozyme (Fig. 11.4A). Neither helper virus nor coexpression of viral replication proteins is required for recovery of infectious virus.

Reovirus can be recovered from cells in which T7 RNA polymerase is delivered transiently by infection with a recombinant vaccinia virus[208] or plasmid transfection[247] or from cells that constitutively express the enzyme[66] (Fig. 11.4B). Since T7 RNA polymerase initiates transcription at a defined guanosine residue and all reovirus RNAs contain the nucleotide sequence, GCUA, at the 5′ terminus of the message-sense strand, T7 RNA polymerase produces transcripts with native reovirus 5′ termini. Self-cleavage of the HDV ribozyme produces RNAs with native 3′ termini.[376] Inclusion of expression plasmids encoding reovirus proteins does not enhance recovery of recombinant reoviruses.[48] However, the efficiency of virus recovery is increased by using baby hamster kidney cells constitutively expressing T7 RNA polymerase,[66] reducing the plasmid number from 10 to 4 by combining reovirus gene segment cDNAs into multicistronic vectors,[242] or incorporating a plasmid encoding the African swine fever virus NP868R capping enzyme[142] or a plasmid encoding a FAST protein from a fusogenic reovirus.[221] Plasmid-derived wild-type virus recapitulates properties of native virus in all cell culture and *in vivo* models of reovirus infection studied to date.[239,242]

Plasmid-based reverse genetics systems also have been developed for fusogenic reoviruses.[226] This technology enabled conclusive demonstration of the importance of FAST protein expression in fusogenic reovirus virulence.[221]

Genetic Complementation

Recombinant reovirus outer-capsid proteins μ1, σ1, and σ3 can bind and "recoat" purified subvirion particles (ISVPs or cores) *in vitro* to yield infectious virion-like particles.[76,77,214] These recoated particles have been used to identify sequences in μ1, σ1, and σ3 proteins that function during cell entry and disassembly.[75,77,213,475]

Reovirus replication is blocked in cell lines stably expressing siRNAs specific for reovirus transcripts.[240] RNAi-mediated inhibition of viral gene expression can be complemented by vectored expression of viral genes in which the siRNA target sequence has been altered to prevent siRNA-mediated degradation. This approach has been used to identify sequences in μ2, μNS, and σNS proteins that function in viral inclusion formation and RNA synthesis.[12,72,240,241] An siRNA trans-complementation strategy also has been used to identify sequence requirements in viral transcripts for efficient translation.[382] Limitations of RNAi trans-complementation include the efficiency of viral RNA knockdown and transfection efficiency of the complementation plasmids.

STAGES OF REPLICATION

Attachment

Reovirus Attachment Protein σ1

The S1-encoded σ1 protein (49 to 51 kDa, 455 to 470 aa) mediates viral binding to cellular receptors[24,79] and influences target cell selection in the infected host.[25,160,426] It is a homotrimer present in 12 trimers per virion.[102,432] Structural information is available for the σ1 proteins of prototype strains T1L and T3D. The σ1 proteins of each strain (T1L, 470 aa, T3D, 455 aa) fold into a filamentous trimer approximately 480 Å long and 90 Å wide at its broadest point, with a globular C-terminal head, a central body, and a slender N-terminal tail[82,130,159,358,427] (Fig. 11.5). Residues 310 to 455 in the T3D σ1 protein comprise the head, which is formed by an 8-stranded β-barrel.[82,389] Residues 169 to 309 in T3D σ1 form the body domain, which is constructed primarily from repeating units of two antiparallel β-strands connected by short loops.[82,130,358] Three such units assemble into a triple β-spiral, which is a motif observed to date only in viral fiber proteins. In T3D σ1, the body domain features four β-spiral repeats at the N-terminus (β1-β4, residues 169 to 235), a short α-helical coiled-coil (residues 236 to 251), and three additional β-spiral repeats (β5-β7, residues 252 to 309) at the C-terminus (Fig. 11.5). The short α-helical coiled coil corresponds to a narrowing in the body domain in a composite image of negative-stained electron micrographs of purified σ1.[159] Residues 1 to 168 in T3D σ1 form the tail domain, with residues 27 to 168 consisting of an elongated α-helical coiled-coil.[130] The extreme N-terminus of σ1 does not contain

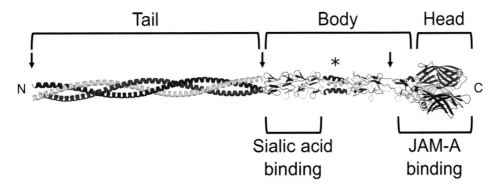

FIGURE 11.5 Structure of reovirus attachment protein σ1. Full-length model of strain type 3 Dearing (T3D) σ1. A full-length depiction of σ1 was produced by linking the structure of N-terminal (residues 27 to 237)[130] and C-terminal (residues 238 to 455)[358] fragments of T3D σ1. The two structures used to produce the model have resolutions of 2.15 and 2.25 Å, respectively. The three monomers are shown in *blue*, *red*, and *yellow*. Tail, body, and head regions are indicated. Discrete regions of flexibility are indicated by *arrows*. A sequence polymorphism that confers susceptibility to cleavage by intestinal proteases is indicated with an *asterisk*. The approximate locations of binding sites for sialic acid and junctional adhesion molecule-A (JAM-A) are shown. Amino (*N*)- and carboxy (*C*)-termini are indicated.

any obvious sequence motifs. It is hydrophobic and anchors the protein into the pentameric turret formed by λ2 in the reovirus virion[139,162,263] (Fig. 11.1). This symmetry mismatch (a trimer of σ1 within a pentamer of λ2) suggests an interaction with limited affinity, which may aid in σ1 release during viral disassembly. Sequence polymorphisms in the extreme N-terminus of σ1 are associated with the numbers of σ1 trimers encapsidated onto virions and may influence σ1-λ2 interactions.[329]

The σ1 molecule possesses discrete regions of flexibility[82,159,358] (Fig. 11.5, arrows). One site of substantial flexibility in T3D σ1 is contributed by a four-residue insertion between the two most C-terminal β-spiral repeats (β6 and β7).[82] This insertion appears to correspond to a region of flexibility observed just below the σ1 head in electron micrographic images.[159] A second region of flexibility is observed at the midpoint of σ1 and corresponds to the transition between the α-helical coiled-coil region of the tail and the β-spiral–containing body. A final region of flexibility close to the N-terminus likely represents the virion insertion domain.[82,159,321] Stabilization of σ1 trimers by introduction of disulfide linkages in the head domain increases the affinity of σ1 for JAM-A,[131] perhaps by locking the protein into a more extended conformation.

Reovirus Uses Sialic Acid as a Serotype-Specific Attachment Factor

Despite similarities in sequence and structure, type 1 (T1) and type 3 (T3) σ1 use different domains to engage distinct sialylated glycans.[357,358] T1 reoviruses specifically bind the terminal α2,3-linked *N*-acetyl-sialic acid on the GM2 glycan (displayed on glycoproteins or GM2 ganglioside) in a shallow groove located on the σ1 head domain[357,426] (e-Fig. 11.2A). In contrast, T3 strains demonstrate more promiscuous glycan engagement and bind terminal α2,3-, α2,6-, or α2,8-linked sialic acid using a groove located in the σ1 body domain[358] (e-Fig. 11.2B). Point mutations engineered in these binding sites specifically abrogate glycan engagement and convert sialic acid-binding strains (referred to as SA+) to non–sialic acid–binding strains (referred to as SA−). For example, alteration of two residues in the sialic acid–binding site of T1L convert a T1SA+ virus to a T1SA− virus.[426] Multiple single amino acid polymorphisms in T3 σ1 produce T3SA− viruses in different genetic backgrounds.[25,358] These non–sialic acid–binding strains are referred to as "glycan-blind" and have been instrumental in defining the contribution of sialic acid engagement to reovirus infection of specific cell types.

Reovirus demonstrates little to no sialic acid requirement for infection of some cell types, such as L929 cells. Diminishing reovirus access to sialic acid on these cells has a negligible effect on binding or infectivity, and different serotypes replicate comparably.[99,357,358] However, infection of other cell types, such as primary murine embryonic fibroblasts (MEFs), is efficient only with T1 or T3 strains that exhibit intact glycan-binding capacity.[99,357] Sialic acid engagement also can allow reovirus infection in a serotype-specific manner. For example, MEL T3cl.2 cells are susceptible only to T3 glycan-binding strains.[358] These cell type–specific differences in glycan requirement for infection are likely attributable to the relative abundance of other reovirus receptors present.[357]

Sialic acid engagement contributes to reovirus pathogenesis and disease outcomes.[25] T1 and T3 glycan-blind viruses induce less severe disease in the CNS relative to the cognate gly-

can-binding viruses (see "Pathogenesis and Pathology—Central Nervous System"). Following intracranial inoculation, T3SA– induces significantly less severe hydrocephalus than T1SA+ but reaches similar peak titers in the brain.[426] Ependymal infection is more localized to the inoculation site for T1SA–, suggesting that the virus may not efficiently disseminate through the ventricles.[426] A similar trend is true for T3 viruses. Following peroral inoculation, both T3SA+ and T3SA– viruses, which contain nine T1L genes and a T3-derived S1 gene that encodes a σ1 protein resistant to cleavage by intestinal proteases (see "Stages of Replication—Cleavage of σ1 by Intestinal Proteases"), establish efficient replication in the intestine, but T3SA+ is detected sooner in peripheral sites like the spleen, liver, and brain, suggesting an advantage in dissemination efficiency.[25] However, T3SA– reaches comparable peak titers at later time points.[25] In the CNS, T3SA+ often replicates to higher titers, induces greater levels of apoptosis, and is more neurovirulent than T3SA–.[25,160] Cultured primary murine cortical neurons also are more susceptible to T3SA+ than T3SA– infection.[160,435] However, while T3SA+ is more neurovirulent, both T3SA+ and T3SA– exhibit comparable CNS tropism.[160] Therefore, although diminished sialic acid–binding capacity alters the virulence of T1 and T3 reovirus, tropism remains unaltered, suggesting that sialic acid functions as an attachment factor and not as a tropism determinant in reovirus CNS infection. Sialic acid–binding capacity also is associated with bile duct injury induced by T3 reovirus in newborn mice and replication in human cholangiocarcinoma cells[25] (see "Pathogenesis and Pathology—Hepatobiliary System").

JAM-A Is Bound by the σ1 Head Domain and Mediates Reovirus Bloodstream Spread

Reovirus strains of all three serotypes use junctional adhesion molecule-A (JAM-A, also known as F11R/JAM/JAM1), a member of the immunoglobulin superfamily, as a receptor.[24,70,349] JAM-A was identified as a reovirus receptor using a genetic screen and subsequently shown to bind directly to the σ1 head domain with nanomolar affinity.[24,389] Human and murine homologs of JAM-A, but not JAM family members JAM-B or JAM-C, serve as receptors for all reovirus serotypes and strains tested to date.[24,70,349] The role of JAM-A as a reovirus receptor *in vivo* has been examined using JAM-A–null mice[9] (see "Pathogenesis and Pathology—Spread of Virus"). Following peroral inoculation, JAM-A is dispensable for reovirus replication in the intestine. However, it is required for infection of vascular endothelial cells and promotes efficient hematogenous dissemination of reovirus to sites of secondary infection. Studies using tissue-specific JAM-A–null mice indicate that endothelial JAM-A but not hematopoietic JAM-A facilitates reovirus T1L bloodstream entry and egress.[251]

The membrane-distal D1 domain of JAM-A is required for high-affinity binding to σ1.[158,184,349] The structure of the σ1–JAM-A complex shows that each σ1 trimer binds three independent JAM-A monomers. Contacts primarily involve the JAM-A dimer interface and a conserved region at the base of the σ1 head[82,235,427] (e-Fig. 11.2C). In addition, the structure of the σ1–JAM-A complex also identifies residues bound by σ1 that are found just outside the dimer interface of JAM-A.[235] These residues may serve as initial contact points for σ1 and facilitate disruption of the JAM-A homodimer to allow interaction of σ1 with the JAM-A dimer interface. The σ1–JAM-A interaction is thermodynamically favored, as the K_D is approximately 1,000-fold lower than the K_D of the JAM-A homodimer interaction.[184,235,462]

The presence of discrete receptor-binding domains in σ1 suggests that reoviruses employ a multiple step binding process. Binding studies using isogenic point mutant viruses T3SA+ and T3SA−, which vary only in the capacity to engage sialic acid,[23] support this hypothesis. Kinetic analyses using inhibitors of sialic acid and JAM-A binding demonstrate that sialic acid is engaged first in the adsorption process, as the inhibitory effect of sialic acid analogs on infection by T3SA+ occurs at early but not late time points.[23] Thus, reovirus binding to sialic acid enhances virus attachment through rapid adhesion of the virus to the cell surface where access to JAM-A is thermodynamically favored. Incubation of T3 reovirus with sialic acid increases affinity of the virus for JAM-A,[243] perhaps by inducing a conformational alteration in σ1. However, sialic acid binding is not required for JAM-A binding, as reoviruses incapable of binding sialic acid can bind JAM-A.[74]

Cleavage of σ1 by Intestinal Proteases

Treatment of virions of some reovirus strains with intestinal proteases *in vitro* to produce ISVPs leads to cleavage of the σ1 protein.[78,320] Strain-specific differences in cleavage susceptibility segregate with a single amino acid polymorphism in the short α-helical coiled-coil in the body domain of σ1 (Fig. 11.5, asterisk). Strains like T3D with a threonine at position 249 in σ1 are susceptible to cleavage by trypsin after Arg245, whereas those with an isoleucine at position 249, like T3SA+ and T3SA−, are resistant to cleavage.[78] It is possible that Thr249 disrupts the α-helical coiled-coil and allows access to sites that otherwise would be shielded from protease.[78,320] Conversion of T3D virions to ISVPs by intestinal proteases leads to loss of the σ1 head domain and a resultant 90% reduction in infectivity.[320] Since cleavage of σ1 occurs C-terminal to the sialic acid–binding pocket, residual infectivity of T3D ISVPs is dependent on this carbohydrate.[320] Susceptibility of the T3D σ1 protein to cleavage likely accounts for the attenuated virulence of this strain after oral inoculation[43,231] (see "Pathogenesis and Pathology—Entry Into the Host").

Determinant of Neutralizing Antibody Responses

In addition to its function in receptor engagement, the σ1 protein is the target of serotype-specific neutralizing antibodies.[68,420] For example, serotype-specific monoclonal antibodies (mAbs) 5C6[463] and 9BG5[68] neutralize infectivity of T1 and T3 reovirus strains, respectively, and bind the σ1 head domain in a serotype-specific fashion.[79] Variants of T1L selected for resistance to neutralizing mAbs have mutations at Ala415, Gln417, Asn445, and Gly447,[193] which are located in the σ1 head. Similarly, variants of T3D selected for resistance to neutralizing mAbs have mutations at Asp340 and Glu419,[27] which also are located in the σ1 head. Structures of the T1 σ1 head domain in complex with mAb 5C6 Fabs and the T3 σ1 head domain in complex with mAb 9BG5 Fabs reveal that each antibody engages its cognate σ1 protein via an epitope that spans two monomers in the σ1 trimer.[129] In each case, the antibody epitope is distinct from the JAM-A binding site,[129] suggesting that the mAbs interfere with JAM-A engagement by steric hindrance. Neutralization-resistant variants of T3D display diminished neurovirulence and altered CNS tropism in mice,[420]

perhaps as a consequence of altered σ1 receptor recognition in the murine CNS.

Nogo-66 Receptor 1 and Reovirus Infection of Neurons

Nogo-66 receptor 1 (NgR1) was discovered as a mediator of reovirus infectivity in an RNA interference screen to identify host genes required for reovirus-induced cytotoxicity.[248] NgR1 is a glycosylphosphatidylinositol-anchored, leucine-rich-repeat protein expressed on the surface of neurons. Ectopic expression of NgR1 allows infection of normally nonsusceptible Chinese hamster ovary (CHO) cells.[248] This infection is mediated by direct interaction of reovirus with NgR1, as evidenced by diminished infectivity following receptor blockade by either preincubation of cells with NgR1-specific antibodies or pre-incubation of virus with soluble NgR1.[248] These competition strategies significantly diminish reovirus infectivity in primary cultures of cortical neurons, suggesting that NgR1 functions as a neural receptor for reovirus (see "Pathogenesis and Pathology—Central Nervous System"). However, it is not known whether NgR1 is required for reovirus neuropathogenesis. Reovirus virions but not ISVPs directly bind and use NgR1 as a receptor, suggesting that either σ3, which is lost during ISVP formation, or a virion conformer of σ1 interacts with NgR1.[248]

The overlapping expression of NgR1 in neural populations targeted by reovirus raises the possibility that NgR1 dictates T3-specific neurotropism. However, expression of NgR1 in CHO cells allows infection by both T1 and T3 strains.[248] Such promiscuous infection by both serotypes is not observed following inoculation of murine cortical neurons in culture.[9,435] T3 infects these neurons in an NgR1-dependent manner, whereas T1 infects neurons poorly, independent of NgR1 expression.[248] Therefore, it is likely that additional host factors, as yet to be identified, promote early steps (attachment and entry) of T3 reovirus infection of neurons.

Entry and Intracellular Trafficking

Internalization by Clathrin-Dependent Endocytosis

Following attachment to cell surface glycans and JAM-A, reovirus is internalized into many types of cells in culture by clathrin-mediated endocytosis (Fig. 11.6). Thin-section electron micrographs show reovirus virions in structures resembling clathrin-coated pits on the cell surface,[276,434] and reovirus virions and clathrin are observed using video fluorescence microscopy to colocalize during internalization.[145] Treatment of cells with chlorpromazine, which impairs clathrin-mediated endocytosis, inhibits reovirus internalization and infection,[276] suggesting a functional role for clathrin in reovirus entry. In addition to clathrin-mediated uptake, reovirus also can be internalized into some cell types using caveolar endocytosis.[392] The mechanism of reovirus endocytosis following binding to NgR1 is not known.

β1 Integrins Promote Entry and Sorting in the Endocytic Compartment

Expression of a JAM-A truncation mutant lacking a cytoplasmic tail allows reovirus to infect nonsusceptible cells,[275] suggesting that molecules other than JAM-A mobilize the

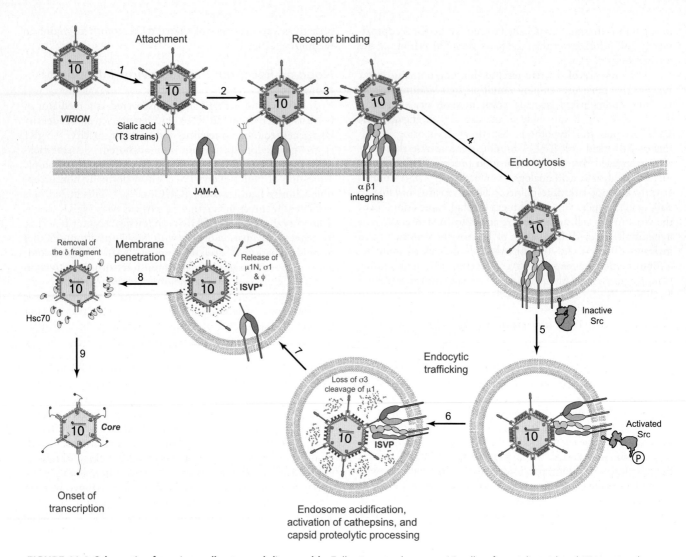

FIGURE 11.6 Schematic of reovirus cell entry and disassembly. Following attachment to (1) cell surface sialic acid and (2) junctional adhesion molecule-A (JAM-A), (3 and 4) virions enter cells by receptor-mediated endocytosis using a mechanism that requires β1 integrin. Following endocytic uptake, (5) activation of Src kinase is required for (6) trafficking of virions to an endocytic compartment where the viral outer-capsid undergoes acid-dependent proteolysis. The first disassembly intermediate is the infectious subvirion particle (ISVP), which is characterized by loss of σ3 and cleavage of μ1C into particle-associated fragments δ and φ. The ISVP then undergoes further conformational changes (7) to form the ISVP*. The ISVP* is characterized by conformational rearrangements of the μ1 fragments to expose hydrophobic residues, release of μ1N and φ, and loss of attachment protein σ1. The μ1 cleavage fragments mediate penetration (8) through the endosomal membrane releasing the transcriptionally active core (9) into the cytoplasm. The cellular chaperone protein Hsc70 participates in the membrane penetration process.

internalization apparatus that promotes reovirus cell entry. The λ2 protein (144 kDa, 1288 to 1289 aa) contains conserved integrin-binding motifs, RGD and KGE,[395] suggesting that reovirus employs integrin-dependent internalization mechanisms to enter cells. The RGD and KGE sequences are displayed on surface-exposed loops of λ2,[356] where they could interact with integrins to promote internalization.

Treatment of cells with antibodies specific for β1 integrin reduces reovirus infection, while antibodies specific for other integrin subunits expressed on susceptible cells, including those specific for α integrin subunits, have no effect.[275] However, antibodies specific for β1 integrin do not alter infection by in vitro–generated ISVPs,[275] which can directly penetrate the plasma membrane and do not require endocytosis for cell entry.[202,271] In comparison to β1 integrin–expressing cells, β1-null cells

are substantially less susceptible to infection by reovirus virions, while infection by ISVPs is equivalent in both cell types.[275] Diminished reovirus replication in β1-null cells correlates with diminished viral uptake, indicating that β1 integrin is required for efficient reovirus cell entry.

Experiments using atomic force microscopy indicate that reovirus virions directly interact with β1 integrin in a cation-dependent manner.[244] While little specific interaction is observed between reovirus and β1 integrin in the presence of Ca^{2+}, the interaction is favored in the presence of Mg^{2+} with a K_D of approximately 350 nM and is maximal in the presence of Mn^{2+}, reaching a K_D of approximately 70 nM, consistent with the effect of these cations on integrin ligand-binding efficiency. In addition to reovirus virions, reovirus cores, which lack σ1, σ3, and μ1, bind integrin with high affinity, suggesting that λ2 is the integrin-binding ligand.[244] Concordantly, a reovirus mutant with alterations in both λ2 integrin-binding motifs fails to bind β1 integrin, highlighting a key function for these sequences in integrin engagement.[244]

NPXY motifs in the β1 integrin cytoplasmic tail play a key role in sorting reovirus within the endocytic compartment. NPXY motifs are found in the cytoplasmic domains of many receptors and function in the recruitment of adaptor proteins to initiate clathrin assembly at the plasma membrane. Substitution of a tyrosine for a phenylalanine residue in either or both β1 integrin NPXY motifs (NPXF) results in inefficient internalization of reovirus virions and diminished infectivity.[276] Infection of cells expressing NPXF β1 integrin results in distribution of virions to lysosomes where they are degraded, suggesting that the β1 integrin NPXY motifs target reovirus to the precise endocytic organelle that permits functional disassembly.

Reovirus Uses Macropinocytosis to Enter Neurons

The major pathway of reovirus internalization in neurons differs from that in nonneuronal cells. In experiments using primary cultures of cortical neurons and dorsal root ganglion neurons,[11] reovirus internalization is blocked by treatment with macropinocytosis inhibitor amiloride, and internalized virions colocalize with high molecular weight dextran, which is taken up by macropinocytosis. These findings suggest that macropinocytosis is the dominant pathway for reovirus internalization in neurons. Moreover, several host factors that mediate macropinocytosis, including actin, dynamin, and phosphoinositide 3-kinase, are required for reovirus internalization and transport in neurons.[11] Inhibiting macropinocytosis diminishes reovirus infectivity in neurons,[11] suggesting that macropinocytosis-mediated entry is essential for productive infection.

Reovirus Sorts to Late Endosomes for Disassembly

Following receptor-mediated endocytosis, reovirus relies on microtubules and dynein-1[281] to traverse the endocytic pathway through early, late, and recycling endosomes.[280] Long-distance axonal transport of reovirus also relies on microtubules and neuronal dynein.[11] Internalized virions remain within nonacidified vesicles during axonal transport until reaching the neuronal cell body for disassembly. Transfection of cells with constitutively active and dominant-negative Rab GTPases that affect early and late endosome biogenesis and maturation influence reovirus infectivity, but reovirus infectivity is not altered in cells expressing mutant Rab GTPases that affect recycling endosomes.[280] Imaging studies are consistent with transient transport of reovirus through early endosomes and accumulation over time in late endosomes,[11,280] where disassembly takes place.[143,434] Therefore, while reovirus virions localize to early, late, and recycling endosomes during entry into host cells, only those that traverse early and late endosomes yield a productive infection. In some types of cells, ISVPs also can be internalized, but these particles appear to escape the endocytic compartment prior to arrival in late endosomes.[54]

Additional host factors are required for reovirus entry. Genistein, a broad-spectrum tyrosine-kinase inhibitor, and PP2, a specific Src-family-kinase inhibitor, diminish reovirus infectivity by inhibiting an early step in the viral life cycle.[279]

Although neither inhibitor impedes internalization of reovirus virions, both inhibitors target virions to lysosomes, suggesting that Src coordinates a signaling network that mediates transport of reovirus to endocytic organelles for viral disassembly and thus promotes functional entry into host cells. Treatment of cells with 5-nonyloxytryptamine (5-NT), a prototype serotonin receptor agonist, inhibits reovirus infection by blocking an early replication step.[278] 5-NT does not impede reovirus attachment but instead alters the distribution of early endosomes with a concomitant impairment of reovirus transit to late endosomes and a delay in viral disassembly. The mechanism by which serotonin signaling mediates these effects is unknown.

Reovirus entry is targeted by cell-intrinsic host defenses. Interferon-inducible transmembrane protein 3 (IFITM3), which localizes to late endosomes,[57] restricts reovirus infection by interfering with viral disassembly.[8] IFITM3 may function either by altering reovirus distribution to late endosomes or modulating the activity of endosomal proteases.

Uncoating

Cleavage of σ3—The First Step in the Reovirus Disassembly Cascade

In cellular endosomes, reovirus virions undergo stepwise disassembly to form discrete intermediates, the first of which is the ISVP[17,434] (Fig. 11.6). ISVPs are characterized by the loss of σ3, a conformational change in σ1, and cleavage of μ1 to form δ and φ. The rate-limiting step in reovirus disassembly is the proteolytic removal of the S4-encoded σ3 protein (41 kDa, 365 aa).[17,434] In some cell types, proteolysis of σ3 is dependent on acidic pH[122,434] and endocytic cysteine proteases.[17] Murine L929 cells treated with inhibitors of endosomal acidification, such as ammonium chloride[434] or bafilomycin A1,[288] or inhibitors of cysteine proteases, such as E64,[17] do not allow reovirus replication when infection is initiated by virions but do so when infection is initiated by ISVPs. Thus, the block to reovirus replication imposed by these inhibitors in murine L929 cells occurs following internalization but prior to disassembly, which is coincident with the proteolysis of σ3.

Cathepsins B and L, which reside in late endosomes and lysosomes, catalyze reovirus disassembly in fibroblasts.[143] Cathepsin S, an acid-independent cysteine protease required for processing internalized antigens, and the acid-independent serine protease neutrophil elastase can mediate uncoating of some reovirus strains in monocyte and macrophage cell lines.[173,175] It is possible that the broad tissue tropism displayed by reovirus is determined in part by the multiple host proteases capable of catalyzing its disassembly.[219]

Proteolytic enzymes also are required for reovirus infection following peroral inoculation of mice[26,44] (see "Pathogenesis and Pathology—Entry into the Host"). Reovirus virions are converted to ISVPs in the intestinal lumen by the resident serine proteases chymotrypsin and trypsin. ISVPs produced in this fashion infect intestinal M cells to allow systemic dissemination of reovirus in the host.[7] ISVPs produced by chymotrypsin or trypsin *in vitro* or in the gut lumen[26,44] display a protein profile (loss of σ3 and cleavage of μ1) indistinguishable from that of ISVPs produced in the endocytic compartment of cells.[18,143]

Sequences in σ3 that influence its susceptibility to proteolysis have been identified through studies of viruses selected during persistent infection (PI viruses) or mutant viruses selected for resistance to either cysteine protease inhibitor E64 (D-EA viruses)[144] or ammonium chloride (ACA-D viruses).[89] These viruses display accelerated kinetics of disassembly and harbor a tyrosine-to-histidine mutation at amino acid 354 (Y354H) near the C-terminus of the protein[89,144,473] (e-Fig. 11.3). Cryo-EM image analysis of a PI virus with an isolated Y354H mutation reveals a structural alteration in σ3 at a hinge region located between its two major domains.[475] These findings suggest that the C-terminus of σ3 influences susceptibility of the protein to cleavage. The Y354H polymorphism also enhances reovirus replication and disease in newborn mice and increases the efficiency of viral transmission between littermates,[137] demonstrating that susceptibility of σ3 to proteolysis is a virulence determinant for reovirus (see "Pathogenesis and Pathology—Cell and Tissue Tropism").

Treatment of reovirus virions *in vitro* with either cathepsin B or cathepsin L leads to an initial cleavage of σ3 at a terminus.[143] Since sequence polymorphisms in the σ3 C-terminus determine susceptibility to proteolysis,[213] the initial cleavage of σ3 probably occurs in this region. During proteolysis by cathepsin L, subsequent cleavages occur between residues 243 to 244 and 250 to 251[143] (e-Fig. 11.3A). These cleavage sites are physically located near the C-terminus in the σ3 crystal structure[335] (e-Fig. 11.3B and C). Because of this proximity, the small end fragment released following initial cathepsin L cleavage likely exposes the cleavage sites between residues 243 to 244 and 250 to 251, rendering them sensitive to proteolysis. The C-terminus therefore appears to control access to internal, proteolytically sensitive sites in σ3. Because reovirus disassembly in some cell types is acid-dependent,[122,434] the C-terminus might be primed for movement at acidic pH. Mutations near the C-terminus, such as Y354H, could alter the conformation of the protein to allow improved access to these cleavage sites and thus accelerate outer capsid disassembly.[475]

Conformational Changes in σ1

The disassembly of reovirus virions to ISVPs is accompanied by a conformational change in σ1. Electron micrographs of negatively stained reovirus virions and ISVPs reveal filamentous projections extending up to 400 Å from the surface of ISVPs but not virions.[162] These images suggest that σ1 adopts a compact form in the virion and a more extended one in the ISVP. Cryo-EM image reconstructions of virions and cores lack a discernable density corresponding to σ1 at the icosahedral vertices[139] (Fig. 11.2). However, cryo-EM image analysis of ISVPs demonstrates discontinuous density for σ1 extending approximately 100 Å from each vertex (Fig. 11.2). Presumably, the full length of σ1 is not visible in reovirus particles because the molecule is flexible, and icosahedral averaging was employed for the cryo-EM image reconstructions, thus minimizing the density for the trimeric σ1 protein. Interdomain regions of flexibility in σ1[159] (Fig. 11.5) may be required to allow such conformational rearrangements. In support of this idea, introduction of cysteine residues at the base of the σ1 head domain to crosslink the protein by establishing disulfide bonds appears to lock the protein into the extended conformation.[131]

Electron micrographs of purified σ1 show molecules with either single- or multilobed head domains,[159] suggesting another type of structural alteration in σ1 in which the head can exist in both "open" and "closed" conformations. A cluster of six conserved aspartic acid residues on a rigid β-hairpin at the base of the σ1 head, sandwiched between hydrophobic residues that block access to solvent, forms the main contact area between monomers in the trimer.[82,389] Of the two aspartic acid residues contributed by each monomer, one (Asp346) is neutralized by a salt-bridge interaction with a nearby residue, while the other (Asp345) is not.[82,389] The three Asp345 side chains closely appose each other at the center of the trimer in an otherwise hydrophobic environment. Since an aspartate-to-asparagine mutation results in σ1 trimers with a structure indistinguishable from wild type,[389] it is likely that Asp345 is protonated in the σ1 crystal structure,[82] thus representing the "closed" conformation of σ1. Using analytical size exclusion chromatography, isolated σ1 head domain becomes monomeric at high pH,[172] confirming protonation of the aspartic acid cluster. The D345N mutation destabilizes the σ1 head domain at low pH,[172] suggesting a function for the aspartic acid cluster during viral traverse through the low pH environment of the stomach and endocytic pathway. Thus, the aspartic acid sandwich motif contributes to σ1 conformational rearrangements by acting as a molecular switch that mediates the oligomeric state of the σ1 head, depending on environmental pH.[172,389]

Membrane Penetration

Critical Function of the μ1 Protein

ISVPs but not virions or cores can penetrate artificial lipid bilayers, model membranes of erythrocytes, or membranes of cells that allow reovirus infection,[73,74,76,202,271,448] indicating that ISVPs or a related subvirion particle is the membrane-active intermediate in the reovirus entry pathway. ISVPs differ from cores by the presence of outer-capsid proteins σ1 and μ1,[102,139] suggesting functions for these proteins in membrane penetration. However, cores recoated with μ1 and σ3 (and not σ1) *in vitro* and then treated with chymotrypsin to remove σ3 are capable of penetrating membranes,[76] indicating that the M2-encoded μ1 protein (76 kDa, 708 aa) is the primary mediator of reovirus membrane penetration. Concordantly, differences in membrane penetration efficiency displayed by reovirus strains T1L and T3D segregate with the M2 gene segment.[73,105,271,387,388,416] Additionally, viruses selected for resistance to denaturants such as ethanol contain mutations in the M2 gene segment and display alterations in membrane penetration capacity.[73,108,202,471]

The μ1 protein is N-terminally myristoylated[325] and folds into four distinct domains[266] (e-Fig. 11.4). Domains I, II, and III are primarily α-helical and serve as the base of the protein. Domain IV forms a jelly-roll β-barrel commonly found in the capsid proteins of many nonenveloped viruses. This domain extends distally and interacts extensively with similar domains of the neighboring μ1 molecules and with σ3. The μ1 protein also contains three proteolytic cleavage sites (e-Fig. 11.4B). These include an autocatalytic cleavage site at amino acid 42, which separates μ1N and μ1C, a cleavage site at approximately amino acid 580, which releases the δ and φ fragments, and a cleavage site at the C-terminus that releases a approximately 10 amino acid peptide.[75,295,322,330] Reovirus cores recoated with a μ1N-μ1C cleavage-resistant μ1 mutant are incapable of membrane penetration, indicating that cleavage of μ1 to yield μ1N and μ1C is required to complete the viral entry steps.[330] Since μ1N is released from viral particles, it is postulated that cleavage of μ1 is required for release of μ1N, which then interacts with membranes as a function of its myristoyl moiety to effect membrane penetration.[210]

Formation of the ISVP*

In the μ1 structure present in virions and ISVPs, the myristoylated μ1N fragment is buried inside a hydrophobic cavity in the α-helical pedestal formed by portions of domains I, II, and III.[266,493] Therefore, massive conformational rearrangements resulting in unwinding of the μ1 trimer must be required to release μ1N during cell entry.[266,492] Exposure of ISVPs to membranes or high salt concentrations leads to formation of an ISVP-like entry intermediate, termed the ISVP*, which is characterized by changes in the conformation of the μ1 δ fragment, loss of the σ1 protein, and an increase in particle hydrophobicity.[73] The autocatalytic cleavage of μ1 to form μ1N and μ1C also occurs in part during ISVP* formation.[324] Thus, the μ1 protein associated with ISVPs is in a metastable state primed to undergo conformational changes and autocatalytic cleavage to assume a more hydrophobic structure capable of interaction with membranes. At high particle concentrations, ISVP* conversion is regulated by a positive feedback mechanism in which μ1N, which is released during ISVP* formation, promotes ISVP-to-ISVP* conversion of the remaining particles.[2] Protease activity during virion-to-ISVP disassembly[274] and endosomal pH[445] also influence the efficiency of ISVP* conversion. There are no high-resolution structures of ISVP*s, perhaps due to the hydrophobicity of these particles.

Genetic studies using ethanol-resistant or thermostable mutants indicate that μ1 residues affecting the overall stability of the virus also regulate membrane penetration efficiency.[73,108,202,471] Several stability-altering residues identified in thermostable reovirus mutants map to either domain IV that forms the jelly-roll β-barrel or the α-helical portions of domain III that lie just below the β-barrel structure.[108,274,297,416] Since these μ1 domains participate in interactions within and between μ1 monomers,[266] these residues may modulate viral stability by preventing unwinding of the μ1 trimer. Polymorphisms in the C-terminal φ fragment also control viral stability[105,186,297] and affect membrane penetration by reducing the efficiency of ISVP-to-ISVP* conversion.[105] While it is not clear how φ residues modulate these properties, since both μ1N and φ are released from the virus particle during ISVP* formation,[210] it is likely that conformational rearrangements in μ1 during ISVP* formation are not restricted to the δ domain but also involve the μ1N and φ domains. Therefore, amino acid substitutions within φ that negatively affect its conformational flexibility would likely prevent the μ1 reorganization required for ISVP* formation. Hyperstable μ1 mutants I442V[108] and K594D[105] produce lower viral loads relative to wild-type virus in newborn mice and are attenuated. These findings indicate that μ1 must balance environmental stability and conformational flexibility to mediate efficient infection.[187]

Pore Formation Mediated by μ1N and φ

Reovirus forms small, size-selective pores in erythrocyte model membranes.[1] Both μ1N and ISVP*s associate with erythrocyte membranes,[1,210] but μ1N is capable of pore formation in the absence of other viral components.[210] The φ domain also associates with membranes.[210] A peptide derived from the first α-helix of φ (residues 582 to 611) induces cytotoxicity in mammalian cells associated with a rapid increase in intracellular calcium

levels and leakage of 10 kDa dextran from small unilamellar liposomes.[233] The increase in intracellular calcium occurs even when cells are incubated in calcium-free medium in the presence of EGTA and does not occur secondary to phospholipase C–mediated signaling, as the calcium increase is not blocked by a phospholipase C inhibitor.[233] In the absence of φ cleavage, establishment of infection is delayed.[417] Although viruses incapable of δ-φ cleavage can penetrate membranes and are infectious,[74,76] collectively, these findings suggest a role for φ during membrane penetration. It is possible that pore formation by μ1N is enhanced by the presence of φ.[210]

Pores formed by released μ1N fragments are considerably smaller than those required to allow the viral intermediate to traverse the membrane.[1] Analogous to erythrocyte membrane rupture, pore formation may result in osmotic lysis of endosomes in which viral particles are present. Alternatively, the initial small pore formed by the virus might recruit cellular factors that produce larger pores or channels through which the viral intermediate can translocate.

Influence of Other Reovirus Structural Proteins on ISVP Stability and Membrane Penetration

In addition to μ1, other reovirus proteins, both in the outer capsid and core, influence viral disassembly and membrane penetration. Sequence polymorphisms in attachment protein σ1 affect ISVP stability and the efficiency of ISVP-to-ISVP* conversion.[446] A candidate σ1 polymorphism responsible for these effects is located in a region of the σ1 tail domain that interacts with λ2 and influences σ1 encapsidation onto virions,[329] suggesting that alterations in σ1 encapsidation or σ1-λ2 interactions may in turn influence μ1 conformational rearrangements during ISVP* formation.[446] Sequence polymorphisms in core proteins σ2 and λ1, which form the bulk of the core shell,[356] also influence ISVP stability and ISVP-to-ISVP* conversion efficiency.[186] These findings indicate that reovirus core proteins can modulate viral entry steps.

Host Factors Required for Membrane Penetration

ISVP-to-ISVP* conversion can be induced *in vitro* by synthetic membranes composed of phosphatidylcholine and phosphatidylethanolamine.[414] The conversion process occurs most efficiently in the presence of lipid-associated μ1N, which recruits ISVP*s to membrane pores.[415] These observations are consistent with the idea that host membranes participate in the entry pathway of reovirus.[266] Particles transitioning from ISVPs to ISVP*s may expose buried regions of μ1 and a small proportion of μ1N, which would allow μ1 to interact with lipid-associated μ1N, thus accelerating formation of ISVP*s.[187] Following ISVP* formation, pores formed by μ1N (and perhaps aided by φ) facilitate core delivery.[1,210,492]

Both the viral core and the δ fragment of μ1 are found in the cytoplasm following reovirus entry.[75] While δ is found distributed diffusely throughout the cytosol, viral cores display a more punctate cytoplasmic localization.[75] These observations suggest that the δ fragment disassociates from the ISVP* either during or immediately after membrane penetration to allow cores to become transcriptionally active. Removal of δ from cores is thought to be accomplished by direct interaction of δ with the host chaperone Hsc70 via an ATP-dependent process.[209] Since chaperones can translocate proteins across membranes, it is possible that concomitant with removal of particle-associated δ, Hsc70 also aids in transport of the viral core across membranes.[209]

Transcription

During infection, transcriptionally active viral core particles produced following proteolytic disassembly and endosomal membrane penetration gain access to the cytosol and produce the initial wave of viral transcripts (primary transcripts) that encode new viral proteins. However, in contrast to transcripts produced by core particles *in vitro*, the primary viral transcriptome synthesized by entering viral particles during the first 4 to 5 hours of infection is biased toward transcripts from the L1, M3, S3, and S4 gene segments.[467] Transcriptionally active core particles in cells may retain remnants of outer-capsid proteins or associate with cellular proteins that differentially influence transcription of some viral gene segments by allostery. Alternatively, the stability of some viral transcripts in cells may depend on the presence of one or more of the λ3, μNS, σNS, or σ3 proteins encoded by the L1, M3, S3, and S4 gene segments, respectively. Wild-type σNS protein, but not a mutant defective in RNA-binding, protects viral mRNA from nuclease digestion and prolongs its half-life.[491] By 10 hours postinfection, all of the viral transcripts are synthesized at frequencies proportional to their length. Primary transcription from particles entering cells peaks around 6 hours postinfection and is replaced by secondary transcription that results from newly assembled transcriptase particles. The large majority of viral mRNA is synthesized as a consequence of secondary transcription.

Cores as Molecular Machines

Viral core particles contain the genome and enzymes required to produce capped viral mRNAs. Each core contains 10 to 12 copies of the viral RNA-dependent RNA polymerase, λ3, and approximately 12 to 24 copies of the polymerase co-factor, μ2. Viral mRNAs exit the core at each of the fivefold symmetry axes, and all 10 gene segments can be transcribed simultaneously. Isolated λ3 polymerase has limited enzymatic activity and likely must interact with its cofactor μ2 and the λ1 shell protein to mediate native catalysis. RNA transcripts synthesized from the [−] strand template of the genomic dsRNA are extruded through a peripentonal channel in the λ1 shell and enter a cavity within the pentameric λ2 turret. Within the λ2 turret, viral transcripts are capped by guanylyltransferase and methyltransferase activities and then released to the cytosol.

Activation of Transcriptase Function

Transcription in virions is repressed. In this state, the 3′ end of each [−] strand template is probably unwound from its complementary [+] strand and held in a preinitiation complex with a polymerase molecule at the active site. Therefore, in virions, the polymerase can only synthesize short abortive transcripts that represent the first 2 to 4 bases complementary to the 5′ end of the [−] strand template. Indeed, approximately 25% of the total RNA found in virions are short ssRNA oligonucleotides that are either abortive transcripts or nontemplated oligoadenylates that are likely synthesized during the last stages of virion morphogenesis as transcription is shut off by assembly of the outer capsid onto nascent cores. Removal of outer-capsid proteins σ3 and μ1 by proteolysis allows a conformational change in the core particle that permits opening of the C-terminal flaps

of the λ2 turret, release of σ1, and activation of the transcriptase. Global changes in the conformation of the RNA gene segments are likely required for activation of transcription.[120] This hypothesis is supported by the observation that the liquid crystalline RNA within transcriptionally active cores is less closely packed than genomic RNA within virions.[296] Structures of transcriptionally primed and quiescent grass carp reovirus particles show changes in the topology of the dsRNA genome segments accompanied by small rearrangements in the core shell protein (VP3; λ1 equivalent) surrounding each transcriptase (VP2; λ3 equivalent) and its cofactor (VP4; μ2 equivalent).[132,466]

The Transcriptional Cycle

Transcription of reovirus dsRNA gene segments is iterative and involves a well-orchestrated series of steps (Figs. 11.7 and 11.8). The dsRNA gene segment is first unwound to allow the 3′ end of the [−] strand template to enter the catalytic site of the polymerase. The 3′ end of the template strand is then specifically recognized and placed in register for priming and initiation of RNA synthesis. After RNA synthesis is initiated, the promoter region of the template is cleared from the active site to allow elongation of the nascent RNA transcript. As elongation proceeds, the transcript is separated from the template and extruded from the polymerase through a different polymerase channel. Upon exit, the template is likely rewound with its cognate [+] strand before having its 3′ end guided back toward the template entry portal to allow efficient reinitiation of synthesis. After the nascent transcript exits the polymerase, the 5′-terminal γ phosphate is removed by an RNA triphosphate phosphohydrolase, and the transcript is passed into a cavity within the λ2 turret where it is guanylated by a guanylyltransferase domain and 7-*N* and 2′-*O* methylated by two, independent methyltransferase domains. Finally, the capped RNA transcript exits the core particle for translation.

Enzymatic Activities Associated With Transcription

(a) RNA-dependent RNA polymerase (λ3). An estimated 10 to 12 copies of the L1-encoded λ3 RNA-dependent RNA polymerase (142 kDa, 1,267 aa) are present within each core particle.[356,498] A 2.5 Å atomic resolution structure of λ3[439] reveals a central RNA-dependent RNA polymerase domain (aa 381 to 890) with canonical right-handed "thumb," "palm," and "fingers" subdomains (Fig. 11.7A). The catalytic cleft is enclosed or "caged" by an N-terminal domain (aa 1 to 380), which bridges the "fingers" and "thumb" subdomains, and a C-terminal "bracelet" domain (aa 891 to 1267) (Fig. 11.7A). The λ3 protein can be modeled as a rounded cube approximately 65 Å in diameter with channels on its front, bottom, rear, and left sides that allow access to the active site (Fig. 11.7B). These channels allow entry of the template and NTPs and exit of the minus-strand template or dsRNA product and the plus-strand transcript (Fig. 11.7C and D).

There is a putative cap-binding site on the outside of the polymerase[439] (Fig. 11.7B). The 5′ cap of the [+] strand RNA likely anchors in this position close to the template entry channel (Fig. 11.7C). This placement would retain the 3′ end of the [−] strand template RNA in a position where it could easily access the polymerase active site. An unusual feature of λ3 is the presence of a priming loop that engages the incoming priming NTP during initiation. This loop is displaced toward

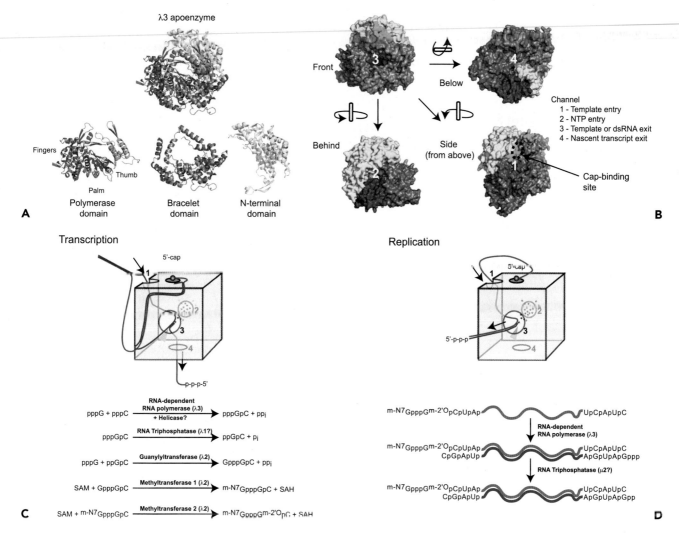

FIGURE 11.7 The reovirus λ3 RNA-dependent RNA polymerase and its enzymatic actions. A: Ribbon diagram of the crystal structure of the λ3 apoenzyme . Access to the central conserved polymerase domain is limited by the N-terminal domain (*yellow*) and C-terminal bracelet domain (*purple*), which form channels. **B:** Space-filling model of the polymerase with the channels indicated that allow (*1*) template entry, (*2*) nucleotide triphosphate entry, (*3*) template or dsRNA exit, and (*4*) nascent transcript exit. The 5′-cap of the template mRNA binds to the polymerase close to the template entry site. The enzymatic activities of λ3, transcription **(C)** and replication **(D)**, and the movement of the template minus-strand RNA (*blue*) during transcription or template positive-strand mRNA (*red*) during replication are shown in the schematic. Other enzymatic activities associated with transcription and replication are indicated below each schematic. (Adapted from Tao Y, Farsetta DL, Nibert ML, et al. RNA synthesis in a cage-structural studies of reovirus polymerase λ3. *Cell* 2002;111:733–745. Copyright © 2002 Elsevier. With permission.)

the "palm" subdomain during elongation. Failure of the loop to move would prevent elongation and might explain the large number of abortive transcripts within viral cores. Thus, the priming loop may be a kinetic barrier to the transition from initiation to elongation during λ3 transcription.[120]

Comparison of the structures of the rotavirus VP1 and reovirus λ3 polymerases suggests that these polymerases exist in two conformers. The first can bind the 3′ end of the [+] strand RNA but not the 3′ end of the [−] strand RNA and potentially mediates assortment and packaging of viral mRNAs. This conformer would be poised for replication. The second represents the transcriptionally active form of the polymerase found within cores. This conformer would not need to specifically recognize the 3′ end, but it would be imperative that initiation begins at the first residue of the template. RNA synthesis is fully conservative and initiates with entry and correct registration of the 3′ end of a template RNA at the active site.[439]

(b) Helicase activity. An unwinding or helicase activity is required to separate the genomic dsRNA [+] and [−] strands prior to transcription and facilitate rewinding of the template [−] strand with the [+] strand after it exits the polymerase. The viral protein responsible for helicase activity during infection is thought to be λ3.[439] The presence of a cap-binding site on λ3 would allow strand separation to occur. In addition, a loop present in the "bracelet" domain of the λ3 polymerase may aid in separation of template and transcript during transcription.[439]

(c) RNA triphosphate phosphohydrolase activity. Following transcription, the terminal γ phosphate at the 5′ end of the transcript is removed, yielding a diphosphate to initiate capping. The L3-encoded λ1 protein (142 kDa, 1275 aa) has

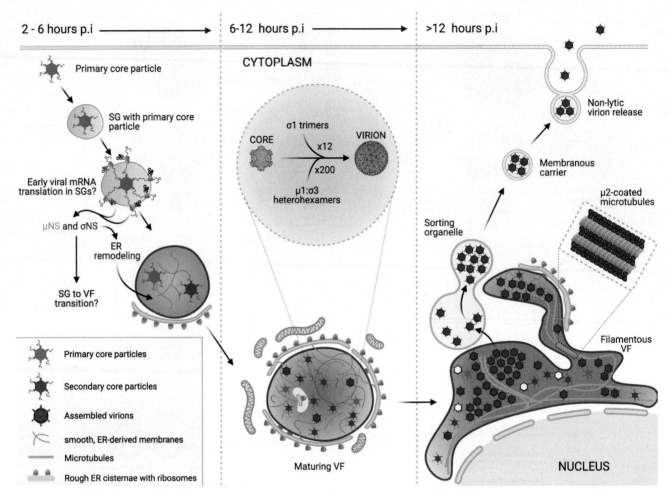

FIGURE 11.8 Schematic of reovirus factory biogenesis and egress. In the first 2 to 6 hours after infection, a transcriptionally active primary core or transcriptase particle is deposited in the cytoplasm and begins synthesis of capped viral transcripts (early or primary transcripts). The onset of transcription leads to particles becoming embedded within stress granules (SGs) in a proportion of cells. Viral transcripts are translated into viral proteins (perhaps *in situ* within SGs). Viral nonstructural proteins μNS and σNS condense around the primary core particle and dissipate or displace SG proteins and lead to formation of a nascent viral factory (VF). Viral proteins continue to be synthesized by ribosomes in close proximity to or within VFs. The μNS and σNS proteins also remodel ER membranes, and by 6 to 12 hours postinfection, thin, fragmented, ER-derived tubular membranes become embedded within VFs. Ribosome-encrusted ER cisternae come to surround and occasionally infiltrate maturing VFs. Assembly of new secondary core or transcriptase particles requires the assortment and packaging of each of 10 primary transcripts into these nascent particles. Mechanisms of genome assortment and packaging are poorly understood. Secondary core or transcriptase particles synthesize the majority of viral transcripts during infection. From 6 hours postinfection, new virions assemble by the addition of viral outer-capsid proteins μ1, σ3, and σ1 onto core particles. From 12 hours postinfection, the VFs of most reovirus strains begin to appear filamentous as a consequence of incorporation of bundles of μ2-coated microtubules. Genome-containing virions may organize in paracrystalline arrays along microtubules. During the late phases of infection in some types of cells, membrane-bound sorting organelles derived from modified lysosomes congregate around VFs. Mature virions are transferred into sorting organelles and then to membranous carriers that transport virions to the plasma membrane where upon fusion of the membranous carrier, progeny virions are released. (Figure prepared using BioRender.com.)

phosphohydrolase activity,[41] and removal of the γ phosphate likely occurs as the transcript is directed out of the core particle through pores in the λ1 shell.[498] The passage of the transcript through λ1 may be facilitated by the RNA-binding activity associated with a λ1 N-terminal domain.[42]

(d) Guanylyltransferase and methyltransferase activity. Following removal of the 5′ γ-phosphate from the transcript, a guanylyltransferase associated with the N-terminal domain of the L2-encoded λ2 protein (144 kDa, 1288 to 1289 aa) adds a

guanylate cap to the 5′ diphosphate of the transcript using GTP as a substrate.[273] The transcript is then further modified by the addition of 7-*N* and 2′-*O* methyl groups by the two methyltransferase subdomains of λ2.[439] The methyl donor comes from *S*-adenosyl methionine (SAM), which is converted to *S*-adenosyl-*L*-homocysteine after the methyl group is transferred to the cap. The long axis of each λ2 monomer within the turret lies at an angle of approximately 45 degrees to the fivefold axis of symmetry. The five λ2 monomers wrap around each other to form a hollow cylinder, approximately 70 Å in diameter at its base, with C-terminal flaps at the top that narrow to approximately 13 Å.[356] The N-terminal guanylyltransferase domains (residues 1 to 385) of the λ2 monomers are located at the base of the turret. Lysine residues at positions 171 and 190 in λ2 are required for enzymatic function and project into the active site.[273] The guanylyltransferase domain is linked by a small domain (residues 386 to 433 and 690 to 802) to two methyltransferase domains (methylase 1, residues 434 to 691, and methylase 2, residues 804 to 1022) that each have a SAM-binding site.[356] It is thought that methylase 1 catalyzes guanosine-7-*N*-methylation and methylase 2 catalyzes guanosine-2′-*O*-methylation. The flap of the λ2 turret is formed by the C-terminal 250 residues that form three immunoglobulin-like folds.[356]

Location of λ3 Within Core Particles

Within viral core particles, each polymerase lies close to but slightly adjacent from the fivefold symmetry axes associated with three λ1A shell proteins.[498] The transcript-exit channel (Fig. 11.7B) faces toward a peripentonal channel between two λ1A conformers. The location of µ2 has not been resolved.[498] However, a homolog of µ2, the VP4 NTPase of grass carp reovirus, lies further radially from the fivefold axis of symmetry than the polymerase, wrapping around its "fingers" subdomain and interacting with helical regions of the N-terminus of core shell protein VP3 (homolog of λ1).[132]

Role of µ2 in Transcription

The M1-encoded µ2 protein (83 kDa, 736 aa) is found in approximately 12 to 24 copies within each core particle. µ2 interacts with and is thought to be a cofactor for the λ3 polymerase and likely also interacts with λ1. µ2 binds ssRNA and dsRNA and has NTPase and RNA 5′ triphosphatase activity.[234] The RNA 5′ triphosphatase activity may be required for removal of the 5′ γ phosphate from newly synthesized [−] strand RNA during dsRNA synthesis. The µ2 NTPase and RTPase activities are required for viral replication, as ectopic expression of mutant µ2 proteins lacking NTPase or RTPase activity (K415A or K419A) fails to complement siRNA-mediated knockdown of wild-type µ2.[241] The structure of µ2 has not been determined. However, the grass carp reovirus µ2 homolog, VP4, has a three-domain structure with an N-terminal nodule, a middle plate-like NTPase domain, and a C-terminal domain.[132] An alanine-to-valine substitution at position 612 in the C-terminus of T3D µ2 impairs NTPase and RNA synthetic activities.[488] Interestingly, this mutation also increases the association of µ2 with µNS. Residue 612 lies in a homologous region of VP4 that contains two lysine residues that are predicted to interact with the dsRNA genome and facilitates the conformational movement of dsRNA associated with the switch from a quiescent to an active state of transcription.

Translation and Viral Factory Formation

Translation of Reovirus mRNAs

Early studies of eukaryotic translation initiation by Marilyn Kozak used reovirus mRNAs synthesized by viral core particles *in vitro* to show an association of mRNA with ribosomes. From these studies, reovirus mRNAs were found to have 5′ terminal sequences blocked or capped by a 7-*N*-methylguanosine linked 5′ to 5′ with a conserved GpCpUpA sequence. The 7-*N*-methylguanosine cap is required for efficient recognition of reovirus

mRNAs by 40S ribosomal subunits. However, nucleotide sequences that vary between gene segments also contain structural information required for efficient association of reovirus mRNAs with ribosomes.[375]

Reovirus mRNAs lack poly(A) tails and have relatively short 3′ NTRs (35 to 83 nucleotides) that terminate with UpCpApUpC-3′. Polyadenylation promotes translation by stabilizing mRNA and facilitating reinitiation by ribosomes as a consequence of mRNA circularization via interactions of the poly(A)-binding protein with the 3′ poly(A) sequence and eIF-4G, which binds the cap-binding protein, eIF-4E. Reovirus mRNAs are thought to also circularize by an unknown mechanism. Translation enhancing and repressing elements are present in the 3′ NTR of the s4 mRNA,[306] which is the most efficiently translated viral transcript. It is likely that such elements also are present in the 3′ NTRs of other segments. The 3′ NTR of s4 mRNA is bound by cellular proteins that may be involved in translational control.[306]

Reovirus core particles synthesize [m7]G-capped viral mRNAs. Capped viral mRNAs are synthesized early after infection by core particles (Fig. 11.8). However, as infection progresses in at least some cell types, such as L929 cells, there is a transition from capped to uncapped viral mRNAs that have the structure [5′-pGpC...].[408] Uncapped viral mRNAs are detected approximately 4 to 6 hours postinfection and peak approximately 12 hours postinfection. The uncapped viral mRNAs are translated much more efficiently than capped viral or host mRNAs in extracts from infected L929 cells collected at 10 hours postinfection.[408] Addition of the σ3 protein to lysates prepared from uninfected L929 cells substantially increases the efficiency of uncapped viral mRNA translation by an unknown mechanism.[261] Core particles also transcribe uncapped viral mRNAs *in vitro* to varying extents depending on the reaction conditions. It is possible that uncapped mRNAs are synthesized in cells by progeny viral core particles, as unlike primary core particles, progeny core particles have repressed guanylyltransferase and methyltransferase activities. Interestingly, the guanylyltransferase and methyltransferase activities of progeny core particles can be stimulated by chymotrypsin,[409] suggesting that these activities are triggered by viral disassembly. Although the evidence for uncapped viral mRNAs in L929 cells is compelling, uncapped viral mRNAs are not found in SC-1 cells.[126] These differences may be attributable to differences in methodology or cell type-specific effects on viral transcription.

The 10 reovirus gene segments encode mRNAs for synthesis of 12 viral proteins (Table 11.2 and Fig. 11.8). Viral protein synthesis gradually increases during infection with a concomitant decrease in cellular protein synthesis[397] (see "Responses of the Host Cell to Infection—Inhibition of Cellular RNA and Protein Synthesis and Induction of Cellular Stress Responses"). Synthesis of viral proteins can be detected as early as 2 to 3 hours after infection. However, because the L1, M3, S3, and S4 gene segments are transcribed before the other gene segments, the λ3, µNS, σNS, and σ3 proteins encoded by these gene segments will be synthesized early.[255] By approximately 10 hours postinfection, most of the proteins synthesized in infected cells are viral in origin. The rates of synthesis of the individual proteins vary, but their relative levels remain constant throughout infection. For example, the µ1 protein, a major outer-capsid protein, is synthesized at 20-fold greater levels than the σ1 protein despite half as much m2 mRNA as s1 mRNA.

Translation of reovirus transcripts is tightly regulated. Some of the factors that influence the differential rates and frequencies of translation of reovirus mRNAs include: (a) nucleotide sequences at the −3 and +4 positions flanking the AUG start codon; (b) length of the 5′ NTRs, which may affect translation rate (those with the longest 5′ NTRs are translated most efficiently); (c) conserved sequence motifs that extend beyond the 5′ and 3′ NTRs within the mRNA, which may recruit specific translation initiation factors; (d) transcript length, which influences translational frequency (shorter transcripts are in general translated at higher levels); and (e) cellular and viral RNA-binding proteins. The viral σNS[168,491] and µNS[10] proteins bind single-stranded RNA and may act to retain the viral transcripts within viral replication and assembly sites.

Stress granules are detected in a proportion of reovirus-infected cells between 2 and 6 hours after infection, with the percentage of infected cells containing stress granules varying with multiplicity of infection, cell type, and viral strain[352] (see "Responses of the Host Cell to Infection—Inhibition of Cellular RNA and Protein Synthesis and Induction of Cellular Stress Responses"). Stress granules are ribonucleoprotein-containing liquid–liquid phase-separated condensates that form as a consequence of stress- or drug-induced inhibition of translational initiation. Stress granules recruit PKR, RIG-I, and MDA-5 and are thought to act as antiviral signaling platforms. Reovirus induction of stress granules requires disassembly of virions but does not require *de novo* synthesis of viral RNA or protein. However, the recruitment of the entering core particles to stress granules requires viral transcription.[352] It is not known how stress granules are induced following viral entry, but the release of dsRNA from damaged core particles or import of dsRNA from endolysosomes into the cytoplasm by RNA transmembrane transporters such as SIDT1 or SIDT2 are possible causes. Reovirus-induced stress granule formation requires phosphorylation of eIF2α.[352] There are five known eIF2α kinases (general control nonderepressible 2 [GCN2], heme-regulated inhibitor kinase [HRI], microtubule-affinity regulating kinase 2 [MARK2], protein kinase R [PKR], and protein kinase R-like ER kinase [PERK]). Reovirus infection induces ribonucleoprotein granules in mouse embryonic fibroblasts lacking GCN2, HRI, PKR, or PERK, suggesting that more than one eIF2α kinase is responsible for phosphorylation of eIF2α following viral entry.[352] However, ribonucleoprotein granules similar to stress granules also form in cells following activation of RNase L. RNase L–dependent granules contain many but not all of the protein markers found in stress granules and form in PKR-null cells treated with poly I:C. Therefore, it is possible that reovirus infection can induce RNase L–dependent granules in infected cells.

Reovirus core particles become embedded within stress granules at early times postinfection.[352] Viral transcripts may be synthesized and retained within stress granules or released into the cytosol. Although stress granules contain stalled 48S ribosomal–mRNA complexes, translation of cellular proteins can occur within stress granules.[289] Therefore, it is possible that reovirus transcripts also are actively translated within stress granules.

By 12 hours postinfection, stress granules within reovirus-infected cells largely disappear, and infected cells are refractory to further induction of stress granules independent of eIF2α phosphorylation status.[351] At later times postinfection, proteins found within stress granules, such as caprin and Ras GTPase-activating protein-binding protein 1 (G3BP1), sometimes distribute around the periphery of viral factories (VFs), particularly in cells infected with strain T2J.[84] This peripheral redistribution of stress granule proteins also is seen in cells coexpressing the viral nonstructural proteins σNS and µNS with G3BP1 and other proteins surrounding or colocalizing with σNS and µNS virus factory–like structures. The viral nonstructural protein σNS associates with G3BP1, a key effector protein involved in formation of stress granules, and coexpression of σNS and µNS interferes with formation of stress granules.[84] These findings suggest that dissipation of stress granules in reovirus-infected cells is in part driven by interactions of σNS and G3BP1 and the association of σNS with µNS. Other viral proteins also may be involved, as the peripheral distribution of stress granule proteins around VFs is less common in cells infected with strains T1L and T3D.

The viral nonstructural protein σ1s enhances protein synthesis in simian virus 40–immortalized endothelial cells, MEFs, human umbilical vein endothelial cells, and T84 human colonic epithelial cells by an unknown mechanism.[344]

Viral Factories

Reovirus transcription, translation, replication, and assembly occur within or on the margins of VFs (Fig. 11.8 and e-Fig. 11.5). VFs first appear as round punctate structures 2 to 4 hours postinfection and increase in size over time. The viral nonstructural protein µNS also colocalizes with SG marker protein TIAR in infected cells between 2 and 6 hours postinfection, suggesting that some VFs may comingle with stress granules.[71] VFs are initially globular, but by approximately 12 hours postinfection, VFs formed by most strains transition to a filamentous morphology as a consequence of their association with stabilized microtubules.[340] VFs are permeated by a meshwork of smooth tubular membrane fragments that derive from the endoplasmic reticulum (ER).[154,442] In addition, from 12 hours postinfection, coated microtubules traverse the VF matrix in cells infected with the majority of viral strains. Viral particles associate with coated microtubules and smooth tubulovesicular membranes within VFs.[124,154]

Reovirus infection perturbs and remodels the ER leading to thinning and fragmentation of ER tubules and collapse and aggregation of the ER, leaving areas of the cytoplasm devoid of ER membranes. Nonstructural proteins σNS and µNS are responsible for ER remodeling. Expression of σNS causes thinning of the tubular ER, while expression of µNS leads to ER fragmentation.[442] The tubulovesicular membranes within VFs are derived from the fragmented ER tubules and make connections with ribosome-encrusted ER cisternae that surround VFs. Occasionally, ribosome-encrusted ER membranes are observed within VFs.[124,442] Mitochondria and lipid droplets also are in close proximity to VFs.[97,154]

Translation of reovirus mRNAs is compartmentalized in infected cells and occurs on the margins or within VFs.[124] Markers for 40S and 60S ribosomes and cellular proteins required for translational initiation, elongation, and termination localize to or concentrate on the margins of VFs. In particular, components of 43S ribosomes associate with nonstructural protein σNS and distribute to the VF margins. σNS colocalizes with ER markers and extends from the VF margins to the surrounding cisternal ER.[124,442] σNS cosediments with 40S and 60S ribosomes and is suggested to recruit ribosomal and translational factors to VFs.[124]

Several hypotheses have been suggested for the biogenesis of VFs. The observation that entering viral core particles become embedded within stress granules and the detection of viral proteins with stress-granule markers early after infection led to the suggestion that stress granules seed VF assembly.[84] The remodeling of ER membranes by σNS and μNS and the close association of VFs with such membranes has led to the suggestion that remodeled ER tubules serve as the organizational scaffold for subsequent factory assembly.[442] VFs are dynamic structures that allow vesicles and membranes to pass through them and show the capacity to split apart and fuse together.[69,124] These observations support a hypothesis that VFs are liquid–liquid phase-separated biomolecular condensates.

The matrix of VFs is formed by the M3-encoded nonstructural protein, μNS (80 kDa, 721 aa) (e-Fig. 11.5). Globular structures similar to VFs in T3D-infected cells form in the cytoplasm of cells expressing μNS.[61] VF-like structures (VFLs) formed by μNS fused to green fluorescent protein are highly dynamic and have properties similar to liquid liquid phase-separated biomolecular condensates.[124] The C-terminal region (aa 471 to 721) of μNS, which is required for formation of VFLs, contains two predicted coiled-coil regions separated by a linker that contains a predicted CCHC Zn-binding motif that is required for formation of VFLs.[58] μNS is a scaffold protein that interacts with and recruits the viral structural proteins found in core particles (λ1, λ2, λ3, μ2, and σ2) and the RNA-binding nonstructural protein σNS[59,61,299,300] (Fig. 11.8). These activities may promote efficient assembly of nascent viral transcriptase particles. Viral RNAs are synthesized within and localize to VFs.[299]

VFs are thought to promote virus replication and assembly by sequestering and concentrating viral RNA and structural proteins (Fig. 11.8). However, they also function to prevent antiviral defenses. VFs sequester phosphorylated IRF3, preventing it from translocating to the nucleus and activating the interferon (IFN) response. The capacity of μNS to form VF-like structures is required for IRF3 sequestration.[421] An N-terminally shortened version of μNS called μNSC that lacks the first 40 amino acids of μNS is synthesized in infected cells.[259] However, μNSC cannot complement siRNA-mediated knockdown of full-length μNS, indicating that interactions of μNS with μ2 and σNS mediated by the N-terminal 40 amino acids is required for viral replication.[241] μNSC is thought to be produced as a consequence of translation initiation from an alternative, in-frame start codon in the m3 mRNA. The function of μNSC in infected cells is not known.

The vast majority of viral transcripts are likely synthesized and extruded from transcriptionally active viral particles buried within the μNS matrix of VFs (Fig. 11.8). Mixing purified viral core particles with purified μNS in vitro leads to condensation of μNS around the core particles, which prevents them from being recoated with outer-capsid proteins but does not affect their transcriptional capacity.[60] As coating of cores with outer-capsid proteins inhibits transcription, μNS may protect transcribing viral core particles from being prematurely inactivated. Core particles rapidly become embedded within μNS VFLs when they enter the cytosol of cells expressing μNS.[59]

μNS contains a conserved C-terminal clathrin-box motif (711-LIDFS-715) that recruits clathrin heavy and light chains to VFs. Clathrin-dependent functions, including endocytosis and secretion, are partially inhibited in cells infected with wild-type reovirus but not a reovirus mutant with a leucine-to-alanine substitution at position 711 of μNS (μNS-L711A).[211] The μNS-L711A mutant displays mildly impaired replication efficiency and normal VF formation. Reovirus-induced inhibition of viral endocytosis and secretion is modest and correlates with VF size. It is possible that sequestration of clathrin in VFs and concomitant inhibition of endocytosis prevents superinfection of cells.[211]

The viral μ2 protein binds to and stabilizes microtubules in vitro and in vivo.[234,340] μ2 is posttranslationally acetylated at its second alanine following removal of the initial methionine residue.[437] μ2 links μNS and thus the VF matrix to the microtubule cytoskeleton.[61] μ2 likely interacts with microtubules as an oligomer, as a self-associative domain (residues 283 to 325) is required for efficient microtubule interaction. The N-terminal residues 1 to 282 are sufficient for interaction with microtubules, and the first 17 residues are essential.[146] Residues 1 to 282 of μ2 correspond to the N-terminal α-helical domain of aquareovirus VP4, and residues 283 to 325 correspond to those within the central plate domain of VP4.[132] Residues 290 to 453 of μ2 are sufficient for interactions with μNS. Point mutants D291A, Y293L, and D299A within this region block the capacity of μ2 to self-associate and bind to microtubules but do not affect interactions with μNS.[146] The isolate of T3D originally derived from the Bernard Fields laboratory forms globular VFs[61] (e-Fig. 11.5). However, most isolates, including T3D isolates from the Patrick Lee laboratory, form filamentous VFs.[307,487] This difference in VF morphology is a consequence of a temperature-sensitive mutation in μ2 (P208S). The Fields T3D strain will form filamentous VFs when cultivated at 31°C, but globular VFs at 37°C. The P208S μ2 mutant has a propensity to aggregate at 37°C, and it is ubiquitylated and targeted for proteasomal degradation.[301] Despite this defect, the Fields T3D μ2 allele appears to function adequately as a cofactor for the λ3 polymerase, as there is no significant impairment of this strain to infect most cultured cells or cause disease in mice. In some cell types, this allele leads to defects in assembly and packaging of the genome, indicating an important function that correlates with microtubule binding.[336,396]

Assortment and Replication of Genomic Nucleic Acid

The process by which the reovirus gene segments are assorted and packaged into nascent viral cores is not fully understood. A common feature of dsRNA viruses is that synthesis of the [−] strand RNA occurs only after packaging of viral [+] strand RNA into a replicase particle. The fidelity of packaging and the lack of evidence of mispackaging suggest a specific mechanism. Members of the dsRNA-containing *Cystoviridae* package three segments of [+] strand RNA into a preassembled procapsid. Packaging of each RNA occurs in a specific order that is regulated by precise recognition of packaging sequences and conformational changes in the procapsid that occur after packaging of each strand. The procapsid conformational change exposes the packaging site for the next segment. Replication occurs after all three viral [+] RNA strands have been packaged. Because viruses in the *Reoviridae* have a larger number of dsRNA gene segments, gene segment assortment and packaging is thought to occur by a different process. One notable difference is that packaging and assortment occur within VFs or viroplasms.

Gene segment assortment is thought to require viral nonstructural ssRNA-binding proteins that have helicase unwinding activity or RNA chaperone activity. Avian and mammalian reovirus σNS proteins have RNA helicase and RNA chaperone activity.[51,491] Moreover, the avian σNS protein can facilitate specific RNA–RNA interactions between two [+] strand RNA segments *in vitro*.[51] A proposed model for assortment is that the 5' and 3' ends of each [+] strand RNA first interact with an RNA-dependent RNA polymerase molecule. The 5' cap would bind to the cap-binding site on the λ3 polymerase, and the 3' terminal sequence would bind to the polymerase template-binding site. Specific intersegment RNA–RNA interactions facilitated by σNS would then drive condensation of the viral [+] strand RNAs. The viral core shell proteins would then assemble on the RNA-polymerase condensate to form a replicase particle. The 5' and 3' UTRs of [+] strand RNA and some portion of the ORF are required for assortment.[119,374,377] The replicase particle then copies the [+] strand RNA to synthesize a [−] strand partner to produce the 10 dsRNA gene segments.[10] The association of core protein λ2 with these RNA–protein complexes occurs concomitantly with the onset of [−] strand synthesis to form a core particle.[10]

Assembly

Reovirus particles are assumed to assemble in VFs. Intact virions, viral core particles, and incomplete viral particles are observed in VFs by electron microscopy.[124,154,442] Assembly of core particles and dsRNA synthesis likely occurs concurrently, as inhibiting polymerase activity yields core-like particles that contain less than complete dsRNA genome complements. Assembly of the outer capsid $\mu 1_3\sigma 3_3$ heterohexamers and σ1 trimers onto core particles occurs after assembly of the core particle (Fig. 11.8). Assembly of the outer-capsid proteins onto cores is likely regulated to prevent premature termination of transcription. Addition of outer-capsid proteins to cores within VFs likely requires the removal of μNS. How this occurs is not known but may involve cellular chaperones. The Hsc70 chaperone distributes to VFs, interacts with μNS, and may function in specific viral assembly steps.[224]

Empty core-like particles assemble in cells that ectopically express the λ1, λ2, and σ2 proteins or the λ1, λ2, λ3, and σ2 proteins, indicating that nonstructural proteins are not required for core assembly. Minimally, a shell will form when λ1 and σ2 are coexpressed and λ3 is incorporated if it is also coexpressed.[482] Assembly of pentameric λ2 turrets requires formation of a shell or partial shell of λ1 and σ2 proteins, as λ2 does not assemble pentamers when expressed alone.[285] Intermediates in the assembly of core particles likely exist but have not been characterized. Host factors may be required for assembly of core particles. The λ2 protein can interact with λ3.[423] Therefore, it is possible that a core assembly intermediate incorporates a complex of μ2 and λ3 (associated with viral [+] strand RNA).

Star-shaped, single-layered icosahedral non–genome-containing particles are seen using cryo-electron tomography in T3D-infected MA104 cells.[436] Based on their structural similarity to cystovirus φ8 procapsids that assemble prior to packaging of the φ8 dsRNA genome, the star-shaped reovirus particles are proposed to be intermediates in the assembly of viral core particles.[436] However, because the T3D strain used for this study has

a defect in assembly of intact genome-containing virions that correlates with a temperature-sensitive mutation in the viral μ2 protein,[336,396] another possibility is that star-shaped particles are defective assemblies.

Association of the reovirus μ2 protein with microtubules may promote viral RNA packaging and assembly by an as yet unknown mechanism.[396] The presence of paracrystalline arrays of genome-containing viral particles within VFs correlates with the capacity of μ2 to bind microtubules.[396] In T1L-infected BSC-1 cells, disruption of microtubules by treatment with nocodazole at 6 hours postinfection leads to loss of paracrystalline arrays of virions in VFs, a decrease in the ratio of full-to-empty particles, and a modest decrease in infectivity.

The reovirus outer capsid consists of 200 heterohexameric assemblies of the μ1 and σ3 proteins arranged in a T = 13 *laevo* lattice.[266] Coexpression of μ1 and σ3 in insect cells leads to formation of $\mu 1_3\sigma 3_3$ heterohexamers that can assemble onto cores *in vitro*.[76] Isolated σ3 purified from insect cells crystallizes as a dimer and is predicted to bind dsRNA as a dimer.[335] The $\mu 1_3\sigma 3_3$ heterohexamer structure (e-Fig. 11.4) indicates that monomers of μ1 must assemble into trimers before monomeric σ3 can bind to each of the three μ1:μ1 interfaces.[266] However, σ3 is found as approximately 140 kDa and 250 kDa homo-oligomers and as an approximately 400 kDa complex that corresponds to $\mu 1_3\sigma 3_3$ heterohexamers in infected cells when immunoprecipitated with a conformation-sensitive mAb. The homo-oligomeric forms of σ3 found in infected cells are larger than dimers. These oligomeric species of σ3 may be dimers bound to dsRNA or assemblies of σ3 larger than dimers in infected cells, potentially with dsRNA acting as a bridge.[237]

Proper folding of σ3 requires the chaperonin T-complex protein 1 (TCP-1) ring complex (TRiC).[237,238] TRiC is a barrel-shaped macromolecular assembly of two back-to-back stacked rings, each consisting of eight subunits. A central cavity within TRiC acts as a folding chamber that is regulated by binding and hydrolysis of ATP. In infected cells, TRiC redistributes to VFs and concentrates on their margins.[237] A network of chaperones interact with σ3, including Hsp70, Hsp90, and prefoldin. Prefoldin is a TRiC co-chaperone that prevents σ3 aggregation and enhances the transfer of unfolded σ3 to TRiC. The assembly of σ3 onto μ1 trimers to form $\mu 1_3\sigma 3_3$ heterohexamers requires TRiC and ATP, with TRiC acting as a holdase for near natively folded σ3 prior to its transfer to μ1 trimers.[238]

Host factors required for assembly of μ1 trimers are not known. However, chaperones are likely to be involved. μ1 associates with lipid droplets, the ER, and mitochondria in infected cells and when expressed alone, but it becomes diffusely distributed throughout the cytosol when coexpressed with σ3.[97] Whether membranes play a role in the assembly of μ1 trimers or the assembly of $\mu 1_3\sigma 3_3$ heterohexamers is unknown.

Assembly of trimers of the σ1 attachment protein requires the cellular chaperones Hsc70 and Hsp90.[169,262] Further assembly of the σ1 trimer onto core particles as part of the outer capsid requires that the λ2 turret initially be open and then close to lock the σ1 tail into place. This assembly reaction also may require cellular chaperones. The encapsidation of σ1 onto virions presumably occurs within VFs.

Release

Mechanisms governing reovirus egress from infected cells are not fully understood. It is likely that the virus is released from at least some types of cells following lysis by as yet unknown mechanisms. A large quantity of infectious virus remains associated with cellular debris following cell death, perhaps in association with VF matrices. Reovirus-induced apoptosis also may promote virus release from infected cells,[287] although the mechanism of release is unclear.

In some infected cells, virions are nonlytically released.[149,153,252] Nonlytic release of virions occurs from the apical surfaces of polarized human respiratory epithelial cells[149] and human brain microvascular endothelial cells.[252] Detailed ultrastructural and confocal microscopy studies of nonpolarized human brain microvascular endothelial cells found virions are released from regions of the basal membrane. This mechanism of nonlytic release involves the movement of genome-containing virions from the margins of VFs into modified lysosome-derived vesicular structures called sorting organelles (Fig. 11.8). Sorting organelles are recruited to the periphery of VFs during late phases of infection, where they collect mature genome-containing virions for transport to the plasma membrane. The genome-containing virions are attached to filaments that may facilitate virion transport into sorting organelles by an unknown mechanism. From the sorting organelle, virions bud into vesicles called membranous carriers that traffic to the plasma membrane, where they appear to fuse and release virions into the extracellular medium.[153] How virions breach the topological barrier and enter the sorting organelle is unclear.

RESPONSES OF THE HOST CELL TO INFECTION

Induction of Interferon and Effects on Viral Replication

Many types of viruses activate cellular sensors that recruit adaptor proteins to stimulate transcription factors ATF-2/c-Jun, interferon regulatory factor-3 (IRF3), and NF-κB, resulting in transcription and secretion of type I IFNs (IFN-α4 and IFN-β). Similar signal transduction networks stimulating IRF1 and IRF3 induce type III IFNs (IFN-λ1, -λ2, and -λ3) (Fig. 11.9). Secreted type I and type III IFNs bind to IFN-α/β and IFN-λ receptors, respectively, on the surface of infected and surrounding cells and, by so doing, activate Jak1 and Tyk2 kinases that phosphorylate and activate the transcription factors, STAT1 and STAT2. Activated STAT1 and STAT2 associate with IRF9 to form the heterotrimeric ISGF3 transcription complex, which translocates to the nucleus to induce transcription of hundreds of overlapping but distinct type I or type III IFN-stimulated genes (ISGs), some of which are antiviral, and one of which (IRF7) is a latent transcription factor (Fig. 11.9). When IRF7 is activated by virus-induced phosphorylation, it can form homodimers or heterodimers with IRF3 to induce multiple IFN-α subtypes and further induce other type I IFNs in a positive amplification loop.

Reovirus induction of IFN requires virion RNA, as fully assembled double-layered viral particles lacking the dsRNA genome (empty particles) fail to activate IRF3/7 or induce IFN.[200] Reovirus disassembly is required for induction of IFN,[222,433] but viral replication is dispensable.[200,433] The 2′-diphosphate found at the 5′-terminus of reovirus genomic RNA binds to and activates RIG-I to induce IFN.[183] However, RIG-I and MDA-5 can be activated by reovirus dsRNA gene segments of different lengths.[223] It remains unclear how the viral gene segments might be exposed during reovirus replication.

Reovirus can activate IRF3 but may sequester this transcription factor in viral factories to prevent its induction of IFN.[421] Such suppression is likely virus strain-specific.[433] While IRF3 is required for reovirus induction of IFN-β in at least some cell types,[199,327] IRF1 is not.[16] Multiple studies suggest cell type–specific requirements. For example, reovirus activation of IRF3/7 may require the sensor RIG-I and its adaptor MAVS[200] or may be mediated by either RIG-I or the related sensor MDA-5.[223,269] In myeloid dendritic cells (DCs), reovirus induction of IFN requires the helicase DHX9[500] or DHX33[267] or a complex of the helicases DDX1, DDX21, and DHX36 and the adaptor molecule TRIF.[495] In addition, reovirus can induce expression of some ISGs independent of IFN by activation of the PI3/Akt pathway.[447]

Reovirus induces secretion of IFN-β in immortalized cells[412] and primary cell cultures.[179,401] Reovirus induces significantly more IFN-β in cardiac myocytes than in cardiac fibroblasts in vitro[429] and in vivo,[264] likely as a consequence of differences in the basal expression of components of the IFN response, the resistance to activation in these cells, or a combination of both.[364,366,504] Reovirus induces detectable levels of only a subset of IFN-α subtypes in cardiac cells.[265]

The induction of IFN by reovirus also is regulated by viral proteins and may be virus strain-specific. The reovirus nonstructural protein σ1s does not affect induction of IFN.[344] Reovirus T3D induces significantly more IFN than does T1L, and this difference segregates with the M1, S2, and L2 gene segments.[401] The M1-encoded μ2 protein may modulate IFN levels by repressing IFN induction of IRF7, as mutation of this repressor function alters reovirus induction of IFN-β.[207] Variants of the T3D strain also can differ in the capacity to induce IFN and ISGs.[308] T3D variant–specific differences in induction of IFN segregate with the M1 and L3 gene segments.[254] Finally, the μ2 protein contains an immunoreceptor tyrosine-based activation motif (ITAM), which is essential for recruitment of the ITAM-signaling intermediate Syk to VFs for maximal activation of NF-κB and induction of IFN.[424]

The sensitivity of reovirus to the antiviral effects of IFN also is regulated by viral proteins and may be virus strain-specific. The reovirus nonstructural protein σ1s does not affect IFN signaling.[344] Reovirus T3D is more sensitive than T1L to the antiviral effects of IFN, and this phenotype also segregates with the M1, S2, and L2 gene segments.[401] The M1-encoded μ2 protein from T1L but not from T3D represses IFN signaling and is associated with nuclear accumulation of the transcription factor, IRF9.[505] A single amino acid polymorphism at μ2 residue 208 (proline in T1L, serine in T3D) determines the capacity of these viruses to repress IFN signaling.[207] Closely related T3D variants can vary in sensitivity to IFN, and this difference segregates with the S1 gene,[253] M1 and L2 genes,[254] and even a single L2-encoded amino acid.[385]

The reovirus S4-encoded σ3 protein binds dsRNA[335] and can modulate the type I IFN response.[38] The reovirus σ3 protein can prevent dsRNA-mediated activation of the antiviral ISG protein kinase R (PKR), which phosphorylates and inactivates eukaryotic translation initiation factor eIF2α.[490] However, PKR is activated by reovirus in IFN-treated cells[189] and is required to protect mice against reovirus-induced disease.[428] Interestingly, activation of PKR does not inhibit reovirus replication[497] and may benefit the virus.[413] Viral dsRNA also indirectly activates the ssRNA endonuclease RNase L, another antiviral ISG, in IFN-treated cells.[326] However, as for PKR, RNase L does not inhibit and may augment reovirus replication.[413]

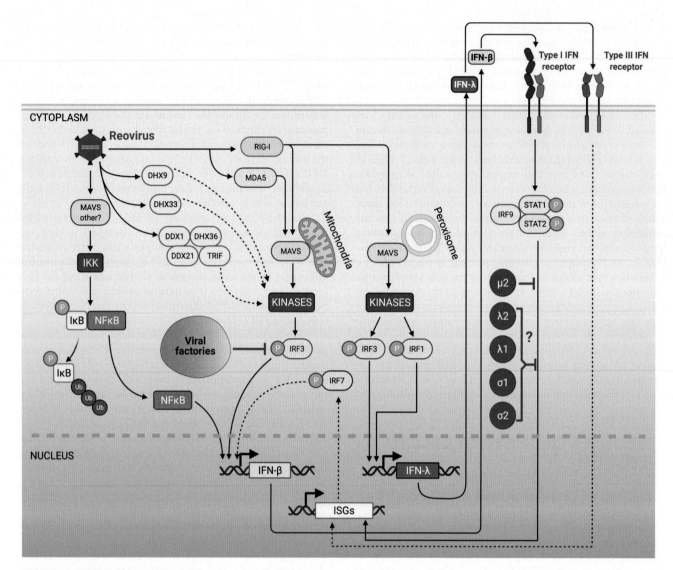

FIGURE 11.9 Reovirus induces interferon expression and represses interferon signaling. Reovirus activation of IRF3 and NF-κB for induction of interferon (IFN) is cell type–specific and uses several pathways. Reovirus 2'-diphosphate found at the 5' terminus of genomic RNA activates RIG-I or an undefined stimulus activates MDA-5. Activated mitochondria-associated MAVS induces phosphorylation of transcription factor IRF3 for induction of IFN-β. Activated peroxisome-associated MAVS induces phosphorylation of transcription factors IRF1 and IRF3 for induction of IFN-λ. Reovirus can sequester IRF3 in VFs to repress induction of IFN. Reovirus activation of NF-κB does not require RIG-I or MAVS, may use the classical or a novel NF-κB activation pathway, and can be regulated by μ1 and enhanced by μ2 ITAM recruitment of cellular Syk. Reovirus also activates DHX9, DHX33, or a complex of DDX1/DDX21/DHX36 and TRIF to induce IFN. Depending on cell type and virus strain, reovirus strain-specific differences in the induction of IFN are associated with the M1, L2, L3, and S2 gene segments, which encode μ2, λ2, λ1, and σ2, respectively. Reovirus strain-specific differences in sensitivity to IFN are associated with the M1, L2, L3, S1, and S2 gene segments. A single amino acid polymorphism in μ2 determines the capacity of this protein to repress IFN signaling, which affects induction of antiviral genes and further induction of IFN through a positive amplification loop. The σ3 protein is an RNA-binding protein that influences viral induction of IFN. The ISG IFITM3 inhibits reovirus infection by inhibiting viral disassembly in endosomes or endosomal membrane penetration. *Dotted arrows* indicate indirect pathways (TRIF, kinases) or pathways that occur later in infection for induction of additional IFN (amplification loop). *Question marks* indicate unknown proteins or unknown functions. (Figure prepared using BioRender.com.)

Inhibition of Cellular RNA and Protein Synthesis and Induction of Cellular Stress Responses

Some strains of reovirus inhibit the synthesis of cellular RNA and protein. The mechanism is not known, but viral replication is required. Reovirus strain-specific differences in this inhibition segregate with the σ3-encoding S4 gene segment. Reovirus inhibition of protein synthesis involves PKR and RNase L,[413] and virus strain-specific differences likely reflect the capacity of the σ3 protein to repress dsRNA-mediated activation of PKR.[206,268,490] The σ3 protein cannot bind dsRNA when complexed with the μ1 protein.[38,266,335,391,398,490] Thus, strain-specific differences in the efficiency of assembly of μ1:σ3 complexes could determine the intracellular distribution of free σ3 in infected cells and consequently inhibition of PKR.[391,489] In addition to inhibition of cellular protein synthesis, the preferential translation of reovirus mRNAs likely requires other mechanisms (see "Replication—Translation and Viral Factory Formation").

For example, reovirus transcripts produced later in infection may lack 5′ caps, although it is not clear whether this influences the preferential translation of reovirus transcripts. Reovirus infection also induces the formation of stress granules,[84,351,352,412] which sequester mRNAs and may prevent their translation. Finally, reovirus recruits ribosomal subunits and cell proteins required for translation into VFs, thus compartmentalizing reovirus translation from suppressed host cell translation.[124]

Reovirus T1L and one T3D strain[53] but not another T3D strain[365] alters the splicing of host cell mRNAs encoded by genes involved in mRNA posttranscriptional modifications. The μ2 protein from T1L, but not T3D strains that encode a serine at μ2 amino acid 208, forms a complex with the cellular mRNA splicing factor SRSF2 and alters its distribution within the nucleus.[365] Depletion of SRSF2 enhances reovirus replication, suggesting that reovirus modulation of SRSF2 benefits the virus.[365] The mechanism by which altered splicing might augment reovirus replication remains unclear, but the IFN pathway is not involved.[53,365]

Reovirus modulates other cellular RNA processes and proteins, likely to benefit viral replication. A potently myocarditic reovirus strain induces the degradation of heat-shock protein HSP25 in cardiac myocytes,[264] and reovirus induces expression of cellular secretogranin II, which enhances viral replication.[34] Reovirus induction and stabilization of host cell transcripts in the TGF-β signaling pathway is virus strain-specific and may influence host cell survival, but effects on viral replication are unclear.[188,422]

Inhibition of Cellular DNA Synthesis and Cell Cycle Progression

Some reovirus strains inhibit cellular DNA synthesis. Differences in the capacity of strains T1L and T3D to inhibit cellular DNA synthesis segregate with the S1 gene segment, which encodes the σ1 and σ1s proteins. Purified σ1 can arrest G_1-to-S progression, presumably by transducing signals following ligation of cell surface receptors.[306] While strain-specific differences in G_2/M arrest similarly segregate with the S1 gene segment,[347] this linkage reflects σ1s rather than σ1 stimulation of the inhibitory hyper-phosphorylation of cell cycle control kinase p34 (cdc2)[346] and requires the N-terminal domain of σ1s.[47] Analysis of strain-specific differences in reovirus-induced cellular gene expression by transcriptional profiling identify several genes that may be involved in reovirus modulation of G_1-to-S, G_2-to-M, as well as the mitotic spindle checkpoint.[345]

Activation of NF-κB and Induction of Apoptosis or Necroptosis

Apoptosis induced by reovirus is a major pathogenic mechanism underlying disease in infected mice (see "Pathogenesis and Pathology"). Reovirus infection leads to apoptosis in many cell lines[93,101,368,457] and primary cell cultures.[116] Although apoptosis can facilitate reovirus release from cells,[287] artificial lysis of cells in most studies may obscure the effects of apoptosis on viral yield.[116,368,457]

Reovirus strains vary in the capacity to induce apoptosis both in cell lines and primary cell cultures. For example, strains T3A and T3D induce greater apoptosis than does T1L, and this difference segregates with the S1 and M2 gene segments.[368,456,457] The failure of T1L to induce apoptosis in immortalized endothelial cells is not remedied by removal of the S1-encoded σ1s protein,[344] and a variant (T3C84) that does not express σ1s nonetheless

induces apoptosis in L929 cells.[369] Together, these data implicate the other S1-encoded protein, σ1, in the cell death response. Concordantly, ectopically expressed σ1[110] or μ1[97,105,418,477] can induce apoptosis. However, σ1s enhances reovirus T3D-induced apoptosis in multiple cell types,[47] suggesting that there may be cell type–specific requirements for the S1 gene products in evoking cell death. Cell type also may determine the effect of reovirus gene polymorphisms, as the M1 and M2 genes determine the capacity of reovirus to induce apoptosis in intestinal epithelial cells.[64] Reovirus induces apoptosis in ribavirin-treated cells,[100] and UV-inactivated virus[457] and empty particles[100] can induce apoptosis, demonstrating that neither viral RNA synthesis nor virion genomic dsRNA are required for apoptosis. Together, these data suggest that attachment, disassembly, and penetration are important steps in cell death induction by reovirus.

The S1-encoded σ1 protein of some reovirus strains binds to sialic acid as a first step in cell engagement,[23] which is followed by subsequent binding to JAM-A.[24] Sialic acid binding increases the efficiency of reovirus-induced caspase-independent cell death[197] and apoptosis,[99] likely by enhancing delivery of viral particles to the cytoplasm. Regardless of sialic acid–binding capacity, reovirus binding to JAM-A is required for apoptosis during infection.[24] However, uptake of antibody-coated reovirus into cells expressing Fc receptors leads to apoptosis,[106] suggesting that σ1 functions in reovirus-induced apoptosis by providing strong cell binding or routing the virus to an endocytic compartment where apoptotic signaling is initiated.

Apoptosis induced by reovirus virions is blocked by drugs that inhibit acid-dependent proteolytic disassembly, an effect that can be bypassed by *in vitro*–generated ISVPs.[100] These findings indicate that apoptosis induction requires virion-to-ISVP disassembly. Membrane penetration by the reovirus disassembly intermediate also is required for apoptosis.[108] However, membrane penetration likely serves primarily to deliver the μ1 effectors of apoptosis to the cytoplasm. A mutation in the ϕ domain of μ1 that does not affect membrane penetration decreases the strength of the proapoptotic signal, indicating that the ϕ domain of μ1 regulates apoptosis following penetration.[105] Concordantly, plasmid-based expression of the μ1 ϕ domain is sufficient to induce apoptosis.[97]

Apoptosis can be elicited by mitochondrial damage via the intrinsic pathway or activation of death receptors via the extrinsic pathway. In many cell types, reovirus infection activates both intrinsic and extrinsic apoptotic pathways (e-Fig. 11.6), although in some cell types, one mechanism may predominate.[115] The intrinsic apoptotic pathway requires activation of pro-apoptotic Bcl-2 family members Bak and Bax, which induce permeabilization of the outer mitochondrial membrane, resulting in release into the cytosol of cytochrome *c* and Smac/DIABLO. Cytochrome *c* couples with dATP in the cytosol to trigger oligomerization of Apaf-1 to form the apoptosome, which recruits and activates caspase-9. Caspase-9 proteolytically processes and activates effector caspase-3 and caspase-7. Smac/DIABLO represses inhibitor of apoptosis proteins (IAPs), which prevent activation of effector caspases. The extrinsic pathway is stimulated by ligand binding to cell surface death receptors. Death receptor oligomerization following ligand binding leads to recruitment of adaptor proteins (such as FADD) that form the death-inducing signaling complex (DISC). The DISC leads to activation of initiator caspase-8, which in turn activates effector caspase-3 and caspase-7. In some cells, activated caspase-8 also activates the intrinsic pathway by cleaving pro-apoptotic Bcl-2 family member Bid to form a truncated version of the molecule, called tBid, which associates with the outer mitochondrial membrane and stimulates oligomerization of Bak and Bax.

Reovirus infection induces the release of cytochrome *c* and Smac/DIABLO,[245] indicating intrinsic pathway activation. Moreover, overexpression of the antiapoptotic mitochondrial protein Bcl-2 blocks reovirus-induced apoptosis.[245,368] Reovirus infection also induces expression of TRAIL (a death receptor ligand) and DR5, a TRAIL receptor,[93] indicating extrinsic pathway activation. Treatment of cells with soluble TRAIL receptor or overexpression of a dominant-negative form of the adaptor protein FADD inhibits reovirus-induced apoptosis.[93,246] However, activation of the extrinsic pathway alone is insufficient for induction of apoptosis during reovirus infection and must be accompanied by activation of the intrinsic pathway to elicit a full response.[109,246]

The μ1 φ domain associates with the ER and mitochondria and can induce apoptosis in the absence of reovirus infection.[97] Apoptosis induced by either μ1 or reovirus infection occurs in cells lacking Bak and Bax, suggesting that in the presence of μ1, tBid is sufficient to disrupt mitochondrial membranes.[477] Interestingly, a peptide corresponding to the region of φ responsible for apoptosis can autonomously destabilize membranes,[233] raising the possibility that φ together with tBid directly mediates mitochondrial release of pro-apoptotic factors.

Reovirus-induced apoptosis requires the activation of NF-κB in most cell types[101,107] (e-Fig. 11.6). Interestingly, reovirus strains that induce apoptosis efficiently (e.g., T3A) or poorly (e.g., T1L) activate NF-κB early in infection, but efficiently apoptotic strains inhibit NF-κB activation late in infection,[91] at least in some cell types. Moreover, a poorly apoptotic strain (T1L) can induce apoptosis efficiently when NF-κB is inhibited late in infection.[94] Inhibition of NF-κB late in infection sensitizes cells to TRAIL-mediated apoptosis, linking NF-κB activation to the extrinsic pathway of apoptosis induction.[94] Additionally, NF-κB–induced expression of cFLIP, which inhibits caspase-8 activity, parallels reovirus early stimulation and late inhibition of NF-κB activation and attenuates apoptosis induced by T1L.[91] However, NF-κB also is required for reovirus-induced cleavage of Bid, which provides a plausible mechanism to connect NF-κB activation to the intrinsic pathway for reovirus-induced apoptosis.[109] Reovirus activation of NF-κB also likely regulates other events in both the extrinsic and intrinsic pathways.[113,333]

The mechanism by which reovirus activates NF-κB is likely dependent on virus strain and cell type. In unstimulated cells, NF-κB is sequestered in the cytoplasm by one of several isoforms of the repressor IκB. Following stimulation of the classical pathway of NF-κB activation, the heterotrimeric IκB kinase (IKK) complex, which is composed of IKKα, IKKβ, and IKKγ (Nemo), phosphorylates IκBα, leading to its ubiquitylation and degradation for release of active NF-κB. Following stimulation of the alternative pathway of NF-κB activation, a complex composed of IKKα and NIK phosphorylates an NF-κB latent component, p100, resulting in its cleavage to the activated NF-κB moiety p52. Expression of dominant-negative forms of IκB inhibit NF-κB activation and apoptosis induced by reovirus,[94,101] suggesting stimulation of the classical NF-κB activation pathway. However, reovirus-induced NF-κB activation and apoptosis require IKKα and IKKγ/Nemo and not the

third component of the classical pathway, IKKβ,[192] suggesting a novel mechanism for regulation of NF-κB by reovirus. Reovirus also can inhibit activation of NF-κB.[294] The φ domain of μ1 is thought to play a role in the activation of NF-κB, as recombinant viruses with mutations in φ (I595K and K594D) have reduced capacity to activate NF-κB.[105] These mutant viruses also are deficient in apoptosis induction. The mechanism by which the μ1 φ domain activates NF-κB is unknown. Finally, an ITAM in μ2 is essential for recruitment of the ITAM-signaling intermediate Syk to VFs, and the μ2 ITAM and Syk are both required for maximal activation of NF-κB.[424]

In contrast to most cells, reovirus-induced apoptosis in cardiac myocytes does not require NF-κB. Reovirus-induced apoptosis increases in cardiac myocytes when NF-κB is inhibited,[91] likely reflecting a requirement for NF-κB in the induction of antiviral cytokine IFN-β by reovirus. Similarly, reovirus-induced apoptosis increases in the heart of NF-κB p50-null mice relative to wild-type mice, and this effect can be ameliorated by treatment with IFN-β.[332] However, apoptosis is decreased in the brain of NF-κB p50-null mice, indicating that the role of NF-κB in reovirus-induced apoptosis *in vivo* is tissue-specific.[332]

Reovirus-induced apoptosis is regulated by additional cellular factors. Reovirus stimulates MEKK1 to activate c-Jun N-terminal kinase (JNK), resulting in phosphorylation and activation of transcription factor c-Jun.[95] JNK activation is required for efficient release of proapoptotic factors cytochrome *c* and Smac/DIABLO from mitochondria. Inhibitors of JNK block or delay reovirus-induced apoptosis.[95] However, c-Jun is not required for reovirus-induced apoptosis, and activated JNK can directly modulate the activities of mitochondrial proapoptotic and antiapoptotic proteins such as Bad, Bid, and Bim.[127] Thus, JNK may directly influence intrinsic apoptotic pathway activation in reovirus-infected cells.

Reovirus increases p53 levels and p53 translocation to mitochondria where it binds Bak and induces apoptosis in *ex vivo* brain slice cultures.[502] Reovirus also stimulates the innate immune response sensor MAVS for activation of transcription factor IRF3, and these signaling events are required for induction of maximum levels of apoptosis.[200] IRF3 and NF-κB, independently of IFN-β, induce Noxa, a proapoptotic BH3-only domain Bcl-2 family protein, and Noxa expression markedly enhances reovirus-induced apoptosis.[222,228,236] Reovirus activates the cellular protease calpain, and apoptosis is reduced by a calpain inhibitor.[117] Reovirus stimulates TGF-β signaling, and inhibition of this pathway reduces apoptosis.[30] Noxa, calpain, and TGF-β pathways also are modulated *in vivo*.[30,117,228] Reovirus induces Ras translocation to fragmented Golgi bodies in Ras-transformed cells to induce apoptosis.[166] In some cell types, reovirus can inhibit MAPK/ERK signaling, which results in a noncanonical, caspase-3–independent form of cell death.[371] Finally, reovirus stabilizes host cell transcripts encoded by multiple genes in the apoptosis pathway, offering another mechanism by which the virus may modulate cell death.[188]

Reovirus T3D also can induce the caspase-independent cell death pathway that leads to necroptosis.[36,37] Reovirus-induced necroptosis does not require activation of NF-κB but instead requires the kinase activity of receptor-interacting protein 1 (RIP1)[36] or RIP3.[37] In contrast to reovirus-induced apoptosis, which does not require viral RNA synthesis,[100] reovirus-induced necroptosis requires both cell sensing of incoming genomic

RNA for IFN signaling and efficient synthesis of dsRNA at later stages of infection.[37] Necroptosis does not alter reovirus replication, presumably because necroptosis occurs long after replication events are complete.[37] Knockdown of the reovirus μ1 protein enhances necroptosis.[372] Knockdown of the reovirus σ3 protein also enhances both induction of IFN and necroptosis, but surprisingly, this effect does not require the dsRNA-binding domain of σ3.[373]

PATHOGENESIS AND PATHOLOGY

Reovirus pathogenesis and host immune responses have been studied most extensively using neonatal mice (Fig. 11.10). These studies provide most of the information in this section.

Entry Into the Host

Reovirus infections in nature initiate in the enteric and respiratory tracts. Reoviruses bind to intestinal M (microfold) cells[178] or pulmonary M cells[313] in the epithelia and replicate and transit through these cells to reach underlying intestinal Peyer's patches or bronchus-associated lymphoid tissue. Concordantly, reovirus replication in the intestine is markedly reduced in the absence of M cells.[178] Reovirus binding to intestinal M cells requires interactions of the σ1 protein with glycoconjugates containing α2-3–linked sialic acid.[194] However, viral replication in the intestine is not dependent on binding to sialic acid[25] or JAM-A.[9] Binding to intestinal M cells by reovirus requires conversion of virions to ISVPs by intestinal proteases[7] (Fig. 11.10). Interestingly, ISVPs are formed efficiently in the intestine[44] but not the lung.[328] In comparison to intact virions, ISVPs inoculated perorally or intranasally lead to higher viral titers in the intestine[26] and the lung,[328] respectively. Moreover, pharmacologic inhibition of intestinal proteases blocks reovirus replication in the intestine.[7,26] However, while proteolytic enzymes resident in host tissues facilitate infection by many reovirus strains,[7,26,44,174,175] tissue proteases cleave the σ1 protein of some strains, including T3D, and thereby compromise infectivity.[320,329] Sequence polymorphisms that govern σ1 cleavage offer one likely mechanism for strain-specific differences in reovirus replication in the intestine[78] (see "Replication—Mechanism of Attachment"), although polymorphisms in the L2-encoded λ2 protein also are involved.[43] The L2 gene segment is similarly associated with the efficiency of reovirus shedding from the intestine and transmission to new hosts.[231]

Site of Primary Replication

Reovirus replicates in epithelial cells in the ileum[64] and the respiratory tract.[149] Virus infects intestinal epithelial cells in the crypts,[46] along the sides of the villi,[64] and at the villus tips[9,46] (Fig. 11.10). Reovirus preferentially infects respiratory epithelial cells basolaterally and is released apically,[149] ensuring egress of virus into the environment for host-to-host dissemination.

Antibiotic treatment of mice reduces reovirus replication in the intestine, suggesting that the intestinal microbiota enhance reovirus replication.[250] Interaction of the virus with bacterial surface polysaccharides may augment virus binding and infection of cells.[250] Indeed, reovirus plaque size is increased by the addition of positively charged moieties including the antibiotic neomycin, offering a mechanism by which antibiotics might increase rather than decrease reovirus replication in the intestine.[479] Finally, reovirus replication is enhanced by butyrate, an abundant metabolite produced by intestinal microbiota that represses type I IFN induction of ISGs, offering an alternative mechanism for bacterial enhancement of reovirus replication in the intestine.[83]

Spread of Virus

Reovirus can disseminate from a site of entry to distant sites within the host by hematogenous or neural routes. Access to lymphoid cells in Peyer's patches and bronchus-associated lymphoid tissue offers one potential mechanism for virus spread. T1 reoviruses access the CNS and other tissues primarily by hematogenous routes, perhaps by adhering to the lymphocyte surface.[454] However, these viruses also can infect and replicate in sensory neurons.[156] Hematogenous spread requires JAM-A expression on endothelial cells but not hematopoietic cells.[251] Reovirus is released preferentially from the apical surface of endothelial cells in the absence of lysis or apoptosis, providing a mechanism for viral entry into the bloodstream to facilitate hematogenous spread.[252] Reoviruses also can spread directly from Peyer's patches to the CNS. Reovirus strain type 3 clone 9 (T3C9) transits from Peyer's patches to adjacent neurons of the myenteric plexus and then through vagal autonomic nerves to the vagal dorsal motor nucleus in the brainstem.[315] In addition, T3 reoviruses can use hematogenous routes to access the CNS and other tissues.[9,45]

Neural spread of T3 reoviruses from a site of intramuscular inoculation to the spinal cord is inhibited by the type I IFN response,[272] although hematogenous dissemination from this site of inoculation also occurs.[45] Reovirus neural spread is not uniformly consistent with either fast or slow axonal transport.[45,454]

Spread by hematogenous or neural routes following intramuscular inoculation is dictated by the viral S1 gene segment,[454] which encodes viral attachment protein σ1 and nonstructural protein σ1s. The σ1 proteins of T1 and T3 reovirus strains bind JAM-A with similar affinities,[427] and both use JAM-A as a receptor.[24,70] Moreover, JAM-A is required for infection of endothelial cells by both serotypes.[9] Therefore, a difference in JAM-A usage does not explain virus strain-specific differences in hematogenous spread. Similarly, preference for hematogenous routes by viruses with a T1 S1 gene segment is not explained by the greater replication of T1L than T3D in cultured endothelial cells, as that capacity segregates with the T1L M1 rather than the S1 gene segment.[291] The σ1s protein is required for viremia and hematogenous spread of both T1 and T3 reoviruses,[45,46,49] likely reflecting both its inhibition of the type I IFN response in lymphatic cells[343] and its enhancement of viral protein expression.[344] However, σ1s is dispensable for neural spread.[45] Therefore, σ1s polymorphisms are not likely to explain preference for hematogenous spread. Instead, it is possible that differential binding of T1 and T3 reoviruses to a neural receptor yet to be identified determines the preference for neural spread. The capacity of T3 σ1 to bind sialic acid enhances the efficiency of viral dissemination[25] but does not significantly affect hematogenous spread.[160]

Cell and Tissue Tropism

Depending on the route of inoculation, reoviruses first replicate in the intestine, lung, or skeletal muscle and then spread to and replicate in the liver, spleen, heart, brain, and other

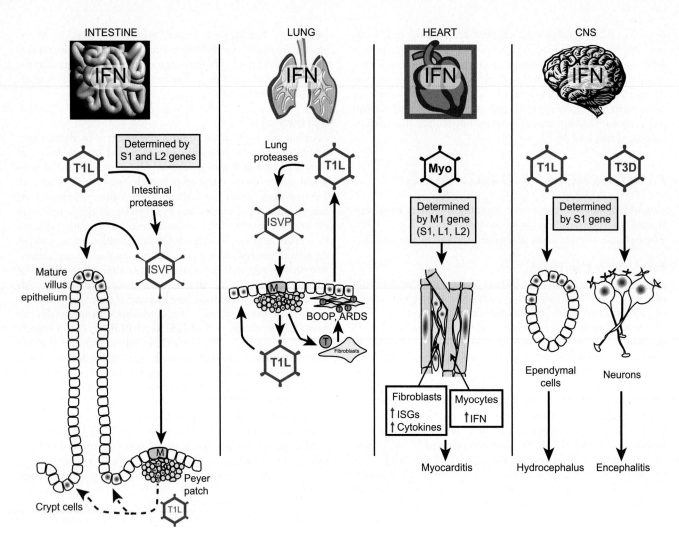

FIGURE 11.10 Viral and host factors determine reovirus tissue tropism. *Intestine.* Reovirus replication in the intestine requires conversion of virions to infectious subvirion particles (ISVPs), which is catalyzed by intestinal proteases. ISVPs can infect epithelial cells at the villus tips or infect and transit through M cells to underlying Peyer's patches to infect epithelial cells in the villus crypts. Virus can spread systemically by hematogenous or neural routes from Peyer's patch cells. Strain-specific differences in reovirus replication in the intestine segregate with the S1 and L2 genes. Virus-induced type I and type III interferons (IFNs) are essential for protection of intestinal tissue against reovirus infection. *Lung.* Reovirus replication in the lung also requires virion-to-ISVP disassembly, which is catalyzed by airway-resident proteases. Following infection and transport through M cells to underlying bronchus-associated lymphoid tissue, virus infects epithelial cells basally and is released apically. Virus-stimulated T cells induce epithelial cell apoptosis and fibrosis, resulting in either bronchiolitis obliterans organizing pneumonia (BOOP) or acute respiratory distress syndrome (ARDS). *Heart.* Some reovirus strains infect and damage cardiac myocytes, leading to myocarditis. Strain-specific polymorphisms in the M1 gene segment dictate differences in virus induction of, and sensitivity to type I IFN, which consequently influence the capacity of reovirus to cause myocarditis. Cardiac myocytes synthesize high levels of type I IFN, while cardiac fibroblasts synthesize high levels of antiviral IFN-stimulated genes (ISGs) and cytokines, offering an integrated network for organ protection. The S1, L1, and L2 genes are also determinants of strain-specific differences in myocarditic potential. *Central nervous system (CNS).* Reovirus infects the CNS, but strains of different serotypes vary in the capacity to infect discrete populations of cells in the brain. The reovirus S1 gene segment, which encodes attachment protein σ1 and nonstructural protein σ1s, determines cell tropism within the CNS. The capacity of reovirus to infect ependymal cells and neurons, leading to hydrocephalus or encephalitis, respectively, is likely influenced by both σ1 and σ1s.

organs. Tissue tropism in mice is influenced by both age and virus strain.[167] In addition, host factors required for reovirus replication influence pathogenesis. For example, reovirus intracellular disassembly is mediated by endosomal cathepsins B,[143] L,[143] or S,[173] depending on the cell type (see "Replication— Uncoating"). In comparison to wild-type mice, peak reovirus titers in cathepsin B-null mice following peroral inoculation are similar in the intestine but lower in the heart and brain and thus mortality is decreased.[219] Similarly, compared with wild-type mice, peak reovirus titers in perorally inoculated mice lacking cathepsins L or S also are diminished at sites of secondary replication, but mortality is increased,[219] consistent with the requirement for these enzymes in cell-mediated immunity.

Capsid stability can profoundly affect reovirus pathogenesis.[137] A Y354H mutation in σ3 decreases capsid stability but dramatically increases myocarditis and inflammatory cytokines in cardiac tissue and increases viral transmission to littermates. Together, these results demonstrate the significant effect of uncoating efficiency on reovirus pathogenesis.

Central Nervous System

T1 reoviruses infect the ependymal cells lining the ventricles in neonatal mice, which results in ependymitis and hydrocephalus.[468] In contrast, T3 reoviruses infect neurons in these animals, replicate to high titers in the brain, and induce a lethal meningoencephalitis.[468] T3 reoviruses also damage spinal cord neurons resulting in acute flaccid paralysis.[181] T3 reoviruses use macropinocytosis of vesicles containing multiple virions for entry into neurons followed by primarily retrograde fast axonal transport to reach the soma for replication.[11] The capacity to bind and infect ependymal cells[440] or neurons[128] and the resulting disease phenotypes are determined by the S1 gene segment (Fig. 11.10). T1 and T3 reoviruses use different glycans as coreceptors. T1 reovirus infection of ependymal cells and induction of hydrocephalus requires T1-specific σ1 engagement of the GM2 glycan on those cells.[426] Infection of neurons in the brain does not require JAM-A[9] or sialic acid,[75] although binding to sialylated glycans as coreceptors enhances reovirus replication in neural tissues and neurovirulence.[160] Instead, infection of neurons requires the Nogo receptor NgR1.[248] Interestingly, ISVPs do not bind NgR1, suggesting that binding is mediated by either σ3, which is lost during formation of ISVPs, or a virion-associated conformer of σ1.[248] Variants selected for resistance to σ1-specific mAbs are attenuated, and one mutant (variant K) retains tropism for the hippocampus but has reduced tropism for the cortex[362,420] (see "Stages of Replication—Determinant of Neutralizing Antibody Responses"). The σ1s protein is dispensable for reovirus replication in the brain,[46,203] but it influences apoptosis and tissue damage in that organ[203] and is required for full neurovirulence.[47] Therefore, it is likely that both σ1 and σ1s contribute to S1-determined differences in reovirus-induced CNS disease.

T3 reoviruses induce apoptosis in neuronal cultures, brain slice cultures, and the brain.[29,105,109,134,179,180,203,362,363] A reovirus mutant lacking the capacity to induce apoptosis is less neurovirulent,[350] and a reovirus mutant with a single amino acid substitution in the φ domain of the M2-encoded μ1 protein that has diminished proapoptotic signaling also is less neurovirulent.[105] Although the majority of apoptotic cells in the CNS are infected, the presence of uninfected apoptotic cells nearby suggests that reovirus also can cause death in bystander cells.[361]

Reovirus-induced apoptosis involves both extrinsic and intrinsic pathways (see "Responses of the Host Cell to Infection—Activation of NF-κB and Induction of Apoptosis or Necroptosis"). Reovirus activates NF-κB in the brain, and apoptosis is significantly diminished in the CNS of NF-κB p50-null mice.[332] Activation of NF-κB is required for reovirus-induced cleavage and activation of the proapoptotic protein, Bid, and reovirus replication and histopathologic injury in brain are substantially reduced in Bid-deficient mice.[109] Additionally, reovirus-induced apoptosis, but not viral replication, is diminished in the CNS of mice lacking the pro-apoptotic Bcl-2 protein, Bax.[35] Reovirus induces p53 translocation to mitochondria and binding to Bak to induce apoptosis in neurons in brain slice cultures and mouse brains.[502] Reovirus replication, CNS injury, and spread within the CNS also are reduced and survival enhanced in mice lacking effector caspase-3,[31] and

a pan-caspase inhibitor decreases reovirus-induced apoptosis in brain slice cultures.[134] Reovirus also activates JNK, which up-regulates Fas, and chemical inhibitors of JNK attenuate reovirus-induced encephalitis.[29,90] Finally, reovirus-induced type I IFN up-regulates Daxx in murine cortical neurons, which can be pro- or antiapoptotic depending on its intracellular location.[135]

Reoviruses induce multiple protective responses in the CNS. Gene expression associated with type I IFN signaling is induced early in infection, while other cytokines and apoptotic pathways are induced later in infection.[92,133,134,452] Reovirus activates the JAK-STAT pathway[179] and induces ISGs[201] in the brain, and type I IFN signaling determines reovirus tropism in the brain and lethality.[133,179] Reovirus-induced secretion of IFN from infected neurons activates and induces apoptosis in astrocytes,[96] but activation of microglia and their increased expression of inflammatory mediators is IFN-independent.[390] The type I IFN response contributes to age-dependent susceptibility to encephalitis.[480] Reovirus increases nitric oxide (NO) production and expression of inducible nitric oxide synthase (iNOS), which regulate reovirus replication in CNS tissue.[180] Reovirus-induced type II IFN (IFN-γ) induces cytoskeletal changes that compromise the blood–brain barrier.[50] Finally, reovirus activates TGF-β receptor I and its signaling effector SMAD3 as well as another TGF-β superfamily member, bone morphogenetic protein (BMP) receptor I, and its effector SMAD1 in CNS tissue, and both pathways inhibit reovirus induced apoptosis in the CNS.[30]

Heart

Reovirus-induced cardiac damage in neonatal mice is caused by a direct cytopathic effect on cardiac cells[28,400] (Fig. 11.10). Reovirus myocarditis is not mediated by adaptive immunity, as reovirus infection causes myocarditis in nude mice, which lack T cells, and in SCID mice, which lack both B and T cells.[400] Studies of reoviruses that vary in myocarditic potential indicate that the extent of myocardial damage correlates with cytopathic effect in primary cultures of cardiac myocytes,[28] and viral replication is required for disease.[232] Reoviruses that fail to induce myocarditis in immunocompetent mice also fail to do so in SCID mice,[400] indicating that cardiac pathology is not induced by an adaptive immune response but instead reflects virus interactions with cardiac cells.

The type I IFN response regulates reovirus-induced myocarditis. Cardiac myocytes express higher basal levels of type I IFN than do cardiac fibroblasts, likely as a prearming protective mechanism.[364] The capacity of reovirus strains to induce myocarditis correlates inversely with induction of and sensitivity to type I IFN in cardiac myocytes.[401] Moreover, nonmyocarditic reovirus strains induce cardiac pathology in mice when type I IFN induction[199,332,401] or IFN-induced gene expression[16,428] is inhibited. Myocarditic capacity segregates primarily with the reovirus M1 gene segment but also is influenced by the S1, L1, and L2 gene segments.[399] The M1 gene segment determines reovirus strain-specific differences in replication in cardiac myocytes,[292] which is regulated by type I IFN responses.[207,401] The M1-encoded μ2 protein can repress IFN signaling,[505] a property determined by a single sequence polymorphism in μ2 at amino acid 208.[207] Substitution at that position modulates reovirus induction of type I IFN, replication in cardiac myocytes, and myocardial injury.[207] Therefore, the strength of the type I

IFN response and viral subversion of IFN effects are critical determinants of virus strain–specific differences in damage to the heart.

Reovirus strain–specific differences in apoptosis induction in primary cardiac myocyte cultures correlate with the capacity to induce myocarditis.[91,114–116,304] Myocarditic reovirus strains activate the extrinsic apoptotic pathway much more than they do the intrinsic pathway,[115] and calpain or caspase inhibitors dramatically reduce reovirus-induced cardiac damage in neonatal mice.[114,116] As is the case in the CNS, the σ1s protein is dispensable for reovirus replication in the heart, but it influences apoptosis and tissue damage in that organ.[203] Thus, death of cardiac myocytes during reovirus-induced myocarditis appears to occur as a consequence of apoptosis.

Patterns of reovirus-induced gene expression in the heart vary according to virus strain and cardiac cell type. The capacity to induce cardiac lesions correlates with cytopathic effect in primary cultures of cardiac myocytes but not cardiac fibroblasts.[28] Myocarditic reovirus strains preferentially induce apoptosis of cardiac myocytes relative to cardiac fibroblasts, while nonmyocarditic reoviruses induce the converse.[304] Nonmyocarditic reoviruses also induce cytokines in cardiac fibroblasts that likely contribute to disease outcome *in vivo*.[304] Reovirus activation of NF-κB[366] and induction of type I IFN and ISG[265,429,504] expression also differs between cardiac myocytes and cardiac fibroblasts (Fig. 11.10). Reovirus-induced changes in the cardiac myocyte proteome also differ between virus strains and correlate with the capacity to induce myocarditis.[265] Finally, a mutation that does not affect reovirus replication in the heart nonetheless increases expression of inflammatory mediators and dramatically increases cardiac tissue damage, indicating that immune-mediated mechanisms can be damaging during reovirus infection.[137] Thus, reovirus cardiac damage reflects an array of host responses determined by both viral and cardiac cell factors.

Hepatobiliary System and Diabetes

Neonatal mice infected with some T3 reovirus strains develop oily fur syndrome, appearing as though they have been dipped in oil.[25,123,474] This condition is associated with viral replication in intrahepatic bile duct epithelium, leading to biliary obstruction and fat malabsorption that in some respects resembles human infantile biliary atresia. For at least one reovirus strain, this disease reflects immune-mediated injury to the bile duct.[319] Differences in the capacity of reovirus strains to induce oily fur syndrome segregate with the S1 gene segment,[474] and reovirus binding to sialic acid is required for biliary tract damage and oily fur syndrome.[25] Mutations in the M2 gene segment can abrogate the capacity to induce this disease, although the mechanism underlying this effect is unclear.[123] Finally, type III IFN protects bile ducts and can influence tissue tropism.[277]

Nonobese diabetic (NOD) mice provide a model system for investigation of type I diabetes mellitus, an autoimmune disease resulting from destruction of pancreatic β cells. In neonatal NOD mice, reovirus strain T3A infects pancreatic islet cells and prevents the development of diabetes but not insulitis (the recruitment of CD8+ T cells and macrophages to pancreatic islets by autoreactive CD4+ T cells).[472] These findings suggest that T3A-induced cytopathic effect and release of antigens from β cells leads to tolerance by induction of regulatory T cells, thereby delaying the onset of diabetes.

Lung

Reovirus strain T1L inoculated intranasally into adult mice induces two different types of pulmonary tissue damage and fibrosis, which model distinct forms of lung disease in humans (Fig. 11.10). T1L can induce bronchiolitis obliterans organizing pneumonia (BOOP), which is characterized by inflammation and intra-alveolar fibrosis.[282] However, a 10-fold higher dose of T1L induces acute respiratory distress syndrome (ARDS), which is characterized by an acute phase with severe inflammation and a chronic phase with persistent intra-alveolar and interstitial fibrosis.[15,282] T1L stimulates infiltration of T cells, which induce apoptosis of epithelial cells in both BOOP and ARDS.[270] However, the Fas/FasL pathway is required only for the development of BOOP, not ARDS.[270]

Juvenile rats inoculated intratracheally with T1L also develop an acute pneumonia, characterized by degeneration of terminally differentiated type I alveolar epithelial cells, type II alveolar epithelial cell hyperplasia to replace the destroyed type I cells, and infiltration of leukocytes.[314] Inoculation with T3D induces a similar pattern of pneumonia but with a more prominent neutrophil infiltrate. Both reovirus strains replicate in type I epithelial cells, but T1L achieves higher titers. The capacity to induce neutrophil infiltration segregates with the T3D S1 gene segment, while replication to high titers segregates with the T1L S1 gene segment.[314] In mice, T3D promotes EpA2-dependent phosphorylation of the NLRP3 inflammasome, preventing its activation and reducing viral clearance.[499] The capacity to replicate to high titers in the lung can be determined by σ1 sensitivity to lung protease-mediated loss (rather than enhancement) of infectivity, while the capacity to disseminate to secondary sites can be influenced by the σ1s protein.[329]

Reovirus infection of primary human airway epithelial cell cultures is more efficient following basolateral as opposed to apical adsorption of virus and is dependent on JAM-A.[149] Despite a preference for basolateral entry, reovirus is released from the apical surface of respiratory epithelial cells and does not disrupt tight junctions.[149] These results suggest that epithelial cells are not the primary cell type responsible for systemic spread of reovirus from the respiratory tract to distant sites within the host.

Airway-resident proteases capable of catalyzing reovirus disassembly enhance infection in the lung. Type II transmembrane serine proteases expressed in human airways facilitate reovirus uncoating and infection *in vitro*. However, murine homologs of these enzymes are inefficient *in vivo*, likely reflecting repression by endogenous protease inhibitors.[328] Reovirus induces neutrophil infiltration in the lung,[314] and the serine protease neutrophil elastase[175] as well as other inflammatory proteases facilitate reovirus uncoating and infection *in vitro*.[328]

Reovirus Genetic Determinants of Tropism and Tissue Injury

Reovirus strains differ in the capacity to infect specific organs and produce tissue-specific disease in neonatal mice. Gene segments that segregate with such differences in reovirus pathogenesis have been identified in many cases (Fig. 11.10). The S1 and L2 gene segments determine the magnitude of reovirus replication in the intestine and efficiency of viral shedding in the stool. The S1 gene segment determines whether reovirus infects CNS neurons resulting in encephalitis or ependymal cells resulting in hydrocephalus, although the M2 gene segment influences neurovirulence. The M1 gene segment is the predominant determinant of the capacity of reovirus to cause myocarditis, although the S1, L1, and L2 gene segments influence the extent of cardiac damage. Results of experiments using adult SCID mice, which lack B cells and T cells, are largely consistent with studies using neonatal mice but provide several additional associations between specific reovirus gene segments and infection in the intestine, heart, and CNS and identify the M1, L1, and L2 gene segments as determinants of liver damage.[191]

Innate Immune Responses

Cells infected by reovirus express an array of innate protective responses, including cytokines, chemokines, and iNOS (see "Responses of the Host Cell to Infection"). Reovirus induces mast cell secretion of cytokines including IFNs[334] to recruit cytotoxic T cells[293] and recruit and activate natural killer (NK) cells.[348] Reovirus σ1 binds human NKp46 and the mouse homolog NCR1 on NK cells resulting in activation of these cells for oncolytic activity.[22] However, NK cells appear neither necessary[218] nor sufficient[190,441] to clear the virus. Neutrophils are recruited to reovirus-infected tissues,[314] but their importance in reovirus clearance has not been defined.

The type I IFN response is essential for protection against reovirus infection (see "Responses of the Host Cell to Infection—Interferon Induction and Effects on Viral Replication, and Tissue Tropism, Damage, and Disease"). Reovirus T3D replication is decreased in multiple organs in mice lacking tripartite motif-29 (TRIM29), a negative regulator of the IFN response.[481] Following peroral inoculation with strain T1L, type I IFN produced by DCs in Peyer's patches protects the intestinal mucosa and lymphoid cells, clears the virus, and prevents death.[218] Consistent with studies implicating RIG-I in reovirus induction of IFN[200] but in contrast to those implicating MDA-5,[223,269] reovirus replicates to higher titers in many tissues of mice lacking MAVS but not mice lacking MDA-5.[183] Also consistent with a requirement for RIG-I–like receptor (RLR) sensing, mice lacking either TLR3 or MyD88, which is an effector molecule for non-TLR3 Toll-like receptors, do not differ from wild-type mice in response to peroral T1L infection.[218] While infection of the T84 intestinal epithelial cell line suggests that intact reovirus virions can be sensed by both TLRs and RLRs, ISVPs are the natural viral form in the intestine and likely sensed exclusively by RLRs,[422] consistent with results gathered from *in vivo* studies. Interestingly, ISVPs induce the prosurvival cytokine TGF-β in T84 cells, suggesting that reovirus induces responses that prolong viral enteric replication and transmission.[422]

The type III IFN (IFN-λ) response also plays an essential protective role against reovirus infection.[258] After reovirus is sensed by RLRs, subsequent activation of mitochondria-associated MAVS induces type I IFN, while activation of peroxisome-associated MAVS induces IFN-λ[331] (Fig. 11.9). As intestinal epithelial cells differentiate, they express a greater number of peroxisomes and, accordingly, yield a more robust IFN-λ response.[331] While type I and type III IFNs induce expression of distinguishable but overlapping sets of antiviral genes, their effects differ dramatically as the type I IFN receptor is expressed on most cells, while the IFN-λ receptor is expressed primarily on epithelial cells. In the intestine, this IFN receptor expression pattern results in a compartmentalized protective IFN response, where the type III IFN receptor on intestinal epithelial cells provides a first barrier to infection, while type I IFN signaling prevents subsequent spread from the intestinal lamina propria.[19,277,342,348]

Activation of NF-κB by reovirus is required for the induction of IFN-β, which in turn protects against reovirus-induced encephalitis[133,179] and myocarditis.[199,332,401,424] However, in reovirus-infected mice, the role of NF-κB in disease pathogenesis is organ-specific. Apoptosis following reovirus infection is reduced in the brains of mice lacking the NF-κB p50 subunit,[332] consistent with a pro-apoptotic role for NF-κB in reovirus infection of the CNS. In contrast, reovirus replication and apoptosis are increased in the hearts of p50-deficient mice, and these effects are prevented by treatment with IFN-β.[332] These observations are consistent with induction of NF-κB–independent apoptosis by reovirus in cardiac myocytes[91] and the importance of IFN-β in protection against reovirus-induced myocarditis.[401] In transformed cells, Ras enhances reovirus replication at least in part by suppressing RIG-I–mediated induction of IFN-β[403] (see "Reovirus Oncolytics").

Adaptive Immune Responses

Reovirus replicates to high titers in neonatal mice, but replication in adult immunocompetent mice is modest and requires inoculation with high doses of virus. In contrast, reovirus replicates to high titers and is lethal in adult SCID mice (B-cell– and T-cell–deficient), and passive transfer of lymphocytes protects these animals against lethal infection.[21,190,441] Together, these results suggest that the adaptive immune response influences the age-dependent restriction of reovirus replication and disease in mice. However, reovirus also can induce immune cell–mediated pathology.

Reovirus strains T1L and T3D do not replicate in peripheral blood mononuclear cells (PBMCs) or DCs derived from PBMCs *in vitro*,[136,147,157] although these strains do replicate in THP-1 human monocyte cells.[151] Instead, DCs adsorbed with reovirus *in vitro* become loaded with viral antigen[157] and express cell surface markers and cytokines characteristic of DC activation.[147] Reovirus-exposed DCs, but not reovirus alone, activate a majority of T cells for antigen-independent cytolytic activity and NK cells for perforin/granzyme-mediated cytolysis.[147] Activation of T cells requires direct cell-to-cell contact with DCs, while activation of NK cells is mediated by DC-secreted soluble factors[147] or reovirus σ1 binding to NKp46/NCR1 on NK cells.[22]

The intestinal immune system includes inductive (Peyer's patches and mesenteric lymph nodes) and effector (lamina propria and intraepithelial lymphocytes [IEL]) sites. Following peroral inoculation, reovirus T1L infects epithelial cells in the intestine resulting in activation of DCs in Peyer's patches.[218] Peyer's patch DCs exposed to reovirus T1L *in vivo* can activate reovirus-primed CD4+ T cells *in vitro*[157] and likely also activate T cells in the intestine. Reovirus T1L-activated T cells in Peyer's patches migrate to the lamina propria and intraepithelial sites.[40] These activated T cells use perforin, Fas-FasL, and TRAIL pathways for cytolysis, but effector utilization is dependent on the mucosal site from which the T cells are harvested.[40] Depletion experiments indicate that CD8+Thy-1+ T cells expressing the αβ TCR mediate IEL CTL activity.[104]

The humoral immune response to reovirus is important in protection of the intestine, mediating clearance following primary infection and prevention of secondary infection. Reovirus is cleared from the intestines of adult wild-type and β2 microglobulin-null (CD8+ T-cell–deficient) mice but not SCID (B-cell– and T-cell–deficient) and MuMT (B-cell– and antibody-deficient) mice.[21,190,284,441] Reovirus T1L inoculated perorally into adult mice induces intestinal IgA and serum IgG.[406] Viable or UV-inactivated reovirus T3D induces polymeric immunoglobulin receptor expression in HT29 human intestinal epithelial cells,[338] suggesting a possible mechanism for intestinal IgA secretion. During primary infection, reovirus T1L is cleared equally well from the intestines of IgA-null mice and wild-type mice. However, following subsequent challenge, reovirus T1L invades Peyer's patches of IgA-null but not wild-type animals,[406] consistent with a protective role for IgA during reinfection. However, the secretory antibody response also can enhance reovirus replication in the intestine by controlling the intestinal microbiota and microbiota-induced inflammatory cytokines.[449]

Studies using exogenous effectors offer additional insights into the importance of antibodies in protection of the intestine against reovirus infection. Oral introduction of IgA or IgG specific for the σ1 protein protects Peyer's patches from reovirus T1L infection.[204,406] Adoptive transfer of splenic lymphocytes derived from reovirus immune mice inhibits reovirus strain T3C9 replication in the intestine, but the efficacy is diminished if B cells are depleted prior to transfer, indicating that antibody responses are important for protection.[21] Intraperitoneal introduction of reovirus-specific polyclonal antiserum or IgG2a mAb into MuMT mice leads to clearance of T3C9.[21]

Antibody and immune cells protect against reovirus infection at distinct stages of the virus–host encounter. Following systemic administration, neutralizing mAbs specific for the σ1 protein do not inhibit primary replication of reovirus T3C9 in the intestine or T3D in skeletal muscle. However, these antibodies potently inhibit viral spread from both of those sites to the spinal cord.[458] Even when administered after virus has reached the spinal cord, antibody prevents viral spread to the brain. Antibody also inhibits replication in the brain following intracranial inoculation of T3D[458,463] and spread from the brain to the eye, spinal cord, and muscle.[458] Similarly, mAbs that do not inhibit T1L replication in skeletal muscle inhibit viremia and replication in the brain.[453] Together, these results indicate that antibody can mediate protection by blocking steps in viral pathogenesis following primary replication.

Adoptive transfer of adult immune spleen cells protects neonatal mice from T3C9 inoculated perorally, T3D inoculated parenterally, and T1L (but not T3D) inoculated intracranially.[464] Depletion of CD4+ or CD8+ T cells leads to significantly increased replication of T3C9 and T3D. Adoptive transfer of immune cells is more effective than mAbs in inhibiting viral replication, while the converse is true for inhibiting reovirus neural spread.[464]

The route of reovirus inoculation is an important determinant of both humoral and cell-mediated immune responses. Peroral inoculation of reovirus T1L induces predominantly IgA in Peyer's patches, while parenteral inoculation of that strain induces predominantly IgG2a in peripheral lymph nodes.[283] However, peroral inoculation of T1L induces IFN-γ and other Th1 cytokines but minimal Th2 cytokines.[150] Peroral inoculation of T1L also induces serum IgG2a, characteristic of a Th1 response, while parenteral inoculation induces both IgG1 and IgG2a, although this effect is MHC haplotype-specific.[283] Finally, peroral inoculation of T1L suppresses the expression of Th2 cytokines IL-4 and IL-10 in draining lymphatic tissues early in infection, and treatment with IL-4 or IL-10 decreases serum IgG2a relative to IgG1.[290] Thus, peroral inoculation of reovirus suppresses Th2 cytokines and promotes a Th1-biased cell-mediated immune response. Concordantly, PBMCs from volunteers presumed to have been infected with reovirus in the past express recall responses when exposed to reovirus that are dominated by strong Th1-like and minimal Th2-like cytokine expression.[136] Interestingly, the requirements for specific PBMC subsets and ligand interactions to elicit cytokine responses are dependent on the virus strain used for stimulation.[136] The route of inoculation also is a determinant of TCR use by CD8+ T cells. Inoculation of reovirus T1L perorally or parenterally favors the use of TCR variable gene segment Vβ6. However, peroral inoculation restricts TCR Jβ gene segment usage, suggesting an even greater limitation on TCR specificity.[161]

Reovirus can induce immune cell-mediated pathology, as noted in mouse models of reovirus-associated lung disease, bile duct damage, and autoimmune insulitis. Reovirus virulence in mice is modulated by LRRK2, which is genetically linked to inflammatory disorders.[404] In mice, reovirus can cause loss of immunological tolerance to dietary antigens that is similar to the immune disruption observed in persons with celiac disease[56] (see "Clinical Features—Celiac Disease"). The underlying mechanism likely reflects reovirus induction of IRF1 in lamina propria DCs causing secretion of cytokines that stimulate differentiation of T_H1 cells that recognize dietary antigen. Type I IFN further induces IRF1 to inhibit maturation of the regulatory T cells that normally block development of T_H1 responses to mediate oral tolerance.

EPIDEMIOLOGY

Epidemiologic surveys for the presence of reovirus antibodies in diverse populations suggest that most humans have been exposed to reovirus and that infection occurs early in childhood. However, reovirus infections are rarely symptomatic. In one study of healthy European volunteers ranging in age from 6 months to over 60 years, the frequency of individuals with detectable IgG antibodies specific for reovirus rose with increasing age.[394] Prevalence was approximately 35% in infants 6 months to 1 year, approximately 60% in individuals 11 to 19 years, and approximately 75% to 85% in individuals 20 years and older with no apparent decline after 60 years of age. In a study of healthy U.S. children ranging in age from birth to 6 years, there was rapid loss of maternal antibody as evidenced by declining seroprevalence from 75% (6 of 8) in infants 0 to 3 months of age to 11% (1 of 9) in those from 3 to 6 months of age.[438] In contrast to the earlier study, none of the individuals 6 months to 1 year of age were seropositive. Seroprevalence increased in the remaining individuals, ranging from 8% (4/49) in 1- to 2-year-olds to 50% (11/22) in 5- to 6-year-olds. Thus, while results from individual studies vary, reovirus infections are common before adulthood.

Nonfusogenic mammalian orthoreoviruses infect a wide variety of species including swine[103,496] and cattle.[103] However, the significance of reovirus as a food animal pathogen is unclear. Reovirus infections also are common in dogs,[118,205] and reoviruses can be isolated from dogs with respiratory or enteric symptoms. However, experimental infections have not provided conclusive evidence that these viruses are pathogenic in dogs,[67] suggesting that concomitant infections with other agents are required to produce disease. Reovirus infections are common in both wild[341] and domesticated[103,393] cats, and reoviruses can be mildly pathogenic in experimentally infected feline species.[305,393] Reovirus was isolated from a white-tailed deer fawn with enteric symptoms,[3] but the significance and prevalence remains unclear.

Fusogenic orthoreoviruses infect birds, mammals, and reptiles. Fusogenic bat reoviruses can be isolated from humans with clinical symptoms[85–87] and, in one study, 13% of individuals frequently exposed to fruit bats were seropositive[85] (see "Clinical Features—Pneumonia"). Additional studies will be required to clarify the prevalence and clinical importance of these zoonotic events.

CLINICAL FEATURES

Reovirus Infections of Humans

Despite its broad host range, reovirus infections in humans and other animals are rarely symptomatic. When reoviruses do produce symptoms, the most common manifestations are coryza, pharyngitis, and cough[85,212,465] and gastroenteritis.[170,298,430] Human challenge studies conducted in the 1960s demonstrated that inoculation of reovirus strains representing each of the three serotypes by nasal instillation led to seroconversion in most cases, but only T1 reovirus was associated with significant disease.[380] Three of eight previously seronegative individuals infected with T1 reovirus developed headache, pharyngitis, sneezing, rhinorrhea, cough, and malaise. A fourth individual developed loose stools but was otherwise asymptomatic. Eight of nine individuals infected with T3 reovirus had positive stool cultures.[380] One infected individual developed mild rhinitis, but the others remained well.

Biliary Atresia

Reovirus infection has been associated with neonatal biliary atresia, which occurs in about 1 in 10,000 live births in the United States. Biliary atresia is characterized by progressive inflammatory obliteration of extrahepatic and intrahepatic bile ducts hypothesized to be precipitated by an environmental insult like a viral infection that triggers inflammatory destruction of bile duct epithelium. In a study conducted in Denver, Colorado, reovirus RNA was detected by RT-PCR in fresh-frozen liver biopsy specimens in 78% (seven of nine) of tissue specimens from infants with choledochal cysts, a condition related to biliary atresia, and 55% (11 of 20) of those from infants with extrahepatic biliary atresia. However, reovirus RNA was detected in only 21% (seven of 33) of those with other liver diseases and 12% (two of 17) of autopsy controls without known hepatic or biliary disease.[455] The differences were statistically significant and support an association between reovirus infection and choledochal cysts and biliary atresia. A second study conducted in Hanover, Germany, detected reovirus RNA in 33% (21 of 64) of fresh liver biopsies taken during Kasai portoenterostomy procedures.[355] No other virus was detected in this study at a frequency of greater than 11%.

Studies to examine the prevalence of reovirus-specific antibodies in infants with biliary atresia have yielded conflicting results. Some have found increased reovirus seroprevalence in such children,[171,311,360] while others have not.[62,65,141,303] Since reovirus infections are nearly universal by adulthood[360,394,438] (see "Epidemiology"), most infants will acquire reovirus-specific antibodies passively from their mothers. Therefore, it is not surprising that levels of reovirus-specific antibodies do not differ between infants with biliary atresia and healthy controls.

It is possible that only certain reovirus strains possess the appropriate combination of virulence determinants to induce biliary atresia. Following peroral inoculation of newborn mice, strain T3SA+, which binds sialic acid, causes bile duct injury. However, strain T3SA−, which does not bind sialic acid, does not harm bile ducts[25] (see "Pathogenesis and Pathology—Hepatobiliary System"). These strains also differ in the capacity to bind cholangiocarcinoma cells,[25] suggesting that sialic acid–binding capacity serves as a reovirus tropism determinant for biliary epithelium. Reovirus type 2 strain BN-77 causes T-helper cell type 1–dependent injury to bile ducts in newborn mice,[319] analogous to the biliary injury in human neonatal biliary atresia. It is possible that biliary atresia results only when an infant born to a reovirus antibody-negative mother is infected with a bile duct–tropic reovirus strain in the peripartum period. Additionally, a genetic predisposition toward aberrant inflammatory responses may be a prerequisite for development of the characteristic biliary fibrosis that follows viral infection.

Central Nervous System Disease

There are isolated case reports linking reovirus strains of all three serotypes to neurologic disease in children. For example, a healthy 3-month-old infant developed meningitis associated with a rise in titer of reovirus-specific antibodies and the isolation of T1 reovirus from the cerebrospinal fluid (CSF).[217] In another case, type 2 (T2) reovirus was isolated from CSF and stool of an 8-week-old girl with meningitis.[196] This child was subsequently found to have a congenital immunodeficiency with hypogammaglobulinemia. In a third case of reovirus-associated meningitis, T3 reovirus was isolated from CSF of a 7-week-old child without other known morbidities.[450] This virus was shown to produce encephalitis in mice.

Reovirus also has been associated with acute necrotizing encephalopathy (ANE), a CNS inflammatory condition that occurs a few days after the development of respiratory symptoms, often in association with influenza. Two cousins, a 6-year-old boy and a 22-month-old girl, were hospitalized in Tours, France, with fever and neurologic symptoms following brief illnesses characterized by headache and rhinorrhea in the boy and girl, respectively.[337] MRI scans of both children demonstrated characteristic abnormalities of ANE: high signal intensity on T2-weighted images in the thalami bilaterally, brainstem tegmentum, and cerebral white matter in external capsules. T2 reovirus was isolated from urine of both children and a throat swab from the girl.[337] Culture and PCR tests were negative for other pathogens. Both children also developed reovirus-specific antibodies. Sequence analysis indicated that the reovirus isolates from these patients were identical and that most gene segments closely resembled strains circulating in China. Interestingly, a family member had returned from Indonesia a few days before the onset of symptoms in the children. No illness was reported in the returning traveler.

Myocarditis

Although certain reovirus strains cause myocarditis in new-born mice,[137,332,399] reovirus is an unusual cause of myocarditis in humans. There is one case report of a possible association of reovirus infection with myocarditis in an adult.[443] A 28-year-old man developed fever associated with transient paroxysmal atrial fibrillation and premature ventricular contractions in the absence of cardiac enzyme elevation. Stool culture yielded a reovirus isolate of unspecified serotype. Serological studies and cardiac biopsy were not performed. It is possible that the reovirus strain isolated from stool contributed to the cardiac abnormalities, but this inference is unproven.

Pneumonia

The fusogenic reoviruses have been associated with respiratory infections in humans. Melaka virus was isolated from a 39-year-old man in Melaka, Malaysia, with fever and pneumonia.[85] Two family members developed similar symptoms 1 week after his illness and had serological evidence of infection with the same virus. It is possible that Melaka virus was transmitted to the index case by an infected bat. Melaka virus encodes a FAST protein and produces syncytia in mammalian cells. The genome organization of the Melaka virus polycistronic S1 gene segment most closely resembles that of Pulau virus (another bat-borne fusogenic orthoreovirus) and NBV.[85] A closely related virus, Sikamat virus, was isolated from a 46-year-old man in Sikamat, Malaysia, with fever, pharyngitis, and myalgia.[87] The man and his family had regularly visited an orchard frequented by fruit bats. Two family members had serological evidence of Sikamat virus infection, but neither became ill.

In a study conducted in a suburban setting in Malaysia known to be inhabited by bats, 34 of 200 persons aged ≥12 years with respiratory symptoms (fever, sore throat, and cough) had pteropine orthoreovirus RNA in oropharyngeal swab samples detected by RT-PCR.[465] Of note, nine were coinfected with influenza A virus and one with coronavirus OC43. None of these individuals required admission to a hospital. These cases illustrate the propensity of orthoreoviruses to spillover from bats to humans and suggest that targeted surveillance will reveal additional bat-borne zoonotic reovirus infections.

Celiac Disease

Celiac disease (CD) is an autoimmune enteropathy that occurs in genetically susceptible individuals exposed to dietary gluten. Feeding mice ovalbumin (OVA) as a model antigen results in systemic tolerance to OVA, which is marked by induction of Tregs and absence of OVA-specific inflammatory T_H1 cells. Peroral inoculation of mice with reovirus strain T1L abrogates oral tolerance to OVA, as evidenced by a reduction in Tregs and promotion of OVA-specific T_H1 cells.[56] Furthermore, HLA-DQ8 transgenic mice inoculated with T1L and fed gliadin, a proteolytic derivative of gluten, develop gluten-specific antibodies and a delayed-type hypersensitivity response to fed antigen, indicating that the mice do not establish tolerance to gluten.[56] Persons with CD express higher levels of reovirus antibodies compared with controls,[56] raising the possibility that reovirus infection is linked to the development of CD in humans (see "Pathogenesis and Pathology—Adaptive Immune Responses").

DIAGNOSIS

Reovirus infections can be diagnosed by isolating virus from tissues or body fluids, detecting viral protein or RNA in patient samples, or demonstrating increases in reovirus-specific antibody titer. Reovirus has been isolated from nasal washings, throat swabs, urine, stool, and CSF. Monkey kidney cells generally have been considered optimum for isolating reovirus from clinical specimens, but reovirus infects most cells that are routinely maintained in clinical microbiology laboratories.[451] In addition to characteristic cytopathic effect, the presence of reovirus proteins can be confirmed using either immunofluorescence or immunocytochemistry to detect reovirus proteins in infected cell cultures.[451] Immunohistochemical techniques also can be employed for detection of reovirus proteins in tissue specimens.[451] Determination of viral serotype can be accomplished using plaque-reduction neutralization or hemagglutination-inhibition assays with type-specific antisera. Sequence analysis of the S1 gene segment can be used to confirm the isolate serotype.[121,450]

A variety of RT-PCR protocols have been established to detect reovirus RNA in blood or tissue samples. Primers specific for the L1,[455] L3,[383] M3,[425] and S4[45] gene segments have been used for this purpose. Primers specific for these and other gene segments also have been used to detect reovirus in cultured cells. The sensitivity and specificity of these protocols have not been established.

Reovirus-specific antibodies in serum can be detected by enzyme-linked immunosorbent assays[359,394,407,438] and immunoblotting.[337,394] Results can be confirmed by plaque-reduction neutralization or hemagglutination-inhibition assays.

PREVENTION AND CONTROL

There are no established therapeutic modalities for reovirus infections in humans. Studies using cultured cells and experimental animals suggest that inhibition of either viral RNA synthetic capacity or host functions required for viral infectivity may have efficacy. Ribavirin, a broad-spectrum inhibitor of viral RNA synthesis, has antiviral activity against reovirus in cultured cells.[100,354] The inosine monophosphate dehydrogenase inhibitor, mycophenolic acid, inhibits the replication of both mammalian and avian reovirus strains by blocking viral transcription.[195,367] Guanidine hydrochloride inhibits reovirus replication by blocking viral dsRNA synthesis.[318] There are no reports of these drugs being used to treat reovirus infections *in vivo*.

A variety of pharmacologic inhibitors of host functions required for reovirus internalization and disassembly decrease reovirus yields in cultured cells. For example, chlorpromazine,[276] which impedes clathrin-dependent uptake, chloroquine,[286] which blocks endosomal acidification, and CLIK-148,[219] which inhibits cathepsin L, arrest reovirus infection. Serotonin receptor agonist 5-nonyloxytryptamine blocks reovirus transit to late endosomes during viral entry.[278] Of these inhibitors, only CLIK-148 has been tested for efficacy against reovirus in animals; this drug diminishes reovirus loads and enhances survival in infected mice.[219]

Pharmacologic manipulation of host innate immune and apoptotic pathways dampen disease in mice infected with reovirus. Type I IFNs diminish reovirus infection in cultured cells[401] and ameliorate reovirus-induced myocarditis[332] and encephalitis in mice.[133] Minocycline delays disease onset and mortality in reovirus encephalitis in association with diminished viral loads and virus-induced apoptosis.[363] Caspase inhibitors[116,362] and a cell-permeating JNK inhibitor[29] have similar effects. Such strategies may have efficacy in the treatment of other viral infections in which apoptosis is a major contributor to tissue pathology.

There are no established vaccines to prevent reovirus infections in humans. Passive administration of antiviral antibodies[453,458,463] or virus-specific immune cells[400,464] can protect mice infected with otherwise lethal doses of reovirus. Remarkably, both humoral and cell-mediated immune effectors can protect against lethal challenge even when administered after viral inoculation.

REOVIRUS ONCOLYTICS

The capacity of mammalian reoviruses to produce oncolysis was first noted in 1960.[33] Subsequent work showed that cells with activated Ras signaling pathways are more susceptible to reovirus infection.[98] Together, these observations led to investigation of the utility of a reovirus strain T3D isolate as an oncolytic agent for the treatment of cancer. Several viruses have been tested in clinical trials for efficacy in the treatment of cancer. However, only talimogene laherparepvec (T-VEC; Imlygic™), a genetically modified herpes simplex virus type 1, is currently licensed by the FDA for use to treat advanced melanoma in humans. Reovirus strain T3D (pelareorep, Oncolytics Biotech, Inc.) was granted Orphan drug status by the FDA in 2015 for the treatment of gastric, glial, ovarian, pancreatic, and peritoneal cancers and provided fast-track designation for the treatment of metastatic breast cancer in 2017. As of this writing, pelareorep is listed in over 100 clinical trials in humans (www.clinicaltrials.gov).

Reovirus T3D has been evaluated for oncolytic activity against a broad variety of tumors *in vitro*, in animal models, and clinically in humans (www.clinicaltrials.gov). Antitumor efficacy *in vitro* has been shown for human malignant glioma, human bladder cancer, breast cancer, colonic and ovarian tumors, gastric cancers, lymphoid tumors, medulloblastoma, melanoma, non–small cell lung cancer, pancreatic cancer, pediatric sarcomas, and prostate cancer.[316] In clinical trials, reovirus is remarkably well tolerated in humans when given at doses of up to 3×10^{10} TCID$_{50}$ intravenously.[176] Although effective in preclinical models, reovirus monotherapy has been disappointing in human clinical trials.[55] As a consequence, all current clinical trials involve combinations of pelareorep with other treatment modalities[316] (www.clinicaltrials.gov).

The question of what makes transformed cells more susceptible than untransformed cells to reovirus infection is an area of active investigation. Although transformed cells with activated Ras signaling pathways are more susceptible to reovirus infection,[431] those in which Ras pathways are not activated also are susceptible.[419] The efficiency of viral replication correlates with reovirus oncolysis, but tumor cell killing also is influenced by sensitivity of cells to apoptosis induction.[410] Factors that enhance the susceptibility of transformed cells to reovirus-induced cell killing include a failure of transformed cells to mount a normal IFN response,[403] enhanced proteolytic disassembly of the virus in the tumor microenvironment,[5,287]

increased receptor availability in tumor tissue,[459] decreased particle-to-infectivity ratios of virus produced in transformed cells, and increased virus release associated with caspase-mediated apoptosis.[287] Several cancers have up-regulated levels of reovirus receptor JAM-A on their surface and on cells in the tumor microenvironment, which may enhance reovirus tropism.[256,501] How cellular transformation enhances these processes is not known, but stabilization of the p53 tumor suppressor protein enhances reovirus-induced apoptosis as a consequence of increased activation of NF-κB.[339] Increased reovirus-induced apoptosis of transformed cells also is associated with increased virus release and spread.[287,339]

Reovirus infection can enhance immune cell targeting of tumors. Reovirus infection can increase tumor cell antigen presentation and recruitment of inflammatory cells,[185] activate DCs,[147] and increase bystander toxicity against reovirus-resistant tumor cells.[148] Interestingly, the reovirus σ1 protein can bind to and activate NK cells.[22]

Pelareorep is a wild-type T3D strain. However, the original T3D strain of virus isolated from a human patient has been independently passaged an unknown number of times in multiple different labs such that each lab-derived version of T3D differs significantly in oncolytic properties from the most oncolytic strain, pelareorep.[307] The most oncolytic T3D strain displays more efficient cell attachment, increased rates of RNA transcription, larger burst size, and higher levels of cell death.[309] Genetic modifications of T3D have been selected for enhanced replication or engineered using reverse genetics to allow infection of JAM-A–negative tumor cell lines (JAM-A–independent [jin] mutants), modify tumor tropism,[110,225,461] overcome metalloprotease cleavage of the σ1 protein,[152] select for superior oncolysis,[310,402] enhance killing of specific tumor types,[370] or express heterologous transgenes.[220,229,230,460] Reovirus strains other than T3D also appear to infect and kill transformed cells.[6]

PERSPECTIVE

Since its discovery more than 60 years ago, reovirus has been used to make numerous important contributions to the field of virology. The ability to manipulate the genome of both virus and host makes reovirus a tractable experimental system for studies to precisely define viral and host determinants of pathogenesis. The application of genetics, biochemistry, cell biology, and structural analyses has yielded a wealth of information about mechanisms that govern reovirus tropism, replication, and disease. However, important questions remain (e-Table 11.3). Perhaps most enigmatic is why reovirus infection is so infrequently associated with disease. A crucial corollary question is whether mounting reports of fusogenic orthoreovirus infections of humans in Asia portend the emergence of more virulent reovirus strains in the future. As reovirus shares a number of features with more pathogenic viruses, it is likely that answers to these questions will reveal broadly conserved principles of virus biology and may illuminate new targets for broad-spectrum antiviral therapeutics and vaccines.

Rapidly advancing clinical applications will set future directions for reovirus research. Reovirus infects transformed cells more efficiently than it does nontransformed cells. Based on initial success in using reovirus for tumor killing in animal models,[98,198] reovirus is currently undergoing evaluation in clinical trials as a virotherapeutic for aggressive and treatment-refractory human cancers. Reovirus undergoes primary replication in intestinal tissue with few or no symptoms yet blocks development of immunological tolerance to newly introduced food antigens in mice.[56] If confirmed, linkage between reovirus and CD in humans would establish the rationale to test reovirus vaccines for the capacity to abrogate CD in children at risk for the disease. Ongoing research to understand mechanisms by which reovirus engages host cells and initiates an infectious cycle will guide strategic retargeting of reovirus to selected host cells and tissues to maximize oncolytic potential and may reveal how minimally pathogenic viruses can nonetheless stimulate pathogenic immune responses.

ACKNOWLEDGMENTS

We acknowledge Bernard Fields, Max Nibert, Leslie Schiff, and Ken Tyler for contributions to chapters about reoviruses in previous editions of Fields Virology. We thank Pavithra Aravamudhan, Karl Boehme, Pranav Danthi, Roy Duncan, Geoff Holm, Jelle Matthijnssens, Kristen Ogden, Cristina Risco, and Thilo Stehle, and members of our laboratories for essential discussions and critical review of portions of the text. Our work has been funded by the National Institutes of Health and the Heinz Endowments.

We refer readers to the Sixth Edition of Fields Virology for historical references.

REFERENCES

1. Agosto MA, Ivanovic T, Nibert ML. Mammalian reovirus, a nonfusogenic nonenveloped virus, forms size-selective pores in a model membrane. *Proc Natl Acad Sci U S A* 2006;103:16496–16501.
2. Agosto MA, Myers KS, Ivanovic T, et al. A positive-feedback mechanism promotes reovirus particle conversion to the intermediate associated with membrane penetration. *Proc Natl Acad Sci U S A* 2008;105:10571–10576.
3. Ahasan MS, Subramaniam K, Sayler KA, et al. Molecular characterization of a novel reassortment mammalian orthoreovirus type 2 isolated from a Florida white-tailed deer fawn. *Virus Res* 2019;270:197642.
4. Ahmed R, Canning WM, Kauffman RS, et al. Role of the host cell in persistent viral infection: coevolution of L cells and reovirus during persistent infection. *Cell* 1981;25:325–332.
5. Alain T, Kim TS, Lun X, et al. Proteolytic disassembly is a critical determinant for reovirus oncolysis. *Mol Ther* 2007;15:1512–1521.
6. Alloussi SH, Alkassar M, Urbschat S, et al. All reovirus subtypes show oncolytic potential in primary cells of human high-grade glioma. *Oncol Rep* 2011;26:645–649.
7. Amerongen HM, Wilson GAR, Fields BN, et al. Proteolytic processing of reovirus is required for adherence to intestinal M-cells. *J Virol* 1994;68:8428–8432.
8. Anafu AA, Bowen CH, Chin CR, et al. Interferon-inducible transmembrane protein 3 (IFITM3) restricts reovirus cell entry. *J Biol Chem* 2013;288:17261–17271.
9. Antar AAR, Konopka JL, Campbell JA, et al. Junctional adhesion molecule-A is required for hematogenous dissemination of reovirus. *Cell Host Microbe* 2009;5:59–71.
10. Antczak JB, Joklik WK. Reovirus genome segment assortment into progeny genomes studied by the use of monoclonal-antibodies directed against reovirus proteins. *Virology* 1992;187:760–776.
11. Aravamudhan P, Raghunathan K, Konopka-Anstadt J, et al. Reovirus uses macropinocytosis-mediated entry and fast axonal transport to infect neurons. *PLoS Pathog* 2020;16:e1008380.
12. Arnold MM, Murray KE, Nibert ML. Formation of the factory matrix is an important, though not a sufficient function of nonstructural protein μNS during reovirus infection. *Virology* 2008;375:412–423.
13. Attoui H, Biagini P, Stirling J, et al. Sequence characterization of Ndelle virus genome segments 1, 5, 7, 8, and 10: evidence for reassignment to the genus Orthoreovirus, family Reoviridae. *Biochem Biophys Res Commun* 2001;287:583–588.
14. Attoui H, Mertens PPC, Becnel J, et al. Reoviridae. In: King AMQ, Adams MJ, Carstens EB, et al., eds. *Virus Taxonomy: Classification and Nomenclature of Viruses Ninth Report of the International Committee on Taxonomy of Viruses.* London: Elsevier/Academic Press; 2012:541–637.
15. Avasarala S, Zhang F, Liu G, et al. Curcumin modulates the inflammatory response and inhibits subsequent fibrosis in a mouse model of viral-induced acute respiratory distress syndrome. *PLoS One* 2013;8:e57285.
16. Azzam-Smoak K, Noah DL, Stewart MJ, et al. Interferon regulatory factor-1, interferon-β, and reovirus-induced myocarditis. *Virology* 2002;298:20–29.
17. Baer GS, Dermody TS. Mutations in reovirus outer-capsid protein σ3 selected during persistent infections of L cells confer resistance to protease inhibitor E64. *J Virol* 1997;71:4921–4928.
18. Baer GS, Ebert DH, Chung CJ, et al. Mutant cells selected during persistent reovirus infection do not express mature cathepsin L and do not support reovirus disassembly. *J Virol* 1999;73:9532–9543.
19. Baldridge MT, Lee S, Brown JJ, et al. Expression of Ifnlr1 on intestinal epithelial cells is critical to the antiviral effects of interferon λ against norovirus and reovirus. *J Virol* 2017;91:e02079-16.
20. Banerjee AK, Shatkin AJ. Guanosine-5′-diphosphate at the 5′ termini of reovirus RNA: evidence for a segmented genome within the virion. *J Mol Biol* 1971;61:643–653.
21. Barkon ML, Haller BL, Virgin HW. Circulating immunoglobulin G can play a critical role in clearance of intestinal reovirus infection. *J Virol* 1996;70:1109–1116.
22. Bar-On Y, Charpak-Amikam Y, Glasner A, et al. NKp46 recognizes the σ1 protein of reovirus: implications for reovirus-based cancer therapy. *J Virol* 2017;91:e01045-17.
23. Barton ES, Connolly JL, Forrest JC, et al. Utilization of sialic acid as a coreceptor enhances reovirus attachment by multistep adhesion strengthening. *J Biol Chem* 2001;276:2200–2211.
24. Barton ES, Forrest JC, Connolly JL, et al. Junction adhesion molecule is a receptor for reovirus. *Cell* 2001;104:441–451.
25. Barton ES, Youree BE, Ebert DH, et al. Utilization of sialic acid as a coreceptor is required for reovirus-induced biliary disease. *J Clin Invest* 2003;111:1823–1833.
26. Bass DM, Bodkin D, Dambrauskas R, et al. Intraluminal proteolytic activation plays an important role in replication of type 1 reovirus in the intestines of neonatal mice. *J Virol* 1990;64:1830–1833.
27. Bassel-Duby R, Spriggs DR, Tyler KL, et al. Identification of attenuating mutations on the reovirus type 3 S1 double-stranded RNA segment with a rapid sequencing technique. *J Virol* 1986;60:64–67.
28. Baty CJ, Sherry B. Cytopathogenic effect in cardiac myocytes but not in cardiac fibroblasts is correlated with reovirus-induced acute myocarditis. *J Virol* 1993;67:6295–6298.
29. Beckham JD, Goody RJ, Clarke P, et al. Novel strategy for treatment of viral central nervous system infection by using a cell-permeating inhibitor of c-Jun N-terminal kinase. *J Virol* 2007;81:6984–6992.
30. Beckham JD, Tuttle K, Tyler KL. Reovirus activates transforming growth factor beta and bone morphogenetic protein signaling pathways in the central nervous system that contribute to neuronal survival following infection. *J Virol* 2009;83:5035–5045.
31. Beckham JD, Tuttle KD, Tyler KL. Caspase-3 activation is required for reovirus-induced encephalitis in vivo. *J Neurovirol* 2010;16:306–317.
32. Benavente J, Martinez-Costas J. Avian reovirus: structure and biology. *Virus Res* 2007;123:105–119.
33. Bennette JG. Isolation of a non-pathogenic tumour-destroying virus from mouse ascites. *Nature* 1960;187:72–73.
34. Berard AR, Severini A, Coombs KM. Differential reovirus-specific and herpesvirus-specific activator protein 1 activation of secretogranin II leads to altered virus secretion. *J Virol* 2015;89:11954–11964.
35. Berens HM, Tyler KL. The proapoptotic Bcl-2 protein Bax plays an important role in the pathogenesis of reovirus encephalitis. *J Virol* 2011;85:3858–3871.
36. Berger AK, Danthi P. Reovirus activates a caspase-independent cell death pathway. *mBio* 2013;4:e00178-13.
37. Berger AK, Hiller BE, Thete D, et al. Viral RNA at two stages of reovirus infection is required for the induction of necroptosis. *J Virol* 2017;91:e0204-16.
38. Bergeron J, Mabrouk T, Garzon S, et al. Characterization of the thermosensitive ts453 reovirus mutant: increased dsRNA binding of σ3 protein correlates with interferon resistance. *Virology* 1998;246:199–210.
39. Betancourt WQ, Gerba CP. Rethinking the significance of reovirus in water and wastewater. *Food Environ Virol* 2016;8:161–173.
40. Bharhani MS, Grewal JS, Pilgrim MJ, et al. Reovirus serotype 1/strain Lang-stimulated activation of antigen-specific T lymphocytes in Peyer's patches and distal gut-mucosal sites: activation status and cytotoxic mechanisms. *J Immunol* 2005;174:3580–3589.
41. Bisaillon M, Lemay G. Characterization of the reovirus lambda1 protein RNA 5′-triphosphatase activity. *J Biol Chem* 1997;272:29954–29957.
42. Bisaillon M, Lemay G. Molecular dissection of the reovirus λ1 protein nucleic acids binding site. *Virus Res* 1997;51:231–237.
43. Bodkin DK, Fields BN. Growth and survival of reovirus in intestinal tissue: role of the L2 and S1 genes. *J Virol* 1989;63:1188–1193.
44. Bodkin DK, Nibert ML, Fields BN. Proteolytic digestion of reovirus in the intestinal lumens of neonatal mice. *J Virol* 1989;63:4676–4681.
45. Boehme KW, Frierson JM, Konopka JL, et al. The reovirus σ1s protein is a determinant of hematogenous but not neural virus dissemination in mice. *J Virol* 2011;85:11781–11790.
46. Boehme KW, Guglielmi KM, Dermody TS. Reovirus nonstructural protein σ1s is required for establishment of viremia and systemic dissemination. *Proc Natl Acad Sci U S A* 2009;106:19986–19991.
47. Boehme KW, Hammer K, Tollefson WC, et al. Nonstructural protein σ1s mediates reovirus-induced cell cycle arrest and apoptosis. *J Virol* 2013;87:12967–12979.
48. Boehme KW, Ikizler M, Kobayashi T, et al. Reverse genetics for mammalian reovirus. *Methods* 2011;55:109–113.
49. Boehme KW, Lai CM, Dermody TS. Mechanisms of reovirus bloodstream dissemination. *Adv Virus Res* 2013;87:1–35.
50. Bonney S, Seitz S, Ryan CA, et al. Gamma interferon alters junctional integrity via rho kinase, resulting in blood–brain barrier leakage in experimental viral encephalitis. *MBio* 2019;10:e01675-19.
51. Borodavka A, Ault J, Stockley PG, et al. Evidence that avian reovirus σNS is an RNA chaperone: implications for genome segment assortment. *Nucleic Acids Res* 2015;43:7044–7057.
52. Both GW, Furuichi Y, Muthukrishnan S, et al. Ribosome binding to reovirus mRNA in protein synthesis requires 5′ terminal 7-methylguanosine. *Cell* 1975;6:185–195.

53. Boudreault S, Martenon-Brodeur C, Caron M, et al. Global profiling of the cellular alternative RNA splicing landscape during virus-host interactions. *PLoS One* 2016;11:e0161914.

54. Boulant S, Stanifer M, Kural C, et al. Similar uptake but different trafficking and escape routes of reovirus virions and infectious subvirion particles imaged in polarized Madin Darby canine kidney cells. *Mol Biol Cell* 2013;24:1196–1207.

55. Bourhill T, Mori Y, Rancourt DE, et al. Going (reo)viral: factors promoting successful reoviral oncolytic infection. *Viruses* 2018;10:421.

56. Bouziat R, Hinterleitner R, Brown JJ, et al. Reovirus infection triggers inflammatory responses to dietary antigens and development of celiac disease. *Science* 2017;356:44–50.

57. Brass AL, Huang IC, Benita Y, et al. The IFITM proteins mediate cellular resistance to influenza A H1N1 virus, West Nile virus, and dengue virus. *Cell* 2009;139:1243–1254.

58. Broering TJ, Arnold MM, Miller CL, et al. Carboxyl-proximal regions of reovirus nonstructural protein μNS necessary and sufficient for forming factory-like inclusions. *J Virol* 2005;79:6194–6206.

59. Broering TJ, Kim J, Miller CL, et al. Reovirus nonstructural protein μNS recruits viral core surface proteins and entering core particles to factory-like inclusions. *J Virol* 2004;78:1882–1892.

60. Broering TJ, McCutcheon AM, Centonze VE, et al. Reovirus nonstructural protein μNS binds to core particles but does not inhibit their transcription and capping activities. *J Virol* 2000;74:5516–5524.

61. Broering TJ, Parker JS, Joyce PL, et al. Mammalian reovirus nonstructural protein μNS forms large inclusions and colocalizes with reovirus microtubule-associated protein μ2 in transfected cells. *J Virol* 2002;76:8285–8297.

62. Brown WR. Lack of confirmation of the association of reovirus 3 and biliary atresia: methodological differences. *Hepatology* 1990;12:1254–1255.

63. Brown EG, Nibert ML, Fields BN. The L2 gene of reovirus serotype 3 controls the capacity to interfere, accumulate deletions and establish persistent infection. In: Compans RW, Bishop DHL, eds. *Double-Stranded RNA Viruses.* New York: Elsevier Biomedical; 1983:275–287.

64. Brown JJ, Short SP, Stencel-Baerenwald J, et al. Reovirus-induced apoptosis in the intestine limits establishment of enteric infection. *J Virol* 2018;92:e02062-17.

65. Brown WR, Sokol RJ, Levin MJ, et al. Lack of correlation between infection with reovirus-3 and extrahepatic biliary atresia or neonatal hepatitis. *J Pediatr* 1988;113:670–676.

66. Buchholz UJ, Finke S, Conzelmann KK. Generation of bovine respiratory syncytial virus (BRSV) from cDNA: BRSV NS2 is not essential for virus replication in tissue culture, and the human RSV leader region acts as a functional BRSV genome promoter. *J Virol* 1999;73:251–259.

67. Buonavoglia C, Martella V. Canine respiratory viruses. *Vet Res* 2007;38:355–373.

68. Burstin SJ, Spriggs DR, Fields BN. Evidence for functional domains on the reovirus type 3 hemagglutinin. *Virology* 1982;117:146–155.

69. Bussiere LD, Choudhury P, Bellaire B, et al. Characterization of a replicating mammalian orthoreovirus with tetracysteine-tagged μNS for live-cell visualization of viral factories. *J Virol* 2017;91:e01371-17.

70. Campbell JA, Schelling P, Wetzel JD, et al. Junctional adhesion molecule a serves as a receptor for prototype and field-isolate strains of mammalian reovirus. *J Virol* 2005;79:7967–7978.

71. Carroll K, Hastings C, Miller CL. Amino acids 78 and 79 of mammalian orthoreovirus protein μNS are necessary for stress granule localization, core protein λ2 interaction, and de novo virus replication. *Virology* 2014;448:133–145.

72. Carvalho J, Arnold MM, Nibert ML. Silencing and complementation of reovirus core protein μ2: functional correlations with μ2-microtubule association and differences between virus- and plasmid-derived μ2. *Virology* 2007;364:301–316.

73. Chandran K, Farsetta DL, Nibert ML. Strategy for nonenveloped virus entry: a hydrophobic conformer of the reovirus membrane penetration protein μ1 mediates membrane disruption. *J Virol* 2002;76:9920–9933.

74. Chandran K, Nibert ML. Protease cleavage of reovirus capsid protein μ1/μ1C is blocked by alkyl sulfate detergents, yielding a new type of infectious subvirion particle. *J Virol* 1998;72:467–475.

75. Chandran K, Parker JS, Ehrlich M, et al. The δ region of outer-capsid protein μ1 undergoes conformational change and release from reovirus particles during cell entry. *J Virol* 2003;77:13361–13375.

76. Chandran K, Walker SB, Chen Y, et al. In vitro recoating of reovirus cores with baculovirus-expressed outer-capsid proteins μ1 and σ3. *J Virol* 1999;73:3941–3950.

77. Chandran K, Zhang X, Olson NH, et al. Complete in vitro assembly of the reovirus outer capsid produces highly infectious particles suitable for genetic studies of the receptor-binding protein. *J Virol* 2001;75:5335–5342.

78. Chappell JD, Barton ES, Smith TH, et al. Cleavage susceptibility of reovirus attachment protein σ1 during proteolytic disassembly of virions is determined by a sequence polymorphism in the σ1 neck. *J Virol* 1998;72:8205–8213.

79. Chappell JD, Duong JL, Wright BW, et al. Identification of carbohydrate-binding domains in the attachment proteins of type 1 and type 3 reoviruses. *J Virol* 2000;74:8472–8479.

80. Chappell JD, Goral MI, Rodgers SE, et al. Sequence diversity within the reovirus S2 gene: reovirus genes reassort in nature, and their termini are predicted to form a panhandle motif. *J Virol* 1994;68:750–756.

81. Chappell JD, Gunn VL, Wetzel JD, et al. Mutations in type 3 reovirus that determine binding to sialic acid are contained in the fibrous tail domain of viral attachment protein σ1. *J Virol* 1997;71:1834–1841.

82. Chappell JD, Prota AE, Dermody TS, et al. Crystal structure of reovirus attachment protein σ1 reveals evolutionary relationship to adenovirus fiber. *EMBO J* 2002;21:1–11.

83. Chemudupati M, Kenney AD, Smith AC, et al. Butyrate reprograms expression of specific interferon stimulated genes. *J Virol* 2020;94:e00326-20.

84. Choudhury P, Bussiere L, Miller CL. Mammalian orthoreovirus factories modulate stress granule protein localization by interaction with G3BP1. *J Virol* 2017;91:e01298-17.

85. Chua KB, Crameri G, Hyatt A, et al. A previously unknown reovirus of bat origin is associated with an acute respiratory disease in humans. *Proc Natl Acad Sci U S A* 2007;104:11424–11429.

86. Chua KB, Voon K, Crameri G, et al. Identification and characterization of a new orthoreovirus from patients with acute respiratory infections. *PLoS One* 2008;3:e3803.

87. Chua KB, Voon K, Yu M, et al. Investigation of a potential zoonotic transmission of orthoreovirus associated with acute influenza-like illness in an adult patient. *PLoS One* 2011;6:e25434.

88. Ciechonska M, Duncan R. Reovirus FAST proteins: virus-encoded cellular fusogens. *Trends Microbiol* 2014;22:715–724.

89. Clark KM, Wetzel JD, Gu Y, et al. Reovirus variants selected for resistance to ammonium chloride have mutations in viral outer-capsid protein σ3. *J Virol* 2006;80:671–681.

90. Clarke P, Beckham JD, Leser JS, et al. Fas-mediated apoptotic signaling in the mouse brain following reovirus infection. *J Virol* 2009;83:6161–6170.

91. Clarke P, Debiasi RL, Meintzer SM, et al. Inhibition of NF-κB activity and cFLIP expression contribute to viral-induced apoptosis. *Apoptosis* 2005;10:513–524.

92. Clarke P, Leser JS, Bowen RA, et al. Virus-induced transcriptional changes in the brain include the differential expression of genes associated with interferon, apoptosis, interleukin 17 receptor A, and glutamate signaling as well as flavivirus-specific upregulation of tRNA synthetases. *MBio* 2014;5:e00902-14.

93. Clarke P, Meintzer SM, Gibson S, et al. Reovirus-induced apoptosis is mediated by TRAIL. *J Virol* 2000;74:8135–8139.

94. Clarke P, Meintzer SM, Moffitt LA, et al. Two distinct phases of virus-induced nuclear factor κB regulation enhance tumor necrosis factor-related apoptosis-inducing ligand-mediated apoptosis in virus-infected cells. *J Biol Chem* 2003;278:18092–18100.

95. Clarke P, Meintzer SM, Wang Y, et al. JNK regulates the release of proapoptotic mitochondrial factors in reovirus-infected cells. *J Virol* 2004;78:13132–13138.

96. Clarke P, Zhuang Y, Berens HM, et al. Interferon β contributes to astrocyte activation in the brain following reovirus infection. *J Virol* 2019;93:e02027-18.

97. Coffey CM, Sheh A, Kim IS, et al. Reovirus outer capsid protein μ1 induces apoptosis and associates with lipid droplets, endoplasmic reticulum, and mitochondria. *J Virol* 2006;80:8422–8438.

98. Coffey MC, Strong JE, Forsyth PA, et al. Reovirus therapy of tumors with activated Ras pathway. *Science* 1998;282:1332–1334.

99. Connolly JL, Barton ES, Dermody TS. Reovirus binding to cell surface sialic acid potentiates virus-induced apoptosis. *J Virol* 2001;75:4029–4039.

100. Connolly JL, Dermody TS. Virion disassembly is required for apoptosis induced by reovirus. *J Virol* 2002;76:1632–1641.

101. Connolly JL, Rodgers SE, Clarke P, et al. Reovirus-induced apoptosis requires activation of transcription factor NF-κB. *J Virol* 2000;74:2981–2989.

102. Coombs KM. Stoichiometry of reovirus structural proteins in virus, ISVP, and core particles. *Virology* 1998;243:218–228.

103. Cox P, Griffith M, Angles M, et al. Concentrations of pathogens and indicators in animal feces in the Sydney watershed. *Appl Environ Microbiol* 2005;71:5929–5934.

104. Cuff CF, Cebra CK, Rubin DH, et al. Developmental relationship between cytotoxic α/β T cell receptor-positive intraepithelial lymphocytes and Peyer's patch lymphocytes. *Eur J Immunol* 1993;23:1333–1339.

105. Danthi P, Coffey CM, Parker JS, et al. Independent regulation of reovirus membrane penetration and apoptosis by the μ1 Φ domain. *PLoS Pathog* 2008;4:e1000248.

106. Danthi P, Hansberger MW, Campbell JA, et al. JAM-A-independent, antibody-mediated uptake of reovirus into cells leads to apoptosis. *J Virol* 2006;80:1261–1270.

107. Danthi P, Holm GH, Stehle T, et al. Reovirus receptors, cell entry, and proapoptotic signaling. In: Pöhlmann S, Simmons G, eds. *Viral Entry into Host Cells.* Austin, TX: Landes Bioscience; 2013:42–71.

108. Danthi P, Kobayashi T, Holm GH, et al. Reovirus apoptosis and virulence are regulated by host cell membrane penetration efficiency. *J Virol* 2008;82:161–172.

109. Danthi P, Pruijssers AJ, Berger AK, et al. Bid regulates the pathogenesis of neurotropic reovirus. *PLoS Pathog* 2010;6:e1000980.

110. Dautzenberg IJ, van den Wollenberg DJ, van den Hengel SK, et al. Mammalian orthoreovirus T3D infects U-118 MG cell spheroids independent of junction adhesion molecule-A. *Gene Ther* 2014;21:609–617.

111. Dawe AL, Nuss DL. Hypoviruses and chestnut blight: exploiting viruses to understand and modulate fungal pathogenesis. *Annu Rev Genet* 2001;35:1–29.

112. Day JM. The diversity of the orthoreoviruses: molecular taxonomy and phylogentic divides. *Infect Genet Evol* 2009;9:390–400.

113. DeBiasi RL, Clarke P, Meintzer S, et al. Reovirus-induced alteration in expression of apoptosis and DNA repair genes with potential roles in viral pathogenesis. *J Virol* 2003;77:8934–8947.

114. DeBiasi RL, Edelstein CL, Sherry B, et al. Calpain inhibition protects against virus-induced apoptotic myocardial injury. *J Virol* 2001;75:351–361.

115. DeBiasi RL, Robinson BA, Leser JS, et al. Critical role for death-receptor mediated apoptotic signaling in viral myocarditis. *J Card Fail* 2010;16:901–910.

116. DeBiasi RL, Robinson BA, Sherry B, et al. Caspase inhibition protects against reovirus-induced myocardial injury in vitro and in vivo. *J Virol* 2004;78:11040–11050.

117. Debiasi RL, Squier MKT, Pike B, et al. Reovirus-induced apoptosis is preceded by increased cellular calpain activity and is blocked by calpain inhibitors. *J Virol* 1999;73:695–701.

118. Decaro N, Campolo M, Desario C, et al. Virological and molecular characterization of a mammalian orthoreovirus type 3 strain isolated from a dog in Italy. *Vet Microbiol* 2005;109:19–27.

119. Demidenko AA, Blattman JN, Blattman NN, et al. Engineering recombinant reoviruses with tandem repeats and a tetravirus 2A-like element for exogenous polypeptide expression. *Proc Natl Acad Sci U S A* 2013;110:E1867–E1876.

120. Demidenko AA, Nibert ML. Probing the transcription mechanisms of reovirus cores with molecules that alter RNA duplex stability. *J Virol* 2009;83:5659–5670.

121. Dermody TS, Nibert ML, Bassel-Duby R, et al. Sequence diversity in S1 genes and S1 translation products of 11 serotype 3 reovirus strains. *J Virol* 1990;64:4842–4850.

122. Dermody TS, Nibert ML, Wetzel JD, et al. Cells and viruses with mutations affecting viral entry are selected during persistent infections of L cells with mammalian reoviruses. *J Virol* 1993;67:2055–2063.

123. Derrien M, Hooper JW, Fields BN. The M2 gene segment is involved in the capacity of reovirus type 3Abney to induce the oily fur syndrome in neonatal mice, a S1 gene segment-associated phenotype. *Virology* 2003;305:25–30.

124. Desmet EA, Anguish LJ, Parker JS. Virus-mediated compartmentalization of the host translational machinery. *MBio* 2014;5:e01463-14.

125. Desrosiers RC, Sen GC, Lengyel P. Difference in 5′ terminal structure between the mRNA and the double-stranded virion RNA of reovirus. *Biochem Biophys Res Commun* 1976;73:32–39.

126. Detjen BM, Walden WE, Thach RE. Translational specificity in reovirus-infected mouse fibroblasts. *J Biol Chem* 1982;257:9855–9860.

127. Dhanasekaran DN, Reddy EP. JNK signaling in apoptosis. *Oncogene* 2008;27:6245–6251.

128. Dichter MA, Weiner HL. Infection of neuronal cell cultures with reovirus mimics in vitro patterns of neurotropism. *Ann Neurol* 1984;16:603–610.

129. Dietrich MH, Ogden KM, Katen SP, et al. Structural insights into reovirus σ1 interactions with two neutralizing antibodies. *J Virol* 2017;91:e01621-16.

130. Dietrich MH, Ogden KM, Long JM, et al. Structural and functional features of the reovirus σ1 tail. *J Virol* 2018;92:e00336-18.

131. Diller JR, Halloran SR, Koehler M, et al. Reovirus σ1 conformational flexibility modulates the efficiency of host cell attachment. *J Virol* 2020;94:e01163-20.

132. Ding K, Nguyen L, Zhou ZH. In situ structures of the polymerase complex and RNA genome show how aquareovirus transcription machineries respond to uncoating. *J Virol* 2018;92:e00774-18.

133. Dionne KR, Galvin JM, Schittone SA, et al. Type I interferon signaling limits reoviral tropism within the brain and prevents lethal systemic infection. *J Neurovirol* 2011;17:314–326.

134. Dionne KR, Leser JS, Lorenzen KA, et al. A brain slice culture model of viral encephalitis reveals an innate CNS cytokine response profile and the therapeutic potential of caspase inhibition. *Exp Neurol* 2011;228:222–231.

135. Dionne KR, Zhuang Y, Leser JS, et al. Daxx upregulation within the cytoplasm of reovirus-infected cells is mediated by interferon and contributes to apoptosis. *J Virol* 2013;87:3447–3460.

136. Douville RN, Su RC, Coombs KM, et al. Reovirus serotypes elicit distinctive patterns of recall immunity in humans. *J Virol* 2008;82:7515–7523.

137. Doyle JD, Stencel-Baerenwald JE, Copeland CA, et al. Diminished reovirus capsid stability alters disease pathogenesis and littermate transmission. *PLoS Pathog* 2015;11:e1004693.

138. Drayna D, Fields BN. Genetic studies on the mechanism of chemical and physical inactivation of reovirus. *J Gen Virol* 1982;63(Pt 1):149–159.

139. Dryden KA, Wang G, Yeager M, et al. Early steps in reovirus infection are associated with dramatic changes in supramolecular structure and protein conformation: analysis of virions and subviral particles by cryoelectron microscopy and image reconstruction. *J Cell Biol* 1993;122:1023–1041.

140. Duncan R. Fusogenic reoviruses and their fusion-associated small transmembrane (FAST) proteins. *Annu Rev Virol* 2019;6:341–363.

141. Dussaix E, Hadchouel M, Tardieu T, et al. Biliary atresia and reovirus type 3 infection [letter]. *N Engl J Med* 1984;310:658.

142. Eaton HE, Kobayashi T, Dermody TS, et al. African swine fever virus NP868R capping enzyme promotes reovirus rescue during reverse genetics by promoting reovirus protein expression, virion assembly, and RNA incorporation into infectious virions. *J Virol* 2017;91:e02416-16.

143. Ebert DH, Deussing J, Peters C, et al. Cathepsin L and cathepsin B mediate reovirus disassembly in murine fibroblast cells. *J Biol Chem* 2002;277:24609–24617.

144. Ebert DH, Wetzel JD, Brumbaugh DE, et al. Adaptation of reovirus to growth in the presence of protease inhibitor E64 segregates with a mutation in the carboxy terminus of viral outer-capsid protein σ3. *J Virol* 2001;75:3197–3206.

145. Ehrlich M, Boll W, Van Oijen A, et al. Endocytosis by random initiation and stabilization of clathrin-coated pits. *Cell* 2004;118:591–605.

146. Eichwald C, Kim J, Nibert ML. Dissection of mammalian orthoreovirus μ2 reveals a self-associative domain required for binding to microtubules but not to factory matrix protein μNS. *PLoS One* 2017;12:e0184356.

147. Errington F, Steele L, Prestwich R, et al. Reovirus activates human dendritic cells to promote innate antitumor immunity. *J Immunol* 2008;180:6018–6026.

148. Errington F, White CL, Twigger KR, et al. Inflammatory tumour cell killing by oncolytic reovirus for the treatment of melanoma. *Gene Ther* 2008;15:1257–1270.

149. Excoffon KJDA, Guglielmi KM, Wetzel JD, et al. Reovirus preferentially infects the basolateral surface and is released from the apical surface of polarized human respiratory epithelial cells. *J Infect Dis* 2008;197:1189–1197.

150. Fan JY, Boyce CS, Cuff CF. T-helper 1 and T-helper 2 cytokine responses in gut-associated lymphoid tissue following enteric reovirus infection. *Cell Immunol* 1998;188:55–63.

151. Farone AL, O'Donnell SM, Brooks CS, et al. Reovirus strain-dependent inflammatory cytokine responses and replication patterns in a human monocyte cell line. *Viral Immunol* 2006;19:546–557.

152. Fernandes JP, Cristi F, Eaton HE, et al. Breast tumor-associated metalloproteases restrict reovirus oncolysis by cleaving the σ1 cell attachment protein and can be overcome by mutation of σ1. *J Virol* 2019;93:e01380-19.

153. Fernández de Castro I, Tenorio R, Ortega-González P, et al. A modified lysosomal organelle mediates nonlytic egress of reovirus. *J Cell Biol* 2020;219:e201910131.

154. Fernandez de Castro I, Zamora PF, Ooms L, et al. Reovirus forms neo-organelles for progeny particle assembly within reorganized cell membranes. *MBio* 2014;5:e00931-13.

155. Fields BN, Joklik WK. Isolation and preliminary genetic and biochemical characterization of temperature-sensitive mutants of reovirus. *Virology* 1969;37:335–342.

156. Flamand A, Gagner JP, Morrison LA, et al. Penetration of the nervous systems of suckling mice by mammalian reoviruses. *J Virol* 1991;65:123–131.

157. Fleeton MN, Contractor N, Leon F, et al. Peyer's patch dendritic cells process viral antigen from apoptotic epithelial cells in the intestine of reovirus-infected mice. *J Exp Med* 2004;200:235–245.

158. Forrest JC, Campbell JA, Schelling P, et al. Structure-function analysis of reovirus binding to junctional adhesion molecule 1. Implications for the mechanism of reovirus attachment. *J Biol Chem* 2003;278:48434–48444.

159. Fraser RD, Furlong DB, Trus BL, et al. Molecular structure of the cell-attachment protein of reovirus: correlation of computer-processed electron micrographs with sequence-based predictions. *J Virol* 1990;64:2990–3000.

160. Frierson JM, Pruijssers AJ, Konopka JL, et al. Utilization of sialylated glycans as coreceptors enhances the neurovirulence of serotype 3 reovirus. *J Virol* 2012;86:13164–13173.

161. Fulton JR, Smith J, Cunningham C, et al. Influence of the route of infection on development of T-cell receptor β-chain repertoires of reovirus-specific cytotoxic T lymphocytes. *J Virol* 2004;78:1582–1590.

162. Furlong DB, Nibert ML, Fields BN. Sigma 1 protein of mammalian reoviruses extends from the surfaces of viral particles. *J Virol* 1988;62:246–256.

163. Furuichi Y, LaFiandra A, Shatkin AJ. 5′-Terminal structure and mRNA stability. *Nature* 1977;266:235–239.

164. Furuichi Y, Morgan M, Muthukrishnan S, et al. Reovirus messenger RNA contains a methylated, blocked 5′-terminal structure: m-7G(5′)ppp(5′)G-MpCp. *Proc Natl Acad Sci U S A* 1975;72:362–366.

165. Furuichi Y, Muthukrishnan S, Shatkin AJ. 5′-Terminal M⁷G(5′)ppp(5′)Gᵐp in vivo: identification in reovirus genome RNA. *Proc Natl Acad Sci U S A* 1975;72:742–745.

166. Garant KA, Shmulevitz M, Pan L, et al. Oncolytic reovirus induces intracellular redistribution of Ras to promote apoptosis and progeny virus release. *Oncogene* 2016;35:771–782.

167. Gauvin L, Bennett S, Liu H, et al. Respiratory infection of mice with mammalian reoviruses causes systemic infection with age and strain dependent pneumonia and encephalitis. *Virol J* 2013;10:67.

168. Gillian AL, Schmechel SC, Livny J, et al. Reovirus protein σNS binds in multiple copies to single-stranded RNA and shares properties with single-stranded DNA binding proteins. *J Virol* 2000;74:5939–5948.

169. Gilmore R, Coffey MC, Lee PW. Active participation of Hsp90 in the biogenesis of the trimeric reovirus cell attachment protein σ1. *J Biol Chem* 1998;273:15227–15233.

170. Giordano MO, Martinez LC, Isa MB, et al. Twenty year study of the occurrence of reovirus infection in hospitalized children with acute gastroenteritis in Argentina. *Pediatr Infect Dis J* 2002;21:880–882.

171. Glaser JH, Balistreri WF, Morecki R. Role of reovirus type 3 in persistent infantile cholestasis. *J Pediatr* 1984;105:912–915.

172. Glorani G, Ruwolt M, Holton N, et al. An unusual aspartic acid cluster in the reovirus attachment fiber σ1 mediates stability at low ph and preserves trimeric organization. *J Virol* 2022;96:e0033122.

173. Golden JW, Bahe JA, Lucas WT, et al. Cathepsin S supports acid-independent infection by some reoviruses. *J Biol Chem* 2004;279:8547–8557.

174. Golden JW, Linke J, Schmechel S, et al. Addition of exogenous protease facilitates reovirus infection in many restrictive cells. *J Virol* 2002;76:7430–7443.

175. Golden JW, Schiff LA. Neutrophil elastase, an acid-independent serine protease, facilitates reovirus uncoating and infection in U937 promonocyte cells. *Virol J* 2005;2:48.

176. Gollamudi R, Ghalib MH, Desai KK, et al. Intravenous administration of Reolysin, a live replication competent RNA virus is safe in patients with advanced solid tumors. *Invest New Drugs* 2010;28:641–649.

177. Gomatos PJ, Tamm I, Dales S, et al. Reovirus type 3: physical characteristics and interaction with L cells. *Virology* 1962;17:441–454.

178. Gonzalez-Hernandez MB, Liu T, Payne HC, et al. Efficient norovirus and reovirus replication in the mouse intestine requires microfold (M) cells. *J Virol* 2014;88:6934–6943.

179. Goody RJ, Beckham JD, Rubtsova K, et al. JAK-STAT signaling pathways are activated in the brain following reovirus infection. *J Neurovirol* 2007;13:373–383.

180. Goody RJ, Hoyt CC, Tyler KL. Reovirus infection of the CNS enhances iNOS expression in areas of virus-induced injury. *Exp Neurol* 2005;195:379–390.

181. Goody RJ, Schittone SA, Tyler KL. Experimental reovirus-induced acute flaccid paralysis and spinal motor neuron cell death. *J Neuropathol Exp Neurol* 2008;67:231–239.

182. Goral MI, MochowGrundy M, Dermody TS. Sequence diversity within the reovirus S3 gene: reoviruses evolve independently of host species, geographic locale, and date of isolation. *Virology* 1996;216:265–271.

183. Goubau D, Schlee M, Deddouche S, et al. Antiviral immunity via RIG-I-mediated recognition of RNA bearing 5′-diphosphates. *Nature* 2014;514:372–375.

184. Guglielmi KM, Kirchner E, Holm GH, et al. Reovirus binding determinants in junctional adhesion molecule-A. *J Biol Chem* 2007;282:17930–17940.

185. Gujar SA, Pan DA, Marcato P, et al. Oncolytic virus-initiated protective immunity against prostate cancer. *Mol Ther* 2011;19:797–804.

186. Gummersheimer SL, Danthi P. Reovirus core proteins λ1 and σ2 promote stability of disassembly intermediates and influence early replication events. *J Virol* 2020;94:e00491-20.

187. Gummersheimer SL, Snyder AJ, Danthi P. Control of capsid transformations during reovirus entry. *Viruses* 2021;13:153.

188. Guo L, Smith JA, Abelson M, et al. Reovirus infection induces stabilization and up-regulation of cellular transcripts that encode regulators of TGF-β signaling. *PLoS One* 2018;13:e0204622.

189. Gupta SL, Holmes SL, Mehra LL. Interferon action against reovirus: activation of interferon induced protein kinase in mouse L929 cells upon reovirus infection. *Virology* 1982;12:495–499.

190. Haller BL, Barkon ML, Li XY, et al. Brain- and intestine-specific variants of reovirus serotype 3 strain dearing are selected during chronic infection of severe combined immunodeficient mice. *J Virol* 1995;69:3933–3937.

191. Haller BL, Barkon ML, Vogler GP, et al. Genetic mapping of reovirus virulence and organ tropism in severe combined immunodeficient mice: organ-specific virulence genes. *J Virol* 1995;69:357–364.

192. Hansberger MW, Campbell JA, Danthi P, et al. IκB kinase subunits α and γ are required for activation of NF-κB and induction of apoptosis by mammalian reovirus. *J Virol* 2007;81:1360–1371.

193. Helander A, Miller CL, Myers KS, et al. Protective immunoglobulin A and G antibodies bind to overlapping intersubunit epitopes in the head domain of type 1 reovirus adhesin σ1. *J Virol* 2004;78:10695–10705.
194. Helander A, Silvey KJ, Mantis NJ, et al. The viral σ1 protein and glycoconjugates containing α2-3-linked sialic acid are involved in type 1 reovirus adherence to M cell apical surfaces. *J Virol* 2003;77:7964–7977.
195. Hermann LL, Coombs KM. Inhibition of reovirus by mycophenolic acid is associated with the M1 genome segment. *J Virol* 2004;78:6171–6179.
196. Hermann L, Embree J, Hazelton P, et al. Reovirus type 2 isolated from cerebrospinal fluid. *Pediatr Infect Dis J* 2004;23:373–375.
197. Hiller BE, Berger AK, Danthi P. Viral gene expression potentiates reovirus-induced necrosis. *Virology* 2015;484:386–394.
198. Hirasawa K, Nishikawa SG, Norman KL, et al. Oncolytic reovirus against ovarian and colon cancer. *Cancer Res* 2002;62:1696–1701.
199. Holm GH, Pruijssers AJ, Li L, et al. Interferon regulatory factor 3 attenuates reovirus myocarditis and contributes to viral clearance. *J Virol* 2010;84:6900–6908.
200. Holm GH, Zurney J, Tumilasci V, et al. Retinoic acid-inducible gene-I and interferon-β promoter stimulator-1 augment proapoptotic responses following mammalian reovirus infection via interferon regulatory factor-3. *J Biol Chem* 2007;282:21953–21961.
201. Hood JL, Morabito MV, Martinez CR III, et al. Reovirus-mediated induction of ADAR1 (p150) minimally alters RNA editing patterns in discrete brain regions. *Mol Cell Neurosci* 2014;61:97–109.
202. Hooper JW, Fields BN. Role of the μ1 protein in reovirus stability and capacity to cause chromium release from host cells. *J Virol* 1996;70:459–467.
203. Hoyt CC, Richardson-Burns SM, Goody RJ, et al. Nonstructural protein σ1s is a determinant of reovirus virulence and influences the kinetics and severity of apoptosis induction in the heart and central nervous system. *J Virol* 2005;79:2743–2753.
204. Hutchings AB, Helander A, Silvey KJ, et al. Secretory immunoglobulin A antibodies against the σ1 outer capsid protein of reovirus type 1 Lang prevent infection of mouse Peyer's patches. *J Virol* 2004;78:947–957.
205. Hwang CC, Mochizuki M, Maeda K, et al. Seroepidemiology of reovirus in healthy dogs in six prefectures in Japan. *J Vet Med Sci* 2014;76:471–475.
206. Imani F, Jacobs BL. Inhibitory activity for the interferon-induced protein kinase is associated with the reovirus serotype 1 σ3 protein. *Proc Natl Acad Sci U S A* 1988;85:7887–7891.
207. Irvin SC, Zurney J, Ooms LS, et al. A single-amino-acid polymorphism in reovirus protein μ2 determines repression of interferon signaling and modulates myocarditis. *J Virol* 2012;86:2302–2311.
208. Ishii K, Ueda Y, Matsuo K, et al. Structural analysis of vaccinia virus DIs strain: application as a new replication-deficient viral vector. *Virology* 2002;302:433–444.
209. Ivanovic T, Agosto MA, Chandran K, et al. A role for molecular chaperone Hsc70 in reovirus outer capsid disassembly. *J Biol Chem* 2007;282:12210–12219.
210. Ivanovic T, Agosto MA, Zhang L, et al. Peptides released from reovirus outer capsid form membrane pores that recruit virus particles. *EMBO J* 2008;27:1289–1298.
211. Ivanovic T, Boulant S, Ehrlich M, et al. Recruitment of cellular clathrin to viral factories and disruption of clathrin-dependent trafficking. *Traffic* 2011;12:1179–1195.
212. Jackson GG, Muldoon RL. Viruses causing common respiratory infection in man. IV. Reoviruses and adenoviruses. *J Infect Dis* 1973;128:811–866.
213. Jane-Valbuena J, Breun LA, Schiff LA, et al. Sites and determinants of early cleavages in the proteolytic processing pathway of reovirus surface protein σ3. *J Virol* 2002;76:5184–5197.
214. Jané-Valbuena J, Nibert ML, Spencer SM, et al. Reovirus virion-like particles obtained by recoating infectious subvirion particles with baculovirus-expressed σ3 protein: an approach for analyzing σ3 functions during virus entry. *J Virol* 1999;73:2963–2973.
215. Jansen van Vuren P, Wiley M, Palacios G, et al. Isolation of a novel fusogenic orthoreovirus from *Eucampsipoda africana* bat flies in South Africa. *Viruses* 2016;8:65.
216. Jiang J, Coombs KM. Infectious entry of reovirus cores into mammalian cells enhanced by transfection. *J Virol Methods* 2005;128:88–92.
217. Johansson PJ, Sveger T, Ahlfors K, et al. Reovirus type 1 associated with meningitis. *Scand J Infect Dis* 1996;28:117–120.
218. Johansson C, Wetzel JD, He J, et al. Type I interferons produced by hematopoietic cells protect mice against lethal infection by mammalian reovirus. *J Exp Med* 2007;204:1349–1358.
219. Johnson EM, Doyle JD, Wetzel JD, et al. Genetic and pharmacologic alteration of cathepsin expression influences reovirus pathogenesis. *J Virol* 2009;83:9630–9640.
220. Kanai Y, Kawagishi T, Matsuura Y, et al. In vivo live imaging of oncolytic mammalian orthoreovirus expressing nanoLuc luciferase in tumor xenograft mice. *J Virol* 2019;93:e00401-19.
221. Kanai Y, Kawagishi T, Sakai Y, et al. Cell-cell fusion induced by reovirus FAST proteins enhances replication and pathogenicity of non-enveloped dsRNA viruses. *PLoS Pathog* 2019;15:e1007675.
222. Katayama Y, Terasawa Y, Tachibana M, et al. Proteolytic disassembly of viral outer capsid proteins is crucial for reovirus-mediated type-I interferon induction in both reovirus-susceptible and reovirus-refractory tumor cells. *Biomed Res Int* 2015;2015:468457.
223. Kato H, Takeuchi O, Mikamo-Satoh E, et al. Length-dependent recognition of double-stranded ribonucleic acids by retinoic acid-inducible gene-I and melanoma differentiation-associated gene 5. *J Exp Med* 2008;205:1601–1610.
224. Kaufer S, Coffey CM, Parker JS. The cellular chaperone hsc70 is specifically recruited to reovirus viral factories independently of its chaperone function. *J Virol* 2012;86:1079–1089.
225. Kawagishi T, Kanai Y, Nouda R, et al. Generation of genetically RGD σ1-modified oncolytic reovirus that enhances JAM-A-independent infection of tumor cells. *J Virol* 2020;94:e01703-20.
226. Kawagishi T, Kanai Y, Tani H, et al. Reverse genetics for fusogenic bat-borne orthoreovirus associated with acute respiratory tract infections in humans: role of outer capsid protein σC in viral replication and pathogenesis. *PLoS Pathog* 2016;12:e1005455.
227. Kedl R, Schmechel S, Schiff L. Comparative sequence analysis of the reovirus S4 genes from 13 serotype 1 and serotype 3 field isolates. *J Virol* 1995;69:552–559.
228. Kelly KR, Espitia CM, Mahalingam D, et al. Reovirus therapy stimulates endoplasmic reticular stress, NOXA induction, and augments bortezomib-mediated apoptosis in multiple myeloma. *Oncogene* 2012;31:3023–3038.
229. Kemp V, Dautzenberg IJC, Cramer SJ, et al. Characterization of a replicating expanded tropism oncolytic reovirus carrying the adenovirus E4orf4 gene. *Gene Ther* 2018;25:331–344.
230. Kemp V, van den Wollenberg DJM, Camps MGM, et al. Arming oncolytic reovirus with GM-CSF gene to enhance immunity. *Cancer Gene Ther* 2019;26:268–281.
231. Keroack M, Fields BN. Viral shedding and transmission between hosts determined by reovirus L2-gene. *Science* 1986;232:1635–1638.
232. Kim M, Hansen KK, Davis L, et al. Z-FA-FMK as a novel potent inhibitor of reovirus pathogenesis and oncolysis in vivo. *Antivir Ther* 2010;15:897–905.
233. Kim JW, Lyi SM, Parrish CR, et al. A proapoptotic peptide derived from reovirus outer capsid protein μ1 has membrane-destabilizing activity. *J Virol* 2011;85:1507–1516.
234. Kim J, Parker JS, Murray KE, et al. Nucleoside and RNA triphosphatase activities of orthoreovirus transcriptase cofactor μ2. *J Biol Chem* 2004;279:4394–4403.
235. Kirchner E, Guglielmi KM, Strauss HM, et al. Structure of reovirus σ1 in complex with its receptor junctional adhesion molecule-A. *PLoS Pathog* 2008;4:e1000235.
236. Knowlton JJ, Dermody TS, Holm GH. Apoptosis induced by mammalian reovirus is β interferon (IFN) independent and enhanced by IFN regulatory factor 3- and NF-κB-dependent expression of Noxa. *J Virol* 2012;86:1650–1660.
237. Knowlton JJ, Fernandez de Castro I, Ashbrook AW, et al. The TRiC chaperonin controls reovirus replication through outer-capsid folding. *Nat Microbiol* 2018;3:481–493.
238. Knowlton JJ, Gestaut D, Ma B, et al. Structural and functional dissection of reovirus capsid folding and assembly by the prefoldin-TRiC/CCT chaperone network. *Proc Natl Acad Sci U S A* 2021;118:e2018127118.
239. Kobayashi T, Antar AA, Boehme KW, et al. A plasmid-based reverse genetics system for animal double-stranded RNA viruses. *Cell Host Microbe* 2007;1:147–157.
240. Kobayashi T, Chappell JD, Danthi P, et al. Gene-specific inhibition of reovirus replication by RNA interference. *J Virol* 2006;80:9053–9063.
241. Kobayashi T, Ooms LS, Chappell JD, et al. Identification of functional domains in reovirus replication proteins μNS and μ2. *J Virol* 2009;83:2892–2906.
242. Kobayashi T, Ooms LS, Ikizler M, et al. An improved reverse genetics system for mammalian orthoreoviruses. *Virology* 2010;398:194–200.
243. Koehler M, Aravamudhan P, Guzman-Cardozo C, et al. Glycan-mediated enhancement of reovirus receptor binding. *Nat Commun* 2019;10:4460.
244. Koehler M, Petitjean SJL, Yang J, et al. Reovirus directly engages integrin to recruit clathrin for entry into host cells. *Nat Commun* 2021;12:2149.
245. Kominsky DJ, Bickel RJ, Tyler KL. Reovirus-induced apoptosis requires mitochondrial release of Smac/DIABLO and involves reduction of cellular inhibitor of apoptosis protein levels. *J Virol* 2002;76:11414–11424.
246. Kominsky DJ, Bickel RJ, Tyler KL. Reovirus-induced apoptosis requires both death receptor- and mitochondrial-mediated caspase-dependent pathways of cell death. *Cell Death Differ* 2002;9:926–933.
247. Komoto S, Kawagishi T, Kobayashi T, et al. A plasmid-based reverse genetics system for mammalian orthoreoviruses driven by a plasmid-encoded T7 RNA polymerase. *J Virol Methods* 2014;196:36–39.
248. Konopka-Anstadt JL, Mainou BA, Sutherland DM, et al. The Nogo receptor NgR1 mediates infection by mammalian reovirus. *Cell Host Microbe* 2014;15:681–691.
249. Koonin EV. Evolution of double-stranded RNA viruses: a case for polyphyletic origin from different groups of positive-stranded RNA viruses. *Semin Virol* 1992;3:327–340.
250. Kuss SK, Best GT, Etheredge CA, et al. Intestinal microbiota promote enteric virus replication and systemic pathogenesis. *Science* 2011;334:249–252.
251. Lai CM, Boehme KW, Pruijssers AJ, et al. Endothelial JAM-A promotes reovirus viremia and bloodstream dissemination. *J Infect Dis* 2015;211:383–393.
252. Lai CM, Mainou BA, Kim KS, et al. Directional release of reovirus from the apical surface of polarized endothelial cells. *MBio* 2013;4:e00049-13.
253. Lanoie D, Côté S, Degeorges E, et al. A single mutation in the mammalian orthoreovirus S1 gene is responsible for increased interferon sensitivity in a virus mutant selected in Vero cells. *Virology* 2019;528:73–79.
254. Lanoie D, Lemay G. Multiple proteins differing between laboratory stocks of mammalian orthoreoviruses affect both virus sensitivity to interferon and induction of interferon production during infection. *Virus Res* 2018;247:40–46.
255. Lau RY, Van Alstyne D, Berckmans R, et al. Synthesis of reovirus-specific polypeptides in cells pretreated with cycloheximide. *J Virol* 1975;16:470–478.
256. Lauko A, Mu Z, Gutmann DH, et al. Junctional adhesion molecules in cancer: a paradigm for the diverse functions of cell-cell interactions in tumor progression. *Cancer Res* 2020;80:4878–4885.
257. Leary TP, Erker JC, Chalmers ML, et al. Detection of mammalian reovirus RNA by using reverse transcription-PCR: sequence diversity within the λ3-encoding L1 gene. *J Clin Microbiol* 2002;40:1368–1375.
258. Lee S, Baldridge MT. Interferon-λ: a potent regulator of intestinal viral infections. *Front Immunol* 2017;8:749.
259. Lee PW, Hayes EC, Joklik WK. Characterization of anti-reovirus immunoglobulins secreted by cloned hybridoma cell lines. *Virology* 1981;108:134–146.
260. Leland MM, Hubbard GB, Sentmore HT III, et al. Outbreak of orthoreovirus-induced meningoencephalomyelitis in baboons. *Comp Med* 2000;50:199–205.
261. Lemieux R, Lemay G, Millward S. The viral protein σ3 participates in translation of late viral mRNA in reovirus-infected L cells. *J Virol* 1987;61:2472–2479.
262. Leone G, Coffey MC, Gilmore R, et al. C-terminal trimerization, but not N-terminal trimerization, of the reovirus cell attachment protein is a posttranslational and Hsp70/ATP- dependent process. *J Biol Chem* 1996;271:8466–8471.
263. Leone G, Mah DCW, Lee PWK. The incorporation of reovirus cell attachment protein σ1 into virions requires the amino-terminal hydrophobic tail and the adjacent heptad repeat region. *Virology* 1991;182:346–350.

264. Li L, Sevinsky JR, Rowland MD, et al. Proteomic analysis reveals virus-specific Hsp25 modulation in cardiac myocytes. *J Proteome Res* 2010;9:2460–2471.
265. Li L, Sherry B. IFN-α expression and antiviral effects are subtype and cell type specific in the cardiac response to viral infection. *Virology* 2010;396:59–68.
266. Liemann S, Chandran K, Baker TS, et al. Structure of the reovirus membrane-penetration protein, μ1, in a complex with its protector protein, σ3. *Cell* 2002;108:283–295.
267. Liu Y, Lu N, Yuan B, et al. The interaction between the helicase DHX33 and IPS-1 as a novel pathway to sense double-stranded RNA and RNA viruses in myeloid dendritic cells. *Cell Mol Immunol* 2014;11:49–57.
268. Lloyd RM, Shatkin AJ. Translational stimulation by reovirus polypeptide σ3: substitution for VA1-RNA and inhibition of phosphorylation of the α-subunit of eukaryotic initiation factor-II. *J Virol* 1992;66:6878–6884.
269. Loo YM, Fornek J, Crochet N, et al. Distinct RIG-I and MDA5 signaling by RNA viruses in innate immunity. *J Virol* 2008;82:335–345.
270. Lopez AD, Avasarala S, Grewal S, et al. Differential role of the Fas/Fas ligand apoptotic pathway in inflammation and lung fibrosis associated with reovirus 1/L-induced bronchiolitis obliterans organizing pneumonia and acute respiratory distress syndrome. *J Immunol* 2009;183:8244–8257.
271. Lucia-Jandris P, Hooper JW, Fields BF. Reovirus M2 gene is associated with chromium release from mouse L cells. *J Virol* 1993;67:5339–5345.
272. Luethy LN, Erickson AK, Jesudhasan PR, et al. Comparison of three neurotropic viruses reveals differences in viral dissemination to the central nervous system. *Virology* 2016;487:1–10.
273. Luongo CL, Reinisch KM, Harrison SC, et al. Identification of the mRNA guanylyltransferase region and active site in reovirus λ2 protein. *J Biol Chem* 2000;275:2804–2810.
274. Madren JA, Sarkar P, Danthi P. Cell entry-associated conformational changes in reovirus particles are controlled by host protease activity. *J Virol* 2012;86:3466–3473.
275. Maginnis MS, Forrest JC, Kopecky-Bromberg SA, et al. β1 integrin mediates internalization of mammalian reovirus. *J Virol* 2006;80:2760–2770.
276. Maginnis MS, Mainou BA, Derdowski AM, et al. NPXY motifs in the β1 integrin cytoplasmic tail are required for functional reovirus entry. *J Virol* 2008;82:3181 3191.
277. Mahlakõiv T, Hernandez P, Gronke K, et al. Leukocyte-derived IFN-α/β and epithelial IFN-λ constitute a compartmentalized mucosal defense system that restricts enteric virus infections. *PLoS Pathog* 2015;11:e1004782.
278. Mainou BA, Ashbrook AW, Smith EC, et al. Serotonin receptor agonist 5-nonyloxytryptamine alters the kinetics of reovirus cell entry. *J Virol* 2015;89:8701–8712.
279. Mainou BA, Dermody TS. Src kinase mediates productive endocytic sorting of reovirus during cell entry. *J Virol* 2011;85:3203–3213.
280. Mainou BA, Dermody TS. Transport to late endosomes is required for efficient reovirus infection. *J Virol* 2012;86:8346–8358.
281. Mainou BA, Zamora PF, Ashbrook AW, et al. Reovirus cell entry requires functional microtubules. *MBio* 2013;4:e00405-13.
282. Majeski EI, Paintlia MK, Lopez AD, et al. Respiratory reovirus 1/L induction of intraluminal fibrosis, a model of bronchiolitis obliterans organizing pneumonia, is dependent on T lymphocytes. *Am J Pathol* 2003;163:1467–1479.
283. Major AS, Cuff CF. Effects of the route of infection on immunoglobulin G subclasses and specificity of the reovirus-specific humoral immune response. *J Virol* 1996;70:5968–5974.
284. Major AS, Cuff CF. Enhanced mucosal and systemic immune responses to intestinal reovirus infection in β2-microglobulin-deficient mice. *J Virol* 1997;71:5782–5789.
285. Mao ZX, Joklik WK. Isolation and enzymatic characterization of protein λ2, the reovirus guanylytransferase. *Virology* 1991;185:377–386.
286. Maratos-Flier E, Goodman MJ, Murray AH, et al. Ammonium inhibits processing and cytotoxicity of reovirus, a nonenveloped virus. *J Clin Invest* 1986;78:1003–1007.
287. Marcato P, Shmulevitz M, Pan D, et al. Ras transformation mediates reovirus oncolysis by enhancing virus uncoating, particle infectivity, and apoptosis-dependent release. *Mol Ther* 2007;15:1522–1530.
288. Martinez CG, Guinea R, Benavente J, et al. The entry of reovirus into L cells is dependent on vacuolar proton-ATPase activity. *J Virol* 1996;70:576–579.
289. Mateju D, Eichenberger B, Voigt F, et al. Single-molecule imaging reveals translation of mRNAs localized to stress granules. *Cell* 2020;183:1801–1812.e1813.
290. Mathers AR, Cuff CF. Role of interleukin-4 (IL-4) and IL-10 in serum immunoglobulin G antibody responses following mucosal or systemic reovirus infection. *J Virol* 2004;78:3352–3360.
291. Matoba Y, Colucci WS, Fields BN, et al. The reovirus M1 gene determines the relative capacity of growth of reovirus in cultured bovine aortic endothelial cells. *J Clin Invest* 1993;92:2883–2888.
292. Matoba Y, Sherry B, Fields BN, et al. Identification of the viral genes responsible for growth of strains of reovirus in cultured mouse heart cells. *J Clin Invest* 1991;87:1628–1633.
293. McAlpine SM, Issekutz TB, Marshall JS. Virus stimulation of human mast cells results in the recruitment of CD56+ T cells by a mechanism dependent on CCR5 ligands. *FASEB J* 2012;26:1280–1289.
294. McNamara AJ, Danthi P. Loss of IKK subunits limits NF-κB signaling in reovirus-infected cells. *J Virol* 2020;94:e00382-20.
295. Mendez, II, She YM, Ens W, et al. Digestion pattern of reovirus outer capsid protein σ3 determined by mass spectrometry. *Virology* 2003;311:289–304.
296. Mendez, II, Weiner SG, She YM, et al. Conformational changes accompany activation of reovirus RNA-dependent RNA transcription. *J Struct Biol* 2008;162:277–289.
297. Middleton JK, Agosto MA, Severson TF, et al. Thermostabilizing mutations in reovirus outer-capsid protein μ1 selected by heat inactivation of infectious subvirion particles. *Virology* 2007;361:412–425.
298. Mikuletič T, Steyer A, Kotar T, et al. A novel reassortant mammalian orthoreovirus with a divergent S1 genome segment identified in a traveler with diarrhea. *Infect Genet Evol* 2019;73:378–383.
299. Miller CL, Arnold MM, Broering TJ, et al. Localization of mammalian orthoreovirus proteins to cytoplasmic factory-like structures via nonoverlapping regions of μNS. *J Virol* 2010;84:867–882.
300. Miller CL, Broering TJ, Parker JS, et al. Reovirus σNS protein localizes to inclusions through an association requiring the μNS amino terminus. *J Virol* 2003;77:4566–4576.
301. Miller CL, Parker JS, Dinoso JB, et al. Increased ubiquitination and other covariant phenotypes attributed to a strain- and temperature-dependent defect of reovirus core protein μ2. *J Virol* 2004;78:10291–10302.
302. Millward S, Graham AF. Structural studies on reovirus: discontinuities in the genome. *Proc Natl Acad Sci U S A* 1970;65:422–429.
303. Minuk GY, Rascanin N, Paul RW, et al. Reovirus type 3 infection in patients with primary biliary cirrhosis and primary sclerosing cholangitis. *J Hepatol* 1987;5:8–13.
304. Miyamoto SD, Brown RD, Robinson BA, et al. Cardiac cell-specific apoptotic and cytokine responses to reovirus infection: determinants of myocarditic phenotype. *J Card Fail* 2009;15:529–539.
305. Mochizuki M, Uchizono S. Experimental infections of feline reovirus serotype 2 isolates. *J Vet Med Sci* 1993;55:469–470.
306. Mochow-Grundy M, Dermody TS. The reovirus S4 gene 3′ nontranslated region contains a translational operator sequence. *J Virol* 2001;75:6517–6526.
307. Mohamed A, Clements DR, Gujar SA, et al. Single amino acid differences between closely related reovirus T3D lab strains alter oncolytic potency in vitro and in vivo. *J Virol* 2020;94:e01688-19.
308. Mohamed A, Konda P, Eaton HE, et al. Closely related reovirus lab strains induce opposite expression of RIG-I/IFN-dependent versus -independent host genes, via mechanisms of slow replication versus polymorphisms in dsRNA binding σ3 respectively. *PLoS Pathog* 2020;16:e1008803.
309. Mohamed A, Smiley JR, Shmulevitz M. Polymorphisms in the most oncolytic reovirus strain confer enhanced cell attachment, transcription, and single-step replication kinetics. *J Virol* 2020;94:e01937-19.
310. Mohamed A, Teicher C, Haefliger S, et al. Reduction of virion-associated σ1 fibers on oncolytic reovirus variants promotes adaptation toward tumorigenic cells. *J Virol* 2015;89:4319–4334.
311. Morecki R, Glaser JH, Cho S, et al. Biliary atresia and reovirus type 3 infection. *N Engl J Med* 1982;307:481–484.
312. Morgan EM, Zweerink HJ. Characterization of transcriptase and replicase particles isolated from reovirus-infected cells. *Virology* 1975;68:455–466.
313. Morin MJ, Warner A, Fields BN. A pathway for entry of reoviruses into the host through M cells of the respiratory tract. *J Exp Med* 1994;180:1523–1527.
314. Morin MJ, Warner A, Fields BN. Reovirus infection in rat lungs as a model to study the pathogenesis of viral pneumonia. *J Virol* 1996;70:541–548.
315. Morrison LA, Sidman RL, Fields BN. Direct spread of reovirus from the intestinal lumen to the central nervous system through vagal autonomic nerve fibers. *Proc Natl Acad Sci U S A* 1991;88:3852–3856.
316. Müller L, Berkeley R, Barr T, et al. Past, present and future of oncolytic reovirus. *Cancers (Basel)* 2020;12:3219.
317. Munemitsu SM, Atwater JA, Samuel CE. Biosynthesis of reovirus-specified polypeptides: molecular cDNA cloning and nucleotide sequence of the reovirus serotype 1 Lang strain bicistronic s1 mRNA which encodes the minor capsid polypeptide σ1a and the nonstructural polypeptide σ1bNS. *Biochem Biophys Res Commun* 1986;140:508–514.
318. Murray KE, Nibert ML. Guanidine hydrochloride inhibits mammalian orthoreovirus growth by reversibly blocking the synthesis of double-stranded RNA. *J Virol* 2007;81:4572–4584.
319. Nakashima T, Hayashi T, Tomoeda S, et al. Reovirus type-2-triggered autoimmune cholangitis in extrahepatic bile ducts of weanling DBA/1J mice. *Pediatr Res* 2014;75:29–37.
320. Nibert ML, Chappell JD, Dermody TS. Infectious subvirion particles of reovirus type 3 Dearing exhibit a loss in infectivity and contain a cleaved σ1 protein. *J Virol* 1995;69:5057–5067.
321. Nibert ML, Dermody TS, Fields BN. Structure of the reovirus cell-attachment protein: a model for the domain organization of σ1. *J Virol* 1990;64:2976–2989.
322. Nibert ML, Fields BN. A carboxy-terminal fragment of protein μ1/μ1C is present in infectious subvirion particles of mammalian reoviruses and is proposed to have a role in penetration. *J Virol* 1992;66:6408–6418.
323. Nibert ML, Margraf RL, Coombs KM. Nonrandom segregation of parental alleles in reovirus reassortants. *J Virol* 1996;70:7295–7300.
324. Nibert ML, Odegard AL, Agosto MA, et al. Putative autocleavage of reovirus μ1 protein in concert with outer-capsid disassembly and activation for membrane permeabilization. *J Mol Biol* 2005;345:461–474.
325. Nibert ML, Schiff LA, Fields BN. Mammalian reoviruses contain a myristoylated structural protein. *J Virol* 1991;65:1960–1967.
326. Nilsen TW, Maroney PA, Baglioni C. Synthesis of (2′-5′)oligoadenylate and activation of an endoribonuclease in interferon-treated HeLa-cells infected with reovirus. *J Virol* 1982;42:1039–1045.
327. Noah DL, Blum MA, Sherry B. Interferon regulatory factor 3 is required for viral induction of beta interferon in primary cardiac myocyte cultures. *J Virol* 1999;73:10208–10213.
328. Nygaard RM, Golden JW, Schiff LA. Impact of host proteases on reovirus infection in the respiratory tract. *J Virol* 2012;86:1238–1243.
329. Nygaard RM, Lahti L, Boehme KW, et al. Genetic determinants of reovirus pathogenesis in a murine model of respiratory infection. *J Virol* 2013;87:9279–9289.
330. Odegard AL, Chandran K, Zhang X, et al. Putative autocleavage of outer capsid protein μ1, allowing release of myristoylated peptide μ1N during particle uncoating, is critical for cell entry by reovirus. *J Virol* 2004;78:8732–8745.
331. Odendall C, Dixit E, Stavru F, et al. Diverse intracellular pathogens activate type III interferon expression from peroxisomes. *Nat Immunol* 2014;15:717–726.
332. O'Donnell SM, Hansberger MW, Connolly JL, et al. Organ-specific roles for transcription factor NF-κB in reovirus-induced apoptosis and disease. *J Clin Invest* 2005;115:2341–2350.
333. O'Donnell SM, Holm GH, Pierce JM, et al. Identification of an NF-κB-dependent gene network in cells infected by mammalian reovirus. *J Virol* 2006;80:1077–1086.

334. Oldford SA, Salsman SP, Portales-Cervantes L, et al. Interferon α2 and interferon γ induce the degranulation independent production of VEGF-A and IL-1 receptor antagonist and other mediators from human mast cells. *Immun Inflamm Dis* 2018;6:176–189.

335. Olland AM, Jané-Valbuena J, Schiff LA, et al. Structure of the reovirus outer capsid and dsRNA-binding protein σ3 at 1.8 Å resolution. *EMBO J* 2001;20:979–989.

336. Ooms LS, Jerome WG, Dermody TS, et al. Reovirus replication protein μ2 influences cell tropism by promoting particle assembly within viral inclusions. *J Virol* 2012;86:10979–10987.

337. Ouattara LA, Barin F, Barthez MA, et al. Novel human reovirus isolated from children with acute necrotizing encephalopathy. *Emerg Infect Dis* 2011;17:1436–1444.

338. Pal K, Kaetzel CS, Brundage K, et al. Regulation of polymeric immunoglobulin receptor expression by reovirus. *J Gen Virol* 2005;86:2347–2357.

339. Pan D, Pan LZ, Hill R, et al. Stabilisation of p53 enhances reovirus-induced apoptosis and virus spread through p53-dependent NF-KB activation. *Br J Cancer* 2011;105:1012–1022.

340. Parker JS, Broering TJ, Kim J, et al. Reovirus core protein μ2 determines the filamentous morphology of viral inclusion bodies by interacting with and stabilizing microtubules. *J Virol* 2002;76:4483–4496.

341. Paul-Murphy J, Work T, Hunter D, et al. Serologic survey and serum biochemical reference ranges of the free-ranging mountain lion (Felis concolor) in California. *J Wildl Dis* 1994;30:205–215.

342. Peterson ST, Kennedy EA, Brigleb PH, et al. Disruption of type III interferon (IFN) genes IFNL2 and IFNL3 recapitulates loss of the type III IFN receptor in the mucosal antiviral response. *J Virol* 2019;93:e01073-19.

343. Phillips MB, Dina Zita M, Howells MA, et al. Lymphatic type 1 interferon responses are critical for control of systemic reovirus dissemination. *J Virol* 2021;95:e02167-20.

344. Phillips MB, Stuart JD, Simon EJ, et al. Nonstructural protein σ1s is required for optimal reovirus protein expression. *J Virol* 2018;92:e02259-17.

345. Poggioli GJ, DeBiasi RL, Bickel R, et al. Reovirus-induced alterations in gene expression related to cell cycle regulation. *J Virol* 2002;76:2585–2594.

346. Poggioli GJ, Dermody TS, Tyler KL. Reovirus-induced σ1s-dependent G2/M cell cycle arrest results from inhibition of p34cdc2. *J Virol* 2001;75:7429–7434.

347. Poggioli GJ, Keefer CJ, Connolly JL, et al. Reovirus-induced G2/M cell cycle arrest requires σ1s and occurs in the absence of apoptosis. *J Virol* 2000;74:9562–9570.

348. Portales-Cervantes L, Haidl ID, Lee PW, et al. Virus-infected human mast cells enhance natural killer cell functions. *J Innate Immun* 2017;9:94–108.

349. Prota AE, Campbell JA, Schelling P, et al. Crystal structure of human junctional adhesion molecule 1: implications for reovirus binding. *Proc Natl Acad Sci U S A* 2003;100:5366–5371.

350. Pruijssers AJ, Hengel H, Abel TW, et al. Apoptosis induction influences reovirus replication and virulence in newborn mice. *J Virol* 2013;87:12980–12989.

351. Qin Q, Carroll K, Hastings C, et al. Mammalian orthoreovirus escape from host translational shutoff correlates with stress granule disruption and is independent of eIF2α phosphorylation and PKR. *J Virol* 2011;85:8798–8810.

352. Qin Q, Hastings C, Miller CL. Mammalian orthoreovirus particles induce and are recruited into stress granules at early times postinfection. *J Virol* 2009;83:11090–11101.

353. Racine T, Hurst T, Barry C, et al. Aquareovirus effects syncytiogenesis by using a novel member of the FAST protein family translated from a noncanonical translation start site. *J Virol* 2009;83:5951–5955.

354. Rankin JT Jr, Eppes SB, Antczak JB, et al. Studies on the mechanism of the antiviral activity of ribavirin against reovirus. *Virology* 1989;168:147–158.

355. Rauschenfels S, Krassmann M, Al-Masri AN, et al. Incidence of hepatotropic viruses in biliary atresia. *Eur J Pediatr* 2009;168:469–476.

356. Reinisch KM, Nibert M, Harrison SC. Structure of the reovirus core at 3.6 angstrom resolution. *Nature* 2000;404:960–967.

357. Reiss K, Stencel JE, Liu Y, et al. The GM2 glycan serves as a functional co-receptor for serotype 1 reovirus. *PLoS Pathog* 2012;8:e1003078.

358. Reiter DM, Frierson JM, Halvorson EE, et al. Crystal structure of reovirus attachment protein σ1 in complex with sialylated oligosaccharides. *PLoS Pathog* 2011;7:e1002166.

359. Richardson SC, Bishop RF, Smith AL. Enzyme-linked immunosorbent assays for measurement of reovirus immunoglobulin G, A, and M levels in serum. *J Clin Microbiol* 1988;26:1871–1873.

360. Richardson SC, Bishop RF, Smith AL. Reovirus serotype 3 infection in infants with extrahepatic biliary atresia or neonatal hepatitis. *J Gastroenterol Hepatol* 1994;9:264–268.

361. Richardson-Burns SM, Kominsky DJ, Tyler KL. Reovirus-induced neuronal apoptosis is mediated by caspase 3 and is associated with the activation of death receptors. *J Neurovirol* 2002;8:365–380.

362. Richardson-Burns SM, Tyler KL. Regional differences in viral growth and central nervous system injury correlate with apoptosis. *J Virol* 2004;78:5466–5475.

363. Richardson-Burns SM, Tyler KL. Minocycline delays disease onset and mortality in reovirus encephalitis. *Exp Neurol* 2005;192:331–339.

364. Rivera-Serrano EE, DeAngelis N, Sherry B. Spontaneous activation of a MAVS-dependent antiviral signaling pathway determines high basal interferon-β expression in cardiac myocytes. *J Mol Cell Cardiol* 2017;111:102–113.

365. Rivera-Serrano EE, Fritch EJ, Scholl EH, et al. A cytoplasmic RNA virus alters the function of the cell splicing protein SRSF2. *J Virol* 2017;91:e02488-16.

366. Rivera-Serrano EE, Sherry B. NF-κB activation is cell type-specific in the heart. *Virology* 2017;502:133–143.

367. Robertson CM, Hermann LL, Coombs KM. Mycophenolic acid inhibits avian reovirus replication. *Antiviral Res* 2004;64:55–61.

368. Rodgers SE, Barton ES, Oberhaus SM, et al. Reovirus-induced apoptosis of MDCK cells is not linked to viral yield and is blocked by Bcl-2. *J Virol* 1997;71:2540–2546.

369. Rodgers SE, Connolly JL, Chappell JD, et al. Reovirus growth in cell culture does not require the full complement of viral proteins: identification of a σ1s-null mutant. *J Virol* 1998;72:8597–8604.

370. Rodríguez Stewart RM, Berry JTL, Berger AK, et al. Enhanced killing of triple-negative breast cancer cells by reassortant reovirus and topoisomerase inhibitors. *J Virol* 2019;93:e01411-19.

371. Rodríguez Stewart RM, Raghuram V, Berry JTL, et al. Noncanonical cell death induction by reassortant reovirus. *J Virol* 2020;94:e01613-20.

372. Roebke KE, Danthi P. Cell entry-independent role for the reovirus μ1 protein in regulating necroptosis and the accumulation of viral gene products. *J Virol* 2019;93:e00199-19.

373. Roebke KE, Guo Y, Parker JSL, et al. Reovirus σ3 protein limits interferon expression and cell death induction. *J Virol* 2020;94:e01485-20.

374. Roner MR, Bassett K, Roehr J. Identification of the 5′ sequences required for incorporation of an engineered ssRNA into the reovirus genome. *Virology* 2004;329:348–360.

375. Roner MR, Gaillard RK Jr, Joklik WK. Control of reovirus messenger RNA translation efficiency by the regions upstream of initiation codons. *Virology* 1989;168:292–301.

376. Roner MR, Joklik WK. Reovirus reverse genetics: incorporation of the CAT gene into the reovirus genome. *Proc Natl Acad Sci U S A* 2001;98:8036–8041.

377. Roner MR, Roehr J. The 3′ sequences required for incorporation of an engineered ssRNA into the reovirus genome. *Virol J* 2006;3:1.

378. Roner MR, Steele BG. Localizing the reovirus packaging signals using an engineered m1 and s2 ssRNA. *Virology* 2007;358:89–97.

379. Rosen L. Serologic grouping of reovirus by hemagglutination-inhibition. *Am J Hyg* 1960;71:242–249.

380. Rosen L, Evans HE, Spickard A. Reovirus infections in human volunteers. *Am J Hyg* 1963;77:29–37.

381. Sabin AB. Reoviruses: a new group of respiratory and enteric viruses formerly classified as ECHO type 10 is described. *Science* 1959;130:1387–1389.

382. Sagar V, Murray KE. The mammalian orthoreovirus bicistronic M3 mRNA initiates translation using a 5′ end-dependent, scanning mechanism that does not require interaction of 5′-3′ untranslated regions. *Virus Res* 2014;183:30–40.

383. Saito T, Shinozaki K, Matsunaga T, et al. Lack of evidence for reovirus infection in tissues from patients with biliary atresia and congenital dilatation of the bile duct. *J Hepatol* 2004;40:203–211.

384. Salsman J, Top D, Boutilier J, et al. Extensive syncytium formation mediated by the reovirus FAST proteins triggers apoptosis-induced membrane instability. *J Virol* 2005;79:8090–8100.

385. Sandekian V, Lemay G. A single amino acid substitution in the mRNA capping enzyme λ2 of a mammalian orthoreovirus mutant increases interferon sensitivity. *Virology* 2015;483:229–235.

386. Saragovi HU, Rebai N, Di Guglielmo GM, et al. A G1 cell cycle arrest induced by ligands of the reovirus type 3 receptor is secondary to inactivation of p21ras and mitogen-activated protein kinase. *DNA Cell Biol* 1999;18:763–770.

387. Sarkar P, Danthi P. Determinants of strain-specific differences in efficiency of reovirus entry. *J Virol* 2010;84:12723–12732.

388. Sarkar P, Danthi P. The μ1 72–96 loop controls conformational transitions during reovirus cell entry. *J Virol* 2013;87:13532–13542.

389. Schelling P, Guglielmi KM, Kirchner E, et al. The reovirus σ1 aspartic acid sandwich: a trimerization motif poised for conformational change. *J Biol Chem* 2007;282:11582–11589.

390. Schittone SA, Dionne KR, Tyler KL, et al. Activation of innate immune responses in the central nervous system during reovirus myelitis. *J Virol* 2012;86:8107–8118.

391. Schmechel S, Chute M, Skinner P, et al. Preferential translation of reovirus mRNA by a σ3-dependent mechanism. *Virology* 1997;232:62–73.

392. Schulz WL, Haj AK, Schiff LA. Reovirus uses multiple endocytic pathways for cell entry. *J Virol* 2012;86:12665–12675.

393. Scott FW, Kahn DE, Gillespie JH. Feline viruses: isolation, characterization, and pathogenicity of a feline reovirus. *Am J Vet Res* 1970;31:11–20.

394. Selb B, Weber B. A study of human reovirus IgG and IgA antibodies by ELISA and western blot. *J Virol Methods* 1994;47:15–25.

395. Seliger LS, Zheng K, Shatkin AJ. Complete nucleotide sequence of reovirus L2 gene and deduced amino acid sequence of viral mRNA guanylyltransferase. *J Biol Chem* 1987;262:16289–16293.

396. Shah PNM, Stanifer ML, Höhn K, et al. Genome packaging of reovirus is mediated by the scaffolding property of the microtubule network. *Cell Microbiol* 2017;19.

397. Sharpe AH, Fields BN. Reovirus inhibition of cellular RNA and protein synthesis: role of the S4 gene. *Virology* 1982;122:381–391.

398. Shepard DA, Ehnstrom JG, Skinner PJ, et al. Mutations in the zinc-binding motif of the reovirus capsid protein σ3 eliminate its ability to associate with capsid protein μ1. *J Virol* 1996;70:2065–2068.

399. Sherry B, Blum MA. Multiple viral core proteins are determinants of reovirus-induced acute myocarditis. *J Virol* 1994;68:8461–8465.

400. Sherry B, Li XY, Tyler KL, et al. Lymphocytes protect against and are not required for reovirus-induced myocarditis. *J Virol* 1993;67:6119–6124.

401. Sherry B, Torres J, Blum MA. Reovirus induction of and sensitivity to β interferon in cardiac myocyte cultures correlate with induction of myocarditis and are determined by viral core proteins. *J Virol* 1998;72:1314–1323.

402. Shmulevitz M, Gujar SA, Ahn DG, et al. Reovirus variants with mutations in genome segments S1 and L2 exhibit enhanced virion infectivity and superior oncolysis. *J Virol* 2012;86:7403–7413.

403. Shmulevitz M, Pan LZ, Garant K, et al. Oncogenic Ras promotes reovirus spread by suppressing IFN-β production through negative regulation of RIG-I signaling. *Cancer Res* 2010;70:4912–4921.

404. Shutinoski B, Hakimi M, Harmsen IE, et al. Lrrk2 alleles modulate inflammation during microbial infection of mice in a sex-dependent manner. *Sci Transl Med* 2019;11:eaas9292.

405. Silverstein SC, Astell C, Christman J, et al. Synthesis of reovirus oligoadenylic acid in vivo and in vitro. *J Virol* 1974;13:740–752.

406. Silvey KJ, Hutchings AB, Vajdy M, et al. Role of immunoglobulin A in protection against reovirus entry into murine Peyer's patches. *J Virol* 2001;75:10870–10879.

407. Singh H, Shimojima M, Fukushi S, et al. Serologic assays for the detection and strain identification of Pteropine orthoreovirus. *Emerg Microbes Infect* 2016;5:e44.
408. Skup D, Millward S. Reovirus-induced modification of cap-dependent translation in infected L cells. *Proc Natl Acad Sci U S A* 1980;77:152–156.
409. Skup D, Millward S. mRNA capping enzymes are masked in reovirus progeny subviral particles. *J Virol* 1980;34:490–496.
410. Smakman N, van den Wollenberg DJ, Elias SG, et al. KRAS(D13) promotes apoptosis of human colorectal tumor cells by reovirus T3D and oxaliplatin but not by tumor necrosis factor-related apoptosis-inducing ligand. *Cancer Res* 2006;66:5403–5408.
411. Smith SC, Gribble J, Diller JR, et al. Reovirus RNA recombination is sequence directed and generates internally deleted defective genome segments during passage. *J Virol* 2021;95:e02181-20.
412. Smith JA, Schmechel SC, Raghavan A, et al. Reovirus induces and benefits from an integrated cellular stress response. *J Virol* 2006;80:2019–2033.
413. Smith JA, Schmechel SC, Williams BR, et al. Involvement of the interferon-regulated antiviral proteins PKR and RNase L in reovirus-induced shutoff of cellular translation. *J Virol* 2005;79:2240–2250.
414. Snyder AJ, Danthi P. Lipid membranes facilitate conformational changes required for reovirus cell entry. *J Virol* 2015;90:2628–2638.
415. Snyder AJ, Danthi P. Lipids cooperate with the reovirus membrane penetration peptide to facilitate particle uncoating. *J Biol Chem* 2016;291:26773–26785.
416. Snyder AJ, Danthi P. The loop formed by residues 340 to 343 of reovirus μ1 controls entry-related conformational changes. *J Virol* 2017;91:e00898-17.
417. Snyder AJ, Danthi P. Cleavage of the C-terminal fragment of reovirus μ1 is required for optimal infectivity. *J Virol* 2018;92:e01848-17.
418. Song L, Lu Y, He J, et al. Multi-organ lesions in suckling mice infected with SARS-associated mammalian reovirus linked with apoptosis induced by viral proteins μ1 and σ1. *PLoS One* 2014;9:e92678.
419. Song L, Ohnuma T, Gelman IH, et al. Reovirus infection of cancer cells is not due to activated Ras pathway. *Cancer Gene Ther* 2009;16:382.
420. Spriggs DR, Bronson RT, Fields BN. Hemagglutinin variants of reovirus type 3 have altered central nervous system tropism. *Science* 1983;220:505–507.
421. Stanifer ML, Kischnick C, Rippert A, et al. Reovirus inhibits interferon production by sequestering IRF3 into viral factories. *Sci Rep* 2017;7:10873.
422. Stanifer ML, Rippert A, Kazakov A, et al. Reovirus intermediate subviral particles constitute a strategy to infect intestinal epithelial cells by exploiting TGF-β dependent pro-survival signaling. *Cell Microbiol* 2016;18:1831–1845.
423. Starnes MC, Joklik WK. Reovirus protein λ3 is a poly(C)-dependent poly(G) polymerase. *Virology* 1993;193:356–366.
424. Stebbing RE, Irvin SC, Rivera-Serrano EE, et al. An ITAM in a nonenveloped virus regulates activation of NF-κB, induction of β interferon, and viral spread. *J Virol* 2014;88:2572–2583.
425. Steele MI, Marshall CM, Lloyd RE, et al. Reovirus 3 not detected by reverse transcriptase-mediated polymerase chain reaction analysis of preserved tissue from infants with cholestatic liver disease. *Hepatology* 1995;21:697–702.
426. Stencel-Baerenwald J, Reiss K, Blaum BS, et al. Glycan engagement dictates hydrocephalus induction by serotype 1 reovirus. *MBio* 2015;6:e02356-14.
427. Stettner E, Dietrich MH, Reiss K, et al. Structure of serotype 1 reovirus attachment protein σ1 in complex with junctional adhesion molecule A reveals a conserved serotype-independent binding epitope. *J Virol* 2015;89:6136–6140.
428. Stewart MJ, Blum MA, Sherry B. PKR's protective role in viral myocarditis. *Virology* 2003;314:92–100.
429. Stewart MJ, Smoak K, Blum MA, et al. Basal and reovirus-induced beta interferon (IFN-β) and IFN-β-stimulated gene expression are cell type specific in the cardiac protective response. *J Virol* 2005;79:2979–2987.
430. Steyer A, Gutierrez-Aguire I, Kolenc M, et al. High similarity of novel orthoreovirus detected in a child hospitalized with acute gastroenteritis to mammalian orthoreoviruses found in bats in Europe. *J Clin Microbiol* 2013;51:3818–3825.
431. Strong JE, Coffey MC, Tang D, et al. The molecular basis of viral oncolysis: usurpation of the Ras signaling pathway by reovirus. *EMBO J* 1998;17:3351–3362.
432. Strong JE, Leone G, Duncan R, et al. Biochemical and biophysical characterization of the reovirus cell attachment protein σ1: evidence that it is a homotrimer. *Virology* 1991;184:23–32.
433. Stuart JD, Holm GH, Boehme KW. Differential delivery of genomic double-stranded RNA causes reovirus strain-specific differences in interferon regulatory factor 3 activation. *J Virol* 2018;92:e01947-17.
434. Sturzenbecker LJ, Nibert ML, Furlong DB, et al. Intracellular digestion of reovirus particles requires a low pH and is an essential step in the viral infectious cycle. *J Virol* 1987;61:2351–2361.
435. Sutherland DM, Aravamudhan P, Dietrich MH, et al. Reovirus neurotropism and virulence are dictated by sequences in the head domain of the viral attachment protein. *J Virol* 2018;92:e00974-18.
436. Sutton G, Sun D, Fu X, et al. Assembly intermediates of orthoreovirus captured in the cell. *Nat Commun* 2020;11:4445.
437. Swanson MI, She YM, Ens W, et al. Mammalian reovirus core protein micro 2 initiates at the first start codon and is acetylated. *Rapid Commun Mass Spectrom* 2002;16:2317–2324.
438. Tai JH, Williams JV, Edwards KM, et al. Prevalence of reovirus-specific antibodies in young children in Nashville, Tennessee. *J Infect Dis* 2005;191:1221–1224.
439. Tao Y, Farsetta DL, Nibert ML, et al. RNA synthesis in a cage-structural studies of reovirus polymerase λ3. *Cell* 2002;111:733–745.
440. Tardieu M, Weiner HL. Viral receptors on isolated murine and human ependymal cells. *Science* 1982;215:419–421.
441. Taterka J, Cebra JJ, Rubin DH. Characterization of cytotoxic cells from reovirus-infected SCID mice: activated cells express natural killer- and lymphokine-activated killer-like activity but fail to clear infection. *J Virol* 1995;69:3910–3914.
442. Tenorio R, Fernández de Castro I, Knowlton JJ, et al. Reovirus σNS and μNS proteins remodel the endoplasmic reticulum to build replication neoorganelles. *MBio* 2018;9:e01253-18.
443. Terheggen F, Benedikz E, Frissen PH, et al. Myocarditis associated with reovirus infection. *Eur J Clin Microbiol Infect Dis* 2003;22:197–198.
444. Thalmann CM, Cummins DM, Yu M, et al. Broome virus, a new fusogenic orthoreovirus species isolated from an Australian fruit bat. *Virology* 2010;402:26–40.
445. Thete D, Danthi P. Conformational changes required for reovirus cell entry are sensitive to pH. *Virology* 2015;483:291–301.
446. Thete D, Danthi P. Protein mismatches caused by reassortment influence functions of the reovirus capsid. *J Virol* 2018;92:e00858-18.
447. Tian J, Zhang X, Wu H, et al. Blocking the PI3K/AKT pathway enhances mammalian reovirus replication by repressing IFN-stimulated genes. *Front Microbiol* 2015;6:886.
448. Tosteson MT, Nibert ML, Fields BN. Ion channels induced in lipid bilayers by subvirion particles of the nonenveloped mammalian reoviruses. *Proc Natl Acad Sci U S A* 1993;90:10549–10552.
449. Turula H, Bragazzi Cunha J, Mainou BA, et al. Natural secretory immunoglobulins promote enteric viral infections. *J Virol* 2018;92:e00826-18.
450. Tyler KL, Barton ES, Ibach ML, et al. Isolation and molecular characterization of a novel type 3 reovirus from a child with meningitis. *J Infect Dis* 2004;189:1664–1675.
451. Tyler KL, Fields BN. Reoviridae: the reoviruses. In: Murphy FA, ed. *Laboratory Diagnosis of Infectious Disease: Principles and Practice (vol II) Viral, Rickettsial and Chlamydial Diseases.* New York: Springer-Verlag; 1988:353–374.
452. Tyler KL, Leser JS, Phang TL, et al. Gene expression in the brain during reovirus encephalitis. *J Neurovirol* 2010;16:56–71.
453. Tyler KL, Mann MA, Fields BN, et al. Protective anti-reovirus monoclonal antibodies and their effects on viral pathogenesis. *J Virol* 1993;67:3446–3453.
454. Tyler KL, McPhee DA, Fields BN. Distinct pathways of viral spread in the host determined by reovirus S1 gene segment. *Science* 1986;233:770–774.
455. Tyler KL, Sokol RJ, Oberhaus SM, et al. Detection of reovirus RNA in hepatobiliary tissues from patients with extrahepatic biliary atresia and choledochal cysts. *Hepatology* 1998;27:1475–1482.
456. Tyler KL, Squier MKT, Brown AL, et al. Linkage between reovirus-induced apoptosis and inhibition of cellular DNA synthesis: role of the S1 and M2 genes. *J Virol* 1996;70:7984–7991.
457. Tyler KL, Squier MK, Rodgers SE, et al. Differences in the capacity of reovirus strains to induce apoptosis are determined by the viral attachment protein σ1. *J Virol* 1995;69:6972–6979.
458. Tyler KL, Virgin HW IV, Bassel-Duby R, et al. Antibody inhibits defined stages in the pathogenesis of reovirus serotype 3 infection of the central nervous system. *J Exp Med* 1989;170:887–900.
459. van Houdt WJ, Smakman N, van den Wollenberg DJ, et al. Transient infection of freshly isolated human colorectal tumor cells by reovirus T3D intermediate subviral particles. *Cancer Gene Ther* 2008;15:284–292.
460. van den Wollenberg DJ, Dautzenberg IJ, Ros W, et al. Replicating reoviruses with a transgene replacing the codons for the head domain of the viral spike. *Gene Ther* 2015;22:267–279.
461. van den Wollenberg DJ, Dautzenberg IJ, van den Hengel SK, et al. Isolation of reovirus T3D mutants capable of infecting human tumor cells independent of junction adhesion molecule-A. *PLoS One* 2012;7:e48064.
462. Vedula SR, Lim TS, Kirchner E, et al. A comparative molecular force spectroscopy study of homophilic JAM-A interactions and JAM-A interactions with reovirus attachment protein σ1. *J Mol Recognit* 2008;21:210–216.
463. Virgin HW, Bassel-Duby R, Fields BN, et al. Antibody protects against lethal infection with the neurally spreading reovirus type 3 (Dearing). *J Virol* 1988;62:4594–4604.
464. Virgin HW IV, Tyler KL. Role of immune cells in protection against and control of reovirus infection in neonatal mice. *J Virol* 1991;65:5157–5164.
465. Voon K, Tan YF, Leong PP, et al. Pteropine orthoreovirus infection among out-patients with acute upper respiratory tract infection in Malaysia. *J Med Virol* 2015;87:2149–2153.
466. Wang X, Zhang F, Su R, et al. Structure of RNA polymerase complex and genome within a dsRNA virus provides insights into the mechanisms of transcription and assembly. *Proc Natl Acad Sci U S A* 2018;115:7344–7349.
467. Watanabe Y, Millward S, Graham AF. Regulation of transcription of the reovirus genome. *J Mol Biol* 1968;36:107–123.
468. Weiner HL, Drayna D, Averill DR Jr, et al. Molecular basis of reovirus virulence: role of the S1 gene. *Proc Natl Acad Sci U S A* 1977;74:5744–5748.
469. Wellehan JF, Jr., Childress AL, Marschang RE, et al. Consensus nested PCR amplification and sequencing of diverse reptilian, avian, and mammalian orthoreoviruses. *Vet Microbiol* 2009;133:34–42.
470. Wenske EA, Chanock SJ, Krata L, et al. Genetic reassortment of mammalian reoviruses in mice. *J Virol* 1985;56:613–616.
471. Wessner DR, Fields BN. Isolation and genetic characterization of ethanol-resistant reovirus mutants. *J Virol* 1993;67:2442–2447.
472. Wetzel JD, Barton ES, Chappell JD, et al. Reovirus delays diabetes onset but does not prevent insulitis in non-obese diabetic mice. *J Virol* 2006;80:3078–3082.
473. Wetzel JD, Wilson GJ, Baer GS, et al. Reovirus variants selected during persistent infections of L cells contain mutations in the viral S1 and S4 genes and are altered in viral disassembly. *J Virol* 1997;71:1362–1369.
474. Wilson GA, Morrison LA, Fields BN. Association of the reovirus S1 gene with serotype 3-induced biliary atresia in mice. *J Virol* 1994;68:6458–6465.
475. Wilson GJ, Nason EL, Hardy CS, et al. A single mutation in the carboxy terminus of reovirus outer-capsid protein σ3 confers enhanced kinetics of σ3 proteolysis, resistance to inhibitors of viral disassembly, and alterations in σ3 structure. *J Virol* 2002;76:9832–9843.
476. Wilson GJ, Wetzel JD, Puryear W, et al. Persistent reovirus infections of L cells select mutations in viral attachment protein σ1 that alter oligomer stability. *J Virol* 1996;70:6598–6606.

477. Wisniewski ML, Werner BG, Hom LG, et al. Reovirus infection or ectopic expression of outer capsid protein μ1 induces apoptosis independently of the cellular proapoptotic proteins Bax and Bak. *J Virol* 2011;85:296–304.

478. Wolf JL, Rubin DH, Finberg R, et al. Intestinal M cells: a pathway of entry for reovirus into the host. *Science* 1981;212:471–472.

479. Woods Acevedo MA, Erickson AK, Pfeiffer JK. The antibiotic neomycin enhances coxsackievirus plaque formation. *mSphere* 2019;4:e00632-18.

480. Wu AG, Pruijssers AJ, Brown JJ, et al. Age-dependent susceptibility to reovirus encephalitis in mice is influenced by maturation of the type-I interferon response. *Pediatr Res* 2018;83:1057–1066.

481. Xing J, Zhang A, Minze LJ, et al. TRIM29 negatively regulates the type I IFN production in response to RNA virus. *J Immunol* 2018;201:183–192.

482. Xu P, Miller SE, Joklik WK. Generation of reovirus core-like particles in cells infected with hybrid vaccinia viruses that express genome segments L1, L2, L3, and S2. *Virology* 1993;197:726–731.

483. Yamakawa M, Furuichi Y, Nakashima K, et al. Excess synthesis of viral mRNA 5-terminal oligonucleotides by reovirus transcriptase. *J Biol Chem* 1981;256:6507–6514.

484. Yamamoto SP, Motooka D, Egawa K, et al. Novel human reovirus isolated from children and its long-term circulation with reassortments. *Sci Rep* 2020;10:963.

485. Yan X, Parent KN, Goodman RP, et al. Virion structure of baboon reovirus, a fusogenic orthoreovirus that lacks an adhesion fiber. *J Virol* 2011;85:7483–7495.

486. Yao K, Goodwin MA, Vakharia VN. Generation of a mutant infectious bursal disease virus that does not cause bursal lesions. *J Virol* 1998;72:2647–2654.

487. Yin P, Keirstead ND, Broering TJ, et al. Comparisons of the M1 genome segments and encoded μ2 proteins of different reovirus isolates. *Virol J* 2004;1:6.

488. Yip WKW, Cristi F, Trifonov G, et al. The reovirus μ2 C-terminal loop inversely regulates NTPase and transcription functions versus binding to factory-forming μNS and promotes replication in tumorigenic cells. *J Virol* 2021;95:e02006-20.

489. Yue Z, Shatkin AJ. Regulated, stable expression and nuclear presence of reovirus double-stranded RNA-binding protein σ3 in HeLa cells. *J Virol* 1996;70:3497–3501.

490. Yue Z, Shatkin AJ. Double-stranded RNA-dependent protein kinase (PKR) is regulated by reovirus structural proteins. *Virology* 1997;234:364–371.

491. Zamora PF, Hu L, Knowlton JJ, et al. Reovirus nonstructural protein σNS acts as an RNA-stability factor promoting viral genome replication. *J Virol* 2018;92:e00563-18.

492. Zhang L, Chandran K, Nibert ML, et al. Reovirus μ1 structural rearrangements that mediate membrane penetration. *J Virol* 2006;80:12367–12376.

493. Zhang X, Ji Y, Zhang L, et al. Features of reovirus outer capsid protein μ1 revealed by electron cryomicroscopy and image reconstruction of the virion at 7.0 Å resolution. *Structure* 2005;13:1545–1557.

494. Zhang X, Jin L, Fang Q, et al. 3.3 Å cryo-EM structure of a nonenveloped virus reveals a priming mechanism for cell entry. *Cell* 2010;141:472–482.

495. Zhang Z, Kim T, Bao M, et al. DDX1, DDX21, and DHX36 helicases form a complex with the adaptor molecule TRIF to sense dsRNA in dendritic cells. *Immunity* 2011;34:866–878.

496. Zhang C, Liu L, Wang P, et al. A potentially novel reovirus isolated from swine in northeastern China in 2007. *Virus Genes* 2011;43:342–349.

497. Zhang P, Samuel CE. Protein kinase PKR plays a stimulus- and virus-dependent role in apoptotic death and virus multiplication in human cells. *J Virol* 2007;81:8192–8200.

498. Zhang X, Walker SB, Chipman PR, et al. Reovirus polymerase λ3 localized by cryo-electron microscopy of virions at a resolution of 7.6 Å. *Nat Struct Biol* 2003;10:1011–1018.

499. Zhang A, Xing J, Xia T, et al. EphA2 phosphorylates NLRP3 and inhibits inflammasomes in airway epithelial cells. *EMBO Rep* 2020;21:e49666.

500. Zhang Z, Yuan B, Lu N, et al. DHX9 pairs with IPS-1 to sense double-stranded RNA in myeloid dendritic cells. *J Immunol* 2011;187:4501–4508.

501. Zhao C, Lu F, Chen H, et al. Dysregulation of JAM-A plays an important role in human tumor progression. *Int J Clin Exp Pathol* 2014;7:7242–7248.

502. Zhuang Y, Berens-Norman HM, Leser JS, et al. Mitochondrial p53 contributes to reovirus-induced neuronal apoptosis and central nervous system injury in a mouse model of viral encephalitis. *J Virol* 2016;90:7684–7691.

503. Zou S, Brown EG. Identification of sequence elements containing signals for replication and encapsidation of the reovirus M1 genome segment. *Virology* 1992;186:377–388.

504. Zurney J, Howard KE, Sherry B. Basal expression levels of IFNAR and Jak-STAT components are determinants of cell-type-specific differences in cardiac antiviral responses. *J Virol* 2007;81:13668–13680.

505. Zurney J, Kobayashi T, Holm GH, et al. Reovirus μ2 protein inhibits interferon signaling through a novel mechanism involving nuclear accumulation of interferon regulatory factor 9. *J Virol* 2009;83:2178–2187.

506. Zweerink HJ, Ito Y, Matsuhisa T. Synthesis of reovirus double-stranded RNA within virion-like particles. *Virology* 1972;50:349–358.

12

Rotaviruses

Sue E. Crawford • Siyuan Ding • Harry B. Greenberg • Mary K. Estes

Introduction and history
Classification
Virion structure
Genome structure and organization
Coding assignments
Stages of replication
  Overview of the replication cycle
  Attachment
  Penetration and uncoating
  RNA synthesis
  Kinetics and cellular sites of transcription, translation, and
    replication
  Genomic RNA encapsidation (packaging) and replication
  Virion maturation
  Virus release
  Virus–host interactions
  Reverse genetics
Pathogenesis and pathology
Epidemiology
  Rotavirus serotypes
  Infection in adults
  Nosocomial infections
  Transmission
  Incubation period
  Geographic distribution and seasonal patterns
  Age, sex, race, and socioeconomic status
  Molecular epidemiologic studies
Immunity
  Adaptive immunity
  Innate immunity
Clinical symptoms
Diagnosis
Treatment
Prevention and control
  Vaccines
  Initial monovalent animal rotavirus ("Jennerian") vaccine
    candidates
  Quadrivalent RRV-based reassortant "Jennerian" rotavirus
    vaccine
  Two major currently licensed live rotavirus vaccines
  Postlicensure safety and efficacy studies of Rotarix and
    RotaTeq
  Selected other currently licensed live attenuated rotavirus
    vaccines deployed on a national or restricted multinational
    basis
  Other approaches to vaccination
  Passive immunization
Perspectives

INTRODUCTION AND HISTORY

Rotaviruses are the single most important cause of severe diarrheal illness in infants and young children. Despite the availability of rotavirus vaccines, rotavirus gastroenteritis was responsible for an estimated 130,000 deaths of children less than 5 years of age throughout the world in 2016 with the greatest toll being in low-income countries.[682]

Human rotaviruses were discovered in 1973 when particles were visualized by Bishop et al. in electron micrographs of thin sections of duodenal mucosa taken from children with acute diarrheal disease.[63] Later virus was identified directly in feces by electron microscopy (EM).[64,221,366] The 70 nm particles observed by negative staining[361,366] of children's feces were subsequently designated rotavirus[222] and documented to be an important etiologic agent of severe diarrhea of infants and young children during the first 2 years of life.[60,360]

Although human rotaviruses were discovered in 1973, several animal viruses described during the previous 10 years were later found to be rotaviruses based on exhibiting characteristic rotavirus morphology and sharing a species antigen with human rotaviruses.[222] These animal agents included: (a) the epizootic diarrhea of infant mice (EDIM) virus seen by Adams and Kraft,[4] using thin section EM in intestinal tissue of suckling mice infected with EDIM virus; (b) a 70-nm simian agent 11 (SA11) that was cultivated in vervet monkey kidney cells from a rectal swab obtained from a healthy vervet monkey[437]; (c) the O (offal) agent isolated in vervet monkey kidney cell culture from the mixed washings of intestines of cattle and sheep[438]; and (d) 70-nm virus particles in stools from calves with a diarrheal illness that could be passaged serially in calves and produce disease,[462] as well as cultivated in primary fetal bovine cell cultures, and named the Nebraska calf diarrhea virus (NCDV).[463] Thus, rotaviruses are excreted in stools of many species and frequently associated with diarrheal disease in the young of those species.

CLASSIFICATION

Rotaviruses comprise the genus *Rotavirus* within the family *Reoviridae* and share common morphologic and biochemical properties (Table 12.1). Early studies using negative stain EM techniques underestimated the particle diameter, while

TABLE 12.1   General characteristics of rotaviruses

Structure
  100 nm icosahedral particles (including the spikes)
  Triple-layered protein capsid
  Nonenveloped (resistant to lipid solvents)
  Capsid contains all enzymes for mRNA production

Genome
  11 segments of dsRNA
  Purified RNA segments are not infectious
  Each RNA segment codes for at least one protein
  vRNA segments from different rotaviruses of the same species
    reassort at high frequency during coinfections of cells

Replication
  Cultivation facilitated by proteases
  Cytoplasmic replication
  Inclusion body formation
  Unique morphogenesis involves transient enveloped particles
  Levels of intracellular calcium important for virus assembly,
    stability, and disassembly
  Virus particles released by cell lysis or by nonclassical vesicular
    transport in polarized epithelial cells

mRNA, messenger RNA; dsRNA, double-stranded RNA.

subsequent cryo-EM studies, in which no stains were used, established the particle diameter to be 100 nm including the spikes.

Salient features are that (a) mature virus particles, including spikes, are about 100 nm (1,000 Å) in diameter and possess a triple-layered icosahedral protein capsid composed of an outer layer, an intermediate layer, and an inner core layer (Fig. 12.1); (b) 60 protein spikes extend from the smooth surface of the outer shell; (c) outer capsid integrity requires calcium; (d) particles contain an RNA-dependent RNA polymerase and other enzymes capable of producing capped RNA transcripts; (e) the virus genome contains 11 segments of double-stranded RNA (dsRNA); (f) rotaviruses of the same species (see below) are capable of genetic reassortment; (g) virus replication occurs in the cytoplasm of infected cells; (h) virus cultivation *in vitro* is facilitated by treatment with proteolytic enzymes enhancing viral infectivity by cleavage of the outer capsid spike protein; and (i) the viruses exhibit a unique morphogenic pathway; transiently enveloped virus particles are formed by budding into endoplasmic reticulum (ER)–derived membranes during morphogenesis. Virions are liberated from infected cells by cell lysis or by a nonclassic vesicular transport in polarized epithelial cells. Historically, mature infectious particles were thought to be nonenveloped; however, infectious rotaviruses enclosed in vesicles have recently been reported.[605]

Rotaviruses are classified by the Rotavirus Classification Working Group[448] based on the serologic reactivity and genetic variability of the middle capsid structural protein VP6 and lack of reassortment between species into ten distinct species (formerly called Groups) designated *Rotavirus A* to *Rotavirus J* (RVA, etc.)[41,452,471] RVA, RVB, and RVC strains are found in both humans and animals, whereas rotaviruses of species D to J have been found only in animals to date. Viruses within each species are capable of genetic reassortment, but reassortment does not occur among viruses in different species, thus defining the unique species.[733] A rotavirus species includes viruses that share cross-reacting antigens detectable by several serologic methods, such as immunofluorescence, enzyme-linked

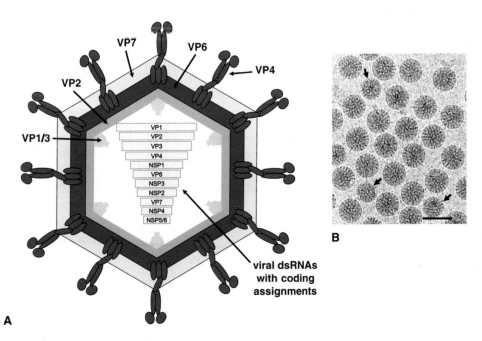

FIGURE 12.1 Schematic diagram and electron micrograph of rotavirus particles. A: The particle is composed of three concentric protein shells (VP7, VP6, VP2, shown in different colors) and the spike protein VP4 that spans the VP6 and VP7 layers and extends out from the particle. Transcription/replication complexes of VP1 and VP3 are located inside the VP2 layer at the fivefold axes of symmetry. The viral dsRNA genome is segmented. **B:** Rotavirus triple-layered particles (TLPs) and a few double-layered particles (DLPs) (*arrows*) are easily visualized by cryogenic electron microscopy (cryo-EM). Bar, 100 nm. (Courtesy of B.V.V. Prasad.)

immunosorbent assay (ELISA), and immune electron micros-copy (IEM). Cross-reactive epitopes on the intermediate capsid protein (VP6) are those usually detected by diagnostic ELISA, primarily because this protein is highly antigenic, and it represents the largest mass of the particle. However, common epitopes among members of RVA species, and presumably other rotavirus species, are found on most (if not all) of the structural proteins and probably on many of the nonstructural proteins as well. This is documented by observing that monospecific antisera and some monoclonal antibodies (mAbs) specific for individual polypeptides cross-react with strains other than those to which they were made.

RVAs cause significant diarrheal disease in infants and in the young of various mammalian and avian species. RVBs have been associated with epidemics of severe diarrhea, primarily in adults in Asia.[30,322,349,651] RVCs have been sporadically reported in fecal specimens from children with diarrhea and in several family outbreaks.[511] Rapid diagnostic tests (ELISA), mAb, and PCR assays to detect non–species-A rotaviruses are available mainly in research laboratories, and these facilitate determining the clinical importance of these viruses[490,734] (also see Diagnosis section below). Very few non–species A rotavirus strains have been successfully propagated in cell culture. The inability to grow most non–species A viruses has hampered obtaining detailed information on these viruses, although gene-coding assignments and sequence data are available. Unless noted otherwise, this chapter focuses on information about the RVA viruses. Reviews on the non–species A rotaviruses and comparisons between the proteins of the species-A and non–species A viruses have been published elsewhere.[81,344,454,596]

RVA viruses are the most extensively studied, and they are further classified based on antigenic and sequence differences of the two outer capsid proteins VP7 and VP4 into G (Glycosylated) and P (Protease-sensitive) types, respectively. To date, there are 57 P-types and 41 G-types.[448] In the infected host, these two outer capsid proteins independently elicit neutralizing antibodies.[272,314] Due to the unavailability of serological reagents for these neutralization antigens, and the increasing ease of sequencing, including whole genome sequencing, each genomic segment of RVA is now classified based on sequencing data.

In 2008, a comprehensive nucleotide sequence-based, complete genome classification system was developed for RVAs.[449] This system assigns a specific genotype to each of the 11 rotavirus genome segments according to established nucleotide percent identity cut-off values. The VP7-VP4-VP6-VP1-VP2-VP3-NSP1-NSP2-NSP3-NSP4-NSP5/6 genes of rotavirus strains are described using the abbreviations Gx-P[x]-Ix-Rx-Cx-Mx-Ax-Nx-Tx-Ex-Hx (x = Arabic numbers starting from 1), respectively (Table 12.2). A Rotavirus Classification Working Group that includes researchers worldwide maintains and evaluates this system. Recent updates are published, and new guidelines recommend uniform nomenclature for individual strains to be: rotavirus species/species of origin/country of identification/common name/year of identification/G- and P-type.[450] The prototype simian agent 11 (SA11) is designated RVA/Simian-tc/ZAF/SA11-H96/1958/G3P5B[2] and the full descriptor of genes is indicated by G3-P[2]-I2-R2-C5-M5-A5-N5-T5-E2-H5. The most common genome constellations worldwide based on analysis of greater than 400 available complete or near-complete rotavirus genome sequences are human Wa-like rotavirus strains and porcine rotavirus strains (Gx-P[x]-I1-R1-C1-M1-A1-N1-T1-E1-H1) and human DS-1–like rotavirus strains and bovine rotaviruses (Gx-P[x]-I2-R2-C2-M2-A2-N2-T2-E2-H2).[449] This analysis reveals close evolutionary links between human and animal rotaviruses. The genetic diversity of RVA strains recently isolated from bats provides evidence of multiple reassortment and host switching events from bats to bats and to other mammals, including unusual human and animal RVA strains. These slowly emerging data suggest that zoonoses of bat rotaviruses might occur more frequently than currently realized.[637]

VIRION STRUCTURE

The morphologic appearance of rotavirus particles is distinctive, and three types of particles can be observed by EM (Fig. 12.2). The complete particles resemble a wheel with

TABLE 12.2 Nucleotide percent identity cut-off values defining genotypes for the 11 rotavirus gene segments

Gene Product	Percentage Identity	Genotypes	Name of Genotypes
VP7	80	41G	**G**lycosylated
VP4	80	57P	**P**rotease-sensitive
VP6	85	31I	**I**nner capsid
VP1	83	27R	**R**NA-dependent RNA polymerase
VP2	84	23C	**C**ore protein
VP3	81	23M	**M**ethyltransferase
NSP1	79	38A	Interferon **A**ntagonist
NSP2	85	27N	**N**TPase
NSP3	85	27T	**T**ranslation enhancer
NSP4	85	31E	**E**nterotoxin
NSP5	91	27H	p**H**osphoprotein

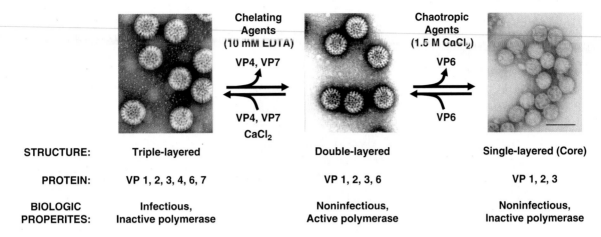

FIGURE 12.2 Structural and biologic properties of rotavirus particles. Electron micrographs show typical triple-layered (TLPs), double-layered (DLPs), and single-layered (SLPs) (core) particles after staining with 1% ammonium molybdate. TLPs, DLPs, and core particles can be produced by sequential capsid protein removal (*top arrows*) or addition (*bottom arrows*) as shown. The proteins and biologic properties of the particles are detailed in the text. Bar, 100 nm.

short spokes and a well-defined, smooth outer rim. The name *rotavirus* (from the Latin *rota*, meaning "wheel") was coined based on this morphology.[222] The complete infectious particles (virions) are also called triple-layered particles (TLPs). These particles are approximately 100 nm in diameter. Double-layered particles (DLPs) lacking the outer shell consisting of VP7 and VP4 are described as *rough particles* because their periphery shows projecting trimeric subunits of the inner capsid. Single-layered particles (SLPs or cores) are seen infrequently; they usually lack genomic RNA and are aggregated.

The structures of triple- and double-layered rotavirus particles are solved to near-atomic resolution based on X-ray crystallography and particle reconstructions of cryo-EM images, and these provide a detailed description of particles[304,402,411,555,623,627,729] (Fig. 12.3). Particles possess icosahedral symmetry with a T = 13*l* (levo) icosahedral surface lattice for the two outer layers, while the innermost layer exhibits a unique T = 1 icosahedral organization. Distinguishing features of the TLP structure include 132 large aqueous channels and 60 spikes.

The channels span the two outer layers and link the outer surface with the inner core. Three types of channels are distinguishable based on their position and size (Fig. 12.3). Twelve type I channels are located at the icosahedral fivefold axes, 60 type II channels are at each of the pentavalent positions surrounding the fivefold axes, and a second set of 60 type III channels are at the six-coordinated positions surrounding the icosahedral threefold axes. Type III channels are about 140 Å in depth and about 55 Å wide at the outer surface of the virus. On entering the particle, these channels constrict before widening to their maximal width, which is close to the surface of the inner shell. Similar features and dimensions are seen in the other two types of channels, except that type I channels have a narrower (~40 Å) opening at the outer surface of the virus. The type I channels are conduits for the export of messenger RNA (mRNA) that first interacts with the enzyme complexes composed of VP1, the RNA-dependent RNA polymerase, and VP3, the capping enzyme,[396] that are present at the inner surface of the fivefold axes of the SLP[400,402,554] (Fig. 12.3). The

VP3 capping enzyme contains five distinct activities (RNA helicase, RNA triphosphatase [RTPase], guanylyltransferase [GTase], methyltransferase [MTase], and 2'-O-methyltransferase [2'O-MTase] activities).[396] VP3 also contains a C-terminal phosphodiesterase domain that functions as an antagonist of the antiviral 2'-5'-oligoadenylate synthetase/ribonuclease L (OAS/RNase L) pathway.[748] Atomic structures of the rotavirus polymerase, alone and in complex with RNA, show VP1 is a compact, globular protein of approximately 70 Å in diameter that has three domains: an N-terminal domain, a polymerase domain, and a C-terminal domain.[429] The polymerase domain exhibits the right-handed architecture (fingers-palm-thumb) typical of polymerases in general as well as canonical motifs (A to F) involved in various aspects of phosphodiester bond formation[429] (Fig. 12.3). Models of how this enzyme functions in coordinated genome replication and packaging are discussed later.

The SLP exhibits a unique T = 1 symmetry and is composed of 120 molecules of VP2 arranged as 60 dimers that surround the genomic dsRNA that is highly ordered[554,623] (Fig. 12.3). X-ray and cryo-EM structures of DLPs show that VP2 has two structural isoforms that interact extensively.[456] One of the subunits in the icosahedral asymmetric unit (VP2A) packs around the icosahedral fivefold axis forming a star-shaped complex with a small pore in the middle lined by conserved basic residues. The other subunit (VP2B) fills in space between the VP2A subunits forming a decameric cap structure at the fivefold axis. Twelve of these decameric complexes make up the VP2 layer that is 25 to 30 Å thick. Many segmented dsRNA viruses contain 120 molecules of a core protein (VP2 for rotavirus, VP3 for bluetongue virus, lambda 1 for reoviruses, the single capsid protein for cypovirus) that surrounds an ordered genome.[317] Although the inner shell protein shares similar features among these dsRNA viruses, rotaviruses and orbiviruses are distinguished by housing their enzymatic functions entirely *within* the inner shell, leading them to be called *nonturreted viruses*, and nascent mRNA transcripts are released through channels penetrating the two capsid layers at the icosahedral vertices.[307,401,402] This capsid architecture contrasts with the structure of the *turreted viruses*,

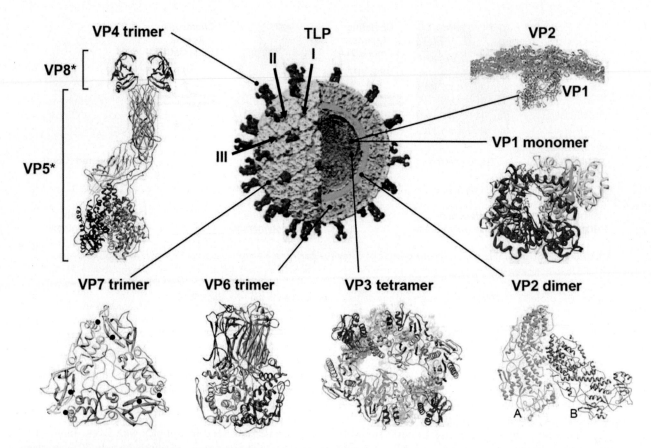

FIGURE 12.3 Rotavirus structures and locations of protein components. A cutaway view of a 9.5 Å cryo-EM of the mature triple-layered rotavirus particle (TLP) shows surface and internal structural features. The TLP is colored with the VP4 spikes (60 trimers) in *red*, the VP7 (260 trimers) surface glycoprotein in *yellow*, the internal (middle) VP6 (260 trimers) layer in *blue*, and the core VP2 (60 dimers) layer in *green*. Atomic structures of the individual proteins also are shown along with their locations in the virion. The ribbon diagram of the VP1/RNA complex shows the N-terminal domain in *yellow*, the C-terminal domain in *magenta*, and the C-terminal plug in *cyan*. The subdomains of the polymerase domain are in *light blue* (fingers), *red* (palm), and *green* (thumb). The VP3 tetramer is viewed along a twofold axis with individual domains colored: KL domain (*red*), guanine-N7 MTase domain (*green*), 2'-O-MTase domain (*orange*), GTase domain (*cyan*), and PDE domain (*magenta*). Two antiparallel VP3 monomers form each dimer, shown in the ribbon (front) and surface (back) representation, respectively. The oligomeric state of VP3 in the particle is unknown. The VP4 spike consists of VP8* (*red*), VP5* β-barrel domain (*orange*), and VP5* foot domain (*blue*).[304] The VP7 trimer is viewed along the threefold axis with three subunits colored in *yellow*, *gold*, and *orange*. The two calcium (Ca²⁺) molecules coordinated between each of the VP7 monomers are shown in *black*. Structures made from the Protein Data Bank (PDB) IDs: PDB 4V7Q (TLP), 6OJ6 (VP1/VP2), 2R7R (VP1), 3KZ4 (VP2), 6O6B (VP3), 4V7Q (VP4), 3KZ4 (VP6), and 3FMG (VP7). (Figure prepared by Liya Hu.)

reoviruses,[569,750] aquareovirus,[749] and cypovirus,[739] where the polymerase enzyme is housed within the core, but the capping enzymes are incorporated as pentameric turret-like projections that extend through the inner capsid layer at each icosahedral vertex.[307]

The VP2 layer is surrounded by 260 trimers of VP6 that form a T = 13 icosahedral lattices (Fig. 12.3) in the DLP. These trimers are located directly below the VP7 trimers in the outer layer so that the channels in the outer layer and the DLP are in register. The DLP is about 705 Å in diameter, and the structure of the VP6 subunit has two domains with an overall structure similar to the VP7 of bluetongue virus[274,445] (Fig. 12.3) and to the μ1 protein of orthoreovirus.[413] The distal domain of rotavirus VP6 has an eight-stranded jelly-roll β-barrel fold that makes contacts with VP7 and VP4, whereas the proximal domain with a cluster of eight α-helices and a conformationally flexible loop structure in VP6 is involved in establishing optimal contacts with the underlying VP2 subunits.[456] Interactions of VP6 with the VP7 layer at the top and the VP2 layer

at the bottom are important in stabilizing the entire rotavirus capsid and integrating the two essential functions of particles: cell entry and endogenous transcription. Structural integrity of the DLP is an essential requirement for endogenous transcription that takes place within the confines of the DLP with capped transcripts exiting through the aqueous type I channels at the fivefold axes.[402] The biophysics of the interaction of different layers of rotavirus particles have recently been studied by atomic force microscopy and revealed (a) the outer capsid layer is stiff and resistant to strain and shields the virus during its travel through the digestive system; (b) the outer and middle layers are strongly connected but are dissociated by the removal of calcium ions, a key step for transcription initiation; (c) the middle layer presents weak hydrophobic interactions with the inner layer that allow conformational dynamics needed for transcription.[346]

Sixty trimeric spikes extend from the smooth surface of the outer shell (Fig. 12.3).[554] These protein spikes are situated at an edge of the type II channels surrounding the fivefold icosahedral axes. The spikes are composed of the protein VP4, as initially shown by seeing that two Fab subunits of a mAb to VP4 bind on the sides near the tips of the spikes.[556] Subsequent cryo-EM studies,[142,186,411,534,627] including the most recent studies at near atomic resolution,[304,623] confirmed that VP4 is the spike protein and showed that the spike has multiple domains with a unique trimeric organization that projects about 120 Å from the surface of the virus with a total radial length of 200 Å. Spikes with well-defined structural features, two distal globular domains, a central body with an approximate twofold symmetry, and a globular domain called the foot domain are only visible in rotavirus particles grown in the presence of trypsin that enhances virus yield.[142,627,728] Proteolysis cleaves VP4 (88 kD) into VP8* (28 kD, aa 1–247) and VP5* (60 kD, aa 248–776), and the cleavage products remain noncovalently associated in the virion (Fig. 12.3; Table 12.3).

Crystallographic structures of VP8* and portions of VP5* as well as cryo-EM analyses at about 3.4 Å resolution indicate that the overall conformation of each VP4 subunit is that of a high loop, with the N-terminal helical segment of VP8* being anchored against the C-terminal domain of VP5* in the foot domain of the same polypeptide chain.[186,304,623] Two β-barrel domains of VP5*, at the central body of the spike, adopt a dimeric appearance above the capsid surface, while another VP5* β-barrel of the third VP4 molecule is positioned closer to the capsid surface interacting with the VP7 capsid layer; the globular domains of each of the VP5* polypeptides form a trimeric base anchored inside the type II channels between the VP7 and VP6 capsid layers.[304,411,534,623,728] Two VP8* molecules are present at the top of two upright VP5* molecules and the third VP8* interacts with the VP5* foot domain.[304] Thus, VP4 subunits undergo extensive rearrangements that resemble conformational transitions of membrane fusion proteins of enveloped viruses during entry into cells.[186,304]

The spike is held in place by interactions with both VP6 and VP7. The spike extends inward about 80 Å where it inserts into the lattice of VP6 trimers at the type II channels that surround the type I channels at the icosahedral fivefold axes. This interaction may facilitate trimerization of cytosolic VP4.[623] The VP7 shell partly covers the base of the VP4 spike and appears to lock VP4 onto the virion within the type II channel.[679]

The outer 35 Å thick capsid layer of rotavirus is formed by 260 trimers of the glycoprotein VP7 (37 kD) (Fig. 12.3). VP7 is a calcium-binding protein[234,593] and consists of two domains: domain I with a disulfide bridge exhibits a Rossmann fold and domain II with three disulfide bridges exhibits a jelly-roll β-sandwich fold. Two Ca^{2+} ions are bound at each subunit interface in the trimer.[17] Three VP7 subunits interact with each other to form a plate-like trimer that sits on top of the VP6 trimers and the N-terminal arms of three VP7 subunits grip the underlying VP6 trimers and intrude into the VP4 foot cavity. These interactions imply that the VP4 spikes must first be attached to the DLPs prior to the addition of VP7 during virus assembly and the addition of VP7 results in a shift in the underlying VP6 trimers.[623] This order of outer capsid assembly is supported by *in vitro* reconstitution studies where sequential addition of recombinant VP4 followed by VP7 onto DLPs can produce infectious virus.[679]

GENOME STRUCTURE AND ORGANIZATION

The viral dsRNA genome is contained within the virus core capsid. Deproteinized rotavirus genomic dsRNA is not infectious, reflecting that virus particles contain their own RNA-dependent RNA polymerase to transcribe the individual RNA segments into active mRNA. The genome RNA is highly ordered within the particle; spherically averaged density shows eight concentric layers of the dsRNA genome with an average spacing of 28 Å between the layers.[554] Several points of contact between the inwardly protruding portion of VP2 as well as VP1 and VP3 interact with the RNA surrounding each fivefold axis[399,554] (Fig. 12.3), and VP2 interactions with VP1 are required for polymerase function during transcriptase and replicase activity.[177,459,522]

The nucleotide sequences of all 11 rotavirus RNA segments for many rotavirus strains are known, and this forms the basis for the classification system discussed above.[449] The prototype simian SA11 strain was the first genome to be completely sequenced. The sequences from different rotavirus strains show similar general features (Fig. 12.4) in each genome segment. Each positive-sense RNA segment starts with a 5′-guanidine followed by a set of conserved sequences that are part of the 5′-noncoding sequences. An open reading frame (ORF) coding for the protein product and ending with the stop codon follows, and then another set of noncoding sequences is found containing a subset of conserved terminal 3′ sequences and ending with two 3′-terminal cytidines. Almost all mRNAs end with the consensus sequence 5′-UGUGACC-3′, and these sequences contain important signals for gene expression and genome replication. The last four nucleotides of the mRNAs function as translation enhancers.[114] The lengths of the 3′- and 5′-noncoding sequences vary for different genes, but the noncoding sequences of homologous strains are highly conserved. No polyadenylation signal is found at the 3′ end of the genes. All of the sequenced genes possess at least one long ORF after the first initiation codon. This is usually a strong initiation codon based on Kozak's rules.[393] Although some of the genes possess additional in-phase (genes 7, 9, and 10) or out-of-phase (gene 11) ORFs, current evidence indicates that all the genes are monocistronic, except gene 11.[455]

The rotavirus gene sequences are A + U rich (60% to 71%), and this bias against CGN and NCC codons is shared with many eukaryotic and viral genes.[471] The dsRNA segments are base-paired end-to-end, and the positive-sense strand contains a 5′ cap sequence $m^7GpppG^{(m)}GC$.[327] Similar features of the RNA termini (capped structures and 5′- and 3′-conserved sequences) are found in the genomes of other segmented viruses (e.g., reovirus, cytoplasmic polyhedrosis virus, orbivirus) in the family *Reoviridae* and in other virus families with segmented RNA genomes (*Orthomyxoviridae*, *Arenaviridae*, and *Bunyaviridae*). One of the most intriguing aspects of the replication cycle of rotaviruses and all segmented dsRNA viruses relates to mechanism(s) of how these viruses coordinately replicate and package the 11 viral mRNAs. The 11 mRNAs must share common cis-acting signals because they are all replicated by the same polymerase, and the UGUG sequence of the consensus sequence is recognized in a base-specific manner by the polymerase, so that its 3′ end overshoots the initiating regis-

TABLE 12.3 Rotavirus proteins

Genome Segment	Protein Product[a]	Nascent Polypeptide (Mol. Wt. × 1,000)[b]	Mature Protein Modified	Location in Virus Particles	Number of Molecules per Virion[c]	ts Mutant Group (Mutation)[d]	Function[e]
1	VP1	125	—	Core	12	C (L138P)	RNA-dependent RNA polymerase, ssRNA binding, complex with VP3
2	VP2	102.4	—	Core	120	F (A387D)	RNA binding, required for replicase activity of VP1
3	VP3	98.1	—	Core	12	B (G527D)	RNA helicase, RNA triphosphatase, guanylyltransferase, methyltransferase, and 2'-O-methyltransferase, ssRNA binding, complex with VP1, inhibit RNase L signaling
4	VP4	86.8	Cleaved VP5* (529) VP8* (247)[f]	Outer capsid	180	A (A401T)	P-type neutralization antigen, viral attachment, homotrimer, protease-enhanced infectivity, virulence, putative fusion region
5	NSP1 (NS53)	58.7	—	Nonstructural		D (L140V)	Interferon antagonist, putative viral E3 ligase, RNA binding
6	VP6	44.8	—	Inner capsid	780	G (T10S, D13H)	Subgroup antigen, trimer, protection (intracellular neutralization), required for transcription
7	NSP3 (NS34)	34.6	—	Nonstructural		NA	Acidic dimer, binds 3' end of viral mRNAs, cellular eIF4G, Hsp90, surrogate of PABP, inhibits host translation
8	NSP2 (NS35)	36.7	—	Nonstructural		E (A152V)	Basic, octamer, RNA binding, NTPase, NDP kinase, RTPase, helix-destabilizing activities, forms viroplasms with VP1 and NSP5
9	VP7	37.4	Cleaved signal peptide glycosylation	Outer capsid	780	K (T280I)	G-type neutralization antigen, glycoprotein calcium-dependent trimer
10	NSP4 (NS20)	20.3	NS29–NS28 uncleaved signal peptide high mannose glycosylation and trimming	Nonstructural		NA	RER transmembrane glycoprotein, viroporin, intracellular receptor for DLPs, role in morphogenesis of TLPs, interacts with viroplasms and autophagy pathway, modulates intracellular calcium and RNA replication, enterotoxin secreted from cells, virulence

Genome Segment	Protein Product[a]	Nascent Polypeptide (Mol. Wt. × 1,000)[b]	Mature Protein Modified	Location in Virus Particles	Number of Molecules per Virion[c]	ts Mutant Group (Mutation)[d]	Function[e]
11	NSP5 (NS26)	21.7	28K, O-glycosylated, phosphorylated (different forms)	Nonstructural		J (A182G)	Basic, phosphoprotein, RNA binding, protein kinase, forms viroplasms with NSP2, interacts with VP2 and NSP6
	NSP6	12	Product of second ORF	Nonstructural			Interacts with NSP5, present in viroplasms and most virus strains, RNA binding

[a]The virion polypeptides are designated as proposed by Mason et al.[443] and modified by Liu et al.[418] and Mattion et al.[454] VP3 is the protein product of gene segment 3, and VP4 is the protein product of gene segment 4. Early studies failed to unequivocally identify a protein product from genome segment 3; hence, the protein product of genome segment 4 was called VP3 in early publications. When the protein product of genome segment 3 was confirmed to be a structural protein located in the inner core, the genome 3 product was designated VP3 and the genome 4 product was renamed VP4.[418] In 1994, the nonstructural proteins were renamed NSP1 to NSP5 to facilitate comparisons among these proteins between different virus strains,[454] and this nomenclature is now accepted. The parentheses in this table show the names of the nonstructural proteins as designated previously (NS followed by a number indicating their apparent molecular weight in thousands determined by electrophoresis in polyacrylamide gels containing sodium dodecyl sulfate). NSP6 has been characterized since 1991.[455]

[b]Molecular weights are for simian agent 11 (SA11) proteins and are calculated from the deduced amino acid sequences from the nucleotide sequence and from the longest potential open reading frame. The gene-protein assignment of segments 7 to 9 is for the SA11 strain.

[c]Calculated from structural studies of purified virions.

[d]NA, no mutant assignment. Two groups of temperature-sensitive mutants (tsH and tsI) are not yet mapped to a genome segment. Data compiled from the following sources.[146,253,254,566]

[e]See text for references.

There are three trypsin cleavage sites in SA11 VP4 at amino acids 231, 241, and 247. The indicated mature products are those based on use of only the preferred second cleavage site.[19]

ssRNA, single-stranded RNA; mRNA, messenger RNA; PABP, poly(A)-binding protein; NTPase, nucleoside triphosphatase; NDP, nucleoside diphosphate; RTPase, RNA triphosphatase; RER, rough endoplasmic reticulum; DLP, double-layered particle; TLP, triple-layered particle.

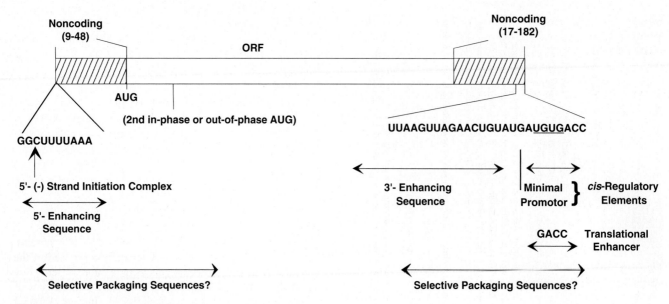

FIGURE 12.4 Major features of rotavirus gene structure. Schematic shows the overall structure of rotavirus genes derived from published sequences of genes 1 through 11. All 11 rotavirus genes have a cap-1 structure at the 5′ end and lack a polyadenylation signal, they are A + U rich, and they contain conserved consensus sequences at their 5′ and 3′ ends. The prototype SA11 genome segments range in size from 667 (segment 11) to 3,302 (segment 1) with a total of 18,556 base pairs. The *bottom arrows* show *cis*-regulatory elements of rotavirus messenger RNA (mRNA) required for replication of transcripts assayed in a cell-free replication system.[524,677,715] The study of viruses with variations in the sequence at the 3′ termini indicates that the minimal promoter is $URN_{0.5}CC$.[715] The 5′ and 3′ noncoding regions at the termini of the mRNA are predicted to interact and stably base pair to form a panhandle structure possibly stabilized by the viral polymerase[327,524,677] and interactions between the 3′ terminus with the nonstructural protein NSP3 may promote translation of viral mRNA.[693] The penultimate 5′-GACC-3′ is a translation enhancer.[114]

ter, producing a stable but catalytically inactive complex.[429] In addition, each mRNA must also contain a signal that is unique to it alone, because the 11 mRNAs must be distinguished from one another during packaging. Generally, the conserved terminal sequences in genome segments contain cis-acting signals that are important for transcription, RNA translation, RNA transport, replication, assembly, or encapsidation of the viral genome segments. Some of the cis-acting signals for rotavirus RNA replication and translation have been identified (Fig. 12.4).[523] Sequence comparisons between rotavirus strains have contributed to identifying conserved sequences and/or secondary structure in the rotavirus genome.[409] Conserved secondary structures in the positive-sense RNAs, including long-range interactions at the 5′ and 3′ terminal regions present in all segments, may facilitate RNA circularization although such structures remain to be detected in cells.[409] Computer modeling and RNAse mapping experiments predict that viral (+)RNAs fold into panhandles through 5′ and 3′ base pairing and the 3′ consensus sequence extends from the panhandle as a single-stranded tail.[108,409,677] Interactions of this extended RNA with different rotavirus and cellular proteins are thought to regulate whether the (+)RNA functions in translation, genome replication or assortment, and packaging.[459]

Rotaviruses are the only known agents of mammals or birds that contain 11 segments of dsRNA. In most cases, the electrophoretic pattern of the genome of the species A viruses is composed of four high molecular weight dsRNA segments (numbered 1 to 4), two middle-sized segments (5 and 6), a distinctive triplet of segments (7 to 9), and two smaller segments (10 and 11). When this basic pattern is not seen, the rotavirus being analyzed may be a species A avian virus, a non–species

A virus, a species A virus that contains rearrangements within individual genome segments (Fig. 12.5A),[167] or a new unique species A virus. Analysis of genomic electropherotypes is a relatively easy, rapid, and popular technique for virus detection and for molecular epidemiology studies to monitor virus outbreaks and transmission. However, because distinct RNA patterns can arise by different mechanisms (reassortment, mutation, rearrangements) and RNA segments of different sequence may comigrate, these profiles are not useful as a definitive criterion for classification of a virus strain.[102] (Also see Molecular Epidemiologic Studies below.) Nucleic acid hybridization combined with Northern blot was initially used to classify viruses based on the relatedness of genome segments[203] (e.g., to classify genetically related viruses into different species)[488] and to identify the origin of specific RNA segments in virus reassortants. This method characterized viruses involved in cross-species transmission[486,487] but is now being replaced by complete genome sequencing. Zoonotic transmission of rotaviruses has been demonstrated by genomic analysis of reassortants derived from rotaviruses from two distinct parental species.[10,224,440,654]

In viruses with genome rearrangements, typical RNA segments are missing or are decreased in concentration in an electrophoretic profile, and are replaced by additional, more slowly (or rarely more rapidly) migrating bands of dsRNA (Fig. 12.5A, lanes 4, 5 and 7). The slowly migrating bands represent concatemeric forms of dsRNA containing sequences specific for the missing RNA segments.[167] The more rapidly migrating bands appear to represent deletions. Viruses with genome rearrangements of this type have been isolated most frequently during infection from immunodeficient, chronically infected children, asymptomatically infected immunocompetent children, and animals (calves, pigs, or rabbits).[167] Viruses with rearranged genomes have also been obtained *in vitro* after serial high multiplicity of infection passage of tissue culture–adapted rotaviruses.[319] Virus isolates with rearrangements in segments 5, 6, 8, 10, and 11 have been characterized, with the greatest number having rearrangements detected in segments 5 and 11. Viruses with a rearranged segment 11 may have some selective advantage (better growth *in vitro* or stability), so they are detected more easily, rather than occurring more frequently.[616]

Viruses that contain rearranged genome segments are generally not defective, and the rearranged segments can reassort and replace normal RNA segments structurally and functionally. These viruses do not have a growth advantage, but they exhibit a selective advantage for being incorporated in viral progeny indicating a preferential packaging of rearranged segments into progeny.[684] In most cases, the profiles of virus-encoded proteins in cells infected with rotaviruses with rearranged genomes are similar to those seen in cells infected with standard rotavirus strains, indicating that the rearrangement of the sequences in a segment leaves the normal ORFs and their expression unaltered. Sequence analyses of rearranged genome segments confirm this and reveal mechanisms by which the rearrangements arise.[381] In most cases, the rearrangements result from a head-to-tail duplication that occurs immediately downstream from the normal ORF and, hence, the rearranged segment retains the capacity to express its normal protein product. Rotaviruses, compared to mammalian reoviruses, are less likely to undergo recombination events and generate defective gene segments.[641]

CODING ASSIGNMENTS

The coding assignments and many properties of the proteins encoded in each of the 11 genome segments are now well established (Fig. 12.5B; Table 12.3), although new protein functions continue to be identified.

The rotavirus genome segments code for six structural proteins found in virus particles and six nonstructural proteins found in infected cells but not present in mature particles; a few tissue culture adapted virus strains lack NSP6 (Table 12.3). Early studies often presented conflicting conclusions concerning the numbers and locations of the rotavirus proteins. Many of these conflicts were resolved, as reviewed elsewhere,[454] when it was recognized that posttranslational modifications (glycosylation, trimming of carbohydrate residues, and proteolytic cleavages) occur after polypeptide synthesis. In addition, strain variations (e.g., the presence of more than one glycosylation site on VP7 in some bovine, equine, porcine, and human rotavirus strains) provide explanations for other differences in polypeptide patterns.

The nomenclature of the viral proteins (as originally proposed for SA11 proteins) designates structural proteins as viral protein-VP followed by a number, with VP1 being the highest molecular weight protein, and proteins generated by cleavage of a larger precursor being indicated by an asterisk (VP4 is cleaved to produce VP5* and VP8*[198,200]). Initial studies referred to the nonstructural proteins as NS followed by a number indicating the protein's molecular weight. This nomenclature has been replaced by NSP1 to NSP6 to facilitate comparisons among cognate nonstructural proteins of different molecular weights[454] (Table 12.3). In fact, much of the literature before 1988 refers

to the genome segment 4 product as "VP3"; before 1994, NS53 and NS35 were the designations used for what is now referred to as NSP1, NSP2, and so forth (Table 12.3). The new nomenclature is used throughout this chapter.

STAGES OF REPLICATION

Overview of the Replication Cycle

Figure 12.6 shows a schematic of the rotavirus replication cycle. Most details of this cycle have been obtained from studies of rotaviruses infecting monkey kidney cell monolayers or, to a lesser degree, polarized intestinal epithelial cells. Other information has come from assays to probe-specific steps in the replication cycle based on the expression and interaction of individual wild-type or mutated proteins and RNA in *in vitro* systems. Conclusions from these studies are generally confirmed in the context of virus replication systems using confocal microscopy and small interfering RNA (siRNA). Recent development of efficient reverse genetics systems allows the incorporation of desired nonlethal mutation into any gene in the rotavirus genome.[357,382–384,603]

In vivo, the natural cell tropism for rotaviruses is for differentiated enterocyte and some enteroendocrine and tuft[68b] cells in the small intestine, suggesting these cells express specific receptor(s) for virus attachment and entry into cells.[68b,289,560,614,615,755] However, extraintestinal spread of rotavirus also occurs in humans and all animal models studied,[33,66,68,143,206,216,516,563] demonstrating a wider range of host cells than previously thought and possible additional receptors. Rotavirus replication in continuous cell cultures derived from monkey kidneys is fairly rapid, with maximal yields of virus occurring after 10 to 12 hours at 37°C or 18 hours at 33°C when cells are infected at high multiplicities of infection (10 to 20 plaque-forming units/cell).[124,457,565] Rotavirus replication in differentiated human intestinal cell lines (Caco-2 cells) grown on permeable filter membranes is slower, with maximal yields of virus detected on the apical surface of cells 20 to 24 hours after infection.[118,119,352] Significantly, EM studies of virus replication in polarized intestinal cells indicate that the replication process in these cells has some distinct differences from the virus replication cycle in nonpolarized cell cultures. These emerging differences are described further below.

The general features of rotavirus replication (based on studies in cultures of monkey kidney cells) are as follows:

1. Cultivation of most virus strains requires the addition of exogenous trypsin or trypsin-like proteases to the culture medium. This ensures the activation of viral infectivity by cleaving the outer capsid protein VP4.
2. Replication is cytoplasmic.
3. Cells do not contain enzymes to replicate dsRNA; hence, the virus must supply the necessary enzymes.
4. Transcripts function both to produce proteins and as a template for the production of negative-strand RNA. Once the complementary negative strand is synthesized, it remains associated with the positive strand.
5. The dsRNA segments are formed within nascent subviral particles, and free dsRNA or free negative-stranded ssRNA is generally not found in infected cells.

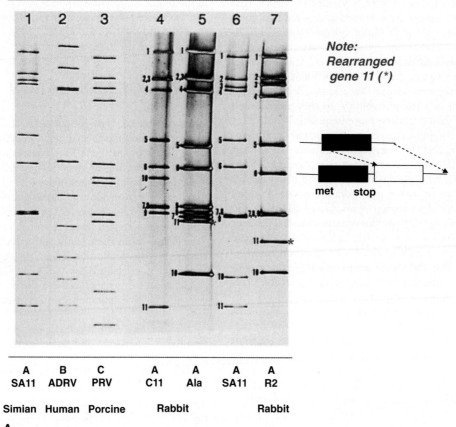

Note: Rearranged gene 11 (*)

met   stop

1	2	3	4	5	6	7
A	B	C	A	A	A	A
SA11	ADRV	PRV	C11	Ala	SA11	R2
Simian	Human	Porcine	Rabbit		Rabbit	

A

1 VP1 — 1 / 1088 / 3302 — **R**NA-dependent RNA polymerase
ss-RNA binding, complexes with VP3

2 VP2 — 1 / 881 / 2690 — **C**ore protein
required for replicase activity of VP1

3 VP3 — 1 / 835 / 2591 — **M**ethyltransferase
guanylyltransferase

4 VP4 — 1 / 776 / 2362 — **P**rotease-sensitive
neutralization antigen, viral attachment protein

5 NSP1 — 1 / 491 / 1581 — Interferon **A**ntagonist

6 VP6 — 1 / 397 / 1356 — **I**nner capsid
required for transcription

7 NSP3 — 1 / 315 / 1104 — **T**ranslation enhancer
binds 3' end of viral mRNAs

8 NSP2 — 1 / 317 / 1059 — **N**TPase
forms viroplasms with NSP5

9 VP7 — 1 / 326 / 1062 — **G**lycosylated
neutralization antigen

10 NSP4 — 1 / 175 / 751 — **E**nterotoxin
viroporin, modulates intracellular calcium

11 NSP6 / NSP5 — 1 / 198 / 667 — p**H**osphoprotein
protein kinase, forms viroplasm with NSP2

B

6. RNA replication occurs within cytoplasmic viroplasms composed of viral and cellular proteins and in complex with lipid droplets (LDs).

7. Subviral particles form in association with viroplasms, and these particles mature by budding through ER-COPII vesicle–derived membranes. In this process, particles acquire their outer capsid proteins.

8. Levels of intracellular calcium are important for controlling virus assembly and particle integrity.

9. Cell lysis releases particles from infected cells grown on monolayers.

In polarized, cultured intestinal cells, virus entry occurs almost exclusively through the apical membrane although some strains enter through both the apical and basolateral membranes (see below). In addition, virus replication in polarized enterocytes alters differentiated enterocyte cell function by perturbing cellular protein trafficking, the cytoskeleton, and tight junctions and by triggering epithelial cell signaling pathways that can activate innate responses and secretion of various chemokines or cytokines[88,251,503] (see below). Finally, the virus is released apically from polarized enterocytes by a novel, Golgi-independent, vesicular transport that does not result in extensive cytopathic effects or cell lysis.[352]

Progress in developmental and stem cell biology has made it possible to establish human intestinal stem cell–derived organoids (HIOs, also called human intestinal enteroids [HIEs]) from adult, pediatric, and fetal intestinal tissue from the different segments of the gastrointestinal tract (see reviews on HIOs/HIEs[560,755]). HIOs recapitulate basic organ structure and maintain the function and genetic diversity of the donor and specific intestinal segment. HIOs have been used as a new model to study human rotavirus infections in nontransformed cultures including host restriction, pathophysiology, and innate epithelial responses to infection[101,614,615] Studies in HIOs show (a) host range restriction; human rotaviruses infect HIOs at higher rates and grow to higher titers than do animal rotaviruses[614]; (b) human rotaviruses infect differentiated enterocytes and also enteroendocrine cells, confirming the tropism for these cell types[614]; (c) rotavirus infection promotes the production of viroplasms and LDs that are classic features of rotavirus replication[614]; (d) three-dimensional HIOs exhibit luminal expansion and fluid secretion following treatment with rotavirus or with the viral enterotoxin NSP4, mimicking the pathophysiological features of diarrhea[614]; (e) rotavirus infection induces intracellular calcium waves by releasing ADP from the infected cells and elevating cytoplasmic calcium in neighboring cells through purinergic paracrine signaling[101]; and (f) infection of HIOs induces a predominant type III interferon (IFN) transcriptional response, while infection of colon carcinoma–derived, Caco-2, cells induces a strong type I IFN response at both the transcriptional and translational levels.[229,615] Unexpectedly in the HIOs, only low levels of type III IFN protein are expressed early after infection indicating a paradox of transcriptional and functional epithelial response to human rotavirus infection. Rotavirus antagonizes this endogenous IFN response at pre- and posttranscriptional levels with the result that homologous rotavirus replication is not substantially restricted by the innate response.[615] HIOs are exciting, advanced models for the study and discovery of new human rotavirus biology and host–pathogen interactions.

Attachment

Rotavirus attachment to epithelial cells is a multistep process involving the interaction of the outer capsid proteins VP4 and VP7 with cellular receptors (Fig. 12.6). Binding to cells does not require cleaved VP4[125,232] or glycosylated VP7,[535] but efficient cell entry requires proteolytic cleavage of VP4 into VP8* and VP5*.

Early studies showed that some rotavirus strains hemagglutinate red blood cells (RBCs) and that sialidase treatment of RBCs reduces virus binding indicating a role for sialic acid (SA) in virus attachment.[48,644] VP8* from the most easily cultivatable animal rotaviruses binds SA, either at a terminal or subterminal position[296] and can infect both surfaces of polarized cells but they preferentially infect polarized cells apically because of the presence of terminal SA.[118,568] Many animal rotaviruses and most strains isolated from humans do not hemagglutinate RBCs but bind to and infect sialidase-treated cells, and preferentially infect polarized intestinal cells through the basolateral surface.[98,118,568] The consequences of efficient infection through the basolateral membrane are not fully understood, but further studies on rotavirus entry into cells likely will reveal other virus–host interactions, including identification of novel cell receptors for the virus, that are relevant for pathogenesis, especially given the extraintestinal spread of virus.

The initial attachment of rotavirus to host cells is mediated by the VP8* domain of the VP4 spike protein to a variety of sialoglycans (such as gangliosides GM1 and GD1a), mucin cores, and histo-blood group antigens (HBGAs).[20,421,561] HBGAs and mucin cores are nonsialylated glycans synthesized by a family of glycosyltransferases expressed on the surface of RBCs (HBGAs alone) and epithelial cells and are present in mucosal secretions.[340,439]

FIGURE 12.5 A: Electropherogram of rotavirus RNA segments. The RNA segments were separated by electrophoresis in a 10% polyacrylamide gel and visualized by staining with silver nitrate. The RNA patterns of a species A rotavirus (SA11, *lane 1*), a species B rotavirus (adult diarrhea rotavirus isolate from China, *lane 2*), and a species C rotavirus (*lane 3*) are shown. The rearranged RNA patterns of three species A rabbit rotavirus strains (C11, *lane 4*, rearrangement in segment 10; Ala, *lane 5* and R2, *lane 7*, rearrangements in segment 11) and their cognate segments compared with those of SA11 (*lane 6*) are also shown. The cognate genes were identified by hybridization with cDNAs for each SA11 RNA segment. *Red asterisks* show rearranged gene 11s in the electropherotypes of Ala and R2 viruses. Schematic on right illustrates features of a rearranged gene 11 that has a duplicated open reading frame but would encode a normal protein because it lacks an initiation site in the duplicated ORF. **B:** Genome structure of rotavirus SA11 virus. RNA segments (in nucleotides) shown in the positive sense and their encoded proteins (in amino acids). The lines at the 5′ and 3′ termini represent the noncoding regions. A few key functions of the proteins are listed with the letter bolded that is used in a new classification system based on the entire genome (see Fig. 12.2). See the text for information on the classification system and more details on gene-coding assignments and locations of known temperature-sensitive mutations. (Reprinted by permission from Springer: Tanaka TN, Conner ME, Graham DY, et al. Molecular characterization of three rabbit rotavirus strains. *Arch Virol* 1988;98(3-4):253–265. Copyright © 1969 Springer-Verlag. Ref.[657])

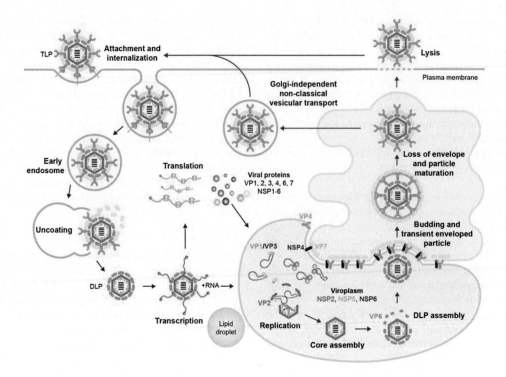

FIGURE 12.6 Schematic of the rotavirus replication cycle. Major features of the rotavirus replication cycle. For details, see section on the replication cycle. Efficient replication requires cleavage of the outer capsid spike protein VP4, which allows the structurally flexible spike protein, VP4, to undergo conformational changes to interact with a series of cellular receptors. The virus is internalized by receptor-mediated endocytosis. The low-calcium environment of the endosome induces the release of the outer capsid VP7 trimers, VP4 penetrates the endosomal membrane, and the transcriptionally active double-layered particle is released into the cytoplasm. Viral mRNAs are used to translate proteins and as templates for RNA genome replication and packaging into newly made DLPs that occur in specialized structures called viroplasms that recruit lipid droplets for formation. TLP assembly is completed by a unique process involving the binding of newly made DLPs to NSP4 that serves as an intracellular receptor, followed by particles budding into ER-COPII–derived autophagy-like membranes. During this process, transient enveloped particles are seen, the outer capsid proteins VP4 and VP7 are assembled, and the transient envelope is lost. The viral glycoproteins do not traffic to the Golgi. In polarized epithelial cells, particles are released both by viral lysis and by a nonclassical vesicular transport mechanism. (Figure prepared by Liya Hu.)

X-ray crystallography and NMR studies show that VP8* from different P-types exhibits a galectin-like fold with two twisted β-sheets separated by a shallow cleft (Fig. 12.7). Galectins are a family of proteins whose natural ligands are carbohydrates. Despite a lack of sequence similarity,[187] the VP8* structure represents one of the first observed cases of a rotavirus protein taking on a fold seen among host proteins and, based on this structural result, it is proposed that VP4 arose from the insertion of a host carbohydrate-binding domain into a viral membrane interaction protein.[187] The sialidase-sensitive animal rotavirus strains, P[3] simian (RRV) VP8* and the P[7] porcine (CRW-8) VP8*, bind SA or the SA–containing ganglioside GM3, respectively, in the shallow cleft between the 2 β-sheets.[187,738] The human P[14] rotavirus, HAL1166, has a narrow VP8* glycan–binding cleft similar to the animal P[3] and P[7] but cannot bind to SA and instead binds to non–sialyated-type A HBGA.[316] In contrast, some rotaviruses, the bovine and human P[11] strains, contain a wider binding cleft and bind precursor HBGAs. This ability to bind a broader spectrum of glycans may be associated with zoonotic transmission of viruses by switching initial binding receptors. The most commonly circulating genotypes associated with human rotavirus infections worldwide, P[4], P[6], and P[8],[419] use a unique site in VP8* not in the cleft to bind H-type 1 glycans. Subtle structural changes in the binding site of the neonatal P[6] VP8* may restrict its ability to bind branched glycans providing a structural basis for the age restriction of these rotaviruses; developmentally regulated unbranched glycans are more abundant in the neonatal gut. Interestingly, epidemiology studies indicate that severe rotavirus gastroenteritis is virtually absent among children lacking functional HBGAs due to genetic polymorphisms affecting expression of the glycosyltransferase FUT2 enzyme.[528] These results indicate that our understanding of rotavirus-glycan interactions remains incomplete. While glycan binding may differ significantly among human rotaviruses, it does not affect susceptibility to infection but rather appears to play a role in the severity of rotavirus disease.[528] In confirmation of this, HIOs from individuals that express or do not express functional FUT2 are susceptible to infection.[614]

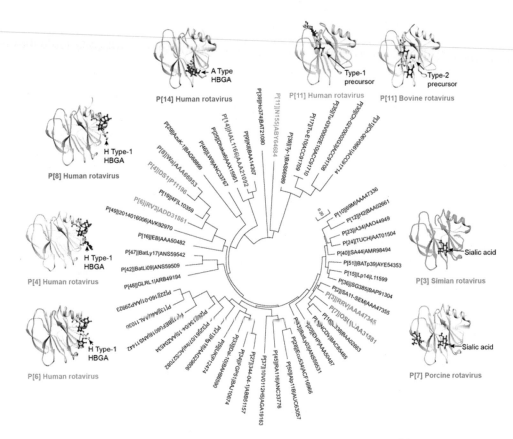

FIGURE 12.7 Phylogenetic analysis of rotavirus VP8* P types was constructed by MEGA6 using the maximum likelihood method.[656] P types with corresponding crystal structures in complex with sialic acid or histo blood group antigens (HBGAs) are colored corresponding to the crystal structures of different VP8*s in complex with specific glycans. Figures were made from the PDB IDs: 1KQR (P[3] simian), 2I2S (P[7] porcine), 5VX5 (P[4] human), 5VX9 (P[6] human), 6K2O (P[8] human), 4DRV (P[14]), 4YFZ (P[11] human), and 4YG6 (P[11] bovine). (Figure prepared by Liya Hu.)

The identification of cellular coreceptor(s) for rotavirus is an active area of research.[18] Early studies and conflicting results are explained by the use of different receptors by different viruses on different cell types (reviewed in Refs. [18,38,421,594]). Several integrins, including $\alpha 2\beta 1$, $\alpha v\beta 3$, $\alpha x\beta 2$, and $\alpha 4\beta 1$, have been implicated as possible receptors for rotavirus cell entry with evidence for $\alpha 2\beta 1$ being the strongest.[137,261,287] Antibodies to these integrins or synthetic peptides that represent integrin-ligand motifs that are present in VP5* or VP7 diminish virus infectivity modestly, and some integrins influence cell binding in an additive manner, suggesting they may play a role at different stages of the cell entry process.[285] Neutralizing antibodies to VP5* and VP7, but not to VP8* and VP6, inhibit virus binding to integrins.[220] Involvement of integrins at a postattachment step is consistent with observations that integrin expression increases infectivity of rotaviruses in poorly permissive cells.[120,305] Integrin usage has been characterized in nonpolarized monkey kidney cells, endothelial and polarized kidney, and intestinal epithelial cells. Integrin and postbinding receptor usage can differ depending on the cell type(s) analyzed and the interactions between sialidase-sensitive and sialidase-resistant rotaviruses with intestinal or extraintestinal cells and may affect the pathogenesis and outcome of infections. Integrins have a polarized distribution and are located at the basolateral plasma membrane (PM),

possibly explaining why sialidase-resistant rotaviruses preferentially infect through the basolateral surface.[118,568] Interesting studies suggested that the addition of VP8* peptides to polarized cells can trigger the movement of basolateral proteins to the apical surface, resulting in another possible mechanism for how rotaviruses might interact with integrins.[495] A DGE sequence in VP5* binds to the α subunit I domain on activated $\alpha 2\beta 1$, and rotavirus binding is eliminated by mutations in activation-responsive helices of this integrin.[219] Despite demonstrated binding of VP5* to integrins, the lack of signaling after this binding leaves open the question of how virus actually penetrates the membrane. VP7 has been proposed to interact with αXβ2 and αvβ3 though GPR and CNP motifs, respectively,[261,743] but the proposed integrin-binding motif (GPR, residues 253–255 on VP7) is questionable because it is located on the inward facing surface of the trimer and would not be available to interact with integrins until after uncoating.[17,261] However, the CPN residues are potentially available for integrin binding. Evaluation of the role of integrin α2 and β3 in rotavirus cell entry using RNA silencing in permissive cells also concluded that these integrins may not play a major role in the rotavirus cell entry process.[330] Other receptors remain to be identified as a porcine rotavirus CRW-8 does not use human or monkey $\alpha 2\beta 1$ as a cellular receptor.[263] The tight junctional protein JAM-A may be a coreceptor for some rotavirus strains, RRV, Wa, and UK, but not YM.[675] Thus, crucial molecules involved in cell entry likely still remain to be identified.

Heat shock cognate protein 70 (hsc70) is another putative coreceptor proposed to bind virus and mediate virus entry into cells based on experiments in which rotavirus entry is blocked by a VP5* synthetic peptide and by antibodies against human recombinant hsc70.[284,421,531] The role of hsc70 is proposed based on observing enhanced virus entry into cells and subsequent enhanced virus infectivity after heating some cells at 45°C.[423] Binding of purified hsc70 to two domains in VP5* as well as to a domain in VP6 is also detected in cell-free assays and may modify the conformation of virus particles to help the virus enter cells.[280,531] To date, however, binding affinities to the proposed post-SA binding receptor molecules have not been determined, and no structures of rotavirus-protein coreceptor complexes are solved. All the implicated rotavirus receptors on cells (GM1 ganglioside, integrin subunits, and hsc70) are associated with detergent-resistant lipid microdomains and infectious rotavirus associates with these domains. Thus, lipid rafts are thought to provide a platform to facilitate efficient interaction of rotavirus receptors with virus particles.[329]

Penetration and Uncoating

After initial binding to cells, rotavirus cell entry is a coordinated, multistep process involving a series of conformational changes in the capsid proteins VP4 and VP7 (Fig. 12.8). Because the initial VP8*-glycan binding has a relatively low affinity, the virus entry event is probably responsible, in part, for cell type and host specificity.[187,328] VP8* mediates the initial binding of the virus to cell surface glycans, whereas VP5* plays a role in host cell membrane penetration.[304]

Efficient entry of rotavirus into cells requires proteolytic cleavage and conformational rearrangements of the spike protein to facilitate membrane penetration. Host type II transmembrane serine proteases TMPRSS2 and TMPRSS11D were shown to mediate trypsin-independent VP4 cleavage and rotavirus infection.[610] Most of our understanding of this processes is based on biochemical, confocal, and cryo-EM to determine the three-dimensional structures of the rhesus rotavirus (RRV) strain of either native TLPs or DLPs recoated with recombinant VP4 and VP7 entering BSC-1 cells.[304] Whether other animal or human strains undergo similar conformational changes for cell entry remains to be determined. Herrmann et al. found VP4 transitions from an upright to a reversed conformation for cell penetration mediated by the following steps (Fig. 12.8).[304]

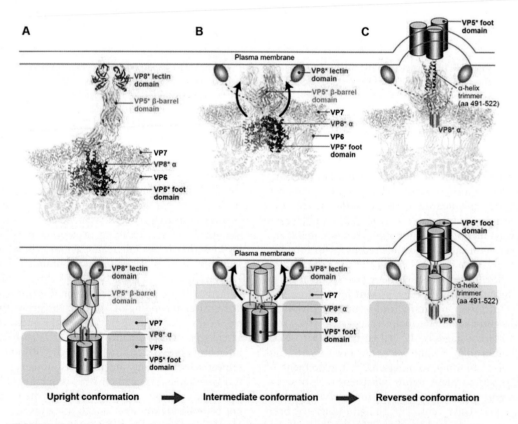

FIGURE 12.8 Model of membrane interaction and the rearrangement of the VP4 spike protein during infection. Atomic models (*top panel*) and cartoon (*bottom panel*) of **(A)** upright (PDB 6WXE), **(B)** intermediate (PDB 6WXF), and **(C)** reversed conformations of the VP4 spike interacting with the plasma or possibly the endosomal membrane (PDB 6WXG). The orientation of the different domains of the VP4 spike protein relative to VP6 and VP7 are shown. See text for details. (Figure prepared by Liya Hu. Modified from Herrmann T, Torres R, Salgado EN, et al. Functional refolding of the penetration protein on a non-enveloped virus. *Nature* 2021;590(7847):666–670.)

(a) The VP8* glycan–binding domains separate from the tips of the twofold clustered VP5* β-barrel domain. While the resolution of the icosahedrally averaged particles was not sufficient to show the VP8*-glycan contacts directly, previous crystallographic analysis indicated minimal conformational changes in VP8* upon SA binding.[474] In the context of the entire rotavirus structure, conformational changes upon VP8* glycan interaction remain to be determined. (b) The unstructured third VP5* β-barrel domain flips outward and interacts with the other two VP5*s to form a reversed conformation β-barrel trimer, exposing the VP5* hydrophobic loops at the surface of the membrane bilayer. This conformational rearrangement translocates a VP5* DGE integrin binding motif to the external surface of the trypsin-primed structural forms of VP5*, making it accessible to bind to an integrin.[219,732] The VP8* glycan–binding domains remain tethered to the VP5* β-barrel trimer by the long N-terminal segment of VP8*. (c) The VP4 foot domain unfolds and is projected toward the membrane by zippering of the central, three-strand, a-helical coiled coil domains. Tomograms show images of RRV TLPs at various stages of engulfment into tightly fitting membrane invaginations entering BSC-1 cells at the rim of the PM, and the extruded VP4 foot appears to be embedded in the membranes that encircle the TLP.[2] The interaction of the VP5* hydrophobic loops at the surface of the membrane bilayer and the extruded foot embedded in the membrane suggest that these are key conformational changes in VP4 for delivery of the DLP into the cytosol.

Internalization of the DLP into the cytosol requires the removal of the outer capsid proteins VP4 and VP7 and does not take place at 0°C to 4°C, indicating that this step requires active cellular processes.[373,536] The outer capsid shell is composed of VP7 trimers held together by calcium (Ca^{2+}) ions and anchors the VP4 spikes onto the particle surface.[623] Ca^{2+} chelation leads to the removal of both VP7 and VP4 and the release of the DLP[126] (see Fig. 12.2). Salgado et al.[599] used live cell imaging of single DLPs recoated with VP4 and VP7, each coupled with distinct fluorescent markers, as well as a fluorescent Ca^{2+} sensor placed on VP5* to monitor the Ca^{2+} concentration, outer capsid protein dissociation, and DLP release from the membrane-bound vesicle enclosing the entering particle. These studies revealed that (a) particles are engulfed in vesicles that are closed off about 5 minutes after initial attachment. (b) This sequestration of the virion from the external cellular environment to the cytosol with a coincident 10,000-fold decrease in the Ca^{2+} concentration leads to a drop in the Ca^{2+} concentration and dissociation and complete loss of VP7 and VP4 from the DLP. Loss of Ca^{2+} (that takes 1 minute) precedes the onset of VP7 dissociation from the TLP (that takes 2 minutes) and DLP release (that takes 7 minutes). Use of the calcium ionophore A23187 to increase the intracellular Ca^{2+} concentration during the early stages of replication can block uncoating,[430] supporting this result that low Ca^{2+} concentrations in the intracellular microenvironment are responsible for TLP uncoating.

Both receptor-mediated endocytosis and direct membrane penetration have been suggested as mechanisms of rotavirus entry into cells, and different rotavirus strains have been shown to enter cells through different endocytic pathways.[287] However, lysosomotropic agents (ammonium chloride, chloroquine, methylamine, and amantadine) that acidify endosomes involved in receptor-mediated endocytosis do not affect rotavirus entry.[233,355,372,430,599] Energy inhibitors (sodium azide and dinitrophenol) have a minimal effect on rotavirus infection, and this has been taken to suggest that rotaviruses do not use endocytosis to enter cells. Other endocytosis inhibitors, such as dansylcadaverine and cytochalasin D, and in some, but not all, cases the vacuolar proton–adenosine triphosphatase (ATPase) inhibitor bafilomycin A1, also do not block rotavirus entry.[602] These results indicate that neither endocytosis nor an intraendosomal acidic pH or a proton gradient is required for rotavirus entry into cells. Most observations are consistent with the model that virus enters cells by endocytoses after direct interactions with a series of receptors on the PM.[493,592,599,719]

Further studies are needed to determine whether the common endocytosis-mediated entry pathway exists for all rotaviruses and in all cell types. Entry of some rotavirus strains with different sialidase sensitivity and integrin dependence into MA104 cells is reported to be dependent on hsc70, dynamin, and cholesterol, but these distinct strains enter cells through clathrin mediated endocytosis pathways.[287,602] In contrast, a genome-wide RNAi screen showed that components of the endosomal sorting complex required for transport (ESCRT) machinery, the small GTPases RHOA and CDC42, and early endosomal antigen 1 (EEA1) were found to be required for clathrin-independent endocytosis of simian and some human rotavirus strains.[633] Some strains escape early endosomes, while others traffic to late endosomes and require the mannose-6-phosphate receptor and endolysosomal proteases from the Golgi complex to exit the vesicular compartment and efficiently start viral replication.[176] The reasons for these differences are not known but might result from the different virus strains or the heterogeneity of raft-type membrane microdomains on different cell types in different differentiation states.[164] Trypsin also has been detected associated with the rotavirus outer capsid and is activated by solubilization of the outer capsid proteins.[49] This activated trypsin is proposed to cleave VP7 and VP4 into fragments capable of disrupting membranes, and this may allow DLPs to gain access to the cytoplasm to begin actively transcribing viral mRNA to complete the next step in the viral life cycle.

RNA Synthesis

Incoming rotavirus DLPs containing the dsRNA genome segments must synthesize mRNAs that direct the synthesis of viral proteins and also serve as templates for the synthesis of the dsRNA genome that becomes encapsidated into newly made particles. The virion polymerase performs these functions as a transcriptase and as a replicase at different times during the replication cycle.

Synthesis of viral transcripts is mediated by the endogenous viral RNA-dependent RNA polymerase complex (PC), VP1 and VP3, which is located in the virion. Robust polymerase activity requires interaction of VP1 with VP2, which takes place via a few key residues.[649] VP1 has a compact cage-like structure with three domains similar to that of the reovirus polymerase[429] (Fig. 12.9A). VP1 contains a putative cap-binding site to anchor the capped 5′ end of the (+)RNA, and the structure has four distinct tunnels that lead to the central catalytic core of VP1. The four distinct tunnels in VP1 are for the entry of the templates [(+)RNA or (−)RNA], the entry of NTPs, the exit of dsRNA/(−)RNA, and the exit of the (+) RNA. Having two distinct product exit tunnels ensures that (+)RNAs are effectively shuttled out of the core, while nascent

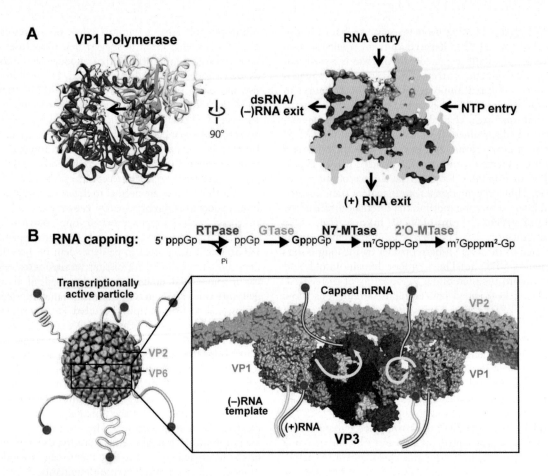

FIGURE 12.9 Structural features of VP1 polymerase, VP3 capping enzymes, and model of RNA capping during endogenous transcription. A: Ribbon diagram of VP1 in complex with ribo-oligonucleotide (PDB ID: 2R7R) (*left panel, arrow* points to RNA oligonucleotide).[429] The N-terminal domain is in *yellow*, the C-terminal domain is in *magenta*, and the C-terminal plug is in *cyan*. The subdomains of the polymerase domain are in *light blue* (fingers), *red* (palm), and *green* (thumb). Cutaway of the surface rendering of the complex showing the four tunnels extending into the central cavity, the catalytic center (*right panel*). There are four tunnels in VP1 for template RNA entry, NTP entry, dsRNA/(−)RNA exit, and (+) RNA exit. **B:** Schematic of the steps and enzymes involved in RNA capping (*top panel*). Reconstruction of an actively transcribing DLP. The *inset* represents the proposed model of transcription and capping by VP1 (*grey*) and VP3 (domains colored as in schematic), respectively (*bottom panel*). The model posits that the base-paired (−)RNA template/(+)RNA product emerges through the template exit channel of VP1 and encounters VP3 for RNA capping, utilizing the modular domains in the tetrameric assembly, which uniquely integrates the five distinct enzymatic steps required for capping the transcripts (shown by *white arrows*): RNA helicase activity required for separating the RNA duplex formed transiently during endogenous transcription, RNA triphosphatase (RTPase), guanylyltransferase (GTase), methyltransferase (MTase), and 2′-O-methyltransferase (2′O-MTase) activities.[396] VP3 has not been identified *in situ* by cryo-EM. (Figure prepared by Liya Hu.)

dsRNA gene segments are directed toward the particle interior. In addition, the (−)RNA exits proximal to the template entry tunnel, which should facilitate its reuse in subsequent rounds of (+)RNA synthesis.

Crystallographic structures of VP1 in complex with the consensus sequences (CS) in the 3′ end of the minus strand (template for (+)RNA synthesis) and in the 3′ end of the (+) RNA (template for (−)RNA synthesis) are also available.[429] These structures indicate that for transcription, sequence-specific recognition of the 3′-CS of the minus strand for (+) strand synthesis is not critical as it takes place within the confines of the capsid.[429] In contrast, sequence-specific interactions are made only with the 3′-CS of the plus strand that is anchored to the template entry site in VP1. This sequence-specific interaction involving the UGUG motif in the 3′-CS (+)RNA confirms biochemical studies that showed this motif is the polymerase recognition signal and is required for high-affinity interactions with VP1 and subsequent replicase activity.[109] Of interest, the VP1 3′-CS (+)RNA complex structure is in an autoinhibited state with a single nucleotide at the 3′ end overshooting the initiation register. For VP1 to initiate (−)RNA synthesis, the over-shot 3′ end of the template must be realigned, a priming loop must be repositioned to allow binding of the priming nucleotide, and a plug formed from the C-terminal domain of the polymerase that is in the dsRNA exit tunnel must be dislodged. While dissociation of the outer capsid layer leads to RNA synthesis without introducing structural changes in VP1, the addition of *S*-adenosyl methionine, Mg^{2+}, and NTPs triggers transcription and induces significant conformational changes in both VP1 and the DLP capsid shell to allow the synthesized transcript to exit the polymerase and the particle.[339]

Cryo-EM and single-particle analysis using asymmetric reconstructions show that VP1 binds stochastically at one of the five possible positions at each of the fivefold vertices; however, VP3 was not visualized.[339] *In vitro* biochemical studies on transcribing particles show that transcripts are capped by the time the sixth or seventh nucleotide is synthesized by VP1, suggesting that VP3 is in close proximity to VP1 during endogenous transcription.[553] The absence of VP3 in the asymmetric reconstructions suggests that VP3 is not firmly anchored to VP1 (or VP2) and that its spatial arrangement inside the particle interior is dynamic.

X-ray crystallography, cryo-EM, and biochemical analyses show that VP3 forms a stable tetrameric assembly with each subunit having a modular domain organization, which uniquely integrates the five distinct enzymatic steps required for capping the transcripts: RNA helicase activity required for separating the RNA duplex formed transiently during endogenous transcription, RTPase, GTase, MTase, and 2′*O*-MTase activities[396] (Fig. 12.9B). The oligomeric state of VP3 in the particle is unknown as the location of VP3 has not been identified *in situ* by cryo-EM, and VP3 tetramers may associate with nonredundant pairs of neighboring VP1 molecules inside the core.

In a proposed model for capping the endogenous transcript[396] (Fig. 12.9B), the duplex formed by the template strand and the nascent transcript that exits from VP1 are separated by the RNA helicase activity associated with VP3. While the transcript continues through the process of capping, the template is returned to form a duplex with the partner positive strand to go through the iterative process of transcription. The γ-phosphate is removed by the RTPase domain of VP3, and the emerging transcript transits through the GTase domain and then through the MTase domains of the twofold related VP3 subunits for subsequent steps of capping. The capped transcript then exits through the closest channel at the fivefold axis in the VP2 capsid layer. Each genome segment is transcribed simultaneously and repeatedly by a specific polymerase complex within the confines of the capsid architecture, and the resulting transcripts exit through the type I channel system at the axis adjacent to its site of synthesis. This mechanism of transcription offers an explanation of why no dsRNA virus contains more than 12 genome segments.

Ultimately, transcription must be inhibited to allow RNA replication to proceed and virus assembly to be completed because transcribing particles will continuously synthesize milligram quantities of mRNAs *in vitro* as long as fresh precursors and an energy-generating system are provided. While not completely understood, transcription can be inhibited by several mechanisms. Cryo-EM studies of DLPs complexed with some monoclonal antibodies to VP6, or the addition of VP7 onto DLPs, indicate a conformational change at the interface of the VP2 to VP6 layers or in the VP6 trimers can inhibit sustained elongation and translocation of transcripts.[213,380,402,671] It is also possible that binding of VP6 to NSP4, which serves as an intracellular receptor for particle assembly (see below), is the key interaction that inhibits transcription. This hypothesis is consistent with the observation that knockdown of NSP4 by siRNA increases viral mRNA synthesis.[635] NSP4 can form pH-dependent pentamers and such structures may interact with VP6 molecules surrounding the type I channels at the fivefold axis of the DLPs as mechanism of inhibiting the transcript exit.[99,612]

Kinetics and Cellular Sites of Transcription, Translation, and Replication

Transcription in cells occurs following the release of DLPs from the endosome. Consistent with this idea, cells are susceptible to infection by liposome-mediated transfection of DLPs, indicating that simple delivery of these particles into the cell cytoplasm permits transcription to proceed.[47] Transcription is asymmetric, and all transcripts are full-length positive strands made off the dsRNA-negative strand.[458] Primary transcription must occur before RNA replication. The synthesis of negative-strand RNA occurs in perinuclear nonmembranous, electron dense cytoplasmic inclusions known as *viroplasms* (see below and Fig. 12.6), concurrently with the packaging of positive-strand RNA into core replication intermediate (RI) particles.[32,634]

The kinetics of synthesis of positive- and negative-stranded RNAs has been studied in rotavirus-infected cells,[646] in a cell-free system using extracts from infected cells,[520] in an electrophoretic system that allows separation of the positive and negative strands of rotavirus RNAs in acid urea agarose gels,[520,521] and by quantitative reverse transcription–PCR.[32] Positive- and negative-stranded RNAs are initially detected during the first 4 hours after infection.[32,646] The amount of mRNA accumulated during the infection period is not equimolar. A small linear increment of plus- and minus-strand RNA synthesis is detected followed by a logarithmic increase at later times of infection. This quantitation indicates that the entering DLPs produce a small amount of mRNA, which is then translated and replicated, producing new DLPs. When these new DLPs are assembled in viroplasms, they then transcribe their genomes, initiating a secondary wave of transcription and replication. Newly assembled DLPs are required for this second wave of transcription as knockdown of any of the viral proteins that constitute the DLP (VP1, VP2, VP3, and VP6) ablates the logarithmic increase in RNA synthesis.[32] The assembly of infectious virus particles parallels the replication of the viral genome.

Viral mRNAs are capped but not polyadenylated, and translation of viral proteins is facilitated by the action of NSP3 and the cellular translation machinery.[264,660] NSP3 function parallels that of the cellular poly(A)-binding protein (PABP). The N-terminus of NSP3 interacts with the 3′-consensus sequence (GACC) of viral mRNAs and the C-terminus of NSP3 interacts with eIF4G as does PABP, but with higher affinity.[264] Although the atomic structure of the full-length NSP3 is not yet determined, atomic structures of N-terminal and C-terminal domains of NSP3 complexed with either ligand indicate that both domains have novel folds and suggest that NSP3 functions as a dimer (Fig. 12.11A and B).[166,277] While the RNA-binding domain forms a rod-shaped symmetric dimer, the N-terminal domain tightly binds to the consensus 3′ end of the mRNAs inside a tunnel formed at the dimeric interface. NSP3 evicts PABP from eIF4G to enhance translation of rotavirus mRNAs and to the concomitant impairment of translation of cellular mRNAs.[512,693] NSP3 mutants that are unable to form dimers can also inhibit host cell translation.[131] PABP evicted from eIF4G accumulates in the nucleus of rotavirus-infected cells, and this relocalization of PABP from the cytoplasm to the nucleus occurs relatively early in the infection cycle (~3 hpi) and requires a limited amount of NSP3.[294,475] The complete depletion of PABP from the cell cytoplasm can reinforce the shutoff of translation of cellular polyadenylated mRNAs and may also enhance translation of viral mRNAs by making available other cellular factors involved in translation termination, RNA stability, or subcellular localization of host mRNAs that would normally be bound to cytoplasmic PABP.[294,544,545]

Rotavirus infection results in a second mechanism to inhibit cellular mRNA translation that involves eIF2α that is phosphorylated early after infection and is maintained throughout the virus replication cycle.[475] This phosphorylation depends on the synthesis of VP2, NSP2, and NSP5, and the continuous phosphorylated status of eIF2α is beneficial for the virus because viral mRNAs are preferentially translated efficiently, while translation of most cellular proteins is stopped. Protein kinase R (PKR) is apparently responsible for this phosphorylation event that is triggered by viral dsRNA detected in the cell cytoplasm outside viroplasms, which is a paradigm shifting result as traditionally it has been assumed that rotaviral dsRNA is hidden from the IFN system by ensuring that genome replication takes place within replicative intermediate particles, such that single-stranded RNA is replicated as it enters these particles.[582] While further work is needed to characterize the nature of the viral dsRNA present in the cytoplasm of infected cells, the multiple mechanisms used by rotaviruses to remodel the host translation machinery in novel ways to assure efficient translation of viral proteins will likely continue to reveal unique regulatory systems.

Most of the rotavirus structural proteins and the nonstructural proteins are synthesized on free ribosomes, although nascent proteins on free ribosomes have not been analyzed. Instead, this conclusion has been drawn based on the absence of signal sequences that would indicate targeting to the ER and lack of protection from digestion in *in vitro* protease protection studies.[196,354] The viral glycoproteins VP7 and NSP4 are synthesized on ribosomes associated with the ER membrane and are cotranslationally inserted into the ER membrane as a result of signal sequences at their N-termini. VP7 has a signal sequence that is cotranslationally cleaved, whereas the signal sequence on NSP4 is not cleaved.[196]

Following translation in the cytoplasm, structural proteins VP1, VP2, VP3, and VP6 and nonstructural proteins NSP2, NSP5 and in some strains NSP6, along with viral (+) RNA form inclusion bodies in the cytoplasm called viroplasms (Fig. 12.6).[256,538,575] Viroplasms, the sites of incorporation of (+) RNA into RIs and virus assembly, first appear 2 to 3 hours after infection. The number of viroplasms initially increases and then decreases with time after infection, whereas the area of each viroplasm increases, suggesting fusion of viroplasms.[191,204] NSP2 and NSP5 are major components of viroplasms, and the expression of these two proteins alone is sufficient to induce the formation of empty viroplasm-like structures (VLS).[204] Viroplasms associate with lipids and proteins (perilipin, ADRP) characteristic of cytoplasmic LDs, and blocking or interfering with LD formation reduces the number of functional viroplasms and production of infectious virus.[112] The proteosome is also essential for early assembly of viroplasms.[130,425] Inhibition

of proteosome activity following virus entry and uncoating reduces accumulation of virus proteins, viroplasm formation, and RNA replication. The requirements of LD and proteasomes for viroplasm function represent examples of a virus hijacking cellular pathways for its own replication and further information of how rotavirus proteins interact or regulate these pathways should help understand the early stages of viroplasm formation and particle assembly.

The key role of NSP2 and NSP5 in viroplasm functions of genome replication and packaging has been demonstrated by studies of temperature-sensitive mutants or knocking-down the expression of NSP2 or NSP5 by RNA interference, antibody treatment, or using a reverse genetics approach, which results in inhibition of viroplasm formation, genome replication, virion assembly, and a general decrease of viral protein synthesis.[96,424,513,688]

NSP2 is an essential multifunctional protein with sequence-independent ssRNA binding as well as enzymatic activities including autokinase,[147] nucleoside triphosphatase (NTPase), nucleoside diphosphate (NDP) kinase,[397] RTPase,[689] and nucleic acid helix destabilizing activities.[659] NSP2 NDP kinase activity may be responsible for homeostasis of the nucleotide pool for replication.[397] NSP2 is the most abundant protein of viroplasms, is essential for viroplasm formation, and exists as an octamer.[661]

The monomeric subunit of NSP2 has two distinct domains separated by a deep, catalytic cleft (Fig. 12.10A and B). The association of monomers results in a doughnut-shaped octamer with a 35 Å central hole along the fourfold axes and grooves that run diagonally across the twofold axes and are lined by basic residues.[338] The C-terminal domain of NSP2 resembles the cellular histidine triad (HIT) family of proteins that hydrolyze nucleotides. The NTP-binding residues are located within the cleft between the two domains. Mutation of the catalytic residue (H225A) abrogates hydrolysis of the γ-phosphate from the 5' end of RNA and dsRNA synthesis.[689] Although the NTPase activity is localized in the monomeric subunit, the ability to bind RNA and other proteins requires the formation of the octamer.[689] Cryo-EM structures of NSP2 octamer complexes show that both ssRNA and NSP5 (the other key component required for viroplasm formation) share the same binding site; NSP5 and ssRNA compete for binding in the NSP2 octamer grooves.[345] Tubulin also binds to these charged grooves.[441] NSP2 also interacts with VP1 and the N-terminal hub of VP2.[704] Taken together, these results indicate that NSP2 is critical for RNA replication and suggest that context-dependent competitive binding of different ligands to the groove may regulate NSP2 function during genome replication and virus assembly.

NSP5 is a dimeric phosphoprotein rich in Ser and Thr residues that undergoes O-linked glycosylation,[6,549,714] as well as phosphorylation that occurs when NSP5 is coexpressed with VP2.[129] NSP5 reportedly exists in several oligomeric forms, and biophysical and structural analyses suggest that the biologically relevant form in cells required for viroplasm formation is a decamer.[442] The self-association of NSP5 may be regulated by NSP6, which is encoded by an alternative reading frame of gene segment 11 in most virus strains and is also associated with viroplasms.[676] However, using the reverse genetics system, NSP6 has been shown to not be essential for viral replication in cell culture.[385]

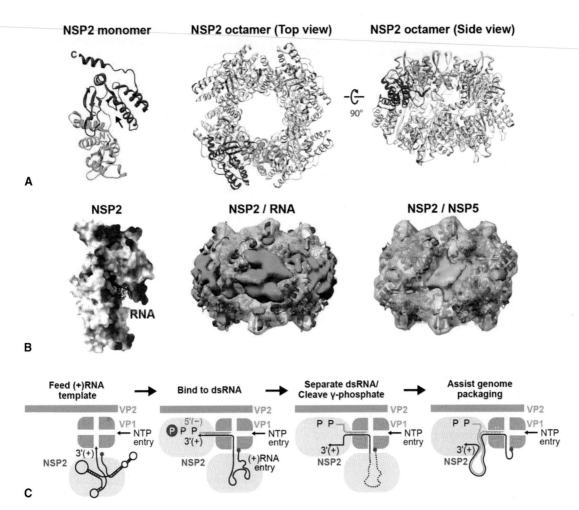

FIGURE 12.10 Structures of NSP2, NSP2 interactions with RNA and NSP5, and model of genome replication. A: Monomeric and octameric structures of NSP2. The N- and C-terminal domains of the monomeric subunits are colored *green* and *red*, respectively, and the rest of the subunits in the functional octamer are shown in *gray*. The donut-shaped octamer is viewed along the fourfold axis (*top middle*) and along one of the two 2-fold axes perpendicular to the groove lined by positively charged residues (*top right*).[338] **B:** Crystal structure of NSP2 monomer in complex with RNA (*left panel*). Cryo-EM reconstruction of NSP2 binding to RNA (RNA in *green, middle panel*) and NSP2 binding to NSP5 (NSP5 in *blue, right panel*) and viewed perpendicular to the groove. These two ligands both bind to the grooves of the NSP2 octamer. **C:** Model of genome replication. Three N-terminal arms of VP2 form a tentacle-like structure and bind VP1 to the inner surface of the VP2 shell.[339] NSP2 also interacts with VP1 and the N-terminal hub of VP2.[704] The catalytic center of NSP2 resembles the histidine triad (HIT) of cellular nucleotidyl hydrolases[338,658] and may function as a molecular motor using energy from NTP hydrolysis to destabilize the mRNA template and feed it to the RNA template to VP1 during genome replication. (Figure prepared by Liya Hu.) (From Jiang X, Jayaram H, Kumar M, et al. Cryoelectron microscopy structures of rotavirus NSP2-NSP5 and NSP2-RNA complexes: implications for genome replication. *J Virol* 2006;80(21):10829–10835.)

Viroplasm assembly is regulated by phosphorylation and involves two forms of NSP2, a cytoplasmically dispersed dNSP2, which interacts with hypophosphorylated NSP5; and a viroplasm-specific vNSP2, which interacts with hyperphosphorylated NSP5.[149] Phosphorylation of NSP2 by the cellular kinase CK1α on serine 313 is required for dNSP2 to traffic to sites of viroplasm formation. NSP5 is also phosphorylated by CK1α, and NSP5 hyperphosphorylation is required for viroplasm assembly.[191,513] Phosphorylation triggers NSP2 octamers, in association with hyperphosphorylated NSP5, to form a lattice structure for viroplasm assembly likely on LDs.[112] Use of a genetically engineered rotavirus phosphomimetic S313D NSP2 mutant showed that vNSP2 interacts with the LD–associated protein PLIN1 prior to the accumulation of other rotavirus proteins indicating NSP2 may be the virus factor that induces LD biogenesis in rotavirus-infected cells.[148]

Genomic RNA Encapsidation (Packaging) and Replication

After its synthesis, dsRNA remains associated with subviral particles, suggesting that free dsRNA is not found in cells. Because of its inherent stiffness,[359] dsRNA is not packaged. The selective packaging mechanism that leads to the presence of equimolar genome segments within rotaviruses, or any of the other members of the family *Reoviridae*, remains a challenging puzzle that is beginning to be unraveled. Several studies provide evidence that viral (+)RNA binds to NSP2, which results in the remodeling of the RNA that is conducive to the formation of stable intersegment contacts.[70] The RNA–RNA interactions follow a sequential order initiated by the small rotavirus segments. These interactions are sequence-specific because targeted specific antisense oligoribonucleotides complementary to short RNA sequences perturb the RNA complexes.[205]

Based on structural and biochemical studies, a model of rotavirus replication includes genome encapsidation and DLP assembly occurring concurrently with the formation of a RI composed of a pentamer of VP2 interacting with VP1 and VP3.[456] The NSP2 octamer feeds unwound RNA, due to its nucleic acid helix destabilizing activity, to the polymerase.[370] NSP2 also interacts with the N-terminal hub of the core capsid protein VP2.[704] These data support a model where NSP2 functions as a molecular motor using energy from NTP hydrolysis to destabilize the mRNA template and feed the RNA template to VP1 during genome replication (Fig. 12.10C).[397] Overall, VP1 replicates the RNA, the (−)RNA exits VP1 and interacts with an octamer of NSP2 so that NSP2, functioning as an RTPase, cleaves the γ-phosphate from the 5′ (−)RNA.[689] This accounts for the absence of the γ-phosphate at the 5′ end of the genomic dsRNA.[327,458] However, how NSP2 recognizes the 5′ (−)RNA CS of the dsRNA product exiting from VP1 is not understood. This knowledge may be important to understand how NSP2 may play a role in facilitating genome packaging. In addition, how NSP2 is excluded from encapsidation is unclear but may involve phosphorylation. Finally, 12 units each composed of pentamers of VP2 dimers, a VP1/VP3 complex, and a dsRNA segment associate to form the VP2 capsid layer, which provides a platform for the subsequent addition of VP6 trimers resulting in the formation of the DLP.[456]

Virion Maturation

Viroplasm maturation and function also require NSP4, the only nonstructural protein that does not bind RNA. Based on siRNA experiments that knocked down NSP4 expression, NSP4 plays a role in the intracellular accumulation and the cellular distribution of several viral proteins, influencing the development of viroplasms, linking genome packaging with particle assembly, and acting as a modulator of viral transcription.[422,635] Precisely, how NSP4 regulates RNA synthesis remains to be determined but NSP4 binding to the nascent DLPs may inhibit transcription.[27,29]

A distinctive feature of rotavirus morphogenesis is that subviral particles, which assemble in the cytoplasmic viroplasms, bud through membranes adjacent to the viroplasms, and maturing particles are transiently enveloped (Fig. 12.6). This is one of the most interesting aspects of rotavirus replication, differing from members of other genera in the family *Reoviridae* and any other viruses. The envelope acquired in this process is lost, and the envelope is replaced by the VP7 outer capsid. Rotavirus particle transport, maturation, and assembly remain an interesting model to understand the transport of protein complexes across membranes as well as envelope particle formation.

NSP4 has multiple domains and an increasing number of functions.[39,611] NSP4 is a 20 kD primary translation product; it is cotranslationally glycosylated to become a 29 kD species, and oligosaccharide processing yields the mature 28 kD protein that is a transmembrane protein of the ER.[195,354] The 175

aa polypeptide backbone of NSP4 consists of an uncleaved signal sequence, three hydrophobic domains with two N-linked high mannose glycosylation sites being in the first hydrophobic domain, a predicted amphipathic α-helix (AAH) that overlaps a folded coiled-coil region, the H_2 transmembrane domain that traverses the ER bilayer, and the C-terminus that is hydrophilic and forms an extended cytoplasmic domain.[73,100,196,354] The carbohydrate moieties remain sensitive to endoglycosidase H digestion, and processing of the Man9GlcNAc carbohydrate added to NSP4 stops at Man8GlcNAc with the mannose-9 species predominating,[73,354] indicating that no further trimming occurs in the Golgi apparatus.[611]

A critical step in virion assembly requires the accumulation of membranes adjacent to viroplasms that involves NSP4-mediated increases in cytoplasmic calcium (Ca^{2+} cyto) and the cellular process of autophagy. In the ER, NSP4 forms a viroporin,[324] a Ca^{2+}-conducting ion channel that releases ER Ca^{2+} into the cytoplasm resulting in decreased ER calcium stores and activation of PM calcium influx channels, ultimately causing a twofold to fourfold elevation in Ca^{2+} cyto.[325,539] Increased Ca^{2+} cyto activates a calcium signaling pathway involving calcium/calmodulin-dependent protein kinase kinase 2 (CAMKK2) and 5′ adenosine monophosphate-activated protein kinase (AMPK) to trigger autophagy.[140] NSP4 exits the ER in COPII vesicles that are hijacked by the cellular autophagy machinery, which mediates the trafficking of NSP4, the outer capsid protein VP7, and the autophagy marker protein LC3 II in these membranes to viroplasms.[138,140] Prior to the discovery that NSP4 exits the ER and forms LC3 II-containing membranes that associate with viroplasms, DLPs were thought to bud through ER membranes.

Morphologic and biochemical data are consistent with rapidly assembling DLPs serving as an intermediate stage in the formation of triple-layered virions. Viroplasms are the sites of synthesis of the DLPs that contain RNA (see above). This conclusion is based on the localization of several of the viral proteins (VP2, NSP2, NSP5, NSP6) to viroplasms, of VP4 and VP6 to the space between the periphery of the viroplasm and the outside of the viroplasm-associated membrane,[256,537] and on the observation that particles emerging from these viroplasms bud directly into the membrane that contains the glycoproteins VP7 and NSP4.

The C-terminal cytoplasmic domain (aa 161 to 175) of NSP4 functions in viral morphogenesis by acting as an intracellular receptor that binds VP6 on the newly made DLPs and mediates the budding of these particles into the viroplasm-associated membranes.[29,666] A receptor role for NSP4 is supported by the observation that DLPs bind to membranes containing only NSP4.[28,29,465] The AAH region, distinct from the receptor domain, is predicted to adopt an α-helical coiled-coil structure and is thought to mediate oligomerization of the virus-binding domains into a homotetramer.[667] A crystal structure of the oligomerization domain of NSP4, which spans aa residues 95 to 137 (NSP4 95 to 137), self-associates into a homotetrameric coiled-coil, with the hydrophobic core interrupted by three polar layers and two of the four Glu120 residues coordinating a divalent cation[74] (Fig. 12.11C, left panel). Crystallization of a similar domain revealed a pentamer that lacks a cation binding site (Fig. 12.11C, right panel).[99,612] Sequence analyses have identified thirty types (30E types) of NSP4 in RVA strains. The highest sequence diversity of NSP4 is located

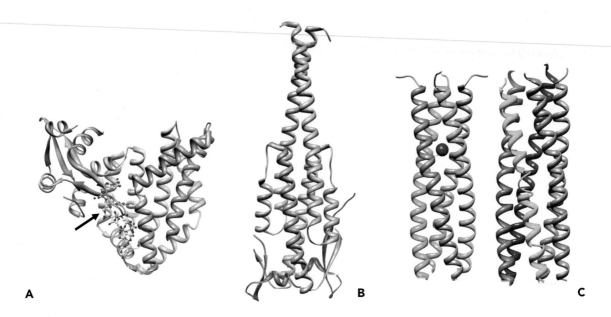

A   **B**   **C**

FIGURE 12.11 X-ray structures of NSP3 and NSP4. A: Structure of the NSP3 N-terminal domain homodimer in complex with the 3' consensus sequence of rotavirus mRNA.[166] The dimeric subunits are shown in *blue* and *golden yellow*. A single 5' RNA segment (shown in ball and stick representation and indicated by an *arrow*) is buried within a basic deep tunnel formed in the asymmetric homodimer. Each subunit participates in different interactions with the mRNA segments. **B:** Structure of NSP3 C-terminal domain homodimer (shown in *blue* and *golden yellow*) in complex with the dimer of the short peptide of eIF4G (shown in *green* and *red*). **C:** Ribbon representation of the homotetramer (*left*) with each dimer shown in *blue* and *green* and the homopentamer (*right*) of NSP4 95–137. The *red circle* indicates the location of the bound calcium in the tetramer.[74,99,612] (Figure prepared by Liya Hu.) (From Groft CM, Burley SK. Recognition of eIF4G by rotavirus NSP3 reveals a basis for mRNA circularization. *Molecular Cell* 2002;9(6):1273–1283.)

in the cytoplasmic domain. It is unclear whether this sequence diversity is important and driven by interactions with specific residues on VP6 or divergent regions on VP4, or both. However, specific combinations of types of VP6 and NSP4 have been found in natural reassortants, suggesting these interactions are biologically important.[332] There also may be host-specific interactions important for function, but these remain to be fully characterized.

Glycosylation of NSP4 is not required for its binding activity to DLP or for oligomerization, but it is required for interaction with calnexin.[29,472,666] NSP4 also has a binding site for VP5* within VP4[29,326] and may play a role in removing the transient envelope.[673] Heterooligomers of NSP4, VP4, and VP7 have been detected in enveloped particles, and calcium has been shown to be important for oligomerization of these proteins in the viroplasm-associated membranes[550] as well as for proper folding of VP7 epitopes and outer capsid assembly.[184,625] The precise mechanisms of how (a) the envelope on particles is removed; (b) the heterooligomeric complexes function in particle budding through the viroplasm-associated membranes; and (c) the outer capsid is assembled onto the newly made DLPs remain poorly understood. However, siRNA experiments indicate that VP4 and VP7 are assembled onto the particle following budding into the membranes adjacent to viroplasms, and VP7 is involved in the removal of the transient envelope.[151,422]

Rotavirus maturation is a calcium-dependent process, and virus yields are decreased when virus is produced in cells maintained in calcium-depleted medium. Viruses produced in absence of calcium are almost exclusively DLPs, and budding

of virus particles into the viroplasm-associated membranes is not observed.[625] The crystal structure of VP7 provides a new understanding of the requirement of calcium in forming TLPs. VP7 forms calcium-dependent trimers (Fig. 12.3); two calcium ions coordinate between each VP7 monomer and stabilize the trimeric interactions. Cryo-EM and single-particle reconstruction of VP7-recoated DLPs showed that the N termini (residues 51–70) of VP7 interact with VP6 and the VP7 trimers clamp onto the VP6 trimer.[110,679] Interestingly, unglycosylated VP7 made in the presence of tunicamycin is relatively stable in a calcium-free environment. The budding process can occur in the absence of calcium, but VP7 is retained within the ER.[7] VP7 does not fold properly unless it is expressed with other rotavirus proteins, and calcium must be present in cells for correct epitope formation.[185] Outer capsid assembly also requires the proper formation of disulfide bonds on VP7.[653] Earlier studies showed that treatment of cells with various agents (tunicamycin, dithiothreitol, or calcium-blocking drugs, such as thapsigargin) results in a buildup of enveloped particles in the viroplasm-associated membranes.[466] These agents may disrupt the proper folding of VP7 that is required for removing the envelope.

Understanding viral morphogenesis has been facilitated by the expression of the rotavirus structural proteins individually or in combinations in insect cells using recombinant baculoviruses.[141,745] This approach first showed that the single-layered VP2 particle shell self-assembles when VP2 is expressed alone and that all of the other capsid proteins can self-assemble into virus-like particles (VLPs) when coexpressed in the proper combinations. VLPs composed of VP2, VP1/2, VP1/2/3, VP2/3, VP2/6, VP2/6/7, VP2/4/6/7, and VP1/2/3/6 can be made.[141,745] The outer and inner capsid proteins of different virus strains can also reassociate and are able to be transcapsidated onto cores isolated from other virus strains and infectious virus is produced.[679] These results demonstrate that the structural proteins contain the intrinsic information required to form particles and that coexpression of mutant proteins is a feasible approach to analyze the domains responsible for the structural interactions between the proteins composing the virus particles. These particles have been useful to (a) analyze the role of cleavage sites in the spike protein in infectivity[243]; (b) investigate the role of individual structural proteins in inducing protective immunity[117,139,499]; (c) probe the inner structure of particles by analyzing difference maps of particles with distinct protein compositions or by X-ray analysis[623]; and (d) analyze RNA transcription and replication[104,107,402,403] and RNA packaging and assembly. Future studies should address questions of which mechanisms control the packaging of the viral genome and virus assembly.

Virus Release

Electron microscopy studies have shown that the infectious cycle ends when the progeny virus is released by host cell lysis in nonpolarized cells.[12,105] Extensive cytolysis late during infection and drastic alterations in the permeability of the PM of infected cells result in the release of cellular and viral proteins.[484] Despite cell lysis, most DLPs and many TLPs remain associated with the cellular debris, suggesting that these particles interact with intracellular structures within cells.[484] Whether the cytoskeleton provides a means of transport of viral proteins and particles to discrete sites in the cell for assembly or acts as a stabilizing element at the assembly site and in the newly budded virions, or whether particles are simply trapped by the cytoskeleton remains to be determined. VP4 interacts with actin and lipid rafts and can remodel microfilaments, and this has been suggested as a mechanism by which the brush border membrane of polarized epithelial cells is destabilized to facilitate rotavirus exit from cells.[236]

Virus–Host Interactions

Rotaviruses, like other obligate intracellular pathogens, are strictly reliant on host factors for replication, multiplication, and perpetuation. Recently, a variety of high throughput genetic screens have revolutionized the study of rotavirus–host interactions.[178,266,633,723] Three siRNA screens were performed to identify rotavirus-associated host factors, using different viral strains and cell types. Several components of the endosomal pathway were found to be important for rotavirus entry in two of these studies, including dynamins, vesicular ATPase, and the ESCRT complex.[266,633] The third study identified distinct genes that support higher growth of several rotavirus vaccine strains.[723] In a separate genome-wide CRISPR/Cas9 loss-of-function screen, deletion of genes in SA and sphingolipid synthesis conferred resistance to rotavirus infection.[178] Of note, UDP-glucose ceramide glucosyltransferase (encoded by *UGCG*) is a top hit in multiple screens, highlighting a critical cell type–independent pro-rotaviral role.

In addition to genetic approaches, host proteins that associate with rotaviral proteins or viral RNA have recently revealed new information on many steps of the rotavirus replication cycle. Drebrin, a cytoskeletal protein that stabilizes actin filaments, interacts with the VP5* fragment of VP4 and impedes rotavirus entry at a postattachment stage.[406] COP-II mediates NSP4 interaction with LC3-II and its localization to viroplasms.[138] In another study, the cellular kinase CK1α phosphorylates NSP2 and contributes to viroplasm formation.[147] In an unbiased proteomics-based screen to identify host proteins that bind to a conserved motif within the species A rotavirus 3′ UTR, Ren et al. identified ATP5B, a core subunit of the mitochondrial ATP synthase, to colocalize with the viral RNA and facilitate the production of infectious viral progeny in HIEs.[570] Multiple host RNA-binding proteins are found at the viroplasm with pro- or antiviral functions.[172,173] It is predictable that deep sequencing, mass spectrometry, and single-cell technology will continue to drive innovation in infectious disease research and shed more light on rotavirus–host interactions.

Reverse Genetics

For RNA viruses, the establishment of a plasmid-only–based cDNA clone to recover infectious viruses represents an important landmark and enables the study of specific mutations and the generation of recombinant reporter viruses, exemplified by recent advances with SARS-CoV-2.[670,725] Influenza A virus, also a segmented RNA virus, has been extensively investigated using a reverse genetics approach.[299,678] Both orthoreovirus and bluetongue virus, also members of the *Reoviridae* family, have been successfully rescued using a plasmid-only–based reverse genetics system.[75,379,557] Until recently, the analysis of rotavirus genes, in contrast, was largely reliant on the use of isolating natural variants and reassortants, helper viruses, synthetic RNA transcripts, and other forms of selection pressure to purposely modify the rotavirus genome.[386,680,683] In 2017, Kanai and colleagues described the first and long-awaited helper virus-free reverse genetics system for rotavirus.[357]

In addition to cDNA clones driven by a T7 RNA polymerase, two important changes were added to the successful helper virus-free reverse genetics system for rotavirus: a Nelson Bay reovirus fusion-associated small transmembrane (FAST) protein that promotes syncytia formation[631] and two subunits of the vaccinia virus capping enzyme to enhance RNA stability.[632] Several modifications and improvements to the original protocol have since been reported (i.e., threefold excess of NSP2- and NSP5-encoding transcription plasmids, an African Swine Fever virus capping enzyme, and inhibition of the IFN signaling in recipient MA104 cells) to further increase the rescue efficiency.[383,541,603]

New discoveries have already been achieved using this recently available tool in three main areas: (a) multiple rotavirus strains have been rescued to date, including simian strains SA11-L2,[357] RRV,[603] human strains KU,[383] Odelia,[371] CDC-9,[603] and murine strain D6/2[603]; (b) point/loss-of-function mutations were introduced to study viral gene/protein functions, including VP3,[643] NSP1,[356,357] NSP2,[148] NSP5,[513] and NSP6,[385] of which NSP1 and NSP6 are shown to be dispensable for rotavirus replication in cell culture; and (c) recombinant viruses with bioluminescent and fluorescent reporters have been generated.[382,540] The utility of a highly efficient rotavirus reverse genetics system holds great promise for the basic study of gene segment compatibility and structure–function relationships as well as more practical studies regarding the insertion capacity as a potential viral vector and targeted attenuated viruses as candidates for next-generation rotavirus vaccines.

PATHOGENESIS AND PATHOLOGY

Our understanding of rotavirus pathogenesis is based primarily on experiments carried out with animal models using homologous viruses (naturally infectious for the experimental host species) and heterologous viruses (naturally isolated from a host species distinct from the experimental species). In animal studies, virus replication can be analyzed in different tissues to obtain precise information about the sites of virus replication and host response to infection. Rotaviruses replicate primarily in the nondividing mature absorptive enterocytes near the tips of the small intestinal villi and enteroendocrine and tuft cells,[68b,289,510,614] suggesting that specific differentiated intestinal epithelial cells express factors required for efficient infection and replication. Although the small intestine is the site of optimal viral replication, several recent studies have demonstrated that antigenemia, viremia, and limited systemic replication likely occurs in a variety of systemic sites, although there is little evidence that this systemic spread and replication is responsible for any specific pathologic findings in normal hosts.[66,207,216,567] Studies have demonstrated, however, that in severely immunocompromised infants, rotaviruses can replicate and cause abnormalities in the liver and other organs.[244] In suckling mice without an intact IFN signaling system, some strains of rotavirus replicate very efficiently in the biliary tree and pancreas, causing biliary atresia and pancreatic disease,[212] and this phenotype may be associated with NSP3.[478] Rotavirus can also efficiently infect human biliary organoids.[111] The genetic basis of this strain-specific predilection to replicate in the biliary tree and pancreas has been assigned to VP4 and NSP1, which mediate viral attachment to host cells and IFN antagonism, respectively.[214] How the virus exits the gastrointestinal tract and gains access to systemic sites is unclear. Whether the ability of certain rotavirus strains to spread and replicate systemically is associated with systemic manifestations such as fever or intussusception is also not known.

The severity, localization, and histological findings of intestinal infection vary among animal species and virus strains (Fig. 12.12A).[71,192,567] However, in virtually all cases, pathologic changes due to rotavirus infection are primarily found in the small intestine.[267,567] In various animal models, infection is associated with either few visible lesions in the intestine, with some lesions such as enterocyte vacuolization (Fig. 12.12C1) and loss, or with significant histopathology changes such as villus blunting[127] and crypt hyperplasia.[756] Rotavirus infection in mice generally does not result in a breach of the intestinal barrier function.[288] Inflammation is mild compared with that observed with many other intestinal pathogens, especially bacterial pathogens. In many cases, no clear correlation exists between the degree of histopathology changes and the severity of the diarrheal disease. Even in species where histopathology is significant, such as cows and pigs, frequently significant diarrhea occurs before histologic signs of intestinal pathology. This dichotomy has been explained by the existence of a variety of mechanisms that cause disease symptoms (primarily vomiting, diarrhea, and fever in humans). More extensive reviews of rotavirus pathogenesis are available.[85,199]

Pathogenesis of rotavirus infection is multifactorial; both host and viral factors and homologous versus heterologous strains affect the outcome of the disease (Fig. 12.12B). For example, the age of inoculation impacts severity of symptoms:

in newborn or suckling IFN signaling-deficient mice, infection results in biliary atresia and death; in 0- to 14-day old normal mice and rats, diarrhea and some extraintestinal replication of virus occur; in adult normal mice, infection occurs in the absence of diarrhea. Genetic analysis of selected virus reassortants identified several viral proteins that are involved in virulence (VP3, VP4, NSP1, VP6, VP7, NSP2, NSP3, and NSP4).[82,214,313,506,567] These proteins are thought to play roles in the efficiency of virus replication (VP3, NSP2, VP6, and NSP3), shut-off of host protein synthesis (NSP3), extraintestinal spread and replication of the virus (NSP1 and NSP3), virus entry into cells (VP4 and VP7), inhibition of IFN signaling (NSP1), and the induction of diarrhea (NSP4).

Interpretation and comparison of various genetic studies of rotavirus pathogenesis and virulence have often been confounded by investigators failing to clearly describe what component(s) of pathogenesis is being examined. For example, some studies have simply examined disease phenotype (diarrhea/no diarrhea), whereas others have attempted to quantify the level of diarrhea by clinical scores. Some studies have focused on the quantity of viral replication in the intestine or shedding in the feces as a surrogate of pathogenesis, and other studies have examined transmissibility between susceptible hosts. Finally, in some studies, disease due to extraintestinal replication was examined as a measure of virulence. Depending on which one of these pathogenicity-associated phenotypes is studied, both the host-associated mechanisms and the viral genes involved are likely to vary. In fact, when the rotavirus pathogenesis literature is examined as a whole, it seems clear that the causes of rotaviral pathology and disease are multifactorial and often dependent on the specific experimental design of the study.

As a more specific example, analysis of the most prominent aspect of rotavirus pathogenesis, rotavirus diarrhea-inducing capacity, has yielded discrepant findings. Rotavirus diarrhea-inducing capacity has been attributed to several different mechanisms, including malabsorption secondary to destruction of enterocytes or alteration of enterocytes' absorptive functions, villus ischemia, virus-encoded enterotoxin NSP4, mislocalization of ion channels, colonic secretion, and activation of the enteric nervous system.[40,160,289,302] Each of these distinct mechanisms would likely be affected by a reduction in viral replication capacity of any cause. In fact, studies in people have directly associated the level of rotavirus shedding in the feces with the diarrheal severity,[358] although recent studies in India failed to find such a correlation in neonates symptomatically or asymptomatically infected with a similar rotavirus strain.[564] Additionally, nonreplicating rotavirus particles can also cause diarrhea.[629] Hence, it is important when studying the basis of rotavirus virulence to be cognizant of the constraints and limitations associated with the specific choice of experimental system or aspect of pathogenesis under examination and to emphasize that the causes of rotavirus disease are multifactorial.

Perhaps one of the most critical determinants of rotavirus virulence is the difference between homologous and heterologous strains for the infected host. Homologous strains tend to replicate efficiently, often cause diarrhea at a very low inoculation dose, and spread efficiently between members of that host species. In general, heterologous strains replicate poorly compared to the homologous strains, only cause diarrhea with large inoculation doses, and do not spread efficiently to other susceptible heterologous

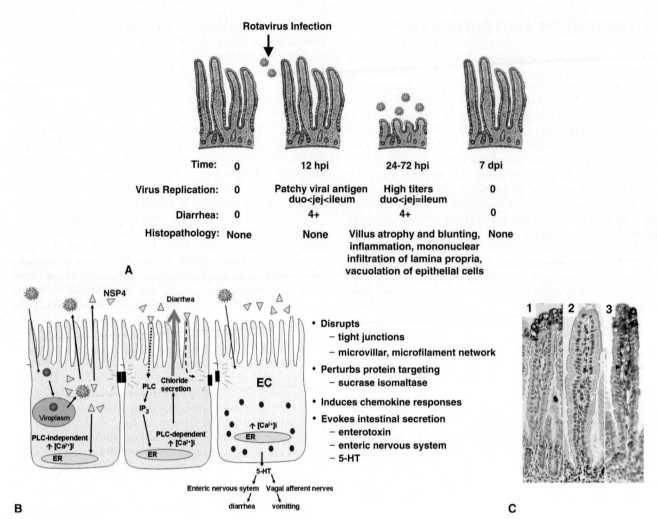

FIGURE 12.12 Rotavirus pathogenesis. A: Schematic of the histopathologic and clinical effects of rotavirus infection of intestinal cells. Rotavirus-induced diarrheal disease begins early after infection prior to significant histopathology of the infected mature enterocytes of the intestine. Diagram based on studies in piglets infected with virulent porcine rotavirus.[707] It is thought that the early, profuse, secretory diarrhea is caused by the action of the rotavirus enterotoxin, NSP4. (See text and Ref. [202].) Histologic changes are seen at later time points when virus titers are high, and loss of the differentiated enterocytes leads to malabsorption. The degree of villus atrophy can vary from species to species. Acute infection and disease normally resolve within 7 days in immunocompetent hosts. **B:** Model of rotavirus-induced diarrhea. Rotavirus infection of a polarized epithelial cell triggers many effects that contribute to pathogenesis. Infection of an initial cell (*left side*) results in virus entry and replication, formation of viroplasms, and release of virus and viral proteins. Intracellular NSP4 mobilizes intracellular calcium from internal stores, primarily the ER by a PLC-independent mechanism that involves NSP4 acting as a viroporin.[324] An NSP4 or NSP4-derived polypeptides (aa 112–175) (*triangles*) are secreted from cells by a nonclassical secretory pathway. Enterocyte function is altered with many cellular mRNAs being shut down, and protein targeting is disrupted.[71,567] Released NSP4-derived polypeptide affects uninfected cells resulting in mobilization of intracellular calcium by a PLC-dependent pathway that activates or regulates chloride secretion.[183] Tight junctions can also be disrupted by rotavirus infection as well as by NSP4 addition to uninfected cells. Rotavirus-infected cells also release extracellular adenosine 5′-diphosphate (ADP) that activates P2Y1 purinergic receptors on neighboring cells inducing intercellular calcium waves; enteroendocrine cells secrete serotonin in response to the ADP signaling. Blocking the ADP signal reduced rotavirus replication, inhibited rotavirus-induced serotonin release and fluid secretion, and reduced diarrhea severity in neonatal mice.[101] Finally, the enteric nervous system can be activated by mediators such as serotonin released from enterochromaffin (EC) cells infected with rotavirus or stimulated by NSP4.[289,432] Disruption of epithelial cell structure and function occurs slowly (at 18 to 24 hours postinfection) and may lead to cell death and alterations of paracellular pathway of fluid movement.[84,350,467,503,655] Rotavirus infection of epithelial cells activates epithelial cell signaling that triggers crosstalk among the diverse types of cells that make up the villus architecture. This results in activation of the enteric nervous system, intestinal secretion, and immune responses.[202,289,431,585] **C:** Viral antigen detection in mouse jejunum. Virus structural proteins are detected in enterocytes at the tips of intestinal villi at 4 days post infection during murine rotavirus infection of neonatal mice (C1), while at the same time, NSP4 is detected in epithelial cells at the tips of the villi, at the epithelial basement membrane, and in noninfected cells further down the villus (C3). NSP4 protein is not detected in uninfected mice (C2).[72]

hosts. Host-range restriction barriers to rotavirus infection, while substantial, are not absolute. There are numerous, generally single case, examples of zoonotic transmission to people.[440] There are, however, few if any examples of an entirely animal origin rotavirus becoming established in the human population. In fact, host-range restriction forms the mechanistic basis for the attenuation of several current rotavirus vaccines. Viral determinants of host-range restriction have not been as thoroughly investigated and studies had been, until the recent development of reverse genetics systems, basically limited to experimental infections of reassortant viruses in pigs and mice. In mice, it appears that NSP1, a gene product involved in suppressing innate immune responses, and probably VP4, the viral attachment protein, are both important factors governing host-range restriction in the gut based on genetic studies.[82,214] In more limited studies in the pig model, NSP1 was not clearly involved.[193,376]

There are factors other than replication that are likely to affect virulence. The discovery of NSP4 as the first viral entero toxin is of interest in this regard because this protein has pleiotropic properties in addition to its intracellular role in viral replication and morphogenesis (see above).[611] NSP4 peptides have been shown to induce age-dependent diarrhea in mice that mimic disease caused by rotavirus infection[40]; this has been confirmed for the NSP4 proteins from several species A and nonspecies A viruses.[269,312] Virulent and avirulent porcine rotaviruses that do or do not cause diarrhea have mutations in NSP4 associated with diarrhea induction. However, analyses of reassortant viruses in gnotobiotic pigs and mice have not identified NSP4 as a host range–specific determinant of diarrheal disease.[313] Analysis of genetically modified viruses should help define these unresolved discrepancies.

A role for the enteric nervous system in rotavirus diarrhea has been shown by the ability to attenuate rotavirus-induced diarrhea in mice and children with drugs that block this pathway.[389,451,598] NSP4 or other factors released from virus-infected cells may mediate this effect directly or by stimulating responses from enteroendocrine cells. These results suggest common mechanisms between diarrheas induced by viruses and bacteria not previously appreciated. Recent studies using human enteroendocrine cells as well as *in vivo* analyses in the mouse model indicate that rotavirus infection induces secretion of serotonin. Serotonin release is also stimulated by NSP4 and could be responsible for the well-documented association of rotavirus infection with vomiting in children.[289] Genetic or pharmacological inhibition of serotonin signaling in mice attenuates rotavirus-induced diarrhea.[290,389] Through the effects of NSP4 on intracellular Ca^{2+} levels, rotaviruses can also exploit paracrine purinergic signaling during intestinal organoid infection to generate intracellular Ca^{2+} waves in both infected and, importantly, uninfected bystander cells. These waves amplify the dysregulation of host cells and alter gastrointestinal physiology to cause diarrhea (Fig. 12.12B).[101]

Rotavirus, as the etiological cause of other enteric diseases, including inflammatory bowel disease and celiac disease, has been reported[297,742] but not well validated or associated in large-scale human studies.[270] In rare cases, rotavirus gastroenteritis was purported to cause central nervous system infection and febrile or nonfebrile seizure.[420] NSP4 has been implicated in the neurological manifestations of rotavirus, and serum anti-NSP4 IgG levels were associated with protection against seizures in patients with rotavirus gastroenteritis.[730] However, there are conflicting data from cohort studies on the possible relationship between rotavirus vaccination and reduction of seizures in children.[86,325,509,537]

EPIDEMIOLOGY

Rotavirus Serotypes

The structural and genetic basis of species A rotavirus classification is covered in the earlier Classification section of this chapter. The two surface proteins, VP4 (Protease-sensitive or P types) and VP7 (Glycosylated or G types), are targets of both homotypic and cross-reactive heterotypic neutralizing antibodies.[485] The serotypic classification of rotavirus is based on a binary system that includes both proteins. There are currently at least 57 G types and 57 P types among species A rotaviruses, but for human rotavirus infections, only a few combinations of G and P types predominate, primarily G1P[8], G2P[4], G3P[8], G4P[8], G9P[8], and G12P[8], which have not changed substantially in the postvaccination era.[153,498] The level of serotypic diversity among rotavirus strains circulating in animal species other than humans has not been as intensively studied.

The initial development of a monoclonal antibody-based ELISA for identification of the G type of clinical isolates and the subsequent application of RT-PCR genotyping and sequencing greatly expanded our understanding of the epidemiology of rotavirus serotypes among people with regard to infection, disease, and immunity.[218,404] The global distribution of common human rotavirus serotypes has been relatively consistent since 1989. VP7 "G" serotypes 1, 2, 3, 4, and more recently 9 and 12 make up the great majority of strains detected, especially in high-income countries. The last comprehensive review encompassing 124 studies published between 1989 and 2004 of the global distribution of rotavirus serotypes and genotypes isolated primarily from humans in 52 countries on five continents, which included 45,571 typed strains, showed that G1 strains were the most frequently detected serotype in each of the continents. G1, G2, G3, and G4 strains accounted for 97.5% of all rotavirus infections studied in Asia, North America, and Europe and 83.5% to 90.4% in South America, Africa, and Australia. G5, G8, G12, and G9 strains appeared focally in several areas, with G9 strains occasionally being predominant.[334,607] Several reviews emphasize the persistent frequency of G1 to G4 strains over the past two decades and the emergence of G9 and G12 strains in a variety of locations around the world.[451,500,601]

Analysis of clinical isolates for their VP4 "P" serotypes has not been widely performed because of the paucity of appropriate, monospecific and highly reactive serologic reagents. Thus, RT-PCR is generally performed for VP4 genotyping rather than serotyping. Based on sequence analysis, P1A[8] strains are the most frequently observed strains in humans, followed in frequency by P1B[4] strains. This is expected because the P1A[8] genotype is most frequently associated with G1, G3, G4, and G9 rotavirus strains. The other major G serotype, G2, characteristically has VP4 P1B[4] specificity. Although various combinations of G and P serotypes or genotypes have been described, a review of 16,474 strains evaluated for both VP7 and VP4 specificities in 124 studies indicated that four predominant combinations, G1P[8], G2P[4], G3P[8], and G4P[8], composed 88.5% of all the strains.[607] A recent analysis indicates G9P[8] strains to be also frequently isolated in humans.[1]

The reason that serotypic classification studies received much attention in the first decade of the 21st century was the assumption that serotypic classifications would correlate with the induction of protective immunity following infection or vaccination. However, current data drawn from a variety of human rotavirus monotypic vaccine studies clearly demonstrate that monotypic vaccines (see Prevention and Control section) protect against multiple rotavirus serotype–associated illnesses in humans as efficiently as multivalent vaccine formulations. Since heterotypic protective immunity is generated after a limited exposure to a restricted number of different serotypes,[89] the intense focus on human rotavirus serotypes has been substantially reduced as a critical determinant of disease prevention as relates to the current group of licensed vaccines. Studies have attempted to correlate rotavirus serotypes with clinical disease severity with limited success.[600]

Infection in Adults

Children and adults are frequently reinfected with rotavirus, but with only moderate, minimal, or no clinical manifestations. In an early study, 22 of 40 adult household contacts of children hospitalized with rotavirus gastroenteritis had serologic evidence of asymptomatic rotavirus reinfection at the time of their child's admission to the hospital.[377] Symptomatic infection in adults is similar to that seen in infants, although diarrhea, vomiting, and dehydration are not usually severe. While subclinical rotavirus infection is the most common outcome in adults, rotavirus gastroenteritis in adults has been described in army recruits in Finland as well as in patients (some geriatric) and staff in hospitals in various countries.[315] In a study from China, rotavirus was second to noroviruses as a cause of viral gastroenteritis in adults.[417] Species A rotavirus outbreaks in adults have been rare and isolated events.[225,415] Rotaviruses are also associated with traveler's diarrhea in certain settings, and a large review of the global etiologies of traveler's diarrhea found that rotavirus infection was responsible for approximately 4% to 7% of cases depending on the location.[624] Symptomatic rotavirus gastroenteritis has also been identified in adults undergoing bone marrow and other transplantations[5,754] as well as in some patients with malignant disease undergoing chemotherapy.[412]

Species B rotaviruses (adult diarrheal rotavirus [ADRV] strain) were implicated in several large outbreaks (involving up to 20,000 individuals) of severe gastroenteritis in adults in various parts of China as well as smaller outbreaks and endemic disease in Bangladesh and India.[321,374] Affected adults often had cholera-like, severe, watery diarrhea, and a few elderly patients died. To date, however, species B rotavirus infections appear to occur primarily as isolated epidemics or sporadic cases, possibly due to contamination of water sources.

Nosocomial Infections

Nosocomial rotavirus infections occur rather frequently. For example, before widespread rotavirus vaccination, 10 of 60 children hospitalized for nondiarrheal disease were subsequently infected by rotavirus and developed diarrheal illness.[595] In studies carried out prior to the availability of rotavirus vaccines, a median of 27% of patients in high-income countries and 32% in low-income to middle-income countries developed diarrhea

and likely acquired rotavirus infections while in the hospital.[217] A review of nosocomial infections in European countries prior to rotavirus vaccine availability showed that infections are mainly associated with young infants (0 to 5 months of age) as opposed to older age groups in the community and that a sizeable proportion of the infections are asymptomatic.[252] Nosocomial infections have also been described in various neonatal nurseries around the world.[61,155] These infections are usually subclinical, although nosocomial outbreaks of rotavirus gastroenteritis have been described in a newborn nursery in Italy.[240] The introduction of rotavirus vaccines has led to a significant reduction in hospital-acquired rotavirus infections.[13,241]

Transmission

Rotaviruses are highly contagious,[260] with as little as one tissue culture infectious dose being able to cause illness in a fully susceptible homologous host. Rotavirus is generally transmitted by the fecal–oral route, is very stable in the environment, and is shed in very large quantities (up to 10^{11} particles per gram) in the feces.[201,311] Oral administration of rotavirus-positive stool filtrate induces diarrheal illness and viral shedding in adult volunteers.[369,711] Some investigators have speculated that rotaviruses might also be transmitted via the respiratory route.[286] However, evidence for this speculation is limited. Shedding of rotavirus from the intestinal tract can occur before onset of diarrhea or following cessation of diarrhea.[543] In one study, the duration of rotavirus shedding ranged from 4 to 29 days, with a median of 7 days, as measured by ELISA, whereas by the more sensitive PCR assay, shedding has been detected for up to 57 days, with a median of 10 days.[574] Shedding in severely immunocompromised children can be even more prolonged.[244]

Exemplary stability of various human and animal rotaviruses in the environment and the low doses required to infect hosts may contribute to the efficient transmission of rotaviruses.[201,375,711] For example, porcine rotavirus present in feces retained infectivity for over 2 years when refrigerated. Although rotaviruses have been detected in both raw and treated sewage, it is unlikely that contaminated water, which is important in species B rotavirus outbreaks, plays an important role in the transmission of species A rotaviruses in high-income countries.[321,640] However, an apparent community-wide water-borne epidemic of species A rotavirus was documented in Turkey in 2011.[390] Effective disinfection of contaminated material and careful hand washing constitute important measures to contain rotavirus infection, especially in hospitals, nurseries, and institutional settings.[718] Rotavirus has been detected on moist surfaces in day care centers, and in one controlled study, rotavirus transmission to volunteers was prevented if a rotavirus contaminate was first sprayed with a disinfectant prior to contact with the volunteer.[93,709]

There has been profound interest in the role of animals as a source of rotavirus infection of humans. This concept gained support from the observation that certain animal rotaviruses share a neutralization antigen with some human rotavirus strains and that some naturally occurring animal rotavirus strains may infect humans and undergo reassortment with human rotaviruses.[453,487] Nonetheless, zoonotic transmission and sustained persistence of animal strains in the human population appear to be rare.[637,731] It should be noted, however, that human–bovine reassortant strains (I321 and 116E) and a human–porcine reassortant strain (serotype G5) have been endemic in selected areas in India and Brazil, respectively.[156] Human–animal rotavirus reassortants have also been detected in Belgium.[31,744] Large-scale full genomic sequencing of rotavirus isolates from around the world demonstrated that genome segments of animal rotavirus origin are present in human isolates at a higher frequency than had been expected.[440] However, to date, such studies focused on sequencing of selected isolates that were unusual from a serologic or electrophoretic perspective, so the actual frequency of such human/animal reassortment in the field remains unclear.

Incubation Period

The incubation period of rotavirus diarrheal illness is estimated to be less than 48 hours in children.[158] The onset of experimentally induced rotavirus diarrhea in adult volunteers occurred 2 to 4 days after experimental challenge.[368,369] From challenge studies, the incubation period of illness under experimental conditions in adults, all of whom are expected to have some level of preexisting immunity, is 1 to 4 days.

Geographic Distribution and Seasonal Patterns

Rotaviruses have been detected throughout the world wherever they have been sought.[562,705] These viruses consistently constitute one of the major etiologic agents of severe infantile diarrhea in every country, despite the existence of several safe and effective rotavirus vaccines for over a decade. Prior to the vaccination program, rotaviruses displayed a marked seasonal pattern of infection in most high-income countries, with epidemic peaks occurring in the cooler winter months of each year.[514] This recurring pattern was observed in the United States, Europe, Australia, and Japan.[152] The cause for this seasonal pattern is not known, but the influence of low relative humidity and increases in indoor activities have been suggested as contributing factors in some studies.[76,387,473] Of note, following the introduction of rotavirus vaccination, the marked seasonality of rotavirus infection declined substantially, and the initiation of the annual epidemic occurs later in the season.[152,664] The usual seasonal pattern of rotavirus infection observed in temperate climates does not occur uniformly in other areas of the world; many locations in the tropics show no, or a diminished, seasonal trend.[306,405] Modeling studies have suggested that the relative lack of rotavirus seasonality observed in many tropical countries may be due to the high birth rates typical of low-income countries.[152]

Age, Sex, Race, and Socioeconomic Status

In high-income countries, rotavirus gastroenteritis of sufficient severity to require hospitalization occurs most frequently in unvaccinated infants and young children from approximately 6 months to 2 years of age.[61] Infants younger than 6 months of age experience the next highest frequency of such illness. In certain studies, especially in low-income countries, the younger than 6-month age group had the highest frequency of severe disease.[145,194,650,686] In one prevaccine study from the United States, the age distribution of patients admitted to the hospital with gastroenteritis of any cause was different for black and nonblack patients; 59% of all black patients admitted for gastroenteritis were younger than 6 months of age, whereas most nonblack patients were older.[78] This difference was also reflected in admissions for rotavirus diarrhea. Because the children were predominantly from inner-city areas, these differences may have reflected the effects of crowded living conditions, which may have allowed earlier and more efficient transmission of the virus.

In low-income countries, in a recent large-scale multicenter surveillance study, despite rotavirus vaccine usage, rotavirus was found to be the second most important diarrheal pathogen within the first 11 months of life and the third between ages 12 and 24 months.[547] In a reanalysis of this study based on the use of RT-PCR, rotavirus ranked number one between 0 and 11 months.[548] In another recent large-scale international epidemiology study, both moderate-to-severe diarrhea and less severe diarrhea were primarily attributed to rotavirus within the first 2 years of age.[391,392] Rotavirus remains the leading cause of severe diarrhea between 0 and 23 months and the second leading cause between 24 and 49 months.[391,392] There were also rotavirus-associated gastroenteric illnesses in children 5 to 13 years of age, and rotavirus was identified as the sole pathogen in 16% of patients in this age group.

The low frequency of clinical illness in most (but not all) normal neonates who shed rotavirus remains unexplained.[60] It seems clear, however, that such asymptomatic neonatal infection is able to induce some protective immunity in the infected children.[248] Malnutrition is considered to play an important role in increasing the severity of clinical manifestations of human rotavirus infections.[157] This phenomenon has been reproduced in experimental mouse and piglet models.[395] Repeated diarrheal infections may precipitate the development of malnutrition as these infections damage the intestinal mucosa, and absorptive enterocytes are compromised over an extended period.[444] Sex difference is not involved in rotavirus susceptibility in either human or mouse studies.

Molecular Epidemiologic Studies

Initial investigations of the molecular epidemiology of human rotaviruses utilized gel electrophoresis and evaluated the individual genomic migration patterns (electropherotypes) of the segmented dsRNA genomes for strain identification, comparison, and epidemiologic correlations.[310] For example, analysis of rotaviruses isolated from 116 children hospitalized with gastroenteritis in Melbourne, Australia, between 1973 and 1979 identified 17 different electropherotypes.[578] In addition to revealing the genetic diversity of human rotaviruses and heterogeneity of circulating rotaviruses, electropherotypes also provided a simple and sensitive method for tracing the spread of rotavirus through a specific population group. The electropherotype cannot be used, however, to predict virulence or serotypic classification.[21,239]

Another early molecular approach to rotavirus epidemiologic studies was RNA/RNA hybridization. This technique employed labeled ssRNA viral transcripts as probes for genomic dsRNA and identified two major families of human rotavirus strains, which had a general lack of homology with animal strains. Occasional human/human and human/animal reassortants and some rare human rotavirus strains were observed using these hybridization techniques.[223,488] In the last 15 years, the availability of full genomic sequencing and reduction in cost have resulted in the general replacement of these two approaches by RT-PCR–based assays coupled to Sanger sequencing or direct RNA sequencing for epidemiologic studies (see Diagnosis section).

IMMUNITY

The mechanisms responsible for generating protective immunity to rotavirus infections and illness following vaccination or natural infection are not yet completely understood. This is particularly true in humans where detailed examination of the acquired immune responses (T and B cells) in young children is limited because of the difficulty in obtaining sufficient amounts of blood in early life. The contribution of innate immunity to the control of rotavirus infection has been examined primarily in animal models. In general, serum antibody levels in animals and people correlate with protection from illness, but this correlation has not been absolute. It seems likely that overall serum antibody levels to rotavirus generally reflect other less easily measured and more specific immune effector functions such as mucosal antibody titers or numbers of virus-specific memory B cells in the gut.[14,226,341] The one circumstance where serum antibody levels directly provide a good correlate of protection is in newborn children where transplacentally acquired humoral immunity appears to provide some protection from illness early in life.[22,169]

There are both inherent and practical complexities to studying the effector mechanisms responsible for the induction and persistence of protective immunity in young children. Therefore, animal models have been instrumental in identifying the respective roles of adaptive and innate immunity, humoral and cellular immune responses, systemic and local immunity, the viral targets of protective immunity, and mechanisms of virus immune evasion.[25,171,226,228] There are, however, several important considerations to keep in mind when evaluating experiments on rotavirus immunity in animal models. Common laboratory and many domestic animals undergo natural infection with homologous rotavirus strains that specifically infect and cause diarrheal disease in the young of that specific species. However, virtually all animal species, except for guinea pigs, studied to date can be experimentally infected with heterologous rotavirus strains (strains initially isolated from another animal species), and in many cases, a high inoculation titer can also cause diarrheal disease in the heterologous host.[525] In general, compared to homologous rotavirus strains, heterologous strains do not spread or spread with reduced efficiency in a heterologous host, do not cause disease at low inoculation titers, replicate less well in the gastrointestinal tract, and are usually attenuated compared to homologous rotavirus strains in the homologous host. In nature, most disease in humans is caused by homologous human rotaviral infection. Studies of the determinants of protective immunity in animal models have used both homologous and heterologous rotavirus strains and thus should be interpreted with caution, especially when heterologous strains have been employed. In addition, most animal models of immunization and subsequent protection are short term (lasting 8 weeks at the most) because of the difficulty of maintaining animals in a nonimmune and rotavirus-susceptible state over long periods of time (years), as is the case with rotavirus disease in humans where some children, even in less developed countries, remain unexposed to rotavirus for at least 3 years after birth.[590] Lastly, once a small animal (primarily mouse) is infected with rotavirus, it is almost completely resistant to subsequent reinfection and symptomatic disease. Humans, on the other hand, remain susceptible to primary infection and disease over a long period of time (at least 3 years) and are susceptible to multiple reinfections and multiple bouts of rotavirus-associated disease in childhood and, to a lesser degree, in later life.[692] Hence, one must approach animal model data on rotavirus immunity with the notion that it may not be directly applicable to the human condition.

Adaptive Immunity

A variety of animal models (mice, rats, rabbits, pigs, calves, lambs, primates, and others) have been used to study rotavirus infection, with the mouse and piglet models being the most common, especially from the standpoint of evaluation of immunity.[208,228,581,737] The protective immunity conferred by serum antibody against rotavirus has been examined in animal studies under various scenarios,[14,54,228] including transplacentally, systemic absorption of colostrum, passive parenteral inoculation with immune serum or purified polyclonal or monoclonal immunoglobulins, or systemic immunization with inactivated virus, VLPs, or recombinant viral proteins with or without an adjuvant. Passively acquired high titers of serum antibody have been associated with protection in a variety of animal studies,[54] but when the level of systemic serum antibody is not sufficiently high, protection is limited.[507] When examined in toto, if present at high levels, enough systemic antibody seems to be able to find its way to be in proximity with intestinal epithelium (whether this is at the basolateral or apical surface is not yet clear) and mediate protection. Recent studies have demonstrated that in several animal species, including humans, there is an active transport mechanism to transcytose systemic immunoglobulin G (IgG) into the intestinal lumen.[37] Of note, the relative sparing of rotavirus infection in the first 2 months of life in children and the correlation of this protection with maternal antibody titers at birth provide indirect support for the notion that serum antibody can, at least under some circumstances, directly mediate local effects in humans as well as animals.[726]

A number of mouse studies have taken advantage of immunologic reagents and gene knockout models to delineate the immune effectors that mediate clearance of primary infection and protection from reinfection.[209] Anatomically, there is an enlargement of Peyer's patches and mesenteric lymph nodes following homologous murine rotavirus infection.[68a,491,626] B cells, and hence antibodies, are critical for the maintenance of long-term, high-level protection from reinfection in mice, and CD8+ T cells mediate short-term reduced susceptibility to reinfection.[227,228] A protective B-cell response can occur in the absence of T-cell help, although it is substantially reduced compared to the response seen in wild-type mice,[68b,228] and T cells can mediate their antirotavirus effects in the absence of perforin, Fas, and IFN-γ.[228] Both B and T cells can clear the primary infection, but T cells appear to do this more quickly and efficiently than B cells. In the mouse, CD8+ T cells can mediate almost complete protection (up to 2 weeks after primary infection) or partial protection (up to 3 months after primary infection) from reinfection; however, this protection diminishes greatly 8 months after primary infection.[211,460] A role for CD8+ T cells in the control of primary rotavirus infection was also demonstrated in a homologous gnotobiotic calf model.[508] The role of CD4+ T cells in rotavirus infection is understudied, and the identities of distinct CD4+ T cell subsets present in the intestinal epithelia and lamina propria are not well delineated. Interestingly, however, in mice, oral vaccination with heterologous rotavirus (simian RRV strain) stimulates regulatory rotavirus-specific CD4+ Latency-Associated Peptide (LAP+) T cells, and depletion of these cells increases vaccine-induced protection against homologous rotavirus (murine EC strain).[573]

Studies using wild-type and various knockout mice have highlighted the importance of intestinal tract homing of both B and T cells, mediated by the $\alpha_4\beta_7$ integrin, CCR9, and CCR10.[336,583] Additional studies using IgA-deficient mice showed that IgA is critical for antirotavirus immunity,[67] and $\alpha v\beta 8$ on type 1 conventional CD103+CD11b− dendritic cells mediated early IgA production to rotavirus.[492] IgG immunity is also dependent on the ability of B cells to traffic to the gut.[394] Lymphotoxin signaling also seems to influence IgA responses to rotavirus antigens.[407] Consistent with the animal findings, people with selective IgA deficiency resolve rotavirus infection normally and appear to develop compensatory increases in antirotavirus IgG during infection.[331] Dietary factors have also been investigated for their influence on the immune response. For example, vitamin A deficiency impairs both serum antibody and cell-mediated immune responses to rotavirus in infant mice.[8] Vitamin A is the precursor of retinoic acid, important for dendritic cell development[746] and microfold cell differentiation in the Peyer's patches,[180] both of which might explain this defect.

There have been less extensive studies of primary T- or B-cell responsiveness to rotavirus infection in people than in animal models, and the functional role these cells play or their correlation to protection has been difficult to evaluate in young children. IFN-γ–secreting circulating rotavirus-specific CD4+ and CD8+ T cells are present in small numbers in children and relatively low amounts in adults. Human antirotavirus T cells express the gut homing receptor $\alpha_4\beta_7$.[336,583] Similarly, circulating human B cells have been examined in a number of human studies using flow cytometry and ELISpot-based assays.[111,584,672] These studies show that human rotavirus–specific B cells also express intestine-specific homing receptors and that both naive and memory rotavirus–specific B cells directed at VP6 are enriched for a CD27+IgD+IgM+ subset of cells. The biological role of rotavirus-specific circulating IgM memory B cells is not yet fully understood.[494]

Several in vitro and animal model systems have been used to identify the viral targets of protective humoral immunity. In vitro neutralization studies using monospecific hyperimmune serum or monoclonal antibodies suggest that VP4 and VP7 are the only two rotavirus targets of neutralizing antibody, although some data indicate that anti-VP6 antibodies and/or nanobodies can also mediate in vitro and in vivo neutralization.[14,90,94,210,447,485,690] These experiments are generally conducted in MA104 cells, which may fail to efficiently detect certain neutralizing antibodies targeted at VP8* that only block rotavirus infection in human intestinal epithelial cells.[210] As discussed in the serotype section, VP4 and VP7 come in a variety of antigenic specificities that are capable of segregating independently by gene reassortment during mixed infections. Many monoclonal and polyclonal antibodies directed at these two surface proteins preferentially react in a serotype-specific manner. On the other hand, both VP4 and VP7 contain heterotypic epitopes, and some antibodies to either protein can specifically mediate heterotypic neutralization.[210,485]

The rules that govern the induction of homotypic versus heterotypic immunity following natural infection or vaccination are poorly understood for rotavirus as they are for many viral infections. This issue has been difficult to evaluate carefully in animal models because of the relatively short window of susceptibility to infection and disease in an experimental setting. Despite these limitations, both homotypic and heterotypic protection have been documented in animal model experiments.[505] More recent vaccine studies in humans make it clear that exposure to infection with a very limited number of VP4 and VP7 serotypes (either from natural infection or vaccination) provides substantial protective immunity to most heterotypic strains.[55] What is still unclear is the basis for this heterotypic immunity. Analysis of monoclonal antibodies derived from resident B cells in adult human intestinal specimens has demonstrated that humans develop both homotypic and heterotypic immunity to VP4 and VP7. The homotypic and heterotypic antibodies to VP4 are primarily directed at VP8* and VP5*, respectively.[210,485]

Two other rotavirus proteins, VP6 and NSP4, have also been implicated as targets of protective immunity following infection. Rare, selected nanobodies specific for VP6 appear to be capable of mediating classic viral neutralization in vitro and passive protection in vivo.[235,436] In addition, in a mouse model, selected anti-VP6 IgAs were protective despite not having traditional in vitro neutralization activity. These antibodies appeared to function intracellularly during transcytosis through intestinal epithelial cells.[90,94,134,213,617] In other studies, CD4+ T cells directed at VP6-mediated protection in mice and rabbits, but not pigs. Systemic immunization with double-layered (VP2 and VP6) particles or VLPs composed of recombinant VP2 and VP6 induced varying levels of resistance to challenge in animal model studies.[639,713] Finally, the viral enterotoxin NSP4 is a potential target of protective immunity, and one study in mice demonstrated protection from disease following administration of antibody to this protein.[115] Whether VP6 or NSP4 immunity plays any protective role in people remains to be explored.

A variety of epidemiologic and serologic studies have provided compelling demonstrations of the development of acquired immunity to rotavirus infection and disease in people over time during early childhood as well as the recurrent nature of asymptomatic or relatively mild symptomatic rotavirus infection over a lifetime (Fig. 12.13). As mentioned above, asymptomatic neonatal infection is associated with a subsequent reduction in severe rotavirus disease, but not with lack of reinfection.[62] A large 2-year prospective study in Mexico showed that one or two natural rotavirus infections were highly effective at preventing further severe infections.[692] In this study, protection was both homo- and heterotypic in nature, although the homotypic response appeared stronger following the first rotavirus exposure than after subsequent reinfections.

Although the precise immunological determinants of protective immunity for rotavirus infection are unclear, some experimental information regarding correlates of rotavirus immunity in people was obtained in an early adult volunteer study. A human rotavirus D strain (serotype G1P[8]) was orally administered to 18 individuals.[368,369] Of them, 5 shed rotavirus and 4 of those 5 developed diarrheal illness. The preexisting level of serum neutralizing antibodies to the homotypic challenge virus or to a heterotypic human rotavirus DS-1 strain (serotype G2P[4]) correlated with resistance to illness. The correlation of levels of neutralizing activity in intestinal fluid to

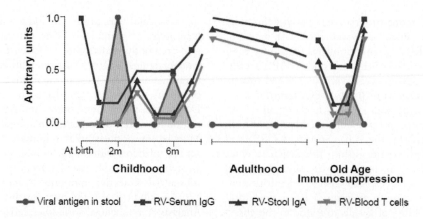

FIGURE 12.13 Relative quantities of rotavirus-specific antibodies and T cells in key periods of natural history of rotavirus infection. In people, rotavirus infections generally occur multiple times over a life span with decreasing frequency as exposures increase. Late in life when exposures are reduced, increased susceptibility can occur. Protection from severe disease can be mediated by passively acquired IgG antibody at birth or from actively acquired IgA or IgG antibody following subsequent infection or vaccination. Protection from subsequent infections or mild disease (indicated by diminished viral shedding and immune boosting) is relative and likely depends on a number of factors but primarily the level of local and systemic antibodies. CD8+ T cells play a role in the timely resolution of rotavirus infection in animal models, but their role in humans is less well documented. Other critical factors like intestinal B and T cells have not been studied. (*Lines* represent a typical set of responses but interindividual variations can exist.)

resistance was not significant. Each of the five ill volunteers developed a serum neutralizing antibody response to the challenge strain and to the heterotypic G2P[4] human DS1 strain as well as to a heterotypic bovine rotavirus NCDV strain (serotype G6P[1]). The prechallenge sera from this study were later reexamined by a competitive epitope-blocking immunoassay for antibody levels against several well-defined VP7 and VP4 neutralization epitopes.[265,628] These studies correlated both homo- and heterotypic blocking activity to VP7 with resistance to disease. In another series of challenge and rechallenge studies, serum rotavirus IgG or jejunal neutralizing antibodies were observed to correlate with protection against infection and illness.[368,369] In a third series of studies, however, serum and jejunal rotavirus antibodies did not correlate with resistance.[710,711]

Rotavirus serum IgA levels have also correlated with resistance to severe rotavirus illness.[308] In a recent vaccination study with 5,074 infants, serum antirotavirus IgA levels correlated with protection against rotavirus gastroenteritis, although the assay used did not distinguish between VP4 and VP7.[36] In a study of infants 1 to 24 months of age and young children residing in an orphanage, a significant correlation was observed between homotypic serum neutralizing antibodies and resistance to disease.[113] The association between fecal IgA and serum IgG antirotavirus antibody titers and protection against infection and illness was also investigated in 100 children younger than 18 months of age attending day care centers in the United States over one or two rotavirus seasons.[446,502] During the two seasons, seven outbreaks of G1 serotype and one of G3 serotype rotaviruses were detected. These studies concluded that (a) a rotavirus-specific fecal IgA titer of at least 1:80 correlated with protection against infection and a titer of at least 1:20 correlated with protection against illness; (b) a preexisting serum antirotavirus IgA titer

of greater than 1:200 or an IgG titer of greater than 1:800 was associated with protection against infection; and (c) a high level of preexisting G type–specific blocking antibody was associated with protection against infection. Similar results were obtained from a study conducted in Australia: a direct correlation was observed between high levels of antirotavirus intestinal IgA antibody and protection against natural rotavirus infection and illness.[135] In a heterologous gnotobiotic piglet model, a direct association was observed between the degree of protection and the level of intestinal IgA antibody–secreting cell response as well as serum IgA, intestinal IgA, and intestinal IgG titers.[674,740] In mice, antirotavirus intestinal or serum IgA correlates with protection against homologous or heterologous rotavirus infection.[208,461]

A large number of animal studies have been carried out that either support or refute the hypothesis that rotavirus immunity is fundamentally homotypic in nature. There are multiple reasons for these contradictory findings including different animal species, different challenge doses and strains, and different measurements of protection (i.e., lack of infection, lack of disease, and reduced disease severity are all possible end points). In any case, from a practical standpoint, it seems clear that a substantial level of heterotypic immunity is induced following primary rotavirus infection in children in high- and middle-income countries, and following immunization with monovalent (G1P[8] or G9P[11]) attenuated human rotavirus vaccines. Both vaccines provide substantial protective immunity from diarrheal disease caused by multiple other strains and serotypes.[55,648] Finally, although serotype-specific neutralizing antibodies have been demonstrated in breast milk, the effect of breast-feeding on the occurrence of rotavirus gastroenteritis is controversial, but the weight of current evidence would indicate a real but generally modest effect.[11,476,496]

Innate Immunity

From *in vitro* and animal model studies, it has become clear that the innate immune system is also deeply involved in the early events of rotavirus immunity and may help shape the outcome of the T- or B-cell responses to infection[335] (Fig. 12.14). Specifically, multiple pieces of evidence have demonstrated a pivotal role of IFN signaling in rotavirus infection. First, a type I IFN response can be detected during active viral replication both *in vivo* and *in vitro*.[255] Second, one of the rotavirus nonstructural proteins, NSP1, functions as an IFN antagonist via the degradation of IFN regulatory factors (IRF) 3, 5, and 7 as well as β-transducin repeat–containing protein (β-TrCP).[44,45,258] Third, this degradation appears to function in a host species and cell type–restricted manner.[619] Fourth, inhibition of IFN signaling in murine models is associated with an enhanced rotavirus replication phenotype for several heterologous strains.[212,215,414] Finally, in human plasmacytoid dendritic cells (pDCs), IFN production is triggered by the exposure to viral particles containing dsRNA.[162] pDC-derived IFN enhances the host B-cell response *in vivo*.[163] Exposure of myeloid dendritic cells (mDCs) to UV-treated rotavirus induces significantly higher-type I IFN levels, suggesting that rotavirus-encoded factors antagonize the IFN response in mDCs, as is the case in fibroblasts and epithelial cells but not in pDCs.[188] There are little data on the innate response to rotavirus in other animal species, but in calves, acute rotavirus infection is also associated with down-regulation of IFN-associated pathways.[9]

Current data support a model indicating that IFNs, at least partially, underlie the molecular basis of host range restriction in the suckling mouse.[215] Mice deficient in type I IFN receptors are substantially more susceptible to heterologous but not homologous rotavirus replication.[212,687] In a mouse model, lethal biliary disease and enhanced rotavirus systemic replication were seen specifically in mice lacking both type I (IFN-α/β) and type II (IFN-γ) IFN receptor signaling or the common adaptor protein STAT1 when infected with the heterologous simian rotavirus RRV strain, and these mice eventually succumb to rotavirus infection.[212] In contrast, murine rotavirus replication was only modestly enhanced in *STAT1* KO mice. The role of type III IFN (IFN-λ1/2/3/4) had not been investigated until recently. Similar to type I IFNs, type III IFNs act to suppress heterologous rotavirus replication in the small intestine.[414,551] In human colonic epithelial cells and HIE cultures, type III IFN is the predominant type of IFN induced by rotavirus infection.[181,615]

Within the infected intestinal epithelial cells, cytosolic RNA sensors RIG-I and MDA5 and the adaptor protein MAVS are key mediators of the IFN expression in response to enteric viruses.[83,410,620,630] At least in human HT-29 cells and murine

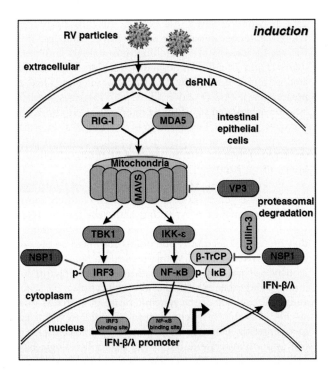
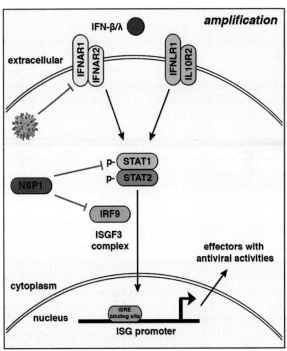

FIGURE 12.14 Rotavirus recognition by and antagonism of the host innate immune system. Rotaviruses interact with both the induction and amplification stages of interferon signaling. Rotaviruses, upon entry into cells, generate pathogen-associated molecular products (PAMPs) that are likely by-products of early viral replication. These viral ligands activate the cytosolic pattern recognition receptors (PRRs) RIG-I and MDA5, leading to MAVS-dependent activation of the transcription factor IRF3 and NF-κB by the kinases TBK1 and IKK-ε, respectively. Phosphorylated IRF3 and NF-κB translocate into the nucleus where they induce the transcription of type I and type III IFNs. Viral replication results in the expression of NSP1, which targets IRF3 and β-TrCP for proteasomal degradation in a virus strain–specific manner. Other IRFs, including IRF5 and IRF7, can also be degraded by NSP1. Rotavirus VP3 targets MAVS for degradation. Secreted type I and type III IFNs engage cognate receptors to amplify the antiviral responses. Rotavirus infection can lead to the degradation of IFN receptors by an unknown mechanism. NSP1 inhibits interferon stimulated gene factor 3 (ISGF3) complex via at least two distinct mechanisms (blocking STAT1 phosphorylation and degrading IRF9), further suppressing ISG expression and associated yet-to-be-identified antiviral activities.

embryonic fibroblasts, both RIG-I and MDA5, which preferentially recognize 5′ppp RNA and long dsRNA molecules, respectively, contribute to rotaviral RNA sensing and subsequent IFN induction. MAVS is also required for IFN induction by rotavirus in macrophages.[174] Rotavirus-encoded RNA capping enzyme VP3 also targets MAVS for degradation, thereby facilitating replication *in vivo*.[181] To efficiently antagonize the IFN induction, rotavirus NSP1 protein mediates the proteasomal degradation of IRF3, 5, 7, and/or 9 depending on the strain,[24] and IRF degradation is associated with the ability of rotaviruses to suppress the host antiviral response.[24,44,45] NSP1 proteins from several human and porcine rotavirus strains mediate the degradation of β-TrCP instead of IRF3 and thereby block NF-κB activation.[175,258] Although TNF-α treatment inhibits rotavirus infection in cell culture,[291] a direct demonstration of the role of NF-κB signaling during rotavirus infection *in vivo* using cytokine or receptor knockouts is lacking.[258] NSP1 targets both IRF3 and β-TrCP via its C-terminal substrate targeting motif.[477,752] NSP1 has been speculated to function as an E3 ubiquitin ligase due to the presence of a putative N-terminal RING finger domain.[259] However, definitive evidence for this hypothesis is missing, and at least in the case of β-TrCP degradation, cullin-3, a host E3 ubiquitin ligase complex, binds to NSP1[433] and is hijacked by human and porcine rotavirus NSP1s.[179]

In addition to targeting the IFN induction pathway, NSP1 also efficiently inhibits the IFN amplification pathway and interferon-independent signaling to facilitate virus infection in vivo.[234a] NSP1 blocks STAT1 phosphorylation and translocation into the nucleus.[309,622] Although the antiviral activities of IFNs are known, the antiviral roles of specific interferon-stimulated genes (ISGs) are less clear. Recent reports showed that 25-hydroxycholesterol, produced by an ISG cholesterol 25-hydroxylase, inhibits rotavirus and reovirus replication.[121,182] Another study showed that the IFN-inducible 2′,5′-oligoadenylate synthetase/ribonuclease L (OAS/RNase L) pathway suppresses rotavirus infection.[748] Rotavirus, as a successful pathogen, also utilizes VP3-dependent and VP3-independent strategies to prevent RNase L activation.[604,643,748] Whether rotavirus also antagonizes a specific ISG mechanism of action remains to be examined.

Pattern recognition signaling other than IFNs also seems to contribute to host control of rotavirus replication *in vivo*. Deletion of either MyD88 or MyD88-independent toll-like receptor 3 (TLR3) enhanced the host susceptibility to rotavirus infection and disease.[552,685] In one study, activation of Nlrc4 inflammasomes by flagellin treatment cleared rotavirus infection in an IL-18-dependent and IL-22-dependent manner.[747] In another study, rotavirus activated an intestinal epithelial cell–specific Nlrp9b inflammasome that restricted virus intestinal replication and pathogenesis.[753] Another NOD-like receptor NLRC5 has been shown to regulate rotavirus-specific T-cell responses.[652] Independent of the inflammasome functions, IL-22 was found to enhance IFN and ISG signaling[303] and IL-18–mediated epithelial cell shedding,[751] both of which exert antirotavirus functions.

The precise mechanisms by which different innate immune responses restrict rotavirus infection at mucosal surfaces versus systemic organs remains to be elucidated. Despite a plethora of strategies that rotaviruses have evolved to inhibit the IFN response, IFN is still actively produced during rotavirus infection *in vivo* in humans, pigs, and other animals.[255] It is also noteworthy that rotavirus pathogenesis, that is, diarrheal disease, may be more directly associated with IFN signaling. Diarrhea development in mice appears to be refractory to exogenous IFN therapy, whereas calves treated with recombinant-type I IFN appear to have attenuated gastrointestinal disease.[15,618] IFN receptor knockout suckling mice do not have enhanced gastrointestinal disease when infected with a murine rotavirus, although rotavirus replication is modestly enhanced by 5- to 10-fold.[414]

The cellular sources of IFN *in vivo* remain an active topic of investigation. In the mouse model, type I IFNs are predominantly produced by CD45+ hematopoietic cells, whereas type III IFNs mainly come from intestinal epithelial cells.[621] This is consistent with the robust-type III IFN induction in HIEs.[181,533,615] Primary human pDCs are highly resistant to rotavirus infection, but they respond to rotavirus exposure with a brisk and substantial IFN response and enhance the mucosal B-cell response to infection.[162,163] The roles of other innate immune cells, such as intestine-resident macrophages and innate lymphoid cells, remain to be fully elucidated.

CLINICAL SYMPTOMS

Rotavirus infections elicit a broad spectrum of clinical responses varying from subclinical infection all the way to severe and fatal dehydrating illness (Table 12.4). An early study from the United States before vaccines were available compared the clinical manifestations of 78 children hospitalized with rotavirus diarrhea and 72 children hospitalized with diarrhea not associated with rotavirus.[579] The majority of both cohorts had a temperature of 37.9°C or above. Those with rotavirus vomited and became dehydrated significantly more often than those who did not have rotavirus. The duration of vomiting was longer in the rotavirus-positive group than in those without rotavirus (2.6 vs. 0.9 days). Rotavirus diarrhea started after vomiting but lasted longer (5 vs. 2.6 days).

Laboratory tests report elevated blood urea nitrogen and urine-specific gravity in rotavirus-infected children and reflect the high frequency of vomiting and dehydration associated with this infection.[579] Recent studies have clearly demonstrated that rotavirus infection is not strictly restricted to the gut and that both viremia and systemic replication are a frequent consequence of natural infection with wild-type rotavirus in both humans and other animals. However, the clinical consequences and the frequency of the systemic phase of rotavirus infection are not clear.[68,206,567] Twenty percent of children with rotavirus gastroenteritis had elevated alanine aminotransferase or aspartate aminotransferase levels.[668] The pathophysiologic basis for these liver function test elevations remains unknown, but rotavirus can actively replicate in both the liver and biliary tree in a mouse model and in children with severe immunodeficiency.[214,244] Before the advent of widespread rotavirus vaccination in developed and many less developed countries, infection was frequently associated with severe dehydration, diarrhea, and death. Greater than 60,000 hospitalizations occurred per year in the United States prior to vaccination.[103] The major factors causing severe illness or death in young children are believed to be dehydration and electrolyte dysregulation. While mortality due to rotavirus infection has decreased by more than 95% in the United States following the widespread administration

TABLE 12.4 Clinical and epidemiological features of human rotavirus infections

Variable	Description
Age predisposition	Primarily affects young children 3 months to 2 years old in high-income countries; younger children affected in low- to middle-income countries. Adults frequently infected, mostly asymptomatic.
Seasonality	Seasonal infection in high-income countries with epidemic peaks in cooler months of each year. No seasonality in tropical climates. Vaccination has diminished/delayed seasonal epidemic in United States/Europe.
Settings	Households, day care centers, hospitals, schools, favoring person-to-person spread. Occasionally waterborne, especially species B rotaviruses.
Asymptomatic infections	Most common in adults and newborns. Can frequently occur in all age groups.
Incubation period	Generally, 24–48 hours.
Symptoms	Sudden onset of vomiting and diarrhea. Diarrheal stools lack blood, mucus, or leukocytes. Fever common in young children.
Severity of illness	Overall, more frequently severe than many other diarrheal etiologies, leading to dehydration and hospitalization. Malnutrition increases disease severity.
Duration of illness	Typically, 3–5 days. Longer illness in immunocompromised individuals.
Viral shedding	Peaks 1–3 days after illness onset. Shedding can be prolonged in immunocompromised individuals. Antigenemia and viremia detectable early after infection.
Mode of transmission and vehicles	Fecal–oral; contact with fomites, food, water less common, environmental contamination.
Immunity	Repeated infections with or without illness can occur with the same or different strains. Increasing levels of immunity occur with each repeated exposures or vaccination.
Treatment	Supportive rehydration (oral preferable) therapy to prevent dehydration. Live, attenuated vaccines are available and highly effective in high-income countries; vaccine effectiveness is lower in children in low-income countries.
Reservoir	Humans primarily; animal reservoirs quite rarely.

of safe and effective vaccines, rotaviruses are still responsible for 128,000 to 215,000 deaths per year around the world in young children in less developed countries, where vaccination is still not yet widely available and the vaccine efficacy is suboptimal.[662,682]

As mentioned above, rotaviruses rarely produce a chronic symptomatic infection that involves diarrhea and hepatic and renal involvement in children with various severe immunodeficiencies.[244,720] Both RV5 and RV1 vaccine-acquired chronic rotavirus infection and prolonged illness have also been observed in infants with severe combined immunodeficiency who were inadvertently vaccinated.[35,519] During chronic infection of immunodeficient children, rotavirus can undergo genomic rearrangements, presumably because of multiple passages at high multiplicity *in vivo*.[167,320] Rotaviruses also pose a special threat to individuals who are immunosuppressed for bone marrow, stem cell, or small bowel transplantation. In one study of a bone marrow transplant unit, 8 of 78 patients with gastroenteritis shed rotavirus as the sole pathogen, and 5 of these individuals died.[736] The rate of severe rotavirus infection in pediatric bone marrow transplantation is no longer this high.[150] Rotavirus infections acquired nosocomially have also rarely been associated with severe diarrhea in adult renal transplant recipients.[529] Rotavirus may cause gastroenteritis in small bowel transplant recipients, often in association with acute episodes of rejection.[5,754] Rotaviruses do not appear to play a disproportionately important role in diarrhea occurring in adults or children infected with human immunodeficiency virus,[647] rein-

forcing the findings that rotavirus immunity is most directly influenced by B cells and antibody-related mechanisms.

Temporal association of rotavirus infection with a variety of other disease conditions, both as isolated illnesses or in a single outbreak, have also been described.[298,638] Because the occurrence of most of these conditions is extremely rare in comparison to the ubiquitous rotavirus infection, it appears that, with the exception of severe disease manifestations in immunocompromised patients, necrotizing enterocolitis and hemorrhagic gastroenteritis in neonates, and pneumatosis intestinalis in infancy, the association of rotavirus infection with most of the reported conditions is likely temporal and not etiologic.[589,727]

Rotavirus infection has also been associated with a number of central nervous system conditions, and the virus has been detected in the cerebrospinal fluid on a number of occasions.[333,378,420,464] However, because viremia is now established to be relatively common, the finding of rotavirus RNA in cerebrospinal fluid does not necessarily imply direct central nervous system replication. Acute rotavirus infection is associated relatively frequently with benign seizures in young children, perhaps due to the elevated temperature seen in many rotavirus infections.[464] In this regard, some publications have observed that following rotavirus vaccination, the incidence of childhood seizures is diminished.[150,527] Finally, there have been several studies attempting to link rotavirus infection to type I diabetes in children, using both mouse model and human studies.[262,532,580] The significance of this notable association is unclear, and likewise, the role of rotavirus vaccination in suppressing type I diabetes remains unclear.[87,246]

An unexpected outcome of widespread rotavirus vaccination programs has been reports of low levels of increased intussusceptions occurring shortly following oral administration of several licensed live attenuated rotavirus vaccines[268,482,517] (see Prevention and Control section). The significance of the temporal association of wild-type rotavirus infection with intussusception deserves further attention. Rotavirus was detected in 20 (33%) of 61 cases of intussusception in two studies, suggesting that wild-type rotavirus might have been the cause.[388,489] Ultrasound examinations of infants with wild-type rotavirus diarrheal illnesses and controls indicated that wild-type rotavirus infections induce a significantly greater number of aggregates of lymph nodes and/or thickening of the ileal wall, both of which may be a prelude to intussusception.[46,577] However, several studies in Australia, France, and Germany failed to find a significant association of intussusception with natural rotavirus infection.[480,497,645] Finally, discussed further in the Prevention Section, several live attenuated rotavirus vaccines licensed by the Food and Drug Administration have been associated with intussusception at low frequencies.[58,92,665] Hence, it seems reasonable to conjecture that virtually any rotavirus infection (including live viral vaccination) in children could be etiologically associated with intussusception if studied in sufficient numbers, but the benefits of the vaccines far outweigh this potential risk.[268]

DIAGNOSIS

The clinical (severe diarrhea, vomiting, dehydration, and fever) and epidemiologic manifestations (seasonality in nontropical areas) of rotavirus illnesses in children generally under 3 years of age are not sufficiently distinctive to permit diagnosis, even during a rotavirus "season." Accurate diagnosis, therefore, requires direct detection of virus particles, antigens, genomes, or virus-specific serologic responses by a laboratory test. Of note, the primary treatment, rehydration, should be administered on clinical grounds alone and is not dependent on the definitive etiologic diagnosis of rotavirus infection.

Since its discovery in 1973, many assays have been developed for the detection of rotavirus in stools,[735] although at present solid-phase immunoassays and RT-PCR–based assays are the primary diagnostic tools.[197] Specimens from the first to the fourth day of illness are optimal for virus detection using traditional assays (e.g., EM or ELISA); however, shedding can continue for up to 3 weeks, depending on the duration of symptoms, and may be detected even longer by RT-PCR. In the 1970s and early 80s, direct visualization of stool material by EM was employed for rotavirus detection.[64,77,221] EM has the advantage of high specificity because rotaviruses have distinctive morphology but suffer from substantial disadvantages such as low throughput and requiring expensive equipment. In early studies, direct EM examination of stools permitted detection of rotavirus in 80% to 90% of the virus-positive specimens when compared to immunoassay techniques.[77] Various methods with higher throughput than EM are now available for the detection of rotaviruses in stool specimens.[479]

The rotavirus detection method of choice in most diagnostic laboratories around the world continues to be based on solid-phase immunoassays and most frequently relies on the detection of widely shared antigenic regions on the species A rotavirus VP6 major structural protein by antibody. These solid-phase immunoassays are reasonably sensitive, do not require highly specialized equipment, are widely available commercially in validated formats, are relatively inexpensive, and often have a built-in control for nonspecific reactions. Other methods for virus detection, such as counterimmunoelectroosmophoresis, gel electrophoresis of rotavirus dsRNA, reverse passive hemagglutination assay, and latex agglutination were used in the past but are no longer widely available.[479] Enzyme immunoassays have also been developed in various research laboratories for detection of noncultivable species B or species C rotavirus and for measurement of antibodies directed against these viruses.[231,434]

Of a variety of research and clinical laboratory techniques that have been used for the detection of species A rotaviruses, the most important and widely used, after the solid-phase immunoassay, is RT-PCR, which is both highly sensitive and specific and has the added advantage of determining rotavirus genotypes.[479] For example, virus shedding could be detected in ELISA-positive children from 4 to 57 days after diarrhea onset using an RT-PCR–based assay.[574] PCR has also been used to detect species B and C rotaviruses.[257]

It is also possible to recover human rotaviruses from stool specimens directly in cell culture with reasonable efficiency,[712] but this approach is not practical except for specific experimental purposes. This method appears to be approximately 75% as efficient as antigen detection assays using conventional procedures.[295] Growth of rotavirus in tissue culture allows the determination of its serotype by neutralization assay, although rotavirus serotype can now also be reliably inferred by nucleotide sequence analysis of the VP7 and VP4 encoding genes. The use of RT-PCR has also enabled the genotyping of rotavirus-positive specimens that could not be serotyped by ELISA or successfully cultivated.[218]

A variety of techniques have been used in the past to measure a serologic response to rotavirus infection, such as IEM, complement fixation (CF) tests, immunofluorescence tests, immune adherence hemagglutination assay, ELISA, neutralization, hemagglutination inhibition, inhibition of reverse passive hemagglutination, enzyme-linked immunospot (ELISpot) assay, and immunocytochemical staining assays. Currently, the most useful serologic assays are IgA and IgG ELISA-based and neutralization assays. In infants and adults, IgG, IgA, and IgM ELISAs are more efficient and sensitive. Because IgA does not cross the placenta, a rotavirus IgA ELISA has been the assay of choice for detecting serologic responses in infants younger than 9 months of age who generally possess passively acquired maternal IgG rotavirus antibodies.[428] This assay is also used for measuring antibodies in saliva, duodenal fluids, and stools[428] and in most studies of seroresponse rates to rotavirus vaccines.[16,165] Fecal rotavirus IgA antibody levels were found to positively correlate with duodenal IgA antibody levels[276] but have been difficult to standardize. It has been suggested that fecal-IgA conversion would be a more sensitive indicator of rotavirus reinfection than seroconversion or detection of virus shedding,[136] but difficulties in accurately and reproducibly monitoring fecal IgA levels have restricted the use of this assay. Based on observations from clinical studies in infants and children, rotavirus IgA responses in serum have been suggested to reflect the immunologic status of the intestinal lumen with respect to rotavirus antibody.[159,308] Several studies have correlated levels of antirotavirus serum IgA with protection, although this association is not absolute.[308,502,692] Acute phase rotavirus infection diagnosis has also been made using a serum IgM response ELISA, which can detect a specific serum IgM response to rotavirus during the acute phase of illness.[159]

The amount of rotavirus neutralizing antibodies can be determined by plaque reduction assays, foci forming unit reduction assays, neutralization of virus as determined by quantitation of viral antigen by ELISA, or inhibition of cytopathic effect.[362] Neutralization assays provide information about the serotype of the infecting rotavirus and the development of a monotypic versus heterotypic antibody response. A competition solid-phase immunoassay that measures epitope-specific immune responses to individual rotavirus epitopes associated with serotypes was shown to be useful in evaluating immune responses at the level of individual epitopes. This technique uses the test serum as the blocking reagent and the individual monoclonal antibodies as the detecting reagent.[428,485]

TREATMENT

The primary aim of treatment of virtually all acute watery diarrheal diseases, including rotaviral gastroenteritis, is to replace fluids and electrolytes lost by vomiting and/or diarrhea. Intravenous fluid and electrolyte administration has been used successfully for many years in treating dehydration from diarrhea. Because facilities and equipment for parenteral administration of fluids and electrolytes are not readily available in many parts of the world, intensive efforts were made to develop effective and easy-to-use oral rehydration solutions (ORS) to substitute for the need for intravenous therapy. ORS is mechanistically based on the specific coupling of sodium and glucose transport in the intestine.[26,504] Various ORS formulations with added glucose or a glucose substitute are effective in treating rotavirus as well as many other enteric pathogens, with some minor variations in their efficacy. Over the years, many variations on the formulation of ORS have been evaluated.[606] These formulations have varied in part based on ease of access to components and reduced cost, but in general, all are quite effective in treating most acute cases of infectious dehydrating diarrheal disease.

More recent studies have examined the value of additional therapeutic approaches to improve the treatment of rotavirus gastroenteritis and diarrhea in general. Atia and Buchman demonstrated that zinc supplementation improves the therapeutic value of ORS for most enteric pathogens, including rotavirus, and this addition has been recommended by the WHO for children with acute diarrhea.[26] Several other additives to the ORS formulation have been investigated including: lactoferrin, lysozyme, and various amino acids such as glycine, alanine, and glutamine. When oral rehydration does not correct the fluid and electrolyte loss, or if the patient is severely dehydrated or in shock, intravenous fluids must be given immediately. Of course, ORS should not be given to patients with depressed consciousness because of the possibility of fluid aspiration.

The American Academy of Pediatrics (AAP) does not currently recommend the use of loperamide, anticholinergic agents, bismuth subsalicylate, adsorbents, or lactobacillus-containing compounds for the management of the acute diarrhea

in children 1 month to 5 years of age. The use of opiates, as well as opiate and atropine combination drugs, for treatment of children with acute diarrhea is also contraindicated by the AAP.[95]

Passive administration of neutralizing antibodies for rotavirus has been studied as a therapeutic intervention. Human milk, containing rotavirus antibodies, has been used successfully to treat children who are immunodeficient and who have chronic rotavirus infection and illness.[613] In contrast, colostrum or milk concentrate from cows immunized with human rotavirus was not highly effective for the treatment of acute rotavirus gastroenteritis in children, although a decrease in the duration of virus shedding was observed.[190] Daily oral administration of rotavirus antibody-containing bovine colostrum appeared to exert a preventative effect during an orphanage outbreak of rotavirus diarrhea.[190] The effect of a single oral dose (300 mg/kg body weight) of gamma globulin in infants hospitalized for gastroenteritis (70% rotavirus associated) was evaluated, and the treatment group had a significantly shorter duration of diarrhea, viral excretion, and hospital stay.[281] In another study, the oral administration of human serum immunoglobulin to two infants with prolonged rotavirus diarrhea of 4 or 7 months' duration was effective in clearing the virus and the associated diarrhea.[282] Also, bovine colostrum prepared by immunizing pregnant cows with human rotavirus strains of G1, G2, G3, or G4 was given orally to patients 4 to 6 months of age with rotavirus diarrhea and was found to significantly reduce the duration and frequency of diarrhea as well as the need for ORS.[292,609] A large review of studies designed to assess the value of treating rotavirus-associated diarrhea with IgY derived from eggs obtained from immunized hens demonstrated significant efficacy in shortening the duration of rotavirus illness.[706] In a porcine model of rotavirus diarrhea, camelid-derived nanobodies directed at the rotavirus VP6 protein were found to be protective from both infection and disease.[690] However, despite the generally positive results observed in the various immunotherapy or microbiome-based studies of rotavirus disease, cost and implementation considerations versus routine vaccination has made these approaches impractical except perhaps in the very rare case of severe or prolonged rotavirus infection associated with immunocompromised individuals.[283]

The efficacy of several pharmacological small-molecule inhibitors of rotavirus replication have also been examined in several model systems. Orally administered nitazoxanide, a broad-spectrum antimicrobial drug, reduced the duration of severe rotavirus diarrhea in two studies of hospitalized pediatric patients.[588,669] Ondansetron, which alleviates murine rotavirus-induced diarrhea in a mouse model,[57] reduces the occurrence of vomiting episodes in infants.[290] However, as noted above, the acute nature of rotavirus-associated illness and the wide success of rotavirus vaccines and ORS has substantially dampened enthusiasm in pursuing a practical antiviral approach to rotavirus illness.

Double-blind, placebo-controlled studies of racecadotril, an enkephalinase inhibitor, found the compound to be effective in the treatment of hospitalized pediatric patients with watery diarrhea (including rotavirus diarrhea) when used in conjunction with ORS.[598] Several preliminary studies provided modest support for a beneficial role for probiotic therapy for rotavirus diarrhea, and one direct comparison of probiotic with nitazoxanide showed that both had modest therapeutic effects, with nitazoxanide being more effective.[587] However, over the last decade, follow-up studies of the use of probiotics were mostly limited to porcine models,[106] likely due to the great success of rotavirus vaccines and ORS, which has dampened enthusiasm for further investigation of other therapeutic or preventative approaches.

PREVENTION AND CONTROL

Vaccines

General Principles and Background

Epidemiologic and hospital-based studies worldwide over the past five decades clearly demonstrate a substantial burden of disease associated with rotavirus infection and strongly support the continued need for prevention in both developed and less developed countries.[34,247] The primary aim of a rotavirus vaccine since inception has been to prevent severe rotavirus gastroenteritis during the first 2 to 3 years of life, the period when rotavirus disease is most serious and takes its greatest toll. As discussed in the Immunity section, while natural infection does not provide sterilizing immunity against reinfections, in general, disease severity is substantially reduced during secondary and subsequent infections.[62,144,692] Considerable evidence from studies in animals indicates that the presence and quantity of rotavirus-specific antibody in the lumen of or close proximity to the gut play a critical role in resistance to rotavirus disease.[16,226] In support of this conclusion, studies from children have associated elevated levels of fecal antirotavirus IgA with resistance to illness.[135] The most reliable and well-documented method of stimulating local intestinal immunity is thought to be a direct infection or immunization in the intestine. For this reason, except in a few cases,[278] most efforts to date have focused on live attenuated vaccines that are administered orally. While reinfection within the first few years of life is common, an infant who has had a primary symptomatic or asymptomatic rotavirus infection usually experiences a milder illness during reinfection. However, the level of protection induced by primary and subsequent reinfections may be less in some poor countries than in the developed world.[245] In one epidemiologic study, neonates who were infected in a newborn nursery during the first 14 days of life experienced almost 50% fewer rotavirus diarrheal episodes during the next 3 years compared to a cohort of infants who had not been infected with rotavirus in the nursery.[62] In a cohort study in Mexico following 200 infants from birth to 24 months of age, many experienced multiple rotavirus infections over this period but no child developed a moderate-to-severe diarrheal illness after their second infection, indicating that wild-type infection effectively "vaccinated" these young children against severe subsequent disease. Protection was greatest against severe disease and considerably less against mild disease or asymptomatic reinfection.[691,692] In general, second infections were caused by a different G serotype ($p = 0.054$), but any primary infection appeared to offer substantial protective efficacy against severe disease on reinfection, irrespective of the serotype of the reinfecting rotavirus. Recently, a similar prospective study from India demonstrated a substantially smaller protective effect from primary natural infection on subsequent reinfection, mirroring what has been observed with rotavirus vaccination in parts of Asia and Africa.[245] In this study, primary rotavirus infection occurred quite early in life, the levels of reinfection were high, and protection against moderate or severe disease increased with the number of reinfections but was only 79% after three infections.

Since wild-type infection in developed and middle-income countries elicits moderate to substantial immunity against subsequent severe diarrheal illness, the key issue that needed to be resolved in designing a live viral vaccine was an effective means of attenuating virulence while retaining immunogenicity. Prior data with several other viruses that infect mucosal surfaces (e.g., influenza A virus and respiratory syncytial virus) indicated that attenuation frequently reflects decreased viral replication in the target organ. However, decreased replication is also frequently associated with decreased immunogenicity. Hence, a delicate balance must be struck between attenuated virulence and desired immunogenicity in the design of live rotavirus vaccines.

A very wide range of serotypically distinct human rotaviruses are currently in circulation, but the majority of infections (over 80%) are caused by viruses with just six G serotypes (1, 2, 3, 4, 9, and 12) and three P serotypes ([4], [6], and [8]).[237,334,559,607,722] The relationship between serotype diversity and protective immunity has been an area of intense investigation almost since the discovery of human rotaviruses. Obviously, the development of an effective vaccine is dependent on its ability to provide significant protection from many, if not all, rotavirus serotypes that infants are likely to encounter. Epidemiologic studies in children have generally provided evidence that both homotypic and heterotypic immunity develop following natural infection with the biggest point of contention being the breadth and duration of the heterotypic response.[14,51,113,169,226,692,708] Unfortunately, experimental studies in animals have not provided a definitive answer vis-à-vis, the design of an optimal human vaccine.[226] In calves and piglets challenge studies, there are conflicting data on the induction of homotypic versus heterotypic immunity.[481,724] Many of these early cross-protection studies did not carefully and quantitatively evaluate the ability of heterotypic immunization to diminish disease severity. Since clinical symptoms are subjective parameters that are difficult to assess in animal models, success was defined as total elimination of disease following challenge. Given that the goal for human vaccines is the reduction of disease severity, this represents an important design defect in some of the animal rotavirus investigations and substantially restricts the utility of these studies to inform the human vaccine design approach.

The early development of live attenuated rotavirus vaccines was deeply influenced by considerations as to whether an effective vaccine would need to contain multiple serotypes or whether a monotypic vaccine could generate sufficient heterotypic immunity to be effective. After multiple studies with different vaccine candidates, we now have extensive field efficacy evidence from around the world that both monotypic and multitypic live attenuated rotavirus vaccines can be successfully used in people and that both approaches substantially reduce morbidly and mortality mediated by different rotavirus serotypes.[55,88,89,165,170,250,275,343,642]

Initial Monovalent Animal Rotavirus ("Jennerian") Vaccine Candidates

The initial rotavirus vaccines employed an approach first reported by Edward Jenner for vaccination against smallpox (see chapter on *Smallpox*). This strategy was based on the well-known tendency of many microbial pathogens to be host-range restricted. As such, viral strains isolated from one species frequently replicate less efficiently in other heterologous species; however, in some cases, this restricted replication capacity is sufficient to induce protective immunity. The usefulness of a *Jennerian* strategy for human rotavirus vaccination was suggested by an early observation that human and animal rotaviruses share a major common antigen.[222,366,721] The potential feasibility of this approach was first shown during animal studies in which calves administered a bovine rotavirus (serotype G6) *in utero* were protected from illness following challenge at birth with an entirely heterotypic human rotavirus (serotype G1).[724] It should always be kept in mind, however, that all licensed live rotavirus vaccines to date are based on cell culture–adapted animal or human strains and that cell culture adaptation itself likely also contributes to an attenuated phenotype *in vivo*.[572]

The initial rotavirus vaccine studies in people involved a cell culture passaged, cold-adapted, bovine rotavirus (NCDV strain, G6P[1], RIT 4237).[694,697] This attenuated, orally administered G6 monovalent vaccine induced over 80% protection to clinically significant diarrhea from serotypically distinct human rotavirus strains in infants and young children in two separate efficacy trials in Finland.[695,696] A two doses of the bovine vaccine had a protective efficacy of 89% against severe rotavirus-induced diarrhea.[703] However, the RIT 4237 vaccine candidate failed to induce significant protection against rotavirus diarrhea in trials in several middle- and low-income countries[161,293] and, as a consequence, further evaluation of this vaccine candidate was not pursued.

Another bovine rotavirus WC3 (Wistar calf) strain, G6P[5], also demonstrated variable protective efficacy in several studies in the United States and overseas.[52,79,122,123] For example, in infants 3 to 12 months of age in Philadelphia, where serotype G1 human strains were predominant, its protective efficacy was 76% against any rotavirus-caused diarrhea and 100% against moderate-to-severe rotavirus diarrhea.[122,123] In contrast, in later studies, the vaccine was less effective in subjects from Cincinnati and the Central African Republic (35% to 41% against moderate-to-severe rotavirus diarrhea) and in China (50% against any rotavirus diarrhea).[52,238] Because of the relatively low and variable levels of protection, this monovalent bovine origin vaccine was withdrawn from further study. However, the WC3 strain later provided the genetic backbone for a safe and effective pentavalent human-bovine reassortant rotavirus vaccine (RotaTeq, RV5, see below) that was first licensed in the United States in 2006 and is now widely available worldwide.

The simian rotavirus RRV strain (G3P[3], MMU 18006) is another animal rotavirus strain and was studied extensively as a monovalent *Jennerian* vaccine candidate in both high-income and middle- and low-income countries.[365,470] In some settings (such as in children over 3 months of age on initial vaccination), it induced mild to moderate transient febrile response in about one-third of the target population of infant vaccines but appeared to be more antigenic than the RIT 4237 vaccine candidate.[427,698] In a field trial in Venezuela, the protective efficacy of the MMU 18006 vaccine in infants 1 to 4 months of age was 83% against any rotavirus diarrhea and 90% against the most severe illnesses. Results of efficacy trials were also encouraging in Sweden and Finland, but the vaccine failed to efficiently protect young infants in New York State or in Arizona; furthermore, it induced only a low level of protection (29%) in infants 2 to 5 months of age in Maryland.[571,702] The basis for the variable protective efficacy of the monovalent RRV vaccine was never clearly determined, but it appeared to work best against homologous G3 strains and less well against heterologous strains.

Quadrivalent RRV-Based Reassortant "Jennerian" Rotavirus Vaccine

Failure of the monovalent RRV vaccine to reproducibly induce high levels of protection in young infants against heterotypic rotavirus strains suggested to some that the strategy for development of a monovalent "*Jennerian*" rotavirus vaccine required modification. The *modified Jennerian* approach led to a quadrivalent (RV4) simian RRV-based vaccine that incorporated each of the four epidemiologically most important human VP7s at the time (G1, G2, G3, and G4) genetically coupled to the simian RRV attenuated in human.[364,365,470] The same approach was also used to create the bovine WC3-based reassortant vaccine currently marketed as RotaTeq (see below). These approaches were enabled by the segmented nature of rotavirus genomes and by the ability of these viruses to undergo gene reassortment at high frequency during mixed infection.[271,273] Virus reassortants for use as vaccine candidates were isolated from cell cultures coinfected with a cultivatable, wild-type animal virus (simian RRV or bovine WC3) and selected human rotaviruses.[301,367,468,469] Antisera against the animal rotavirus parent were sometimes used to select specific virus reassortants with the appropriate human VP7 or VP4. In the case of the simian RRV strain, single human rotavirus gene substitution reassortants were isolated that possessed the human G1, G2, G4, or simian G3 VP7 genes on a background of 10 simian rotavirus genes, creating an RV4 quadrivalent vaccine.[468,469] Of course, if one wished to make a new reassortant-based rotavirus vaccine today, one would take advantage of the newly available reverse genetics techniques (see section on Reverse Genetics).

In large-scale efficacy and safety trials of RV4 in Finland, Native Americans in the United States, and a poor urban population in Venezuela, vaccine efficacy ranged from 48% to 68% against any rotavirus-caused diarrhea and efficacy against severe rotavirus diarrhea reached 91% in Finland, 88% in Venezuela, and 69% in Native Americans.[347,348,530,608] Based on these trial data in 1998, the U.S. Food and Drug Administration granted a biologics license to Wyeth Laboratories for the manufacture and distribution of RV4 (designated RotaShield) for the immunization of infants at 2, 4, and 6 months of age. The vaccine was recommended for universal vaccination in the United States and given to almost 1 million young children. However, in 1999, the Centers for Disease Control (CDC) reported that between September 1, 1998 and July 7, 1999, 15 cases of intussusception had been reported to the Vaccine Adverse Events Reporting System (VAERS) following RV4 administration.[132] Based on a very significant temporal association between RV4 vaccination and intussusception during the first 2 weeks after the first vaccine dose, this observation was translated to an attributable risk of intussusception estimate following vaccination of up to 1 in 2,500, or approximately 1,600 excess cases of intussusception in a full national vaccination program.[3,482] In 1999, after reviewing the available risk estimate data at the time, the Advisory Committee on Immunization Practices[3] withdrew its recommendation[97] and the RV4 vaccine rapidly disappeared from the marketplace.

Years after the withdrawal of RotaShield, controversy persists regarding the level of actual intussusception risk associated with this rotavirus vaccine administration.[249,363,483] Of note, more recent findings demonstrate that two currently licensed and very widely deployed rotavirus vaccines (RV1 and RV5, see below) also are associated with a very small increased risk of intussusception among recipients. These findings have called into question the advisability of the RV4 vaccine withdrawal and the focus on vaccine-associated intussusception as a major rotavirus vaccine safety concern. Further complicating the analysis is the observation that the age at vaccination was likely an important confounding factor in the rare occurrence of intussusception following RV4 use.[367,636] Avoidance of first vaccination of infants over 3 months of age and initial vaccination during the relatively refractory period of the first 2 to 3 months of life might have substantially reduced or eliminated the risk of intussusception with the RV4.

Two Major Currently Licensed Live Rotavirus Vaccines

Despite the safety issues raised by the withdrawal of the RotaShield vaccine, work on other alternative live, attenuated vaccine candidates continued with vigor.[251,300,501] Two separate but parallel approaches were pursued. Initial studies with a monovalent rotavirus vaccine (RV1) derived from a virulent human rotavirus 89–12 strain with G1P[8] serotype specificity was continued. Unlike the *Jennerian* candidates, this vaccine candidate was attenuated only through multiple tissue culture passages.[50,542,591] In a pivotal efficacy study, 17,000 infants and young children received two oral doses of the attenuated human rotavirus vaccine candidate or placebo at 2 and 4 months of age, and the vaccine was highly effective at preventing severe rotavirus gastroenteritis (84.7%) and hospitalization (85%).[591] This vaccine provided high levels of protection (90.8%) against homotypic G1P[8] strains and reasonable protection against G heterotypic, P homotypic G3P[8], G4P[8], and G9P[8] strains. In separate, postlicensure studies, recipients of this G1P[8] vaccine generated protection against the entirely heterotypic G2P[4] strains.[133,353,416,700] Because of the previous increased incidence of intussusception in the two weeks post initial vaccination of the RV4 vaccine, the safety arm of the RV1 pivotal Phase III trials included more than 60,000 infants, of whom one half received the vaccine and the other half the placebo. A temporal link with intussusception was not observed in this very large, randomized trial.[416,591] Given the high level of efficacy and safety profile, this monovalent attenuated human rotavirus vaccine, manufactured by GlaxoSmithKline under the trade name Rotarix, was licensed for use in the United States in 2008 and is currently licensed in more than 110 countries around the world.

While Rotarix was under development, a *Jennerian* bovine rotavirus candidate strain WC3 (G6P[5], described above) was used as the genetic backbone for a series of monoreassortants with selected human strains to create a pentavalent *modified Jennerian* vaccine, RV5. This approach was taken because of the variable protective efficacy achieved using WC3 alone or using single monoreassortants of WC3. Five individual WC3 reassortants were formulated into a pentavalent vaccine containing G1 through G4 VP7s and a single P[8] VP4.[300,301] This approach was similar to that taken for the development of RotaShield except that the genetic backbone was derived from a bovine rotavirus rather than a simian strain and the vaccine contained

an additional component that expressed a human rotavirus VP4 protein as well as the four component reassortant viruses expressing various serotypically distinct (G1-4) VP7 proteins. In a pivotal efficacy study, more than 5,000 infants and young children received three oral doses of RV5 or placebo at 2, 4, and 6 months of age, and the vaccine was highly effective in preventing any rotavirus gastroenteritis (74%) as well as severe gastroenteritis (98%).[701] It provided a high level of protection against G1, 2, 3, 4, and 9 serotypes. Similar to Rotarix, a large safety component of the Phase III trial was undertaken that included more than 68,000 infants, and no risk of intussusception was noted. This *modified Jennerian* pentavalent vaccine (RotaTeq), manufactured by Merck, was licensed for use in the United States in early 2006 and is now licensed in over 100 countries around the world.

Postlicensure Safety and Efficacy Studies of Rotarix and RotaTeq

In the 15 years since the RV5 and RV1 vaccines were licensed in the United States, they have also been broadly introduced in Central and South America, much of Western Europe, Australia, as well as a number of countries in Africa.[242] This has allowed investigators to examine the performance in terms of both safety and efficacy of the two vaccines in actual practice as opposed to controlled clinical trial settings. These Phase IV postlicensure studies in high-income and moderate-income countries confirmed the high efficacy and safety of the Phase III trials[13,69,663,699] (Table 12.5). Of interest, in these and other postlicensure rotavirus vaccine studies, an unanticipated but clear-cut "herd immunity" effect was also observed.[526,546] To date, no apparent difference in vaccine efficacy or safety at the population level has been observed between RV1 and RV5, and there is not yet any compelling data to indicate that vaccine introduction significantly alters the genotype distribution among circulating rotavirus strains.[318]

Studies from middle-income to low-income countries such as Mexico and Nicaragua also showed substantial decreases in hospitalizations.[518,558] In Mexico, where RV1 was primarily used, there was a 41% decrease in diarrhea-related mortality in infants under 11 months of age that was clearly associated with vaccination.[576] Follow-up studies in Latin America show that RV1 remained highly efficacious when coadministered with other childhood vaccines including oral polio.[681] A variety of orally administered vaccines, such as polio and some cholera vaccines, perform less well in very poor countries, such as India and Sub-Saharan Africa. Randomized control trials indicate that this also holds true for both RV1 and RV5.[23,435,741] Compared to an overall efficacy of over 90% in the United States and Western Europe, over 85% in regions of Asia, and 80% in Latin America, studies of RV1 efficacy in South Africa and Malawi demonstrated significantly reduced efficacy of 77% and 49%, respectively.[435] Similarly, a study of RV5 in Ghana, Kenya, and Mali revealed efficacy against severe diarrhea of only 39% but substantially higher overall efficacy during the first year of life (64%); efficacy rates varied by country, being highest in Kenya and lowest in Mali.[23] Finally, a double-blind, placebo-controlled trial of RV5 against severe rotavirus gastroenteritis in low-income countries of Asia (rural Bangladesh and urban Vietnam) demonstrated an overall efficacy rate of 48%.[741] The reason behind the suboptimal performance of the rotavirus vaccines in the poorest countries remains unknown, although there is no shortage of

TABLE 12.5 Comparison of the four major licensed rotavirus vaccines with multinational deployment

	RotaTeq (RV5)	Rotarix (RV1)	Rotasiil	Rotavac
Manufacturer	Merck	GlaxoSmithKline	Serum Institute of India	Bharat Biotech
Genetic backbone	Bovine rotavirus-WC3	Human rotavirus-89-12	Bovine rotavirus-UK	Human rotavirus-116E
Composition	5 human–bovine reassortants	Single human rotavirus	5 human–bovine reassortants	Single human rotavirus
Human VP7/VP4 types	G1, 2, 3, and 4 and P[8]	G1P[8]	G1, 2, 3, 4, and 9 and P[5]	G9P[11]
Dosage schedule	3 doses (2, 4, and 6 months)	2 doses (2 and 4 months)	3 doses (6, 10, and 14 weeks)	3 doses (6, 10, and 14 weeks)
Administration	Oral	Oral	Oral	Oral
Formulation and storage	Liquid 2°C–8°C for 24 months	Liquid 2°C–8°C for 36 months	Lyophilized 25°C for 30 months; <40°C for 18 months	Liquid/frozen 2°C–8°C for 6 months; −20°C for 5 years
Protection against severe disease in:[a]				
Developed countries	90% 100%	85%–96%	NA	NA
Low- and lower-middle-income countries	43%–64%	49%–77%	36% (in India); 67% (in Niger)	56% (in India)
Vaccine shedding	21%	≥50%	NA	NA
First license date	2006	2008	2017	2015
WHO prequalification date	October 2008	March 2009	September 2018	January 2018

[a]Different scoring systems, analyses, and populations were used; efficacy results are not directly comparable.
NA, not available.

hypotheses, and it is likely to be multifactorial.[116,168,426,515] However, because of the considerable beneficial effect of the RV1 and RV5 vaccines, even in the poorest countries where the deleterious health effects of rotavirus infection are greatest, The World Health Organization's Strategic Advisory Group of Experts recommended that health authorities in all nations routinely vaccinate young children against rotavirus.[586]

Both RV1 and RV5 vaccines are shed in readily detectable amounts following vaccination (with RV1 shed at higher levels than RV5), but no significant adverse effects have been linked to vaccine transmission. More recent population-based studies from Mexico, Brazil, and Australia report no serious reactogenicity but a temporal association (as was the case with the original RV4 vaccine) with intussusception.[91,517] The rates of RV1 and RV5 vaccine-associated intussusception appear to be very low (<1 in 50,000) however, and it seems clear that the benefits of these two vaccines substantially exceed the risks based on the data currently available.[268] In addition to intussusception, several reports demonstrate that severely immunocompromised infants are at some risk for vaccine-acquired chronic infection and illness, despite the attenuated nature of the rotavirus vaccines,[519] and this led to a change in the vaccine labeling to exclude administration to children with SCID.

Selected Other Currently Licensed Live Attenuated Rotavirus Vaccines Deployed on a National or Restricted Multinational Basis

Several other regional rotavirus vaccines are currently available. They are attenuated on the basis of reassortment and host range restriction, and/or by natural attenuation. The bovine rotavirus UK strain (G6P[5]) constitutes the backbone of a pentavalent (RV5) human–bovine rotavirus reassortant vaccine composed of individual human rotavirus VP7 specificity for G1, 2, 3, 4, and 9 in a background of 10 bovine rotavirus genes.[468,469] This vaccine, originally developed in the United States at the NIH, is now licensed as "Rotasiil" in India and manufactured by the Serum Institute of India, as a safe and effective intervention to help prevent severe rotavirus disease. Another pure *Jennerian* vaccine, a lamb origin rotavirus LLR strain (G10P[15]), is currently produced by the Lanzhou Institute and was first licensed for human use in China in 2000.[408] The vaccine is currently not included in the national immunization program in China, and its efficacy level has not been well studied outside China.[80,230] Two live neonatal origin human rotavirus strains were first identified in healthy newborns in Indian and Australian newborn nurseries and have subsequently been used as the basis for new rotavirus vaccines. The origin of these vaccines stems from early observations that neonates who experienced subclinical rotavirus infections in newborn nurseries in Australia or India during the first 14 days of life were protected against subsequent clinically significant rotavirus diarrhea for up to 3 years.[56,62] One neonatal vaccine 116E strain (G9P[11]) is a naturally occurring human–bovine rotavirus reassortant originally isolated from an asymptomatically infected baby in a newborn nursery New Delhi.[248] The 116E strain has 10 human origin rotavirus genes and a single bovine rotavirus gene encoding VP4. It was licensed as a safe and effective vaccine (marketed as ROTAVAC and produced by Bharat) and widely adopted for childhood immunization in India, representing the first rotavirus vaccine that was discovered, developed, manufactured, licensed, and heavily utilized in a less developed country. Phase

II clinical studies with the other neonatal strain RV3 (G3P[6]), isolated from an Australian newborn nursery, also suggest that this vaccine candidate is immunogenic, safe, and efficacious.[42,43] Finally, Rotavin-M1 (PolyVac) is yet another rotavirus vaccine based on an attenuated human rotavirus strain (G1P[8]) isolated from a child hospitalized for diarrhea[154] and is now licensed and manufactured in Vietnam.[59,398]

Other Approaches to Vaccination

Due to the restricted efficacies of RV1 and RV5 live attenuated vaccines in very poor countries of Africa and Asia, other strategies for rotavirus immunization continue to be explored. One of the more actively pursued approaches is to use either purified inactivated whole human rotavirus, VLPs, or a recombinant rotaviral protein (the VP8* tryptic fragment of VP4) administered parenterally as a vaccine immunogen.[53,117,128,139,279,342,717] Several types of animal studies in mice, pigs, and primates support the potential of these approaches to induce protective immunity, and studies in primates have shown that systemically administered passively transferred serum antibodies can protect from infectious rotavirus challenge.[716] Phase I and II studies using a monovalent recombinant P[8] VP8* protein have been carried out in people, but it induced a limited homotypic antibody response in a field efficacy trial.[279] A trivalent P[4], P[6], and P[8] VP8* subunit vaccine candidate is currently under assessment in people.[278]

Passive Immunization

Passive immunization, either parenteral or enteral, with some form of rotavirus-enriched antibody preparation has been shown to be effective in preventing or dampening rotavirus illness in both animals and people[189,292,609,716] (also see Treatment section). Various sources of passively administered rotavirus antibodies (e.g., eggs from immunized hens, or milk formula containing bovine milk immunoglobulin from milk of cows hyperimmunized with human rotaviruses) have been considered. However, except in very special circumstances, such as in immunocompromised individuals with severe or chronic rotavirus infection, passive immunization is simply not currently practical for protection against rotavirus illness due to both cost and lack of commercially available licensed product.

PERSPECTIVES

Rotavirus disease has become vaccine preventable with clear and substantial evidence of efficacy for children in high-income, middle-income, and low-income countries and reductions of mortality in children in middle-to-low-income countries. This is an exciting achievement yet other questions remain to be answered regarding vaccines such as: Can the efficacy of the current oral vaccines be improved in children in some middle-income and low-income countries based on understanding why such children do not respond with high rates of induced protective immunity? Is this due to malnutrition, genetic heterogeneity, intestinal microbiota, interference from other oral vaccines, frequent infection with other intestinal pathogens, preexisting maternal antibodies, other health factors of children, or different circulating rotavirus strains that are not part of the current vaccines? Will worldwide vaccination induce changes in the epidemiology of circulating virus strains? Will epidemiology

studies be able to show that vaccination reduces rare childhood diseases, such as biliary atresia, that might be associated with rotavirus infections but where causation has been difficult to prove in children? Can a correlate of protection be identified to facilitate the future development of third-generation vaccines?

Even with successful vaccines, rotaviruses will continue to serve as very useful models to understand enteric mucosal pathogen cell interactions. The interactions of viral and cellular proteins that influence virus entry into cells, trigger epithelial cell responses, and modulate function of the differentiated epithelial cells or neighboring cells in the complex architecture of the intestine remain to be understood. This will require new studies of virus pathogenesis *in vivo* and such studies will require multidisciplinary efforts to understand fully the complex biochemical and physiologic consequences of infection. New discoveries of human rotaviruses and host–pathogen interactions are expected to be revealed from studies using the highly tractable reverse genetics system and physiologically active and biologically relevant HIOs from different individuals, age groups, and segments of the intestine. Rotaviruses also provide a prototypical infection for the study of the local intestinal innate and acquired immune response. Some questions to be asked include the following: Why do rotavirus infections cause minimal intestinal inflammation? How do rotaviruses escape the intestine and cause extraintestinal infections? Do such infections result in currently unrecognized disease in a subset of individuals with specific genetic properties? What is the basis for host range and organ-specific replication restriction? What factors govern the development of homotypic versus heterotypic humoral immunity? Why is the circulating T-cell response so small following rotavirus infection? What role does innate immunity play in determining the clinical outcome of rotavirus infection in people? Continued analysis of cellular responses (both epithelial and immune) by using transcriptomics, proteomics, and metabolomics analyses will help define pathways of cellular signaling that influence the outcome of infection as well as cellular genes important for replication.

More studies on rotaviruses that represent most human and animal rotavirus strains will address whether these viruses have other unexpected cellular receptors or unusual properties that affect their stability or transmission. Successful reverse genetics systems for rotaviruses should facilitate future probing of viral gene function, which is especially needed to fully understand pathogenesis, and potentially the design of new vaccine candidates with targeted attenuation. The application of new techniques in cell biology to understand the structural and biochemical basis of the unusual processes of rotavirus entry into, and exit from, cells can be expected to unravel new mechanisms of intracellular protein and vesicle trafficking. Structural knowledge of rotavirus and its proteins should help lead to new methods and inhibitors to interrupt virus transmission, prevent virus replication, and treat disease.

REFERENCES

1. Abdel-Haq N, Amjad M, McGrath E, et al. Emergence of human rotavirus genotype G9 in metropolitan Detroit between 2007 and 2009. *J Med Microbiol* 2011;60(Pt 6):761–767.
2. Abdelhakim AH, Salgado EN, Fu X, et al. Structural correlates of rotavirus cell entry. *PLoS Pathog* 2014;10(9):e1004355.
3. ACIP. Verbatim transcript of the meeting of the Advisory Committee on Immunization Practices. In: Reporters NLaAC, trans. *Advisory Committee on Immunization Practices.* Vol. 3. Morbidiity Mortality Weekly, CDC, Atlanta, GA; 1999:1–174.
4. Adams WR, Kraft LM. Epizootic diarrhea of infant mice: identification of the etiologic agent. *Science* 1963;141:359–360.

5. Adeyi OA, Costa G, Abu-Elmagd KM, et al. Rotavirus infection in adult small intestine allografts: a clinicopathological study of a cohort of 23 patients. *Am J Transplant* 2010;10(12):2683–2689.
6. Afrikanova I, Miozzo MC, Giambiagi S, et al. Phosphorylation generates different forms of rotavirus NSP5. *J Gen Virol* 1996;77:2059–2065.
7. Ahmadian S, Shahrabadi MS. Morphological study of the role of calcium in the assembly of the rotavirus outer capsid protein VP7. *Biotech Histochem* 1999;74(5):266–273.
8. Ahmed F, Jones DB, Jackson AA. Effect of vitamin A deficiency on the immune response to epizootic diarrhoea of infant mice (EDIM) rotavirus infection in mice. *Br J Nutr* 1991;65(3):475–485.
9. Aich P, Wilson HL, Kaushik RS, et al. Comparative analysis of innate immune responses following infection of newborn calves with bovine rotavirus and bovine coronavirus. *J Gen Virol* 2007;88(Pt 10):2749–2761.
10. Alaoui Amine S, Melloul M, El Alaoui MA, et al. Evidence for zoonotic transmission of species A rotavirus from goat and cattle in nomadic herds in Morocco, 2012–2014. *Virus Genes* 2020;56(5):582–593.
11. Ali A, Kazi AM, Cortese MM, et al. Impact of withholding breastfeeding at the time of vaccination on the immunogenicity of oral rotavirus vaccine—a randomized trial. *PLoS One* 2015;10(6):e0127622.
12. Altenburg BC, Graham DY, Estes MK. Ultrastructural study of rotavirus replication in cultured cells. *J Gen Virol* 1980;46:75–85.
13. Anderson EJ, Rupp A, Shulman ST, et al. Impact of rotavirus vaccination on hospital-acquired rotavirus gastroenteritis in children. *Pediatrics* 2011;127(2):e264–e270.
14. Angel J, Franco MA, Greenberg HB. Rotavirus vaccines: recent developments and future considerations. *Nat Rev Microbiol* 2007;5(7):529–539.
15. Angel J, Franco MA, Greenberg HB, et al. Lack of a role for type I and type II interferons in the resolution of rotavirus-induced diarrhea and infection in mice. *J Interferon Cytokine Res* 1999;19(6):655–659.
16. Angel J, Steele AD, Franco MA. Correlates of protection for rotavirus vaccines: Possible alternative trial endpoints, opportunities, and challenges. *Hum Vaccin Immunother* 2014;10(12):3659–3671.
17. Aoki ST, Settembre EC, Trask SD, et al. Structure of rotavirus outer-layer protein VP7 bound with a neutralizing Fab. *Science* 2009;324(5933):1444–1447.
18. Arias CF, Lopez S. Rotavirus cell entry: not so simple after all. *Curr Opin Virol* 2021;48:42–48.
19. Arias CF, Romero P, Alvarez V, et al. Trypsin activation pathway of rotavirus infectivity. *J Virol* 1996;70(9):5832–5839.
20. Arias CF, Silva-Ayala D, Lopez S. Rotavirus entry: a deep journey into the cell with several exits. *J Virol* 2015;89(2):890–893.
21. Arista S, Giovannelli L, Pistoia D, et al. Electropherotypes, subgroups, and serotypes of human rotavirus strains causing gastroenteritis in infants and young children in Palermo, Italy, from 1985 to 1989. *Res Virol* 1990;141:435–448.
22. Armah GE, Breiman RF, Tapia MD, et al. Immunogenicity of the pentavalent rotavirus vaccine in African infants. *Vaccine* 2012;30(Suppl 1):A86–A93.
23. Armah GE, Sow SO, Breiman RF, et al. Efficacy of pentavalent rotavirus vaccine against severe rotavirus gastroenteritis in infants in developing countries in sub-Saharan Africa: a randomised, double-blind, placebo-controlled trial. *Lancet* 2010;376(9741):606–614.
24. Arnold MM, Barro M, Patton JT. Rotavirus NSP1 mediates degradation of interferon regulatory factors through targeting of the dimerization domain. *J Virol* 2013;87(17):9813–9821.
25. Arnold MM, Sen A, Greenberg HB, et al. The battle between rotavirus and its host for control of the interferon signaling pathway. *PLoS Pathog* 2013;9(1):e1003064.
26. Atia AN, Buchman AL. Oral rehydration solutions in non-cholera diarrhea: a review. *Am J Gastroenterol* 2009;104(10):2596–2604; quiz 2605.
27. Au KS, Chan WK, Burns JW, et al. Receptor activity of rotavirus nonstructural glycoprotein NS28. *J Virol* 1989;63:4553–4562.
28. Au KS, Chan WK, Estes MK. Rotavirus morphogenesis involves an endoplasmic reticulum transmembrane glycoprotein. In: Compans R, Helenius A, Oldstone M, eds. *Cell Biology of Virus Entry, Replication and Pathogenesis.* Vol. 90. New York: Alan R. Liss, Inc.; 1988:257–267.
29. Au KS, Mattion NM, Estes MK. A subviral particle binding domain on the rotavirus nonstructural glycoprotein NS28. *Virology* 1993;194:665–673.
30. Aung MS, Nahar S, Aida S, et al. Distribution of two distinct rotavirus B (RVB) strains in the north-central Bangladesh and evidence for reassortment event among human RVB revealed by whole genomic analysis. *Infect Genet Evol* 2017;47:77–86.
31. Awachat PS, Kelkar SD. Unexpected detection of simian SA11-human reassortant strains of rotavirus G3P[8] genotype from diarrhea epidemic among tribal children of Western India. *J Med Virol* 2005;77(1):128–135.
32. Ayala-Breton C, Arias M, Espinosa R, et al. Analysis of the kinetics of transcription and replication of the rotavirus genome by RNA interference. *J Virol* 2009;83(17):8819–8831.
33. Azevedo AS, Yuan L, Jeong KI, et al. Viremia and nasal and rectal shedding of rotavirus in gnotobiotic pigs inoculated with Wa human rotavirus. *J Virol* 2005;79(9):5428–5436.
34. Badur S, Ozturk S, Pereira P, et al. Systematic review of the rotavirus infection burden in the WHO-EMRO region. *Hum Vaccin Immunother* 2019;15(11):2754–2768.
35. Bakare N, Menschik D, Tiernan R, et al. Severe combined immunodeficiency (SCID) and rotavirus vaccination: reports to the Vaccine Adverse Events Reporting System (VAERS). *Vaccine* 2010;28(40):6609–6612.
36. Baker JM, Tate JE, Leon J, et al. Postvaccination serum antirotavirus immunoglobulin A as a correlate of protection against rotavirus gastroenteritis across settings. *J Infect Dis* 2020;222(2):309–318.
37. Baker K, Qiao SW, Kuo T, et al. Immune and non-immune functions of the (not so) neonatal Fc receptor, FcRn. *Semin Immunopathol* 2009;31(2):223–236.
38. Baker M, Prasad BV. Rotavirus cell entry. *Curr Top Microbiol Immunol* 2010;343:121–148.
39. Ball JM, Mitchell DM, Gibbons TF, et al. Rotavirus NSP4: Aa multifunctional viral enterotoxin. *Viral Immunol* 2005;18(1):27–40.
40. Ball JM, Tian P, Zeng CQ, et al. Age-dependent diarrhea induced by a rotaviral nonstructural glycoprotein. *Science* 1996;272(5258):101–104.
41. Banyai K, Kemenesi G, Budinski I, et al. Candidate new rotavirus species in Schreiber's bats, Serbia. *Infect Genet Evol* 2017;48:19–26.
42. Barnes GL, Lund JS, Adams L, et al. Phase 1 trial of a candidate rotavirus vaccine (RV3) derived from a human neonate. *J Paediatr Child Health* 1997;33(4):300–304.
43. Barnes GL, Lund JS, Mitchell SV, et al. Early phase II trial of human rotavirus vaccine candidate RV3. *Vaccine* 2002;20:2950–2956.
44. Barro M, Patton JT. Rotavirus nonstructural protein 1 subverts innate immune response by inducing degradation of IFN regulatory factor 3. *Proc Natl Acad Sci USA* 2005;102(11):4114–4119.
45. Barro M, Patton JT. Rotavirus NSP1 inhibits expression of type I interferon by antagonizing the function of interferon regulatory factors IRF3, IRF5, and IRF7. *J Virol* 2007;81(9):4473–4481.
46. Bass D, Cordoba E, Dekker C, et al. Intestinal imaging of children with acute rotavirus gastroenteritis. *J Pediatr Gastroenterol Nutr* 2004;39(3):270–274.
47. Bass DM, Baylor MR, Chen C, et al. Liposome-mediated transfection of intact viral particles reveals that plasma membrane penetration determines permissivity of tissue culture cells to rotavirus. *J Clin Invest* 1992;90:2313–2320.
48. Bastardo JW, Holmes IH. Attachment of SA-11 rotavirus to erythrocyte receptors. *Infect Immun* 1980;29:1134–1140.
49. Benureau Y, Huet JC, Charpilienne A, et al. Trypsin is associated with the rotavirus capsid and is activated by solubilization of outer capsid proteins. *J Gen Virol* 2005;86:3143–3151.
50. Bernstein DI, Sack DA, Rothstein E, et al. Efficacy of live, attenuated, human rotavirus vaccine 89–12 in infants: a randomised placebo-controlled trial. *Lancet* 1999;354(9175):287–290.
51. Bernstein DI, Sander DS, Smith VE, et al. Protection from rotavirus reinfection: 2-year prospective study. *J Infect Dis* 1991;164(2):277–283.
52. Bernstein DI, Smith VE, Sander DS, et al. Evaluation of WC3 rotavirus vaccine and correlates of protection in healthy infants. *J Infect Dis* 1990;162:1055–1062.
53. Bertolotti-Ciarlet A, Ciarlet M, Crawford SE, et al. Immunogenicity and protective efficacy of rotavirus 2/6-virus-like particles produced by a dual baculovirus expression vector and administered intramuscularly, intranasally, or orally to mice. *Vaccine* 2003;21:3885–3900.
54. Besser TE, Gay CC, McGuire TC, et al. Passive immunity to bovine rotavirus infection associated with transfer of serum antibody into the intestinal lumen. *J Virol* 1988;62(7):2238–2242.
55. Bhandari N, Rongsen-Chandola T, Bavdekar A, et al. Efficacy of a monovalent human-bovine (116E) rotavirus vaccine in Indian infants: a randomised, double-blind, placebo-controlled trial. *Lancet* 2014;383(9935):2136–2143.
56. Bhandari N, Sharma P, Taneja S, et al. A dose-escalation safety and immunogenicity study of live attenuated oral rotavirus vaccine 116E in infants: a randomized, double-blind, placebo-controlled trial. *J Infect Dis* 2009;200(3):421–429.
57. Bialowas S, Hagbom M, Nordgren J, et al. Rotavirus and serotonin cross-talk in diarrhoea. *PLoS One* 2016;11(7):e0159660.
58. Bines JE. Intussusception and rotavirus vaccines. *Vaccine* 2006;24:3772–3776.
59. Bines JE, At Thobari J, Satria CD, et al. Human neonatal rotavirus vaccine (RV3-BB) to target rotavirus from birth. *N Engl J Med* 2018;378(8):719–730.
60. Bishop RF. Natural history of human rotavirus infections In: Kapikian AZ, ed. *Viral Infections of the Gastrointestinal Tract.* 2nd ed. New York: Marcel Dekker, Inc.; 1994:131–168.
61. Bishop RF. Natural history of human rotavirus infection. *Arch Virol Suppl* 1996;12:119–128.
62. Bishop RF, Barnes GL, Cipriani E, et al. Clinical immunity after neonatal rotavirus infection, a prospective longitudinal study in young children. *N Eng J Med* 1983;309(2):72–76.
63. Bishop RF, Davidson GP, Holmes IH, et al. Virus particles in epithelial cells of duodenal mucosa from children with acute non-bacterial gastroenteritis. *Lancet* 1973;2(841):1281–1283.
64. Bishop RF, Davidson GP, Holmes IH, et al. Detection of a new virus by electron microscopy of faecal extracts from children with acute gastroenteritis. *Lancet* 1974;1(849):149–151.
65. Bluestone CD, Connell JT, Doyle WJ, et al. General discussion. *Pediatr Infect Dis J* 1988;7(3):239–242.
66. Blutt SE, Kirkwood CD, Parreno V, et al. Rotavirus antigenaemia and viraemia: a common event? *Lancet* 2003;362:1445–1449.
67. Blutt SE, Miller AD, Salmon SL, et al. IgA is important for clearance and critical for protection from rotavirus infection. *Mucosal Immunol* 2012;5(6):712–719.
68. Blutt SE, Fenaux M, Warfield KL, et al. Active viremia in rotavirus-infected mice. *J Virol* 2006;80(13):6702–6705.
68a. Blutt SE, Warfield KL, Lewis DE, et al. Early response to rotavirus infection involves massive B cell activation. *J Immunol* 2002:168(11):5716–5721.
68b. Bomidi C, Robertson M, Coarfa C, et al. Single-cell sequencing of rotavirus-infected intestinal epithelium reveals cell-type specific epithelial repair and tuft cell infection. *Proc Natl Acad Sci U S A* 2021;118(45):e2112814118.
69. Boom JA, Tate JE, Sahni LC, et al. Sustained protection from pentavalent rotavirus vaccination during the second year of life at a large, urban United States pediatric hospital. *Pediatr Infect Dis J* 2010;29(12):1133–1135.
70. Borodavka A, Dykeman EC, Schrimpf W, et al. Protein-mediated RNA folding governs sequence-specific interactions between rotavirus genome segments. *Elife* 2017;6:e27453.
71. Boshuizen JA, Reimerink JH, Korteland-van Male AM, et al. Changes in small intestinal homeostasis, morphology, and gene expression during rotavirus infection of infant mice. *J Virol* 2003;77(24):13005–13016.
72. Boshuizen JA, Rossen WA, Sitaram CK, et al. Rotavirus enterotoxin NSP4 binds to the extracellular matrix proteins Laminin-beta3 and fibronectin. *J Virol* 2004;78(18):10045–10053.
73. Both GW, Siegman LJ, Bellamy AR, et al. Coding assignment and nucleotide sequence of simian rotavirus SA11 gene segment 10: location of glycosylation sites suggests that the signal peptide is not cleaved. *J Virol* 1983;48:335–339.
74. Bowman GD, Nodelman IM, Levy O, et al. Crystal structure of the oligomerization domain of NSP4 from rotavirus reveals a core metal-binding site. *J Mol Biol* 2000;304:861–871.

75. Boyce M, Celma CC, Roy P. Development of reverse genetics systems for bluetongue virus: recovery of infectious virus from synthetic RNA transcripts. *J Virol* 2008;82(17):8339–8348.

76. Brandt CD, Kim HW, Rodriguez WJ, et al. Rotavirus gastroenteritis and weather. *J Clin Microbiol* 1982;16(3):478–482.

77. Brandt CD, Kim HW, Rodriguez WJ, et al. Comparison of direct electron microscopy, immune electron microscopy, and rotavirus enzyme-linked immunosorbent assay for detection of gastroenteritis viruses in children. *J Clin Microbiol* 1981;13:976–981.

78. Brandt CD, Kim HW, Yolken RH, et al. Comparative epidemiology of two rotavirus serotypes and other viral agents associated with pediatric gastroenteritis. *Am J Epidemiol* 1979;110(3):243–254.

79. Bresee JS, Glass RI, Ivanoff B, et al. Current status and future priorities for rotavirus vaccine development, evaluation and implementation in developing countries. *Vaccine* 1999;17(18):2207–2222.

80. Bresee JS, Hummelman E, Nelson EA, et al. Rotavirus in Asia: the value of surveillance for informing decisions about the introduction of new vaccines. *J Infect Dis* 2005;192(Suppl 1):S1–S5.

81. Bridger JC, Kapikian AZ. Non-group A rotaviruses. In: Kapikian AZ, ed. *Viral Infections of the Gastrointestinal Tract*. 2nd ed. New York: Marcel Dekker, Inc.; 1994:369–407.

82. Broome RL, Vo PT, Ward RL, et al. Murine rotavirus genes encoding outer capsid proteins VP4 and VP7 are not major determinants of host range restriction and virulence. *J Virol* 1993;67(5):2448–2455.

83. Broquet AH, Hirata Y, McAllister CS, et al. RIG-I/MDA5/MAVS are required to signal a protective IFN response in rotavirus-infected intestinal epithelium. *J Immunol* 2011;186(3):1618–1626.

84. Brunet JP, Cotte-Laffitte J, Linxe C, et al. Rotavirus infection induces an increase in intracellular calcium concentration in human intestinal epithelial cells: role in microvillar actin alteration. *J Virol* 2000;74(5):2323–2332.

85. Burke B, Desselberger U. Rotavirus pathogenicity. *Virology* 1996;218:299–305.

86. Burke RM, Tate JE, Dahl RM, et al. Rotavirus vaccination is associated with reduced seizure hospitalization risk among commercially insured US children. *Clin Infect Dis* 2018;67(10):1614–1616.

87. Burke RM, Tate JE, Jiang B, et al. Rotavirus and type 1 diabetes—is there a connection? A synthesis of the evidence. *J Infect Dis* 2020;222(7):1076–1083.

88. Burke RM, Tate JE, Kirkwood CD, et al. Current and new rotavirus vaccines. *Curr Opin Infect Dis* 2019;32(5):435–444.

89. Burnett E, Parashar UD, Tate JE. Real-world effectiveness of rotavirus vaccines, 2006–19: a literature review and meta-analysis. *Lancet Glob Health* 2020;8(9):e1195–e1202.

90. Burns JW, Siadat-Pajouh M, Krishnaney AA, et al. Protective effect of rotavirus VP6-specific IgA monoclonal antibodies that lack neutralizing activity. *Science* 1996;272:101–104.

91. Buttery JP, Danchin MH, Lee KJ, et al. Intussusception following rotavirus vaccine administration: post-marketing surveillance in the National Immunization Program in Australia. *Vaccine* 2011;29(16):3061–3066.

92. Buttery JP, Standish J, Bines JE. Intussusception and rotavirus vaccines: consensus on benefits outweighing recognized risk. *Pediatr Infect Dis J* 2014;33(7):772–773.

93. Butz AM, Fosarelli P, Dick J, et al. Prevalence of rotavirus on high-risk fomites in day-care facilities. *Pediatrics* 1993;92(2):202–205.

94. Caddy SL, Vaysburd M, Wing M, et al. Intracellular neutralisation of rotavirus by VP6-specific IgG. *PLoS Pathog* 2020;16(8):e1008732.

95. CaJacob NJ, Cohen MB. Update on diarrhea. *Pediatr Rev* 2016;37(8):313–322.

96. Campagna M, Eichwald C, Vascotto F, et al. RNA interference of rotavirus segment 11 mRNA reveals the essential role of NSP5 in the virus replicative cycle. *J Gen Virol* 2005;86:1481–1487.

97. CDC. Withdrawal of rotavirus vaccine recommendation. *Morb Mortal Wkly Rep* 1999;48(43):1007.

98. Cevallos Porta D, Lopez S, Arias CF, et al. Polarized rotavirus entry and release from differentiated small intestinal cells. *Virology* 2016;499:65–71.

99. Chacko AR, Jeyakanthan J, Ueno G, et al. A new pentameric structure of rotavirus NSP4 revealed by molecular replacement. *Acta Crystallogr D Biol Crystallogr* 2012;68(Pt 1):57–61.

100. Chan WK, Au KS, Estes MK. Topography of the simian rotavirus nonstructural glycoprotein (NS28) in the endoplasmic reticulum membrane. *Virology* 1988;164:435–442.

101. Chang-Graham AL, Perry JL, Engevik MA, et al. Rotavirus induces intercellular calcium waves through ADP signaling. *Science* 2020;370(6519):eabc3621.

102. Chanock SJ, Wenske EA, Fields BN. Human rotaviruses and genome RNA. *J Infect Dis* 1983;148(1):49–50.

103. Charles MD, Holman RC, Curns AT, et al. Hospitalizations associated with rotavirus gastroenteritis in the United States, 1993–2002. *Pediatr Infect Dis J* 2006;25(6):489–493.

104. Charpilienne A, Lepault J, Rey F, et al. Identification of rotavirus VP6 residues located at the interface with VP2 that are essential for capsid assembly and transcriptase activity. *J Virol* 2002;76(15):7822–7831.

105. Chasey D. Different particle types in tissue culture and intestinal epithelium infected with rotavirus. *J Gen Virol* 1977;37:443–451.

106. Chattha KS, Vlasova AN, Kandasamy S, et al. Divergent immunomodulating effects of probiotics on T cell responses to oral attenuated human rotavirus vaccine and virulent human rotavirus infection in a neonatal gnotobiotic piglet disease model. *J Immunol* 2013;191(5):2446–2456.

107. Chen D, Estes MK, Ramig RF. Specific interactions between rotavirus outer capsid proteins VP4 and VP7 determine expression of a cross-reactive, neutralizing VP4-specific epitope. *J Virol* 1992;66(1):432–439.

108. Chen D, Patton JT. Rotavirus RNA replication requires a single-stranded 3′ end for efficient minus-strand synthesis. *J Virol* 1998;72(9):7387–7396.

109. Chen D, Patton JT. Reverse transcriptase adds nontemplated nucleotides to cDNAs during 5′-RACE and primer extension. *Biotechniques* 2001;30(3):574–580, 582.

110. Chen JZ, Settembre EC, Aoki ST, et al. Molecular interactions in rotavirus assembly and uncoating seen by high-resolution cryo-EM. *Proc Natl Acad Sci U S A* 2009;106(26):10644–10648.

111. Chen S, Li P, Wang Y, et al. Rotavirus infection and cytopathogenesis in human biliary organoids potentially recapitulate biliary atresia development. *mBio* 2020;11(4):e01968-20.

112. Cheung W, Gill M, Esposito A, et al. Rotaviruses associate with cellular lipid droplet components to replicate in viroplasms, and compounds disrupting or blocking lipid droplets inhibit viroplasm formation and viral replication. *J Virol* 2010;84(13):6782–6798.

113. Chiba S, Yokoyama T, Nakata S, et al. Protective effect of naturally acquired homotypic and heterotypic rotavirus antibodies. *Lancet* 1986;2:417–421.

114. Chizhikov V, Patton JT. A four-nucleotide translation enhancer in the 3′-terminal consensus sequence of the nonpolyadenylated mRNAs of rotavirus. *RNA* 2000;6(6):814–825.

115. Choi NW, Estes MK, Langridge WHR. Oral immunization with a shiga toxin B subunit: rotavirus NSP4(90) fusion protein protects mice against gastroenteritis. *Vaccine* 2005;23(44):5168–5176.

116. Church JA, Parker EP, Kirkpatrick BD, et al. Interventions to improve oral vaccine performance: a systematic review and meta-analysis. *Lancet Infect Dis* 2019;19(2):203–214.

117. Ciarlet M, Crawford SE, Barone C, et al. Subunit rotavirus vaccine administered parenterally to rabbits induces protective immunity. *J Virol* 1998;72:9233–9246.

118. Ciarlet M, Crawford SE, Estes MK. Differential infection of polarized epithelial cell lines by sialic acid-dependent and sialic acid-independent rotavirus strains. *J Virol* 2001;75(23):11834–11850.

119. Ciarlet M, Estes MK. Human and most animal rotavirus strains do not require the presence of sialic acid on the cell surface for efficient infectivity. *J Gen Virol* 1999;80:943–948.

120. Ciarlet M, Ludert JE, Iturriza-Gomara M, et al. Initial interaction of rotavirus strains with N-acetylneuraminic (sialic) acid residues on the cell surface correlates with VP4 genotype, not species of origin. *J Virol* 2002;76(8):4087–4095.

121. Civra A, Francese R, Gamba P, et al. 25-Hydroxycholesterol and 27-hydroxycholesterol inhibit human rotavirus infection by sequestering viral particles into late endosomes. *Redox Biol* 2018;19:318–330.

122. Clark HF, Furukawa T, Bell LM, et al. Immune response of infants and children to low-passage bovine rotavirus (strain WC3). *Am J Dis Child* 1986;140(4):350–356.

123. Clark HF, Offit PA, Ellis RW, et al. WC3 reassortant vaccines in children. *Arch Virol Suppl* 1996;12:S187–S198.

124. Clark SM, Barnett BB, Spendlove RS. Production of high-titer bovine rotavirus with trypsin. *J Clin Microbiol* 1979;9:413–417.

125. Clark SM, Roth JR, Clark ML, et al. Trypsin enhancement of rotavirus infectivity: mechanism of enhancement. *J Virol* 1981;39:816–822.

126. Cohen J, Laporte J, Charpilienne A, et al. Activation of rotavirus RNA polymerase by calcium chelation. *Arch Virol* 1979;60:177–186.

127. Collins J, Starkey WG, Wallis TS, et al. Intestinal enzyme profiles in normal and rotavirus-infected mice. *J Pediatr Gastroenterol Nutr* 1988;7(2):264–272.

128. Conner ME, Crawford SE, Barone C, et al. Rotavirus vaccine administered parenterally induces protective immunity. *J Virol* 1993;67(11):6633–6641.

129. Contin R, Arnoldi F, Campagna M, et al. Rotavirus NSP5 orchestrates recruitment of viroplasmic proteins. *J Gen Virol* 2010;91(Pt 7):1782–1793.

130. Contin R, Arnoldi F, Mano M, et al. Rotavirus replication requires a functional proteasome for effective assembly of viroplasms. *J Virol* 2011;85(6):2781–2792.

131. Contreras-Trevino HI, Reyna-Rosas E, Leon-Rodriguez R, et al. Species A rotavirus NSP3 acquires its translation inhibitory function prior to stable dimer formation. *PLoS One* 2017;12(7):e0181871.

132. Control CfD. https://www.cdc.gov/mmwr/preview/mmwrhtml/mm5334a3.htm Published 1999.

133. Correia JB, Patel MM, Nakagomi O, et al. Effectiveness of monovalent rotavirus vaccine (Rotarix) against severe diarrhea caused by serotypically unrelated G2P[4] strains in Brazil. *J Infect Dis* 2010;201(3):363–369.

134. Corthesy B, Benureau Y, Perrier C, et al. Rotavirus anti-VP6 secretory immunoglobulin A contributes to protection via intracellular neutralization but not via immune exclusion. *J Virol* 2006;80(21):10692–10699.

135. Coulson BS, Grimwood K, Hudson IL, et al. Role of coproantibody in clinical protection of children during reinfection with rotavirus. *J Clin Microbiol* 1992;30(7):1678–1684.

136. Coulson BS, Grimwood K, Masendycz PJ, et al. Comparison of rotavirus immunoglobulin A coproconversion with other indices of rotavirus infection in a longitudinal study in childhood. *J Clin Microbiol* 1990;28(6):1367–1374.

137. Coulson BS, Londrigan SL, Lee DJ. Rotavirus contains integrin ligand sequences and a disintegrin-like domain that are implicated in virus entry into cells. *Proc Natl Acad Sci U S A* 1997;94:5389–5394.

138. Crawford SE, Criglar JM, Liu Z, et al. COPII vesicle transport is required for rotavirus NSP4 interaction with the autophagy protein LC3 II and trafficking to viroplasms. *J Virol* 2019;94(1):e01341-19.

139. Crawford SE, Estes MK, Ciarlet M, et al. Heterotypic protection and induction of a broad heterotypic neutralization response by rotavirus-like particles. *J Virol* 1999;73(6):4813–4822.

140. Crawford SE, Hyser JM, Utama B, et al. Autophagy hijacked through viroporin-activated calcium/calmodulin-dependent kinase kinase-beta signaling is required for rotavirus replication. *Proc Natl Acad Sci U S A* 2012;109(50):E3405–E3413.

141. Crawford SE, Labbe M, Cohen J, et al. Characterization of virus-like particles produced by the expression of rotavirus capsid proteins in insect cells. *J Virol* 1994;68(9):5945–5952.

142. Crawford SE, Mukherjee AK, Estes MK, et al. Trypsin cleavage stabilizes the rotavirus VP4 spike. *J Virol* 2001;75:6052–6061.

143. Crawford SE, Patel DG, Cheng E, et al. Rotavirus viremia and extraintestinal viral infection in the neonatal rat model. *J Virol* 2006;80(10):4820–4832.

144. Crawford SE, Ramani S, Tate JE, et al. Rotavirus infection. *Nat Rev Dis Primers* 2017;3:17083.

145. Crawley JMS, Bishop RF, Barnes GL. Rotavirus gastroenteritis in infants aged 0–6 months in Melbourne, Australia; implications for vaccination. *J Paediatr Child Health* 1993;29:219–221.

146. Criglar J, Greenberg HB, Estes MK, et al. Reconciliation of rotavirus temperature-sensitive mutant collections and assignment of reassortment groups D, J, and K to genome segments. *J Virol* 2011;85(10):5048–5060.
147. Criglar JM, Anish R, Hu L, et al. Phosphorylation cascade regulates the formation and maturation of rotaviral replication factories. *Proc Natl Acad Sci U S A* 2018;115(51):E12 015–E12023.
148. Criglar JM, Crawford SE, Zhao B, et al. A genetically engineered rotavirus NSP2 phosphorylation mutant impaired in viroplasm formation and replication shows an early interaction between vNSP2 and cellular lipid droplets. *J Virol* 2020;94(15):e00972-20.
149. Criglar JM, Hu L, Crawford SE, et al. A novel form of rotavirus NSP2 and phosphorylation-dependent NSP2-NSP5 interactions are associated with viroplasm assembly. *J Virol* 2014;88(2):786–798.
150. Croce E, Hatz C, Jonker EF, et al. Safety of live vaccinations on immunosuppressive therapy in patients with immune-mediated inflammatory diseases, solid organ transplantation or after bone-marrow transplantation—a systematic review of randomized trials, observational studies and case reports. *Vaccine* 2017;35(9):1216–1226.
151. Cuadras MA, Bordier BB, Zambrano J, et al. Dissecting rotavirus particle-raft interaction with small interfering RNAs: insights into rotavirus transit through the secretory pathway. *J Virol* 2006;80(8):3935–3946.
152. Curns AT, Panozzo CA, Tate JE, et al. Remarkable postvaccination spatiotemporal changes in United States rotavirus activity. *Pediatr Infect Dis J* 2011;30(1 Suppl):S54–S55.
153. da Silva MFM, Rose TL, Gomez MM, et al. G1P[8] species A rotavirus over 27 years—pre- and post-vaccination eras—in Brazil: full genomic constellation analysis and no evidence for selection pressure by Rotarix(R) vaccine. *Infect Genet Evol* 2015;30:206–218.
154. Dang DA, Nguyen VT, Vu DT, et al. A dose-escalation safety and immunogenicity study of a new live attenuated human rotavirus vaccine (Rotavin-M1) in Vietnamese children. *Vaccine* 2012;30(Suppl 1):A114–A121.
155. Das BK, Gentsch JR, Cicirello HG, et al. Characterization of rotavirus strains from newborns in New Delhi, India. *J Clin Microbiol* 1994;32(7):1820–1822.
156. Das M, Dunn SJ, Woode GN, et al. Both surface proteins (VP4 and VP7) of an asymptomatic neonatal rotavirus strain (I321) have high levels of sequence identity with the homologous proteins of a serotype 10 bovine rotavirus. *Virology* 1993;194:374–379.
157. Das SK, Chisti MJ, Sarker MHR, et al. Long-term impact of changing childhood malnutrition on rotavirus diarrhoea: two decades of adjusted association with climate and socio-demographic factors from urban Bangladesh. *PLoS One* 2017;12(9):e0179418.
158. Davidson GP, Bishop RF, Townley RR, et al. Importance of a new virus in acute sporadic enteritis in children. *Lancet* 1975;1(7901):242–246.
159. Davidson GP, Hogg RJ, Kirubakaran CP. Serum and intestinal immune response to rotavirus enteritis in children. *Infect Immun* 1983;40(2):447–452.
160. De Marco G, Bracale I, Buccigrossi V, et al. Rotavirus induces a biphasic enterotoxic and cytotoxic response in human-derived intestinal enterocytes, which is inhibited by human immunoglobulins. *J Infect Dis* 2009;200(5):813–819.
161. De Mol P, Zissis G, Butzler J-P, et al. Failure of live, attenuated oral rotavirus vaccine. *Lancet* 1986;2:108.
162. Deal EM, Jaimes MC, Crawford SE, et al. Rotavirus structural proteins and dsRNA are required for the human primary plasmacytoid dendritic cell IFNalpha response. *PLoS Pathog* 2010;6(6):e1000931.
163. Deal EM, Lahl K, Narvaez CF, et al. Plasmacytoid dendritic cells promote rotavirus-induced human and murine B cell responses. *J Clin Invest* 2013;123(6):2464–2474.
164. Delmas O, Breton M, Sapin C, et al. Heterogeneity of Raft-type membrane microdomains associated with VP4, the rotavirus spike protein, in Caco-2 and MA 104 cells. *J Virol* 2007;81(4):1610–1618.
165. Dennehy PH. Rotavirus vaccines: an overview. *Clin Microbiol Rev* 2008;21(1):198–208.
166. Deo RC, Groft CM, Rajashankar KR, et al. Recognition of the rotavirus mRNA 3′ consensus by an asymmetric NSP3 homodimer. *Cell* 2002;108(1):71–81.
167. Desselberger U. Genome rearrangements of rotaviruses. *Adv Virus Res* 1996;46:69–95.
168. Desselberger U. Differences of rotavirus vaccine effectiveness by country: likely causes and contributing factors. *Pathogens* 2017;6(4):65.
169. Desselberger U, Huppertz HI. Immune responses to rotavirus infection and vaccination and associated correlates of protection. *J Infect Dis* 2011;203(2):188–195.
170. Desselberger U, Manktelow E, Li W, et al. Rotaviruses and rotavirus vaccines. *Br Med Bull* 2009;90:37–51.
171. Dharakul T, Rott L, Greenberg HB. Recovery from chronic rotavirus infection in mice with severe combined immunodeficiency: virus clearance mediated by adoptive transfer of immune CD8+ T lymphocytes. *J Virol* 1990;64(9):4375–4382.
172. Dhillon P, Rao CD. Rotavirus induces formation of remodeled stress granules and P bodies and their sequestration in viroplasms to promote progeny virus production. *J Virol* 2018;92(24):e01363-18.
173. Dhillon P, Tandra VN, Chorghade SG, et al. Cytoplasmic relocalization and colocalization with viroplasms of host cell proteins, and their role in rotavirus infection. *J Virol* 2018;92(15):e00612-18.
174. Di Fiore IJ, Holloway G, Coulson BS. Innate immune responses to rotavirus infection in macrophages depend on MAVS but involve neither the NLRP3 inflammasome nor JNK and p38 signaling pathways. *Virus Res* 2015;208:89–97.
175. Di Fiore IJ, Pane JA, Holloway G, et al. NSP1 of human rotaviruses commonly inhibits NF-kappaB signalling by inducing beta-TrCP degradation. *J Gen Virol* 2015;96(Pt 7):1768–1776.
176. Diaz-Salinas MA, Silva-Ayala D, Lopez S, et al. Rotaviruses reach late endosomes and require the cation-dependent mannose-6-phosphate receptor and the activity of cathepsin proteases to enter the cell. *J Virol* 2014;88(8):4389–4402.
177. Ding K, Celma CC, Zhang X, et al. In situ structures of rotavirus polymerase in action and mechanism of mRNA transcription and release. *Nat Commun* 2019;10(1):2216.
178. Ding S, Diep J, Feng N, et al. STAG2 deficiency induces interferon responses via cGAS-STING pathway and restricts virus infection. *Nat Commun* 2018;9(1):1485.
179. Ding S, Mooney N, Li B, et al. Comparative proteomics reveals strain-specific beta-TrCP degradation via rotavirus NSP1 hijacking a host Cullin-3-Rbx1 complex. *PLoS Pathog* 2016;12(10):e1005929.
180. Ding S, Song Y, Brulois KF, et al. Retinoic acid and lymphotoxin signaling promote differentiation of human intestinal M cells. *Gastroenterology* 2020;159(1):214–226e1.
181. Ding S, Zhu S, Ren L, et al. Rotavirus VP3 targets MAVS for degradation to inhibit type III interferon expression in intestinal epithelial cells. *Elife* 2018;7:e39494.
182. Doms A, Sanabria T, Hansen JN, et al. 25-Hydroxycholesterol production by the cholesterol-25-hydroxylase interferon-stimulated gene restricts mammalian reovirus infection. *J Virol* 2018;92(18):e01047-18.
183. Dong Y, Zeng CQ, Ball JM, et al. The rotavirus enterotoxin NSP4 mobilizes intracellular calcium in human intestinal cells by stimulating phospholipase C-mediated inositol 1,4,5-trisphosphate production. *Proc Natl Acad Sci U S A* 1997;94(8):3960–3965.
184. Dormitzer PR, Greenberg HB. Calcium chelation induces a conformational change in recombinant herpes simplex virus-1-expressed rotavirus VP7. *Virology* 1992;189:828–832.
185. Dormitzer PR, Ho DY, Mackow ER, et al. Neutralizing epitopes on herpes simplex virus-1-expressed rotavirus VP7 are dependent on coexpression of other rotavirus proteins. *Virology* 1992;187:18–32.
186. Dormitzer PR, Nason EB, Prasad BVV, et al. 444 Structural rearrangements in the membrane penetration protein of a non-enveloped virus. *Nature* 2004;430(7003):1053–1058.
187. Dormitzer PR, Sun ZYJ, Blixt O, et al. Specificity and affinity of sialic acid binding by the rhesus rotavirus VP8*core. *J Virol* 2002;76(20):10512–10517.
188. Douagi I, McInerney GM, Hidmark AS, et al. Role of interferon regulatory factor 3 in type I interferon responses in rotavirus-infected dendritic cells and fibroblasts. *J Virol* 2007;81(6):2758–2768.
189. Ebina T. Prophylaxis of rotavirus gastroenteritis using immunoglobulin. *Arch Virol Suppl* 1996;12:S217–S223.
190. Ebina T, Sato A, Umezu K, et al. Prevention of rotavirus infection by cow colostrum containing antibody against human rotavirus. *Lancet* 1983;2(8357):1029–1030.
191. Eichwald C, Rodriguez JF, Burrone OR. Characterization of rotavirus NSP2/NSP5 interactions and the dynamics of viroplasm formation. *J Gen Virol* 2004;85:625–634.
192. Eisengart LJ, Chou PM, Iyer K, et al. Rotavirus infection in small bowel transplant: a histologic comparison with acute cellular rejection. *Pediatr Dev Pathol* 2009;12(2):85–88.
193. El-Attar L, Dhaliwal W, Howard CR, et al. Rotavirus cross-species pathogenicity: molecular characterization of a bovine rotavirus pathogenic for pigs. *Virology* 2001;291(1):172–182.
194. Engleberg NC, Holburt EN, Barrett TJ, et al. Epidemiology of diarrhea due to rotavirus on an Indian reservation: risk factors in the home environment. *J Infect Dis* 1982;145(6):894–898.
195. Ericson BL, Graham DY, Mason BB, et al. Identification, synthesis, and modifications of simian rotavirus SA11 polypeptides in infected cells. *J Virol* 1982;42(3):825–839.
196. Ericson BL, Graham DY, Mason BB, et al. Two types of glycoprotein precursors are produced by the Simian rotavirus SA11. *Virology* 1983;127:320–332.
197. Esona MD, Gautam R. Rotavirus. *Clin Lab Med* 2015;35(2):363–391.
198. Espejo RT, Lopez S, Arias C. Structural polypeptides of simian rotavirus SA11 and the effect of trypsin. *J Virol* 1981;37(1):156–160.
199. Estes MK, Atmar RL. Viral pathogens of the intestine. In: Hecht G, ed. *Microbial Pathogenesis and the Intestinal Epithelial Cell.* Washington, DC: ASM Press; 2003:525–545.
200. Estes MK, Graham DY, Mason BB. Proteolytic enhancement of rotavirus infectivity: molecular mechanisms. *J Virol* 1981;39(3):879–888.
201. Estes MK, Graham DY, Smith EM, et al. Rotavirus stability and inactivation. *J Gen Virol* 1979;43:403–409.
202. Estes MK, Morris AP. A viral enterotoxin. A new mechanism of virus-induced pathogenesis. *Adv Exp Med Biol* 1999;473:73–82.
203. Estes MK, Tanaka T. Nucleic acid probes for rotavirus detection and characterization. In: Tenover F, ed. *DNA Probes for Infectious Diseases.* Boca Raton, FL: CRC Press; 1989:79–100.
204. Fabbretti E, Afrikanova I, Vascotto F, et al. Two non-structural rotavirus proteins, NSP2 and NSP5, form viroplasm-like structures in vivo. *J Gen Virol* 1999;80(Pt 2):333–339.
205. Fajardo T, Sung PY, Celma CC, et al. Rotavirus genomic RNA complex forms via specific RNA-RNA interactions: disruption of RNA complex inhibits virus infectivity. *Viruses* 2017;9(7):167.
206. Fenaux M, Cuadras MA, Feng N, et al. Extraintestinal spread and replication of a homologous EC rotavirus strain and a heterologous rhesus rotavirus in BALB/c mice. *J Virol* 2006;80(11):5219–5232.
207. Feneaux M, Cuadras MA, Feng N, et al. Extra-intestinal spread and replication of homologous (EC) and a heterologous (RRV) rotavirus in BALB/c mice. *J Virol* 2006;80(11):5219–5232.
208. Feng N, Burns JW, Bracy L, et al. Comparison of mucosal and systemic humoral immune responses and subsequent protection in mice orally inoculated with a homologous or a heterologous rotavirus. *J Virol* 1994;68(12):7766–7773.
209. Feng N, Franco MA, Greenberg HB. Murine model of rotavirus infection. *Adv Exp Med Biol* 1997;412:233–240.
210. Feng N, Hu L, Ding S, et al. Human VP8* mAbs neutralize rotavirus selectively in human intestinal epithelial cells. *J Clin Invest* 2019;129(9):3839–3851.
211. Feng N, Jaimes MC, Lazarus NH, et al. Redundant role of chemokines CCL25/TECK and CCL28/MEC in IgA+ plasmablast recruitment to the intestinal lamina propria after rotavirus infection. *J Immunol* 2006;176(10):5749–5759.
212. Feng N, Kim B, Fenaux M, et al. Role of interferon in homologous and heterologous rotavirus infection in the intestines and extraintestinal organs of suckling mice. *J Virol* 2008;82(15):7578–7590.
213. Feng N, Lawton JA, Gilbert J, et al. Inhibition of rotavirus replication by a non-neutralizing, rotavirus VP6-specific IgA mAb. *J Clin Invest* 2002;109(9):1203–1213.
214. Feng N, Sen A, Wolf M, et al. Roles of VP4 and NSP1 in determining the distinctive replication capacities of simian rotavirus RRV and bovine rotavirus UK in the mouse biliary tract. *J Virol* 2011;85(6):2686–2694.
215. Feng N, Yasukawa LL, Sen A, et al. Permissive replication of homologous murine rotavirus in the mouse intestine is primarily regulated by VP4 and NSP1. *J Virol* 2013;87(15):8307–8316.

216. Fischer TK, Ashley D, Kerin T, et al. Rotavirus antigenemia in patients with acute gastroenteritis. *J Infect Dis* 2005;192(5):913–919.

217. Fischer TK, Bresee JS, Glass RI. Rotavirus vaccines and the prevention of hospital-acquired diarrhea in children. *Vaccine* 2004;22(Suppl 1):S49–S54.

218. Fischer TK, Gentsch JR. Rotavirus typing methods and algorithms. *Rev Med Virol* 2004;14:71–82.

219. Fleming FE, Graham KL, Takada Y, et al. Determinants of the specificity of rotavirus interactions with the alpha2beta1 integrin. *J Biol Chem* 2011;286(8):6165–6174.

220. Fleming FE, Graham KL, Taniguchi K, et al. Rotavirus-neutralizing antibodies inhibit virus binding to integrins alpha 2 beta 1 and alpha 4 beta 1. *Arch Virol* 2007;152(6):1087–1101.

221. Flewett TH, Bryden AS, Davies H. Letter: virus particles in gastroenteritis. *Lancet* 1973;2(844):1497.

222. Flewett TH, Bryden AS, Davies H. Relation between viruses from acute gastroenteritis of children and newborn calves. *Lancet* 1974;2:61–63.

223. Flores J, Perez I, White L, et al. Genetic relatedness among human rotaviruses as determined by RNA hybridization. *Infect Immun* 1982;37(2):648–655.

224. Flores PS, Costa FB, Amorim AR, et al. Rotavirus A, C, and H in Brazilian pigs: potential for zoonotic transmission of RVA. *J Vet Diagn Invest* 2021;33(1):129–135.

225. Foster SO, Palmer EL, Gary GW Jr, et al. Gastroenteritis due to rotavirus in an isolated Pacific Island group: an epidemic of 3,439 cases. *J Infect Dis* 1980;141(1):32–39.

226. Franco MA, Angel J, Greenberg HB. Immunity and correlates of protection for rotavirus vaccines. *Vaccine* 2006;24(15):2718–2731.

227. Franco MA, Greenberg HB. Role of B cells and cytotoxic T lymphocytes in clearance of and immunity to rotavirus infection in mice. *J Virol* 1995;69(12):7800–7806.

228. Franco MA, Greenberg HB. Immunity to rotavirus in T cell deficient mice. *Virology* 1997;238(2):169–179.

229. Frias AH, Jones RM, Fifadara NH, et al. Rotavirus-induced IFN-beta promotes anti-viral signaling and apoptosis that modulate viral replication in intestinal epithelial cells. *Innate Immun* 2012;18(2):294–306.

230. Fu C, Tate JE, Jiang B. Effectiveness of Lanzhou lamb rotavirus vaccine against hospitalized gastroenteritis: further analysis and update. *Hum Vaccin* 2010;6(11):953.

231. Fujii R, Kuzuya M, Hamano M, et al. Detection of human group C rotaviruses by an enzyme-linked immunosorbent assay using monoclonal antibodies. *J Clin Microbiol* 1992;30(5):1307–1311.

232. Fukuhara N, Yoshie O, Kitaoka S, et al. Role of VP3 in human rotavirus internalization after target cell attachment via VP7. *J Virol* 1988;62(7):2209–2218.

233. Fukuhara N, Yoshie O, Kitaoka S, et al. Evidence for endocytosis-independent infection by human rotavirus. *Arch Virol* 1987;97:93–99.

234. Gajardo R, Vende P, Poncet D, et al. Two proline residues are essential in the calcium-binding activity of rotavirus VP7 outer capsid protein. *J Virol* 1997;71(3):2211–2216.

234a. Gaopeng H, Qiru Z, Jelle M, Greenberg HB, Siyuan D. Rotavirus NSP1 contributes to intestinal viral replication, pathogenesis, and transmission. *mBio* 2021;12(6):e0320821.

235. Garaicoechea L, Olichon A, Marcoppido G, et al. Llama-derived single-chain antibody fragments directed to rotavirus VP6 protein possess broad neutralizing activity in vitro and confer protection against diarrhea in mice. *J Virol* 2008;82(19):9753–9764.

236. Gardet A, Breton M, Fontages P, et al. Rotavirus spike protein VP4 binds to and remodels actin bundles of the epithelial brush order into actin bodies. *J Virol* 2006;80(8):3947–3956.

237. Gentsch JR, Laird AR, Bielfelt B, et al. Serotype diversity and reassortment between human and animal rotavirus strains: implications for rotavirus vaccine programs. *J Infect Dis* 2005;192(Suppl 1):S146-S159.

238. Georges-Courbot MC, Monges J, Siopathis MR, et al. Evaluation of the efficacy of a low-passage bovine rotavirus (strain WC3) vaccine in children in Central Africa. *Res Virol* 1991;142:405–411.

239. Gerna G, Arista S, Passarani N, et al. Electropherotype heterogeneity within serotypes of human rotavirus strains circulating in Italy. *Arch Virol* 1987;95:129–135.

240. Gerna G, Forster J, Parea M, et al. Nosocomial outbreak of neonatal gastroenteritis caused by a new serotype 4, subtype 4B human rotavirus. *J Med Virol* 1990;31(3):175–182.

241. Gervasi G, Capanna A, Mita V, et al. Nosocomial rotavirus infection: an up to date evaluation of European studies. *Hum Vaccin Immunother* 2016;12(9):2413–2418.

242. Giaquinto C, Dominiak-Felden G, Van Damme P, et al. Summary of effectiveness and impact of rotavirus vaccination with the oral pentavalent rotavirus vaccine: a systematic review of the experience in industrialized countries. *Hum Vaccin* 2011;7(7):734–748.

243. Gilbert JM, Greenberg HB. Cleavage of rhesus rotavirus VP4 after arginine 247 is essential for rotavirus-like particle-induced fusion from without. *J Virol* 1998;72(6):5323–5327.

244. Gilger MA, Matson DO, Conner ME, et al. Extraintestinal rotavirus infections in children with immunodeficiency. *J Pediatr* 1992;120:912–917.

245. Gladstone BP, Ramani S, Mukhopadhya I, et al. Protective effect of natural rotavirus infection in an Indian birth cohort. *N Engl J Med* 2011;365(4):337–346.

246. Glanz JM, Clarke CL, Xu S, et al. Association between rotavirus vaccination and type 1 diabetes in children. *JAMA Pediatr* 2020;174(5):455–462.

247. Glass RI. Perceived threats and real killers. *Science* 2004;304:927.

248. Glass RI, Bhan MK, Ray P, et al. Development of candidate rotavirus vaccines derived from neonatal strains in India. *J Infect Dis* 2005;192(Suppl 1):S30–S35.

249. Glass RI, Bresee JS, Parashar UD, et al. The future of rotavirus vaccines: a major setback leads to new opportunities. *Lancet* 2004;363:1547–1550.

250. Glass RI, Parashar UD. The promise of new rotavirus vaccines. *N Engl J Med* 2006;354(1):75–77.

251. Glass RI, Parashar UD, Bresee JS, et al. Rotavirus vaccines: current prospects and future challenges. *Lancet* 2006;368(9532):323–332.

252. Gleizes O, Desselberger U, Tatochenko V, et al. Nosocomial rotavirus infection in European countries: a review of the epidemiology, severity and economic burden of hospital-acquired rotavirus disease. *Pediatr Infect Dis J* 2006;25(1 Suppl):S12–S21.

253. Gombold JL, Estes MK, Ramig RF. Assignment of simian rotavirus SA11 temperature-sensitive mutant groups B and E to genome segments. *Virology* 1985;143:309–320.

254. Gombold JL, Ramig RF. Assignment of simian rotavirus SA11 temperature-sensitive mutant groups A, C, F, and G to genome segments. *Virology* 1987;161:463–473.

255. Gonzalez AM, Azevedo MS, Jung K, et al. Innate immune responses to human rotavirus in the neonatal gnotobiotic piglet disease model. *Immunology* 2010;131(2):242–256.

256. Gonzalez RA, Espinosa R, Romero P, et al. Relative localization of viroplasmic and endoplasmic reticulum-resident rotavirus proteins in infected cells. *Arch Virol* 2000;145(9):1963–1973.

257. Gouvea V, Allen JR, Glass RI, et al. Detection of group B and C rotaviruses by polymerase chain reaction. *J Clin Microbiol* 1991;29(3):519–523.

258. Graff JW, Ettayebi K, Hardy ME. Rotavirus NSP1 inhibits NFkappaB activation by inducing proteasome-dependent degradation of beta-TrCP: a novel mechanism of IFN antagonism. *PLoS Pathog* 2009;5(1):e1000280.

259. Graff JW, Ewen J, Ettayebi K, et al. Zinc-binding domain of rotavirus NSP1 is required for proteasome-dependent degradation of IRF3 and autoregulatory NSP1 stability. *J Gen Virol* 2007;88(Pt 2):613–620.

260. Graham DY, Dufour GR, Estes MK. Minimal infective dose of rotavirus. *Arch Virol* 1987;92:261–271.

261. Graham KL, Halasz P, Tan Y, et al. Integrin-using rotaviruses bind alpha 2 beta 1 integrin alpha 2 I domain via VP4 DGE sequence and recognize alpha X beta 2 and alpha V beta 3 by using VP7 during cell entry. *J Virol* 2003;77(18):9969–9978.

262. Graham KL, Sanders N, Tan Y, et al. Rotavirus infection accelerates type 1 diabetes in mice with established insulitis. *J Virol* 2008;82(13):6139–6149.

263. Graham KL, Takada Y, Coulson BS. Rotavirus spike protein VP5* binds alpha2beta1 integrin on the cell surface and competes with virus for cell binding and infectivity. *J Gen Virol* 2006;87(Pt 5):1275–1283.

264. Gratia M, Vende P, Charpilienne A, et al. Challenging the roles of NSP3 and untranslated regions in rotavirus mRNA translation. *PLoS One* 2016;11(1):e0145998.

265. Green KY, Kapikian AZ. Identification of VP7 epitopes associated with protection against human rotavirus illness or shedding in volunteers. *J Virol* 1992;66(1):548–553.

266. Green VA, Pelkmans L. A systems survey of progressive host-cell reorganization during rotavirus infection. *Cell Host Microbe* 2016;20(1):107–120.

267. Greenberg H, Clark H, Offit P. Rotavirus pathology and pathophysiology. In: Lille AC, Compans RW, Cooper M, et al., eds. *Current Topics in Microbiology and Immunology*. Vol. 185. Berlin, Heidelberg, New York, London, Paris, Tokyo, Hong Kong, Barcelona, Budapest: Springer-Verlag; 1994:255–283.

268. Greenberg HB. Rotavirus vaccination and intussusception—act two. *N Engl J Med* 2011;364(24):2354–2355.

269. Greenberg HB, Estes MK. Rotaviruses: from pathogenesis to vaccination. *Gastroenterology* 2009;136(6):1939–1951.

270. Greenberg HB, Gebhard RL, McClain CJ, et al. Antibodies to viral gastroenteritis viruses in Crohn's disease. *Gastroenterology* 1979;76(2):349–350.

271. Greenberg HB, Kalica AR, Wyatt RG, et al. Rescue of noncultivatable human rotavirus by gene reassortment during mixed infection with ts mutants of a cultivatable bovine rotavirus. *Proc Natl Acad Sci USA* 1981;78(1):420–424.

272. Greenberg HB, Valdesuso J, Van Wyke K, et al. Production and preliminary characterization of monoclonal antibodies directed at two surface proteins of rhesus rotavirus. *J Virol* 1983;47(2):267–275.

273. Greenberg HB, Wyatt RG, Kapikian AZ, et al. Rescue and serotypic characterization of noncultivable human rotavirus by gene reassortment. *Infect Immun* 1982;37(1):104–109.

274. Grimes JM, Burroughs JN, Gouet P, et al. The atomic structure of the bluetongue virus core. *Nature* 1998;395(6701):470–478.

275. Grimwood K, Lambert SB, Milne RJ. Rotavirus infections and vaccines: burden of illness and potential impact of vaccination. *Paediatr Drugs* 2010;12(4):235–256.

276. Grimwood K, Lund JCS, Coulson BS, et al. Comparison of serum and mucosal antibody responses following severe acute rotavirus gastroenteritis in young children. *J Clin Microbiol* 1988;26(4):732–738.

277. Groft CM, Burley SK. Recognition of eIF4G by rotavirus NSP3 reveals a basis for mRNA circularization. *Molecular Cell* 2002;9(6):1273–1283.

278. Groome MJ, Fairlie L, Morrison J, et al. Safety and immunogenicity of a parenteral trivalent P2-VP8 subunit rotavirus vaccine: a multisite, randomised, double-blind, placebo-controlled trial. *Lancet Infect Dis* 2020;20(7):851–863.

279. Groome MJ, Koen A, Fix A, et al. Safety and immunogenicity of a parenteral P2-VP8-P[8] subunit rotavirus vaccine in toddlers and infants in South Africa: a randomised, double-blind, placebo-controlled trial. *Lancet Infect Dis* 2017;17(8):843–853.

280. Gualtero DF, Guzman F, Acosta O, et al. Amino acid domains 280–297 of VP6 and 531–554 of VP4 are implicated in heat shock cognate protein hsc70-mediated rotavirus infection. *Arch Virol* 2007;152(12):2183–2196.

281. Guarino A, Canani RB, Russo S, et al. Oral immunoglobulins for treatment of acute rotaviral gastroenteritis. *Pediatrics* 1994;93(1):12–16.

282. Guarino A, Guandalini S, Albano F, et al. Enteral immunoglobulins for treatment of protracted rotaviral diarrhea. *Pediatr Infect Dis J* 1991;10(8):612–614.

283. Guarino A, Russo S, Castaldo A, et al. Passive immunotherapy for rotavirus-induced diarrhoea in children with HIV infection [letter]. *AIDS* 1996;10(10):1176–1178.

284. Guerrero CA, Bouyssounade D, Zarate S, et al. Heat shock cognate protein 70 is involved in rotavirus cell entry. *J Virol* 2002;76(8):4096–4102.

285. Guerrero CA, Mendez E, Zarate S, et al. Integrin alpha(v)beta(3) mediates rotavirus cell entry. *Proc Natl Acad Sci USA* 2000;97:14644–14649.

286. Gurwith M, Wenman W, Hinde D, et al. A prospective study of rotavirus infection in infants and young children. *J Infect Dis* 1981;144(3):218–224.

287. Gutierrez M, Isa P, Sanchez-San Martin C, et al. Different rotavirus strains enter MA104 cells through different endocytic pathways: the role of clathrin-mediated endocytosis. *J Virol* 2010;84(18):9161–9169.

288. Hagbom M, De Faria FM, Winberg ME, et al. Neurotrophic factors protect the intestinal barrier from rotavirus insult in mice. *mBio* 2020;11(1):e02834-19.

289. Hagbom M, Istrate C, Engblom D, et al. Rotavirus stimulates release of serotonin (5-HT) from human enterochromaffin cells and activates brain structures involved in nausea and vomiting. *PLoS Pathog* 2011;7(7):e1002115.

290. Hagbom M, Novak D, Ekstrom M, et al. Ondansetron treatment reduces rotavirus symptoms—a randomized double-blinded placebo-controlled trial. *PLoS One* 2017;12(10):e0186824.

291. Hakim MS, Ding S, Chen S, et al. TNF-alpha exerts potent anti-rotavirus effects via the activation of classical NF-kappaB pathway. *Virus Res* 2018;253:28–37.
292. Hammarstrom L. Passive immunity against rotavirus in infants. *Acta Paediatr Suppl* 1999;88(430):127–132.
293. Hanlon P, Hanlon L, Marsh V, et al. Trial of an attenuated bovine rotavirus vaccine (RIT 4237) in Gambian infants. *Lancet* 1987;1(8546):1342–1345.
294. Harb M, Becker MM, Vitour D, et al. Nuclear localization of cytoplasmic poly(A)-binding protein upon rotavirus infection involves the interaction of NSP3 with eIF4G and RoXaN. *J Virol* 2008;82(22):11283–11293.
295. Hasegawa A, Matsuno S, Inouye S, et al. Isolation of human rotaviruses in primary cultures of monkey kidney cells. *J Clin Microbiol* 1982;16(2):387–390.
296. Haselhorst T, Fleming FE, Dyason JC, et al. Sialic acid dependence in rotavirus host cell invasion. *Nat Chem Biol* 2009;5(2):91–93.
297. Hashavya S, Wilscrhanski M, Averbuch D, et al. Rotavirus-associated colitis in a six-month-old baby. *Pediatr Int* 2010;52(4):e204–e206.
298. Hattori H, Torii S, Nagafuji H, et al. Benign acute myositis associated with rotavirus gastroenteritis. *J Pediatr* 1992;121:748–749.
299. Heaton NS, Moshkina N, Fenouil R, et al. Targeting viral proteostasis limits influenza virus, HIV, and dengue virus infection. *Immunity* 2016;44(1):46–58.
300. Heaton PM, Ciarlet M. Vaccines: the pentavalent rotavirus vaccine: discovery to licensure and beyond. *Clin Infect Dis* 2007;45(12):1618–1624.
301. Heaton PM, Goveia MG, Miller JM, et al. Development of a pentavalent rotavirus vaccine against prevalent serotypes of rotavirus gastroenteritis. *J Infect Dis* 2005;192(Suppl 1): S17–S21.
302. Hempson SJ, Matkowskyj K, Bansal A, et al. Rotavirus infection of murine small intestine causes colonic secretion via age restricted galanin-1 receptor expression. *Gastroenterology* 2010;138(7):2410–2417.
303. Hernandez PP, Mahlakoiv T, Yang I, et al. Interferon-lambda and interleukin 22 act synergistically for the induction of interferon-stimulated genes and control of rotavirus infection. *Nat Immunol* 2015;16(7):698–707.
304. Herrmann T, Torres R, Salgado EN, et al. Functional refolding of the penetration protein on a non-enveloped virus. *Nature* 2021;590(7847):666–670.
305. Hewish MJ, Takada Y, Coulson BS. Integrins alpha2beta1 and alpha4beta1 can mediate SA11 rotavirus attachment and entry into cells. *J Virol* 2000;74(1):228–236.
306. Hieber JP, Shelton S, Nelson JD, et al. Comparison of human rotavirus disease in tropical and temperate settings. *Am J Dis Child* 1978;132(9):853–858.
307. Hill CL, Booth TF, Prasad BV, et al. The structure of a cypovirus and the functional organization of dsRNA viruses. *Nat Struct Biol* 1999;6(6):565–568.
308. Hjelt K, Grauballe PC, Paerregaard A, et al. Protective effect of preexisting rotavirus-specific immunoglobulin A against naturally acquired rotavirus infection in children. *J Med Virol* 1987;21:39–47.
309. Holloway G, Dang VT, Jans DA, et al. Rotavirus inhibits IFN-induced STAT nuclear translocation by a mechanism that acts after STAT binding to importin-alpha. *J Gen Virol* 2014;95(Pt 8):1723–1733.
310. Holmes IH. Development of rotavirus molecular epidemiology: electropherotyping. *Arch Virol Suppl* 1996;12:87–91.
311. Holmes IH, Ruck BJ, Bishop RF, et al. Infantile enteritis viruses: morphogenesis and morphology. *J Virol* 1975;16(4):937–943.
312. Horie Y, Nakagomi O, Koshimura Y, et al. Diarrhea induction by rotavirus NSP4 in the homologous mouse model system. *Virology* 1999;262(2):398–407.
313. Hoshino Y, Saif LJ, Kang SY, et al. Identification of group A rotavirus genes associated with virulence of a porcine rotavirus and host range restriction of a human rotavirus in the gnotobiotic piglet model. *Virology* 1995;209(1):274–280.
314. Hoshino Y, Sereno MM, Midthun K, et al. Independent segregation of two antigenic specificities (VP3 and VP7) involved in neutralization of rotavirus infectivity. *PNAS* 1985;82:8701–8704.
315. Hrdy DB. Epidemiology of rotaviral infection in adults. *Rev Infect Dis* 1987;9(3):461–469.
316. Hu L, Crawford SE, Czako R, et al. Cell attachment protein VP8* of a human rotavirus specifically interacts with A-type histo-blood group antigen. *Nature* 2012;485(7397):256–259.
317. Hu L, Estes MK, Prasad BVV. *Reoviruses (Reoviridae) and Their Structural Relatives.* 4th ed. Oxford: Academic Press; 2021.
318. Hull JJ, Teel EN, Kerin TK, et al. United States rotavirus strain surveillance from 2005 to 2008: genotype prevalence before and after vaccine introduction. *Pediatr Infect Dis J* 2011;30(1 Suppl):S42–S47.
319. Hundley F, Biryahwaho B, Gow M, et al. Genome rearrangements of bovine rotavirus after serial passage at high multiplicity of infection. *Virology* 1985;143:88–103.
320. Hundley F, McIntyre M, Clark B, et al. Heterogeneity of genome rearrangements in rotaviruses isolated from a chronically infected immunodeficient child. *J Virol* 1987;61:3365–3372.
321. Hung T. Rotavirus and adult diarrhea. *Adv Virus Res* 1988;35:193–218.
322. Hung T, Chen GM, Wang CG, et al. Rotavirus-like agent in adult non-bacterial diarrhoea in China. *Lancet* 1983;2(8358):1078–1079.
323. Hungerford DJ, French N, Iturriza-Gomara M, et al. Reduction in hospitalisations for acute gastroenteritis-associated childhood seizures since introduction of rotavirus vaccination: a time-series and change-point analysis of hospital admissions in England. *J Epidemiol Community Health* 2019;73(11):1020–1025.
324. Hyser JM, Collinson-Pautz MR, Utama B, et al. Rotavirus disrupts calcium homeostasis by NSP4 viroporin activity. *mBio* 2010;1(5):e00265-10.
325. Hyser JM, Utama B, Crawford SE, et al. Activation of the endoplasmic reticulum calcium sensor STIM1 and store-operated calcium entry by rotavirus requires NSP4 viroporin activity. *J Virol* 2013;87(24):13579–13588.
326. Hyser JM, Zeng CQ, Beharry Z, et al. Epitope mapping and use of epitope-specific antisera to characterize the VP5* binding site in rotavirus SA11 NSP4. *Virology* 2008;373(1): 211–228.
327. Imai M, Akatani K, Ikegami N, et al. Capped and conserved terminal structures in human rotavirus genome double-stranded RNA segments. *J Virol* 1983;47:125–136.
328. Isa P, Arias CF, Lopez S. Role of sialic acids in rotavirus infection. *Glycon J* 2006;23:27–37.
329. Isa P, Realpe M, Romero P, et al. Rotavirus RRV associates with lipid membrane microdomains during cell entry. *Virology* 2004;322(2):370–381.
330. Isa P, Sanchez-Aleman MA, Lopez S, et al. Dissecting the role of integrin subunits alpha 2 and beta 3 in rotavirus cell entry by RNA silencing. *Virus Res* 2009;145(2):251–259.
331. Istrate C, Hinkula J, Hammarstrom L, et al. Individuals with selective IgA deficiency resolve rotavirus disease and develop higher antibody titers (IgG, IgG1) than IgA competent individuals. *J Med Virol* 2008;80(3):531–535.
332. Iturriza-Gomara M, Anderton E, Kang G, et al. Evidence for genetic linkage between the gene segments encoding NSP4 and VP6 proteins in common and reassortant human rotavirus strains. *J Clin Microbiol* 2003;41(8):3566–3573.
333. Iturriza-Gomara M, Auchterlonie IA, Zaw W, et al. Rotavirus gastroenteritis and central nervous system (CNS) infection: characterization of the VP7 and VP4 genes of rotavirus strains isolated from paired fecal and cerebrospinal fluid samples from a child with CNS disease. *J Clin Microbiol* 2002;40(12):4797–4799.
334. Iturriza-Gomara M, Dallman T, Banyai K, et al. Rotavirus genotypes co-circulating in Europe between 2006 and 2009 as determined by EuroRotaNet, a pan-European collaborative strain surveillance network. *Epidemiol Infect* 2011;139(6):895–909.
335. Iwasaki A, Medzhitov R. Control of adaptive immunity by the innate immune system. *Nat Immunol* 2015;16(4):343–353.
336. Jaimes MC, Rojas OL, Gonzalez AM, et al. Frequencies of virus-specific CD4(+) and CD8(+) T lymphocytes secreting gamma interferon after acute natural rotavirus infection in children and adults. *J Virol* 2002;76(10):4741–4749.
337. Jaimes MC, Rojas OL, Kunkel EJ, et al. Maturation and trafficking markers on rotavirus-specific B cells during acute infection and convalescence in children. *J Virol* 2004; 78(20):10967–10976.
338. Jayaram H, Taraporewala Z, Patton JT, et al. Rotavirus protein involved in genome replication and packaging exhibits a HIT-like fold. *Nature* 2002;417(6886):311–315.
339. Jenni S, Salgado EN, Herrmann T, et al. In situ structure of rotavirus VP1 RNA-dependent RNA polymerase. *J Mol Biol* 2019;431(17):3124–3138.
340. Jensen PH, Kolarich D, Packer NH. Mucin-type O-glycosylation—putting the pieces together. *FEBS J* 2010;277(1):81–94.
341. Jiang B, Gentsch JR, Glass RI. The role of serum antibodies in the protection against rotavirus disease: an overview. *Clin Infect Dis* 2002;34(10):1351–1361.
342. Jiang B, Gentsch JR, Glass RI. Inactivated rotavirus vaccines: a priority for accelerated vaccine development. *Vaccine* 2008;26(52):6754–6758.
343. Jiang B, Patel M, Parashar U. Rotavirus vaccines for global use: what are the remaining issues and challenges? *Hum Vaccin* 2010;6(5):425–427.
344. Jiang B, Tsunemitsu H, Gentsch JR, et al. Nucleotide sequence of gene 5 encoding the inner capsid protein (VP6) of bovine group C rotavirus: comparison with corresponding genes of group C, A, and B rotaviruses. *Virology* 1992;190:542–547.
345. Jiang X, Jayaram H, Kumar M, et al. Cryoelectron microscopy structures of rotavirus NSP2-NSP5 and NSP2-RNA complexes: implications for genome replication. *J Virol* 2006;80(21):10829–10835.
346. Jimenez-Zaragoza M, Yubero MP, Martin-Forero E, et al. Biophysical properties of single rotavirus particles account for the functions of protein shells in a multilayered virus. *Elife* 2018;7:e37295.
347. Joensuu J, Koskenniemi E, Pang X-L, et al. Randomised placebo-controlled trial of rhesus-human reassortant rotavirus vaccine for prevention of severe rotavirus gastroenteritis. *Lancet* 1997;350:1205–1209.
348. Joensuu J, Koskenniemi E, Vesikari T. Prolonged efficacy of rhesus-human reassortant rotavirus vaccine. *Pediatr Infect Dis J* 1998;17(5):427–429.
349. Joshi MS, Lole KS, Barve US, et al. Investigation of a large waterborne acute gastroenteritis outbreak caused by group B rotavirus in Maharashtra state, India. *J Med Virol* 2019;91(10):1877–1881.
350. Jourdan N, Brunet JP, Sapin C, et al. Rotavirus infection reduces sucrase-isomaltase expression in human intestinal epithelial cells by perturbing protein targeting and organization of microvillar cytoskeleton. *J Virol* 1998;72(9):7228–7236.
351. Jourdan N, Cotte LJ, Forestier F, et al. Infection of cultured human intestinal cells by monkey RRV and human Wa rotavirus as a function of intestinal epithelial cell differentiation. *Res Virol* 1995;146(5):325–331.
352. Jourdan N, Maurice M, Delautier D, et al. Rotavirus is released from the apical surface of cultured human intestinal cells through nonconventional vesicular transport that bypasses the Golgi apparatus. *J Virol* 1997;71(11):8268–8278.
353. Justino MC, Linhares AC, Lanzieri TM, et al. Effectiveness of the monovalent G1P[8] human rotavirus vaccine against hospitalization for severe G2P[4] rotavirus gastroenteritis in Belem, Brazil. *Pediatr Infect Dis J* 2011;30(5):396–401.
354. Kabcenell AK, Atkinson PH. Processing of the rough endoplasmic reticulum membrane glycoproteins of rotavirus SA11. *J Cell Biol* 1985;101:1270–1280.
355. Kaljot KT, Shaw RD, Rubin DH, et al. Infectious rotavirus enters cells by direct cell membrane penetration, not be endocytosis. *J Virol* 1988;62(4):1136–1144.
356. Kanai Y, Kawagishi T, Nouda R, et al. Development of stable rotavirus reporter expression systems. *J Virol* 2019;93(4):e01774-18.
357. Kanai Y, Komoto S, Kawagishi T, et al. Entirely plasmid-based reverse genetics system for rotaviruses. *Proc Natl Acad Sci U S A* 2017;114(9):2349–2354.
358. Kang G, Iturriza-Gomara M, Wheeler JG, et al. Quantitation of group A rotavirus by real-time reverse-transcription-polymerase chain reaction: correlation with clinical severity in children in South India. *J Med Virol* 2004;73(1):118–122.
359. Kapahnke R, Rappold W, Desselberger U, et al. The stiffness of dsRNA: hydrodynamic studies on fluorescence-labelled RNA segments of bovine rotavirus. *Nucleic Acids Res* 1986; 14:3215–3228.
360. Kapikian A. Viral gastroenteritis. *JAMA* 1993;269(5):627–629.
361. Kapikian AZ. Acute viral gastroenteritis. *Prev Med* 1974;3(4):535–542.
362. Kapikian AZ. Viral gastroenteritis In: Evans K, Kaslow R, eds. *Viral Infections in Humans.* New York: Plenum Press; 1997:293–340.
363. Kapikian AZ. Ecological studies, rotavirus vaccination, and intussusception. *Lancet* 2002;359(9311):1065–1066; author reply 1066.

364. Kapikian AZ, Flores J, Hoshino Y, et al. Prospects for development of a rotavirus vaccine against rotavirus diarrhea in infants and young children. *Rev Infect Dis* 1989;11(Suppl 3):S539–S546.
365. Kapikian AZ, Hoshino Y, Chanock RM, et al. Efficacy of a quadrivalent rhesus rotavirus-based human rotavirus vaccine aimed at preventing severe rotavirus diarrhea in infants and young children. *J Infect Dis* 1996;174(Suppl 1):S65–S72.
366. Kapikian AZ, Kim HW, Wyatt RG, et al. Reoviruslike agent in stools: association with infantile diarrhea and development of serologic tests. *Science* 1974;185(156):1049–1053.
367. Kapikian AZ, Simonsen L, Vesikari T, et al. A hexavalent human rotavirus-bovine rotavirus (UK) reassortant vaccine designed for use in developing countries and delivered in a schedule with the potential to eliminate the risk of intussusception. *J Infect Dis* 2005;192(Suppl 1):S22–S29.
368. Kapikian AZ, Wyatt RG, Levine MM, et al. Studies in volunteers with human rotaviruses. *Develop Biol Standard* 1983;53:209–218.
369. Kapikian AZ, Wyatt RG, Levine MM, et al. Oral administration of human rotavirus to volunteers: induction of illness and correlates of resistance. *J Infect Dis* 1983;147(1):95–106.
370. Kattoura MD, Chen X, Patton JT. The rotavirus RNA-binding protein NS35 (NSP2) forms 10S multimers and interacts with the viral RNA polymerase. *Virology* 1994;202(2):803–813.
371. Kawagishi T, Nurdin JA, Onishi M, et al. Reverse genetics system for a human group A rotavirus. *J Virol* 2020;94(2):e00963-19.
372. Keljo DJ, Kuhn M, Smith A. Acidification of endosomes is not important for the entry of rotavirus into the cell. *J Pediatr Gastroenterol Nutr* 1988;7:257–263.
373. Keljo DJ, Smith AK. Characterization of binding of simian rotavirus SA-11 to cultured epithelial cells. *J Pediatr Gastroenterol Nutr* 1988;7:249–256.
374. Kelkar SD, Zade JK. Group B rotaviruses similar to strain CAL-1, have been circulating in Western India since 1993. *Epidemiol Infect* 2004;132(4):745–749.
375. Keswick BH, Pickering LK, DuPont HL, et al. Survival and detection of rotaviruses on environmental surfaces in day care centers. *Appl Environ Microbiol* 1983;46(4):813–816.
376. Kim HJ, Park JG, Matthijnssens J, et al. Intestinal and extra-intestinal pathogenicity of a bovine reassortant rotavirus in calves and piglets. *Vet Microbiol* 2011;152(3–4):291–303.
377. Kim HW, Brandt CD, Kapikian AZ, et al. Human reovirus-like agent infection. Occurrence in adult contacts of pediatric patients with gastroenteritis. *JAMA* 1977;238(5):404–407.
378. Kobayashi S, Negishi Y, Ando N, et al. Two patients with acute rotavirus encephalitis associated with cerebellar signs and symptoms. *Eur J Pediatr* 2010;169(10):1287–1291.
379. Kobayashi T, Antar AA, Boehme KW, et al. A plasmid-based reverse genetics system for animal double-stranded RNA viruses. *Cell Host Microbe* 2007;1(2):147–157.
380. Kohli E, Pothier P, Tosser G, et al. Inhibition of in vitro reconstitution of rotavirus transcriptionally active particles by anti-VP6 monoclonal antibodies. *Arch Virol* 1994;135(1–2):193–200.
381. Kojima K, Taniguchi K, Urasawa T, et al. Sequence analysis of normal and rearranged NSP5 genes from human rotavirus strains isolated in nature: implications for the occurrence of the rearrangement at the step of plus strand synthesis. *Virology* 1996;224(2):446–452.
382. Komoto S, Fukuda S, Ide T, et al. Generation of recombinant rotaviruses expressing fluorescent proteins by using an optimized reverse genetics system. *J Virol* 2018;92(13):e00588-18.
383. Komoto S, Fukuda S, Kugita M, et al. Generation of infectious recombinant human rotaviruses from just 11 cloned cDNAs encoding the rotavirus genome. *J Virol* 2019; 93(8):e02207-18.
384. Komoto S, Fukuda S, Murata T, et al. Reverse genetics system for human rotaviruses. *Microbiol Immunol* 2020;64(6):401–406.
385. Komoto S, Kanai Y, Fukuda S, et al. Reverse genetics system demonstrates that rotavirus nonstructural protein NSP6 is not essential for viral replication in cell culture. *J Virol* 2017;91(21):e00695-17.
386. Komoto S, Sasaki J, Taniguchi K. Reverse genetics system for introduction of site-specific mutations into the double-stranded RNA genome of infectious rotavirus. *Proc Natl Acad Sci USA* 2006;103(12):4646–4651.
387. Konno T, Suzuki H, Katsushima N, et al. Influence of temperature and relative humidity on human rotavirus infection in Japan. *J Infect Dis* 1983;147(1):125–128.
388. Konno T, Suzuki H, Kutsuzawa T, et al. Human rotavirus infection in infants and young children with intussusception. *J Med Virol* 1978;2:265–269.
389. Kordasti S, Sjövall H, Lundgren O, et al. Serotonin and vasoactive intestinal peptide antagonists attenuate rotavirus diarrhoea. *Gut* 2004;53:952–957.
390. Koroglu M, Yakupogullari Y, Otlu B, et al. A waterborne outbreak of epidemic diarrhea due to group A rotavirus in Malatya, Turkey. *New Microbiol* 2011;34(1):17–24.
391. Kotloff KL, Nasrin D, Blackwelder WC, et al. The incidence, aetiology, and adverse clinical consequences of less severe diarrhoeal episodes among infants and children residing in low-income and middle-income countries: a 12-month case–control study as a follow-on to the Global Enteric Multicenter Study (GEMS). *Lancet Glob Health* 2019;7(5):e568–e584.
392. Kotloff KL, Nataro JP, Blackwelder WC, et al. Burden and aetiology of diarrhoeal disease in infants and young children in developing countries (the Global Enteric Multicenter Study, GEMS): a prospective, case–control study. *Lancet* 2013;382(9888):209–222.
393. Kozak M. Structural features in eukaryotic mRNAs that modulate the initiation of translation. *J Biol Chem* 1991;266(30):19867–19870.
394. Kuklin NA, Rott L, Feng N, et al. Protective intestinal anti-rotavirus B cell immunity is dependent on alpha 4 beta 7 integrin expression but does not require IgA antibody production. *J Immunol* 2001;166(3):1894–1902.
395. Kumar A, Vlasova AN, Deblais L, et al. Impact of nutrition and rotavirus infection on the infant gut microbiota in a humanized pig model. *BMC Gastroenterol* 2018;18(1):93.
396. Kumar D, Yu X, Crawford SE, et al. 2.7 A cryo-EM structure of rotavirus core protein VP3, a unique capping machine with a helicase activity. *Sci Adv* 2020;6(16):eaay6410.
397. Kumar M, Jayaram H, Vasquez-Del Carpio R, et al. Crystallographic and biochemical analysis of rotavirus NSP2 with nucleotides reveals a nucleoside diphosphate kinase-like activity. *J Virol* 2007;81(22):12272–12284.
398. Kumar P, Shukla RS, Patel A, et al. Formulation development of a live attenuated human rotavirus (RV3-BB) vaccine candidate for use in low- and middle-income countries. *Hum Vaccin Immunother* 2021;17(7):2298–2310.
399. Labbe M, Baudoux P, Charpilienne A, et al. Identification of the nucleic acid binding domain of the rotavirus VP2 protein. *J Gen Virol* 1994;75:3423–3430.
400. Lawton JA, Estes MK, Prasad BV. Comparative structural analysis of transcriptionally competent and incompetent rotavirus-antibody complexes. *Proc Natl Acad Sci U S A* 1999;96(10):5428–5433.
401. Lawton JA, Estes MK, Prasad BV. Mechanism of genome transcription in segmented dsRNA viruses. *Adv Virus Res* 2000;55:185–229.
402. Lawton JA, Estes MK, Prasad BVV. Three-dimensional visualization of mRNA release from actively transcribing rotavirus particles. *Nature Struct Biol* 1997;4(2):118–121.
403. Lawton JA, Zeng CQ, Mukherjee SK, et al. Three-dimensional structural analysis of recombinant rotavirus-like particles with intact and amino-terminal-deleted VP2: implications for the architecture of the VP2 capsid layer. *J Virol* 1997;71(10):7353–7360.
404. Leshem E, Lopman B, Glass R, et al. Distribution of rotavirus strains and strain-specific effectiveness of the rotavirus vaccine after its introduction: a systematic review and meta-analysis. *Lancet Infect Dis* 2014;14(9):847–856.
405. Levy K, Hubbard AE, Eisenberg JN. Seasonality of rotavirus disease in the tropics: a systematic review and meta-analysis. *Int J Epidemiol* 2009;38(6):1487–1496.
406. Li B, Ding S, Feng N, et al. Drebrin restricts rotavirus entry by inhibiting dynamin-mediated endocytosis. *Proc Natl Acad Sci U S A* 2017;114(18):E3642–E3651.
407. Li C, Lam E, Perez-Shibayama C, et al. Early-life programming of mesenteric lymph node stromal cell identity by the lymphotoxin pathway regulates adult mucosal immunity. *Sci Immunol* 2019;4(42):eaax1027.
408. Li J, Zhang Y, Yang Y, et al. Effectiveness of Lanzhou lamb rotavirus vaccine in preventing gastroenteritis among children younger than 5 years of age. *Vaccine* 2019;37(27):3611–3616.
409. Li W, Manktelow E, von Kirchbach JC, et al. Genomic analysis of codon, sequence and structural conservation with selective biochemical-structure mapping reveals highly conserved and dynamic structures in rotavirus RNAs with potential cis-acting functions. *Nucleic Acids Res* 2010;38(21):7718–7735.
410. Li Y, Yu P, Qu C, et al. MDA5 against enteric viruses through induction of interferon-like response partially via the JAK-STAT cascade. *Antiviral Res* 2020;176:104743.
411. Li Z, Baker ML, Jiang W, et al. Rotavirus architecture at subnanometer resolution. *J Virol* 2009;83(4):1754–1766.
412. Liakopoulou E, Mutton K, Carrington D, et al. Rotavirus as a significant cause of prolonged diarrhoeal illness and morbidity following allogeneic bone marrow transplantation. *Bone Marrow Transplant* 2005;36(8):691–694.
413. Liemann S, Chandran K, Baker TS, et al. Structure of the reovirus membrane-penetration protein, Mu1, in a complex with is protector protein, Sigma3. *Cell* 2002;108(2):283–295.
414. Lin JD, Feng N, Sen A, et al. Distinct roles of type I and type III interferons in intestinal immunity to homologous and heterologous rotavirus infections. *PLoS Pathog* 2016;12(4):e1005600.
415. Linhares AC, Pinheiro FP, Freitas RB, et al. An outbreak of rotavirus diarrhea among a non-immune isolated South American Indian community. *Am J Epidemiol* 1981;113(6):703–710.
416. Linhares AC, Velazquez FR, Perez-Schael I, et al. Efficacy and safety of an oral live attenuated human rotavirus vaccine against rotavirus gastroenteritis during the first 2 years of life in Latin American infants: a randomised, double-blind, placebo-controlled phase III study. *Lancet* 2008;371(9619):1181–1189.
417. Liu LJ, Liu W, Liu YX, et al. Identification of norovirus as the top enteric viruses detected in adult cases with acute gastroenteritis. *Am J Trop Med Hyg* 2010;82(4):717–722.
418. Liu M, Offit PA, Estes MK. Identification of the simian rotavirus SA11 genome segment 3 product. *Virology* 1988;163:26–32.
419. Liu Y, Huang P, Tan M, et al. Rotavirus VP8*: phylogeny, host range, and interaction with histo-blood group antigens. *J Virol* 2012;86(18):9899–9910.
420. Lloyd MB, Lloyd JC, Gesteland PH, et al. Rotavirus gastroenteritis and seizures in young children. *Pediatr Neurol* 2010;42(6):404–408.
421. Lopez S, Arias CF. Multistep entry of rotavirus into cells: a Versaillesque dance. *Trends Microbiol* 2004;12(6):271–278.
422. Lopez T, Camacho M, Zayas M, et al. Silencing the morphogenesis of rotavirus. *J Virol* 2005;79(1):184–192.
423. Lopez T, Lopez S, Arias CF. Heat shock enhances the susceptibility of BHK cells to rotavirus infection through the facilitation of entry and post-entry virus replication steps. *Virus Res* 2006;121(1):74–83.
424. Lopez T, Rojas M, Ayala-Breton C, et al. Reduced expression of the rotavirus NSP5 gene has a pleiotropic effect on virus replication. *J Gen Virol* 2005;86(Pt 6):1609–1617.
425. Lopez T, Silva-Ayala D, Lopez S, et al. Replication of the rotavirus genome requires an active ubiquitin-proteasome system. *J Virol* 2011;85(22):11964–11971.
426. Lopman BA, Pitzer VE, Sarkar R, et al. Understanding reduced rotavirus vaccine efficacy in low socio-economic settings. *PLoS One* 2012;7(8):e41720.
427. Losonsky GA, Rennels MB, Lim Y, et al. Systemic and mucosal immune responses to rhesus rotavirus vaccine MMU 18006. *Pediatr Infect Dis J* 1988;7(6):388–393.
428. Losonsky GA, Reymann M. The immune response in primary asymptomatic and symptomatic rotavirus infection in newborn infants. *J Infect Dis* 1990;161(2):330–332.
429. Lu X, McDonald SM, Tortorici MA, et al. Mechanism for coordinated RNA packaging and genome replication by rotavirus polymerase VP1. *Structure* 2008;16(11):1678–1688.
430. Ludert JE, Michelangeli F, Gil F, et al. Penetration and uncoating of rotaviruses in cultured cells. *Intervirology* 1987;27:95–101.
431. Lundgren O, Peregrin AT, Persson K, et al. Role of the enteric nervous system in the fluid and electrolyte secretion of rotavirus diarrhea. *Science* 2000;287(5452):491–495.
432. Lundgren O, Svensson L. The enteric nervous system and infectious diarrhea. In: Desselberger U, Gray J, eds. *Viral Gastroenteritis*. Amsterdam: Elsevier Science; 2003:51–68.
433. Lutz LM, Pace CR, Arnold MM. Rotavirus NSP1 associates with components of the cullin RING ligase family of E3 ubiquitin ligases. *J Virol* 2016;90(13):6036–6048.
434. Mackow ER. Group B and C rotaviruses. In: Blaser MJ, Smith PD, Ravdin JI, eds. *Infections of the Gastrointestinal Tract*. New York: Raven Press, Ltd.; 1995:983–1008, Chapt. 65.
435. Madhi SA, Cunliffe NA, Steele D, et al. Effect of human rotavirus vaccine on severe diarrhea in African infants. *N Engl J Med* 2010;362(4):289–298.

436. Maffey L, Vega CG, Mino S, et al. Anti-VP6 VHH: an experimental treatment for rotavirus A-associated disease. *PLoS One* 2016;11(9):e0162351.
437. Malherbe H, Harwin R. The cytopathic effects of vervet monkey viruses. *S A Med J* 1963;37:407–411.
438. Malherbe HH, Strickland-Cholmley M. Simian virus SA11 and the related O agent. *Arch Ges Virusforsch* 1967;22(1):235–245.
439. Marionneau S, Cailleau-Thomas A, Rocher J, et al. ABH and Lewis histo-blood group antigens, a model for the meaning of oligosaccharide diversity in the face of a changing world. *Biochimie* 2001;83(7):565–573.
440. Martella V, Banyai K, Matthijnssens J, et al. Zoonotic aspects of rotaviruses. *Vet Microbiol* 2010;140(3–4):246–255.
441. Martin D, Duarte M, Lepault J, et al. Sequestration of free tubulin molecules by the viral protein NSP2 induces microtubule depolymerization during rotavirus infection. *J Virol* 2010;84(5):2522–2532.
442. Martin D, Ouldali M, Menetrey J, et al. Structural organisation of the rotavirus nonstructural protein NSP5. *J Mol Biol* 2011;413(1):209–221.
443. Mason BB, Graham DY, Estes MK. Biochemical mapping of the simian rotavirus SA11 genome. *J Virol* 1983;46(2):413–423.
444. Mata L, Simhom A, Urrutia J. Diseases and disabilities In: Scrimshaw NS, ed. *The Children of Santa Maria Cauque: A Prospective Field Study of Health and Growth.* Cambridge, MA: MIT Press; 1983:254–292.
445. Mathieu M, Petitpas I, Navaza J, et al. Atomic structure of the major capsid protein of rotavirus: implications for the architecture of the virion. *EMBO J* 2001;20(7):1485–1497.
446. Matson DO, O'Ryan ML, Herrera I, et al. Fecal antibody responses to symptomatic and asymptomatic rotavirus infections. *J Infect Dis* 1993;167:577–583.
447. Matsui SM, Offit PA, Vo PT, et al. Passive protection against rotavirus-induced diarrhea by monoclonal antibodies to the heterotypic neutralization domain of VP7 and the VP8 fragment of VP4. *J Clin Microbiol* 1989;27(4):780–782.
448. Matthijnssens J. Rotavirus Classification Working Group: RCWG. https://rega.kuleuven.be/cev/viralmetagenomics/virus-classification/rcwg
449. Matthijnssens J, Ciarlet M, Heiman E, et al. Full genome-based classification of rotaviruses reveals a common origin between human Wa-like and porcine rotavirus strains and human DS-1-like and bovine rotavirus strains. *J Virol* 2008;82(7):3204–3219.
450. Matthijnssens J, Ciarlet M, McDonald SM, et al. Uniformity of rotavirus strain nomenclature proposed by the Rotavirus Classification Working Group (RCWG). *Arch Virol* 2011;156(8):1397–1413.
451. Matthijnssens J, Heylen E, Zeller M, et al. Phylodynamic analyses of rotavirus genotypes G9 and G12 underscore their potential for swift global spread. *Mol Biol Evol* 2010;27(10):2431–2436.
452. Matthijnssens J, Otto PH, Ciarlet M, et al. VP6-sequence-based cutoff values as a criterion for rotavirus species demarcation. *Arch Virol* 2012;157(6):1177–1182.
453. Matthijnssens J, Rahman M, Martella V, et al. Full genomic analysis of human rotavirus strain B4106 and lapine rotavirus strain 30/96 provides evidence for interspecies transmission. *J Virol* 2006;80(8):3801–3810.
454. Mattion NM, Cohen J, Estes MK, et al. The rotavirus proteins. In: Kapikian AZ, ed. *Viral Infections of the Gastrointestinal Tract.* 2nd ed. New York: Marcel Dekker, Inc.; 1994: 169–249.
455. Mattion NM, Mitchell DB, Both GW, et al. Expression of rotavirus proteins encoded by alternative open reading frames of genome segment 11. *Virology* 1991;181:295–304.
456. McClain B, Settembre E, Temple BR, et al. X-ray crystal structure of the rotavirus inner capsid particle at 3.8 A resolution. *J Mol Biol* 2010;397(2):587–599.
457. McCrae MA, Faulkner-Valle GP. Molecular biology of rotaviruses. I. Characterization of basic growth parameters and pattern of macromolecular synthesis. *J Virol* 1981;39: 490–496.
458. McCrae MA, McCorquodale JG. Molecular biology of rotaviruses. V. Terminal structure of viral RNA species. *Virology* 1983;126:204–212.
459. McDonald SM, Patton JT. Rotavirus VP2 core shell regions critical for viral polymerase activation. *J Virol* 2011;85(7):3095–3105.
460. McNeal MM, Barone KS, Rae MN, et al. Effector functions of antibody and CD8+ cells in resolution of rotavirus infection and protection against reinfection in mice. *Virology* 1995;214(2):387–397.
461. McNeal MM, Broome RL, Ward RL. Active immunity against rotavirus infection in mice is correlated with viral replication and titers of serum rotavirus IgA following vaccination. *Virology* 1994;204(2):642–650.
462. Mebus C, Underdahl N, Rhodes M, et al. Calf diarrhea (scours): reproduced with a virus from a field outbreak. *Res Bull* 1969;233(March 1969):1–16.
463. Mebus CA, Kono M, Underdahl NR, et al. Cell culture propagation of neonatal calf diarrhea (scours) virus. *Can Vet J* 1971;12(3):69–72.
464. Medici MC, Abelli LA, Guerra P, et al. Case report: detection of rotavirus RNA in the cerebrospinal fluid of a child with rotavirus gastroenteritis and meningism. *J Med Virol* 2011;83(9):1637–1640.
465. Meyer JC, Bergmann CC, Bellamy AR. Interaction of rotavirus cores with the nonstructural glycoprotein NS28. *Virology* 1989;171:98–107.
466. Michelangeli F, Liprandi F, Chemello ME, et al. Selective depletion of stored calcium by thapsigargin blocks rotavirus maturation but not the cytopathic effect. *J Virol* 1995; 69(6):3838–3847.
467. Michelangeli F, Ruiz MC, Del Castillo JR, et al. Effect of rotavirus infection on intracellular calcium homeostasis in cultured cells. *Virology* 1991;181:520–527.
468. Midthun K, Greenberg HB, Hoshino Y, et al. Reassortant rotaviruses as potential live rotavirus vaccine candidates. *J Virol* 1985;53(3):949–954.
469. Midthun K, Hoshino Y, Kapikian AZ, et al. Single gene substitution rotavirus reassortants containing the major neutralization protein (VP7) of human rotavirus serotype 4. *J Clin Microbiol* 1986;24(5):822–826.
470. Midthun K, Kapikian AZ. Rotavirus vaccines: an overview. *Clin Microbiol Rev* 1995;9(3):423–434.
471. Mihalov-Kovacs E, Gellert A, Marton S, et al. Candidate new rotavirus species in sheltered dogs. Hungary. *Emerg Infect Dis* 2015;21(4):660–663.
472. Mirazimi A, Nilsson M, Svensson L. The molecular chaperone calnexin interacts with the NSP4 enterotoxin of rotavirus in vivo and in vitro. *J Virol* 1998;72(11):8705–8709.
473. Moe K, Shirley JA. The effects of relative humidity and temperature on the survival of human rotavirus in faeces. *Arch Virol* 1982;72:179–186.
474. Monnier N, Higo-Moriguchi K, Sun ZYJ, et al. High-resolution molecular and antigen structure of the VP8*core of a sialic acid-independent human rotavirus strain. *J Virol* 2006;80(3):1513–1523.
475. Montero H, Rojas M, Arias CF, et al. Rotavirus infection induces the phosphorylation of eIF2alpha but prevents the formation of stress granules. *J Virol* 2008;82(3):1496–1504.
476. Moon SS, Wang Y, Shane AL, et al. Inhibitory effect of breast milk on infectivity of live oral rotavirus vaccines. *Pediatr Infect Dis J* 2010;29(10):919–923.
477. Morelli M, Dennis AF, Patton JT. Putative E3 ubiquitin ligase of human rotavirus inhibits NF-kappaB activation by using molecular mimicry to target beta-TrCP. *mBio* 2015;6(1).
478. Mossel EC, Ramig RF. Rotavirus genome segment 7 (NSP3) is a determinant of extraintestinal spread in the neonatal mouse. *J Virol* 2002;76(13):6502–6509.
479. Mukhopadhya I, Sarkar R, Menon VK, et al. Rotavirus shedding in symptomatic and asymptomatic children using reverse transcription-quantitative PCR. *J Med Virol* 2013;85(9):1661–1668.
480. Mulcahy DL, Kamath KR, de Silva LM, et al. A two-part study of the aetiological role of rotavirus in intussusception. *J Med Virol* 1982;9:51–55.
481. Murakami Y, Nishioka N, Watanabe T, et al. Prolonged excretion and failure of cross-protection between distinct serotypes of bovine rotavirus. *Vet Microbiol* 1986;12:7–14.
482. Murphy TV, Gargiullo PM, Massoudi MS, et al. Intussusception among infants given an oral rotavirus vaccine. *N Engl J Med* 2001;344(8):564–572.
483. Murphy TV, Smith PJ, Gargiullo PM, et al. The first rotavirus vaccine and intussusception: epidemiological studies and policy decisions. *JID* 2003;187:1309–1313.
484. Musalem C, Espejo RT. Release of progeny virus from cells infected with simian rotavirus SA11. *J Gen Virol* 1985;66:2715–2724.
485. Nair N, Feng N, Blum LK, et al. VP4- and VP7-specific antibodies mediate heterotypic immunity to rotavirus in humans. *Sci Transl Med* 2017;9(395):eaam5434.
486. Nakagomi O, Nakagomi T. Genetic diversity and similarity among mammalian rotaviruses in relation to interspecies transmission of rotavirus. *Arch Virol* 1991;120:43–55.
487. Nakagomi O, Nakagomi T. Interspecies transmission of rotaviruses studied from the perspective of genogroup. *Microbiol Immunol* 1993;37:337–348.
488. Nakagomi O, Nakagomi T. Molecular epidemiology of human rotaviruses: genogrouping by RNA-RNA hybridization. *Arch Virol Suppl* 1996;12:93–98.
489. Nakagomi T. Rotavirus infection and intussusception: a view from retrospect. Minireview. *Microbiol Immunol* 2000;44:619–628.
490. Nakata S, Estes MK, Graham DY, et al. Antigenic characterization and ELISA detection of adult diarrhea rotaviruses. *J Infect Dis* 1986;154(3):448–455.
491. Nakawesi J, Konjit GM, Dasoveanu DC, et al. Rotavirus infection causes mesenteric lymph node hypertrophy independently of type I interferon or TNF-alpha in mice. *Eur J Immunol* 2021;51(5):1143–1152.
492. Nakawesi J, This S, Hutter J, et al. alphavbeta8 integrin-expression by BATF3-dependent dendritic cells facilitates early IgA responses to Rotavirus. *Mucosal Immunol* 2021;14(1):53–67.
493. Nandi P, Charpilienne A, Cohen J. Interaction of rotavirus particles with liposomes. *J Virol* 1992;66(6):3363–3367.
494. Narvaez CF, Feng N, Vasquez C, et al. Human rotavirus-specific IgM Memory B cells have differential cloning efficiencies and switch capacities and play a role in antiviral immunity in vivo. *J Virol* 2012;86(19):10829–10840.
495. Nava P, Lopez S, Arias CF, et al. The rotavirus surface protein VP8 modulates the gate and fence function of tight junctions in epithelial cells. *J Cell Sci* 2004;117(23):5509–5519.
496. Newburg D, Peterson J, Ruiz-Palacios G, et al. Role of human-milk lactadherin in protection against symptomatic rotavirus infection. *Lancet* 1998;351:1160–1164.
497. Nicolas JC, Ingrand D, Fortier B, et al. A one-year virological survey of acute intussusception in childhood. *J Med Virol* 1982;9:267–271.
498. Novikova NA, Sashina TA, Epifanova NV, et al. Long-term monitoring of G1P[8] rotaviruses circulating without vaccine pressure in Nizhny Novgorod, Russia, 1984–2019. *Arch Virol* 2020;165(4):865–875.
499. O'Neal CM, Clements JD, Estes MK, et al. Rotavirus 2/6 viruslike particles administered intranasally with cholera toxin, *Escherichia coli* heat-labile toxin (LT), and LT-R192G induce protection from rotavirus challenge. *J Virol* 1998;72(4):3390–3393.
500. O'Ryan M. The ever-changing landscape of rotavirus serotypes. *Pediatr Infect Dis J* 2009;28(3 Suppl):S60–S62.
501. O'Ryan M, Linhares AC. Update on Rotarix: an oral human rotavirus vaccine. *Expert Rev Vaccines* 2009;8(12):1627–1641.
502. O'Ryan ML, Matson DO, Estes MK, et al. Anti-rotavirus G type-specific and isotype-specific antibodies in children with natural rotavirus infections. *J Infect Dis* 1994;169(3):504–511.
503. Obert G, Peiffer I, Servin AL. Rotavirus-induced structural and functional alterations in tight junctions of polarized intestinal Caco-2 cell monolayers. *J Virol* 2000;74(10):4645–4651.
504. Ofei SY, Fuchs GJ III. Principles and practice of oral rehydration. *Curr Gastroenterol Rep* 2019;21(12):67.
505. Offit PA. Rotaviruses: immunologic determinants of protection against infection and disease. *Adv Virus Res* 1994;44:161–202.
506. Offit PA, Blavat G, Greenberg HB, et al. Molecular basis of rotavirus virulence: role of gene segment 4. *J Virol* 1986;57(1):46–49.
507. Offit PA, Clark HF. Protection against rotavirus-induced gastroenteritis in a murine model by passively acquired gastrointestinal but not circulating antibodies. *J Virol* 1985;54(1): 58–64.
508. Oldham G, Bridger JC, Howard CJ, et al. In vivo role of lymphocyte subpopulations in the control of virus excretion and mucosal antibody responses of cattle infected with rotavirus. *J Virol* 1993;67(8):5012–5019.
509. Orrico-Sanchez A, Lopez-Lacort M, Munoz-Quiles C, et al. Lack of impact of rotavirus vaccines on seizure-related hospitalizations in children under 5 years old in Spain. *Hum Vaccin Immunother* 2018;14(6):1534–1538.

510. Osborne MP, Haddon SJ, Spencer AJ, et al. An electron microscopic investigation of time-related changes in the intestine of neonatal mice infected with murine rotavirus. *J Pediatr Gastroenterol Nutr* 1988;7(2):236–248.

511. Oseto M, Yamashita Y, Hattori M, et al. Successful propagation of human group C rotavirus in a continuous cell line and characterization of the isolated virus. *Abstracts of 27th Joint Viral Diseases Meeting of the US-Japan Cooperative Medical Sciences Program* 1993:46.

512. Padilla-Noriega L, Paniagua M, Guzman-Leon S. Rotavirus protein NSP3 shuts off host cell protein synthesis. *Virology* 2002;298(1):1–7.

513. Papa G, Venditti L, Arnoldi F, et al. Recombinant rotaviruses rescued by reverse genetics reveal the role of NSP5 hyperphosphorylation in the assembly of viral factories. *J Virol* 2019;94(1).

514. Parashar U, Bresee J, Gentsch J, et al. Rotavirus. *Emerg Infect Dis* 1998;4(4):561–570.

515. Parker EP, Ramani S, Lopman BA, et al. Causes of impaired oral vaccine efficacy in developing countries. *Future Microbiol* 2018;13:97–118.

516. Patel M, Rench MA, Boom JA, et al. Detection of rotavirus antigenemia in routinely obtained serum specimens to augment surveillance and vaccine effectiveness evaluations. *Pediatr Infect Dis J* 2010;29(9):836–839.

517. Patel MM, Lopez-Collada VR, Bulhoes MM, et al. Intussusception risk and health benefits of rotavirus vaccination in Mexico and Brazil. *N Engl J Med* 2011;364(24):2283–2292.

518. Patel MM, Parashar UD. Assessing the effectiveness and public health impact of rotavirus vaccines after introduction in immunization programs. *J Infect Dis* 2009;200(Suppl 1):S291–S299.

519. Patel NC, Hertel PM, Estes MK, et al. Vaccine-acquired rotavirus in infants with severe combined immunodeficiency. *N Engl J Med* 2010;362(4):314–319.

520. Patton JT. Synthesis of simian rotavirus SA11 double-stranded RNA in a cell-free system. *Virus Res* 1986;6(3):217 233.

521. Patton JT, Carpi RVD, Spencer E. Replication and transcription of the rotavirus genome. *Curr Pharm Des* 2004;10(30):3769–3777.

522. Patton JT, Jones MT, Kalbach AN, et al. Rotavirus RNA polymerase requires the core shell protein to synthesize the double-stranded RNA genome. *J Virol* 1997;71(12):9618 9626.

523. Patton JT, Spencer E. Genome replication and packaging of segmented double-stranded RNA viruses. *Virology* 2000;277(2):217–225.

524. Patton JT, Wentz M, Xiaobo J, et al. Cis-acting signals that promote genome replication in rotavirus mRNA. *J Virol* 1996;70(6):3961–3971.

525. Paul PS, Lyoo YS. Immunogens of rotaviruses. *Vet Microbiol* 1993;37(3–4):299–317.

526. Paulke-Korinek M, Kundi M, Rendi-Wagner P, et al. Herd immunity after two years of the universal mass vaccination program against rotavirus gastroenteritis in Austria. *Vaccine* 2011;29(15):2791–2796.

527. Payne DC, Baggs J, Zerr DM, et al. Protective association between rotavirus vaccination and childhood seizures in the year following vaccination in US children. *Clin Infect Dis* 2014;58(2):173–177.

528. Payne DC, Currier RL, Staat MA, et al. Epidemiologic association between FUT2 secretor status and severe rotavirus gastroenteritis in children in the United States. *JAMA Pediatr* 2015;169(11):1040–1045.

529. Peigue-Lafeuille H, Henquell C, Chambon M, et al. Nosocomial rotavirus infections in adult renal transplant recipients. *J Hosp Infect* 1991;18(1):67–70.

530. Perez-Schael I, Guntinas MJ, Perez M, et al. Efficacy of the rhesus rotavirus-based quadrivalent vaccine in infants and young children in Venezuela. *N Engl J Med* 1997;337(17):1181–1187.

531. Perez-Vargas J, Romero P, Lopez S, et al. The peptide-binding and ATPase domains of recombinant hsc70 are required to interact with rotavirus and reduce its infectivity. *J Virol* 2006;80(7):3322–3331.

532. Perrett KP, Jachno K, Nolan TM, et al. Association of rotavirus vaccination with the incidence of type 1 diabetes in children. *JAMA Pediatr* 2019;173(3):280–282.

533. Pervolaraki K, Stanifer ML, Munchau S, et al. Type I and type III interferons display different dependency on mitogen-activated protein kinases to mount an antiviral state in the human gut. *Front Immunol* 2017;8:459.

534. Pesavento JB, Crawford SE, Roberts E, et al. pH-induced conformational change of the rotavirus VP4 spike: implications for cell entry and antibody neutralization. *J Virol* 2005;79(13):8572–8580.

535. Petrie BL, Compans RW, Bishop DHL. Biologic activity of rotavirus particles lacking glycosylated proteins. In: *Double-Stranded RNA Viruses*. New York: Elsevier; 1983:146–156.

536. Petrie BL, Graham DY, Estes MK. Identification of rotavirus particle types. *Intervirology* 1981;16:20–28.

537. Petrie BL, Graham DY, Hanssen H, et al. Localization of rotavirus antigens in infected cells by ultrastructural immunocytochemistry. *J Gen Virol* 1982;63:457–467.

538. Petrie BL, Greenberg HB, Graham DY, et al. Ultrastructural localization of rotavirus antigens using colloidal gold. *Virus Res* 1984;1:133–152.

539. Pham T, Perry JL, Dosey TL, et al. The rotavirus NSP4 viroporin domain is a calcium-conducting ion channel. *Sci Rep* 2017;7:43487.

540. Philip AA, Patton JT. Expression of separate heterologous proteins from the rotavirus NSP3 genome segment using a translational 2A stop-restart element. *J Virol* 2020;94(18):e00959-20.

541. Philip AA, Perry JL, Eaton HE, et al. Generation of recombinant rotavirus expressing NSP3-UnaG fusion protein by a simplified reverse genetics system. *J Virol* 2019;93(24).

542. Phua KB, Quak SH, Lee BW, et al. Evaluation of RIX4414, a live, attenuated rotavirus vaccine, in a randomized, double-blind, placebo-controlled phase 2 trial involving 2464 Singaporean infants. *J Infect Dis* 2005;192(Suppl 1):S6–S16.

543. Pickering LK, Bartlett AV, Reves RR, et al. Asymptomatic excretion of rotavirus before and after rotavirus diarrhea in children in day care centers. *J Pediatr* 1988;112:361–365.

544. Piron M, Delaunay T, Grosclaude J, et al. Identification of the RNA-binding, dimerization, and eIF4GI-binding domains of rotavirus nonstructural protein NSP3. *J Virol* 1999;73(7):5411–5421.

545. Piron M, Vende P, Cohen J, et al. Rotavirus RNA-binding protein NSP3 interacts with eIF4GI and evicts the poly(A) binding protein from eIF4F. *EMBO J* 1998;17(19):5811–5821.

546. Pitzer VE, Viboud C, Simonsen L, et al. Demographic variability, vaccination, and the spatiotemporal dynamics of rotavirus epidemics. *Science* 2009;325(5938):290–294.

547. Platts-Mills JA, Babji S, Bodhidatta L, et al. Pathogen-specific burdens of community diarrhoea in developing countries: a multisite birth cohort study (MAL-ED). *Lancet Glob Health* 2015;3(9):e564–e575.

548. Platts-Mills JA, Liu J, Rogawski ET, et al. Use of quantitative molecular diagnostic methods to assess the aetiology, burden, and clinical characteristics of diarrhoea in children in low-resource settings: a reanalysis of the MAL-ED cohort study. *Lancet Glob Health* 2018;6(12):e1309–e1318.

549. Poncet D, Lindenbaum P, L'Haridon R, et al. In vivo and in vitro phosphorylation of rotavirus NSP5 correlates with its localization in viroplasms. *J Virol* 1997;71(1):34–41.

550. Poruchynsky MS, Maass DR, Atkinson PH. Calcium depletion blocks the maturation of rotavirus by altering the oligomerization of virus-encoded proteins in the ER. *J Cell Biol* 1991;114:651–661.

551. Pott J, Mahlakoiv T, Mordstein M, et al. IFN-lambda determines the intestinal epithelial antiviral host defense. *Proc Natl Acad Sci U S A* 2011;108(19):7944–7949.

552. Pott J, Stockinger S, Torow N, et al. Age-dependent TLR3 expression of the intestinal epithelium contributes to rotavirus susceptibility. *PLoS Pathog* 2012;8(5):e1002670.

553. Prasad BV, Crawford S, Lawton JA, et al. Structural studies on gastroenteritis viruses. *Novartis Found Symp* 2001;238:26–37; discussion 37–46.

554. Prasad BV, Rothnagel R, Zeng CQ, et al. Visualization of ordered genomic RNA and localization of transcriptional complexes in rotavirus. *Nature* 1996;382(6590):471–473.

555. Prasad BV, Wang GJ, Clerx JP, et al. Three-dimensional structure of rotavirus. *J Mol Biol* 1988;199(2):269–275.

556. Prasad BVV, Burns JW, Marietta E, et al. Localization of VP4 neutralization sites in rotavirus by three-dimensional cryo-electron microscopy. *Nature* 1990;343(6257):476–479.

557. Pretorius JM, Huismans H, Theron J. Establishment of an entirely plasmid-based reverse genetics system for Bluetongue virus. *Virology* 2015;486:71–77.

558. Quintanar-Solares M, Yen C, Richardson V, et al. Impact of rotavirus vaccination on diarrhea-related hospitalizations among children < 5 years of age in Mexico. *Pediatr Infect Dis J* 2011;30(1 Suppl):S11–S15.

559. Rakau KG, Nyaga MM, Gededzha MP, et al. Genetic characterization of G12P[6] and G12P[8] rotavirus strains collected in six African countries between 2010 and 2014. *BMC Infect Dis* 2021;21(1):107.

560. Ramani S, Crawford SE, Blutt SE, et al. Human organoid cultures: transformative new tools for human virus studies. *Curr Opin Virol* 2018;29:79–86.

561. Ramani S, Hu L, Venkataram Prasad BV, et al. Diversity in rotavirus-host glycan interactions: a "sweet" spectrum. *Cell Mol Gastroenterol Hepatol* 2016;2(3):263–273.

562. Ramani S, Kang G. Burden of disease & molecular epidemiology of group A rotavirus infections in India. *Indian J Med Res* 2007;125(5):619–632.

563. Ramani S, Paul A, Saravanabavan A, et al. Rotavirus antigenemia in Indian children with rotavirus gastroenteritis and asymptomatic infections. *Clin Infect Dis* 2010;51(11):1284–1289.

564. Ramani S, Sankaran P, Arumugam R, et al. Comparison of viral load and duration of virus shedding in symptomatic and asymptomatic neonatal rotavirus infections. *J Med Virol* 2010;82(10):1803–1807.

565. Ramig RF. Isolation and genetic characterization of temperature-sensitive mutants of simian rotavirus SA11. *Virology* 1982;120:93–105.

566. Ramig RF. Isolation and genetic characterization of temperature-sensitive mutants that define five additional recombination groups in simian rotavirus SA11. *Virology* 1983;130:464–473.

567. Ramig RF. Pathogenesis of intestinal and systemic rotavirus infection. *J Virol* 2004;78(19):10213–10220.

568. Realpe M, Espinosa R, Lopez S, et al. Rotaviruses require basolateral molecules for efficient infection of polarized MDCKII cells. *Virus Res* 2010;147(2):231–241.

569. Reinisch KM, Nibert ML, Harrison SC. Structure of the reovirus core at 3.6 A resolution. *Nature* 2000;404(6781):960–967.

570. Ren L, Ding S, Song Y, et al. Profiling of rotavirus 3'UTR-binding proteins reveals the ATP synthase subunit ATP5B as a host factor that supports late-stage virus replication. *J Biol Chem* 2019;294(15):5993–6006.

571. Rennels MB, Losonsky GA, Young AE, et al. An efficacy trial of the rhesus rotavirus vaccine in Maryland. The Clinical Study Group. *Am J Dis Child* 1990;144(5):601–604.

572. Resch TK, Wang Y, Moon S, et al. Serial passaging of the human rotavirus CDC-9 strain in cell culture leads to attenuation: characterization from in vitro and in vivo studies. *J Virol* 2020;94(15).

573. Rey LM, Gil JA, Mateus J, et al. LAP(+) cells modulate protection induced by oral vaccination with rhesus rotavirus in a neonatal mouse model. *J Virol* 2019;93(19):e00882-19.

574. Richardson SC, Grimwood K, Gorrell R, et al. Extended excretion of rotavirus after severe diarrhoea in young children. *Lancet* 1998;351(9119):1844–1848.

575. Richardson SC, Mercer LE, Sonza S, et al. Intracellular localization of rotaviral proteins. *Arch Virol* 1986;88:251–264.

576. Richardson V, Hernandez-Pichardo J, Quintanar-Solares M, et al. Effect of rotavirus vaccination on death from childhood diarrhea in Mexico. *N Engl J Med* 2010;362(4):299–305.

577. Robinson CG, Hernanz-Schulman M, Zhu Y, et al. Evaluation of anatomic changes in young children with natural rotavirus infection: is intussusception biologically plausible? *J Infect Dis* 2004;189:1382–1387.

578. Rodger SM, Bishop RF, Birch C, et al. Molecular epidemiology of human rotaviruses in Melbourne, Australia, from 1973 to 1979, as determined by electrophoresis of genome ribonucleic acid. *J Clin Microbiol* 1981;13(2):272–278.

579. Rodriguez WJ, Kim HW, Arrobio JO, et al. Clinical features of acute gastroenteritis associated with human reovirus-like agent in infants and young children. *J Pediatr* 1977;91(2):188–193.

580. Rogers MAM. Percentage of children who developed type 1 diabetes after rotavirus vaccination. *JAMA Pediatr* 2020;174(9):909.

581. Rojas AM, Boher Y, Guntinas MJ, et al. Homotypic immune response to primary infection with rotavirus serotype G1. *J Med Virol* 1995;47(4):404–409.

582. Rojas M, Arias CF, Lopez S. Protein kinase R is responsible for the phosphorylation of eIF2alpha in rotavirus infection. *J Virol* 2010;84(20):10457–10466.
583. Rojas OL, Gonzalez AM, Gonzalez R, et al. Human rotavirus specific T cells: quantification by ELISPOT and expression of homing receptors on CD4+ T cells. *Virology* 2003;314(2):671–679.
584. Rojas OL, Narvaez CF, Greenberg HB, et al. Characterization of rotavirus specific B cells and their relation with serological memory. *Virology* 2008;380(2):234–242.
585. Rollo EE, Kumar KP, Reich NC, et al. The epithelial cell response to rotavirus infection. *J Immunol* 1999;163(8):4442–4452.
586. Rotavirus Rotavirus vaccines WHO position paper: January 2013—recommendations. *Vaccine* 2013;31(52):6170–6171.
587. Rossignol JF. Nitazoxanide: a first-in-class broad-spectrum antiviral agent. *Antiviral Res* 2014;110:94–103.
588. Rossignol JF, Abu-Zekry M, Hussein A, et al. Effect of nitazoxanide for treatment of severe rotavirus diarrhoea: randomised double-blind placebo-controlled trial. *Lancet* 2006;368(9530):124–129.
589. Rotbart HA, Nelson WL, Glode MP, et al. Neonatal rotavirus-associated necrotizing enterocolitis: case control study and prospective surveillance during an outbreak. *J Pediatr* 1988;112:87–93.
590. Ruiz-Gomez J, Alvarez MT, Silva-Acosta C, et al. Rotavirus. I. Hemagglutination and complement fixation inhibitor antibodies in individuals of Mexico city. *Arch Invest Med (Mex)* 1981;12(1):121–131.
591. Ruiz-Palacios GM, Perez-Schael I, Velazquez FR, et al. Safety and efficacy of an attenuated vaccine against severe rotavirus gastroenteritis. *N Engl J Med* 2006;354(1):11–22.
592. Ruiz MC, Alonso-Torre SR, Charpilienne A, et al. Rotavirus interaction with isolated membrane vesicles. *J Virol* 1994;68(6):4009–4016.
593. Ruiz MC, Charpilienne A, Liprandi F, et al. The concentration of Ca2+ that solubilizes outer capsid proteins from rotavirus particles is dependent on the strain. *J Virol* 1996;70(8):4877–4883.
594. Ruiz MC, Leon T, Diaz Y, et al. Molecular biology of rotavirus entry and replication. *ScientificWorldJournal* 2009;9:1476–1497.
595. Ryder RW, McGowan JE, Hatch MH, et al. Reovirus-like agent as a cause of nosocomial diarrhea in infants. *J Pediatr* 1977;90(5):698–702.
596. Saif LJ. Nongroup A rotaviruses of humans and animals. In: Jiang B, Ramig RF, eds. *Current Topics in Microbiology and Immunology*. Vol. 185. Berlin: Springer-Verlag; 1994:339–371.
597. Salas A, Pardo-Seco J, Cebey-Lopez M, et al. Impact of rotavirus vaccination on childhood hospitalizations for seizures: heterologous or unforeseen direct vaccine effects? *Vaccine* 2019;37(25):3362–3368.
598. Salazar-Lindo E, Santisteban-Ponce J, Chea-Woo E, et al. Racecadotril in the treatment of acute watery diarrhea in children. *N Engl J Med* 2000;343(7):463–467.
599. Salgado EN, Garcia Rodriguez B, Narayanaswamy N, et al. Visualization of calcium ion loss from rotavirus during cell entry. *J Virol* 2018;92(24).
600. Saluja T, Dhingra MS, Sharma SD, et al. Association of rotavirus strains and severity of gastroenteritis in Indian children. *Hum Vaccin Immunother* 2017;13(3):711–716.
601. Sanchez-Padilla E, Grais RF, Guerin PJ, et al. Burden of disease and circulating serotypes of rotavirus infection in sub-Saharan Africa: systematic review and meta-analysis. *Lancet Infect Dis* 2009;9(9):567–576.
602. Sanchez-San Martin C, Lopez T, Arias CF, et al. Characterization of rotavirus cell entry. *J Virol* 2004;78(5):2310–2318.
603. Sanchez-Tacuba L, Feng N, Meade NJ, et al. An optimized reverse genetics system suitable for efficient recovery of simian, human, and murine-like rotaviruses. *J Virol* 2020;94(18):e01294-20.
604. Sanchez-Tacuba L, Rojas M, Arias CF, et al. Rotavirus controls activation of the 2′-5′-oligoadenylate synthetase/RNase L pathway using at least two distinct mechanisms. *J Virol* 2015;89(23):12145–12153.
605. Santiana M, Ghosh S, Ho BA, et al. Vesicle-cloaked virus clusters are optimal units for inter-organismal viral transmission. *Cell Host Microbe* 2018;24(2):208–220 e8.
606. Santillanes G, Rose E. Evaluation and management of dehydration in children. *Emerg Med Clin North Am* 2018;36(2):259–273.
607. Santos N, Hoshino Y. Global distribution of rotavirus serotypes/genotypes and its implication for the development and implementation of an effective rotavirus vaccine. *Rev Med Virol* 2005;15(1):29–56.
608. Santosham M, Moulton LH, Reid R, et al. Efficacy and safety of high-dose rhesus-human reassortant rotavirus vaccine in Native American populations. *J Pediatr* 1997;131(4):632–638.
609. Sarker SA, Casswall TH, Mahalanabis D, et al. Successful treatment of rotavirus diarrhea in children with immunoglobulin from immunized bovine colostrum. *Pediatr Infect Dis J* 1998;17(12):1149–1154.
610. Sasaki M, Itakura Y, Kishimoto M, et al. Host serine proteases TMPRSS2 and TMPRSS11D mediate proteolytic activation and trypsin-independent infection in group A rotaviruses. *J Virol* 2021;95(11):e00398-21.
611. Sastri NP, Crawford SE, Estes MK. *Pleiotropic Properties of Rotavirus Nonstructural Protein 4 (NSP4) and Their Effects on Viral Replication and Pathogenesis*. In: Viral Gastroenteritis: Molecular Epidemiology and Pathogenesis. Elsevier Amsterdam; 2016.
612. Sastri NP, Viskovska M, Hyser JM, et al. Structural plasticity of the coiled-coil domain of rotavirus NSP4. *J Virol* 2014;88(23):13602–13612.
613. Saulsbury FT, Winkelstein JA, Yolken RH. Chronic rotavirus infection in immunodeficiency. *J Pediatr* 1980;97(1):61–65.
614. Saxena K, Blutt SE, Ettayebi K, et al. Human intestinal enteroids: a new model to study human rotavirus infection, host restriction, and pathophysiology. *J Virol* 2016;90(1):43–56.
615. Saxena K, Simon LM, Zeng XL, et al. A paradox of transcriptional and functional innate interferon responses of human intestinal enteroids to enteric virus infection. *Proc Natl Acad Sci U S A* 2017;114(4):E570–E579.
616. Schnepf N, Deback C, Dehee A, et al. Rearrangements of rotavirus genomic segment 11 are generated during acute infection of immunocompetent children and do not occur at random. *J Virol* 2008;82(7):3689–3696.
617. Schwartz-Cornil I, Benureau Y, Greenberg H, et al. Heterologous protection induced by the inner capsid proteins of rotavirus requires transcytosis of mucosal immunoglobulins. *J Virol* 2002;76(16):8110–8117.
618. Schwers A, Broecke CV, Maenhoudt M, et al. Experimental rotavirus diarrhoea in colostrum-deprived newborn calves: assay of treatment by administration of bacterially produced human interferon (Hu-IFN 2). *Ann Rech Vet* 1985;16(3):213–218.
619. Sen A, Feng N, Ettayebi K, et al. IRF3 inhibition by rotavirus NSP1 is host cell and virus strain dependent but independent of NSP1 proteasomal degradation. *J Virol* 2009;83(20):10322–10335.
620. Sen A, Pruijssers AJ, Dermody TS, et al. The early interferon response to rotavirus is regulated by PKR and depends on MAVS/IPS-1, RIG-I, MDA-5, and IRF3. *J Virol* 2011;85(8):3717–3732.
621. Sen A, Rothenberg ME, Mukherjee G, et al. Innate immune response to homologous rotavirus infection in the small intestinal villous epithelium at single-cell resolution. *Proc Natl Acad Sci U S A* 2012;109(50):20667–20672.
622. Sen A, Rott L, Phan N, et al. Rotavirus NSP1 protein inhibits interferon-mediated STAT1 activation. *J Virol* 2014;88(1):41–53.
623. Settembre EC, Chen JZ, Dormitzer PR, et al. Atomic model of an infectious rotavirus particle. *EMBO J* 2011;30(2):408–416.
624. Shah N, DuPont HL, Ramsey DJ. Global etiology of travelers' diarrhea: systematic review from 1973 to the present. *Am J Trop Med Hyg* 2009;80(4):609–614.
625. Shahrabadi MS, Babiuk LA, Lee PW. Further analysis of the role of calcium in rotavirus morphogenesis. *Virology* 1987;158:103–111.
626. Sharma S, Hagbom M, Nordgren J, et al. Detection of rotavirus- and norovirus-specific IgG memory B cells in tonsils. *J Med Virol* 2019;91(2):326–329.
627. Shaw AL, Rothnagel R, Chen D, et al. Three-dimensional visualization of the rotavirus hemagglutinin structure. *Cell* 1993;74:693–701.
628. Shaw RD, Fong KJ, Losonsky GA, et al. Epitope-specific immune responses to rotavirus vaccination. *Gastroenterology* 1987;93:941–950.
629. Shaw RD, Hempson SJ, Mackow ER. Rotavirus diarrhea is caused by nonreplicating viral particles [published erratum appears in *J Virol* 1996 Aug;70(8):5740]. *J Virol* 1995;69(10):5946–5950.
630. Shekarian T, Sivado E, Jallas AC, et al. Repurposing rotavirus vaccines for intratumoral immunotherapy can overcome resistance to immune checkpoint blockade. *Sci Transl Med* 2019;11(515):eaat5025.
631. Shmulevitz M, Duncan R. A new class of fusion-associated small transmembrane (FAST) proteins encoded by the non-enveloped fusogenic reoviruses. *EMBO J* 2000;19(5):902–912.
632. Shuman S, Moss B. Purification and use of vaccinia virus messenger RNA capping enzyme. *Methods Enzymol* 1990;181:170–180.
633. Silva-Ayala D, Lopez T, Gutierrez M, et al. Genome-wide RNAi screen reveals a role for the ESCRT complex in rotavirus cell entry. *Proc Natl Acad Sci U S A* 2013;110(25):10270–10275.
634. Silvestri LS, Taraporewala ZF, Patton JT. Rotavirus replication: plus-sense templates for double-stranded RNA synthesis are made in viroplasms. *J Virol* 2004;78(14):7763–7774.
635. Silvestri LS, Tortorici AA, Vasquez-Del Carpio R, et al. Rotavirus glycoprotein NSP4 is a modulator of viral transcription in the infected cell. *J Virol* 2005;79(24):15165–15174.
636. Simonsen L, Viboud C, Elixhauser A, et al. More on RotaShield and intussusception: the role of age at the time of vaccination. *J Infect Dis* 2005;192(Suppl 1):S36–S43.
637. Simsek C, Corman VM, Everling HU, et al. At least seven distinct rotavirus genotype constellations in bats with evidence of reassortment and zoonotic transmissions. *mBio* 2021;12(1).
638. Smeets CCJM, Brussel W, Leyton QH, et al. First report of Guillain-Barre syndrome after rotavirus-induced gastroenteritis in a very young infant. *Eur J Pediatr* 2000;159:224.
639. Smiley KL, McNeal MM, Basu M, et al. Association of gamma interferon and interleukin-17 production in intestinal CD4+ T cells with protection against rotavirus shedding in mice intranasally immunized with VP6 and the adjuvant LT(R192G). *J Virol* 2007;81(8):3740–3748.
640. Smith EM, Gerba CP. Development of a method for detection of human rotavirus in water and sewage. *Appl Environ Microbiol* 1982;43(6):1440–1450.
641. Smith SC, Gribble J, Diller JR, et al. Reovirus RNA recombination is sequence directed and generates internally deleted defective genome segments during passage. *J Virol* 2021;95(8):e02181-20.
642. Soares-Weiser K, Bergman H, Henschke N, et al. Vaccines for preventing rotavirus diarrhoea: vaccines in use. *Cochrane Database Syst Rev* 2019;2019(10):CD008521.
643. Song Y, Feng N, Sanchez-Tacuba L, et al. Reverse genetics reveals a role of rotavirus VP3 phosphodiesterase activity in inhibiting RNase L signaling and contributing to intestinal viral replication in vivo. *J Virol* 2020;94(9):e01952-19.
644. Spence L. Haemagglutinin from rotavirus. *Lancet* 1976;2:1023.
645. Staatz G, Alzen G, Heimann G. Gastrointestinal infection, most common cause of intussusception in childhood: results of a 10-year study. *Klin Padiatr* 1998;210:61–64.
646. Stacy-Phipps S, Patton JT. Synthesis of plus- and minus-strand RNA in rotavirus-infected cells. *J Virol* 1987;61:3479–3484.
647. Steele AD, Cunliffe N, Tumbo J, et al. A review of rotavirus infection in and vaccination of human immunodeficiency virus-infected children. *J Infect Dis* 2009;200(Suppl 1):S57–S62.
648. Steele AD, Neuzil KM, Cunliffe NA, et al. Human rotavirus vaccine Rotarix provides protection against diverse circulating rotavirus strains in African infants: a randomized controlled trial. *BMC Infect Dis* 2012;12:213.
649. Steger CL, Brown ML, Sullivan OM, et al. In vitro double-stranded RNA synthesis by rotavirus polymerase mutants with lesions at core shell contact sites. *J Virol* 2019;93(20):e01049-19.
650. Stoll BJ, Glass RI, Huq MI, et al. Surveillance of patients attending a diarrhoeal disease hospital in Bangladesh. *Brit Med J* 1982;285:1185–1188.
651. Su CQ, Wu YL, Shen HK, et al. An outbreak of epidemic diarrhoea in adults caused by a new rotavirus in Anhui Province of China in the summer of 1983. *J Med Virol* 1986;19:167–173.

652. Sun T, Ferrero RL, Girardin SE, et al. NLRC5 deficiency has a moderate impact on immunodominant CD8(+) T-cell responses during rotavirus infection of adult mice. *Immunol Cell Biol* 2019;97(6):552–562.
653. Svensson L, Dormitzer PR, von Bonsdorff CH, et al. Intracellular manipulation of disulfide bond formation in rotavirus proteins during assembly. *J Virol* 1994;68(8):5204–5215.
654. Tacharoenmuang R, Komoto S, Guntapong R, et al. Characterization of a G10P[14] rotavirus strain from a diarrheic child in Thailand: evidence for bovine-to-human zoonotic transmission. *Infect Genet Evol* 2018;63:43–57.
655. Tafazoli F, Zeng CQY, Estes MK, et al. The NSP4 enterotoxin of rotavirus induces paracellular leakage in polarized epithelial cells. *J Virol* 2001;75(3):1540–1546.
656. Tamura K, Stecher G, Peterson D, et al. MEGA6: Molecular Evolutionary Genetics Analysis version 6.0. *Mol Biol Evol* 2013;30(12):2725–2729.
657. Tanaka TN, Conner ME, Graham DY, et al. Molecular characterization of three rabbit rotavirus strains. *Arch Virol* 1988;98:253–265.
658. Taraporewala Z, Chen D, Patton JT. Multimers formed by the rotavirus nonstructural protein NSP2 bind to RNA and have nucleoside triphosphatase activity. *J Virol* 1999;73(12):9934–9943.
659. Taraporewala ZF, Patton JT. Identification and characterization of the helix-destabilizing activity of rotavirus nonstructural protein NSP2. *J Virol* 2001;75(10):4519–4527.
660. Taraporewala ZF, Patton JT. Nonstructural proteins involved in genome packaging and replication of rotaviruses and other members of the *Reoviridae*. *Virus Res* 2004;101(1): 57–66.
661. Taraporewala ZF, Schuck P, Ramig RF, et al. Analysis of a temperature-sensitive mutant rotavirus indicates that NSP2 octamers are the functional form of the protein. *J Virol* 2002; 76(14):7082–7093.
662. Tate JE, Burton AH, Boschi-Pinto C, et al.; World Health Organization-Coordinated Global Rotavirus Surveillance Network. Global, regional, and national estimates of rotavirus mortality in children <5 years of age, 2000–2013. *Clin Infect Dis* 2016;62(Suppl 2):S96–S105.
663. Tate JE, Cortese MM, Payne DC, et al. Uptake, impact, and effectiveness of rotavirus vaccination in the United States: review of the first 3 years of postlicensure data. *Pediatr Infect Dis J* 2011;30(1 Suppl):S56–S60.
664. Tate JE, Panozzo CA, Payne DC, et al. Decline and change in seasonality of US rotavirus activity after the introduction of rotavirus vaccine. *Pediatrics* 2009;124(2):465–471.
665. Tate JE, Yen C, Steiner CA, et al. Intussusception rates before and after the introduction of rotavirus vaccine. *Pediatrics* 2016;138(3):e20161082.
666. Taylor JA, O'Brien JA, Lord VJ, et al. The RER-localized rotavirus intracellular receptor: a truncated purified soluble form is multivalent and binds virus particles. *Virology* 1993;194:807–814.
667. Taylor JA, O'Brien JA, Yeager M. The cytoplasmic tail of NSP4, the endoplasmic reticulum-localized non-structural glycoprotein of rotavirus, contains distinct virus binding and coiled coil domains. *EMBO J* 1998;15(17):4469–4476.
668. Teitelbaum JE, Daghistani R. Rotavirus causes hepatic transaminase elevation. *Dig Dis Sci* 2007;52(12):3396–3398.
669. Teran CG, Teran-Escalera CN, Villarroel P. Nitazoxanide vs. probiotics for the treatment of acute rotavirus diarrhea in children: a randomized, single-blind, controlled trial in Bolivian children. *Int J Infect Dis* 2009;13(4):518–523.
670. Thi Nhu Thao T, Labroussaa F, Ebert N, et al. Rapid reconstruction of SARS-CoV-2 using a synthetic genomics platform. *Nature* 2020;582(7813):561–565.
671. Thouvenin E, Schoehn G, Rey F, et al. Antibody inhibition of the transcriptase activity of the rotavirus DLP: a structural view. *J Mol Biol* 2001;307(1):161–172.
672. Tian C, Luskin GK, Dischert KM, et al. Immunodominance of the VH1-46 antibody gene segment in the primary repertoire of human rotavirus-specific B cells is reduced in the memory compartment through somatic mutation of nondominant clones. *J Immunol* 2008;180(5):3279–3288.
673. Tian P, Ball JM, Zeng CQY, et al. The rotavirus nonstructural glycoprotein NSP4 possesses membrane destabilization activity. *J Virol* 1996;70(10):6973–6981.
674. To TL, Ward LA, Yuan L, et al. Serum and intestinal isotype antibody responses and correlates of protective immunity to human rotavirus in a gnotobiotic pig model of disease *J Gen Virol* 1998;79(Pt 11):2661–2672.
675. Torres-Flores JM, Silva-Ayala D, Espinoza MA, et al. The tight junction protein JAM-A functions as coreceptor for rotavirus entry into MA104 cells. *Virology* 2015;475:172–178.
676. Torres-Vega MA, Gonzalez RA, Duarte M, et al. The C-terminal domain of rotavirus NSP5 is essential for its multimerization, hyperphosphorylation and interaction with NSP6. *J Gen Virol* 2000;81:821–830.
677. Tortorici MA, Shipiro BA, Patton JT. A base-specific recognition signal in the 5′ consensus sequence of rotavirus plus-strand RNAs promotes replication of the double-stranded RNA genome segments. *RNA* 2006;12(2):133–146.
678. Tran V, Moser LA, Poole DS, et al. Highly sensitive real-time in vivo imaging of an influenza reporter virus reveals dynamics of replication and spread. *J Virol* 2013;87(24): 13321–13329.
679. Trask SD, Dormitzer PR. Assembly of highly infectious rotavirus particles recoated with recombinant outer capsid proteins. *J Virol* 2006;80(22):11293–11304.
680. Trask SD, Taraporewala ZF, Boehme KW, et al. Dual selection mechanisms drive efficient single-gene reverse genetics for rotavirus. *Proc Natl Acad Sci U S A* 2010;107(43): 18652–18657.
681. Tregnaghi MW, Abate HJ, Valencia A, et al. Human rotavirus vaccine is highly efficacious when coadministered with routine expanded program of immunization vaccines including oral poliovirus vaccine in Latin America. *Pediatr Infect Dis J* 2011;30(6):e103–e108.
682. Troeger C, Khalil IA, Rao PC, et al. Rotavirus vaccination and the global burden of rotavirus diarrhea among children younger than 5 years. *JAMA Pediatr* 2018;172(10):958–965.
683. Troupin C, Dehee A, Schnuriger A, et al. Rearranged genomic RNA segments offer a new approach to the reverse genetics of rotaviruses. *J Virol* 2010;84(13):6711–6719.
684. Troupin C, Schnuriger A, Duponchel S, et al. Rotavirus rearranged genomic RNA segments are preferentially packaged into viruses despite not conferring selective growth advantage to viruses. *PLoS One* 2011;6(5):e20080.
685. Uchiyama R, Chassaing B, Zhang B, et al. MyD88-mediated TLR signaling protects against acute rotavirus infection while inflammasome cytokines direct Ab response. *Innate Immun* 2015;21(4):416–428.
686. Urasawa S, Urasawa T, Djoko Y, et al. A survey of rotavirus infection in the tropics. *Jap J Med Sci Biol* 1981;34:293–298.
687. Vancott JL, McNeal MM, Choi AHC, et al. The role of interferons in rotavirus infections and protection. *J Interferon Cytokine Res* 2003;23:163–170.
688. Vascotto F, Visintin M, Cattaneo A, et al. Design and selection of an intrabody library produced de-novo for the non-structural protein NSP5 of rotavirus. *J Immunol Methods* 2005;301(1–2):31–40.
689. Vasquez-Del Carpio R, Gonzalez-Nilo FD, Riadi G, et al. Histidine triad-like motif of the rotavirus NSP2 octamer mediates both RTPase and NTPase activities. *J Mol Biol* 2006;362(3):539–554.
690. Vega CG, Bok M, Vlasova AN, et al. Recombinant monovalent llama-derived antibody fragments (VHH) to rotavirus VP6 protect neonatal gnotobiotic piglets against human rotavirus-induced diarrhea. *PLoS Pathog* 2013;9(5):e1003334.
691. Velazquez FR. Protective effects of natural rotavirus infection. *Pediatr Infect Dis J* 2009;28(3 Suppl):S54–S56.
692. Velazquez FR, Matson DO, Calva JJ, et al. Rotavirus infections in infants as protection against subsequent infections. *N Engl J Med* 1996;335(14):1022–1028.
693. Vende P, Piron M, Castagne N, et al. Efficient translation of rotavirus mRNA requires simultaneous interaction of NSP3 with the eukaryotic translation initiation factor eIF4G and the mRNA 3′ end. *J Virol* 2000;74(15):7064–7071.
694. Vesikari T. Trials of oral bovine and rhesus rotavirus vaccines in Finland: a historical account and present status. *Arch Virol Suppl* 1996;12:177–186.
695. Vesikari T, Isolauri E, D'Hondt E, et al. Protection of infants against rotavirus diarrhoea by RIT 4237 attenuated bovine rotavirus strain vaccine. *Lancet* 1984;1(8384):977–981.
696. Vesikari T, Isolauri E, Delem A, et al. Clinical efficacy of the RIT 4237 live attenuated bovine rotavirus vaccine in infants vaccinated before a rotavirus epidemic. *J Pediatr* 1985;107:189–194.
697. Vesikari T, Joensuu J. Review of rotavirus vaccine trials in Finland. *J Infect Dis* 1996;174 (Suppl 1):S81–S87.
698. Vesikari T, Kapikian AZ, Delem A, et al. A comparative trial of rhesus monkey (RRV-1) and bovine (RIT 4237) oral rotavirus vaccines in young children. *J Infect Dis* 1986; 153(5):832–839.
699. Vesikari T, Karvonen A, Ferrante SA, et al. Sustained efficacy of the pentavalent rotavirus vaccine, RV5, up to 3.1 years following the last dose of vaccine. *Pediatr Infect Dis J* 2010;29(10):957–963.
700. Vesikari T, Karvonen A, Prymula R, et al. Efficacy of human rotavirus vaccine against rotavirus gastroenteritis during the first 2 years of life in European infants: randomised, double-blind controlled study. *Lancet* 2007;370(9601):1757–1763.
701. Vesikari T, Matson DO, Dennehy P, et al. Safety and efficacy of a pentavalent human-bovine (WC3) reassortant rotavirus vaccine. *N Engl J Med* 2006;354(1):23–33.
702. Vesikari T, Rautanen T, Varis T, et al. Rhesus rotavirus candidate vaccine—clinical trial in children vaccinated between 2 and 5 months of age. *Am J Dis Child* 1990;144:285–289.
703. Vesikari T, Ruuska T, Delem A, et al. Efficacy of two doses of RIT 4237 bovine rotavirus vaccine for prevention of rotavirus diarrhoea. *Acta Paediatr Scand* 1991;80(2):173–180.
704. Viskovska M, Anish R, Hu L, et al. Probing the sites of interactions of rotaviral proteins involved in replication. *J Virol* 2014;88(21):12866–12881.
705. Waggie Z, Hawkridge A, Hussey GD. Review of rotavirus studies in Africa: 1976–2006. *J Infect Dis* 2010;202(Suppl):S23–S33.
706. Wang X, Song L, Tan W, et al. Clinical efficacy of oral immunoglobulin Y in infant rotavirus enteritis: systematic review and meta-analysis. *Medicine (Baltimore)* 2019;98(27):e16100.
707. Ward LA, Rosen BI, Yuan L, et al. Pathogenesis of an attenuated and a virulent strain of group A human rotavirus in neonatal gnotobiotic pigs. *J Gen Virol* 1996;77(Pt 7): 1431–1441.
708. Ward RL, Bernstein DI. Rotarix: a rotavirus vaccine for the world. *Clin Infect Dis* 2009;48(2):222–228.
709. Ward RL, Bernstein DI, Knowlton DR, et al. Prevention of surface-to-human transmission of rotaviruses by treatment with disinfectant spray. *J Clin Microbiol* 1991;29(9): 1991–1996.
710. Ward RL, Bernstein DI, Shukla R, et al. Effects of antibody to rotavirus on protection of adults challenged with a human rotavirus. *J Infect Dis* 1989;159(1):79–88.
711. Ward RL, Bernstein DI, Young EC, et al. Human rotavirus studies in volunteers: determination of infectious dose and serological response to infection. *J Infect Dis* 1986;154(5): 871–880.
712. Ward RL, Knowlton DR, Pierce MJ. Efficiency of human rotavirus propagation in cell culture. *J Clin Microbiol* 1984;19(6):748–753.
713. Ward RL, McNeal MM. VP6: a candidate rotavirus vaccine. *J Infect Dis* 2010; 202(Suppl):S101–S107.
714. Welch SK, Crawford SE, Estes MK. Rotavirus SA11 genome segment 11 protein is a nonstructural phosphoprotein. *J Virol* 1989;63:3974–3982.
715. Wentz MJ, Patton JT, Ramig RF. The 3′-terminal consensus sequence of rotavirus mRNA is the minimal promoter of negative-strand RNA synthesis. *J Virol* 1996;70(11): 7833–7841.
716. Westerman LE, McClure HM, Jiang B, et al. Serum IgG mediates mucosal immunity against rotavirus infection. *Proc Natl Acad Sci U S A* 2005;102(20):7268–7273.
717. Westerman LE, Xu J, Jiang B, et al. Experimental infection of pigtailed macaques with a simian rotavirus, YK-1. *J Med Virol* 2005;75(4):616–625.
718. Wilde J, Van R, Pickering L, et al. Detection of rotaviruses in the day care environment by reverse transcriptase polymerase chain reaction. *J Infect Dis* 1992;166:507–511.
719. Wolf M, Vo PT, Greenberg HB. Rhesus rotavirus entry into a polarized epithelium is endocytosis dependent and involves sequential VP4 conformational changes. *J Virol* 2011;85(6):2492–2503.
720. Wood DJ, David TJ, Chrystie IL, et al. Chronic enteric virus infection in two T-cell immunodeficient children. *J Med Virol* 1988;24:435–444.

721. Woode GN. Morphological and antigenic relationships between viruses (Rotaviruses) from acute gastroenteritis of children, calves, piglets, mice and foals. *Infect Immun* 1976;14:804–810.

722. Woods PA, Gentsch J, Gouvea V, et al. Distribution of serotypes of human rotavirus in different populations. *J Clin Microbiol* 1992;30(4):781–785.

723. Wu W, Orr-Burks N, Karpilow J, et al. Development of improved vaccine cell lines against rotavirus. *Sci Data* 2017;4:170021.

724. Wyatt RG, Mebus CA, Yolken RH, et al. Rotaviral immunity in gnotobiotic calves: heterologous resistance to human virus induced by bovine virus. *Science* 1979;203(4380):548–550.

725. Xie X, Muruato A, Lokugamage KG, et al. An infectious cDNA clone of SARS-CoV-2. *Cell Host Microbe* 2020;27(5):841–848 e3.

726. Xu J, Dennehy P, Keyserling H, et al. Serum antibody responses in children with rotavirus diarrhea can serve as proxy for protection. *Clin Diagn Lab Immunol* 2005;12(2):273–279.

727. Yeager AM, Kanof ME, Kramer SS, et al. Pneumatosis intestinalis in children after allogeneic bone marrow transplantation. *Pediatr Radiol* 1987;17(1):18–22.

728. Yeager M, Berriman JA, Baker TS, et al. Three-dimensional structure of the rotavirus haemagglutinin VP4 by cryo-electron microscopy and difference map analysis. *EMBO J* 1994;13:1011–1018.

729. Yeager M, Dryden KA, Olson NH, et al. Three-dimensional structure of rhesus rotavirus by cryoelectron microscopy and image reconstruction. *J Cell Biol* 1990;110:2133–2144.

730. Yeom JS, Kim YS, Jun JS, et al. NSP4 antibody levels in rotavirus gastroenteritis patients with seizures. *Eur J Paediatr Neurol* 2017;21(2):367–373.

731. Yinda CK, Zeller M, Conceicao-Neto N, et al. Novel highly divergent reassortant bat rotaviruses in Cameroon, without evidence of zoonosis. *Sci Rep* 2016;6:34209.

732. Yoder JD, Dormitzer PR. Alternative intermolecular contacts underlie the rotavirus VP5* two- to three-fold rearrangement. *EMBO J* 2006;25:1558–1568.

733. Yolken R, Arango-Jaramillo A, Eiden J, et al. Lack of genomic reassortment following infection of infant rats with group A and group B rotavirus. *J Infect Dis* 1988;158(5):1120–1123.

734. Yolken R, Wee SB, Eiden J, et al. Identification of a group-reactive epitope of group B rotaviruses recognized by monoclonal antibody and application to the development of a sensitive immunoassay for viral characterization. *J Clin Microbiol* 1988;26:1853–1858.

735. Yolken R, Wilde J. Assays for detecting human rotavirus. In: Kapikian AZ, ed. *Viral Infections of the Gastro Intestinal Tract*. 2nd ed. New York: Marcel Dekker, Inc; 1994:251–278.

736. Yolken RH, Bishop CA, Townsend TR, et al. Infectious gastroenteritis in bone-marrow-transplant recipients. *N Engl J Med* 1982;306(17):1009–1012.

737. Youngman KR, Franco MA, Kuklin NA, et al. Correlation of tissue distribution, developmental phenotype, and intestinal homing receptor expression of antigen-specific B cells during the murine anti-rotavirus immune response. *J Immunol* 2002;168(5):2173–2181.

738. Yu X, Coulson BS, Fleming FE, et al. Novel structural insights into rotavirus recognition of ganglioside glycan receptors. *J Mol Biol* 2011;413(5):929–939.

739. Yu X, Jin L, Zhou ZH. 3.88 A structure of cytoplasmic polyhedrosis virus by cryo-electron microscopy. *Nature* 2008;453(7193):415–419.

740. Yuan L, Kang SY, Ward LA, et al. Antibody-secreting cell responses and protective immunity assessed in gnotobiotic pigs inoculated orally or intramuscularly with inactivated human rotavirus. *J Virol* 1998;72(1):330–338.

741. Zaman K, Dang DA, Victor JC, et al. Efficacy of pentavalent rotavirus vaccine against severe rotavirus gastroenteritis in infants in developing countries in Asia: a randomised, double-blind, placebo-controlled trial. *Lancet* 2010;376(9741):615–623.

742. Zanoni G, Navone R, Lunardi C, et al. In celiac disease, a subset of autoantibodies against transglutaminase binds toll-like receptor 4 and induces activation of monocytes. *PLoS Med* 2006;3(9):e358.

743. Zarate S, Romero P, Espinosa R, et al. VP7 mediates the interaction of rotaviruses with integrin alpha v beta 3 through a novel integrin-binding site. *J Virol* 2004;78(20):10839–10847.

744. Zeller M, Nuyts V, Heylen E, et al. Emergence of human G2P[4] rotaviruses containing animal derived gene segments in the post-vaccine era. *Sci Rep* 2016;6:36841.

745. Zeng CQY, Wentz MJ, Cohen J, et al. Characterization and replicase activity of double-layered and single-layered rotavirus-like particles expressed from baculovirus recombinants. *J Virol* 1996;70(5):2736–2742.

746. Zeng R, Oderup C, Yuan R, et al. Retinoic acid regulates the development of a gut-homing precursor for intestinal dendritic cells. *Mucosal Immunol* 2013;6(4):847–856.

747. Zhang B, Chassaing B, Shi Z, et al. Viral infection. Prevention and cure of rotavirus infection via TLR5/NLRC4-mediated production of IL-22 and IL-18. *Science* 2014;346(6211):861–865.

748. Zhang R, Jha BK, Ogden KM, et al. Homologous 2',5'-phosphodiesterases from disparate RNA viruses antagonize antiviral innate immunity. *Proc Natl Acad Sci U S A* 2013;110(32):13114–13119.

749. Zhang X, Jin L, Fang Q, et al. 3.3 A cryo-EM structure of a nonenveloped virus reveals a priming mechanism for cell entry. *Cell* 2010;141(3):472–482.

750. Zhang X, Walker SB, Chipman PR, et al. Reovirus polymerase lambda 3 localized by cryo-electron microscopy of virions at a resolution of 7.6 A. *Nat Struct Biol* 2003;10(12):1011–1018.

751. Zhang Z, Zou J, Shi Z, et al. IL-22-induced cell extrusion and IL-18-induced cell death prevent and cure rotavirus infection. *Sci Immunol* 2020;5(52).

752. Zhao B, Shu C, Gao X, et al. Structural basis for concerted recruitment and activation of IRF-3 by innate immune adaptor proteins. *Proc Natl Acad Sci U S A* 2016;113(24):E3403–E3412.

753. Zhu S, Ding S, Wang P, et al. Nlrp9b inflammasome restricts rotavirus infection in intestinal epithelial cells. *Nature* 2017;546(7660):667–670.

754. Ziring D, Tran R, Edelstein S, et al. Infectious enteritis after intestinal transplantation: incidence, timing, and outcome. *Transplant Proc* 2004;36(2):379–380.

755. Zou WY, Blutt SE, Crawford SE, et al. Human intestinal enteroids: new models to study gastrointestinal virus infections. *Methods Mol Biol* 2019;1576:229–247.

756. Zou WY, Blutt SE, Zeng XL, et al. Epithelial WNT ligands are essential drivers of intestinal stem cell activation. *Cell Rep* 2018;22(4):1003–1015.

Polly Roy

History
Classification
Virion structure
    Virion particle and outer capsid
    Core particle and proteins
    Structural arrangement of internal minor proteins
    RNA genome seen in x-ray structure of the core
Genome structure and organization
Molecular genetics
Stages of virus replication
    Virus entry
    Transcription and replication
    Protein synthesis and virus replication
    Capsid assembly
    Maturation, trafficking, and egress of progeny virions
    Virus egress
Effects on host cells
Clinical signs and pathogenesis
Epidemiology
Immune response
Vaccines
    Classical, subunit/VLP, and reverse genetics-based vaccines
Perspective

HISTORY

Two important orbivirus diseases, African horse sickness (AHS) and bluetongue (BT) disease of sheep and cattle, led to their initial identification on the continent of Africa.[73,197] A major outbreak of AHS occurred in 1719 when approximately 1,700 animals died, and a further significant outbreak occurred in 1854 to 1855, affecting some 70,000 horses. AHS mainly appeared in years of unusually high rainfall and warm weather, and it was speculated that insect vectors were involved in the spread of the disease. Only in 1900 was it demonstrated that AHS was caused by a virus, African horse sickness virus (AHSV), when M'Fadyean succeeded in transmitting the disease by a bacteria-free filtrate from an infected animal to a healthy one.[116] The major vertebrate reservoir for the virus was believed to be Zebra.[5] To date, AHSV occurs in multiple serotypes (AHSV-1 to AHSV-9) and is endemic in eastern and central Africa and many parts of sub-Saharan Africa. From 1943 onward, AHS outbreaks have been reported in other parts of the world including Palestine, Turkey, Israel, Pakistan, the Indian subcontinent, Spain, Portugal, and more recently in Thailand and Malaysia.[25,43,101]

In the late 18th century, BT disease was observed in domestic animals as well as in wild ruminants (e.g., blesbuck, white-tailed deer, elk, and pronghorn antelope) and, as for AHS, BT was confined to Africa for many decades. For BT, distinctive lesions in the mouths of the infected animals and a dark blue tongue were the characteristic symptoms. A detailed description of the disease was first published in 1905[180] when it was named malarial catarrhal fever,[44] and Theiler demonstrated that the causative agent was a filterable virus, now called bluetongue virus (BTV).[198] The first confirmed outbreak outside of Africa occurred in Cyprus in 1924, followed by further outbreaks in 1943 to 1944, which killed 2,500 sheep with a mortality rate reaching 70%. In the United States, BT disease in sheep was first recognized in 1948, while a major epizootic began in Portugal and extended into Spain in 1956. Further outbreaks of the disease in the Middle East, Southeast Asia, Southern Europe, and the United States in the early 1940s and 1950s led to its description as an emerging disease.[79] Virus isolates, of 25 different serotypes, have been made in tropical, semitropical, and temperate zones of the world, including North and South America, Australia, Southern Europe, Israel, Africa, and Southeast Asia. In 1998, significant outbreaks of BT occurred in Europe, initially in Greece and then in many other Mediterranean countries, causing the death of over a million sheep by 2005.[156] In 2006 and 2007, BT emerged in Northwestern Europe eventually expanding into the United Kingdom, Denmark, and the Netherlands.[37,68,117,193] In recent years, several new serotypes have been isolated from various parts of the world.[22,179,225] An important factor in the distribution of BTV worldwide is the availability of suitable vectors, usually biting midges (gnats) of the *Culicoides* species.

CLASSIFICATION

The orbivirus genus is 1 of 15 genera within the *Reoviridae* family, which includes vertebrate, arthropod, and plant pathogens. Despite a basic similarity with other family members, orbiviruses differ greatly in their structure, physicochemical properties, replication cycle, pathogenesis, and epidemiology. Orbiviruses are arthropod-borne with 170 distinct species that are transmitted by mosquitoes, gnats, and ticks. Each species has multiple serotypes, which are differentiated by virus neutralization tests.[139] Orbiviruses infect a wide range of vertebrate hosts, including ruminants (domesticated and wild), equids (domesticated and wild), rodents, bats, marsupials, birds, sloths, and primates, including humans. In addition to AHSV and BTV, one other closely related orbivirus, epizootic hemorrhagic disease virus (EHDV) of deer, is an important animal pathogen, and all three viruses are transmitted by biting midges (gnats) of the genus *Culicoides*. The orbivirus serogroups, serotypes, principal vectors, and main hosts are listed in Table 13.1 with their assigned abbreviations.[139] BTV, with 28 serotypes, is the prototype of the genus and is one of the most widespread animal pathogens, periodically causing serious outbreaks among sheep and cattle. Consequently, BTV has been studied extensively and acts as an important representative of this class of large nonenveloped viruses. In recent years, considerable progress has been made in determining the BTV structure at the atomic level, and the introduction of mutations into the replicating viral genome by reverse genetics (RG) systems, developed first for BTV,[17] has opened up new opportunities to dissect the various stages of virus replication, assembly, and egress as well as the nature of host–virus interactions. In addition, the development of several novel technologies has revealed key aspects of the genome packaging mechanism and allowed the generation of new types of vaccine strains. Thus, BTV represents one of the best characterized viruses and key aspects of its replication, assembly, egress, and its interaction with hosts are reviewed here.

VIRION STRUCTURE

BTV and other orbiviruses are nonenveloped, icosahedral particles containing segmented, double-stranded RNA (dsRNA) genomes[217] (Fig. 13.1). The BTV particle is architecturally complex, has a diameter of 88 nm, and consists of two capsids of concentric protein layers, comprising 7 structural proteins and a genome of 10 dsRNA segments (S1 to S10), which are divided into three different size classes, large, medium, and small.[75,148,217] The outer capsid is made up of two proteins, VP2 and VP5, and surrounds the inner capsid otherwise called the "core."[82,208] The core is composed of VP7 and VP3 in two concentric layers, which encapsidate the dsRNA genome and the viral replicase complex of three minor proteins, VP1, VP4, and VP6.

Virion Particle and Outer Capsid

Early electron micrographs (EM) of BTV revealed characteristically fuzzy particles, suggesting BTV is sensitive to preparation conditions.[42] However, later cryo-electron microscopy (cryo-EM) and image analysis of BTV particles revealed the well-ordered structural arrangement of the virion particle, a diameter of approximately 880 Å and the accurate positioning of VP2 and VP5 proteins in relation to each other and to the underlying core surface. Sixty triskelion spike-like structures formed by VP2 trimers surrounded 120 globular structures made up of VP5 trimers, and both attach to the underlying core surface layer independently of each other.[74,76,148,226] Further, cryo-EM of the whole particle has resulted in near-atomic resolution (3.5 Å) not only confirming the structural interactions but also suggesting how VP2 and VP5 may function during virus entry

into the cell (Fig. 13.2).[227] The monomer of the receptor-binding protein, VP2, is divided in four distinct domains, hub, hairpin, pyramidal body, and highly flexible tip. The hub domain has a 10-stranded lectin-like β-barrel flanked by three helices and drives the monomer–monomer interactions of the trimer. A unique zinc finger motif, located at the interface of the hub and the body domains, is responsible for pH-triggered conformational change of VP2.[223] Each VP2 trimer contacts the VP7 layer of the core through the hub base, the body, and the hairpin domains. The body domain extends to the highly flexible external tip domain containing at least four helices and a β-sheet, which likely makes direct contact with the cell surface receptor. In contrast to VP2, VP5 has a highly compact globular fold predominated by α-helices with a central coiled-coil motif facilitating trimerization, analogous to viral membrane fusion proteins.[153] The structure of each VP5 monomer is a near-rectangular shape with three distinct domains, the flexible N-terminal dagger domain, sequestered in the canyons underlying the VP7 core surface, a helix-rich unfurling domain with two parallel strands and a stem helix, and the C-terminal anchoring domain with membrane interaction elements (Fig. 13.3). Notably, a β-meander motif in the anchoring domain contains a histidine cluster that senses the late-endosomal pH to induce membrane interaction. Three stem helices in the middle of a VP5 trimer form a coiled-coil. The interaction between VP5 and core protein VP7 is extensive with all three VP5 domains involved, but VP5 interaction with VP2 is relatively weak, via only two regions, the VP2 hub domain, which interacts with the N-terminal helices of the VP5 trimer, and the VP2 hairpin loop, which interacts with the anchoring domain of an adjacent VP5 trimer (Figs. 13.2 and 13.3).

Core Particle and Proteins

Unlike the whole particle, the core (470S) is very robust and can be generated by proteolytic treatment of purified virus preparations. The core particle has been studied extensively at the structural level, initially by cryo-EM (at various resolutions between 22 and 40 Å), subsequently by a 3.6 Å atomic structure of crystallized cores, and recently again by cryo-EM. The 3D structure of the icosahedral core shows a triangulation number of 13 (T = 13) and an early atomic structure of recombinant VP7 protein revealed an unusual organization that provided a paradigm in the field.[65,66,74,75,154] The core surface is formed of 260 VP7 (38 kDa) trimers, arranged around 132 channels as six-membered rings, with five-member rings at the vertices (Fig. 13.4A). Surrounded by VP7 trimers, these aqueous channels (or pores) can be grouped into three types; type I channels run along the icosahedral fivefold axes, type II channels surround the fivefold axes, and type III channels are located around the icosahedral threefold axes. They are small (7 Å diameter) at the icosahedral threefold axes (class III) and slightly larger (9 Å diameter) at the fivefold axes (class I), and act as portals to release newly synthesized transcripts once virus entry is complete. The five quasi-equivalent trimers form a visible protomeric unit with each trimer consisting of an "upper" (an antiparallel β-sandwich formed by the centre domain) and "lower" (mainly α-helical and formed by the N and the C termini of the molecule) domain (Fig. 13.4B).[66] The top domain of one monomer sits on the lower domain of the adjacent monomer, and the interactions between monomers are

TABLE 13.1   Orbiviruses: serogroups, serotypes, vectors, and vertebrate hosts

Serogroup	Serotype	Vectors	Hosts
African horse sickness (AHS)	AHSV 1–9	*Culicoides*	Equids (horses, mules, donkeys), dogs, elephants, camels, cattle, sheep, goats, predatory carnivores
Bluetongue (BT)	BTV 1–28	*Culicoides*	Sheep, cattle, goats, camels, elephants, ruminants (domestic and wild), predatory carnivores, wild ungulates
Changuinola	Almeirim, Altamira, Caninde, Changuinola, Gurupi, Iratuia, Jamanxi, Jari, Monte Dourado, Ourem, Purus, Saraca	Phlebotomines Culicine mosquitoes	Humans, rodents, sloths
Chenuda	Baku, Chenuda, Essaouira, Huncho, Kala Iris, Mono Lake, Six Gun City	Ticks	Seabirds
Chobar Gorge	Chobar Gorge, Fomede	Ticks	Bats
Corriparta	Acado, Corriparta 1–4, Jacareacanga	Phlebotomines Culicine mosquitoes	Humans, rodents
Epizootic hemorrhagic disease (EHD)	EHDV 1–9, Ibaraki	*Culicoides*	Cattle, sheep, deer, camels, llamas, wild ruminants, marsupials
Equine encephalosis (EE)	EEV 1–7	*Culicoides*	Equids
Eubenangee	Eubenangee, Ngoupe, Pata, Tilgerry	*Culicoides*, anopheline, and culicine mosquitoes	Unknown
Ieri virus	Ieri, Gomoko, Arkonam	Mosquitoes	Birds
Great Island	Above Maiden, Arbroath, Bauline, Broadhaven, Cape Wrath, Colony, Colony B North, Ellidaey, Foula, Great Island, Great Saltee Island, Grimsey, Inner Farne, Kemerovo, Kenai, Kharagysh, Lipovnik, Lundy, Maiden, Mill Door, Mykines, North Clett, North End, Nugget, Okhotsk, Poovoot, Rost Islands, Saint Abb's Head, Shiant Islands, Thormodseyjarlettur, Tillamook, Tindholmur, Tribec, Vearoy, Wexford, Yaquina Head	Ticks	Seabirds, rodents, humans
Lebombo	Lebombo	Culicine mosquitoes	Humans, rodents
Orungo	ORU 1–4	Culicine mosquitoes	Humans, camels, cattle, goats, sheep, monkeys
Palyam	Abadina, Bunyip Creek, CSIRO village, D'Aguilar, Gweru, Kasba (Chuzan), Kindia, Marrakai, Marondera, Nyabira, Palyam, Petevo, Vellore	*Culicoides* Culicine mosquitoes	Cattle, sheep
Peruvian horse sickness	PHSV–1	Mosquitoes	Horses
St. Croix River	St. Croix River	Ticks	Unknown
Umatilla	Llano Seco, Minnal, Netivot, Umatilla	Culicine mosquitoes	Humans, birds
Wad Medani	Seletar, Wad Medani	*Boophilus*, *Rhipicephalus*, *Hyalomma*, *Argas*	Domesticated animals
Wallal	Mudjinbarry, Wallal, Wallal K	*Culicoides*	Wallabies, kangaroos
Warrego	Mitchell River, Warrego, Warrego K	*Culicoides* Anopheline and culicine mosquitoes	Wallabies, kangaroos
Wongorr virus	Paroo River, Picola, Wongorr 1–6	*Culicoides*, anopheline, and culicine mosquitoes	Cattle, macropods

Adapted from Mertens et al. *Virus Taxonomy: VIIIth Report of the International Committee on Taxonomy of Viruses.* London: Elsevier Academic Press; 2005:447–483. Please also see for further reading.

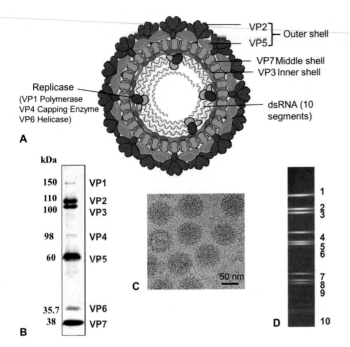

A

B

C

D

FIGURE 13.1 Bluetongue virus particles and components.
A: Schematic diagram of bluetongue virus (BTV) showing the positions and structural organization of BTV components. **B:** Gel electrophoresis profile of 7 BTV structural proteins. **C:** Electron micrographs of purified BTV particles. **D:** Gel electrophoresis profile of 10 BTV genomic segments.

extensive. Two other x-ray structures of upper VP7 domains, from BTV and AHSV, have confirmed these structural arrangements.[6,65] The VP7 trimer layer interacts tightly with the VP3 layer underneath via extensive lower domain interactions.

The inner core layer of 59 nm diameter is made up of 60 VP3 (103 kDa) dimers with T = 2 symmetry (Fig. 13.4C).[66,67,74,154] The dimers occur in an "A" or "B" type conformation, each with three domains, the carapace, apical, and dimerization domains (Fig. 13.4D). Five of the "A" conformers arrange as a five-pointed star around each fivefold axis, while five "B" conformers are positioned one between each of the points of the star, to produce a decamer. The icosahedral organization of the VP3 inner shell is shared by all members of *Reoviridae* and other viruses with segmented dsRNA genomes. It may be preserved for similar biological functions, for example, keeping the transcriptional complex and genome correctly configured across the different viruses. The inner surface of the VP3 shell has relatively few charged residues and has a series of shallow grooves.

Structural Arrangement of Internal Minor Proteins

The remaining three minor enzymatic proteins, VP1, VP4, and VP6, are closely associated with the dsRNA genomic segments, and together with the VP3 layer, they form the subcore particle. Their organization in relation to each other and to the genome within the core are less well defined than the core itself, although the structures of VP1 and VP4 are known and the entire genome of 10 dsRNAs comprising 19,218 base pairs has been modeled

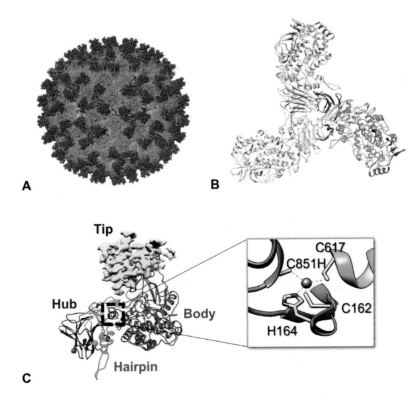

A **B** **C**

FIGURE 13.2 Structure of BTV virion particle. A: Cryo-EM density map of BTV virion at 3.5 Å resolution, shown as radially colored surface representation. **B:** VP2 triskelion formed by three VP2 monomers. **C:** Side view of VP2 monomer showing four distinct domains (hub, hairpin, body, and tip) and a zinc finger motif (CCCH tetrahedron) located at the junction of hub and body domains. (Panels **A** and **C** adapted by permission from Nature: Zhang X, Patel A, Celma CC, et al. Atomic model of a nonenveloped virus reveals pH sensors for a coordinated process of cell entry. *Nat Struct Mol Biol* 2016;23(1):74–80. Copyright © 2015 Springer Nature.)

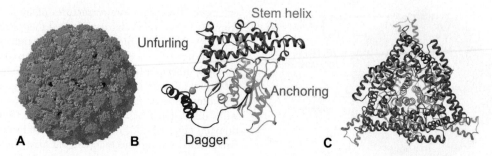

FIGURE 13.3 Structure of BTV particle without the VP2 layer. A: The particle showing the VP5 layer in two different trimer conformers (*green* and *cyan*) on the top of the VP7 layer (*yellow*). **B:** Side view of a VP5 monomer showing three distinct domains (dagger, unfurling, and anchoring). **C:** Top view of a VP5 trimer as a helical globular complex with an embedded ribbon model showing the central coiled-coil helix bundle formed by stem helices (*cyan blue*).[227] (Panels **B** and **C** adapted by permission from Nature: Zhang X, Patel A, Celma CC, et al. Atomic model of a nonenveloped virus reveals pH sensors for a coordinated process of cell entry. *Nat Struct Mol Biol* 2016;23(1):74–80. Copyright © 2015 Springer Nature.)

as four internal concentric layers.[59,60,66] Reconstruction of recombinant core-like particles (CLPs) made of VP3 and VP7 with VP1 and VP4, but lacking the genome, exhibited a flower-shaped density directly beneath the icosahedral fivefold axes and attached to the underside of the VP3 layer indicating that VP1 and VP4 may interact with each other.[75,148] However, more recent high-resolution cryo-EM structures of the BTV core itself have revealed VP1, but not VP4, anchored to the inner surface of the capsid shell (Figs. 13.5 and 13.6A). The interaction occurs with the five asymmetrically arranged N termini of the VP3 "A"

conformer, which clusters at fivefold axis.[72] The virus polymerase, VP1, has the universal "hand-shaped" core domain but two additional unique motifs not found in other viral RdRps, a "fingernail" attached to the conserved fingers subdomain, and a helix bundle formed by three novel helices, one from the palm subdomain and two from the N-terminal subdomain, and engagement with VP3 occurs via the fingernail (Fig. 13.6B). VP1 has two further unique terminal domains: an N-terminal domain and a C-terminal domain, both of which are essential for the initiation of transcription activity by the core.[72]

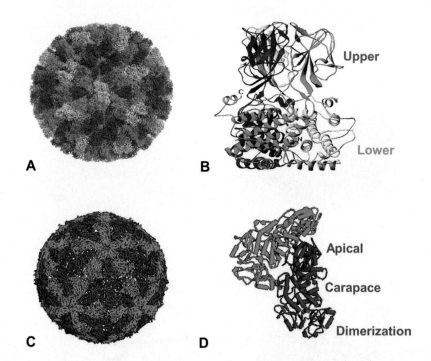

FIGURE 13.4 Crystal structure of BTV core particle and two major core proteins. A: BTV core surface at 3.5 Å resolutions, showing 13 copies of VP7, arranged as 5 trimers (colored *red, orange, green, yellow,* and *blue*) form an icosahedral asymmetric unit. **B:** Trimer image of the VP7 atomic structure at 2.8 Å resolutions. Two domains of the molecule (*upper* and *lower*) and the carboxyl and amino termini indicated. Note the flat base of the trimer lies in a horizontal plane in this view. **C:** The subcore particle showing the arrangements of two different VP3 conformers (*green* and *red*) in each of the 12 decamers. **D:** VP3 dimer unit, each monomer with three distinct domains (apical, carapace, and dimerization). (Panels **A, C** and **D** adapted by permission from Nature: Grimes JM, Burroughs JN, Gouet P, et al. The atomic structure of the bluetongue virus core. *Nature* 1998;395(6701):470–478. Copyright © 1998 Springer Nature; Panel **B** adapted from Basak AK, Grimes JM, Gouet P, et al. Structures of orbivirus VP7: implications for the role of this protein in the viral life cycle. *Structure* 1997;5(7):871–883. Copyright © 2002 Elsevier Science Ltd. With permission.)

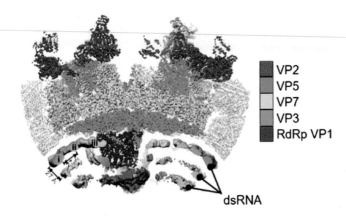

FIGURE 13.5 Cryo-EM reconstruction of the vertex region of BTV virion. The icosahedral reconstruction of BTV vertex (*gray*) showing the relative locations of the genomic RNA and individual proteins. The RNA densities are low-pass filtered and radially colored. (Adapted with permission from He Y, Shivakoti S, Ding K, et al. In situ structures of RNA-dependent RNA polymerase inside bluetongue virus before and after uncoating. *Proc Natl Acad Sci U S A* 2019;116(33):16535–16540.)

Although the exact location of VP4 has not been confirmed, the protein can be incorporated into CLPs, either alone or in complex with VP1, indicating it is likely to interact with the VP3 layer. In isolation, VP4 catalyses the formation of cap1 structures at the 5′ termini of the core-generated RNA transcripts, suggesting it may be located close to the channels through which newly synthesized transcripts must exit.[159,160] VP4 orchestrates a series of reactions, including RNA triphosphatase, guanylyltransferase, and two methyltransferase activities.[126,158–160] The x-ray

structure of VP4 shows an elongated hourglass morphology with defined domains along the length of the protein (Fig. 13.6C).[192] Two of these domains have significant structural homology to known methyltransferases and have been assigned as OMTase and N7MTase based on their structural similarity to vaccinia virus VP39 (OMTase) and Ecm1 (mRNAcap N7MTase), respectively.[46,77] A C-terminal domain of unique architecture is putatively assigned the GTase domain and is the most highly conserved region of VP4 between different orbivirus species. The functional assignment of these domains was further substantiated by direct site-directed mutagenesis *in vitro* and *in vivo* virus replication using reverse genetics.[186] An additional domain with kinase-like structural homology is present at the N terminus but lacks catalytic residues and the kinase P-loop.

The smallest core protein VP6 (36 kDa) has RNA-binding properties, resembles an RNA helicase, and is essential for RNA packaging but is not incorporated into recombinant CLPs. However, a recent study demonstrated that VP6 directly interacts with VP3 via its C-terminus *in vitro* and that perturbation of this interaction abolished RNA packaging *in vivo*, indicating the interaction with VP3 is essential for recruitment of RNA during virus assembly *in vivo*.[134,191] A nuclear magnetic resonance analysis has revealed that VP6 has a large structured domain with two large loops that exhibit significant flexibility consistent with a molecule that expands to accommodate variously sized RNAs.[133]

RNA Genome Seen in X-ray Structure of the Core

The electron density in the centre of the x-ray structure of the core is consistent with layers of highly ordered RNA.[63]

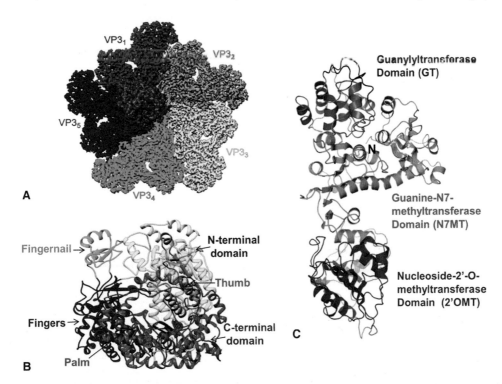

FIGURE 13.6 Three-dimensional atomic structures of BTV polymerase and capping enzyme. A: Cryo-EM density map of five copies of VP3 dimers (VP3A+VP3B) and RdRp VP1, viewed from the inside of the inner capsid. **B:** Ribbon representation of the atomic model of BTV RdRp VP1, with different domains colored as indicated. **C:** Ribbon representation of the atomic model of BTV VP4, with active sites colored as indicated. (Adapted with permission from He Y, Shivakoti S, Ding K, et al. In situ structures of RNA-dependent RNA polymerase inside bluetongue virus before and after uncoating. *Proc Natl Acad Sci U S A* 2019;116(33):16535–16540.)

Approximately 80% of the genome can be modeled as four concentric layers that have center-to-center spacing between the RNA strands of 26 to 30 Å. Grooves in the inner surface of the VP3 shell form a spiral around the fivefold axis with which the dsRNA layers appear to interact. The topography of the RNA molecules is uncertain, as the density detected in the inner layers of RNA gets progressively weaker, although each layer maintains an overall spiral organization.

GENOME STRUCTURE AND ORGANIZATION

The complete sequence of all 10 dsRNA segments was initially determined for BTV-10[60] and subsequently for a number of BTV serotypes as well as for many other orbiviruses (see Refs.[140,170]). For BTV-10, the sizes of the RNA segments range from 3,954 (segment 1) to 822 base pairs (bp) (segment 10), and the total genome is 19,220 bp long (Table 13.2). Each segment varies in sequence but shares common complementary untranslated regions (UTRs) of variable length, which include highly conserved hexanucleotides at both ends. The 5′ terminus of the coding strand of each duplex is capped and methylated, as are BTV messenger RNA (mRNA) transcripts. Apart from seg-

ment 1, the first AUG initiation codon in the mRNA strand of each segment initiates a single main open reading frame (ORF). However, there are two methionine codons in the same reading frame in the S9 and S10 RNA sequences. S9 codes VP6 and a small protein NS4,[161,186] while S10 codes for two related proteins with alternate starts NS3 and NS3A.[55,137] The encoded structural proteins are numbered VP1 to VP7 in the order of their migration on polyacrylamide gels following analysis of purified virions while the five nonstructural proteins (NS1, NS2, NS3, NS3A, and NS4) are synthesized in infected cells.[171]

MOLECULAR GENETICS

In early 1980s, the genetic diversity of the different BTV genome segments was identified by RNA oligonucleotide fingerprint analyses of field samples, and both genetic drift and shift were shown to contribute to BTV evolution.[171] In some segments, variability was clearly linked to serotype (e.g., segments 2 and 5 encoding outer capsid proteins VP2 and VP5). Further, genome segment reassortment occurred readily between different BTV serotypes but not between viruses belonging to different groups.[62,170] Partly as a result of these data, individual orbivirus serogroups are now recognized as distinct virus species.[140] Early hybridization studies confirmed

TABLE 13.2   Proteins encoded by BTV segments and their functions

Genome Segment	No. of bp[a]	Proteins	No. of aa	Predicted Size (dalton)	Estimated no. of Molecules	Location in Virion	Function
S1	3,954	VP1	1,302	149,588	12	Inner core	RNA-dependent RNA polymerase
S2	2,926	VP2	956	111,112	180	Outer capsid	Receptor binding, virus entry, hemagglutinin, type-specific neutralization
S3	2,772	VP3	901	103,344	120	Core	Scaffold for VP7 trimers
S4	2,011	VP4	654	76,433	24	Inner core	Capping enzyme with guanylyltransferase, methyltransferases 1 and 2, RNA 5′ triphosphatase, inorganic pyrophosphatase NTPase activity
S5	1,639	VP5	526	59,163	360	Outer capsid	Membrane penetration, virus entry
S6	1,770	NS1	552	64,445	NA	Nonstructural	Up-regulates viral protein translation, forms tubules
S7	1,156	VP7	349	38,548	780	Core surface layer	Viral core protein, group-specific antigenic determinant
S8	1,123	NS2	357	40,999	NA	Nonstructural	Phosphorylated, recruits viral ssRNA and core components, forms cytoplasmic VIBs, site of viral core assembly
S9	1,046	VP6	328	35,750	60–72	Inner core	Involved in viral genomic RNA packaging, has hexameric configuration, helicase
		NS4	~79	~10,000	NA	Nonstructural	Host–virus interaction, regulates interferon response
S10	822	NS3	229	25,572	NA	Nonstructural	Glycoprotein, responsible for virus trafficking and egress
		NS3A	216	24,020			

[a]Based on BTV-10 genome sequence.

that genome segments 2 and 5 (encoding the two outer capsid proteins) exhibited little or no cross-hybridization between serotypes, whereas the other eight RNA segments consistently showed some level of relatedness. Segments 1, 3, 4, 6, and 8 are relatively conserved, whereas segments 7 and 10 vary somewhat. Thus, genome segment reassortment may be an important factor in the generation of genetic diversity in orbivirus populations in nature. These results were initially confirmed by sequence comparisons of segments encoding VP5 and VP2 from six different serotypes.[171] Apart from segment 10 of

AHSV, which appears to be even more variable than that of BTV, similar results have been obtained for AHSV.[34,213] Recent extensive phylogenetic analyses of more than 200 different isolates of BTV have confirmed these early studies. The accumulating data suggested that while VP5 showed up to 70% sequence identity, VP2 sequences varied from 22% to 73% between serotypes.[118,163] Based on this analysis, 28 serotypes were identified forming 10 distinct groups based on the fact that some serotypes are more closely related than others[118,119] (Fig. 13.7A). Isolates within each serotype can also be separated

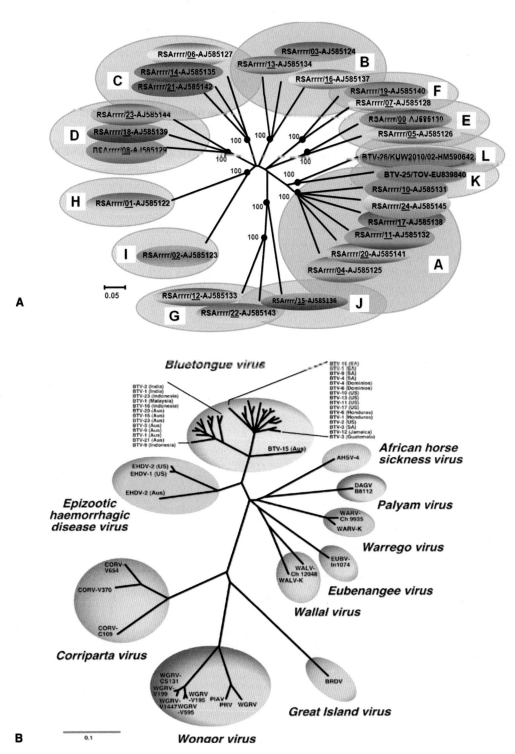

FIGURE 13.7 Phylogenetic trees of BTV serotypes **(A)** and orbiviruses **(B)**.

into two major geographical groups, Eastern (endemic in Asia, Indonesia, and Australia) and Western (endemic in Africa, the Caribbean, and the Americas). Serotypes have additionally been classified into distinct nucleotypes based on phylogenetic analysis of segment 2 (VP2) and segment 5 (VP5). VP2 was classified into 12 nucleotypes: A to L that correlates with BTV serotypes, while VP5 was classified into 10 nucleotypes: A to J and have partial correlation with BTV serotypes.

A close genetic relationship has also been demonstrated among the three *Culicoides* transmitted orbiviruses, BTV, EHDV, and AHSV. Segments encoding the core proteins, for example, VP3, are the most conserved, whereas VP2 is the most variable[90,164,219] (Fig. 13.7B). Despite as little as 17% to 23% identity, however, the VP2 protein of the three orbiviruses has a similar predicted secondary structure. Unlike VP2, the other outer capsid protein VP5 is more conserved among the three viruses, clearly indicating that these viruses share strong phylogenetic relationships.

STAGES OF VIRUS REPLICATION

The basic features of replication cycles of orbiviruses are similar to those of reoviruses and rotaviruses. However, unlike these viruses, orbiviruses multiply in arthropods as well as in vertebrate hosts, and so some stages of orbivirus replication and morphogenesis are unique. Each replication stage is described below, and the overall information available on the BTV replication cycle and assembly is summarized in a schematic diagram (Fig. 13.8).

Virus Entry

Infection by an orbivirus is established when the "core" translocates across the endosomal membrane following virus uptake, a process performed by the outer capsid proteins.[36,40,52,70,71,84] For BTV and closely related viruses, the larger VP2 protein binds to surface glycoproteins and facilitates clathrin-mediated endocytosis of the virion, while the smaller VP5 protein penetrates the host cell membrane and delivers the 470S core particle into the host cytosol.[40,53,70] Compounds that raise the lysosomal or endosomal pH (e.g., ammonium chloride) prevent endocytosis of virus particles and the subsequent release of the uncoated cores into the cytoplasm.[52] The process has two distinct stages: VP2 senses the pH in the early endosome (6.5 to 6.0) and detaches, while the remaining particle continues to the late endosome, where VP5 senses a lower pH (5.5) and gains membrane "fusion" activity, allowing the core to escape through the endosomal membrane (Fig. 13.9). This stepwise and concerted entry mechanism requires the ability to accurately sense the relative pH at each location.

It is known that BTV particles agglutinate ruminant erythrocytes[38] and the outermost spike-like VP2 protein that attaches to the cell surface during virus entry is alone responsible for such hemagglutination activity.[70] However, no definitive receptor has yet been assigned for BTV or any other orbiviruses. Recent high-resolution cryo-EM structure and biological data suggested that VP2 is likely to interact with sialic acids (SAs).[11,226] This was confirmed by probing glycan arrays with nanoparticles displaying multivalent VP2, which showed VP2 not only binds α2,3-linked SA with high affinity but also binds α2,6-linked SA. Further, in the presence of specific SA inhibitors, BTV infection and virus growth in susceptible sheep cells

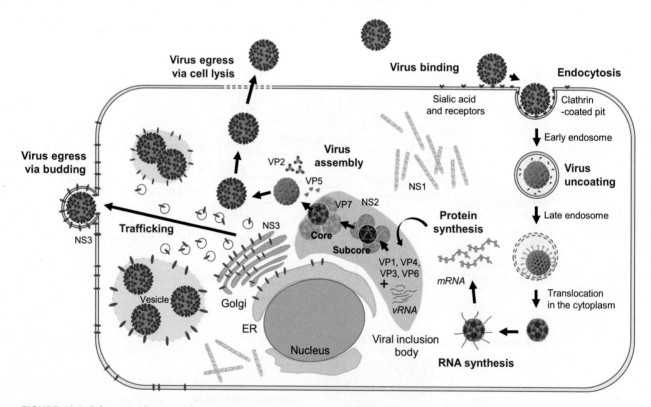

FIGURE 13.8 Schematic diagram of an orbivirus replication cycle (deduced from bluetongue virus data). The schematic shows each stage of virus replication from host cell attachment to egress of the progeny virus particles from the cell.

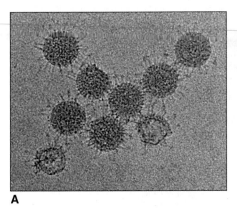 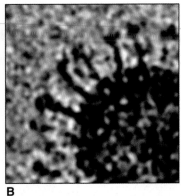 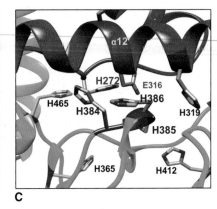

A **B** **C**

FIGURE 13.9 Cryo-EM image (~9 Å resolution) of the BTV virion at low pH environment. A and B: VP2 detached entirely, and VP5 conformation changes substantially to an extended filament structure at low pH. **C:** The core β-sheet of the anchor with a pH-sensing histidine cluster and the residues that are responsible to sense the low pH. (Panels **B** and **C** adapted by permission from Nature: Zhang X, Patel A, Celma CC, et al, Atomic model of a nonenveloped virus reveals pH sensors for a coordinated process of cell entry. *Nat Struct Mol Biol* 2016;23(1):74–80. Copyright © 2015 Springer Nature.)

is retarded confirming specific SAs act as receptors for BTV attachment.[221]

High-resolution cryo-EM structure has also made it possible to deduce how the outer capsid proteins VP2 and VP5 of BTV coordinate the process of cell entry.[227] VP2 possesses 28 His residues, several of which are highly conserved across the BTV serotypes, indicating they may play an important functional role during virus entry. However, a comprehensive structure–function analysis of residues in VP2 revealed that no one His residue is critical for pH-sensing activity. Rather, a cluster of residues making up a zinc finger (CCCH), which includes a His residue, acts to sense the low pH that triggers VP2 detachment (see Fig. 13.2C). Both the conformation of the zinc finger and its correct position are critical for function during virus entry.[223]

The disengagement of VP2 from the complete virion in the early endosome is followed by the activation of the now exposed VP5 in the late endosome. VP5 shares certain structural features with the fusion proteins of enveloped viruses, consistent with membrane penetration activity. In particular, peptides representing the two amino-terminal amphipathic helices of VP5 were shown to cause leakiness of the membrane, and the full-length protein triggers strong syncytia and multinuclear cell formation when localized to the plasma membrane and treated with low pH.[53,73] The VP5 trimer also contains clusters of histidine residues, mainly dispersed in the unfurling domain and the anchoring domain and potentially could sense the low pH environment (6.0 to 5.0) for cell entry. Of the total of 19 His residues, 13 are clustered at the interface of the anchoring domain (see Fig. 13.3) and the helices of the unfurling domain. Even a single substitution at selected sites leads to loss of virus recovery, indicating that these residues are critical for the change of VP5 conformation that facilitates membrane penetration. Further, an isolated recombinant VP5 anchoring domain alone recapitulates the sensing of low pH. VP5 function is the result of dramatic refolding of the dagger and unfurling domains in the low pH of the late endosome (Fig. 13.9),[152,223,227] but in the absence of direct observation of high-resolution structures in low pH conditions and membrane attachment intermediates, the details of the exact mechanism remained undefined until very recently. However, a combination of integrative single-particle cryo-EM, cryo-electron tomography (cryo-ET), and structure-guided mutagenesis have now shown the step-wise conformational changes that occur in the endosome, including membrane inser-

tion by the VP5 dagger domain, pore formation, and viral passage through the pore.[224] The virion structure at low pH is drastically different from that at pH 8.8 and causes global structural changes in VP2, VP5, and VP7, the three capsid proteins. At low pH, VP2 is no longer visible and of the three domains of VP5 interacting with VP7 at high pH, only the anchoring domain interacts at low pH. The VP5 trimer transforms into an elongated shape with a stalk protruding from a triangular base and a loop from the anchor domain of each monomer inserts into a cleft formed between two adjacent VP7 trimers, which appears to act like a root to anchor VP5 to the core. The near-atomic resolution structures of BTV at four low-pH-triggered states reveal three drastic VP5 actions; the launch of the hidden dagger domain, the formation of the "anchor loops" already noted, and a refolding of the "unfurling domains" into a six-helix stalk. Further, 3D structures of BTV interacting with liposomes show that the length of the VP5 stalk decreases from 19.5 to 15.5 nm after insertion into membrane.[224] This stalk, along with the dagger domain and a "WHXL" motif (membrane-binding motif) in the anchoring domain, breaks the endosomal membrane, leading to core release into cell cytosol as shown in the schematic cartoon (Fig. 13.10).

In summary, VP2 initiates contact with the mammalian host cell, and VP5 mediates the penetration of the host cell membrane by breaking the endosomal membrane. Core particles lacking both VP2 and VP5 proteins are released into the cytoplasm from the endosomal vesicles. In contrast to mammalian cells, BTV cores lacking VP2 and VP5 are reportedly infectious for invertebrate cells[138] with the integrin binding "RGD" motif of VP7 involved in entry into cells of *Culicoides* species.[195] The mechanism of membrane penetration in this host remains to be determined.

Transcription and Replication

Upon release into the cytoplasm, the core becomes transcriptionally active and serves as a compartment within which the 10 genome segments are repeatedly transcribed by the core-associated enzymes VP1, VP4, and VP6.[208,216] Ten capped non-polyadenylated mRNAs are synthesized from the 10 genome segments and are released from the core particle into the host cell cytoplasm (Fig. 13.11). Transcripts are not produced at equimolar amounts from the 10 segments of BTV,[84] the smaller genome segments being generally the most abundant, although segment 6 RNA (encoding NS1) is made in greater amounts

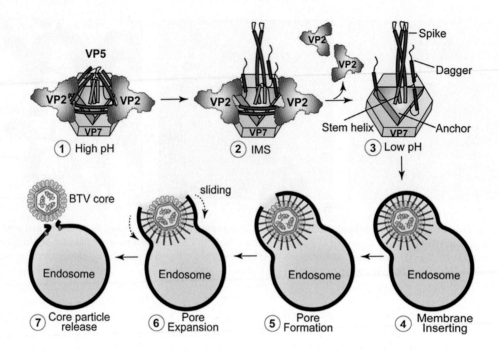

FIGURE 13.10 A schematic of BTV membrane penetration. The **upper panel** shows the conformational changes of a VP5 trimer and its neighboring VP2 and VP7 upon exposure to the low pH condition. Different domains of VP5 are colored with dagger domain in *blue*, stem helices in *cyan*, unfurling domain in *red*, and anchoring domain in *green*. Arrows show the process of structure transition and membrane penetration. The **lower panel** shows the structural rearrangements of BTV stepwise inside the late endosome, leading to the formation of a pore, enlargement of the pore, and eventually the passage of the BTV core through the pore. (Reprinted by permission from Nature: Xia X, Wu W, Cui Y, et al. Bluetongue virus capsid protein VP5 perforates membranes at low endosomal pH during viral entry. *Nat Microbiol* 2021;6(11):1424–1432. Copyright © 2021 Springer Nature.)

than the smallest segment, segment 10 RNA (encoding NS3/NS3A). The 10 transcripts act as templates both for the translation of viral proteins and for negative-strand viral RNA synthesis to generate more genomic dsRNAs.[137,208,209] The replication of BTV, like other members of the family, uses a packaged plus-strand RNA as template for the synthesis of a "minus" strand, resulting in genomic dsRNA, which remains within nascent progeny particles. The basis of copy choice between the plus-

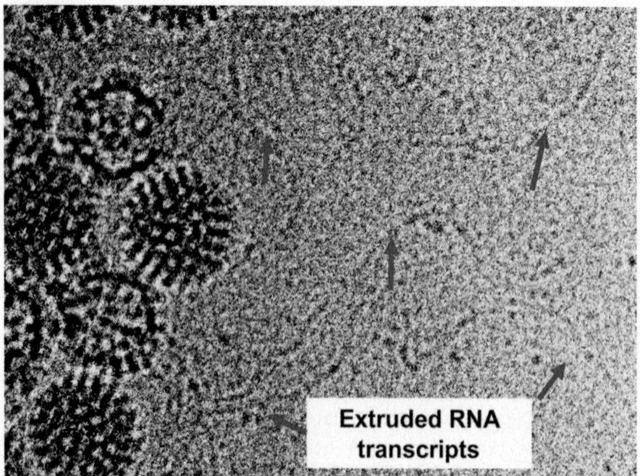

and minus-strand RNAs and the full roles of each protein in the process remain to be defined. Transfection of mammalian cells with *in vitro* BTV transcripts also leads to generation of viral proteins and infectious virus particles as demonstrated by the passage of infectivity in BSR cells.[17] These findings underpinned the development of a helper virus–independent reverse genetics system for BTV and other orbiviruses.[17,128]

When intact cores isolated from virus particles are activated *in vitro* in the presence of magnesium ions and NTP substrates, distinct conformational changes can be seen around the fivefold axis.[63,72] This is interpreted as an outward movement of VP3 and VP7, allowing opening of a pore in the VP3 layer at the fivefold axes through which the mRNAs are extruded. The structural integrity of the core particle appears to be essential for efficient transcriptional activity *in vivo*, but it has been possible to use *in vitro* assays with the three minor proteins of the core to delineate the specific roles of each (see Ref.[165]).

The Largest Protein VP1 Is the RNA-Dependent RNA Polymerase

The first indication that the largest BTV protein, VP1 (149.5 kD), is the virus polymerase protein came from sequence comparison with other DNA and RNA polymerases and from an *in vitro* polymerase assay that used a crude extract of insect cells infected with a recombinant baculovirus expressing only BTV VP1.[60,205] Subsequent *in vitro* studies with purified recombinant VP1 protein have shown that it exhibits a processive replicase activity in the absence of any other viral proteins and initiates BTV minus-strand synthesis *de novo*.[19] Recombinant

Extruded RNA transcripts

FIGURE 13.11 Electron micrographs of transcribing core particles. Transcription takes place at the vertices of the cores extruding mRNA through the apices.

VP1 copies each of the plus-strand RNA segments fully, from the smallest (822 nt) to the largest (3,954 nt), either individually or simultaneously in a single *in vitro* reaction, to produce a dsRNA duplex that is RNase I resistant and RNase III sensitive. Synthesis of dsRNAs from capped single-stranded RNA (ssRNA) templates is significantly higher than from uncapped ssRNA templates and could be mimicked by priming with complementary terminal dinucleotides (Ref.[131] and unpublished findings). Some evidence for template specificity was suggested by the fact that dsRNAs were not synthesized from nonviral ssRNA templates unless they were fused to specific BTV sequences. These data contrast those of rotavirus and reovirus where the assigned polymerase protein (VP1) is only active in the context of the inner shell protein VP2[202] and where recombinant reovirus polymerase λ3 is generally incapable of synthesizing *de novo* reovirus RNA, although short RNA transcripts have been observed.[181,196]

Of the three domains, the polymerase domain (PD), N-terminal domain (NTD), and C-terminal domain (CTD) of VP1, only the purified PD fragment, not the NTD or CTD fragments, bound NTPs, but only when all three were mixed together, RdRp activity was reconstituted *in vitro*. Further, the activity depended on the signature catalytic GDD motif (aa763 to 765) within the PD domain.[218] These data are consistent with the structural data obtained more recently, which has shown that the detachment of VP2 and VP5 during viral entry induces global movement in the core and local conformational changes of the N termini of the VP3 "A" conformer, which primes the polymerase within the capsid for transcription.[72] The N-terminal domain of VP1 opens the genome duplex to isolate the template strand, while the C-terminal domain splits the emerging template–transcript product, guiding genome reannealing to form a transcription bubble. At the same time, the VP3 layer is wedged open to allow release of the newly synthesized transcripts through the channels at the five field axis of the particle (see Fig. 13.6A and B). The interaction with the N-terminal helix of the VP3 A conformer, which was noted earlier as a docking site for VP1 within the core, thus acts as a latch to control RdRp activity. However, the mechanistic detail of this transcription switch and, importantly, how the polymerase subsequently switches to replication are still unclear.

The Minor Protein VP4 Is the mRNA Capping Enzyme

Although VP1 has been shown to be active as the viral RdRp, it does not form the methylated cap structure found at the 5′ end of all BTV mRNAs. Rather, the cap results from the three key enzymatic activities noted earlier as associated with VP4; (a) an RNA triphosphatase (RTase) that hydrolyzes the 5′-triphosphate terminus of the mRNA to a diphosphate, (b) a guanylyltransferase (GTase) that caps the diphosphate terminus with GMP via a 5′-5′ triphosphate linkage, and (c) a guanine-*N*7-methyltransferase (N7MTase) that adds a methyl group to the N7 position of the blocking guanosine (see Fig. 13.6C). An additional nucleoside-2′-*O*-methyltransferase (2′OMTase) is also required for BTV to methylate the 2′-hydroxyl group of the ribose of the first nucleotide (namely type 1 cap). Recombinant, purified VP4 (76.4 kD) synthesizes type 1–like "cap" structures *in vitro* that are identical to those found on authentic BTV mRNA.[126,159,160] This is notably different from other viral capping enzymes, for example, those of vaccinia virus, where

completion of capping is dependent on a complex of three proteins.[214] The atomic structure of the protein shows how a single protein orchestrates all of these activities via different domains (see Fig. 13.6C),[192] and the catalytic activity of each domain has also been confirmed by individual domain expression and site-specific mutagenesis.[186]

The Minor Protein VP6 Is the Helicase and RNA Packaging Enzyme

Genome replication in the *Reoviridae* is fully conservative and logically requires helicase activity, either to unwind the dsRNA ahead of transcription or to separate the parental and newly synthesized RNAs after. For BTV, VP6 has a strong binding affinity for both ssRNAs and dsRNAs, possesses nucleoside triphosphatase activity, and unwinds dsRNA substrates *in vitro*.[182] Similar to other helicases, VP6 is hexameric and forms ring-like structures in the presence of BTV RNAs.[98] Using reverse genetics, it was confirmed that VP6 is an integral part of the transcription complex.[130] How substrates pass from one component of the transcription complex to the next remains a significant question however. A recent proteomic (RNA cross-linking and peptide fingerprinting, RCAP) approach has identified the VP6 domains responsible for RNA binding. Both recombinant VP6 and core-associated VP6 proteins have multiple distinct RNA-binding regions, but only one region is shared between them. A combination of targeted mutagenesis in VP6 and reverse genetics identified this RNA-binding region as essential for virus replication, and *in vitro* assembly assays have further suggested that this region plays a specific role in ssRNA recruitment during capsid assembly, strengthening a role for VP6 in genome packaging as well as in replication.[191]

Protein Synthesis and Virus Replication

BTV-specific proteins are detectable within 2 to 4 hours postinfection, and the rate of protein synthesis increases rapidly until 11 to 13 hours postinfection.[83] In addition to the seven structural proteins of the virion, four virus-encoded nonstructural proteins, NS1, NS2, NS3/NS3A, and NS4, are synthesized in BTV-infected cells. Infection of mammalian cells with BTV, in contrast to insect cells, leads to a rapid inhibition of cellular macromolecular synthesis and the induction of a robust apoptotic response triggered by multiple apoptotic pathways.[147,185] Of the four NS proteins, NS1 (64 kD) and NS2 (41 kD) are produced abundantly, and each forms a distinct structure found in infected cells, indicating these two proteins are involved in early virus replication. NS1 forms a large number of unique tubular structures, hallmarks of BTV and other orbivirus infection (Fig. 13.12A).[81,206] It also selectively upregulates viral protein synthesis by binding to the conserved 3′ terminal hexanucleotide sequence (5′ ACUUAC 3′) of viral mRNAs.[18] It could be that NS1 interacts with the viral RNA and host translational factors to recruit ribosomes to the viral mRNA. NS1 is essential for virus replication, as NS1 knockout and point mutants introduced by reverse genetics are lethal.[132] A near-atomic resolution structure of NS1 tubules has been reported, showing them to be helical assemblies of NS1 monomers (Fig. 13.12C).[99] Individual NS1 monomers have three domains, an amino-terminal "foot," a "head," and a carboxyl-terminal "body" with an unusual extended carboxyl-terminal arm (Fig. 13.12D). The structure also revealed two putative zinc fingers whose function is not yet clear. The C-ter-

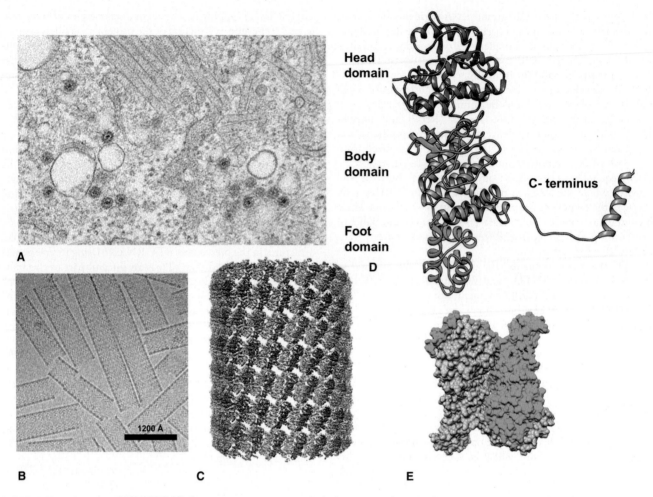

FIGURE 13.12 Images of BTV NS1 tubules. A: Negative staining of tubules in BTV-infected cells. **B:** Negative staining of purified BTV tubules isolated from insect cells infected with recombinant baculovirus expressing NS1. **C:** Cryo-EM reconstruction of BTV tubule at 4.0 Å showing helical assemblies of NS1. **D:** Atomic model (shown as ribbon diagram) of an NS1 monomer showing three distinct domains (head, body, and foot) and the extended C-terminal arm handshake. **E:** Space-filling surface rendering of an NS1 dimeric building subunit of tubular form. Note the hydrophobic groove in the head domain and the hydrophobic inner surface of the C-terminal arm. Note that the monomers are arranged in the tubule in an alternating head-to-foot orientation. (Panels **B**, **C** and **D** adapted by permission from Nature: Kerviel A, Ge P, Lai M, et al. Atomic structure of the translation regulatory protein NS1 of bluetongue virus. *Nat Microbiol* 2019;4(5):837–845. Copyright © 2019 Springer Nature.)

minal arm of one monomer wraps around the head domain of another through hydrophobic interactions, and deletion of the C terminus prevents tubule formation, though not viral replication (Fig. 13.12E). This suggests that NS1 monomers, not tubules, are the active form stimulating viral mRNA translation. Whether there is a role for the tubular form, other than as a repository for excess protein, remains to be determined.

NS2 (41 kDa), which is the only phosphorylated protein of BTV, forms the second structure in infected cells, viral inclusion bodies (VIBs, Fig. 13.13A).[21,39,86,97] Expression of phosphorylated NS2 alone results in the formation of inclusion bodies (Fig. 13.13B) similar to the VIBs.[142,200] NS2 is phosphorylated by cellular casein kinase II (CKII) via two serine residues at positions 249 and 259.[142] It also possesses nucleotide triphosphatase (NTP) phosphohydrolase activity.[78] In addition, NS2 binds Ca^{2+} efficiently via an EF-hand–like Ca^{2+}-binding motif located in the carboxyl-terminal region, and Ca^{2+} binding is perturbed when the Asp and Glu residues in the motif were substituted by alanine (Fig. 13.13C).[157] Further, Ca^{2+} binding by NS2 triggered a helix-to-coil secondary structure transition forming helical oligomers, which, when visualized

by cryo-EM, suggested that Ca^{2+} caused the NS2 N-terminal domain to wrap around the C-terminal domain in the oligomer (Fig. 13.13D). The presence of Ca^{2+} also enhanced the phosphorylation of NS2 significantly, and mutations at the Ca^{2+}-binding site in the viral genome failed in virus recovery. The protein has a high content of positively charged residues and has affinity for viral ssRNA over host RNAs, but phosphorylation is not necessary for either of these RNA-binding properties.[60,124,199] Chemical and enzymatic structure probing of the preferentially bound RNAs has suggested that NS2 recognizes unique hairpin loop secondary structures,[115] which could be part of a mechanism of how BTV mRNAs are selected from the pool of cellular messages for incorporation into assembling virus particles. NS2 also recruits newly synthesized core proteins, consistent with this model.

NS1 and NS2 Are Essential Components of the Primary Replication Complex

The assembly of a distinct early replicase complex in BTV-infected cells was suggested by the opportunistic finding that repeated transfection of *in vitro* generated BTV RNA

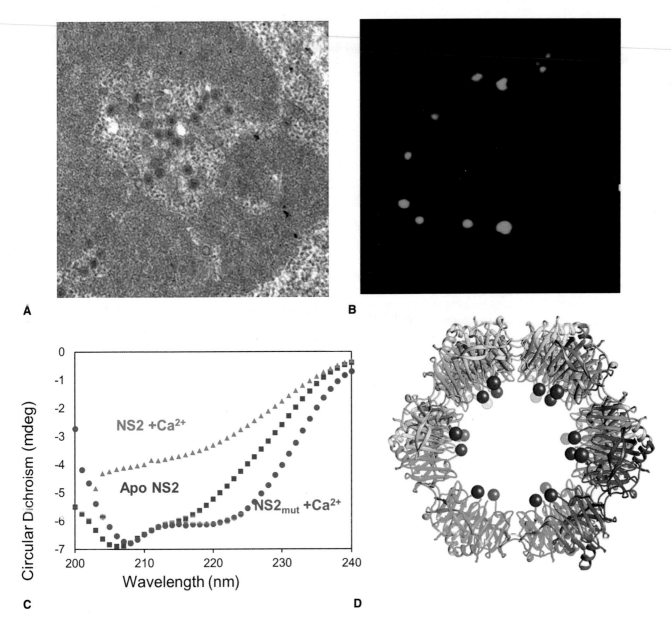

FIGURE 13.13 NS2, the predominant component of inclusion bodies. A: Virus inclusion body in BTV-infected cells containing immature virus particles. (Adapted from Kar AK, Bhattacharya B, Roy P. Bluetongue virus RNA binding protein NS2 is a modulator of viral replication and assembly. *BMC Mol Biol* 2007;8:4. https://creativecommons.org/licenses/by/2.0.) **B:** Inclusion bodies formed by baculovirus-expressed GFP-tagged NS2. **C:** NS2–calcium interaction. Circular dichroism analysis of NS2 in the presence of Ca^{2+} showing helix to coil transition in contrast to NS2 in the absence of Ca^{2+}. Mutation at Ca^{2+}-binding site shows no change of NS2 helix. **D:** Cryo-EM of NS2 oligomer model in the presence of Ca^{2+} showing NS2 N-terminal helical domain[23] wrapping around the C-terminal domain (labeled as *purple spheres*).

transcripts improved the recovery of infectious BTV by approximately 50-fold when compared to single transfection.[17] Stimulation did not require the complete set of transcripts, only those encoding the inner capsid proteins VP1, VP3, VP4, and VP6 but also NS1 and NS2, the two NS proteins associated with VIBs and BTV protein synthesis.[132] The same study also suggested that helicase VP6 acted early in replication and that "capped" transcripts were not essential for packaging, as the second transfection could use capped or uncapped transcripts with the same level of rescue. Interestingly, the addition of a transcript encoding VP7 to the primary transfection mix, which would allow completion of the core particle, did not further

stimulate virus recovery, suggesting that a fully competent replicase complex required only a VP3-based substructure.

VIBs and Virus Assembly

VIBs are large globular inclusion bodies that are a signature feature of all other members of the *Reoviridae* including orbiviruses.[21] VIBs initially appear as granular material scattered throughout the cell, but then coalesce to form a prominent perinuclear inclusion.[21,39,86,97,171] RNA packaging and assembly of subviral particles for all orbiviruses occur within these VIBs, which are also known as "virus factories."[97,132,142] The phosphorylated NS2, the major component, is essential for VIB

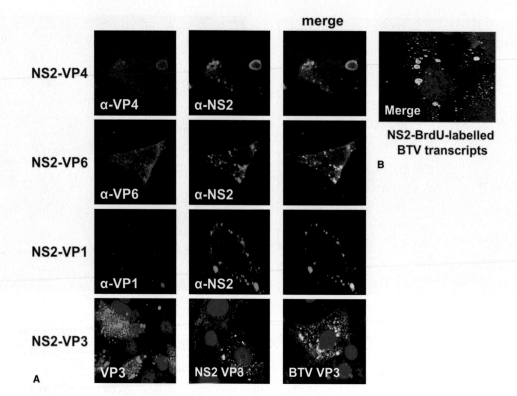

FIGURE 13.14 Interaction of NS2 and viral proteins. A: Confocal microscopy showing the colocalization of three polymerase complex proteins and NS2 in BTV-infected cells. **B:** Same showing the interactions of NS2 and 5-bromo-2′-deoxyuridine–labeled BTV ssRNA transcripts.

formation (Fig. 13.14).[142,171,200] Various analyses have led to the discovery of cellular enzymes including CK2, phosphatase 2A, and heat-shock (Hsp90) protein within VIBs, in addition to the viral components.[142–145] Further, coexpression of core structural proteins has shown that although VP1, VP3, VP4, and VP6 all colocalize with NS2 inclusions in the absence of viral replication, the core surface protein VP7 requires the presence of VP3 to be recruited (Fig. 13.14A and B). Electron microscopy using recombinant NS2 and virion proteins in different combinations has revealed that NS2 associates with assembling core particles.[97,142] Consistent with this, when a cell line constitutively expressing NS2 was infected with BTV followed by first treatment with actinomycin D and subsequent addition of bromouridine, the newly synthesized labeled BTV transcripts were identified within the VIBs.[97] Since nonphosphorylated NS2 fails to assemble into VIBs, the modification of NS2 may control the level of VIBs formation to provide the matrix for viral assembly.[142] The accumulating data suggest that the assembly of VIBs is reversible, and a working hypothesis is that NS2 coordinates VIB assembly and disassembly, and so virus assembly and release, through phosphorylation/dephosphorylation and Ca^{2+} signaling. Experimental perturbation of Ca^{2+} binding inhibits virus replication, supporting this model.[157]

Since VIBs lack membranes, these structures may be liquid–liquid phase separation (LLP) structures, which typically condense RNA and proteins into defined but dynamic structures within the cell.[93,189,228] This would explain their known regulation by external factors such as temperature, osmotic potential, and ionic composition in addition to posttranslational modifications such as phosphorylation. Recent studies

on the CKII-mediated *in vitro* phosphorylation of NS2 demonstrated that phosphorylation of NS2 triggers phase separation of NS2 with the level of enzyme activity corresponding to the extent of NS2 phase separation, implying that the phosphorylated population of NS2 phase separates while nonphosphorylated NS2 does not (Rahman & Roy, 2022; Manuscript in preparation). Thus, NS2 may recruit viral components to their assembly site[142] (Figs. 13.13 and 13.14) and control the assembly and release of virus particles via phosphorylation of NS2 and guide the emergence of immature virus particles from their site of synthesis into the cytoplasm.

Capsid Assembly
BTV structural proteins have an inherent capacity to self-assemble into CLPs and virus-like particles (VLPs) that lack the viral genome[56,57] (Fig. 13.15A), and their assembly by expression of viral structural proteins in insect cells (see Ref.[172]) has shed much light on the assembly pathway. Further, a combination of recent high-resolution structural information of BTV particles together with the development of reverse genetics has contributed significantly to the understanding of the virus assembly pathway as discussed below.

VP3 Assembly and Subcore Formation
A key question in virus assembly is whether the VP3 decamer observed in the core structure[66] is an identifiable intermediate in the assembly process. As the dimerization domain present in the VP3 AB conformers is known, it could be deleted, leading to the abolition of the subcore, yet decamer formation was retained (Fig. 13.15B). This indicates that decamers are the first

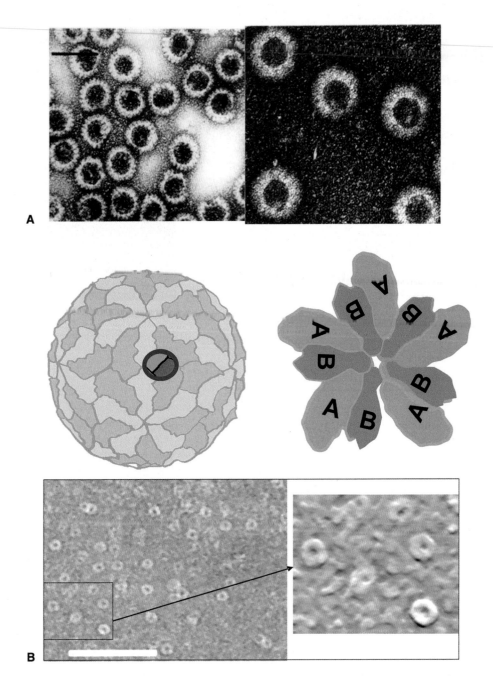

FIGURE 13.15 Assembly of recombinant BTV proteins. A: Recombinant baculoviruses expressing VP3 and VP7 forming core-like particles, CLPs (*left panel*), and VP2, VP3, VP5, and VP7 expression forming virus-like particles, VLPs (*right panel*). **B:** *Upper panel* is a schematic presentation of VP3 layer of BTV indicating the dimerization site between the two subunits A and B (*left*) and the schematic of a VP3 decamer (*right*). *Lower panel* is the dimerization domain deletion mutant of recombinant VP3, which generates VP3 decamers, the subunit of VP3 layer. (Panel **B** adapted from Kar AK, Ghosh M, Roy P. Mapping the assembly pathway of Bluetongue virus scaffolding protein VP3. *Virology* 2004;324(2):387–399. Copyright © 2004 Elsevier. With permission.)

stable assembly intermediate and that decamer–decamer interactions then proceed via the dimerization domain and drive the assembly of the complete VP3 subcore.

Based on CLP assembly, both VP1 and VP4 have been shown to associate independently with the VP3 layer[110,148] and a VP1-VP4 complex also interacts directly with the VP3 decamer in solution.[98] By contrast, while BTV RNAs interact with VP3 *in vitro*, they fail to associate with VP3 decamers under the same conditions. BTV cores may thus initiate with the complex formed by VP1 and VP4 with VP3 decamers, which subsequently recruits the RNA segments prior to completion of their assembly. However, current high-resolution structural analysis of virus cores by cryo-EM has failed to locate VP6 and the location of VP4 is uncertain, although both are likely to be at the fivefold axis with VP1. There may be some flexibility in their precise arrangements or they could be obscured by the genomic RNA within the core.[72] More recent molecular analysis, using recombinant VP6 and VP3 and pull-down experiments, has

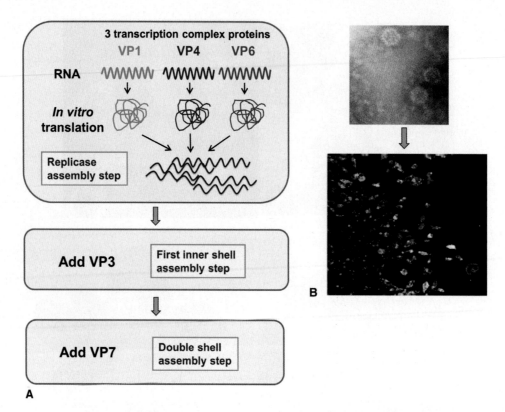

FIGURE 13.16 *In vitro* **reconstitution of BTV core. A:** Cartoon of the cell-free assembly assay of BTV cores showing the sequential inclusion and incubation of BTV proteins and 10 ssRNA transcripts (shown in *purple*). **B:** EM analysis of assembled particles (**upper panel**) purified by sucrose gradient. **Lower panel** shows *in vitro* generated cores are infectious in *Culicoides* insect cells and expressing BTV proteins, NS1 (*green*) and VP5 (*red*). (Adapted with permission from Lourenco S, Roy P. In vitro reconstitution of Bluetongue virus infectious cores. *Proc Natl Acad Sci U S A* 2011;108(33):13746–13751.)

indicated that VP6 has direct interaction with VP3. Newly synthesized mRNAs are also probably packaged during the assembly of subcores, and it is likely that RNA replication takes place after subcore or core formation. Using an *in vitro* translation cell-free assembly system (CFA), evidence has been obtained of the assembly of BTV RNA–protein complexes *de novo* showing that no host protein is required (Fig. 13.16).[112] Following translation of the core replicase components, the addition of 10 ssRNAs representing noncapped positive-strand copies of each genomic segment leads to assembly of a complete BTV core. Such *in vitro* assembled cores are functional, as the 10 packaged ssRNA molecules convert to 10 dsRNA genomic segments when the necessary nucleotides are added. Furthermore, reconstituted cores isolated from sucrose velocity gradients were infectious in *Culicoides* insect vector cell culture, generating all the viral proteins and subsequently leading to the recovery of fully infectious particles. The *in vitro* virus assembly system makes it possible to delineate the role and order of each component in the assembly pathway as well as the requirements for genome packaging.

Assembly of Genomic RNA and Packaging

The mechanism by which BTV and related viruses with multipartite genomes package their genomes into capsids has proved elusive. However, use of the CFA assay has shown that the sorting of the segmented RNA genome starts the process and that marked individual segments, as well as mutant RNAs, could

be incorporated.[112] Subsequently, it was demonstrated that a set of smaller segments (S7 to S10) could be packaged in the absence of larger segments but that larger segments required smaller segments in order to be packaged. Excluding one segment individually from a packaging reaction of 9 versus all 10 ssRNA segments in the CFA has confirmed an essential role for the smaller segments as initiators, as measured by quantitative RT-PCR (qRT-PCR). Exclusion of the smallest segment S10 abolished RNA packaging, but exclusion of the three larger segments (S1 to S3) still allowed packaging of the remaining seven segments with a 50% efficiency (Fig. 13.17A). Further, the secondary structure of the smallest segment, S10, was important for packaging, and it has a high affinity for RNA–RNA interaction with three small ssRNAs (S7 to S9) but not with larger segments or with unrelated rotavirus segments.[190] A series of pull-down experiments with different combinations of ssRNA segments has confirmed that complex formation starts with the smaller segments, which form a complex that binds the medium segments, forming a larger complex which in turn interacts with the larger segments (Fig. 13.17B).

An electrophoretic mobility shift assay (EMSA) has shown distinct retarded bands when RNA products representing the interacting segments were cotranscribed rather than coincubated, suggesting that RNA segments interact during or soon after synthesis. Further, short antisense nuclease-resistant oligoribonucleotides (ORNs) that are complementary to the 3′UTR of S10 disrupted complex formation by EMSA, and

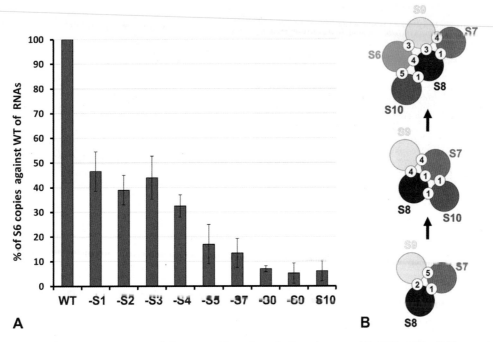

FIGURE 13.17 Packaging of 10 ssRNA segments follows specific orders. A: Complete set of 10 BTV ssRNAs (WT) or exclusion of one ssRNA segment at a time (-S1, -S2, etc.) in the cell-free assembly assay demonstrating RNA segments are packaged sequentially and larger segments packaging depends on smaller RNA segments. (Adapted from Sung PY, Roy P. Sequential packaging of RNA genomic segments during the assembly of Bluetongue virus. *Nucleic Acids Res* 2014;42(22):13824–13838. https://creativecommons.org/licenses/by/4.0/.) **B:** The cartoon showing predicted BTV S6 to S10 *trans* network at three stages of RNA complex assembly during RNA packaging; individual segments are color-coded, and the numbers of putative interaction sites among different segments in different stages are shown in the *white circles*. (Adapted from AlShaikhahmed K, Leonov G, Sung PY, et al. Dynamic network approach for the modelling of genomic sub-complexes in multi-segmented viruses. *Nucleic Acids Res* 2018;46(22):12087–12098. https://creativecommons.org/licenses/by/4.0/.)

their inclusion in the CFA assay inhibited packaging and reduced virus replication in cell culture.[48] These data have confirmed that RNA–RNA interactions are required to trigger BTV RNA segment packaging into the assembling capsid and that specific sequences are involved in such interactions. The same interactions occur in another related orbivirus, EHDV, and in rotavirus, an 11-segmented RNA genome, supporting the view that these classes of viruses utilize similar mechanisms for packaging their segmented RNA genomes.[47,49] The RNA–RNA interactions between different genomic segments appear to occur *transiently* at multiple specific sites, termed segment assortment signals (SASs), that are dispersed across each segment (Fig. 13.17B) prior to formation of the *cis*-acting RNA networks required for packaging.[2] The deduction of the packaging mechanism has uncovered a unique aspect of the virus replication cycle that could be exploited as a drug target to inhibit assembly or for designing defective interfering particles containing an incomplete set of genomic segments that may act as effective vaccines.

VP7 Assembly and Core Formation

The mismatch between the number of subunits in the VP3 and VP7 layers of the core poses an interesting problem for an icosahedral structure. Core assembly has been shown to depend on the VP7 trimer, the precise "shape" of the trimers being sufficient to drive the formation of the tight lattice of 260 trimers on the VP3 core surface.[107,108] The VP7 trimers probably form around different nucleation sites instead of a cascade of trimer associations originating from a single nucleation site, as

originally suggested by structural studies.[66] A likely pathway of core assembly is therefore that a number of strong VP7 trimer–VP3 contacts act as multiple equivalent initiation sites and that a second set of weaker interactions then "fill in the gaps" to complete the outer layer of the core. The "T" trimers (of a complete set of P, Q, R, S, and T trimers noted in the structure) at the threefold axes of symmetry have the strongest interactions and act as nucleation, whereas the "P" trimers, which are farthest from the threefold axis and closer to the fivefold axis are the last to attach. This variation in attachment allows assembly even of nonicosahedral matched layers.[108]

Interactions Between Core and Outer Capsid Proteins

Following the assembly of the core particle, the viral outer capsid proteins, VP2 and VP5, are added. Cryo-EM experiments have aided our understanding of how the outer capsid proteins interact with the outer VP7 layer of the core,[148,226,227] showing that although the triangular shaped top of VP7 serves as a platform for the deposition of the VP2 and VP5, the resulting structural interaction is mismatched.[226,227] Each VP2 trimer contacts four VP7 trimers through the base of the VP2 hub, body, and hairpin domains via a loop, which interacts with the jelly-roll top domain of the VP7 trimer (Fig. 13.18).

The interaction between VP5 and VP7 are extensive with all three VP5 domains involved (Fig. 13.18). By contrast, the VP2 interaction with VP5 is relatively weak, via only two regions, the VP2 hub domain, which interacts with the N-terminal helices of the VP5 trimer, and the VP2 hairpin loop,

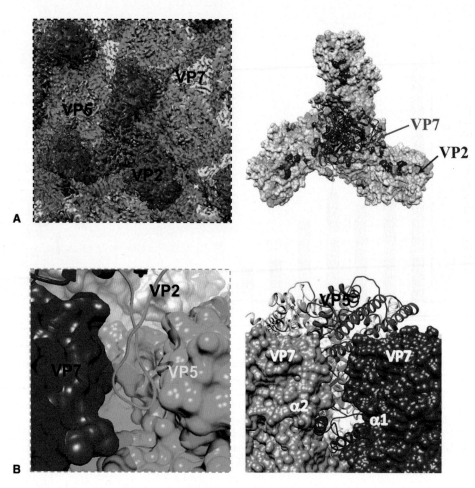

FIGURE 13.18 Interactions between VP2, VP5, and VP7 proteins. A: Cryo-EM of a cut-off portion of virion surface showing interaction of a VP2 trimer with VP7 and VP5 (*left panel*) and the ribbon model (*red*) shows a VP7 trimer interacting with the hub domains of a VP2 trimer (*right panel*). **B:** The hairpin loop region of VP2 interacting with VP7 and VP5 (*left panel*) and interactions of two helices (α1 and α2) of the VP5 dagger domain with two adjacent VP7 trimers (*right panel*). (Adapted by permission from Nature: Zhang X, Patel A, Celma CC, et al. Atomic model of a nonenveloped virus reveals pH sensors for a coordinated process of cell entry. *Nat Struct Mol Biol* 2016;23(1):74–80. Copyright © 2015 Springer Nature.)

which interacts with the anchoring domain of an adjacent VP5 trimer. These weak interactions are consistent with the requirements for VP2 detachment during cell entry when VP2 must dissociate to permit the conformational change of VP5 discussed above.[152,223,224]

Despite the detailed understanding of protein–protein interactions, how and where VP2 and VP5 are added to the core in infected cells remains unclear. Visualized by microscopy, assembled cores within the VIBs appear to recruit VP5, although the major VIB protein, NS2, does not interact with it directly.[146] A loose arrangement may be necessary at this time as VP5 addition may occlude the channels through which replication substrates (ATP and nucleotides) pass in order to complete core transcription. This would shut down the core and prevent the completion of replication. Each VP5 trimer bridges the channel formed by six underlying VP7 trimers,[227] and its binding would be consistent with the lock that freezes the virus in a primed state for the next round of infection. The assembly of VP2 protein, however, clearly does not occur in the VIBs,[64,146] and localization of its assembly site remains to be determined. Given their weak lateral interactions, it is likely that VP2 attaches to the core independently of VP5. There may be no

particular site for VP2 attachment, more a gradual coating as the VP5-coated core exits the VIB. Such view would be consistent with the fact that VP2 and VP5 interaction with the core occurs easily in either baculovirus expression systems (to form a VLP) or by *in vitro* transcription–translation systems.[56,74,109,111]

Maturation, Trafficking, and Egress of Progeny Virions

Electron microscopy of BTV- and AHSV-infected cell sections shows a striking vesicular distribution of virus particles, indicating that vesicular structures are involved in virus maturation.[9,12,215] Further, disruption of lipid rafts with methyl-beta-cyclodextrin decreases the BTV viral titer.[11] A conserved membrane-docking domain similar to a motif in synaptotagmin, a protein belonging to the SNARE (soluble *N*-ethylmaleimide–sensitive fusion attachment protein receptor) family, was identified in the VP5 sequence.[11] Site-directed mutagenesis of this motif, followed by flotation and confocal analyses, has confirmed a raft association for VP5 that is essential for BTV replication. SNARE domains interact with the negatively charged lipid phosphatidylinositol (4,5) bisphosphate [PI(4,5)P2] in membrane rafts, and both VP5 and BTV nonstructural

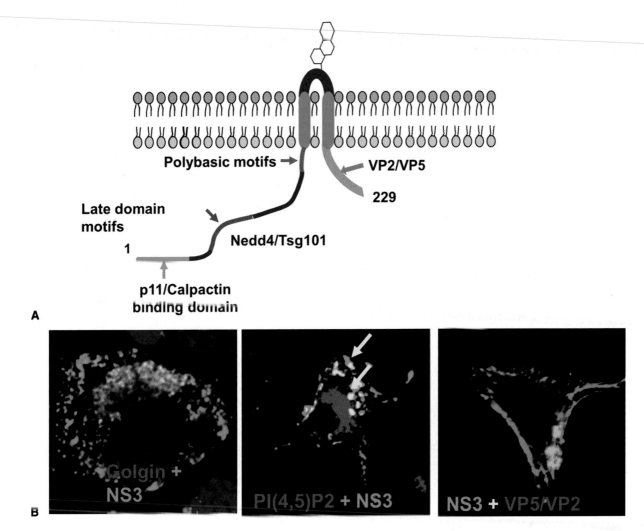

FIGURE 13.19 BTV NS3 protein. A: Schematic diagram showing the organization of BTV NS3 protein domains and its interacting sites with BTV outer capsid proteins and various host proteins during virus egress. **B:** Confocal microscopy showing the colocalization of NS3 and Golgi body, and interactions of NS3, PI(4,5)P2(D) (indicated by *arrows*), and two outer capsid proteins.[13]

protein NS3 colocalizes with PI(4,5)P2 in infected cells[14] (Fig. 13.19B). Depletion of PI(4,5)P2 or its relocation to endosomal-like structures inhibits BTV, emphasizing the importance of these membrane microdomains for BTV virion maturation and egress.[8,10,26,88,103] The data are consistent with a role of internal vesicular membranes in providing a scaffold for virus assembly and the use of those vesicles for trafficking assembled virus to the plasma membrane.

Role of NS3 in Virus Trafficking

NS3, a 229aa protein of molecular mass 25.5 kDa, and its shorter form, NS3A (24 kDa), which lacks the N-terminal 13 amino acids, are the major regulatory proteins of virus maturation, trafficking, and egress.[27,87,220] NS3/NS3A is the only glycoprotein containing membrane domains synthesized by BTV. NS3/NS3A is synthesized in the endoplasmic reticulum (ER) and transits through the Golgi apparatus, where it becomes glycosylated, prior to reaching the plasma membrane.[4,222] To date, no molecular structure of NS3 is available. The protein consists of a long N-terminal and a shorter C-terminal cytoplasmic domain, linked by two transmembrane hydrophobic domains (aa118 to 141; aa162 to 182) and a short 21aa extracellular loop with a single N-linked glycosylation site at asparagine 150 (Fig. 13.19A).[4,8,222] Although NS3 is highly conserved across all BTV serotypes,[85,155] certain amino acids have been linked to variation in BTV virulence, consistent with its role in virus spread.[58]

NS3 can be visualized at the periphery of the VIBs indicating that it may facilitate the export of core particles, possibly already covered in VP5, from the VIBs to the site of release.[146] The C-terminal domain of NS3 interacts with both VP5 and VP2.[8,11] The NS3 C-terminal cytoplasmic domain directly binds VP2, and floatation experiments have confirmed that NS3, the two outer capsid proteins VP2 and VP5, as well as the core proteins all are associated with lipid raft domains.[12,14] BTV also uses the cell cytoskeleton in virus particles maturation, as it has been demonstrated that VP2 is able to interact with the vimentin intermediate filaments.[10]

BTV infection of mammalian cells was shown to induce autophagy, while exogenous induction of autophagy has been shown to promote BTV infection. Conversely, inhibition of autophagy inhibits BTV replication, delaying the accumulation of NS3 and the outer capsid protein VP2, to reduce virus maturation overall.[104] Together, these findings demonstrate a clear link between intracellular vesicles and virus maturation and egress.

A recent study revealed that NS3 possesses two polybasic motifs (PBM1 and PMB2) located upstream of the first transmembrane domain, which are conserved among the orbiviruses. While PBM1 acts as an ER retention signal, PBM2 is a membrane export signal.[103] Deletion of these motifs attenuates the virus, such that the majority of released particles are immature cores that are released due to cell lysis, again indicating that NS3 is also essential for the maturation of BTV particles. As noted, VP5 protein possesses an independent membrane export signal, but the depletion of the PBM domains in NS3 inhibits VP5 export to the plasma membrane.[146] The C-terminal domain of NS3 interacts with the outer capsid proteins of BTV, while the N-terminal domain hijacks several host factors of the exocytic and vesicular sorting pathways (Fig. 13.19A). Among them, 13 residues at the N terminus of NS3 form an amphipathic helix acting as an annexin II protein-binding motif.[8,11] Annexin II is involved in Ca++-dependent exocytosis[175] and is often involved in the maturation and egress of enveloped viruses.[100,177] In the case of BTV, inhibition of the NS3–annexin II interaction decreases the release of progeny particles. Moreover, mutant virus with a truncated NS3 lacking the annexin II interaction domain are highly attenuated, with progeny virions scattered in the cytoplasm of infected cells. The NS3 N-terminal domain also harbors the PPRY motif, which is responsible for binding the NEDD4 ubiquitin ligase, and its deletion reduces virus shedding, with the majority of particles remaining outside intracellular vesicles rather than inside, as is found for WT BTV.[9] NS3 is thus a key mediator of virus maturation and egress by interacting with immature cores at the interface of the ER and the VIBs and by driving complete particles to egress at the plasma membrane as detailed below.

Virus Egress

Orbiviruses use multiple mechanisms for egress from infected host cells as summarized below (Fig. 13.20).

Lytic Release

Classically, nonenveloped viruses were thought to rely on lytic strategies for release, killing the infected cell in the process. Correspondingly, orbiviruses and several other members of the *Reoviridae* family trigger cellular apoptosis[32,33,35,147,204] with the BTV outer capsid proteins alone being sufficient to trigger

it.[35,147] The mitogen-activated protein kinase/extracellular signal–regulated kinase (MAPK/ERK) pathway, a key mediator of apoptosis, is modulated by BTV in a strain-dependent manner.[102,143] Moreover, it has been shown that, with VP2, NS3 is a major determinant of BTV virulence.[29,91] NS3 is also responsible for activation of proinflammatory pathways.[102] The suggestion that oligomers of BTV and AHSV NS3 are viroporins[31,69] and induce plasma membrane permeation would be in keeping with this activity. BTV-induced apoptosis and the activation of the proinflammatory pathways are the main events leading to BTV lytic release from infected mammalian cells. However, several studies on NS3 mutant viruses revealed that when lytic release of BTV is inhibited, BTV is still able to spread from cell to cell, albeit highly attenuated, suggesting that lytic release is not the only mode of BTV egress (Fig. 13.20).[26,103,210]

Nonlytic Egress

Observations from the 1960s showed that purified BTV particles could sometimes be found surrounded by an envelope.[16] Direct observation of infected cells by electron microscopy later revealed that BTV particles can be released by budding at the plasma membrane, where particles acquire an envelope, in contrast to the naked particles that are released by lysis.[87] The localization of NS3 protein by immunogold labeling and electron microscopy in such cells revealed it to be present at the plasma membrane, surrounding budding virus particles.[89] Budding of BTV has also been observed in insect cells. Expression of the BTV inner and outer capsid protein using a baculovirus expression system stimulated the release of VLPs via budding, but this was dependent on the coexpression of the NS3 protein, further implicating NS3 in nonlytic BTV morphogenesis and release.[88]

In addition to the late domain motif PPRY discussed, NS3 possesses a second late domain motif PSAP, which is responsible for binding the human tumor-susceptibility gene 101 (TSG101) proteins.[220] TSG101 is a component of the ESCRT-I complex, regulating vesicular trafficking and the formation of multivesicular bodies (MVBs).[3] Many enveloped viruses such as Ebola virus or HIV recruit TSG101 to enable virus budding at the plasma membrane, suggesting a significant similarity in the egress mechanisms used by the nonenveloped BTV and the enveloped viruses.[125] In the case of BTV, depletion of the TSG101-binding motif in NS3 inhibits virus budding at the plasma membrane but does not interfere with the replication cycle of the virus.[26,220] Similar effects were seen with a mutant virus in which the VP2 interacting C-terminal sequences of NS3 were altered. NS3 is thus a key mediator of virus maturation

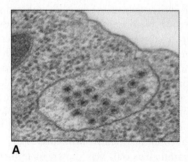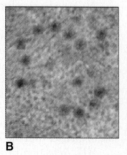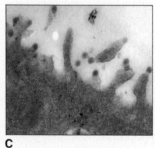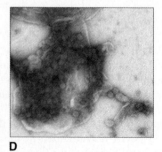

A   **B**   **C**   **D**

FIGURE 13.20 Electron microscope analysis of BTV-infected cell sections. A: Intracellular vesicular trafficking of virion particles. **B:** Release of naked virus particles via cell lysis. **C:** Budding of virus particles at the plasma membrane. **D:** Release of multiple virus particles in extracellular vesicles (EVs) at the plasma membrane.

and egress, by interacting with immature cores at the interface of the ER and the VIBs and by driving complete particles into egress by one of two mechanisms, lysis that follows the induction of apoptosis or nonlytic budding at the plasma membrane (Fig. 13.21). The relative balance of these routes determines the level of pathology associated with different serotypes and possibly with the level of NS3 expression.

Recently, it has been shown that BTV particles egress within extracellular vesicles (EV).[104] The presence of BTV in EVs was initially confirmed by electron microscopy of EVs purified from infected cell culture's supernatants and blood from BTV-infected cattle. EVs showed enhanced infectivity when compared to free virus in cell culture, although their importance to pathogenesis *in vivo* remains to be confirmed. Biochemically, BTV infection triggers an increase of the lysosomal membrane protein LAMP1 at the plasma membrane and increase in the pH of lysosomes, from acidic to neutral range, both of which are indicative of an increase in the exocytosis of secretory lysosomes.[120,141] In contrast, inhibition of the MVBs or autophagous lysosomes was shown to decrease the release of infectious EVs. Together, these data suggest a model in which nascent BTV particles transiting in MVBs toward the lysosomes

and redirected to the cell membrane and subsequently released as extracellular vesicles (Fig. 13.21).

EFFECTS ON HOST CELLS

BTV infection causes hemorrhagic disease in ruminants and induces cell death through apoptosis. In BTV-infected mammalian cells, both the biochemical and morphologic hallmarks of apoptosis are observed within 24 hours of infection, including activation of nuclear factor kappa B (NF-kB), caspase-3, DNA fragmentation, membrane blebbing, and cellular shrinkage. No such changes are observed in insect (*Culicoides*) cells, despite efficient BTV replication.[147] In cell culture, both extrinsic (caspase-8 activation) and intrinsic (caspase-9 activation) pathways play a role in BTV apoptosis, and a correlation may exist between apoptosis, cytopathic effect, and pathogenesis.[185] Analysis of primary sheep and bovine lung endothelial cells infected with BTV suggests that apoptosis may contribute to the pathogenesis of bluetongue disease in the mammal.[35] BTV infection induces an early and transient NF-kB response, and virus titres are higher in the presence of an NF-kB inhibitor (SN50). BTV

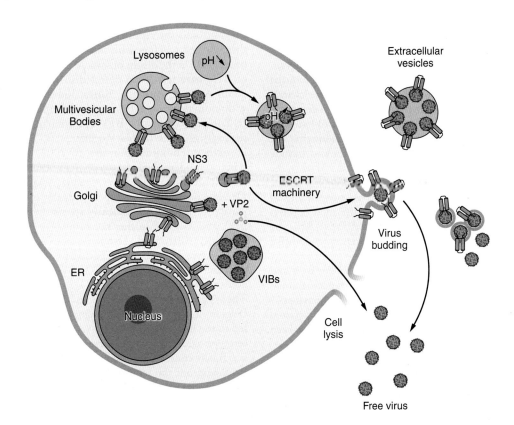

FIGURE 13.21 A cartoon of the BTV egress pathways from infected mammalian cells. NS3 is responsible for trafficking BTV particles toward MVBs. Virions are then moved to secretory lysosomes where the pH is increased from acidic to neutral, thereby preventing virion degradation. Lysosomes containing BTV particles are then secreted as EVs cloaked virus, which is then transmitted to a next cell. Progeny BTV virions are also exported to the plasma membrane mediated by interactions between NS3 and outer capsid proteins of BTV and members of the cellular ESCRT machinery. BTV virions are then released by budding at the plasma membrane, but only a fraction of virions retains a transient envelope. In addition, apoptosis triggered by BTV infection leads to cell death, fragmentation, and free virus particle release between 12 and 24 hours postinfection. ER, endoplasmic reticulum; Golgi, Golgi apparatus; VIBs, viral inclusion bodies; and NS3 is represented in *blue*. (Reprinted from Labadie T, Sullivan E, Roy P. Multiple routes of bluetongue virus egress. *Microorganisms* 2020;8(7):965. https://creativecommons.org/licenses/by/4.0/.)

infection also induces the translocation of interferon regulatory factors (IRF-3 and IRF-7) into the nucleus, although as with the NF-kB response, they are not sustained. The morphology of cellular microfilaments changes extensively during infection (see Ref.[105]), in keeping with the observations previously noted that BTV proteins, virus particles, VIBs, and tubules are intimately associated with the intermediate filaments of the cytoskeleton.

CLINICAL SIGNS AND PATHOGENESIS

Orbiviruses produce a spectrum of disease during an incubation period of 4 to 12 days, from subclinical infection to high morbidity and mortality, depending on virus strain and host species.[24,122,174] Following its introduction by insect bite, the regional lymphatic system underlying the infected skin laceration mediates the dissemination of the virus to local endothelial cells and peripheral blood mononuclear phagocytes (PBMs). The virus proliferates in the PBMs and lymph nodes and is further disseminated by PBM migration to the spleen, thymus, and other lymph nodes. In the final phase of infection, the virus is viremic, circulating in the bloodstream from where it can be transmitted by further *Culicoides* bite.

BTV and related orbiviruses (e.g., AHSV and EHDV) result in disease with pathophysiological features resembling other viral hemorrhagic fevers.[50,106,123,203] Infection of endothelial cells is followed by infection of vascular smooth muscle cells and pericytes, which then undergo lytic infections, resulting in virus-induced vascular injury and a cascade of pathophysiologic events characterized by capillary leakage, hemorrhage, and disseminated intravascular coagulation. Clinically, these events are manifested by edemas, hemorrhages of blood vessels (in the conjunctiva and skin), hypotension, and shock. Other clinical features include fever, lameness, excessive salivation, and congestion. However, the swollen cyanotic tongue symptom that gives bluetongue its name is rare in infected animal. The mortality rate varies depending on host breed and species, but there is a general correlation between endothelial destruction and severity of disease; sheep show the most severe clinical signs and generally have extensive endothelial infections, but cattle, where infections are often subclinical, generally have only minimal endothelial cell damage.[121] Both BTV and EHDV can cross the placenta, and infection of pregnant animals can result in fetal infection, abortion, or congenital anomalies.[121] Practically, this causes concern as live attenuated BTV vaccines and BTV contamination of vaccines for other animals have been shown to be a principal cause of teratogenesis.[20]

The different pathologies seen when BTV and EHDV infect sheep, cattle, goats, and deer are paralleled by AHSV, which affects members of the *Equidae* family. Horses exhibit the most severe disease, whereas donkeys and mules generally show mild clinical signs. Zebra, a natural reservoir for AHSV, exhibits viremia but no clinical signs of infection. The severity of AHS disease in horse ranges from a pulmonary form with close to 100% mortality to AHS fever, which is characterized by high temperature for 1 to 3 days but 100% recovery.

EPIDEMIOLOGY

Evidence for antigenic strain variation and varied virulence for BTV were first reported in 1948,[149] and the epidemiology of

BTV that followed was focused on animals with clinical signs. However, the introduction of simple serologic tests for the presence of the virus in the 1970s led to the recognition of the high prevalence of subclinical infections by BTV and other orbiviruses in ruminants throughout the tropics and subtropics. As with many arbovirus transmitted diseases, outbreaks are highly dependent on the density of vector and vertebrate hosts and whether the vertebrate host is immunologically naive. In endemic zones, infections are generally subclinical, but in naive populations, large epizootic outbreaks with severe disease are observed. The global distribution of BTV, EHDV, and AHSV has undergone drastic expansion in recent years. Changes in climate and increased travel and trade have expanded the global distribution of BTV, EHDV (and to some extent AHSV), and of *Culicoides* species able to transmit them. Molecular epidemiology studies indicate that individual strains can move large distances due to the windborne movements of infected insects and that a single bite from a fully infected adult *Culicoides* is sufficient to reliably transmit the virus to a susceptible mammalian host.

Although BTV has been detected worldwide, in the past, Europe has experienced only infrequent and short-lived incursions of the disease. In recent years, however, different BTV serotypes have emerged in Europe with some now considered endemic, and the repeated introduction and establishment of these viruses, together with their persistence over several years, has resulted in the deaths of several million animals.[136] Serotypes of BTV have now been detected in Europe, North America, South America, Australia, Korea, India, and the Middle East with more than one BTV serotype identified in many regions. In Europe, particularly, BTV epidemiology has changed dramatically since 1998 when six different BTV serotypes emerged in southern European countries. By 2002, different BTV serotypes were identified in Greece, Italy, Bulgaria, Kosovo, Serbia, Montenegro, Macedonia, Croatia, Albania, and Bosnia and Herzegovina. Several serotypes gradually spread north, and in particular, BTV-8 subsequently spread across southern European countries and further north into Luxembourg, the Czech Republic, Switzerland, Denmark, and the United Kingdom. New outbreaks were also reported in Hungary, Austria, Sweden, and Norway. By 2008, BTV-6 was identified in Germany and the Netherlands, and BTV-11 was identified in Belgium. The high number of cases reported for the BTV-8 outbreak in Belgium, Germany, the Netherlands, France, and Luxembourg led to the implementation of a vaccination strategy against the serotype across several countries in Europe, and the outbreak was finally controlled in 2009. The origin of the outbreak virus is unclear, but the sequence of the strain shows most similarity to one found in sub-Saharan Africa.[117] The persistence and spread of such strains has provided evidence for an epidemiological "step-change" in virus distribution.[156] Climate change may have contributed by changes in the period of activity and size of vector populations,[61] and the earlier assumption that *Culicoides obsoletus* and *Culicoides pulicaris*, which are more common in North and Central Europe than the African vector *Culicoides imicola*, were unable to transmit virus sufficiently to sustain a large outbreak has proved wrong. AHSV remains confined mainly to the African continent, although as with BTV prior to 1998, AHSV has caused sporadic, short-lived outbreaks of disease in Europe and the Middle East. An outbreak of AHS (1987–1991), caused by an infected zebra, was limited to the south west of the Iberian Peninsula, but elsewhere, there have been outbreaks in Thailand[201] and Malaysia,[150] both of which had severe economic impacts due to the loss of livestock and restrictions on animal movement. Molecular epidemiology has improved hugely the analyses of geographic variants among the orbiviruses and their relationship to ecosystems and arthropod vectors. It is clear that weather patterns play an important role in transmission and that BTV (and probably other orbiviruses) can be transmitted by a wider range of vector species than previously realized.

IMMUNE RESPONSE

Neutralizing antibodies to BTV are produced within 8 to 14 days of infection,[54] and there is a very good correlation between the induction of neutralizing antibodies against VP2 and the protection of sheep against homologous challenge.[80,173] Infection of sheep and cattle with two serotypes confers protection against other serotypes that had not been included in the inoculum.[188] Similarly, antibodies raised to a mixture of recombinant VP2 proteins of various serotypes not only neutralized the infectivity of the homologous strains but also cross-neutralized certain heterologous viruses.[207] It is possible that cross-reactive epitopes exist on VP2, but other mechanisms may also be involved in this cross protection. In addition to the antibody response, cell-mediated immunity (CMI) also plays a role in recovery from infection and protection against reinfection. Cytotoxic (CD8+) cells responsive *in vitro* to BTV antigen were demonstrated in the blood of cattle and sheep during the first week of infection and peaked 2 weeks later.[41,162] Cell-mediated immunity in sheep was evident by demonstrating cytotoxic T lymphocyte (CTL) responses and further confirmed as an active component of protection in recipient twins by the passive transfer of immune lymphocytes that had been depleted of B cells.[95,194] Despite this, the specificity and overall role of T cells in protection are poorly understood. Antibody-dependent, cell-mediated cytotoxicity may also play a role in protective immunity.[95]

VACCINES

Classical, Subunit/VLP, and Reverse Genetics-Based Vaccines

Live Virus and Inactivated Vaccines

Live attenuated BTV vaccines have been developed by serial passage in embryonated hen's eggs, and to deal with the multiple serotypes, multivalent vaccination has generally been used in endemic areas.[1] Similarly, live attenuated virus vaccines for the nine serotypes of AHSV have been developed.[45] In South Africa, the country where BT and AHS diseases were first characterized, live attenuated virus vaccines have been used for over 50 years and are known to induce an effective and lasting immunity. But although multivalent vaccines are used, optimal immunity and protection from disease is best provided by serotype-specific vaccines.[45] Live attenuated virus vaccines have also had some drawbacks, including abortion/embryonic death and teratogenesis in fetuses of pregnant females.[92,94,135,151,178] In addition, the strength of the

protective antibody response to attenuated vaccines correlates directly with their ability to replicate in vaccinated animals, and when those responses are suboptimal, viremia still occurs and is sufficient for the vaccine strain to be transmitted to biting midges.[51,178] A knock-on effect is that reversion to virulence and/or reassortment of the vaccine strain with wild-type viruses is likely.[188] In the field, a BTV-16 strain circulating in Italy in 2002 was found to be a reassortment between BTV-2 and BTV-16 live attenuated vaccine strains.[7] Consequently, while attenuated vaccines for BTV may offer a route to immediate disease control, they are not suitable for a program designed to eradicate the disease in an area. Chemically, inactivated BTV vaccines were used for mass vaccination of sheep and cattle in European countries during the BTV-8 and BTV-1 outbreaks. While these have been demonstrated to be safe and immunogenic in animals, they are only available for a limited number of serotypes,[176] and in some cases, adverse reactions have been associated with them. Inactivated vaccines generally induce relatively transient immunity in comparison to live attenuated vaccines and require booster immunizations. The high cost of vaccine production, due to the need for large amounts of the antigens required for each vaccination, is another major drawback.

A major limitation to the use of both the live attenuated and inactivated vaccines is the significant economic impact they have on agricultural trade as their use does allow discrimination between infected versus vaccinated animals (DIVA). Neither of these vaccine types is DIVA compliant, and restrictions are imposed on animal trade and movement if an animal is diagnosed positive, even if that positivity is the result of vaccination. Further, due to the presence of genomic RNA after vaccination and short-term BTV viremia in animals in the case of the live attenuated vaccine, a genetic-based DIVA test is not always feasible.

Subunit/VLP Vaccines

To circumvent these issues, a number of recombinant protein technologies have been used to develop DIVA compliant vaccine candidates and to reduce the potential adverse effects associated with inactivated and attenuated vaccines. Recombinant BTV proteins have predominantly been assessed in sheep in experimental vaccine and challenge trials and have been shown to afford protection, although they have yet to be commercialized. Recombinant outer capsid protein VP2, the serotype determining protein, elicits protective neutralizing antibody in vaccinated animals, but combinations of both outer capsid proteins (VP2+VP5) result in better protection. VP2 alone is nonetheless an attractive candidate; for AHSV for example, when horses vaccinated with as little as 5 µg of baculovirus expressed recombinant AHSV-4 VP2, they were fully protected.[96,127,167] VP2-based vaccines have also been developed using virus vector systems (i.e., poxviruses, herpesvirus, and adenovirus) and have been designed to express either a single or multiple proteins in animals following vaccination.[15,187] Enhanced protective immunity has been shown for recombinant VLPs vaccines containing VP2 and VP5 and the two core proteins (VP3 and VP7), mimicking the whole virus particle but without the viral genome or replicase proteins.[166,169] VLPs have the characteristic icosahedral structure with the four recombinant structural proteins present in the same position and molar ratios as native particles.[76] Multiple vaccination studies with homologous and heterologous

VLPs (~10 μg per dose) resulted in complete protection against virulent virus challenges in sheep.[183] In contrast, vaccination of sheep with CLPs (only VP3 and VP7) mitigated against disease but did not afford complete protection and lacked neutralizing antibodies. Extensive trials with VLPs of the European serotypes have been undertaken in European breeds of sheep.[184] These trials assessed VLPs delivered singly or as a cocktail, as well as the evolutionary lineage of the virus strain used, in order to assess their potential for commercialization. Evolutionary divergence was clearly highlighted as a factor with the development of serotype-specific neutralizing antibodies being found to be more critical than the phylogenetic relationship *per se*. The delivery of VLPs as a cocktail of different serotypes did not limit the ability of each serotype to raise a serotype-specific neutralizing antibody response or interfere with the protective efficacy of the vaccine when animals were challenged (Fig. 13.22). Thus, multiple serotype vaccines based on a limited number of VLPs could represent a "universal" vaccine for BTV rather than generating new vaccines for each new outbreak. Most importantly, as nonstructural proteins are absent, it is possible to distinguish between VLP-vaccinated animals and those that are infected with the virus, thus addressing one of the major problems with current vaccines. As entirely protein-based vaccines, VLPs have no genetic component avoiding all issues of reversion or recombination.

Reverse Genetics-Based Vaccines

The use of reverse genetics has allowed direct introduction of mutations/deletions in the viral genome and recovery of replication-abortive virus strains using specific helper cell lines for both BTV and AHSV. Entry competent replication abortive (ECRA) vaccines, formerly known as disabled infectious single-cycle (DISC) vaccines were designed based on this principle. The ECRA vaccines are modified particles that lack the VP6 coding region, an essential part of the replicase complex as discussed above.[130] These strains can enter permissive cells,

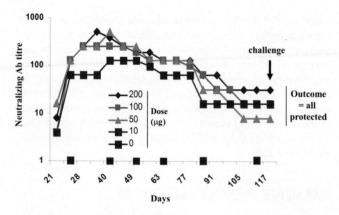

FIGURE 13.22 VLPs are highly immunogenic and protective against virulent virus challenge. Groups of sheep were vaccinated with BTV-10 VLPs in different doses and were challenged with virulent viruses. All vaccinated sheep were completely protected.[168,169]

disassemble, and synthesize all other viral proteins but are incapable of replication due to the absence of VP6, which is necessary to complete replication of the dsRNA genome. As the "core" elements of such ECRA vaccines are conserved, the same basic design allows the rapid generation of multiple vaccine strains simply by substituting the segments that encode the two outer capsid proteins. Vaccination trials in sheep and cattle with ECRA vaccines have shown very promising results.[28,30,129] A single dose was sufficient to confer complete protection against challenge in sheep 42 days after vaccination, while a cocktail of six different vaccines protected animals as early as 21 days against challenge with any virulent strain and protective immunity extended to 5 months before challenge, the latest time point assessed (Fig. 13.23). ECRA vaccines for all nine serotypes of the closely related AHSV were also developed.[113,114] Initially, their protective efficacy was established using an IFNAR-

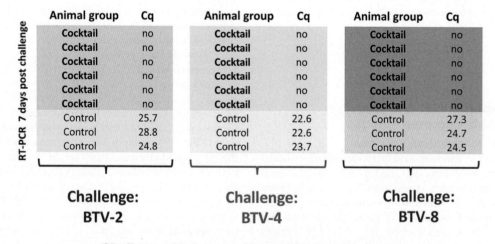

Challenge 42 days or 154 days postvaccination

FIGURE 13.23 Multivalent ECRA vaccines in a cocktail confer protection in sheep against virus infection. Groups of sheep (six animals of each test group or three animals of each control group) were vaccinated with a cocktail of six different ECRA vaccines (BTV-1, BTV-2, BTV-4, BTV-8, BTV-13, and BTV-21) and challenged at 21 days (early) or 154 days (5 months, late) post vaccination with virulent viruses; all vaccinated animals, both in the early challenge or the late challenge group, were protected and had no signs of clinical disease or virus replication.

knockout mouse model, and subsequently, they were assessed in ponies, the natural hosts. The data obtained showed complete protection, by both monovalent and multivalent cocktails (four or five strains) vaccine strains, against virulent virus challenges with protective neutralization antibodies sustained for up to 5 months postvaccination. ECRA vaccines are cost-effective as no formal inactivation is required, and the ECRA RNA segments of the inoculums are present in the bloodstream for a very short period, minimizing the risk of transmission via an insect vector, genome segment reassortment, or reversion to virulence. A DIVA test is also possible, based on the lack of VP6. Although still experimental, ECRA vaccines appear a promising alternative to those currently available for BTV and AHSV.

Further RG-based vaccine candidates for both BTV and AHSV, known as a disabled infectious single-animal (DISA) vaccine, in which segment 10 encoding NS3/NS3A has been deleted, have also been described. Unlike the ECRA strains, the DISA strain still replicates in normal cells and in sheep, although it is significantly attenuated, as discussed earlier, NS3 is a significant pathogenicity factor. Despite the possibility of reacquisition of NS3 from a concurrent virus infection, DISA vaccines have shown protection in vaccinated animals and an inability to replicate in the *Culicoides* vector, which would likely block animal transmission.[211,212] While such vaccine candidates, which show promising levels of efficacy and safety, have been developed, they are not yet in commercial production. The voluntary vaccination policy adopted in Europe and the acceptance of endemic disease in many parts of the world have resulted in a dearth of commercial interest in new vaccines, although, given the likelihood of new BTV outbreaks in Europe, vaccines that can be produced safely and efficiently remain the best option to control future outbreaks.

PERSPECTIVE

Significant progress in understanding the structure and biochemistry of the BTV replication cycle has resulted in a number of new findings and applied outcomes. The function of BTV proteins as enzymes in the transcription complex, as structural proteins in capsid assembly, and as mediators of host–virus interaction, especially in virus entry, egress, and pathogenicity, have all been described. BTV is thus very well characterized, genetically and structurally, and it is reasonable to suppose that other related viruses will have similar core functions. Significant challenges remain however. Most of what has been learned of BTV and related orbiviruses has focused on the replication in mammalian cells, principally cells in culture. The replication and spread of BTV in whole animals is less well studied, and the replication and spread in *Culicoides* species even less so. These should improve with the development of tractable small animal models for the former and annotation of the whole genome sequence of *Culicoides* for the latter. The identification of further host cell factors critical to BTV replication may be important here as they could inform the construction of suitable transgenic models and indicate why certain species of *Culicoides* are preferred for transmission. Assuming developments in these areas, the whole biology of BTV infection, including pathogenesis, breed susceptibility, and transmission, should become as well understood as the molecular aspects described. When they do, the mechanisms of virus evolution

and emergence, and the roles played by each host in the process should become apparent. As for the application of basic virology, it is likely that these developments too will result in better future control of orbivirus disease.

REFERENCES

1. Alexander RA, Haig DA, Adelaar TF. The attenuation of bluetongue virus by serial passage through fertile eggs. *Onderstepoort J Vet Sci Anim Ind* 1947;21(2):231–241.
2. AlShaikhahmed K, et al. Dynamic network approach for the modelling of genomic subcomplexes in multi-segmented viruses. *Nucleic Acids Res* 2018;46(22):12087–12098.
3. Banfer S, et al. Molecular mechanism to recruit galectin-3 into multivesicular bodies for polarized exosomal secretion. *Proc Natl Acad Sci U S A* 2018;115(19):E4396–E4405.
4. Bansal OB, et al. Membrane organization of bluetongue virus nonstructural glycoprotein NS3. *J Virol* 1998;72(4):3362–3369.
5. Barnard BJ. Epidemiology of African horse sickness and the role of the zebra in South Africa. *Arch Virol Suppl* 1998;14:13–19.
6. Basak AK, et al. Structures of orbivirus VP7: implications for the role of this protein in the viral life cycle. *Structure* 1997;5(7):871–883.
7. Batten CA, et al. A European field strain of bluetongue virus derived from two parental vaccine strains by genome segment reassortment. *Virus Res* 2008;137(1):56–63.
8. Beaton AR, et al. The membrane trafficking protein calpactin forms a complex with bluetongue virus protein NS3 and mediates virus release. *Proc Natl Acad Sci U S A* 2002;99(20):13154–13159.
9. Bhattacharya B, Celma CC, Roy P. Influence of cellular trafficking pathway on bluetongue virus infection in ovine cells. *Viruses* 2015;7(5):2378–2403.
10. Bhattacharya B, Noad R, Roy P. Interaction between Bluetongue virus outer capsid protein VP2 and vimentin is necessary for virus egress. *Virol J* 2007;4:7.
11. Bhattacharya B, Roy P. Bluetongue virus outer capsid protein VP5 interacts with membrane lipid rafts via a SNARE domain. *J Virol* 2008;82(21):10600–10612.
12. Bhattacharya B, Roy P. Role of lipids on entry and exit of bluetongue virus, a complex non-enveloped virus. *Viruses* 2010;2(5):1218–1235.
13. Bhattacharya B, Roy P. Cellular phosphoinositides and the maturation of bluetongue virus, a non-enveloped capsid virus. *Virol J* 2013;10:73.
14. Bhattacharya B, Roy P. Cellular phosphoinositides and the maturation of bluetongue virus, a non-enveloped capsid virus. *Virol J* 2013;10:73.
15. Boone JD, et al. Recombinant canarypox virus vaccine co-expressing genes encoding the VP2 and VP5 outer capsid proteins of bluetongue virus induces high level protection in sheep. *Vaccine* 2007;25(4):672–678.
16. Bowne JG, Ritchie AE. Some morphological features of bluetongue virus. *Virology* 1970;40(4):903–911.
17. Boyce M, Celma CC, Roy P. Development of reverse genetics systems for bluetongue virus: recovery of infectious virus from synthetic RNA transcripts. *J Virol* 2008;82(17):8339–8348.
18. Boyce M, Celma CC, Roy P. Bluetongue virus non-structural protein 1 is a positive regulator of viral protein synthesis. *Virol J* 2012;9(1):178.
19. Boyce M, et al. Purified recombinant bluetongue virus VP1 exhibits RNA replicase activity. *J Virol* 2004;78(8):3994–4002.
20. Breard E, et al. Transient adverse effects of an attenuated bluetongue virus vaccine on the quality of ram semen. *Vet Rec* 2007;160(13):431–435.
21. Brookes SM, Hyatt AD, Eaton BT. Characterization of virus inclusion bodies in bluetongue virus infected cells. *J Gen Virol* 1993;74(3):525–530.
22. Bumbarov V, et al. Characterization of bluetongue virus serotype 28. *Transbound Emerg Dis* 2020;67(1):171–182.
23. Butan C, Van Der Zandt H, Tucker PA. Structure and assembly of the RNA binding domain of bluetongue virus non-structural protein 2. *J Biol Chem* 2004;279(36):37613–37621.
24. Carpenter S, et al. African horse sickness virus: history, transmission, and current status. *Annu Rev Entomol* 2017;62:343–358.
25. Castillo-Olivares J. African horse sickness in Thailand: challenges of controlling an outbreak by vaccination. *Equine Vet J* 2021;53(1):9–14.
26. Celma CC, Roy P. A viral nonstructural protein regulates bluetongue virus trafficking and release. *J Virol* 2009;83(13):6806–6816.
27. Celma CC, Roy P. Interaction of calpactin light chain (S100A10/p11) and a viral NS protein is essential for intracellular trafficking of nonenveloped bluetongue virus. *J Virol* 2011;85(10):4783–4791.
28. Celma CC, et al. Rapid generation of replication-deficient monovalent and multivalent vaccines for bluetongue virus: protection against virulent virus challenge in cattle and sheep. *J Virol* 2013;87(17):9856–9864.
29. Celma CC, et al. Pathogenicity study in sheep using reverse-genetics-based reassortant bluetongue viruses. *Vet Microbiol* 2014;174(1–2):139–147.
30. Celma CC, et al. Replication-deficient particles: new insights into the next generation of bluetongue virus vaccines. *J Virol* 2017;91(1):e01892-16.
31. Chacko N, et al. A coiled-coil motif in non-structural protein 3 (NS3) of bluetongue virus forms an oligomer. *Virus Genes* 2015;51(2):244–251.
32. Chaibi C, et al. Rotavirus induces apoptosis in fully differentiated human intestinal Caco-2 cells. *Virology* 2005;332(2):480–490.
33. Clarke P, et al. Reovirus-induced apoptosis is mediated by TRAIL. *J Virol* 2000;74(17):8135–8139.
34. de Sal RO, Zellner M, Grubman MJ. Phylogenetic analysis of segment 10 from African horsesickness virus and cognate genes from other orbiviruses. *Virus Res* 1994;33(2):157–165.
35. DeMaula CD, et al. Infection kinetics, prostacyclin release and cytokine-mediated modulation of the mechanism of cell death during bluetongue virus infection of cultured

ovine and bovine pulmonary artery and lung microvascular endothelial cells. *J Gen Virol* 2001;82(Pt 4):787–794.

36. Du J, et al. Trafficking of bluetongue virus visualized by recovery of tetracysteine-tagged virion particles. *J Virol* 2014;88(21):12656–12668.
37. Ducheyne E, et al. A stochastic predictive model for the natural spread of bluetongue. *Prev Vet Med* 2011;99(1):48–59.
38. Eaton BT, Crameri GS. The site of bluetongue virus attachment to glycophorins from a number of animal erythrocytes. *J Gen Virol* 1989;70(Pt 12):3347–3353.
39. Eaton BT, Hyatt AD. Association of bluetongue virus with the cytoskeleton. *Subcell Biochem* 1989;15:233–273.
40. Eaton BT, Hyatt AD, Brookes SM. The replication of bluetongue virus. *Curr Top Microbiol Immunol* 1990;162:89–118.
41. Ellis JA, et al. T lymphocyte subset alterations following bluetongue virus infection in sheep and cattle. *Vet Immunol Immunopathol* 1990;24(1):49–67.
42. Els HJ, Verwoerd DW. Morphology of bluetongue virus. *Virology* 1969;38(2):213–219.
43. Erasmus BJ. The pathogenesis of African horse sickness. In: *Third International Conference on Equine Infectious Diseases.* Basel, Paris: Karger; 1973.
44. Erasmus BJ. Bluetongue in sheep and goats. *Aust Vet J* 1975;51(4):165–170.
45. Erasmus BJ. A new approach to polyvalent immunization against African horsesickness. In: *Fourth International Conference on Equine Infectious Diseases.* New York: Veterinary Publication Incorporation; 1978.
46. Fabrega C, et al. Structure and mechanism of mRNA cap (guanine-N7) methyltransferase. *Mol Cell* 2004;13(1):77–89.
47. Fajardo T Jr, AlShaikhahmed K, Roy P. Generation of infectious RNA complexes in Orbiviruses: RNA-RNA interactions of genomic segments. *Oncotarget* 2016;7(45):72559–72570.
48. Fajardo T Jr, Sung PY, Roy P. Disruption of specific RNA-RNA interactions in a double-stranded RNA virus inhibits genome packaging and virus infectivity. *PLoS Pathog* 2015;11(12):e1005321.
49. Fajardo T, et al. Rotavirus genomic RNA complex forms via specific RNA-RNA interactions: disruption of RNA complex inhibits virus infectivity. *Viruses* 2017;9(7):167.
50. Favero CM, et al. Epizootic hemorrhagic disease in brocket deer, *Brazil. Emerg Infect Dis* 2013;19(2):346–348.
51. Ferrari G, et al. Active circulation of bluetongue vaccine virus serotype-2 among unvaccinated cattle in central Italy. *Prev Vet Med* 2005;68(2–4):103–113.
52. Forzan M, Marsh M, Roy P. Bluetongue virus entry into the cells. *J Virol* 2007;81(9):4819–4827.
53. Forzan M, Wirblich C, Roy P. A capsid protein of nonenveloped Bluetongue virus exhibits membrane fusion activity. *Proc Natl Acad Sci U S A* 2004;101(7):2100–2105.
54. Foster NM, et al. Temporal relationships of viremia, interferon activity, and antibody responses of sheep infected with several bluetongue virus strains. *Am J Vet Res* 1991;52(2):192–196.
55. French TJ, Inumaru S, Roy P. Expression of two related nonstructural proteins of bluetongue virus (BTV) type 10 in insect cells by a recombinant baculovirus: production of polyclonal ascitic fluid and characterization of the gene product in BTV-infected BHK cells. *J Virol* 1989;63(8):3270–3278.
56. French TJ, Marshall JJ, Roy P. Assembly of double-shelled, virus-like particles of bluetongue virus by the simultaneous expression of four structural proteins. *J Virol* 1990;64(12):5695–5700.
57. French TJ, Roy P. Synthesis of bluetongue virus (BTV) corelike particles by a recombinant baculovirus expressing the two major structural core proteins of BTV. *J Virol* 1990;64(4):1530–1536.
58. Ftaich N, et al. Turnover rate of NS3 proteins modulates bluetongue virus replication kinetics in a host-specific manner. *J Virol* 2015;89(20):10467–10481.
59. Fukusho A, Ritter GD, Roy P. Variation in the bluetongue virus neutralization protein VP2. *J Gen Virol* 1987;68(Pt 11):2967–2973.
60. Fukusho A, et al. Completion of the sequence of bluetongue virus serotype 10 by the characterization of a structural protein, VP6, and a non-structural protein, NS2. *J Gen Virol* 1989;70(Pt 7):1677.
61. Gloster J, et al. Bluetongue in the United Kingdom and northern Europe in 2007 and key issues for 2008. *Vet Rec* 2008;162(10):298–302.
62. Gorman BM. The bluetongue viruses. *Curr Top Microbiol Immunol* 1990;162:1–19.
63. Gouet P, et al. The highly ordered double-stranded RNA genome of bluetongue virus revealed by crystallography. *Cell* 1999;97(4):481–490.
64. Gould AR, Hyatt AD, Eaton BT. Morphogenesis of a bluetongue virus variant with an amino acid alteration at a neutralization site in the outer coat protein, VP2. *Virology* 1988;165(1):23–32.
65. Grimes J, et al. The crystal structure of bluetongue virus VP7. *Nature* 1995;373(6510):167–170.
66. Grimes JM, et al. The atomic structure of the bluetongue virus core. *Nature* 1998;395:470–478.
67. Grimes JM, et al. An atomic model of the outer layer of the bluetongue virus core derived from X-ray crystallography and electron cryomicroscopy. *Structure* 1997;5(7):885–893.
68. Haider N, et al. Quantifying the potential for bluetongue virus transmission in Danish cattle farms. *Sci Rep* 2019;9(1):13466.
69. Han Z, Harty RN. The NS3 protein of bluetongue virus exhibits viroporin-like properties. *J Biol Chem* 2004;279(41):43092–43097.
70. Hassan SH, Roy P. Expression and functional characterization of bluetongue virus VP2 protein: Role in cell entry. *J Virol* 1999;73(12):9832–9842.
71. Hassan SH, et al. Expression and functional characterization of bluetongue virus VP5 protein: role in cellular permeabilization. *J Virol* 2001;75(18):8356–8367.
72. He Y, et al. In situ structures of RNA-dependent RNA polymerase inside bluetongue virus before and after uncoating. *Proc Natl Acad Sci U S A* 2019;116(33):16535–16540.
73. Henning MW. *Animal diseases in South Africa.* 3rd ed. Cape Town, South Africa: Central News Agency Ltd.; 1956:785–808.
74. Hewat EA, et al. Three-dimensional reconstruction of baculovirus expressed bluetongue virus core-like particles by cryo-electron microscopy. *Virology* 1992;189(1):10–20.
75. Hewat EA, Booth TF, Roy P. Structure of bluetongue virus particles by cryoelectron microscopy. *J Struct Biol* 1992;109(1):61–69.
76. Hewat EA, Booth TF, Roy P. Structure of correctly self-assembled bluetongue virus-like particles. *J Struct Biol* 1994;112(3):183–191.
77. Hodel AE, et al. The 1.85 A structure of vaccinia protein VP39: a bifunctional enzyme that participates in the modification of both mRNA ends. *Cell* 1996;85(2):247–256.
78. Horscroft NJ, Roy P. Thermal denaturation of proteins for SDS-PAGE analysis by microwave irradiation. *Biotechniques* 1997;22:224–226.
79. Howell PG. Bluetongue. In: *Emerging Diseases of Animals.* Rome, Italy: FAO Agricultural Studies; 1963.
80. Huismans H, Cloete M, le Roux A. The genetic relatedness of a number of individual cognate genes of viruses in the bluetongue and closely related serogroups. *Virology* 1987;161(2):421–428.
81. Huismans H, Els HJ. Characterization of the tubules associated with the replication of three different orbiviruses. *Virology* 1979;92(2):397–406.
82. Huismans H, et al. Isolation of a capsid protein of bluetongue virus that induces a protective immune response in sheep. *Virology* 1987;157(1):172–179.
83. Huismans H, Van Dijk AA. Bluetongue virus structural components. *Curr Top Microbiol Immunol* 1990;162:21–41.
84. Huismans H, van Dijk AA, Els HJ. Uncoating of parental bluetongue virus to core and subcore particles in infected L cells. *Virology* 1987;157(1):180–188.
85. Hwang GY, et al. Sequence conservation among the cognate nonstructural NS3/3A protein genes of six bluetongue viruses. *Virus Res* 1992;23(1–2):151–161.
86. Hyatt AD, Eaton BT. Ultrastructural distribution of the major capsid proteins within bluetongue virus and infected cells. *J Gen Virol* 1988;69(Pt 4):805–815.
87. Hyatt AD, Eaton BT, Brookes SM. The release of bluetongue virus from infected cells and their superinfection by progeny virus. *Virology* 1989;173(1):21–34.
88. Hyatt AD, Zhao Y, Roy P. Release of bluetongue virus-like particles from insect cells is mediated by BTV nonstructural protein NS3/NS3A. *Virology* 1993;193(2):592–603.
89. Hyatt AD, et al. Localization of the non-structural protein NS3 in bluetongue virus-infected cells. *J Gen Virol* 1991;72(Pt 9):2263–2267.
90. Iwata H, Yamagawa M, Roy P. Evolutionary relationships among the gnat-transmitted orbiviruses that cause African horse sickness, bluetongue, and epizootic hemorrhagic disease as evidenced by their capsid protein sequences. *Virology* 1992;191(1):251–261.
91. Janowicz A, et al. Multiple genome segments determine virulence of bluetongue virus serotype 8. *J Virol* 2015;89(10):5238–5249.
92. Jimenez-Cabello L, et al. Viral vector vaccines against bluetongue virus. *Microorganisms* 2020;9(1):42.
93. Jobe F, et al. Respiratory syncytial virus sequesters NF-kappaB subunit p65 to cytoplasmic inclusion bodies to inhibit innate immune signaling. *J Virol* 2020;94(22):e01380-20.
94. Johnson SJ, et al. Clinico-pathology of Australian bluetongue virus serotypes for sheep. In: Walton TE, Osburn BI, eds. *Bluetongue, African Horse Sickness and Related Orbiviruses.* Boca Raton, FL: CRC Press; 1992:737–743.
95. Jones LD, et al. The non-structural proteins of bluetongue virus are a dominant source of cytotoxic T cell peptide determinants. *J Gen Virol* 1996;77(Pt 5):997–1003.
96. Kaname Y, et al. Recovery of African horse sickness virus from synthetic RNA. *J Gen Virol* 2013;94(Pt 10):2259–2265.
97. Kar AK, Bhattacharya B, Roy P. Bluetongue virus RNA binding protein NS2 is a modulator of viral replication and assembly. *BMC Mol Biol* 2007;8:4.
98. Kar AK, Ghosh M, Roy P. Mapping the assembly of Bluetongue virus scaffolding protein VP3. *Virology* 2004;324(2):387–399.
99. Kerviel A, et al. Atomic structure of the translation regulatory protein NS1 of bluetongue virus. *Nat Microbiol* 2019;4(5):837–845.
100. Koga R, et al. Annexin A2 mediates the localization of measles virus matrix protein at the plasma membrane. *J Virol* 2018;92(10):e00181-18.
101. Komarov A, Goldsmit L. A disease similar to bluetongue in cattle and sheep in Israel. *Ref Vet* 1951;8:96–100.
102. Kundlacz C, et al. Novel function of bluetongue virus NS3 protein in regulation of the MAPK/ERK signaling pathway. *J Virol* 2019;93(16):e00336-19.
103. Labadie T, Jegouic S, Roy P. Bluetongue virus nonstructural protein 3 orchestrates virus maturation and drives non-lytic egress via two polybasic motifs. *Viruses* 2019;11(12):1107.
104. Labadie T, Roy P. A non-enveloped arbovirus released in lysosome-derived extracellular vesicles induces super-infection exclusion. *PLoS Pathog* 2020;16(10):e1009015.
105. Labadie T, Sullivan E, Roy P. Multiple routes of bluetongue virus egress. *Microorganisms* 2020;8(7):965.
106. Laegreid W. African horse sickness. In: Studdert M, ed. *Virus Infections of Equines.* New York: Elsevier; 1996:101–123.
107. Limn C-H, et al. Functional dissection of the major structural protein of bluetongue virus: identification of key residues within VP7 essential for capsid assembly. *J Virol* 2000;74(18):8658–8669.
108. Limn CK, Roy P. Intermolecular interactions in a two-layered viral capsid that requires a complex symmetry mismatch. *J Virol* 2003;77(20):11114–11124.
109. Liu HM, Booth TF, Roy P. Interactions between bluetongue virus core and capsid proteins translated in vitro. *J Gen Virol* 1992;73(Pt 10):2577–2584.
110. Loudon PT Roy P. Interaction of nucleic acids with core-like and subcore-like particles of bluetongue virus. *Virology* 1992;191(1):231–236.
111. Loudon PT, et al. Expression of the outer capsid protein VP5 of two bluetongue viruses, and synthesis of chimeric double-shelled virus-like particles using combinations of recombinant baculoviruses. *Virology* 1991;182(2):793–801.
112. Lourenco S, Roy P. In vitro reconstitution of Bluetongue virus infectious cores. *Proc Natl Acad Sci U S A* 2011;108:13746–13751.
113. Lulla V, et al. Assembly of replication-incompetent African horse sickness virus particles: rational design of vaccines for all serotypes. *J Virol* 2016;90(16):7405–7414.

114. Lulla V, et al. Protective efficacy of multivalent replication-abortive vaccine strains in horses against African horse sickness virus challenge. *Vaccine* 2017;35(33):4262–4269.
115. Lymperopoulos K, et al. Sequence specificity in the interaction of bluetongue virus non structural protein 2 (NS2) with viral RNA. *J Biol Chem* 2003;278(34):31722–31730.
116. M'Fadyean J. The ultravisible viruses. *J Comp Pathol Therap* 1908;21:58–68, 168–175, 232–242.
117. Maan S, et al. Sequence analysis of bluetongue virus serotype 8 from the Netherlands 2006 and comparison to other European strains. *Virology* 2008;377(2):308–318.
118. Maan S, et al. Analysis and phylogenetic comparisons of full-length VP2 genes of the 24 bluetongue virus serotypes. *J Gen Virol* 2007;88(Pt 2):621–630.
119. Maan S, Maan NS, Nomikou K, et al. Identification of a novel bluetongue virus serotype (BTV-26) from Kuwait. *Emerg Infect Dis* 2011;17(5):886–889. doi: 10.3201/eid1705.101742.
120. Machado E, et al. Regulated lysosomal exocytosis mediates cancer progression. *Sci Adv* 2015;1(11):e1500603.
121. MacLachlan NJ. The pathogenesis and immunology of bluetongue virus infection of ruminants. *Comp Immunol Microbiol Infect Dis* 1994;17(3–4):197–206.
122. Maclachlan NJ, et al. Epizootic haemorrhagic disease. *Rev Sci Tech* 2015;34(2):341–351.
123. Mahrt CR, Osburn BI. Experimental bluetongue virus infection of sheep; effect of vaccination: pathologic, immunofluorescent, and ultrastructural studies. *Am J Vet Res* 1986;47(6):1198–1203.
124. Markotter W, Theron J, Nel LH. Segment specific inverted repeat sequences in bluetongue virus mRNA are required for interaction with the virus non structural protein NS2. *Virus Res* 2004;105(1):1–9.
125. Martin-Serrano J, Zang T, Bieniasz PD. HIV-1 and Ebola virus encode small peptide motifs that recruit Tsg101 to sites of particle assembly to facilitate egress. *Nat Med* 2001;7(12):1313–1319.
126. Martinez Costas J, et al. Guanylyltransferase and RNA 5′-triphosphatase activities of the purified expressed VP4 protein of bluetongue virus. *J Mol Biol* 1998;280(5):859–866.
127. Martinez-Torrecuadrada JL, et al. Full protection against African horsesickness (AHS) in horses induced by baculovirus-derived AHS virus serotype 4 VP2, VP5 and VP7. *J Gen Virol* 1996;77(Pt 6):1211–1221.
128. Matsuo E, Celma CC, Roy P. A reverse genetics system of African horse sickness virus reveals existence of primary replication. *FEBS Lett* 2010;584(15):3386–3391.
129. Matsuo E, et al. Generation of replication-defective virus-based vaccines that confer full protection in sheep against virulent bluetongue virus challenge. *J Virol* 2011;85(19):10213–10221.
130. Matsuo E, Roy P. Bluetongue virus VP6 acts early in the replication cycle and can form the basis of chimeric virus formation. *J Virol* 2009;83(17):8842–8848.
131. Matsuo E, Roy P. Bluetongue virus VP1 polymerase activity in vitro: template dependency, dinucleotide priming and cap dependency. *PLoS One* 2011;6(11):e27702.
132. Matsuo E, Roy P. Minimum requirements for bluetongue virus primary replication in vivo. *J Virol* 2013;87(2):882–889.
133. Matsuo E, et al. Structure based modification of bluetongue virus helicase protein VP6 to produce a viable VP6-truncated BTV. *Biochem Biophys Res Commun* 2014;451(4):603–608.
134. Matsuo E, et al. Interaction between a unique minor protein and a major capsid protein of bluetongue virus controls virus infectivity. *J Virol* 2018;92(3):e01784-17.
135. Mayo C, et al. A review of potential bluetongue virus vaccine strategies. *Vet Microbiol* 2017;206:84–90.
136. Mellor PS, et al. Bluetongue in Europe and the Mediterranean Basin: history of occurrence prior to 2006. *Prev Vet Med* 2008;87(1–2):4–20.
137. Mertens PP, Brown F, Sangar DV. Assignment of the genome segments of bluetongue virus type 1 to the proteins which they encode. *Virology* 1984;135(1):207–217.
138. Mertens PP, et al. Enhanced infectivity of modified bluetongue virus particles for two insect cell lines and for two Culicoides vector species. *Virology* 1996;217(2):582–593.
139. Mertens PPC. Orbiviruses and coltiviruses. In: Webster RG, Granoff A, eds. *Encyclopedia of Virology*. 2nd ed. London: Academic Press; 1999:1043–1061.
140. Mertens PPC, et al. Orbivirus, Reoviridae. In: Fauquet CM, et al., eds. *Virus Taxonomy, VIIIth Report of the ICTV*. London: Elsevier/Academic Press; 2005:466–483.
141. Miao Y, et al. A TRP channel senses lysosome neutralization by pathogens to trigger their expulsion. *Cell* 2015;161(6):1306–1319.
142. Modrof J, Lymperopoulos K, Roy P. Phosphorylation of bluetongue virus nonstructural protein 2 is essential for formation of viral inclusion bodies. *J Virol* 2005;79(15):10023–10031.
143. Mohl BP, Emmott E, Roy P. Phosphoproteomic analysis reveals the importance of kinase regulation during orbivirus infection. *Mol Cell Proteomics* 2017;16(11):1990–2005.
144. Mohl BP, Roy P. Cellular casein kinase 2 and protein phosphatase 2A modulate replication site assembly of bluetongue virus. *J Biol Chem* 2016;291(28):14566–14574.
145. Mohl BP, Roy P. Hsp90 chaperones bluetongue virus proteins and prevents proteasomal degradation. *J Virol* 2019;93(20).
146. Mohl BP, et al. Differential localization of structural and non-structural proteins during the bluetongue virus replication cycle. *Viruses* 2020;12(3):343.
147. Mortola E, Noad R, Roy P. Bluetongue virus outer capsid proteins are sufficient to trigger apoptosis in mammalian cells. *J Virol* 2004;78(6):2875–2883.
148. Nason E, et al. Interactions between the inner and outer capsids of bluetongue virus. *J Virol* 2004;78(15):8059–8067.
149. Neitz WO. Immunological studies on bluetongue in sheep. *Onderstepoort J Vet Sci Anim Ind* 1948;23(1–2):93–136.
150. Noor NM. African horse sickness—Malaysia: (Terengganu) Serotype Pending, OIE. 2020 [cited 2020 16/11]. Information received on [and dated] 2 Sep 2020 from Dr. Dato'Dr Norlizan Mohd Noor, Deputy Director General, Veterinary Services, Ministry of Agriculture and Agro-Based Industry, Putrajaya, Malaysia. 2020.
151. Osburn BI, et al. Experimental viral-induced congenital encephalopathies. I. Pathology of hydranencephaly and porencephaly caused by bluetongue vaccine virus. *Lab Invest* 1971;25(3):197–205.
152. Patel A, Mohl BP, Roy P. Entry of bluetongue virus capsid requires the late endosome-specific lipid lysobisphosphatidic acid. *J Biol Chem* 2016;291(23):12408–12419.
153. Patel A, Roy P. The molecular biology of Bluetongue virus replication. *Virus Res* 2014;182:5–20.
154. Prasad BVV, Yamaguchi S, Roy P. Three-dimensional structure of single-shelled bluetongue virus. *J Virol* 1992;66(4):2135–2142.
155. Pudupakam RS, et al. Genetic characterization of the non-structural protein-3 gene of bluetongue virus serotype-2 isolate from India. *Vet World* 2017;10(3):348–352.
156. Purse BV, et al. Climate change and the recent emergence of bluetongue in Europe. *Nat Rev Microbiol* 2005;3(2):171–181.
157. Rahman SK, et al. A calcium sensor discovered in Bluetongue virus nonstructural protein 2 is critical for virus replication. *J Virol* 2020;94(20):e01099-20.
158. Ramadevi N, Rodriguez J, Roy P. A leucine zipper-like domain is essential for dimerization and encapsidation of bluetongue virus nucleocapsid protein VP4. *J Virol* 1998;72(4):2983–2990.
159. Ramadevi N, Roy P. Bluetongue virus core protein VP4 has nucleoside triphosphate phosphohydrolase activity. *J Gen Virol* 1998;79(Pt 10):2475–2480.
160. Ramadevi N, et al. Capping and methylation of mRNA by purified recombinant VP4 protein of bluetongue virus. *Proc Natl Acad Sci U S A* 1998;95:13537–13542.
161. Ratinier M, et al. Identification and characterization of a novel non-structural protein of bluetongue virus. *PLoS Pathog* 2011;7(12):e1002477.
162. Rojas JM, Rodriguez-Calvo T, Sevilla N. Recall T cell responses to bluetongue virus produce a narrowing of the T cell repertoire. *Vet Res* 2017;48(1):38.
163. Roy P. Bluetongue virus genetics and genome structure. *Virus Res* 1989;13(3):179–206.
164. Roy P. Bluetongue virus proteins. *J Gen Virol* 1992;73(Pt 12):3051–3064.
165. Roy P. Bluetongue virus: dissection of the polymerase complex. *J Gen Virol* 2008;89(Pt 8):1789–1804.
166. Roy P, et al. Long-lasting protection of sheep against bluetongue challenge after vaccination with virus-like particles: evidence for homologous and partial heterologous protection. *Vaccine* 1994;12(9):805–811.
167. Roy P, et al. Recombinant baculovirus-synthesized African horsesickness virus (AHSV) outer-capsid protein VP2 provides protection against virulent AHSV challenge. *J Gen Virol* 1996;77(Pt 9):2053–2057.
168. Roy P, Callis J, Erasmus BJ. Protection of sheep against Bluetongue disease after vaccination with core-like and virus-like particles: evidence for homologous and partial heterologous proteins. In: *97th Annual Meeting* Las Vegas, NV: United States Animal Health Association; 1993:88–93.
169. Roy P, French T, Erasmus BJ. Protective efficacy of virus-like particles for bluetongue disease. *Vaccine* 1992;10(1):28–32.
170. Roy P, Gorman BM. Bluetongue viruses. In: Roy P, Gorman BM, eds. *Current Topics in Microbiology and Immunology*. Heidelberg: Springer-Verlag; 1990:1–200.
171. Roy P, Marshall JJ, French TJ. Structure of the bluetongue virus genome and its encoded proteins. *Curr Top Microbiol Immunol* 1990;162:43–87.
172. Roy P, Noad R. Virus-like particles as a vaccine delivery system: myths and facts. *Hum Vaccin* 2008;4(1):5–8.
173. Roy P, et al. Recombinant virus vaccine for bluetongue disease in sheep. *J Virol* 1990;64(5):1998–2003.
174. Saminathan M, et al. An updated review on bluetongue virus: epidemiology, pathobiology, and advances in diagnosis and control with special reference to India. *Vet Q* 2020;40(1):258–321.
175. Sarafian T, et al. The participation of annexin II (calpactin I) in calcium-evoked exocytosis requires protein kinase C. *J Cell Biol* 1991;114(6):1135–1147.
176. Savini G, et al. Assessment of efficacy of a bivalent BTV-2 and BTV-4 inactivated vaccine by vaccination and challenge in cattle. *Vet Microbiol* 2009;133(1–2):1–8.
177. Saxena V, et al. Annexin A2 is involved in the formation of hepatitis C virus replication complex on the lipid raft. *J Virol* 2012;86(8):4139–4150.
178. Schultz G, Delay PD. Losses in newborn lambs associated with bluetongue vaccination of pregnancy ewes. *J Am Vet Med Assoc* 1955;127(942):224–226.
179. Schulz C, et al. Bluetongue virus serotype 27: detection and characterization of two novel variants in Corsica, France. *J Gen Virol* 2016;97(9):2073–2083.
180. Spreull J. Malarial catarrhal fever (bluetongue) of sheep in South Africa. *J Comp Pathol Ther* 1905;18:321–337.
181. Starnes MC, Joklik WK. Reovirus protein lambda 3 is a poly(C)-dependent poly(G)polymerase. *Virology* 1993;193(1):356–366.
182. Stauber N, et al. Bluetongue virus VP6 protein binds ATP and exhibits an RNA-dependent ATPase function and a helicase activity that catalyze the unwinding of double-stranded RNA substrates. *J Virol* 1997;71(10):7220–7226.
183. Stewart M, et al. Validation of a novel approach for the rapid production of immunogenic virus-like particles for bluetongue virus. *Vaccine* 2010;28(17):3047–3054.
184. Stewart M, et al. Bluetongue virus serotype 8 virus-like particles protect sheep against virulent virus infection as a single or multi-serotype cocktail immunogen. *Vaccine* 2013;31(3):553–558.
185. Stewart ME, Roy P. Role of cellular caspases, nuclear factor-kappa B and interferon regulatory factors in Bluetongue virus infection and cell fate. *Virol J* 2010;7:362.
186. Stewart ME, Roy P. Structure-based identification of functional residues in the nucleoside-2′-*O*-methylase domain of Bluetongue virus VP4 capping enzyme. *FEBS Open Bio* 2015;5:138–146.
187. Stone-Marschat MA, et al. Immunization with VP2 is sufficient for protection against lethal challenge with African horsesickness virus Type 4. *Virology* 1996;220(1):219–222.
188. Stott JL, et al. Genome segment reassortment between two serotypes of bluetongue virus in a natural host. *J Virol* 1987;61(9):2670–2674.
189. Su JM, et al. Formation and function of liquid-like viral factories in negative-sense single-stranded RNA virus infections. *Viruses* 2021;13(1):126.
190. Sung PY, Roy P. Sequential packaging of RNA genomic segments during the assembly of bluetongue virus. *Nucleic Acids Res* 2014;42(22):13824–13838.
191. Sung PY, et al. The interaction of bluetongue virus VP6 and genomic RNA is essential for genome packaging. *J Virol* 2019;93(5).
192. Sutton G, et al. Bluetongue virus VP4 is an RNA-capping assembly line. *Nat Struct Mol Biol* 2007;14(5):449–451.

193. Szmaragd C, et al. The spread of bluetongue virus serotype 8 in Great Britain and its control by vaccination. *PLoS One* 2010;5(2):e9353.

194. Takamatsu H, Jeggo MH. Cultivation of bluetongue virus-specific ovine T cells and their cross-reactivity with different serotype viruses. *Immunology* 1989;66(2):258–263.

195. Tan B, et al. RGD tripeptide of bluetongue virus VP7 protein is responsible for core attachment to Culicoides cells. *J Virol.* 2001;75(8):3937–3947.

196. Tao Y, et al. RNA synthesis in a cage-structural studies of reovirus polymerase lambda3. *Cell* 2002;111(5):733–745.

197. Theal GM. *Records of South-Eastern Africa collected in various libraries and archive departments in Europe.* Government of Cape Colony; 1899:224.

198. Theiler A. The immunization of mules with polyvalent serum and virus. In: *Transvaal Department of Agricultural Report in Veterinary Bacteriology 1906–1907.* Pretoria, South Africa: Transvaal Department of Agriculture; 1908:192–213.

199. Theron J, Nel LH. Stable protein-RNA interaction involves the terminal domains of bluetongue virus mRNA, but not the terminally conserved sequences. *Virology* 1997;229(1):134–142.

200. Thomas CP, Booth TF, Roy P. Synthesis of bluetongue virus-encoded phosphoprotein and formation of inclusion bodies by recombinant baculovirus in insect cells: it binds the single-stranded RNA species. *J Gen Virol* 1990;71(Pt 9):2073–2083.

201. Toh X, et al. Use of nanopore sequencing to characterize African horse sickness virus (AHSV) from the African horse sickness outbreak in Thailand in 2020. *Transbound Emerg Dis* 2021. doi: 10.1111/tbed.14056.

202. Tortorici MA, et al. Template recognition and formation of initiation complexes by the replicase of a segmented double-stranded RNA virus. *J Biol Chem* 2003;3:3.

203. Tsai KS, Karstad L. Epizootic hemorrhagic disease virus of deer: an electron microscopic study. *Can J Microbiol* 1970;16(6):427–432.

204. Tyler KL, et al. Differences in the capacity of reovirus strains to induce apoptosis are determined by the viral attachment protein sigma 1. *J Virol* 1995;69(11):6972–6979.

205. Urakawa T, Ritter DG, Roy P. Expression of largest RNA segment and synthesis of VP1 protein of bluetongue virus in insect cells by recombinant baculovirus: association of VP1 protein with RNA polymerase activity. *Nucleic Acids Res* 1989;17(18):7395–7401.

206. Urakawa T, Roy P. Bluetongue virus tubules made in insect cells by recombinant baculoviruses: expression of the NS1 gene of bluetongue virus serotype 10. *J Virol* 1988;62(11):3919–3927.

207. Urakawa T, et al. Synthesis of recombinant baculoviruses expressing the outer capsid protein VP2 of five BTV serotypes and the induction of neutralizing antibodies to homologous and heterologous BTV serotypes [published errata appear in Virus Res 1994 Oct;34(1):93 and 1994 Nov;34(2):187]. *Virus Res* 1994;31(2):149–161.

208. Van Dijk AA, Huismans H. The in vitro activation and further characterization of the bluetongue virus-associated transcriptase. *Virology* 1980;104(2):347–356.

209. Van Dijk AA, Huismans H. In vitro transcription and translation of bluetongue virus mRNA. *J Gen Virol* 1988;69(Pt 3):573–581.

210. van Gennip RG, van de Water SG, van Rijn PA. Bluetongue virus nonstructural protein NS3/NS3a is not essential for virus replication. *PLoS One* 2014;9(1):e85788.

211. van Rijn PA, et al. Bluetongue Disabled Infectious Single Animal (DISA) vaccine: studies on the optimal route and dose in sheep. *Vaccine* 2017;35(2):231–237.

212. van Rijn PA, et al. African horse sickness virus (AHSV) with a deletion of 77 amino acids in NS3/NS3a protein is not virulent and a safe promising AHS Disabled Infectious Single Animal (DISA) vaccine platform. *Vaccine* 2018;36(15):1925–1933.

213. van Staden V, Stoltz MA. Expression of nonstructural protein NS3 of African horsesickness virus (AHSV): evidence for a cytotoxic effect of NS3 in insect cells, and characterization of the gene products in AHSV infected Vero cells. *Arch Virol* 1995;140(2):289–306.

214. Venkatesan S, Gershowitz A, Moss B. Modification of the 5′ end of mRNA. Association of RNA triphosphatase with the RNA guanylyltransferase-RNA (guanine-7-)methyltransferase complex from vaccinia virus. *J Biol Chem* 1980;255(3):903–908.

215. Venter E, et al. Comparative ultrastructural characterization of African horse sickness virus-infected mammalian and insect cells reveals a novel potential virus release mechanism from insect cells. *J Gen Virol* 2014;95(Pt 3):642–651.

216. Verwoerd DW, Huismans H. Studies on the in vitro and the in vivo transcription of the bluetongue virus genome. *Onderstepoort J Vet Res* 1972;39(4):185–191.

217. Verwoerd DW, et al. Structure of the bluetongue virus capsid. *J Virol* 1972;10(4):783–794.

218. Wehrfritz JM, et al. Reconstitution of bluetongue virus polymerase activity from isolated domains based on a three-dimensional structural model. *Biopolymers* 2007;86(1):83–94.

219. Williams CF, et al. The complete sequence of four major structural proteins of African horse sickness virus serotype 6: evolutionary relationships within and between the orbiviruses. *Virus Res* 1998;53(1):53–73.

220. Wirblich C, Bhattacharya B, Roy P. Nonstructural protein 3 of bluetongue virus assists virus release by recruiting ESCRT-I protein Tsg101. *J Virol* 2006;80(1):460–473.

221. Wu W, Roy P. Sialic acid binding sites in VP2 of bluetongue virus and their use during virus entry. *J Virol* 2022;96(1):e01677-21.

222. Wu X, et al. Multiple glycoproteins synthesized by the smallest RNA segment (S10) of bluetongue virus. *J Virol* 1992;66(12):7104–7112.

223. Wu W, et al. Mapping the pH sensors critical for host cell entry by a complex nonenveloped virus. *J Virol* 2019;93(4).

224. Xia X, et al. Bluetongue virus capsid protein VP5 perforates membranes at low endosomal pH during viral entry. *Nat Microbiol* 2021;6(11):1424–1432. doi: 10.1038/s41564-021-00988-8.

225. Yang H, et al. Novel putative bluetongue virus serotype 29 isolated from inapparently infected goat in Xinjiang of China. *Transbound Emerg Dis* 2020;68(4):2543–2555.

226. Zhang X, et al. Bluetongue virus coat protein VP2 contains sialic acid-binding domains, and VP5 resembles enveloped virus fusion proteins. *Proc Natl Acad Sci U S A* 2010;107(14):6292–6297.

227. Zhang X, et al. Atomic model of a nonenveloped virus reveals pH sensors for a coordinated process of cell entry. *Nat Struct Mol Biol* 2016;23(1):74–80.

228. Zhou Y, et al. Measles virus forms inclusion bodies with properties of liquid organelles. *J Virol* 2019;93(21).

Robert LeDesma • Alexander Ploss

History
Classification
   Animal reservoirs and animal hepeviruses
Virion structure
Genome structure and organization
   ORF1
   ORF2
   ORF3
   ORF4
Stages of replication
   HEV attachment and entry
   HEV replication
   HEV viral assembly
   HEV virion release
Pathogenesis and pathology
   Histopathology
   Extrahepatic manifestations
Epidemiology
Pregnancy
Diagnosis
Prevention and control
   Treatment
   Vaccination and prevention
Perspective
Acknowledgments

HISTORY

Prior to the discovery of hepatitis E virus (HEV), hepatitis B virus (HBV) was thought to be the only cause of transfusion-associated hepatitis and hepatitis A virus (HAV) the sole etiologic agent of enterically transmitted hepatitis. This remained the prevalent theory—with HEV unrecognized as a distinct clinical entity—until the late 1970s, when an epidemic of waterborne hepatitis in the Kashmir region of India affected more than 50,000 individuals and resulted in nearly 2,000 deaths. Although a large proportion of these patients presented with hepatitis, their sera tested negative for HAV and HBV, leading to the conclusion that a novel agent was responsible.[116,242] This all changed in 1983, when a similar epidemic of non-A non-B (NANB) hepatitis occurred among Soviet troops in Afghanistan. Investigating the responsible agent and its pathogenesis, Russian virologist Mikhail Balayan ingested filtered fecal extracts, which resulted in acute hepatitis 36 days post inoculation and his subsequent identification of virus-like particles from his own stool by immune electron microscopy (IEM).[12] This finding led to the characterization of what would come to be known as HEV and led to collaborative studies between Russian scientists and the United States Centers for Disease Control (CDC).[21]

The epidemiological and clinical similarities between HAV and HEV infections, such as their ability to be transmitted via the fecal–oral route, are now known to be high, but these are more recent discoveries. In regions where hepatitis was endemic—caused by the known viruses HAV, HBV, and hepatitis C virus (HCV)—sporadic cases caused by this new etiological agent were also observed,[10,117] leading to its classification as epidemic or enterically transmitted NANB hepatitis. During this period, the only means of studying this novel entity was by transmitting this agent to primates and visualizing virions via IEM. However, in 1990, HEV was cloned and (partially) sequenced, opening avenues for the development of virus-specific diagnostics.[199] Since these early endeavors to demystify this new clinical agent, 659 complete genomic sequences have been deposited and enterically transmitted NANB hepatitis was renamed and classified as HEV.[199]

CLASSIFICATION

HEV is a single-stranded, positive-sense RNA virus originally classified based on genome organization in the family *Caliciviridae*. However, in 1992, the first bioinformatic analysis revealed a loose relationship with several divergent viruses including rubella virus (RuV), alphaviruses of the *Togaviridae* family, and the plant furovirus beet necrotic yellow vein virus.[127] Subsequently, the new family *Hepeviridae* was formed and has two distinct genera: *Orthohepevirus* and *Piscihepevirus*. The latter has one member, cutthroat trout virus,[14] while the former is subdivided into four species (*Orthohepevirus A–D*) based on sequence identity and host range, encompassing HEVs that infect avian species and mammals[192] (Fig. 14.1).

Orthohepevirus A currently contains eight genotypes (HEV-1 through HEV-8), with genotypes 1 to 4 all belonging to the same serotype.[224] Infections with genotypes 1 to 4 and 7 have been observed in humans, with genotypes 1 and 2 restricted to humans and nonhuman primates, while genotypes 3 and 4 can infect humans and several other animal species

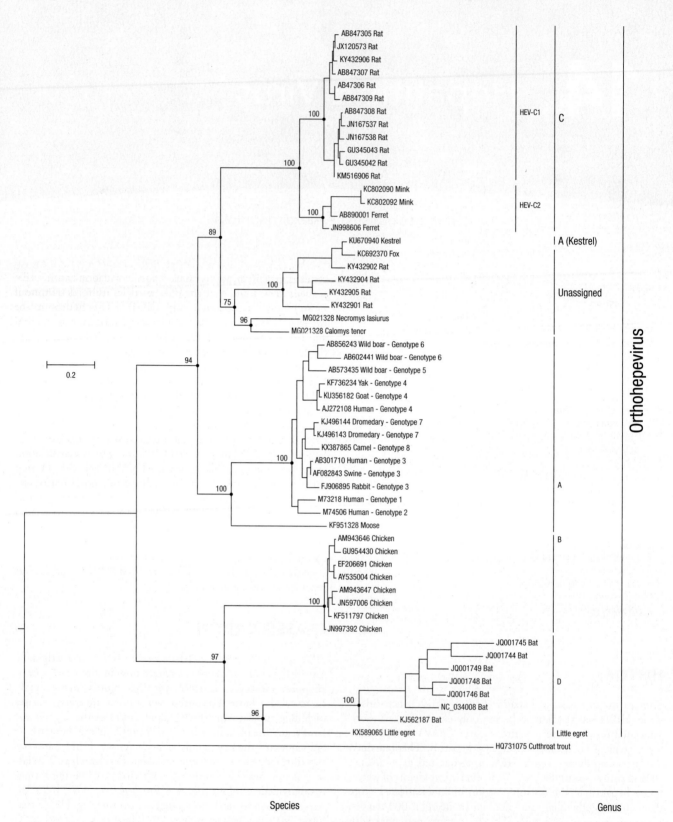

FIGURE 14.1 Phylogenetic tree of *Hepeviridae*. Maximum likelihood midpoint rooted phylogenetic tree depicting the evolutionary relationships of viruses within the *Hepeviridae* family. The *scale bar* indicates evolutionary distances in numbers of substitutions per amino acid site. Bootstrap values of 1,000 replicates are shown in principal nodes. (Adapted from de Souza WM, Romeiro MF, Sabino-Santos G Jr, et al. Novel orthohepeviruses in wild rodents from São Paulo State, Brazil. *Virology* 2018;519:12–16. https://creativecommons.org/licenses/by/4.0/.)

such as rabbit, dolphin, deer, and boar.[37,77,157,191,208,209,220,244] Although recent work found that rabbits could be experimentally infected with swine HEV (genotype 3), disease was mild.[71] Genotypes 5 and 6 are restricted to wild boar,[219] and genotype 7, although first identified in camelids, has been reported in a human patient and caused severe disease in a separate liver transplant patient (Fig. 14.2).[134,243] Lastly, genotypes 7 and 8 have been experimentally shown to infect rhesus monkeys[238]; it is still unknown whether genotype 8 HEV has been able to infect humans or not, and this remains an open question in the zoonosis of HEV.

Orthohepevirus B primarily infects chickens, causing decreased egg production and hepatitis–splenomegaly syndrome,[72] and has also been detected in wild birds such as the egret.[198,258] The viruses in this species experimentally cannot infect nonhuman primates (reviewed in Ref.[255]).

Orthohepevirus C species are known to infect mammals, rodents, and marsupials, including minks, ferrets, Asian musk shrews, rats, and the greater bandicoot rat.[210,213] Although rarely reported in humans, a few cases of HEV in this species, such as HEV-C1, have been found to zoonotically transmit between rats and humans.[212,213]

Orthohepevirus D species have only been isolated from bats.[192] As surveillance and sequencing efforts continue, more members of the *Hepeviridae* family are likely to be discovered, expanding the known host range, and with it, the taxonomy of

HEV will likely change again, as it has several times in its past (Fig. 14.1).

Animal Reservoirs and Animal Hepeviruses

As described above, a wide array of HEVs have been genetically identified from over a dozen distinct animal species. Of the currently known HEV species, some have been proven zoonotic, others proven not zoonotic, and the zoonotic potential for the remaining majority has not been fully determined. Further, additional species have been found in which HEV RNA has not been isolated but have been shown to possess antibodies to HEV (such as dogs, cats, goats, buffalo, sheep, and work horses), demonstrating an exposure to HEV or a closely related agent[87,202,261] (reviewed in Ref.[112]). It is difficult to determine if the aforementioned animal species harbor currently undiscovered strains of HEV, or if they are susceptible to currently identified strains (e.g., some dairy cows in China have been shown to act as an intermediate host of genotype 4 zoonotic HEV between swine and humans).[78] The only way to determine if these animals harbor new species of HEV would require the collection and analysis of the animals' metagenomic data and viromes; however, the transient viremia and low level of viral RNA during HEV infection complicates this process.

The dynamics of HEV spread and the discovery of new animal reservoirs of the virus are an active area of investigation. For example, how genotypes 3 and 4 of HEV spread to

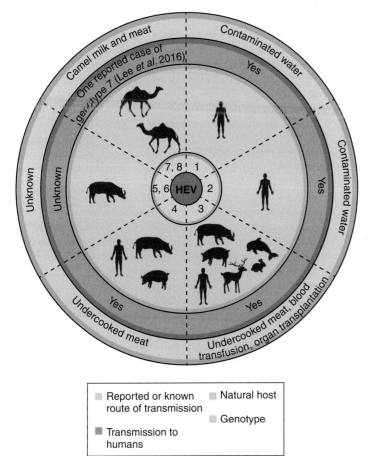

FIGURE 14.2 Host range of hepatitis E virus. The *Orthohepevirus A* genus consists of hepatitis E virus (HEV) genotypes 1 to 8. Genotypes 1 and 2 are known to only infect humans and are transmitted via the fecal–oral route, typically through contaminated water. Genotypes 3 and 4 have a wider host range and can be transmitted to humans through the consumption of undercooked meats, especially pork. Genotypes 5 and 6 infect wild boar; however, it is unknown whether these genotypes can be transmitted to humans (though wild boar genotype 3 HEV has been reported being transmitted to humans). Genotypes 7 and 8 infect dromedary and Bactrian camels, respectively. There has been one case reported of genotype 7 HEV transmission to a liver transplant patient who consumed camel meat and milk. (Reprinted by permission from Nature: Nimgaonkar I, Ding Q, Schwartz RE, et al. Hepatitis E virus: advances and challenges. *Nat Rev Gastroenterol Hepatol* 2018;15(2):96–110. Copyright © 2017 Springer Nature.)

their diverse host range remains incompletely understood, but some progress has been made. For instance, it is known that genotypes 3 and 4 are zoonotically transmitted from swine, wild boar, and deer to humans via undercooked meat consumption. Phylogenetic and molecular analysis of genotype 3 and 4 HEV sequences from humans and pigs have shown high identity between the two populations and a lack of species clustering, suggesting that these strains were not required to adapt to a new host species before jumping between swine and humans.[19] In contrast, it is unclear if other genotype 3 and 4 HEV viruses found in other animals, such as rabbits, can cross the species barrier. It has been demonstrated that cynomolgus macaques can be experimentally infected with rabbit genotype 3 HEV,[147] suggesting a potential ability of this HEV strain to infect humans, though this remains to be elucidated. The zoonotic ability of wild boar HEV genotypes 5 and 6, and the interspecies transmissibility of camelid genotypes 7 and 8 remain incompletely understood; while it is known that camelid genotype 7 has infected humans, it is not known if camelid genotype 7 can infect other potential animal reservoirs such as rabbits and swine, the ways swine genotypes 3 and 4 can infect a wide variety of animal species. Further, it has been experimentally determined that avian HEV from chickens can infect turkeys; however, avian HEV cannot infect rhesus monkeys, shedding light on a potential species barrier for this genus of HEV.[80]

Surprisingly and enigmatically, other animals consumed by humans that harbor HEV but not known to be actively infected have been identified. Specifically, genotypes 3 and 4 HEV have been identified in mussels, oysters, bivalves, and shellfish, and experimental bioaccumulation studies have shown that some oysters, clams, and mussels can concentrate HEV (reviewed in Ref.[50]). It is important to note that while novel zoonotic HEV transmission between shellfish and humans has not been recorded, consuming shellfish has been linked to a case of genotype 4 HEV in a Japanese patient travelling to Vietnam,[125] and an outbreak of HEV on a cruise ship.[203] The prevailing theory as to how shellfish may act as an intermediary is likely due to proximity to contaminated surface and irrigation water with animal sewage and is an ongoing area of investigation (reviewed in Ref.[50]). Teasing out the dynamics of cross-species spread of HEV and discovering the new and emerging species of HEV is vital in order to fully understand and combat the virus.

VIRION STRUCTURE

HEV particles exist in a quasi-enveloped state as small, spherical virions measuring 39.6 ± 1.0 nm in diameter when covered in a lipid membrane or 26.9 ± 0.9 nm in diameter when the envelope has been disrupted via detergents and proteases as imaged by transmission electron microscopy (TEM).[167,221] These particles can be distinguished via sucrose-gradient ultracentrifugation, with enveloped HEV (eHEV) at a density of 1.15 to 1.16 g/mL and HEV collected from feces—largely nonenveloped likely due to stripping of the lipid-associated membrane by the harsh conditions of the digestive tract—at a density of 1.27 to 1.28 g/mL.[221] Supporting these findings, negative contrast electron micrographs measure HEV between 27 and 34 nm in diameter[192] (Fig. 14.3). The nonenveloped HEV virion

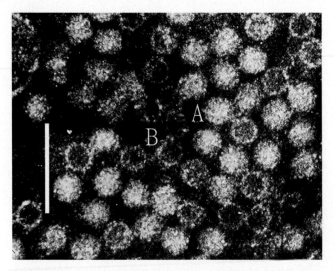

FIGURE 14.3 Negative contrast electron micrograph of human hepatitis E virus virions from a patient's stool collected in Nepal. Virion (*A*); empty capsid (*B*). *Scale bar* represents 100 nm. (Photograph from M. Purdy. Reprinted from Purdy MA, Harrison TJ, Jameel S, et al. ICTV virus taxonomy profile: *Hepeviridae. J Gen Virol* 2017;98(11):2645–2646.)

as visualized via IEM is a spherical particle approximately 30 to 34 nm in diameter[12] with a capsid that can be subdivided into three major functional domains: the shell (S), middle (M), and protruding (P) domains.[251] The S domain is composed of a continuous capsid, which adopts a jelly-roll fold seen in other small RNA viruses. The P domain is made up of a P1 domain of threefold protrusions and a P2 domain of twofold spikes.[68] Both the P1 and P2 domains adopt β-barrel folds and are hypothesized to be involved in receptor binding. The P domain of the capsid contains C-terminal residues that form dimer contacts comprising the protrusions[144] (reviewed in Ref.[113]). While advancements toward visualizing the HEV particle at even finer resolutions have been made, it remains an experimental challenge to produce enough replication-competent viral particles for structural study.

Due to this limitation, self-assembled empty viral-like particles (VLPs) have been produced via overexpression of open reading frame 2 (ORF2) proteins in insect cells (ORF2 encodes the capsid protein and is likely responsible for binding/encapsidation of the viral RNA genome and virion formation)[68,142,247,251] (Fig. 14.4). The icosahedral symmetry of the VLPs differs depending on where ORF2 is truncated. If the ORF2 protein is limited to amino acids (AAs) 112 to 660, VLPs are generated with T = 1 symmetry of 60 protein copies.[142,247] This is similar to the crystal structure of the truncated ORF2 (AAs 112 to 608) of HEV genotypes 3 and 4, which also has T = 1 symmetry[68,251] (Fig. 14.4A and B). However, none of the aforementioned VLPs are thought to bind RNA, which is not surprising considering these studies were carried out via heterologous systems due to technical issues. Strikingly, the diameter of a T = 1 VLP is 23.7 nm, whereas native particles collected from infected monkeys have a diameter of 27 nm.[142] VLPs made of ORF2 AAs 112 to 608 lacking portions of the N and C termini have T = 3 icosahedral symmetry and are thought to be closer to the full-sized RNA-binding virion[248,263] (Fig. 14.4C and D).

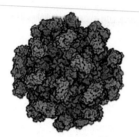

PDB Accession: 2ZTN
Genotype: 3 (2712 strain)
Amino Acids: 112 - 608
Icosahedral Symmetry: T=1

A

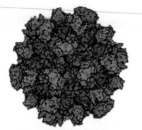

PDB Accession: 3HAG
Genotype: 4 (China T1 Isolate)
Amino Acids: 112 - 608
Icosahedral Symmetry: T=1

B

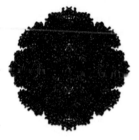

PDB Accession: 3IYO
Genotype: 3
Amino Acids: 14 - 608
Icosahedral Symmetry: T=3

C

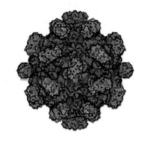

PDB Accession: 6LAT
Genotype: 1
Amino Acids: 112 - 606
Icosahedral Symmetry: T=3

D

FIGURE 14.4 Structure of HEV virion and viral-like particles (VLPs). A: HEV VLP of genotype 3 2712 strain resolved at 3.50 Å. **B:** HEV VLP of genotype 4 China T1 isolate resolved at 3.50 Å. **C:** HEV virion-sized VLP of genotype 3 HEV unknown strain resolved at 10.5 Å. **D:** Virion model of genotype 1 HEV unknown strain determined via antibody 8C11 structure overlaid to T = 3 icosahedral symmetry virion-sized VLP (EMDB no. 5173).

GENOME STRUCTURE AND ORGANIZATION

As mentioned, HEV has a positive-sense, single-stranded RNA genome [(+) ssRNA] approximately 7.2 kb in length with 5′ and 3′ untranslated regions (UTRs). *Cis*-acting elements within both UTRs are vital for HEV replication, translation, and/or assembly. The RNA genome has a 5′ 7-methylguanosine cap and a 3′ polyadenylated tail, thus resembling host mRNAs.[92,260]

The HEV genome encodes three ORFs, with the exception of genotype 1, which has an ORF4[168,249] (Fig. 14.5). ORFs 1 to 3 encode the viral replicase, capsid, and a multifunctional phosphoprotein/viroporin necessary for viral egress, respectively, and are each discussed below (Fig. 14.5).

ORF1

Initial sequence alignments with other viruses suggested that ORF1 consisted of seven putative regions, listed here in order from 5′ to 3′: a methyltransferase, Y domain of unknown function, putative papain-like cysteine protease (PCP), hypervariable/proline-rich hinge region, X/macrodomain, helicase, and RNA-dependent RNA polymerase (RdRp)[127] (Fig. 14.5). Functional testing of many of these regions are still ongoing;

however, it is known that the methyltransferase, helicase, and RdRp domains do in fact exhibit their predicted functions, with some caveats, as detailed below.

Methyltransferase

Competitive binding experiments and binding assays with monoclonal antibodies initially demonstrated that the HEV genome has a 5′ 7-methylguanosine cap.[92] AAs 26 to 240 of ORF1 were originally predicted to be responsible for the viral methyltransferase activity,[127,150] but later work showed that AAs 1 to 979 comprise the 110-kD methyltransferase/guanylyltransferase that caps the viral genome.[150] This 110-kD protein exhibits a tight membrane-bound association that mimics integral membrane proteins, persisting in the presence of high salt concentration, EDTA treatment, and elevated pH.[150] Shorter peptides derived from this region are incapable of performing the requisite capping functions, suggesting a likely multidomain functionality of the ORF1 protein. The methyltransferase/guanylyltransferase domains of over 50 viral genera have a core region followed by a structurally conserved (not sequence conserved) region known as an "iceberg region" that is thought to contain membrane binding sites, as demonstrated in better understood viruses.[3] For HEV, this region is thought to be the poorly understood Y-domain, which is included in a region necessary for methyltransferase/guanylyltransferase activity in HEV (AAs 1 to 979).

Y-Domain

Currently, there is still very little known about the HEV Y-domain, though certain sequence motifs are conserved across all HEV genotypes and with other viruses; a palmitoylation site is predicted at AAs C336-C337 and an alpha-helix predicted from L410-E416, which might interact with the cytoplasmic membrane.[181] Mutation of the conserved C336, C337, or W413 to alanine in the Y-domain of genotype 1 HEV renders the virus replication deficient in HepG2/C3A hepatoma cells,[181] potentially by disrupting the genome's secondary structure at the aforementioned "iceberg region" necessary for methyltransferase/guanylyltransferase activity.[3] Regardless, there is still much to be learned about this important viral region.

Putative Papain-Like Cysteine Protease

This enigmatic region of HEV remains a source of debate. First suggested based on loose sequence alignment with rubella virus,[127] this region has been explored via several heterologous expression systems, and a consensus in the field has yet to be reached. Currently, it is not known whether this domain acts as a true virally encoded protease with viral and/or host targets or if it has been misidentified and serves other, yet-to-be elucidated functions. Both hypotheses are outlined below.

Evidence for proteolytic activity of the PCP region

The studies arguing for the existence of a protease domain within ORF1 disagree on how many subunits the ORF1 polyprotein is processed into and the type of protease this region encodes. Furthermore, these studies have largely been conducted in heterologous, nonauthentic infection systems, further muddling the results.

Evidence presented arguing that the PCP region is a cysteine protease suggested that ORF1 is processed into nine subunits, and *in silico* analysis predicted a papain-like β-barrel fold with C434 and H443 acting as the catalytic dyad as well as three potential

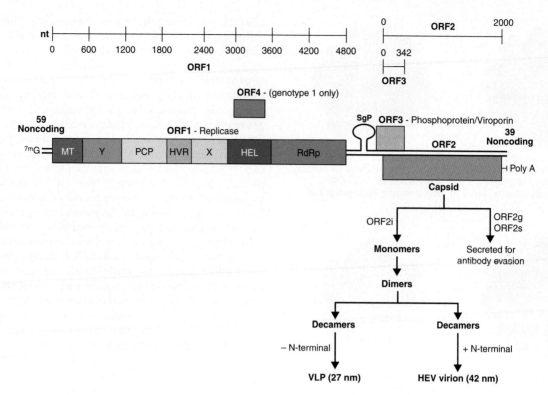

FIGURE 14.5 HEV genome organization and protein products. The HEV genome is a (+) sense single-stranded RNA approximately 7.2 kb in length, possesses a 5′ 7-methylguanosine cap (⁷mG) and a 3′ poly-A tail. The RNA has 5′ and 3′ noncoding regions and 3 open reading frames (ORFs). ORF1 encodes the nonstructural proteins that comprise the viral replicase, which includes a methyltransferase (MT), Y domain of unknown function (Y), putative protease (PCP), hypervariable region (HVR), X domain/macro domain (X), helicase (Hel), and an RNA-dependent RNA polymerase (RdRp). ORF2 encodes the capsid (ORF2i) and two secreted forms (ORF2g and ORF2s) that interfere with antibody neutralization. ORF3 encodes a multifunctional phosphoprotein/viroporin necessary for viral egress. *Cis*-reactive elements include the 5′ and 3′ UTRs, and subgenomic promoter (SgP). Virion assembly begins with capsid monomers oligomerizing into decamers. Full-length decamers encapsidate viral RNA into virions, while N-terminally truncated decamers form viral-like particles (VLPs). nt, nucleotides.

disulfide bridges and a putative zinc-binding motif.[183] In an attempt to experimentally characterize this region, baculovirus was used to express ORF1 within insect cells, a nonnatural host, and nine distinct protein species were observed via matrix-assisted laser desorption ionization–time-of-flight (MALDI-TOF) mass spectrometry. Samples treated with a cysteine protease inhibitor lost this processing of the ORF1 polyprotein.[204]

A separate study suggested that ORF1 is processed into two subunits. Utilizing a genotype 1 (SAR55) reporter replicon harboring GFP as a proxy for viral replication, mutating C457A, C459A, C471A, C472A, C481A, C483A, H443L, H497L, or H590L abrogated viral replication.[179] Further, HA- or histidine-tagged *in vitro* translated ORF1 transfected into Huh7 S10-3 human hepatoma cells suggested that the 186 kDa ORF1 polyprotein is processed into 78 kDa and 38 kDa subspecies.[179]

A chymotrypsin-like protease was suggested by a study that incubated purified and dialyzed fragments of ORF1 and ORF2 with AAs 440 to 610 of the PCP region (suggested by sequence alignments to be AAs 430 to 590). ORF1 and ORF2 were processed into smaller fragments that was stopped by treatment with a chymotrypsin inhibitor.[177]

Lastly, a recent study predicted two putative cleavage sites for cellular thrombin and one for cellular factor Xa in ORF1 conserved across all genotypes. When these sites were mutated

in a genotype 1 reporter replicon, viral replication was impeded in Huh S10-3 cells. Treating these same cells with either a serine protease inhibitor or siRNA interfering with the aforementioned cellular factors also impeded replication.[100]

All the above studies were unable to show HEV polyprotein processing in the context of a natural infection cycle or in systems that accurately mimic HEV infection. As such, it is difficult to conclude whether or not this putative protease domain exists and if so, what type of protease it is and what the cellular or viral protein targets, if any, are.

Evidence against proteolytic activity of the PCP region

Conversely, transfection of an ORF1 encoding vector did not exhibit evidence of processing in human cells. Expression of ORF1 in Huh7 human hepatoma cells or HeLa cells did not result in proteolytic cleavage, and the full-length protein localized with the endoplasmic reticulum (ER) membrane.[187] Epitope-tagged genotype 1 and/or genotype 3 ORF1 in 293T cells or HEP293TT cells did not show processing via Western blot.[215,218] Importantly, the latter study was able to show that the epitope-tagged replicon was replication competent. Furthermore, immunopurification of epitope-tagged ORF1 from human-derived HepG2 cells also demonstrated a lack of processing.[8] Finally, a study expressing truncated versions of ORF1 containing the putative protease domain in HepG2 human hepatoma cells was also unable to find evidence of cleavage, although the authors did observe deubiquitination activity in this domain.[105]

The results of these studies are as varied as the strategies used to investigate the functionality of this highly contested domain, but it remains clear that further rigorous study is needed to deconvolute the activity (if any) of this domain.

Hypervariable Region

The hypervariable region (HVR) of HEV—also known as the polyproline region due to its abundance of proline residues[211]—is bordered by the highly conserved sequences TLYTRTWS at its 5′ end and RRLLXTYPDG at the 3′ end. However, the intervening HVR, as its name suggests, is the most divergent across all HEV genotypes.[193] This region's amino acid sequence identity varies by 71% across all the known HEV genotypes and up to 31% among genotype 1, 41% among genotype 3, 46% among genotype 4, and 30% among avian HEV.[162,189] This region is also responsible for the size differences seen across the HEV genotypes due to varied insertions and/or deletions. The HVR was initially thought to span 105 AAs, but as more HEV genotypes were discovered and sequenced, the highly conserved nature of the flanking 5′ and 3′ sequences emerged. As such, the HVR is now thought to typically be 70 to 72 AAs in length for genotype 1 HEV, 68 AAs for genotype 2, 80 to 86 AAs for genotype 3, and 84 AAs for genotype 4 as well as avian HEV.[189]

Functionally speaking, it is proposed that this region serves a structural role, acting as a proline-rich hinge between adjoined ORF1 regions.[127] This is supported by the fact that the HVR overlaps with an intrinsically disordered region (IDR), which has a high proportion of polar, charged, and structure-breaking amino acids (i.e., proline and glycine).[193] These observations, combined with the conserved absence of bulky hydrophobic amino acids and presence of small amino acids such as glycine, proline, alanine, and serine across the HEV genotypes suggests that the HVR may govern key interviral protein–protein interactions.[193]

The HVR may also affect host tropism as it is required for viral replication in a genotype-specific manner. Swapping HVRs between HEV genotypes or deleting regions of the HVR both drastically reduce viral replication efficiency.[190] The sequence divergence within the HVR of the zoonotic HEV genotypes 3 and 4 is more than twofold higher than that of human-tropic genotype 1, suggesting that greater sequence heterogeneity may play a role in greater species tropism.[193] *In vitro* studies demonstrating that insertions within the HVR can expand the host range of HEV genotypes 1 and 3 lend credence to the above hypothesis.[208]

The HVR is also capable of acquiring and tolerating insertions, both naturally and artificially, leading to the development of vital tools for studying HEV. Six sites within the HVR were recently identified via an unbiased transposon-mediated insertion screen that can tolerate various insertions, allowing for the development of a new epitope-tagged ORF1.[218] Analyses of isolates from chronically infected patients show insertions within the HVR of other parts of the HEV viral genome or human host genes.[88,136] While it is unknown how these natural insertions originated, they have nonetheless been important for the study of HEV. Two HEV genotype 3 strains with human ribosomal protein sequences inserted into the HVR have increased replicative capacity in cell culture, overcoming a previous barrier to the study of this deadly pathogen. These strains, LBPR-0379 and Kernow-C1, acquired S19 and S17 ribosomal protein sequences, respectively.[172,207] Virus containing these HVR insertions were initially discovered as minor species within the total HEV quasi-species isolated from clinical fecal samples. Through serial passage in cell culture, however, these initially minor species became dominant, indicating a replicative advantage. The Kernow-C1 strain after six passages in cell culture (Kernow-C1 p6) is one of the most robustly replicating HEV strains *in vitro*, and the S17 insertion has expanded the host range of this isolate in cell culture to swine, thus suggesting a role in tropism.[207] However, these insertions did not expand HEV host tropism in swine *in vivo*.[226] Interestingly, the S17 insertion includes a nuclear localization signal allowing for nuclear import of the ORF1 protein, but the significance of this remains to be elucidated.[111] Furthermore, seven new insertions within the HVR of genotype 3 strains were recently discovered, three of which were reported during the acute phase of infection.[138] The novel insertions included both virus–host recombinant variants and duplications of HEV sequences; the latter were found to have statistically significant increases in net viral load and post-translational modifications (PTMs) such as ubiquitination, phosphorylation, and acetylation.[138] Altogether, the finding of insertions in the HVR that promote robust replication in cell culture has been a boon to the study of HEV.

X/Macro Domain

The X domain, or macro domain, was named due to its weak sequence homology with human macro domain–containing proteins, which are known to bind ADP-ribose.[106] Bacteria and higher-order organisms use mono- and poly-ADP-ribosylation PTMs for numerous vital biological processes such as transcription, regulation of chromatin structure, and DNA repair.[5,36,106] Several viral macro domains bind ADP-ribose metabolites, including the macro domain of HEV, which binds poly-ADP-ribose with high affinity.[140,171] The presence of the HEV helicase in *cis* drastically increases the binding of the macro domain to poly-ADP-ribose, stimulating poly-ADP-ribose chain removal from host proteins.[140]

The HEV X domain shares sequence homology with the active site of coronavirus cellular X domain–associated macro domain protein/ADP-ribose-1″-monophosphatase (CoV Appr-1″-pase); mutating the putative catalytic site within the HEV X domain severely diminished replication of an SAR55 genotype 1 reporter replicon.[180] The X domain may also have *cis* interactions with the methyltransferase domain and ORF3 protein. A study utilizing a yeast two-hybrid system found that the HEV X domain binds the ORF1 methyltransferase (MTase) N terminus (which includes the MTase catalytic pocket) and also the ORF3 protein at both the N and C termini via X domain residues conserved across all HEV genotypes.[6] The HEV MTase and ORF3 protein appear to compete in binding the X domain, suggesting that this domain may function in a regulatory capacity, as the virus likely needs to focus on replication early in infection (MTase activity to cap newly synthesized genomes) and viral egress later in infection, which is mediated in part by the ORF3 protein.[6,47] Whether the HEV X/macro domain has additional activities remains to be determined.

Helicase

RNA viruses utilize virally encoded helicases to unwind RNA duplex structures; this process is typically coupled with NTP hydrolysis and is responsible for most viral helicase activities (reviewed in Refs.[93,214]). The HEV helicase has NTPase activity, can hydrolyze ATP,[158] and has 5′-3′ polarity.[104] Deletion of conserved helicase superfamily motifs[93] identified within the HEV helicase have varied effects, ranging from increased or reduced NTPase activity, decreased RNA unwinding activity, or both.[158] Additionally, the point mutations A1213V in genotype 1 SAR55 and V1213A in genotype 3 SHEV3 replicons reduce viral replication efficiency.[26] Purified partial HEV helicase domain (AAs 960 to 1204) can hydrolyze all rNTPs but demonstrates a preference for dATP and dCTP.[104] This fragment also exhibits 5′ NTPase activity, suggesting a role in RNA cap formation,[104] which may be why AAs 1 to 979 of the ORF1 protein are needed for successful methyltransferase activity.

RNA-Dependent RNA Polymerase

Like most RNA viruses, HEV encodes an RdRp, which synthesizes (+) and (−) viral RNA transcripts using as templates the viral antisense product of transcription and (+) sense genome, respectively. The HEV RdRp is located downstream of the helicase at the 3′ end of ORF1 in all genotypes, but spans different nucleotide ranges due to the varying sizes of the HEV genotypes. Of the phylogenetically defined RdRp supergroups, the HEV RdRp is classified in supergroup III, which also includes the RdRp of RuV and plant furoviruses.[126] These RdRps contain a highly conserved catalytic GDD motif; when mutated in HEV, the replicative activity is abolished.[48] Unfortunately, structural information for many supergroup III RdRps, including that of HEV, is still lacking[233] (reviewed in Ref.[84]).

Viral RdRps often utilize host or other viral proteins to exert their activity. As demonstrated by a yeast two-hybrid screen, the RdRp of HEV can self-interact,[176] as also seen with other (+) RNA viruses such as HCV and polio virus.[75] However, the stoichiometry of this self-interaction is unknown. The HEV RdRp likely interacts with the helicase and methyltransferase, as the activities of these two domains are complementary to the RNA transcription activity of the RdRp.[176]

Regarding interactions with host factors, the HEV RdRp binds the antitranslational, interferon-induced host protein IFIT1,[188] likely inhibiting its activity. Additionally, the RdRp of genotypes 1 and 3 replicates the HEV genome more robustly when the microRNA miR-122 is overexpressed; the opposite effect is observed when miR-122 is knocked out, suggesting a pro-viral role similar to that seen with HCV, though the specifics of this interaction remain unknown.[70,90]

Cis-Acting Regulatory Elements

The HEV RNA genome requires several cis-acting regulatory elements (CREs) to complete its replication cycle: the 3′ UTR (also known as the noncoding region [NCR]), the subgenomic promoter (SgP), and two recently discovered uncharacterized regions, one within ORF1 and one within ORF2 (Fig. 14.5). These elements likely exert their regulatory activities via RNA secondary structures, as they contain highly conserved sequences across HEV genotypes[25] and form RNA stem–loops in the 3′ region.[2] Swapping the 3′ UTR among strains of genotypes 1, 2, and 3 does not decrease viral replication, despite sequence heterogeneity,[64] suggesting that RNA structure versus a conserved sequence motif is necessary for RdRp binding. Alphaviruses such as Sindbis virus and Semliki Forest virus that replicate their genomes in an asymmetric manner like HEV

also have sequences similar to these HEV regulatory regions.[67,173] During the asymmetric replication of HEV, the viral genome serves as a template for generating a (−) ssRNA antigenome from which more (+) ssRNA viral genomes can be made for packaging into virions. The RdRp (or higher-order replication complex) first binds the 3′ UTR of the viral genome to initiate transcription of the full-length antigenome. From this antigenome, the SgP is bound by the RdRp and is transcribed into the capped, approximately 2.2 kb bicistronic subgenomic RNA from which ORF2 (viral capsid) and ORF3 (phosphoproteins) are translated.[25,27,48] The SgP is located primarily downstream of the ORF1 coding region (but begins slightly within ORF1), ending just before the transcriptional start site of ORF3. Mutating specific regions in the SgP prevents translation of ORF2 and ORF3.[79,81] The SgP also contains a highly conserved RNA stem–loop structure that, unlike the 3′ UTR, seems to require both structural and sequence elements for infectivity.[79]

Regarding the two not fully characterized CREs located in ORF1 and ORF2, synonymous mutations in these elements abolished replication of HEV replicons, suggesting that an alteration in RNA secondary structure prevents these CREs from exerting their function.[91] Taken together, it seems that the tool-box for delving deeper into the full function of the SgP and other CREs is still lacking.[25] More efficient cell culture systems, kinetics assays of subgenome and antigenome production, and detection assays of viral protein products are needed to further understand the interplay between these CREs and HEV replication.

ORF2

ORF2 encodes the capsid protein and is necessary for genome packaging.[7,216] The ORF2 protein is translated from the 2.2 kb subgenomic RNA (see "cis-Acting Regulatory Elements"), which is transcribed from the (−) antigenome[66] (Fig. 14.5). In patients, ORF2 protein is found in three forms: ORF2i (the ORF2 found in infectious particles), ORF2g (glycosylated ORF2), and ORF2c (cleaved ORF2).[7] ORF2g and ORF2c are not associated with viral particles but are both secreted, are the dominant HEV antigens in patient sera, and are known to be N-glycosylated and targeted by patient antibodies.[7,161] These secreted forms of ORF2 are translated from the original presumed AUG start codon, while ORF2i is translated from an AUG 15 codons downstream of the first AUG in the subgenomic RNA. Interestingly, the secreted forms of ORF2 do not include the putative receptor-binding motif and can interfere with antibody-mediated neutralization without inhibiting cell receptor binding and uptake.[254]

The ORF2 capsid protein colocalizes with ORF3 protein and the apical cellular marker dipeptidyl peptidase-4 in HepG2/C3A subclone F2 cells, while secreted ORF2 is observed both apically and basally in these cells.[28] Full-length ORF2 protein can inhibit RIG-I–like receptor–mediated innate immune signaling[74] and, via its N-terminal arginine-rich domain, can prevent TANK-binding kinase-1 (TBK1)-mediated activation of interferon regulatory factor 3 (IRF3) within the mitochondrial antiviral signaling protein–TBK1–IRF3 complex.[145] ORF2 is also vital for the assembly of HEV virions, as discussed in detail below.

ORF3

The ORF3 protein is a multifunctional phosphoprotein, though its phosphorylation is not required for HEV genome replication or infectious particle production in rhesus macaques[65] (Fig. 14.5). The ORF3 protein was first identified as a phosphorylated 13-kDa protein associated with the host cytoskeleton.[256] Further study found that the ORF3 protein is not required for replication of the HEV genome, assembly of infectious virions, or infection of human hepatoma cells *in vitro*.[54] Viral particles isolated from feces do not contain ORF3 protein,[53,222] unlike those isolated from sera[222] or produced in cell culture.[53,222] Of note, HEV virions derive envelopes from host cells during egress and are quasi-enveloped. While these membranes that conceivably contain ORF3 are retained while quasi-enveloped HEV circulates in the blood stream, they are shed in the feces presumably due to the high concentration of bile salts. The ORF3 protein also affects several cellular processes: it activates mitogen-activated protein kinase (MAPK),[128,182] inhibits the MAPK phosphatase,[107] decreases fibrinogen secretion,[195] and increases interferon induction in human hepatoma cells.[169] Evidence also suggests that ORF3 serves as a viroporin, an ion channel necessary for viral egress.[47] Furthermore, ORF3 interacts with the nonglycosylated form of the ORF2 protein[230] and expedites export of α1-microglobulin from hepatocytes.[231]

ORF4

HEV genotype 1 encodes a novel ORF, ORF4, that overlaps with ORF1 (Fig. 14.5). This protein's expression is regulated via an internal ribosomal entry site (IRES) and can be induced by ER stress.[168,249] ORF4 assembles a protein complex consisting of the HEV RdRp, helicase, and X domain as well as host β-tubulin and eukaryotic translation elongation factor 1 alpha 1, the latter of which stimulates HEV RdRp activity when in association with ORF4 protein.[168] Ectopic expression of HEV genotype 1 ORF4 can also enhance HEV genotype 3 replication.[249]

ORF4 was also detected in rat HEV, but its role in this related virus is largely unknown. ORF4 protein was not detected in sera from experimentally infected rats, and deletion of ORF4 from the rat HEV genome did not affect ORF1 protein levels or viral replication.[275]

STAGES OF REPLICATION

HEV Attachment and Entry

HEV entry remains an enigmatic area of study. The entry factors, including the cellular receptor(s) HEV depends upon for entry into host cells remain(s) unknown. Although several host factors are known to play a role in HEV attachment/entry, the mechanisms nonenveloped versus (quasi)enveloped HEV use remain entangled. What is known about the route of entry for each is outlined below.

Nonenveloped (Naked) HEV Entry

Nonenveloped HEV is prominently found in the bile and feces of infected individuals[222] and is largely transmitted enterically, though how it traverses the gut–blood barrier remains unknown. During the course of a natural infection, HEV is highly hepatotropic. However, like HAV, *in vitro* studies of HEV suggest a wider tissue tropism, including human lung epithelial cells (A549), colon epithelial cells (Caco-2), neuronally derived cells, and placental cells.[52,62,124,156,208,264] Whether these experimental findings in immortalized/cancer-derived cell lines, which harbor genetic abnormalities and phenotypic differences compared to healthy cells, figure in clinical infection remains to be seen.

With this caveat in mind, work with HEV VLPs in hepatoma cell lines suggests that syndecans, a subset of heparan sulfate proteoglycans (HSPGs), play a role in binding the viral ORF3 protein[94] (Fig. 14.6). HPSGs are ubiquitous to almost all cell surfaces across all domains of life and feature in the

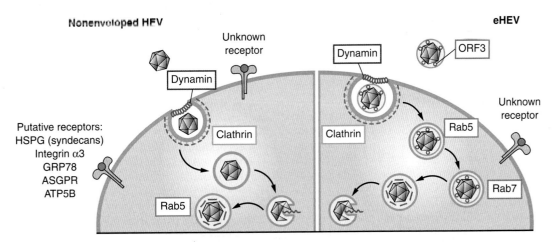

FIGURE 14.6 Nonenveloped (naked) HEV and enveloped HEV (eHEV) attachment and entry. The cellular receptor for both naked HEV and eHEV remains unknown. Though, nonenveloped (naked) HEV is thought to bind one or more of the following cellular factors on the surface of the cell to facilitate entry (*left*): heparin sulfate proteoglycans (HSPGs), integrin α3, glucose-regulated protein 78 (GRP78), asialoglycoprotein receptor (ASGPR), and/or ATP synthase subunit 5β (ATP5B). Once attached, naked HEV enters the cell via clathrin- and dynamin 2–dependent endocytosis. The HEV genome is released into the cytoplasm via unknown mechanism(s), potentially by capsid rearrangement. Once the genome is released, the capsid is degraded in Rab5+ endosomal compartments. eHEV attachment and entry mechanisms are currently unknown (*right*). eHEV, like naked HEV, is internalized via clathrin- and dynamin 2–dependent endocytosis but is further trafficked through the early (Rab5+) and late (Rab7+) endosomes and enters the lysosome to allow release of the HEV genome into the cytoplasm by an unknown mechanism. (Adapted from Oechslin N, Moradpour D, Gouttenoire J. On the host side of the hepatitis E virus life cycle. *Cells* 2020;9(5):1294. https://creativecommons.org/licenses/by/4.0/.)

attachment of many enveloped and nonenveloped viruses. However, as discussed further below, HSPGs are not involved in the binding of enveloped HEV.[252] Other cellular host factors implicated in the binding of naked HEV include glucose-regulated protein 78, asialoglycoprotein receptor, ATP synthase subunit 5β, and integrin alpha-3 (extensively reviewed in Ref.[253]).

Nonenveloped, fluorescently tagged HEV VLPs can bind Huh7 human hepatoma cells with high affinity, entering via clathrin-mediated endocytosis.[76,102] These VLPs were degraded after being trafficked to acidic lysosomal compartments via Rab5-positive compartments, and important factors for this HEV internalization included membrane cholesterol, actin, and members of the PI3K pathway[76] (Fig. 14.6). Surprisingly, low pH was not required, suggesting that uncoating of naked HEV particles occurs before entering Rab5-positive compartments. Currently, the actual uncoating process of naked HEV remains opaque.

eHEV Entry

eHEV does not have viral proteins that extrude from the envelope, begging the questions: how does cell binding occur and how is cellular tropism determined? Does eHEV entry involve membrane fusion and/or a separate attachment, entry, and uncoating process distinctive from that of naked HEV? eHEV membranes do contain phosphatidylserine (similar to exosomes), which may bind to the protein T-cell immunoglobulin mucin family member 1 on host cells.[83] eHEV does enter cells less efficiently than naked HEV, presumably due to poorer attachment that, as mentioned above, is not mediated via HSPGs[252] (Fig. 14.6).

eHEV initially enters the host cell the same way naked HEV does: via clathrin- and dynamin-mediated endocytosis.[102] Once inside the host cell, eHEV is transported into Rab5- and Rab7-positive endosomal compartments, eventually entering the lysosome where, unlike naked HEV, acidification is necessary for infectivity.[76,252] Our understanding of how quasi-enveloped viruses enter host cells and are subsequently trafficked has been greatly increased by the study of enveloped HAV (reviewed in Ref.[200]), but whether or not these findings also hold true for eHEV remains to be elucidated.

It is likely that the HEV viral envelope would need to be degraded within the lysosome to allow the capsid to bind elements within the lysosomal membrane to trigger rearrangement and formation of a pore for genome delivery; depletion of a critical component of the lipid membrane degradation process, Niemann-Pick disease type C1 protein, decreased eHEV infectivity by 50%.[252] Additionally, pretreating cells with an inhibitor of lysosomal acid lipase, an enzyme essential in lipid metabolism, led to a dose-dependent decrease in eHEV, but not naked HEV, infectivity.[252] These results are consistent with enveloped HAV entry,[200] suggesting a shared entry mechanism for these distantly related viruses.

After the membrane of eHEV is shed, the capsid would now be free to potentially interact with elements within the lysosomal membrane and the viral genome subsequently released into the cytoplasm. These elements in the lysosomal membrane could be the same ones that naked HEV interacts with on the cell surface, although this hypothesis remains unverified. Further, other viruses (such as coxsackieviruses) are known to utilize different receptors during the entry process,[38] so this could also be a mechanism utilized by eHEV.

HEV Replication

Since the generation of the first infectious HEV cDNA clone,[223] many strides have been made in understanding how HEV replicates in host cells. Host factor heat-shock protein 90 (HSP90) has been implicated early in infection during intracellular transport of the HEV capsid,[262] and inhibition of HSP90 can suppress HEV replication[174] (Fig. 14.7). Once released into the cytoplasm from the capsid, the HEV genome, being (+), capped at its 5′ end, and polyadenylated at the 3′ end, is translated directly by host ribosomes.[55,92,150,260] Upon ribosomal binding, ORF1 is translated into a protein with methyltransferase, helicase, and RdRp activity (all necessary for HEV genome synthesis), but it is unclear whether this protein is processed into discreet functional units (see "Genome Structure and Organization" for further information). The RdRp binds the poly-A tail and RNA secondary stem–loop structures at the 3′ end of HEV genome,[2] using the genome as a template to produce a full-length, (−) antigenome. From this antigenome, more full-length, (+) genome is made as well as the smaller subgenomic RNA encoding ORF2 and ORF3 proteins[66,235] (Fig. 14.7). There is a temporal and quantitative separation between (+) and (−) RNA production. (−) RNA is produced approximately 1,000-fold less than (+) RNA, with (−) antigenome production peaking approximately 8 hours post transfection of HEV genomic RNA *in vitro*.[235]

HEV replication and genomic RNA synthesis likely occurs at intracellular membranes. Studies have shown that the HEV replicase within ORF1 localizes with ER membrane markers,[196] and the ORF1 protein can be recovered from the membrane fraction of ultracentrifugation gradients.[218]

HEV Viral Assembly

To date, little is known about how infectious HEV virions are assembled. Only full-length, (+) genomic HEV RNA is packaged within HEV virions. The viral genome is distinguished from host RNA by a sequence at the N-terminal domain of the ORF2 capsid protein that specifically binds a 76 nucleotide region at the 5′ end of the HEV RNA genome[216,223] (Fig. 14.8).

HEV ORF2 protein can self-oligomerize into VLPs, a process mediated by disulfide bonds formed between cysteine residues at the C terminus.[146] Further, the C-terminal 52 amino acids are dispensable for capsid formation, but absolutely vital for infectivity, suggesting a role in encapsidation and stabilization of encapsidated particles.[205]

Much remains to be discovered about the assembly process of HEV, including the intracellular location of viral assembly, whether HEV has a temporal viral "switch" that promotes assembly/egress over replication, and whether host factors are involved in HEV particle assembly.

HEV Virion Release

Once HEV has successfully entered a host cell, undergone replication, and assembled new virions, these virions must exit the cell in order to infect new host cells. Virion release is accomplished not through cell lysis but rather through the multifunctional, ca. 114 AA ORF3 phosphoprotein. This protein is not necessary for viral replication, assembly, or entry[54] but is essential for egress.[47,250] Phosphorylated ORF3 protein interacts with the nonglycosylated form of the ORF2 protein[230] (see "Genome Structure and Organization") and could contribute to the mechanism by which virions are "chosen" for egress, but this has yet to be definitively shown.

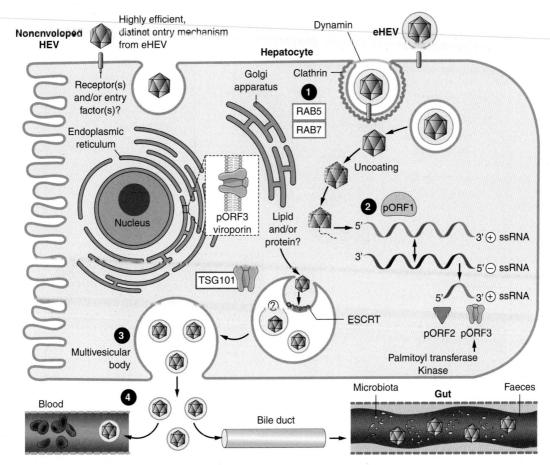

FIGURE 14.7 Life cycle of hepatitis E virus. HEV begins its replication cycle either as naked HEV or enveloped HEV (eHEV); each bind to a host cell via an unknown receptor. Each enter the cell via clathrin- and dynamin-dependent receptor mediated endocytosis. Via mechanisms not fully understood but involve Rab 5 and Rab 7 endosomal compartments (step 1) (see Fig. 14.6), the HEV capsid deposits the HEV positive sense single-stranded RNA ((+) ssRNA) into the cytoplasm, where it is immediately translated by host ribosomes. The ORF1 protein (pORF1) encodes an RNA-dependent RNA polymerase (RdRp) that uses the (+) ssRNA genome as a template to transcribe full-length negative-sense (−) single-stranded RNA ((−) ssRNA) (step 2). From this (−) ssRNA antigenome, the RdRp can subsequently transcribe both new full-length HEV template for packing into virions, and shorter subgenomic RNA (sgRNA) that encodes ORF2 capsid protein (pORF2) and ORF3 phosphoprotein/viroporin (pORF3). pORF3 is known to bind tumor susceptibility gene 101 protein (TSG101), which is a member of the endosomal sorting complexes required for transport (ESCRT) pathway to bud from cell membranes (step 3). pORF3 likely interacts with TSG101 to promote budding of progeny virions into multivesicular bodies (MVBs), which fuse with the cellular plasma membrane for virion release. eHEV envelopes are likely derived from the *trans*-Golgi network, and viral particles within eHEV have been shown to associate with pORF3; pORF3 has also been shown to exhibit ion channel activity, suggesting a transmembrane localization. eHEV virions released from the apical membrane of the cell enter the bile duct, where the envelope is likely stripped away by detergents, proteases, and bile salts (step 4), explaining why only naked (nonenveloped) HEV is shed in feces. Alternatively, if eHEV is released from the basal membrane of hepatocytes, it enters the serum in its enveloped form, where it is protected from neutralizing antibodies, but less efficient at infecting new cells. (Adapted by permission from Nature: Nimgaonkar I, Ding Q, Schwartz RE, et al. Hepatitis E virus: advances and challenges. *Nat Rev Gastroenterol Hepatol* 2018;15(2):96–110. Copyright © 2017 Springer Nature.)

Egress of HEV particles occurs via the host cellular exosomal pathway: the N-terminal hydrophobic domains of ORF3 were shown to interact with host microtubules,[256] and the PSAP late domain amino acid motif in the ORF3 C-terminal domain with the tumor susceptibility gene 101, a component in the endosomal sorting complexes required for transport (ESCRT) machinery.[101,114,217] Altering this PSAP domain via mutagenesis reduces virus release into culture media, and swapping it with a heterologous late domain motif or supplying WT ORF3 *in trans* cannot rescue virus release, demonstrating the necessity of this domain in virus release[115] (Figs. 14.7 and 14.8). Further, host cellular exosomal components, including tetraspanins (specifically CD63, CD9, and CD81), phosphatidylserine, trans-Golgi network protein 2, and epithelial cellular adhesion molecule, copurify with eHEV, indicating the presence of these host proteins on the virion's surface[165–167] (Fig. 14.8).

HEV egress is also known to be mediated by multivesicular bodies (MVBs), which fuse with the plasma membrane of the host cell to release eHEV. This process involves Rab27, as evidenced by eHEV release decreasing with Rab27 knockdown.[165]

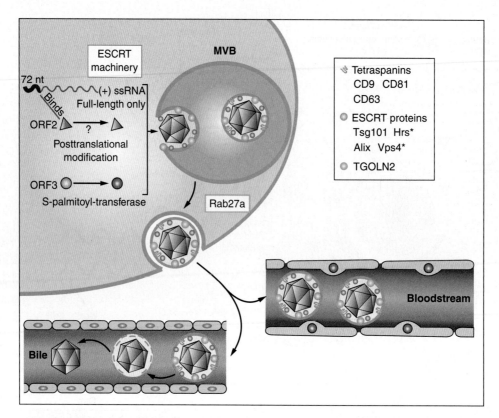

FIGURE 14.8 Proposed assembly and release mechanisms for naked HEV and enveloped HEV. Encapsidation of the viral genome is thought to occur by binding of an N-terminal motif of 76-nucleotides on the HEV genome by pORF2; the nonglycosylated form of pORF2 also spontaneously self-assembles into a protective capsid. eHEV particle formation involves phosphorylation and palmitoylation of ORF3 protein and components of the endosomal sorting complexes required for transport (ESCRT) pathway: tumor susceptibility gene 101 (TSG101), hepatocyte growth factor–regulated tyrosine kinase substrate (Hrs), vacuolar protein sorting 4 (Vps4), and apoptosis-linked gene 2–interacting protein X (Alix). The virion is enveloped by the exosomal membrane that harbors the tetraspanins CD9, CD63, and CD81, as well as *trans*-Golgi network protein 2 (TGOLN2), Alix, and TSG101. eHEV release involves Rab-27a–dependent trafficking of multivesicular bodies (MVBs) and fusion with the cellular plasma membrane. Released virions remain associated with the exosomal envelope during circulation unless they are delipidated in the bile duct. *Asterisks* note host factors not found on eHEV. (Adapted from Oechslin N, Moradpour D, Gouttenoire J. On the host side of the Hepatitis E virus life cycle. *Cells* 2020;9(5):1294. https://creativecommons.org/licenses/by/4.0/.)

Once an eHEV virion within an MVB is poised for release, ORF3 oligomerizes into an ion channel (see "Genome Structure and Organization"), which is required for virus release.[47] However, how this ion channel provides a conducive environment for virion egress remains unknown.

Besides phosphorylation, ORF3 is palmitoylated by an unknown palmitoyltransferase, and this PTM is necessary for membrane association of ORF3 and infectious particle release[63] (Fig. 14.8). It is likely that these distinct PTMs allow ORF3 to play the disparate roles mentioned above in HEV infection, and other functionalities may come to light with more study.

In vivo, HEV infection primarily takes place in and among hepatocytes. Hepatocytes are polarized epithelial cells with an apical surface that within the context of the liver abuts the bile canaliculi and a basolateral surface that abuts the hepatic sinusoid.[59] Newly formed HEV virions can be released at either of these surfaces, but the vast majority are released apically into the bile canaliculi and subsequently shed into the feces.[28] The small proportion of virions that are released basolaterally go into the bloodstream and thus spread throughout the body.

PATHOGENESIS AND PATHOLOGY

Although often asymptomatic, HEV can present as acute hepatitis and result in fever, reduced appetite, nausea, vomiting, abdominal pain, joint pain, dark urine, and jaundice (reviewed in Refs.[137,239]). In approximately 5% to 30% of patients, infection is self-limiting and does not require hospitalization, with symptoms resolving in no more than 6 weeks; in a subset of patients, however, infections can become chronic. In rare cases, HEV causes fulminant hepatitis, which is usually fatal.[240]

According to the CDC, the incubation period for HEV ranges from 15 to 60 days post exposure. Fecal shedding and viremia are often first detected approximately 21 days post exposure and about 7 days prior to symptom onset[12,30] but can both wane approximately 7 to 8 weeks post exposure. In infected patients, liver enzymes, such as alanine aminotransferase, aspartate aminotransferase, and bilirubin, typically rise approximately 4 to 5 weeks post exposure, peak approximately 7 to 8 weeks post exposure, and can last up to 13 weeks. Concurrently, approximately 7 to 8 weeks post exposure, levels of immunoglobulin G (IgG) and M (IgM) specific to HEV rise to detectable levels.[118] IgM antibodies against HEV disappear after several months, whereas anti-HEV IgG rapidly declines soon after infection but can remain detectable for years post exposure (Fig. 14.9).

HEV needs to pass through the gut and intestinal–blood barrier in order to reach the liver where the virus replicates in hepatocytes.[130] HEV has been found to replicate in human intestinal epithelial cells as well as intestinal explants,[154] helping to explain the virus' ability to complete its journey to the liver.

Patients with chronic liver disease not caused by HEV are at a higher risk of life-threatening hepatitis E if infected with HEV concomitantly.[110,131,259]

Histopathology

The histopathology of HEV infection is less well characterized compared to other viral hepatitis infections. The typical pattern of liver injury seen in patients with HEV overlaps with that observed in other forms of acute viral hepatitis, including lymphocyte infiltration of the portal tract, hepatocyte ballooning, scattered apoptotic (acidophilic) bodies, and cholestasis.[186] Severe cases of HEV infection are associated with cholangiolitis, parenchymal injury, portal inflammation, and fulminant hepatic failure[151,185] (reviewed in Ref.[39]). In addition, widespread necrosis of hepatocytes and collapse of the parenchyma have been observed[39] (Fig. 14.10).

HEV infection in human patients may be accompanied by comorbidities, so experimental and natural infection by HEV in animals have improved our understanding of the nature of injuries solely attributed to HEV infection (reviewed in Ref.[112]). For instance, macaques inoculated with HEV displayed elevated liver enzyme levels in their serum, had antibodies reactive to HEV, developed liver lesions, and excreted HEV in their feces.[77] Swine are naturally susceptible to genotypes 3 and 4 of HEV, and upon necropsy of naturally or experimentally infected pigs, histopathological lesions were observed, including portal inflammation, focal hepatocellular necrosis, and multifocal lymphoplasmacytic hepatitis.[20] Avian HEV infection in chickens is known to be associated with hepatitis–splenomegaly syndrome, and chickens experimentally infected with HEV developed gross and microscopic liver

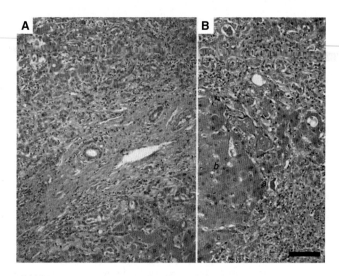

FIGURE 14.10 Histopathology of HEV in an HEV-infected patient. A: Hematoxylin and eosin (H&E) stain. The periportal parenchyma contains a marked ductular reaction characterized by a proliferation of small-caliber ducts lined with pale basophilic epithelial cells extending from the margin of the portal tract. Prominent extracellular matrix separates the ductules. Neighboring hepatocytes are in disarray, and prominent bile plugs are seen in distended canaliculi and ductules. A mild lymphocytic infiltrate is dispersed throughout the portal tract and adjacent parenchyma. **B:** H&E stain. Higher-magnification image from the same patient. Prominent cholestasis is seen in distended canaliculi with formation of small bile lake at the interface of a prominent ductular reaction on the right and a focus of hepatocytes (*a*) that are lightly vacuolated and lack normal sinusoidal arrangement. (*b*) Focus of hypertrophic hepatocytes lacking vacuoles indicative of early liver regeneration against a background of a damaged parenchyma. *Scale bar*—100 μm. (Courtesy of M. Sjogren.) (Reprinted from Purcell RH, Emerson SU. Hepatitis E. In: Mandel GL, Bennett JE, Dolin R, eds. *Principles and Practice of Infectious Diseases.* 6th ed. Philadelphia, PA: Elsevier; 2005:2204–2217. Copyright © 2005 Elsevier. With permission.)

lesions, including subcapsular hemorrhages and lymphocytic periphlebitis and phlebitis, respectively.[16] Rabbits experimentally infected with genotype 1 and genotype 4 HEV developed elevated serum levels of ALT and microscopic lesions characterized by local hepatocellular necrosis.[148] Finally, rats pose

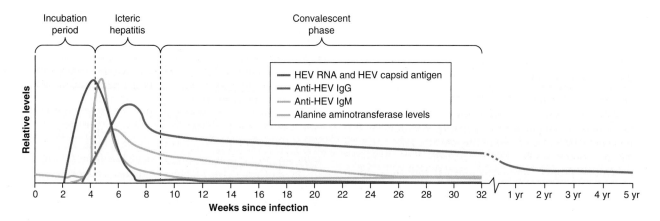

FIGURE 14.9 Clinical course of HEV disease. Appearance and relative levels of hepatitis E virus (HEV) RNA, capsid proteins, and antibodies during HEV infection. IgG, immunoglobulin G; IgM, immunoglobulin M. (Reprinted by permission from Nature: Kamar N, Izopet J, Pavio N, et al. Hepatitis E virus infection. *Nat Rev Dis Primers* 2017;3:17086. Copyright © 2017 Springer Nature.)

an interesting case. On one hand, rats infected with rat HEV developed large amounts of viral RNA copies in liver tissue but did not develop noticeable liver damage.[45] However, Wistar rats inoculated with human stool suspensions from genotype 1 HEV became infected and showed histopathological changes in the liver, spleen, and lymph nodes[153]; however, inoculation of swine genotypes 1 to 3 and boar genotype 4 HEV did not infect Wistar or Sprague Dawley rats[143,191] (reviewed in Ref.[112]). Further discovery and characterization of HEV in animals will be instrumental in increasing our understanding of HEV histopathology.

Extrahepatic Manifestations

The liver is the primary site of HEV replication and the organ predominantly affected, but there is evidence of extrahepatic virus and symptoms. HEV RNA has been detected in numerous swine tissues, such as stomach, heart, lung, salivary gland, pancreas, colon, small intestine, tonsil, lymph node, muscle, spleen, and kidney tissues.[31,241] However, it is unclear whether some of these extrahepatic manifestations could be due to contamination during postmortem sampling or active HEV replication. Negative-strand HEV RNA, indicative of replicating HEV, was detected primarily in the small intestine, lymph nodes, colon, and liver, demonstrating active infection of those tissues.[241] In pregnant women, HEV has been detected in the placenta,[17] and these clinical observations have been corroborated by *ex vivo* infections of decidua basalis and placenta.[62] HEV has also been shown to replicate in cultured neurons, and HEV RNA and protein have been found in the brain tissues of infected monkeys as well as in the cerebrospinal fluid of HEV-infected patients.[264] Notably, HEV infection has been correlated with neurological disorders, such as Bell palsy, polyradiculopathy, neuralgic amyotrophy, and Guillain-Barré syndrome[35,96,232] (reviewed in Ref.[137]). HEV can also affect the kidneys, leading to impaired renal function, glomerular disease, membranoproliferative glomerulonephritis, membranous glomerulonephritis, cryoglobulinemia, and may also increase risk of an IgA nephropathy flare-up in patients with this condition (reviewed in Ref.[223]). Several other extrahepatic conditions have been attributed to HEV infection including pancreatitis, thrombocytopenia, and cutaneous CD30+ T-cell lymphoproliferative disorder[152] (reviewed in Ref.[15]). Although HEV RNA was recently detected in porcine semen, there is currently no evidence that HEV is sexually transmittable among humans.[42,73,141]

EPIDEMIOLOGY

HEV infects an estimated 20 million individuals annually. Approximately 3.4 million develop clinically symptomatic disease and about 70,000 succumb to the infection, subsequently leading to approximately 3,000 stillbirths.[197,240] Although fatality among healthy, immunocompetent individuals does not surpass 2%, HEV-infected pregnant women and their babies—both *in utero* and shortly after birth—are disproportionately at risk of death, with maternal fatality rates as high as 30%[197] (reviewed in Ref.[129,132]). Furthermore, immunocompromised individuals—such as organ transplant recipients and

individuals with concurrent, untreated HIV infection—are at a higher risk for developing chronic hepatitis E (reviewed in Refs.[34,40,237]).

Since HEV is transmissible via the fecal–oral route,[12] excrement-contaminated water sources account for many of the infections in developing countries. This is evidenced by the frequency of HEV outbreaks following floods (when sewage water mixes with drinking water) as well as water shortages (when the concentration of preexisting excrement increases in sources of drinking water) (reviewed in Refs.[1,121]). HEV is also a public health concern in industrialized countries, where transmission primarily occurs zoonotically, through the consumption of undercooked pork products,[33,139] or nosocomially, from contaminated blood and organ donations (reviewed in Ref.[160]). Together, the multiple routes of transmission and nearly global endemicity make HEV a worldwide health concern (Fig. 14.11).

In the United States, some studies estimate human HEV seroprevalence to be 6% (such as Ref.[49]), while others estimate it to have risen to 8.1% for U.S.-born individuals, and in subsets of the population such as non-Hispanic Asian males, as high as 16.8% since 2016[24]; though only 0.002% of plasma donations screen positive for HEV RNA.[201] In Europe, HEV seroprevalence is generally higher and can differ considerably across countries and regions, with the most alarming seroprevalence reaching 71.3% in a French subpopulation (reviewed in Ref.[32]). In response, many European countries are debating or have begun screening blood donations for HEV RNA (reviewed in Ref.[51]). It is important to note that HEV is not routinely considered when patients present with hepatitis, and the assays used in seroprevalence studies are of varying sensitivity and accuracy.[11,163,236] Consequently, HEV infection is likely more common than portrayed by the literature, and seroprevalence statistics must be interpreted with caution, especially when comparing data derived from different assays.

PREGNANCY

For reasons that remain largely opaque, HEV rarely results in fulminant hepatitis in nonpregnant patients,[133] though pregnant women infected with HEV are especially at risk of severe outcomes, including miscarriage, stillbirth, fulminant hepatic failure in the mother, vertical transmission to the fetus, and maternal death[18,85,119,120,122] (reviewed in Ref.[184]). The risk of mortality from HEV infection increases with every trimester, reaching as high as 30% and is a phenomenon not seen with other hepatitis viruses (reviewed in Refs.[132,159,245]) (Fig. 14.12). Pregnant women typically succumb to HEV infection via eclampsia and/or hemorrhage, and stillbirths and newborn morbidity and mortality after birth are also common due to vertical transmission of HEV and/or the death of the mother.[120] Up to 56% of fetuses and newborns who acquire HEV from the mother do not survive the infection (reviewed in Ref.[129]); liveborn neonates often suffer from the same clinical manifestations of HEV as adults, although they typically clear the infection (Fig. 14.11). The mechanisms behind the increased severity of HEV during pregnancy

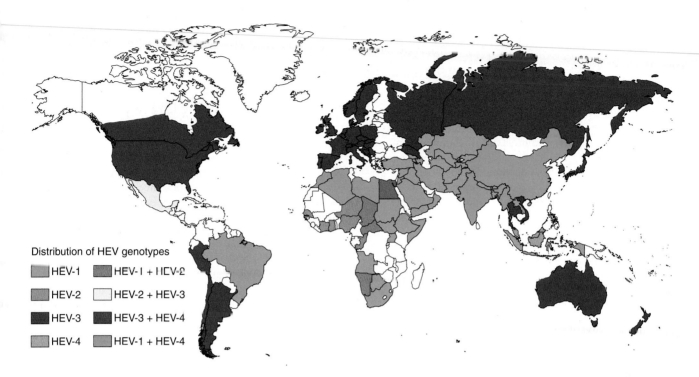

FIGURE 14.11 Global distribution of HEV by human-tropic genotypes. The different colors on the map indicate the distribution of HEV genotypes (HEV-1 through HEV-4) across the globe (HEV-7 was confirmed in a human patient in the United Arab Emirates, not colored on this map). The figure was created with SimpleMappr, an online tool to produce publication-quality point maps (Reprinted from Pallerla SR, Harms D, Johne R, et al. Hepatitis E virus infection: circulation, molecular epidemiology, and impact on global health. *Pathogens* 2020;9(10):856. https://creativecommons.org/licenses/by/4.0/.)

remain unknown, but high viral load, dysregulation of the progesterone signaling pathway, changing hormone levels, and altered immunity, may attribute to this enhanced mortality[18,85,103] (reviewed in Ref.[745]).

Experimental infection in animal models would ideally help elucidate the mechanisms behind the increased severity of HEV during pregnancy, though there has been mixed success in this endeavor. For instance, infection of pregnant rhesus macaques during any trimester did not exhibit a difference between pregnant- or non–pregnant-infected animals when comparing serological, biochemical, or histopathological profiles. Furthermore, no vertical transmission to offspring or increased mortality in pregnant macaques was observed.[229] Similarly, pregnant pigs infected with swine genotype 3 hepatitis did not show an effect on fetal size, piglet viability, birth weight, weight gain, or result in vertical transmission of infection, despite the pregnant pigs showing active infection.[100] Alternatively, pregnant rabbits infected with genotype 3 rabbit HEV showed a wide array of pregnancy-associated disease; two rabbits experienced miscarriage, three died, and positive- and negative-strand HEV RNA was detected in placental tissues in infected rabbits. Furthermore, vertical transmission to offspring was detected via RNA present in the feces and seroconversion with HEV IgG antibodies,[246] though these studies require further study and replication.

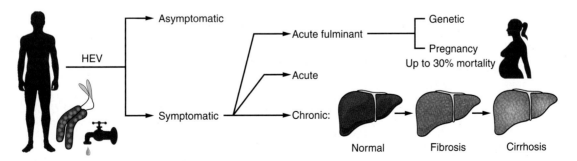

FIGURE 14.12 Pathogenesis and disease progression of HEV. The primary routes of transmission of HEV are through contaminated water sources or the consumption of undercooked pork. Asymptomatic infection is the result for the majority of cases; however, chronic infections and cirrhosis in immunocompromised individuals such as solid-organ transplant recipients can occur. Further, acute fulminate liver failure leading to death in pregnant women can be as high as 30%. (From Nimgaonkar I, Ploss A. A porcine model for chronic hepatitis E. *Hepatology.* 2018;67(2):787–790. Copyright © 2017 by the American Association for the Study of Liver Diseases. Reprinted by permission of John Wiley & Sons, Inc.)

DIAGNOSIS

The European Association for the Study of the Liver suggests testing for HEV in patients with hepatitis (irrespective of travel history), presenting with suspected drug-induced liver injury, with abnormal liver function tests after receiving blood products, or exhibiting unexplained flares of chronic liver disease.[56] HEV testing is further warranted in all immunosuppressed patients with unexplained abnormal liver function tests and in travelers returning from areas endemic for HEV who are presenting with hepatitis. Testing is also recommended in patients presenting with neuralgic amyotrophy and Guillain-Barré syndrome regardless of whether they have elevated liver enzyme levels and also for patients with encephalitis/myelitis.

To accurately diagnose acute or chronic HEV, a combination of molecular approaches and serological tests are employed. Specific tests for IgM and IgG HEV antibodies have been developed and are commercially available in Europe, Asia, and several other geographic regions, though an FDA-approved diagnostic test is currently unavailable in the United States, likely leading to HEV being underdiagnosed. Serological tests can detect anti-HEV IgM in up to 90% of acute infections if serum is collected between 1 and 4 weeks following the onset of disease.[23,57,61,164] However, anti-HEV IgM is a less reliable marker for chronically infected individuals as it is no longer detectable in greater than 50% of patients 3 months after disease onset.[9,12] Anti-HEV IgG increases 2 to 4 weeks following the onset of hepatitis and can also be used as a serological

biomarker.[9,23,43] RT-PCR is arguably the most sensitive method for detecting HEV RNA in the blood and feces of patients with acute or chronic hepatitis E.

PREVENTION AND CONTROL

Treatment

Currently, there is no specific treatment for acute hepatitis E. Since the majority of cases are self-limiting, patients are usually given supportive care.[29] If viral clearance is not achieved, clinical guidelines for treating chronic infections stipulate lowering the dose of immunosuppressive drugs and, subsequently, giving up to two courses of ribavirin (RBV). If both treatment courses with RBV fail, pegylated interferon (IFN) α has been reported to be effective in some patients, particularly organ-transplant recipients, as well as in an immunocompromised patient with no history of immune suppressive therapy or HIV[56,69,95,99] (Fig. 14.13). Although RBV is the treatment of choice, it only clears HEV in 80% of treated patients[97] and is not recommended for pregnant women due to its teratogenic potential. Furthermore, HEV strains isolated from patients nonresponsive to RBV treatment were found to have mutations in the polymerase region of the viral genome (Y1320H, G1634R, and K1383N), with the former two mutations increasing replication efficiency and decreasing susceptibility to RBV.[44,46]

Given these shortcomings, there is an urgent need for new therapeutic approaches (reviewed in Ref.[123]). Several compounds

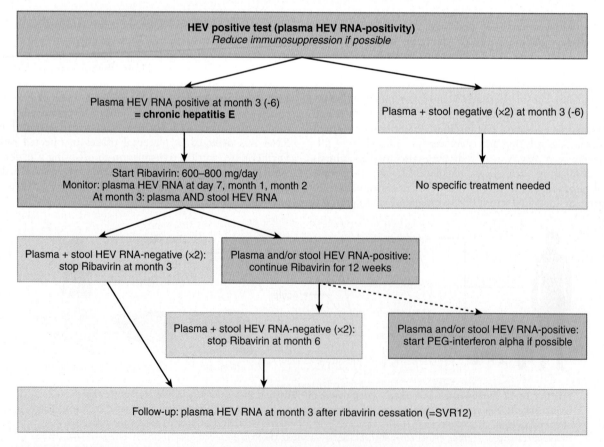

FIGURE 14.13 Treatment algorithm for chronic hepatitis E. (Adapted with permission from Colson P, Decoster C. Recent data on hepatitis E. *Curr Opin Infect Dis* 2019;32(5):475–481.)

have shown anti-HEV activity *in vitro* (Fig. 14.14), including 2′-C-methylcytidine (2-CMC, also known as NM107),[194] 66E2,[149] GPC-N114, and NITD008[170] (Fig. 14.14), all presumably via inhibition of the RdRP. Ciprofloxacin and IFN-λ1-3, identified in a screen of FDA-approved compounds, inhibited replication of an HEV reporter genome,[175] but none of these molecules progressed into clinical development. Combination therapy of pegylated IFN-α and sofosbuvir, a potent, clinically approved inhibitor of the HCV RdRP, has also been used to treat chronic hepatitis E, but it is still under debate whether the addition of sofosbuvir has any therapeutic effect.[4,41,95,98,155,234] Silvestrol was shown to block translation of the HEV capsid protein and decrease RNA loads in the feces of infected humanized mice and in cell cultures. However, silvestrol is not a direct-acting antiviral (DAA) compound and inhibits translation of essential host proteins, diminishing its attractiveness as a potential therapeutic option.[60,227] Recently, a screen of over 60,000 compounds identified isocotoin as an inhibitor of HEV replication through inhibition of HSP90.[174] A few other modalities, such as zinc salts[109] and ethanol extracts from the plants *Lysimachia mauritiana*[86] and *Liriope platyphylla*,[178] appear to also suppress HEV replication, but more stringent testing (including, but not limited to, pharmacokinetics, toxicity, and efficacy in animal models) is necessary to evaluate their true therapeutic

potential. Discovering HEV-specific DAAs[4] and/or an antiviral targeting a host factor is a major goal and would be considerably accelerated by a better understanding of the functional domains within ORF1 and the host factors essential for HEV replication.

Vaccination and Prevention

An HEV vaccine (Hecolin, Xiamen Innovax Biotech) composed of adjuvanted recombinant HEV capsid successfully prevented infection against genotype 4 HEV in 100% of patients who received three doses[265] (Table 14.1). While this vaccine is currently only licensed in China and is therefore unavailable to the vast majority of at-risk individuals,[240] a phase IV clinical trial is currently underway in rural Bangladesh in women of childbearing age,[257] expanding our efforts to safely protect severely at-risk populations. A second vaccine also based on a recombinant HEV capsid protein was shown to be safe and effective in a phase II clinical trial but was not further developed.[206,228]

Proper sewage disposal so that water supplies are not contaminated with fecal material is critical in areas where HEV is endemic. Hepatitis E has been reported to be effectively prevented by chlorination of drinking water, which can inactivate HEV virions,[58] although some studies suggest chlorination

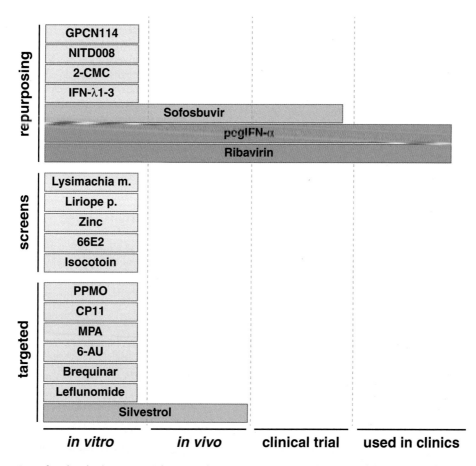

FIGURE 14.14 Overview of molecules/extracts with antiviral activity against HEV. Overview of drugs, molecules, and extracts with demonstrated antiviral activity against HEV. The depicted molecules are classified according to the strategy used to identify them. So far only Sofosbuvir, pegylated IFN-α, ribavirin, and silvestrol have been used in experimental settings outside of *in vitro* cell systems. (Adapted from Kinast V, Burkard TL, Todt D, et al. Hepatitis E virus drug development. *Viruses* 2019;11(6):485. https://creativecommons.org/licenses/by/4.0/.)

TABLE 14.1 Vaccines against HEV

Vaccine Manufacturer	Antigen (Genotype 1)	Expression System	Dose	HEV Genotype in Vaccinated Population	Efficacy (95% CI)
GlaxoSmithKline (Belgium)	Recombinant capsid protein (AAs 112–607)	Baculovirus in insect cells	20 µg with alum	1	95.5% (89–99)
Xiamen Innovax Biotech (China)	Recombinant capsid protein (AAs 368–606)	*Escherichia coli*	30 µg with alum	4	100% (72–100)

may be inadequate for heavily contaminated water supplies.[135] However, this approach has practical limitations due to financial constraints and inadequate infrastructure in the developing countries that would most benefit from such interventions. For stopping zoonotic transmission of HEV, the arguably most effective approach is proper food preparation. Prior to consumption, meat products from HEV reservoir species (e.g., swine) should be cooked at no less than 70°C for at least 5 minutes to fully inactivate the virus.[13,82,89]

PERSPECTIVE

Hepatitis E remains a major global medical problem. The disease burden is likely considerably larger than current estimates since idiopathic hepatitis is often not correctly attributed to HEV. HEV transmission remains high not only between individuals via the fecal–oral route in undeveloped countries and during water contamination events but also due to the vast zoonotic reservoirs of this virus. HEV causes a broad range of clinically apparent symptoms, and disease outcome varies considerably across the patient population, making correct diagnosis, timely intervention, and accurate reporting difficult. It is particularly pressing to determine the cause of the uniquely high mortality rate in pregnant women. Although an effective vaccine has been developed, it is not widely available, limiting its impact on containing global spread. Undoubtedly, efforts need to be taken to seek broad regulatory approval of the HEV vaccine, especially considering the disastrous impact of HEV on fetal and maternal health in developing countries. Furthermore, treatment options remain inadequate, and RBV is contraindicated in one of the most affected patient populations: pregnant women. Recent work has highlighted some new avenues for suppressing HEV in cell culture, but there is a still a long way to go toward achieving the critical goal of effective DAAs or host-targeting antivirals.

Since the virus was first identified in 1983, our understanding of the molecular virology and interactions between HEV and its mammalian hosts have improved considerably. However, the precise functions for many of the different domains within ORF1 remain unclear. Likewise, a more complete set of host factors essential for the HEV life cycle have yet to be identified.

To address these and other questions, experimental tools need to be further refined. Cell systems are now available for some HEV genotypes but are lacking for others. The scarcity of small animal models that closely mimic human disease poses challenges for mechanistically dissecting the complex interplay of this virus with its host at the organismal level. Fortunately, the global scientific community has significantly increased HEV research in the past two decades, leading to the many exciting discoveries listed above, with many more undoubtedly on the way. The days of HEV as an understudied and enigmatic pathogen are numbered.

ACKNOWLEDGMENTS

We thank our colleagues and members of the Ploss Lab, especially Jenna Gaska, Ila Nimgaonkar, and Nicholas Archer, for fruitful discussions. Research in Ploss laboratory is funded in part by grants from the National Institutes of Health (R01 AI138797, R01AI107301, R01AI146917, R01AI153236), a Research Scholar Award from the American Cancer Society (RSG-15-048-01-MPC to A.P.), a Burroughs Wellcome Fund Award for Investigators in Pathogenesis (101539), and funds from the U.S. Department of Defense (W81XWH1810237) and Princeton University. R.L. is supported by NIGMS of the National Institutes of Health under grant number T32GM007388 and is also a recipient of a predoctoral fellowship from the National Science Foundation. We apologize to all colleagues whose work could not be cited due to space constraints.

REFERENCES

1. Aggarwal R. *The Global Prevalence of Hepatitis E Virus Infection and Susceptibility: A Systematic Review Immunization, Vaccines and Biologicals—World Health Organization.* 2010. www.who.int/vaccines-documents/
2. Agrawal S, Gupta D, Panda SK. The 3' end of hepatitis E virus (HEV) genome binds specifically to the viral RNA-dependent RNA polymerase (RdRp). *Virology* 2001;282:87–101.
3. Ahola T, Karlin DG. Sequence analysis reveals a conserved extension in the capping enzyme of the alphavirus supergroup, and a homologous domain in nodaviruses. *Biol Direct* 2015;10:16.
4. Alric L, Bonnet D, Laurent G, et al. Chronic hepatitis E virus infection: successful virologic response to pegylated interferon-alpha therapy. *Ann Intern Med* 2010;153:135–136.
5. Ame JC, Spenlehauer C, de Murcia G. The PARP superfamily. *Bioessays* 2004;26:882–893.
6. Anang S, Subramani C, Nair VP, et al. Identification of critical residues in Hepatitis E virus macro domain involved in its interaction with viral methyltransferase and ORF3 proteins. *Sci Rep* 2016;6:25133.
7. Ankavay M, Montpellier C, Sayed IM, et al. New insights into the ORF2 capsid protein, a key player of the hepatitis E virus lifecycle. *Sci Rep* 2019;9:6243.
8. Ansari IH, Nanda SK, Durgapal H, et al. Cloning, sequencing, and expression of the hepatitis E virus (HEV) nonstructural open reading frame 1 (ORF1). *J Med Virol* 2000;60:275–283.
9. Arankalle VA, Chadha MS, Tsarev SA, et al. Seroepidemiology of water-borne hepatitis in India and evidence for a third enterically-transmitted hepatitis agent. *Proc Natl Acad Sci U S A* 1994;91:3428–3432.
10. Arankalle VA, Chobe LP, Jha J, et al. Aetiology of acute sporadic non-A, non-B viral hepatitis in India. *J Med Virol* 1993;40:121–125.
11. Avellon A, Morago L, Garcia-Galera del Carmen M, et al. Comparative sensitivity of commercial tests for hepatitis E genotype 3 virus antibody detection. *J Med Virol* 2015;87:1934–1939.
12. Balayan MS, Andjaparidze AG, Savinskaya SS, et al. Evidence for a virus in non-A, non-B hepatitis transmitted via the fecal-oral route. *Intervirology* 1983;20:23–31.
13. Barnaud E, Rogee S, Garry P, et al. Thermal inactivation of infectious hepatitis E virus in experimentally contaminated food. *Appl Environ Microbiol* 2012;78:5153–5159.

14. Batts W, Yun S, Hedrick R, et al. A novel member of the family Hepeviridae from cutthroat trout (Oncorhynchus clarkii). *Virus Res* 2011;158:116–123.

15. Bazerbachi F, Haffar S, Garg SK, et al. Extra-hepatic manifestations associated with hepatitis E virus infection: a comprehensive review of the literature. *Gastroenterol Rep (Oxf)* 2016;4:1–15.

16. Billam P, Huang FF, Sun ZF, et al. Systematic pathogenesis and replication of avian hepatitis E virus in specific-pathogen-free adult chickens. *J Virol* 2005;79:3429–3437.

17. Bose PD, Das BC, Hazam RK, et al. Evidence of extrahepatic replication of hepatitis E virus in human placenta. *J Gen Virol* 2014;95:1266–1271.

18. Bose PD, Das BC, Kumar A, et al. High viral load and deregulation of the progesterone receptor signaling pathway: association with hepatitis E-related poor pregnancy outcome. *J Hepatol* 2011;54:1107–1113.

19. Bouquet J, Tesse S, Lunazzi A, et al. Close similarity between sequences of hepatitis E virus recovered from humans and swine, France, 2008–2009. *Emerg Infect Dis* 2011;17: 2018–2025.

20. Bouwknegt M, Rutjes SA, Reusken CB, et al. The course of hepatitis E virus infection in pigs after contact-infection and intravenous inoculation. *BMC Vet Res* 2009;5:7.

21. Bradley D, Andjaparidze A, Cook EH Jr, et al. Aetiological agent of enterically transmitted non-A, non-B hepatitis. *J Gen Virol* 1988;69(Pt 3):731–738.

22. Bradley DW, Krawczynski K, Cook EH Jr, et al. Enterically transmitted non-A, non-B hepatitis: serial passage of disease in cynomolgus macaques and tamarins and recovery of disease-associated 27- to 34-nm viruslike particles. *Proc Natl Acad Sci U S A* 1987;84:6277–6281.

23. Bryan JP, Tsarev SA, Iqbal M, et al. Epidemic hepatitis E in Pakistan: patterns of serologic response and evidence that antibody to hepatitis E virus protects against disease. *J Infect Dis* 1994;170:517–521.

24. Cangin C, Focht B, Harris R, et al. Hepatitis E seroprevalence in the United States: Results for immunoglobulins IGG and IGM. *J Med Virol* 2019;91:124–131.

25. Cao D, Huang YW, Meng XJ. The nucleotides on the stem loop RNA structure in the junction region of the hepatitis E virus genome are critical for virus replication. *J Virol* 2010;84:13040–13044.

26. Cao D, Ni YY, Meng XJ. Substitution of amino acid residue V1213 in the helicase domain of the genotype 3 hepatitis E virus reduces virus replication. *Virol J* 2018;15:32.

27. Cao D, Ni YY, Walker M, et al. Roles of the genomic sequence surrounding the stem-loop structure in the junction region including the 3′ terminus of open reading frame 1 in hepatitis E virus replication. *J Med Virol* 2018;90:1524–1531.

28. Capelli N, Marion O, Dubois M, et al. Vectorial release of hepatitis E virus in polarized human hepatocytes. *J Virol* 2019;93(4):e01207-18.

29. Centers for Disease Control and Prevention. Hepatitis E Questions and Answers for Health Professionals. 2018. https://www.cdc.gov/hepatitis/hev/hevfaq.htm#section1. Accessed

30. Chauhan A, Jameel S, Dilawari JB, et al. Hepatitis E virus transmission to a volunteer. *Lancet* 1993;341:149–150.

31. Choi C, Chae C. Localization of swine hepatitis E virus in liver and extrahepatic tissues from naturally infected pigs by in situ hybridization. *J Hepatol* 2003;38:827–832.

32. Clemente-Casares P, Ramos-Romero C, Ramirez-Gonzalez E, et al. Hepatitis E virus in industrialized countries: the silent threat. *Biomed Res Int* 2016;2016:9838041.

33. Colson P, Borentain P, Queyriaux B, et al. Pig liver sausage as a source of hepatitis E virus transmission to humans. *J Infect Dis* 2010;202:825–834.

34. Colson P, Dhiver C, Poizot-Martin I, et al. Acute and chronic hepatitis E in patients infected with human immunodeficiency virus. *J Viral Hepat* 2011;18:227–228.

35. Comont T, Bonnet D, Sigur N, et al. [Acute hepatitis E infection associated with Guillain-Barre syndrome in an immunocompetent patient]. *Rev Med Interne* 2014;35:333–336.

36. Corda D, Di Girolamo M. Functional aspects of protein mono-ADP-ribosylation. *EMBO J* 2003;22:1953–1958.

37. Cossaboom CM, Cordoba L, Dryman BA, et al. Hepatitis E virus in rabbits, Virginia, USA. *Emerg Infect Dis* 2011;17:2047–2049.

38. Coyne CB, Bergelson JM. Virus-induced Abl and Fyn kinase signals permit coxsackievirus entry through epithelial tight junctions. *Cell* 2006;124:119–131.

39. Cullen JM, Lemon SM. Comparative pathology of hepatitis A virus and hepatitis E virus infection. *Cold Spring Harb Perspect Med* 2019;9(4):a033456.

40. Dalton HR, Bendall RP, Keane FE, et al. Persistent carriage of hepatitis E virus in patients with HIV infection. *N Engl J Med* 2009;361:1025–1027.

41. Dao Thi VL, Debing Y, Wu X, et al. Sofosbuvir inhibits hepatitis E virus replication in vitro and results in an additive effect when combined with ribavirin. *Gastroenterology* 2016;150:82–85 e4.

42. Dauby N, Suin V, Jacques M, et al. Hepatitis E virus (HEV): seroprevalence and HEV RNA detection in subjects attending a sexually transmitted infection clinic in Brussels, Belgium. *Epidemiol Infect* 2017;145:3370–3374.

43. Dawson GJ, Chau KH, Cabal CM, et al. Solid-phase enzyme-linked immunosorbent assay for hepatitis E virus IgG and IgM antibodies utilizing recombinant antigens and synthetic peptides. *J Virol Methods* 1992;38:175–186.

44. Debing Y, Gisa A, Dallmeier K, et al. A mutation in the hepatitis E virus RNA polymerase promotes its replication and associates with ribavirin treatment failure in organ transplant recipients. *Gastroenterology* 2014;147:1008–1011.e7; quiz e15–e6.

45. Debing Y, Mishra N, Verbeken E, et al. A rat model for hepatitis E virus. *Dis Model Mech* 2016;9:1203–1210.

46. Debing Y, Ramiere C, Dallmeier K, et al. Hepatitis E virus mutations associated with ribavirin treatment failure result in altered viral fitness and ribavirin sensitivity. *J Hepatol* 2016;65:499–508.

47. Ding Q, Heller B, Capuccino JM, et al. Hepatitis E virus ORF3 is a functional ion channel required for release of infectious particles. *Proc Natl Acad Sci U S A* 2017;114:1147–1152.

48. Ding Q, Nimgaonkar I, Archer NF, et al. Identification of the intragenomic promoter controlling hepatitis E virus subgenomic RNA transcription. *mBio* 2018;9(3): e00769-18.

49. Ditah I, Ditah F, Devaki P, et al. Current epidemiology of hepatitis E virus infection in the United States: low seroprevalence in the National Health and Nutrition Evaluation Survey. *Hepatology* 2014;60:815–822.

50. Doceul V, Bagdassarian E, Demange A, et al. Zoonotic hepatitis E virus: classification, animal reservoirs and transmission routes. *Viruses* 2016;8:270.

51. Domanovic D, Tedder R, Blumel J, et al. Hepatitis E and blood donation safety in selected European countries: a shift to screening? *Euro Surveill* 2017;22(16).30514.

52. Drave SA, Debing Y, Walter S, et al. Extra-hepatic replication and infection of hepatitis E virus in neuronal-derived cells. *J Viral Hepat* 2016;23:512–521.

53. Emerson SU, Nguyen HT, Torian U, et al. Release of genotype 1 hepatitis E virus from cultured hepatoma and polarized intestinal cells depends on open reading frame 3 protein and requires an intact PXXP motif. *J Virol* 2010;84:9059–9069.

54. Emerson SU, Nguyen H, Torian U, et al. ORF3 protein of hepatitis E virus is not required for replication, virion assembly, or infection of hepatoma cells in vitro. *J Virol* 2006;80:10457–10464.

55. Emerson SU, Zhang M, Meng XJ, et al. Recombinant hepatitis E virus genomes infectious for primates: importance of capping and discovery of a cis-reactive element. *Proc Natl Acad Sci U S A* 2001;98:15270–15275.

56. European Association for the Study of the Liver; Electronic address: easloffice@easloffice. eu; European Association for the Study of the Liver. EASL Clinical Practice Guidelines on hepatitis E virus infection. *J Hepatol* 2018;68:1256–1271.

57. Favorov MO, Fields HA, Purdy MA, et al. Serologic identification of hepatitis E virus infections in epidemic and endemic settings. *J Med Virol* 1992;36:246–250.

58. Girones R, Carratala A, Calgua B, et al. Chlorine inactivation of hepatitis E virus and human adenovirus 2 in water. *J Water Health* 2014;12:436–442.

59. Gissen P, Arias IM. Structural and functional hepatocyte polarity and liver disease. *J Hepatol* 2015;63:1023–1037.

60. Glitscher M, Himmelsbach K, Woytinek K, et al. Inhibition of hepatitis E virus spread by the natural compound silvestrol. *Viruses* 2018;10(6):301.

61. Goldsmith R, Yarbough PO, Reyes GR, et al. Enzyme-linked immunosorbent assay for diagnosis of acute sporadic hepatitis E in Egyptian children. *Lancet* 1992;339:328–331.

62. Gouilly J, Chen Q, Siewiera J, et al. Genotype specific pathogenicity of hepatitis E virus at the human maternal-fetal interface. *Nat Commun* 2018;9:4748.

63. Gouttenoire J, Pollan A, Abrami L, et al. Palmitoylation mediates membrane association of hepatitis E virus ORF3 protein and is required for infectious particle secretion. *PLoS Pathog* 2018;14:e1007471.

64. Graff J, Nguyen H, Kasorndorkbua C, et al. In vitro and in vivo mutational analysis of the 3′-terminal regions of hepatitis e virus genomes and replicons. *J Virol* 2005;79:1017–1026.

65. Graff J, Nguyen H, Yu C, et al. The open reading frame 3 gene of hepatitis E virus contains a cis-reactive element and encodes a protein required for infection of macaques. *J Virol* 2005;79:6680–6689.

66. Graff J, Torian U, Nguyen H, et al. A bicistronic subgenomic mRNA encodes both the ORF2 and ORF3 proteins of hepatitis E virus. *J Virol* 2006;80:5919–5926.

67. Grakoui A, Levis R, Raju R, et al. A cis-acting mutation in the Sindbis virus junction region which affects subgenomic RNA synthesis. *J Virol* 1989;63:5216–5227.

68. Guu TS, Liu Z, Ye Q, et al. Structure of the hepatitis E virus-like particle suggests mechanisms for virus assembly and receptor binding. *Proc Natl Acad Sci U S A* 2009;106:12992–12997.

69. Haagsma EB, Riezebos-Brilman A, van den Berg AP, et al. Treatment of chronic hepatitis E in liver transplant recipients with pegylated interferon alpha-2b. *Liver Transpl* 2010;16:474–477.

70. Haldipur B, Bhukya PL, Arankalle V, et al. Positive regulation of hepatitis E virus replication by MicroRNA-122. *J Virol* 2018;92(11):e01999-17.

71. Han SH, Park BJ, Ahn HS, et al. Cross-species transmission of swine hepatitis E virus genotype 3 to rabbits. *Viruses* 2020;12(1):53.

72. Haqshenas G, Shivaprasad HL, Woolcock PR, et al. Genetic identification and characterization of a novel virus related to human hepatitis E virus from chickens with hepatitis-splenomegaly syndrome in the United States. *J Gen Virol* 2001;82:2449–2462.

73. Heil J, Hoebe C, Loo I, et al. Hepatitis E prevalence in a sexual high-risk population compared to the general population. *PLoS One* 2018;13:e0191798.

74. Hingane S, Joshi N, Surjit M, et al. Hepatitis E virus ORF2 inhibits RIG-I mediated interferon response. *Front Microbiol* 2020;11:656.

75. Hobson SD, Rosenblum ES, Richards OC, et al. Oligomeric structures of poliovirus polymerase are important for function. *EMBO J* 2001;20:1153–1163.

76. Holla P, Ahmad I, Ahmed Z, et al. Hepatitis E virus enters liver cells through a dynamin-2, clathrin and membrane cholesterol-dependent pathway. *Traffic* 2015;16:398–416.

77. Hoofnagle JH, Nelson KE, Purcell RH. Hepatitis E. *N Engl J Med* 2012;367:1237–1244.

78. Huang F, Li Y, Yu W, et al. Excretion of infectious hepatitis E virus into milk in cows imposes high risks of zoonosis. *Hepatology* 2016;64:350–359.

79. Huang YW, Opriessnig T, Halbur PG, et al. Initiation at the third in-frame AUG codon of open reading frame 3 of the hepatitis E virus is essential for viral infectivity in vivo. *J Virol* 2007;81:3018–3026.

80. Huang FF, Sun ZF, Emerson SU, et al. Determination and analysis of the complete genomic sequence of avian hepatitis E virus (avian HEV) and attempts to infect rhesus monkeys with avian HEV. *J Gen Virol* 2004;85:1609–1618.

81. Ichiyama K, Yamada K, Tanaka T, et al. Determination of the 5′-terminal sequence of subgenomic RNA of hepatitis E virus strains in cultured cells. *Arch Virol* 2009;154: 1945–1951.

82. Imagawa T, Sugiyama R, Shiota T, et al. Evaluation of heating conditions for inactivation of hepatitis E virus genotypes 3 and 4. *J Food Prot* 2018;81:947–952.

83. Jemielity S, Wang JJ, Chan YK, et al. TIM-family proteins promote infection of multiple enveloped viruses through virion-associated phosphatidylserine. *PLoS Pathog* 2013;9:e1003232.

84. Jia H, Gong P. A structure-function diversity survey of the RNA-dependent RNA polymerases from the positive-strand RNA viruses. *Front Microbiol* 2019;10:1945.

85. Jilani N, Das BC, Husain SA, et al. Hepatitis E virus infection and fulminant hepatic failure during pregnancy. *J Gastroenterol Hepatol* 2007;22:676–682.

86. Jin SE, Kim JE, Kim SY, et al. An ethanol extract of Lysimachia mauritiana exhibits inhibitory activity against hepatitis E virus genotype 3 replication. *J Microbiol* 2017;55:984–988.

87. Johne R, Plenge-Bonig A, Hess M, et al. Detection of a novel hepatitis E-like virus in faeces of wild rats using a nested broad-spectrum RT-PCR. *J Gen Virol* 2010;91:750–758.

88. Johne R, Reetz J, Ulrich RG, et al. An ORF1-rearranged hepatitis E virus derived from a chronically infected patient efficiently replicates in cell culture. *J Viral Hepat* 2014;21:447–456.

89. Johne R, Trojnar E, Filter M, et al. Thermal stability of hepatitis E virus as estimated by a cell culture method. *Appl Environ Microbiol* 2016;82:4225–4231.

90. Jopling CL, Yi M, Lancaster AM, et al. Modulation of hepatitis C virus RNA abundance by a liver-specific MicroRNA. *Science* 2005;309:1577–1581.

91. Ju X, Xiang G, Gong M, et al. Identification of functional cis-acting RNA elements in the hepatitis E virus genome required for viral replication. *PLoS Pathog* 2020;16:e1008488.

92. Kabrane-Lazizi Y, Meng XJ, Purcell RH, et al. Evidence that the genomic RNA of hepatitis E virus is capped. *J Virol* 1999;73:8848–8850.

93. Kadare G, Haenni AL. Virus-encoded RNA helicases. *J Virol* 1997;71:2583–2590.

94. Kalia M, Chandra V, Rahman SA, et al. Heparan sulfate proteoglycans are required for cellular binding of the hepatitis E virus ORF2 capsid protein and for viral infection. *J Virol* 2009;83:12714–12724.

95. Kamar N, Abravanel F, Garrouste C, et al. Three-month pegylated interferon-alpha-2a therapy for chronic hepatitis E virus infection in a haemodialysis patient. *Nephrol Dial Transplant* 2010;25:2792–2795.

96. Kamar N, Izopet J, Cintas P, et al. Hepatitis E virus-induced neurological symptoms in a kidney-transplant patient with chronic hepatitis. *Am J Transplant* 2010;10:1321–1324.

97. Kamar N, Izopet J, Tripon S, et al. Ribavirin for chronic hepatitis E virus infection in transplant recipients. *N Engl J Med* 2014;370:1111–1120.

98. Kamar N, Pan Q. No clear evidence for an effect of sofosbuvir against hepatitis E virus in organ transplant patients. *Hepatology* 2019;69:1846–1847.

99. Kamar N, Rostaing L, Abravanel F, et al. Pegylated interferon-alpha for treating chronic hepatitis E virus infection after liver transplantation. *Clin Infect Dis* 2010;50:e30–e33.

100. Kanade GD, Pingale KD, Karpe YA. Activities of thrombin and factor Xa are essential for replication of hepatitis E virus and are possibly implicated in ORF1 polyprotein processing. *J Virol* 2018;92(6):e01853-17.

101. Kannan H, Fan S, Patel D, et al. The hepatitis E virus open reading frame 3 product interacts with microtubules and interferes with their dynamics. *J Virol* 2009;83:6375–6382.

102. Kapur N, Thakral D, Durgapal H, et al. Hepatitis E virus enters liver cells through receptor-dependent clathrin-mediated endocytosis. *J Viral Hepat* 2012;19:436–448.

103. Kar P, Jilani N, Husain SA, et al. Does hepatitis E viral load and genotypes influence the final outcome of acute liver failure during pregnancy? *Am J Gastroenterol* 2008;103:2495–2501.

104. Karpe YA, Lole KS. RNA 5′-triphosphatase activity of the hepatitis E virus helicase domain. *J Virol* 2010;84:9637–9641.

105. Karpe YA, Lole KS. Deubiquitination activity associated with hepatitis E virus putative papain-like cysteine protease. *J Gen Virol* 2011;92:2088–2092.

106. Karras GI, Kustatscher G, Buhecha HR, et al. The macro domain is an ADP-ribose binding module. *EMBO J* 2005;24:1911–1920.

107. Kar-Roy A, Korkaya H, Oberoi R, et al. The hepatitis E virus open reading frame 3 protein activates ERK through binding and inhibition of the MAPK phosphatase. *J Biol Chem* 2004;279:28345–28357.

108. Kasorndorkbua C, Thacker BJ, Halbur PG, et al. Experimental infection of pregnant gilts with swine hepatitis E virus. *Can J Vet Res* 2003;67:303–306.

109. Kaushik N, Subramani C, Anang S, et al. Zinc salts block hepatitis E virus replication by inhibiting the activity of viral RNA-dependent RNA polymerase. *J Virol* 2017;91(21):e00754-17.

110. Kc S, Sharma D, Basnet BK, et al. Effect of acute hepatitis E infection in patients with liver cirrhosis. *JNMA J Nepal Med Assoc* 2009;48:226–229.

111. Kenney SP, Meng XJ. The lysine residues within the human ribosomal protein S17 sequence naturally inserted into the viral nonstructural protein of a unique strain of hepatitis E virus are important for enhanced virus replication. *J Virol* 2015;89:3793–3803.

112. Kenney SP, Meng XJ. Hepatitis E virus: animal models and zoonosis. *Annu Rev Anim Biosci* 2019;7:427–448.

113. Kenney SP, Meng XJ. Hepatitis E virus genome structure and replication strategy. *Cold Spring Harb Perspect Med* 2019;9(1):a031724.

114. Kenney SP, Pudupakam RS, Huang YW, et al. The PSAP motif within the ORF3 protein of an avian strain of the hepatitis E virus is not critical for viral infectivity in vivo but plays a role in virus release. *J Virol* 2012;86:5637–5646.

115. Kenney SP, Wentworth JL, Heffron CL, et al. Replacement of the hepatitis E virus ORF3 protein PxxP motif with heterologous late domain motifs affects virus release via interaction with TSG101. *Virology* 2015;486:198–208.

116. Khuroo MS. Study of an epidemic of non-A, non-B hepatitis. Possibility of another human hepatitis virus distinct from post-transfusion non-A, non-B type. *Am J Med* 1980;68:818–824.

117. Khuroo MS, Duermeyer W, Zargar SA, et al. Acute sporadic non-A, non-B hepatitis in India. *Am J Epidemiol* 1983;118:360–364.

118. Khuroo MS, Kamili S, Dar MY, et al. Hepatitis E and long-term antibody status. *Lancet* 1993;341:1355.

119. Khuroo MS, Kamili S, Jameel S. Vertical transmission of hepatitis E virus. *Lancet* 1995;345:1025–1026.

120. Khuroo MS, Kamili S, Khuroo MS. Clinical course and duration of viremia in vertically transmitted hepatitis E virus (HEV) infection in babies born to HEV-infected mothers. *J Viral Hepat* 2009;16:519–523.

121. Khuroo MS, Khuroo MS, Khuroo NS. Hepatitis E: discovery, global impact, control and cure. *World J Gastroenterol* 2016;22:7030–7045.

122. Khuroo MS, Teli MR, Skidmore S, et al. Incidence and severity of viral hepatitis in pregnancy. *Am J Med* 1981;70:252–255.

123. Kinast V, Burkard TL, Todt D, et al. Hepatitis E virus drug development. *Viruses* 2019;11(6):485.

124. Knegendorf L, Drave SA, Dao Thi VL, et al. Hepatitis E virus replication and interferon responses in human placental cells. *Hepatol Commun* 2018;2:173–187.

125. Koizumi Y, Isoda N, Sato Y, et al. Infection of a Japanese patient by genotype 4 hepatitis e virus while traveling in Vietnam. *J Clin Microbiol* 2004;42:3883–3885.

126. Koonin EV. The phylogeny of RNA-dependent RNA polymerases of positive-strand RNA viruses. *J Gen Virol* 1991;72(Pt 9):2197–2206.

127. Koonin EV, Gorbalenya AE, Purdy MA, et al. Computer-assisted assignment of functional domains in the nonstructural polyprotein of hepatitis E virus: delineation of an additional group of positive-strand RNA plant and animal viruses. *Proc Natl Acad Sci U S A* 1992;89:8259–8263.

128. Korkaya H, Jameel S, Gupta D, et al. The ORF3 protein of hepatitis E virus binds to Src homology 3 domains and activates MAPK. *J Biol Chem* 2001;276:42389–42400.

129. Krain LJ, Atwell JE, Nelson KE, et al. Fetal and neonatal health consequences of vertically transmitted hepatitis E virus infection. *Am J Trop Med Hyg* 2014;90:365–370.

130. Krawczynski K, Bradley DW. Enterically transmitted non-A, non-B hepatitis: identification of virus-associated antigen in experimentally infected cynomolgus macaques. *J Infect Dis* 1989;159:1042–1049.

131. Kumar A, Aggarwal R, Naik SR, et al. Hepatitis E virus is responsible for decompensation of chronic liver disease in an endemic region. *Indian J Gastroenterol* 2004;23:59–62.

132. Kumar S, Subhadra S, Singh B, et al. Hepatitis E virus: the current scenario. *Int J Infect Dis* 2013;17:e228–e233.

133. Kuwada SK, Patel VM, Hollinger FB, et al. Non-A, non-B fulminant hepatitis is also non-E and non-C. *Am J Gastroenterol* 1994;89:57–61.

134. Lee GH, Tan BH, Teo EC, et al. Chronic infection with camelid hepatitis E Virus in a liver transplant recipient who regularly consumes camel meat and milk. *Gastroenterology* 2016;150:355–357 e3.

135. Lenglet A, Ehlkes L, Taylor D, et al. Does community-wide water chlorination reduce hepatitis E virus infections during an outbreak? A geospatial analysis of data from an outbreak in Am Timan, Chad (2016–2017). *J Water Health* 2020;18:556–565.

136. Lhomme S, Abravanel F, Dubois M, et al. Characterization of the polyproline region of the hepatitis E virus in immunocompromised patients. *J Virol* 2014;88:12017–12025.

137. Lhomme S, Marion O, Abravanel F, et al. Clinical manifestations, pathogenesis and treatment of hepatitis E virus infections. *J Clin Med* 2020;9(2):331.

138. Lhomme S, Nicot F, Jeanne N, et al. Insertions and duplications in the polyproline region of the hepatitis E virus. *Front Microbiol* 2020;11:1.

139. Li TC, Chijiwa K, Sera N, et al. Hepatitis E virus transmission from wild boar meat. *Emerg Infect Dis* 2005;11:1958–1960.

140. Li C, Debing Y, Jankevicius G, et al. Viral macro domains reverse protein ADP-ribosylation. *J Virol* 2016;90:8478–8486.

141. Li H, Wu J, Sheng Y, et al. Prevalence of hepatitis E virus (HEV) infection in various pig farms from Shaanxi Province, China: First detection of HEV RNA in pig semen. *Transbound Emerg Dis* 2019;66:72–82.

142. Li TC, Yamakawa Y, Suzuki K, et al. Expression and self-assembly of empty virus-like particles of hepatitis E virus. *J Virol* 1997;71:7207–7213.

143. Li TC, Yoshizaki S, Ami Y, et al. Susceptibility of laboratory rats against genotypes 1, 3, 4, and rat hepatitis E viruses. *Vet Microbiol* 2013;163:54–61.

144. Li SW, Zhang J, He ZQ, et al. Mutational analysis of essential interactions involved in the assembly of hepatitis E virus capsid. *J Biol Chem* 2005;280:3400–3406.

145. Lin S, Yang Y, Nan Y, et al. The capsid protein of hepatitis E virus inhibits interferon induction via its N-terminal arginine-rich motif. *Viruses* 2019;11(11):1050.

146. Liu Z, Behloul N, Baha S, et al. Role of the C-terminal cysteines in virus-like particle formation and oligomerization of the hepatitis E virus ORF2 truncated proteins. *Virology* 2020;544:1–11.

147. Liu P, Bu QN, Wang L, et al. Transmission of hepatitis E virus from rabbits to cynomolgus macaques. *Emerg Infect Dis* 2013;19:559–565.

148. Ma H, Zheng L, Liu Y, et al. Experimental infection of rabbits with rabbit and genotypes 1 and 4 hepatitis E viruses. *PLoS One* 2010;5:e9160.

149. Madhvi A, Hingane S, Srivastav R, et al. A screen for novel hepatitis C virus RdRp inhibitor identifies a broad-spectrum antiviral compound. *Sci Rep* 2017;7:5816.

150. Magden J, Takeda N, Li T, et al. Virus-specific mRNA capping enzyme encoded by hepatitis E virus. *J Virol* 2001;75:6249–6255.

151. Malcolm P, Dalton H, Hussaini HS, et al. The histology of acute autochthonous hepatitis E virus infection. *Histopathology* 2007;51:190–194.

152. Mallet V, Bruneau J, Zuber J, et al. Hepatitis E virus-induced primary cutaneous CD30(+) T cell lymphoproliferative disorder. *J Hepatol* 2017;67:1334–1339.

153. Maneerat Y, Clayson ET, Myint KS, et al. Experimental infection of the laboratory rat with the hepatitis E virus. *J Med Virol* 1996;48:121–128.

154. Marion O, Lhomme S, Nayrac M, et al. Hepatitis E virus replication in human intestinal cells. *Gut* 2020;69:901–910.

155. Mazzola A, Tran Minh M, Charlotte F, et al. Chronic hepatitis E viral infection after liver transplantation: a regression of fibrosis after antiviral therapy. *Transplantation* 2017;101:2083–2087.

156. Meister TL, Bruening J, Todt D, et al. Cell culture systems for the study of hepatitis E virus. *Antiviral Res* 2019;163:34–49.

157. Meng XJ. From barnyard to food table: the omnipresence of hepatitis E virus and risk for zoonotic infection and food safety. *Virus Res* 2011;161:23–30.

158. Mhaindarkar V, Sharma K, Lole KS. Mutagenesis of hepatitis E virus helicase motifs: effects on enzyme activity. *Virus Res* 2014;179:26–33.

159. Mishra L, Seeff LB. Viral hepatitis, A though E, complicating pregnancy. *Gastroenterol Clin North Am* 1992;21:873–887.

160. Miyamura T. Hepatitis E virus infection in developed countries. *Virus Res* 2011;161:40–46.

161. Montpellier C, Wychowski C, Sayed IM, et al. Hepatitis E virus lifecycle and identification of 3 forms of the ORF2 capsid protein. *Gastroenterology* 2018;154:211–223 e8.

162. Munoz-Chimeno M, Cenalmor A, Garcia-Lugo MA, et al. Proline-rich hypervariable region of hepatitis E virus: arranging the disorder. *Microorganisms* 2020;8(9):1417.

163. Murrison LB, Sherman KE. The enigma of hepatitis E virus. *Gastroenterol Hepatol (N Y)* 2017;13:484–491.

164. Mushahwar IK, Dawson GJ, Bile KM, et al. Serological studies of an enterically transmitted non-A, non-B hepatitis in Somalia. *J Med Virol* 1993;40:218–221.

165. Nagashima S, Jirintai S, Takahashi M, et al. Hepatitis E virus egress depends on the exosomal pathway with secretory exosomes derived from multivesicular bodies. *J Gen Virol* 2014;95:2166–2175.
166. Nagashima S, Takahashi M, Jirintai S, et al. The membrane on the surface of hepatitis E virus particles is derived from the intracellular membrane and contains trans-Golgi network protein 2. *Arch Virol* 2014;159:979–991.
167. Nagashima S, Takahashi M, Kobayashi T, et al. Characterization of the quasi-enveloped hepatitis E virus particles released by the cellular exosomal pathway. *J Virol* 2017;91(22):e00822-17.
168. Nair VP, Anang S, Subramani C, et al. Endoplasmic reticulum stress induced synthesis of a novel viral factor mediates efficient replication of genotype-1 hepatitis E virus. *PLoS Pathog* 2016;12:e1005521.
169. Nan Y, Ma Z, Wang R, et al. Enhancement of interferon induction by ORF3 product of hepatitis E virus. *J Virol* 2014;88:8696–8705.
170. Netzler NE, Enosi Tuipulotu D, Vasudevan SG, et al. Antiviral candidates for treating hepatitis E virus infection. *Antimicrob Agents Chemother* 2019;63(6):e00003-19.
171. Neuvonen M, Ahola T. Differential activities of cellular and viral macro domain proteins in binding of ADP-ribose metabolites. *J Mol Biol* 2009;385:212–225.
172. Nguyen HT, Torian U, Faulk K, et al. A naturally occurring human/hepatitis E recombinant virus predominates in serum but not in faeces of a chronic hepatitis E patient and has a growth advantage in cell culture. *J Gen Virol* 2012;93:526–530.
173. Niesters HG, Strauss JH. Mutagenesis of the conserved 51-nucleotide region of Sindbis virus. *J Virol* 1990;64:1639–1647.
174. Nimgaonkar I, Archer NF, Becher I, et al. Isocotoin suppresses hepatitis E virus replication through inhibition of heat shock protein 90. *Antiviral Res* 2021;185:104997
175. Nishiyama T, Kobayashi T, Jirintai S, et al. Screening of novel drugs for inhibiting hepatitis E virus replication. *J Virol Methods* 2019;270:1–11.
176. Osterman A, Stellberger T, Gebhardt A, et al. The hepatitis E virus intraviral interactome. *Sci Rep* 2015;5:13872.
177. Paliwal D, Panda SK, Kapur N, et al. Hepatitis E virus (HEV) protease: a chymotrypsin-like enzyme that processes both non-structural (pORF1) and capsid (pORF2) protein. *J Gen Virol* 2014;95:1689–1700.
178. Park G, Parveen A, Kim JE, et al. Spicatoside A derived from Liriope platyphylla root ethanol extract inhibits hepatitis E virus genotype 3 replication in vitro. *Sci Rep* 2019;9:4397.
179. Parvez MK. Molecular characterization of hepatitis E virus ORF1 gene supports a papain-like cysteine protease (PCP)-domain activity. *Virus Res* 2013;178:553–556.
180. Parvez MK. The hepatitis E virus ORF1 'X-domain' residues form a putative macrodomain protein/Appr-1''-pase catalytic-site, critical for viral RNA replication. *Gene* 2015;566:47–53.
181. Parvez MK. Mutational analysis of hepatitis E virus ORF1 "Y-domain": Effects on RNA replication and virion infectivity. *World J Gastroenterol* 2017;23:590–602.
182. Parvez MK, Al-Dosari MS. Evidence of MAPK-JNK1/2 activation by hepatitis E virus ORF3 protein in cultured hepatoma cells. *Cytotechnology* 2015;67:545–550.
183. Parvez MK, Khan AA. Molecular modeling and analysis of hepatitis E virus (HEV) papain-like cysteine protease. *Virus Res* 2014;179:220–224.
184. Perez-Gracia MT, Suay-Garcia B, Mateos-Lindemann ML. Hepatitis E and pregnancy: current state. *Rev Med Virol* 2017;27:e1929.
185. Peron JM, Bureau C, Poirson H, et al. Fulminant liver failure from acute autochthonous hepatitis E in France: description of seven patients with acute hepatitis E and encephalopathy. *J Viral Hepat* 2007;14:298–303.
186. Peron JM, Danjoux M, Kamar N, et al. Liver histology in patients with sporadic acute hepatitis E: a study of 11 patients from South-West France. *Virchows Arch* 2007;450:405–410.
187. Perttila J, Spuul P, Ahola T. Early secretory pathway localization and lack of processing for hepatitis E virus replication protein pORF1. *J Gen Virol* 2013;94:807–816.
188. Pingale KD, Kanade GD, Karpe YA. Hepatitis E virus polymerase binds to IFIT1 to protect the viral RNA from IFIT1-mediated translation inhibition. *J Gen Virol* 2019;100:471–483.
189. Pudupakam RS, Huang YW, Opriessnig T, et al. Deletions of the hypervariable region (HVR) in open reading frame 1 of hepatitis E virus do not abolish virus infectivity: evidence for attenuation of HVR deletion mutants in vivo. *J Virol* 2009;83:384–395.
190. Pudupakam RS, Kenney SP, Cordoba L, et al. Mutational analysis of the hypervariable region of hepatitis e virus reveals its involvement in the efficiency of viral RNA replication. *J Virol* 2011;85:10031–10040.
191. Purcell RH, Engle RE, Rood MP, et al. Hepatitis E virus in rats, Los Angeles, California, USA. *Emerg Infect Dis* 2011;17:2216–2222.
192. Purdy MA, Harrison TJ, Jameel S, et al. ICTV virus taxonomy profile: Hepeviridae. *J Gen Virol* 2017;98:2645–2646.
193. Purdy MA, Lara J, Khudyakov YE. The hepatitis E virus polyproline region is involved in viral adaptation. *PLoS One* 2012;7:e35974.
194. Qu C, Xu L, Yin Y, et al. Nucleoside analogue 2′-C-methylcytidine inhibits hepatitis E virus replication but antagonizes ribavirin. *Arch Virol* 2017;162:2989–2996.
195. Ratra R, Kar-Roy A, Lal SK. ORF3 protein of hepatitis E virus interacts with the Bbeta chain of fibrinogen resulting in decreased fibrinogen secretion from HuH-7 cells. *J Gen Virol* 2009;90:1359–1370.
196. Rehman S, Kapur N, Durgapal H, et al. Subcellular localization of hepatitis E virus (HEV) replicase. *Virology* 2008;370:77–92.
197. Rein DB, Stevens GA, Theaker J, et al. The global burden of hepatitis E virus genotypes 1 and 2 in 2005. *Hepatology* 2012;55:988–997.
198. Reuter G, Boros A, Matics R, et al. A novel avian-like hepatitis E virus in wild aquatic bird, little egret (Egretta garzetta), in Hungary. *Infect Genet Evol* 2016;46:74–77.
199. Reyes GR, Purdy MA, Kim JP, et al. Isolation of a cDNA from the virus responsible for enterically transmitted non-A, non-B hepatitis. *Science* 1990;247:1335–1339.
200. Rivera-Serrano EE, Gonzalez-Lopez O, Das A, et al. Cellular entry and uncoating of naked and quasi-enveloped human hepatoviruses. *Elife* 2019;8:e43983.
201. Roth NJ, Schafer W, Alexander R, et al. Low hepatitis E virus RNA prevalence in a large-scale survey of United States source plasma donors. *Transfusion* 2017;57:2958–2964.
202. Saad MD, Hussein HA, Bashandy MM, et al. Hepatitis E virus infection in work horses in Egypt. *Infect Genet Evol* 2007;7:368–373.
203. Said B, Ijaz S, Kafatos G, et al.; Hepatitis E Incident Investigation Team. Hepatitis E outbreak on cruise ship. *Emerg Infect Dis* 2009;15:1738–1744.
204. Sehgal D, Thomas S, Chakraborty M, et al. Expression and processing of the Hepatitis E virus ORF1 nonstructural polyprotein. *Virol J* 2006;3:38.
205. Shiota T, Li TC, Yoshizaki S, et al. The hepatitis E virus capsid C-terminal region is essential for the viral life cycle: implication for viral genome encapsidation and particle stabilization. *J Virol* 2013;87:6031–6036.
206. Shrestha MP, Scott RM, Joshi DM, et al. Safety and efficacy of a recombinant hepatitis E vaccine. *N Engl J Med* 2007;356:895–903.
207. Shukla P, Nguyen HT, Faulk K, et al. Adaptation of a genotype 3 hepatitis E virus to efficient growth in cell culture depends on an inserted human gene segment acquired by recombination. *J Virol* 2012;86:5697–5707.
208. Shukla P, Nguyen HT, Torian U, et al. Cross-species infections of cultured cells by hepatitis E virus and discovery of an infectious virus-host recombinant. *Proc Natl Acad Sci U S A* 2011;108:2438–2443.
209. Smith DB, Simmonds P, Izopet J, et al. Proposed reference sequences for hepatitis E virus subtypes. *J Gen Virol* 2016;97:537–542.
210. Smith DB, Simmonds P, Members Of The International Committee On The Taxonomy Of Viruses Study Group, Jameel S, et al. Consensus proposals for classification of the family Hepeviridae. *J Gen Virol* 2014;95:2223–2232.
211. Smith DB, Vanek J, Ramalingam S, et al. Evolution of the hepatitis E virus hypervariable region. *J Gen Virol* 2012;93:2408–2418.
212. Sridhar S, Yip CCY, Wu S, et al. Rat hepatitis E virus as cause of persistent hepatitis after liver transplant. *Emerg Infect Dis* 2018;24:2241–2250
213. Sridhar S, Yip CC, Wu S, et al. Transmission of rat hepatitis E virus infection to humans in Hong Kong: a clinical and epidemiological analysis. *Hepatology* 2021;73:10–22.
214. Steimer L, Klostermeier D. RNA helicases in infection and disease. *RNA Biol* 2012;9:751–771.
215. Suppiah S, Zhou Y, Frey TK. Lack of processing of the expressed ORF1 gene product of hepatitis E virus. *Virol J* 2011;8:245.
216. Surjit M, Jameel S, Lal SK. The ORF2 protein of hepatitis E virus binds the 5′ region of viral RNA. *J Virol* 2004;78:320–328.
217. Surjit M, Oberoi R, Kumar R, et al. Enhanced alpha1 microglobulin secretion from Hepatitis E virus ORF3-expressing human hepatoma cells is mediated by the tumor susceptibility gene 101. *J Biol Chem* 2006;281:8135–8142.
218. Szkolnicka D, Pollan A, Da Silva N, et al. Recombinant hepatitis E viruses harboring tags in the ORF1 protein. *J Virol* 2019;93(19):e00459-19.
219. Takahashi M, Nishizawa T, Sato Y, et al. Prevalence and genotype/subtype distribution of hepatitis E virus (HEV) among wild boars in Japan: identification of a genotype 5 HEV strain. *Virus Res* 2020;287:198106.
220. Takahashi H, Tanaka T, Jirintai S, et al. A549 and PLC/PRF/5 cells can support the efficient propagation of swine and wild boar hepatitis E virus (HEV) strains: demonstration of HEV infectivity of porcine liver sold as food. *Arch Virol* 2012;157:235–246.
221. Takahashi M, Tanaka T, Takahashi H, et al. Hepatitis E virus (HEV) strains in serum samples can replicate efficiently in cultured cells despite the coexistence of HEV antibodies: characterization of HEV virions in blood circulation. *J Clin Microbiol* 2010;48:1112–1125.
222. Takahashi M, Yamada K, Hoshino Y, et al. Monoclonal antibodies raised against the ORF3 protein of hepatitis E virus (HEV) can capture HEV particles in culture supernatant and serum but not those in feces. *Arch Virol* 2008;153:1703–1713.
223. Tam AW, Smith MM, Guerra ME, et al. Hepatitis E virus (HEV): molecular cloning and sequencing of the full-length viral genome. *Virology* 1991;185:120–131.
224. Tang X, Yang C, Gu Y, et al. Structural basis for the neutralization and genotype specificity of hepatitis E virus. *Proc Natl Acad Sci U S A* 2011;108:10266–10271.
225. Tanggis, Kobayashi T, Takahashi M, Jirintai S, et al. An analysis of two open reading frames (ORF3 and ORF4) of rat hepatitis E virus genome using its infectious cDNA clones with mutations in ORF3 or ORF4. *Virus Res* 2018;249:16–30.
226. Tian D, Yugo DM, Kenney SP, et al. Dissecting the potential role of hepatitis E virus ORF1 nonstructural gene in cross-species infection by using intergenotypic chimeric viruses. *J Med Virol* 2020. doi:10.1002/jmv.26226. https://pubmed.ncbi.nlm.nih.gov/32589758/
227. Todt D, Moeller N, Praditya D, et al. The natural compound silvestrol inhibits hepatitis E virus (HEV) replication in vitro and in vivo. *Antiviral Res* 2018;157:151–158.
228. Tsarev SA, Tsareva TS, Emerson SU, et al. Recombinant vaccine against hepatitis E: dose response and protection against heterologous challenge. *Vaccine* 1997;15:1834–1838.
229. Tsarev SA, Tsareva TS, Emerson SU, et al. Experimental hepatitis E in pregnant rhesus monkeys: failure to transmit hepatitis E virus (HEV) to offspring and evidence of naturally acquired antibodies to HEV. *J Infect Dis* 1995;172:31–37.
230. Tyagi S, Korkaya H, Zafrullah M, et al. The phosphorylated form of the ORF3 protein of hepatitis E virus interacts with its non-glycosylated form of the major capsid protein, ORF2. *J Biol Chem* 2002;277:22759–22767.
231. Tyagi S, Surjit M, Roy AK, et al. The ORF3 protein of hepatitis E virus interacts with liver-specific alpha1-microglobulin and its precursor alpha1-microglobulin/bikunin precursor (AMBP) and expedites their export from the hepatocyte. *J Biol Chem* 2004;279:29308–29319.
232. van den Berg B, van der Eijk AA, Pas SD, et al. Guillain-Barre syndrome associated with preceding hepatitis E virus infection. *Neurology* 2014;82:491–497.
233. van der Heijden MW, Bol JF. Composition of alphavirus-like replication complexes: involvement of virus and host encoded proteins. *Arch Virol* 2002;147:875–898.
234. van der Valk M, Zaaijer HL, Kater AP, et al. Sofosbuvir shows antiviral activity in a patient with chronic hepatitis E virus infection. *J Hepatol* 2017;66:242–243.
235. Varma SP, Kumar A, Kapur N, et al. Hepatitis E virus replication involves alternating negative- and positive-sense RNA synthesis. *J Gen Virol* 2011;92:572–581.
236. Vollmer T, Diekmann J, Eberhardt M, et al. Monitoring of anti-hepatitis E virus antibody seroconversion in asymptomatically infected blood donors: systematic comparison of nine commercial anti-HEV IgM and IgG Assays. *Viruses* 2016;8(8):232.

237. Wang Y, Metselaar HJ, Peppelenbosch MP, et al. Chronic hepatitis E in solid-organ transplantation: the key implications of immunosuppressants. *Curr Opin Infect Dis* 2014;27:303–308.

238. Wang L, Teng JLL, Lau SKP, et al. Transmission of a novel genotype of hepatitis E virus from Bactrian Camels to Cynomolgus Macaques. *J Virol* 2019;93(7):e02014-18.

239. Wedemeyer H, Pischke S, Manns MP. Pathogenesis and treatment of hepatitis e virus infection. *Gastroenterology* 2012;142:1388–1397 e1.

240. WHO. Hepatitis E. 2017. https://www.who.int/en/news-room/fact-sheets/detail/hepatitis-e. Accessed

241. Williams TP, Kasorndorkbua C, Halbur PG, et al. Evidence of extrahepatic sites of replication of the hepatitis E virus in a swine model. *J Clin Microbiol* 2001;39:3040–3046.

242. Wong DC, Purcell RH, Sreenivasan MA, et al. Epidemic and endemic hepatitis in India: evidence for a non-A, non-B hepatitis virus aetiology. *Lancet* 1980;2:876–879.

243. Woo PC, Lau SK, Teng JL, et al. New hepatitis E virus genotype in camels, the Middle East. *Emerg Infect Dis* 2014;20:1044–1048.

244. Woo PC, Lau SK, Teng JL, et al. New hepatitis E virus genotype in Bactrian Camels, Xinjiang, China, 2013. *Emerg Infect Dis* 2016;22:2219–2221.

245. Wu C, Wu X, Xia J. Hepatitis E virus infection during pregnancy. *Virol J* 2020;17:73.

246. Xia J, Liu L, Wang L, et al. Experimental infection of pregnant rabbits with hepatitis E virus demonstrating high mortality and vertical transmission. *J Viral Hepat* 2015;22: 850–857.

247. Xing L, Kato K, Li T, et al. Recombinant hepatitis E capsid protein self-assembles into a dual-domain T = 1 particle presenting native virus epitopes. *Virology* 1999;265:35–45.

248. Xing L, Li TC, Mayazaki N, et al. Structure of hepatitis E virion-sized particle reveals an RNA-dependent viral assembly pathway. *J Biol Chem* 2010;285:33175–33183.

249. Yadav KK, Boley PA, Fritts Z, et al. Ectopic expression of genotype 1 hepatitis E virus ORF4 increases genotype 3 HEV viral replication in cell culture. *Viruses* 2021;13(1):75.

250. Yamada K, Takahashi M, Hoshino Y, et al. ORF3 protein of hepatitis E virus is essential for virion release from infected cells. *J Gen Virol* 2009;90:1880–1891.

251. Yamashita T, Mori Y, Miyazaki N, et al. Biological and immunological characteristics of hepatitis E virus-like particles based on the crystal structure. *Proc Natl Acad Sci U S A* 2009;106:12986–12991.

252. Yin X, Ambardekar C, Lu Y, et al. Distinct entry mechanisms for nonenveloped and quasi-enveloped hepatitis E viruses. *J Virol* 2016;90:4232–4242.

253. Yin X, Feng Z. Hepatitis E virus entry. *Viruses* 2019;11(10):883.

254. Yin X, Ying D, Lhomme S, et al. Origin, antigenicity, and function of a secreted form of ORF2 in hepatitis E virus infection. *Proc Natl Acad Sci U S A* 2018;115:4773–4778.

255. Yugo DM, Cossaboom CM, Meng XJ. Naturally occurring animal models of human hepatitis E virus infection. *ILAR J* 2014;55:187–199.

256. Zafrullah M, Ozdener MH, Panda SK, et al. The ORF3 protein of hepatitis E virus is a phosphoprotein that associates with the cytoskeleton. *J Virol* 1997;71:9045–9053.

257. Zaman K, Dudman S, Stene-Johansen K, et al. HEV study protocol: design of a cluster-randomised, blinded trial to assess the safety, immunogenicity and effectiveness of the hepatitis E vaccine HEV 239 (Hecolin) in women of childbearing age in rural Bangladesh. *BMJ Open* 2020;10:e033702.

258. Zhang J, Gu Y, Ge SX, et al. Analysis of hepatitis E virus neutralization sites using monoclonal antibodies directed against a virus capsid protein. *Vaccine* 2005;23:2881–2892.

259. Zhang X, Ke W, Xie J, et al. Comparison of effects of hepatitis E or A viral superinfection in patients with chronic hepatitis B. *Hepatol Int* 2010;4:615–620.

260. Zhang M, Purcell RH, Emerson SU. Identification of the 5′ terminal sequence of the SAR-55 and MEX-14 strains of hepatitis E virus and confirmation that the genome is capped. *J Med Virol* 2001;65:293–295.

261. Zhang W, Shen Q, Mou J, et al. Hepatitis E virus infection among domestic animals in eastern China. *Zoonoses Public Health* 2008;55:291–298.

262. Zheng ZZ, Miao J, Zhao M, et al. Role of heat-shock protein 90 in hepatitis E virus capsid trafficking. *J Gen Virol* 2010;91:1728–1736.

263. Zheng Q, Jiang J, He M, et al. Viral neutralization by antibody-imposed physical disruption. *Proc Natl Acad Sci U S A* 2019;116(52):26933–26940. doi:10.1073/pnas.1916028116.

264. Zhou X, Huang F, Xu L, et al. Hepatitis E virus infects neurons and brains. *J Infect Dis* 2017;215:1197–1206.

265. Zhu FC, Zhang J, Zhang XF, et al. Efficacy and safety of a recombinant hepatitis E vaccine in healthy adults: a large-scale, randomised, double-blind placebo-controlled, phase 3 trial. *Lancet* 2010;376:895–902.

Stephen P. Goff • Monica J. Roth

Introduction to retroviruses
Taxonomic classification
  Alpharetroviruses
  Betaretroviruses
  Gammaretroviruses
  Deltaretroviruses
  Epsilonretroviruses
  Lentiviruses
  Spumaviruses
  Evolutionary relationships
  Transforming viruses
Virion structure
  Virion proteins
Organization of the RNA genome
Overview of the life cycle
  Changes in the viral genome
Virus transmission
The virus receptors
  Alpharetrovirus receptors
  Betaretrovirus receptors
  Gammaretrovirus receptors
  Deltaretrovirus receptors
  Lentivirus receptors
Penetration and uncoating
Reverse transcription
  Steps in reverse transcription of the retroviral genome
  Biochemistry and structure of reverse transcriptase
Recombination
  Models for recombination
Integration of the proviral DNA
  Unintegrated DNA forms
  Entry into the nucleus
  Structure of the provirus
  Biochemistry of integration
  Viral att sites
  Structure of the integrase
  Preintegration complex
  Host proteins and integration
  Distribution of integration sites
Expression of viral RNAs
  Overview of viral RNA synthesis
  Initiation of transcription
  Beginning and ending the RNA
  RNA processing
Translation and protein processing
  Gag gene expression

Pro gene expression
Pol gene expression
Env gene expression
Other viral gene products
Virion assembly
  Assembly of C-type virions
  Assembly of B- and D-type virions
  Gag and virion assembly
  Virion assembly in vitro
  Virion size
  Incorporation of other proteins into assembling virions
  Host proteins in the virion
RNA packaging
  Gag sequences important for packaging
  RNA sequences important for packaging
  Dimerization of the viral genome
  Incorporation of tRNA primer
  tRNA primer placement
Protein processing and virion maturation
  Activation of the protease
  Protease structure and function
  Protease inhibitors
  Processing of the Gag precursor
  Processing of the Gag-Pro-Pol precursor
  Processing of the Env precursor
  Morphological changes upon virion maturation
  Structure of virion core: CA packing
Resistance to retrovirus infection: host restriction factors
  Replication blocks mediated by endogenous retrovirus genes
  Early block to infection by Trim5a
  Deamination of viral DNA by the APOBECs
  Blocking early events in monocyte lineage cells by SAMHD1
  Elimination of viral RNAs by ZAP
  Trapping virion particles on the cell surface by tetherin
  Blocking envelope by the SERINC proteins
Retroviral diseases
  The varied effects of retroviral infection
  Diseases caused by the replication-competent retroviruses
  Host determinants of retroviral disease
Acute transforming retroviruses: transduction of cellular pro-tooncogenes
Endogenous viruses and virus-like sequences
  Endogenous elements in chickens, mice, pigs, and humans
  Properties of the endogenous provirus-like elements
Retroviral vectors, packaging lines, and gene therapy
Perspectives

INTRODUCTION TO RETROVIRUSES

The retrovirus family, the *Retroviridae*, are a large and diverse group of viruses found in all vertebrates. These viruses replicate through an extraordinary and unique life cycle, differentiating them sharply from other viruses. The virion particles generally contain a genomic RNA, but upon entry into the host cell, this RNA is reverse transcribed into a DNA form of the genome that is integrated into the host chromosomal DNA. The integrated form of the viral DNA, the provirus, then serves as the template for the formation of viral RNAs and proteins that assemble progeny virions. These features of life cycle—especially, the reverse flow of genetic information from RNA to DNA, and the establishment of the DNA in an integrated form in the host genome—are the defining hallmarks of the retroviruses. This life cycle also accounts for many of their diverse biological activities. The creation of the proviral DNA confers on the viruses a powerful ability to maintain a persistent infection in the face of a host immune response and to enter the germ line, permitting the vertical transmission of virus.

The retroviruses have played a unique role in the history of molecular biology. They have attracted attention on several grounds.

- Biochemistry: The viral replication enzymes, including the reverse transcriptase (RT) and integrase (IN), are extraordinarily useful tools in manipulating nucleic acids *in vitro* and *in vivo*. Through the preparation of cDNAs, RT has been crucial for studies of mRNA synthesis and gene regulation.
- Pathogenicity: Retroviruses are known as major pathogens affecting nearly all vertebrates. HIV-1, the agent of the AIDS pandemic, will probably cause more human death and suffering than all but a handful of pathogens in recorded history.
- Markers of evolutionary history: The insertion of a provirus into the germ line provides a mendelian tag that marks an event at a particular time in evolution. The inheritance of that tag can then be used to follow speciation, population migrations, and evolution of species.
- Insertional activation of oncogenes: The integration of retroviral DNA is inherently mutagenic, and retrovirus replication thus can cause gross alterations of host genes and patterns of gene expression. When insertions lead to tumor formation, the locations serve to identify new oncogenes.
- Transduction: Retroviruses can acquire host sequences in the formation of acutely transforming genomes. The identity, structure, and expression of these genes has provided much of our current knowledge of the routes by which normal growth control can be subverted by genetic alterations.
- Gene delivery vectors: The structure of transforming viruses provided a model for the use of retroviruses to deliver therapeutic genes efficiently and cleanly into cells. Retroviruses now serve as major tools in the medical black bag of gene therapists.

This chapter will describe the replication and molecular biology of the retroviruses, concentrating on the most broadly conserved aspects of the life cycle. Because of the magnitude of the retroviral literature, citations here cannot be comprehensive, and referencing has been selective and concentrated on more recent publications. The distinctive features of the human retroviruses, especially the lentiviruses and spumaviruses, will be addressed in much more detail in later chapters.

TAXONOMIC CLASSIFICATION

The retroviruses were originally classified by the morphology of the virion core as visualized in the electron microscope. Examples of the appearance of the virions in these micrographs are presented in Figure 15.1. The virion particles are typically spherical and are surrounded by an envelope consisting of a lipid membrane bilayer. The surface is studded by projections of an envelope glycoprotein. There is a spherical layer of protein under the membrane and an internal nucleocapsid whose shape varies characteristically from virus to virus. The shape and position of the nucleocapsid core was historically used as the major classifying feature of the retroviral genera. A-type particles were defined as those forming intracellular structures with a characteristic morphology, a thick shell with a hollow, electron-lucent center. These particles are now appreciated as representing an immature capsid on route toward the formation of other structures. This term is thus no longer in use to denote a virus classification, though it is used to describe the structures formed by some virus-related intracellular retrotransposons (the intracisternal A-type particles, or IAPs).[376,434] B-type viruses show a round but eccentrically positioned inner core. C-type viruses assemble at the plasma membrane and contain a central, symmetrically placed spherical inner core. The D-type viruses assemble in the cytoplasm, via an A-type intermediate, and upon budding exhibit a distinctive cylindrical core.

These older classifications have been useful in partially defining the various genera of the family *Retroviridae*, but the number of genera have now been expanded on the basis of new criteria. The genera have been formalized and given new names by the International Committee on Taxonomy of Viruses. The alpharetroviruses and gammaretroviruses are considered "simple" retroviruses; the deltaretroviruses, epsilonretroviruses, lentiviruses, and spumaviruses are considered "complex"; and the betaretroviruses could be considered as intermediate between these. The simple viruses encode only the Gag, Pro, Pol, and Env gene products; the complex viruses encode these same gene products but also an array of small regulatory proteins with a range of functions. The properties of the viruses belonging to each of these genera are summarized briefly below. Representative members of each genus are listed (Table 15.1).

Alpharetroviruses

The alpharetroviruses are simple retroviruses characterized by a C-type morphology and are typified by the avian leukosis–sarcoma viruses (ALSV). The genome contains *gag*, *pro*, *pol*, and *env* genes, with no additional known viral genes; *pro* is at the 3′ end of *gag* and in the same reading frame. The tRNA primer is tRNAtrp. The viruses are widespread in many avian host species. The ALV members are classified into 10 subgroups (termed A–J) by their distinct receptor utilization. The first four subgroups represent exogenous viruses of chickens; the subgroup E includes a family of endogenous chicken viruses; and subgroups F and G include endogenous viruses of pheasants. One member, the avian sarcoma virus, is unique in containing an active oncogene, v-*src*, at its 3′ end.

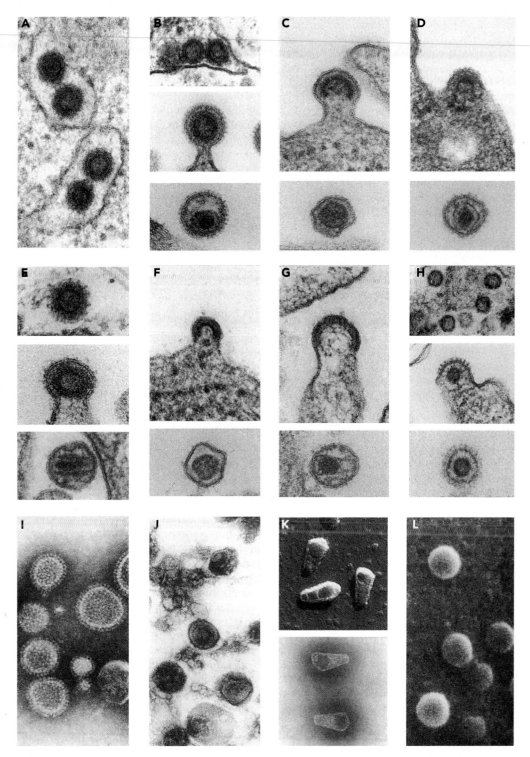

FIGURE 15.1 Electron micrographs of representative virion particles. The diameters of all the particles are approximately 100 nm. **A:** Type A particles. Intracisternal A particles in the endoplasmic reticulum. **B:** Betaretrovirus. Mouse mammary tumor virus, MMTV; type B morphology (*top*, intracytoplasmic particles; *middle*, budding particles; *bottom*, mature extracellular particles). **C:** Gammaretrovirus. Murine leukemia virus, MuLV; type C morphology (*top*, budding; *bottom*, mature extracellular particles). **D:** Alpharetrovirus. Avian leukosis virus; type C morphology (*top*, budding; *bottom*, mature extracellular particles). **E:** Betaretrovirus. Mason-Pfizer monkey virus; MPMV; type D morphology (*top*, intracytoplasmic A–type particles; *middle*, budding; *bottom*, mature extracellular particles). **F:** Deltaretrovirus. Bovine leukemia virus, BLV (*top*, budding; *bottom*, mature extracellular particles). **G:** Lentivirus. Bovine immunodeficiency virus (*top*, budding; *bottom*, mature extracellular particles). **H:** Spumavirus. Bovine syncytial virus (*top*, intracytoplasmic particles; *middle*, budding; *bottom*, mature extracellular particles). **I:** Betaretrovirus. Mouse mammary tumor virus, MMTV; type B morphology, visualized by negative staining with phosphotungstic acid. **J:** Gammaretrovirus, visualized as pseudoreplica stained with uranyl acetate. **K:** Lentivirus. Purified cone-shaped cores of equine infectious anemia virus (*top*, cores visualized by shadow casting technique; *bottom*, cores visualized by negative staining with phosphotungstic acid). **L:** Budding retroviral particles visualized by scanning electron microscopy. (Micrographs courtesy of Dr. Matthew Gonda, and reproduced from Coffin JM, Hughes SH, Varmus HE, eds. *Retroviruses.* Cold Spring Harbor, NY: Cold Spring Harbor Press; 1997.)

TABLE 15.1 *Retroviridae* family

Subfamily	Name (Genus)	Examples (Species)	Morphology
Orthoretrovirinae	Alpharetrovirus	Avian leukosis virus (ALV)	C-type
		Rous sarcoma virus (RSV)	
	Betaretrovirus	Mouse mammary tumor virus (MMTV)	B, D-type
		Mason-Pfizer monkey virus (M-PMV)	
		Jaagsiekte sheep retrovirus (JSRV)	
	Gammaretrovirus	Murine leukemia viruses (MuLV)	C-type
		Feline leukemia virus (FeLV)	
		Gibbon ape leukemia virus (GaLV)	
		Reticuloendotheliosis virus (RevT)	
	Deltaretrovirus	Human T-lymphotropic virus (HTLV) type 1, 2	Rod-shaped core
		Bovine leukemia virus (BLV)	
		Simian T-lymphotropic virus (STLV) type 1, 2, 3	
	Epsilonretrovirus	Walleye dermal sarcoma virus (WDSV)	—
		Walleye epidermal hyperplasia virus 1	
	Lentivirus	Human immunodeficiency virus type 1 (HIV-1)	Rod/Cone-shaped cores
		Human immunodeficiency virus type 2 (HIV-2)	
		Simian immunodeficiency virus (SIV)	
		Equine infectious anemia virus (EIAV)	
		Feline immunodeficiency virus (FIV)	
		Caprine arthritis–encephalitis virus (CAEV)	
		Visna/maedi virus (VMV)	
Spumaretrovirinae	Spumavirus	Prototype foamy virus (PFV)	Immature

Betaretroviruses

The betaretroviruses are simple retroviruses characterized by either a "B-type" morphology, with a round eccentric core, or "D-type" morphology, with a cylindrical core. The best-known examples are the mouse mammary tumor virus (MMTV) and the Mason-Pfizer monkey virus (M-PMV). Assembly occurs in the cytoplasm via an "A-type" intermediate, and the completed immature particle is then transported to the plasma membrane and budded. The genomes contain *gag*, *pro*, *pol*, and *env* genes, and the *gag*, *pro*, and *pol* genes are all in different reading frames. The genome of MMTV contains an additional gene termed the *sag* gene, for superantigen, and a regulator of RNA export termed *rem*.[480] The viruses also contain a dUTPase region as part of the *pro* ORF.[187] The tRNA primer is tRNALys3 or tRNALys1,2. There are both exogenous and endogenous viruses in this genus. Examples are found in mice, primates, sheep, and many other mammals.

Gammaretroviruses

The gammaretroviruses are simple viruses characterized by a C-type morphology. This genus has the largest number of members known, including the murine leukemia viruses (MuLVs), the feline leukemia viruses (FeLVs), and the gibbon ape leukemia virus (GALV). The genome contains only *gag*, *pro*, *pol*, and *env* genes; the *gag*, *pro*, and *pol* sequences are in the same reading frame, and the Gag-Pro-Pol protein is expressed by translational readthrough of a stop codon at the end of *gag*. The genome primer is most often tRNApro or tRNAglu, though others have been found. The murine viruses are divided into subgroups by their distinct receptor utilization. Many exogenous and endogenous viruses are found in diverse mammals, and examples have been isolated from reptiles and birds.

Deltaretroviruses

The deltaretroviruses are complex viruses characterized by a C-type morphology. The most famous examples are the human T-lymphotropic viruses (HTLVs) and the bovine leukemia virus (BLV). The genome contains *gag*, *pro*, *pol*, and *env* genes; the *gag*, *pro*, and *pol* genes are present in three different reading frames, and expression of the Gag-Pro-Pol protein requires two successive frameshifts. In addition, the genomes contain regulatory genes termed *rex* and *tax* that are expressed from an alternatively spliced mRNA. These gene products control the synthesis, transport, and processing of the viral RNAs. The tRNA primer is tRNApro. The HTLV-1 genome is notable in containing an antisense gene, termed *hbz*, encoding a bZIP protein, which promotes antisense transcription and represses sense transcription driven by *tax*.[464]

Epsilonretroviruses

The epsilonretroviruses are complex viruses characterized by a C-type morphology. The prototype is the walleye dermal sarcoma virus. The genomes contain *gag*, *pro*, *pol*, and *env* genes; the *gag*, *pro*, and *pol* genes are in the same reading frame. They also contain one to three additional genes termed ORFs A, B, and C. The ORFa gene is a viral homologue of the host cyclin D gene and so may regulate the cell cycle. The viruses use tRNAHis or Arg as primers. The only known examples are exogenous viruses in fish and reptiles.

Lentiviruses

The lentiviruses are complex viruses characterized by a unique virion morphology, with cylindrical or conical cores. The most important example is the human immunodeficiency virus type 1 (HIV-1), but nonprimate viruses in the genus include the caprine arthritis–encephalitis virus (CAEV), visna virus, and feline immunodeficiency virus (FIV). The genomes express *gag*, *pro*, *pol*, and *env* genes; *gag* is in one reading frame and *pro-pol* in another. A single frameshift is used to express Gag-Pro-Pol. The Pol region of the nonprimate lentiviruses includes a domain for dUTPase. A number of accessory genes are also expressed. In HIV-1, these genes are *vif*, *vpr*, *vpu*, *tat*, *rev*, and *nef*; these genes control transcription, RNA processing, virion assembly, host gene expression, and a number of other replication functions. The tRNA primer is tRNALys1,2. A large number of exogenous viruses in this genus have been found in diverse mammals, but the only endogenous sequences are relatively distant from the extant viruses.

Spumaviruses

The spumaviruses are complex viruses with a unique virion morphology, containing prominent spikes on the surface and a central but uncondensed core. The prototype example is the prototype foamy virus (PFV). The virion is assembled in the cytoplasm and budded into the ER and plasma membrane. There is probably only a single cleavage of the Gag protein near the C terminus and no major change in morphology during maturation. The genomes express *gag*, *pro*, *pol*, and *env* genes and also at least two accessory genes known as *tas/bel-1* and *bet*.[214,478] The *tas* gene encodes a transcriptional transactivator. Unique features are the separate expression of the Pol protein from a spliced mRNA and the presence of large amounts of reverse-transcribed DNA in the virion.[490] The genome contains a start site for antisense transcription within the LTR. The tRNA primer is tRNALys1,2. A number of exogenous viruses have been found in diverse mammals, and distantly related sequences are present as endogenous elements in the human genome.

Evolutionary Relationships

Sequences of various retroviral genomes have been compared and used to determine the relatedness of any pair.[470] A number of phylogenetic trees can be constructed using *gag*, *pro*, *pol*, or *env* genes, and in most aspects, these trees are similar. A tree based on comparisons of the *pol* gene (Fig. 15.2) shows the

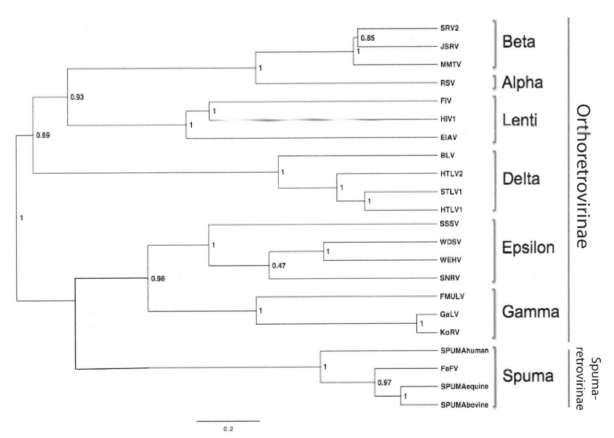

FIGURE 15.2 Phylogenetic reconstruction of representative exogenous retroviruses using reverse transcriptase sequences. The BEASTv1.6.1 tree[178] was created using two independent Bayesian MCMC chains (length of 1 million, 20% burn) run under relaxed clock (uncorrelated exp[177]) and rate heterogeneity among sites (gamma distribution with 8 categories). Monophyletic taxon sets consisting of alpha, beta, delta, epsilon, gamma, lenti, and spuma were also used in the model. The posterior probabilities label each node and branch lengths are scaled to expected substitutions per site. (Modified from a figure provided courtesy of Marcella McClure, Montana State University, Bozeman, MT.)

clustering of viruses within each of the main genera. However, it is important to realize that a phylogenetic tree is not necessarily identical to an evolutionary history and that the history that led to the formation of the known genera is not necessarily simple. It is noteworthy that there is no obvious clustering of all the simple viruses into a group apart from all the complex viruses. Thus, complex viruses probably arose from the simple ones more than once, with many evolving through the independent acquisition of separate genes. Trees based on the envelope genes are divergent from other trees, suggesting frequent exchanges by recombination. Various of the betaretroviruses in particular contain very dissimilar *env* genes.

Retroviruses are related to viruses of some other families. The retroviral RTs show close sequence similarity to the polymerases of the hepadnaviruses and the caulimoviruses, which also replicate by reverse transcription. The retroviruses also show extensive similarity in both *gag* and *pol* gene sequences to the retrotransposons, endogenous mobile elements with LTRs, and to retroposons, elements without LTRs such as the human LINE-1 elements. Retroviral RTs show more distant similarity to proteins encoded by the group II mitochondrial introns and by the retrons, elements in myxobacteria and rare isolates of *Escherichia coli*; to telomerase, a reverse transcriptase responsible for maintenance of the chromosomal termini in eukaryotes; and even slight similarity to the DNA polymerases of viruses and hosts.[469] The evolutionary history implied by these relationships has yet to be deciphered.

Transforming Viruses

During the replication of any retrovirus, replication-defective variants can arise through deletion or recombination events. Such mutants or variants can be propagated as a mixed virus culture along with the wild-type parent. In these mixtures of two genomes, the replication-competent parent acts as a helper virus to provide the missing replication functions in *trans* for the replication-defective virus, seen most often for alpha- and gammaretroviruses. Viral genomes can acquire host genes through recombination. If a newly acquired gene product is mitogenic or antiapoptotic for the host cell, or in more subtle ways alters the growth of the cell, the recombinant may become a potent oncogenic virus. A large number of such transducing viruses have been isolated and characterized as derivatives of one or another of the replication-competent parent viruses. A partial listing of the most intensively studied of these viruses is presented in Table 15.2. Study of the host-derived oncogenes provided the key insights leading to our current understanding of the molecular basis of cancer as well as to new targets for treatment.

VIRION STRUCTURE

Retrovirus virions are initially assembled and released from infected cells as immature particles containing unprocessed Gag and Gag-Pol precursors of the proteins that eventually make up the mature virus. The immature virion morphology is spherical, with a characteristic electron-lucent center. The immature virions have been described as a "protein vesicle," to suggest some fluidity in the interactions between the individual Gag proteins that make up the particle. Upon maturation, the precursor proteins are cleaved, and the structure and morphology of the virion changes profoundly. The mature retrovirus particle is a spherical structure, roughly 100 nm in diameter. The size of the virions in a given preparation is not highly homogeneous

TABLE 15.2	Examples of acute transforming retroviruses	
Parental Virus	**Transforming Virus**	**Transduced Gene(s)**
ALV	Rous sarcoma virus	c-src
	Avian myeloblastosis virus	c-myb
	Avian erythroblastosis virus	c-erbA,B
	Avian sarcoma virus CT10	c-crk
	Fujinami sarcoma virus	c-fps
	Y73 avian sarcoma virus	c-yes
	Avian sarcoma virus 17	c-jun
Moloney MuLV	Abelson murine leukemia virus	c-abl
	Harvey sarcoma virus	H-ras
	Kirsten sarcoma virus	Ki-ras
	Moloney murine sarcoma virus	c-mos
	FBJ murine sarcoma virus	c-fos
	3611-MSV	c-raf
Feline leukemia virus	Snyder-Theilen feline sarcoma virus	c-fes
	Gardner-Arnstein feline sarcoma virus	c-fes
	McDonough feline sarcoma virus	c-fms
Simian sarcoma–associated virus	Wooly monkey sarcoma virus	c-sis

but rather varies over a fairly wide range. After processing of the Gag precursor during virion maturation, one of the cleavage products, the CA protein, collapses to form a more ordered paracrystalline core. The virions exhibit a buoyant density in sucrose in the range of 1.16 to 1.18 g/mL. The sedimentation rate of the particles is typically about 600 **S**. The virions are sensitive to heat, detergent, and formaldehyde.

Virion Proteins

The stoichiometry of the various viral gene products in the virion is not very firmly established, but estimates suggest that about 1,500 to perhaps 2,000 Gag precursors are present per particle. After processing, all cleavage products are thought to be retained, suggesting equimolar presence of these proteins in the mature virions. The levels of the Pol proteins are typically about one-tenth to one-twentieth those of the Gag proteins, corresponding to about 100 to 200 molecules per virion. The levels of the Env proteins are quite variable among the viruses. For the gammaretroviruses, the levels of Env are close to that of Gag; perhaps, 1,200 monomers, or 400 trimers, are present per virion. For the lentiviruses, the levels of Env per virion are much lower, possibly as low as 10 trimers per virion.[837]

Nomenclature

The cleavage of Gag, Pro, Pol, and Env precursors forms the products in the mature infectious virions. These proteins are named by convention by a two-letter code: MA for matrix or membrane-associated protein; CA for capsid; NC for

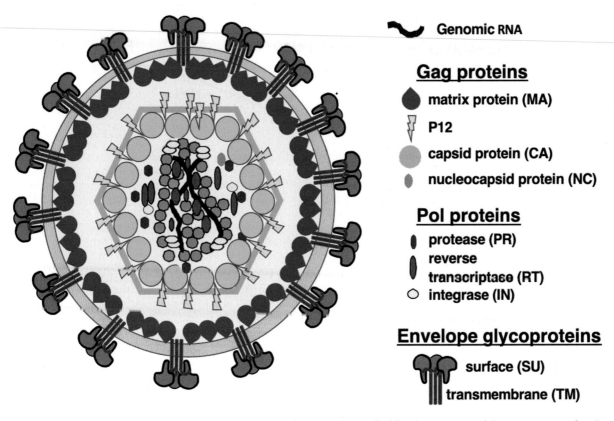

Genomic RNA

Gag proteins

- matrix protein (MA)
- P12
- capsid protein (CA)
- nucleocapsid protein (NC)

Pol proteins

- protease (PR)
- reverse transcriptase (RT)
- integrase (IN)

Envelope glycoproteins

- surface (SU)
- transmembrane (TM)

FIGURE 15.3 Generalized gammaretrovirion structure and components. A highly schematic view of the arrangement of viral gene products within the virion particle. The two-letter nomenclature for each protein is indicated, when assigned.

nucleocapsid; PR for protease; RT for reverse transcriptase; IN for integrase; SU for surface protein; and TM for transmembrane protein.[396] A highly schematic version of the generic retrovirion can be drawn (Fig. 15.3).

Arrangement of Virion Components

The genomic RNA is highly condensed in the virion by its association with the nucleocapsid protein, NC. The complex is contained within a protein core largely composed of the capsid protein CA, another Gag gene product. The shape of the core is different among the various retroviral genera and indeed is a distinguishing feature of the genera. In most of the viruses, the core is roughly spherical, but in some cases, it can be either conical or cylindrical. In all the viruses, the core is surrounded by a roughly spherical shell consisting of MA, which in turn is surrounded by the lipid bilayer of the virion envelope. The virion membrane contains the envelope glycoprotein, with the TM subunit present as a single-pass transmembrane protein anchor, and the SU subunit as an entirely extravirion protein bound to TM. The envelope proteins for those viruses examined closely have been found to reside in the membrane as trimers.

ORGANIZATION OF THE RNA GENOME

The viral genome is a dimer of linear, positive sense, single-stranded RNA, with each monomer 7 to 13 kb in size. The viral genomic RNA is present as a homodimer of two identical sequences, and thus, the virions are functionally diploid. Dimer formation is initiated by interactions between the two 5′ ends

of the RNAs in a self-complementary region termed the dimer initiation site (DIS). The RNA genome is generated by normal host transcriptional machinery and thus exhibits many of the features of a normal mRNA. The RNA is capped at the 5′ end, using the common m7G5′ppp5′G_mp structure, and contains a string of poly(A) sequence, about 200 nt long, at the 3′ end. The RNAs carry some posttranscriptional modifications, most prominently 2′O-methylation and adenosine N-6-methylation.[352]

A number of noncoding sequences are so important that they have been named to facilitate descriptions of their functions in the life cycle (Fig. 15.4). These key sequences are clustered at the termini of the RNA. A short sequence, the R (for repeated) region, is so-called because it is present twice in the RNA: once immediately after the cap at the 5′ end and again at the 3′ end, just before the poly(A) tail. Downstream of the 5′ R lies another sequence, termed U5 for unique 5′ sequence, which includes one of the *att* sites required for proviral integration. The U5 region is followed by the primer binding site, an 18-nt sequence at which a host tRNA is hybridized to the genome and the site of initiation of minus strand DNA synthesis.

The region downstream from the pbs contains the major signals for the encapsidation of the viral RNA into the virion particle, in sequences called the Psi element. The region also often contains the major splice donor site for the formation of subgenomic mRNAs. The bulk of the RNA sequences that follow are coding regions for the viral proteins. The genomes of all the replication-competent retroviruses contain at a minimum three genes or open reading frames: from 5′ to 3′ along the

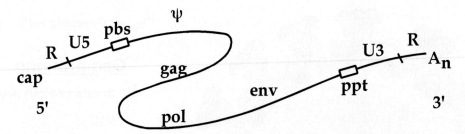

FIGURE 15.4 The organization of the retroviral RNA genome. The single-stranded RNA genome is depicted as a *curved line*. From 5′ to 3′ along the RNA, the features include a 5′ cap structure; R, a sequence block repeated at both 5′ and 3′ ends; U5, a unique 5′ sequence block; pbs, the primer binding site and site of initiation of minus strand DNA synthesis; Y, the major recognition site for the packaging of the viral RNA into the virion particle; the *gag*, *pol*, and *env* genes; ppt, the polypurine tract and site of initiation of the plus strand DNA synthesis; U3, a unique 3′ sequence block; the second copy of the R sequence; and finally, a 3′ poly(A) sequence.

genome, the genes are termed *gag* (from group-specific *a*ntigen), encoding internal structural proteins; *pol*, for polymerase; and *env*, for envelope. The three genes in the simple retroviruses occupy nearly all the available space in the center of the genome.

Downstream of the genes lies a short polypurine tract (ppt), a run of at least nine A and G residues. The ppt is the site of initiation of plus strand DNA synthesis. The ppt is followed by a sequence block termed U3 for unique 3′ sequence; this region contains a number of key cis-acting elements for viral gene expression and one of the *att* sites required for DNA integration.

The U3 abuts the 3′ copy of the R region, which is followed by the poly(A) tail. As we shall see, the R, U5, U3, pbs, and ppt sequences all play important roles in reverse transcription.

OVERVIEW OF THE LIFE CYCLE

Retroviruses replicate through a complex life cycle. A short summary of the steps of the cycle is as follows (a schematic view is shown in Fig. 15.5):

Retroviral Replication Cycle

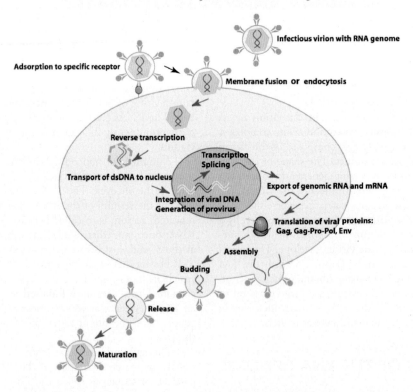

FIGURE 15.5 A schematic overview of the retrovirus life cycle. The major steps in the replication of a typical retrovirus are indicated, including those in the early phase of the life cycle, extending from the infecting virion (*top*) to the formation of the integrated provirus, and those in the late phase of the life cycle, extending from the provirus to the formation of mature progeny virus (*bottom left*).

- Receptor binding and membrane fusion
- Internalization
- Reverse transcription of the RNA genome within the capsid to form double-stranded linear DNA
- Nuclear entry of the DNA
- Integration of the linear DNA to form the provirus
- Transcription of the provirus to form viral RNAs
- Splicing and nuclear export of the RNAs
- Translation of the RNAs to form precursor proteins
- Assembly of the virion and packaging of the viral RNA genome
- Budding and release of the virions
- Proteolytic processing of the precursors and maturation of the virions

Changes in the Viral Genome

A quick perusal of this list reveals that the life cycle begins with an RNA genome, passes through an intracellular DNA intermediate, and is completed with a return to an RNA form in the progeny virus particle. An overview of the structures of the genome at various times in this cycle is presented in Figure 15.6. The RNA genome of the virion contains short terminal repeats (the R region) near its termini. During reverse transcription, as we shall see below, sequence blocks termed U5 and U3 are duplicated, so that the resulting double-stranded DNA is longer at both ends than the RNA template. This DNA thus contains long terminal repeats (the LTRs, consisting of sequence blocks U3, R, and U5) at both ends. The next step is the integration of the DNA to form the provirus; the integrated provirus is collinear with the unintegrated DNA and retains the LTRs (except for one or two base pairs lost at the termini during the

course of integration). Finally, the DNA is forward transcribed by the RNA polymerase II system to produce the progeny RNA genome. Transcription is initiated at the U3-R boundary of the 5′ LTR and extends down the genome, and the transcripts are processed and polyadenylated at the R-U5 boundary of the 3′ LTR, recreating the exact structure of the input RNA, complete with its short terminal repeats. This RNA is packaged and exported in virion particles. Each step will be described in more detail below.

VIRUS TRANSMISSION

Three distinct modes of virus transmission have been identified *in vitro* and *in vivo*.[671] These include cell-free infection, cell-to-cell infection, and transinfection. For cell-free infection, the virus directly transfers from a producer cell to a recipient cell through the extracellular space, whereas for cell-to-cell infection, the virus transfers via a virological synapse requiring close cell contacts. For transinfection, the virus particles are transmitted from a donor to a recipient cell via an intermediate cell (the "Trojan horse" mechanism). Here, the viruses do not actually infect the intermediate cells but rather are taken up and then presented to the target cell through an infectious synapse.[296] In one example, Friend MuLV can be transmitted by transinfection *in vivo*, using CD169/Siglec-1 on intermediate cells for capture and subsequent delivery of the virus to permissive lymphocytes.[669,670,745] HIV-1 and some other retroviruses can be captured and internalized by dendritic cells (DCs), macrophages, and other cells using Siglec-1, or perhaps gangliosides, and then ultimately delivered by transinfection to recipient T cells.[316,577] DC-SIGN may or may not be required.[70,241] The

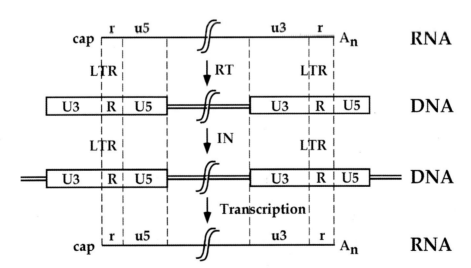

FIGURE 15.6 Structures of the termini of the viral RNA and DNA genomes at various stages of the viral life cycle. Sequence blocks in RNA are indicated by lower case and those in DNA by upper case. The structure of the RNA genome in the virion particle is indicated at the *top*. Reverse transcription of the RNA soon after infection involves the duplication and translocation of u5 and u3 sequence blocks and results in the formation of a double-stranded DNA molecule containing two terminal LTRs. The integration of the DNA genome occurs at the terminal sequences, establishing a provirus that is collinear with the preintegrative DNA. The forward transcription of the provirus is initiated at the U3/R border in the provirus; the resulting RNAs are cleaved and polyadenylated at the r/u5 border, recreating a viral RNA genome (*bottom*) identical to the infecting RNA.

relative importance of the pathways utilized *in vivo* for the various retroviruses remains controversial.[102] Productive viral infections in all cases utilize the viral Env proteins and their cognate receptors and are sensitive to inhibition by agents that block Env–receptor interactions.

THE VIRUS RECEPTORS

To enter a cell and initiate infection, all retroviruses require an interaction between a cell surface molecule—a receptor—and the envelope protein on the virion surface. The interactions are complex, involving an initial binding, drastic conformational changes in the envelope protein, an induced fusion of the viral and cellular membranes, and the internalization of the virion core into the cytoplasm. The SU subunit of Env makes the major initial contacts with receptor, and the TM subunit is responsible for membrane fusion. The reorganization of the two lipid bilayers—one on the virion and one on the cell—to join them and evert the core into the cell is a remarkable process (Fig. 15.7). The key steps involve the exposure of a hydrophobic fusion peptide that inserts into the target cell membrane and the drawing together of the two membranes by formation of a bundle of alpha-helices. Through x-ray crystallography, cryo-electron microscopy, cryo-electron tomography, total internal reflection fluorescence microscopy, and additional structural studies, snapshots of the intermediates formed during this complex process of entry, from prereceptor(s) binding through membrane fusion, have been obtained.[56,110,288,322,378,414,611,767,768,774] Similar events are probably utilized by many enveloped viruses of other families.

An important tool in the analysis of receptor utilization is the phenomenon of virus interference or superinfection resistance. Cells chronically infected by a particular virus cannot be infected by any virus that must enter by the same receptor as used by the first virus, though they are readily infected by viruses that utilize a distinct receptor. The reason is that the expression of the Env protein by the first virus binds to the receptor intracellularly, preventing its export to the cell surface or its function as a receptor for newly applied virus. This phenomenon allows for the rapid classification of those viruses that use a common receptor.

There is a great deal of information about the identity and structures of the receptors used by various retroviruses. The properties of the receptors of the major retroviral genera are summarized below. It is immediately apparent that these viruses utilize an extraordinarily diverse set of cell surface molecules as receptors (Table 15.3; see Refs.[50,717,773] for reviews). For many retroviruses, the receptors can be divided into various functional types, including phosphate transporters, amino acid transporters, and vitamin transporters.[260]

Alpharetrovirus Receptors

The receptor for the A subgroup of avian viruses was identified as encoding a membrane-anchored glycoprotein with sequence similarity to the ligand-binding repeat of the low-density lipoprotein receptor (LDLR),[42,811] and its identity as the true receptor has been confirmed by correlating its genetic map position with the genetically identified *tv-a* locus.[41] Tv-a is reported to transport transcobalamin-bound vitamin B_{12}.[373] The *tv-b* locus, encoding the receptor for both the B and D subgroups of the ASLV, encodes a protein termed CAR1, unrelated to *tv-a* but with sequence similarity to the receptors for tumor necrosis factor (TNF) and the Fas death receptors.[84] The intracellular portion of the molecule contains the sequence of a "death domain," present on other cytotoxic receptors and can trigger the apoptotic death of the cell upon ligand binding. The *tv-c* locus is closely linked to *tv-a* but encodes an unrelated surface protein, one with strong sequence similarity to mammalian butyrophilins, members of the immunoglobulin family.[189] The *tv-e* locus is present in turkey but not chicken and allows for infection by the subgroup E viruses. The gene is orthologous to and was cloned by its sequence similarity to the chicken *tv-b* locus.[5] The receptor for ALV-J receptor is chNHE1, a Na+/H+ exchanger type 1, a multi-membrane pass protein similar to the receptor used for gammaretroviruses.[109]

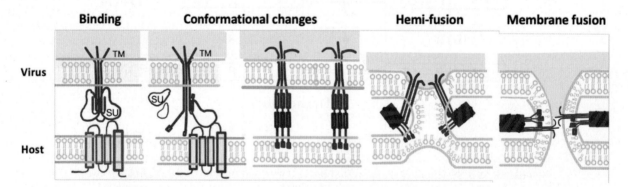

| Binding | Conformational changes | Hemi-fusion | Membrane fusion |

FIGURE 15.7 Intermediate steps in virus entry. Stages of entry from binding to content transfer (membrane fusion) are shown schematically for fusion at the cell surface. Material inside the virus is colored *turquoise*. The Env SU and TM subunits are labeled. Host viral receptor is shown as a multiple membrane pass protein (*brown*). Membranes are colored *orange*. Components of the leucine zippers in TM are boxed in *red* and *purple*. Entry begins with binding of the trimeric Env protein, containing SU and TM subunits, to cell surface receptor. Conformational changes, often associated with eviction of the SU subunit, result in the insertion of a fusion peptide into the cell membrane. Further conformational changes bring the two membranes into proximity and mediate first hemifusion and then full fusion of the bilayers. Expansion of the opening allows entry of the virion core into the cytoplasm.

TABLE 15.3 Retrovirus receptors

Virus(es)	Receptor Name(s)	Function	References
MuLV, ecotropic	CAT-1 (SLC7A1)	Basic amino acid transporter	185,342,486,534,749
MuLV, amphotropic/10A1	Ram-1/GLVR2/PiT-2/ (SLC20A2)	Phosphate transporter	185,342,486,534,749
MuLV 10A1; FeLV-B/T, KoRV-A, GALV	GLVR1/PiT-1 (SLC20A1)	Phosphate transporter	17,324,535,786,801
MuLV, xenotropic; polytropic	Rmc1/XPR1	G-coupled receptor Phosphate exporter	43,412,718,807
M813 ecotropic	SMIT-1 (SLC5A3)	Na/inositol transporter	286,600
GLN MuLV, FeLV TG35-2	RFC (SLC19A1)	Reduced folate/thiamine transporter	489,627
FeLV-A, KoRV-B	THTR1 (SLC19A2)	Thiamine transporter	477,680,802
FeLV-C	Flvcr (SLC49A1/2)	Heme exporter	606,607
MMTV	TfR1	Transferrin receptor	638
ASLV-A	tv-a	LDLR-like Uptake of TCN1 bound Vitamin B$_{12}$	42,134,373,811
ALV-B, -D, -E	tv-b, e	Fas receptor-like	4,5,83,84,688
ALV-C	tv-c	Butyrophilin-like	189
ALV-J	chNHE1	Na+/H+ exchanger type 1	109
PERV-A	HuPAR-1, -2/GPR172A (SLC52A1)	Riboflavin transporter	133,192
PERV-B	SMVT/SLC5A6	Sodium-dependent vitamin transporter	685
RD114, BaEV, MPMV, SNV HERV-W	RDR, RDR2/ASCT1, 2 SLC1A4/5	Glutamate/neutral amino acid transporter	388,613,719
BLV	Blvr-SLC7A1	Cationic amino acid transporter	28,314
JSRV	HYAL2	Hyaluronidase receptor	484,609
HTLV-1	GLUT-1	Glucose transporter	452
HIV-1, HIV-2, SIVs	CD4 plus, CCR5, CXCR4	T-cell differentiation markers; chemokine receptors	183,205,362,442,682
FIV	CD134 plus, CXCR4	T-cell activation/differentiation markers	147,678

Betaretrovirus Receptors

The receptor for MMTV was cloned by cosegregation of DNA markers with virus susceptibility in mouse/hamster radiation chimeric cell lines and so identified as the transferrin receptor tfr1 on mouse chromosome 16.[638] A second receptor for the betaretroviruses was also identified. The type D simian viruses, including MPMV and SRV-1, -2, -4, and -5, show cross-interference with three type C viruses: feline endogenous virus (RD114), baboon endogenous virus (BaEV), and avian reticuloendotheliosis virus (REV), suggesting that they all utilize a common cell surface receptor. Gene transfer of a human cDNA library into nonpermissive mouse cells was used to identify a gene that conferred susceptibility to infection by RD114.[719] The cDNA encoded a protein nearly identical to the previously cloned human Na$^+$–dependent neutral amino acid transporter named Bo.[350,613] Consistent with this similarity, expression of the RD114 receptor in NIH 3T3 cells resulted in enhanced cellular uptake of L-[^{3}H]alanine and L-[^{3}H]glutamine.

Gammaretrovirus Receptors

Several receptors for various gammaretroviruses are known.[717] The mouse gammaretroviruses have been classified on the basis of their receptor usage as ecotropic (eco-, for same), infecting rodent cells; or xenotropic (xeno-, for other), infecting only other species; or amphotropic (ampho-, for other), infecting rodent and more species; or polytropic (poly-, for many), infecting many species like amphotropics but with different interference properties. The first example, the mouse receptor used by the ecotropic MuLVs, was identified by gene transfer to nonpermissive human cells, selecting for susceptibility to MuLV infection.[11] The gene encodes a membrane glycoprotein of 67 kDa containing a total of 14 membrane spanning domains. The normal function of the protein has been identified as a transporter or permease for cationic, basic amino acids.[358] The receptor, termed mCAT-1, was shown to be identical to y+, the previously characterized transporter in mammalian cells. The gene for mCAT-1 is now known as *Atrc1*.

The amphotropic receptor is utilized by a group of murine leukemia viruses derived from wild mice able to infect a wide range of mammalian species, including humans. The receptor was cloned by selection for susceptibility to virus infection after transfection of cDNA libraries into nonpermissive CHO cells[185,486] and by its homology to the gene for the previously identified GALV receptor.[749] The gene, known variously as *Ram1* or GLVR2 or rPiT-2, encodes a sodium-dependent phosphate symporter.[342] The synthesis and stability of the receptor is regulated by phosphate levels, and its down-regulation by virus infection results in substantial reduction in phosphate uptake by cells.

The receptor utilized in common by the gibbon ape leukemia virus, the simian sarcoma-associated helper virus, and the feline leukemia virus subgroup B is widely expressed in many mammals, including primates, cat, dog, mink, rabbit, and rat (but not mouse), as well as in some avian species. The human receptor is termed GLVR1 or hPiT-1.[324,528] The sequence of the gene predicts the existence of 10 membrane-spanning segments and a large third intracellular loop. The protein is a sodium-dependent phosphate symporter.[342,534] Specific amino acid changes introduced into the fourth extracellular loop can block FeLV-B and SSAV infection without affecting GALV, suggesting that these various viruses interact in slightly different ways with the receptor. A remarkable feature of infection by FeLV-B via feline PiT-1 is a requirement for the coexpression of an endogenous Env-like protein dubbed FeLIX.[16]

The xenotropic MuLVs are viruses present as proviruses in the mouse germ line but unable to infect inbred mouse cells. The polytropic MuLVs are also endogenous viruses with a wide host range that includes many mammalian species. Xenotropic and polytropic murine leukemia viruses cross-interfere to various extents in nonmouse species and in wild Asian mice, suggesting that they might use a common receptor for infection. The mouse receptor for the polytropic viruses was cloned by gene transfer and was identified with the *Rmc1* gene.[807] The human xenotropic receptor, XPR1, mediates infection by both the xenotropic and polytropic viruses.[804] The gene encodes a membrane protein related to the yeast Syg1p protein (suppressor of yeast G alpha deletion). XPR1 functions as a phosphate exporter, regulated by $InsP_8$, a member of the inositol pyrophosphate signaling family.[412]

The receptor utilized by the subgroup C feline leukemia viruses (FeLV-C), FLVCR1, encodes a protein with 12 membrane-spanning domains that functions as a heme exporter.[606,607] The binding of virus to this receptor blocks erythroid differentiation and results in red blood cell aplasia, correlating with the pathogenesis of the virus.[606] The FeLV-A receptor is the thiamine transporter THTR1.[477]

Additional receptors for other gammaretroviruses are known to exist. Three characterized porcine endogenous retroviruses (PERV-A, -B, and -C) have been tested in interference assays with each other and with murine viruses using the known receptors, and all three apparently utilize distinct and novel receptors.[20,722] The human PERV-A receptor has been identified as HuPAR1 and -2, known riboflavin transporters.[133,192] Interestingly, screening a library of variant FeLV Envs with random insertions within the receptor-binding domain resulted in convergent receptor utilization for the novel Env CP isolate to similarly utilize HuPAR1, -2 as its receptor.[466,467] PERV-B receptor is the sodium-dependent vitamin transporter (SMVT) (SLC5A6).[685]

Deltaretrovirus Receptors

The receptor for the bovine leukemia virus, BLV, is the CAT1/SLC7A1 protein, a cationic amino acid transporter,[28,314] although it was previously reported to be a protein highly similar to the delta subunit of the AP-3 complex.[34,711] HTLV-1 utilizes the Glut1 glucose transporter as the receptor.[452]

Lentivirus Receptors

The first receptor identified for any retrovirus was the CD4 molecule, established as essential for infection by HIV-1.[151,362,442] CD4 is an important surface protein on T cells and with few exceptions serves to define the helper subset of T cells. CD4 is also expressed at significant levels on dendritic cells, macrophages, and on certain cells in the brain, likely microglia and astrocytes rather than cells of neural origin. The limited distribution of expression of CD4 accounts well for the tropism of HIV-1, largely restricted to helper T cells and macrophages. There may be other routes of entry utilized at lower efficiency: antibody to virus, for example, can promote virus entry into cells by the Fc receptor. Receptor-negative dendritic cells can take up virions and deliver them efficiently to T cells to promote their infection, but even here, infection of the recipient cells requires their expression of the CD4 receptor.[241,379]

Early work established that although CD4 was sufficient to mediate virus binding to a cell surface, it was not sufficient to mediate virus infection and entry. For example, rodent cells and other cells of nonprimate origin could not be successfully infected by HIV-1 even if they were engineered to express human CD4. Searches for genes that would render such cells sensitive to virus infection ultimately led to the identification of various members of the chemokine receptor family, notably CCR5 and CXCR4, as co-receptors needed to mediate the postbinding steps of membrane fusion and virus entry.[183,205,682] Antibodies to the co-receptor as well as the natural ligand for these molecules, the chemokines themselves, can block virus entry. Variants of SIV and HIV-1 have been identified that are CD4 independent, needing only a chemokine receptor for infection; these viruses suggest that the chemokine receptors might have been the primary receptor for a primordial virus. A further proof of the importance of the chemokine receptor is the existence of a mutant allele of the gene encoding CCR5 in the human population, a 32-bp deletion, that confers dramatic virus resistance to homozygous individuals. Relatedly, the feline immunodeficiency virus (FIV) utilizes the CD134 protein, a T-cell activation marker, as the primary receptor, with CXCR4 as the co-receptor.[157,678] More discussion of the roles of CD4 and the co-receptors in virus entry will be presented in the following chapters on HIV-1.

PENETRATION AND UNCOATING

Once virus particles have bound to the receptor, the virion and host membranes fuse together, and the virion core is delivered into the cytoplasm of the infected cell. Entry may require, or be promoted by, membrane regions of special lipid composition termed lipid "rafts".[418,453,596] Virus particles may "surf" or slide across the outside of the cell to preferred locations where fusion or entry inside the cell can occur.[395] For many retroviruses, the processes of fusion and entry are thought to be pH independent; that is, they are not dependent on an endosomal acidification step to induce a pH-dependent change in the conformation of the envelope. Thus, for these viruses, fusion can occur at the cell surface. However, many MuLVs and all avian retroviruses are inhibited by drugs that block acidification, and these viruses thus likely enter by passage through endosomes and low pH-mediated fusion.

The process of fusion involves major rearrangements of the Env proteins and especially includes the exchange of disulfide bonds that exist within or between the TM and SU subunits of Env. The process for the MuLVs seems to be controlled by Ca^{+2} levels and involves TM-SU intersubunit disulfide-bond isomerization and SU dissociation.[761] Entry by HIV-1 probably also involves the removal or shedding of SU. The TM and SU subunits of HIV-1 Env are not held together by disulfide bonds.

The processes of uncoating or opening of the core and its relationship to reverse transcription are poorly understood. It is clear that the previous processing of the Gag precursor to the mature Gag proteins is required for infection; immature virions are uninfectious and cannot initiate reverse transcription, and mutants that prevent particular cleavages of the Gag protein are similarly blocked. A large number of mutant viruses with other alterations in the *gag* gene have been shown to be defective in early steps of infection, before reverse transcription. The course of reverse transcription takes place inside of largely intact core particle. Mutant virions that are fragile and uncoat prematurely or, conversely, are resistant to disassembly, are both poorly infectious, suggesting that the timing of uncoating may be critical.[715] The particles must allow for the deoxynucleotides to enter, and some model structures of the HIV-1 cores suggest that dXTPs may enter through the apices at the sixfold axes, which display pores ringed by positively charged residues. There has been much controversy as to the timing and location of uncoating or disassembly of the virion core. It is likely that there are significant differences among the viruses. The gammaretrovirus cores may shed much of the capsid before their DNA accesses the nucleus during cell mitosis. HIV-1 cores, however, are transported through nuclear pores as intact conical structures, and reverse transcription is only completed after nuclear entry. Uncoating only occurs very late, immediately before integration into the host genome.[403]

Small molecule inhibitors have been used to demonstrate a role of the cytoskeleton in virus entry and furthermore to suggest that viruses may utilize different entry pathways in different cell lines.[361] Biochemical analyses of these early events are made difficult by the presence of large numbers of defective particles that are probably not on the infectious pathway and that tend to obscure the properties of the rare particles that are on this pathway. Nevertheless, examination by fluorescence microscopy of GFP-tagged virion particles during infection has indicated that intracellular movement likely occurs along cytoskeletal fibers.[472]

The TRIM proteins restrict virus infection early in infection, roughly at the time of core transport (see below), and recent studies document a competition between cyclophilin A and TRIM5a for binding to the HIV-1 capsid.[359]

REVERSE TRANSCRIPTION

The reverse transcription of the viral RNA genome into a double-stranded DNA form is the defining hallmark of the retroviruses, and the step from which these viruses derive their name. The course of reverse transcription is complex and highly ordered, involving the initiation of DNA synthesis at precise positions and translocations of DNA intermediates that result in duplication of sequence blocks in the final product (for reviews, see Refs.[246,729]). The major steps in the reaction are relatively well-established, largely through the analysis of reactions carried out *in vitro* in purified virion particles (the so-called endogenous reaction). These *in vitro* reactions have traditionally been very inefficient, with very low yields of double-stranded DNA relative to input RNA genomes. Recently, dramatic improvements in the efficiency of the reactions have been achieved,[122] and a major factor is the inclusion of inositol hexakisphosphate (IP6) in the reactions, which binds to the capsid and stabilizes the core particle.[321]

Reverse transcription normally begins soon after entry of the virion core into the cytoplasm of the infected cell. The reaction takes place in a large complex, roughly resembling the virion core, and containing Gag proteins including CA, NC, RT, IN, and the viral RNA.[76] The signal that triggers the onset of DNA synthesis is not known, though it may be as simple as the exposure of the viral core to the relatively high levels of deoxyribonucleotides present in the cytoplasm. This notion is consistent with the observation that simply stripping or permeabilizing the virion membrane with detergents in the presence of deoxyribonucleotides is sufficient to induce DNA synthesis. This may also be at least part of the explanation for the difficulty HIV has in completing reverse transcription and infection in quiescent cells. In some cells, notably cells arrested by starvation, triphosphate levels may be low and limiting for reverse transcriptase, so that addition of exogenous nucleosides can stimulate viral DNA synthesis. But the events that initiate reverse transcription may be more complicated. Indeed, conformational changes in the RNA genome at the tRNA primer site may trigger DNA synthesis.[46]

DNA synthesis can be initiated "prematurely" during virion assembly and release, such that virion preparations can be shown to contain small amounts of the early DNA intermediates. In most cases, the levels of these DNAs are very low, indicating that only a very small minority of the virion particles have carried out any significant synthesis. However, some circumstances affecting the rate of production and release of virions may enhance this synthesis. In addition, in some particular retroviruses, notably the spumaviruses, substantial DNA synthesis occurs during assembly, such that the major form of the genome found in mature virions is a partially or even completely reverse-transcribed DNA molecule.[490,815] These viruses thus resemble the hepadnaviruses more closely than the conventional retroviruses in the relative timing of assembly and reverse transcription.

Reverse transcription has traditionally been considered to occur strictly in the cytoplasm, and indeed, very early work showed that enucleated cells—with no nucleus—could support reverse transcription of incoming retroviral RNA into DNA.[750] Furthermore, when cells arrested in the cell cycle by aphidicolin are infected with MuLVs, viral pre-integrative complexes (PICs) containing full-length viral DNAs are formed in the cytoplasm, and these PICs are capable of integration when extracted and tested *in vitro*.[634] But recent results suggest that at least for HIV-1, reverse transcription is completed only later, after entry into the nucleus.[166,216] This finding raises the implication that an intact or largely intact PIC must pass through a nuclear pore to enter the nucleus.

Steps in Reverse Transcription of the Retroviral Genome

The course of reverse transcription is complex. The reaction can be broken down into a series of discrete steps,[246] as presented in Figure 15.8.

Formation of Minus Strand Strong Stop DNA

The process of reverse transcription is initiated from the paired 3′ OH of a primer tRNA annealed to the viral RNA genome at a complementary sequence termed the primer binding site (pbs). DNA is first synthesized from this primer, using the plus strand RNA genome as template, to form minus strand DNA sequences. Synthesis occurs toward the 5′ end of the RNA to generate U5 and R sequences. The intermediate formed in this step is termed minus strand strong stop DNA. The primer tRNA remains attached to its 5′ end.

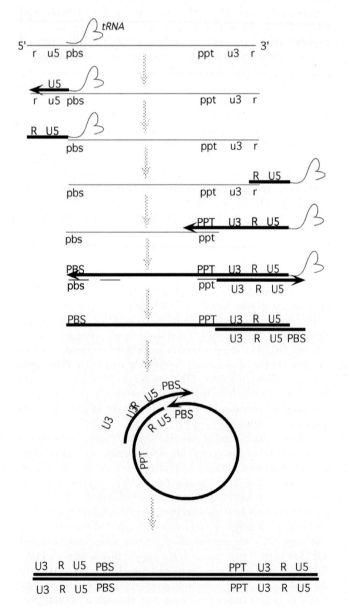

FIGURE 15.8 The reverse transcription of the retroviral genome. *Thin lines* represent RNA; *thick lines* represent DNA. See text for details. (Modified drawing courtesy of A. Telesnitsky.)

First Translocation

The next step involves the translocation, or "jump," of the strong stop DNA from the 5′ to the 3′ end of the genome. This translocation requires the degradation of those 5′ RNA sequences that were placed in RNA:DNA hybrid form by the formation of strong stop DNA. The degradation is mediated by the RNase H activity of RT, separate from its DNA polymerase activity, and specifically able to degrade RNA present in RNA:DNA hybrid form. RT mutants with altered RNase H activity do not mediate the translocation. This step exposes the single-stranded DNA and facilitates its annealing to the r sequences at the 3′ end of the genome.[117] Normally, a full-length strong stop DNA, synthesized by copying to the 5′ cap of the RNA, performs the translocation, though incomplete molecules can jump at low efficiency. The NC protein may facilitate the transfer step. Although there have been reports that jumping is always in *trans*, from one RNA template to the other RNA in the virion, the best evidence is that minus strand strong stop jumping goes randomly to either RNA.

Long Minus Strand DNA Synthesis

The annealing of minus strand strong stop DNA recreates a suitable primer–template structure for DNA synthesis, and RT can now continue to elongate the minus strand strong stop DNA to form long minus strand products. Synthesis ends in the vicinity of the pbs. As the genome enters RNA:DNA hybrid form, the RNA becomes susceptible to RNase H action and is degraded.

Initiation of Plus Strand DNA Synthesis

The primer for plus strand synthesis is created by the digestion of the genomic RNA by RNase H. A particular short purine-rich sequence near the 3′ end of the genome, the polypurine tract (ppt), is relatively resistant to the activity of RNase H. The ppt remains hybridized to the minus strand DNA and serves as the primer for synthesis of the plus strand DNA, using the minus strand DNA as template. The sequence of the ppt, an unusual structure of the nucleic acid at the ppt, and residues of the RNase H domain of RT have all been implicated in defining the cleavages that form the primer. Sequences upstream of the polypurine tract, an AT-rich region called the T-box, are also important for proper priming. The primer, once it has served to initiate DNA synthesis, is removed from the DNA. Synthesis proceeds toward the 5′ end of the minus strand, first copying the U3, R, and U5 sequences and then extending further to copy a portion of the primer tRNA still present at its 5′ end. Elongation stops at a modified base (1-methyladenosine, m1A) normally found at position 19 of the tRNA. The resulting intermediate is termed plus strand strong stop DNA.

In some viruses, secondary plus strand initiation sites are used. There may be multiple RNA primers generated from the RNA genome by the nuclease action of RNase H that can initiate DNA synthesis at dispersed heterogeneous sites. In the case of the lentiviruses and spumaviruses, a second copy of the ppt sequence near the center of the genome is used at high efficiency and is important for proper completion of reverse transcription.[112]

Removal of tRNA

In the next step, the primer tRNA at the 5′ end of the minus strand DNA is removed by RNase H. Its removal may occur in two stages: with an initial cleavage near the RNA–DNA junction and a second one within the tRNA. The cleavage need not occur exactly at the RNA–DNA junction, and a single ribonucleotide base (A) is normally left on the 5′ terminus of the HIV-1 minus strand without affecting subsequent processes. The posttranscriptional modifications present in the natural tRNA are probably important for proper recognition by RT and for plus strand strong stop translocation.

The Second Translocation

The removal of the tRNA exposes the 3′ end of the plus strand strong stop DNA to permit its pairing with the 3′ end of the minus strand DNA. The sequences anneal via the shared pbs sequences. This annealing forms a circular intermediate, with both 3′ termini in a suitable structure for elongation.

Completion of Both Strands

Both strands are now elongated. The final extension of the minus strand DNA is coupled to displacement of the plus strand strong stop DNA from the 5′ end of the minus strand; as minus strand elongation occurs, the plus strand strong stop is peeled away and transferred to the 3′ end of the minus strand. At the end of this elongation, the circle is opened up into a linear DNA. The plus strands are then extended. When multiple plus strand initiation events have occurred, the completed plus strand will consist of adjacent fragments and so contain nicks or discontinuities. Displacement synthesis by an upstream fragment can slowly displace downstream RNAs and DNAs, leading to longer plus strands. However, some nicks, gaps, or overlapping flaps may persist in the final double-stranded product. These breaks may be at heterogeneous positions, though strong sites of plus strand initiation, such as the one at the central ppt of lentiviruses, can lead to specific sites for such discontinuities. Sequences near the central ppt of the lentiviruses cause termination of synthesis during elongation from upstream primers, thus ensuring the maintenance of a discontinuity at this site.[113] This site retains a partially displaced sequence or overlap of a few nucleotides—99 nt in the case of HIV-1. The structure has been shown to persist even to the time of integration of the DNA into the cell. Host DNA repair processes ultimately correct all such discontinuities.

Although most of the viral DNA is made in the cytoplasm, it may not always be completed in the cytoplasm. For some viruses (including, notably, HIV-1), completion of the two DNA strands may occur only after entry into the nucleus. Specific mutants with alterations in the Cys-His residues of the NC protein show an interesting phenotype: the formation of linear DNA with heterogeneous and truncated ends.[253] These experiments suggest that NC plays a role in the completion, or the stabilization of the ends, of the viral DNA.

A key consequence of the two translocation events that occur during reverse transcription is the duplication of sequences—duplication of U5 during minus strand strong stop DNA translocation and of U3 during plus strand strong stop DNA translocation. The resulting DNA thus contains two long terminal repeats, or LTRs, that have been assembled during reverse transcription. Each LTR consists of the sequence blocks U3-R-U5. The positions of the LTR edges—the left edge of U3 and the right edge of U5—are determined by the sites of initiation of DNA synthesis for the two DNA strands. Thus,

the terminal sequences of the complete DNA molecule are also determined by these sites of initiation. These sequences for most viruses are perfect or imperfect inverted repeats and serve an important role during integration of the DNA (see below).

Biochemistry and Structure of Reverse Transcriptase

The enzyme that mediates the complex series of events outlined above is reverse transcriptase (RT), one of the most famous of the viral polymerases[33]; for review, see Ref.[686]. All RTs contain two separate activities present in two separate domains: a DNA polymerase able to incorporate deoxyribonucleotides on either an RNA or a DNA template, and an RNase H activity able to degrade RNA only in duplex form. These two activities are responsible for the various steps of reverse transcription. Two distinct domains of the enzyme contain these two activities: an amino-terminal domain contains the DNA polymerase and a carboxy-terminal domain contains the RNase H activity.[724] While isolated domains can be shown to exhibit either one of the two activities separately, an intact enzyme is required for full activity and specificity. However, for the MuLVs, the two functions can be provided by two mutant RT molecules, each defective in either the polymerase or the RNAseH domain, so long as they are co-incorporated into a single virion.

DNA Polymerase

The DNA polymerase activity is similar to that of all host and viral polymerases in requiring a primer, which can be either RNA or DNA, and a template—but unlike most DNA polymerases, the template can also be either RNA or DNA. RTs incorporate dXTPs to a growing 3′OH end with release of PPi and require divalent cations, usually Mg++. The primer must contain a 3′ OH end that is paired with the template. RTs cannot perform nick translation reactions, but they can efficiently perform strand displacement synthesis. Strand displacement is stimulated by the addition of the nucleocapsid protein (NC). The only fundamental way in which RTs are unusual among the DNA polymerases is that they exhibit comparable specific activity on either DNA or RNA templates.

RTs are readily isolated from purified virion particles and can be even more easily prepared as recombinant proteins expressed in bacteria. RTs are relatively slow DNA polymerases, under standard conditions only incorporating 1 to 100 nucleotides per second, depending on the template. Further, they exhibit poor processivity and tend to release primer–template frequently *in vitro*. The enzyme must then rebind to the substrate to continue synthesis. Secondary structures in RNA templates can strongly enhance the pausing of RT and its tendency to release from the template.[279] The enzyme also exhibits low fidelity, and though the error rates vary widely with the primer, template and type of assay, the misincorporation rate of most RTs under physiological conditions *in vitro* is on the order of 10^{-4} errors per base incorporated. This rate suggests that during replication, there would be approximately one mutation per genome per reverse transcription cycle. Indeed, the mutation rate observed *in vivo* is roughly consistent with this high error rate, though fidelity *in vivo* may be somewhat better than *in vitro*. Drug-resistant variants of HIV-1 RT that do not incorporate chain-terminating analogues are often found to exhibit higher fidelity, perhaps because they require a more precise fit for the correct incoming triphosphate to allow for discrimination against the analogue. A wide range of types of mutations are created by RT errors, and both the type and the frequency of appearance of each type of mutation exhibit a complex dependence on sequences and structures in the template.

Reverse transcriptases do not generally exhibit a proofreading nuclease activity,[44] and misincorporated bases are not removed efficiently by most RTs as they are by host DNA polymerases. However, mutants of the HIV-1 RT resistant to 5′ azido-thymidine (AZT) have been shown to exhibit an enhanced ability to remove the incorporated AZT moiety at the 3′ end through an ATP-mediated excision pathway that releases AZTppppA, with AZT resistance mutations favoring the excision pathway.[482,740] Thus, it is possible for RT to remove some such analogues and rescue a terminated chain for continued elongation.

RNase H

The RNase H activity of RT is an endonuclease that releases oligonucleotides with a 3′ OH and a 5′ PO_4. This property allows the products of RNase H action to serve as primers for initiation of DNA synthesis by the DNA polymerase function of RT. There is an obligate requirement that the RNA be in duplex form, normally an RNA-DNA hybrid. However, retroviral RTs are also able to degrade some RNA-RNA duplexes, an activity termed RNaseH*.[298] The RNase H enzyme is capable of acting on the RNA of a template in concert with the polymerase as it moves along a nucleic acid and as it does so its active site is located about 17 to 18 bp behind the growing 3′ end.[251] RNase H can also act independently of polymerization. All RNase H activity requires a divalent cation, usually Mg^{++}.

Subunit Structures

RT is incorporated into the virion particle during assembly in the form of a large Gag-Pol precursor (see below) and is released by proteolytic processing of the precursor during virion maturation. Different viruses make somewhat different cleavages in the precursor, and thus, the RTs exhibit several different subunit structures (see below). In the gammaretroviruses, RT is a simple monomer in solution, corresponding only to the amino-terminal DNA polymerase and the carboxy-terminal RNase H domains. These two domains can be expressed separately, and the isolated proteins exhibit their respective activities,[724] though the specificity of the RNase H is affected by this separation. In the alpharetroviruses, the RT is present as an ab heterodimer, comprised of a smaller a subunit containing the DNA polymerase and RNase H domains; and a larger b subunit containing these two domains but also retaining the integrase domain. In the lentiviruses, RT is again a heterodimer with a larger subunit (p66) containing the DNA polymerase and RNase H domains, and a smaller subunit (p51) lacking RNase H. The properties of the different enzymes as DNA polymerases are very similar in spite of these different subunit structures, and so the significance of these various compositions for RT function is unclear. A curious observation was made that some RT inhibitors—the so-called nonnucleoside RT inhibitors—can enhance the association of p66 and p51, locking them into an inactive dimer.[716]

Crystal Structures of RTs

The three-dimensional structure of a number of RTs have been determined by x-ray crystallographic studies and electron microscopy with over 190 unique structures deposited into the Protein Data Bank (www.rcsb.org). These structures include the unliganded HIV-1 RT,[302,632] drug-resistant mutants of RT, RT bound to nucleoside RT inhibitors (NRTIs), nonnucleoside RT inhibitors (NNRTIs), dsRNA initiation complexes, duplex DNA and RNA:DNA hybrid elongation complexes, RNA:DNA hybrid substrates poised and at a distance for RNase H hydrolysis, RNA pseudoknot inhibitors, and tertiary complexes of nucleotide substrates with template–primers (for review, see Ref.[799]). The two subunits of HIV-1 RT are folded quite differently so that the overall structure is highly asymmetric. The structure of the p66 is similar to that of a right hand, with fingers, palm, and thumb domains named on the basis of their position in the structure (Fig. 15.9). The nucleic acid lies in the grip of the hand, held by the fingers and thumb. The YXDD motif present at the active site for the DNA polymerase lies at the base of the palm. The RNase H domain is attached to the hand at the wrist. The p51 subunit, while made up of the same domains as the amino-terminal part of p66, is folded differently and lies under the hand, not making direct contact to the nucleic acid and so thought to serve a structural role, but not to participate in chemistry. The structure of p66 with and without a liganded nucleic acid is quite different, with the thumb domain flexing to allow substrate binding. Compilation of these structures reveals the complex movement of the individual fingers, palm, connection, thumb, and RNase H domains to accommodate the distinct substrates required for reverse transcription as well as the coordination between the polymerase and RNase H domains. Additional studies are currently focusing on the structure of the p66 homodimer and the process of unwinding/exposing the protease cleavage site for generation of p51.[799]

Structures of the fingers and palm subdomain and of the complete Moloney MuLV RT at very high resolution have also been determined.[155,243] The monomeric protein is broadly similar to the p66 subunit of HIV-1 RT.

RT Inhibitors

RT is a major target of antiviral drugs useful in the treatment of retroviral diseases such as AIDS. All FDA-approved drugs targeting RT used to date are inhibitors of the DNA polymerase activity and fall into two classes: nucleoside analogue inhibitors (NRTIs, chain terminators) and nonnucleoside RT inhibitors (NNRTIs).[201] The nucleoside analogues are typically unphosphorylated precursors or prodrugs and need to be activated by phosphorylation to the triphosphate form. These are then incorporated by RT into the growing chain and serve to block further elongation. Early inhibitors included dideoxyinosine (ddI) and dideoxycytosine (ddC). Examples of current clinically approved NRTIs include abacavir (ABC), emtricitabine (FTC), lamivudine (3TC), tenofovir disoproxil fumarate (tenofovir DF, TDF), stavudine (d4T), and zidovudine (AZT, azidothymidine). Islatravir (EFdA) is an NRTI that shows promise for acting as a long-acting drug with high potency and long half-life, functioning as a translocation inhibitor.[648,683,809]

The NNRTIs are a group of compounds that are structurally diverse but nevertheless interact with a common binding pocket (NNIBP) located at the base of the RT p66 thumb domain, changing the conformation of the protein to an extended conformation.[683,726,742] FDA-approved NNRTIs include rilpivirine (RPV), etravirine (ETR), delavirdine (DLV), doravirine (DOR), efavirenz (EFV), and nevirapine (NVP).

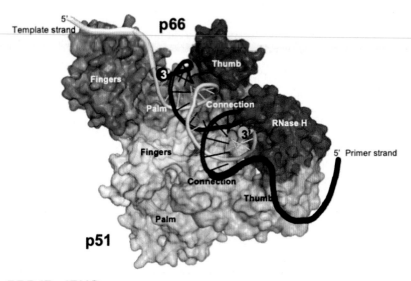

PDB ID: 4PUO

FIGURE 15.9 Schematic image of the heterodimeric p66 p51RT reverse transcriptase of human immunodeficiency virus type 1 (HIV-1, PDB ID 4PUO). The molecule is arranged in the conventional orientation to show its similarity to the human right hand, palm up. Fingers, thumb, palm, connection, and RNase H domains of each subunit are indicated (p66 *top*, individual domains labeled in *white*) and p51 (*bottom*, individual domains labeled in *black*). An RNA template strand (*grey line*) and a DNA primer strand (*black line*) are modeled into the polymerase (Pol) and RNase H (RH) active sites.

Nevirapine has been developed in an extended-release formulation. Long-acting NNRTIs under investigation include dapivirine (DPV), rilpivirine (RPV), and elsulfavirine.

Monotherapy with a single drug selects for drug-resistant variants that quickly predominate in the virus population. These variants typically exist before treatment in the swarm of replicating virus in a patient, termed the viral quasispecies, due to the high mutation rate of RT and, importantly, to the large population size and large number of replication cycles that characterize HIV-1 infection. For each drug, a pattern of mutations has been identified that serves to indicate the appearance of drug resistance[386] and provide insight into the mechanism of action of the drug as well as of escape. In many cases, these mutations alter the binding side for the nucleoside or NNRTI such that the drug cannot bind and so cannot inhibit the enzyme. In the case of AZT, however, the mutations do not prevent the binding and incorporation of AZTTP into the growing chain but rather activate a reverse reaction in which the AZT nucleotide is removed from the chain, subsequently permitting normal elongation.[482,740] Combination therapy, typically involving the simultaneous treatment with three different drugs, can suppress virus replication to such an extent that variants resistant to all the drugs do not appear, at least for months or years. Preexposure prophylaxis (PrEP) regimens contain single or double antiviral combinations.

RECOMBINATION

The process of reverse transcription could in principle take place using a single template RNA molecule. In fact, however, retrovirions contain two copies of the RNA genome co-packaged into one particle, and the course of reverse transcription typically makes use of both RNAs.[303,707] Recombination occurs between homologous sequences in the two RNAs, and it happens at surprisingly high frequencies, more than once—even a dozen times or more—per replication cycle per genome on average.[626,831] These events allow for successful virus infection even when there are breaks in the RNA genomes, because RT can translocate to the other genome to complete the minus DNA strand. Normally, the two RNAs in a virion are identical, so that homologous recombination events are invisible and without genetic consequence. When the two co-packaged RNAs are distinct, however, as when they derive from two viruses or viral strains expressed in the same cell, the result is a very high frequency of recombination between them in the resulting proviral DNAs. Thus, physical markers and genetic markers recombine rapidly whenever the two genomes are co-packaged into one virion and so are coextant during a single round of reverse transcription. The frequency is highly dependent on the sequence and structure of the RNA in the region undergoing recombination. Similar recombination does not occur at high frequency when cells are coinfected simultaneously with two separate virus preparations, suggesting that each incoming virus particle performs its own reverse transcription reaction in *cis* and does not freely exchange RNAs with other reactions happening in the same cell.

Models for Recombination

High-frequency recombination mainly occurs during minus strand synthesis by a copy choice mechanism.[830] As RT proceeds along an RNA, it has the potential to carry out a template switch in which an incomplete DNA copied from one template serves to prime further elongation on the other RNA molecule.[436,573] Pausing may enhance this transfer, and so secondary structures in the RNA may act as hot spots for such recombination. Breaks in the RNA genome, which may be encountered often, cause a "forced copy choice": transfer to the other RNA. This rescues an otherwise dead virus and may represent the major evolutionary basis for the diploid genome. The RNase H activity of RT may help release an incomplete DNA and so promote its serving as primer on the new template, and NC also facilitates the reaction.[517]

The translocation of the strong stop DNAs provides a special opportunity for recombination between the two viral genomes. When the minus strand strong stop DNA is formed, it has the potential to translocate from the 5' end of its template to the 3' end of either RNA molecule; though this event has been reported to occur strictly in *cis*, or strictly in *trans*, it most likely occurs randomly. Similarly, when plus strand strong stop DNA is formed, it too could in principle translocate to the 3' end of either minus strand. However, this translocation seems most often to occur in *cis*, perhaps simply because the frequency with which two long minus strand DNAs are successfully formed, and so are available to serve as acceptors, is low.

Recombination between two RNAs during reverse transcription can also occur between nonhomologous sites at lower frequency. Reconstructions suggest that these events are perhaps 100 to 1,000 times less frequent than homologous recombination. These events can result in duplications or deletions in the DNA product of the reaction. Furthermore, if nonviral RNAs or chimeric RNAs containing viral and nonviral sequences are packaged into virions, such nonhomologous recombination events can create new joints and link a viral sequence to the nonviral sequences. These events are thought to play a central role in the process of transduction of cellular genes and most importantly during the formation of acute oncogenic retroviral genomes (see below).

INTEGRATION OF THE PROVIRAL DNA

The integration of the linear retroviral DNA, like reverse transcription, is a crucial and defining feature of the retroviral life cycle. Integration is required for efficient replication of most retroviruses; mutants that are unable to integrate do not establish a spreading infection. The orderly and efficient integration of viral DNA is unique to the retroviruses. Although infection by some DNA viruses can result in the integration of viral DNA fragments into the host genome at low efficiency, these events are not the result of specific viral functions. Further, the establishment of the integrated provirus is responsible for much of retroviral biology. It accounts for the ability of the viruses to persist in the infected cell; for their ability to permanently enter the germ line; and for the mutagenic and oncogenic activities of some viruses. It also establishes a reservoir of latently infected cells in HIV-1–infected individuals that resists antiviral drug therapy and that can be reactivated to induce virus replication.

Once the provirus is established, the DNA is permanently incorporated into the genome of the infected cell. There is no mechanism by which it can be efficiently eliminated. At very low frequencies, homologous recombination between the two LTRs can delete most of the provirus, but even here, a single ("solo") LTR remains.[752] As the host cell divides, the provirus is transmitted to daughter cells as a new mendelian locus. Thus, it is likely to persist in the cell for its normal life span, and, if the integrated provirus is intact, to convert the cell permanently to a chronic producer of progeny virus.

Unintegrated DNA Forms

The product of the reverse transcription reaction, as outlined above, is a full-length double-stranded linear DNA version of the genome, flanked at each end by copies of the LTR. The next step is the movement of the DNA into the nucleus and the appearance of two new DNA forms: closed circular molecules containing either one or two tandem copies of the LTR (Fig. 15.10). A small amount of the one-LTR circle may be formed during reverse transcription (see above), but the bulk is thought to be formed by homologous recombination between the two LTRs of the linear DNA. The tandem two-LTR circles are formed by the blunt-end ligation of the termini of the linear DNA using nonhomologous end-joining machinery of the host. This event creates a unique sequence, termed the LTR-LTR junction, that is often used as a hallmark of nuclear entry of the viral DNA. The joints are often imperfect, with loss of nucleotides from one or both termini at the joint.[689,776] There are also some circles that arise by autointegration of the ends of the linear DNA into internal sites, forming DNAs with deletions or inversions[679]; these circles are generally nonfunctional in terms of generating progeny virus.

Three distinct unintegrated DNA forms—one linear and two circular—coexist in the nucleus. It is now clear that circles are not efficient substrates in the integration reaction and that the immediate precursor for the integration reaction is the linear duplex DNA. The circles are apparently dead-end products of a side reaction, formed by host enzymes acting on linear DNAs that have failed to integrate. There are settings and cell types in which unintegrated viral DNAs are observed to accumulate to high levels; various tissues in human HIV disease show considerable amounts of circular DNAs. While this DNA may reflect some unusual processing of the DNA, much of it is probably formed simply by massive infection occurring shortly before the DNA is harvested.

Unintegrated retroviral DNAs are not efficiently expressed[645] but rather are heavily silenced at the level of transcription.[511,594] The silencing is largely relieved by the histone deacetylase trichostatin A, suggesting that it involves chromatin modifications.[572,656] The viral DNAs are loaded with nucleosomes upon entry into the nucleus, and the histones are rapidly marked with covalent modifications characteristic of silent chromatin, including high levels of trimethylation on H3 lysine 9 (H3K9me3) and low levels of acetylation (H3Ac).[242,764] Screens have identified several host factors involved in mediating the silencing.[180,838] Mutant viruses that cannot integrate are unable to establish an efficient spreading infection, although low levels of virus can be produced,[664] and integrase inhibitors are very effective at blocking HIV-1 replication *in vivo*. A very small subset of cells infected with such integration-defective mutants do integrate viral sequences through nonviral means, creating oligomeric tandem repeats similar to those formed after naked DNA-mediated transformation.[272] Including an SV40 origin of DNA replication on a retroviral genome, and driving the initiation of DNA replication of the unintegrated circular forms in cells expressing SV40 T antigen, can allow for viral expression and spread.[432] The HIV-1 Vpr protein, brought into cells by HIV-1 virion particles, can significantly relieve the silencing.[593,594] Curiously, cells expressing the HTLV-1 Tax protein also promote expression from unintegrated HIV-1 DNAs.[311]

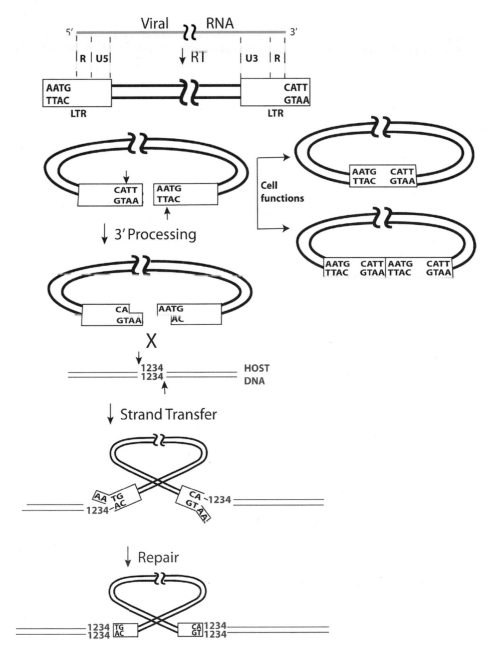

FIGURE 15.10 Schematic of the integration process. *Top:* Unintegrated DNA structures formed after retroviral infection. The incoming RNA genome (*top*) is converted by RT to a double-stranded linear DNA containing two LTRs (*boxes*). The termini of the DNA consist of short inverted repeats and always contain a conserved CA dinucleotide near the 3' ends; the 3' terminal sequences of the MuLVs (CATT) are shown. The linear DNA is then localized to the nucleus, and two circular double-stranded DNAs are formed: a circle containing one LTR, and a circle containing two tandem LTRs. The LTR-LTR junction contains a unique inverted repeat sequence. The linear double-stranded DNA is also processed by the viral integrase with the endonucleolytic removal of dinucleotides at the 3' termini to serve as precursor of the integrated provirus. The target site in the host DNA is here indicated by the arbitrary sequence block denoted 1234. Integration occurs by joining the 3' CA dinucleotides in a strand transfer reaction in which the 3' OH ends attack phosphodiester bonds of the target site DNA to make staggered breaks in the two strands. The reaction is associated with loss of two base pairs at the termini of the viral DNA and with duplication of a small number of base pairs (four shown here) initially present only once in the target DNA. *Bottom:* The resulting gapped intermediate is subsequently repaired by host enzymes.

Entry Into the Nucleus

A key step that must take place before integration can occur is the entry of the viral DNA into the nucleus. The mechanisms of nuclear entry are not fully understood, but there are at least two distinct routes used by different retroviruses. The simple retroviruses show a profound requirement for the infected cell to pass through mitosis for successful establishment of the integrated provirus,[402,485,634,751] and the block in nondividing cells is at or close to the step of nuclear entry. Tests of the state of the viral DNA in nondividing cells are consistent with the notion that the preintegration complex must await the breakdown of the nuclear membrane in order to have access to the cellular DNA. Infection of nondividing cells results in the accumulation of linear double-stranded DNA in the cytoplasm and no further signs of infection. The viral DNA will persist in the cell for some time, and if the cell is stimulated to undergo division, the viral DNA will integrate and infection will proceed. However, the DNA loses its capacity to become activated in this way fairly rapidly.[18,485] Some simple retroviruses are not strongly dependent on mitosis,[281] and some postmitotic cell types may be somewhat susceptible to infection.[422] For many viruses, the restriction is quantitatively very significant and profoundly limits the utility of simple retroviral vectors for gene therapy. The restriction can be beneficial in some settings, allowing specific targeting of mitotic cells.

In contrast, the lentiviruses and spumaviruses are able to successfully infect nondividing cells, suggesting that there must be an active transport of the viral DNA through an intact nuclear membrane.[91,401,402,513,772] This capability has made lentiviruses, especially HIV-1, very attractive as gene delivery vectors for gene therapy applications. The molecular basis for this capability is becoming much clearer. Experiments suggest that the CA protein of the incoming PIC defines competence for nuclear import.[803] The lentiviral CA may serve to deliver the PIC to particular Nups, nuclear pore components, to initiate import. Studies of HIV-1 mutants with single changes in CA suggest that PICs can be imported via either of two alternative pathways, with wild-type virus using Nup153 and TNP03, and the CA-N74D mutant using Nup155.[120,375,392,462,463] Other studies have implicated Nup98 in HIV-1 PIC entry into the nucleus.[182] Motor proteins may also be involved: studies have shown that motor Kif5B and pore protein Nup358 work together to mediate nuclear import.[167] Another study of import *in vitro* has suggested that another specific importer protein, importin 7, is required for PIC entry,[200,822] though this has been disputed.[839] Fractionation of extracts using similar *in vitro* import assays showed, remarkably, that tRNAs can promote uptake of PICS into nuclei.[823] Whether tRNAs mediate import *in vivo* remains uncertain.

The timing and mechanisms of nuclear import of HIV-1 PICs, and especially the relationship of import to the timing of completion of reverse transcription and virion uncoating, has recently been brought into sharper focus. The host factor CPSF6 regulates the efficiency and timing of nuclear entry for HIV-1 PICs through direct interactions of CPSF6 and the capsid.[47] This interaction is also affected by the host factor cyclophilin A (CypA), which binds to a similar site on CA and may delay or inhibit nuclear import.[835] Super-resolution imaging and other methods indicate that a large conical particle, perhaps a nearly intact core, is imported through the nuclear pores[840] and that uncoating of the viral core is accomplished only within the nucleus.[92,403,500,668] The process of HIV-1 reverse transcription itself has been shown to be completed only after nuclear entry, finishing immediately before integration.[166,668] These recent findings are provoking redrafting of many figures in textbooks presenting the course of early events of infection.

The foamy viruses may have a distinctive route of nuclear entry involving microtubular transport by dynein and centrosomal association, but the mechanism is not yet well understood.[583,644]

Structure of the Provirus

An important aspect of retroviral integration that distinguishes the process from nonviral or other viral mechanisms of DNA integration is the fact that the insertions create a consistent provirus structure. The integrated provirus is collinear with the product of reverse transcription and consists of a 5′ LTR, the intervening viral sequences, and a 3′ LTR, inserted cleanly into host sequences. The joints between host and viral DNA are always at the same sites, very near the edges of the viral LTRs. As compared to the unintegrated linear DNA, there is a loss of a small number of base pairs, usually two, from each terminus of the viral DNA, and there is a duplication of a small number of base pairs of host DNA initially present once at the site of insertion that flank the provirus (Fig. 15.10). The number of base pairs duplicated is characteristic of each virus and ranges from 4 to 6 bp.

Biochemistry of Integration

The integration of the viral DNA into a target is mediated by the viral integrase protein, IN,[558,608,664] which is brought into the cell inside the virion and acts to insert the linear DNA into the host chromosome. Some aspects of IN function have been studied by analysis of viral DNA formed *in vivo*.[639] Most of our understanding of IN function, however, has been obtained through analysis of *in vitro* integration reactions, using complexes extracted from infected cells,[86,226] or using recombinant IN protein. Efforts have led to the identification of conditions and factors that promote the formation of an active PIC and that enhance concerted joining.[8,212,759] Once such a protein–nucleic acid complex is formed, it is quite stable. Recently, dramatic improvements in the efficiency of coupled reverse transcription–integration reactions carried out *in vitro* have allowed much more detailed study of the requirements for both steps and demonstrate the retention of the CA protein as a key player.[122]

The integration reaction proceeds in two steps: 3′ end processing and strand transfer. A schematic view of these reactions is shown in Figure 15.10.

3′ End Processing

In the first step, the two terminal nucleotides at the 3′ ends of the blunt-ended linear DNA are removed by the integrase to produce recessed 3′ ends and correspondingly protruding 5′ ends. This cleavage occurs endonucleolytically at a highly conserved CA sequence and releases a dinucleotide. For most viruses, the terminal sequence is such that a TT dinucleotide is released, though this rule has exceptions. The ends do not remain covalently bound to protein, and the energy of the hydrolyzed phosphodiester bond is not retained.

Strand Transfer

In the second step, the 3′ OH ends created by processing are used in a strand transfer reaction to attack the phosphodiester bonds of the target DNA.[226] The formation of the new phosphodiester bond between the viral end and the host DNA displaces one of the phosphodiester bonds in the host DNA, leaving a nick. The protruding 5′ end of the viral DNA is not joined to the host DNA by IN. The reaction is a direct transesterification, and so no ATP or other energy source is required. Mutational studies strongly suggest that the two activities—processing and joining—utilize the same active site residues. In fact, the two steps involve similar chemistry: 3′ end processing is an attack on DNA by a hydroxyl residue of water, while joining is an attack on DNA by a 3′ hydroxyl residue of another DNA.

The integrase has been a highly successful target of inhibitors that have provided a major class of antiviral therapies in the treatment of AIDS (for review, see Ref.[692]). Current inhibitors of IN block the strand transfer reactions, named integrase strand transfer inhibitors (INSTIs). All INSTIs contain a metal-chelating component that binds to the metals within the IN active in the presence of the viral LTR DNA. The presence of the INSTI displaces the terminal A of the vDNA and blocks the binding of the host target DNA.[193,264] FDA-approved drugs include raltegravir (RAL), dolutegravir (DTG), elvitegravir and bictegravir (as a combination treatment), and cabotegravir (CAB). CAB is a long-acting INSTI, currently approved by the FDA as a once-monthly injection along with the NNRTI rilpivirine (https://www.fda.gov/drugs/drug-approvals-and-databases/drug-trials-snapshot-cabenuva).[715] Figure 15.11 shows the structures of three viral integrases (PFV,[481] RSV,[555] and HIV-1[406]) in the context of the cleaved synaptic complex in the presence of INSTIs.

Disintegration

The IN protein exhibits a third enzymatic activity *in vitro*: a reversal of the integration reaction known as disintegration.[119] This activity releases DNA from a branched structure and seals the nick at the site of the branch. Once the integration reaction is complete at both ends and gaps are repaired, this structure is no longer available, and the significance of the activity *in vivo* is uncertain.

Target Site Duplication

In a wild-type virus, when the two ends are joined to the two strands of the target DNA, the two sites of attack are staggered by a few (4 to 6) base pairs. After the joining, the resulting structure contains short gaps in the host DNA and unpaired bases from each 5′ end of the viral DNA. The 5′ ends of the viral DNA are not joined to host DNA by any known activities of IN. However, they are very quickly repaired *in vivo*, almost as quickly as the initial integration reaction.[633] The processing and filling in the gaps creates a short duplication of sequence that was present only once at the target site; these duplications flank the integrated provirus. The number of bases duplicated is characteristic of each virus. Thus, the gammaretroviruses cause a 4 bp duplication; HIV-1 causes a 5 bp duplication; and the alphretroviruses cause a 6 bp duplication.

Viral att Sites

The sequences at the termini of the viral DNA, the *att* sites, are recognized by the viral IN protein and are important for end processing and joining.[94,127,132,754] These terminal sequences are imperfect inverted repeats. The most conserved residues are a CA dinucleotide pair that lies near the 3′ terminus and determines the site of 3′ processing. Sequences upstream from

the CA for perhaps 10 to 12 bp are needed for efficient integration, but these sequences are different for different viruses, with no indication of broadly conserved sequence motifs. Since the two termini of any given virus are somewhat different, they usually show differential efficiency of utilization in various assays. The fact that two distinct ends are bound together in a complex may be important for the concerted integration of these ends into the target.[758]

Both 3′ processing and strand transfer reactions are concerted reactions *in vivo*. The processing step occurs simultaneously at both termini of the viral DNA and requires the correct sequences at both termini. Indeed, for MuLV, a mutation altering the sequence at one end of the viral DNA was found to block the processing reaction at both ends.[508] This result suggests that the reaction requires both termini to be loaded into a complex before hydrolysis proceeds.

Structure of the Integrase

The IN protein consists of three distinct domains: an N-terminal region containing an HHCC zinc finger motif, a central catalytic core, and a less well-conserved C-terminal region containing an SH3 fold. Many of the residues important for enzymatic activities have been identified by mutagenesis. The most crucial residues for catalysis are the acidic amino acids in the D,D-35-E motif, a highly conserved array of three residues in the core region of many integrases and transposases.[377] Mutants indicate that both the N and C terminus are also important for function. Perhaps surprisingly, pairs of IN mutants with alterations in different regions of the molecule can often complement to restore normal integration. The separate N-terminal domains can even complement a nonoverlapping fragment, suggesting that these domains can still coassemble into a functional oligomeric complex.

For HIV-1, a large set of mutations affect a secondary function of IN in virion assembly and morphogenesis. These affect the ability of IN to bind RNA, resulting ultimately in mislocalization of the ribonucleoprotein complex outside the viral capsid lattice.[190,354] Allosteric IN inhibitors (ALLINIs, also named LEDGINs[121]) are reported to result in similar aberrant viral particles with eccentrically positioned RNPs.[29,164,333]

The IN protein is a multimer whose oligomeric state varies among the retrovirus genera (Fig. 15.11). The minimal function oligomer consists of a core tetramer (the conserved intasome core). Understanding of the assembly of the intasome in the presence of DNA as well as nucleosomes has greatly been advanced through x-ray crystallographic and cryo-EM structure studies. For the spumavirus PFV IN, the structure of the intact tetramer (a dimer of dimers) with two viral LTRs assembled on a mononucleosome presents the most detailed view of the enzyme and has even allowed for the positioning of the viral complex on the target DNA wrapped around the nucleosome.[461] This builds on the crystal structures of PFV IN, providing models of the PFV intasome tetramer named the target capture (TCC) and strand transfer complex (STC).[445] For other retroviral IN molecules within intasomes, the degree of multimerization is varied, with HTLV/STLV (deltaretrovirus) assembling as a tetramer,[39,60] MMTV (betaretrovirus) and RSV (alpharetrovirus) assembling as an octamer,[30,555,808] and MVV (a lentivirus) assembling as a hexadecamer.[31] For HIV and other lentiviral complexes (SIVrcm), the multimerization states have varied from tetramers through hexadecamers, depending

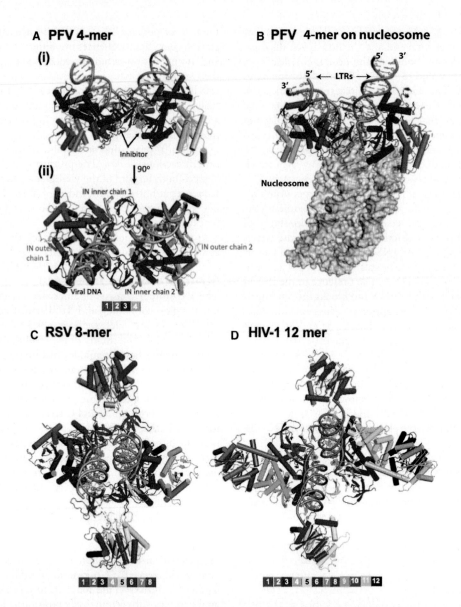

A PFV 4-mer

(i)

Inhibitor

(ii) 90°

IN inner chain 1

IN outer chain 1

IN outer chain 2

Viral DNA   IN inner chain 2

1 2 3 4

B PFV 4-mer on nucleosome

5′ 3′

5′ ← LTRs

3′

Nucleosome

C RSV 8-mer

1 2 3 4 5 6 7 8

D HIV-1 12 mer

1 2 3 4 5 6 7 8 9 10 11 12

FIGURE 15.11 Comparison of the structures of retroviral intasome complexes. Architecture of the intasome structures of PFV (PDB ID 4BDZ and 6RNY), RSV (PDB ID 7KU7), and HIV-1 (PDB ID 6U8Q) are shown with alpha helixes represented as cylinders. For all panels, the relative coloring of the monomer chains are numbered and indicated in the key, with the conserved intasome core colored in solid *red* and *blue*. **A:** Panel shows the PFV tetramer. Orientation of the complex is rotated 90 degrees in A(ii) with the IN inner and outer chains labeled. **B:** Panel shows the Cryo-EM structure of the PFV intasome in a strand transfer complex on a mononucleosome. The structure is shown in the same orientation for the PFV shown in panel A (i). vDNA (*gray*) is depicted as a cartoon with 5′ and 3′ termini labeled and nucleosomal DNA (*light pink*) and histones (*light gray*) are depicted as a space-filling model. **C and D:** Panels present the RSV-8-mer and HIV-12-mer, respectively. The inhibitors (XZ-259, MK-2048, and dolutegravir) for all the PFV **(panel A)**, RSV **(panel C)**, and HIV-1 **(panel D)** complexes, respectively, are shown as spheres in *green*. No integrase inhibitor is within **panel B**.

on variations in the constructs and the presence of substrates/inhibitors.[136,406,567,568] Many structures have been resolved in complex with integrase inhibitors.[274–276,481] Figure 15.11 presents examples of the divergent multimerization states of three viral INs in the presence of various INSTIs. PFV forms a stable tetramer in the presence of the strand transfer inhibitor XZ-90 (structure in PDB:ID 4BDZ),[481] RSV forms an octamer in the

presence of the inhibitor MK-2048 (PDB: ID 7KU7),[555] and HIV is here shown as a 12-mer in the presence of dolutegravir (DLU) (PDB: ID 6U8Q).[406]

Preintegration Complex

Integrase does not normally act alone, and a large complex of proteins and nucleic acid is responsible for mediating the formation of the provirus *in vivo*.[76,115] The full nature and components of the preintegration complex (PIC), or intasome, are not known in any detail for either the simple or the complex viruses. The PIC of the simple viruses contain CA, NC, RT, and IN, but other viral proteins may be present.[76,601] The PICs of the complex viruses may be different from those of the simple viruses,[198,199] consistent with their distinctive ability to infect nondividing cells.[401,402] Many of these proteins probably stay with the DNA in an intact capsid after entry into the nucleus, and the course of uncoating is under intense investigation. The PICS contain a large structure protecting the two ends of the DNA, and the integrase is likely holding them in proximity. The formation of this structure, detected as a footprint in a modified nuclease sensitivity assay,[770] requires both IN and the correct sequences at the termini of the DNA.[771]

Host Proteins and Integration

A number of host proteins have been identified as potentially involved in the establishment of the provirus. One such protein is BAF-1, a low molecular weight protein recovered from the MuLV PIC for its ability to inhibit autointegration of the LTR edges into internal sites in the viral DNA.[393] By inhibiting this reaction, BAF-1 can enhance normal integration into target DNAs in *trans*. However, infection of BAF-1–deficient cells occurs normally, suggesting that BAF-1 is not an essential player in the early events of the viral life cycle.

Many host factors that specifically interact with the retroviral IN proteins have been identified. For lentiviruses and gammaretroviruses, the host factors binding IN have direct influence on the characteristics of the integration sites. HIV-1 IN interacts with LEDGF (for lens epithelial-derived growth factor, a misnomer), a nuclear protein of uncertain function, which dramatically enhances its integration activity,[118,423,443] and directs integration broadly into expressed genic regions.[459,681] LEDGF is also reported to target HIV integration to highly spliced genes through its interaction with mRNA splicing factors.[684] Additional determinants for HIV target-site selection are associated with the CA protein, through its interaction with the host polyadenylation specificity factor 6 (CPSF6),[392,696] which promotes passage of the capsid through the nuclear pore and directs integration to active epigenetic marks and away from gene-sparse lamin-associated regions near the inside of the nuclear envelope.[1,696]

The IN protein of MuLV and likely other gammaretroviruses binds to the host bromodomain and extra-terminal domain (BET) proteins through an interaction between a conserved sequence within the IN C terminus (the ET-binding motif [ETBM] or tail peptide [TP])[9,10,143] and the ET domain of the BET proteins Brd2, 3, and 4.[9,159,227,269,674] Through their N-terminal bromodomains, BET proteins bind to acetylated histone marks[494,825] present at regions of active transcription.[399] and thereby biases MuLV integration to active promoter/enhancer regions.[158,381] In the absence of the IN tail peptide, MuLV integration occurs within quiescent chromatin and can delay virus replication and tumor activation in a mouse model.[430]

Host factors that bind to other retroviral IN proteins have been identified, including the FAcilitates Chromatin Transcription (FACT) complex binding to the ALV IN[789] and the B56 regulatory subunit of PP2A binding to the HTLV IN.[39,60,444]

The integration of retroviral DNA has been shown to activate an apoptotic program in cells deficient in the DNA-stimulated protein kinase (DNA-PK), an enzyme implicated in the DNA damage response[154]; the related kinase ATR and other components of the nonhomologous end-joining repair machinery may also be involved.[152,153] While it is not clear whether these kinases play any direct role in integration, they are likely involved in sensing the products of active integrase and responding to the damage. Their absence leads to substantial cell death in cells taking up the PIC at high multiplicity of infection.

Distribution of Integration Sites

An important issue affecting the ability of the retroviruses to create mutations is the distribution of integration sites in the host genome. Proviruses are inserted at very approximately random locations in the genome and thus have the opportunity to create mutations in any gene. Various studies, however, have uncovered significant deviations from a completely random distribution. At the sequence level, examination of large numbers of integration sites has revealed weak but statistically highly significant preferences for shared nonpalindromic target sequences.[756,794,360,797] Large scale surveys of thousands of integration sites cloned from pools of infected cells have allowed analysis of the frequency of insertions into the 5′ upstream regions of genes, transcribed regions, and nontranscribed regions. Different viruses display distinct biases for their target sites.[38,158,381,488,657,796] For HIV-1 and MuLV, the biases have been attributed to the host proteins (LEDGF, CPSF6, and BET proteins) that interact with IN, CA, and other components in the PIC. HIV-1 tends to insert into transcribed regions, more or less equally along such regions[459,681]; MuLV tends to selectively insert its DNA in sequences upstream from the 5′ end of transcribed regions, near transcriptional start sites; ASLV showed only very weak preference for active genes and none for 5′ regions. PFV integrates into low-transcription gene poor regions and lamin-A/B–associated genomic regions.[266,526,738] These studies collectively show that various retroviruses have evolved mechanisms to choose aspects of their integration sites, perhaps in support of their chosen lifestyles during infection.

The integration site preferences may also depend on the internal structures of the infected cell nucleus and the transport systems that move the PIC within the nucleus. Visualizing the location of PICs has shown that PICs can mediate integration either near the nuclear membrane or alternatively deeper into the nucleus, depending on the interaction of CA with the CPSF6 host factor.[1] HIV-1 PICs are directed to nuclear "speckles," large structures of uncertain function visualized by specific antisera.[217,411]

EXPRESSION OF VIRAL RNAs

The integration of the provirus signals a dramatic change in the lifestyle of the retroviruses; it marks the end of the early phase of the life cycle and the beginning of the late phase. The early phase is driven by viral enzymes performing unique events such as reverse transcription and DNA integration, while the late phase is mediated by host enzymes performing such relatively normal processes as transcription and translation. This late phase of gene expression may begin immediately following integration with the synthesis of viral RNAs and proteins, and the assembly of progeny virions (see Fig. 15.12 for an overview). For many viruses, the transcriptional promoters that

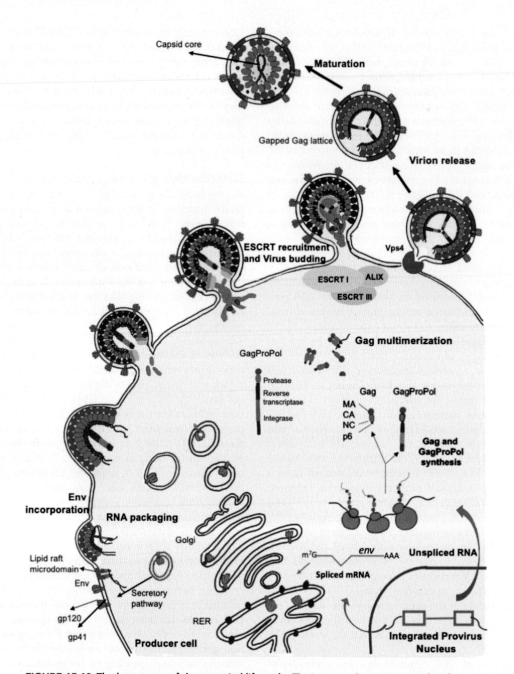

FIGURE 15.12 The late stages of the retroviral life cycle. The integrated provirus is used as the template for the expression of viral RNAs. A subset of the transcripts are spliced, and the unspliced and spliced mRNAs are exported to the cytoplasm. The unspliced RNA is used to make Gag and Gag-Pro-Pol proteins and also serves as the genome; spliced mRNA is used to make Env proteins. For lentiviruses, the Gag precursor, containing the MA, CA, and NC domains, and the Gag-Pro-Pol precursor, containing the MA, CA, NC, PR, RT, and IN domains, are transported to the inner leaflet of the plasma membrane. The proteins bind the viral genomic RNA (*thin line*). Curvature is induced in the membrane as the virion grows, and the roughly spherical particle is finally pinched off and released from the cell. The proteins and RNA associate under the membrane to form the budding progeny virion. Host proteins involved in budding, including the ESCRT 1, ESCRT III, ALIX, and Vps4 are indicated. The virion proteins are reorganized upon processing by the viral protease to form the mature, infectious virus (*top*).

drive this expression are constitutively active and cause the production of virions in a relatively unregulated way. In other viruses, the activity of the promoter may be regulated, either by viral or host factors. We will review the basic phenomenology of proviral gene expression and mention briefly the regulation exhibited by the complex retroviruses.

Overview of Viral RNA Synthesis

The synthesis of viral RNA from the viral DNA leads to the formation of a long primary transcript, which is then processed and may be spliced to form a small number of stable transcripts. The U3 region of the LTR contains a promoter recognized by the RNA polymerase II system, and these sequences direct the initiation of transcription starting at the U3-R border. Cellular machinery then caps the 5′ end of the RNA with m7G5′ppp5′G_mp. The first G residue after the cap is a templated base in the provirus. Transcription proceeds through the genome and continues through the 3′ LTR and into the downstream flanking host DNA. Finally, the RNA is cleaved and polyadenylated at the R-U5 border of the 3′ LTR, generating a complete unspliced viral genomic RNA suitable for incorporation into the virion particle (see Fig. 15.4). An AAUAAA sequence serves as the signal for this 3′ processing. The sequence normally lies in the R region, but the complete sequence needed for recognition can be complex, lying upstream or downstream, and may even be discontinuous, brought together by RNA folding to create the functional signal. The exact site of polyadenylation is not critical for virus replication. Some longer RNAs that extend into downstream flanking sequences are produced normally,[289] and these can be intermediates in the transduction of host genes. Mutants in which the polyadenylation signal is inactivated generate longer RNAs,[712,832] and these RNAs are quite efficiently able to mediate normal replication.[712]

A subset of the full-length RNAs is spliced to give rise to one or more subgenomic RNAs. The patterns of spliced mRNAs can be simple or exceedingly complex. Both the unspliced and spliced RNAs are then exported from the nucleus for translation.

Initiation of Transcription

The efficiency of transcription initiation at the U3-R boundary of the 5′ LTR is the major determinant of the levels of viral RNA formed in the cell. The promoter in the LTR is typically a very potent one, and the levels of viral RNA are often constitutively high. However, the cell type, the physiological state, and the integration site[203] can all result in substantial variation in the efficiency of transcription. In some viruses, the promoter is not constitutively active but depends on the activity of specific regulatory factors such as the glucocorticoid receptors.

Positive Regulatory Elements in U3

The transcriptional elements in the U3 region of the simple viruses contain both core promoter sequences and enhancers. The core promoters contain a TATA box, bound by TFIIB; a CCAAT box, bound by CEBP[643]; and sometimes an initiator sequence near the U3-R border. The U3 regions of even closely related retroviruses are very diverse and can evolve rapidly during viral replication. The enhancers are similar to those found in many host promoters in containing multiple short sequence motifs, arranged in very close packing; often, there are tandemly repeated copies of some of these motifs. These short sequences are the binding sites for a large number of host factors that regulate transcription (e.g., see Ref.[698]). Different cells and cell types will make use of distinct arrays of these factors to mediate transcription from a given viral LTR.[257] The factors are not simply additive but may interact in complex ways on particular viral sequences. A partial list of these factors used by various retrovirus LTRs include Sp1; USF-1; the Ets family of factors, which include more than 20 members in vertebrates; the core-binding factor (CBF), consisting of an a-b heterodimer; nuclear factor 1 (NF1); and a mammalian type C retrovirus enhancer factor (MCREF-1). Specific viruses may often contain recognition sites for other more specific positive regulatory factors. Major examples of such factors include the glucocorticoid

receptors, driving expression of the MMTV genome, and to a much lesser extent, MuLVs; NF-kB, important for expression from the HIV-1 LTR in certain cell types; the GATA factors for Cas-BR-E and other MuLVs; and the c-Myb protein. Evidence has been obtained that the STAT factors, DNA-binding proteins normally activated the Janus kinases (Jaks), may also be important for MMTV transcription.[605]

Negative Regulatory Elements

A number of negative regulatory factors that reduce viral expression have been identified. Embryonic carcinoma cells, and true embryonic cells, are the best-characterized examples of cell types that strongly repress LTR-mediated transcription through expression of negative regulatory proteins. The murine leukemia viruses are silenced via a stem cell–specific repressor that binds to a site overlapping almost perfectly with the proline tRNA primer binding site.[351,582] The proteins responsible for this silencing in mouse embryonic stem cells have recently been identified as TRIM28 (Kap-1) and the zinc finger protein ZFP809.[791,792] Viruses that use an alternate primer tRNA and so lack the PBS recognition site for these proteins can escape the repression.[293] Other negative factors include one known variously as UCRBP, NF-E1 or YY1,[213] and a cellular embryonal LTR-binding protein (ELP[739]).

Trans-Acting Viral Regulatory Factors

The complex retroviruses encode an array of small regulatory proteins that can activate transcription from the viral LTR in *trans*. Examples of these transactivators include the HTLV-1 Tax protein[162] and the HIV-1 Tat protein.[144] The Tax protein acts in concert with a complex of host proteins, the activating transcription factor/CRE-binding protein (ATF/CREB), and binds to three cAMP response elements in the viral LTR. Tax thus sets up a positive feedback loop that results in high levels of viral transcripts. The Tat protein is unusual among transcriptional activators in that it binds to a structure in the 5′ end of nascent viral RNA, rather than to DNA.[170,675] Tat binds to a bulged hairpin structure, the TAR element, and recruits a pair of host proteins, cyclin T/Cdk9, to the RNA. These proteins enhance the ability of RNA polymerase to elongate beyond the LTR and down the genome with high processivity, probably by phosphorylation of the C-terminal repeat domain (CTD) of the polymerase. Again, the result is a strong positive feedback loop that results in high levels of viral RNA. For more detailed discussion of Tat function, see Ref.[144] and Chapter 17 of this book.

Beginning and Ending the RNA

Because proviruses contain two identical LTRs, transcription can be initiated at both 5′ LTR and 3′ LTR. However, the 5′ LTR is generally much more efficiently utilized than the 3′ LTR.[289] One possible mechanism is promoter interference, in which transcription initiated at the upstream promoter suppresses the utilization of the downstream promoter. It is also possible that elements near the 3′ LTR may restrict use of the downstream LTR, so that generally transcripts initiating at the 5′ LTR predominate. These restraints may be lost in virally induced tumors, in which transcription from the 3′ LTR into neighboring oncogenes can be significantly enhanced.[69] Similarly, since there are two LTRs, transcripts might in principle be subject to 3′ end processing at either the 5′ LTR or the 3′ LTR, but most of the RNAs formed extend from the 5′ LTR to the 3′ LTR.

At least one retrovirus, HTLV-1, is known to encode an antisense transcript that is formed by RNA polymerase II initiation in the 3′ LTR and elongating toward the 5′ LTR.[36] This transcript encodes a single protein, termed bZIP or HBZ, that plays a role in the oncogenic transforming activity of the virus and also acts to antagonize the viral Tax protein, the activator of transcription in the sense direction.[244] The formation and function of the HBZ protein will be discussed in the chapter on HTLV-1 (Chapter 16).

RNA Processing

The full-length polyadenylated transcript of the retroviral genome is directed into several pathways. A portion of the transcripts is exported directly from the nucleus and serves as the genome to be packaged into the progeny virion particle, assembling either at the plasma membrane or in the cytoplasm. Another portion is also exported but is used instead for translation to form the Gag and Gag-Pol polyproteins. What determines the routing and distribution of the RNAs into these two pathways has been highly debated. Recent work in HIV-1 has revealed that the precise site of transcriptional initiation, defining the sequence at the 5′ terminus of the capped RNA, is a major determinant of the distribution of the RNA between these two pathways. The 5′ ends of HIV-1 RNAs can contain either one, two, or three G residues; RNAs with two or three Gs are folded into a conformation that is preferentially recognized by initiation factors including eIF4E and are destined for translation, while RNAs with one G fold so as to sequester the 5′ cap and are preferentially dimerized and used for packaging.[85,355] The MuLVs do not seem to utilize this same system.

A third portion of the transcripts is spliced to yield subgenomic mRNAs. For the simple retroviruses, there is a single spliced mRNA encoding the Env glycoprotein. For the complex viruses, there can be multiple alternatively spliced mRNAs, encoding both Env and an array of auxiliary proteins. Examples of the complicated array of mRNAs that are formed for both simple and complex viruses are shown in Figure 15.13. The protein products of these multiply spliced mRNAs will be discussed in following chapters.

The splicing and subsequent export from the nucleus of only a portion of an initially transcribed RNA is an unusual process; normally splicing goes to completion, and only then is the mRNA exported. The export of a precursor mRNA is usually prevented until splicing is complete. At least three aspects of the retroviral genome may promote the export of unspliced mRNAs. First, the splice sites of the viral RNA may have quite poor overall efficiency of utilization by the splicing machinery in the cell.[340] Indeed, the sequences at the splice donor and acceptor regions are often poor matches to the consensus sequences for splice sites, and mutations that make the sites better matches increase splicing and are actually deleterious to virus replication. These mutations can be suppressed by secondary mutations that reduce splicing efficiency. The overall folding of the RNA may affect the efficiency of splicing, and thus, sequences at some distance, as in the *gag* gene, may modulate splicing.[700]

Secondly, studies of ASLV have identified specific sequences that act as negative regulators of splicing (NRS) through their interaction with host factors.[14,247,473,474,532] These elements can

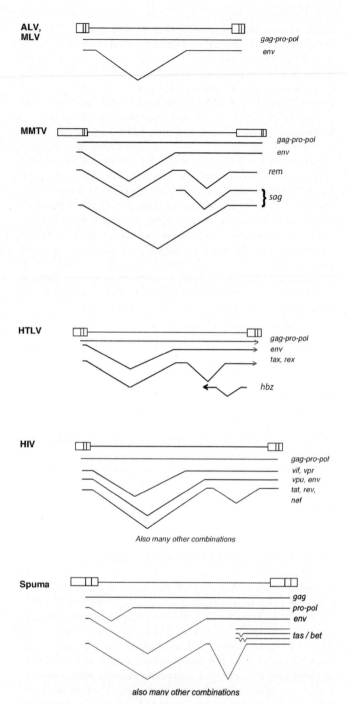

FIGURE 15.13 Splicing patterns of representative retroviral RNAs. All retroviruses direct the synthesis of an unspliced RNA transcript, as well as a variable array of subgenomic mRNAs. Examples of the splicing patterns of the mRNAs of various retroviruses are shown. The complex viruses like HIV-1 also encode a larger array of mRNAs containing various combinations of exons. Orientation of transcription is indicated with *forward* or *reverse* arrows.

be important for the expression of transduced genes in some viruses.[691] The HIV-1 genome includes several sequences that act as inhibitors of splicing to specific acceptor sites, thereby controlling the ratios of formation of the many subgenomic mRNAs.[195] Many of these sequences are embedded within coding regions for viral proteins, suggesting they arose in the face of a complex selective pressure for maintenance of both RNA splicing ratios and protein structures.[592] Similar signals may exist in other viruses; mutations in the Gag region of MuLV can affect genomic and mRNA processing in complex ways.

In addition, unspliced mRNAs contain cis-acting elements that promote the export of the RNA out of the nucleus, the so-called constitutive transport elements (CTEs).[79] These sequences are located near the 3′ end of the genomic RNA of MPMV and in similar regions of the alpharetroviruses. The CTE is recognized by one or more host proteins that assemble a complex onto the RNA to mediate its export, including Tap and its cofactor Nxt.[390] In the complex viruses, RNA export is regulated through complex interactions of the Rex or Rev gene products with cis-acting sites, the RRE elements that promote RNA export, and of various host factors with the CRS/INS elements that prevent it (see Ref.[145] for review). The key players include Crm1, a cellular nuclear export factor, and DDX3, an RNA helicase (see Chapter 17 for detailed discussion of the mechanism of Rev action). MMTV encodes a Rem protein with analogous function to Rev.

Viral RNAs are subject to other modifications common to cellular mRNAs. Like cellular mRNAs, the N6 position on specific A residues can be methylated,[336] and other sites can be modified by double-stranded RNA adenosine deaminase. Several other modifications have recently been identified, including 5-methyl cytosine.[788] These modifications can regulate the stability of the viral RNAs, affect the extent and specificity of RNA splicing,[352,353] and also prevent recognition of the RNA by the innate immune system.[116]

TRANSLATION AND PROTEIN PROCESSING

All replication-competent retroviral genomes, at a minimum, contain open reading frames designated the *gag, pro, pol,* and *env* genes. These genes are expressed by complex mechanisms to form precursor proteins, which are then processed during and after virion assembly to form the mature, infectious virus particle. The expression of the various proteins as large precursors that are subsequently cleaved provides several advantages: it allows for many proteins to be made from one ORF; it ensures that the proteins are made at proper ratios; and it allows for many proteins to be targeted to the virion during assembly as a single entity. The *gag, pro,* and *pol* genes are expressed in a complex way from the full-length unspliced mRNA. The arrangement of these genes, and especially the way *pro* is expressed, is different in different viruses. A summary of the arrangement of the ORFs of various viruses is shown in Figure 15.14.

Gag Gene Expression

The *gag* gene is present at the 5′ proximal position on all retroviral genomes. A full-length mRNA, identical in sequence to the genomic RNA, is translated in the cytoplasm to form a Gag precursor protein, in the 50 to 80 kDa range. Translation begins with an AUG initiator codon and proceeds to a terminator codon at the 3′ end of the ORF. The viral RNA typically contains long 5′ untranslated region, and it has been uncertain whether ribosomes could scan from the 5′ cap to the start codon for Gag translation. These 5′ RNA sequences are

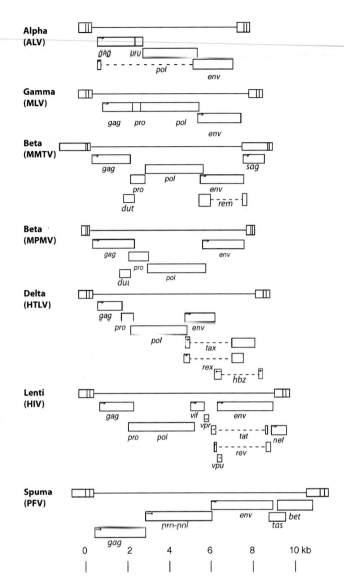

FIGURE 15.14 Arrangements of the open reading frames (ORFs) encoded by various retroviruses. The major ORFs of each virus are indicated by the *open boxes*. ORFs in the same reading frame are in the same line, and ORFs in different frames are on different lines. Translational starts are indicated by the *small arrows*. Spliced introns are indicated by the *dashed lines*.

predicted to contain stable secondary structures that would inhibit scanning. Furthermore, the long 5′ UTRs often contain AUG codons in contexts that are favorable for translation, that are not in frame with the *gag* ORF, and presumably would inhibit successful translation of Gag. Experiments suggest that for the MuLVs and related endogenous RNAs, an internal ribosome entry site (IRES) is present near the start of the *gag* ORF and is used to initiate translation in a cap-independent mechanism.[54,55,427] Thus, at least in these viruses, ribosomes can bind directly near the *gag* gene and do not need to scan the mRNA. Although the suggestion is not without controversy,[483] it is likely that many other viruses, including HIV-1, also utilize IRES elements for translation of Gag.[160,161,533] In the case of HIV-1, the IRES is remarkable in that critical sequences extend downstream of the AUG, lying within the Gag coding region.[90]

Some gammaretroviruses encode an additional Gag protein besides the major product, termed gPr80^{gag} or "glycoGag." This Gag protein is longer than the major product and derives from infrequent translational initiation at a nonconventional CUG codon upstream from the initiating AUG codon. Translation beginning at this codon first forms an N-terminal leader sequence and then proceeds in the same reading frame through the normal AUG and the rest of the Gag protein. Thus, where the proteins overlap their sequences are identical. The leader sequence contains a functional signal peptide directing the translation machinery to the endoplasmic reticulum and specifying that the Gag protein be cotranslationally inserted into the secretory pathway. The Gag become glycosylated at several sites, is transported via the Golgi to the cell surface, and persists for some time as a membrane-bound glycoprotein, with the carboxy-terminal domain exposed on the cell surface.[585] The protein is processed into several fragments and has a relatively short half-life. It is not required for virus replication in some cells.[663] However, the protein can facilitate release of virus at lipid rafts,[524] apparently acting in concert with the host La protein[525], and perhaps most importantly, it can mimic the function of the HIV-1 Nef protein in antagonizing the SERINC restriction factor and thereby promote virion release.[588]

The major Gag product is often modified by the addition of myristic acid, a relatively rare 14-carbon fatty acid, to the penultimate amino-terminal residue, a glycine.[287] The addition is mediated by a myristyl CoA transferase that cotranslationally transfers myristate from a myristyl CoA donor to the amino group of the glycine residue, forming an amide bond. The fatty acid is important for the membrane localization and binding of the Gag precursor, increasing the hydrophobicity of the amino-terminal domain. Mutant Gags in which the glycine is altered are not modified; these Gags do not associate with membrane properly and do not aggregate to form virions.[87,255,615] It should be noted that although the myristate is important, it is not sufficient for membrane targeting; hydrophobic residues in the MA domain are also required. Furthermore, basic residues further downstream in the MA of some viruses form a patch of positive charge that interact with negatively charged phospholipids in the membrane.

An amino-terminal myristate is not found on the Gags of lentiviruses, BIV, EIAV, visna, or alpharetroviruses. For the alpharetroviruses, the amino terminus is not myristoylated but rather acetylated. The Gag protein of these viruses is apparently sufficiently hydrophobic to be targeted to the membrane without the fatty acid in avian cells, though, curiously, not in mammalian cells. Alteration of the alpharetrovirus Gag to allow its myristoylation permits virion assembly in mammalian cells[785] and does not block its function in avian cells.

Pro Gene Expression

The relative position of the *pro* gene on retroviral genomes is always the same—in between *gag* and *pol*. However, *pro* is expressed in very different ways in different viruses. Sometimes it is fused in frame onto the 3′ end of *gag*, sometimes it is fused to the 5′ end of *pol*, and sometimes it is present as a separate reading frame (Fig. 15.15). These various patterns have led to confusion in the literature; sometimes *pro* is considered a portion of *gag*, or sometimes of *pol*. Because of these different patterns of expression, it is best to consider this ORF as a separate gene.

The various arrangements of the *pro* gene and its mode of expression are as follows. For the alpharetroviruses, *gag* and *pro*

are fused and expressed as a single protein; *pol* is in a different reading frame, and a frameshift is used to express the Gag-Pro-Pol polyprotein. For the betaretroviruses and deltaretroviruses, *gag*, *pro*, and *pol* are all in different frames, and successive frameshifts are used to express Gag-Pro and Gag-Pro-Pol polyproteins. For the gammaretroviruses and epsilonretroviruses, *gag* and a *pro-pol* fusion are in the same reading frame and separated by a stop codon, and translational readthrough is used to make Gag-Pro-Pol. For the lentiviruses, *gag* and a *pro-pol* fusion are in different reading frames, and frameshifting is used to make Gag-Pro-Pol. Finally, for the spumaviruses, *pro* is fused to *pol* in the same frame, and the Pro-Pol protein is expressed without Gag, from a spliced mRNA. We will say more about these varied mechanisms of expression in the following section.

Pol Gene Expression

The *pol* gene encodes several proteins needed at lower levels than the Gag proteins for the replication of the virus, including the reverse transcriptase and integrase enzymes. The *pol* ORF is not expressed as a separate protein in most retroviruses but rather is expressed as a part of a larger Gag-Pro-Pol fusion protein. The Gag-Pro-Pol protein must be made at the correct abundance, in proportion to the amount of Gag protein, for efficient assembly of infectious virus; expression of only Gag-Pro-Pol does not result in virion assembly.[204,565] The formation of this protein is mediated by either one of two mechanisms, depending on the virus.

Translational Readthrough

In the gammaretroviruses and epsilonretroviruses, the Gag and Pro-Pol ORFs are in the same reading frame and are separated by a single UAG stop codon at the boundary between Gag and Pro-Pol. The translation of Gag-Pro-Pol in these viruses occurs by translational readthrough—that is, by suppression of termination—at the UAG stop codon.[810] Most of the time translation of the RNA results simply in the formation of the Gag protein. But approximately 5% to 10% of the time, ribosomes translating the RNA do not terminate at the UAG codon and instead utilize a normal aminoacyl tRNA, usually a glutamine tRNA, to insert an amino acid at the position of the stop codon. Translation then continues, in frame, through the entire long *pro-pol* ORF, resulting in the formation of a long Gag-Pro-Pol precursor protein. The high-level suppression of termination is specified by a specific structure in the RNA immediately downstream of the UAG stop codon.[295,557] The precise features of this structure that are required for suppression are not completely known, but they include a purine-rich sequence immediately downstream of the stop codon and a pseudoknot formed from the next 60 or so nucleotides.[208] The RNA structure is likely dynamic and may interconvert between conformations that either do or do not promote readthrough. The distribution of conformations, and the corresponding efficiency of readthrough, was found to be exquisitely sensitive to pH *in vitro*, and it is plausible that cellular proteins could control readthrough by similar effects on RNA conformation.[299] The structure may slow translation, and it may also in some other way alter the balance between termination, which requires binding of termination factors eRF1 and eRF3 by the ribosome, versus incorporation of an amino acid, which requires misreading of the codon by an aminoacyl tRNA. No changes in the tRNA pool occur during infection. The signals in the RNA can operate to mediate suppression of both UAA and UGA termination codons as well as UAG.[206,207]

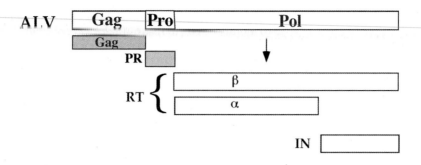

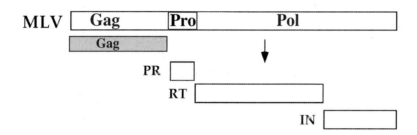

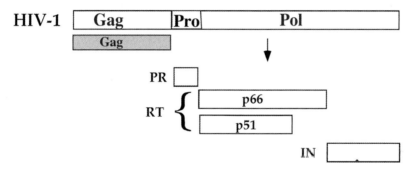

FIGURE 15.15 Cleavage patterns during the processing of the Gag-Pro-Pol fusion proteins of various retroviruses. The structure of the mature cleavage products found in the virion particles are shown aligned with their location in the precursor. Gag proteins are colored in *gray*.

A screen for proteins interacting with the MuLV RT resulted in the identification of the eukaryotic termination factor eRF-1, and subsequent studies showed that ectopic overexpression of RT could inhibit termination and promote translational readthrough of the Gag stop codon *in vivo*.[541] Mutant viruses with point mutations in RT blocking the interaction with eRF-1 were unable to express normal levels of Gag-Pro-Pol and failed to replicate. These results suggest that RT, likely in the context of the nascent Gag-Pro-Pol protein, can bind and inhibit eRF-1 and thereby increase the level of readthrough to increase its own synthesis. The final level of Gag-Pro-Pol produced in this positive feedback loop is presumably ultimately limited by other factors.

Translational Frameshifting

In the alpharetroviruses and lentiviruses, the *gag* and *pol* ORFs lie in different reading frames, and the formation of the Gag-Pro-Pol fusion is mediated by a translational frameshift mechanism.[317] Most of the time, translation again results in the simple formation of the Gag protein. But approximately 10% of the time, as the translation approaches a specific site near the end of the *gag* ORF, the ribosome slips back one nucleotide (a −1 frameshift) and proceeds onward in the new reading frame. The ribosome passes through the stop codon out of frame and so continues to synthesize protein using the codons of the *pol* ORF. As for readthrough, the determinants of frameshifting lie in the RNA sequence and structure near the site of the event. The requirements for frameshifting include a "slippery site," a string of homopolymeric bases where the frameshift occurs; these are oligo U or oligo A in different viruses. In addition, the frameshifting requires either a very large and near-perfect hairpin or stem–loop structure (as for HIV-1 group M viruses), or a large pseudoknot structure (as for HIV-1 group O viruses), similar to those used in readthrough, though apparently containing a distinctive bend at the junction of the two paired sequences. Recently, a host protein, dubbed Shiftless, has been identified as regulating the efficiency of frameshifting.[766] As for readthrough, the proper frameshifting efficiency is crucial for normal virus replication.

In the betaretroviruses (e.g., MMTV) and deltaretroviruses (e.g., BLV, HTLV-1), the *pro* gene is present as a separate ORF, in a different reading frame from that of *gag* or *pol*. Two successive frameshifts are utilized to make the long Gag-Pro-Pol fusion protein. Near the 3′ end of the *gag* ORF, ribosomes carry out a first (−1) frameshift and continue into the *pro* ORF; near the 3′ end of the *pro* ORF, they perform a second (−1) frameshift and continue on into the *pol* ORF. These two frameshifts occur at extremely high frequencies—as much as 30% of the time that the ribosome transits through each site—so that the overall frequency of formation of the Gag-Pro-Pol protein is perhaps 10% that of formation of Gag.

Separate Pol Expression

The spumaviruses are unique among the retroviruses in that the synthesis of the Pol protein is not mediated by the formation of a Gag-Pro-Pol fusion protein. Instead, a subgenomic spliced mRNA is translated directly to form a separate Pro-Pol protein.[191,424] This protein must be directed to the assembling virion by distinct domains rather than by the Gag portion of a Gag-Pro-Pol fusion.

Env Gene Expression

In all retroviruses, the *env* gene is expressed from a distinct subgenomic mRNA. The *env* message is a singly spliced mRNA, in which a 5′ leader is joined to the coding region of *env*. Thus, the bulk of the *gag* and *pol* genes are removed as an intron from the mRNA. The resulting message is exported to the cytoplasm and translated from a conventional AUG initiator codon. In the alpharetroviruses, the AUG is actually the same one used for Gag translation; it lies in the leader, and the splicing brings this AUG and the first six codons into frame with the *env* coding region. The first translated amino acids constitute a hydrophobic signal peptide and direct the nascent protein to the rough endoplasmic reticulum. The leader is removed by a cellular protease (the signal peptidase) in the ER, and the protein is heavily glycosylated by transfer of oligosaccharide from a dolichol carrier to asparagine residues on Env. These residues lie in the conventional Asn-X-Ser/Thr motifs recognized by the modification enzymes. Near the end of the cotranslational insertion of Env into the ER, a highly hydrophobic sequence acts as a stop transfer signal to anchor the protein in the membrane. The remaining C-terminal portion of the protein stays on the cytoplasmic side of the membrane.

Before the Env proteins are transported to the cell surface, they are folded and oligomerized in the ER. The formation of oligomers is required for stable expression of the protein and is sensitive to overall conformation; many mutants of Env show defects in oligomerization.[741] Envelope proteins generally form trimers in the mature virus.[431] The folding of the protein is presumably catalyzed by chaperone proteins in the ER, and the formation of disulfide bonds between various pairs of cysteine residues by disulfide interchange enzymes.

The Env protein is then exported to the Golgi and cleaved by furin proteases to form the separate SU and TM subunits. This cleavage is essential for the normal function of the Env protein. The cleavage occurs at a dibasic pair of amino acids[173,222,397,575] and produces a hydrophobic N terminus for the TM protein that is required to mediate fusion of the viral and host membranes during virus entry. In the Golgi, the sugar residues are modified by the sequential removal of mannose residues and addition of *N*-acetyl glucosamine and other sugars to many of the oligosaccharide. *O*-linked glycosylation and sulfation of Env glycoproteins have also been documented.[587] The pathway by which Env is transported to the cell surface is not fully understood, but presumably, host vesicular transport systems are utilized. The protein typically becomes a prominent cell surface protein on the infected cell.

In polarized epithelial cells, Env proteins are often restricted to the basolateral surface of the cell.[548] This localization is mediated by a tyrosine-based motif, Yxxf, present in the cytoplasmic tail of Env[549] (x, any amino acid; f, hydrophobic residue). Remarkably, this targeting of Env can redirect the budding of HIV-1 Gag proteins to this surface.

Other Viral Gene Products

The complex retroviruses express a number of small proteins with a range of functions. The proteins are translated from subgenomic mRNAs, usually resulting from multiple splicing events that join a 5′ LTR to a number of small exons encoding the protein. These gene products will be discussed in greater detail in later chapters (see Refs.[144,259,591] for reviews).

Betaretroviruses

- Sag: The MMTV genome encodes a small protein functioning as a superantigen to stimulate lymphocyte activation by interacting with the beta chain of the T-cell receptor, providing a suitable tissue for virus replication.[604]
- Rem: MMTV encodes a Rev-like protein expressed as a precursor protein. Its Rev-like function is encoded in the N-terminal signal peptide region, which is cleaved by translocon-associated signal peptidase, allowing for release of SP into the cytosol.[96,97,310]
- dUTPase: The *pol* region of several betaretroviruses, as well as some nonprimate lentiviruses, includes a *dut* gene, encoding dUTPase, a deoxyribonucleotidase catalyzing the conversion of dUTP to dUMP and PPi. Its activity lowers the frequency of incorporation of uridine bases in the viral DNA by RT, which would trigger excision by uracil *N*-glycosidase and breakage at the resulting apurinic site.

Deltaretroviruses

- Tax: The Tax gene product is a positive regulator of transcription from the viral LTR. Tax functions in association with the activating transcription factor/CRE-binding protein (ATF/CREB) by binding to three cAMP response elements in the viral LTR. Tax also plays a role in transformation, perhaps through Rb destruction, E2F-1 activation, or through effects on the cell cycle.[349]
- Rex: The Rex gene product facilitates the export of unspliced and singly spliced viral mRNAs from the nucleus. Its action is probably similar to that of the lentiviral rev protein.
- HBZ: A product of an antisense ORF encoded by HTLV-1, HBX or bZIP, is a transcriptional regulatory protein with oncogenic activity.

Epsilonretroviruses

- Orf a: The Orf a product of the piscine retroviruses is a cyclin D homologue that functions as a cyclin in yeast.[385] The function of the protein in virus replication or tumor formation is uncertain.
- Orfs b, c: The function of these Orfs is unknown.

Lentiviruses

- Tat: The Tat protein is a potent transactivator of transcription from the viral LTR. The protein acts by binding to a hairpin structure, the TAR element, encoded in the R region of nascent viral RNA, and recruiting host factors cyclin T and Cdk9 to the RNA. Tat does not increase the rate of RNA polymerase II initiation but enhances its processivity or elongation by Cdk9-mediated phosphorylation of the CTD of pol II.

- Rev: The Rev protein mediates the export of the unspliced and singly spliced viral RNAs from the nucleus, thus permitting the expression of the Gag, Pol, and Env gene products. Viral RNAs contain multiple sequences, called CRS or INS elements, which bind several proteins—PTB/hnRNP I, hnRNP A1, PABP1, and p54nrb/PSF—that retain the RNAs in the nucleus.[6,842] Rev binds to the Rev-responsive element (RRE) present in the HIV-1 *env* gene, and by interacting with the importin Crm1, it acts to export the viral RNAs through the nuclear pore, overriding the retention signals.

- Nef: The Nef protein is a multifunctional protein not essential for replication in some cells in culture but important for efficient replication *in vivo*. Nef-defective viruses do not induce high-level viremia in infected animals, and progression to disease is delayed or prevented. Nef down-regulates the CD4 receptor from the cell surface,[239] facilitating virus release, probably by bridging CD4 to adapter proteins (APs).[584] Nef also down-regulates MHC class I levels, thereby inhibiting the CTL-mediated lysis of HIV-1–infected cells. HIV-1 Nef also down-regulates the SERINC3 and 5 restriction factors, which target Envelope proteins, and thereby enhances replication. The Nef of certain SIVs antagonize the antiviral protein tetherin[828] and thus promote virion assembly and release.

- Vpr: The Vpr protein, as noted below, is packaged at high levels into virion particles through an interaction with the p6 domain of Gag.[27,320,667] Vpr may facilitate the import of the preintegration complex into the nucleus in nondividing cells. Vpr also causes a strong cell cycle arrest in the G2 stage of the cell cycle, perhaps through an indirect inhibition of Cdc25 phosphatase activity. Vpr binds *via* VprBP/DCAF1 to a ubiquitin ligase complex containing Cullin-4A and DDB1, to promote the ubiquitinylation and degradation of many targets,[261] perhaps including the cell cycle regulator Ctd1.[300,658] Recently, the most critical target of Vpr in inducing G2 arrest has been identified as a protein known as cPERP-B or CCDC137.[826] The functions of this protein are not characterized.

- Vif: The Vif protein is expressed at high levels in the cytoplasm and is packaged into virion particles of both homologous and heterologous viruses. Vif enhances infectivity by degrading or sequestering members of the APOBEC3 family of cytidine deaminases that attack the minus strand DNA and mutate C to U during reverse transcription.[64,277]

- Vpu: The Vpu gene product, found only in HIV-1, is a membrane protein that enhances virion production by antagonizing tetherin, which traps virions on the cell surface and prevents their spread to neighboring cells.[518] Vpu also mediates the degradation of CD4 by the ubiquitin-conjugating pathway.[660]

- Vpx: HIV-2 and specific SIVs (from sooty mangabeys, SIVsmm, and from red-capped mangabeys, SIVrcm) encode a small protein, Vpx, which enhances early steps of infection and overcomes a block to infection of monocyte-derived macrophages and dendritic cells. Vpx acts by targeting the antiviral protein SAMHD1, a nucleotidase, for degradation.[301,382]

Spumaviruses

- Tas: The Tas (or Bel1) protein is a transactivator of transcription from the viral LTR, acting at sequences near the 5′ end of the genome. Its mechanism of action may be similar to that of the lentiviral Tat protein.

- Bet: The Bet protein, like HIV-1 Vif, inhibits APOBEC3G.[425,642]

VIRION ASSEMBLY

As the Gag, Gag-Pro-Pol, and Env proteins are synthesized, they come together to form progeny virions (for reviews, see Refs.[307,646,714,784]). The assembly of the retrovirus particle is driven primarily by the Gag precursor protein. Gag is required for the formation of a virion and indeed is sufficient to mediate the assembly and release of an immature "bald" particle—lacking infectivity and the "hair" of the Env protein. The Gag protein that is responsible for assembly is the uncleaved Gag precursor. This form of the protein is thus targeted for assembly and export—the "way out" of the cell. The trafficking routes that deliver Gag to the site of assembly and budding are not established with certainty for any retrovirus. Once the Gag proteins are processed by the viral protease, changes in virion structure occur to promote virus entry—the "way in" to the next cell.

There are two major routes by which the various retroviruses assemble their virions.

Assembly of C-Type Virions

For most of the retroviruses, including lentiviruses and those with the C-type morphology, assembly occurs at the plasma membrane; in these cases, the Gag precursor protein is targeted to the cytoplasmic face of the plasma membrane by hydrophobic sequences, basic residues, and sometimes by a myristic acid moiety,[287] present at the amino terminus. It is not clear if monomeric or dimeric or higher-order structures of Gag are transported to the membrane to begin assembly. The Gag proteins aggregate, presumably by side-to-side contacts, and create a patch under the membrane. As the patch of protein grows, curvature is induced in the membrane, causing the nascent virus to bud outward. The bud eventually grows to a complete sphere, attached to the cell by a narrow stalk. The stalk is then pinched off with the help of the cellular ESCRT machinery, the virion is released, and the host membrane is sealed. The structure of the immature virion is roughly spherical, with Gag arranged radially.[781] The various steps are depicted in Figure 15.12.

The route of transport of Gag from the cytoplasm to the cell membrane may not be simple or direct and differs among virus genera. A substantial amount of Gag protein is found in the nucleus,[515,653] and in some viruses, including the alpharetroviruses, the Gag in this compartment may be a precursor to the molecules on the plasma membrane.[562] Whether this is an obligatory step in virion assembly is unclear, but genomic RNA for packaging may be bound in the nucleus.[238] There is also evidence that Gags, perhaps bound to the genomic RNAs that they will package into particles, are trafficked to the plasma membrane on endosomal vesicles.[40] In other cases, including HIV-1, high-resolution imaging indicates that a few Gag precursors assemble at the cell membrane and then bind a (probable dimer) RNA to initiate particle formation there.

Assembly of B- and D-Type Virions

In the alternative lifestyle exhibited by viruses with B- and D-type morphology, the betaretrovirus and the spumavirus capsids assemble in the cytoplasm and then are subsequently transported to the plasma membrane for envelopment and release.[622] These two pathways would seem relatively distinct, and one might have supposed that the two groups of viruses would have evolved very different requirements for assembly and that the details of the Gag-Gag interactions would be different. But these two mechanisms are not so far apart. Indeed, a single amino acid substitution in the MA protein of M-PMV can change the morphogenetic pathway of this betaretrovirus from a cytoplasmic site of assembly to a membrane site of assembly.[624] Thus, the main difference may be the timing of exposure of determinants for membrane transport; in the C-types, such a determinant might be constitutively available, while for the B- and D-types, the determinant may not be exposed until assembly occurs. For both mechanisms, the nascent virions consist of a spherical particle surrounded by a lipid bilayer, which is pinched off from the cell and then released into the extracellular space.

MPMV Gag does not seem to assemble at the site of translation; the protein apparently first travels in a microtubule-dependent process to the pericentriolar region of the cytoplasm through interactions between a short peptide signal, known as the cytoplasmic targeting-retention signal, and the dynein/dynactin motor. The Gag precursors are assembled to form immature capsids in pericentriolar microdomains. Env may effect release of Gag from the centriolar region. Mutants of Rab11 that inhibit efflux of transferrin from the recycling endosome and Env localization also inhibited Gag transport.[672,673] The mechanism of the subsequent movement to the cell surface is uncertain.

Gag and Virion Assembly

For most retroviruses, the expression of the Gag precursor is sufficient to mediate virion assembly and release, earning the protein the name of the "particle making machine." (An exception to this rule is the foamy viruses, which also require the presence of the Env glycoprotein for efficient budding.) Because of its central role in virion assembly, the Gag proteins have been subjected to intense mutational analyses to define the domains required for various steps in the process.[273,784] Surprisingly, small portions of Gag, containing only a few critical regions, can still assemble virions.[763] Three domains, at least, seem to be crucial: a membrane-binding (M) domain, an interaction (I) domain, and a late assembly (L) domain. It is important to remember that the form of the Gag protein that is mediating assembly is the uncleaved precursor; thus, the assembly domains need not lie neatly within any of the cleavage products that form later and can span cleavage sites.

The M Domain

The M domain, or membrane-binding domain, ranging from 30 to 90 residues in length, is located in MA at the amino terminus of Gag. Mutations affecting this domain abolish assembly, but M mutants retain their ability to interact with other Gags and can be rescued into particles by the coexpression of a wild-type protein. The region seems to contain both hydrophobic and basic residues that are needed for proper interaction with lipid and with the acidic moieties of phospholipids. Structural information for the isolated M domain is consistent with this role. How Gag finds specific membranes is unclear, but M domains seem to be involved.[654] There is evidence that budding is enhanced at membrane regions of unusual lipid composition termed lipid "rafts",[101,514,521,522,538] defined by high levels of phosphatidylinositol (4,5) bisphosphate.[536]

For many retroviruses, myristoylation of Gag, along with specific residues in MA, is required for membrane binding. This interaction with membrane, in turn, is important for virion assembly of the C-type viruses and for their proper subsequent Gag processing.[661] Mutational studies have led to the notion of a "myristyl switch," in which the myristic acid is exposed to mediate plasma membrane binding during virion assembly but then can be sequestered in the compact globular core of MA after Gag processing.[537,551,697,836] Although this region is generally considered important for virion assembly, surprisingly, much of the RSV MA and almost the entire HIV-1 MA domain can be deleted from Gag without preventing assembly, so long as a functional membrane-binding signal, even from a nonviral source, is retained. In the latter case, there are some effects on assembly: virions are budded indiscriminately into both intracellular membranes as well as at the cell surface. The amino-terminal sequences of Gag can be replaced with a heterologous membrane-binding signal, such as that present at the amino terminus of the Src kinase. It should be noted that the interaction of Gag with membrane is not required for assembly of the B- or D-type viruses *per se*. For these viruses, mutations in the myristate addition signals do not affect the cytoplasmic assembly of the virions but rather block the transport of the assembled particles to the plasma membrane.[623]

The I Domain

The I or interaction domain is defined as a major region of Gag-Gag interaction, largely contained in the CA and NC regions. Although the major I domain has been suggested to lie in NC, analyses have suggested that the C-terminal half of CA and NC are equally important for normal assembly. Mutations in the I domain block or reduce assembly,[505] and those particles produced by these mutants have aberrantly low density, indicating fewer and poorly packed Gag proteins. The key feature of the I domains is not the zinc-binding residues of the Cys-His box, but rather basic residues flanking the boxes that interact with nucleic acid. RNA bridging between NCs is likely a critical step in virion assembly. The assembly functions of NC can be replaced by foreign proteins, and the key activity seems to be the formation of protein–protein contacts.[325,833] Mutations in this region can also affect particle size as well as yield. It has been noted that the poor virion production by deletion mutants of HIV-1 can be suppressed by mutation of the protease,[543] suggesting that some of the defects of I domain mutations could be caused by inappropriate or premature processing of Gag by the viral protease. There are other hints that controlling the timing of protease activation is very important to formation of infectious virions.

Assembly of HIV-1 virions *in vivo* has also more recently been shown to be highly dependent on the presence of inositol hexakisphosphate (IP6). Depletion of IP6 by genetic manipulations of the biosynthetic pathways in the host causes accumulation of intracellular Gag, decreased yield of virions, formation of aberrant structures, and slow virus spread.[449,695] IP6 acts to stabilize the assembling Gags and so enhances the course of assembly. It additionally plays a key role in the reassembly of the condensed virion core after maturation of Gag to CA proteins, forming structures essential for proper reverse transcription upon entry into the infected cell. About 300 copies of IP6 are incorporated per HIV-1 virion particles. For a review of IP6 involvement, see Ref.[168]

The L Domain

The third assembly domain is the L or late domain.[783,800] Mutants affected in this function fail to produce and release particles efficiently, and though the mutant Gag proteins form spherical structures, they accumulate under the membrane and do not progress normally. The buds remain tethered to the cell surface by a membrane stalk, suggesting that the function of the L domain is to mediate virus cell separation. L domains lie at different locations in the Gag proteins of different viruses. In ASLV, MPMV, and the MuLVs, the L domain lies in the amino terminal third of the protein, and its critical residues are PPPY. In HIV-1, the domain lies in p6, at the C terminus, and instead contains the motif PTAP. In EIAV, the domain lies in p9 and contains the motif YPDL. Many viruses contain more than one L domain, and in such cases, each domain can provide partial function. Remarkably, many (though not all) of these L domain motifs are interchangeable among the various retroviruses and show a substantial position independence for their function.[404,544,563,818] L domains have been shown to be important for the release of many budding viruses, including VSV, rabies virus, and Ebola.

The L domains are now appreciated as serving as the binding sites for various components of a host machinery normally involved in protein sorting and delivery into late endosomal compartments, the multivesicular bodies.[240,495,510,706,727] The complex that carries out these trafficking events contains more than 20 distinct proteins held together through a network of protein–protein interactions.[757] Most show strong similarity to the so-called VPS proteins of the yeast ESCRT complexes, for endosomal sorting complexes required for transport, identified genetically as involved in vacuolar protein sorting in yeast.[25,26] The proteins have been divided into three groups: the ESCRT-I complex, containing Vps28, Vps37C,[181] and Tsg101, a gene first identified as a tumor suppressor locus[405]; ESCRT-II, containing Eap20, 30, and 45; and ESCRT-III, containing a large number of CHMPs (for charged MVB proteins). Other key proteins include Alix/AIP-1 and the release factor Vps4A. The PTAP/PSAP class of L domains is bound by Tsg101; the PPPY class of L domains is recognized by various members of the Nedd4 family, a group of ubiquitin ligases that interact with Tsg101, and the YPxL class is bound by Alix/AIP-1. Other proteins associated with the ESCRT complexes, including the

vesicle-associated endophilins, may also bind Gag and play a role in virus budding.[765] Depletion of many of the ESCRT homologues, or overexpression of dominant-acting negative fragments of these proteins, can potently inhibit retroviral budding and release.[240,326]

Virion Assembly *In Vitro*

Early work showed that Gag proteins and fragments of Gag are competent to assemble *in vitro* to form various structures, spherical or tubular, that recreate some features of virion cores.[186,364,647] The formation of these structures is dramatically enhanced by addition of RNA or oligonucleotides,[440,441] and in some settings, the length of the tubes can be determined by the length of the RNA.[100] Larger Gag fragments that include more amino-terminal regions can assemble into spherical particles,[265,331] and this assembly is stimulated by RNA[211,440,441] and host cell extracts.[99] A critical component in these extracts was identified as IP6.[98] Virus-like particles have also been formed with the Gag proteins of MPMV in cell-free protein synthesis systems and in bacteria.[519]

Much progress has been made in the assembly of mature-like HIV-1 virion core structures *in vitro*. The amino-terminal residue of CA, a proline, is critical for proper folding and assembly.[641] HIV-1 Gag CA-NC fragments can assemble into conical structures,[232] with a pitch that falls into discrete values. Image reconstruction of these cones has allowed the formation of a model for the packing of the CA protein into hexagonal arrays.[410] These assembly reactions are promoted by IP6, which binds to a ring of positively charged basic residues that form a pore in the center of capsid lattice and thereby stabilizes the structure.[450,619] The overall shape of the particle is then determined by the placement of CA pentamers in the hexamer array, allowing for the formation of a closed sphere, cylinder, or cone (see Fig. 15.16).

Virion Size

The number of Gag proteins per virion particle is estimated to be in the range of 1,200 to 1,800, though this number may vary somewhat from virus to virus (and has been disputed[80]). The number of Gag-Pro-Pol proteins is roughly 10 to 20 times lower, approximately 100 to 200 per virion. The proteins in the immature virus do not form a completely homogeneous, ordered crystalline array, but rather they may form a "protein micelle" that is somewhat fluid like a lipid micelle. The diameter of even wild-type virus preparations is not tightly homogeneous but shows a distribution that suggests some flexibility in the structures during assembly. However, the average size of the particle is determined by the Gag protein, and mutants with alterations in Gag often show abnormal or excessively heterogeneous diameters.[374] Mutations in the CA domain commonly show this phenotype. Thus, CA-CA contacts may play a role in determining the angle between Gags during their packing into a spherical shape.

Gag proteins of one virus are sometimes able to interact with the Gags of another virus to coassemble and form mixed virion particles. Various mutants with alterations in the Gag proteins of the MuLVs can coassemble into particles that show phenotypes of both parental Gags.[337,614] Viruses of very different genera can even form mixed particles in some cases.

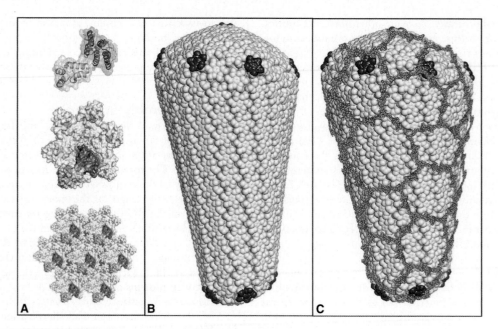

FIGURE 15.16 Structures of HIV-1 CA and virion cores. **A:** CA monomer (PDB ID 3MGE) with the NTD colored in *dark blue* and CTD in *light blue* (*top*). *Middle view* shows the CA hexamer (*cyan*) and the *bottom* shows the assembly into larger complex. **B and C:** Reconstruction of the conical core of a single HIV-1 virion in the absence (**B**) and presence (**C**) of the Trim5a cage. Hexamers of the HIV-1 CA protein (*cyan*) is organized in a folded array. Curvature is introduced by the asymmetric placement of pentameric defects (*dark blue*) at each end of the cone (**B**). Trim5 α is indicated in *magenta* (**C**) overlayed over the CA core. Models were generated based on https://github.com/alvinyu33/trim5-public/, files cg_capsd_core1.pdb and cg_trim5_trimer-of-dimer.pdb.[812] (Figures generated using PyMol and Powerpoint courtesy of Swapna Gurla.)

Incorporation of Other Proteins Into Assembling Virions

During assembly, other proteins are incorporated into the particle by contacts to Gag; these include Gag-Pro-Pol, Env, and auxiliary proteins encoded by the complex viruses. The Gag-Pol precursor is incorporated into the assembling bud by virtue of the Gag protein present at the amino terminus. Gag to Gag-Pro-Pol contacts can in some cases lead to the incorporation of mutants of Gag-Pro-Pol that do not retain the myristate modification to the amino terminus,[566] suggesting that the interaction is quite strong. Gag fusions to foreign proteins can be similarly incorporated into particles formed by Gag[330]; this process can even be used to target antiviral proteins into virions. Consistent with this notion, many mutations that block assembly of Gag, when tested in the context of Gag-Pol, are found to have similar effects on the incorporation of Gag-Pol.[141,665] However, some mutations in HIV-1 Gag have also been identified that specifically affect the incorporation of Gag-Pol, suggesting that Gag-Pol utilizes some distinctive contacts not important for Gag-Gag interactions.[687] Further, in the spumaviruses, Pol is incorporated without an appended Gag region, suggesting that distinct interactions must be utilized for its incorporation.[191]

The Env protein is concentrated at the sites of budding and incorporated into the virions by virtue of contacts between the cytoplasmic tail of Env and the amino-terminal MA portion of Gag. These interactions have been difficult to document directly, though there are some biochemical[138,798] and cross-linking studies in support of these contacts. Genetics has provided good evidence for this interaction. Selected mutants of MA show defects in Env incorporation,[175,221] and some mutants of the cytoplasmic tail of TM are not efficiently incorporated.[503,504,817] In addition, HIV-1 Env proteins, specifically delivered to the basolateral surface of polarized epithelial cells, can redirect the sites of budding of Gag from a nonspecific assembly on both membranes to the exclusive assembly at basolateral membranes and can similarly redirect Gag in neurons. Finally, mutants and revertants of these mutants with second-site suppressors in the binding partner have provided strong evidence for these interactions.[220,221] However, it should be noted that the envelope proteins of viruses very distant from retroviruses, including VSV and influenza, can be functionally incorporated into retrovirus particles (a process known as pseudotyping) without any obvious sequence similarity in their cytoplasmic tails. Furthermore, truncating the tail of ASLV Env does not prevent its incorporation or function.[574] Thus, there may be mechanisms to direct Env proteins to assembling virions without these specific contacts to Gag—a default pathway or a pathway using other interactions.

The HIV-1 protein Vpr is efficiently incorporated into assembling virions at very high levels, approaching equimolarity with Gag. This incorporation requires the presence of the p6 domain of Gag[667] and is likely mediated by a direct interaction.[27] The binding can be used to direct foreign proteins into the particle; a fusion between Vpr and a foreign protein will be targeted to virions. Furthermore, Vpr can be used to direct separately expressed versions of RT or IN to particles in a functional form, to complement mutations in the RT or IN domains of the Gag-Pol fusion.

Host Proteins in the Virion

A number of host proteins have been shown to be present inside the virion particle; in most cases, the significance of the protein is unknown. Prominent among the virion-associated factors are a number of cytoskeletal proteins. These include actin[22,546,780] and various members of the ezrin–radixin–moesin (ERM) family, specifically including ezrin, moesin, and cofilin.[545,546] Gag and especially the NC protein of HIV-1 have been shown to directly bind to actin,[621,780] perhaps offering a mechanism for its incorporation into the particle. A complication in analyzing virion-associated proteins is that virion preparations tend to be contaminated with substantial amounts of microvesicles, entities released by cells that exhibit a density and size very similar to that of virions and containing an array of host proteins.[58]

The virions of HIV-1 contain substantial levels of cyclophilin A, a protein proline isomerase of uncertain function but implicated in protein folding and signal transduction.[218,455,752] The role of the virion-associated form is uncertain. Several other proteins have also been found in virions: a translational elongation factor, eIF-1a,[123] and a protein known as H03,[383] with similarity to histidyl-tRNA synthetase, are additional examples. An intriguing protein present in HIV-1 virions is lysyl-tRNA synthetase (LysRS), the cognate synthetase responsible for the charging of tRNA (Lys), the primer tRNA for HIV-1.[105,107,318] The incorporation of lysyl-tRNA synthetase is mediated by a direct interaction with Gag, specifically the C-terminal portion of CA, and does not require the tRNA itself. The synthetase may facilitate tRNA incorporation.[105]

Host proteins may also be attracted into virion cores by mechanisms other than Gag. The host uracil DNA glycosidase, responsible for removing uracil bases from DNA, was shown to be incorporated into virions by contacts to IN.[782] The Ini1/Snf5 protein is also incorporated into virions through binding to IN.[821] Another protein, the RNA transporter staufen, is incorporated into virions, perhaps through contact with viral RNA.[498]

There are also substantial levels of host membrane proteins in the virion envelope. The mechanism of incorporation of these proteins into the virion is not clear, and in most cases, again the significance is uncertain. However, one such molecule, MHC class I, is present at levels approaching those of the Env protein and can be functionally significant, in that xenogeneic antibodies targeted to MHC can neutralize the infectivity of viruses such as HIV-1.[22]

RNA PACKAGING

The RNA genome is incorporated into virions by virtue of interactions between specific RNA sequences near the 5′ end of the genome, termed the packaging or Psi sequences, and specific residues in the NC domain of Gag (see Refs.[52,149]). Direct binding is readily observed *in vitro* (e.g.,[53,147]), though specificity is hard to demonstrate. Both partners in this interaction have been intensively studied.

Gag Sequences Important for Packaging

The Gag precursor is the form of the protein that is responsible for packaging viral RNA,[531] and the NC portion of the precursor plays the largest role. Mutations affecting the NC protein often reduce the incorporation of the genomic RNA into the virion particle (see Ref.[52] for review). The most crucial sequences are the Cys-His boxes, short sequence blocks resembling zinc fingers and containing the motif Cys-X2-Cys-X4-His-X4-Cys[254]; but basic residues elsewhere in the NC molecule are also important. Structures of the HIV-1 NC bound to various RNAs have been resolved by NMR, revealing specific contacts between both hydrophobic and basic residues of NC and nucleotides in the stem–loop of the RNA.[13,156] The NC protein of various viruses contains either one or two copies of the Cys-His box. When two copies are present, they are not equivalent or interchangeable, suggesting that they mediate distinct interactions with RNA.[252] Some viral cores can cross-package heterologous viral RNAs, suggesting good binding to the heterologous Psi region, and sometimes, there is a strong preference for the homologous RNA. Exchanging the NC domains between viruses can sometimes transfer the preferential selectivity of a Gag protein for its cognate RNA, though the specificity of these hybrid Gags is often poor.

Although Gags can definitely package RNAs in *trans*—that is, RNAs such as vector genomes that do not encode Gag—there may be enhanced encapsidation of the RNAs that encode Gag in *cis*, perhaps by the interaction of nascent Gag with RNA during its translation.[262,343,415,595]

RNA Sequences Important for Packaging

The packaging or Psi regions on the viral RNA genome that are recognized for incorporation are quite distinct in nucleic acid sequence among the various viruses (e.g., see Ref.[509]). The key Psi regions lie near the 5′ end of the RNA, generally between the LTR and Gag.[344,457,468,824] However, other regions of the genome can affect RNA packaging, including sequences upstream in R and in U5, downstream in Gag coding regions, and even near the 3′ end of the genome. In the case of ASLV, a region of 270 nt is necessary and sufficient to mediate the packaging of a foreign RNA.[341] In the case of the MuLVs, sequences that are at least partially sufficient to mediate selective packaging have been similarly identified.[2,45] These Psi regions are relatively autonomous; Psi can be moved to ectopic positions in the genome with at least some retention of function.[456]

Considerable effort has been focused on the structures of the 5′ RNA of various viruses (e.g.,[35,124–126,345,389,550,813,824]). Sophisticated methods have recently been applied to the study of the HIV-1 packaging elements, facilitated by improvements in NMR methods for probing of RNA structures (see Fig. 15.17). They reveal sequences involved in initiation of dimerization (DIS), as well as structures utilized for other purposes, including TAR, the PBS (before annealing of the tRNA), the major splice donor, and the translation start for Gag synthesis. These studies have revealed alternative structures that expose or sequester sites for NC binding,[77,169] depending on the fate of the RNA for either packaging or for translation. Mutational studies show that stem–loops, often containing GACG in the loops[146,156,389] that may serve as Gag binding sites, contribute to the efficiency of packaging of the RNA.[210,497] One of the stem–loop structures of the HIV-1 Psi could be replaced by a completely foreign sequence that was selected on the basis of its binding activity with NC, and the resulting RNA was efficiently packaged and utilized for replication, strongly suggesting that the binding to Gag is the key function of Psi.[125]

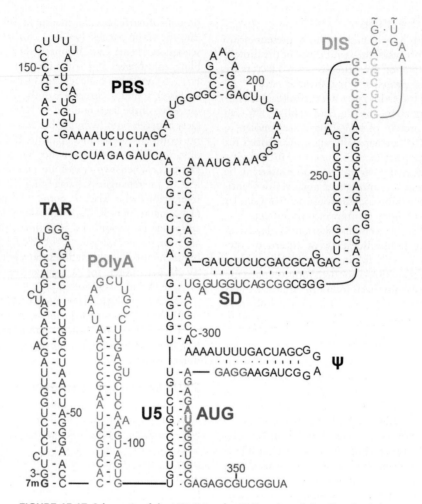

FIGURE 15.17 Schematic of the HIV 5′-Leader (5-L) region of the dimeric viral RNA. Individual *cis*- and *trans*-acting functional RNA sequences are highlighted including 7ᵐG cap (*red*) trans-activation response regions (TAR, *brown*), polyadenylation signal (polyA, *blue*), U5 (*dark blue*), primer binding site for initiation of reverse transcription (PBS, *black*), dimer initiation sites for genome dimerization (DIS, shown as a dimer in *orange/yellow*), major splice donor site (SD, *magenta*), the hairpin included within the psi packaging sequence (Ψ, *black symbol*), and the *gag* start codon (AUG, *green*). The transcription start sites are heterogeneous, and schematic numbering starts at the 2-G position. (Adapted with permission from Kharytonchyk S, Monti S, Smaldino PJ, et al. Transcriptional start site heterogeneity modulates the structure and function of the HIV-1 genome. *Proc Natl Acad Sci U S A* 2016;113(47):13378–13383.)

Virions also contain a number of host RNAs of uncertain significance. There are substantial levels of 7S RNA, a low molecular weight RNA normally involved in host RNA splicing.[348] In addition, there are low levels of host mRNA. Particles released without efficient packaging of the viral genome (as are produced by Psi mutant genomes) may carry enhanced levels of host RNAs, and various mutants with alterations in NC can show selective enhancement of both endogenous viral and host RNAs,[479] including ribosomal RNA and even intact ribosomes.[507] A variant avian leukosis virus, SE21Q1b, packages unusually high levels of host RNA[228,421] and is capable of transducing these host sequences into new cells by reverse transcription.[435] This phenotype of high-efficiency transduction is associated with an unusually high level of proviral expression and particle production rather than any specific alteration in a viral protein.[15]

Dimerization of the Viral Genome

Mature virions contain a dimeric RNA that is highly condensed into a stable, compactly folded structure referred to as the 70S dimer on the basis of its sedimentation rate. Specific sequences in the 5′ end of the RNA,[292] termed dimerization initiation sequences (DIS), are required for RNA dimerization *in vitro* and for the formation of the dimeric virion RNA *in vivo*.[51,346,438,499] A model for the process of dimerization, the "kissing loop" model, suggests that duplex formation between two RNAs is initiated between loops on the two RNAs and propagates outward through the stems through the action of NC.[126,171,271,437,491,506,552,553,629,720] Though the sequences of various retroviruses can vary widely, some structural features are conserved.[737]

Viral and even virus–host chimeric RNAs are normally always packaged as a dimer.[291] A high-affinity binding site for

NC is sequestered by base pairing in the monomeric MLV and HIV-1 RNAs, and dimerization of the RNA exposes this and other binding sites, allowing tight binding by NC.[148,165] This strongly suggests that dimerization is a prerequisite for packaging. Further studies support this idea and suggest that many mutations in the virus affect packaging by altering the monomer–dimer equilibrium and thus the amount of dimer available for NC binding.[540] However, some ASLV mutants can apparently package monomeric RNA.[542,564] Even here, it remains possible that dimers are packaged but dissociate later.

The viral RNA in newly budded virions is present as a relatively "unstable" dimer, dissociated by heat at relatively low temperatures, and becomes condensed to a more stable dimer during virion maturation.[225,590] This condensation requires the proteolytic processing of Gag[223] and may be mediated by the free NC upon its release from the precursor. It is likely that the paired regions of an unstable dimer are extended by NC.[184,629,790] Dimerization may sometimes, but not always, require mature Pol proteins; RT and IN seem to be required for stable dimerization of HIV-1 RNA but not MuLV or MPMV.[95,677] The dimerization of viral RNAs can be induced *in vitro* and is stimulated by addition of NC or the Gag precursor. However, it is uncertain to what extent these reactions reflect dimerization *in vivo*.

Incorporation of tRNA Primer

A key aspect of RNA packaging is the incorporation of a host tRNA along with the genome to serve as the initiating primer for minus strand DNA synthesis (for review, see Ref.[446]). Virions contain a substantial pool of free tRNA, perhaps 50 to 100 copies per particle. The bulk of these tRNAs are not associated with the genomic RNA and are present in virions that lack the genome. In some viruses, these tRNAs are largely representative of the pool of tRNAs in the cell, while in others, they are enriched for the tRNAs needed for priming DNA synthesis, though even here many other tRNAs are present. Viruses prepared without the Pol proteins do not show this enrichment, suggesting that Pol, and most probably the RT domain of Gag-Pro-Pol, is responsible for bringing these tRNAs into the virion.[356,581] In accord with this notion, the RT of ASLV has been shown to preferentially bind tRNAtrp from a mixture of tRNAs, accounting for its enrichment in the virion.[556] Similarly, HIV-1 RT preferentially binds tRNAlys3, and the interaction domain has been shown to at least include the anticodon loop of the tRNA. The incorporation of tRNAlys3 and its placement onto the HIV-1 genome are likely also catalyzed by the copackaged lysyl-tRNA synthetase.[105,363] However, no similar preference for the natural primer tRNApro has been detected for the MuLV RT, nor is a tRNA synthetase apparently copackaged in MuLV particles.[104] It may be significant that the MuLVs have been shown to be able to utilize a range of different primer tRNAs when only the complementary sequence in the genome (the pbs) is altered to promote their use.

tRNA Primer Placement

A very small subset of the virion-associated tRNAs—two per virion—are annealed to the primer binding site (pbs), an 18-nt sequence near the 5′ end of the genome with perfect complementarity to the 3′ sequences of a specific primer tRNA. The pbs sequences are, as one would expect, essential for normal reverse transcription of the virus.[625] The sequence of the pbs can

determine the primer tRNA that is utilized,[814] but changes in the pbs tend to revert back to the wild type,[777] suggesting that alternate tRNAs do not function well. An interesting aspect of reverse transcription provides for an efficient mechanism for this reversion: the use of the original tRNA even once during replication will convert the pbs back to the original sequence, because the tRNA itself is the template for the DNA copy of the pbs. Other sequence blocks of the tRNA are also paired with complementary sequences in R and U5 to form a large, complex structure required for proper tRNA primer placement and utilization.[7,128,306,312,496] These other sequences are presumably responsible for the selectivity for the natural tRNA primer. In the alpharetroviruses, *pol* gene products are required to mediate the placement of the tRNA on the genome; but in the gammaretroviruses, *pol* is not required.[224] In the case of HIV-1, Gag and Pol proteins and the copackaged lysyl-tRNA synthetase are all required.[103,106,306,356,416,637] The Gag precursor, and especially the NC domain, is thought to play a major role in promoting the annealing of the tRNA to the genome. While NC can promote annealing of complementary RNAs and DNAs *in vitro*, its role and the mechanism by which it may act *in vivo* remain uncertain.

PROTEIN PROCESSING AND VIRION MATURATION

As retrovirions are budded from the cell surface, the Gag and Gag-Pro-Pol precursor proteins are proteolytically cleaved to release the smaller proteins present in the infectious virions (for review, see Ref.[756]). The cleavage of Gag and Gag-Pro-Pol is mediated by the viral protease PR, which is expressed in Gag, Gag-Pol, or Gag-Pro-Pol fusion proteins. Thus, PR is responsible for cleaving itself out of a precursor protein and then making a number of other cleavages in these proteins.

Activation of the Protease

The processing of Gag and Gag-Pro-Pol precursors is intimately linked to assembly and budding and is controlled so that the precursors are not cleaved until they are assembled. It is not certain how PR is regulated during assembly to begin cleaving its substrates. The structure of PR has revealed that the active enzyme is a homodimer (see below), and thus, its activation could be promoted by dimerization of the Gag or Gag-Pro-Pol precursor associated with assembly. As the virions form, one could imagine the high concentrations of the protein generating an active PR that would begin to cleave Gag and Gag-Pro-Pol and would release the mature PR dimer as well. However, for the betaretroviruses like MPMV, this mechanism cannot explain the delay in processing. For these viruses, assembly occurs in the cytoplasm and should result in the establishment of a high concentration of Gag-Pro-Pol at that time. Yet cleavage does not begin in the cytoplasm but rather is restrained until budding and export of the preformed virion particle. Thus, other unknown mechanisms, perhaps coupled to membrane association, must be responsible.

Various domains of Gag have been suggested to inhibit PR, and conformational changes could relieve this inhibition. In the alpharetroviruses, a cleavage at the NC-PR boundary is required to release active PR, so activating this cleavage could serve as a trigger.[93] Similar cleavages at the p6*-PR boundary are important for full activation of the HIV-1 PR. Another possibility is the activation of the PR by a drop in the pH associated with virion release. It should be noted that the overexpression of PR in many artificial settings, both in bacteria and in animal cells, as a Gag-PR fusion or alone, can result in formation of highly active enzyme. The high level expression of PR is often toxic for cells, presumably due to its inappropriate action on many host proteins.

Protease Structure and Function

The retroviral proteases are aspartyl proteases with clear sequence similarity to members of the cellular family of aspartyl proteases.[338,426] The three-dimensional structures of many proteases, including those from ASLV, HIV-1, HIV-2, SIV, FIV, and EIAV, have been determined by x-ray crystallography.[384,487,516,769] The viral enzymes are small, typically containing about 100 amino acids and are homodimers as isolated from virions. Each subunit contributes to the active site a single aspartate residue, lying in a loop near the center of the molecule. There is a long cleft at the interface between the subunits where the substrate lies; there are pockets to interact with each of the side chains of the substrate, conferring specificity to the enzyme. Each subunit has a flap consisting of an antiparallel sheet with a b-turn that covers the cleft, and this flap moves out of the way to permit the binding of the substrate into the active site.

Retroviral proteases have a complex specificity for substrate peptides. The enzyme makes contact with approximately seven or eight side chains on the substrate and thus can select its cleavage sites on the basis of at least these amino acids. The cleavage sites tend to be within hydrophobic sequences and yet must lie in accessible and extended conformations. Some analyses of the various sites in Gag and Gag-Pol that are recognized by PR suggest that either one of two sequence motifs constitute a consensus site: one set has an aromatic residue or proline flanking the cleavage site, and the other set has aliphatic residues at these positions. Mutational analyses have allowed further definition of the residues on PR that make specific contacts to the substrate.

Protease Inhibitors

Studies of mutant viruses lacking PR demonstrated that the protease is essential for virus replication. Viruses lacking a functional PR can still express Gag and Gag-Pol precursors and can mediate the assembly and release of immature virion particles. Thus, PR is not required for the process of virion assembly *per se*. However, these particles are noninfectious and are blocked at an early step prior to the initiation of reverse transcription.[142,339,368] Because of its essential role in virus infectivity, PR was appreciated early in the course of the AIDS epidemic as an attractive target for antiviral therapy. A number of molecules have been generated that can bind and inhibit PR, including peptide mimetics with uncleavable, nonsessile bonds at the cleavage site. Some are transition state analogues and may have inhibition constants (Ki) in the nanomolar or subnanomolar range. These inhibitors have been extremely effective antiviral agents, and because they target a distinct enzyme and distinct step in the life cycle from the RT inhibitors, they have been particularly effective in combination with earlier drugs targeted at RT.

Processing of the Gag Precursor

During and after release from the cell, the Gag precursor is cleaved by the protease into a series of products present at equimolar levels in the virion. The number and size of the products vary considerably among the various viruses; the spumaretroviral Gag is exceptional in undergoing the fewest cleavages.

The Matrix Protein, MA

Beginning at the amino terminus, most Gags are processed to form a membrane-associated or matrix protein termed MA. The MA protein is thought to remain bound to the inner face of the membrane as a peripheral membrane protein and can be cross-linked to lipid. MA may make contacts with the cytoplasmic tail of the envelope protein. When the precursor Gag is myristoylated at the amino terminus, the corresponding MA protein retains that myristate and so is presumably bound tightly into the membrane. The compact structure of the MPMV MA protein has been elucidated by NMR.[135] The MA proteins of HIV-1 and SIV have been shown to form trimers in crystallization studies[48,612] and can contribute to the ability of a larger Gag precursor to form trimers in solution.[493] The protein can form extended sheets of trimers, with a large opening in the network. If similar structures were to form in a sphere, the surface could have openings into which the envelope tail may fit.

The Capsid Protein, CA

Gag proteins are cleaved to generate a large product serving as the major capsid protein, CA, in the virion core. The sequence of the CA protein is relatively well conserved among Gags and contains the most highly conserved motif among Gags, the so-called major homology region (MHR). The function of this motif remains uncertain; although mutations in the region affect virion assembly in some viruses,[140,451,602,704] it is not absolutely required. The three-dimensional structure of CA is highly conserved. CA forms the shell of the condensed inner core of the mature virus and thus makes a spherical, cylindrical, or conical structure, depending on the virion morphology. Image reconstruction of electron micrographs, coupled to the subdomain structures, has lead to models for the packing of CA to form these large assemblies. The major CA-CA contacts must form after processing during the condensation of the virion core and are very different from the contacts that exist in the immature virion particle.

The CA protein can form dimers in solution, and recombinant proteins containing CA, or CA plus NC, can assemble to form higher-order structures consisting of either tubes, spheres, and, in the case of HIV-1, cones.[232] CA has also been studied after tethering sheets of the protein to membrane.[37,231] The CA protein has proved difficult to crystallize. Structures of the N-terminal and C-terminal fragments of the HIV-1, RSV, and EIAV CA were first determined,[230,248,323,370] and only later were complete CA proteins visualized.[234] Mutants of HIV-1 CA with engineered potential to form disulfide cross-links have allowed isolation and crystallization of stable hexamers,[597] and later work defined a similar arrangement of CA proteins in the pentamers that introduce curvature into the hexamers array.[598] The structure of mature cones in HIV-1 virions has been revealed by cryo-EM tomography.[465]

The Nucleocapsid Protein, NC

All Gag proteins except for those of the spumaviruses are cleaved to produce a nucleocapsid protein, NC, located near the carboxy terminus of the precursor. NC proteins are small, highly basic proteins containing one or two copies of the Cys-His motif, $Cys-X_2-Cys-X_4-His-X_4-Cys$. These sequences bind a single Zn^{++} ion avidly and fold around the ion into a characteristic structure that is smaller and rather different from the better-known zinc finger structure. The structures of NC proteins in solution have been studied by NMR, revealing a tightly folded knuckle with disordered flanking sequences.[367,492] The interaction with zinc results in the incorporation of substantial levels of Zn^{++} into all retrovirus virion particles.

The NC protein in virions is closely associated with the viral RNA, probably coating the entire RNA molecule; the stoichiometry of binding is such that each NC molecule can bind to about six nucleotides of RNA. NC proteins bind nonspecifically to heteropolymeric single-stranded nucleic acid with moderate affinity.[746] However, NCs also exhibit specificity. Tests of binding to nucleic acids of defined sequence have shown that NCs bind poorly to poly(A) and most tightly to nucleic acids containing GT dinucleotides, especially alternating (GT)n polymers.[211] In addition, NC has been shown to exhibit sequence-specific binding activity *in vitro* for nucleic acids containing the Psi region, required for packaging of the viral RNA.[53] A specific complex of the HIV-1 NC with a stem–loop derived from Psi has been studied by NMR, and the resulting structure shows a number of specific contacts between hydrophobic residues of NC and bases in the four-nucleotide loop and between basic residues and specific phosphates in the stem and loop.[156]

NC proteins change the base-pairing properties of nucleic acids and thus can have profound effects on the kinetics and thermodynamics of annealing. Under various conditions *in vitro*, NC can stimulate the dimerization of RNAs and duplex formation between tRNA and its complementary sequences at the primer binding site.[72] Thus, NC can help promote primer tRNA placement during virion assembly.[618] NC can also help melt out secondary structures and may facilitate the movement of RT along the template during reverse transcription. In addition, it is clear that NC can bind to double-stranded nucleic acid and thus is probably retained on the viral DNA after its synthesis by reverse transcriptase. NC mutants have been found that affect the course of DNA synthesis or DNA stability during the early stages of virus infection, suggesting a role in the processing of the DNA and protection of DNA from degradation.[253,723]

Potent inactivators of virus infectivity targeting the NC protein have been identified.[628,743] These compounds, disulfide-substituted benzamides (DIBAs), eject the zinc ion from NC and cross-link the cysteines via disulfide bonds. Virions treated with these compounds are potently inactivated without disrupting the virion structure, and the course of virion assembly in infected cells is similarly blocked. Drug-resistant variants are not readily recovered. The compounds are too cytotoxic for therapeutic use.

Other Gag Products

Some retroviral Gag proteins, including those of the alpharetroviruses, betaretroviruses, and gammaretroviruses, contain one or more poorly conserved domains of 10 to 24 kDa lying in between MA and CA. The functions of many of these proteins are still unclear. The ASLV p2 protein, the MuLV p12 protein, and the MPMV p24 protein contain a PPPY motif that plays an important role in late stages of virion assembly (see above). The MuLV p12 protein is a phosphoprotein[88,725,753,762,819,820] with roles in late stages but most notably also in early stages of infection.[141,819] The N terminus of p12 binds to CA and stabilizes the CA lattice.[762,779] In the absence of the p12 NTD, gammaretroviruses are unable to abrogate host restriction factors (TRIM5a/Fv-1[778]), also supporting a need for p12 to interact with CA. Analysis of chimeric Gags made between different MuLVs further indicates specificity in the p12-CA pairing.[394] Gammaretrovirus PICs are not imported to the nucleus through pores but rather require cells to pass through mitosis to access host chromatin,[634] and the major role of p12 seems to be to tether the incoming PIC to host chromatin during this process. This is mediated by the C-terminal domain of p12, which in M-MuLV encodes minimally an 11-amino acid sequence (SP(M/I)ASRLRGRR)[89] that tethers the PIC to the host mitotic chromosomes,[89,188,655,762,778] resulting in the postmitotic localization or retention of the PIC in the nucleus. Subsequent release of the PIC from the mitotic chromosomes allows viral integration to proceed through the IN functions.[655] For PFV and SFV_{mac}, a chromatin-binding sequence directing the PIC to bind to an acidic patch on H2A-H2B is located at the C terminus of Gag.[400]

In the lentiviruses, a p6 domain is present at the carboxy terminus of the Gag precursor. The HIV-1 p6 contains the PTAP sequence, serving as the late or L domain that interacts with the host Tsg101 protein, and mutations affecting the sequence drastically impair virus production. Particle production by such p6 mutants can be largely restored by mutation of the viral PR protease, suggesting that some of the effects are mediated by premature proteolysis of Gag.[304] p6 is also required to mediate the incorporation of Vpr into virion particles, likely by providing a direct docking site.

Processing of the Gag-Pro-Pol Precursor

At roughly the same time that the Gag precursors are cleaved during virion maturation, the Pro and Pol regions of the Gag-Pro-Pol precursor are also cleaved, giving rise to the PR, RT, and IN products. The Pro- and Pol-containing precursors of different viruses are cleaved in diverse patterns (Fig. 15.15). The functional significance of the different subunit structures of these various RTs is unclear, since they all perform a very similar set of reactions during virus replication.

The Gag-Pro-Pol precursor of the betaretroviruses and the nonprimate lentiviruses is also processed to produce the dUTPase protein, DU. In the betaretroviruses, the *pro* ORF encodes both DU and PR; in the nonprimate lentiviruses, the enzyme is encoded in the *pol* ORF, and DU lies in between RT and IN in the polyprotein. This enzyme acts to reduce the levels of dUTP that could otherwise be incorporated into viral DNA. Mutants of FIV lacking the function indeed show increased rates of mutation during replication,[398] and similar mutants of CAEV tend to accumulate G-to-A substitution mutations[744] presumably due to incorporation of dU residues.

Processing of the Env Precursor

The major proteolytic cleavage of the Env protein to form the SU and TM subunits is performed during its transport through the ER and Golgi by host proteases termed furins. This cleavage is essential for virus infectivity[471,575] and is thought to induce substantial rearrangements of the polypeptide chain. The TM subunit remains embedded in the membrane and contains an extracellular domain, a membrane-spanning segment, and a cytoplasmic tail. The SU subunit lies wholly outside the cell, and after its incorporation into the virion particle, wholly on the extravirion surface. It is held onto the virion by contacts to TM, and most often by noncovalent bonds, though disulfide links may occur in some viruses. SU is heavily glycosylated, and the presence of at least some of these sugars is important for virus infectivity. Perhaps, the most important function of this heavy glycosylation is to hide the peptides on the surface of Env from neutralizing antibodies that would otherwise have access to the virion surface. In addition, palmitoylation of the Env proteins of many viruses is essential for function.[407,530,640]

The Surface Subunit, SU

For most viruses, the major receptor-binding site is located in hypervariable sequences on the SU subunit, so that SU is a major determinant of host range. Chimeric SU proteins can be generated to demonstrate that the receptor utilization function maps to specific regions of the protein. The key regions of the avian retroviral Env proteins have been similarly defined by selecting for changes in host range *in vivo*; these studies show that very small changes can result in the use of new receptors. The structures of two SU proteins have been determined at high resolution: a fragment of murine leukemia virus SU,[196] and a fragment of the HIV-1 SU bound to its receptor CD4.[380,630] These structures suggest that the receptors make contacts to the envelope in shallow pockets that may not be readily bound by antibodies.

The Transmembrane Subunit, TM

The major contacts for oligomer formation of Env are thought to lie in TM; isolated TM proteins form trimers in solution and in crystals.[196,197,366,447] The trimer is held together by a modified leucine zipper motif that bridges the monomers via hydrophobic interactions. The TM subunit contains the so-called fusion peptide at or near its amino terminus, and TM plays the major role in fusion of the virion and host membrane. Many TM mutations are defective for membrane fusion. The key role of the fusion peptide of TM is to insert into the host membrane.

It is possible to separate the two major functions of the Env protein onto two different molecules that cooperate to mediate these steps. Thus, the receptor-binding function can be mediated by one Env protein, and the membrane fusion function can be mediated by another Env. This is apparent in the ability of two Env proteins to complement in mixed trimers.[617] It is also demonstrated by the ability of a wild-type Env to provide the membrane fusion function for a chimeric Env that on its own can only mediate cell surface binding.

The TM subunit of the murine leukemia viruses undergoes a second cleavage during virion assembly that is mediated by the viral protease, PR. This step removes a short sequence called p2E, or the R peptide, from the carboxy terminus of TM.[258] The cleavage step may require presentation of the tail to the protease, or some conformational change in the tail, that is mediated by Gag proteins; alterations in the MA or p12 Gag proteins can modulate the cleavage of TM.[357,819] Astonishingly, the cleavage is necessary to active the fusogenic activity of the envelope protein and thus promote virus entry.[82,616] Mutants

in which the tail is truncated at the site of cleavage are constitutively activated for fusion, and these viruses induce dramatic syncytia in receptor-positive cells. Mutants in which the tail is not removed are inhibited for fusion, and particular residues can be shown to be required.[805] How the cytoplasmic tail inhibits the fusogenic activity of Env is very much unclear.

In a similar way, the cytoplasmic tails of the TM of M-PMV and EIAV are processed by the protease. In the case of M-PMV, the presence of the intact tail is necessary for efficient incorporation of Env into the virion. The replication of some viruses in host cells of foreign species (such as SIV in human cells) can select for alterations and truncations of the TM tails. The selective advantage conferred by this truncation is not well understood, though various aspects of Env function seem to be enhanced by this truncation.[841]

Morphological Changes Upon Virion Maturation

The maturation of retrovirus particles is a complex process that is required for the formation of an infectious virus. The particles that are initially assembled either at the plasma membrane (by most retroviruses) or in the cytoplasm (by the betaretroviruses) have a characteristic immature morphology: the particles are round and stain with an electron-dense ring and a relatively electron-lucent center. After release from the cell, the morphology changes to a more condensed structure, with a central core largely detached from the surrounding envelope. In the alpharetroviruses, gammaretroviruses, and deltaretroviruses, the core is roughly spherical and concentric with the envelope; in the betaretrovirus, the core is spherical but eccentrically placed within the envelope; in the lentiviruses, the core is cylindrical or conical. In the spumaviruses, the morphology does not change dramatically after assembly.

Mutant viruses lacking PR show little change from the immature morphology. Thus, cleavage of Gag and Gag-Pol is required for the restructuring of the virion into the mature form.[339] The changes in morphology visible in electron micrographs are associated with major rearrangements of the Gag proteins. Indeed, the physical properties of the virion change dramatically upon maturation. Whereas the immature core is quite stable to nonionic detergents and harsh conditions, the mature virion core is relatively labile. This change may be reflected in the inability of the immature virion, and the acquired ability of the mature virion, to uncoat upon infection of new cells and initiate reverse transcription.

Structure of Virion Core: CA Packing

After maturation, the Gag proteins rearrange to form the distinctive virion core, composed of the CA protein surrounding the dimeric viral RNA condensed with the NC protein. The core is visible by electron microscopy as an electron-dense structure inside an electron-lucent area surrounded by a spherical shell and lipid envelope. The shape of the core is characteristic of the virus genera: round for the alpha- and gammaretroviruses, cylindrical for the betaretroviruses, and conical for the lentiviruses. Image reconstruction and x-ray crystallography studies of CA assemblies reveal that CA forms a hexameric array.[232,370,410]

Much work has been done on the *in vitro* assembly of CA into large structures. The hexamers can form a two-dimensional lattice,[231] or long helical tubes or cones[232,265] *in vitro*. The N-terminal domains of CA form external hexameric rings, and the C-terminal domain forms internal dimer contacts to link together adjacent hexamers. While hexamers can form tubes without distortion, the curvature needed to close the ends of a cylinder or cone, or to form a sphere, is generated by introducing pentamers into the otherwise hexameric array.[236,410] The various structures can be built with exactly 12 pentamers distributed around the particle. Flexibility in the NTD-CTD interactions between CA proteins allow for the formation of pentamers and for their accommodation into the hexamer array. Asymmetric placement of the pentamers can create the cone-shaped core of the HIV-1 virion (Fig. 15.16).

RESISTANCE TO RETROVIRUS INFECTION: HOST RESTRICTION FACTORS

Several loci in the mouse genome have long been known to provide dominant resistance to the murine leukemia viruses, including Fv1[420,586] and Fv4.[703] Recently, a number of novel host genes have been identified that also confer virus resistance to otherwise sensitive cells (for reviews, see Refs.[62,249]). In some cases, particularly HIV-1, these genes were identified as the targets of viral proteins that serve to inactivate the host restriction system; mutation of the viral functions then revealed the underlying restriction. In other cases, they were identified as the basis for a species-specific virus resistance—for example, the resistance to HIV-1 exhibited by various nonhuman primates. Collectively, these restriction systems target nearly all steps in the virus life cycle (Fig. 15.18). Although these factors are typically not effective in blocking wild-type viruses in humans, there is hope that they can somehow be activated or enhanced and so provide antiviral protection.

Replication Blocks Mediated by Endogenous Retrovirus Genes

One gene present in Japanese wild mice, identified as conferring resistance to Friend MuLV, has a simple mode of action: the *Fv4* gene restricts virus replication by blocking the ecotropic virus receptor.[709,728] The *Fv4* locus corresponds to a defective endogenous provirus that encodes an Env protein fragment; the product down-regulates the receptor and renders mice resistant to infection by exogenous viruses.[308,371] Similar blocks have been identified by envelope genes in chicken and primates.[631,708]

The *Fv1* gene was identified in several inbred mice in the early 1970s as mediating resistance to leukemogenesis by the Friend MuLV.[420,586] Two naturally occurring alleles provide resistance: the Fv1[b] allele (in Balb/c mice) allows replication of so-called B-tropic viruses but blocks N-tropic viruses, while the Fv1[n] allele (in NIH Swiss mice) allows replication of N-tropic viruses but blocks B-tropic viruses. Resistance is dominant in heterozygous animals. The tropism of the MuLVs can be characterized by their ability to replicate on cells of particular genotypes: N-tropic viruses grow only on Fv1[nn] cells, B-tropic viruses grow only on FV1[bb] cells, and NB-tropic viruses grow on both. The determinants of viral tropism lie in a small sequence of the CA protein.[73,297,547,636,699] The block to infection in resistant cells is at an interesting stage: largely after reverse transcription and before nuclear entry and provirus integration.[329,806] Curiously, the block to integration that is observed for a particular virus

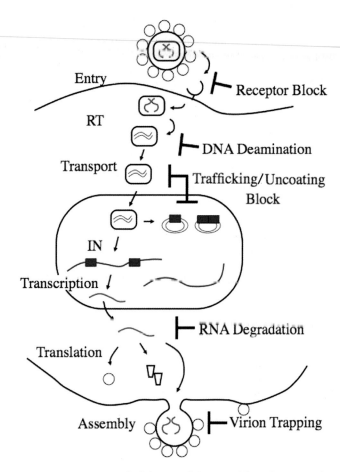

FIGURE 15.18 Sites of inhibition of the virus life cycle imposed by various restriction factors. A schematic of the virus life cycle is shown with steps in replication indicated on the *left*. Timing of blocks by different restriction factors is indicated on the *right*.

and cell combination *in vivo* is lost when the PIC is extracted and tested for its ability to integrate *in vitro*.[603] The *Fv1* gene was identified as a unique member of an endogenous retrovirus gene family, with close similarity to the *gag* genes of the HERV-L family.[59] The intracellular expression of this variant Gag protein can interact with the incoming PIC and its associated CA protein to block infection. Blocks have also been identified that target the JSRV Gag.[502]

Early Block to Infection by Trim5a

Human and many other mammals are resistant to N-tropic MuLVs via an activity originally dubbed Ref1.[57,735] This block is similar to that induced by the murine Fv1[b] gene (both are determined by residue 110 of the CA protein), although it acts earlier, before viral DNA synthesis. Rhesus macaques and other nonhuman primates manifest a similar block to HIV-1 infection in the early steps of the life cycle, also determined by CA, and originally called Lv1.[139,501] As with Fv1, these blocks were saturable: exposing cells to high levels of a restricted virus could overcome, or "abrogate," the block to infection by a second virus.[57,280,369] The gene responsible for these blocks encodes TRIM5a, a member of a large protein family known as the RBCC (for ring, B box, coiled-coil) or TRIM (for tripartite sequence motif) proteins.[283,347,578,705] The mechanism of action of TRIM5a in blocking virus infection involves specific binding to the CA protein of the incoming virus.[666] TRIM5a forming a hexameric lattice superimposed over hexameric tubes or cones CA protein has been visualized[233,413] (see Fig. 15.16). Formation of these lattices requires the coiled-coil region and the SPRY region.[635,760] For a review of TRIM5a restriction, see Ref.[235]

The critical residues of HIV-1 CA for TRIM5a recognition lie in the cyclophilin A binding loop,[229,747] and indeed, complex interactions between CA, TRIM5a, and cyclophilin A may determine virus sensitivity.[282,736] A major role of CypA in regulating HIV-1 infection may be in its ability to compete with and prevent binding of TRIM5a to CA. A remarkable confirmation of the functional interrelationships between these proteins is the finding that in a new world primate, the owl monkey, the TRIM5 gene is interrupted by the transposition of a cyclophilin A pseudogene and expresses a TRIM-Cyp fusion protein.[523,652] A similar, but independently arising gene fusion has been found in other primate lineages.[417,755] These fusion proteins confer potent resistance to viruses that retain a cyclophilin A binding site in their CA proteins. A plausible model for the action of all these factors is a premature disruption of the capsid soon after viral entry. A further complication is that restriction by TRIM5a may occur in two steps, with an initial proteasome-dependent step before reverse transcription and then a proteasome-independent one after reverse transcription.[795]

TRIM5a has also been shown to play a role in the induction of interferon production by stimulating synthesis of unlinked polyubiquitin chains.[580] Thus, another antiviral function of TRIM5a may be to signal interferon production in response to an incoming viral core; this function seems to be independent of its direct antiviral activity.

Deamination of Viral DNA by the APOBECs

A major mechanism of resistance to HIV-1 is provided by the deamination of cytosine residues in the minus strand of the viral DNA formed during reverse transcription.[278,676] The main enzymes responsible for this activity in primates are APOBEC3G and F, members of a family of cytidine deaminases that includes APOBEC1 (standing for apolipoprotein B mRNA-editing enzyme, catalytic polypeptide, a regulator of ApoB mRNA expression) and AID (for activation-induced cytidine deaminase, used in immunoglobulin class switching and hypermutation of immunoglobulin genes during affinity maturation). APOBEC3G is packaged into virions, and during subsequent infection, it can deaminate as many as 4% of the C residues of the viral DNA minus strand, resulting in both DNA destruction and G-to-A hypermutation of the surviving plus strand DNAs.[277,391,455,829] In addition to its deaminase activity, APOBEC3G may independently trap or inhibit viral DNA synthesis during infection.[520]

This potent block to infection mediated by the APOBECs is counteracted in human cells by the HIV-1 Vif protein, which drastically reduces the levels of APOBEC3G and F in the infected cell and prevents their incorporation into virions. Vif binds APOBEC3G and F and blocks them either by inducing their proteasomal degradation via the Cullin-5–SCF ubiquitin ligase complex, by inhibiting them directly or by blocking their translation. The APOBECs of many nonhuman primates are not recognized by HIV-1 Vif, and as a result, these species can block HIV-1 infection. In addition, the family member APOBEC3B, which has potent antiviral activity in cell lines, is resistant to HIV-1 Vif.[172] It is not clear why this isoform is not expressed adequately in lymphocytes to protect humans from infection.

Another host enzyme, uracil *N*-glycosylase (UNG), may collaborate with the APOBECs to promote degradation of the viral DNA. This enzyme is also packaged into virions and recognizes and removes uracils in the DNA, the product of deamination of cytidines, leaving an abasic site. This would block normal reverse transcription and lead to destruction of the viral DNA. However, the HIV-1 gene product Vpr can mediate the inactivation of UNG and the related SMUG enzymes, again probably via ubiquitin ligase-triggered proteasomal degradation.[659]

Blocking Early Events in Monocyte Lineage Cells by SAMHD1

Dendritic and myeloid cells exhibit a potent restriction of HIV-1 replication that prevents the normal accumulation of viral DNAs in the cytoplasm in the early phase of infection. The block can be counteracted by delivery of the Vpx protein encoded by HIV-2 and certain strains of SIVs. Recent work has identified SAMHD1 as the mediator of the block.[301,382] Remarkably, SAMHD1 is a nucleotidase, which reduces dXTPs to such low levels that reverse transcription of the viral RNA by RT cannot occur. It is most effective in monocytes or quiescent cells, which naturally have low levels of dXTPs. Vpx induces proteasomal degradation of SAMHD1, increases the cellular dXTP levels, and thereby allows virus infection.

Elimination of Viral RNAs by ZAP

A block to MuLV infection was initially identified in a screen of cDNA overexpression libraries for genes that confer virus resistance. The product of a rat gene, dubbed ZAP (for zinc finger antiviral protein), blocks viral gene expression by eliminating viral RNAs from the cytoplasm of the infected cell.[237] ZAP contains four CCCH-type zinc fingers that bind directly to viral RNA[267] and targets the RNA for destruction by the RNA exosome.[268] Remarkably, ZAP expression also renders cells resistant to infection by a number of alphaviruses, including Sindbis, Semliki Forest virus, and Venezuelan equine encephalitis virus,[61] and by Ebola virus. ZAP has recently been demonstrated to selectively bind RNAs containing clustered CpG dinucleotides often present at high levels on viral RNAs and at low levels on host RNAs.[721] Its activity requires a variety of cofactors, including KHNYN, TRIM25, and components of the RNA exosome.[209,408,649,834]

Trapping Virion Particles on the Cell Surface by Tetherin

HIV-1 mutants lacking the Vpu gene are poorly able to replicate in certain cell lines, with the major block being at the time of virion release from the infected cell surface. The inhibition was traced to the cell surface expression of a protein dubbed tetherin or BST-2, which traps the virion particles and prevents viral spread to neighboring cells.[518,576] Tetherin can similarly inhibit spreading infections by many enveloped viruses.[332] The Vpu protein of wild-type HIV-1 binds to tetherin and inactivates it; this may be achieved by sequestering it, by preventing its delivery to the cell surface, or by directing its ubiquitinylation and degradation.[176,179,284,315,454]

Some strains of HIV-1 and other primate lentiviruses use different proteins (e.g., Nef or Env) to achieve the same result.[21,245,365,651,827,828]

Blocking Envelope by the SERINC Proteins

The serine incorporator (**SERINC**) proteins are multipass transmembrane proteins involved in lipid synthesis. Some members of the SERINC family, notably SERINC3 and 5, are potent lentiviral restriction factors. These proteins are incorporated into nascent virions and inhibit their subsequent fusion capability and infectivity.[694,733] The SERINCs inhibit the formation of small fusion pores between viruses and cells normally created by the Env protein. The viral Env protein determines sensitivity to SERINCs. The antiviral activity is also counteracted by the Nef proteins of several lentiviruses,[150] by the MuLV glycoGag protein,[409] and by the EIAV S2 protein.[111]

RETROVIRAL DISEASES

The Varied Effects of Retroviral Infection

Retroviruses cause an extremely wide range of responses in infected animal hosts. We begin discussion of retroviral pathogenesis with a little-appreciated but important point: retroviruses in general are surprisingly benign. The vast majority of the replication-competent retroviruses are not cytopathic, and the infection of cells cause remarkably little impact on their replication or physiology. The morphology, the control of cell division, and the doubling time of cells in culture are not significantly changed after infection. Once a chronic infection is established, only a relatively small amount of the cellular metabolism is committed to virus expression: typically, a few percent of the cellular mRNA and protein are viral, and so the cell can perform its normal functions and survive for its normal lifespan. Indeed, animals show few acute affects upon infection. The animals do become viremic, and a vigorous immune response is often mounted that can reduce the levels of virus production. However, infected mice or birds may live relatively normal lives for many months or years, and so it is appropriate to consider the viruses as relatively benign parasites. It is noteworthy that the virus is not eliminated but only suppressed by the immune response, and low-level viremia usually persists in infected animals for life.

Retroviruses often do, however, cause disease. The chronic viremia of the replication-competent retroviruses is tantamount to high-level mutagenesis of infected cells, for each infection event is associated with a proviral insertion that constitutes a mutation. Eventually, the odds are that a cell will suffer an insertion that alters the normal control of cell division or cell survival, and abnormal proliferation of this cell results in tumorigenesis. Many retroviruses cause disease in this way, including the so-called slow leukemia viruses and agents such as MMTV. A few retroviruses, however, are more pathogenic: a small minority of the retroviruses are directly cytopathic, and many of the infected cells are killed. These agents can thus destroy the infected tissues and directly damage their function. Examples include the cytopathic avian viruses and the AIDS virus, HIV-1. Finally, a special class of retroviruses exists, the so-called acute transforming viruses, that can induce a rapid tumor formation. These viruses were among the first filterable

oncogenic agents ever discovered, and their dramatic effects were a major motivation for the intense study of all the tumor viruses throughout the 20th century. We now understand that these agents are transducing viruses; the replication of retroviruses allows for recombination events between viral and host sequences that move genes onto the viral genome. These viruses carry and express host genes at inappropriate levels, in inappropriate cells, and often with drastic alterations in gene structure. If the gene product so expressed by the virus is mitogenic or antiapoptotic, the result can be a potent alteration in the physiology of the infected cell. These acute transforming viruses can thus initiate a highly aggressive tumor very efficiently and with minimal latency, because each infection of a cell has the high potential to initiate an oncogenic transformation event. Most often, the acquisition of the host gene comes with a loss of a viral gene essential for its replication; as a result, these viruses are often replication-defective and depend on a helper virus, usually a related replication-competent leukemia virus, for their transmission to new cells. We will discuss each of these various classes of pathogenic viruses in turn.

Diseases Caused by the Replication-Competent Retroviruses

The typical pathology of many of the simple replication-competent retroviruses is the development of leukemia or lymphoma after a very long latency. For this reason, these agents are often called the slow leukemia viruses; examples are found in rodents, including the many murine leukemia viruses, and in birds, including the avian leukemia–leukosis viruses. The symptoms eventually begin with a lymphoid hyperplasia,[701] which may be directly attributed to the immune response; not all the affected cells are infected, and the proliferating cells may be stimulated by cytokines that are released in response to the infection.[81] A subset of these expanding cells progress to frank leukemia, which ultimately can be fatal in susceptible animals. The cell type transformed by the virus can be very narrowly defined, or more broadly variable, but will depend strongly on viral determinants. For example, the ASLV group of viruses typically cause a bursal or B-cell lymphoma in birds; the Moloney MuLV causes a T-cell leukemia; the Friend helper MuLV causes an erythroleukemia; and MMTV causes a mammary epithelial tumor.

In some species and settings, the infecting virus is the proximal agent of disease; such is the case with infection of rats by the Moloney MuLV. However, the course of leukemogenesis in mice and other animals is often associated with the appearance of recombinant retroviruses derived from the parental infecting virus and endogenous sequences present in the germ line.[114,194] Some of the viruses arising in mice can be detected through an expanded host range, as an ecotropic virus acquires *env* sequences that allow infection through the polytropic receptors; these viruses are often termed MCF viruses, for *m*ink *c*ell *f*ocus forming viruses. The presence or absence of suitable endogenous proviruses in the germ line that provide the sequences needed for recombination can control the severity and course of disease.

Oncogenesis by Insertional Mutagenesis

The most common mechanism of action of the replication-competent viruses in initiating tumors is termed proviral insertional mutagenesis, leading to the misexpression of endogenous protooncogenes.[285,527,571] During replication in the infected animal, an enormous number of cells are infected and so acquire new proviral DNA insertions at near-random sites. Each of these insertions constitutes a somatic mutation, and thus, retrovirus infection can be thought of as similar to a massive exposure to a potent mutagen. The vast majority of the insertions are harmless. But very rarely a provirus insertion can create a dominant-acting mutation that profoundly alters the physiology of the cell. When a provirus integrates near a gene that controls growth and so alters its expression, the cell may proliferate and ultimately form a clonal tumor in which all cells contain the provirus integrated at the same site.

A large number of cellular genes have been identified as potential targets for insertional activation in retrovirus-induced tumors. Among the most notable are an array of transcription factors, including c-myc, N-myc, c-myb, Fli1, Fli2, Ets1 (Tpl1), Evi-1 (Fim3), Bmi1 (Flvi2), and Spi1 (PU.1); a number of secreted growth factors, such as Wnt1 (Int1), Wnt3 (Int4), Int2 (Fgf3), and Fgf8; growth factor receptors, including c-erbB, Int3 (Notch4), Mis6 (Notch1), c-fms (Fim2), the prolactin receptor, and Fit1; and genes implicated in intracellular signal transduction pathways, such as the serine/threonine kinases Pim1 and Pim2. Many of these genes are also known to be involved in or implicated in tumorigenesis in other settings, either when transduced on retroviral genomes or when activated by nonviral mutations, including point mutations and chromosomal rearrangements. However, a number of the protooncogenes have only been identified by virtue of their having served as target sites during tumorigenesis by leukemia viruses, and thus, this route has made important contributions to our list of known protooncogenes.

The patterns of activation of these protooncogenes by retroviral insertion are quite varied. At least four distinct mechanisms have been observed (Fig. 15.19).

1. Promoter insertion. The provirus may insert upstream of the gene or within the gene and in the same transcriptional orientation as the gene. Transcription beginning in the 3′ LTR reads into the gene and results in high-level expression of a transcript with R-U5 sequences at the 5′ end. The resulting transcripts may be similar to the natural transcripts but may be longer or truncated relative to the normal mRNAs, and the encoded proteins may be of wild-type structure.

2. Enhancer insertion. The provirus may insert either upstream or downstream of the gene or in introns, and in either orientation relative to the gene. The insertion brings the powerful transcriptional enhancers present in the U3 regions of the two LTRs into close proximity of the gene and so activates the endogenous promoter elements. While the levels are inappropriately high, the structure of the resulting transcript is normal. The HTLV-1 genome contains a binding site for the CCCTC-binding factor (CTCF), providing the potential to cause long-distance looping with CTCF sites elsewhere in the host genome and thereby alter chromatin and gene expression.[475,650]

3. Posttranscriptional stimulation of expression. The provirus may insert downstream of the coding region and stabilize the formation of an mRNA. The provirus may provide a polyadenylation signal that enhances the formation of stable transcripts, or the insertion may remove RNA destabilization

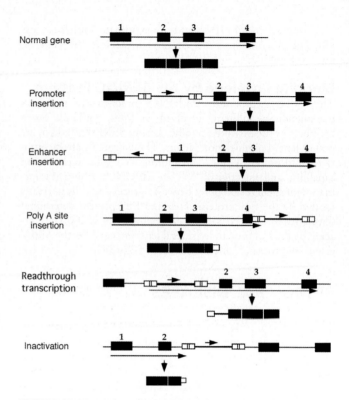

FIGURE 15.19 Genetic alterations in target gene expression induced by retroviral insertional mutagenesis. Various changes in normal gene expression that have been observed upon insertion of retroviral DNA are diagrammed. A target gene containing four exons is used in these examples (*top*). Promoter insertion: insertion of the provirus in the same transcriptional orientation in the first intron is shown to result in the formation of a new mRNA initiated in the 3′ LTR and extending into the downstream exons. Enhancer insertion: insertion upstream of the gene, in this case in reverse orientation, is shown enhancing the expression from the natural promoter. PolyA site insertion: insertion at the 3′ end of the gene in the forward orientation is shown providing a polyA addition signal and thereby increasing the levels of a prematurely truncated mRNA. Leader insertion: insertion of the provirus in the same transcriptional orientation is shown to result in the formation of an RNA initiating in the 5′ LTR, extending through the provirus, and into downstream exons. Splicing results in the retention of only the viral leader on the chimeric mRNA. Inactivation: insertion is shown causing premature end formation of the mRNA, resulting in the formation of an inactive fragment.

signals in the 3′ UTR that would normally mediate the rapid turnover of the RNA. Mutations affecting the coding sequences can result in abnormal stabilization of the protein product. These mechanisms can result in inappropriately high steady-state levels of the mRNA and protein products.

4. Readthrough transcription. The provirus inserts upstream or in the gene, but transcription initiates in the 5′ LTR, reads through the provirus, and continues into the gene. The formation of such transcripts is often enhanced by mutations in the provirus, such as loss of the 3′ LTR. The transcripts may be spliced aberrantly in complex patterns.

Insertional activation of a protooncogene by a provirus is not sufficient on its own to fully transform a cell but only represents the first step in a progression to a frank leukemia or tumor. ALV insertions cause visible overgrowth in bursal follicles, and subsequent mutations are needed for the growths to become malignant.[24] In insertional leukemogenesis by MLV, additional mutations are usually required for full transformation; these mutations can be point mutations in other protooncogenes or loss-of-function mutations of tumor suppressor genes. In some retroviral tumors, more than one oncogene can be activated by insertion of separate proviruses. Similarly, an acute transforming genome is often not sufficient to transform a cell in one step, and additional mutations must arise subsequently. In some tumors induced by a replication-defective transforming virus, the helper virus may provide such mutations by its own insertional activation event. For HIV-1, insertions at a limited number of genes are reported to result in clonal expansion, growth, persistence, and/or survival advantages but generally do not result in cancer.[108,131,309,448] HIV-1 integration in one gene, however, is found in AIDS-associated T-cell lymphomas, likely coupled to additional mutations.[476]

Gene inactivation, as opposed to gene activation, is also an important event in some tumors. Retrovirus insertion can frequently disrupt gene expression to effectively produce a null or hypomorphic mutation. These mutations are normally silent, since a second allele would be expected to continue to express a functional gene product. However, if the host animal is already heterozygous due to an inherited germ-line mutation in one allele, or if the insertional inactivation is coupled to a loss of the other allele by other means such as sister chromatid exchange, the net result can be homozygous loss of function. When the target gene is a tumor suppressor, the consequence is the promotion of tumorigenesis.

Viral Determinants of Pathogenicity

Several viral genes and sequences can affect the incidence and severity of retroviral disease. The viral LTR contains the most important determinants of leukemogenicity and of the cell tropism for transformation. The enhancer and promoter elements of the LTR are responsible for protooncogene activation, and their relative transcriptional activity thus controls the transforming ability of many viruses. If these elements are strongly tissue- or cell type–specific, the virus will be most competent for transformation of those cells in which the LTR is most active. A variety of viruses show profound tropisms for transformation that are controlled in this way.[74,428,559] For example, the promoter of the Moloney MuLV is most active in T cells, and the virus shows strong tropism for the formation of T-cell leukemias. The Friend helper virus LTR contains an enhancer that is most active in erythroid cells, and the virus is correspondingly highly tropic for erythroid cells.[75] The promoter of MMTV contains glucocorticoid response elements that provide high-level expression only in cells with high levels of the glucocorticoid receptor and only when exposed to glucocorticoids; as a result, MMTV is specific for mammary tumors.[263] Variant betaretroviruses, such as the thymotropic DMBA-LV virus, show selectivity for T cells that is probably attributable to changes in the LTR. Determinants of leukemogenicity have also been mapped to *gag*, *pol*, and *env* genes, though it is not clear what aspects of their functions is required in most cases. It may be that vigorous replication *in vivo* is the simple key feature of a highly transforming leukemia virus. There may also be trans-acting functions encoded by the leukemia viruses that modulate expression of specific host genes, but their roles are uncertain. The murine and feline leukemia virus LTRs encode short RNAs that can activate host genes in *trans*, apparently through activation of an AP-1–like activity.

Cytopathic Viruses

Some viruses show distinctive pathogenicity mediated by specific gene products. Cas-Br-E MuLV is a well-studied murine virus that induces a hindlimb paralysis with significant neuronal loss in the absence of an inflammatory response.[599] Both neurons and glial cells accumulate vacuoles. The virus targets endothelial cells and microglial cells in the brain, and it is likely that the infection of the microglial cells is most crucial to disease induction. Infection may impair or block the neuronal support function of these cells, resulting in loss of neurons, though the mechanism of neuronal cell death is unclear. It is possible that the expression of the Env protein is toxic. The major determinant of pathogenicity is in the SU subunit of the Env protein.[439,560] A number of other MuLVs, such as the ts1 mutant of the Moloney MuLV TB strain,[794] can cause neurological symptoms, including hindlimb paralysis and spongiform encephalomyelopathy,[63] and in these cases too, the SU protein is thought to be important. TR1.3, a Friend-related MuLV, is a neuropathogenic virus that induces fusion of capillary endothelial cells, leading to a hemorrhagic stroke syndrome. The crucial determinant in the virus is a tryptophan residue at position 102 of the SU protein. In some viruses, the LTR is also likely to play a role in disease specificity,[163,561] perhaps by determining the level of expression and the ability to spread efficiently and access the primary target cell.

A number of the ASLV group of viruses are cytopathic[775] and can cause an acute wasting disease characterized by poor growth, anemia, and immunosuppression associated with atrophy of the bursa and thymus.[620] The disease probably reflects the ability of these viruses to lyse infected cells. The isolation of the ALV receptor for the subgroup B viruses and its identification as a member of the TNF receptor family suggests the possibility that the binding of Env to the receptor is directly triggering an apoptotic response. The cytopathic and noncytopathic viruses seem both to be able to trigger similar responses, however, so it is not clear what aspect of the interaction might be necessary and sufficient for cell killing. The vigorous replication of the virus, and an ability to mediate high-level reinfection before superinfection resistance appears, may also be significant determinants of cytopathology (see Ref.[610] for further discussion).

Yet another disease caused by a variant virus is the feline-acquired immunodeficiency syndrome, or FAIDS. This disease was originally associated with a complex mixture of FeLV isolates. The agent responsible was shown to be an FeLV with mutations affecting the SU subunit of the *env* gene. The mutant FeLV is incapable of establishing superinfection resistance, and so large amounts of unintegrated viral DNA accumulate during superinfection, ultimately leading to high expression of viral gene products and causing cell lysis.

The lentiviruses cause an array of important diseases in animals and humans, most notably AIDS. The major cause of disease is probably cell killing. The very high level of gene expression mediated by HIV-1 infection in some cell types may be a crucial aspect of the cell killing,[693] but the key viral gene products remain obscure. HIV-1 infection eventually leads to depletion of CD4-positive cells and thus to immunodeficiency, culminating in severe opportunistic infections. The lentiviruses also cause a number of other pathologies, including anemia, and neurological disease, that are poorly understood. These diseases will be discussed in later chapters.

Stimulation of Host Cell Proliferation

MMTVs lead to the formation of mammary tumors through the insertional activation of a number of protooncogenes. However, unlike other simple retroviruses, MMTVs carry an additional gene termed *sag*, for superantigen, that is important for disease induction (see Ref.[130] for review). Sag proteins bind to MHC class II molecules in regions that are common to molecules with many different binding specificities and so can activate as many as 10% of all T cells.

The *sag* gene is located in the U3 region of the MMTV LTR and encodes a low-abundance glycosylated membrane protein.[78] The protein must be proteolytically processed for proper export to the cell surface. Importantly, expression of a functional Sag protein by MMTV is required to establish infection in an animal. The virus is normally transmitted in mother's milk to newborn mice, infects B cells in the Peyer patch, and induces a vigorous Sag-mediated stimulation of T cells. There follows a B-cell response that provides a large pool of susceptible B cells for the virus,[19] and it is these cells that then carry the virus to the mammary gland. Following infection of the mammary epithelial cells, the provirus is transcriptionally silent until the LTR is activated by hormonal signals into high-level expression and secretion of large amounts of virus in milk to complete the cycle of infecting the next generation. In a few infected cells, this process ultimately, following two or more pregnancies, leads to transformation by insertional activation. This pattern of viral spread through one intermediate cell type to ultimately lead to disease in another cell type is a paradigm for complex viral pathologies, such as that exhibited by polioviruses.

The *sag* gene of MMTV was also appreciated as acting as a host gene important in disease progression when a number of mouse genes, termed Mls for minor lymphocyte-stimulating antigen, were shown to map to endogenous MMTV proviruses and ultimately were identified as the *sag* genes. The expression of Mls during development results in the clonal deletion of many T cells in mice carrying the gene. Thus, mice carrying endogenous proviruses will often lose T cells needed for virus replication and so will be resistant to exogenous MMTV disease.

A number of other viruses carry variants of the normal replication genes that cause specific pathologies in the infected host. One MuLV, spleen focus-forming virus, SFFV-P, causes a severe polycythemia; infection leads to a massive expansion of erythroid precursors (BFU-E and CFU-E) and a concomitant loss of mature red cells. This agent consists of a complex of a replication-defective variant and a Friend MuLV helper virus to propagate it. The defective genomes carry a mutant *env* gene encoding a shorter SU molecule, termed gp55, that no longer functions to mediate virus entry. However, gp55 can bind directly to the erythropoietin receptor (EpoR) and stimulate the mitogenic and differentiative responses normally triggered by ligand binding to the receptor. This activity allows the virus to infect these dividing preerythroid cells, and the continued expression of the envelope protein in these cells promotes their factor-independent growth and expansion in an autocrine loop.

Ultimately, a frank erythroleukemia results and may be associated with proviral activation of protooncogenes occurring as a result of the continuing infections. It is clear that the *env* gene of the virus is sufficient to cause the disease.[793] A very similar virus, the SFFV-A, causes a severe splenomegaly and anemia. This virus is closely related to SFFV-P and also activates the Epo receptor to expand immature cells. Variation in the envelope between these two strains alters the target cell and the consequences of its expansion.[334] It should be noted that this mitogenic activity of gp55 is not a completely novel property of the deleted Env. The parental F-MuLV helper Env protein has a weak ability to bind and send mitogenic signals through the Epo receptor, presumably resulting in expansion of Epo receptor–positive cells. This increase in target cell number is presumably able to enhance virus spread and so serves as a positively selected trait for the virus. Other Env proteins, including those of the MCF viruses, may activate the IL-2 receptor.

Another replication-defective variant, the murine-acquired immune deficiency syndrome or MAIDS virus, causes a relatively acute hyperproliferation of B-lineage cells in infected mice.[23,305] There is a subsequent proliferation of macrophages and CD4⁺ T cells. The expansion of these cells displaces many other cell types, including T cells, and the animals eventually show a significantly defective immune response. The mechanism of the immunodeficiency is not fully clear, and there is some indication that an antigen-driven stimulation leads to an anergic state. However, the immunosuppression occurs, the disease is in reality a lymphoproliferative disorder and is quite distinct from human AIDS in its pathology. The causative agent is again a replication-defective variant carried by a replication-competent helper virus. The defective genome encodes a mutant Gag precursor in which the central portion, including the p12 region, is replaced by a foreign Gag derived from endogenous retrovirus sequences. The altered Gag has been shown to interact with the c-Abl protein, a tyrosine kinase first identified as the transduced oncogene of the Abelson murine leukemia virus, in that virus expressed as a Gag-Abl fusion protein. Thus, the MAIDS virus seems to act by forming a noncovalent interaction with the c-Abl protein as an approximate mimic of the Gag-Abl protein formed by transduction on the Abelson virus.

An ovine disease has attracted attention as a potential model for human lung cancer. Sheep pulmonary adenomatosis (SPA) is a contagious bronchioloalveolar carcinoma of sheep associated with an exogenous type betaretrovirus, Jaagsiekte sheep retrovirus (JSRV). Epithelial tumor cells are sites of large amounts of viral DNA.[554]

Two of the epsilonretroviruses, the piscine (fish) retroviruses, cause a dermal sarcoma of freshwater fish that shows a remarkable seasonal appearance and regression. The mechanism of transformation of cells by the virus is not totally clear but seems to reflect the activity of the cyclin D homologue encoded the orf A gene, which may induce inappropriate entry of the cells into cycle by activation of a cyclin-dependent kinase (cdk).

Host Determinants of Retroviral Disease

A number of genes have been identified that determine sensitivity or resistance to retroviral diseases. Some of these genes act at the level of virus replication, directly controlling the ability of the virus to enter and spread. The Fv1 locus described above is a good example of a gene that acts in a cell-autonomous way to restrict the replication of various murine leukemia viruses.[328]

A large set of those genes that affect sensitivity to viral disease modify the availability of target cells for virus growth, or the immune response to virus infection, and therefore indirectly control the levels of viremia. The *Fv2* gene is an example of such a gene.[419] Virus susceptibility (Fv2^s) is dominant over virus resistance (Fv2^r) at this locus. The virus-susceptible allele encodes a truncated form of the stem cell kinase receptor (Stk), which promotes virus-induced erythroleukemia[579]; expansion of the Fv2^s-expressing cells may provide increased target cells for virus replication. The Fv2^{rr} homozygous mice are resistant due to a limited expansion of BFU-E clones, and a reduced ability of the Friend MuLV to find sensitive targets.[71,710] Finally, mutations in certain genes can sensitize or predispose organisms to oncogenic transformation by retroviruses. Because transformation is almost always a multistep process, mutations in one of the genes in a transforming pathway can increase the frequency with which a virus-mediated loss of another gene becomes manifest as a frank tumor. Thus, knockout mutations of such tumor suppressors as the p53 or p73 genes can sensitize to transformation by a number of oncogenic retroviruses. Similarly, a preexisting transgene such as a regulated version of the myc oncogene expressed in B-cell lineages, Emu-Myc, can predispose these cells to insertional activation of other protooncogenes in viremic animals.[748] New integration sites that would not normally be detected in wild-type mice are often utilized in such mice.

ACUTE TRANSFORMING RETROVIRUSES: TRANSDUCTION OF CELLULAR PROTOONCOGENES

Many potent transforming retroviruses, which can initiate rapid tumor formation with a quickly fatal outcome, have been isolated and characterized. These viruses are recombinant transducing viruses, which have acquired portions of cellular genes that are responsible for the transforming activity. The prototype of these viruses is the Rous sarcoma virus, which carries a transforming version of the c-src gene. In the exceptional case of some RSV strains, the viral replication functions, including the coding regions for the Gag, Pol, and Env proteins, are all intact so that the resulting transducing genome is replication-competent. In all other cases, the acquisition of the transforming gene from the host has occurred with a loss of one or more of the viral replication functions, so that the resulting virus is replication-defective. However, these genomes retain all the cis-acting elements needed for their replication and thus can be transmitted from one cell to another by coinfection with a replication-competent helper virus. The concerted replication of two viral genomes in a complex—a replication-competent helper virus and a replication-defective acute transforming virus—is a common feature of most of the transforming viruses.

Transforming viral genomes exhibit a range of different structures but have some features in common. Those segments required in cis for viral replication are always retained: the LTRs, the PBS, and the PPT are present because they are required for reverse transcription and forward transcription. The RNA packaging signals are retained. Much of the regions required in *trans* are often deleted, since these functions can be provided by the helper, and are replaced with the host sequences. The host

gene may be expressed separately or, more often, is joined to Gag, Pol, or Env sequences to form a fusion protein.

The formation of a transducing virus is thought to involve a complex series of events that results in the acquisition of the coding regions of a host gene by the replication-competent parental virus.[713] Several models have been proposed to account for the observed structures including DNA-based events (e.g.,[662]), but more often, RNA-based events (summarized in Ref.[734]). The most commonly accepted model includes the following steps (Fig. 15.20):

- The process begins with the insertion of a provirus upstream of the gene to be transduced. An insertion in the middle of a gene can initiate the transduction of the downstream portion of that gene.
- Next, readthrough transcription beginning in the 5′ LTR generates a large RNA containing viral sequences fused to downstream sequences. Such transcripts are seen in a significant fraction of ALV-infected cells. This event can be enhanced by lesions in the 3′ LTR that prevent normal RNA processing and polyadenylation at this site.
- In either mechanism, the chimeric RNA can be spliced and is then packaged into virions along with a wild-type RNA or the RNA of a helper virus.[290,712]
- Finally, nonhomologous recombination occurs during reverse transcription to append 3′ viral sequences to the chimeric genome. A template switch by RT from the helper to the chimeric RNA and back during minus strand synthesis can mediate such a nonhomologous event at low but easily detected frequencies.[250,731,831] The completion of reverse transcription on this template would result in the generation of a provirus with host sequences flanked by viral termini, similar to those seen in transforming retroviral genomes. Consistent with this model is the appearance of poly(A) sequences at the 3′ junction between host and viral sequences in some viruses; if the translocation by RT from viral to host RNA occurs in the host poly(A) sequences, a portion will be retained in the final genome.

A key feature of the resulting genome is the presence of only the mRNA sequences—that is, only the exons—and not the introns of the host gene. Thus, very large genes can be transduced by retroviruses because they only carry the exonic coding regions of the gene. Most transforming retroviral genomes are not only a result of these relatively simple recombination events but rather have also undergone multiple rearrangements thereafter. The RNAs encoded by these genomes often exhibit complex patterns of splicing, which can involve cryptic splice sites in both virus and host sequences. Several of the known rodent viruses carry segments of endogenous retroviral or virus-like sequences, especially the virus-like 30S (VL30) elements.

The genes that have been identified on the many acute transforming viruses are wildly diverse in their sequence and functions. These genes are among the most intensively studied of all known genes; their clear involvement in oncogenesis has focused enormous attention on their structures and function. The genes include growth factors (v-Sis), growth factor receptors (v-erbB), intracellular tyrosine kinases (v-src, v-fps, v-fes, v-abl), members of the G protein family (H-ras, Ki-ras), transcription factors (v-myc, v-erbA), and many others. The genes

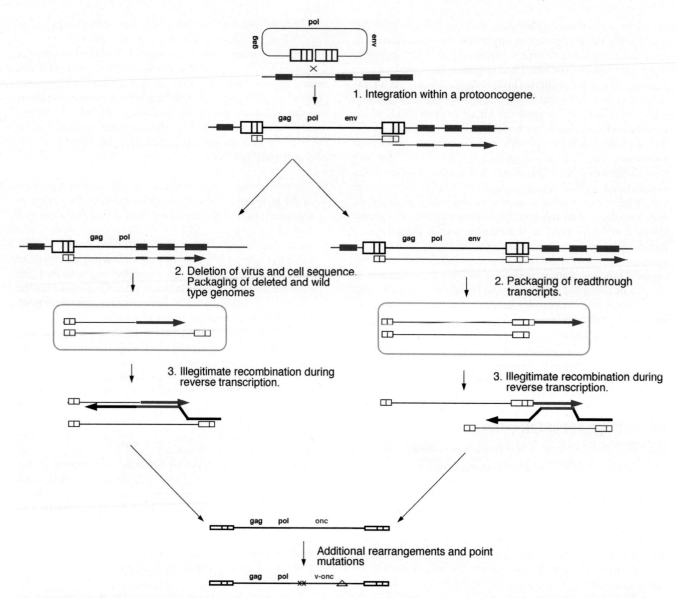

FIGURE 15.20 Two pathways for the acquisition of host oncogenes by a replication-competent retroviruses in the formation of an acute transforming genome. Integration is shown establishing a provirus within a protooncogene in the same transcriptional orientation (*top*). Either of two processes then occurs. In one mechanism (*left*), a deletion of the chromosomal DNA fuses the 5′ half of the provirus to the downstream portion of the gene. The fused DNA then encodes a fused RNA, which may be spliced and packaged into virion particles along with wild-type helper RNA. During reverse transcription, RT switches from the helper to the fusion RNA to append the 3′ portion of the helper onto the hybrid RNA. The completed reverse-transcribed DNA is integrated and transmitted thereafter as a replication-defective viral genome. In the other mechanism (*right*), a readthrough RNA extending from the 5′ LTR through the provirus and into the downstream portion of the gene is formed. The RNA is packaged into virion particles along with wild-type helper RNA. During reverse transcription, RT switches from helper to host and back to helper RNAs to form the hybrid genome. As before, the completed reverse-transcribed DNA is integrated and transmitted thereafter as a replication-defective viral genome. In either scenario, the transducing genome may undergo additional rearrangements and mutations under selective pressure for more efficient transforming activity and transmission.

are now appreciated as playing major roles in mitogenic signaling pathways, in the control of the cell cycle, and in anti-apoptotic pathways that act to limit cell survival. There is no indication that all such genes have been identified, and it is likely that new transforming viruses will continue to provide new examples of genes that can be activated by transduction to initiate tumor formation.

The acquisition of these genes, as noted above, is often associated with fusion of the coding region to Gag, Pol, or Env

sequences. Thus, the expression of the oncogene results in a fusion protein that may exhibit dramatically altered biochemical activity, intracellular localization, or stability. These changes are often a key aspect of the perversion of the normal function of the protooncogene to create the fully transforming viral oncogene. In other cases, or in addition to these alterations, there may be specific mutations that arise during or after the transduction process. These mutations, which may be as simple as a point mutation, or as drastic as a frameshift or deletion mutation, can be the major cause of activation of the onco-gene. Presumably, the high mutation rate of viral replication allows for the appearance of such mutations, and a selection for tumor formation in enhancing virus spread, is responsible for the appearance of these mutations.

ENDOGENOUS VIRUSES AND VIRUS-LIKE SEQUENCES

Virtually, all animals contain a large number of retroviral or retrovirus-like DNA elements integrated into the germ line (for comprehensive reviews, see Refs.[68,429,570,702]). These endogenous retroviral elements can represent a substantial fraction of the total DNA in a genome; while the sequences most closely related to the exogenous retroviruses may only represent a percent or so of the total DNA in many species, the LTR retroelements in total can occupy 10% or more of the genome.[730]

The retroviral provirus is closely related in structure and mode of replication to transposable elements—the retroelements—found in the genomes of all living things, from bacteria to humans.[67] Many of these elements are remarkably similar to proviruses, with LTRs that function similarly and with sequence similarity to *gag* and *pol* genes. The retroviruses have probably existed as parasites of cells from very ancient times and evolved together with transposable elements.[174]

Endogenous Elements in Chickens, Mice, Pigs, and Humans

Many endogenous retrovirus sequences have been characterized in chickens and other birds and can be grouped into at least four families. The ALV-related elements were among the first to be discovered, including the replication-competent provirus RAV-0. Most of the other family members are replication-defective and lack *env* sequences. The newer families of such viruses continue to be characterized.[690]

A vast literature describes the endogenous retrovirus sequences in inbred mice.[49,137,313,372,703] Phylogenic trees based on sequence suggest as many as eight groups, though only four have been studied in detail: class I, gammaretrovirus-like; class II, betaretrovirus-like; and classes III and IV, not similar to exogenous viruses. Those similar to the gammaretroviruses are present at 50 to 100 copies per genome.[703] These proviruses are all very similar to one another but can be grouped according to their similarity to exogenous viruses that utilize particular receptors into four groups: the ecotropic, xenotropic, polytropic, and modified polytropic. The distribution of these sequences among different murine species and subspecies can help reveal their evolution and spread. Replication-competent members of the family are found in many but not all inbred mice.[129] For reviews of the properties of the murine endogenous retrovirus genomes, see.[219,319] The class II or betaretrovirus-like elements are present in low copy number (0 to 4 per genome).

Other elements more distantly related to exogenous viruses are present at high copy number. The VL30 (for virus-like 30S) elements are present in the genome at a copy number of perhaps 100 to 200[5]; these elements encode a 30S RNA that is packaged efficiently into the virion particles of exogenous viruses and so contaminates most virion RNAs. They presumably represent a parasitic RNA that spreads by exploiting exogenous

viruses. The IAP (for intracisternal A-type particle) elements are present at about 1,000 to 2,000 copies in the genome.[434,529,539] These elements can express intracellular particles containing RT, but the particles are budded into the ER and not released from cells. Most but not all lack *env* genes and so cannot form infectious particles by themselves but could be pseudotyped with those that do. Some IAPs can transpose intracellularly at low frequencies.

The potential to use pig organs or cells in xenotransplantation into humans has raised considerable interest in the presence of endogenous retroviral elements in the pig. Although viruses can be rescued from porcine cells, and while these viruses can infect human cells quite efficiently,[569,787] preliminary studies suggest that they are not easily transmitted to humans in transplant settings. There remains a real possibility for their transfer to humans, however, and the consequences could be significant.

Retroviral elements are also abundant in the human genome.[66,429,458,460] These elements are collectively termed HERVs, for human endogenous retroviruses, and subgroups are denoted by a letter indicating the amino acid specificity of the tRNA primer. All are defective, but a very small number of these elements are still actively transcribed in somatic cells. The distribution of the HERV-K (HML-2) family in various primates has been surveyed to help build evolutionary trees of these species.[327] There are also provirus families distantly related to the lentiviruses in a few nonhuman mammalian genomes; some have the potential to encode rev-like elements that could, in principle, be pathogenic.

Properties of the Endogenous Provirus-Like Elements

The distribution of elements in a given species is relatively stable over the course of a few generations. Thus, most individuals in an inbred population show a constant, characteristic pattern of endogenous elements. The rate of loss of a given provirus is very low, primarily occurring by LTR-LTR recombination do give "solo" LTRs, and the appearance of new proviruses is rare in most animals. However, the pattern is quite different in different species, and even in different strains of animals, suggesting that rearrangements happen often over longer evolutionary times. It is known that new copies of MuLVs can appear at higher frequency if newborn females are viremic. Thus, early infection of germ cells can introduce new proviruses into the germ line. This route has even been used to create mutations *de novo* in laboratory mice at reasonable frequencies.

Most endogenous proviruses are transcriptionally silent; the DNA is often heavily methylated at CpG sites and so repressed. Subsets are activated for transcription at specific developmental stages or in specific tissues. These may reflect the mechanisms by which the transcription of many exogenous viruses are repressed *in vivo*. Expression of many of the endogenous viral RNAs is induced by agents causing DNA damage, such as UV light, and by agents affecting DNA methylation, such as BrdU and other halogenated pyrimidines. The expression of others is stimulated by glucocorticoids. The IAPs are often induced during the differentiation of various cell types and even more often in immortalized tumor cell lines.

The bulk of the endogenous retroviruses are fossil DNAs, grossly defective, and no longer capable of encoding proteins;

the ORFs contain numerous stop codons and frameshifts that would preclude the formation of any functional viral gene products. However, these elements can often give rise to RNAs, and these RNAs can be packaged efficiently by virions encoded by exogenous viruses and thus can give rise to new proviruses. Furthermore, these copackaged RNAs can then recombine with the exogenous viral RNAs and so contribute small sequence blocks to these viruses, potentially altering the host range and replication properties of the virus. The continuous contribution of endogenous sequences to virus evolution is a fact that needs to be considered whenever genetic selections are imposed on a virus. In addition, a few of the elements are functional and can transpose intracellularly or can even give rise to replication-competent viruses. Even when viruses are induced from the elements, however, the viruses are most often not highly pathogenic for the host in which they reside. Thus, many of the inducible elements in the mouse are xenotropic and cannot spread in the animal, and those that can do not cause an acute disease. The LTRs of the endogenous elements are often quite weak as transcriptional promoters as compared to those of exogenous viruses. This may reflect selections against highly pathogenic agents either before or after their introduction into the germ line.

The creation of a new provirus in the germ line by necessity creates a mutation, and while most such insertions probably have no significant effect, occasionally deleterious germ-line mutations occur. A number of ancient, "spontaneous" mutations, upon analysis, have been found to have been caused by a proviral insertion. In mice, these include such classic mutations as the *rd1* allele, causing a slow retinal degeneration, and which includes an insertion affecting the beta subunit of the retinal cGMP phosphodiesterase; the *hr* mutation, causing a hairless phenotype; the dilute coat-color allele *d*; and a mutation termed *Slp* (for sex-limited protein) in the C4 complement gene, in which an insertion of a viral LTR renders the gene androgen responsive.

Many of the endogenous elements may be positively selected in their host species. This may be due to advantageous mutations that are created by the insertion or to antiviral effects mediated by the gene products encoded by the endogenous proviruses. The *Fv1* and *Fv4* genes are examples of such elements. These virus-like elements confer resistance to exogenous viruses and so may serve to protect the host from leukemia induced by infection. The MMTV sag gene, if present on an endogenous provirus, acts to delete T cells that would respond to the superantigen; thus, subsequent infection by an exogenous MMTV cannot use sag to induce the proliferation of cells needed for its vigorous replication. Thus, the inherited provirus protects the host from MMTV disease.

An extreme version of the utilization of endogenous retroviral sequences for positive purposes is the case of the syncytins, proteins mediating cell–cell fusion into syncytia during formation of the placenta. The sequences of these proteins are highly similar to retroviral envelope sequences, and phylogenetics suggest that they arose from viral genomes, a process called exaptation, several times during the evolution of placental mammals.[387]

RETROVIRAL VECTORS, PACKAGING LINES, AND GENE THERAPY

The structure and mechanism of transmission of the naturally arising replication-defective transforming viral genomes provide a clear model for the directed use of retroviruses to mediate gene transfer. Retroviral vectors that mimic the structure of the transforming viruses can readily be generated, and these vectors can be engineered to carry the cDNA sequences of virtually any gene. These genomes can then be propagated with wild-type virus as helper. However, it is also possible to generate helper-free preparations of particles that transduce the vector genome via the early steps of the life cycle, without delivering the helper genome, and thereby preventing subsequent spread of the vector. These helper-free particles are generated in packaging cell lines: cells engineered to express the *gag*, *pol*, and *env* genes but not expressing packageable helper viral RNAs. The first such lines simply carried a provirus lacking the Psi site, the RNA packaging signal.[457] These cells produce virions deficient in the helper genome, and introducing a Psi+ vector construct with all necessary cis-acting sequences into these cells results in the encapsidation and release of the vector RNA into those particles. These particles can then be harvested and used to deliver the vector and its gene into susceptible cells. It is also possible to generate transducing virus preparations by transiently transfecting cells with DNAs that encode the helper functions and DNAs that encode the vector. This approach is preferable in instances where the viral gene products are toxic and therefore difficult to express stably in a packaging cell line. A limitation of these packaging systems is that small amounts of the Psi-minus helper RNA are encapsidated along with the vector. Endogenous retroviral genomes, such as the endogenous MuLVs in mouse cells,[3] are also encapsidated efficiently, and recombination events between these RNAs during reverse transcription can recreate a replication-competent virus. These events are probably similar to recombinational repair of mutations in genomes that occur during growth in cell culture. This issue has raised considerable fears that gene therapy vectors intended for therapeutic use could initiate a viremia, and perhaps a viral leukemia, in patients. More elaborate cell lines, in which the *gag*, *pol*, or *env* genes are expressed via separate RNAs, can reduce the frequency with which such recombination events occur to very low levels. Additionally, the use of so-called self-inactivating (SIN) vector genomes with deletion of transcriptional promoter sequences in the 3′ U3 region—such that the 5′ U3 region in the resulting provirus acquires the deletion during reverse transcription—can reduce insertional activation of host protooncogenes.[816] The use of internal tissue-specific promoters can also reduce or eliminate generalized enhancer activation by the integrating vector.[270]

Retrovirus particles transducing a desirable gene can be directed to target cells through the use of many distinct envelope proteins. This method is possible because retrovirus particles can readily form pseudotypes; that is, they can incorporate and use the envelope proteins of a wide array of different viruses. The wide range of pseudotypes that can be formed presumably reflects the flexibility of the core–envelope interaction. The host range can be further expanded or restricted by the engineering of envelopes with new binding specificities. Chimeric envelope molecules have been particularly popular tools in targeting virions to new receptors. Another approach is to engineer animals that express a foreign receptor in a tissue-specific manner and deliver genes with a virus envelope that only recognizes the transgenic receptor.[202] The envelope–receptor interaction can even be reversed: it is possible to express a particular virus receptor molecule on the virion surface and thereby target the virus to those cells expressing the corresponding viral envelope.[32]

A major limitation of early retroviral gene therapy efforts was the inability of most helper viruses to mediate the infection and transduction of nondividing cells. The major block is during the early stages of infection, when there is a strong requirement for cell division for infection by most viruses.[634] However, the ability of lentiviruses to infect nondividing cells has largely overcome this limitation (for review, see Ref.[12]). Delivery to strictly nondividing neurons, and to poorly dividing primary lymphocyte cultures, has been demonstrated with vectors based on HIV-1[65,335,512,513] as well as FIV.[589] HIV-1–based vectors (euphemistically called "lentivirus vectors") are the most widely used for gene therapy applications today.

PERSPECTIVES

The study of retroviruses has led not only to a detailed characterization of many steps of virus replication but also to important fundamental discoveries concerning host physiology, genetics, and disease. The viruses have served as entrees into such phenomena as cell surface receptors, cell division, DNA synthesis, the cell cycle, mechanisms of gene expression, and intracellular transport. The value of focusing on retrovirus functions in unraveling cellular functions is clear: these agents have evolved over huge periods of time to exploit key aspects of the cell, and we should make use of their success to help identify those aspects. There is every reason to believe that their continued study will yet reveal new aspects of cell physiology.

REFERENCES

1. Achuthan V, Perreira JM, Sowd GA, et al. Capsid-CPSF6 interaction licenses nuclear HIV-1 trafficking to sites of viral DNA integration. *Cell Host Microbe* 2018;24(3):392–404.e8.
2. Adam MA, Miller AD. Identification of a signal in a murine retrovirus that is sufficient for packaging of nonretroviral RNA into virions. *J Virol* 1988;62:3802–3806.
3. Adams SE, Rathjen PD, Stanway CA, et al. Complete nucleotide sequence of a mouse VL30 retro-element. *Mol Cell Biol* 1988;8:2989–2998.
4. Adkins HB, Blacklow SC, Young JA. Two functionally distinct forms of a retroviral receptor explain the nonreciprocal receptor interference among subgroups B, D, and E avian leukosis viruses. *J Virol* 2001;75(8):3520–3526.
5. Adkins HB, Brojatsch J, Naughton J, et al. Identification of a cellular receptor for subgroup E avian leukosis virus. *Proc Natl Acad Sci U S A* 1997;94(21):11617–11622.
6. Afonina E, Neumann M, Pavlakis GN. Preferential binding of poly(A)-binding protein 1 to an inhibitory RNA element in the human immunodeficiency virus type 1 gag mRNA. *J Biol Chem* 1997;272(4):2307–2311.
7. Aiyar A, Cobrinik D, Ge Z, et al. Interaction between retroviral U5 RNA and the TψC loop of the tRNATrp primer is required for efficient initiation of reverse transcription. *J Virol* 1992;66:2464–2472.
8. Aiyar A, Hindmarsh P, Skalka AM, et al. Concerted integration of linear retroviral DNA by the avian sarcoma virus integrase in vitro: dependence on both long terminal repeat termini. *J Virol* 1996;70(6):3571–3580.
9. Aiyer S, Swapna GV, Malani N, et al. Altering murine leukemia virus integration through disruption of the integrase and BET protein family interaction. *Nucleic Acids Res* 2014;42(9):5917–5928.
10. Aiyer S, Swapna GVT, Ma LC, et al. A common binding motif in the ET domain of BRD3 forms polymorphic structural interfaces with host and viral proteins. *Structure* 2021;29(8):886–898.e6.
11. Albritton LM, Tseng L, Scadden D, et al. A putative murine ecotropic retrovirus receptor gene encodes a multiple membrane-spanning protein and confers susceptibility to virus infection. *Cell* 1989;57:659–666.
12. Amado RG, Chen ISY. Lentiviral vectors-the promise of gene therapy within reach? *Science* 1999;285:674–676.
13. Amarasinghe GK, De Guzman RN, Turner RB, et al. NMR structure of the HIV-1 nucleocapsid protein bound to stem-loop SL2 of the psi-RNA packaging signal. Implications for genome recognition. *J Mol Biol* 2000;301(2):491–511.
14. Amendt BA, Simpson SB, Stoltzfus CM. Inhibition of RNA splicing at the Rous sarcoma virus src 3' splice site is mediated by an interaction between a negative cis element and a chicken embryo fibroblast nuclear factor. *J Virol* 1995;69(8):5068–5076.
15. Anderson DJ, Stone J, Lum R, et al. The packaging phenotype of the SE21Q1b provirus is related to high proviral expression and not trans-acting factors. *J Virol* 1995;69(11):7319–7323.
16. Anderson MM, Lauring AS, Burns CC, et al. Identification of a cellular cofactor required for infection by feline leukemia virus. *Science* 2000;287(5459):1828–1830.
17. Anderson MM, Lauring AS, Robertson S, et al. Feline Pit2 functions as a receptor for subgroup B feline leukemia viruses. *J Virol* 2001;75(22):10563–10572.
18. Andreadis ST, Brott D, Fuller AO, et al. Moloney murine leukemia virus-derived retroviral vectors decay intracellularly with a half-life in the range of 5.5 to 7.5 hours. *J Virol* 1997;71(10):7541–7548.
19. Ardavin C, Martin P, Ferrero I, et al. B cell response after MMTV infection: extrafollicular plasmablasts represent the main infected population and can transmit viral infection. *J Immunol* 1999;162(5):2538–2545.
20. Argaw T, Wilson CA. Detailed mapping of determinants within the porcine endogenous retrovirus envelope surface unit identifies critical residues for human cell infection within the proline-rich region. *J Virol* 2012;86(17):9096–9104.
21. Arias JF, Colomer-Lluch M, von Bredow B, et al. Tetherin Antagonism by HIV-1 group M Nef proteins. *J Virol* 2016;90(23):10701–10714.
22. Arthur LO, Bess JWJ, Sowder RCI, et al. Cellular proteins bound to immunodeficiency viruses: implications for pathogenesis for vaccines. *Science* 1992;258:1935–1938.
23. Aziz DC, Hanna Z, Jolicoeur P. Severe immunodeficiency disease induced by a defective murine leukaemia virus. *Nature* 1989;338:505–508.
24. Baba TW, Humphries EH. Formation of a transformed follicle is necessary but not sufficient for development of an avian leukosis virus-induced lymphoma. *Proc Natl Acad Sci U S A* 1985;82(1):213–216.
25. Babst M, Katzmann DJ, Estepa-Sabal EJ, et al. Escrt-III: an endosome-associated heterooligomeric protein complex required for mvb sorting. *Dev Cell* 2002;3(2):271–282.
26. Babst M, Katzmann DJ, Snyder WB, et al. Endosome-associated complex, ESCRT-II, recruits transport machinery for protein sorting at the multivesicular body. *Dev Cell* 2002;3(2):283–289.
27. Bachand F, Yao XJ, Hrimech M, et al. Incorporation of Vpr into human immunodeficiency virus type 1 requires a direct interaction with the p6 domain of the p55 gag precursor. *J Biol Chem* 1999;274(13):9083–9091.
28. Bai L, Sato H, Kubo Y, et al. CAT1/SLC7A1 acts as a cellular receptor for bovine leukemia virus infection. *FASEB J* 2019;33(12):14516–14527.
29. Balakrishnan M, Yant SR, Tsai L, et al. Non-catalytic site HIV-1 integrase inhibitors disrupt core maturation and induce a reverse transcription block in target cells. *PLoS One* 2013;8(9):e74163.
30. Ballandras-Colas A, Brown M, Cook NJ, et al. Cryo-EM reveals a novel octameric integrase structure for betaretroviral intasome function. *Nature* 2016;530(7590):358–361.
31. Ballandras-Colas A, Maskell DP, Serrao E, et al. A supramolecular assembly mediates lentiviral DNA integration. *Science* 2017;355(6320):93–95.
32. Balliet JW, Bates P. Efficient infection mediated by viral receptors incorporated into retroviral particles. *J Virol* 1998;72(1):671–676.
33. Baltimore D. RNA-dependent DNA polymerase in virions of RNA tumour viruses. *Nature* 1970;226:1209–1211.
34. Ban J, Portetelle D, Altaner C, et al. Isolation and characterization of a 2.3-kilobase-pair cDNA fragment encoding the binding domain of the bovine leukemia virus cell receptor. *J Virol* 1993;67:1050–1057.
35. Banks JD, Linial ML. Secondary structure analysis of a minimal avian leukosis-sarcoma virus packaging signal. *J Virol* 2000;74(1):456–464.
36. Barbeau B, Mesnard JM. Making sense out of antisense transcription in human T-cell lymphotropic viruses (HTLVs). *Viruses* 2011;3(5):456–468.
37. Barklis E, McDermott J, Wilkens S, et al. Structural analysis of membrane-bound retrovirus capsid proteins. *EMBO J* 1997;16(6):1199–1213.
38. Barr SD, Leipzig J, Shinn P, et al. Integration targeting by avian sarcoma-leukosis virus and human immunodeficiency virus in the chicken genome. *J Virol* 2005;79(18):12035–12044.
39. Barski MS, Minnell JJ, Hodakova Z, et al. Cryo-EM structure of the deltaretroviral intasome in complex with the PP2A regulatory subunit B56gamma. *Nat Commun* 2020;11(1):5043.
40. Basyuk E, Galli T, Mougel M, et al. Retroviral genomic RNAs are transported to the plasma membrane by endosomal vesicles. *Dev Cell* 2003;5(1):161–174.
41. Bates P, Rong L, Varmus HE, et al. Genetic mapping of the cloned subgroup A avian sarcoma and leukosis virus receptor gene to the TVA locus. *J Virol* 1998;72(3):2505–2508.
42. Bates P, Young JA, Harmus HE. A receptor for subgroup A Rous sarcoma virus is related to the low density lipoprotein receptor. *Cell* 1993;74:1043–1051.
43. Battini JL, Rasko JE, Miller AD. A human cell-surface receptor for xenotropic and polytropic murine leukemia viruses: possible role in G protein-coupled signal transduction. *Proc Natl Acad Sci U S A* 1999;96(4):1385–1390.
44. Battula N, Loeb LA. On the fidelity of DNA replication. Lack of exodeoxyribonuclease activity and error-correcting function in avian myeloblastosis virus DNA polymerase. *J Biol Chem* 1976;251(4):982–986.
45. Beasley BE, Hu WS. cis-Acting elements important for retroviral RNA packaging specificity. *J Virol* 2002;76(10):4950–4960.
46. Beerens N, Berkhout B. The tRNA primer activation signal in the human immunodeficiency virus type 1 genome is important for initiation and processive elongation of reverse transcription. *J Virol* 2002;76(5):2329–2339.
47. Bejarano DA, Peng K, Laketa V, et al. HIV-1 nuclear import in macrophages is regulated by CPSF6-capsid interactions at the nuclear pore complex. *Elife* 2019;8:e41800.
48. Belyaev AS, Stuart D, Sutton G, et al. Crystallization and preliminary X-ray investigation of recombinant simian immunodeficiency virus matrix protein. *J Mol Biol* 1994;241(5):744–746.
49. Benit L, Lallemand JB, Casella JF, et al. ERV-L elements: a family of endogenous retrovirus-like elements active throughout the evolution of mammals. *J Virol* 1999;73(4):3301–3308.

50. Berger EA, Murphy PM, Farber JM. Chemokine receptors as HIV-1 coreceptors: roles in viral entry, tropism, and disease. *Annu Rev Immunol* 1999;17:657–700.
51. Berkhout B, van Wamel JL. The leader of the HIV-1 RNA genome forms a compactly folded tertiary structure. *RNA* 2000;6(2):282–295.
52. Berkowitz R, Fisher J, Goff SP. RNA packaging. *Curr Top Microbiol Immunol* 1996;214:177–218.
53. Berkowitz RD, Luban J, Goff SP. Specific binding of human immunodeficiency virus type 1 gag polyprotein and nucleocapsid protein to viral RNAs detected by RNA mobility shift assays. *J Virol* 1993;67(12):7190–7200.
54. Berlioz C, Darlix JL. An internal ribosomal entry mechanism promotes translation of murine leukemia virus gag polyprotein precursors. *J Virol* 1995;69(4):2214–2222.
55. Berlioz C, Torrent C, Darlix JL. An internal ribosomal entry signal in the rat VL30 region of the Harvey murine sarcoma virus leader and its use in dicistronic retroviral vectors. *J Virol* 1995;69(10):6400–6407.
56. Berndsen ZT, Chakraborty S, Wang X, et al. Visualization of the HIV-1 Env glycan shield across scales. *Proc Natl Acad Sci U S A* 2020;117(45):28014–28025.
57. Besnier C, Ylinen L, Strange B, et al. Characterization of murine leukemia virus restriction in mammals. *J Virol* 2003;77(24):13403–13406.
58. Bess JW Jr, Gorelick RJ, Bosche WJ, et al. Microvesicles are a source of contaminating cellular proteins found in purified HIV-1 preparations. *Virology* 1997;230(1):134–144.
59. Best S, Le Tissier P, Towers G, et al. Positional cloning of the mouse retrovirus restriction gene Fv1. *Nature* 1996;382(6594):826–829.
60. Bhatt V, Shi K, Salamango DJ, et al. Structural basis of host protein hijacking in human T-cell leukemia virus integration. *Nat Commun* 2020;11(1):3121.
61. Bick MJ, Carroll JW, Gao G, et al. Expression of the zinc-finger antiviral protein inhibits alphavirus replication. *J Virol* 2003;77(21):11555–11562.
62. Bieniasz PD. Intrinsic immunity: a front-line defense against viral attack. *Nat Immunol* 2004;5(11):1109–1115.
63. Bilello JA, Pitts OM, Hoffman PM. Characterization of a progressive neurodegenerative disease induced by a temperature-sensitive Moloney murine leukemia virus infection. *J Virol* 1986;59:234–241.
64. Bishop KN, Holmes RK, Sheehy AM, et al. APOBEC-mediated editing of viral RNA. *Science* 2004;305(5684):645.
65. Blomer U, Naldini L, Kafri T, et al. Highly efficient and sustained gene transfer in adult neurons with a lentivirus vector. *J Virol* 1997;71(9):6641–6649.
66. Blond JL, Beseme F, Duret L, et al. Molecular characterization and placental expression of HERV-W, a new human endogenous retrovirus family. *J Virol* 1999;73(2):1175–1185.
67. Boeke JD, Garfinkel DJ, Styles CA, et al. Ty elements transpose through an RNA intermediate. *Cell* 1985;40:491–500.
68. Boeke JD, Stoye JP. Retrotransposons, endogenous retroviruses, and the evolution of retroelements. In: Coffin JM, Hughes SH, Varmus HE, eds. *Retroviruses*. Cold Spring Harbor, NY: Cold Spring Harbor Press; 1997:343–436.
69. Boerkoel CF, Kung H-J. Transcriptional interaction between retroviral long terminal repeats (LTRs): Mechanism of 5′ LTR suppression and 3′ LTR promoter activation of *c-myc* in avian B-cell lymphomas. *J Virol* 1992;66:4814–4823.
70. Boggiano C, Manel N, Littman DR. Dendritic cell-mediated trans-enhancement of human immunodeficiency virus type 1 infectivity is independent of DC-SIGN. *J Virol* 2007;81(5):2519–2523.
71. Bondurant MC, Koury MJ, Krantz SB. The Fv-2 gene controls induction of erythroid burst formation by Friend virus infection in vitro: studies of growth regulators and viral replication. *J Gen Virol* 1985;66(Pt 1):83–96.
72. Bonnet-Mathoniere B, Girard PM, Muriaux D, et al. Nucleocapsid protein 10 activates dimerization of the RNA of Moloney murine leukaemia virus in vitro. *Eur J Biochem* 1996;238(1):129–135.
73. Boone LR, Glover PL, Innes CL, et al. Fv-1 N- and B-tropism-specific sequences in murine leukemia virus and related endogenous proviral genomes. *J Virol* 1988;62:2644–2650.
74. Boral AL, Okenquist SA, Lenz J. Identification of the SL3-3 virus enhancer core as a T-lymphoma cell-specific element. *J Virol* 1988;63:76–84.
75. Bosze Z, Thiesen H-J, Charnay P. A transcriptional enhancer with specificity for erythroid cells is located in the long terminal repeat of the Friend murine leukemia virus. *EMBO J* 1986;5:1615–1624.
76. Bowerman B, Brown PO, Bishop JM, et al. A nucleoprotein complex mediates the integration of retroviral DNA. *Genes Dev* 1989;3:469–478.
77. Boyd PS, Brown JB, Brown JD, et al. NMR studies of retroviral genome packaging. *Viruses* 2020;12(10):1115.
78. Brandt-Carlson C, Butel JS. Detection and characterization of a glycoprotein encoded by the mouse mammary tumor virus long terminal repeat gene. *J Virol* 1991;65:6051–6060.
79. Bray M, Prasad S, Dubay JW, et al. A small element from the Mason-Pfizer monkey virus genome makes human immunodeficiency virus type 1 expression and replication Rev-independent. *Proc Natl Acad Sci U S A* 1994;91(4):1256–1260.
80. Briggs JA, Simon MN, Gross I, et al. The stoichiometry of Gag protein in HIV-1. *Nat Struct Mol Biol* 2004;11(7):672–675.
81. Brightman BK, Davis BR, Fan H. Preleukemic hematopoietic hyperplasia induced by Moloney murine leukemia virus is an indirect consequence of viral infection. *J Virol* 1990;64:4582–4584.
82. Brody BA, Rhee SS, Hunter E. Postassembly cleavage of a retroviral glycoprotein cytoplasmic domain removes a necessary incorporation signal and activates fusion activity. *J Virol* 1994;68(7):4620–4627.
83. Brojatsch J, Naughton J, Adkins HB, et al. TVB receptors for cytopathic and noncytopathic subgroups of avian leukosis viruses are functional death receptors. *J Virol* 2000;74(24):11490–11494.
84. Brojatsch J, Naughton J, Rolls MM, et al. CAR1, a TNFR-related protein, is a cellular receptor for cytopathic avian leukosis-sarcoma viruses and mediates apoptosis. *Cell* 1996;87(5):845–855.
85. Brown JD, Kharytonchyk S, Chaudry I, et al. Structural basis for transcriptional start site control of HIV-1 RNA fate. *Science* 2020;368(6489):413–417.
86. Brown PO, Bowerman B, Varmus HE, et al. Correct integration of retroviral DNA in vitro. *Cell* 1987;49:347–356.
87. Bryant M, Ratner L. Myristoylation-dependent replication and assembly of human immunodeficiency virus 1. *Proc Natl Acad Sci U S A* 1990;87:523–527.
88. Brzezinski JD, Felkner R, Modi A, et al. Phosphorylation requirement of murine leukemia virus p12. *J Virol* 2016;90(24):11208–11219.
89. Brzezinski JD, Modi A, Liu M, et al. Repression of the chromatin-tethering domain of murine leukemia virus p12. *J Virol* 2016;90(24):11197–11207.
90. Buck CB, Shen X, Egan MA, et al. The human immunodeficiency virus type 1 gag gene encodes an internal ribosome entry site. *J Virol* 2001;75(1):181–191.
91. Bukrinsky MI, Sharova N, Dempsey MP, et al. Active nuclear import of human immunodeficiency virus type 1 preintegration complexes. *Proc Natl Acad Sci U S A* 1992;89:6580–6584.
92. Burdick RC, Li C, Munshi M, et al. HIV-1 uncoats in the nucleus near sites of integration. *Proc Natl Acad Sci U S A* 2020;117(10):5486–5493.
93. Burstein H, Bizub D, Kotler M, et al. Processing of avian retroviral *gag* polyprotein precursors is blocked by a mutation at the NC-PR cleavage site. *J Virol* 1992;66:1781–1785.
94. Bushman FD, Craigie R. Sequence requirements for integration of Moloney murine leukemia virus DNA in vitro. *J Virol* 1990;64:5645–5648.
95. Buxton P, Tachedjian G, Mak J. Analysis of the contribution of reverse transcriptase and integrase proteins to retroviral RNA dimer conformation. *J Virol* 2005;79(10):6338–6348.
96. Byun H, Das P, Yu H, et al. Mouse mammary tumor virus signal peptide uses a novel p97-dependent and derlin-independent retrotranslocation mechanism to escape proteasomal degradation. *mBio* 2017;8(2):e00328-17.
97. Byun H, Halani N, Gou Y, et al. Requirements for mouse mammary tumor virus Rem signal peptide processing and function. *J Virol* 2012;86(1):214–225.
98. Campbell S, Fisher RJ, Towler EM, et al. Modulation of HIV-like particle assembly in vitro by inositol phosphates. *Proc Natl Acad Sci U S A* 2001;98(19):10875–10879.
99. Campbell S, Rein A. In vitro assembly properties of human immunodeficiency virus type 1 Gag protein lacking the p6 domain. *J Virol* 1999;73(3):2270–2279.
100. Campbell S, Vogt VM. Self-assembly in vitro of purified CA-NC proteins from Rous sarcoma virus and human immunodeficiency virus type 1. *J Virol* 1995;69(10):6487–6497.
101. Campbell SM, Crowe SM, Mak J. Lipid rafts and HIV-1: from viral entry to assembly of progeny virions. *J Clin Virol* 2001;22(3):217–227.
102. Cavrois M, Neidleman J, Greene WC. The Achilles heel of the Trojan horse model of HIV-1 trans-infection. *PLoS Pathog* 2008;4(6):e1000051.
103. Cen S, Huang Y, Khorchid A, et al. The role of Pr55(gag) in the annealing of tRNA3Lys to human immunodeficiency virus type 1 genomic RNA. *J Virol* 1999;73(5):4485–4488.
104. Cen S, Javanbakht H, Kim S, et al. Retrovirus-specific packaging of aminoacyl-tRNA synthetases with cognate primer tRNAs. *J Virol* 2002;76(24):13111–13115.
105. Cen S, Javanbakht H, Niu M, et al. Ability of wild-type and mutant lysyl-tRNA synthetase to facilitate tRNA(Lys) incorporation into human immunodeficiency virus type 1. *J Virol* 2004;78(3):1595–1601.
106. Cen S, Khorchid A, Gabor J, et al. Roles of Pr55(gag) and NCp7 in tRNA(3)(Lys) genomic placement and the initiation step of reverse transcription in human immunodeficiency virus type 1. *J Virol* 2000;74(22):10796–10800.
107. Cen S, Khorchid A, Javanbakht H, et al. Incorporation of lysyl-tRNA synthetase into human immunodeficiency virus type 1. *J Virol* 2001;75(11):5043–5048.
108. Cesana D, Santoni de Sio FR, Rudilosso L, et al. HIV-1-mediated insertional activation of STAT5B and BACH2 trigger viral reservoir in T regulatory cells. *Nat Commun* 2017;8(1):498.
109. Chai N, Bates P. Na+/H+ exchanger type 1 is a receptor for pathogenic subgroup J avian leukosis virus. *Proc Natl Acad Sci U S A* 2006;103(14):5531–5536.
110. Chan DC, Fass D, Berger JM, et al. Core structure of gp41 from the HIV envelope glycoprotein. *Cell* 1997;89(2):263–273.
111. Chande A, Cuccurullo EC, Rosa A, et al. S2 from equine infectious anemia virus is an infectivity factor which counteracts the retroviral inhibitors SERINC5 and SERINC3. *Proc Natl Acad Sci U S A* 2016;113(46):13197–13202.
112. Charneau P, Alizon M, Clavel F. A second origin of DNA plus-strand synthesis is required for optimal human immunodeficiency virus replication. *J Virol* 1992;66:2814–2820.
113. Charneau P, Mirambeau G, Roux P, et al. HIV-1 reverse transcription. A termination step at the center of the genome. *J Mol Biol* 1994;241(5):651–662.
114. Chattopadhyay SK, Cloyd MW, Linemeyer DL, et al. Cellular origin and role of mink cell focus-forming viruses in murine thymic lymphomas. *Nature* 1982;295:25–31.
115. Chen H, Wei SQ, Engelman A. Multiple integrase functions are required to form the native structure of the human immunodeficiency virus type I intasome. *J Biol Chem* 1999;274(24):17358–17364.
116. Chen S, Kumar S, Espada CE, et al. N6-methyladenosine modification of HIV-1 RNA suppresses type-I interferon induction in differentiated monocytic cells and primary macrophages. *PLoS Pathog* 2021;17(3):e1009421.
117. Chen Y, Balakrishnan M, Roques BP, et al. Mechanism of minus strand strong stop transfer in HIV-1 reverse transcription. *J Biol Chem* 2003;278(10):8006–8017.
118. Cherepanov P, Maertens G, Proost P, et al. HIV-1 integrase forms stable tetramers and associates with LEDGF/p75 protein in human cells. *J Biol Chem* 2003;278(1):372–381.
119. Chow SA, Vincent KA, Ellison V, et al. Reversal of integration and DNA splicing mediated by integrase of human immunodeficiency virus. *Science* 1992;255:723–726.
120. Christ F, Thys W, De Rijck J, et al. Transportin-SR2 imports HIV into the nucleus. *Curr Biol* 2008;18(16):1192–1202.
121. Christ F, Voet A, Marchand A, et al. Rational design of small-molecule inhibitors of the LEDGF/p75-integrase interaction and HIV replication. *Nat Chem Biol* 2010;6(6):442–448.
122. Christensen DE, Ganser-Pornillos BK, Johnson JS, et al. Reconstitution and visualization of HIV-1 capsid-dependent replication and integration in vitro. *Science* 2020;370(6513):eabc8420.
123. Cimarelli A, Luban J. Translation elongation factor 1-alpha interacts specifically with the human immunodeficiency virus type 1 Gag polyprotein. *J Virol* 1999;73(7):5388–5401.

124. Clever JL, Mirandar D Jr, Parslow TG. RNA structure and packaging signals in the 5′ leader region of the human immunodeficiency virus type 1 genome. *J Virol* 2002;76(23):12381–12387.
125. Clever JL, Taplitz RA, Lochrie MA, et al. A heterologous, high-affinity RNA ligand for human immunodeficiency virus Gag protein has RNA packaging activity. *J Virol* 2000;74(1):541–546.
126. Clever JL, Wong ML, Parslow TG. Requirements for kissing-loop-mediated dimerization of human immunodeficiency virus RNA. *J Virol* 1996;70(9):5902–5908.
127. Cobrinik D, Katz R, Terry R, et al. Avian sarcoma and leukosis virus pol-endonuclease recognition of the tandem long terminal repeat junction: minimum site required for cleavage is also required for viral growth. *J Virol* 1987;61:1999–2008.
128. Cobrinik D, Soskey L, Leis J. A retroviral RNA secondary structure required for efficient initiation of reverse transcription. *J Virol* 1988;62:3622–3630.
129. Coffin JM. Endogenous viruses. In: Weiss R, Teich N, Varmus H, Coffin J, eds. *RNA Tumor Viruses.* Cold Spring Harbor, NY: Cold Spring Harbor Laboratory; 1982:1109–1204.
130. Coffin JM. Superantigens and endogenous retroviruses: a confluence of puzzles. *Science* 1992;255:411–413.
131. Coffin JM, Bale MJ, Wells D, et al. Integration in oncogenes plays only a minor role in determining the in vivo distribution of HIV integration sites before or during suppressive antiretroviral therapy. *PLoS Pathog* 2021;17(4):e1009141.
132. Colicelli J, Goff SP. Mutants and pseudorevertants of Moloney murine leukemia virus with alterations at the integration site. *Cell* 1985;42:573–580.
133. Colon-Moran W, Argaw T, Wilson CA. Three cysteine residues of SLC52A1, a receptor for the porcine endogenous retrovirus-A (PERV-A), play a critical role in cell surface expression and infectivity. *Virology* 2017;507:140–150.
134. Connolly L, Zingler K, Young JA. A soluble form of a receptor for subgroup A avian leukosis and sarcoma viruses (ALSV-A) blocks infection and binds directly to ALSV-A. *J Virol* 1994;68(4):2760–2764.
135. Conte MR, Klikova M, Hunter E, et al. The three-dimensional solution structure of the matrix protein from the type D retrovirus, the Mason-Pfizer monkey virus, and implications for the morphology of retroviral assembly. *EMBO J* 1997;16(19):5819–5826.
136. Cook NJ, Li W, Berta D, et al. Structural basis of second-generation HIV integrase inhibitor action and viral resistance. *Science* 2020;367(6479):806–810.
137. Copeland NG, Hutchinson KW, Jenkins NA. Excision of the DBA ecotropic provirus in dilute coat-color revertants of mice occurs by homologous recombination involving the viral LTRs. *Cell* 1983;33:379–387.
138. Cosson P. Direct interaction between the envelope and matrix proteins of HIV-1. *EMBO J* 1996;15(21):5783–5788.
139. Cowan S, Hatziioannou T, Cunningham T, et al. Cellular inhibitors with Fv1-like activity restrict human and simian immunodeficiency virus tropism. *Proc Natl Acad Sci U S A* 2002;99(18):11914–11919.
140. Craven RC, Leure-duPree AE, Weldon RA Jr, et al. Genetic analysis of the major homology region of the Rous sarcoma virus Gag protein. *J Virol* 1995;69(7):4213–4227.
141. Crawford S, Goff SP. Mutations in gag proteins p12 and p15 of Moloney murine leukemia virus block early stages of infection. *J Virol* 1984;49:909–917.
142. Crawford S, Goff SP. A deletion mutation in the 5′ part of the pol gene of Moloney murine leukemia virus blocks proteolytic processing of the gag and pol polyproteins. *J Virol* 1985;53(3):899–907.
143. Crowe BL, Larue RC, Yuan C, et al. Structure of the Brd4 ET domain bound to a C-terminal motif from gamma-retroviral integrases reveals a conserved mechanism of interaction. *Proc Natl Acad Sci U S A* 2016;113(8):2086–2091.
144. Cullen BR. HIV-1 auxiliary proteins: making connections in a dying cell. *Cell* 1998;93(5):685–692.
145. Cullen BR. Nuclear mRNA export: insights from virology. *Trends Biochem Sci* 2003;28(8):419–424.
146. D'Souza V, Dey A, Habib D, et al. NMR structure of the 101-nucleotide core encapsidation signal of the Moloney murine leukemia virus. *J Mol Biol* 2004;337(2):427–442.
147. D'Souza V, Melamed J, Habib D, et al. Identification of a high affinity nucleocapsid protein binding element within the Moloney murine leukemia virus Psi-RNA packaging signal: implications for genome recognition. *J Mol Biol* 2001;314(2):217–232.
148. D'Souza V, Summers MF. Structural basis for packaging the dimeric genome of Moloney murine leukaemia virus. *Nature* 2004;431(7008):586–590.
149. D'Souza V, Summers MF. How retroviruses select their genomes. *Nat Rev Microbiol* 2005;3(8):643–655.
150. Dai W, Usami Y, Wu Y, et al. A long cytoplasmic loop governs the sensitivity of the anti-viral host protein SERINC5 to HIV-1 Nef. *Cell Rep* 2018;22(4):869–875.
151. Dalgleish AG, Beverly PCL, Clapham PR, et al. The CD4 (T4) antigen is an essential component of the receptor for the AIDS retrovirus. *Nature* 1984;312:763–767.
152. Daniel R, Greger JG, Katz RA, et al. Evidence that stable retroviral transduction and cell survival following DNA integration depend on components of the nonhomologous end joining repair pathway. *J Virol* 2004;78(16):8573–8581.
153. Daniel R, Kao G, Taganov K, et al. Evidence that the retroviral DNA integration process triggers an ATR-dependent DNA damage response. *Proc Natl Acad Sci U S A* 2003;100(8):4778–4783.
154. Daniel R, Katz RA, Skalka AM. A role for DNA-PK in retroviral DNA integration. *Science* 1999;284(5414):644–647.
155. Das D, Georgiadis MM. The crystal structure of the monomeric reverse transcriptase from Moloney murine leukemia virus. *Structure* 2004;12(5):819–829.
156. De Guzman RN, Wu ZR, Stalling CC, et al. Structure of the HIV-1 nucleocapsid protein bound to the SL3 psi-RNA recognition element. *Science* 1998;279(5349):384–388.
157. de Parseval A, Chatterji U, Sun P, et al. Feline immunodeficiency virus targets activated CD4+ T cells by using CD134 as a binding receptor. *Proc Natl Acad Sci U S A* 2004;101(35):13044–13049.
158. De Ravin SS, Su L, Theobald N, et al. Enhancers are major targets for murine leukemia virus vector integration. *J Virol* 2014;88(8):4504–4513.
159. De Rijck J, de Kogel C, Demeulemeester J, et al. The BET family of proteins targets Moloney murine leukemia virus integration near transcription start sites. *Cell Rep* 2013;5(4):886–894.
160. Deffaud C, Darlix JL. Characterization of an internal ribosomal entry segment in the 5′ leader of murine leukemia virus env RNA. *J Virol* 2000;74(2):846–850.
161. Deffaud C, Darlix JL. Rous sarcoma virus translation revisited: characterization of an internal ribosome entry segment in the 5′ leader of the genomic RNA. *J Virol* 2000;74(24):11581–11588.
162. Derse D. Bovine leukemia virus transcription is controlled by a virus-encoded trans-acting factor and by cis-acting response elements. *J Virol* 1987;61:2462–2471.
163. DesGroseillers L, Rassart E, Robitaille Y, et al. Retrovirus-induced spongiform encephalopathy: The 3′-end long terminal repeat-containing viral sequences influence the incidence of the disease and the specificity of the neurological syndrome. *Proc Natl Acad Sci U S A* 1985;82:8818–8822.
164. Desimmie BA, Schrijvers R, Demeulemeester J, et al. LEDGINs inhibit late stage HIV-1 replication by modulating integrase multimerization in the virions. *Retrovirology* 2013;10:57.
165. Dey A, York D, Smalls-Mantey A, et al. Composition and sequence-dependent binding of RNA to the nucleocapsid protein of Moloney murine leukemia virus. *Biochemistry* 2005;44(10):3735–3744.
166. Dharan A, Bachmann N, Talley S, et al. Nuclear pore blockade reveals that HIV-1 completes reverse transcription and uncoating in the nucleus. *Nat Microbiol* 2020;5(9):1088–1095.
167. Dharan A, Talley S, Tripathi A, et al. KIF5B and Nup358 cooperatively mediate the nuclear import of HIV-1 during infection. *PLoS Pathog* 2016;12(6):e1005700.
168. Dick RA, Mallery DL, Vogt VM, et al. IP6 Regulation of HIV capsid assembly, stability, and uncoating. *Viruses* 2018;10(11):640.
169. Ding P, Kharytonchyk S, Waller A, et al. Identification of the initial nucleocapsid recognition element in the HIV-1 RNA packaging signal. *Proc Natl Acad Sci U S A* 2020;117(30):17737–17746.
170. Dingwall C, Ernberg I, Gait MJ, et al. HIV-1 *tat* protein stimulates transcription by binding to a U-rich bulge in the stem of the TAR RNA structure. *EMBO J* 1990;9:4145–4154.
171. Dirac AM, Huthoff H, Kjems J, et al. The dimer initiation site hairpin mediates dimerization of the human immunodeficiency virus, type 2 RNA genome. *J Biol Chem* 2001;276(34):32345–32352.
172. Doehle BP, Schafer A, Cullen BR. Human APOBEC3B is a potent inhibitor of HIV-1 infectivity and is resistant to HIV-1 Vif. *Virology* 2005;339(2):281–288.
173. Dong J, Dubay JW, Perez LG, et al. Mutations within the proteolytic cleavage site of the Rous sarcoma virus glycoprotein define a requirement for dibasic residues for intracellular cleavage. *J Virol* 1992;66:865–874.
174. Doolittle RF, Feng D-F. Tracing the origin of retroviruses. *Curr Top Microbiol Immunol* 1992;176:195–212.
175. Dorfman T, Mammano F, Haseltine WA, et al. Role of the matrix protein in the virion association of the human immunodeficiency virus type 1 envelope glycoprotein. *J Virol* 1994;68(3):1689–1696.
176. Douglas JL, Viswanathan K, McCarroll MN, et al. Vpu directs the degradation of the human immunodeficiency virus restriction factor BST-2/Tetherin via a beta-TrCP-dependent mechanism. *J Virol* 2009;83(16):7931–7947.
177. Drummond AJ, Ho SY, Phillips MJ, et al. Relaxed phylogenetics and dating with confidence. *PLoS Biol* 2006;4(5):e88.
178. Drummond AJ, Rambaut A. BEAST: bayesian evolutionary analysis by sampling trees. *BMC Evol Biol* 2007;7:214.
179. Dube M, Roy BB, Guiot-Guillain P, et al. Antagonism of tetherin restriction of HIV-1 release by Vpu involves binding and sequestration of the restriction factor in a perinuclear compartment. *PLoS Pathog* 2010;6(4):e1000856.
180. Dupont L, Bloor S, Williamson JC, et al. The SMC5/6 complex compacts and silences unintegrated HIV-1 DNA and is antagonized by Vpr. *Cell Host Microbe* 2021;29(5):792–805 e6.
181. Eastman SW, Martin-Serrano J, Chung W, et al. Identification of human VPS37C, a component of endosomal sorting complex required for transport-I important for viral budding. *J Biol Chem* 2005;280(1):628–636.
182. Ebina H, Aoki J, Hatta S, et al. Role of Nup98 in nuclear entry of human immunodeficiency virus type 1 cDNA. *Microbes Infect* 2004;6(8):715–724.
183. Edinger AL, Hoffman TL, Sharron M, et al. An orphan seven-transmembrane domain receptor expressed widely in the brain functions as a coreceptor for human immunodeficiency virus type 1 and simian immunodeficiency virus. *J Virol* 1998;72(10):7934–7940.
184. Egele C, Schaub E, Ramalanjaona N, et al. HIV-1 nucleocapsid protein binds to the viral DNA initiation sequences and chaperones their kissing interactions. *J Mol Biol* 2004;342(2):453–466.
185. Eglitis MA, Kadan MJ, Wonilowicz E, et al. Introduction of human genomic sequences renders CHO-K1 cells susceptible to infection by amphotropic retroviruses. *J Virol* 1993;67:1100–1104.
186. Ehrlich LS, Agresta BE, Carter CA. Assembly of recombinant human immunodeficiency virus type 1 capsid protein in vitro. *J Virol* 1992;66:4874–4883.
187. Elder JH, Lerner DL, Hasselkus-Light CS, et al. Distinct subsets of retroviruses encode dUTPase. *J Virol* 1992;66:1791–1794.
188. Elis E, Ehrlich M, Prizan-Ravid A, et al. p12 tethers the murine leukemia virus pre-integration complex to mitotic chromosomes. *PLoS Pathog* 2012;8(12):e1003103.
189. Elleder D, Stepanets V, Melder DC, et al. The receptor for the subgroup C avian sarcoma and leukosis viruses, Tvc, is related to mammalian butyrophilins, members of the immunoglobulin superfamily. *J Virol* 2005;79(16):10408–10419.
190. Elliott JL, Eschbach JE, Koneru PC, et al. Integrase-RNA interactions underscore the critical role of integrase in HIV-1 virion morphogenesis. *Elife* 2020;9:e54311.
191. Enssle J, Jordan I, Mauer B, et al. Foamy virus reverse transcriptase is expressed independently from the Gag protein. *Proc Natl Acad Sci U S A* 1996;93(9):4137–4141.

192. Ericsson TA, Takeuchi Y, Templin C, et al. Identification of receptors for pig endogenous retrovirus. *Proc Natl Acad Sci U S A* 2003;100(11):6759–6764.
193. Espeseth AS, Felock P, Wolfe A, et al. HIV-1 integrase inhibitors that compete with the target DNA substrate define a unique strand transfer conformation for integrase. *Proc Natl Acad Sci U S A* 2000;97(21):11244–11249.
194. Evans LH, Cloyd MW. Generation of mink cell focus-forming viruses by Friend murine leukemia virus: recombination with specific endogenous proviral sequences. *J Virol* 1984;49:772–781.
195. Exline CM, Feng Z, Stoltzfus CM. Negative and positive mRNA splicing elements act competitively to regulate human immunodeficiency virus type 1 vif gene expression. *J Virol* 2008;82(8):3921–3931.
196. Fass D, Davey RA, Hamson CA, et al. Structure of a murine leukemia virus receptor-binding glycoprotein at 2.0 angstrom resolution. *Science* 1997;277(5332):1662–1666.
197. Fass D, Harrison SC, Kim PS. Retrovirus envelope domain at 1.7 angstrom resolution. *Nat Struct Biol* 1996;3(5):465–469.
198. Fassati A, Goff SP. Characterization of intracellular reverse transcription complexes of Moloney murine leukemia virus. *J Virol* 1999;73(11):8919–8925.
199. Fassati A, Goff SP. Characterization of intracellular reverse transcription complexes of human immunodeficiency virus type 1. *J Virol* 2001;75(8):3626–3635.
200. Fassati A, Gorlich D, Harrison I, et al. Nuclear import of HIV-1 intracellular reverse transcription complexes is mediated by importin 7. *EMBO J* 2003;22(14):3675–3685.
201. FDA. https://www.fda.gov/consumers/free-publications-women/hiv-and-aids-medicines-help-you#nucleo. Published 2021.
202. Federspiel MJ, Bates P, Young JA, et al. A system for tissue-specific gene targeting: transgenic mice susceptible to subgroup A avian leukosis virus-based retroviral vectors. *Proc Natl Acad Sci U S A* 1994;91(23):11241–11245.
203. Feinstein SC, Ross SR, Yamamoto KR. Chromosomal position effects determine transcriptional potential of integrated mammary tumor virus DNA. *J Mol Biol* 1982;156:549–566.
204. Felsenstein KM, Goff SP. Expression of the gag-pol fusion protein of Moloney murine leukemia virus without gag protein does not induce virion formation or proteolytic processing. *J Virol* 1988;62:2179–2182.
205. Feng Y, Broder CC, Kennedy PE, et al. HIV-1 entry cofactor: functional cDNA cloning of a seven-transmembrane, G protein-coupled receptor. *Science* 1996;272(5263):872–877.
206. Feng YX, Copeland TD, Oroszlan S, et al. Identification of amino acids inserted during suppression of UAA and UGA termination codons at the gag-pol junction of Moloney murine leukemia virus. *Proc Natl Acad Sci U S A* 1990;87(22):8860–8863.
207. Feng YX, Levin JG, Hatfield DL, et al. Suppression of UAA and UGA termination codons in mutant murine leukemia viruses. *J Virol* 1989;63(6):2870–2873.
208. Feng YX, Yan H, Rein A, et al. Bipartite signal for read-through suppression in murine leukemia virus mRNA: an eight-nucleotide purine-rich sequence immediately downstream of the *gag* termination codon followed by an RNA pseudoknot. *J Virol* 1992;66:5127–5132.
209. Ficarelli M, Wilson H, Pedro Galao R, et al. KHNYN is essential for the zinc finger antiviral protein (ZAP) to restrict HIV-1 containing clustered CpG dinucleotides. *Elife* 2019;8:e46767.
210. Fisher J, Goff SP. Mutational analysis of stem-loops in the RNA packaging signal of the Moloney murine leukemia virus. *Virology* 1998;244(1):133–145.
211. Fisher RJ, Rein A, Fivash M, et al. Sequence-specific binding of human immunodeficiency virus type 1 nucleocapsid protein to short oligonucleotides. *J Virol* 1998;72(3):1902–1909.
212. Fitzgerald ML, Vora AC, Zeh WG, et al. Concerted integration of viral DNA termini by purified avian myeloblastosis virus integrase. *J Virol* 1992;66:6257–6263.
213. Flanagan JR, Becker KG, Ennist DL, et al. Cloning of a negative transcription factor that binds to the upstream conserved region of Moloney murine leukemia virus. *Mol Cell Biol* 1992;12:38–44.
214. Flugel RM, Rethwilm A, Maurer B, et al. Nucleotide sequence of the env gene and its flanking regions of the human spumaretrovirus reveals two novel genes. *EMBO J* 1987;6:2077–2084.
215. Forshey BM, von Schwedler U, Sundquist WI, et al. Formation of a human immunodeficiency virus type 1 core of optimal stability is crucial for viral replication. *J Virol* 2002;76(11):5667–5677.
216. Francis AC, Marin M, Prellberg MJ, et al. HIV-1 uncoating and nuclear import precede the completion of reverse transcription in cell lines and in primary macrophages. *Viruses* 2020;12(11):1234.
217. Francis AC, Marin M, Singh PK, et al. HIV-1 replication complexes accumulate in nuclear speckles and integrate into speckle-associated genomic domains. *Nat Commun* 2020;11(1):3505.
218. Franke EK, Yuan HE, Luban J. Specific incorporation of cyclophilin A into HIV-1 virions. *Nature* 1994;372(6504):359–362.
219. Frankel WN, Stoye JP, Taylor BA, et al. A linkage map of endogenous murine leukemia proviruses. *Genetics* 1990;124:221–236.
220. Freed EO, Martin MA. Virion incorporation of envelope glycoproteins with long but not short cytoplasmic tails is blocked by specific, single amino acid substitutions in the human immunodeficiency virus type 1 matrix. *J Virol* 1995;69(3):1984–1989.
221. Freed EO, Martin MA. Domains of the human immunodeficiency virus type 1 matrix and gp41 cytoplasmic tail required for envelope incorporation into virions. *J Virol* 1996;70(1):341–351.
222. Freed EO, Risser R. The role of envelope glycoprotein processing in murine leukemia virus infection. *J Virol* 1987;61(9):2852–2856.
223. Fu W, Gorelick RJ, Rein A. Characterization of human immunodeficiency virus type 1 dimeric RNA from wild-type and protease-defective virions. *J Virol* 1994;68(8):5013–5018.
224. Fu W, Ortiz-Conde BA, Gorelick RJ, et al. Placement of tRNA primer on the primer-binding site requires pol gene expression in avian but not murine retroviruses. *J Virol* 1997;71(9):6940–6946.
225. Fu W, Rein A. Maturation of dimeric viral RNA of Moloney murine leukemia virus. *J Virol* 1993;67(9):5443–5449.
226. Fujiwara T, Mizuuchi K. Retroviral DNA integration: structure of an integration intermediate. *Cell* 1988;54:497–504.
227. Gallay K, Blot G, Chahpazoff M, et al. In vitro, in cellulo and structural characterizations of the interaction between the integrase of Porcine Endogenous Retrovirus A/C and proteins of the BET family. *Virology* 2019;532:69–81.
228. Gallis B, Linial M, Eisenmann R. An avian oncovirus mutant deficient in genomic RNA: Characterization of the packaged RNA as cellular messenger RNA. *Virology* 1979;94:146–161.
229. Gamble TR, Vajdos FF, Yoo S, et al. Crystal structure of human cyclophilin A bound to the amino-terminal domain of HIV-1 capsid. *Cell* 1996;87(7):1285–1294.
230. Gamble TR, Yoo S, Vajdos FF, et al. Structure of the carboxyl-terminal dimerization domain of the HIV-1 capsid protein. *Science* 1997;278(5339):849–853.
231. Ganser BK, Cheng A, Sundquist WI, et al. Three-dimensional structure of the M-MuLV CA protein on a lipid monolayer: a general model for retroviral capsid assembly. *EMBO J* 2003;22(12):2886–2892.
232. Ganser BK, Li S, Klishko VY, et al. Assembly and analysis of conical models for the HIV-1 core. *Science* 1999;283(5398):80–83.
233. Ganser-Pornillos BK, Chandrasekaran V, Pornillos O, et al. Hexagonal assembly of a restricting TRIM5alpha protein. *Proc Natl Acad Sci U S A* 2011;108(2):534–539.
234. Ganser-Pornillos BK, Cheng A, Yeager M. Structure of full-length HIV-1 CA: a model for the mature capsid lattice. *Cell* 2007;131(1):70–79.
235. Ganser-Pornillos BK, Pornillos O. Restriction of HIV-1 and other retroviruses by TRIM5. *Nat Rev Microbiol* 2019;17(9):546–556.
236. Ganser-Pornillos BK, von Schwedler UK, Stray KM, et al. Assembly properties of the human immunodeficiency virus type 1 CA protein. *J Virol* 2004;78(5):2545–2552.
237. Gao G, Guo X, Goff SP. Inhibition of retroviral RNA production by ZAP, a CCCH-type zinc finger protein. *Science* 2002;297(5587):1703–1706.
238. Garbitt-Hirst R, Kenney SP, Parent LJ. Genetic evidence for a connection between Rous sarcoma virus gag nuclear trafficking and genomic RNA packaging. *J Virol* 2009;83(13):6790–6797.
239. Garcia JV, Miller AD. Serine phosphorylation-independent downregulation of cell-surface CD4 by nef. *Nature* 1991;350:508–511.
240. Garrus JE, von Schwedler UK, Pornillos OW, et al. Tsg101 and the vacuolar protein sorting pathway are essential for HIV-1 budding. *Cell* 2001;107(1):55–65.
241. Geijtenbeek TB, Kwon DS, Torensma R, et al. DC-SIGN, a dendritic cell-specific HIV-1-binding protein that enhances trans-infection of T cells. *Cell* 2000;100(5):587–597.
242. Geis FK, Goff SP. Unintegrated HIV-1 DNAs are loaded with core and linker histones and transcriptionally silenced. *Proc Natl Acad Sci U S A* 2019;116(47):23735–23742.
243. Georgiadis MM, Jessen SM, Ogata CM, et al. Mechanistic implications from the structure of a catalytic fragment of Moloney murine leukemia virus reverse transcriptase. *Structure* 1995;3:879–892.
244. Giam CZ, Semmes OJ. HTLV-1 infection and adult T-cell leukemia/lymphoma-A tale of two proteins: Tax and HBZ. *Viruses* 2016;8(6):161.
245. Giese S, Lawrence SP, Mazzon M, et al. The Nef protein of the macrophage tropic HIV-1 strain AD8 counteracts human BST-2/Tetherin. *Viruses* 2020;12(4):459.
246. Gilboa E, Mitra SW, Goff S, et al. A detailed model of reverse transcription and tests of crucial aspects. *Cell* 1979;18:93–100.
247. Giles KE, Beemon KL. Retroviral splicing suppressor sequesters a 3′ splice site in a 50S aberrant splicing complex. *Mol Cell Biol* 2005;25(11):4397–4405.
248. Gitti RK, Lee BM, Walker J, et al. Structure of the amino-terminal core domain of the HIV-1 capsid protein. *Science* 1996;273:231–235.
249. Goff SP. Retrovirus restriction factors. *Mol Cell* 2004;16(6):849–859.
250. Goldfarb MP, Weinberg RA. Generation of novel, biologically active Harvey sarcoma viruses via apparent illegitimate recombination. *J Virol* 1981;38:136–150.
251. Gopalakrishnan V, Peliska JA, Benkovic SJ. Human immunodeficiency virus type 1 reverse transcriptase: spatial and temporal relationship between the polymerase and RNase H activities. *Proc Natl Acad Sci U S A* 1992;89:10763–10767.
252. Gorelick RJ, Chabot DJ, Rein A, et al. The two zinc fingers in the human immunodeficiency virus type 1 nucleocapsid protein are not functionally equivalent. *J Virol* 1993;67(7):4027–4036.
253. Gorelick RJ, Fu W, Gagliardi TD, et al. Characterization of the block in replication of nucleocapsid protein zinc finger mutants from Moloney murine leukemia virus. *J Virol* 1999;73:8185–8195.
254. Gorelick RJ, Henderson LE, Hanser JP, et al. Point mutants of Moloney murine leukemia virus that fail to package viral RNA: evidence for specific RNA recognition by a "zinc finger-like" protein sequence. *Proc Natl Acad Sci U S A* 1988;85:8420–8424.
255. Gottlinger HG, Sodroski JG, Haseltine WA. Role of capsid precursor processing and myristoylation in morphogenesis and infectivity of human immunodeficiency virus type 1. *Proc Natl Acad Sci U S A* 1989;86:5781–5785.
256. Grandgenett DP. Symmetrical recognition of cellular DNA target sequences during retroviral integration. *Proc Natl Acad Sci U S A* 2005;102(17):5903–5904.
257. Granger SW, Fan H. In vivo footprinting of the enhancer sequences in the upstream long terminal repeat of Moloney murine leukemia virus: differential binding of nuclear factors in different cell types. *J Virol* 1998;72(11):8961–8970.
258. Green N, Shinnick TM, Witte O, et al. Sequence-specific antibodies show that maturation of Moloney leukemia virus envelope polyprotein involves removal of a COOH-terminal peptide. *Proc Natl Acad Sci U S A* 1981;78(10):6023–6027.
259. Green PL, Chen IS. Regulation of human T cell leukemia virus expression. *FASEB J* 1990;4(2):169–175.
260. Greenwood AD, Ishida Y, O'Brien SP, et al. Transmission, evolution, and endogenization: lessons learned from recent retroviral invasions. *Microbiol Mol Biol Rev* 2018;82(1):e00044-17.
261. Greenwood EJD, Williamson JC, Sienkiewicz A, et al. Promiscuous targeting of cellular proteins by Vpr drives systems-level proteomic remodeling in HIV-1 infection. *Cell Rep* 2019;27(5):1579–1596 e7.
262. Griffin SD, Allen JF, Lever AM. The major human immunodeficiency virus type 2 (HIV-2) packaging signal is present on all HIV-2 RNA species: cotranslational RNA encapsidation and limitation of Gag protein confer specificity. *J Virol* 2001;75(24):12058–12069.
263. Grimm SL, Nordeen SK. Mouse mammary tumor virus sequences responsible for activating cellular oncogenes. *J Virol* 1998;72(12):9428–9435.

264. Grobler JA, Stillmock K, Hu B, et al. Diketo acid inhibitor mechanism and HIV-1 integrase: implications for metal binding in the active site of phosphotransferase enzymes. *Proc Natl Acad Sci U S A* 2002;99(10):6661–6666.

265. Gross I, Hohenberg H, Huckhagel C, et al. N-Terminal extension of human immunodeficiency virus capsid protein converts the in vitro assembly phenotype from tubular to spherical particles. *J Virol* 1998;72(6):4798–4810.

266. Guelen L, Pagie L, Brasset E, et al. Domain organization of human chromosomes revealed by mapping of nuclear lamina interactions. *Nature* 2008;453(7197):948–951.

267. Guo X, Carroll JW, Macdonald MR, et al. The zinc finger antiviral protein directly binds to specific viral mRNAs through the CCCH zinc finger motifs. *J Virol* 2004;78(23):12781–12787.

268. Guo X, Ma J, Sun J, et al. The zinc-finger antiviral protein recruits the RNA processing exosome to degrade the target mRNA. *Proc Natl Acad Sci U S A* 2007;104(1):151–156.

269. Gupta SS, Maetzig T, Maertens GN, et al. Bromo- and extraterminal domain chromatin regulators serve as cofactors for murine leukemia virus integration. *J Virol* 2013;87(23):12721–12736.

270. Hacein-Bey-Abina S, Pai SY, Gaspar HB, et al. A modified gamma-retrovirus vector for X-linked severe combined immunodeficiency. *N Engl J Med* 2014;371(15):1407–1417.

271. Haddrick M, Lear AL, Cann AJ, et al. Evidence that a kissing loop structure facilitates genomic RNA dimerisation in HIV-1. *J Mol Biol* 1996;259(1):58–68.

272. Hagino-Yamagishi K, Donehower LA, Varmus HE. Retroviral DNA integrated during infection by an integration-deficient mutant of murine leukemia virus is oligomeric. *J Virol* 1987;61:1964–1971.

273. Hansen M, Jelinek L, Whiting S, et al. Transport and assembly of gag proteins into Moloney murine leukemia virus. *J Virol* 1990;64:5306–5316.

274. Hare S, Gupta SS, Valkov E, et al. Retroviral intasome assembly and inhibition of DNA strand transfer. *Nature* 2010;464(7286):232–236.

275. Hare S, Maertens GN, Cherepanov P. 3'-processing and strand transfer catalysed by retroviral integrase in crystallo. *EMBO J* 2012;31(13):3020–3028.

276. Hare S, Vos AM, Clayton RF, et al. Molecular mechanisms of retroviral integrase inhibition and the evolution of viral resistance. *Proc Natl Acad Sci U S A* 2010;107(46):20057–20062.

277. Harris RS, Bishop KN, Sheehy AM, et al. DNA deamination mediates innate immunity to retroviral infection. *Cell* 2003;113(6):803–809.

278. Harris RS, Liddament MT. Retroviral restriction by APOBEC proteins. *Nat Rev Immunol* 2004;4(11):868–877.

279. Harrison GP, Mayo MS, Hunter E, et al. Pausing of reverse transcriptase on retroviral RNA templates is influenced by secondary structures both 5' and 3' of the catalytic site. *Nucleic Acids Res* 1998;26(14):3433–3442.

280. Hatziioannou T, Cowan S, Goff SP, et al. Restriction of multiple divergent retroviruses by Lv1 and Ref1. *EMBO J* 2003;22(3):385–394.

281. Hatziioannou T, Goff SP. Infection of nondividing cells by Rous sarcoma virus. *J Virol* 2001;75(19):9526–9531.

282. Hatziioannou T, Perez-Caballero D, Cowan S, et al. Cyclophilin interactions with incoming human immunodeficiency virus type 1 capsids with opposing effects on infectivity in human cells. *J Virol* 2005;79(1):176–183.

283. Hatziioannou T, Perez-Caballero D, Yang A, et al. Retrovirus resistance factors Ref1 and Lv1 are species-specific variants of TRIM5alpha. *Proc Natl Acad Sci U S A* 2004;101(29):10774–10779.

284. Hauser H, Lopez LA, Yang SJ, et al. HIV-1 Vpu and HIV-2 Env counteract BST-2/tetherin by sequestration in a perinuclear compartment. *Retrovirology* 2010;7:51.

285. Hayward WS, Neel BG, Astrin SM. Activation of a cellular onc gene by promoter insertion in ALV-induced lymphomas. *Nature* 1981;290:475–480.

286. Hein S, Prassolov V, Zhang Y, et al. Sodium-dependent myo-inositol transporter 1 is a cellular receptor for Mus cervicolor M813 murine leukemia virus. *J Virol* 2003;77(10):5926–5932.

287. Henderson LE, Krutzsch HC, Oroszlan S. Myristyl amino-terminal acylation of murine retrovirus proteins: an unusual post-translational protein modification. *Proc Natl Acad Sci U S A* 1983;80:339–343.

288. Henderson R, Lu M, Zhou Y, et al. Disruption of the HIV-1 envelope allosteric network blocks CD4-induced rearrangements. *Nat Commun* 2020;11(1):520.

289. Herman SA, Coffin JM. Differential transcription from the long terminal repeats of integrated avian leukosis virus DNA. *J Virol* 1986;60:497–505.

290. Herman SA, Coffin JM. Efficient packaging of readthrough RNA in ALV: implications for oncogene transduction. *Science* 1987;236:845–848.

291. Hibbert CS, Mirro J, Rein A. mRNA molecules containing murine leukemia virus packaging signals are encapsidated as dimers. *J Virol* 2004;78(20):10927–10938.

292. Hibbert CS, Rein A. Preliminary physical mapping of RNA-RNA linkages in the genomic RNA of Moloney murine leukemia virus. *J Virol* 2005;79(13):8142–8148.

293. Hilberg F, Stocking C, Ostertag W, et al. Functional analysis of a retroviral host-range mutant: altered long terminal repeat sequences allow expression in embryonal carcinoma cells. *Proc Natl Acad Sci U S A* 1987;84:5232–5236.

294. Holman AG, Coffin JM. Symmetrical base preferences surrounding HIV-1, avian sarcoma/leukosis virus, and murine leukemia virus integration sites. *Proc Natl Acad Sci U S A* 2005;102(17):6103–6107.

295. Honigman A, Wolf D, Yaish S, et al. *cis* acting RNA sequences control the gag-pol translation readthrough in murine leukemia virus. *Virology* 1991;183:313–319.

296. Hope TJ. VIROLOGY. Visualizing trans-infection. *Science* 2015;350(6260):511–512.

297. Hopkins N, Schindler J, Hynes R. Six NB-tropic murine leukemia viruses derived from a B-tropic virus of BALB/c have altered p30. *J Virol* 1977;21:309–318.

298. Hostomsky Z, Hughes SH, Goff SP, et al. Redesignation of the RNase D activity associated with retroviral reverse transcriptase as RNase H. *J Virol* 1994;68(3):1970–1971.

299. Houck-Loomis B, Durney MA, Salguero C, et al. An equilibrium-dependent retroviral mRNA switch regulates translational recoding. *Nature* 2011;480(7378):561–564.

300. Hrecka K, Gierszewska M, Srivastava S, et al. Lentiviral Vpr usurps Cul4-DDB1[VprBP] E3 ubiquitin ligase to modulate cell cycle. *Proc Natl Acad Sci U S A* 2007;104(28):11778–11783.

301. Hrecka K, Hao C, Gierszewska M, et al. Vpx relieves inhibition of HIV-1 infection of macrophages mediated by the SAMHD1 protein. *Nature* 2011;474(7353):658–661.

302. Hsiou Y, Ding J, Das K, et al. Structure of unliganded HIV-1 reverse transcriptase at 2.7 A resolution: implications of conformational changes for polymerization and inhibition mechanisms. *Structure* 1996;4(7):853–860.

303. Hu W-S, Temin HM. Retroviral recombination and reverse transcription. *Science* 1990;250:1227–1233.

304. Huang M, Orenstein JM, Martin MA, et al. p6Gag is required for particle production from full-length human immunodeficiency virus type 1 molecular clones expressing protease. *J Virol* 1995;69(11):6810–6818.

305. Huang M, Simard C, Kay DG, et al. The majority of cells infected with the defective murine AIDS virus belong to the B-cell lineage. *J Virol* 1991;65:6562–6571.

306. Huang Y, Khorchid A, Gabor J, et al. The role of nucleocapsid and U5 stem/A-rich loop sequences in tRNA(3Lys) genomic placement and initiation of reverse transcription in human immunodeficiency virus type 1. *J Virol* 1998;72(5):3907–3915.

307. Hunter E. Macromolecular interactions in the assembly of HIV and other retroviruses. *Semin Virol* 1994;5:71–83.

308. Ikeda H, Sugimura H. Fv-4 resistance gene: a truncated endogenous murine leukemia virus with ecotropic interference properties. *J Virol* 1989;63:5405–5412.

309. Ikeda T, Shibata J, Yoshimura K, et al. Recurrent HIV-1 integration at the BACH2 locus in resting CD4+ T cell populations during effective highly active antiretroviral therapy. *J Infect Dis* 2007;195(5):716–725.

310. Indik S, Gunzburg WH, Salmons B, et al. A novel, mouse mammary tumor virus encoded protein with Rev-like properties. *Virology* 2005;337(1):1–6.

311. Irwan ID, Karnowski HL, Bogerd HP, et al. Reversal of epigenetic silencing allows robust HIV-1 replication in the absence of integrase function. *mBio* 2020;11(3):e01038-20.

312. Isel C, Westhof E, Massire C, et al. Structural basis for the specificity of the initiation of HIV-1 reverse transcription. *EMBO J* 1999;18(4):1038–1048.

313. Itin A, Keshet E. A novel retroviruslike family in mouse DNA. *J Virol* 1986;59:301–307.

314. Ivanova Svilena (FR), Giovannini Donatella (FR), Bellis Julien (FR), Lezaar Jawida (FR), Petit Vincent (FR), Battini Jean-Luc (FR), Sitbon Marc (FR), Courgnaud Valérie (FR). *Use of Receptor-Binding Domain Derived from Bovine Leukemia Virus for the Diagnosis or Treatment of Cationic l-Amino Acid Transporter-Related Diseases.* Metafora Biosystems (FR), Centre Nat Rech Scient (FR), Université de Montpellier (FR), Université Paris Descartes —PARIS V (FR). WO/2017/085271. https://www.freepatentsonline.com/WO2017085271.html

315. Iwabu Y, Fujita H, Tanaka Y, et al. Direct internalization of cell-surface BST-2/tetherin by the HIV-1 accessory protein Vpu. *Commun Integr Biol* 2010;3(4):366–369.

316. Izquierdo-Useros N, Lorizate M, McLaren PJ, et al. HIV-1 capture and transmission by dendritic cells: the role of viral glycolipids and the cellular receptor Siglec-1. *PLoS Pathog* 2014;10(7):e1004146.

317. Jacks T, Varmus HE. Expression of the Rous sarcoma virus pol gene by ribosomal frameshifting. *Science* 1985;230:1237–1242.

318. Javanbakht H, Halwani R, Cen S, et al. The interaction between HIV-1 Gag and human lysyl-tRNA synthetase during viral assembly. *J Biol Chem* 2003;278(30):27644–27651.

319. Jenkins NA, Copeland NG, Taylor BA, et al. Organization, distribution and stability of endogenous ecotropic murine leukemia virus DNA in chromosomes of *Mus musculus*. *J Virol* 1982;43:26–36.

320. Jenkins Y, Pornillos O, Rich RL, et al. Biochemical analyses of the interactions between human immunodeficiency virus type 1 Vpr and p6(Gag). *J Virol* 2001;75(21):10537–10542.

321. Jennings J, Shi J, Varadarajan J, et al. The host cell metabolite inositol hexakisphosphate promotes efficient endogenous HIV-1 reverse transcription by stabilizing the viral capsid. *mBio* 2020;11(6):e02820-20.

322. Jette CA, Barnes CO, Kirk SM, et al. Cryo-EM structures of HIV-1 trimer bound to CD4-mimetics BNM-III-170 and M48U1 adopt a CD4-bound open conformation. *Nat Commun* 2021;12(1):1950.

323. Jin Z, Jin L, Peterson DL, et al. Model for lentivirus capsid core assembly based on crystal dimers of EIAV p26. *J Mol Biol* 1999;286(1):83–93.

324. Johann SV, Gibbons JJ, O'Hara B. GLVR1, a receptor for gibbon ape leukemia virus, is homologous to a phosphate permease of *Neurospora crassa* and is expressed at high levels in the brain and thymus. *J Virol* 1992;66:1635–1640.

325. Johnson MC, Scobie HM, Ma YM, et al. Nucleic acid-independent retrovirus assembly can be driven by dimerization. *J Virol* 2002;76(22):11177–11185.

326. Johnson MC, Spidel JL, Ako-Adjei D, et al. The C-terminal half of TSG101 blocks Rous sarcoma virus budding and sequesters Gag into unique nonendosomal structures. *J Virol* 2005;79(6):3775–3786.

327. Johnson WE, Coffin JM. Constructing primate phylogenies from ancient retrovirus sequences. *Proc Natl Acad Sci U S A* 1999;96:10254–10260.

328. Jolicoeur P. The Fv-1 gene of the mouse and its control of murine leukemia virus replication. *Curr Top Microbiol Immunol* 1979;86:67–122.

329. Jolicoeur P, Rassart E. Effect of Fv-1 gene product on synthesis of linear and supercoiled viral DNA in cells infected with murine leukemia virus. *J Virol* 1980;33:183–195.

330. Jones TA, Blaug G, Hansen M, et al. Assembly of gag-b-galactosidase proteins into retrovirus particles. *J Virol* 1990;64:2265–2279.

331. Joshi SM, Vogt VM. Role of the Rous sarcoma virus p10 domain in shape determination of gag virus-like particles assembled in vitro and within Escherichia coli. *J Virol* 2000;74(21):10260–10268.

332. Jouvenet N, Neil SJ, Zhadina M, et al. Broad-spectrum inhibition of retroviral and filoviral particle release by tetherin. *J Virol* 2009;83(4):1837–1844.

333. Jurado KA, Wang H, Slaughter A, et al. Allosteric integrase inhibitor potency is determined through the inhibition of HIV-1 particle maturation. *Proc Natl Acad Sci U S A* 2013;110(21):8690–8695.

334. Kabat D. Molecular biology of Friend viral erythroleukemia. *Curr Top Microbiol Immunol* 1989;148:1–42.

335. Kafri T, van Praag H, Ouyang L, et al. A packaging cell line for lentivirus vectors. *J Virol* 1999;73(1):576–584.

336. Kane SE, Beemon K. Precise localization of m6A in Rous sarcoma virus RNA reveals clustering of methylation sites: implications for RNA processing. *Mol Cell Biol* 1985;5:2298–2306.

337. Kashmiri SVS, Rein A, Bassin RH, et al. Donation of N- or B-tropic phenotype to NB-tropic murine leukemia virus during mixed infections. *J Virol* 1977;22:626–633.

338. Katoh I, Ikawa Y, Yoshinaka Y. Retrovirus protease characterized as a dimeric aspartic proteinase. *J Virol* 1989;63:2226–2232.

339. Katoh I, Yoshinaka Y, Rein A, et al. Murine leukemia virus maturation: protease region required for conversion from "immature" to "mature" core form and for virus infectivity. *Virology* 1985;145:280–292.

340. Katz RA, Skalka AM. Control of retroviral RNA splicing through maintenance of suboptimal processing signals. *Mol Cell Biol* 1990;10:696–704.

341. Katz RA, Terry RW, Skalka AM. A conserved cis-acting sequence in the 5′ leader of avian sarcoma virus RNA is required for packaging. *J Virol* 1986;59:163–167.

342. Kavanaugh MP, Miller DG, Zhang W, et al. Cell-surface receptors for gibbon ape leukemia virus and amphotropic murine retrovirus are inducible sodium-dependent phosphate symporters. *Proc Natl Acad Sci U S A* 1994;91(15):7071–7075.

343. Kaye JF, Lever AM. Human immunodeficiency virus types 1 and 2 differ in the predominant mechanism used for selection of genomic RNA for encapsidation. *J Virol* 1999;73(4):3023–3031.

344. Kaye JF, Richardson JH, Lever AM. cis-acting sequences involved in human immunodeficiency virus type 1 RNA packaging. *J Virol* 1995;69(10):6588–6592.

345. Keane SC, Heng X, Lu K, et al. RNA structure. Structure of the HIV-1 RNA packaging signal. *Science* 2015;348(6237):917–921.

346. Keane SC, Van V, Frank HM, et al. NMR detection of intermolecular interaction sites in the dimeric 5′-leader of the HIV-1 genome. *Proc Natl Acad Sci U S A* 2016;113(46):13033–13038.

347. Keckesova Z, Ylinen LM, Towers GJ. The human and African green monkey TRIM5alpha genes encode Ref1 and Lv1 retroviral restriction factor activities. *Proc Natl Acad Sci U S A* 2004;101(29):10780–10785.

348. Keene SE, King SR, Telesnitsky A. 7SL RNA is retained in HIV-1 minimal virus-like particles as an S-domain fragment. *J Virol* 2010;84(18):9070–9077.

349. Kehn K, Fuente Cde L, Strouss K, et al. The HTLV-I Tax oncoprotein targets the retinoblastoma protein for proteasomal degradation. *Oncogene* 2005;24(4):525–540.

350. Kekuda R, Prasad PR, Fei YJ, et al. Cloning of the sodium-dependent, broad-scope, neutral amino acid transporter Bo from a human placental choriocarcinoma cell line. *J Biol Chem* 1996;271:18657–18661.

351. Kempler G, Freitag B, Berwin B, et al. Characterization of the Moloney murine leukemia virus stem cell-specific repressor binding sites. *Virology* 1993;193:690–699.

352. Kennedy EM, Bogerd HP, Kornepati AV, et al. Posttranscriptional m(6)A editing of HIV-1 mRNAs enhances viral gene expression. *Cell Host Microbe* 2016;19(5):675–685.

353. Kennedy EM, Bogerd HP, Kornepati AVR, et al. Posttranscriptional m(6)A editing of HIV-1 mRNAs enhances viral gene expression. *Cell Host Microbe* 2017;22(6):830.

354. Kessl JJ, Kutluay SB, Townsend D, et al. HIV-1 integrase binds the viral RNA genome and is essential during virion morphogenesis. *Cell* 2016;166(5):1257–1268 e12.

355. Kharytonchyk S, Monti S, Smaldino PJ, et al. Transcriptional start site heterogeneity modulates the structure and function of the HIV-1 genome. *Proc Natl Acad Sci U S A* 2016;113(47):13378–13383.

356. Khorchid A, Javanbakht H, Wise S, et al. Sequences within Pr160gag-pol affecting the selective packaging of primer tRNA(Lys3) into HIV-1. *J Mol Biol* 2000;299(1):17–26.

357. Kiernan RE, Freed EO. Cleavage of the murine leukemia virus transmembrane env protein by human immunodeficiency virus type 1 protease: transdominant inhibition by matrix mutations. *J Virol* 1998;72(12):9621–9627.

358. Kim JW, Closs EI, Albritton LM, et al. Transport of cationic amino acids by the mouse ecotropic retrovirus receptor. *Nature* 1991;352:725–728.

359. Kim K, Dauphin A, Komurlu S, et al. Cyclophilin A protects HIV-1 from restriction by human TRIM5alpha. *Nat Microbiol* 2019;4(12):2044–2051.

360. Kirk PD, Huvet M, Melamed A, et al. Retroviruses integrate into a shared, non-palindromic DNA motif. *Nat Microbiol* 2016;2:16212.

361. Kizhatil K, Albritton LM. Requirements for different components of the host cell cytoskeleton distinguish ecotropic murine leukemia virus entry via endocytosis from entry via surface fusion. *J Virol* 1997;71(10):7145–7156.

362. Klatzman D, Champagne E, Chamaret S, et al. T-lymphocyte T4 molecule behaves as the receptor for human retrovirus LAV. *Nature* 1984;312:767–768.

363. Kleiman L, Halwani R, Javanbakht H. The selective packaging and annealing of primer tRNALys3 in HIV-1. *Curr HIV Res* 2004;2(2):163–175.

364. Klikova M, Rhee SS, Hunter E, et al. Efficient in vivo and in vitro assembly of retroviral capsids from Gag precursor proteins expressed in bacteria. *J Virol* 1995;69(2):1093–1098.

365. Kluge SF, Mack K, Iyer SS, et al. Nef proteins of epidemic HIV-1 group O strains antagonize human tetherin. *Cell Host Microbe* 2014;16(5):639–650.

366. Kobe B, Center RJ, Kemp BE, et al. Crystal structure of human T cell leukemia virus type 1 gp21 ectodomain crystallized as a maltose-binding protein chimera reveals structural evolution of retroviral transmembrane proteins. *Proc Natl Acad Sci U S A* 1999;96(8):4319–4324.

367. Kodera Y, Sato K, Tsukahara T, et al. High-resolution solution NMR structure of the minimal active domain of the human immunodeficiency virus type-2 nucleocapsid protein. *Biochemistry* 1998;37(51):17704–17713.

368. Kohl NE, Emini EA, Schleif WA, et al. Active human immunodeficiency virus protease is required for viral infectivity. *Proc Natl Acad Sci U S A* 1988;85:4686–4690.

369. Kootstra NA, Munk C, Tonnu N, et al. Abrogation of postentry restriction of HIV-1-based lentiviral vector transduction in simian cells. *Proc Natl Acad Sci U S A* 2003;100(3):1298–1303.

370. Kovari LC, Momany CA, Miyagi F, et al. Crystals of Rous sarcoma virus capsid protein show a helical arrangement of protein subunits. *Virology* 1997;238(1):79–84.

371. Kozak CA, Gromet NJ, Ikeda H, et al. A unique sequence related to the ecotropic murine leukemia virus is associated with the Fv-4 restriction gene. *Proc Natl Acad Sci U S A* 1984;81:834–837.

372. Kozak CA, O'Neill RR. Diverse wild mouse origins of xenotropic, mink-cell focus-forming, and two types of ecotropic proviral genes. *J Virol* 1987;61:3082–3088.

373. Krchlikova V, Mikesova J, Geryk J, et al. The avian retroviral receptor Tva mediates the uptake of transcobalamin bound vitamin B12 (cobalamin). *J Virol* 2021;95(8):e02136-20.

374. Krishna NK, Campbell S, Vogt VM, et al. Genetic determinants of Rous sarcoma virus particle size. *J Virol* 1998;72(1):564–577.

375. Krishnan L, Matreyek KA, Oztop I, et al. The requirement for cellular transportin 3 (TNPO3 or TRN-SR2) during infection maps to human immunodeficiency virus type 1 capsid and not integrase. *J Virol* 2010;84(1):397–406.

376. Kuff EL, Leuders KK. The intracisternal A-particle gene family: structure and functional aspects. *Adv Cancer Res* 1988;51:183–276.

377. Kulkosky J, Jones KS, Katz RA, et al. Residues critical for retroviral integrative recombination in a region that is highly conserved among retroviral/retrotransposon integrases and bacterial insertion sequences transposases. *Mol Cell Biol* 1992;12:2331–2338.

378. Kumar S, Sarkar A, Pugach P, et al. Capturing the inherent structural dynamics of the HIV-1 envelope glycoprotein fusion peptide. *Nat Commun* 2019;10(1):763.

379. Kwon DS, Gregorio G, Bitton N, et al. DC-SIGN-mediated internalization of HIV is required for trans-enhancement of T cell infection. *Immunity* 2002;16(1):135–144.

380. Kwong PD, Wyatt R, Robinson J, et al. Structure of an HIV gp120 envelope glycoprotein in complex with the CD4 receptor and a neutralizing human antibody. *Nature* 1998;393(6686):648–659.

381. LaFave MC, Varshney GK, Gildea DE, et al. MLV integration site selection is driven by strong enhancers and active promoters. *Nucleic Acids Res* 2014;42(7):4257–4269.

382. Laguette N, Sobhian B, Casartelli N, et al. SAMHD1 is the dendritic- and myeloid-cell-specific HIV-1 restriction factor counteracted by Vpx. *Nature* 2011;474(7353):654–657.

383. Lama J, Trono D. Human immunodeficiency virus type 1 matrix protein interacts with cellular protein HO3. *J Virol* 1998;72(2):1671–1676.

384. Lapatto R, Blundell T, Hemmings A, et al. X-ray analysis of HIV-1 proteinase at 2.7 Å resolution confirms structural homology among retroviral enzymes. *Nature* 1989;342:299–302.

385. LaPierre LA, Casey JW, Holzschu DL. Walleye retroviruses associated with skin tumors and hyperplasias encode cyclin D homologs. *J Virol* 1998;72(11):8765–8771.

386. Larder BA, Kemp SD. Multiple mutations in HIV-1 reverse transcriptase confer high-level resistance to Zidovudine (AZT). *Science* 1989;246:1155–1158.

387. Lavialle C, Cornelis G, Dupressoir A, et al. Paleovirology of 'syncytins', retroviral env genes exapted for a role in placentation. *Philos Trans R Soc Lond B Biol Sci* 2013;368(1626):20120507.

388. Lavillette D, Marin M, Ruggieri A, et al. The envelope glycoprotein of human endogenous retrovirus type W uses a divergent family of amino acid transporters/cell surface receptors. *J Virol* 2002;76(13):6442–6452.

389. Lawrence DC, Stover CC, Noznitsky J, et al. Structure of the intact stem and bulge of HIV-1 Psi-RNA stem-loop SL1. *J Mol Biol* 2003;326(2):529–542.

390. LeBlanc JJ, Uddowla S, Abraham B, et al. Tap and Dbp5, but not Gag, are involved in DR-mediated nuclear export of unspliced Rous sarcoma virus RNA. *Virology* 2007;363(2):376–386.

391. Lecossier D, Bouchonnet F, Clavel F, et al. Hypermutation of HIV-1 DNA in the absence of the Vif protein. *Science* 2003;300(5622):1112.

392. Lee K, Ambrose Z, Martin TD, et al. Flexible use of nuclear import pathways by HIV-1. *Cell Host Microbe* 2010;7(3):221–233.

393. Lee MS, Craigie R. A previously unidentified host protein protects retroviral DNA from autointegration. *Proc Natl Acad Sci U S A* 1998;95(4):1528–1533.

394. Lee SK, Nagashima K, Hu WS. Cooperative effect of gag proteins p12 and capsid during early events of murine leukemia virus replication. *J Virol* 2005;79(7):4159–4169.

395. Lehmann MJ, Sherer NM, Marks CB, et al. Actin- and myosin-driven movement of viruses along filopodia precedes their entry into cells. *J Cell Biol* 2005;170(2):317–325.

396. Leis J, Baltimore D, Bishop JM, et al. Standardized and simplified nomenclature for proteins common to all retroviruses. *J Virol* 1988;62:1808–1809.

397. Lenz J, Crowther R, Straceski A, et al. Nucleotide sequence of the Akv env gene. *J Virol* 1982;42(2):519–529.

398. Lerner DL, Wagaman PC, Phillips TR, et al. Increased mutation frequency of feline immunodeficiency virus lacking functional deoxyuridine-triphosphatase. *Proc Natl Acad Sci U S A* 1995;92(16):7480–7484.

399. LeRoy G, Rickards B, Flint SJ. The double bromodomain proteins Brd2 and Brd3 couple histone acetylation to transcription. *Mol Cell* 2008;30(1):51–60.

400. Lesbats P, Serrao E, Maskell DP, et al. Structural basis for spumavirus GAG tethering to chromatin. *Proc Natl Acad Sci U S A* 2017;114(21):5509–5514.

401. Lewis P, Hensel M, Emerman M. Human immunodeficiency virus infection of cells arrested in the cell cycle. *EMBO J* 1992;11:3053–3058.

402. Lewis PF, Emerman M. Passage through mitosis is required for oncoretroviruses but not for the human immunodeficiency virus. *J Virol* 1994;68(1):510–516.

403. Li C, Burdick RC, Nagashima K, et al. HIV-1 cores retain their integrity until minutes before uncoating in the nucleus. *Proc Natl Acad Sci U S A* 2021;118(10):e2019467118.

404. Li F, Chen C, Puffer BA, et al. Functional replacement and positional dependence of homologous and heterologous L domains in equine infectious anemia virus replication. *J Virol* 2002;76(4):1569–1577.

405. Li L, Cohen SN. Tsg101: a novel tumor susceptibility gene isolated by controlled homozygous functional knockout of allelic loci in mammalian cells. *Cell* 1996;85(3):319–329.

406. Li M, Chen X, Wang H, et al. A peptide derived from lens epithelium-derived growth factor stimulates HIV-1 DNA integration and facilitates intasome structural studies. *J Mol Biol* 2020;432(7):2055–2066.

407. Li M, Yang C, Tong S, et al. Palmitoylation of the murine leukemia virus envelope protein is critical for lipid raft association and surface expression. *J Virol* 2002;76(23):11845–11852.

408. Li MM, Lau Z, Cheung P, et al. TRIM25 enhances the antiviral action of zinc-finger antiviral protein (ZAP). *PLoS Pathog* 2017;13(1):e1006145.

409. Li S, Ahmad I, Shi J, et al. Murine leukemia virus glycosylated gag reduces murine SERINC5 protein expression at steady-state levels via the endosome/lysosome pathway to counteract SERINC5 antiretroviral activity. *J Virol* 2019;93(2):e01651-18.

410. Li S, Hill CP, Sundquist WI, et al. Image reconstructions of helical assemblies of the HIV-1 CA protein. *Nature* 2000;407(6802):409–413.

411. Li W, Singh PK, Sowd GA, et al. CPSF6-dependent targeting of speckle-associated domains distinguishes primate from nonprimate lentiviral integration. *mBio* 2020;11(5):e02254-20.

412. Li X, Gu C, Hostachy S, et al. Control of XPR1-dependent cellular phosphate efflux by InsP8 is an exemplar for functionally-exclusive inositol pyrophosphate signaling. *Proc Natl Acad Sci U S A* 2020;117(7):3568–3574.

413. Li YL, Chandrasekaran V, Carter SD, et al. Primate TRIM5 proteins form hexagonal nets on HIV-1 capsids. *Elife* 2016;5:e16269.

414. Li Z, Li W, Lu M, et al. Subnanometer structures of HIV-1 envelope trimers on aldrithiol-2 inactivated virus particles. *Nat Struct Mol Biol* 2020;27(8):726–734.

415. Liang C, Hu J, Russell RS, et al. Translation of Pr55(gag) augments packaging of human immunodeficiency virus type 1 RNA in a cis-acting manner. *AIDS Res Hum Retroviruses* 2002;18(15):1117–1126.

416. Liang C, Rong L, Morin N, et al. The roles of the human immunodeficiency virus type 1 Pol protein and the primer binding site in the placement of primer tRNA(3Lys) onto viral genomic RNA. *J Virol* 1997;71:9075–9086.

417. Liao CH, Kuang YQ, Liu HL, et al. A novel fusion gene, TRIM5-Cyclophilin A in the pig-tailed macaque determines its susceptibility to HIV-1 infection. *AIDS* 2007;21(Suppl 8):S19–S26.

418. Liao Z, Graham DR, Hildreth JE. Lipid rafts and HIV pathogenesis: virion-associated cholesterol is required for fusion and infection of susceptible cells. *AIDS Res Hum Retroviruses* 2003;19(8):675–687.

419. Lilly F. Fv-2: Identification and location of a second gene governing the spleen focus response to Friend leukemia virus in mice. *J Natl Cancer Inst* 1970;45:163–169.

420. Lilly F, Pincus T. Genetic control of murine viral leukemogenesis. *Adv Cancer Res* 1973;17:231–277.

421. Linial M, Medeiros E, Hayward WS. An avian oncovirus mutant (SE 21Q1b) deficient in genomic RNA: biological and biochemical characterization. *Cell* 1978;15:1371–1381.

422. Liu XH, Xu W, Russ J, et al. The host range of gammaretroviruses and gammaretroviral vectors includes post-mitotic neural cells. *PLoS One* 2011;6(3):e18072.

423. Llano M, Saenz DT, Meehan A, et al. An essential role for LEDGF/p75 in HIV integration. *Science* 2006;314(5798):461–464.

424. Lochelt M, Flugel RM. The human foamy virus pol gene is expressed as a Pro-Pol polyprotein and not as a Gag-Pol fusion protein. *J Virol* 1996;70(2):1033–1040.

425. Lochelt M, Romen F, Bastone P, et al. The antiretroviral activity of APOBEC3 is inhibited by the foamy virus accessory Bet protein. *Proc Natl Acad Sci U S A* 2005;102(22):7982–7987.

426. Loeb DD, Hutchinson III CA, Edgell MH, et al. Mutational analysis of human immunodeficiency virus type 1 protease suggests functional homology with aspartic proteinases. *J Virol* 1989;63:111–121.

427. Lopez-Lastra M, Ulrici S, Gabus C, et al. Identification of an internal ribosome entry segment in the 5′ region of the mouse VL30 retrotransposon and its use in the development of retroviral vectors. *J Virol* 1999;73(10):8393–8402.

428. LoSardo JE, Boral AL, Lenz J. Relative importance of elements within the SL3-3 virus enhancer for T-cell specificity. *J Virol* 1990;64:1756–1763.

429. Lower R, Lower J, Kurth R. The viruses in all of us: characteristics and biological significance of human endogenous retrovirus sequences. *Proc Natl Acad Sci U S A* 1996;93(11):5177–5184.

430. Loyola L, Achuthan V, Gilroy K, et al. Disrupting MLV integrase:BET protein interaction biases integration into quiescent chromatin and delays but does not eliminate tumor activation in a MYC/Runx2 mouse model. *PLoS Pathog* 2019;15(12):e1008154.

431. Lu M, Blacklow SC, Kim PS. A trimeric structural domain of the HIV-1 transmembrane glycoprotein. *Nat Struct Biol* 1995;2(12):1075–1082.

432. Lu R, Nakajima N, Hofmann W, et al. Simian virus 40-based replication of catalytically inactive human immunodeficiency virus type 1 integrase mutants in nonpermissive T cells and monocyte-derived macrophages. *J Virol* 2004;78(2):658–668.

433. Luban J, Bossolt KA, Franke EK, et al. Human immunodeficiency virus type 1 gag protein binds to cyclophilins A and B. *Cell* 1993;73:1067–1078.

434. Lueders KK, Kuff EL. Sequences associated with intracisternal A particles are repeated in the mouse genome. *Cell* 1977;12:963–972.

435. Lum R, Linial ML. Retrotransposition of nonviral RNAs in an avian packaging cell line. *J Virol* 1998;72(5):4057–4064.

436. Luo G, Taylor J. Template switching by reverse transcriptase during DNA synthesis. *J Virol* 1990;64:4321–4328.

437. Ly H, Nierlich DP, Olsen JC, et al. Moloney murine sarcoma virus genomic RNAs dimerize via a two-step process: a concentration-dependent kissing-loop interaction is driven by initial contact between consecutive guanines. *J Virol* 1999;73(9):7255–7261.

438. Ly H, Parslow TG. Bipartite signal for genomic RNA dimerization in Moloney murine leukemia virus. *J Virol* 2002;76(7):3135–3144.

439. Lynch WP, Brown WJ, Spangrude GJ, et al. Microglial infection by a neurovirulent murine retrovirus results in defective processing of envelope protein and intracellular budding of virus particles. *J Virol* 1994;68(5):3401–3409.

440. Ma YM, Vogt VM. Rous sarcoma virus Gag protein-oligonucleotide interaction suggests a critical role for protein dimer formation in assembly. *J Virol* 2002;76(11):5452–5462.

441. Ma YM, Vogt VM. Nucleic acid binding-induced Gag dimerization in the assembly of Rous sarcoma virus particles in vitro. *J Virol* 2004;78(1):52–60.

442. Maddon PJ, Dalgleish AG, McDougal JS, et al. The T4 gene encodes the AIDS virus receptor and is expressed in the immune system and the brain. *Cell* 1986;47:333–348.

443. Maertens G, Cherepanov P, Pluymers W, et al. LEDGF/p75 is essential for nuclear and chromosomal targeting of HIV-1 integrase in human cells. *J Biol Chem* 2003;278(35):33528–33539.

444. Maertens GN. B′-protein phosphatase 2A is a functional binding partner of delta-retroviral integrase. *Nucleic Acids Res* 2016;44(1):364–376.

445. Maertens GN, Hare S, Cherepanov P. The mechanism of retroviral integration through X-ray structures of its key intermediates. *Nature* 2010;468:326–329.

446. Mak J, Kleiman L. Primer tRNAs for reverse transcription. *J Virol* 1997;71(11):8087–8095.

447. Malashkevich VN, Chan DC, Chutkowski CT, et al. Crystal structure of the simian immunodeficiency virus (SIV) gp41 core: conserved helical interactions underlie the broad inhibitory activity of gp41 peptides. *Proc Natl Acad Sci U S A* 1998;95(16):9134–9139.

448. Maldarelli F, Wu X, Su L, et al. HIV latency. Specific HIV integration sites are linked to clonal expansion and persistence of infected cells. *Science* 2014;345(6193):179–183.

449. Mallery DL, Faysal KMR, Kleinpeter A, et al. Cellular IP6 levels limit HIV production while viruses that cannot efficiently package IP6 are attenuated for infection and replication. *Cell Rep* 2019;29(12):3983–3996 e4.

450. Mallery DL, Kleinpeter AB, Renner N, et al. A stable immature lattice packages IP6 for HIV capsid maturation. *Sci Adv* 2021;7(11):eabe4716.

451. Mammano F, Ohagen A, Hoglund S, et al. Role of the major homology region of human immunodeficiency virus type 1 in virion morphogenesis. *J Virol* 1994;68(8):4927–4936.

452. Manel N, Kim FJ, Kinet S, et al. The ubiquitous glucose transporter GLUT-1 is a receptor for HTLV. *Cell* 2003;115(4):449–459.

453. Manes S, del Real G, Lacalle RA, et al. Membrane raft microdomains mediate lateral assemblies required for HIV-1 infection. *EMBO Rep* 2000;1(2):190–196.

454. Mangeat B, Gers-Huber G, Lehmann M, et al. HIV-1 Vpu neutralizes the antiviral factor Tetherin/BST-2 by binding it and directing its beta-TrCP2-dependent degradation. *PLoS Pathog* 2009;5(9):e1000574.

455. Mangeat B, Turelli P, Caron G, et al. Broad antiretroviral defence by human APOBEC3G through lethal editing of nascent reverse transcripts. *Nature* 2003;424(6944):99–103.

456. Mann R, Baltimore D. Varying the position of a retrovirus packaging sequence results in the encapsidation of both unspliced and spliced RNAs. *J Virol* 1985;54:401–407.

457. Mann RS, Mulligan RC, Baltimore D. Construction of a retrovirus packaging mutant and its use to produce helper-free defective retrovirus. *Cell* 1983;32:871–879.

458. Mariani-Costantini R, Horn TM, Callahan R. Ancestry of a human endogenous retrovirus family. *J Virol* 1989;63:4982–4985.

459. Marshall HM, Ronen K, Berry C, et al. Role of PSIP1/LEDGF/p75 in lentiviral infectivity and integration targeting. *PLoS One* 2007;2(12):e1340.

460. Martin J, Herniou E, Cook J, et al. Human endogenous retrovirus type I-related viruses have an apparently widespread distribution within vertebrates. *J Virol* 1997;71(1):437–443.

461. Maskell DP, Renault L, Serrao E, et al. Structural basis for retroviral integration into nucleosomes. *Nature* 2015;523(7560):366–369.

462. Matreyek KA, Engelman A. The requirement for nucleoporin NUP153 during human immunodeficiency virus type 1 infection is determined by the viral capsid. *J Virol* 2011;85(15):7818–7827.

463. Matreyek KA, Yucel SS, Li X, et al. Nucleoporin NUP153 phenylalanine-glycine motifs engage a common binding pocket within the HIV-1 capsid protein to mediate lentiviral infectivity. *PLoS Pathog* 2013;9(10):e1003693.

464. Matsuoka M, Green PL. The HBZ gene, a key player in HTLV-1 pathogenesis. *Retrovirology* 2009;6:71.

465. Mattei S, Glass B, Hagen WJ, et al. The structure and flexibility of conical HIV-1 capsids determined within intact virions. *Science* 2016;354(6318):1434–1437.

466. Mazari PM, Argaw T, Valdivieso L, et al. Comparison of the convergent receptor utilization of a retargeted feline leukemia virus envelope with a naturally-occurring porcine endogenous retrovirus A. *Virology* 2012;427(2):118–126.

467. Mazari PM, Linder-Basso D, Sarangi A, et al. Single-round selection yields a unique retroviral envelope utilizing GPR172A as its host receptor. *Proc Natl Acad Sci U S A* 2009;106(14):5848–5853.

468. McCann EM, Lever AM. Location of cis-acting signals important for RNA encapsidation in the leader sequence of human immunodeficiency virus type 2. *J Virol* 1997;71(5):4133–4137.

469. McClure MA. Evolutionary history of reverse transcriptase. In: Skalka AM, Goff SP, eds. *Reverse transcriptase.* Cold Spring Harbor, NY: Cold Spring Harbor Press; 1993:425–444.

470. McClure MA, Johnson MS, Feng D-F, et al. Sequence comparisons of retroviral proteins: relative rates of change and general phylogeny. *Proc Natl Acad Sci U S A* 1988;85:2469–2473.

471. McCune JM, Rabin LB, Feinberg MB, et al. Endoproteolytic cleavage of gp160 is required for activation of human immunodeficiency virus. *Cell* 1988;53:55–67.

472. McDonald D, Vodicka MA, Lucero G, et al. Visualization of the intracellular behavior of HIV in living cells. *J Cell Biol* 2002;159(3):441–452.

473. McNally LM, McNally MT. U1 small nuclear ribonucleoprotein and splicing inhibition by the Rous sarcoma virus negative regulator of splicing element. *J Virol* 1999;73(3):2385–2393.

474. McNally MT, Beemon K. Intronic sequences and 3′ splice sites control Rous sarcoma virus RNA splicing. *J Virol* 1992;66:6–11.

475. Melamed A, Yaguchi H, Miura M, et al. The human leukemia virus HTLV-1 alters the structure and transcription of host chromatin in cis. *Elife* 2018;7:e36245.

476. Mellors JW, Guo S, Naqvi A, et al. Insertional activation of STAT3 and LCK by HIV-1 proviruses in T cell lymphomas. *Sci Adv* 2021;7(42):eabi8795.

477. Mendoza R, Anderson MM, Overbaugh J. A putative thiamine transport protein is a receptor for feline leukemia virus subgroup A. *J Virol* 2006;80(7):3378–3385.

478. Mergia A, Shaw KES, Pratt-Lowe E, et al. Identification of the simian foamy virus transcriptional transactivator gene (taf). *J Virol* 1991;65:2903–2909.

479. Meric C, Goff SP. Characterization of Moloney murine leukemia virus mutants with single-amino-acid substitutions in the cys-his box of the nucleocapsid protein. *J Virol* 1989;63:1558–1568.

480. Mertz JA, Simper MS, Lozano MM, et al. Mouse mammary tumor virus encodes a self-regulatory RNA export protein and is a complex retrovirus. *J Virol* 2005;79(23):14737–14747.

481. Metifiot M, Maddali K, Johnson BC, et al. Activities, crystal structures, and molecular dynamics of dihydro-1H-isoindole derivatives, inhibitors of HIV-1 integrase. *ACS Chem Biol* 2013;8(1):209–217.

482. Meyer PR, Matsuura SE, So AG, et al. Unblocking of chain-terminated primer by HIV-1 reverse transcriptase through a nucleotide-dependent mechanism. *Proc Natl Acad Sci U S A* 1998;95(23):13471–13476.

483. Miele G, Mouland A, Harrison GP, et al. The human immunodeficiency virus type 1 5′ packaging signal structure affects translation but does not function as an internal ribosome entry site structure. *J Virol* 1996;70(2):944–951.

484. Miller AD. Identification of Hyal2 as the cell-surface receptor for jaagsiekte sheep retrovirus and ovine nasal adenocarcinoma virus. *Curr Top Microbiol Immunol* 2003;275:179–199.

485. Miller DG, Adam MA, Miller AD. Gene transfer by retrovirus vectors occurs only in cells that are actively replicating at the time of infection. *Mol Cell Biol* 1990;10:4239–4242.

486. Miller DG, Edwards RH, Miller AD. Cloning of the cellular receptor for amphotropic murine retroviruses reveals homology to that for gibbon ape leukemia virus. *Proc Natl Acad Sci U S A* 1994;91(1):78–82.

487. Miller M, Jaskolski M, Mohana Rao JK, et al. Crystal structure of a retroviral protease proves relationship to aspartic protease family. *Nature* 1989;337:576–579.
488. Mitchell RS, Beitzel BF, Schroder AR, et al. Retroviral DNA integration: ASLV, HIV, and MLV show distinct target site preferences. *PLoS Biol* 2004;2(8):E234.
489. Miyake A, Kawasaki J, Ngo H, et al. Reduced folate carrier: an entry receptor for a novel feline leukemia virus variant. *J Virol* 2019;93(13):e00269-19.
490. Moebes A, Enssle J, Bieniasz PD, et al. Human foamy virus reverse transcription that occurs late in the viral replication cycle. *J Virol* 1997;71(10):7305–7311.
491. Monie TP, Greatorex JS, Zacharias M, et al. The human T-cell lymphotropic virus type-I dimerization initiation site forms a hairpin loop, unlike previously characterized retroviral dimerization motifs. *Biochemistry* 2004;43(20):6085–6090.
492. Morellet N, Jullian N, Derocquingny H, et al. Determination of the structure of the nucleocapsid protein NCp7 from the human immunodeficiency virus type-1 by H-1 NMR. *EMBO J* 1992;11:3059–3065.
493. Morikawa Y, Zhang WH, Hockley DJ, et al. Detection of a trimeric human immunodeficiency virus type 1 Gag intermediate is dependent on sequences in the matrix protein, p17. *J Virol* 1998;72(9):7659–7663.
494. Moriniere J, Rousseaux S, Steuerwald U, et al. Cooperative binding of two acetylation marks on a histone tail by a single bromodomain. *Nature* 2009;461(7264):664–668.
495. Morita E, Sundquist WI. Retrovirus budding. *Annu Rev Cell Dev Biol* 2004;20:395–425.
496. Morris S, Johnson M, Stavnezer E, et al. Replication of avian sarcoma virus in vivo requires an interaction between the viral RNA and the TpsiC loop of the tRNA(Trp) primer. *J Virol* 2002;76(15):7571–7577.
497. Mougel M, Zhang Y, Barklis E. cis-active structural motifs involved in specific encapsidation of Moloney murine leukemia virus RNA. *J Virol* 1996;70(8):5043–5050.
498. Mouland AJ, Mercier J, Luo M, et al. The double-stranded RNA-binding protein Staufen is incorporated in human immunodeficiency virus type 1: evidence for a role in genomic RNA encapsidation. *J Virol* 2000;74(12):5441–5451.
499. Mujeeb A, Clever JL, Billeci TM, et al. Structure of the dimer initiation complex of HIV-1 genomic RNA. *Nat Struct Biol* 1998;5(6):432–436.
500. Muller TG, Zila V, Peters K, et al. HIV-1 uncoating by release of viral cDNA from capsid-like structures in the nucleus of infected cells. *Elife* 2021;10:e64776.
501. Munk C, Brandt SM, Lucero G, et al. A dominant block to HIV-1 replication at reverse transcription in simian cells. *Proc Natl Acad Sci U S A* 2002;99(21):13843–13848.
502. Mura M, Murcia P, Caporale M, et al. Late viral interference induced by transdominant Gag of an endogenous retrovirus. *Proc Natl Acad Sci U S A* 2004;101(30):11117–11122.
503. Murakami T, Freed EO. Genetic evidence for an interaction between human immunodeficiency virus type 1 matrix and alpha-helix 2 of the gp41 cytoplasmic tail. *J Virol* 2000;74(8):3548–3554.
504. Murakami T, Freed EO. The long cytoplasmic tail of gp41 is required in a cell type-dependent manner for HIV-1 envelope glycoprotein incorporation into virions. *Proc Natl Acad Sci U S A* 2000;97(1):343–348.
505. Muriaux D, Costes S, Nagashima K, et al. Role of murine leukemia virus nucleocapsid protein in virus assembly. *J Virol* 2004;78(22):12378–12385.
506. Muriaux D, De Rocquigny H, Roques BP, et al. NCp7 activates HIV-1Lai RNA dimerization by converting a transient loop-loop complex into a stable dimer. *J Biol Chem* 1996;271(52):33686–33692.
507. Muriaux D, Mirro J, Nagashima K, et al. Murine leukemia virus nucleocapsid mutant particles lacking viral RNA encapsidate ribosomes. *J Virol* 2002;76(22):11405–11413.
508. Murphy JE, Goff SP. A mutation at one end of Moloney murine leukemia virus DNA blocks cleavage of both ends by the viral integrase in vivo. *J Virol* 1992;66:5092–5095.
509. Mustafa F, Lew KA, Schmidt RD, et al. Mutational analysis of the predicted secondary RNA structure of the Mason-Pfizer monkey virus packaging signal. *Virus Res* 2004;99(1):35–46.
510. Myers EL, Allen JF. Tsg101, an inactive homologue of ubiquitin ligase e2, interacts specifically with human immunodeficiency virus type 2 gag polyprotein and results in increased levels of ubiquitinated gag. *J Virol* 2002;76(22):11226–11235.
511. Nakajima N, Lu R, Engelman A. Human immunodeficiency virus type 1 replication in the absence of integrase-mediated DNA recombination: definition of permissive and nonpermissive T-cell lines. *J Virol* 2001;75(17):7944–7955.
512. Naldini L, Blomer U, Gage FH, et al. Efficient transfer, integration, and sustained long-term expression of the transgene in adult rat brains injected with a lentiviral vector. *Proc Natl Acad Sci U S A* 1996;93(21):11382–11388.
513. Naldini L, Blomer U, Gallay P, et al. In vivo gene delivery and stable transduction of nondividing cells by a lentiviral vector. *Science* 1996;272(5259):263–267.
514. Narayan S, Barnard RJ, Young JA. Two retroviral entry pathways distinguished by lipid raft association of the viral receptor and differences in viral infectivity. *J Virol* 2003;77(3):1977–1983.
515. Nash MA, Meyer MK, Decker GL, et al. A subset of $Pr65^{gag}$ is nucleus associated in murine leukemia virus-infected cells. *J Virol* 1993;67:1350–1356.
516. Navia MA, Fitzgerald PMD, McKeever BM, et al. Three-dimensional structure of aspartyl protease from human immunodeficiency virus HIV-1. *Nature* 1989;337:615–620.
517. Negroni M, Buc H. Recombination during reverse transcription: an evaluation of the role of the nucleocapsid protein. *J Mol Biol* 1999;286(1):15–31.
518. Neil SJ, Zang T, Bieniasz PD. Tetherin inhibits retrovirus release and is antagonized by HIV-1 Vpu. *Nature* 2008;451(7177):425–430.
519. Nermut MV, Bron P, Thomas D, et al. Molecular organization of Mason-Pfizer monkey virus capsids assembled from Gag polyprotein in *Escherichia coli*. *J Virol* 2002;76(9):4321–4330.
520. Newman EN, Holmes RK, Craig HM, et al. Antiviral function of APOBEC3G can be dissociated from cytidine deaminase activity. *Curr Biol* 2005;15(2):166–170.
521. Nguyen DG, Booth A, Gould SJ, et al. Evidence that HIV budding in primary macrophages occurs through the exosome release pathway. *J Biol Chem* 2003;278(52):52347–52354.
522. Nguyen DH, Hildreth JE. Evidence for budding of human immunodeficiency virus type 1 selectively from glycolipid-enriched membrane lipid rafts. *J Virol* 2000;74(7):3264–3272.
523. Nisole S, Lynch C, Stoye JP, et al. A Trim5-cyclophilin A fusion protein found in owl monkey kidney cells can restrict HIV-1. *Proc Natl Acad Sci U S A* 2004;101(36):13324–13328.
524. Nitta T, Kuznetsov Y, McPherson A, et al. Murine leukemia virus glycosylated Gag (gPr80gag) facilitates interferon-sensitive virus release through lipid rafts. *Proc Natl Acad Sci U S A* 2010;107(3):1190–1195.
525. Nitta T, Tam R, Kim JW, et al. The cellular protein La functions in enhancement of virus release through lipid rafts facilitated by murine leukemia virus glycosylated Gag. *MBio* 2011;2(1):e00341-10.
526. Nowrouzi A, Dittrich M, Klanke C, et al. Genome-wide mapping of foamy virus vector integrations into a human cell line. *J Gen Virol* 2006;87(Pt 5):1339–1347.
527. Nusse R. The activation of cellular oncogenes by retroviral insertion. *Trends Genet* 1986;2:244–247.
528. O'Hara B, Johann SV, Klinger HP, et al. Characterization of a human gene conferring sensitivity to infection by gibbon ape leukemia virus. *Cell Growth Differ* 1990;1:119–127.
529. Obata MM, Khan AS. Structure, distribution and expression of an ancient murine endogenous retroviruslike DNA family. *J Virol* 1988;62:4381–4386.
530. Ochsenbauer-Jambor C, Miller DC, Roberts CR, et al. Palmitoylation of the Rous sarcoma virus transmembrane glycoprotein is required for protein stability and virus infectivity. *J Virol* 2001;75(23):11544–11554.
531. Oertle S, Spahr P-F. Role of the gag polyprotein precursor in packaging and maturation of Rous sarcoma virus genomic RNA. *J Virol* 1990;64:5757–5763.
532. Ogert RA, Lee LH, Beemon KL. Avian retroviral RNA element promotes unspliced RNA accumulation in the cytoplasm. *J Virol* 1996;70(6):3834–3843.
533. Ohlmann T, Lopez-Lastra M, Darlix JL. An internal ribosome entry segment promotes translation of the simian immunodeficiency virus genomic RNA. *J Biol Chem* 2000;275(16):11899–11906.
534. Olah Z, Lehel C, Anderson WB, et al. The cellular receptor for gibbon ape leukemia virus is a novel high affinity sodium-dependent phosphate transporter. *J Biol Chem* 1994;269(41):25426–25431.
535. Oliveira NM, Farrell KB, Eiden MV. In vitro characterization of a koala retrovirus. *J Virol* 2006;80(6):3104–3107.
536. Ono A, Ablan SD, Lockett SJ, et al. Phosphatidylinositol (4,5) bisphosphate regulates HIV-1 Gag targeting to the plasma membrane. *Proc Natl Acad Sci U S A* 2004;101(41):14889–14894.
537. Ono A, Freed EO. Binding of human immunodeficiency virus type 1 Gag to membrane: role of the matrix amino terminus. *J Virol* 1999;73(5):4136–4144.
538. Ono A, Freed EO. Plasma membrane rafts play a critical role in HIV-1 assembly and release. *Proc Natl Acad Sci U S A* 2001;98(24):13925–13930.
539. Ono M, Cole MD, White AT, et al. Sequence organization of cloned intracisternal A particle genes. *Cell* 1980;21:465–473.
540. Ooms M, Huthoff H, Russell R, et al. A riboswitch regulates RNA dimerization and packaging in human immunodeficiency virus type 1 virions. *J Virol* 2004;78(19):10814–10819.
541. Orlova M, Yueh A, Leung J, et al. Reverse transcriptase of Moloney murine leukemia virus binds to eukaryotic release factor 1 to modulate suppression of translational termination. *Cell* 2003;115(3):319–331.
542. Ortiz-Conde BA, Hughes SH. Studies of the genomic RNA of leukosis viruses: implications for RNA dimerization. *J Virol* 1999;73:7165–7174.
543. Ott DE, Coren LV, Chertova EN, et al. Elimination of protease activity restores efficient virion production to a human immunodeficiency virus type 1 nucleocapsid deletion mutant. *J Virol* 2003;77(10):5547–5556.
544. Ott DE, Coren LV, Gagliardi TD, et al. Heterologous late-domain sequences have various abilities to promote budding of human immunodeficiency virus type 1. *J Virol* 2005;79(14):9038–9045.
545. Ott DE, Coren LV, Johnson DG, et al. Actin-binding cellular proteins inside human immunodeficiency virus type 1. *Virology* 2000;266(1):42–51.
546. Ott DE, Coren LV, Kane BP, et al. Cytoskeletal proteins inside human immunodeficiency virus type 1 virions. *J Virol* 1996;70(11):7734–7743.
547. Ou C-Y, Boone LR, Koh CK, et al. Nucleotide sequences of gag-pol regions that determine the *Fv-1* host range property of BALB/c N-tropic and B-tropic murine leukemia viruses. *J Virol* 1983;48:779–784.
548. Owens RJ, Compans RW. Expression of the human immunodeficiency virus envelope glycoprotein is restricted to basolateral surfaces of polarized epithelial cells. *J Virol* 1989;63:978–982.
549. Owens RJ, Dubay JW, Hunter E, et al. Human immunodeficiency virus envelope protein determines the site of virus release in polarized epithelial cells. *Proc Natl Acad Sci U S A* 1991;88:3987–3991.
550. Paillart JC, Dettenhofer M, Yu XF, et al. First snapshots of the HIV-1 RNA structure in infected cells and in virions. *J Biol Chem* 2004;279(46):48397–48403.
551. Paillart JC, Gottlinger HG. Opposing effects of human immunodeficiency virus type 1 matrix mutations support a myristyl switch model of gag membrane targeting. *J Virol* 1999;73(4):2604–2612.
552. Paillart JC, Skripkin E, Ehresmann B, et al. A loop-loop "kissing" complex is the essential part of the dimer linkage of genomic HIV-1 RNA. *Proc Natl Acad Sci U S A* 1996;93(11):5572–5577.
553. Paillart JC, Westhof E, Ehresmann C, et al. Non-canonical interactions in a kissing loop complex: the dimerization initiation site of HIV-1 genomic RNA. *J Mol Biol* 1997;270(1):36–49.
554. Palmarini M, Dewar P, De las Heras M, Inglis NF, Dalziel RG, Sharp JM. Epithelial tumour cells in the lungs of sheep with pulmonary adenomatosis are major sites of replication for Jaagsiekte retrovirus. *J Gen Virol* 1995;76(Pt 11):2731–2737.
555. Pandey KK, Bera S, Shi K, et al. Cryo-EM structure of the Rous sarcoma virus octameric cleaved synaptic complex intasome. *Commun Biol* 2021;4(1):330.
556. Panet A, Haseltine WA, Baltimore D, et al. Specific binding of tryptophan transfer RNA to avian myeloblastosis virus RNA-dependent DNA polymerase (reverse transcriptase). *Proc Natl Acad Sci U S A* 1975;72(7):2535–2539.
557. Panganiban AT. Retroviral gag gene amber codon suppression is caused by an intrinsic cis-acting component of the viral mRNA. *J Virol* 1988;62:3574–3580.
558. Panganiban AT, Temin HM. The retrovirus *pol* gene encodes a product required for DNA integration: identification of a retrovirus *int* locus. *Proc Natl Acad Sci U S A* 1984;81:7885–7889.
559. Pantginis J, Beaty RM, Levy LS, et al. The feline leukemia virus long terminal repeat contains a potent genetic determinant of T-cell lymphomagenicity. *J Virol* 1997;71(12):9786–9791.

560. Paquette Y, Hanna Z, Savard P, et al. Retrovirus-induced murine motor neuron disease: Mapping the determinant of spongiform degeneration within the envelope gene. *Proc Natl Acad Sci U S A* 1989;86:3896–3900.
561. Paquette Y, Kay DG, Rassart E, et al. Substitution of the U3 long terminal repeat region of the neurotropic Cas-Br-E retrovirus affects its disease-inducing potential. *J Virol* 1990;64:3742–3752.
562. Parent LJ. New insights into the nuclear localization of retroviral Gag proteins. *Nucleus* 2011;2(2):92–97.
563. Parent LJ, Bennett RP, Craven RC, et al. Positionally independent and exchangeable late budding functions of the Rous sarcoma virus and human immunodeficiency virus Gag proteins. *J Virol* 1995;69(9):5455–5460.
564. Parent LJ, Cairns TM, Albert JA, et al. RNA dimerization defect in a Rous sarcoma virus matrix mutant. *J Virol* 2000;74(1):164–172.
565. Park J, Morrow CD. Overexpression of the *gag-pol* precursor from human immunodeficiency virus type 1 proviral genomes results in efficient proteolytic processing in the absence of virion production. *J Virol* 1991;65:5111–5117.
566. Park J, Morrow CD. The nonmyristylated Pr160gag-pol polyprotein of human immunodeficiency virus type 1 interacts with Pr55gag and is incorporated into viruslike particles. *J Virol* 1992;66:6304–6313.
567. Passos DO, Li M, Jozwik IK, et al. Structural basis for strand-transfer inhibitor binding to HIV intasomes. *Science* 2020;367(6479):810–814.
568. Passos DO, Li M, Yang R, et al. Cryo-EM structures and atomic model of the HIV-1 strand transfer complex intasome. *Science* 2017;355(6320):89–92.
569. Patience C, Takeuchi Y, Weiss RA. Infection of human cells by an endogenous retrovirus of pigs. *Nat Med* 1997;3(3):282–286.
570. Patience C, Wilkinson DA, Weiss RA. Our retroviral heritage. *Trends Genet* 1997;13(3):116–120.
571. Payne GS, Courtneidge SA, Crittenden LB, et al. Analysis of avian leukosis virus DNA and RNA in bursal tumours: viral gene expression is not required for maintenance of the tumor state. *Cell* 1981;23(2):311–322.
572. Pelascini LP, Janssen JM, Gonçalves MA. Histone deacetylase inhibition activates transgene expression from integration-defective lentiviral vectors in dividing and non-dividing cells. *Hum Gene Ther* 2013;24(1):78–96.
573. Peliska JA, Benkovic SJ. Mechanism of DNA strand transfer reactions catalyzed by HIV-1 reverse transcriptase. *Science* 1992;258:1112–1118.
574. Perez LG, Davis GL, Hunter E. Mutants of the Rous sarcoma virus envelope glycoprotein that lack the transmembrane anchor and cytoplasmic domains: Analysis of intracellular transport and assembly into virions. *J Virol* 1987;61:2981–2988.
575. Perez LG, Hunter E. Mutations within proteolytic cleavage site of the Rous sarcoma virus glycoprotein that block processing to gp85 and gp37. *J Virol* 1987;61:1609–1614.
576. Perez-Caballero D, Zang T, Ebrahimi A, et al. Tetherin inhibits HIV-1 release by directly tethering virions to cells. *Cell* 2009;139(3):499–511.
577. Perez-Zsolt D, Cantero-Perez J, Erkizia I, et al. Dendritic Cells From the Cervical Mucosa Capture and Transfer HIV-1 via Siglec-1. *Front Immunol* 2019;10:825.
578. Perron MJ, Stremlau M, Song B, et al. TRIM5alpha mediates the postentry block to N-tropic murine leukemia viruses in human cells. *Proc Natl Acad Sci U S A* 2004;101(32):11827–11832.
579. Persons DA, Paulson RF, Loyd MR, et al. Fv2 encodes a truncated form of the Stk receptor tyrosine kinase. *Nat Genet* 1999;23(2):159–165.
580. Pertel T, Hausmann S, Morger D, et al. TRIM5 is an innate immune sensor for the retrovirus capsid lattice. *Nature* 2011;472(7343):361–365.
581. Peters GG, Hu J. Reverse transcriptase as the major determinant for selective packaging of tRNA's into avian sarcoma virus particles. *J Virol* 1980;36:692–700.
582. Petersen R, Kempler G, Barklis E. A stem-cell specific silencer in the primer-binding site of a retrovirus. *Mol Cell Biol* 1991;11:1214–1221.
583. Petit C, Giron ML, Tobaly-Tapiero J, et al. Targeting of incoming retroviral Gag to the centrosome involves a direct interaction with the dynein light chain 8. *J Cell Sci* 2003;116(Pt 16):3433–3442.
584. Piguet V, Gu F, Foti M, et al. Nef-induced CD4 degradation: a diacidic-based motif in Nef functions as a lysosomal targeting signal through the binding of beta-COP in endosomes. *Cell* 1999;97(1):63–73.
585. Pillemer EA, Kooistra DA, Witte ON, et al. Monoclonal antibody to the amino-terminal L sequence of murine leukemia virus glycosylated gag poly proteins demonstrates their unusual orientation in the cell membrane. *J Virol* 1986 57:413–421.
586. Pincus T, Hartley JW, Rowe WP. A major genetic locus affecting resistance to infection with murine leukemia viruses. IV. Dose–response relationships in *Fv-1* sensitive and resistant cell cultures. *Virology* 1975;65:333–342.
587. Pinter A, Honnen WJ. O-linked glycosylation of retroviral envelope gene products. *J Virol* 1988;62:1016–1021.
588. Pizzato M. MLV glycosylated-Gag is an infectivity factor that rescues Nef-deficient HIV-1. *Proc Natl Acad Sci U S A* 2010;107(20):9364–9369.
589. Poeschla EM, Wong-Staal F, Looney DJ. Efficient transduction of nondividing human cells by feline immunodeficiency virus lentiviral vectors. *Nat Med* 1998;4(3):354–357.
590. Polge E, Darlix JL, Paoletti J, et al. Characterization of loose and tight dimer forms of avian leukosis virus RNA. *J Mol Biol* 2000;300(1):41–56.
591. Pollard VW, Malim MH. The HIV-1 Rev protein. *Annu Rev Microbiol* 1998;52:491–532.
592. Pollom E, Dang KK, Potter EL, et al. Comparison of SIV and HIV-1 genomic RNA structures reveals impact of sequence evolution on conserved and non-conserved structural motifs. *PLoS Pathog* 2013;9(4):e1003294.
593. Poon B, Chang MA, Chen IS. Vpr is required for efficient Nef expression from unintegrated human immunodeficiency virus type 1 DNA. *J Virol* 2007;81(19):10515–10523.
594. Poon B, Chen IS. Human immunodeficiency virus type 1 (HIV-1) Vpr enhances expression from unintegrated HIV-1 DNA. *J Virol* 2003;77(7):3962–3972.
595. Poon DT, Chertova EN, Ott DE. Human immunodeficiency virus type 1 preferentially encapsidates genomic RNAs that encode Pr55(Gag): functional linkage between translation and RNA packaging. *Virology* 2002;293(2):368–378.
596. Popik W, Alce TM, Au WC. Human immunodeficiency virus type 1 uses lipid raft-colocalized CD4 and chemokine receptors for productive entry into CD4(+) T cells. *J Virol* 2002;76(10):4709–4722.
597. Pornillos O, Ganser-Pornillos BK, Kelly BN, et al. X-ray structures of the hexameric building block of the HIV capsid. *Cell* 2009;137(7):1282–1292.
598. Pornillos O, Ganser-Pornillos BK, Yeager M. Atomic-level modelling of the HIV capsid. *Nature* 2011;469(7330):424–427.
599. Portis JL, Lynch WP. Dissecting the determinants of neuropathogenesis of the murine oncornaviruses. *Virology* 1998;247(2):127–136.
600. Prassolov V, Hein S, Ziegler M, et al. Mus cervicolor murine leukemia virus isolate M813 belongs to a unique receptor interference group. *J Virol* 2001;75(10):4490–4498.
601. Prizan-Ravid A, Elis E, Laham-Karam N, et al. The Gag cleavage product, p12, is a functional constituent of the murine leukemia virus pre-integration complex. *PLoS Pathog* 2010;6(11):e1001183.
602. Provitera P, Goff A, Harenberg A, et al. Role of the major homology region in assembly of HIV-1 Gag. *Biochemistry* 2001;40(18):5565–5572.
603. Pryciak PM, Varmus HE. Fv-1 restriction and its effects on murine leukemia virus integration in vivo and in vitro. *J Virol* 1992;66:5959–5966.
604. Pucillo CE, Palmer LD, Hodes RJ. Superantigenic characteristics of mouse mammary tumor viruses play a critical role in susceptibility to infection in mice. *Immunol Res* 1995;14(1):58–68.
605. Qin W, Golovkina TV, Peng T, et al. Mammary gland expression of mouse mammary tumor virus is regulated by a novel element in the long terminal repeat. *J Virol* 1999;73(1):368–376.
606. Quigley JG, Burns CC, Anderson MM, et al. Cloning of the cellular receptor for feline leukemia virus subgroup C (FeLV-C), a retrovirus that induces red cell aplasia. *Blood* 2000;95:1093–1099.
607. Quigley JG, Yang Z, Worthington MT, et al. Identification of a human heme exporter that is essential for erythropoiesis. *Cell* 2004;118(6):757–766.
608. Quinn TP, Grandgenett DP. Genetic evidence that the avian retrovirus DNA endonuclease domain of pol is necessary for viral integration. *J Virol* 1988;62:2307–2312.
609. Rai SK, Duh FM, Vigdorovich V, et al. Candidate tumor suppressor HYAL2 is a glycosylphosphatidylinositol (GPI)-anchored cell-surface receptor for jaagsiekte sheep retrovirus, the envelope protein of which mediates oncogenic transformation. *Proc Natl Acad Sci U S A* 2001;98(8):4443–4448.
610. Rainey GJ, Coffin JM. Evolution of broad host range in retroviruses leads to cell death mediated by highly cytopathic variants. *J Virol* 2006;80(2):562–570.
611. Rantalainen K, Berndsen ZT, Antanasijevic A, et al. HIV-1 envelope and MPER antibody structures in lipid assemblies. *Cell Rep* 2020;31(4):107583.
612. Rao Z, Belyaev AS, Fry E, et al. Crystal structure of SIV matrix antigen and implications for virus assembly. *Nature* 1995;378(6558):743–747.
613. Rasko JE, Battini JL, Gottschalk RJ, et al. The RD114/simian type D retrovirus receptor is a neutral amino acid transporter. *Proc Natl Acad Sci U S A* 1999;96(5):2129–2134.
614. Rein A, Kashmiri SV, Bassin RH, et al. Phenotypic mixing between N- and B-tropic murine leukemia viruses: infectious particles with dual sensitivity to Fv-1 restriction. *Cell* 1976;7(3):373–379.
615. Rein A, McClure MR, Rice NR, et al. Myristylation site in Pr65gag is essential for virus particle formation by Moloney murine leukemia virus. *Proc Natl Acad Sci U S A* 1986;83:7246–7250.
616. Rein A, Mirro J, Haynes JG, et al. Function of the cytoplasmic domain of a retroviral transmembrane protein: p15E-p2E cleavage activates the membrane fusion capability of the murine leukemia virus Env protein. *J Virol* 1994;68(3):1773–1781.
617. Rein A, Yang C, Haynes JA, et al. Evidence for cooperation between murine leukemia virus Env molecules in mixed oligomers. *J Virol* 1998;72(4):3432–3435.
618. Remy E, de Rocquigny H, Petitjean P, et al. The annealing of tRNA3Lys to human immunodeficiency virus type 1 primer binding site is critically dependent on the NCp7 zinc fingers structure. *J Biol Chem* 1998;273(9):4819–4822.
619. Renner N, Mallery DL, Faysal KMR, et al. A lysine ring in HIV capsid pores coordinates IP6 to drive mature capsid assembly. *PLoS Pathog* 2021;17(2):e1009164.
620. Resnick-Roguel N, Burstein H, Hamburger J, et al. Cytocidal effect caused by the envelope glycoprotein of a newly isolated avian hemangioma-inducing retrovirus. *J Virol* 1989;63:4325–4330.
621. Rey O, Canon J, Krogstad P. HIV-1 Gag protein associates with F-actin present in microfilaments. *Virology* 1996;220(2):530–534.
622. Rhee SS, Hui H, Hunter E. Preassembled capsids of type D retroviruses contain a signal sufficient for targeting specifically to the plasma membrane. *J Virol* 1990;64:3844–3852.
623. Rhee SS, Huner E. Myristylation is required for intracellular transport but not for assembly of D-type retrovirus capsids. *J Virol* 1987;61:1045–1053.
624. Rhee SS, Hunter E. A single amino acid substitution within the matrix protein of a type D retrovirus converts its morphogenesis to that of a type C retrovirus. *Cell* 1990;63:77–86.
625. Rhim H, Park J, Morrow CD. Deletions in the tRNALys primer-binding site of human immunodeficiency virus type 1 identify essential regions for reverse transcription. *J Virol* 1991;65:4555–4564.
626. Rhodes T, Wargo H, Hu WS. High rates of human immunodeficiency virus type 1 recombination: near-random segregation of markers one kilobase apart in one round of viral replication. *J Virol* 2003;77(20):11193–11200.
627. Ribet D, Harper F, Esnault C, et al. The GLN family of murine endogenous retroviruses contains an element competent for infectious viral particle formation. *J Virol* 2008;82(9):4413–4419.
628. Rice WG, Schaeffer CA, Harten B, et al. Inhibition of HIV-1 infectivity by zinc-ejecting aromatic C-nitroso compounds. *Nature* 1993;361:473–475.
629. Rist MJ, Marino JP. Mechanism of nucleocapsid protein catalyzed structural isomerization of the dimerization initiation site of HIV-1. *Biochemistry* 2002;41(50):14762–14770.
630. Rizzuto CD, Wyatt R, Hernandez-Ramos N, et al. A conserved HIV gp120 glycoprotein structure involved in chemokine receptor binding. *Science* 1998;280(5371):1949–1953.

631. Robinson HL, Astrin SM, Senior AM, et al. Host Susceptibility to endogenous viruses: defective, glycoprotein-expressing proviruses interfere with infections. *J Virol* 1981;40(3):745–751.
632. Rodgers DW, Gamblin SJ, Harris BA, et al. The structure of unliganded reverse transcriptase from the human immunodeficiency virus type 1. *Proc Natl Acad Sci U S A* 1995;92(4):1222–1226.
633. Roe T, Chow SA, Brown PO. 3′-end processing and kinetics of 5′-end joining during retroviral integration in vivo. *J Virol* 1997;71(2):1334–1340.
634. Roe T, Reynolds TC, Yu G, et al. Integration of murine leukemia virus DNA depends on mitosis. *EMBO J* 1993;12(5):2099–2108.
635. Roganowicz MD, Komurlu S, Mukherjee S, et al. TRIM5alpha SPRY/coiled-coil interactions optimize avid retroviral capsid recognition. *PLoS Pathog* 2017;13(10):e1006686.
636. Rommelaere J, Donis-Keller H, Hopkins N. RNA sequencing provides evidence for allelism of determinants of the N-, B-, or NB-tropism of murine leukemia viruses. *Cell* 1979;16:43–50.
637. Rong L, Liang C, Hsu M, et al. Roles of the human immunodeficiency virus type 1 nucleocapsid protein in annealing and initiation versus elongation in reverse transcription of viral negative-strand strong-stop DNA. *J Virol* 1998;72(11):9353–9358.
638. Ross SR, Schofield JJ, Farr CJ, et al. Mouse transferrin receptor 1 is the cell entry receptor for mouse mammary tumor virus. *Proc Natl Acad Sci U S A* 2002;99(19):12386–12390.
639. Roth MJ, Schwartzberg PL, Goff SP. Structure of the termini of DNA intermediates in the integration of retroviral DNA: dependence on IN function and terminal DNA sequence. *Cell* 1989;58:47–54.
640. Rousso I, Mixon MB, Chen BK, et al. Palmitoylation of the HIV-1 envelope glycoprotein is critical for viral infectivity. *Proc Natl Acad Sci U S A* 2000;97(25):13523–13525.
641. Rumlova-Klikova M, Hunter E, Nermut MV, et al. Analysis of Mason-Pfizer monkey virus Gag domains required for capsid assembly in bacteria: role of the N-terminal proline residue of CA in directing particle shape. *J Virol* 2000;74(18):8452–8459.
642. Russell RA, Wiegand HL, Moore MD, et al. Foamy virus Bet proteins function as novel inhibitors of the APOBEC3 family of innate antiretroviral defense factors. *J Virol* 2005;79(14):8724–8731.
643. Ryden TA, Beemon K. Avian retroviral long terminal repeats bind CCAAT/enhancer-binding protein. *Mol Cell Biol* 1989;9:1155–1164.
644. Saib A, Puvion-Dutilleul F, Schmid M, et al. Nuclear targeting of incoming human foamy virus Gag proteins involves a centriolar step. *J Virol* 1997;71(2):1155–1161.
645. Sakai H, Kawamura M, Sakuragi J, et al. Integration is essential for efficient gene expression of human immunodeficiency virus type 1. *J Virol* 1993;67:1169–1174.
646. Sakalian M, Hunter E. Molecular events in the assembly of retrovirus particles. *Adv Exp Med Biol* 1998;440:329–339.
647. Sakalian M, Parker SD, Weldon RA Jr, et al. Synthesis and assembly of retrovirus Gag precursors into immature capsids in vitro. *J Virol* 1996;70(6):3706–3715.
648. Salie ZL, Kirby KA, Michailidis E, et al. Structural basis of HIV inhibition by translocation-defective RT inhibitor 4′-ethynyl-2-fluoro-2′-deoxyadenosine (EFdA). *Proc Natl Acad Sci U S A* 2016;113(33):9274–9279.
649. Sanchez JG, Sparrer KMJ, Chiang C, et al. TRIM25 binds RNA to modulate cellular antiviral defense. *J Mol Biol* 2018;430(24):5280–5293.
650. Satou Y, Miyazato P, Ishihara K, et al. The retrovirus HTLV-1 inserts an ectopic CTCF-binding site into the human genome. *Proc Natl Acad Sci U S A* 2016;113(11):3054–3059.
651. Sauter D, Kirchhoff F. Tetherin antagonism by primate lentiviral nef proteins. *Curr HIV Res* 2011;9(7):514–523.
652. Sayah DM, Sokolskaja E, Berthoux L, et al. Cyclophilin A retrotransposition into TRIM5 explains owl monkey resistance to HIV-1. *Nature* 2004;430(6999):569–573.
653. Scheifele LZ, Garbitt RA, Rhoads JD, et al. Nuclear entry and CRM1-dependent nuclear export of the Rous sarcoma virus Gag polyprotein. *Proc Natl Acad Sci U S A* 2002;99(6):3944–3949.
654. Scheifele LZ, Rhoads JD, Parent LJ. Specificity of plasma membrane targeting by the Rous sarcoma virus gag protein. *J Virol* 2003;77(1):470–480.
655. Schneider WM, Brzezinski JD, Aiyer S, et al. Viral DNA tethering domains complement replication-defective mutations in the p12 protein of MuLV Gag. *Proc Natl Acad Sci U S A* 2013;110(23):9487–9492.
656. Schneider WM, Wu DT, Amin V, et al. MuLV IN mutants responsive to HDAC inhibitors enhance transcription from unintegrated retroviral DNA. *Virology* 2012;426(2):188–196.
657. Schroder AR, Shinn P, Chen H, et al. HIV-1 integration in the human genome favors active genes and local hotspots. *Cell* 2002;110(4):521–529.
658. Schrofelbauer B, Hakata Y, Landau NR. HIV-1 Vpr function is mediated by interaction with the damage-specific DNA-binding protein DDB1. *Proc Natl Acad Sci U S A* 2007;104(10):4130–4135.
659. Schrofelbauer B, Yu Q, Zeitlin SG, et al. Human immunodeficiency virus type 1 Vpr induces the degradation of the UNG and SMUG uracil-DNA glycosylases. *J Virol* 2005;79(17):10978–10987.
660. Schubert U, Anton LC, Bacik I, et al. CD4 glycoprotein degradation induced by human immunodeficiency virus type 1 Vpu protein requires the function of proteasomes and the ubiquitin-conjugating pathway. *J Virol* 1998;72(3):2280–2288.
661. Schultz AM, Rein A. Unmyristylated Moloney murine leukemia virus Pr65gag is excluded from virus assembly and maturation events. *J Virol* 1989;63:2370–2372.
662. Schwartz JR, Duesberg S, Duesberg PH. DNA recombination is sufficient for retroviral transduction. *Proc Natl Acad Sci U S A* 1995;92(7):2460–2464.
663. Schwartzberg P, Colicelli J, Goff SP. Deletion mutants of Moloney murine leukemia virus which lack glycosylated gag protein are replication competent. *J Virol* 1983;46(2):538–546.
664. Schwartzberg P, Colicelli J, Goff SP. Construction and analysis of deletion mutations in the pol gene of Moloney murine leukemia virus: a new viral function required for productive infection. *Cell* 1984;37:1043–1052.
665. Schwartzberg P, Colicelli J, Gordon ML, et al. Mutations in the gag gene of Moloney murine leukemia virus: effects on production of virions and reverse transcriptase. *J Virol* 1984;49:918–924.
666. Sebastian S, Luban J. TRIM5alpha selectively binds a restriction-sensitive retroviral capsid. *Retrovirology* 2005;2:40.
667. Selig L, Pages JC, Tanchou V, et al. Interaction with the p6 domain of the gag precursor mediates incorporation into virions of Vpr and Vpx proteins from primate lentiviruses. *J Virol* 1999;73(1):592–600.
668. Selyutina A, Persaud M, Lee K, et al. Nuclear import of the HIV-1 core precedes reverse transcription and uncoating. *Cell Rep* 2020;32(13):108201.
669. Sewald X, Gonzalez DG, Haberman AM, et al. In vivo imaging of virological synapses. *Nat Commun* 2012;3:1320.
670. Sewald X, Ladinsky MS, Uchil PD, et al. Retroviruses use CD169-mediated trans-infection of permissive lymphocytes to establish infection. *Science* 2015;350(6260):563–567.
671. Sewald X, Motamedi N, Mothes W. Viruses exploit the tissue physiology of the host to spread in vivo. *Curr Opin Cell Biol* 2016;41:81–90.
672. Sfakianos JN, Hunter E. M-PMV capsid transport is mediated by Env/Gag interactions at the pericentriolar recycling endosome. *Traffic* 2003;4(10):671–680.
673. Sfakianos JN, LaCasse RA, Hunter E. The M-PMV cytoplasmic targeting-retention signal directs nascent Gag polypeptides to a pericentriolar region of the cell. *Traffic* 2003;4(10):660–670.
674. Sharma A, Larue RC, Plumb MR, et al. BET proteins promote efficient murine leukemia virus integration at transcription start sites. *Proc Natl Acad Sci U S A* 2013;110(29):12036–12041.
675. Sharp PA, Marciniak RA. HIV TAR: an RNA enhancer? *Cell* 1989;59:229–230.
676. Sheehy AM, Gaddis NC, Choi JD, et al. Isolation of a human gene that inhibits HIV-1 infection and is suppressed by the viral Vif protein. *Nature* 2002;418(6898):646–650.
677. Shehu-Xhilaga M, Hill M, Marshall JA, et al. The conformation of the mature dimeric human immunodeficiency virus type 1 RNA genome requires packaging of pol protein. *J Virol* 2002;76(9):4331–4340.
678. Shimojima M, Miyazawa T, Ikeda Y, et al. Use of CD134 as a primary receptor by the feline immunodeficiency virus. *Science* 2004;303(5661):1192–1195.
679. Shoemaker CS, Goff S, Gilboa E, et al. Structure of a cloned circular Moloney murine leukemia virus molecule containing an inverted segment: implications for retrovirus integration. *Proc Natl Acad Sci U S A* 1980;77:3932–3936.
680. Shojima T, Yoshikawa R, Hoshino S, et al. Identification of a novel subgroup of Koala retrovirus from Koalas in Japanese zoos. *J Virol* 2013;87(17):9943–9948.
681. Shun MC, Raghavendra NK, Vandegraaff N, et al. LEDGF/p75 functions downstream from preintegration complex formation to effect gene-specific HIV-1 integration. *Genes Dev* 2007;21(14):1767–1778.
682. Simmons G, Reeves JD, McKnight A, et al. CXCR4 as a functional coreceptor for human immunodeficiency virus type 1 infection of primary macrophages. *J Virol* 1998;72(10):8453–8457.
683. Singh K, Sarafianos SG, Sonnerborg A. Long-acting anti-HIV drugs targeting HIV-1 reverse transcriptase and integrase. *Pharmaceuticals (Basel)* 2019;12(2):62.
684. Singh PK, Plumb MR, Ferris AL, et al. LEDGF/p75 interacts with mRNA splicing factors and targets HIV-1 integration to highly spliced genes. *Genes Dev* 2015;29(21):2287–2297.
685. Sitbon Marc (FR), Petit Vincent (FR), Ivanova Svilena (CH), Battini Jean-Luc (FR), Courgnaud Valérie (FR), Giovannini Donatella (FR), Lezaar Jawida (FR). *Use of Ligands Derived from Receptor-Binding Domain of Porcine Endogenous Retrovirus Type B for Diagnosing SMVT-Related Diseases.* Metafora Biosystems (FR), Centre Nat Rech Scient (FR), Univ Montpellier (FR), Univ Paris Descartes Paris V (FR). WO/2020/070330. https://www.freepatentsonline.com/WO2020070330.html.
686. Skalka AM, Goff SP, eds. *Reverse Transcriptase.* Cold Spring Harbor, NY: Cold Spring Harbor Press; 1993.
687. Smith AJ, Srinivasakumar N, Hammarskjold M-L, et al. Requirements for incorporation of Pr160[gag-pol] from human immunodeficiency virus type 1 into virus-like particles. *J Virol* 1993;67:2266–2275.
688. Smith EJ, Brojatsch J, Naughton J, et al. The CAR1 gene encoding a cellular receptor specific for subgroup B and D avian leukosis viruses maps to the chicken tvb locus. *J Virol* 1998;72(4):3501–3503.
689. Smith JS, Kim S, Roth MJ. Analysis of long terminal repeat circle junctions of human immunodeficiency virus type 1. *J Virol* 1990;64:6286–6290.
690. Smith LM, Toye AA, Howes K, et al. Novel endogenous retroviral sequences in the chicken genome closely related to HPRS-103 (subgroup J) avian leukosis virus. *J Gen Virol* 1999;80(Pt 1):261–268.
691. Smith MR, Smith RE, Dunkel I, et al. Genetic determinant of rapid-onset B-cell lymphoma by avian leukosis virus. *J Virol* 1997;71(9):6534–6540.
692. Smith SJ, Zhao XZ, Passos DO, et al. Integrase strand transfer inhibitors are effective anti-HIV drugs. *Viruses* 2021;13(2):205.
693. Somasundaran M, Robinson HL. Unexpectedly high levels of HIV-1 RNA and protein synthesis in a cytocidal infection. *Science* 1988;242:1554–1557.
694. Sood C, Marin M, Chande A, et al. SERINC5 protein inhibits HIV-1 fusion pore formation by promoting functional inactivation of envelope glycoproteins. *J Biol Chem* 2017;292(14):6014–6026.
695. Sowd GA, Aiken C. Inositol phosphates promote HIV-1 assembly and maturation to facilitate viral spread in human CD4+ T cells. *PLoS Pathog* 2021;17(1):e1009190.
696. Sowd GA, Serrao E, Wang H, et al. A critical role for alternative polyadenylation factor CPSF6 in targeting HIV-1 integration to transcriptionally active chromatin. *Proc Natl Acad Sci U S A* 2016;113(8):E1054–E1063.
697. Spearman P, Horton R, Ratner L, et al. Membrane binding of human immunodeficiency virus type 1 matrix protein in vivo supports a conformational myristyl switch mechanism. *J Virol* 1997;71(9):6582–6592.
698. Speck NA, Baltimore D. Six distinct nuclear factors interact with the 75-base-pair repeat of the Moloney murine leukemia virus enhancer. *Mol Cell Biol* 1987;7:1101–1110.
699. Stevens A, Bock M, Ellis S, et al. Retroviral capsid determinants of Fv1 NB and NR tropism. *J Virol* 2004;78(18):9592–9598.
700. Stoltzfus CM, Fogarty CJ. Multiple regions in the Rous sarcoma virus src gene intron act in cis to affect the accumulation of unspliced RNA. *J Virol* 1989;63:1669–1676.

701. Storch TG, Arnstein GP, Manohar V, et al. Proliferation of infected lymphoid precursors before Moloney murine leukemia virus-induced T-cell lymphoma. *J Natl Cancer Inst* 1985;74:137–143.
702. Stoye JP, Coffin JM. Endogenous viruses. In: Weiss R, Teich N, Varmus H, et al., eds. *RNA Tumor Viruses.* Vol 2/supplements and appendixes. Cold Spring Harbor, NY: Cold Spring Harbor Laboratory; 1985:357–404.
703. Stoye JP, Coffin JM. The four classes of endogenous murine leukemia virus: Structural relationships and potential for recombination. *J Virol* 1987;61:2659–2669.
704. Strambio-de-Castilla C, Hunter E. Mutational analysis of the major homology region of Mason-Pfizer monkey virus by use of saturation mutagenesis. *J Virol* 1992;66:7021–7032.
705. Stremlau M, Owens CM, Perron MJ, et al. The cytoplasmic body component TRIM5alpha restricts HIV-1 infection in Old World monkeys. *Nature* 2004;427(6977):848–853.
706. Stuchell MD, Garrus JE, Muller B, et al. The human endosomal sorting complex required for transport (ESCRT-I) and its role in HIV-1 budding. *J Biol Chem* 2004;279(34):36059–36071.
707. Stuhlmann H, Berg P. Homologous recombination of copackaged retrovirus RNAs during reverse transcription. *J Virol* 1992;66:2378–2388.
708. Sugimoto J, Sugimoto M, Bernstein H, et al. A novel human endogenous retroviral protein inhibits cell-cell fusion. *Sci Rep* 2013;3:1462.
709. Suzuki S. *Fv-4,* a new gene affecting the splenomegaly induction by Friend leukemia virus. *J Exp Med* 1975;45:473–478.
710. Suzuki S, Axelrad AA. Fv-2 locus controls the proportion of erythropoietic progenitor cells (BFU-E) synthesizing DNA in normal mice. *Cell* 1980;19(1):225–236.
711. Suzuki T, Ikeda H. The mouse homolog of the bovine leukemia virus receptor is closely related to the delta subunit of adaptor-related protein complex AP-3, not associated with the cell surface. *J Virol* 1998;72(1):593–599.
712. Swain A, Coffin JM. Polyadenylation at correct sites in genome RNA is not required for retrovirus replication or genome encapsidation. *J Virol* 1989;63:3301–3306.
713. Swain A, Coffin JM. Mechanism of transduction by retroviruses. *Science* 1992;255:841–845.
714. Swanstrom R, Wills JW. Synthesis, assembly, and processing of viral proteins. In: Coffin JM, Hughes SH, Varmus HE, eds. *Retroviruses.* Cold Spring Harbor, NY: Cold Spring Harbor Press; 1997:263–334.
715. Swindells S, Andrade-Villanueva JF, Richmond GJ, et al. Long-Acting Cabotegravir and Rilpivirine for Maintenance of HIV-1 Suppression. *N Engl J Med* 2020;382(12):1112–1123.
716. Tachedjian G, Orlova M, Sarafianos SG, et al. Nonnucleoside reverse transcriptase inhibitors are chemical enhancers of dimerization of the HIV type 1 reverse transcriptase. *Proc Natl Acad Sci U S A* 2001;98(13):7188–7193.
717. Tailor CS, Lavillette D, Marin M, et al. Cell surface receptors for gammaretroviruses. *Curr Top Microbiol Immunol* 2003;281:29–106.
718. Tailor CS, Nouri A, Lee CG, et al. Cloning and characterization of a cell surface receptor for xenotropic and polytropic murine leukemia viruses. *Proc Natl Acad Sci U S A* 1999;96(3):927–932.
719. Tailor CS, Nouri A, Zhao Y, et al. A sodium-dependent neutral-amino-acid transporter mediates infections of feline and baboon endogenous retroviruses and simian type D retroviruses. *J Virol* 1999;73(5):4470–4474.
720. Takahashi K, Baba S, Koyanagi Y, et al. Two basic regions of NCp7 are sufficient for conformational conversion of HIV-1 dimerization initiation site from kissing-loop dimer to extended-duplex dimer. *J Biol Chem* 2001;276(33):31274–31278.
721. Takata MA, Goncalves-Carneiro D, Zang TM, et al. CG dinucleotide suppression enables antiviral defence targeting non-self RNA. *Nature* 2017;550(7674):124–127.
722. Takeuchi Y, Patience C, Magre S, et al. Host range and interference studies of three classes of pig endogenous retrovirus. *J Virol* 1998;72(12):9986–9991.
723. Tanchou V, Decimo D, Pechoux C, et al. Role of the N-terminal zinc finger of human immunodeficiency virus type 1 nucleocapsid protein in virus structure and replication. *J Virol* 1998;72(5):4442–4447.
724. Tanese N, Goff SP. Domain structure of the Moloney murine leukemia virus reverse transcriptase: Mutational analysis and separate expression of the DNA polymerase and RNase H activities. *Proc Natl Acad Sci U S A* 1988;85:1777–1781.
725. Tanese N, Roth MJ, Goff SP. Analysis of retroviral pol gene products with antisera raised against fusion proteins produced in *Escherichia coli. J Virol* 1986;59(2):328–340.
726. Tantillo C, Ding J, Jacobo-Molina A, et al. Locations of anti-AIDS drug binding sites and resistance mutations in the three-dimensional structure of HIV-1 reverse transcriptase. Implications for mechanisms of drug inhibition and resistance. *J Mol Biol* 1994;243(3):369–387.
727. Tanzi GO, Piefer AJ, Bates P. Equine infectious anemia virus utilizes host vesicular protein sorting machinery during particle release. *J Virol* 2003;77(15):8440–8447.
728. Taylor GM, Gao Y, Sanders DA. Fv-4: identification of the defect in Env and the mechanism of resistance to ecotropic murine leukemia virus. *J Virol* 2001;75(22):11244–11248.
729. Telesnitsky A, Goff SP. Reverse transcription and the generation of retroviral DNA. In: Coffin JM, Hughes SH, Varmus HE, eds. *Retroviruses.* Cold Spring Harbor, NY: Cold Spring Harbor Press; 1997:121–160.
730. Temin HM. Reverse transcription in the eukaryotic genome: Retroviruses, pararetroviruses, retro transposons, and retrotranscripts. *Mol Biol Evol* 1985;6:455–468.
731. Temin HM, Zhang J. 3′ junctions of oncogene-virus sequences and the mechanisms for formation of highly oncogenic retroviruses. *J Virol* 1993;67:1747–1751.
732. Thali M, Bukovsky A, Kondo E, et al. Functional association of cyclophilin A with HIV-1 virions. *Nature* 1994;372(6504):363–365.
733. Timilsina U, Umthong S, Lynch B, et al. SERINC5 potently restricts retrovirus infection in vivo. *mBio* 2020;11(4):e00588-20.
734. Topping R, Demoitie MA, Shin NH, et al. Cis-acting elements required for strong stop acceptor template selection during Moloney murine leukemia virus reverse transcription. *J Mol Biol* 1998;281(1):1–15.
735. Towers G, Bock M, Martin S, et al. A conserved mechanism of retrovirus restriction in mammals. *Proc Natl Acad Sci U S A* 2000;97(22):12295–12299.
736. Towers GJ, Hatziioannou T, Cowan S, et al. Cyclophilin A modulates the sensitivity of HIV-1 to host restriction factors. *Nat Med* 2003;9(9):1138–1143.
737. Tran T, Liu Y, Marchant J, et al. Conserved determinants of lentiviral genome dimerization. *Retrovirology* 2015;12:83.
738. Trobridge GD, Miller DG, Jacobs MA, et al. Foamy virus vector integration sites in normal human cells. *Proc Natl Acad Sci U S A* 2006;103(5):1498–1503.
739. Tsukiyama T, Niwa O, Yokoro K. Characterization of the negative regulatory element of the 5′ noncoding region of Moloney murine leukemia virus in mouse embryonal carcinoma cells. *Virology* 1990;177:772–776.
740. Tu X, Das K, Han Q, et al. Structural basis of HIV-1 resistance to AZT by excision. *Nat Struct Mol Biol* 2010;17(10):1202–1209.
741. Tucker SP, Srinivas RV, Compans RW. Molecular domains involved in oligomerization of the Friend murine leukemia virus envelope glycoprotein. *Virology* 1991;185:710–720.
742. Tucker TJ, Lumma WC, Culberson JC. Development of nonnucleoside HIV reverse transcriptase inhibitors. *Methods Enzymol* 1996;275:440–472.
743. Tummino PJ, Scholten JD, Harvey PJ, et al. The in vitro ejection of zinc from human immunodeficiency virus (HIV) type 1 nucleocapsid protein by disulfide benzamides with cellular anti- HIV activity. *Proc Natl Acad Sci U S A* 1996;93(3):969–973.
744. Turelli P, Guiguen F, Mornex JF, et al. dUTPase-minus caprine arthritis-encephalitis virus is attenuated for pathogenesis and accumulates G-to-A substitutions. *J Virol* 1997;71(6):4522–4530.
745. Uchil PD, Pi R, Haugh KA, et al. A protective role for the lectin CD169/Siglec-1 against a pathogenic murine retrovirus. *Cell Host Microbe* 2019;25(1):87–100 e10.
746. Urbaneja MA, Kane BP, Johnson DG, et al. Binding properties of the human immunodeficiency virus type 1 nucleocapsid protein p7 to a model RNA: elucidation of the structural determinants for function. *J Mol Biol* 1999;287(1):59–75.
747. Vajdos FF, Yoo S, Houseweart M, et al. Crystal structure of cyclophilin A complexed with a binding site peptide from the HIV-1 capsid protein. *Protein Sci* 1997;6(11):2297–2307.
748. van Lohulzen M, Verbeek S, Scheijen B, et al. Identification of cooperating oncogenes in Em-myc transgenic mice by provirus tagging. *Cell* 1991;65:737–752.
749. van Zeijl M, Johann SV, Closs E, et al. A human amphotropic retrovirus receptor is a second member of the gibbon ape leukemia virus receptor family. *Proc Natl Acad Sci U S A* 1994;91(3):1168–1172.
750. Varmus HE, Guntaka RV, Fan WJ, et al. Synthesis of viral DNA in the cytoplasm of duck embryo fibroblasts and in enucleated cells after infection by avian sarcoma virus. *Proc Natl Acad Sci U S A* 1974;71(10):3874–3878.
751. Varmus HE, Padgett T, Heasley S, et al. Cellular functions are required for the synthesis and integration of avian sarcoma virus-specific DNA. *Cell* 1977;11(2):307–319.
752. Varmus HE, Quintrell NE, Ortiz S. Retroviruses as mutagens: insertion and excision of a non-transforming provirus alters expression of a resident transforming provirus. *Cell* 1981;25:23–26.
753. Versteegen RJ, Copeland TD, Oroszlan S. Complete amino acid sequence of the group-specific antigen gene-encoded phosphorylated proteins of mouse leukemia viruses. *J Biol Chem* 1982;257(6):3007–3013.
754. Vink C, van Gent DC, Elgersma Y, et al. Human immunodeficiency virus integrase protein requires a subterminal position of its viral DNA recognition sequence for efficient cleavage. *J Virol* 1991;65:4636–4644.
755. Virgen CA, Kratovac Z, Bieniasz PD, et al. Independent genesis of chimeric TRIM5-cyclophilin proteins in two primate species. *Proc Natl Acad Sci U S A* 2008;105(9):3563–3568.
756. Vogt VM. Proteolytic processing and particle maturation. *Curr Top Microbiol Immunol* 1996;214:95–131.
757. von Schwedler UK, Stuchell M, Muller B, et al. The protein network of HIV budding. *Cell* 2003;114(6):701–713.
758. Vora AC, Chiu R, McCord M, et al. Avian retrovirus U3 and U5 DNA inverted repeats. Role of nonsymmetrical nucleotides in promoting full-site integration by purified virion and bacterial recombinant integrases. *J Biol Chem* 1997;272(38):23938–23945.
759. Vora AC, Grandgenett DP. Assembly and catalytic properties of retrovirus integrase-DNA complexes capable of efficiently performing concerted integration. *J Virol* 1995;69(12):7483–7488.
760. Wagner JM, Christensen DE, Bhattacharya A, et al. General model for retroviral capsid pattern recognition by TRIM5 proteins. *J Virol* 2018;92(4):e01563-17.
761. Wallin M, Ekstrom M, Garoff H. Isomerization of the intersubunit disulphide-bond in Env controls retrovirus fusion. *EMBO J* 2004;23(1):54–65.
762. Wanaguru M, Barry DJ, Benton DJ, et al. Murine leukemia virus p12 tethers the capsid-containing pre-integration complex to chromatin by binding directly to host nucleosomes in mitosis. *PLoS Pathog* 2018;14(6):e1007117.
763. Wang CT, Lai HY, Li JJ. Analysis of minimal human immunodeficiency virus type 1 gag coding sequences capable of virus-like particle assembly and release. *J Virol* 1998;72(10):7950–7959.
764. Wang GZ, Wang Y, Goff SP. Histones are rapidly loaded onto unintegrated retroviral DNAs soon after nuclear entry. *Cell Host Microbe* 2016;20(6):798–809.
765. Wang MQ, Kim W, Gao G, et al. Endophilins interact with Moloney murine leukemia virus Gag and modulate virion production. *J Biol* 2003;3(1):4.
766. Wang X, Xuan Y, Han Y, et al. Regulation of HIV-1 Gag-Pol expression by shiftless, an inhibitor of programmed-1 ribosomal frameshifting. *Cell* 2019;176(3):625–635 e14.
767. Ward AB, Wilson IA. The HIV-1 envelope glycoprotein structure: nailing down a moving target. *Immunol Rev* 2017;275(1):21–32.
768. Ward AE, Kiessling V, Pornillos O, et al. HIV-cell membrane fusion intermediates are restricted by Serincs as revealed by cryo-electron and TIRF microscopy. *J Biol Chem* 2020;295(45):15183–15195.
769. Weber IT, Miller M, Jaskolski M, et al. Molecular modeling of the HIV-1 protease and its substrate binding site. *Science* 1989;243:928–931.
770. Wei SQ, Mizuuchi K, Craigie R. A large nucleoprotein assembly at the ends of the viral DNA mediates retroviral DNA integration. *EMBO J* 1997;16(24):7511–7520.
771. Wei SQ, Mizuuchi K, Craigie R. Footprints on the viral DNA ends in Moloney murine leukemia virus preintegration complexes reflect a specific association with integrase. *Proc Natl Acad Sci U S A* 1998;95(18):10535–10540.
772. Weinberg JB, Matthews TJ, Cullen BR, et al. Productive human immunodeficiency virus type 1 (HIV-1) infection of nonproliferating human monocytes. *J Exp Med* 1991;174(6):1477–1482.

773. Weiss RA, Tailor CS. Retrovirus receptors. *Cell* 1995;82(4):531–533.

774. Weissenhorn W, Dessen A, Harrison SC, et al. Atomic structure of the ectodomain from HIV-1 gp41. *Nature* 1997;387(6631):426–430.

775. Weller SK, Temin HM. Cell killing by avian leukosis viruses. *J Virol* 1981;39:713–721.

776. Whitcomb JM, Kumar R, Hughes SH. Sequence of the circle junction of human immunodeficiency virus type 1: implications for reverse transcription and integration. *J Virol* 1990;64:4903–4906.

777. Whitcomb JM, Ortiz-Conde BA, Hughes SH. Replication of avian leukosis viruses with mutations at the primer binding site: use of alternative tRNAs as primers. *J Virol* 1995;69(10):6228–6238.

778. Wight DJ, Boucherit VC, Nader M, et al. The gammaretroviral p12 protein has multiple domains that function during the early stages of replication. *Retrovirology* 2012;9:83.

779. Wight DJ, Boucherit VC, Wanaguru M, et al. The N-terminus of murine leukaemia virus p12 protein is required for mature core stability. *PLoS Pathog* 2014;10(10):e1004474.

780. Wilk T, Gowen B, Fuller SD. Actin associates with the nucleocapsid domain of the human immunodeficiency virus Gag polyprotein. *J Virol* 1999;73(3):1931–1940.

781. Wilk T, Gross I, Gowen BE, et al. Organization of immature human immunodeficiency virus type 1. *J Virol* 2001;75(2):759–771.

782. Willetts KE, Rey F, Agostini I, et al. DNA repair enzyme uracil DNA glycosylase is specifically incorporated into human immunodeficiency virus type 1 viral particles through a Vpr-independent mechanism. *J Virol* 1999;73(2):1682–1688.

783. Wills JW, Cameron CE, Wilson CB, et al. An assembly domain of the Rous sarcoma virus Gag protein required late in budding. *J Virol* 1994;68(10):6605–6618.

784. Wills JW, Craven RC. Form, function and use of retroviral gag proteins. *AIDS* 1991;5:639–654.

785. Wills JW, Craven RC, Achacoso JA. Creation and expression of myristylated forms of Rous sarcoma virus gag protein in mammalian cells. *J Virol* 1989;63:4331–4343.

786. Wilson CA, Eiden MV, Anderson WB, et al. The dual-function hamster receptor for amphotropic murine leukemia virus (MuLV), 10A1 MuLV, and gibbon ape leukemia virus is a phosphate symporter. *J Virol* 1995;69(1):534–537.

787. Wilson CA, Wong S, Muller J, et al. Type C retrovirus released from porcine primary peripheral blood mononuclear cells infects human cells. *J Virol* 1998;72(4):3082–3087.

788. Winans S, Beemon K. m(5)C goes viral. *Cell Host Microbe* 2019;26(2):154–155.

789. Winans S, Larue RC, Abraham CM, et al. The FACT complex promotes avian leukosis virus DNA integration. *J Virol* 2017;91(7):e00082-17.

790. Windbichler N, Werner M, Schroeder R. Kissing complex-mediated dimerisation of HIV-1 RNA: coupling extended duplex formation to ribozyme cleavage. *Nucleic Acids Res* 2003;31(22):6419–6427.

791. Wolf D, Goff SP. TRIM28 mediates primer binding site-targeted silencing of murine leukemia virus in embryonic cells. *Cell* 2007;131(1):46–57.

792. Wolf D, Goff SP. Embryonic stem cells use ZFP809 to silence retroviral DNAs. *Nature* 2009;458(7242):1201–1204.

793. Wolff L, Ruscetti S. The spleen focus-forming virus (SFFV) envelope gene, when introduced into mice in the absence of other SFFV genes, induces acute erythroleukemia. *J Virol* 1988;62:2158–2163.

794. Wong PKY, Knupp C, Yuen PH, et al. ts1, a paralytogenic mutant of Moloney murine leukemia virus TB, has an enhanced ability to replicate in the central nervous system and primary nerve cell culture. *J Virol* 1985;55:760–767.

795. Wu X, Anderson JL, Campbell EM, et al. Proteasome inhibitors uncouple rhesus TRIM5alpha restriction of HIV-1 reverse transcription and infection. *Proc Natl Acad Sci U S A* 2006;103(19):7465–7470.

796. Wu X, Li Y, Crise B, et al. Transcription start regions in the human genome are favored targets for MLV integration. *Science* 2003;300(5626):1749–1751.

797. Wu X, Li Y, Crise B, et al. Weak palindromic consensus sequences are a common feature found at the integration target sites of many retroviruses. *J Virol* 2005;79(8):5211–5214.

798. Wyma DJ, Kotov A, Aiken C. Evidence for a stable interaction of gp41 with Pr55(Gag) in immature human immunodeficiency virus type 1 particles. *J Virol* 2000;74(20):9381–9387.

799. Xavier Ruiz F, Arnold E. Evolving understanding of HIV-1 reverse transcriptase structure, function, inhibition, and resistance. *Curr Opin Struct Biol* 2020;61:113–123.

800. Xiang Y, Cameron CE, Wills JW, et al. Fine mapping and characterization of the Rous sarcoma virus Pr76gag late assembly domain. *J Virol* 1996;70(8):5695–5700.

801. Xu W, Gorman K, Santiago JC, et al. Genetic diversity of koala retroviral envelopes. *Viruses* 2015;7(3):1258–1270.

802. Xu W, Stadler CK, Gorman K, et al. An exogenous retrovirus isolated from koalas with malignant neoplasias in a US zoo. *Proc Natl Acad Sci U S A* 2013;110(28):11547–11552.

803. Yamashita M, Emerman M. Capsid is a dominant determinant of retrovirus infectivity in nondividing cells. *J Virol* 2004;78(11):5670–5678.

804. Yan Y, Liu Q, Wollenberg K, et al. Evolution of functional and sequence variants of the mammalian XPR1 receptor for mouse xenotropic gammaretroviruses and the human-derived retrovirus XMRV. *J Virol* 2010;84(22):11970–11980.

805. Yang C, Compans RW. Analysis of the murine leukemia virus R peptide: delineation of the molecular determinants which are important for its fusion inhibition activity. *J Virol* 1997;71(11):8490–8496.

806. Yang WK, Kiggins JO, Yang DM, et al. Synthesis and circularization of N- and B-tropic retroviral DNA in Fv-1 permissive and restrictive mouse cells. *Proc Natl Acad Sci U S A* 1980;77:2994–2998.

807. Yang YL, Guo L, Xu S, et al. Receptors for polytropic and xenotropic mouse leukaemia viruses encoded by a single gene at Rmc1. *Nat Genet* 1999;21(2):216–219.

808. Yin Z, Shi K, Banerjee S, et al. Crystal structure of the Rous sarcoma virus intasome. *Nature* 2016;530(7590):362–366.

809. Yoshida Y, Honma M, Kimura Y, et al. Structure, synthesis and inhibition mechanism of nucleoside analogues as HIV-1 reverse transcriptase inhibitors (NRTIs). *ChemMedChem* 2021;16(5):743–766.

810. Yoshinaka Y, Katoh I, Copeland TD, et al. Murine leukemia virus protease is encoded by the gag-pol gene and is synthesized through suppression of an amber termination codon. *Proc Natl Acad Sci U S A* 1985;82:1618–1622.

811. Young JAT, Bates P, Varmus HE. Isolation of a chicken gene that confers susceptibility to infection by subgroup A avian leukosis and sarcoma viruses. *J Virol* 1993;67:1811–1816.

812. Yu A, Skorupka KA, Pak AJ, et al. TRIM5alpha self-assembly and compartmentalization of the HIV-1 viral capsid. *Nat Commun* 2020;11(1):1307.

813. Yu E, Fabris D. Direct probing of RNA structures and RNA-protein interactions in the HIV-1 packaging signal by chemical modification and electrospray ionization Fourier transform mass spectrometry. *J Mol Biol* 2003;330(2):211–223.

814. Yu Q, Morrow CD. Complementarity between 3′ terminal nucleotides of tRNA and primer binding site is a major determinant for selection of the tRNA primer used for initiation of HIV-1 reverse transcription. *Virology* 1999;254(1):160–168.

815. Yu SF, Sullivan MD, Linial ML. Evidence that the human foamy virus genome is DNA. *J Virol* 1999;73(2):1565–1572.

816. Yu SF, von Ruden T, Kantoff PW, et al. Self-inactivating retroviral vectors designed for transfer of whole genes into mammalian cells. *Proc Natl Acad Sci U S A* 1986;83(10):3194–3198.

817. Yu X, Yuan X, McLane MF, et al. Mutations in the cytoplasmic domain of human immunodeficiency virus type 1 transmembrane protein impair the incorporation of env proteins into mature virions. *J Virol* 1993;67:213–221.

818. Yuan B, Campbell S, Bacharach E, et al. Infectivity of Moloney murine leukemia virus defective in late assembly events is restored by late assembly domains of other retroviruses. *J Virol* 2000;74(16):7250–7260.

819. Yuan B, Li X, Goff SP. Mutations altering the Moloney murine leukemia virus p12 Gag protein affect virion production and early events of the virus life cycle. *EMBO J* 1999;18(4700–4710).

820. Yueh A, Goff SP. Phosphorylated serine residues and an arginine-rich domain of the Moloney murine leukemia virus p12 protein are required for early events of viral infection. *J Virol* 2003;77(3):1820–1829.

821. Yung E, Sorin M, Pal A, et al. Inhibition of HIV-1 virion production by a transdominant mutant of integrase interactor 1. *Nat Med* 2001;7(8):920–926.

822. Zaitseva L, Cherepanov P, Leyens L, et al. HIV-1 exploits importin 7 to maximize nuclear import of its DNA genome. *Retrovirology* 2009;6:11.

823. Zaitseva L, Myers R, Fassati A. tRNAs promote nuclear import of HIV-1 intracellular reverse transcription complexes. *PLoS Biol* 2006;4(10):e332.

824. Zeffman A, Hassard S, Varani G, et al. The major HIV-1 packaging signal is an extended bulged stem loop whose structure is altered on interaction with the Gag polyprotein. *J Mol Biol* 2000;297(4):877–893.

825. Zeng L, Zhou MM. Bromodomain: an acetyl-lysine binding domain. *FEBS Lett* 2002;513(1):124–128.

826. Zhang F, Bieniasz PD. HIV-1 Vpr induces cell cycle arrest and enhances viral gene expression by depleting CCDC137. *Elife* 2020;9:e55806.

827. Zhang F, Landford WN, Ng M, et al. SIV Nef proteins recruit the AP-2 complex to antagonize Tetherin and facilitate virion release. *PLoS Pathog* 2011;7(5):e1002039.

828. Zhang F, Wilson SJ, Landford WC, et al. Nef proteins from simian immunodeficiency viruses are tetherin antagonists. *Cell Host Microbe* 2009;6(1):54–67.

829. Zhang H, Yang B, Pomerantz RJ, et al. The cytidine deaminase CEM15 induces hypermutation in newly synthesized HIV-1 DNA. *Nature* 2003;424(6944):94–98.

830. Zhang J, Tang LY, Li T, et al. Most retroviral recombinations occur during minus-strand DNA synthesis. *J Virol* 2000;74(5):2313–2322.

831. Zhang J, Temin HM. Rate and mechanism of nonhomologous recombination during a single cycle of retroviral replication. *Science* 1993;259:234–238.

832. Zhang QY, Clausen PA, Yatsula BA, et al. Mutation of polyadenylation signals generates murine retroviruses that produce fused virus-cell RNA transcripts at high frequency. *Virology* 1998;241(1):80–93.

833. Zhang Y, Qian H, Love Z, et al. Analysis of the assembly function of the human immunodeficiency virus type 1 gag protein nucleocapsid domain. *J Virol* 1998;72(3):1782–1789.

834. Zheng X, Wang X, Tu F, et al. TRIM25 is required for the antiviral activity of zinc finger antiviral protein. *J Virol* 2017;91(9):e00088-17.

835. Zhong Z, Ning J, Boggs EA, et al. Cytoplasmic CPSF6 regulates HIV-1 capsid trafficking and infection in a cyclophilin A-dependent manner. *mBio* 2021;12(2):e03142-20.

836. Zhou W, Resh MD. Differential membrane binding of the human immunodeficiency virus type 1 matrix protein. *J Virol* 1996;70(12):8540–8548.

837. Zhu P, Liu J, Bess J Jr, et al. Distribution and three-dimensional structure of AIDS virus envelope spikes. *Nature* 2006;441(7095):847–852.

838. Zhu Y, Wang GZ, Cingoz O, et al. NP220 mediates silencing of unintegrated retroviral DNA. *Nature* 2018;564(7735):278–282.

839. Zielske SP, Stevenson M. Importin 7 may be dispensable for human immunodeficiency virus type 1 and simian immunodeficiency virus infection of primary macrophages. *J Virol* 2005;79(17):11541–11546.

840. Zila V, Margiotta E, Turonova B, et al. Cone-shaped HIV-1 capsids are transported through intact nuclear pores. *Cell* 2021;184(4):1032–1046 e18.

841. Zingler K, Littmann DR. Truncation of the cytoplasmic domain of the simian immunodeficiency virus envelope glycoprotein increases env incorporation into particles and fusogenicity and infectivity. *J Virol* 1993;67:2824–2831.

842. Zolotukhin AS, Michalowski D, Bear J, et al. PSF acts through the human immunodeficiency virus type 1 mRNA instability elements to regulate virus expression. *Mol Cell Biol* 2003;23(18):6618–6630.

Human T-Cell Leukemia Virus Types 1 and 2

Charles R. M. Bangham • Masao Matsuoka

History
    Discovery of ATL
    Discovery of HTLV 1
    History of HAM
HTLV-1: the virus
    Genetic structure; main features and functions of Gag, Pol, Env
    Sequence variation and evolution
    Tax and Rex: main physiological actions
    HBZ: physiological actions
    Accessory genes
    Genomic instability in ATL cells
Pathogenesis and persistence *in vivo*
    Entry into cells and host
    Cell and tissue tropism
    Integration and clonality
    Site of replication and spread
    Proviral load: correlation with disease
    Immune response
    Within-host evolution: selection *in vivo*
    Pathogenesis of ATL
    Pathogenesis of inflammatory diseases
Epidemiology
    Age
    Morbidity/Mortality
    Origin and spread of epidemics
    Prevalence and seroepidemiology
    Genetic diversity of HTLV-1
Clinical features
    ATL
    HTLV-1–associated myelopathy/tropical spastic paraparesis
        (HAM/TSP)
    HTLV-1 uveitis
    Infective dermatitis
Prevention and treatment
    Prevention
    Treatment
    Vaccines

HISTORY

Discovery of ATL

In the 1970s, T cells and B cells were identified as distinct subsets of lymphocytes. While the frequency of B-cell lymphoid malignancies was higher than that of T-cell malignancies in western countries, T-cell neoplasms were frequently observed in Japan. Based on this finding and the distinct clinical features, the disease entity of adult T-cell leukemia–lymphoma (ATL) was described in Japan.[376] ATL is characterized by several clinical features, including skin lesions, hypercalcemia, the presence of leukemic cells with multilobulated nuclei, and an aggressive clinical course.[354] Patients with ATL were clustered in a limited area of southern Japan including the islands of Kyushu and Okinawa, an observation that suggested a pathogen(s) as a causative agent.[376]

Discovery of HTLV-1

The discovery of oncogenic retroviruses in animals led to a search for retroviruses in human cancer cells. In 1980, the first human retrovirus was found in a T-cell line established from a patient who had a diagnosis of mycosis fungoides, and the retrovirus was named human T-cell leukemia virus (HTLV).[298,349] In 1981, it was reported that ATL patients had antibodies that reacted with ATL cell lines,[125] suggesting that ATL was associated with a new antigen, possibly derived from an unknown virus. Thereafter, it became evident that the sequence of the provirus in ATL cells was almost identical to that of HTLV. The clinical features of ATL resemble those of mycosis fungoides. Therefore, the patient from whom the HTLV-infected cell line was established might have been misdiagnosed. The diagnosis should probably have been ATL.

History of HAM

In 1984, the disease known as tropical spastic paraparesis (TSP), formerly called Jamaican neuropathy,[251] was found to be associated with HTLV-1,[88] and the same disease was reported in Japan as HTLV-1–associated myelopathy (HAM).[284] Occasional cases have been reported of a similar condition in HTLV-1–seronegative individuals, but the association with HTLV-1 is secure, and the condition, formerly designated HAM/TSP, is now generally known as HAM. Other inflammatory diseases were also found to be linked with this virus, including HTLV-1–associated uveitis, myositis, alveolitis, and infective dermatitis.[197,249,252,266,343]

HTLV-2 was discovered in a cell line that was established from a patient with T-cell variant hairy cell leukemia.[316] Thereafter, infection with this virus was found in the native Amerindian population of North, Central, and South America, people in Central and West Africa, and drug abusers in the United States and Europe.[73] HTLV-2 has been reported to cause a neurodegenerative disease resembling HAM/TSP.[132] However, no definite associations with lymphoproliferative diseases have been reported.

In addition to HTLV-1 and -2, HTLV-3 and -4 were isolated from bushmeat hunters in Cameroon.[398] Since the numbers of HTLV-3 or -4 infected individuals are limited, their pathological roles in human diseases remain unknown.

HTLV-1: THE VIRUS

Genetic Structure; Main Features and Functions of Gag, Pol, Env

HTLV is a delta-type retrovirus, and an HTLV virion contains two copies of single-stranded genomic RNA. Upon viral entry into a host cell, the viral RNA is reverse transcribed (using the proline transfer-RNA as a primer), and the viral genome becomes integrated into the host cellular DNA as a provirus. The genetic structure of the provirus is shown in Figure 16.1.

Most HTLV-1–infected cells contain a single copy of the provirus.[53] The provirus encodes the structural (Gag, Env), enzymatic (protease, reverse transcriptase, integrase), nonstructural regulatory (Tax, Rex), and accessory proteins (p12, p30, p13, HBZ) (Fig. 16.1).[319] Of these proteins, only HBZ is encoded by the minus strand of the HTLV-1 provirus.[83] In addition to genomic unspliced mRNA, HTLV-1 expresses multiple other mRNAs by differential splicing (Figs. 16.1 and 16.2).[320] After infection of host cells, the initial dominant mRNA is the default doubly spliced *tax/rex* mRNA encoding the x-III and the x-IV ORF. Since the protein product Tax is a transcriptional activator of HTLV-1 transcription, Tax further amplifies the HTLV-1 transcripts, especially *tax/rex* mRNA, and their protein products. Once the other product, Rex, accumulates in a sufficient amount, it inhibits the nuclear export of *tax/rex* mRNA, instead increasing the export of singly spliced *env* mRNA and unspliced genomic RNA encoding *gag/pro-pol* (Fig. 16.2), resulting in formation of viral particles. Thus, Tax and Rex are essential for efficient HTLV-1 replication and production.

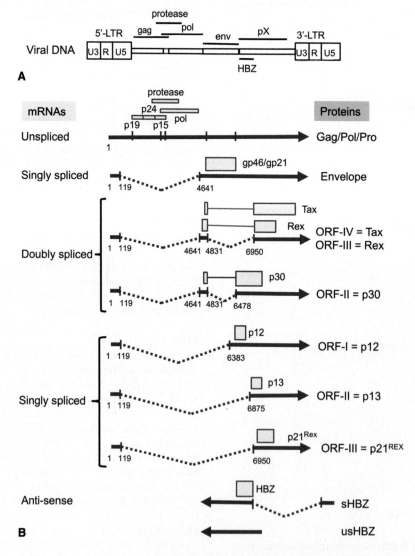

FIGURE 16.1 HTLV-1 genome organization, transcripts, and products.
A: Schematic organization of HTLV-1 proviral DNA. **B:** Structure, splicing, and orientation of HTLV-1 transcripts and their corresponding products.

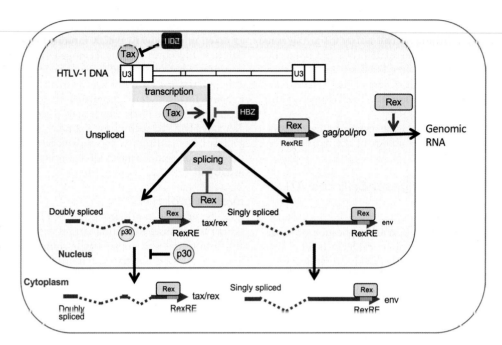

FIGURE 16.2 Flowchart of HTLV-1 gene regulation. HTLV-1 encodes three major transcripts: an unspliced genomic one, a singly spliced one, and a doubly spliced one, and these encode the Gag/Pro/Pol, Env, and Tax/Rex proteins, respectively. After initial infection, HTLV-1 dominantly expresses the default doubly spliced *tax/rex* transcript. Tax further augments viral transcription through the HTLV-1 long terminal repeat (LTR) promoter, and this activity is negatively regulated by HBZ. Upon accumulation of Rex, Rex inhibits the splicing of transcripts, thereby increasing the amounts of unspliced and singly spliced transcripts and their products (Gag, Pro, Pol, Env), resulting in HTLV-1 production. p30 inhibits the nuclear export of *tax/rex* transcripts to repress HTLV-1 gene expression. RxRE, Rex-response element.

Roles of Viral Genes in Viral Replication and Proliferation of Infected Cells

HTLV-1 transmits only through cell-to-cell contact: transmission needs living infected cells, and free virus shows poor infectivity.[237] Therefore, the virus increases the number of infected cells *in vivo*, which facilitates viral transmission.[21] This virus spreads *in vivo* by two different routes: (a) *de novo* replication and (b) mitotic division of infected cells. During the chronic stage of infection, mitotic division is predominant, since reverse transcriptase inhibitors (RTIs) and integrase inhibitors do not significantly alter the number of infected cells (proviral load [PVL]) *in vivo*.[200,362,373] *De novo* infection depends on proviral plus-strand transcription (leading to expression of *gag*, *pol*, *env*, *tax* and *rex*), which is undetectable in the majority of circulating HTLV-1–infected cells at a given time. Thus, the pattern of viral gene transcription differs between the plus strand and minus strands, and their respective products have different roles in viral spreading. Plus-strand transcription is essential for *de novo* infection, whereas minus-strand transcription (leading to expression of the *HBZ* gene) is critical for the sustained preferential proliferation of infected cells (mitotic division).

Sequence Variation and Evolution

Causes of Sequence Variation

The chief cause of sequence variation in HTLV-1 is point mutation resulting from nucleotide misincorporation by the error-prone viral reverse transcriptase (RT). Like other RNA-dependent polymerases, HTLV-1 RT introduces frequent mutations: about 7×10^{-6} mutations per base pair per replication cycle.[231] G to A mutations introduced by the cytidine deaminase enzyme APOBEC3G are also observed, with a higher frequency in ATL clones, but the impact of APOBEC3G on HTLV-1 is limited by a C-terminal peptide motif in the nucleocapsid domain of HTLV-1 Gag, which inhibits APOBEC3G incorporation into virions.[61] Rare instances of recombination in HTLV-1 have also been reported.[62]

As in other retroviruses, RT also makes frequent insertions and deletions, and abortive transcripts are common. Defective (incomplete) proviruses lack either an internal region (type 1 defective) or the 5′ LTR and part of the 5′ end of the provirus (type 2 defective).[358] The proportion of defective proviruses is about 20% in nonmalignant HTLV-1 infection,[172] considerably lower than in HIV infection (>90%).

Extent of Sequence Variation

There is detectable within-host sequence variation, resulting partly from immune-mediated selection.[271] However, because HTLV-1 persists during chronic infection mainly through sustained replication of long-lived infected T-cell clones,[200,394] RT contributes little to viral replication, and the extent of sequence variation, both within one host and at the population level, is consequently very small compared with HIV-1. In ATL, mutations that silence the Tax protein are observed in approximately 50% of cases, and type 2 proviruses are found in approximately 30%.[172]

Significance of Sequence Variation

No single sequence is specifically associated with the manifestations of HTLV-1 infection: an identical sequence may result in either asymptomatic carriage, inflammatory disease, or ATL,[55,189,285] although there is a small difference in the risk of HAM associated with two different HTLV-1 genotypes in southern Japan.[80] Mutations that alter T-cell epitopes[271] or that result in the loss of Tax expression or loss of the 5′ LTR may confer a selective advantage on the infected T cell clone and can contribute to oncogenesis in ATL.[2,172,246,334]

Sequence variation in HTLV-1 has been of great importance in understanding the epidemiology of the virus[2,334]; see "Epidemiology."

HTLV-1 Provirus in Nonmalignant Cells and ATL Cells

After infection, the HTLV-1 provirus exists in the cellular genome and causes clonal proliferation and replication of virus. Since the HTLV-1 provirus is the direct evidence of HTLV-1 infection in the cells, analyses of HTLV-1 proviruses provide important information on the pathogenesis of HTLV-1. HTLV-1 proviruses in ATL cases are divided into three subtypes: (a) complete, (b) type 1 defective, and (c) type 2 defective.[358] Type 1 defective provirus retains the 5′ and 3′ LTRs but lacks internal sequences including *gag*, *pol*, and *env*. Type 2 defective provirus lacks the 5′ LTR and part of the internal region of the provirus. Importantly, approximately half of type 2 defective proviruses have a six-bp repeat at both ends. This short repeat is generated during integration of the viral DNA into the genome: its presence in such cases, therefore, indicates that this defective provirus is generated before proviral integration.[246] This type of defective provirus is also present in HTLV-1 carriers.[172,246] Since the 5′ LTR is the promoter/enhancer for plus-strand transcription of the provirus, this type of provirus lacks expression of viral genes encoded by the plus strand, including the *tax* gene.

APOBEC3G (A3G) is antiretroviral factor, which changes cytosine to uracil of single-stranded DNA by deamination during reverse transcription. A3G causes G-to-A mutations in the plus strand of the provirus, resulting in generation of nonsense mutations in the provirus. HTLV-1 proviruses in ATL cases frequently contain nonsense mutations, which correspond to target sequences of A3G.[70] A hot-spot of nonsense mutation is observed in the *tax* gene. Approximately 10% of ATL cases have a nonsense mutation in the *tax* gene.[79,356] Furthermore, this nonsense mutation of the *tax* gene is also observed in some HTLV-1–infected cells in asymptomatic carriers.[70] These findings indicate that HTLV-1–infected cells containing the *tax* gene with nonsense mutation transform to ATL cells.

DNA methylation of the HTLV-1 provirus silences transcription of viral genes. In particular, DNA methylation is detected in the 5′ LTR, whereas the 3′ LTR is not methylated in ATL cells.[188] DNA methylation first occurs in the *gag*, *pol*, and *env* regions and then extends in the 5′ and 3′ directions *in vivo*, and when the 5′ LTR becomes methylated, viral transcription is silenced.[360] Heavy DNA methylation of the 5′ LTR silences transcription of plus-strand genes. In contrast, the 3′ LTR is not methylated, which is constant with continuous expression of the *HBZ* gene.

Tax expression is disrupted approximately in half of ATL cases by any of three mechanisms: (a) deletion of 5′ LTR, (b) nonsense mutation of the *tax* gene, and (c) DNA methylation of 5′ LTR.[356] Importantly, about 25% of ATL cases do not

express Tax at the stage of infection, due to nonsense mutation or deletion of 5′ LTR, which indicates that Tax is not essential for HTLV-1–induced leukemogenesis.[274] The *tax* gene transcription is barely detected in the remaining half of ATL cases, although the 5′ LTR is not heavily methylated and the *tax* gene remains intact.[221] It is speculated that Tax is intermittently expressed in these cases, which may, therefore, depend on both Tax and HBZ. In such cases, Tax may contribute to leukemogenesis by impairing the DNA damage response pathway and the repair of double-strand DNA breaks, resulting in genomic instability.[224,425]

Evolution of HTLV-1

Like the other human retroviruses, HTLV-1 had its origins in simian retroviruses in nonhuman primates[190,387] and was probably introduced into humans by bushmeat hunting and animal bites.[74,175] At least 4 interspecies transmission events are thought to have occurred,[2] although the host nonhuman primate species has not always been clearly identified. HTLV-2 is similarly derived from closely related simian T-cell leukemia viruses (STLVs) in West Africa.[388]

HTLV-1 is thought to have been endemic in humans for tens of thousands of years.[2,334,387] The most divergent sequences of HTLV-1 are found in Papua New Guinea and Melanesia[91] and Australia[41]: since there are no native nonhuman primates in Australia, it is assumed that the virus was introduced by the humans who arrived on the continent between 10,000 and 60,000 years ago. The rate of evolution of HTLV-1 is significantly slower than that of other RNA viruses such as influenza A virus.[137,347] The rate of evolution is constrained by the mode of within-host persistence by clonal proliferation and by the presence of overlapping reading frames in the provirus; it is also likely that there is strong selection during transmission between individuals, that is, a transmission bottleneck.

A key target of the host immune response to HTLV-1 is HBZ protein (see "Cell-mediated immune response"). *HBZ* is expressed by a nonmalignant infected T cell approximately 50% of the time,[243] and an effective host CTL response to HBZ is associated with a lower PVL and a lower risk of HAM. Consequently, HTLV-1 has evolved to minimize its exposure to CTL surveillance by restricting *HBZ* expression to a minimal level—typically 1 to 5 mRNA copies per *HBZ*-expressing cell,[32] and by limiting the export of *HBZ* mRNA to the cytoplasm.[299] As a result, HBZ protein is expressed at a very low level. The low affinity of HBZ peptides for binding to HLA class 1 proteins[215] also limits the effectiveness of the CTL response.

Tax and Rex: Main Physiological Actions

Most T-cell lines immortalized *in vitro* by HTLV-1 express high levels of Tax.[216] However, the *tax* transcript is barely detected *in vivo*,[356] indicating that T-cell lines with higher Tax expression do not reflect the physiological pattern of Tax expression. By contrast, several ATL cell lines derived from ATL patients (e.g., MT-1, KK-1), and HTLV-1–infected T-cell lines established from HTLV-1 carriers and HAM/TSP patients, express Tax sparsely.[221] Furthermore, some ATL cell lines derived from primary ATL cells do not express Tax.[356] Single-cell analyses showed that, at any given time, only a small number of T cells express *tax* and other viral genes encoded on the proviral plus strand,[32,221] which likely corresponds with the *in vivo* expression pattern of the *tax* gene.

Tax

Tax is a protein of 353 amino acids, localized in both the nucleus and cytoplasm.[97] The main functions of Tax are (a) trans-activation of plus-strand transcription of viral genes and (b) modulation of cell signaling pathways through its interaction with host factors.

Tax activates plus-strand transcription of the HTLV-1 provirus

Like the majority of mammalian genes, the HTLV-1 proviral plus strand is not continuously expressed but rather is expressed in intermittent, self-limiting bursts.[32,221] The plus-strand bursts are infrequent, in contrast with the minus-strand (*HBZ*) bursts: the great majority of HTLV-1–infected cells freshly isolated from peripheral blood are *tax*-negative at a given instant, whereas approximately 50% express *HBZ* at a low level.[243] Because of the positive feedback exerted by the Tax protein, the plus-strand burst is intense, producing several hundred transcripts within approximately 3 hours.[243] The burst is regulated like a cellular immediate-early stress-response gene (such as *c-fos*): it is triggered by cellular stress, depends on p38-MAPK, and is not inhibited by protein synthesis inhibitors.[194] The promoter/enhancer in the 5′ LTR is maintained in a poised state by ubiquitylation of histone H2A at lysine 119 by polycomb repressive complex 1 (PRC1); the onset of the plus-strand burst is accompanied by loss of this inhibitory epigenetic mark.[194]

The duration of the plus-strand burst in fresh PBMCs is approximately 6 to 10 hours[243]; it is likely to be similar *in vivo*, but direct evidence is lacking. A major factor responsible for terminating the burst is the action of Rex protein on mRNA splicing and transport; it is not known whether additional factors contribute to the active termination of the burst.

Molecular mechanism of Tax-mediated transcriptional activation

Tax activates HTLV-1 transcription through the long terminal repeat (LTR)[71,278,322,323,335] (Fig. 16.2). The HTLV-1 LTR is divided into three regions: U3, R, and U5. Three repetitive 21-bp sequences in the U3 region act as Tax-responsive enhancers (TREs).[326] Each 21-bp TRE is in turn composed of three elements: the core element and two elements that lie, respectively, 5′ and 3′ to the core element, all three elements are indispensable for efficient Tax activation of HTLV-1 transcription. The core sequence of a TRE is highly similar to a cyclic AMP response element (CRE) and indeed acts as a binding site for the CRE-binding protein/activating transcription factor (ATF) family of transcription factors (CREB/ATFs).[29,415,421,422] Thus, the TRE is also called a viral cAMP response element (vCRE) and is responsive to cAMP. The 5′ and 3′ elements within a TRE are GC-rich. While Tax itself does not interact directly with TRE DNA, it can do so in concert with DNA-bound CREB protein.[421,422] When this happens, DNA-bound Tax interacts with the minor groove of the adjacent GC-rich sequences to stabilize the protein–DNA complex.[205,206]

CREB is ubiquitously expressed and regulates a number of cellular genes, especially cAMP-induced genes.[396] A cAMP-initiated signal phosphorylates CREB at serine 133, recruiting two transcriptional coactivators, CREB-binding protein (CBP) and p300. An *in vitro* chromatin-based transcription study indicated that phosphorylation of CREB is essential for Tax activity, through stabilizing the Tax/CREB/CBP/DNA complex. Tax by itself induces the phosphorylation of CREB.[180] CBP/p300 is a histone acetyltransferase that acetylates histone tails, thereby changing chromatin structures to activate transcription. *In vitro* and *in vivo* studies showed that p300 is crucial for Tax-dependent transcriptional activation, where p300, interacting with Tax and CREB, induces the acetylation of nucleosome histones over the TRE DNA.[86,87,95,116,196,203,206] Interestingly, p300 recruitment by Tax to an integrated HTLV-1 promoter reduces the amount of histone H1 and H3 proteins on the promoter DNA and stimulates the recruitment of RNA polymerase II.[204] These results suggest that recruitment of CBP/p300 to the integrated promoter acetylates histone tails, thereby removing histone octamers from the HTLV-1 promoter.

TORCs and P-TEFb (CDK-9/cyclin T1) are additional positive regulators of Tax-dependent HTLV-1 promoter activation.[46,47,153,18,335,427] Both proteins interact with Tax, and the knockdown of either by siRNA reduces Tax-dependent activation. On the other hand, Bcl-3, by interacting with TORC3, acts as a negative transcriptional regulator of the HTLV-1 LTR.[129]

Tax-Mediated Cellular Signaling Pathways

Tax not only activates plus-strand transcription of viral genes but also possesses pleiotropic effects on signaling pathways of host cells (Fig. 16.3). Tax is intermittently expressed in approximately half of ATL cases; it is probably also expressed—again intermittently—in most HTLV-1–infected cells in both asymptomatic carriers and patients with HAM. Sporadic Tax expression enhances transcription of NF-κB–associated genes and antiapoptotic genes[221] but suppresses the cell cycle transition from S to G2/M.

Activation of NF-κB by Tax

Tax activates the transcription factor NF-κB, thereby inducing the expression of a number of cellular genes, and this activity is crucial for many aspects of the HTLV-1 life cycle.[16,207,233,303,344] Several NF-κB inhibitors induce apoptosis in HTLV-1–infected T cells, indicating that NF-κB is crucial for survival of HTLV-1–infected T cells. NF-κB is a family of transcription factors including NF-κB1 (p50), p65, c-Rel, NF-κB2 (p52), RelB, and Bcl-3, and these factors are divided into two groups belonging to the canonical (NF-κB1/p50, p65, c-Rel) and the noncanonical (NF-κB2/p52, RelB, Bcl-3) pathways. Both NF-κB pathways are activated by Tax in T cells.[400]

To activate the canonical pathway, Tax interacts with several NF-κB regulators. IKKγ is essential for Tax activation of NF-κB, since the mutation of IKKγ in fibroblasts or T cells totally abrogates Tax activation of NF-κB.[48,85,114,406] IKKγ is a scaffold component of the IκB kinase (IKK) complex, IKKα/IKKβ/IKKγ. Through interacting with IKKγ, Tax activates IKKβ to induce phosphorylation and degradation of IκBs (IκBα, IκBβ), thereby allowing nuclear translocation of p50/p65.[219,345]

Tax also activates the noncanonical NF-κB pathway.[400] Tax simultaneously binds to the IKK complex (IKKγ, IKKα) and NF-κB2/p100, but not IKKβ, and thus induces

Tax

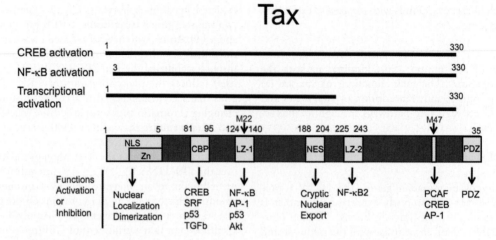

FIGURE 16.3 Functional domains of Tax. Regions of Tax required for activation of the cyclic adenosine monophosphate response element binding protein/activating transcription factor (CREB/ATF) pathway, activation of the NF-κB pathway, and transcriptional activation function of Tax measured by a Tax fusion protein with the yeast DNA-binding protein GAL4 are indicated. Positions of substitution mutations in the Tax mutants M22 and M47 are also indicated. M22 is active in the CREB pathway but inactive in the NF-κB pathway, whereas M47 is the reverse. LZ-2 and PDZ motifs distinguish Tax1 from Tax2. NLS, nuclear localization signal; NES, cryptic nuclear export signal; Zn, zinc finger motif; LZ-1 and LZ-2, leucine zipper-like structures.

IKKα-mediated phosphorylation of p100, its processing into p52, and the subsequent translocation of p52/RelB into the nucleus. Knockdown of NF-κB2/p100 by short hairpin RNA reduces Tax-induced IL-2–independent growth induction in CTLL-2 cells.[121] Thus, the noncanonical NF-κB pathway is also crucial for the transforming activity of Tax.

In half of ATL cases, *tax* is either silenced or only transiently transcribed, although the NF-κB pathway is activated in all ATL cases. This suggests that NF-κB is activated by other mechanisms. Overexpression of NF-κB–inducing kinase (NIK) is associated with constitutive activation of NF-κB.[306] Furthermore, microRNA-31 (miR-31) negatively regulates the non-canonical NF-κB pathway by targeting NIK. Therefore, the suppression of miR-31 that is observed in ATL cells leads to activation of the NF-κB pathway.[403]

Apoptosis inhibition by Tax

HTLV-1–infected T cells are resistant to various types of apoptosis, and this resistance is mostly mediated by Tax.[173,258] Tax inhibits apoptosis of T cells induced by IL-2 withdrawal in an IL-2–dependent T-cell line (CTLL-2). Studies of Tax mutants (M47, M22) indicate that inhibition of apoptosis is mediated through the NF-κB pathway.[146] Tax activates the expression of several antiapoptotic genes in T cells, including CTLL-2 cells, through the NF-κB pathway. These genes include *Bcl-xL*, *xIAP*, *cIAP*, and *cFLIP*.[375]

Activation of the PI3K/AKT pathway by Tax

IL-2 activates PI3K and its downstream kinase, Akt, in normal T cells—events which are essential for apoptosis inhibition and cell growth. However, even in the absence of IL-2, HTLV-1–transformed T-cell lines show constitutive activation of the PI3K/Akt pathway. Moreover, several inhibitors of this pathway, such as LY294002 (an inhibitor for PI3K), induce growth arrest of HTLV-1–transformed T-cell lines and then induce

apoptosis, suggesting that continuous activation of this pathway is essential for maintaining survival of HTLV-1–infected T cells.[136,152] To do this, Tax directly interacts with PI3K. PI3K consists of two subunits: the catalytic p110α subunit and the inhibitory p85α subunit. Tax directly binds to the p85α inhibitory subunit, causing the release of the active p110α catalytic subunit.[291] Activation of the PI3K/Akt pathway by Tax results in activation of the downstream target mammalian target of rapamycin (mTOR) in HTLV-1–infected T cells as well as Tax-expressing cells.[416]

Physiological Functions of Tax

T-cell lines transformed *in vitro* by HTLV-1 express Tax at a high level, which does not reflect the physiological expression pattern of Tax. Tax expression *in vivo* is suppressed at a low level. It is speculated that Tax is intermittently expressed, so that at a given instant Tax is present in only a small number of infected cells and ATL cells.[32,221] Intermittent Tax expression (Tax burst) promotes transcription of the plus-strand of the provirus, which leads to *de novo* infection. Simultaneously, the Tax burst generates T cells with higher expression of antiapoptotic genes, which is important to maintain the whole cell population.[221] Since Tax is a highly immunogenic viral protein, restriction of Tax expression to an intermittent pattern is beneficial for survival of non-malignant HTLV-1–infected cells and ATL cells *in vivo*.

Rex

HTLV-1 has two posttranscriptional regulators, Rex and p30.[169,412] The role of p30 in posttranscriptional mRNA regulation is described below.

In addition to unspliced genomic mRNA encoding *gag/pro-pol*, HTLV-1 produces singly spliced *env* mRNA and doubly spliced *tax/rex* and *p30* mRNAs. RNAs with introns generally undergo splicing by the cellular RNA machinery; otherwise they are degraded. Thus, upon initial infection of host cells, HTLV-1 dominantly expresses doubly spliced *tax/rex* and *p30* mRNA. Once the Rex protein is produced, Rex controls the ratio of spliced forms of HTLV-1 mRNAs[119,139] (Fig. 16.2). Rex increases the amount of singly spliced (*env*) and unspliced (*gag/pro-pol*) mRNAs and reduces the amount of its own doubly spliced mRNA. Rex does this by inhibiting the splicing of singly spliced (*env*) and unspliced (*gag/pro-pol*) mRNAs, stabilizing them, and promoting their transport to the cytoplasm. In the absence of Rex, unspliced HTLV-1 mRNAs are retained in the nucleus due to two cis-acting repressive sequences (CRS) in the 5′ and 3′ LTRs,[182,321] but Rex overcomes the inhibitory activity of the CRSs and induces the translocation of the unspliced RNAs into the cytoplasm.

These Rex functions are achieved through at least three activities. The first is sequence-specific RNA binding. Rex interacts specifically with the HTLV-1 RNA, at the Rex-responsive element (RxRE) located in the U3 and R regions of the 3′ LTR.[3,38,379] RNA binding by Rex is accomplished by an arginine-rich highly basic region in Rex (aa1-19).[109] This domain also contains a nuclear localization signal (NLS) and a nucleolus targeting signal, which allow Rex to enter the nucleolus where it can interact with the RNA.[276,332] The RxRE RNA forms a long stem loop structure, and one stem loop (called stem loop D) is essential for Rex binding and function.[103] The second Rex function (multimerization) is mediated through aa32-133.[395] Rex mutants that cannot form multimers behave as dominant-negative proteins.[37,395] The third Rex function is interaction with the nuclear export receptor, CRM1/exportin 1, which mediates the transport of viral mRNAs from the nucleus to the cytoplasm. Interaction with CRM1 is also required for multimerization of Rex, since a Rex mutant defective for CRM1 interaction failed to form a multimer. Rex contains a typical leucine-rich nuclear export signal (NES) (aa81-94) that mediates its interaction with CRM1. HTLV-1 production is less efficient in rat cells than human cells, because Rex is less active in rat cells than human cells. The rat CRM1 is impaired in promoting Rex to form multimers, which may explain the reduced activity of Rex in rat cells.[106,420]

Rex is activated by phosphorylation.[177] While PMA (phorbol myristate acetate), an activator of PKC (protein kinase C), transiently enhances phosphorylation of Rex, treatment of HTLV-1–infected cell lines with a PKC inhibitor reduces the amount of unspliced *gag-pol* mRNA.[1] Liquid chromatography tandem mass spectrometry analysis showed that Rex is phosphorylated at multiple sites, and mutation analysis indicated that phosphorylations at Ser-97 and Thr-174 are critical for its function.[177] Rex also suppresses nonsense-mediated mRNA decay, which ensures the stability of viral genomic RNA.[265]

Tax Expression and Its Suppression by HBZ and Rex

High expression of Tax induces senescence and suppresses the S phase of the cell cycle.[195,221] Thus, Tax overexpression is harmful to infected cells. Therefore, HTLV-1 has redundant mechanisms to alleviate detrimental effects of Tax and reduce Tax expression. Rex inhibits splicing of the *tax* gene and promotes generation of unspliced RNA. Furthermore, HBZ suppresses Tax expression through inhibition of the binding of CREB-2 to TREs.[83] In addition, *HBZ* RNA impairs the interaction of RNA polymerase II with LTR by displacing TATA-box binding protein (TBP), resulting in suppression of the basal transcription machinery.[84] Since *HBZ* is transcribed from a TATA-less promoter, this sup-

pressive effect of HBZ RNA does not influence *HBZ* transcription. Hyperactivation of NF-κB by Tax causes up-regulation of cyclin-dependent kinase inhibitors, p21 and p27, which leads to cellular senescence.[426] HBZ protein hinders the onset of Tax-induced senescence through inhibition of the canonical NF-κB pathway.[424] Thus, when Tax expression is predominant during a plus-strand burst, Rex progressively suppresses Tax expression via altered splicing. Then, HBZ (RNA and protein) maintains latency by suppression of sense-transcription.[293]

HBZ: Physiological Actions

Transcription of the HBZ Gene

Two major forms of the *HBZ* RNA have been reported: a spliced form (*sHBZ*) and an unspliced form (*usHBZ*). The first exon of the *sHBZ* gene transcript is located in the U3 and R regions of the 3′ LTR (Figs. 16.1 and 16.2). Transcriptional start sites for *sHBZ* are scattered in the U5 and R regions of the 3′ LTR, an observation which is consistent with the finding that the predicted promoter was TATA-less.[413] Three Sp1 binding sites are critical for transcription of the *HBZ* gene. Since Sp1 is a well-known regulator of housekeeping genes, transcription of the sHBZ gene may be constitutive and relatively constant. The levels of *HBZ* gene transcript are better correlated with provirus load than those of the *tax* gene transcript,[305] confirming that the *HBZ* gene is frequently expressed in HTLV-1–infected cells. Thus, transcription from the minus strand stands in contrasts to that from the plus strand, which is highly inducible by Tax. RNA-FISH analyses show that *HBZ* is expressed in most cells at a much lower level of transcription.[32,243] Importantly, *HBZ* expression is strongly associated with the S and G2/M phases of the cell cycle, suggesting that *HBZ* promotes mitosis in expressing cells.

The difference between sHBZ and usHBZ is only a few amino acids, as shown in Figure 16.1. The spliced transcript of *HBZ* is translated into a polypeptide of 206 amino acids, while the protein product of unspliced *HBZ* is a polypeptide of 209 amino acids. The expression level of *sHBZ* RNA is much higher than that of *usHBZ* RNA,[381] and the half-life of sHBZ protein is much longer than that of usHBZ.[413] These data indicate that expression levels of sHBZ are much higher than those of usHBZ, suggesting that sHBZ is more important than usHBZ for HTLV-1–infected cells and ATL cells.

Functions of HBZ

HBZ has important functions in both its protein and mRNA forms[242,313] (Fig. 16.4). RNA-FISH showed that *HBZ* mRNA is mainly localized in the nucleus whereas *tax* is exported from the nucleus.[32]

Function of HBZ protein

HBZ protein is localized in the nucleus with a speckled pattern.[131] HBZ has three domains: the activation, central, and bZIP domains (Fig. 16.4). HBZ was originally reported to suppress Tax-mediated viral gene transcription from the 5′ LTR via interaction with CREB2 and c-Jun.[24,83] Indeed, many actions of HBZ act in opposition to those of Tax (Fig. 16.5). Further, HBZ interacts with various host factors that contain a bZIP domain, including CREB, JunB, ATF-1, and ATF-3, and hinders their transcriptional activation.[24,104,130,202] Conversely, interaction of HBZ with JunD activates transcription of target genes.[365] As a mechanism, HBZ modulates translational control

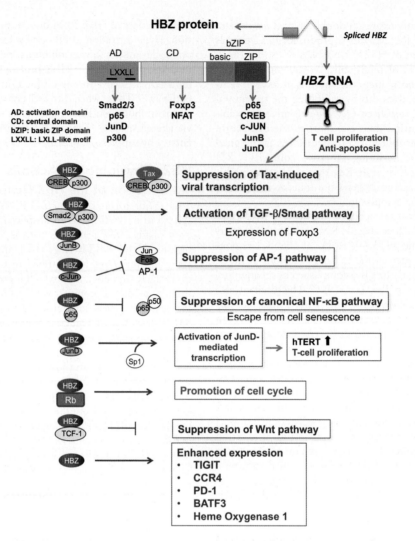

FIGURE 16.4 Functions of HBZ. HBZ has three domains: activation, central, and bZIP. The HBZ protein exerts a variety of functions by interacting with host factors. On the other hand, HBZ RNA promotes proliferation via up-regulation of the E2F1 gene.

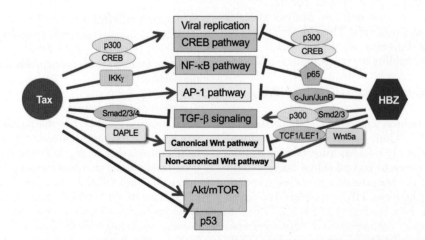

FIGURE 16.5 Interplay between Tax and HBZ. Interplays between Tax and HBZ on various pathways are shown. In most pathways, HBZ has opposite effects to Tax.

of JunD, inducing expression of the truncated isoform, Delta JunD,[363] Furthermore, HBZ enhances TGF-β/Smad pathway by interaction with Smad2/3 and p300.[423]

In most ATL cases, ATL cells express Foxp3,[122] a master molecule of regulatory T (Treg) cells. Furthermore, in HTLV-1–infected individuals, the proportion of HTLV-1–infected cells is higher in Treg populations,[312] indicating that HTLV-1 is associated with Treg cells. HBZ induces Foxp3 expression in T cells, and its induction is enhanced in the presence of TGF-β.[314] Thus, activation of TGF-β/Smad by HBZ induces Foxp3 expression in infected cells. This accounts for why HTLV-1 is associated with Treg cells. Furthermore, HBZ interacts with Foxp3 protein and impairs its functions.[314] Thus, HBZ increases the number of functionally impaired Treg cells and may lead to the development of malignancy derived from Treg cells. HBZ also induces expression of Treg-associated molecules including CCR4 and T-Cell Immunoglobulin and ITIM Domain (TIGIT).[340,410] Thus, HBZ determines the immunophenotype of HTLV-1–infected cells and ATL cells.

HBZ also selectively inhibits the classical NF-κB pathway by inhibiting DNA binding of p65 and promoting the degradation of p65.[424] Although Tax expression is reported to induce cell senescence by hyperactivation of NFκB, inhibition of classical pathway of NFκB by HBZ attenuates senescence caused by Tax.[293]

shRNA library screening identified IRF4 and BATF3 as master regulators of proliferation of ATL cells. HBZ binds to a superenhancer of the *BATF3* locus, leading to up-regulation of BATF3 and its downstream target, *MYC*.[263] Thus, HBZ promotes proliferation of expressing T cells.

Function of HBZ RNA
Suppression of *HBZ* gene expression by shRNA inhibits proliferation of ATL cell lines.[13,313] Expression of *HBZ* in transgenic mice increases the number of T cells, while suppression of *HBZ* expression decreases tumor formation and infiltration of ATL cells.[13] Thus, HBZ expression is associated with proliferation of ATL cells *in vivo* and *in vitro*. Mutation analysis of the *HBZ* gene showed that *HBZ* RNA, rather than HBZ protein, has a growth promoting effect on T cells whereas HBZ protein rather suppresses proliferation.[242,313] The 5′ region of the *sHBZ* transcript is critical for this activity.[242,413] Kinetic analysis of viral mRNA shows strong nuclear retention of *HBZ* mRNA.[299] Poor polyadenylation of *HBZ* mRNA causes this nuclear retention.[213] An antisense transcript of HIV-1 is also poorly polyadenylated and localized in the nucleus, suggesting that this is a common feature of antisense transcripts of retroviruses.

APH-2
An antisense transcript similar to *HBZ* has been discovered in HTLV-2 and named antisense protein of HTLV-2 (APH-2).[107] The *APH-2* gene encodes a 183 amino acid polypeptide that is localized in the nucleus. Although APH-2 does not have a bZIP domain, APH-2 interacts with CREB and represses Tax2-mediated transcription from the 5′ LTR of HTLV-2. Both HBZ and APH-2 have suppressive effects on transcription of sense viral genes, although any other functions of APH-2 remain to be elucidated.

Accessory Genes
p12/p8
p12 is encoded by the singly spliced mRNA of HTLV-1 ORFI.[49,192] p12 is a highly hydrophobic membrane protein of 99 amino acids, and it is localized in the endoplasmic reticulum (ER) and Golgi complex.[64,191] p12 has a noncanonical ER retention/retrieval motif, two putative transmembrane (TM) domains, four putative proline-rich (PXXP) Src-homology 3 (SH3)-binding domains, two putative leucine zipper (LZ) motifs, and a putative adaptin motif[77,269] (Fig. 16.6). When

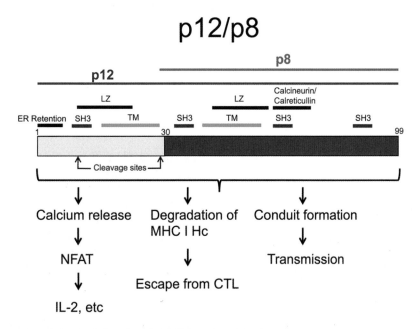

FIGURE 16.6 Schematic structure, functional domains, and functions of p12/p8. The protease cleavage sites are indicated. The known functions of p12/p8 are summarized. p8 induces cellular conduit formation, which is involved in HTLV-1 transmission. TM, putative transmembrane domain; LZ, leucine zipper-like structure; SH3, Src-homology 3; ER retention, endoplasmic reticulum retention signal.

ectopically expressed in HeLa cells, p12 forms a homodimer through its TM domains.[374]

A p12-deficient HTLV-1 mutant (p12 mutation of Met-1 to Leu and an HBZ mutation of His-151 to Gln) had reduced infectivity of DCs, and when rhesus macaques were infected with it, viral propagation and persistent infection were poorly established.[383] On the other hand, this mutant HTLV-1 produced infectious viruses comparable to wild type HTLV-1, immortalized primary human T cells *in vitro*, and established persistent infection in rabbits. Thus, DC infection with HTLV-1 appears to be critical for persistent infection in macaques, and p12 may play a role in this process.

Effect of p12 on T-cell activation and proliferation

p12 activates Ca^{2+} signaling in T cells.[63,64] Ectopic overexpression of p12 in a T-cell line increases intracellular Ca^{2+} levels, stimulating the phosphatase calcineurin to dephosphorylate NFAT and then NFAT to activate transcription of genes such as IL-2.[4,179] p12 increases intracellular Ca^{2+} concentration by interacting with two ER resident proteins, calnexin and calreticulin, which regulate Ca^{2+} release from the ER.[64] In addition, p12 interacts directly with calcineurin. Since HTLV-1–transformed T-cell lines do not generally exhibit constitutive NFAT binding to the IL-2 promoter,[272] NFAT appears to be only transiently activated by p12 at a particular phase of HTLV-1 infection such as an initial infection.

p12 in T cells can stimulate the IL-2 signaling pathway downstream of the IL-2R. p12 interacts with the beta and gamma chains of the IL-2R and enhances the phosphorylation of STAT5 and its DNA binding, thereby augmenting transcription.[257] Expression of p12 in a human T-cell line transformed by a p12-defective HTLV-1 mutant augments colony formation in soft agar in conditions of low IL-2.

p12-induced attenuation of the host immune response

p12 is implicated in reduced host immunity to HTLV-1–infected cells. HTLV-1–infected primary CD4+ T cells are resistant to autologous NK cell–mediated killing.[16a] Such killing is initiated by binding of NK to target cells via adhesion molecules such as the ICAMs. HTLV-1 infection reduces the expression of ICAM1 and ICAM2 in primary CD4+ T cells, thereby reducing NK cell binding. Lentivirus-mediated expression of p12 in primary CD4+ T cells downmodulates expression of ICAM1 and ICAM2. In addition, p12 can reduce CTL-mediated killing.[157] p12, through interaction with the MHC class I heavy chain, inhibits its interaction with β2-microglobulin, thereby inducing the proteasome-dependent degradation of MHC class I.

Functions of p8

Proteolytic cleavage of p12 generates the C-terminal product p8, which may promote HTLV-1 transmission.[385] The cleavage of p12 removes the ER retention/retrieval motifs, and thus p8 is localized to the T-cell membrane (Fig. 16.6). Upon T-cell receptor activation, p8 is recruited into the immunological synapse. Comparison of p8-positive and negative HTLV-1 indicates that p8 increases cell-to-cell contact and induces lymphocyte function–associated antigen-1 (LFA-1) mediated cell clustering, augmenting the number and length of conduits (filopodia-like

membrane extensions) and thereby enhancing HTLV-1 transmission.

p13

p13 is encoded by the singly spliced monocistronic mRNA of the HTLV-1 x-II ORF.[329] p13 is a highly basic protein of 87 amino acids and is identical to the C-terminal 87 amino acids of p30. p13 has the following domains: an amphipathic alpha helix (residues 20 to 35), a mitochondrial targeting signal (MTS) (residues 21 to 30), a transmembrane region (residues 30 to 40), and several PXXP motifs (Fig. 16.7).

A p13-defective HTLV-1 virus (with a mutation of the p13 initiation codon) showed comparable infectivity of rabbit PBMC to that of wild type virus, but the mutant virus could not establish infection in rabbits *in vivo*, as measured by viral loads and antibody responses, indicating that p13 plays a still-unknown role in establishing HTLV-1 infection *in vivo*.[126]

p13 is localized mostly in the inner mitochondrial membrane, and its ectopic expression in isolated mitochondria induces mitochondrial swelling, depolarization, increased respiratory chain activity, and production of ROS, through activation of the inward K^+ current.[30,330] p13 also induces ROS production in primary quiescent T cells.

p30

p30 is encoded by the doubly spliced mRNA of x-II ORF and is a protein of 241 amino acids.[115,250] It is unusually rich in Ser (23%) and Arg (12%) and localized in the nucleus and the nucleolus.

Posttranscriptional regulation of viral RNA by p30

p30 inhibits the nuclear export of doubly spliced *tax/rex* mRNA through retaining the mRNA in the nucleus.[268] p30 binds to the splice junction region (*env* exon) of *tax/rex* mRNA. Although both Rex and p30 interact with HTLV-1 RNA and decrease the amount of *tax/rex* mRNA exported from the nucleus, they generally have opposite functions in virus production. Whereas Rex stimulates virus production through augmenting the expression of structural proteins (Gag, Pol, Env), p30 inhibits

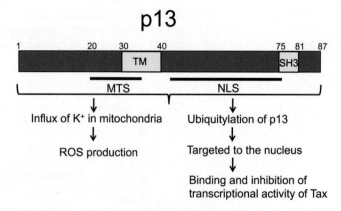

FIGURE 16.7 Schematic structure, functional domains, and functions of p13. The functions of p13 are summarized. TM, putative transmembrane domain; MTS, mitochondrial targeting signal; SH3, Src-homology 3; NLS, nuclear localization signal; LZ, leucine zipper-like structure.

virus production through reducing the expression of Tax and Rex. Interestingly, the Rex and p30 proteins interact with each other, and their interaction is augmented by the presence of the viral mRNAs.[56,331] While p30 has little effect on Rex activity, Rex counteracts p30 activity and induces the expression of Tax and Rex proteins. Thus, the ratio of p30:Rex may control the transition between virus latency and virus production. Since Tax is transiently expressed in HTLV-1–infected cells and ATL cells, and transcription of genes encoded in the sense strand of the provirus depends on Tax, it follows that expression of p30 is also transient, which may contribute to the fine-tuning of viral replication.

An HTLV-1 infectious clone with a nonsense mutation in *p30* was inoculated into four Rhesus macaques. Reversion to wild type was observed in two macaques, indicating that p30 is necessary for infectivity *in vivo*.[383] Furthermore, viral replication of the HTLV-1 infectious clone with the p30 mutant was severely impaired in human dendritic cells.

Transcriptional and posttranscriptional regulation of cellular genes by p30

p30 also interacts with several cellular factors. p30 interacts with the Ets domain of PU.1, which leads to suppression of TLR4.[57] Furthermore, p30 suppresses the expression of interferon-responsive genes.[72] These functions of p30 account for impaired viral infectivity to myeloid cells in a p30-deficient infectious clone. p30 also suppresses proliferation of T cells by inhibiting their entry into the S phase of the cell cycle and causing accumulation of cells in the G2 and M phases.[25,56] These effects are caused by p30 interacting with cyclin E and CDK2, resulting in inhibition of cyclin E-CDK2 complex. Similar to Tax, p30 also impairs homologous recombination repair.[26] Thus, Tax and p30 possess similar effects on cell cycling and DNA repair of expressing cells. It is possible that these functions play critical roles in *de novo* infection when *tax* undergoes a transcriptional burst.

Genomic Instability in ATL Cells

ATL cells have numerous genetic abnormalities such as DNA mutations, chromosomal translocations, deletions and duplications, and aneuploidy, and these genetic aberrations are linked to ATL development. For example, homozygous deletions of p16 (CDNN2A) and p15 (CDKN2B) genes, tumor suppressor genes that regulate the cell cycle, were frequently observed in aggressive acute and lymphoma-type ATL.[117] Both Tax and HBZ are implicated in the genomic instability of ATL cells.

p53

The tumor suppressor p53 is the "guardian of the genome" in DNA damage responses. p53 is functionally inactivated by Tax.[407] Tax interacts with the p53 coactivator CBP/p300 and blocks its access to p53, thereby reducing the transcriptional activation function of p53.[346]

Defective DNA Repair

DNA repair activity is attenuated by Tax in HTLV-1–infected T-cell lines.[150,165,224,245,295] Tax represses transcription of the DNA polymerase β gene, which plays a crucial role in DNA repair.[150] Ataxia telangiectasia mutated (ATM), a member of the PI3K-like kinase family, is activated by various DNA damaging agents, and its activation is essential in initiating signaling cascades that stop DNA replication and allow the repair of damaged DNA. ATM activation by ionizing radiation and signals downstream of ATM activation are diminished in HTLV-1–infected T-cell lines as well as cells expressing Tax alone.[43] Upon treatment with ionizing radiation, both normal and Tax-expressing cells stop DNA replication, but the interval before replication resumes is shorter in Tax-expressing cells than in the parental control cells; simultaneously, the cells expressing Tax are defective for DNA repair activity. Although the precise mechanism by which Tax blocks DNA repair has not been fully elucidated, Tax is known to interact with several host factors involved in DNA repair, such as DNA-dependent protein kinase, Ku, Chk1, and Chk2.[65,288,289]

Constitutive NF-κB activation by Tax induces cell cycle arrest or senescence.[212,293,408] Activation of NF-κB by Tax induces an R-loop structure—a three-stranded nucleic acid structure consisting of an RNA–DNA hybrid and a single-strand DNA—which induces senescence.[118] Two transcription-coupled nucleotide excision-repair endonucleases, xeroderma pigmentosum F (XPF) and XPG, are important for excision of R-loops. In ATL cells, expression of these two endonucleases is suppressed, indicating that such ATL cells proliferate regardless of accumulated R-loops.

HBZ induces DNA-strand breaks, which are caused by activated miR17 and miR22. These microRNAs suppress expression of hSSB2, which encodes a single-stranded DNA-binding protein associated with genome stability.[391] hSSB2 is implicated in reduced efficiency in HR-dependent repair of DSBs and defective ATM-dependent phosphorylation.[211] Thus, HBZ is also associated with genome instability, which is linked to oncogenesis.

Chromosomal Instability

The centrosome is a microtubule organizing center during cell division and plays a crucial role in the precise duplication and segregation of chromosomes. While normal T cells have one centrosome during interphase, in HTLV-1–infected cell lines, around 30% of the cell population has more than two centrosomes, indicating that a centrosomal aberration may contribute to the chromosomal abnormalities observed in HTLV-1–infected cells.[45] Such abnormal centrosomes are induced by the ectopic expression of Tax in human T cells.

This activity of Tax is mediated through its interaction with several host proteins such as TAX1BP2 and RanBP1.[45] Endogenous TAX1BP2 is localized in the centrosome, and its knockdown induces centrosome amplification. Furthermore, overexpression of Tax1BP2 reduces Tax-induced centrosome amplification. These results indicate that Tax induces centrosome aberrations by inactivating TAX1BP2. In contrast, the knockdown of RanBP1 abrogates centrosome amplification by Tax as well as centrosome localization of Tax, indicating that RanBP1 targets Tax to centrosomes. MAD1 is another Tax-interacting protein localized in the centrosome during metaphase. While the knockdown of MAD1 induces multinucleated cells, its overexpression inhibits induction of multinuclear cells by Tax.[154] Thus, MAD1 is also involved in the genomic instability induced by Tax in HTLV-1–infected cells.

PATHOGENESIS AND PERSISTENCE *IN VIVO*

Entry Into Cells and Host

Entry Into the Host

Transmission of HTLV-1 between individuals requires transfer of infected lymphocytes, because lymphocytes naturally infected with the virus produce few if any cell-free virions. There are three main routes of transmission: breast-feeding and sexual intercourse are the two natural routes, by which the virus is maintained in the population. Breast milk contains lymphocytes[210]; seminal fluid also contains lymphocytes and appears to enhance HTLV-1 replication.[255] The risk of mother-to-child transmission of HTLV-1 is associated with a high PVL,[380] with the presence of anti-Tax antibodies in the mother,[127] and with prolonged breast-feeding.[397] Transfusion of blood products that contain lymphocytes was an important source of HTLV-1 infections in countries with endemic HTLV-1 infection before screening of blood products was introduced,[280] and transplantation of solid organs from HTLV-1–infected donors is a persistent but rare cause of infection.[361]

In a host infected by sexual intercourse, the portal of entry is the genital mucosa. In the breast-fed infant, infection probably enters in the oropharynx, which is surrounded by the lymphoid tissue of Waldeyer ring, including the tonsils. It is unlikely that the virus enters in the infant's stomach. Although the pH of the stomach of neonates is not strongly acidic, because of ingestion of amniotic fluid, which has a pH of about 7, the pH drops quickly in the first few days after birth, reaching pH 3 by 1 week.[12] The precise site and mechanism of the entry of infected T cells across the epithelial barrier in either portal of entry are not well understood.[292] It is often assumed that dendritic cells play a part in the initial acquisition of infection at the portal of entry, but direct evidence is lacking.

Entry Into the Cell

HTLV-1 is unusual among viruses in its almost exclusive reliance on cell-to-cell contact for transmission of infection between cells: naturally infected cells release few—if any—cell-free infectious virions, and HTLV-1 relies instead on the mobility of the host cell to spread both within and between hosts.[19] Since the virus can infect a very broad range of human cell types, other mammalian cells, and some avian cells (see "Cell and "Tissue Tropism"), the cellular receptor for the virus was inferred to be widely distributed. Early attempts to identify the receptor exploited the ability of HTLV-1–producing T cell lines to induce multinucleate syncytia by fusion of the plasma membrane of the infected cell with a cell that is brought into contact.[261] Sommerfelt et al.[336] used human–mouse somatic cell hybrids to identify the chromosome responsible for conferring susceptibility to infection by VSV pseudotypes carrying the HTLV-1 envelope glycoprotein. Their results indicated a region on the long arm of chromosome 17. Tajima et al.[351] similarly used HTLV-1 Env-induced fusion with somatic cell hybrid lines, with a recombinant vaccinia virus expression system, to localize the putative receptor to 17q21-23. However, subsequent studies identified the two key cellular receptor molecules GLUT-1 and Neuropilin-1 (NRP-1), encoded respectively on chromosomes 1 and 10. The identity of the putative additional factors encoded on chromosome 17 remains unknown.

The GLUT-1 glucose transporter was the first identified cellular receptor for HTLV-1 (Fig. 16.8A).[54,158,181,229] GLUT-1 interacts with the receptor-binding domain (RBD) (the first 215 aa) of HTLV-1 Env and HTLV-2 Env. Knockdown of GLUT-1 by siRNA results in reduced binding of the HTLV-1 and HTLV-2 RBD to the cells as well as reduced infection by HTLV-2-env pseudotype virus, and the binding is rescued by overexpression of GLUT-1 but not GLUT-3, another glucose-transporter family member. In addition, polyclonal chicken antibody against the extracellular loop domain of GLUT-1 inhibits Env-mediated fusion as well as infection.[156] Specific regions of GLUT-1 mediate the binding to HTLV-1 Env and virus entry into cells.[227]

NRP-1 also functions as an HTLV-1 receptor.[93] Overexpression of NRP-1 in cells with a low endogenous expression of NRP-1 augments HTLV-1 Env-mediated infection, and NRP-1 knockdown by siRNA in 293T cells reduces HTLV-1 Env-mediated infection. NRP-1 colocalizes with the

Virus entry and receptors

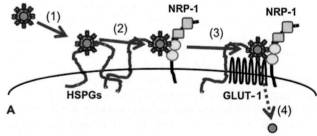

Virological synapse

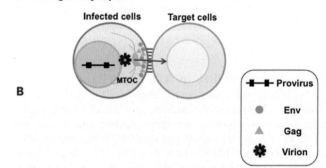

FIGURE 16.8 The HTLV-1 receptor complex and the current model of HTLV-1 entry. A: (*1*) The HTLV-1 envelope protein (Env) attaches to heparan sulfate proteoglycans (HSPGs) on the target cell, which increases the local concentration of the viruses at the cell surface. (*2*) HTLV-1 Env then binds to neuropilin-1 (NRP-1), and this binding induces a conformational change of Env that facilitates its interaction with glucose transporter 1 (GLUT-1). (*3*) The formation of a ternary complex of Env, NRP-1, and GLUT-1 induces a conformational change of Env that triggers the fusion of the viral and cell membranes. **B:** The contact site between an HTLV-1–infected cell and a target cell forms a special structure referred to as the virological synapse (VS). VS formation involves polarization of the microtubule-organizing center near the site of cell-to-cell contact in the infected cell. Complete, enveloped infectious virions can pass from the infected cell to the target cell either in pockets between the two cells' plasma membranes in the center of the VS or in an extracellular carbohydrate-rich assembly at the periphery of the VS.

Env protein at the cell membrane and forms a complex with GLUT-1. This complex formation is augmented by the expression of Env protein, suggesting that NRP-1 and GLUT-1 make an HTLV-1 receptor complex that mediates HTLV-1 binding and entry (Fig. 16.8A), just as the CD4 molecule and chemokine receptors do for HIV infection. In addition, the relative importance of GLUT1 and NRP-1 for HTLV-1 infection may differ between cell types. For instance, knockdown of GLUT1 reduced Env-mediated fusion in HeLa cells but not in U87 glioblastoma/astroglyoma cells.[155]

While the primary cellular receptors for HTLV-1 are GLUT-1 and NRP-1, infection is also enhanced by the surface adhesion molecules ICAM-1, ICAM-3, and VCAM-1. Heparan sulfate proteoglycans (HSPGs), cofactors in many viral infections, also promote HTLV-1 binding and infection of CD4+ T cells.[158,296] HTLV-1 virions as well as purified gp46 proteins bind to HSPGs on CD4+ T cells, and the binding is abrogated by treatment of target cells with heparan sulfate lyase. Moreover, soluble heparin blocks HTLV-1 infection of susceptible cells.

HTLV-1 entry into susceptible cells begins with the binding of the HTLV-1 envelope proteins to a viral receptor on the membrane of the host cell, and it is followed by the fusion of viral and cell membranes.[17,92,228] The HTLV-1 envelope protein (Env) is synthesized as a 68 kD polyprotein precursor and is cleaved to produce two subunits, the surface glycoprotein (SU) of 46 kD (gp46) and the transmembrane (TM) glycoprotein of 21 kD (gp21). Mature Env proteins on the virion are trimers, consisting of three SUs and three TMs linked by disulfide bonds. The cytoplasmic domain of gp21 controls envelope-mediated syncytium formation and cell-to-cell HTLV-1 entry.[178,297] The C-terminus of gp21 contains a PDZ-domain protein binding motif, and the deletion of this motif reduces the stability of Env.[35] In addition, the Y-S-L-I motif in the cytoplasmic domain of gp21 is crucial for cell-to-cell HTLV-1 transmission.[58]

Virological Synapse

Since the discovery of HTLV-1 in 1980, it was recognized that efficient transmission of HTLV-1 between cells required cell-to-cell contact, but the reasons for this requirement were unknown. An important clue came from the observation that HTLV-1 preferentially infects T cells that are themselves specific for HTLV-1 antigens—both CD8+ T cells[112] and CD4+ T cells.[102] This observation led to the hypothesis that HTLV-1 is transmitted between cells through the immunological synapse, the specialized area of cell-to-cell contact that is formed between a T cell and an antigen-presenting cell.[66] Confocal microscopy of two-cell conjugates that are formed spontaneously between PBMCs from infected individuals[135] indeed revealed a structure (Fig. 16.8B) that closely resembles the immunological synapse, with organized microdomains of proteins forming an annular adhesion domain surrounding a central domain containing the viral Gag protein instead of the signaling molecules and cytokines present in the center of the immunological synapse. However, there is a crucial difference between this HTLV-1–induced structure and the immunological synapse: the microtubule organizing center (MTOC), which comes to lie near the cell-to-cell contact in both HTLV-1 transmission and in the immunological synapse, is polarized inside the HTLV-1–infected cell toward the responding antigen-specific T cell. By contrast, in the immunological synapse, the MTOC is polarised in the

responding T cell toward the antigen-presenting cell. It, therefore, became clear that the polarization of a microtubule cytoskeleton is driven by the virus itself, and not by T-cell receptor recognition of antigen as in the immunological synapse. The integrity of the microtubule cytoskeleton is required for cell-to-cell transmission of infection.[135] The structure is, therefore, named a virological synapse[135]; subsequent work by other groups showed that HIV and MLV can also be transmitted between cells via a virological synapse.

The two chief molecular signals that trigger formation of the HTLV-1 virological synapse are engagement of ICAM-1 on the surface of the infected T cell by LFA-1 on the target cell (Barnard et al., 2005) and activation of the CREB pathway by HTLV-1 Tax protein present at the MTOC.[267]

Although HTLV-1–infected cells regularly cause syncytia *in vitro* by fusion with many different cell types, cell fusion is not involved in the virological synapse and does not appear to occur *in vivo*. HTLV-1, therefore, relies on the Env glycoprotein to fuse the virion envelope with the plasma membrane of the target cell.[59,60] Electron tomography reveals the ultrastructure of the HTLV-1 virological synapse: large areas of the plasma membranes of the donor (infected) and target (recipient) cells are closely apposed with a separation of approximately 24 nM.[225] But the closely apposed membranes are interrupted by several pockets of 100 to 200 nM, isolated from the extracellular fluid. Immunostaining reveals HTLV-1 Gag protein both lining the plasma membrane in the vicinity of the pocket and in particles resembling virions in the lumen of the pocket.

These observations led to the current picture of the mechanism of transmission of HTLV-1 between cells.[19] When a cell expressing LFA-1 engages ICAM-1 on the surface of a cell expressing HTLV-1 Tax protein, the plasma membranes of the two cells form a large, close contact, with an annular adhesion structure containing LFA-1 and Talin. The microtubule cytoskeleton in the infected cell is then reoriented to bring the MTOC next to the virological synapse, and the microtubules are used to transport the viral material to the synapse. Enveloped virions are formed in the isolated pockets within the synapse[225] and traverse the short distance, of the order of a few virion diameters, to fuse with the plasma membrane of the target cell. Cell-to-cell transmission of HTLV-1 can also occur at the periphery of the synapse, in carbohydrate-rich, extracellular matrix containing virions[286] (Fig. 16.8B). *In vitro*, HTLV-1 transfer between cells has also been observed via cellular conduits named tunnelling nanotubes,[385] whose formation is promoted by the HTLV-1 accessory protein p8, which is expressed by certain strains of HTLV-1.

Propagation of HTLV-1 *in vitro*, even by cell contact with a strong HTLV-1–producing T cell line, is surprisingly inefficient. It is likely that specific conditions *in vivo*, yet unidentified, make this process more efficient.

Cell and Tissue Tropism

The cell types infected by HTLV-1 are determined in part by the expression of the three molecules identified as cellular receptors or cofactors: GLUT-1, NRP-1, and heparan sulphate proteoglycans (HSPGs). However, HTLV-1 can infect most types of nucleated human cells *in vitro*,[193,261,336] whereas *in vivo* it is almost wholly confined to T lymphocytes: typically approximately 95% of the PVL is present in CD4+ T cells, and approximately 5% in CD8+ T cells.[238] Most HTLV-1–infected T cells also carry the key marker of the memory phenotype, CD45RO[300]; the infected CD4+CD45RO+ and CD8+CD45RO+ cells proliferate *in vivo* significantly faster than uninfected cells.[15] It is not known whether the CD45RO molecule itself enhances infection; it is more likely that the infected cells preferentially survive *in vivo* in the long-lived memory (CD45RO+) clones. HTLV-1 cannot be propagated efficiently *in vitro* in cell types other than T lymphocytes.

By contrast, HTLV-2 is present almost exclusively in CD8+ T cells *in vivo*.[240] Both HTLV-1 and HTLV-2 use GLUT-1 and NRP-1 as their primary cellular receptors, and the two molecules can be expressed on both CD4+ and CD8+ T cells. *In vitro*, both HTLV-1 and HTLV-2 can infect both CD4+ and CD8+ T cells.[163] However, the two viruses differ in their ability to transform T cells *in vitro*: whereas HTLV-2 transforms CD4+ T cells, HTLV-2 transforms CD8+ T cells. The distinct transforming abilities of the two viruses *in vitro* are due to the respective envelope glycoprotein,[163,164,401] but the molecular details of this action of Env are not known. These observations imply that the cell-type specificity of both virus propagation and subsequent cellular transformation by HTLV-1 and HTLV-2 is determined by postentry factors, rather than by distinct mechanisms of cell entry.[232] At present, these putative postentry factors are not well understood.

HTLV-3 uses GLUT-1 as a viral receptor, but neither NRP-1 nor HSPG is required for infection, and HTLV-3 binds not only activated primary T cells but also resting ones.[401] These results suggest that these three HTLVs acquired distinct entry mechanisms after diversification from their common ancestor.

Both HTLV-1 and HTLV-2 are exquisitely adapted to persist *in vivo* in T lymphocytes. Since they depend on the virological synapse to spread, it is possible that T-cell–specific factors involved in the virological synapse, such as the unusually high mobility of the MTOC in T cells, contribute to the selective propagation of these viruses in T lymphocytes.

Integration and Clonality

Integration of HTLV-1 in the host cell genome as a double-stranded DNA provirus is an essential part of the viral life cycle, as in other retroviruses.[19] The site of integration in host DNA is not random, but rather is determined by factors at a succession of different spatial scales (Fig. 16.9). Each of these factors imposes a statistically significant but small effect on the choice of integration site, and as a result the virus is widely dispersed throughout the genome (see "Clonality of HTLV-1 and HTLV-2"). Each infected T cell carries a single copy of the provirus[53]: the mechanisms of resistance to superinfection by HTLV-1 are not known. Unlike HIV-1 infection, there are no hotspots of HTLV-1 integration in the human genome.

At the smallest scale, there is preferential integration of HTLV-1 in a primary DNA sequence motif of about eight nucleotides.[184] It was previously thought that retroviral insertion site motifs were palindromic, but it is now known that the palindromicity in the consensus sequence was due to the presence

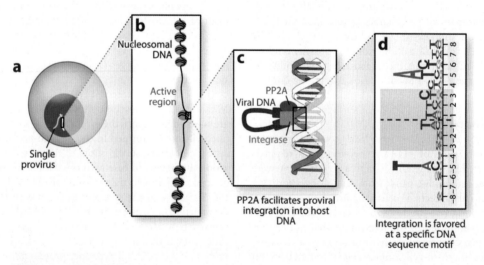

Bangham CRM. 2018.
Annu. Rev. Immunol. 36:43–71

FIGURE 16.9 The genomic integration site of HTLV-1 is specified at different spatial scales. (*a*) Most HTLV-1–infected cells contain a single provirus. Initial integration of the provirus does not favor a particular chromosome, but a provirus integrated in an acrocentric chromosome has a significant survival advantage *in vivo*. (*b*) Integration in the host genome preferentially occurs in nucleosomal DNA in transcriptionally active regions, near certain transcription factors and other chromatin-associated proteins. (*c*) Protein phosphatase 2A (PP2A) facilitates the integration of the provirus, possibly by tethering the preintegration complex or intasome to the host chromatin. (*d*) There is a weak but reproducible preference, as in other exogenous retroviruses, to integrate at a specific, nonpalindromic DNA sequence motif. Initial targeting of the integration does not favor any one chromosome, but strong *in vivo* selection results in preferential survival of clones carrying a provirus in one of the five acrocentric chromosomes, especially chromosome 13. The reason for this preferential survival *in vivo* is not known. (Republished with permission of Annual Reviews, Inc. from Bangham CRM. Human T cell leukemia virus type 1: persistence and pathogenesis. *Annu Rev Immunol* 2018;36:43–71; permission conveyed through Copyright Clearance Center, Inc. Copyright © 2018 by Annual Reviews, https://www.annualreviews.org.)

of the short (nonpalindromic) motif on either the plus-strand or the minus-strand of the host genome.[184] The integration site motif that is used by both HTLV-1 and HTLV-2 closely resembles that of HIV-1.[184]

The mechanism of integration is shared by other retroviruses.[218] The virus-encoded integrase forms a preintegration complex or "intasome" with the newly reverse-transcribed double-stranded DNA of the virus, the viral integrase makes a six base pair staggered cut in the host genome, and the free ends are ligated respectively to the 5′ and 3′ ends of the double-stranded viral DNA. The 6-nucleotide gap left at each end by the staggered cut in the genome is then filled in, generating a 6-base pair repeat flanking the integration provirus.

The abundant host phosphatase PP2A associates with the HTLV-1 integrase and participates in the process of proviral integration.[217] The tetrameric structure of the integrase of the closely related simian virus STLV-1, in complex with the B56g regulatory subunit of PP2A, has been determined by cryo-EM.[23] PP2A does not directly bind chromatin, and the molecular details of its cooperation with the integrase are not yet known. HTLV-1 also shows a bias toward integration into open chromatin near certain transcription factor binding sites, especially STAT-1, HDAC6, and TP53.[239]

Clonality of HTLV-1 and HTLV-2

A cardinal difference between HTLV-1 and HIV-1 lies in the direct impact of the virus on the infected T cell: HIV-1 expression usually kills the host cell, whereas HTLV-1 expression is nonlytic. This difference is reflected in the distinct modes of persistence of the viruses *in vivo*: while HIV-1 persists in the absence of antiretroviral therapy by constant *de novo* infection, HTLV-1 persists during the long chronic phase of infection chiefly by continued proliferation of clones of infected T

cells.[15,200] Each infected T-cell clone can be identified by the sequence of the host genome flanking the single-copy provirus; this sequence is shared by each cell in that clone.

In chronic infection, an equilibrium is established in each host between the immune response to the virus (see "Immune Response") and the number and abundance of HTLV-1–infected T cell clones (Fig. 16.10). At this equilibrium, a small number of infected clones can reach a high abundance in the peripheral blood: this phenomenon is known as oligoclonal expansion. Early, semiquantitative methods of detection (Southern blot and PCR-based protocols) could identify only the most abundant clones, and these techniques led to the misapprehension of two fundamental aspects. First, it appeared that oligoclonal expansion was associated with the inflammatory disease, and by implication might be involved in causing the inflammatory tissue damage. Second, the number of infected T-cell clones in each host was estimated at about 100.[394] The introduction of a sensitive high-throughput method to map and quantify the proviral integration sites[96] corrected these misunderstandings. First, the results showed that a typical host had over 10^4 distinct clones of HTLV-1–infected T cells. Second, the PVL, which is the strongest correlate of the risk of both the inflammatory and malignant diseases associated with HTLV-1, is proportional to the number of distinct clones present in the individual, not to the degree of oligoclonal expansion. The degree of oligoclonality, which is rigorously quantified by the oligoclonality index,[96] does not differ between patients with HAM and asymptomatic carriers. The oligoclonal expansion is more easily detected in samples from patients with HAM simply because of the greater absolute abundance of the largest clones in these individuals.

These observations show that the risk of HTLV-1–associated disease is correlated with the number of HTLV-1–infected clones, not to the degree of oligoclonal expansion. In ATL, one

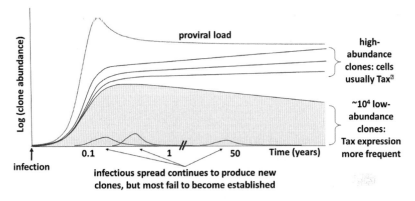

FIGURE 16.10 Schematic depiction of the dynamics of proviral load and clone abundance in one individual over time. The trajectory of the proviral load is inferred from data on the early stage of infection and the long-term stability of the load in the chronic stage of infection. Many HTLV-1–infected clones persist for years; the number of cells in each high-abundance clone (i.e., a clone that contains many sister cells) tends to increase progressively over time, whereas each low-abundance clone decreases in number; these changes result in a progressive rise in the oligoclonality index. Each infected cell expresses Tax in uncommon, intermittent bursts[32,221]: the frequency of expression appears to be greater in the low-abundance clones than in the high-abundance clones, perhaps owing to cytotoxic T-lymphocyte–mediated selection. The contribution of infectious spread to the maintenance of an individual's set point proviral load is not known. (Modified from Bangham CRM, Matsuoka M. Human T-cell leukaemia virus type 1: parasitism and pathogenesis. *Philos Trans R Soc Lond B Biol Sci* 2017;372(1732):20160272. https://creativecommons.org/licenses/by/4.0/.)

or more clones undergo malignant transformation, and the oligoclonality index quickly exceeds the normal range.[302]

Although HTLV-1 persists in the chronic phase mainly by mitotic spread—proliferation of existing clones—there are two reasons why infectious spread of the virus must continue throughout the infection. First, the immune response is persistently activated, indicating constant synthesis of viral antigens. Second, the virus itself does not change between the primary infection and the persistent phase. Longitudinal data on clonal abundance in individuals with nonmalignant infection indicate that, in the chronic phase, mitotic spread exceeds infectious spread by at least 10^7 to 1.[200] But since the number of CD4$^+$ T cells in the body is very large, on average it can be estimated that about 5×10^9 new infected cells are produced per day, of which between 100 and 200 result from *de novo* infection, and the remainder from mitotic proliferation of existing clones.[200] Thus, in a typical infected individual, an average of 6×10^5 new clones are created over 10 years. Since the infection (in nonmalignant cases) is in quasi-equilibrium, and the oligoclonality index and PVL change slowly (if at all) over time, this figure implies that an approximately equal number of clones must be destroyed over the same period, either by the immune response (see "Immune Response") or by being out-competed by faster-growing clones. Many newly infected cells are likely to fail to establish a long-lived clone. However, some newly created clones may become established, if they possess a strong growth or survival advantage.

Whereas mitotic spread of HTLV-1 dominates during the chronic phase of infection, infectious spread must have been abundant during the early phase, to establish the large number of infected clones observed in each host (Fig. 16.10). In the early stages of infection in recipients of solid organ transplants from HTLV-1–infected individuals, the PVL can double in 1.4 days,[51] leading to a 1,000-fold increase in the PVL within 14 days, but the ratio of mitotic to infectious spread at this stage has not been measured.

By contrast with HTLV-1, HTLV-2—which infects virtually only CD8$^+$ T cells *in vivo*—generates a much smaller number of clones of infected host cells in the steady-state chronic infection.[240] As in HTLV-1 infection, the infected T-cell clones are long-lived and stable. Each infected clone, however, can reach a high abundance in the circulation. The resulting high value of the oligoclonality index[96] in HTLV-2 does not carry the same implications for disease as in HTLV-1, because HTLV-2 does not cause malignant disease.

Site of Replication and Spread

After transmission by breast milk, sexual contact, or blood transfusion, HTLV-1 infects DCs and T cells *in vivo* and spreads through cell-to-cell contact. HTLV-1–infected cells proliferate and spread in the body. In experimentally infected squirrel monkeys (*Saimiri sciureus*), the HTLV-1 provirus was detected first in peripheral blood mononuclear cells (PBMCs) and then in lymphoid organs including lymph node, spleen, and bone marrow.[176] This shows that HTLV-1 spreads in lymphoid tissues. In HTLV-1–infected individuals, bone marrow has been identified as a reservoir of HTLV-1.[208] The identification of the HTLV-1 provirus integrated in precisely the same genomic site in different hematopoietic cell types[81] suggests that hematopoietic stem cells can be infected with HTLV-1.

HTLV-1 virions cannot be detected in HTLV-1–infected individuals. Instead, HTLV-1–infected cells proliferate *in vivo*: HTLV-1 copy number increases by mitosis of infected cells, while HTLV remains in the form of a provirus integrated in the host genome. Expression of adhesion molecules, including ICAM-1 and LFA-1, is up-regulated on HTLV-1–infected cells.[76] In HAM/TSP patients and HTLV-1 carriers, infected cells not only circulate in the blood but also infiltrate into the skin, lung, and intestine. Thus, HTLV-1–infected cells persist and spread *in vivo*. If infected cells have proinflammatory properties, their proliferation and activation might induce inflammatory diseases.

Proviral Load: Correlation With Disease

HTLV-1 infection is almost wholly intracellular, and most infected T cells *in vivo* do not express the provirus at a given instant, so the appropriate measure of the viral burden is the PVL, the average number of proviral copies per 100 PBMCs. Since the great majority of infected cells carry a single copy of the provirus,[53] the PVL may be approximated by the percentage of infected PBMCs.

The PVL is the strongest correlate of the risk of both the inflammatory disease HAM[260] and the malignant disease ATL[145] caused by HTLV-1. The PVL reaches a steady state value or fixed point in each infected individual: this value can fluctuate by about fivefold over time within the individual host[236] but typically does not progress unless ATL supervenes. But the PVL set point can differ between infected people by several orders of magnitude.[260] What determines a person's set point PVL? Since the virus varies little in sequence between individuals, and there is wide variation in the PVL between hosts infected with an identical virus, this variation is attributable to differences in the host, rather than the virus. Further, since the PVL in a given individual usually returns to the same set point after perturbation by drug treatment, the set point is likely to be determined at least in part by genetic mechanisms. The highly polymorphic gene complexes of the major histocompatibility complex (human leukocyte antigen [HLA]) and the killer immunoglobulin-like receptors (KIRs) play a significant part in determining a person's PVL set point[151,318] (see "Immune Response"). However, these genetic effects account for only a fraction of the observed variation between people in the PVL of HTLV-1[318]; it is likely that the remaining variation is due to the additive effects of many genetic polymorphisms in the host, each polymorphism contributing a small proportion to the total observed variation.

The reasons for the strong correlation observed between PVL and the risk of ATL are not known with certainty, but two factors are likely to contribute. First, the PVL is correlated with the number of different clones of HTLV-1–infected T cell,[96] and the probability that one or more clones accumulates replicative mutations that lead to malignant transformation is likely to rise in proportion. Second, a high PVL results partly from an inefficient T-cell–mediated immune response to the virus[18]; this inefficient response will also reduce the rate at which HTLV-1–expressing cells are killed *in vivo*, so enhancing the survival of potentially malignant clones.

The reasons for the observed correlation between the PVL and the risk of HAM are discussed below (see "Pathogenesis of Inflammatory Diseases").

Immune Response

Innate Immune Response

Primary infection with HTLV-1 is asymptomatic, and consequently it has not been possible to study the impact of the innate immune response in the early stages of infection. However, certain components of the innate immune response have been shown to affect the virus even during chronic infection. The cytidine deaminase APOBEC3G, which plays a significant part in HIV-1 infection, produces uncommon mutations in the plus strand of the provirus of HTLV-1.[70] A clone carrying such mutations may survive indefinitely, because the *HBZ* gene, which is necessary for clonal survival, is encoded on the minus strand of the provirus and so is not mutated by the APOBEC3G. The contribution of cytokines to both the innate and the acquired immune response is diminished by the HTLV-1 Tax protein, which induces the expression of the gene SOCS1, which encodes a suppressor of cytokine signaling.[44,281] The deoxynucleotide triphosphate (dNTP) triphosphohydrolase SAMHD1 again has important activity against certain lentiviruses.[98] The enzyme acts by depleting the intracellular concentration of dNTPs, thereby inhibiting viral replication. SAMHD1 limits HTLV-1 replication in macrophages,[348] resulting in apoptosis induced by STING. However, since the macrophage carries a very small proportion of the HTLV-1 PVL, the importance of SAMHD1 in HTLV-1 infection is limited.

Type 1 interferons can suppress HTLV-1 in replication both *in vitro* and *in vivo*.[160,183] However, the impact of type 1 interferon in natural infection is limited by two factors. First, Tax protein inhibits the kinase TBK1,[418] which normally phosphorylates the interferon regulatory factor IRF3, so diminishing interferon production. Second, the induction of SOCS1 may reduce the impact of interferon-induced cytokines.

While type 1 interferon alone has little impact on HTLV-1 infection *in vivo*, sustained treatment with a combination of IFNα and the nucleoside analogue AZT has been shown to prevent the progression of ATL in certain cases[28]; see Treatment.

The three main cell types in the innate immune response to viruses are the dendritic cell (DC), the natural killer (NK) cell, and the regulatory T cell (Treg). DCs can be infected with HTLV-1,[149,159,193,214] and these cells may play a significant part in the earliest stage of the acquisition of the infection. HTLV-1–infected DCs can immortalize CD4+ T cells, indicating that DCs can transmit the virus to CD4+ T cells. DCs can also infect other cells through the virological synapse.[27] Cell-free HTLV-1 infection of DCs has been demonstrated *in vitro*: this process is enhanced by DC-specific ICAM-3–grabbing nonintegrin (DC-SIGN), which interacts with ICAM-2 and ICAM-3 but not HTLV-1 Env. However, since infectious cell-free HTLV-1 virions are rare or absent *in vivo*, the physiological importance of cell-free infection is doubtful. HSPG and NRP-1 are involved in the transfer of HTLV-1 from DCs to CD4+ T cells.

DCs are also the most important producer of type 1 interferons. The small numbers of DCs compared with T cells in both the circulation and the tissues may limit the importance of this cell type during chronic infection. However, DCs efficiently elicit a cytotoxic T-lymphocyte response, and DCs treated with HTLV-1 Tax peptides can elicit a CTL response that causes at least a temporary reduction in the PVL of HTLV-1 in both rats[7] and humans.[339]

The role of the NK cell in HTLV-1 infection is also poorly understood. Both NK and NK-T cells are reduced in frequency in the blood in HTLV-1 infection,[75,304,417] especially in patients with HAM, but the importance of this phenomenon is unknown.

HTLV-1 induces the expression of the transcription factor FoxP3, which is characteristic of Tregs[312]; in addition, infected cells frequently express the surface markers CD25, GITR, CTLA4, and CCR4 that are also found on Tregs. These molecules are also frequently expressed in ATL clones: FoxP3 is found in approximately 36% of cases.[167] However, HTLV-1–infected FoxP3+ cells lack regulatory function,[5,370] so the infected cell is not a true regulatory T cell, and ATL is not necessarily a tumor of Tregs.[371] HTLV-1 also induces expression of the chemokine CCL22,[120,372] which binds the receptor CCR4 that is found on true Tregs. By this means, HTLV-1 maintains a high frequency of CCR4+ cells in the host, which have Treg function. This may represent an adaptation by the virus to reduce the efficacy of the cell-mediated immune response, thereby favoring its persistence in the host.

Acquired Immune Response

Antibody response

In primary infection, antibodies to the core (Gag) protein of HTLV-1 are the first to appear, and they predominate the first 2 months.[230] Antibodies to Env appear later, and finally antibodies to the Tax protein are detected in about 50% of individuals.[230,256] The titre of HTLV-1–specific antibodies can reach very high levels in chronic infection, consistent with the notion that viral antigen synthesis persists indefinitely *in vivo*. It is likely that a high titre of HTLV-1–specific antibody simply results from a high PVL. But the role of antibody in either protection against infection or the pathogenesis of the associated diseases remains uncertain. Passively transferred antibody can inhibit milk-borne transmission of HTLV-1 in rabbits[315] and *in vitro* infection of cord blood lymphocytes by co-culture with HTLV-1–infected cells can be prevented by HTLV-1 seropositive plasma from cord blood.[352] However, there is no strong evidence that antibodies provide effective protection against HTLV-1 infection in the human.

Cell-mediated immune response

HTLV-1 infection elicits a strong cell-mediated immune response, with abundant circulating CD8+ (cytotoxic) T lymphocytes (CTLs)[148,290] and CD4+ (helper) T cells[100] specific to the viral antigens. Activated CTLs kill virus-infected, MHC-matched target cells. By contrast, memory CTLs, which persist for months or years following an active infection, are not directly cytolytic but require reexposure to their cognate viral antigen to restimulate the cell and render it capable of cell-mediated killing. However, CTLs isolated from the peripheral blood of a person with nonmalignant HTLV-1 infection—both patients with HAM and asymptomatic carriers—can kill HLA-matched HTLV-1–infected target cells immediately *ex vivo*.[112,290] This observation implied that HTLV-1 antigens are frequently expressed *in vivo*: the implications for the understanding of the regulation of HTLV-1 latency are discussed in Clonality of HTLV-1 and HTLV-2.

The HTLV-1 Tax protein is highly immunodominant in the CTL response to the virus[99,148,162]; activated CTLs specific to Gag and Pol are also frequently detectable in freshly isolated PBMCs.

CTLs are usually necessary to eradicate a transient virus from the body: in the absence of CTLs, a normally short-lived virus becomes persistent. CTLs also play a central part in limiting the replication of persistent viruses, such as Epstein-Barr virus or cytomegalovirus. Evidence that CTLs determine the outcome of HTLV-1 infection came from immunogenetic studies of a population with endemic HTLV-1 infection in Japan.[151,392] In this population, individuals carrying either of the class 1 HLA genes *HLA-A*02* or *HLA-Cw*08* had a significant reduction in both the PVL and the risk of HAM[151] compared with those who lacked both these alleles. Since class HLA proteins determine the specificity and activity of CTLs, these observations show that the genetically determined efficiency or "quality" of the HTLV-1–specific CTL response limits HTLV-1 replication *in vivo*.[18,277] Calculation of the prevented fraction of disease shows that the HLA class 1 protective effect prevents about 50% of potential cases of HAM in this population in southern Japan.[151]

Further evidence of the protective role of CTLs came from two observations. First, heterozygosity in HLA class 1 genes, which is associated with a broader antigenic repertoire of CTLs, is associated with a lower PVL in the southern Japanese population.[151] Second, it was discovered that inhibitory genes of the KIR complex enhance the effectiveness of the CTL response to persistent viruses. This effect was discovered in HTLV-1 infection and then generalized to hepatitis C virus and HIV-1 infections.[36,318]

Because Tax is the dominant target antigen recognized by the abundant, chronically activated HTLV-1–specific CTLs present in the circulation, it was natural to assume that the anti-Tax CTL response restricted by the common allele *HLA-A*0201* was critical in this protective response. However, Boelen et al.[36] showed that the protective effect of the A*02-restricted CTLs was effected via the *HLA-A*0207* allele, not the more frequent *HLA*-A*0201 allele.

The most important determinant of the PVL and the risk of HAM is the CTL response not to the immunodominant Tax protein, but rather to the HBZ protein.[123,215,341] This observation is counterintuitive, because HBZ is a weak CTL antigen, and is expressed at a very low level in the infected cell. However, it is now known that whereas each HTLV-1–infected cell expresses *tax* in uncommon, intermittent bursts,[32,221] it expresses *HBZ* about 50% of the time.[243] Further, *HBZ* expression is required for clonal persistence *in vivo*.[359] It appears that HTLV-1 has evolved to limit the expression of this critical gene to the minimal level required for survival *in vivo*, while minimizing its exposure to immune surveillance.

In addition to the intermittent plus-strand expression and the low level and low immunogenicity of the HBZ protein, HTLV-1 uses further tactics that may contribute to immune evasion. First, the HTLV-1 accessory protein p12, which is expressed by some strains of HTLV-1, physically interacts with the free human MHC class I heavy chain and induces its degradation,[157] facilitating the escape of HTLV-1–infected cells from destruction by CTLs. Second, Tax induces the production of CCL22 by infected T cells,[372] which maintains a higher frequency of circulating FoxP3+ Tregs; in turn, the high FoxP3+ Treg frequency is correlated with reduced efficiency of CTL-mediated killing of HTLV-1–infected cells by CTLs.[370]

Study of the helper T-cell response to HTLV-1 is complicated by the fact that it is the dominant host cell for the virus, and expression of the virus alters the function of the infected cell. However, a short-term ELISpot assay made it possible to distinguish between activation of the cell by exogenous viral antigen from activation by the expression of Tax inside the cell.[100,101] The results show that the frequency of HTLV-1–specific CD4+ T cells was significantly higher in patients with HAM than in asymptomatic carriers with a similar PVL.[100] Two further observations corroborate the implication that CD4+ T cells play a part in the pathogenesis of HAM. First, these cells predominate in the early stage of the inflammatory lesion in the central nervous system.[377] Second, the class 2 MHC allele *DRB1*0101* is associated with a higher risk of HAM.[151,185,273,337,382]

Immunodeficiency and HTLV-1-Associated Diseases

Thus, the host immune system controls the dynamics of HTLV-1 infection and the development of disease. This idea is supported by the clinical observation that ATL occurs more commonly in immunocompromised hosts. Among 24 patients with posttransplantation lymphoproliferative disorders (PTLPDs) after renal transplantation in Japan, five ATL cases were reported.[133] In these cases, HTLV-1 was probably transmitted by blood transfusion during hemodialysis. Of eight HTLV-1 carriers who received living-donor liver transplants and subsequent immunosuppressive treatment, three developed ATL.[174] These findings indicate that the host immune system commonly suppresses the development of ATL, while an impaired immune system may allow HTLV-1–infected cells to transform into ATL cells.

The impairment of cell-mediated immunity is profound in ATL patients, who frequently succumb to opportunistic infections with various pathogens, including various fungi, cytomegalovirus, *Pneumocystis jirovecii*, and mycobacteria.[355] Thus, immune impairment is both a cause and a consequence of ATL.

Individuals with nonmalignant HTLV-1 infection, both asymptomatic and those with inflammatory diseases such as HAM, also show a degree of impairment of cell-mediated immunity, as evidenced by a higher incidence of a range of opportunistic infections and malignancies.[317] The associated infections include severe *Strongyloides stercoralis* infection[390]; tuberculosis[389]; infective dermatitis[33]; bronchiectasis[67]; and infections of the lung, kidney, and bladder.[317] The associated malignant diseases include liver cancer, cervical cancer, and lymphoma (distinct from ATL).[317]

Within-Host Evolution: Selection *In vivo*

In a persistent infection, the immune response exerts a strong selection pressure on the infectious agent, which in turn develops adaptations that lessen its susceptibility to immune-mediated destruction. In HTLV-1 infection, the strong CTL response (see "Immune Response") selects immune escape variants,[270,271] but the inability of HTLV-1 to tolerate major sequence change limits the outgrowth of such variant sequences. Instead of immune escape, HTLV-1 relies more for its persistence *in vivo* on the regulation of its transcriptional latency (see "Clonality of HTLV-1 and HTLV-2") to minimize its exposure to the immune system.

Each clone of infected T cells possesses characteristics of HTLV-1 expression that depend in part on the genomic integration site of the provirus.[37,289] Consequently, there is selection in the host for the survival of HTLV-1–infected clones with particular characteristics, which are only beginning to be understood. Initial integration of HTLV-1 occurs in each chromosome in proportion to the size of the chromosome, but survival of that clone *in vivo* is favored if the provirus is integrated in one of the acrocentric chromosomes, especially chromosome 13.[52] It is possible that this selective survival is associated with the intranuclear location of acrocentric chromosomes, which are characteristically found during interphase at the periphery of the nucleolus, which is a transcriptionally repressive region.

Expression of the *tax* gene is lost in the malignant clone in approximately 60% of cases of ATL.[356] Three mechanisms by which *tax* expression was disrupted were identified: (a) deletion of the 5′LTR,[246,358] (b) DNA methylation of the 5′LTR,[188,360] and (c) genetic changes in the *tax* gene (nonsense mutations, deletion, and insertion).[70,79] In all cases, the pX region and the 3′LTR remained intact, suggesting the importance of the *HBZ* gene in the survival of the malignant clone.

Analysis of whole HTLV-1 proviruses in ATL cells shows that all the viral genes can contain nonsense mutations except the *HBZ* gene.[70] Most nonsense mutations were generated in a tryptophan codon (TGG) by G-to-A mutation (TGG to TGA, or TGG to TAG). The sequences of these G-to-A mutations in HTLV-1 proviruses correspond to the target sequences of APOBEC3G.[70] APOBEC3G is a host factor that generates G-to-A mutations during reverse transcription. In the case of HIV-1, an accessory protein, Vif, promotes the degradation of APOBEC3G, which enables HIV-1 to escape fatal nonsense mutations. By contrast, HTLV-1 does not encode an accessory gene that counteracts APOBEC3G. The Gag protein of HTLV-1 suppresses the incorporation of APOBEC3G into the virion,[61] but this inhibitory activity is not strong enough to completely suppress all G-to-A mutations.[308] If nonsense mutations are generated in viral genes that are not essential for cellular proliferation, HTLV-1–infected cells can still proliferate and transform to leukemic cells. This result indicates that nonsense mutations of all viral genes except the *HBZ* gene can be generated before integration and ATL can still ensue, suggesting that *HBZ* is an essential gene for leukemogenesis.

Pathogenesis of ATL

HTLV-1 infection is a necessary cause of ATL, but it is not sufficient: the lifetime risk of ATL in HTLV-1–infected people is about 5%,[142] and the disease usually presents clinically after several decades of HTLV-1 infection. The median age at diagnosis is between 40 and 50 years in the Caribbean and South America.[128] In Japan, the median age at presentation has risen progressively from 56.9 years in the mid-1980s to 67.5 years in 2020,[144] suggesting that a cohort of the population developed a high prevalence of HTLV-1 infection in the 1920s and 1930s.

Two broad types of oncogenic mechanism must be considered in ATL: first, insertional mutagenesis, and second, transactivation by viral gene products. HTLV-1 usually infects approximately 10^4 clones in each individual host; in some cases, this number exceeds 10^6.[199] Since each clone contains a provirus in a unique genomic location, the potential for insertional mutagenesis is great. The provirus may disrupt host gene expression *in cis* in three ways. First, if the provirus is inserted inside a host gene, the resulting disruption of gene expression may be oncogenic, if the gene acts as a tumor suppressor. However, there is no evidence of this mechanism in ATL. Second, the provirus can deregulate host transcription immediately adjacent to the integration site.[241] Third, the provirus can alter the pattern of chromatin looping of the host genome. HTLV-1 binds the zinc finger protein CTCF,[311] which plays a central part in forming the chromatin loops that regulate the structure and expression of the genome.[294] CTCF binds to a DNA motif of approximately 20 nucleotides at approximately 50,000 sites in the human genome. By dimerizing with CTCF bound to a nearby site in the host chromatin, HTLV-1–bound CTCF brings the provirus near host genes that are distant (up to several Mb) from the integration site in the linear genome and can alter host transcription at these distant sites.[241]

Which of these three types of proviral mutagenesis might contribute to the oncogenesis of ATL? There are no hotspots of HTLV-1 integration in the host genome in ATL,[52] so direct insertional mutagenesis of host genes is not a major cause of ATL. However, integration within 10 kb upstream of a group of 11 host genes was significantly overrepresented in a study of 197 ATL cases, accounting for 6% of the cases.[52] These 11 genes are associated with three ontological categories: cell morphology, immune cell trafficking, and hematological system development and function, and they have been implicated in other malignancies. Thus, deregulation of nearby host genes by the provirus may contribute to oncogenesis in some cases. It is not yet known whether the observed deregulation of more distant host genes *in cis* that are brought into proximity by CTCF-mediated chromatin looping also plays a part in ATL oncogenesis.

Most attention in the study of ATL oncogenesis has been focused on the two chief regulatory genes of HTLV-1, *tax* and *HBZ*, because the products of these genes exert profound diverse effects on gene expression and function of the host cell (see "Tax and Rex: Main Physiological Actions"). Transgenic mice expressing either *tax* or *HBZ* develop tumors, and *tax* can immortalize T cells *in vitro*. However, neither *tax* nor *HBZ* is an acutely transforming oncogene such as *myc*, *ras*, or *src*. Further, as mentioned, *tax* is expressed in each infected cell in uncommon, intermittent bursts.[32,221] In approximately 25% of ATL cases, Tax expression is disabled by nonsense mutations of the *tax* gene or loss of the 5′ LTR at the time of HTLV-1 infection.[356] These ATL cells are transformed and persist without Tax; they depend on HBZ expression. In approximately 50% of ATL cases, Tax is transiently expressed: these ATL cells depend on both Tax and HBZ. Taken together, these findings indicate two different types of requirement for viral genes for leukemogenesis in ATL: one is HBZ dependent, and the other type needs both Tax and HBZ.[274]

Kataoka et al.[170] identified the host genes that are most commonly mutated in ATL, in a study of 426 cases. The most frequent mutations were found in genes (including *PLCG1*, *PRKCB*, *CARD11*, etc.) that participate in pathways highly active in T cells, including T-cell receptor–NF-κB signaling and T-cell trafficking. These putative oncogenic driver mutations can be detected in the circulation in some cases several years before clinical presentation.[301] The mutational burden in infected T cells 1 year before diagnosis of ATL is significantly greater than in age-matched HTLV-1 carriers who remained healthy during 10 years of follow-up.[301]

These observations suggest that the dominant mechanism of oncogenesis in ATL is the accumulation of replicative mutations due to the continued proliferation of HTLV-1–infected T-cell clones over many years. The risk of oncogenesis in a given cell type is proportional to the total number of cell divisions that a given cell lineage has undergone.[367,368] HTLV-1–infected T-cell clones typically survive indefinitely[96] and proliferate faster than uninfected T cells.[15] While specific actions of *tax* and *HBZ* (see "Tax and Rex: Main Physiological Actions") may exacerbate the risk of malignant transformation, their fundamental function is to promote the survival and transmission of the virus by maintaining the longevity of the infected T-cell clone. Thus, their chief contribution to oncogenesis is indirect, by promoting the accumulation of replicative mutations in long-lived clones.[21]

Pathogenesis of Inflammatory Diseases

Up to 5% of HTLV-1–infected people develop a chronic inflammatory disease. The most frequently diagnosed of these conditions is HAM[20] (see 'History of HAM' above). HTLV-1 also causes chronic inflammatory conditions in many other tissues, in particular uveitis,[248] infective dermatitis,[201] polymyositis,[252] and bronchiectasis,[67] which also has an infective component in its pathogenesis.

The risk of these inflammatory diseases is strongly correlated with the PVL of HTLV-1.[260,317] Certain strains of HTLV-1 are associated with a slightly higher risk of HAM in Japan,[78] but the bulk of the variation in individual risk is attributable to the host. The reason for the correlation between PVL and the risk of HAM is likely to be the less efficient cytotoxic T-cell response to HTLV-1 in these individuals[18] (see "Immune Response"), which is associated with both a higher PVL, a higher risk of HAM[151] and a greater number of HTLV-1–expressing cells at a given time.[14]

Helper (CD4+) T cells predominate in early lesions of HAM.[143,147,377] As the disease progresses, the proportion of CD8+ T cells in the lesion increases. It is not understood what initiates the infiltration of T cells across the blood–brain barrier or into other tissues. However, HTLV-1 Tax induces strong expression of ICAM-1, which increases the adhesion and migration of T cells across epithelial barriers. In HAM, a mechanism of self-perpetuating inflammation has been proposed.[6] The secretion of IFNγ by T cells stimulates the secretion by astrocytes of the chemokine CXCL10 (IP-10), which attracts more T cells that express the cognate receptor CXCR3. It is not known whether a similar mechanism operates in the other inflammatory conditions associated with HTLV-1.

The mechanism of tissue damage is not known with certainty. There is no convincing evidence that the resident cells in the inflamed tissues are themselves infected with HTLV-1, and antibodies that cross-react between Tax protein and a self-antigen[209] are not specific to HAM.[419] The cell damage is thought to be caused by inflammatory substances, in particular IFNγ, secreted by the invading T cells. HTLV-1–infected CD4+ T cells express high levels of IFNγ,[111] and the frequency of IFNγ+CD4+ T cells is especially high in patients with HAM.[100] In mature lesions in HAM, it is likely that the invading CD8+ T cells contribute further inflammatory substances such as IFNγ and TNFα.

EPIDEMIOLOGY

Age

A high risk of mother-to-child transmission is associated with prolonged breast-feeding (>12 months), a high PVL (>1% PBMCs) and seropositivity in more than one child of the same mother.[287] In adults, HTLV-1 seroprevalence rises with age, and the seropositivity rate in females is higher than that in males,[34] because sexual transmission of this virus is more efficient from male to female than from female to male.[134,338] Sexual transmission may occur even in old HTLV-1 discordant couples, which can account for the continuous increase in seropositivity rate in the older population. As mentioned, the average age of ATL patients at diagnosis was 63 years in Japan, which is 15 years older than the average age of ATL patients at presentation in the Caribbean islands,[355] suggesting that genetic background or environmental factors—or both—influence the development of ATL. The mean age at onset of HAM/TSP patients in Japan was 43 years.[283] In addition, HAM/TSP can develop within a few months after infection,[369] whereas ATL typically develops after a long clinically latent period in nonimmunosuppressed individuals.

Morbidity/Mortality

HTLV-1 establishes a persistent infection. There are geographical differences in the incidences of these HTLV-1–associated diseases.[128] The cumulative lifetime risk of ATL among HTLV-1 carriers in Japan is about 6.6% for men and 2.1% for women; most HTLV-1 carriers remain asymptomatic throughout their lives.[11] By contrast, the risk of ATL is four times lower in Jamaicans. The lifetime risk of HAM/TSP in HTLV-1 carriers has been estimated as 0.25% in southern Japan,[166] but the risk in populations of Afro-Caribbean descent is about 10 times greater (1.9% to 3.7%).[226,282] The reasons for these surprisingly large differences between populations in the risk of ATL and HAM/TSP are not well understood. In addition to ATL and HAM/TSP, HTLV-1 is associated with a significantly increased risk of a wide range of diseases,[317] especially seborrheic dermatitis, Sjögren syndrome, and lung disease (bronchiectasis, bronchitis, and bronchiolitis). HTLV-1 infection also predisposes to a number of infections with other pathogens, notably TB and *Strongyloides stercoralis*, and to infections of the kidney and bladder. Finally, the risk of liver cancer, cervical cancer, and lymphoma (other than ATL) is greater in HTLV-1–seropositive persons, but the risk of gastric cancer is reduced. The adjusted risk of death from any cause is approximately 1.57 times higher in HTLV-1–infected individuals than in seronegative individuals.[317]

Origin and Spread of Epidemics

HTLV and STLV are thought to originate from common ancestors and share molecular, virological, and epidemiological features. Therefore, they have been designated primate T-cell leukemia viruses (PTLVs). Phylogenetic analyses have revealed that HTLV-1c first diverged from STLV around 50,000 ± 10,000 years ago, while the spread of HTLV-1 in Africa is estimated to have occurred at least 27,300 ± 8,200 years ago. Subsequently, HTLV-1a, which is the most common subtype in Japan, diverged from the African strain 12,300 ± 4,900 years ago.[384] Thus, these viruses have had a long history with humans after the initial interspecies transmission. By contrast, HIV-1 is thought to originate from simian immunodeficiency virus in chimpanzees (SIV$_{CPZ}$),[82] and the interspecies transmission to humans is estimated to have occurred about one hundred years ago.[399] Recently, new retroviruses have been identified in bushmeat hunters in central Africa. HTLV-3 has been found in asymptomatic carriers in Cameroon.[40,398] HTLV-3 is highly homologous to its simian counterpart, STLV-3, which was detected in monkeys in Africa. The genome organization of HTLV-3 is similar to HTLV-1.[222] No diseases have been reported to be associated with HTLV-3.

Prevalence and Seroepidemiology

It is estimated that at least 5 to 10 million people live with HTLV-1 worldwide.[89] However, this number remains highly uncertain, because systematic epidemiological studies have not been carried out in some regions endemic for the virus. The chief known endemic areas are southwestern Japan, the Caribbean basins, Central and West Africa, and South America. In addition, epidemiological studies of HTLV-1 have revealed high seroprevalence rates in Melanesia, Papua New Guinea, and the Solomon islands, as well as among Australian aborigines.[34,68] In Japan, approximately 1.08 million individuals were estimated to be infected with HTLV-1 in 2009, and among them, 1,000 carriers develop ATL each year. The rate of mother-to-child transmission of HTLV-1 in Japan has declined, following the introduction of a nationwide policy of discouraging breast-feeding by seropositive mothers. However, the rate of sexual transmission among adolescents and adults has maintained the annual number of new cases of infection at >4000.[309]

The epidemiology of HTLV-2 is quite distinct.[108] The main populations where HTLV-2 is endemic are in North America, where it is prevalent in certain Native American groups and intravenous drug user groups,[259] and in Brazil.[69] The total number of people infected with HTLV-2 in the world is estimated to be 6- to 12-fold lower than the number infected with HTLV-1,[259] although as in HTLV-1, this estimate is somewhat uncertain, because many areas have not been systematically studied.

Genetic Diversity of HTLV-1

Several subtypes of HTLV-1 have been identified: the cosmopolitan HTLV-1a subtype[244]; the Central African subtypes HTLV-1b,[105,386] HTLV-1d,[225] HTLV-1e,[334] and HTLV-1f[307]; and the Australo-Melanesian subtype HTLV-1c.[91,324] These subtypes are closely linked with interspecies transmission and human migration events. The sequence of HTLV-1 does not differ systematically between asymptomatic carriers and those with ATL or HAM/TSP,[55] although small differences in the risk of HAM/TSP have been associated with certain genotypes.[78]

CLINICAL FEATURES

During chronic infection with HTLV-1, the PVL remains relatively constant within an individual but can differ between infected individuals by over 1,000-fold. Most individuals remain asymptomatic during their entire lives, while a small fraction of carriers develop either ATL or one of the HTLV-1–associated inflammatory diseases (Fig. 16.11) ([317]; see "Morbidity/Mortality").

ATL

ATL develops more frequently in males (the male to female ratio is 1.5:1). The age at onset ranges from 25 to 94 years. The predominant physical findings are peripheral lymph node enlargement (72% of cases), hepatomegaly (47%), splenomegaly (25%), and skin lesions (53%).[355] ATL cells infiltrate into various organs/tissues, including skin, liver, lung, the gastrointestinal tract, the central nervous system, and bone. Various skin lesions, such as papules, erythema, and nodules are

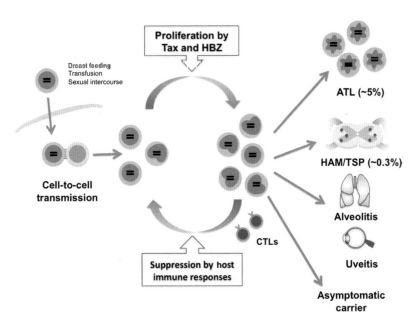

FIGURE 16.11 The natural course of HTLV-1 infection. After transmission of HTLV-1, infected cells proliferate owing to the actions of HBZ and Tax. The growth of HTLV-1–infected cells is suppressed by cytotoxic T lymphocytes *in vivo*. The number of HTLV-1–infected cells is thus determined by balance between viral gene expression and the host immune system. About 5% of HTLV carriers develop adult T-cell leukemia after a long latent period. A smaller fraction of carriers present with inflammatory diseases, such as HTLV-1–associated myelopathy/tropical spastic paraparesis (HAM/TSP), uveitis, or alveolitis. Most carriers remain asymptomatic.

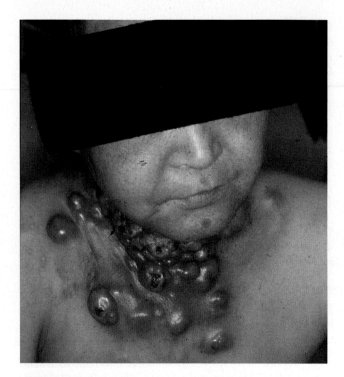

FIGURE 16.12 Skin lesion of an adult T-cell leukemia (ATL) patient. ATL cells frequently involve skin and form various lesions. In this patient, ATL cells form a tumor lesion.

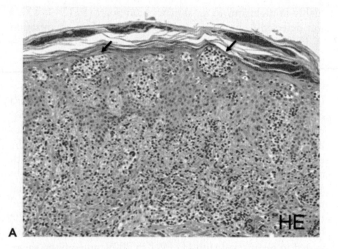

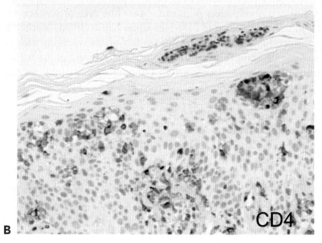

FIGURE 16.13 Skin involvement of adult T-cell leukemia (ATL). A: ATL cells infiltrate into epidermis and form Pautrier microabscesses (*arrows*). **B:** CD4+ cells are identified by the immunohistochemical staining.

frequently observed in ATL patients (Fig. 16.12). ATL cells densely infiltrate the dermis and epidermis, forming Pautrier microabscesses in the epidermis (Fig. 16.13).

ATL cells in the peripheral blood have characteristic indented or lobulated nuclei (Fig. 16.14): such cells are known as "flower cells." Anemia and thrombocytopenia are rare since involvement of bone marrow is not severe. The typical surface phenotype of ATL cells is CD4+CD8-CD25+, which is similar to that of Treg cells. ATL cells frequently express FoxP3[168] (Fig. 16.15) and other markers characteristic of Treg cells or activated T cells; however, the phenotype is somewhat variable, and ATL should not be regarded as a tumor of Treg cells.[371] ATL cells often express CD25 (IL-2 receptor alpha chain) on the cell surface and secrete its soluble form; consequently, the concentration of soluble IL-2 receptor is abnormally high in ATL and is correlated with the tumor mass and clinical course.[409] ATL cells elaborate various cytokines that can affect the immune response and influence the pathophysiology of ATL. For example, eosinophilia, caused by elevated IL-5 levels, is frequently observed in patients with ATL.

Hypercalcemia is a complication in about 70% of ATL patients at some point during the clinical course of the disease, particularly during the aggressive stage.[186] Pathological studies of ATL patients with hypercalcemia have shown that high serum Ca^{2+} levels are due to an increased number of osteoclasts and accelerated bone resorption (Fig. 16.16). During differentiation of osteoclasts, precursor cells sequentially express c-Fms (the receptor for M-CSF) followed by receptor activator nuclear factor kB (RANK).[9] M-CSF and RANK ligand (RANKL) have been shown to be critical factors for the differentiation of osteoclasts and are physiologically produced by stromal cells and osteoblasts. ATL cells from patients with hypercalcemia have

high RANKL transcript levels and induce the differentiation of hematopoietic stem cells into osteoclasts *in vitro* in the presence of M-CSF.[275] In addition, parathyroid hormone–related protein (PTH-rP) elaborated from ATL cells activates osteoclasts and promotes bone resorption.[393]

HTLV-1–Associated Myelopathy/Tropical Spastic Paraparesis (HAM/TSP)

HAM/TSP is characterized by a slow progressive spastic paraparesis, urinary dysfunction, and sensory disturbances.[20,283] HAM/TSP patients also often have other organ disorders such as leukoencephalopathy (69%), abnormal findings on chest X-ray (50%), Sjögren syndrome (25%), and arthropathy (17%).[262] In contrast to ATL, HAM/TSP develops predominantly in females (the male to female ratio is 1:2.9).

Pathological studies of HAM/TSP patients demonstrate severe involvement of the thoracic spinal cord, in which T cells cause perivascular cuffing and infiltrate into the parenchyma.[283] In HAM/TSP, the PVL is typically higher than in asymptomatic carriers,[260] and HTLV-1–infected CD4+ T cells infiltrate into the spinal cord.[42,234,254] The number of HTLV-1–specific

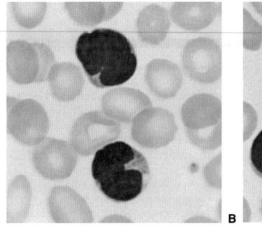
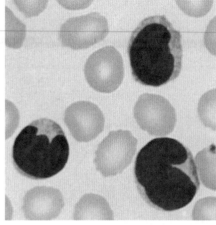

FIGURE 16.14 Adult T-cell leukemia (ATL) cells in the peripheral blood. A and B: ATL cells in an acute ATL case show the characteristic morphology.

HLA class I restricted CD8+ T cells is also increased in HAM/TSP patients,[22] Among viral antigens, Tax has a dominant epitope that is recognized by CTLs.[99,162] Tax-reacting CD8+ T cells also migrate into the spinal cord along with HTLV-1–infected CD4+ T cells.[378] These HTLV-1–infected cells and reacting CTLs produce proinflammatory cytokines (TNFα, IFNγ, IL-1β), leading to demyelination and axonal damage.

HTLV-1 Uveitis

HTLV-1 infection induces uveitis, an inflammatory disorder of the intraocular tissues. The most characteristic findings in HTLV-1 uveitis are vitreous opacities associated with mild iritis and mild retinal vasculitis: this type is classified as intermediate uveitis, since the intermediate part of the eyeball is affected by the inflammation.[249] Infiltrating HTLV-1–infected cells are implicated in the pathogenesis of this uveitis. The standard treatment of the condition is topical or systemic corticosteroids.

Infective Dermatitis

Infective dermatitis (ID), a severe, chronic, relapsing dermatitis first described in Jamaican children, was found to be associated with HTLV-1 infection.[197] ID is characterized by a severe exudative dermatitis with crusting of the scalp, neck, external ears, axillae, and groin. In the affected skin region, *Staphylococcus aureus* or beta-hemolytic *Streptococcus* infection is typically

detected. Oral trimethoprim–sulfamethoxazole is the treatment of choice because of low cost and effectiveness.[220] Patients with ID tend to have an elevated provirus load. ID has been reported prior to the development of ATL and HAM/TSP; ID is, therefore, implicated as an indicator for other HTLV-1–associated diseases.

PREVENTION AND TREATMENT

Prevention

Transmission of HTLV-1 between individuals requires the transfer of living infected cells. All routes are preventable. Mother-to-infant transmission can be reduced by bottle-feeding or freeze–thaw processing of breast milk,[8] which kills the infected cells in the breast milk. However, HTLV-1 transmission still occurs in about 5% of infants who do not drink breast milk, indicating the presence of a route of transmission other than breast-feeding.[350] As a mechanism, HTLV-1 infection was found in placental villous tissues, suggesting that infected trophoblast cells serve as viral reservoirs.[364] The risk of transmission by breast-feeding was found to increase with the degree of concordance of the HLA genotype between mother and child,[31] suggesting that immunological responses influence the transmission from mother to child. Blood screening almost

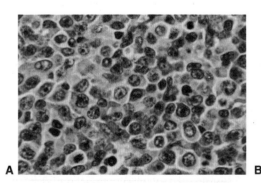
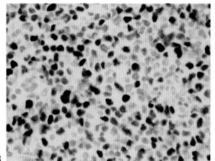

FIGURE 16.15 Lymph node lesion of an adult T-cell leukemia (ATL) patient. A: Histological analysis (hematoxylin–eosin staining) shows monotonous proliferation of ATL cells. **B:** Immunohistochemical analysis shows that ATL cells are FoxP3 positive.

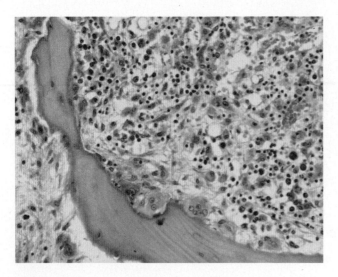

FIGURE 16.16 Increased number of osteoclasts in a hypercalcemic adult T-cell leukemia patient. In a hypercalcemic patient, the number of osteoclasts increases in the bone and accelerates bone resorption.

completely prevents viral transmission by blood transfusion.[138] RTIs should be useful for preventing *de novo* infection by accidental exposure to contaminated blood, although no clinical evidence has yet been reported.

Treatment

Diagnosis

HTLV-1 infection can be diagnosed by the presence of antibody to HTLV-1. The presence of serum antibodies against HTLV-1 can be demonstrated by enzyme-linked immunosorbance assay (ELISA), gelatin particle hemagglutination, indirect immunofluorescence, and western blot assays. The provirus load, which represents the percentage of PBMCs infected with HTLV-1, is measured by real-time PCR or droplet digital PCR (ddPCR). In HTLV-1–infected individuals, the provirus load ranges from less than 0.01% up to more than 50% PBMCs (each cell typically carries a single copy of the HTLV-1 provirus[53]).

The diagnostic criteria for ATL have been defined as follows[50,327]: (a) histologically and/or cytologically proved lymphoid malignancy with T-cell surface antigens; (b) abnormal T cells present in the peripheral blood (except for lymphoma-type ATL). These abnormal T lymphocytes can include not only typical ATL cells, the so-called flower cells, but also the small and mature T lymphocytes with incised or lobulated nuclei that are characteristic of the chronic or smoldering type of ATL; (c) antibody to HTLV-1 present in the serum at diagnosis; and (d) demonstration of monoclonal integration of HTLV-1 provirus by the Southern blot method.

ATL is a poorly treatable neoplastic disease due to its resistance to anticancer drugs and the complication of immunodeficiency. Patients with acute or lymphoma-type ATL are usually treated with combination chemotherapy. With the most commonly used combination chemotherapy in Japan (VCAP-AMP-VECP therapy: vincristine, cyclophosphamide, doxorubicin, and prednisone (VCAP), doxorubicin, ranimustine, and prednisone [AMP], and vindesine, etoposide, carboplatin, and prednisone [VECP]),[402] 81% of the 93 eligible patients responded, with 33 patients obtaining complete response (35.5%) and 42

obtaining partial response (45.2%). The median survival time of patients was 13 months. Thus, the prognosis of ATL patients treated by chemotherapy remains poor.[171]

The major impediments in therapy for ATL patients are the drug resistance of ATL cells to chemotherapeutic agents and the profoundly immunodeficient state of patients.[328] Cell-mediated immunity is impaired in ATL patients, whereas humoral immunity remains intact. The immunodeficiency of ATL patients may be caused by the immunosuppressive function of ATL cells, since they express immunosuppressive molecules,[359] frequently including many molecules that are characteristic of Tregs. The immunodeficiency of ATL patients often leads to opportunistic fungal, viral, and bacterial infections, which worsens the prognosis.[355]

Successful allogeneic bone marrow transplantation was reported for an acute ATL patient in 1996.[39,366] In a recent systematic review of 18 studies, the overall survival rate after transplantation was approximately 40% and the relapse rate was 36%.[140] ATL patients with chronic graft versus host disease (GVHD) show a better prognosis than those without chronic GVHD, indicating that host immune responses play critical roles.[161] Thus, immune responses are critical for treatment of ATL.

The HTLV-1 provirus load decreased remarkably in many patients who received an allogeneic stem-cell transplant,[279] suggesting that cell-mediated immunity to HTLV-1 was enhanced in these patients, an observation which might account for the efficacy of this therapy. ATL cells express high levels of cell-surface Fas antigen and are susceptible to Fas-mediated signaling.[357,411] These findings suggest that ATL cells are vulnerable to CTLs, which accounts for the good therapeutic responses. In individuals who received alloSCT, CTLs to Tax peptides were activated in the recipients; the provirus load became profoundly suppressed, suggesting a role of anti-HTLV-1 immune responses in the efficacious outcome.[113] Tax-peptide pulsed dendritic cells could suppress ATL.[339] Thus, Tax is a promising target for treatment of ATL in the approximately 50% of cases in which Tax is expressed by the malignant clone.

ATL cells express CCR4 on their surfaces.[414] ATL cells resemble Treg cells, which is because HBZ induces Foxp3. Treg cells express CCR4. Furthermore, HBZ also induces transcription of the *CCR4* gene,[340] and HTLV-1–infected cells express CCR4.[405] Mogamulizumab, a defucosylated humanized anti-CCR4 antibody, has shown to be effective in ATL patients.[141,404] Mogamulizumab not only kills ATL cells via enhanced antibody-dependent cell-mediated cytotoxicity (ADCC) but also enhances antiviral immunity through suppression of Treg cells.[342]

Previous studies reported that the prognosis of patients with aggressive subtypes of ATL (acute and lymphoma types) was less than 1 year, whereas that of indolent types (chronic and smoldering types) was much longer.[327] Later studies indicated that the prognosis of the indolent subtypes of ATL, chronic and smoldering ATL, is poorer than previously thought: the mean survival time of patients was only 4.1 years.[353] Therapy using IFN-α combined with zidovudine has been reported to be highly effective for these indolent ATL patients.[28] However, viral replication has not been demonstrated in ATL cells. Instead, many nonsense mutations, deletion, and insertions of HTLV-1 provirus were reported in ATL cells.[70,356] These data suggest that IFN-α combined with zidovudine may suppress the growth of ATL cells without any effects on viral replication.

A systematic review of therapies for HAM/TSP[10] concluded that corticosteroids can provide significant benefit: pulsed, high-dose methylprednisolone may be effective in induction therapy, and low-dose oral prednisolone can be used in maintenance therapy. However, the benefit of other types of treatment is less clear. HAM/TSP is associated with a high PVL. Since nonmalignant HTLV-1–infected cells also include CCR4-like ATL cells,[405] the anti-CCR4 monoclonal antibody mogamulizimab was used to treat HAM/TSP. The treatment decreased the number of HTLV-1–infected cells, with an associated reduction of spasticity.[310] However, the clinical benefit of this treatment may be short lived.

As expected, RTIs can suppress replication of HTLV-1 *in vitro*, although the efficacy of various RTIs against HTLV-1 differs from that against HIV-1.[124] RTIs can also block HTLV-1 infection if they are administrated at the time of HTLV-1 exposure.[235] However, RTIs cannot suppress HTLV-1 infection if they are administered 1 week later.[247] This finding suggests that clonal proliferation of infected cells is predominant after the initial *in vivo* spread of HTLV-1[200]; it is consistent with the observation that RTIs do not change provirus load in patients with HAM.[367] Thus, the clinical use of inhibitors against HTLV-1 replication is limited to preventive administration after accidental exposure to HTLV-1–positive blood.

Vaccines

The passive transfer of immunoglobulin derived from HTLV-1–infected individuals could block HTLV-1 infection,[253,315] suggesting that a vaccine to HTLV-1 is capable of inhibiting its transmission. Indeed, immunization with peptide derived from envelope protein[264] and vaccines expressing envelope protein[325] can block transmission of HTLV-1 in rabbits and monkeys. These findings show that a preventive vaccine for HTLV-1 is possible, in contrast with HIV-1 infection.

Tax might be a target for a therapeutic vaccine due to its high immunogenicity. In a rat model, a Tax peptide based vaccine inhibited the growth of a Tax expressing rat T-cell line *in vivo*.[110] However, the fact that Tax expression is frequently lost in ATL cells limits the value of Tax for a therapeutic vaccine for ATL.

REFERENCES

1. Adachi Y, Copeland TD, Takahashi C, et al. Phosphorylation of the Rex protein of human T-cell leukemia virus type I. *J Biol Chem* 1992;267:21977–21981.
2. Afonso PV, Cassar O, Gessain A. Molecular epidemiology, genetic variability and evolution of HTLV-1 with special emphasis on African genotypes. *Retrovirology* 2019;16:39.
3. Ahmed YF, Hanly SM, Malim MH, et al. Structure-function analyses of the HTLV-1 Rex and HIV-1 Rev RNA response elements: insights into the mechanism of Rex and Rev action. *Genes Dev* 1990;4:1014–1022.
4. Albrecht B, DSouza CD, Ding W, et al. Activation of nuclear factor of activated T cells by human T-lymphotropic virus type 1 accessory protein p12(I). *J Virol* 2002;76:3493–3501.
5. Anderson MR, Enose-Akahata Y, Massoud R, et al. Epigenetic modification of the FoxP3 TSDR in HAM/TSP decreases the functional suppression of Tregs. *J Neuroimmune Pharmacol* 2014;9:522–532.
6. Ando H, Sato T, Tomaru U, et al. Positive feedback loop via astrocytes causes chronic inflammation in virus-associated myelopathy. *Brain* 2013;136:2876–2887.
7. Ando S, Hasegawa A, Murakami Y, et al. HTLV-1 tax-specific CTL epitope-pulsed dendritic cell therapy reduces proviral load in infected rats with immune tolerance against tax. *J Immunol* 2017;198:1210–1219.
8. Ando Y, Ekuni Y, Matsumoto Y, et al. Long-term serological outcome of infants who received frozen-thawed milk from human T-lymphotropic virus type-I positive mothers. *J Obstet Gynaecol Res* 2004;30:436–438.
9. Arai F, Miyamoto T, Ohneda O, et al. Commitment and differentiation of osteoclast precursor cells by the sequential expression of c-Fms and receptor activator of nuclear factor kappaB (RANK) receptors. *J Exp Med* 1999;190:1741–1754.
10. Araujo A, Bangham CRM, Casseb J, et al. Management of HAM/TSP: systematic review and consensus-based recommendations 2019. *Neurol Clin Pract* 2021;11:49–56.
11. Arisawa K, Soda M, Endo S, et al. Evaluation of adult T-cell leukemia/lymphoma incidence and its impact on non-Hodgkin lymphoma incidence in southwestern Japan. *Int J Cancer* 2000;85:319–324.
12. Armand M, Hamosh M, Mehta NR, et al. Effect of human milk or formula on gastric function and fat digestion in the premature infant. *Pediatr Res* 1996;40:429–437.
13. Arnold J, Zimmerman B, Li M, et al. Human T-cell leukemia virus type-1 antisense-encoded gene, Hbz, promotes T-lymphocyte proliferation. *Blood* 2008;112:3788–3797.
14. Asquith B, Bangham CR. Quantifying HTLV-I dynamics. *Immunol Cell Biol* 2007;85:280–286.
15. Asquith B, Zhang Y, Mosley AJ, et al. In vivo T lymphocyte dynamics in humans and the impact of human T-lymphotropic virus 1 infection. *Proc Natl Acad Sci U S A* 2007;104:8035–8040.
16. Ballard DW, Bohnlein E, Lowenthal JW, et al. HTLV-I tax induces cellular proteins that activate the kappa B element in the IL-2 receptor alpha gene. *Science* 1988;241:1652–1655.
16a. Banerjee P, Feuer G, Barker E. Human T-cell leukemia virus type 1 (HTLV-1) p12I down-modulates ICAM-1 and -2 and reduces adherence of natural killer cells, thereby protecting HTLV-1-infected primary CD4+ T cells from autologous natural killer cell-mediated cytotoxicity despite the reduction of major histocompatibility complex class I molecules on infected cells. *J Virol* 2007;81:9707–9717.
17. Bangham CRM. The immune control and cell-to-cell spread of human T-lymphotropic virus type 1. *J Gen Virol* 2003;84:3177–3189.
18. Bangham CRM. CTL quality and the control of human retroviral infections. *Eur J Immunol* 2009;39:1700–1712.
19. Bangham CRM. Human T cell leukemia virus type 1: persistence and pathogenesis. *Annu Rev Immunol* 2018;36:43–71.
20. Bangham CRM, Araujo A, Yamano Y, et al. HTLV-1-associated myelopathy/tropical spastic paraparesis. *Nat Rev Dis Primers* 2015;1:15012.
21. Bangham CRM, Matsuoka M. Human T-cell leukemia virus type 1: parasitism and pathogenesis. *Philos Trans R Soc Lond B Biol Sci* 2017;372:20160272.
22a. Barnard AL, Igakura T, Tanaka Y, et al. Engagement of specific T-cell surface molecules regulates cytoskeletal polarization in HTLV-1-infected lymphocytes. *Blood* 2005;106:988–995.
22. Bangham CRM, Osame M. Cellular immune response to HTLV-1. *Oncogene* 2005;24:6035–6046.
23. Barski MS, Minnell JJ, Hodakova Z, et al. Cryo-EM structure of the deltaretroviral intasome in complex with the PP2A regulatory subunit B56gamma. *Nat Commun* 2020;11:5043.
24. Basbous J, Arpin C, Gaudray G, et al. The HBZ factor of human T-cell leukemia virus type I dimerizes with transcription factors JunB and c-Jun and modulates their transcriptional activity. *J Biol Chem* 2003;278:43620–43627.
25. Baydoun HH, Pancewicz J, Bai X, et al. HTLV-I p30 inhibits multiple S phase entry checkpoints, decreases cyclin E-CDK2 interactions and delays cell cycle progression. *Mol Cancer* 2010;9:302.
26. Baydoun HH, Pancewicz J, Nicot C. Human T-lymphotropic type 1 virus p30 inhibits homologous recombination and favors unfaithful DNA repair. *Blood* 2011;117:5897–5906.
27. Bayliss RJ, Piguet V. Masters of manipulation: viral modulation of the immunological synapse. *Cell Microbiol* 2018;20:e12944.
28. Bazarbachi A, Plumelle Y, Carlos Ramos J, et al. Meta-analysis on the use of zidovudine and interferon-alfa in adult T-cell leukemia/lymphoma showing improved survival in the leukemic subtypes. *J Clin Oncol* 2010;28:4177–4183.
29. Beimling P, Moelling K. Direct interaction of CREB protein with 21 bp Tax-response elements of HTLV-ILTR. *Oncogene* 1992;7:257–262.
30. Biasiotto R, Aguiari P, Rizzuto R, et al. The p13 protein of human T cell leukemia virus type 1 (HTLV-1) modulates mitochondrial membrane potential and calcium uptake. *Biochim Biophys Acta* 2010;1797:945–951.
31. Biggar RJ, Ng J, Kim N, et al. Human leukocyte antigen concordance and the transmission risk via breast-feeding of human T cell lymphotropic virus type I. *J Infect Dis* 2006;193:277–282.
32. Billman MR, Rueda D, Bangham CRM. Single-cell heterogeneity and cell-cycle-related viral gene bursts in the human leukaemia virus HTLV-1. *Wellcome Open Res* 2017;2:87.
33. Bittencourt AL, de Oliveira M. Cutaneous manifestations associated with HTLV-1 infection. *Int J Dermatol* 2010;49:1099–1110.
34. Blattner WA, Gallo RC. Epidemiology of HTLV-I and HTLV-II infection. In Takahashi K, ed. *Adult T-cell Leukemia*. New York: Oxford University Press; 1994.
35. Blot V, Delamarre L, Perugi F, et al. Human Dlg protein binds to the envelope glycoproteins of human T-cell leukemia virus type 1 and regulates envelope mediated cell-cell fusion in T lymphocytes. *J Cell Sci* 2004;117:3983–3993.
36. Boelen L, Debebe B, Silveira M, et al. Inhibitory killer cell immunoglobulin-like receptors strengthen CD8(+) T cell-mediated control of HIV-1, HCV, and HTLV-1. *Sci Immunol* 2018;3:eaao2892.
37. Bogerd H, Greene WC. Dominant negative mutants of human T-cell leukemia virus type I Rex and human immunodeficiency virus type 1 Rev fail to multimerize in vivo. *J Virol* 1993;67:2496–2502.
38. Bogerd HP, Huckaby GL, Ahmed YF, et al. The type I human T-cell leukemia virus (HTLV-I) Rex trans-activator binds directly to the HTLV-I Rex and the type 1 human immunodeficiency virus Rev RNA response elements. *Proc Natl Acad Sci U S A* 1991;88:5704–5708.
39. Borg A, Yin JA, Johnson PR, et al. Successful treatment of HTLV-1-associated acute adult T-cell leukaemia lymphoma by allogeneic bone marrow transplantation. *Br J Haematol* 1996;94:713–715.
40. Calattini S, Chevalier SA, Duprez R, et al. Discovery of a new human T-cell lymphotropic virus (HTLV-3) in Central Africa. *Retrovirology* 2005;2:30.
41. Cassar O, Einsiedel L, Afonso PV, et al. Human T-cell lymphotropic virus type 1 subtype C molecular variants among indigenous australians: new insights into the molecular epidemiology of HTLV-1 in Australo-Melanesia. *PLoS Negl Trop Dis* 2013;7:e2418.

42. Cavrois M, Gessain A, Gout O, et al. Common human T cell leukemia virus type 1 (HTLV-1) integration sites in cerebrospinal fluid and blood lymphocytes of patients with HTLV-1-associated myelopathy/tropical spastic paraparesis indicate that HTLV-1 crosses the blood-brain barrier via clonal HTLV-1-infected cells. *J Infect Dis* 2000;182:1044–1050.

43. Chandhasin C, Ducu RI, Berkovich E, et al. Human T-cell leukemia virus type 1 tax attenuates the ATM-mediated cellular DNA damage response. *J Virol* 2008;82:6952–6961.

44. Charoenthongtrakul S, Zhou Q, Shembade N, et al. Human T cell leukemia virus type 1 tax inhibits innate antiviral signaling via NF-{kappa}B-dependent induction of SOCS1. *J Virol* 2011;85:6955–6962.

45. Ching YP, Chan SF, Jeang KT, et al. The retroviral oncoprotein Tax targets the coiled-coil centrosomal protein TAX1BP2 to induce centrosome overduplication. *Nat Cell Biol* 2006;8:717–724.

46. Cho WK, Jang MK, Huang K, et al. Human T-lymphotropic virus type 1 Tax protein complexes with P-TEFb and competes for Brd4 and 7SK snRNP/HEXIM1 binding. *J Virol* 2010;84:12801–12809.

47. Cho WK, Zhou M, Jang MK, et al. Modulation of the Brd4/P-TEFb interaction by the human T-lymphotropic virus type 1 tax protein. *J Virol* 2007;81:11179–11186.

48. Chu ZL, Shin YA, Yang JM, et al. IKKgamma mediates the interaction of cellular IkappaB kinases with the tax transforming protein of human T cell leukemia virus type 1. *J Biol Chem* 1999;274:15297–15300.

49. Ciminale V, Pavlakis GN, Derse D, et al. Complex splicing in the human T-cell leukemia virus (HTLV) family of retroviruses: novel mRNAs and proteins produced by HTLV type I. *J Virol* 1992;66:1737–1745.

50. Cook L, Melamed A, Yaguchi H, et al. The impact of HTLV-1 on the cellular genome. *Curr Opin Virol* 2017;26:125–131.

51. Cook LB, Melamed A, Demontis MA, et al. Rapid dissemination of human T-lymphotropic virus type 1 during primary infection in transplant recipients. *Retrovirology* 2016;13:3.

52. Cook LB, Melamed A, Niederer H, et al. The role of HTLV-1 clonality, proviral structure, and genomic integration site in adult T-cell leukemia/lymphoma. *Blood* 2014;123:3925–3931.

53. Cook LB, Rowan AG, Melamed A, et al. HTLV-1-infected T cells contain a single integrated provirus in natural infection. *Blood* 2012;120:3488–3490.

54. Coskun AK, Sutton RE. Expression of glucose transporter 1 confers susceptibility to human T-cell leukemia virus envelope-mediated fusion. *J Virol* 2005;79:4150–4158.

55. Daenke S, Nightingale S, Cruickshank JK, et al. Sequence variants of human T-cell lymphotropic virus type I from patients with tropical spastic paraparesis and adult T-cell leukemia do not distinguish neurological from leukemic isolates. *J Virol* 1990;64:1278–1282.

56. Datta A, Silverman L, Phipps AJ, et al. Human T-lymphotropic virus type-1 p30 alters cell cycle G2 regulation of T lymphocytes to enhance cell survival. *Retrovirology* 2007;4:49.

57. Datta A, Sinha-Datta U, Dhillon NK, et al. The HTLV-I p30 interferes with TLR4 signaling and modulates the release of pro- and anti-inflammatory cytokines from human macrophages. *J Biol Chem* 2006;281:23414–23424.

58. Delamarre L, Pique C, Rosenberg AR, et al. The Y-S-L-I tyrosine-based motif in the cytoplasmic domain of the human T-cell leukemia virus type 1 envelope is essential for cell-to-cell transmission. *J Virol* 1999;73:9659–9663.

59. Delamarre L, Rosenberg AR, Pique C, et al. A novel human T-leukemia virus type 1 cell-to-cell transmission assay permits definition of SU glycoprotein amino acids important for infectivity. *J Virol* 1997;71:259–266.

60. Derse D, Hill SA, Lloyd PA, et al. Examining human T-lymphotropic virus type 1 infection and replication by cell-free infection with recombinant virus vectors. *J Virol* 2001;75:8461–8468.

61. Derse D, Hill SA, Princler G, et al. Resistance of human T cell leukemia virus type 1 to APOBEC3G restriction is mediated by elements in nucleocapsid. *Proc Natl Acad Sci U S A* 2007;104:2915–2920.

62. Desrames A, Cassar O, Gout O, et al. Northern African strains of human T-lymphotropic virus type 1 arose from a recombination event. *J Virol* 2014;88:9782–9788.

63. Ding W, Albrecht B, Kelley RE, et al. Human T-cell lymphotropic virus type 1 p12(I) expression increases cytoplasmic calcium to enhance the activation of nuclear factor of activated T cells. *J Virol* 2002;76:10374–10382.

64. Ding W, Albrecht B, Luo R, et al. Endoplasmic reticulum and cis-Golgi localization of human T-lymphotropic virus type 1 p12(I): association with calreticulin and calnexin. *J Virol* 2001;75:7672–7682.

65. Durkin SS, Guo X, Fryrear KA, et al. HTLV-1 Tax oncoprotein subverts the cellular DNA damage response via binding to DNA-dependent protein kinase. *J Biol Chem* 2008;283:36311–36320.

66. Dustin ML, Cooper JA. The immunological synapse and the actin cytoskeleton: molecular hardware for T cell signaling. *Nat Immunol* 2000;1:23–29.

67. Einsiedel L, Fernandes L, Spelman T, et al. Bronchiectasis is associated with human T-lymphotropic virus 1 infection in an Indigenous Australian population. *Clin Infect Dis* 2012;54:43–50.

68. Einsiedel L, Pham H, Wilson K, et al. Human T-Lymphotropic Virus type 1c subtype proviral loads, chronic lung disease and survival in a prospective cohort of Indigenous Australians. *PLoS Negl Trop Dis* 2018;12:e0006281.

69. Eiraku N, Novoa P, da Costa Ferreira M, et al. Identification and characterization of a new and distinct molecular subtype of human T-cell lymphotropic virus type 2. *J Virol* 1996;70:1481–1492.

70. Fan J, Ma G, Nosaka K, et al. APOBEC3G generates nonsense mutations in human T-cell leukemia virus type 1 proviral genomes in vivo. *J Virol* 2010;84:7278–7287.

71. Felber BK, Paskalis H, Kleinman-Ewing C, et al. The pX protein of HTLV-I is a transcriptional activator of its long terminal repeats. *Science* 1985;229:675–679.

72. Fenizia C, Fiocchi M, Jones K, et al. Human T-cell leukemia/lymphoma virus type 1 p30, but not p12/p8, counteracts toll-like receptor 3 (TLR3) and TLR4 signaling in human monocytes and dendritic cells. *J Virol* 2014;88:393–402.

73. Feuer G, Green PL. Comparative biology of human T-cell lymphotropic virus type 1 (HTLV-1) and HTLV-2. *Oncogene* 2005;24:5996–6004.

74. Filippone C, Betsem E, Tortevoye P, et al. A severe bite from a nonhuman primate is a major risk factor for HTLV-1 infection in hunters from Central Africa. *Clin Infect Dis* 2015;60:1667–1676.

75. Fujihara K, Itoyama Y, Yu F, et al. Cellular immune surveillance against HTLV-I infected T lymphocytes in HTLV-I associated myelopathy/tropical spastic paraparesis (HAM/TSP). *J Neurol Sci* 1991;105:99–107.

76. Fukudome K, Furuse M, Fukuhara N, et al. Strong induction of ICAM-1 in human T cells transformed by human T-cell-leukemia virus type 1 and depression of ICAM-1 or LFA-1 in adult T-cell-leukemia-derived cell lines. *Int J Cancer* 1992;52:418–427.

77. Fukumoto R, Andresen V, Bialuk I, et al. In vivo genetic mutations define predominant functions of the human T-cell leukemia/lymphoma virus p12I protein. *Blood* 2009;113:3726–3734.

78. Furukawa Y, Bangham CR, Taylor GP, et al. Frequent reversible membrane damage in peripheral blood B cells in human T cell lymphotropic virus type I (HTLV-I)-associated myelopathy/tropical spastic paraparesis (HAM/TSP). *Clin Exp Immunol* 2000;120:307–316.

79. Furukawa Y, Kubota R, Tara M, et al. Existence of escape mutant in HTLV-I tax during the development of adult T-cell leukemia. *Blood* 2001;97:987–993.

80. Furukawa Y, Yamashita M, Usuku K, et al. Phylogenetic subgroups of human T cell lymphotropic virus (HTLV) type I in the tax gene and their association with different risks for HTLV-I-associated myelopathy/tropical spastic paraparesis. *J Infect Dis* 2000;182:1343–1349.

81. Furuta R, Yasunaga JI, Miura M, et al. Human T-cell leukemia virus type 1 infects multiple lineage hematopoietic cells in vivo. *PLoS Pathog* 2017;13:e1006722.

82. Gao F, Bailes E, Robertson DL, et al. Origin of HIV-1 in the chimpanzee Pan troglodytes troglodytes. *Nature* 1999;397:436–441.

83. Gaudray G, Gachon F, Basbous J, et al. The complementary strand of the human T-cell leukemia virus type 1 RNA genome encodes a bZIP transcription factor that down-regulates viral transcription. *J Virol* 2002;76:12813–12822.

84. Gazon H, Chauhan PS, Porquet F, et al. Epigenetic silencing of HTLV-1 expression by the HBZ RNA through interference with the basal transcription machinery. *Blood Adv* 2020;4:5574–5579.

85. Geleziunas R, Ferrell S, Lin X, et al. Human T-cell leukemia virus type 1 Tax induction of NF-kappaB involves activation of the IkappaB kinase alpha (IKKalpha) and IKKbeta cellular kinases. *Mol Cell Biol* 1998;18:5157–5165.

86. Georges SA, Giebler HA, Cole PA, et al. Tax recruitment of CBP/p300, via the KIX domain, reveals a potent requirement for acetyltransferase activity that is chromatin dependent and histone tail independent. *Mol Cell Biol* 2003;23:3392–3404.

87. Georges SA, Kraus WL, Luger K, et al. p300-mediated tax transactivation from recombinant chromatin: histone tail deletion mimics coactivator function. *Mol Cell Biol* 2002;22:127–137.

88. Gessain A, Barin F, Vernant JC, et al. Antibodies to human T-lymphotropic virus type-I in patients with tropical spastic paraparesis. *Lancet* 1985;2:407–410.

89. Gessain A, Cassar O. Epidemiological aspects and world distribution of HTLV-1 infection. *Front Microbiol* 2012;3:388.

90. Gessain A, Gallo RC, Franchini G. Low degree of human T-cell leukemia/lymphoma virus type I genetic drift in vivo as a means of monitoring viral transmission and movement of ancient human populations. *J Virol* 1992;66:2288–2295.

91. Gessain A, Yanagihara R, Franchini G, et al. Highly divergent molecular variants of human T-lymphotropic virus type I from isolated populations in Papua New Guinea and the Solomon Islands. *Proc Natl Acad Sci U S A* 1991;88:7694–7698.

92. Ghez D, Lepelletier Y, Jones KS, et al. Current concepts regarding the HTLV-1 receptor complex. *Retrovirology* 2010;7:99.

93. Ghez D, Lepelletier Y, Lambert S, et al. Neuropilin-1 is involved in human T-cell lymphotropic virus type 1 entry. *J Virol* 2006;80:6844–6854.

94. Ghorbel S, Sinha-Datta U, Dundr M, et al. Human T-cell leukemia virus type I p30 nuclear/nucleolar retention is mediated through interactions with RNA and a constituent of the 60 S ribosomal subunit. *J Biol Chem* 2006;281:37150–37158.

95. Giebler HA, Loring JE, van Orden K, et al. Anchoring of CREB binding protein to the human T-cell leukemia virus type 1 promoter: a molecular mechanism of Tax transactivation. *Mol Cell Biol* 1997;17:5156–5164.

96. Gillet NA, Malani N, Melamed A, et al. The host genomic environment of the provirus determines the abundance of HTLV-1-infected T-cell clones. *Blood* 2011;117:3113–3122.

97. Goh WC, Sodroski J, Rosen C, et al. Subcellular localization of the product of the long open reading frame of human T-cell leukemia virus type I. *Science* 1985;227:1227–1228.

98. Goldstone DC, Ennis-Adeniran V, Hedden JJ, et al. HIV-1 restriction factor SAMHD1 is a deoxynucleoside triphosphate triphosphohydrolase. *Nature* 2011;480:379–382.

99. Goon PK, Biancardi A, Fast N, et al. Human T cell lymphotropic virus (HTLV) type-1-specific CD8+ T cells: frequency and immunodominance hierarchy. *J Infect Dis* 2004;189:2294–2298.

100. Goon PK, Hanon E, Igakura T, et al. High frequencies of Th1-type CD4(+) T cells specific to HTLV-1 Env and Tax proteins in patients with HTLV-1-associated myelopathy/tropical spastic paraparesis. *Blood* 2002;99:3335–3341.

101. Goon PK, Igakura T, Hanon E, et al. High circulating frequencies of tumor necrosis factor alpha- and interleukin-2-secreting human T-lymphotropic virus type 1 (HTLV-1)-specific CD4+ T cells in patients with HTLV-1-associated neurological disease. *J Virol* 2003;77:9716–9722.

102. Goon PK, Igakura T, Hanon E, et al. Human T cell lymphotropic virus type I (HTLV-I)-specific CD4+ T cells: immunodominance hierarchy and preferential infection with HTLV-I. *J Immunol* 2004;172:1735–1743.

103. Grone M, Hoffmann E, Berchtold S, et al. A single stem-loop structure within the HTLV-1 Rex response element is sufficient to mediate Rex activity in vivo. *Virology* 1994;204:144–152.

104. Hagiya K, Yasunaga J, Satou Y, et al. ATF3, an HTLV-1 bZip factor binding protein, promotes proliferation of adult T-cell leukemia cells. *Retrovirology* 2011;8:19.

105. Hahn BH, Shaw GM, Popovic M, et al. Molecular cloning and analysis of a new variant of human T-cell leukemia virus (HTLV-ib) from an African patient with adult T-cell leukemia-lymphoma. *Int J Cancer* 1984;34:613–618.

106. Hakata Y, Yamada M, Shida H. Rat CRM1 is responsible for the poor activity of human T-cell leukemia virus type 1 Rex protein in rat cells. *J Virol* 2001;75:11515–11525.
107. Halin M, Douceron E, Clerc I, et al. Human T-cell leukemia virus type 2 produces a spliced antisense transcript encoding a protein that lacks a classic bZIP domain but still inhibits Tax2-mediated transcription. *Blood* 2009;114:2427–2438.
108. Hall WW, Ishak R, Zhu SW, et al. Human T lymphotropic virus type II (HTLV-II): epidemiology, molecular properties, and clinical features of infection. *J Acquir Immune Defic Syndr Hum Retrovirol* 1996;13(Suppl 1):S204–S214.
109. Hammes SR, Greene WC. Multiple arginine residues within the basic domain of HTLV-I Rex are required for specific RNA binding and function. *Virology* 1993;193:41–49.
110. Hanabuchi S, Ohashi T, Koya Y, et al. Regression of human T-cell leukemia virus type I (HTLV-I)-associated lymphomas in a rat model: peptide-induced T-cell immunity. *J Natl Cancer Inst* 2001;93:1775–1783.
111. Hanon E, Goon P, Taylor GP, et al. High production of interferon gamma but not interleukin-2 by human T-lymphotropic virus type I-infected peripheral blood mononuclear cells. *Blood* 2001;98:721–726.
112. Hanon E, Hall S, Taylor GP, et al. Abundant tax protein expression in CD4+ T cells infected with human T-cell lymphotropic virus type I (HTLV-I) is prevented by cytotoxic T lymphocytes. *Blood* 2000;95:1386–1392.
113. Harashima N, Kurihara K, Utsunomiya A, et al. Graft-versus-Tax response in adult T-cell leukemia patients after hematopoietic stem cell transplantation. *Cancer Res* 2004;64:391–399.
114. Harhaj EW, Sun SC. IKKgamma serves as a docking subunit of the IkappaB kinase (IKK) and mediates interaction of IKK with the human T-cell leukemia virus Tax protein. *J Biol Chem* 1999;274:22911–22914.
115. Harrod R. Silencers of HTLV-1 and HTLV-2: the pX-encoded latency-maintenance factors. *Retrovirology* 2019;16:25.
116. Harrod R, Tang Y, Nicot C, et al. An exposed KID-like domain in human T-cell lymphotropic virus type 1 Tax is responsible for the recruitment of coactivators CBP/p300. *Mol Cell Biol* 1998;18:5052–5061.
117. Hatta Y, Hirama T, Miller CW, et al. Homozygous deletions of the p15 (MTS2) and p16 (CDKN2/MTS1) genes in adult T-cell leukemia. *Blood* 1995;85:2699–2704.
118. He Y, Pasupala N, Zhi H, et al. NF-kappaB-induced R-loop accumulation and DNA damage select for nucleotide excision repair deficiencies in adult T cell leukemia. *Proc Natl Acad Sci U S A* 2021;118(10):e2005568118.
119. Hidaka M, Inoue J, Yoshida M, et al. Post-transcriptional regulator (rex) of HTLV-1 initiates expression of viral structural proteins but suppresses expression of regulatory proteins. *EMBO J* 1988;7:519–523.
120. Hieshima K, Nagakubo D, Nakayama T, et al. Tax-inducible production of CC chemokine ligand 22 by human T cell leukemia virus type 1 (HTLV-1)-infected T cells promotes preferential transmission of HTLV-1 to CCR4-expressing CD4+ T cells. *J Immunol* 2008;180:931–939.
121. Higuchi M, Tsubata C, Kondo R, et al. Cooperation of NF-kappaB2/p100 activation and the PDZ domain binding motif signal in human T-cell leukemia virus type 1 (HTLV-1) Tax1 but not HTLV-2 Tax2 is crucial for interleukin-2-independent growth transformation of a T-cell line. *J Virol* 2007;81:11900–11907.
122. Higuchi Y, Yasunaga JI, Mitagami Y, et al. HTLV-1 induces T cell malignancy and inflammation by viral antisense factor-mediated modulation of the cytokine signaling. *Proc Natl Acad Sci U S A* 2020;117:13740–13749.
123. Hilburn S, Rowan A, Demontis MA, et al. In vivo expression of human T-lymphotropic virus type 1 basic leucine zipper protein generates specific CD8+ and CD4+ T lymphocyte responses that correlate with clinical outcome. *J Infect Dis* 2011;203:529–536.
124. Hill SA, Lloyd PA, McDonald S, et al. Susceptibility of human T cell leukemia virus type I to nucleoside reverse transcriptase inhibitors. *J Infect Dis* 2003;188:424–427.
125. Hinuma Y, Nagata K, Hanaoka M, et al. Adult T-cell leukemia: antigen in an ATL cell line and detection of antibodies to the antigen in human sera. *Proc Natl Acad Sci U S A* 1981;78:6476–6480.
126. Hiraragi H, Kim SJ, Phipps AJ, et al. Human T-lymphotropic virus type 1 mitochondrion-localizing protein p13(II) is required for viral infectivity in vivo. *J Virol* 2006;80:3469–3476.
127. Hirata M, Hayashi J, Noguchi A, et al. The effects of breastfeeding and presence of antibody to p40tax protein of human T cell lymphotropic virus type-I on mother to child transmission. *Int J Epidemiol* 1992;21:989–994.
128. Hisada M, Stuver SO, Okayama A, et al. Persistent paradox of natural history of human T lymphotropic virus type I: parallel analyses of Japanese and Jamaican carriers. *J Infect Dis* 2004;190:1605–1609.
129. Hishiki T, Ohshima T, Ego T, et al. BCL3 acts as a negative regulator of transcription from the human T-cell leukemia virus type 1 long terminal repeat through interactions with TORC3. *J Biol Chem* 2007;282:28335–28343.
130. Hivin P, Basbous J, Raymond F, et al. The HBZ-SP1 isoform of human T-cell leukemia virus type I represses JunB activity by sequestration into nuclear bodies. *Retrovirology* 2007;4:14.
131. Hivin P, Frederic M, Arpin-Andre C, et al. Nuclear localization of HTLV-I bZIP factor (HBZ) is mediated by three distinct motifs. *J Cell Sci* 2005;118:1355–1362.
132. Hjelle B, Appenzeller O, Mills R, et al. Chronic neurodegenerative disease associated with HTLV-II infection. *Lancet* 1992;339:645–646.
133. Hoshida Y, Li T, Dong Z, et al. Lymphoproliferative disorders in renal transplant patients in Japan. *Int J Cancer* 2001;91:869–875.
134. Iga M, Okayama A, Stuver S, et al. Genetic evidence of transmission of human T cell lymphotropic virus type 1 between spouses. *J Infect Dis* 2002;185:691–695.
135. Igakura T, Stinchcombe JC, Goon PK, et al. Spread of HTLV-I between lymphocytes by virus-induced polarization of the cytoskeleton. *Science* 2003;299:1713–1716.
136. Ikezoe T, Nishioka C, Bandobashi K, et al. Longitudinal inhibition of PI3K/Akt/mTOR signaling by LY294002 and rapamycin induces growth arrest of adult T-cell leukemia cells. *Leuk Res* 2007;31(5):673–682.
137. Ina Y, Gojobori T. Molecular evolution of human T-cell leukemia virus. *J Mol Evol* 1990;31:493–499.
138. Inaba S, Okochi K, Sato H, et al. Efficacy of donor screening for HTLV-I and the natural history of transfusion-transmitted infection. *Transfusion* 1999;39:1104–1110.
139. Inoue J, Seiki M, Yoshida M. The second pX product p27 chi-III of HTLV-1 is required for gag gene expression. *FEBS Lett* 1986;209:187–190.
140. Iqbal M, Reljic T, Klocksieben F, et al. Efficacy of allogeneic hematopoietic cell transplantation in human T cell lymphotropic virus type 1-associated adult t cell leukemia/lymphoma: results of a systematic review/meta-analysis. *Biol Blood Marrow Transplant* 2019;25:1695–1700.
141. Ishida T, Jo T, Takemoto S, et al. Dose-intensified chemotherapy alone or in combination with mogamulizumab in newly diagnosed aggressive adult T-cell leukaemia-lymphoma: a randomized phase II study. *Br J Haematol* 2015;169:672–682.
142. Ishitsuka K, Tamura K. Human T-cell leukaemia virus type I and adult T-cell leukaemia-lymphoma. *Lancet Oncol* 2014;15:e517–e526.
143. Iwai K, Mori N, Oie M, et al. Human T-cell leukemia virus type 1 tax protein activates transcription through AP-1 site by inducing DNA binding activity in T cells. *Virology* 2001;279:38–46.
144. Iwanaga M. Epidemiology of HTLV-1 infection and ATL in Japan: an update. *Front Microbiol* 2020;11:1124.
145. Iwanaga M, Watanabe T, Utsunomiya A, et al. Human T-cell leukemia virus type I (HTLV-1) proviral load and disease progression in asymptomatic HTLV-1 carriers: a nationwide prospective study in Japan. *Blood* 2010;116:1211–1219.
146. Iwanaga Y, Tsukahara T, Ohashi T, et al. Human T-cell leukemia virus type 1 tax protein abrogates interleukin-2 dependence in a mouse T-cell line. *J Virol* 1999;73:1271–1277.
147. Izumo S. Neuropathology of HTLV-1-associated myelopathy (HAM/TSP): the 50th Anniversary of Japanese Society of Neuropathology. *Neuropathology* 2010;30(5):480–485.
148. Jacobson S, Shida H, McFarlin DE, et al. Circulating CD8+ cytotoxic T lymphocytes specific for HTLV-I pX in patients with HTLV-I associated neurological disease. *Nature* 1990;348:245–248.
149. Jain P, Manuel SL, Khan ZK, et al. DC-SIGN mediates cell-free infection and transmission of human T-cell lymphotropic virus type 1 by dendritic cells. *J Virol* 2009;83:10908–10921.
150. Jeang KT, Widen SG, Semmes OJ IV, et al. HTLV-I trans-activator protein, tax, is a trans-repressor of the human beta-polymerase gene. *Science* 1990;247:1082–1084.
151. Jeffery KJ, Usuku K, Hall SE, et al. HLA alleles determine human T-lymphotropic virus-I (HTLV-I) proviral load and the risk of HTLV-I-associated myelopathy. *Proc Natl Acad Sci U S A* 1999;96:3848–3853.
152. Jeong SJ, Pise-Masison CA, Radonovich MF, et al. Activated AKT regulates NF-kappaB activation, p53 inhibition and cell survival in HTLV-1-transformed cells. *Oncogene* 2005;24:6719–6728.
153. Jiang S, Inada T, Tanaka M, et al. Involvement of TORC2, a CREB co-activator, in the in vivo-specific transcriptional control of HTLV-1. *Retrovirology* 2009;6:73.
154. Jin DY, Spencer F, Jeang KT. Human T cell leukemia virus type 1 oncoprotein Tax targets the human mitotic checkpoint protein MAD1. *Cell* 1998;93:81–91.
155. Jin Q, Agrawal L, VanHorn-Ali Z, et al. Infection of CD4+ T lymphocytes by the human T cell leukemia virus type 1 is mediated by the glucose transporter GLUT-1: evidence using antibodies specific to the receptors large extracellular domain. *Virology* 2006;349:184–196.
156. Jin Q, Agrawal L, Vanhorn-Ali Z, et al. GLUT-1-independent infection of the glioblastoma/astroglioma U87 cells by the human T cell leukemia virus type 1. *Virology* 2006;353:99–110.
157. Johnson JM, Nicot C, Fullen J, et al. Free major histocompatibility complex class I heavy chain is preferentially targeted for degradation by human T-cell leukemia/lymphotropic virus type 1 p12(I) protein. *J Virol* 2001;75:6086–6094.
158. Jones KS, Akel S, Petrow-Sadowski C, et al. Induction of human T cell leukemia virus type I receptors on quiescent naive T lymphocytes by TGF-beta. *J Immunol* 2005;174:4262–4270.
159. Jones KS, Petrow-Sadowski C, Huang YK, et al. Cell-free HTLV-1 infects dendritic cells leading to transmission and transformation of CD4(+) T cells. *Nat Med* 2008;14:429–436.
160. Journo C, Mahieux R. HTLV-1 and innate immunity. *Viruses* 2011;3:1374–1394.
161. Kanda J, Hishizawa M, Utsunomiya A, et al. Impact of graft-versus-host disease on outcomes after allogeneic hematopoietic cell transplantation for adult T-cell leukemia: a retrospective cohort study. *Blood* 2012;119:2141–2148.
162. Kannagi M, Harada S, Maruyama I, et al. Predominant recognition of human T cell leukemia virus type I (HTLV-I) pX gene products by human CD8+ cytotoxic T cells directed against HTLV-I-infected cells. *Int Immunol* 1991;3:761–767.
163. Kannian P, Fernandez S, Jones KS, et al. Human T lymphotropic virus type 1 SU residue 195 plays a role in determining the preferential CD4+ T cell immortalization/transformation tropism. *J Virol* 2013;87:9344–9352.
164. Kannian P, Yin H, Doueiri R, et al. Distinct transformation tropism exhibited by human T lymphotropic virus type 1 (HTLV-1) and HTLV-2 is the result of postinfection T cell clonal expansion. *J Virol* 2012;86:3757–3766.
165. Kao SY, Marriott SJ. Disruption of nucleotide excision repair by the human T-cell leukemia virus type 1 Tax protein. *J Virol* 1999;73:4299–4304.
166. Kaplan JE, Osame M, Kubota H, et al. The risk of development of HTLV-I-associated myelopathy/tropical spastic paraparesis among persons infected with HTLV-I. *J Acquir Immune Defic Syndr* 1990;3:1096–1101.
167. Karube K, Aoki R, Sugita Y, et al. The relationship of FOXP3 expression and clinicopathological characteristics in adult T-cell leukemia/lymphoma. *Mod Pathol* 2008;21:617–625.
168. Karube K, Ohshima K, Tsuchiya T, et al. Expression of FoxP3, a key molecule in CD4CD25 regulatory T cells, in adult T-cell leukaemia/lymphoma cells. *Br J Haematol* 2004;126:81–84.
169. Kashanchi F, Brady JN. Transcriptional and post-transcriptional gene regulation of HTLV-1. *Oncogene* 2005;24:5938–5951.
170. Kataoka K, Nagata Y, Kitanaka A, et al. Integrated molecular analysis of adult T cell leukemia/lymphoma. *Nat Genet* 2015;47:1304–1315.
171. Katsuya H, Ishitsuka K, Utsunomiya A, et al. TL-Prognostic Index Project. Treatment and survival among 1594 patients with ATL. *Blood* 2015;126:2570–2577.

172. Katsuya H, Islam S, Tan BJY, et al. The nature of the HTLV-1 provirus in naturally infected individuals analyzed by the viral DNA-capture-Seq approach. *Cell Rep* 2019;29:724–735 e4.
173. Kawakami A, Nakashima T, Sakai H, et al. Inhibition of caspase cascade by HTLV-I tax through induction of NF-kappaB nuclear translocation. *Blood* 1999;94:3847–3854.
174. Kawano N, Shimoda K, Ishikawa F, et al. Adult T-cell leukemia development from a human T-cell leukemia virus type I carrier after a living-donor liver transplantation. *Transplantation* 2006;82:840–843.
175. Kazanji M, Mouinga-Ondeme A, Lekana-Douki-Etenna S, et al. Origin of HTLV-1 in hunters of nonhuman primates in Central Africa. *J Infect Dis* 2015;211:361–365.
176. Kazanji M, Ureta-Vidal A, Ozden S, et al. Lymphoid organs as a major reservoir for human T-cell leukemia virus type 1 in experimentally infected squirrel monkeys (*Saimiri sciureus*): provirus expression, persistence, and humoral and cellular immune responses. *J Virol* 2000;74:4860–4867.
177. Kesic M, Doueiri R, Ward M, et al. Phosphorylation regulates human T-cell leukemia virus type 1 Rex function. *Retrovirology* 2009;6:105.
178. Kim FJ, Manel N, Boublik Y, et al. Human T-cell leukemia virus type 1 envelope-mediated syncytium formation can be activated in resistant Mammalian cell lines by a carboxy-terminal truncation of the envelope cytoplasmic domain. *J Virol* 2003;77:963–969.
179. Kim SJ, Ding W, Albrecht B, et al. A conserved calcineurin-binding motif in human T lymphotropic virus type 1 p12I functions to modulate nuclear factor of activated T cell activation. *J Biol Chem* 2003;278:15550–15557.
180. Kim YM, Ramirez JA, Mick JE, et al. Molecular characterization of the tax-containing HTLV-1 enhancer complex reveals a prominent role for CREB phosphorylation in tax transactivation. *J Biol Chem.* 2007;282(26):18750–18757.
181. Kinet S, Swainson L, Lavanya M, et al. Isolated receptor binding domains of HTLV-1 and HTLV-2 envelopes bind Glut-1 on activated CD4+ and CD8+ T cells. *Retrovirology* 2007;4:31.
182. King JA, Bridger JM, Lochelt M, et al. Nucleocytoplasmic transport of HTLV-1 RNA is regulated by two independent LTR encoded nuclear retention elements. *Oncogene* 1998;16:3309–3316.
183. Kinpara S, Hasegawa A, Utsunomiya A, et al. Stromal cell-mediated suppression of human T-cell leukemia virus type 1 expression in vitro and in vivo by type I interferon. *J Virol* 2009;83:5101–5108.
184. Kirk PD, Huvet M, Melamed A, et al. Retroviruses integrate into a shared, non-palindromic DNA motif. *Nat Microbiol* 2016;2:16212.
185. Kitze B, Usuku K, Yamano Y, et al. Human CD4+ T lymphocytes recognize a highly conserved epitope of human T lymphotropic virus type 1 (HTLV-1) env gp21 restricted by HLA DRB1*0101. *Clin Exp Immunol* 1998;111:278–285.
186. Kiyokawa T, Yamaguchi K, Takeya M, et al. Hypercalcemia and osteoclast proliferation in adult T-cell leukemia. *Cancer* 1987;59:1187–1191.
187. Koga H, Ohshima T, Shimotohno K. Enhanced activation of tax-dependent transcription of human T-cell leukemia virus type I (HTLV-I) long terminal repeat by TORC3. *J Biol Chem* 2004;279:52978–52983.
188. Koiwa T, Hamano-Usami A, Ishida T, et al. 5-long terminal repeat-selective CpG methylation of latent human T-cell leukemia virus type 1 provirus in vitro and in vivo. *J Virol* 2002;76:9389–9397.
189. Komurian F, Pelloquin F, de The G. In vivo genomic variability of human T-cell leukemia virus type I depends more upon geography than upon pathologies. *J Virol* 1991;65:3770–3778.
190. Koralnik IJ, Boeri E, Saxinger WC, et al. Phylogenetic associations of human and simian T-cell leukemia/lymphotropic virus type I strains: evidence for interspecies transmission. *J Virol* 1994;68:2693–2707.
191. Koralnik IJ, Fullen J, Franchini G. The p12I, p13II, and p30II proteins encoded by human T-cell leukemia/lymphotropic virus type I open reading frames I and II are localized in three different cellular compartments. *J Virol* 1993;67:2360–2366.
192. Koralnik IJ, Gessain A, Klotman ME, et al. Protein isoforms encoded by the pX region of human T-cell leukemia/lymphotropic virus type I. *Proc Natl Acad Sci U S A* 1992;89:8813–8817.
193. Koyanagi Y, Itoyama Y, Nakamura N, et al. In vivo infection of human T-cell leukemia virus type I in non-T cells. *Virology* 1993;196:25–33.
194. Kulkarni A, Taylor GP, Klose RJ, et al. Histone H2A monoubiquitylation and p38-MAPKs regulate immediate-early gene-like reactivation of latent retrovirus HTLV-1. *JCI Insight* 2018;3(20):e123196.
195. Kuo YL, Giam CZ. Activation of the anaphase promoting complex by HTLV-1 tax leads to senescence. *EMBO J* 2006;25:1741–1752.
196. Kwok RP, Laurance ME, Lundblad JR, et al. Control of cAMP-regulated enhancers by the viral transactivator Tax through CREB and the co-activator CBP. *Nature* 1996;380:642–646.
197. LaGrenade L, Hanchard B, Fletcher V, et al. Infective dermatitis of Jamaican children: a marker for HTLV-I infection. *Lancet* 1990;336:1345–1347.
198. Larocca D, Chao LA, Seto MH, et al. Human T-cell leukemia virus minus strand transcription in infected T-cells. *Biochem Biophys Res Commun* 1989;163:1006–1013.
199. Laydon DJ, Melamed A, Sim A, et al. Quantification of HTLV-1 clonality and TCR diversity. *PLoS Comput Biol* 2014;10:e1003646.
200. Laydon DJ, Sunkara V, Boelen L, et al. The relative contributions of infectious and mitotic spread to HTLV-1 persistence. *PLoS Comput Biol* 2020;16:e1007470.
201. Lee R, Schwartz RA. Human T-lymphotrophic virus type 1-associated infective dermatitis: a comprehensive review. *J Am Acad Dermatol* 2011;64:152–160.
202. Lemasson I, Lewis MR, Polakowski N, et al. Human T-cell leukemia virus type 1 (HTLV-1) bZIP protein interacts with the cellular transcription factor CREB to inhibit HTLV-1 transcription. *J Virol* 2007;81:1543–1553.
203. Lemasson I, Polakowski NJ, Laybourn PJ, et al. Transcription factor binding and histone modifications on the integrated proviral promoter in human T-cell leukemia virus-I-infected T-cells. *J Biol Chem* 2002;277:49459–49465.
204. Lemasson I, Polakowski NJ, Laybourn PJ, et al. Tax-dependent displacement of nucleosomes during transcriptional activation of human T-cell leukemia virus type 1. *J Biol Chem* 2006;281:13075–13082.
205. Lenzmeier BA, Baird EE, Dervan PB, et al. The tax protein-DNA interaction is essential for HTLV-I transactivation in vitro. *J Mol Biol* 1999;291:731–744.
206. Lenzmeier BA, Giebler HA, Nyborg JK. Human T-cell leukemia virus type 1 Tax requires direct access to DNA for recruitment of CREB binding protein to the viral promoter. *Mol Cell Biol* 1998;18:721–731.
207. Leung K, Nabel GJ. HTLV-1 transactivator induces interleukin-2 receptor expression through an NF-kappa B-like factor. *Nature* 1988;333:776–778.
208. Levin MC, Krichavsky M, Fox RJ, et al. Extensive latent retroviral infection in bone marrow of patients with HTLV-I-associated neurologic disease. *Blood* 1997;89:346–348.
209. Levin MC, Lee SM, Kalume F, et al. Autoimmunity due to molecular mimicry as a cause of neurological disease. *Nat Med* 2002;8:509–513.
210. Li HC, Biggar RJ, Miley WJ, et al. Provirus load in breast milk and risk of mother-to-child transmission of human T lymphotropic virus type I. *J Infect Dis* 2004;190:1275–1278.
211. Li Y, Bolderson E, Kumar R, et al. HSSB1 and hSSB2 form similar multiprotein complexes that participate in DNA damage response. *J Biol Chem* 2009;284:23525–23531.
212. Liu M, Yang L, Zhang L, et al. Human T-cell leukemia virus type 1 infection leads to arrest in the G1 phase of the cell cycle. *J Virol* 2008;82:8442–8455.
213. Ma G, Yasunaga JI, Shimura K, et al. Human retroviral antisense mRNAs are retained in the nuclei of infected cells for viral persistence. *Proc Natl Acad Sci U S A* 2021;118(17):e2014783118.
214. Macatonia SE, Cruickshank JK, Rudge P, et al. Dendritic cells from patients with tropical spastic paraparesis are infected with HTLV-1 and stimulate autologous lymphocyte proliferation. *AIDS Res Hum Retroviruses* 1992;8:1699–1706.
215. MacNamara A, Rowan A, Hilburn S, et al. HLA class I binding of HBZ determines outcome in HTLV-1 infection. *PLoS Pathog* 2010;6:e1001117.
216. Maeda M, Tanabe-Shibuya J, Miyazato P, et al. IL-2/IL-2 receptor pathway plays a crucial role in the growth and malignant transformation of HTLV-1-infected T cells to develop adult T-cell leukemia. *Front Microbiol* 2020;11:356.
217. Maertens GN. B-protein phosphatase 2A is a functional binding partner of delta-retroviral integrase. *Nucleic Acids Res* 2016;44:364–376.
218. Maertens GN, Hare S, Cherepanov P. The mechanism of retroviral integration from X-ray structures of its key intermediates. *Nature* 2010;468:326–329.
219. Maggirwar SB, Harhaj E, Sun SC. Activation of NF-kappa B/Rel by Tax involves degradation of I kappa B alpha and is blocked by a proteasome inhibitor. *Oncogene* 1995;11:993–998.
220. Mahe A, Chollet-Martin S, Gessain A. HTLV-I-associated infective dermatitis. *Lancet* 1999;354:1386.
221. Mahgoub M, Yasunaga JI, Iwami S, et al. Sporadic on/off switching of HTLV-1 Tax expression is crucial to maintain the whole population of virus-induced leukemic cells. *Proc Natl Acad Sci U S A* 2018;115:E1269–E1278.
222. Mahieux R, Gessain A. The human HTLV-3 and HTLV-4 retroviruses: new members of the HTLV family. *Pathol Biol (Paris)* 2009;57:161–166.
223. Mahieux R, Ibrahim F, Mauclere P, et al. Molecular epidemiology of 58 new African human T-cell leukemia virus type 1 (HTLV-1) strains: identification of a new and distinct HTLV-1 molecular subtype in Central Africa and in Pygmies. *J Virol* 1997;71:1317–1333.
224. Majone F, Jeang KT. Clastogenic effect of the human T-cell leukemia virus type I Tax oncoprotein correlates with unstabilized DNA breaks. *J Biol Chem* 2000;275:32906–32910.
225. Majorovits E, Nejmeddine M, Tanaka Y, et al. Human T-lymphotropic virus-1 visualized at the virological synapse by electron tomography. *PLoS One* 2008;3:e2251.
226. Maloney EM, Cleghorn FR, Morgan OS, et al. Incidence of HTLV-I-associated myelopathy/tropical spastic paraparesis (HAM/TSP) in Jamaica and Trinidad. *J Acquir Immune Defic Syndr Hum Retrovirol* 1998;17:167–170.
227. Manel N, Battini JL, Sitbon M. Human T cell leukemia virus envelope binding and virus entry are mediated by distinct domains of the glucose transporter GLUT1. *J Biol Chem* 2005;280:29025–29029.
228. Manel N, Battini JL, Taylor N, et al. HTLV-1 tropism and envelope receptor. *Oncogene* 2005;24:6016–6025.
229. Manel N, Kim FJ, Kinet S, et al. The ubiquitous glucose transporter GLUT-1 is a receptor for HTLV. *Cell* 2003;115:449–459.
230. Manns A, Murphy EL, Wilks R, et al. Detection of early human T-cell lymphotropic virus type I antibody patterns during seroconversion among transfusion recipients. *Blood* 1991;77:896–905.
231. Mansky LM. In vivo analysis of human T-cell leukemia virus type 1 reverse transcription accuracy. *J Virol* 2000;74:9525–9531.
232. Martinez MP, Al-Saleem J, Green PL. Comparative virology of HTLV-1 and HTLV-2. *Retrovirology* 2019;16:21.
233. Maruyama M, Shibuya H, Harada H, et al. Evidence for aberrant activation of the interleukin-2 autocrine loop by HTLV-1-encoded p40x and T3/Ti complex triggering. *Cell* 1987;48:343–350.
234. Matsuoka E, Takenouchi N, Hashimoto K, et al. Perivascular T cells are infected with HTLV-I in the spinal cord lesions with HTLV-I-associated myelopathy/tropical spastic paraparesis: double staining of immunohistochemistry and polymerase chain reaction in situ hybridization. *Acta Neuropathol* 1998;96:340–346.
235. Matsushita S, Mitsuya H, Reitz MS, et al. Pharmacological inhibition of in vitro infectivity of human T lymphotropic virus type I. *J Clin Invest* 1987;80:394–400.
236. Matsuzaki T, Nakagawa M, Nagai M, et al. HTLV-I proviral load correlates with progression of motor disability in HAM/TSP: analysis of 239 HAM/TSP patients including 64 patients followed up for 10 years. *J Neurovirol* 2001;7:228–234.
237. Mazurov D, Ilinskaya A, Heidecker G, et al. Quantitative comparison of HTLV-1 and HIV-1 cell-to-cell infection with new replication dependent vectors. *PLoS Pathog* 2010;6:e1000788.
238. Melamed A, Laydon DJ, Al Khatib H, et al. HTLV-1 drives vigorous clonal expansion of infected CD8(+) T cells in natural infection. *Retrovirology* 2015;12:91.
239. Melamed A, Laydon DJ, Gillet NA, et al. Genome-wide determinants of proviral targeting, clonal abundance and expression in natural HTLV-1 infection. *PLoS Pathog* 2013;9:e1003271.

240. Melamed A, Witkover AD, Laydon DJ, et al. Clonality of HTLV-2 in natural infection. *PLoS Pathog* 2014;10:e1004006.
241. Melamed A, Yaguchi H, Miura M, et al. The human leukemia virus HTLV-1 alters the structure and transcription of host chromatin in cis. *Elife* 2018;7:e36245.
242. Mitobe Y, Yasunaga J, Furuta R, et al. HTLV-1 bZIP factor RNA and protein impart distinct functions on T-cell proliferation and survival. *Cancer Res* 2015;75: 4143–4152.
243. Miura M, Dey S, Ramanayake S, et al. Kinetics of HTLV-1 reactivation from latency quantified by single-molecule RNA FISH and stochastic modelling. *PLoS Pathog* 2019;15:e1008164.
244. Miura T, Fukunaga T, Igarashi T, et al. Phylogenetic subtypes of human T-lymphotropic virus type I and their relations to the anthropological background. *Proc Natl Acad Sci U S A* 1994;91:1124–1127.
245. Miyake H, Suzuki T, Hirai H, et al. Trans-activator Tax of human T-cell leukemia virus type 1 enhances mutation frequency of the cellular genome. *Virology* 1999;253:155–161.
246. Miyazaki M, Yasunaga J, Taniguchi Y, et al. Preferential selection of human T-cell leukemia virus type 1 provirus lacking the 5 long terminal repeat during oncogenesis. *J Virol* 2007;81:5714–5723.
247. Miyazato P, Yasunaga J, Taniguchi Y, et al. De novo human T-cell leukemia virus type 1 infection of human lymphocytes in NOD-SCID, common gamma-chain knockout mice. *J Virol* 2006;80:10683–10691.
248. Mochizuki M, Watanabe T, Yamaguchi K, et al. Uveitis associated with human T lymphotropic virus type I:seroepidemiologic, clinical, and virologic studies. *J Infect Dis* 1992;166:943–944.
249. Mochizuki M, Yamaguchi K, Takatsuki K, et al. HTLV-I and uveitis. *Lancet* 1992;339:1110.
250. Moles R, Sarkis S, Galli V, et al. p30 protein: a critical regulator of HTLV-1 viral latency and host immunity. *Retrovirology* 2019;16:42.
251. Montgomery RD, Cruickshank EK, Robertson WB, et al. Clinical and pathological observations on Jamaican neuropathy, a report on 206 cases. *Brain* 1964;87:425–462.
252. Morgan OS, Rodgers-Johnson P, Mora C, et al. HTLV-1 and polymyositis in Jamaica. *Lancet* 1989;2:1184–1187.
253. Morishita N, Ishii K, Tanaka Y, et al. Immunoglobulin prophylaxis against human T cell lymphotropic virus type II in rabbits. *J Infect Dis* 1994;169:620–623.
254. Moritoyo T, Reinhart TA, Moritoyo H, et al. Human T-lymphotropic virus type I-associated myelopathy and tax gene expression in CD4+ T lymphocytes. *Ann Neurol* 1996;40:84–90.
255. Moriuchi M, Moriuchi H. Seminal fluid enhances replication of human T-cell leukemia virus type 1: implications for sexual transmission. *J Virol* 2004;78:12709–12711.
256. Mueller NE, Blattner WA. Retroviruses: HTLV. In: Evans AS, Kaslow R, eds. *Viral Infections of Humans: Epidemiology and Control.* New York: Plenum Medical Press; 1997.
257. Mulloy JC, Crownley RW, Fullen J, et al. The human T-cell leukemia/lymphotropic virus type 1 p12I proteins bind the interleukin-2 receptor beta and gamma chains and affects their expression on the cell surface. *J Virol* 1996;70:3599–3605.
258. Mulloy JC, Kislyakova T, Cereseto A, et al. Human T-cell lymphotropic/leukemia virus type 1 Tax abrogates p53-induced cell cycle arrest and apoptosis through its CREB/ATF functional domain. *J Virol* 1998;72:8852–8860.
259. Murphy EL, Cassar O, Gessain A. Estimating the number of HTLV-2 infected persons in the world. *Retrovirology* 2015;12:O5.
260. Nagai M, Usuku K, Matsumoto W, et al. Analysis of HTLV-I proviral load in 202 HAM/TSP patients and 243 asymptomatic HTLV-I carriers: high proviral load strongly predisposes to HAM/TSP. *J Neurovirol* 1998;4:586–593.
261. Nagy K, Clapham P, Cheingsong-Popov R, et al. Human T-cell leukemia virus type I: induction of syncytia and inhibition by patients sera. *Int J Cancer* 1983;32:321–328.
262. Nakagawa M, Izumo S, Ijichi S, et al. HTLV-I-associated myelopathy: analysis of 213 patients based on clinical features and laboratory findings. *J Neurovirol* 1995;1:50–61.
263. Nakagawa M, Shaffer AL III, Ceribelli M, et al. Targeting the HTLV-I-regulated BATF3/IRF4 transcriptional network in adult T cell leukemia/lymphoma. *Cancer Cell* 2018;34:286–297 e10.
264. Nakamura H, Hayami M, Ohta Y, et al. Protection of cynomolgus monkeys against infection by human T-cell leukemia virus type-I by immunization with viral env gene products produced in Escherichia coli. *Int J Cancer* 1987;40:403–407.
265. Nakano K, Watanabe T. HTLV-1 Rex tunes the cellular environment favorable for viral replication. *Viruses* 2016;8:58.
266. Nakao K, Matsumoto M, Ohba N. Seroprevalence of antibodies to HTLV-I in patients with ocular disorders. *Br J Ophthalmol* 1991;75:76–78.
267. Nejmeddine M, Negi VS, Mukherjee S, et al. HTLV-1-Tax and ICAM-1 act on T-cell signal pathways to polarize the microtubule-organizing center at the virological synapse. *Blood* 2009;114:1016–1025.
268. Nicot C, Dundr M, Johnson JM, et al. HTLV-1-encoded p30II is a post-transcriptional negative regulator of viral replication. *Nat Med* 2004;10:197–201.
269. Nicot C, Harrod RL, Ciminale V, et al. Human T-cell leukemia/lymphoma virus type 1 nonstructural genes and their functions. *Oncogene* 2005;24:6026–6034.
270. Niewiesk S, Daenke S, Parker CE, et al. The transactivator gene of human T-cell leukemia virus type I is more variable within and between healthy carriers than patients with tropical spastic paraparesis. *J Virol* 1994;68:6778–6781.
271. Niewiesk S, Daenke S, Parker CE, et al. Naturally occurring variants of human T-cell leukemia virus type I Tax protein impair its recognition by cytotoxic T lymphocytes and the transactivation function of Tax. *J Virol* 1995;69:2649–2653.
272. Niinuma A, Higuchi M, Takahashi M, et al. Aberrant activation of the interleukin-2 autocrine loop through the nuclear factor of activated T cells by nonleukemogenic human T-cell leukemia virus type 2 but not by leukemogenic type 1 virus. *J Virol* 2005;79:11925–11934.
273. Nishimura Y, Okubo R, Minato S, et al. A possible association between HLA and HTLV-I-associated myelopathy (HAM) in Japanese. *Tissue Antigens* 1991;37:230–231.
274. Nosaka K, Matsuoka M. Adult T-cell leukemia-lymphoma as a viral disease: subtypes based on viral aspects. *Cancer Sci* 2021;112(5):1688–1694.
275. Nosaka K, Miyamoto T, Sakai T, et al. Mechanism of hypercalcemia in adult T-cell leukemia: overexpression of receptor activator of nuclear factor kappaB ligand on adult T-cell leukemia cells. *Blood* 2002;99:634–640.
276. Nosaka T, Siomi H, Adachi Y, et al. Nucleolar targeting signal of human T-cell leukemia virus type I rex-encoded protein is essential for cytoplasmic accumulation of unspliced viral mRNA. *Proc Natl Acad Sci U S A* 1989;86:9798–9802.
277. Nowak MA, Bangham CR. Population dynamics of immune responses to persistent viruses. *Science* 1996;272:74–79.
278. Nyborg JK, Egan D, Sharma N. The HTLV-1 Tax protein: revealing mechanisms of transcriptional activation through histone acetylation and nucleosome disassembly. *Biochim Biophys Acta* 2010;1799:266–274.
279. Okamura J, Utsunomiya A, Tanosaki R, et al. Allogeneic stem-cell transplantation with reduced conditioning intensity as a novel immunotherapy and antiviral therapy for adult T-cell leukemia/lymphoma. *Blood* 2005;105:4143–4145.
280. Okochi K, Sato H. Transmission of ATLV (HTLV-I) through blood transfusion. *Princess Takamatsu Symp* 1984;15:129–135.
281. Oliere S, Hernandez E, Lezin A, et al. HTLV-1 evades type I interferon antiviral signaling by inducing the suppressor of cytokine signaling 1 (SOCS1). *PLoS Pathog* 2010;6:e1001177.
282. Orland JR, Engstrom J, Fridey J, et al. Prevalence and clinical features of HTLV neurologic disease in the HTLV Outcomes Study. *Neurology* 2003;61:1588–1594.
283. Osame M, Nakagawa M, Izumo S. HTLV-1-associated myelopathy/tropical spastic paraparesis (HAM/TSP). In: Takatsuki K, ed. *Adult T-cell Leukemia.* New York: Oxford University Press; 1994.
284. Osame M, Usuku K, Izumo S, et al. HTLV-I associated myelopathy, a new clinical entity. *Lancet* 1986;1:1031–1032.
285. Paine E, Garcia J, Philpott TC, et al. Limited sequence variation in human T-lymphotropic virus type 1 isolates from North American and African patients. *Virology* 1991;182:111 123.
286. Pais-Correia AM, Sachse M, Guadagnini S, et al. Biofilm-like extracellular viral assemblies mediate HTLV-1 cell-to-cell transmission at virological synapses. *Nat Med* 2010;16:83–89.
287. Paiva AM, Assone T, Haziot MEJ, et al. Risk factors associated with HTLV-1 vertical transmission in Brazil: longer breastfeeding, higher maternal proviral load and previous HTLV-1-infected offspring. *Sci Rep* 2018;8:7742.
288. Park HU, Jeong JH, Chung JH, et al. Human T-cell leukemia virus type 1 Tax interacts with Chk1 and attenuates DNA-damage induced G2 arrest mediated by Chk1. *Oncogene* 2004;23:4966–4974.
289. Park HU, Jeong SJ, Jeong JH, et al. Human T-cell leukemia virus type 1 Tax attenuates gamma-irradiation-induced apoptosis through physical interaction with Chk2. *Oncogene* 2006;25:438–447.
290. Parker CE, Daenke S, Nightingale S, et al. Activated, HTLV-1-specific cytotoxic T-lymphocytes are found in healthy seropositives as well as in patients with tropical spastic paraparesis. *Virology* 1992;188:628–636.
291. Peloponese JM Jr, Jeang KT. Role for Akt/protein kinase B and AP-1 in cellular proliferation induced by the human T-cell leukemia virus type 1 (HTLV-1) tax oncoprotein. *J Biol Chem* 2006;281:8927–8938.
292. Percher F, Jeannin P, Martin-Latil S, et al. Mother-to-child transmission of HTLV-1 epidemiological aspects, mechanisms and determinants of mother-to-child transmission. *Viruses* 2016;8(2):40.
293. Philip S, Zahoor MA, Zhi HJ, et al. Regulation of human T-lymphotropic virus type I latency and reactivation by HBZ and Rex. *PLoS Pathog* 2014;10(4):e1004040.
294. Phillips JE, Corces VG. CTCF: master weaver of the genome. *Cell* 2009;137: 1194–1211.
295. Philpott SM, Buehring GC. Defective DNA repair in cells with human T-cell leukemia/bovine leukemia viruses: role of tax gene. *J Natl Cancer Inst* 1999;91:933–942.
296. Pinon JD, Klasse PJ, Jassal SR, et al. Human T-cell leukemia virus type 1 envelope glycoprotein gp46 interacts with cell surface heparan sulfate proteoglycans. *J Virol* 2003;77:9922–9930.
297. Pique C, Pham D, Tursz T, et al. The cytoplasmic domain of the human T-cell leukemia virus type I envelope can modulate envelope functions in a cell type-dependent manner. *J Virol* 1993;67:557–561.
298. Poiesz BJ, Ruscetti FW, Gazdar AF, et al. Detection and isolation of type C retrovirus particles from fresh and cultured lymphocytes of a patient with cutaneous T-cell lymphoma. *Proc Natl Acad Sci U S A* 1980;77:7415–7419.
299. Rende F, Cavallari I, Corradin A, et al. Kinetics and intracellular compartmentalization of HTLV-1 gene expression: nuclear retention of HBZ mRNAs. *Blood* 2011;117: 4855–4859.
300. Richardson JH, Edwards AJ, Cruickshank JK, et al. In vivo cellular tropism of human T-cell leukemia virus type 1. *J Virol* 1990;64:5682–5687.
301. Rowan AG, Dillon R, Witkover A, et al. Evolution of retrovirus-infected premalignant T-cell clones prior to adult T-cell leukemia/lymphoma diagnosis. *Blood* 2020;135:2023–2032.
302. Rowan AG, Witkover A, Melamed A, et al. T cell receptor Vbeta staining identifies the malignant clone in adult t cell leukemia and reveals killing of leukemia cells by autologous CD8+ T cells. *PLoS Pathog* 2016;12:e1006030.
303. Ruben S, Poteat H, Tan TH, et al. Cellular transcription factors and regulation of IL-2 receptor gene expression by HTLV-I tax gene product. *Science* 1988;241:89–92.
304. Saito M, Braud VM, Goon P, et al. Low frequency of CD94/NKG2A+ T lymphocytes in patients with HTLV-1-associated myelopathy/tropical spastic paraparesis, but not in asymptomatic carriers. *Blood* 2003;102:577–584.
305. Saito M, Matsuzaki T, Satou Y, et al. In vivo expression of the HBZ gene of HTLV-1 correlates with proviral load, inflammatory markers and disease severity in HTLV-1 associated myelopathy/tropical spastic paraparesis (HAM/TSP). *Retrovirology* 2009;6:19.
306. Saitoh Y, Yamamoto N, Dewan MZ, et al. Overexpressed NF-kappaB-inducing kinase contributes to the tumorigenesis of adult T-cell leukemia and Hodgkin Reed-Sternberg cells. *Blood* 2008;111:5118–5129.

307. Salemi M, Desmyter J, Vandamme AM. Tempo and mode of human and simian T-lymphotropic virus (HTLV/STLV) evolution revealed by analyses of full-genome sequences. *Mol Biol Evol* 2000;17:374–386.
308. Sasada A, Takaori-Kondo A, Shirakawa K, et al. APOBEC3G targets human T-cell leukemia virus type 1. *Retrovirology* 2005;2:32.
309. Satake M, Iwanaga M, Sagara Y, et al. Incidence of human T-lymphotropic virus 1 infection in adolescent and adult blood donors in Japan: a nationwide retrospective cohort analysis. *Lancet Infect Dis* 2016;16:1246–1254.
310. Sato T, Coler-Reilly ALG, Yagishita N, et al. Mogamulizumab (Anti-CCR4) in HTLV-1-associated myelopathy. *N Engl J Med* 2018;378:529–538.
311. Satou Y, Miyazato P, Ishihara K, et al. The retrovirus HTLV-1 inserts an ectopic CTCF-binding site into the human genome. *Proc Natl Acad Sci U S A* 2016;113:3054–3059.
312. Satou Y, Utsunomiya A, Tanabe J, et al. HTLV-1 modulates the frequency and phenotype of FoxP3+CD4+ T cells in virus-infected individuals. *Retrovirology* 2012;9:46.
313. Satou Y, Yasunaga J, Yoshida M, et al. HTLV-I basic leucine zipper factor gene mRNA supports proliferation of adult T cell leukemia cells. *Proc Natl Acad Sci U S A* 2006;103:720–725.
314. Satou Y, Yasunaga J, Zhao T, et al. HTLV-1 bZIP factor induces T-cell lymphoma and systemic inflammation in vivo. *PLoS Pathog* 2011;7:e1001274.
315. Sawada T, Iwahara Y, Ishii K, et al. Immunoglobulin prophylaxis against milkborne transmission of human T cell leukemia virus type I in rabbits. *J Infect Dis* 1991;164:1193–1196.
316. Saxon A, Stevens RH, Quan SG, et al. Immunologic characterization of hairy cell leukemias in continuous culture. *J Immunol* 1978;120:777–782.
317. Schierhout G, McGregor S, Gessain A, et al. Association between HTLV-1 infection and adverse health outcomes: a systematic review and meta-analysis of epidemiological studies. *Lancet Infect Dis* 2020;20:133–143.
318. Seich al Basatena NK, MacNamara A, Vine AM, et al. KIR2DL2 enhances protective and detrimental HLA class I-mediated immunity in chronic viral infection. *PLoS Pathog* 2011;7:e1002270.
319. Seiki M, Hattori S, Hirayama Y, et al. Human adult T-cell leukemia virus: complete nucleotide sequence of the provirus genome integrated in leukemia cell DNA. *Proc Natl Acad Sci U S A* 1983;80:3618–3622.
320. Seiki M, Hikikoshi A, Taniguchi T, et al. Expression of the pX gene of HTLV-I: general splicing mechanism in the HTLV family. *Science* 1985;228:1532–1534.
321. Seiki M, Hikikoshi A, Yoshida M. The U5 sequence is a cis-acting repressive element for genomic RNA expression of human T cell leukemia virus type I. *Virology* 1990;176:81–86.
322. Seiki M, Inoue J, Takeda T, et al. The p40x of human T-cell leukemia virus type I is a trans-acting activator of viral gene transcription. *Jpn J Cancer Res* 1985;76:1127–1131.
323. Seiki M, Inoue J, Takeda T, et al. Direct evidence that p40x of human T-cell leukemia virus type I is a trans-acting transcriptional activator. *EMBO J* 1986;5:561–565.
324. Sherman MP, Saksena NK, Dube DK, et al. Evolutionary insights on the origin of human T-cell lymphoma/leukemia virus type I (HTLV-I) derived from sequence analysis of a new HTLV-I variant from Papua New Guinea. *J Virol* 1992;66:2556–2563.
325. Shida H, Tochikura T, Sato T, et al. Effect of the recombinant vaccinia viruses that express HTLV-I envelope gene on HTLV-I infection. *EMBO J* 1987;6:3379–3384.
326. Shimotohno K, Takano M, Teruuchi T, et al. Requirement of multiple copies of a 21-nucleotide sequence in the U3 regions of human T-cell leukemia virus type I and type II long terminal repeats for trans-acting activation of transcription. *Proc Natl Acad Sci U S A* 1986;83:8112–8116.
327. Shimoyama M. Diagnostic criteria and classification of clinical subtypes of adult T-cell leukaemia-lymphoma. A report from the Lymphoma Study Group (1984–87). *Br J Haematol* 1991;79:428–437.
328. Shimoyama M. Chemotherapy of ATL. In: Takatsuki K, ed. *Adult T-cell leukemia*. New York: Oxford University Press; 1994.
329. Silic-Benussi M, Biasiotto R, Andresen V, et al. HTLV-1 p13, a small protein with a busy agenda. *Mol Aspects Med* 2010;31:350–358.
330. Silic-Benussi M, Cavallari I, Vajente N, et al. Redox regulation of T-cell turnover by the p13 protein of human T-cell leukemia virus type 1: distinct effects in primary versus transformed cells. *Blood* 2010;116:54–62.
331. Sinha-Datta U, Datta A, Ghorbel S, et al. Human T-cell lymphotrophic virus type I rex and p30 interactions govern the switch between virus latency and replication. *J Biol Chem* 2007;282:14608–14615.
332. Siomi H, Shida H, Nam SH, et al. Sequence requirements for nucleolar localization of human T cell leukemia virus type I pX protein, which regulates viral RNA processing. *Cell* 1988;55:197–209.
333. Siu YT, Chin KT, Siu KL, et al. TORC1 and TORC2 coactivators are required for tax activation of the human T-cell leukemia virus type 1 long terminal repeats. *J Virol* 2006;80:7052–7059.
334. Slattery JP, Franchini G, Gessain A. Genomic evolution, patterns of global dissemination, and interspecies transmission of human and simian T-cell leukemia/lymphotropic viruses. *Genome Res* 1999;9:525–540.
335. Sodroski JG, Rosen CA, Haseltine WA. Trans-acting transcriptional activation of the long terminal repeat of human T lymphotropic viruses in infected cells. *Science* 1984;225:381–385.
336. Sommerfelt MA, Williams BP, Clapham PR, et al. Human T cell leukemia viruses use a receptor determined by human chromosome 17. *Science* 1988;242:1557–1559.
337. Sonoda S, Fujiyoshi T, Yashiki S. Immunogenetics of HTLV-I/II and associated diseases. *J Acquir Immune Defic Syndr Hum Retrovirol* 1996;13(Suppl 1):S119–S123.
338. Stuver SO, Tachibana N, Okayama A, et al. Heterosexual transmission of human T cell leukemia/lymphoma virus type I among married couples in southwestern Japan: an initial report from the Miyazaki Cohort Study. *J Infect Dis* 1993;167:57–65.
339. Suehiro Y, Hasegawa A, Iino T, et al. Clinical outcomes of a novel therapeutic vaccine with Tax peptide-pulsed dendritic cells for adult T cell leukaemia/lymphoma in a pilot study. *Br J Haematol* 2015;169:356–367.
340. Sugata K, Yasunaga J, Kinosada H, et al. HTLV-1 viral factor HBZ induces CCR4 to promote T-cell migration and proliferation. *Cancer Res* 2016;76:5068–5079.
341. Sugata K, Yasunaga J, Mitobe Y, et al. Protective effect of cytotoxic T lymphocytes targeting HTLV-1 bZIP factor. *Blood* 2015;126:1095–1105.
342. Sugata K, Yasunaga J, Miura M, et al. Enhancement of anti-STLV-1/HTLV-1 immune responses through multimodal effects of anti-CCR4 antibody. *Sci Rep* 2016;6:27150.
343. Sugimoto M, Nakashima H, Watanabe S, et al. T-lymphocyte alveolitis in HTLV-I-associated myelopathy. *Lancet* 1987;2:1220.
344. Sun SC, Yamaoka S. Activation of NF-kappaB by HTLV-I and implications for cell transformation. *Oncogene* 2005;24:5952–5964.
345. Suzuki T, Hirai H, Murakami T, et al. Tax protein of HTLV-1 destabilizes the complexes of NF-kappa B and I kappa B-alpha and induces nuclear translocation of NF-kappa B for transcriptional activation. *Oncogene* 1995;10:1199–1207.
346. Suzuki T, Uchida-Toita M, Yoshida M. Tax protein of HTLV-1 inhibits CBP/p300-mediated transcription by interfering with recruitment of CBP/p300 onto DNA element of E-box or p53 binding site. *Oncogene* 1999;18:4137–4143.
347. Suzuki Y, Gojobori T. The origin and evolution of human T-cell lymphotropic virus types I and II. *Virus Genes* 1998;16:69–84.
348. Sze A, Belgnaoui SM, Olagnier D, et al. Host restriction factor SAMHD1 limits human T cell leukemia virus type 1 infection of monocytes via STING-mediated apoptosis. *Cell Host Microbe* 2013;14:422–434.
349. Tagaya Y, Matsuoka M, Gallo R. 40 years of the human T-cell leukemia virus: past, present, and future. *F1000Res* 2019;8:F1000 Faculty Rev-228.
350. Tajima K, Inoue M, Takezaki T, et al. Ethnoepidemiology of ATL in Japan with special reference to the Mongoloid dispersal. In: Takatsuki K, ed. *Adult T-cell Leukemia* New York: Oxford University Press; 1994.
351. Tajima Y, Tashiro K, Camerini D. Assignment of the possible HTLV receptor gene to chromosome 17q21-q23. *Somat Cell Mol Genet* 1997;23:225–227.
352. Takahashi K, Takezaki T, Oki T, et al. Inhibitory effect of maternal antibody on mother-to-child transmission of human T-lymphotropic virus type I. The Mother-to-Child Transmission Study Group. *Int J Cancer* 1991;49:673–677.
353. Takasaki Y, Iwanaga M, Imaizumi Y, et al. Long-term study of indolent adult T-cell leukemia-lymphoma. *Blood* 2010;115:4337–4343.
354. Takatsuki K. Discovery of adult T-cell leukemia. *Retrovirology* 2005;2:16.
355. Takatsuki K, Yamaguchi K, Matsuoka M. ATL and HTLV-I-related diseases. In: Takatsuki K, ed. *Adult T-cell Leukemia*. New York: Oxford University Press; 1994.
356. Takeda S, Maeda M, Morikawa S, et al. Genetic and epigenetic inactivation of tax gene in adult T-cell leukemia cells. *Int J Cancer* 2004;109:559–567.
357. Tamiya S, Etoh K, Suzushima H, et al. Mutation of CD95 (Fas/Apo-1) gene in adult T-cell leukemia cells. *Blood* 1998;91:3935–3942.
358. Tamiya S, Matsuoka M, Etoh K, et al. Two types of defective human T-lymphotropic virus type I provirus in adult T-cell leukemia. *Blood* 1996;88:3065–3073.
359. Tanaka A, Matsuoka M. HTLV-1 alters T cells for viral persistence and transmission. *Front Microbiol* 2018;9:461.
360. Taniguchi Y, Nosaka K, Yasunaga J, et al. Silencing of human T-cell leukemia virus type I gene transcription by epigenetic mechanisms. *Retrovirology* 2005;2:64.
361. Taylor GP. Human T-lymphotropic virus type 1 infection and solid organ transplantation. *Rev Med Virol* 2018;28.
362. Taylor GP, Goon P, Furukawa Y, et al. Zidovudine plus lamivudine in Human T-Lymphotropic Virus type-I-associated myelopathy: a randomised trial. *Retrovirology* 2006; 3:63.
363. Terol M, Gazon H, Lemasson I, et al. HBZ-mediated shift of JunD from growth suppressor to tumor promoter in leukemic cells by inhibition of ribosomal protein S25 expression. *Leukemia* 2017;31:2235–2243.
364. Tezuka K, Fuchi N, Okuma K, et al. HTLV-1 targets human placental trophoblasts in seropositive pregnant women. *J Clin Invest* 2020;130:6171–6186.
365. Thebault S, Basbous J, Hivin P, et al. HBZ interacts with JunD and stimulates its transcriptional activity. *FEBS Lett* 2004;562:165–170.
366. Tholouli E, Liu Yin JA. Successful treatment of HTLV-1-associated acute adult T-cell leukemia lymphoma by allogeneic bone marrow transplantation: a 12 year follow-up. *Leuk Lymphoma* 2006;47:1691–1692.
367. Tomasetti C, Li L, Vogelstein B. Stem cell divisions, somatic mutations, cancer etiology, and cancer prevention. *Science* 2017;355:1330–1334.
368. Tomasetti C, Vogelstein B. Cancer etiology. Variation in cancer risk among tissues can be explained by the number of stem cell divisions. *Science* 2015;347:78–81.
369. Toro C, Rodes B, Poveda E, et al. Rapid development of subacute myelopathy in three organ transplant recipients after transmission of human T-cell lymphotropic virus type I from a single donor. *Transplantation* 2003;75:102–104.
370. Toulza F, Heaps A, Tanaka Y, et al. High frequency of CD4+FoxP3+ cells in HTLV-1 infection: inverse correlation with HTLV-1-specific CTL response. *Blood* 2008;111:5047–5053.
371. Toulza F, Nosaka K, Takiguchi M, et al. FoxP3+ regulatory T cells are distinct from leukemia cells in HTLV-1-associated adult T-cell leukemia. *Int J Cancer* 2009;125:2375–2382.
372. Toulza F, Nosaka K, Tanaka Y, et al. Human T-lymphotropic virus type 1-induced CC chemokine ligand 22 maintains a high frequency of functional FoxP3+ regulatory T cells. *J Immunol* 2010;185:183–189.
373. Trevino A, Parra P, Bar-Magen T, et al. Antiviral effect of raltegravir on HTLV-1 carriers. *J Antimicrob Chemother* 2012;67:218–221.
374. Trovato R, Mulloy JC, Johnson JM, et al. A lysine-to-arginine change found in natural alleles of the human T-cell lymphotropic/leukemia virus type 1 p12(I) protein greatly influences its stability. *J Virol* 1999;73:6460–6467.
375. Tsukahara T, Kannagi M, Ohashi T, et al. Induction of Bcl-x(L) expression by human T-cell leukemia virus type 1 Tax through NF-kappaB in apoptosis-resistant T-cell transfectants with Tax. *J Virol* 1999;73:7981–7987.
376. Uchiyama T, Yodoi J, Sagawa K, et al. Adult T-cell leukemia: clinical and hematologic features of 16 cases. *Blood* 1977;50:481–492.
377. Umehara F, Izumo S, Nakagawa M, et al. Immunocytochemical analysis of the cellular infiltrate in the spinal cord lesions in HTLV-I-associated myelopathy. *J Neuropathol Exp Neurol* 1993;52:424–430.
378. Umehara F, Nakamura A, Izumo S, et al. Apoptosis of T lymphocytes in the spinal cord lesions in HTLV-I-associated myelopathy: a possible mechanism to control viral infection in the central nervous system. *J Neuropathol Exp Neurol* 1994;53:617–624.

379. Unge T, Solomin L, Mellini M, et al. The Rex regulatory protein of human T-cell lymphotropic virus type I binds specifically to its target site within the viral RNA. *Proc Natl Acad Sci U S A* 1991;88:7145–7149.

380. Ureta-Vidal A, Angelin-Duclos C, Tortevoye P, et al. Mother-to-child transmission of human T-cell-leukemia/lymphoma virus type I: implication of high antiviral antibody titer and high proviral load in carrier mothers. *Int J Cancer* 1999;82:832–836.

381. Usui T, Yanagihara K, Tsukasaki K, et al. Characteristic expression of HTLV-1 basic zipper factor (HBZ) transcripts in HTLV-1 provirus-positive cells. *Retrovirology* 2008;5:34.

382. Usuku K, Nishizawa M, Matsuki K, et al. Association of a particular amino acid sequence of the HLA-DR beta 1 chain with HTLV-I-associated myelopathy. *Eur J Immunol* 1990;20:1603–1606.

383. Valeri VW, Hryniewicz A, Andresen V, et al. Requirement of the human T-cell leukemia virus p12 and p30 products for infectivity of human dendritic cells and macaques but not rabbits. *Blood* 2010;116:3809–3817.

384. Van Dooren S, Salemi M, Vandamme AM. Dating the origin of the African human T-cell lymphotropic virus type-i (HTLV-I) subtypes. *Mol Biol Evol* 2001;18:661–671.

385. Van Prooyen N, Gold H, Andresen V, et al. Human T-cell leukemia virus type 1 p8 protein increases cellular conduits and virus transmission. *Proc Natl Acad Sci U S A* 2010;107:20738–20743.

386. Vandamme AM, Liu HF, Goubau P, et al. Primate T-lymphotropic virus type I LTR sequence variation and its phylogenetic analysis: compatibility with an African origin of PTLV-I. *Virology* 1994;202:212–223.

387. Vandamme AM, Salemi M, Desmyter J. The simian origins of the pathogenic human T-cell lymphotropic virus type I. *Trends Microbiol* 1998;6:477–483.

388. Vandamme AM, Salemi M, Van Brussel M, et al. African origin of human T-lymphotropic virus type 2 (HTLV-2) supported by a potential new HTLV-2d subtype in Congolese Bambuti Efe Pygmies. *J Virol* 1998;72:4327–4340.

389. Verdonck K, Gonzalez E, Schrooten W, et al. HTLV-1 infection is associated with a history of active tuberculosis among family members of HTLV-1-infected patients in Peru. *Epidemiol Infect* 2008;136:1076–1083.

390. Verdonck K, Gonzalez E, Van Dooren S, et al. Human T-lymphotropic virus 1: recent knowledge about an ancient infection. *Lancet Infect Dis* 2007;7:266–281.

391. Vernin C, Thenoz M, Pinatel C, et al. HTLV-1 bZIP factor HBZ promotes cell proliferation and genetic instability by activating OncomiRs. *Cancer Res* 2014;74:6082–6093.

392. Vine AM, Witkover AD, Lloyd AL, et al. Polygenic control of human T lymphotropic virus type I (HTLV-I) provirus load and the risk of HTLV-I-associated myelopathy/tropical spastic paraparesis. *J Infect Dis* 2002;186:932–939.

393. Watanabe T, Yamaguchi K, Takatsuki K, et al. Constitutive expression of parathyroid hormone-related protein gene in human T cell leukemia virus type 1 (HTLV-1) carriers and adult T cell leukemia patients that can be trans-activated by HTLV-1 tax gene. *J Exp Med* 1990;172:759–765.

394. Wattel E, Cavrois M, Gessain A, et al. Clonal expansion of infected cells: a way of life for HTLV-I. *J Acquir Immune Defic Syndr Hum Retrovirol* 1996;13(Suppl 1):S92–S99.

395. Weichselbraun I, Farrington GK, Rusche JR, et al. Definition of the human immunodeficiency virus type 1 Rev and human T-cell leukemia virus type I Rex protein activation domain by functional exchange. *J Virol* 1992;66:2583–2587.

396. Wen AY, Sakamoto KM, Miller LS. The role of the transcription factor CREB in immune function. *J Immunol* 2010;185:6413–6419.

397. Wiktor SZ, Pate EJ, Rosenberg PS, et al. Mother-to-child transmission of human T-cell lymphotropic virus type I associated with prolonged breast-feeding. *J Hum Virol* 1997;1:37–44.

398. Wolfe ND, Heneine W, Carr JK, et al. Emergence of unique primate T-lymphotropic viruses among central African bushmeat hunters. *Proc Natl Acad Sci U S A* 2005;102:7994–7999.

399. Worobey M, Gemmel M, Teuwen DE, et al. Direct evidence of extensive diversity of HIV-1 in Kinshasa by 1960. *Nature* 2008;455:661–664.

400. Xiao G, Cvijic ME, Fong A, et al. Retroviral oncoprotein Tax induces processing of NF-kappaB2/p100 in T cells: evidence for the involvement of IKKalpha. *EMBO J* 2001;20:6805–6815.

401. Xie L, Green PL. Envelope is a major viral determinant of the distinct in vitro cellular transformation tropism of human T-cell leukemia virus type 1 (HTLV-1) and HTLV-2. *J Virol* 2005;79:14536–14545.

402. Yamada Y, Tomonaga M, Fukuda H, et al. A new G-CSF-supported combination chemotherapy, LSG15, for adult T-cell leukaemia-lymphoma: Japan Clinical Oncology Group Study 9303. *Br J Haematol* 2001;113:375–382.

403. Yamagishi M, Nakano K, Miyake A, et al. Polycomb-mediated loss of miR-31 activates NIK-dependent NF-kappaB pathway in adult T cell leukemia and other cancers. *Cancer Cell* 2012;21:121–135.

404. Yamamoto K, Utsunomiya A, Tobinai K, et al. Phase I study of KW-0761, a defucosylated humanized anti-CCR4 antibody, in relapsed patients with adult T-cell leukemia-lymphoma and peripheral T-cell lymphoma. *J Clin Oncol* 2010;28:1591–1598.

405. Yamano Y, Araya N, Sato T, et al. Abnormally high levels of virus-infected IFN-gamma+ CCR4+ CD4+ CD25+ T cells in a retrovirus-associated neuroinflammatory disorder. *PLoS One* 2009;4:e6517.

406. Yamaoka S, Courtois G, Bessia C, et al. Complementation cloning of NEMO, a component of the IkappaB kinase complex essential for NF-kappaB activation. *Cell* 1998;93:1231–1240.

407. Yamato K, Oka T, Hiroi M, et al. Aberrant expression of the p53 tumor suppressor gene in adult T-cell leukemia and HTLV-1-infected cells. *Jpn J Cancer Res* 1993;84:4–8.

408. Yang L, Kotomura N, Ho YK, et al. Complex cell cycle abnormalities caused by human T-lymphotropic virus type 1 Tax. *J Virol* 2011;85:3001–3009.

409. Yasuda N, Lai PK, Ip SH, et al. Soluble interleukin 2 receptors in sera of Japanese patients with adult T cell leukemia mark activity of disease. *Blood* 1988;71:1021–1026.

410. Yasuma K, Yasunaga J, Takemoto K, et al. HTLV-1 bZIP factor impairs anti-viral immunity by inducing co-inhibitory molecule, T cell immunoglobulin and ITIM domain (TIGIT). *PLoS Pathog* 2016;12:e1005372.

411. Yasunaga J, Taniguchi Y, Nosaka K, et al. Identification of aberrantly methylated genes in association with adult T-cell leukemia. *Cancer Res* 2004;64:6002–6009.

412. Yoshida M. Multiple viral strategies of HTLV-1 for dysregulation of cell growth control. *Annu Rev Immunol* 2001;19:475–496.

413. Yoshida M, Satou Y, Yasunaga J, et al. Transcriptional control of spliced and unspliced human T-cell leukemia virus type 1 bZIP factor (HBZ) gene. *J Virol* 2008;82:9359–9368.

414. Yoshie O, Fujisawa R, Nakayama T, et al. Frequent expression of CCR4 in adult T-cell leukemia and human T-cell leukemia virus type 1-transformed T cells. *Blood* 2002;99:1505–1511.

415. Yoshimura T, Fujisawa J, Yoshida M. Multiple cDNA clones encoding nuclear proteins that bind to the tax-dependent enhancer of HTLV-1: all contain a leucine zipper structure and basic amino acid domain. *EMBO J* 1990;9:2537–2542.

416. Yoshita M, Higuchi M, Takahashi M, et al. Activation of mTOR by human T-cell leukemia virus type 1 Tax is important for the transformation of mouse T cells to interleukin-2-independent growth. *Cancer Sci* 2012;103(2):369–374.

417. Yu F, Itoyama Y, Fujihara K, et al. Natural killer (NK) cells in HTLV-I-associated myelopathy/tropical spastic paraparesis-decrease in NK cell subset populations and activity in HTLV-I seropositive individuals. *J Neuroimmunol* 1991;33:121–128.

418. Yuen CK, Chan CP, Fung SY, et al. Suppression of type I interferon production by human T-cell leukemia virus type 1 oncoprotein tax through inhibition of IRF3 phosphorylation. *J Virol* 2016;90:3902–3912.

419. Yukitake M, Sueoka E, Sueoka-Aragane N, et al. Significantly increased antibody response to heterogeneous nuclear ribonucleoproteins in cerebrospinal fluid of multiple sclerosis patients but not in patients with human T-lymphotropic virus type I-associated myelopathy/tropical spastic paraparesis. *J Neurovirol* 2008;14:130–135.

420. Zhang X, Hakata Y, Tanaka Y, et al. CRM1, an RNA transporter, is a major species-specific restriction factor of human T cell leukemia virus type 1 (HTLV-1) in rat cells. *Microbes Infect* 2006;8:851–859.

421. Zhao LJ, Giam CZ. Interaction of the human T-cell lymphotrophic virus type I (HTLV-I) transcriptional activator Tax with cellular factors that bind specifically to the 21-base-pair repeats in the HTLV-I enhancer. *Proc Natl Acad Sci U S A* 1991;88:11445–11449.

422. Zhao LJ, Giam CZ. Human T-cell lymphotropic virus type I (HTLV-I) transcriptional activator, Tax, enhances CREB binding to HTLV-I 21-base-pair repeats by protein-protein interaction. *Proc Natl Acad Sci U S A* 1992;89:7070–7074.

423. Zhao T, Satou Y, Sugata K, et al. HTLV-1 bZIP factor enhances TGF-{beta} signaling through p300 coactivator. *Blood* 2011;118:1865–1876.

424. Zhao T, Yasunaga J, Satou Y, et al. Human T-cell leukemia virus type 1 bZIP factor selectively suppresses the classical pathway of NF-kappaB. *Blood* 2009;113:2755–2764.

425. Zhi H, Guo X, Ho YK, et al. RNF8 dysregulation and down-regulation during HTLV-1 infection promote genomic instability in adult T-Cell leukemia. *PLoS Pathog* 2020;16:e1008618.

426. Zhi H, Yang L, Kuo YL, et al. NF-kappaB hyper-activation by HTLV-1 tax induces cellular senescence, but can be alleviated by the viral anti-sense protein HBZ. *PLoS Pathog* 2011;7:e1002025.

427. Zhou M, Lu H, Park H, et al. Tax interacts with P-TEFb in a novel manner to stimulate human T-lymphotropic virus type 1 transcription. *J Virol* 2006;80:4781–4791.

Human Immunodeficiency Viruses: Replication

Melanie Ott • Eric O. Freed

Introduction
Classification and origins of HIVs
Genomic organization of HIVs
Biology of HIV infections
    HIV replication and tropism
    HIV transmission
HIV-1 animal models
    Chimpanzees
    SIV models in nonhuman primates
    Humanized mouse models
Molecular biology of HIV-1 replication
    Overview
    Virus binding and entry: the Env glycoproteins
    Postentry trafficking of the HIV capsid
    Reverse transcription
    Nuclear import
    Postentry blocks to lentiviral infection
    Integration
    Viral gene expression
    Virus assembly and release: the Gag proteins
    Env glycoprotein incorporation into virions
    Protease (PR) and virus maturation
    The accessory proteins
Perspectives
Acknowledgments

INTRODUCTION

In the late 1970s and early 1980s, previously healthy individuals in the United States and Europe presented with symptoms of immunologic dysfunction, including generalized lymphadenopathy, opportunistic infections, and a variety of unusual cancers (non-Hodgkin lymphoma and Kaposi's sarcoma). A common accompanying laboratory finding in affected individuals was marked depletion of the CD4+ T lymphocyte subset in the peripheral blood. The disease was first brought to the attention of the general medical community in June 1981.[489] Within several months, it became clear that a similar immunodeficiency syndrome, which came to be known as acquired immunodeficiency syndrome, or AIDS, was also affecting other groups, including hemophiliacs, blood transfusion recipients, recent Haitian immigrants, and, most significantly, sexual partners or children of members of the various risk groups.

The emerging epidemiological pattern suggested that the new disease was transmitted by a novel pathogen in contaminated blood or following sexual intercourse with an affected individual. In the spring of 1983, Montagnier, Barre-Sinoussi, and their colleagues at the Pasteur Institute in Paris reported the isolation of a virus from the lymph nodes of an individual who presented with generalized lymphadenopathy of unknown origin.[30] During its replication in cultured cells, the virus, termed lymphadenopathy-associated virus (LAV), released high titers of progeny virions that contained magnesium-dependent reverse transcriptase (RT) activity and exhibited electron microscopic (EM) features typical of retroviruses. However, unlike the commonly studied retroviruses, LAV was highly cytopathic in human peripheral blood mononuclear cells (PBMCs), specifically killing CD4+ T lymphocytes in cell cultures.[493] Gallo and colleagues at the National Institutes of Health subsequently reported the isolation of a nearly identical retrovirus from tissue culture samples obtained from the Pasteur Institute group. Gallo and colleagues named this virus human T-cell leukemia virus type III (HTLV-III) to distinguish it from the noncytopathic HTLV-1 and HTLV-2 and obtained the first serological evidence linking exposure to LAV-like retroviruses and immunodeficient individuals from the various groups at risk.[565,623] The new retrovirus, associated with AIDS in the United States, Europe, and central Africa, and exhibiting morphologic and genetic characteristics typical of the lentivirus genus (Fig. 17.1), was named human immunodeficiency virus, or HIV[136] (and subsequently HIV-1). In 1986, a related but immunologically distinct human retrovirus (now called HIV-2) was recovered from individuals residing in several West African countries.[134]

CLASSIFICATION AND ORIGINS OF HIVs

The observation of particle-associated RT activity placed the new agent in the *Retroviridae* family. EM analysis showed that the mature HIV-1 particles contained a cone-shaped, cylindrical core reminiscent of that previously described for visna virus (Fig. 17.1).[259] The cloning and sequencing of proviral DNA, initially purified from productively infected cultures of PBMC/T-cell leukemia lines (T-cell lines), indicated that HIV-1 not only possessed a genomic organization related to that of other replication–competent retroviruses but placed it taxonomically

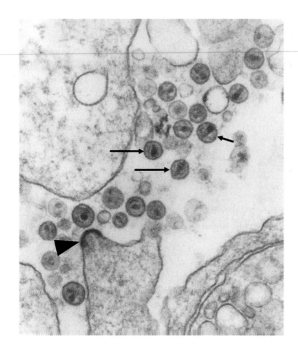

FIGURE 17.1 Morphology of HIV-1 particles. Electron micrograph showing an HIV-1 particle in the process of budding from infected cultured human peripheral blood mononuclear cells (PBMCs) (*arrowhead*) and several particles containing the conical core characteristic of mature, infectious HIV-1 virions (*arrows*) (100,000× magnification). (Courtesy of Dr. Jan Orenstein.).

in the lentivirus genus.[584,724] This relationship is shown diagrammatically in Figure 2 of Chapter 15. As their name suggests, lentiviruses (*lenti*, slow) were known to cause slow, unremitting disease in sheep, goats, and horses, and to target various lineages of hematopoietic cells, particularly monocytes/macrophages and lymphocytes.

After the isolation, molecular cloning, and initial classification of HIV-1, several genetically distinct primate lentiviruses were discovered and their phylogenetic relationships to HIV-1 were determined. For example, viruses isolated from captive macaques or feral monkey species in Africa were shown to possess particle morphologies and genomic organizations similar to those of HIV-1 (described in Chapter 19). Because inoculation of Asian macaque species, such as rhesus monkeys, with some of these newly discovered viruses recovered from African monkeys induced an AIDS-like illness,[157] these viruses were named simian immunodeficiency virus (SIV) to distinguish them from the human viruses, HIV-1 and HIV-2. The detailed genetic interrelationships of members of the primate lentivirus genus are presented in Figure 1 of Chapter 19. HIV-2 is more closely related to SIV_{smm},[299] a virus indigenous to African sooty mangabey monkeys, than to HIV-1; HIV-2 likely arose through a zoonotic transmission of SIV_{smm} from monkeys to humans.[248,649]

Based on previously studied replication–competent retroviruses, it was originally anticipated that HIV-1 would be genetically homogeneous. However, early comparisons of proviral DNAs from Europe, North America, and Africa revealed extensive genetic heterogeneity even among sequences derived

from a single individual.[41] Although nucleotide changes were distributed throughout the HIV-1 genome, the greatest variability occurred in the gene encoding the envelope (Env) glycoprotein, gp160. The term "quasispecies" was subsequently coined to describe the pool of diverse and changing populations of virus present in an HIV-1–infected individual.[487] Several factors contribute to the extraordinary genetic heterogeneity of HIV-1: (a) error-prone viral DNA synthesis during reverse transcription, (b) high recombination frequencies accompanying reverse transcription, (c) large population size *in vivo*, and (d) continuous pressure from the host to select for new variants.

The earliest phylogenetic analyses of HIV-1 isolates focused on samples from Europe, North America, and Africa; discrete clusters of viruses were identified from these geographical regions. Distinct genetic subtypes or clades of HIV-1 were subsequently defined and classified into four groups: M (main); O (outlier); N (non-M, non-O); and P (Fig. 17.2A).[291] The M group of HIV-1, which comprises greater than 99% of the global virus isolates, consists of nine subtypes (A, B, C, D, F, G, H, J, and K) and several dozen circulating recombinant forms (CRFs), which arose by the intermixing of viruses cocirculating in a particular geographical locale.[443,480,547,600] Subtype B viruses, the most intensively studied HIV-1 subtype, are the most prevalent isolates in Europe, North America, and Australia. Subtype C strains are responsible for greater than 50% of infections globally. HIV-1 group O isolates were recovered from individuals living in Cameroon, Gabon, and Equatorial Guinea.[691] The overall prevalence of this group has declined over time. Group N and P isolates are extremely rare.

A primate lentivirus designated SIV_{cpz} has a genomic structure very similar to that of HIV-1, including its signature *vpu* gene. SIV_{cpz} was isolated from two chimpanzee subspecies, *Pan troglodytes troglodytes* (*ptt*) and *Pan troglodytes schweinfurthii* (*pts*). The prevalence of SIV_{cpz} recovered from *ptt* animals (SIV_{cpzPtt}) in the wild varies widely compared to the more even and higher distribution of SIVs infecting sooty mangabeys and African green monkeys. Phylogenetically, the SIV_{cpzPtt} strains are related to HIV-1 groups M and N but not to group O or SIV_{cpzPts} (Fig. 17.2B) and geographically separated chimpanzee populations carry distinct genetic lineages of SIV_{cpzPtt}.[369] Cross-species transmission of SIV_{cpz} to humans in Central Africa and SIV_{sm} in West Africa gave rise to HIV-1 and HIV-2, respectively.[247,248] Based on nucleotide substitutions over time, a common ancestor of HIV-1 group M has been proposed to have emerged in the 1920s,[742] whereas progenitors for HIV-2 groups A and B have been dated to the 1940s.[415] The SIV_{cpz} strains giving rise to HIV-1 have been introduced into humans at least four times (as reflected in groups M, N, O, and P). It is thought that the source of HIV-1 group M, the cause of the worldwide AIDS epidemic, originated in *ptt* chimpanzees living in southeast Cameroon.[369] SIV_{cpz} is itself a recombinant between two other SIVs, SIV_{rcm} and SIV_{gsn}, which likely coinfected a chimpanzee.[650] Because of the high degree of genetic relatedness between chimpanzees and humans, the propagation of SIV_{cpz} in chimpanzees likely increased its ability to replicate in humans when the subsequent interspecies jump occurred.

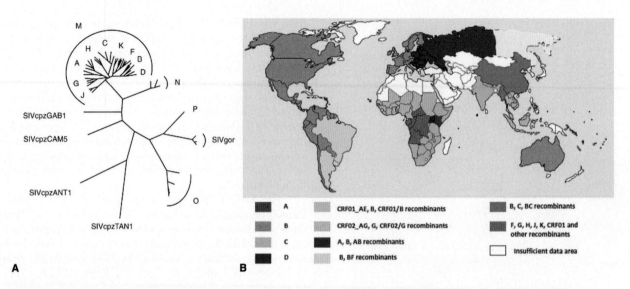

A   **B**

FIGURE 17.2 HIV-1 genetic subtypes and their worldwide distribution. A: Phylogenetic relationships of HIV-1 groups M, N, O, and P with different SIV (SIV$_{cpz}$ and SIV$_{gpr}$) isolates. (Reprinted from Hemelaar J. The origin and diversity of the HIV-1 pandemic. *Trends Mol Med* 2012;18(3):182–192. Copyright © 2011 Elsevier. With permission.) **B:** The global prevalence of HIV-1 subgroups with the predominant clades or circulating recombinant forms (CRFs) in each geographical region indicated. (Provided by Dr. Sodsai Tovanabutra, U.S. Military HIV Research Program, Henry Jackson Foundation.)

GENOMIC ORGANIZATION OF HIVs

Nucleotide sequencing of several of the original HIV-1 isolates revealed that in contrast to the well-characterized and intensively studied prototypical retroviruses, whose genomes often contain only three genes (*gag*, *pol*, and *env*) encoding the structural proteins and enzymes required for productive infection, the HIV-1 genome included several additional and overlapping open reading frames (ORFs) of unknown function (Fig. 17.3). Not only did HIV-1 and HIV-2 contain multiple additional ORFs but also their genomic organizations appeared to be very similar. Further analyses revealed that HIV-1 contained the distinguishing *vpu* gene[141,681] and HIV-2 carried a signature *vpx*[361] gene.

Like all replication–competent orthoretroviruses, the three primary translation products from the *gag*, *pol*, and *env* genes are initially synthesized as polyprotein precursors, which are subsequently processed by viral or cellular proteases into mature, particle-associated proteins (Fig. 17.4). The 55-kDa Gag precursor, Pr55^{Gag}, is cleaved into the matrix (MA), capsid (CA), nucleocapsid (NC), and p6 proteins, and the two spacer peptides SP1 and SP2 during or shortly after the release of progeny virions. Autocatalysis of the 160 kDa Gag–Pol polyprotein, Pr160^{GagPol}, gives rise to the protease (PR), the heterodimeric RT, and integrase (IN) enzymes, whereas proteolytic digestion by a cellular enzyme in the Golgi converts the glycosylated 160-kDa Env precursor, gp160, into the gp120 surface (SU) and gp41 transmembrane (TM) cleavage products. The remaining six HIV-1–encoded proteins (Vif, Vpr, Tat, Rev, Vpu, and Nef) are the primary translation products of spliced mRNAs, as is the Env glycoprotein.

HIV-1 and HIV-2 have incorporated multiple sequence elements into their genomic RNAs that direct the balanced and coordinated production of progeny virions.[55,72] The 5' approximately 400 nucleotide untranslated region of HIV-1 genomic RNA is highly structured and contains multiple elements that mediate transcriptional elongation of viral RNA transcripts,

splicing, genomic RNA dimerization, packaging of full-length viral RNA, and reverse transcription (Fig. 17.5A). These include the dimerization initiation signal (DIS), a palindromic sequence that promotes RNA dimerization and packaging into virions (Fig. 17.5A and B).

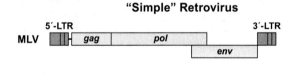

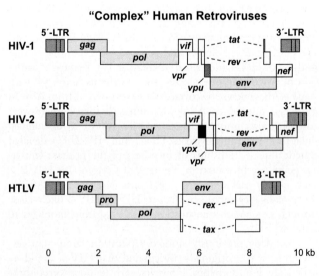

FIGURE 17.3 Genomic organization of simple and complex retroviruses. The genes of murine leukemia virus (MLV), human T-cell leukemia virus (HTLV), HIV-1, and HIV-2 are depicted as they are arranged in their respective proviral DNA. The sizes of the different proviral DNAs are shown in proportion to the 9.7-kb HIV provirus.

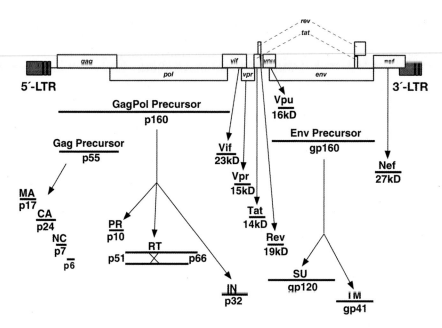

FIGURE 17.4 HIV-1–encoded proteins. The location of the HIV genes, the molecular masses (in kDa) of primary translation products (in some cases, polyproteins), and the processed mature viral proteins are indicated.

Three regions encompassing the primer binding site (PBS) stem participate in the placement and stabilization of the tRNA^{Lys3} primer, which is incorporated into HIV-1 particles and is required for the initiation of reverse transcription. These regions include the PBS itself, which can base pair with the 3′-terminal 18 nucleotides of tRNA^{Lys3}; the primer activation signal (PAS), which interacts with the thymidine-pseudouridine-cytidine (TψC) arm of the tRNA to trigger the reverse transcription reaction; and the A-loop, which is complementary to the anticodon loop of tRNA^{Lys3} (Reviewed in Ref.[57]). The unwinding of both the tRNA primer and the PBS stem within the 5′ untranslated region of the HIV-1 genome, as well as the incorporation of the primer into nascent virions, is facilitated by the NC domain of the Gag polyprotein, which plays the role of a molecular chaperone in this process. This topic, and genomic RNA packaging, will be discussed in more detail below. Lysyl-tRNA synthetase has been reported to bind Gag and facilitate tRNA^{Lys3} incorporation into virions.[334]

The viral genomic RNA contains a heptameric UUUUUUA "slippery" sequence within the *gag* gene where ribosomal frameshifting (FS) can occur during translation of the full-length viral RNA (Fig. 17.5C). This sequence functions in conjunction with a downstream 8-nt spacer and hairpin to mediate (−)1 translational frameshifting at a frequency of about 5%.[329] The viral RNA folds into other structures including the transactivation response region (TAR, near the 5′ end

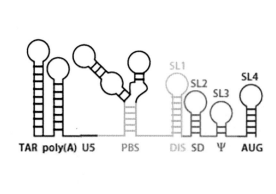

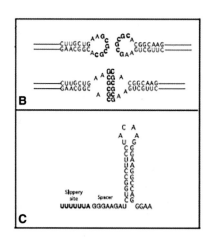

FIGURE 17.5 A: Model of the secondary structure at the 5′ terminus of HIV-1 genomic RNA. The positions of the TAR stem-loop, poly(A) stem-loop, primer binding site (PBS), dimerization initiation sequence (DIS), major splice donor (SD) (stem loop 2), ψ stem-loop (SL3), and AUG stem loop (SL4). The AUG serves as translation initiation codon for Gag. **B:** The self-complementary dimerization initiation sequence (DIS), located at the crown of stem-loop 1, participates in the formation of "kissing loop" intermediates, an initial step in the RNA dimerization reaction. **C:** RNA stem-loop structure downstream of the UUUUUUA frameshifting sequence. (**Penal A** adapted with permission of Annual Reviews, Inc. from Bieniasz P, Telesnitsky A. Multiple, switchable protein: RNA interactions regulate human immunodeficiency virus type 1 assembly. *Annu Rev Virol* 2018;5(1):165–183; permission conveyed through Copyright Clearance Center, Inc.)

of the viral RNA) and Rev-responsive element (RRE, within the *env* gene), which are involved in RNA synthesis and RNA nuclear-to-cytoplasmic transport, respectively. Multiple inhibitory sequences (INS), associated with the instability or nuclear retention of HIV transcripts, are scattered throughout genes encoding the *gag*, *pol*, and *env* genes.[452,604] Finally, although not strictly considered a *cis*-acting element, HIV-1 genomic RNA contains a significantly higher adenosine (A) content (~39%) than does mammalian DNA; this bias contributes to an unusual codon usage.[45]

BIOLOGY OF HIV INFECTIONS

The main cellular targets of HIV-1 in infected individuals are CD4+ T lymphocytes, which bear a high surface density of CD4. CD4+ cells of the macrophage lineage are efficiently infected by evolutionary variants of HIV-1 selected for the ability to use a low density of surface CD4 for entry. A quintessential property of HIV-1 and the other primate lentiviruses is to sequentially use CD4 and a second receptor (the coreceptor) during entry into susceptible cells.

HIV Replication and Tropism

Two coreceptors are predominantly used by primate lentiviruses to infect CD4+ cells: the CC chemokine receptor CCR5 and the CXC chemokine receptor CXCR4. Virus isolates that use CCR5 are classified as "R5-tropic," viruses that use CXCR4 are designated "X4-tropic," and strains that can use either coreceptor are referred to as "X4/R5-tropic" or "dual-tropic". Because X4-tropic viruses evolve from R5-tropic viruses the dual-tropic designation is somewhat artificial in that these are viruses that are evolving to use CXCR4 with few primary isolates ever being exclusively X4-tropic. Primary T cells express both CCR5 and CXCR4 and can be infected by all three groups of virus isolates. In contrast to primary CD4+ T cells, many immortalized T-cell lines, which are used extensively to study HIV-1 replication in tissue culture, express CXCR4 but not CCR5. Most T-cell line adapted HIV-1 strains thus use CXCR4 as their coreceptor. Activated PBMCs in culture are highly susceptible to HIV-1 infection. In contrast, resting PBMCs are largely refractory to HIV-1 infection[676,774] at least in part due to inefficient reverse transcription resulting from low dNTP pools in these cells.

R5-tropic strains are the predominant viruses detected in recently infected individuals and throughout the asymptomatic phase of untreated HIV-1 infection; in addition, the transmitted/asymptomatic virus requires a high density of CD4 for efficient entry and thus can be called R5 T cell-tropic. In approximately 50% of untreated individuals infected with subtype B HIV-1, X4-tropic variants eventually emerge, often coincident with accelerated CD4+ T-cell depletion and more rapid progression to AIDS.

The role that macrophages play in HIV-1 infection remains incompletely understood. Although macrophages express CCR5, they are inefficiently infected by most R5-tropic strains of HIV-1 (i.e., the R5 T cell-tropic form of HIV-1), in part because of low surface expression of CD4 in this cell type. Viruses capable of infecting macrophages are thus adapted to use low CD4 levels during infection and can be referred to as macrophage-tropic (or M-tropic).[351] In addition, macrophages

express the restriction factor sterile alpha motif and histidine-aspartate domain–containing protein 1 (SAMHD1), which blocks efficient reverse transcription. Members of the HIV-2/SIV$_{smm}$/SIV$_{mac}$ lineage of primate lentiviruses express Vpx, which counteracts SAMHD1, but HIV-1 isolates do not encode a *vpx* gene (see section "Vpx"). In infected individuals, macrophage infection is relatively rare, except in the brain and central nervous system (CNS) and late in disease in untreated individuals when CD4+ T cells have been severely depleted (for review, see Ref.[490]). HIV-1 can be found in the CNS very soon after transmission initially via the trafficking of infected lymphocytes, which release R5 T cell-tropic virus. HIV-1 does not productively infect neurons but instead targets perivascular macrophages and parenchymal microglial cells, which also express a low density of surface CD4. The establishment of persistent infection within the CNS appears to require the evolution of M-tropic virus given the dearth of CD4+ T cells in the CNS compartment.

Under some circumstances, DCs can be infected with (or at least capture) HIV-1. DCs are antigen-presenting cells that capture, transport, and present antigens to CD4+ and CD8+ T lymphocytes. Three main subtypes of DCs have been identified: plasmacytoid DCs (PDCs) and conventional DCs (cDCs) (previously called myeloid DCs), which are further classified into cDC1 and cDC2 subsets. cDCs reside in multiple tissues including the skin (where they are called Langerhans cells) and the intestinal and genital tract mucosa. PDCs are found in the blood, T-cell zones of lymph nodes, and thymus and can be recruited to sites of inflammation. cDCs present near mucosal surfaces may represent the first line of defense against sexually transmitted HIV-1, transporting virus particles from this portal of entry to draining lymph nodes where they are degraded into antigenic peptides for presentation to CD4+ T lymphocytes. Paradoxically, this critical initial response exacerbates the HIV-1 acute infection; although productive HIV-1 infection of DCs is very inefficient, vigorous virus replication is observed when DCs are first pulsed with virus and then cocultivated with CD4+ T lymphocytes, a process called transinfection.[253] During this process, HIV-1 particles bound to the DC surface are internalized and then "presented" to susceptible CD4+ T cells at points of close cell–cell contact, utilizing adhesion molecules involved in the formation of the immunologic synapse.[395]

HIV Transmission

HIV can spread through two general mechanisms: (a) cell-free infection and (b) cell–cell transfer across points of close cell–cell contact, referred to as the virological synapse (VS). Early studies reported that cell-to-cell transmission of HIV-1 is orders of magnitude more efficient than cell-free infection.[185] The formation of a VS with T cells, first reported for HTLV-1,[321] utilizes some of the components of the immunological synapse machinery involved in the interaction between lymphocytes and antigen-presenting cells.[6] The formation of the HIV-1 VS is initiated by the binding of gp120 on the surface of the infected cell to CD4 molecules on the target cell.[347] This conjugate is further stabilized by interactions between cellular adhesion molecules, for example, lymphocyte function associated antigen (LFA) and intercellular adhesion molecules (ICAMs), which promote additional recruitment of actin, viral proteins (Gag and Env), CD4, and integrins to cell–cell contact regions.

Cytoskeletal remodeling drives virus assembly in the infected cell to the plasma membrane and toward the target cell. Progeny particles released into the synaptic space are then able to directly enter the target cell.[625] The copolarization of clustered viral proteins in the donor cell with receptors in multiple adjacent recipients can also lead to the formation of polysynaptic structures.[358] Inhibitors of HIV-1 replication, including neutralizing antibodies, are able to block both cell-free and cell-to-cell infection, but transfer across the VS may allow the virus to be less susceptible to inhibition.[118,782,783] Consistent with this hypothesis, Env mutations that enhance the efficiency of cell–cell transfer reduce the susceptibility of HIV-1 to antiretroviral drugs, at least in cell culture.[714]

The genetic diversity of HIV-1 isolates in most newly infected individuals is quite low, indicating that transmission from one individual to another is mediated by a single virus, or a small number of viruses.[739] Over time, in the absence of ART, viral diversity increases markedly as a result of high levels of ongoing, error-prone virus replication and evasion of the host immune response. When ART is initiated, viral loads (as measured by the number of viral RNA copies per ml of plasma) rapidly undergo a multi log decline to levels below the detection limit of standard clinical assays. The development of highly sensitive PCR-based assays to measure viral loads revealed a low level of viremia in the majority of individuals on ART; this low-level viremia is highly stable over many years on therapy.[536] The viral genetic diversity in individuals on suppressive ART does not change over time, and drug resistance mutations typically do not arise. These observations suggest that the low-level viremia that persists during suppressive ART is not a result of ongoing rounds of virus replication but rather is generated by a population of latently infected cells that produce virion-associated viral RNA that can be measured in the plasma. This latent reservoir is thought to reside primarily in resting memory CD4+ T cells[133,217,741]; for review see Ref.[645] Most latently infected cells harbor defective integrated viral genomes (integrated viral DNA is often referred to as a provirus) but some contain intact proviruses capable of producing replication-competent virus. Latently infected cells have been shown to clonally expand,[142,453,723] with every cell in an expanded clone containing a single provirus integrated at an identical site in the human genome. In relatively rare cases, by integrating in host cell genes that control cell proliferation, the integrated provirus contributes to the expansion of the infected cell clone. In the majority of instances, however, clonal expansion is driven not by the integrated provirus but by homeostatic proliferation or antigen stimulation.[139,658] Expanded cell clones containing intact proviruses provide a source of replication-competent HIV-1 that can rapidly restore viral loads to pretherapy levels if ART is discontinued. It may be that all proviruses in latently infected cells are maintained by cell replication/expansion, although this is a difficult point to prove with existing technologies.

HIV-1 ANIMAL MODELS

Chimpanzees

In the search for an HIV-1 animal model during the early phase of the AIDS epidemic, cell suspensions from virus-infected individuals were inoculated into a variety of mammalian species including nonhuman primates, but only chimpanzees consistently became infected. It was subsequently shown that asymptomatic HIV-1 infection could readily be established in chimpanzees, but viremia was not maintained and no long-standing impairment to the immune system occurred.[19] This could reflect genetic changes that occurred in the SIV_cpz progenitor of HIV-1 following its transmission from chimpanzees and adaptation to humans.[626] The failure of chimpanzees to develop disease in a timely fashion following inoculation with tissue culture–adapted or patient-derived HIV-1 isolates, coupled with their endangered-species status, has stopped their use as an animal model of HIV-1–induced immunodeficiency.

SIV Models in Nonhuman Primates

When it became apparent that humans and chimpanzees were the only mammalian species that could be infected by HIV-1, attention turned to the SIV/Asian macaque model. Infection of some macaque species with SIV causes a persistent pathogenic infection with similar progression to AIDS as observed in HIV-infected patients and is today widely used for cure-based studies. Rhesus macaques infected with either the reference swarm SIVmac251 or with the SIVmac251-derived infectious molecular clone SIVmac239 reproduce several aspects of human HIV infections, including sustained, high viral loads, progressive depletion of mucosal CD4+ T cells, and chronic immune activation.[273,399] But despite these similarities, several limitations exist. The most critical for cure research are the overall higher viral loads, and the natural resistance to nonnucleoside RT inhibitors exhibited by SIV strains.[171,592,736] Due to these features, SIV infection is more difficult to control with ART in macaques compared to HIV infection.[284,656,686] Other inherent differences between HIV and SIV include Vpx, an accessory protein encoded in SIV, but not HIV. As noted above, Vpx antagonizes the host SAMHD1 protein, which restricts replication of lentiviruses by depleting the deoxynucleotriphosphate pool during reverse transcription.[74]

In addition to different macaque species, HIV-1 research has also utilized African NHPs that are natural hosts of SIVs, such as African green monkeys, sooty mangabeys, and mandrills. SIV infection of these species with their naturally occurring SIV strains generally does not progress to AIDS, therefore, permitting comparative studies aimed at identifying the correlates of immune protection and the lack of disease progression.[106,538,663]

Viruses that contain both SIV and HIV gene segments have been used in many studies in NHPs. The earliest versions of these SIV/HIV chimeric viruses (SHIVs) consisted of the genetic backbone of SIV_mac239, into which the HIV-1 *tat, rev, vpu, env,* and, in some instances, portions of *vpr* and *nef* genes were inserted. Infection with this virus causes a very aggressive disease phenotype with death from immunodeficiency within 3 to 6 months of inoculation; it was widely used for vaccine studies from 2000 to 2004.[322,342,590] Simian-tropic HIV-1 clones have also been developed that are adapted to replicate in monkey cells both in culture and in animals.[630]

Humanized Mouse Models

As mice are inherently nonpermissive to HIV infection due to several blocks in the viral replication cycle including transcription, mice engrafted with human cells and tissue have been utilized as a small-animal model for studies of HIV-1 pathogenesis and vaccine development. In very early studies, severe combined immunodeficiency (SCID) mice, engrafted with human PBMC or fragments of human fetal thymus and fetal liver engrafted under the renal capsule, were shown to support HIV-1 replication and exhibit moderate to profound depletions of CD4+ T lymphocytes but generated no immune responses to the virus.[502,518] Relatively low levels of human cell engraftment were achieved in these first-generation humanized mice.

Although the subsequent development of nonobese diabetic (NOD)-SCID animals resulted in improved human PBMC engraftment, the relatively short lifespan of the mice and residual murine NK-cell activity limited their usefulness. Targeted mutations of the mouse interleukin-2-receptor-γ chain ($\gamma_c^{-/-}$) and reconstitutions with PBMC, hematopoietic stem cells (HSC), or human cord blood greatly increased engraftment of human tissue.[325] Inoculation of these mice with HIV-1 by parenteral and mucosal routes resulted in sustained disseminated infections.[26,44]

A common engraftment method of human cells is the intravenous or intrahepatic injection of CD34+ HSCs[546] into adult or newborn immunodeficient mice, respectively, after myeloablative irradiation or administration of myeloablative doses of drugs.[287] The unique engraftment method using surgical implantation of human fetal liver and thymus tissues followed by injection of matched CD34+ HSCs gave rise to the bone marrow liver thymus (BLT) model.[73,363,402] The human thymic tissue allows for T-cell education in the context of human cells,[660] and the BLT model has become the current gold standard for studying HIV-1 immune responses.[250,363] However, limitations include postengraftment graft versus host disease that reduces the lifespan of these mice, the lack of functional B-cell populations, and the technical expertise required to establish and maintain the BLT mice. Humanized mouse models are being continuously improved through genetic manipulations and "further humanization" including knock-in of human HLA alleles, the thymic stromal cell–derived lymphopoietin, and human myeloid–promoting cytokines.[254]

MOLECULAR BIOLOGY OF HIV-1 REPLICATION

Overview

The HIV-1 replication cycle (Fig. 17.6) begins with the binding of Env on the surface of virus particles to CD4 molecules on susceptible target cells. Although binding of Env to CD4 is generally essential for HIV infectivity, as noted above the subsequent interaction of Env with a coreceptor—CCR5 or CXCR4—is required for membrane fusion and entry (Reviewed in Ref.[113]). Unlike some other enveloped viruses that enter cells by receptor-mediated endocytosis, HIV-1 and many other retroviruses fuse directly with the plasma membrane under most conditions. After membrane fusion, the capsid core traffics along the microtubule network where reverse transcription is initiated during movement to the nucleus (Reviewed in Ref.[98]). The partially double-stranded DNA reverse transcription product is transported through the cytoplasm and to the nucleus as a component of a reverse transcription complex (RTC), which contains the viral enzymes RT and IN and the Gag proteins CA and NC. As noted earlier, lentiviruses are unique among retroviruses in generating RTCs that are actively transported by the nuclear import machinery across nuclear pores in an intact nuclear envelope. Recent evidence has suggested that reverse transcription is completed within the nucleus.[420] After the import of the RTC into the nucleus, newly synthesized full-length, linear, double-stranded viral DNA is integrated into the chromosomal DNA of the target cell. The integrated viral DNA—the provirus—remains part of the genetic makeup of the infected cell for the lifetime of that cell.

The proviral DNA serves as the template for RNA polymerase II (Pol II)-directed viral RNA synthesis. The coordinated interaction of the HIV-encoded Tat protein and the cellular NF-κB and Sp1 transcriptional transactivating proteins with the RNA Pol II transcriptional apparatus ensures the production of high levels of viral RNA. Unspliced or partially spliced HIV transcripts are exported from the nucleus to the cytoplasm by a unique transport mechanism mediated by the virus-encoded Rev protein that allows viral RNAs with introns to exit the nucleus. The subsequent translation of the gp160 Env precursor occurs on the endoplasmic reticulum (ER); gp160 is cleaved by a cellular protease to gp120 and gp41 during its trafficking through the secretory pathway to the plasma membrane. The Gag and Gag–Pol polyprotein precursors are synthesized on free cytoplasmic ribosomes and then move to the cell surface. The Gag and Gag–Pol polyproteins, in association with dimers of genomic RNA, condense at the plasma membrane to form an electron-dense "bud" that gives rise to a spherical, immature particle containing heterotrimeric gp120 and gp41. Proteolytic processing of the Gag and Pol proteins by the viral PR during or immediately after particle release generates the cone-shaped core characteristic of mature HIV virions.

Many of the basic replicative steps described above and illustrated in Figure 17.6 are shared with the so-called "simple" retroviruses encoding only the Gag, Pol, and Env proteins. However, during its evolution, HIV acquired additional genes—the regulatory proteins Tat and Rev and the accessory proteins Vif, Vpu, Vif, Vpr, and Nef (and Vpx in the case of HIV-2)—to carry out functions that are either (a) performed by cellular proteins already present in the cells infected by the simple retroviruses or (b) uniquely required for virus replication, transmission, and survival in hematopoietic cells targeted by the primate lentiviruses. In some laboratory cell lines, the HIV-1 accessory proteins are not required for replication—hence the term "accessory"—however, these additional genes are required for replication to high levels and pathogenesis *in vivo*.

HIV-1 encodes only 15 proteins and thus, like all other viruses, must utilize a large number of cellular proteins for successful replication. Over the years, a variety of techniques have been used to identify virus–host protein interactions and proteins required for HIV-1 replication (often referred to as HIV "dependency factors"). A number of cellular factors—in some cases referred to as restriction factors—have also been identified that disrupt virus replication. Many of these inhibitory factors are induced by interferon (IFN) and constitute part of the innate immune defense against invading viral pathogens. A primary function of the HIV accessory proteins is to counteract these cellular inhibitory factors.

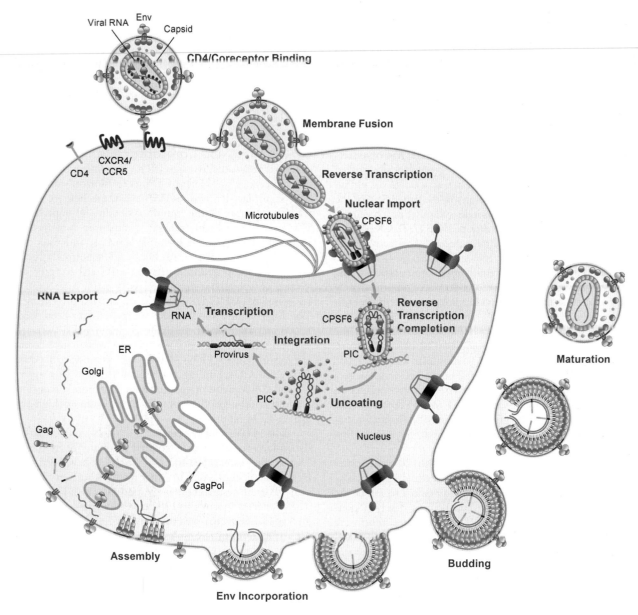

FIGURE 17.6 The HIV-1 replication cycle. Productive HIV-1 infection begins with the binding of the viral Env glycoprotein complex to CD4 on the target cell, and subsequent interaction between Env and coreceptor. Conformational changes in Env trigger a membrane fusion reaction between the viral envelope and target cell plasma membrane. The core particle is then released into the cytosol where reverse transcription, mediated by the viral reverse transcriptase (RT), initiates. The core then traffics along microtubules to the nuclear envelope where it docks and is transported across a nuclear pore into the nucleus. Reverse transcription is completed and capsid uncoating occurs. The newly synthesized viral DNA, as part of the preintegration complex (PIC), integrates into cellular chromosomal DNA. Integration is catalyzed by the viral integrase (IN). The integrated viral DNA—the provirus—serves as the template for DNA-dependent RNA polymerase (pol II) transcription. Unspliced, singly spliced, and multiply spliced viral RNAs are exported to the cytoplasm, where they are translated into viral proteins or, in the case of a population of unspliced viral RNA, used for packaging. The Env glycoprotein precursor is translated in the ER and the Gag and Gag–Pol polyprotein precursors are translated in the cytosol. Env, Gag, and Gag–Pol are transported to the plasma membrane, where progeny virus particles coassemble with full-length, dimeric viral RNA. The mature Env glycoprotein complex, a heterotrimer of gp120 and gp41, is incorporated into the assembling Gag lattice. The nascent particle buds from the plasma membrane in an immature state. Concomitant with release of the virus particle from the infected cell, the viral protease (PR) cleaves the Gag and Gag–Pol precursors, triggering conformational rearrangements that lead to the formation of a mature, infectious virus particle containing a characteristic conical core.

Virus Binding and Entry: The Env Glycoproteins

The HIV Env glycoproteins are translated from the singly spliced, 4.3-kb Vpu/Env bicistronic mRNA on ribosomes associated with the rough ER. The Env glycoprotein precursor, gp160, is an integral membrane protein that is anchored to cell membranes by the gp41 transmembrane domain (TMD) (Fig. 17.7) (for review see Ref.[112]). gp160 is cotranslationally glycosylated and undergoes trimerization in the lumen of the ER before it is transported to the Golgi, where, like other retroviral Env precursor glycoproteins, it is proteolytically cleaved by cellular furin or furin-like proteases at a polybasic amino acid sequence. Gp160 cleavage results in the generation of the mature gp120 and gp41 glycoprotein subunits, which remain associated via noncovalent interactions (Fig. 17.7). Cleavage of gp160 is strictly required for Env-induced fusion activity and virus infectivity.[232,479]

The HIV Env glycoprotein complex, in particular the gp120 component, is very heavily glycosylated; approximately half the molecular mass of gp160 is composed of N-linked oligosaccharide side chains. During transport of Env from its site of synthesis in the ER to the plasma membrane, many of the side chains are modified by the addition of complex sugars. The numerous oligosaccharide side chains form a sugar "cloud" obscuring much of the surface of gp120 from host immune recognition. As shown in Figure 17.7, gp120 contains interspersed conserved (C1 to C5) and variable (V1 to V5) domains. The Cys residues present in the gp120 proteins of different isolates are highly conserved and form disulfide bonds that link the first four variable regions in large loops.[416]

After its arrival at the cell surface, the gp120-gp41 trimer of heterodimers complex is rapidly internalized. A Tyr-X-X-Leu (YxxL) sequence in the membrane-proximal region of the HIV-1 gp41 cytoplasmic tail (see Fig. 17.7) is largely responsible for this rapid internalization.[398,608] Analogous motifs are also present in the TM Env glycoproteins of HIV-2, SIV, and several other retroviruses. Tyr-based motifs are known to mediate endocytosis of cellular plasma membrane proteins by binding the μ2 chain of the clathrin-associated adapter protein 2 (AP-2) complex, and these interactions have been observed with gp41 cytoplasmic tails.[66,526] A dileucine motif at the C-terminus of the gp41 cytoplasmic tail also participates in Env internalization and trafficking via interactions with the AP-1 complex[46,92,751] (Fig. 17.7).

CD4 Binding and Coreceptor Interactions

As noted above, the first step in HIV/SIV infection is the interaction between gp120 and CD4, the major cell-surface receptor for primate lentiviruses (for review, see Ref.[113]). CD4 is a 55-kDa member of the immunoglobulin (Ig) superfamily; it is composed of a highly charged cytoplasmic domain, a single hydrophobic membrane-spanning domain, and four distinct extracellular domains, D1 to D4.[446] CD4 normally functions to stabilize the interaction between the T-cell receptor on the surface of T lymphocytes and class II major histocompatibility complex (MHC-II) molecules on antigen-presenting cells. The high-affinity binding site for gp120 has been localized to a small segment of the CD4 N-terminal D1 extracellular domain, analogous to the second complementarity-determining region (CDR-2) loop of an Ig light chain variable domain. Important CD4 binding determinants in gp120 map to the C3 and C4 domains of gp120, although a more discontinuous, conformation-dependent domain is involved in high-affinity gp120–CD4 binding.

The HIV-1 Env trimer is highly conformationally dynamic, a feature that is required for many of its functions. Distinct conformational states of the trimer have been revealed by structural studies and by other methods such as single-molecule Förster resonance energy transfer (FRET) analyses.[510] The crystallization of a gp120 "core" domain—an unglycosylated gp120 derivative lacking the V1/V2 and V3 loops and the N- and C-termini—complexed with fragments of CD4 and a

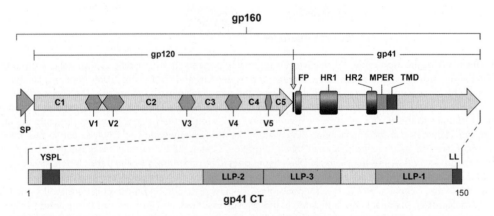

FIGURE 17.7 Linear representation of the HIV-1 Env glycoprotein. The *vertical yellow arrow* indicates the site of gp160 cleavage to gp120 and gp41; SP denotes the signal peptide. In gp120, variable (V1–V5) and conserved (C1–C5) domains are indicated. The gp41 ectodomain contains the N-terminal fusion peptide (FP), the two heptad repeats (HR1 and HR2), and the membrane-proximal external region (MPER). The transmembrane domain (TMD) is represented by a *purple box*. In the approximately 150 amino acid gp41 cytoplasmic tail (CT), the Tyr-Ser-Pro-Leu (YSPL) and Leu-Leu (LL) motifs implicated in Env trafficking and internalization are indicated. The putative helical motifs—or lentiviral lytic peptides (LLP-1, LLP-2, and LLP-3)—are shown. (Adapted from Checkley MA, Luttge BG, Freed EO. HIV-1 envelope glycoprotein biosynthesis, trafficking, and incorporation. *J Mol Biol* 2011;410(4):582-608. Copyright © 2011 Elsevier. With permission.)

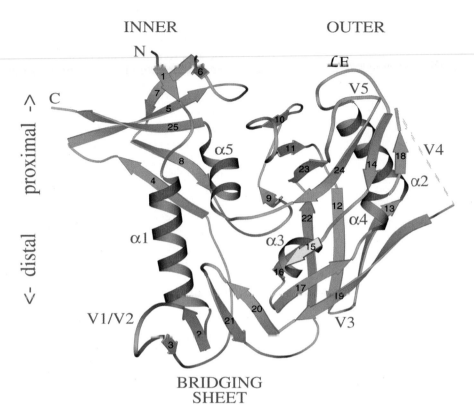

INNER   OUTER

FIGURE 17.8 Ribbon diagram of the gp120 core. In this orientation, the viral membrane would be at the top, the target cell membrane at the bottom. The inner and outer domains are connected by a four-stranded β-bridging sheet. The remnants of variable loops V1/V2, V3, V4, and V5 are shown. (Adapted by permission from Nature: Kwong PD, Wyatt R, Robinson J, et al. Structure of an HIV gp120 envelope glycoprotein in complex with the CD4 receptor and a neutralizing human antibody. *Nature* 1998;393(6686):648–659. Copyright © 1998 Springer Nature.)

neutralizing antibody contributed substantially to our understanding of the gp120–CD4 interaction.[397,748] The core structure revealed two major domains (referred to as the "inner" and "outer" domains) connected by a so-called "bridging sheet" (see Fig. 17.8). The latter is composed of a four-stranded, antiparallel β-sheet derived from sequences in the V1/V2 stem and portions of C4. Comparison of the CD4-bound HIV-1 gp120 structure with that of the non–CD4-bound (unliganded) gp120 from SIVmac and HIV-1 reveals that gp120, the inner domain in particular, undergoes a remarkably extensive conformational change upon CD4 binding.[114,534] This shift in conformation leads to a more open gp120 structure, creating the bridging sheet, which is absent in the unliganded structure. High-resolution structures of the Env trimer have been challenging to obtain, but a recent study used cryoelectron tomography of chemically inactivated virus particles to obtain subnanometer structures of unliganded, antibody-bound or CD4-bound intact Env trimers[430] (Fig. 17.9).

Soon after the identification of CD4 as the major HIV/SIV receptor, it was recognized that this protein is not sufficient for HIV-induced membrane fusion and virus entry. In the mid-1990s, a number of studies demonstrated that members of the G protein–coupled receptor superfamily of seven-transmembrane domain proteins provided the long-sought coreceptor function.[12,113,126,175] As mentioned above, the two major coreceptors for HIV/SIV infection are CXCR4 and CCR5

(for review see Ref.[119]) and virus isolates are classified based on their coreceptor usage: X4, R5, and X4/R5 (dual-tropic), with CCR5 being the most commonly used coreceptor and the one used by the vast majority of transmitted viruses.

Several domains within gp120 contribute to Env–coreceptor interactions. As mentioned above, gp120 undergoes extensive conformational changes upon binding to CD4 on the target cell membrane, essentially creating the coreceptor binding site,[114] which would be highly susceptible to neutralizing antibodies and thus forms only transiently and close to the host cell membrane.[537] The structure of the gp120-CCR5 complex, solved by cryoEM, shows two primary interaction interfaces between the two proteins: the V3 loop of gp120 inserts into the chemokine binding pocket of CCR5 and the bridging sheet of gp120 binds the N-terminus of the coreceptor.[646]

Certain laboratory-adapted isolates of HIV-1, HIV-2, and SIV use coreceptors in a CD4-independent manner, that is, as primary receptors.[206,470,572] The coreceptor-binding surface is highly exposed in variants selected to replicate in a CD4-independent fashion.[301,384] Because their coreceptor-binding surface is constitutively exposed, CD4-independent isolates tend to be hypersensitive to neutralization.

It was noted that certain individuals, despite persistent high-risk behavior, remain HIV-1 uninfected. The discovery of CCR5 and CXCR4 as HIV-1 coreceptors raised the possibility that some of these individuals might encode mutant coreceptor

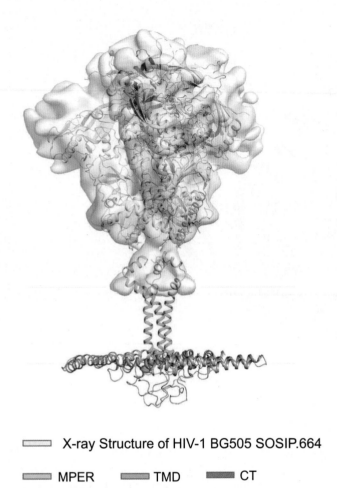

X-ray Structure of HIV-1 BG505 SOSIP.664

MPER   TMD   CT

FIGURE 17.9 Model of the HIV-1 Env trimer. The ectodomain structure is based on fitting cryoEM densities[437] into the crystal structure of HIV-1 BG505 SOSIP.664 (PDB ID code 5T3Z).[268] The membrane-proximal external region (MPER) is shown in *blue*, the transmembrane domain (TMD) in *green* and the cytoplasmic tail (CT) in *magenta*. (Adapted with permission from Piai A, Fu Q, Sharp AK, et al. NMR model of the entire membrane-interacting region of the HIV-1 fusion protein and its perturbation of membrane morphology. *J Am Chem Soc* 2021;143(17):6609–6615. Copyright © 2021 American Chemical Society.)

alleles. Indeed, a mutant CCR5 allele, referred to as CCR5/Δ32, contains a 32-bp deletion that leads to the expression of a truncated protein that is not efficiently expressed at the cell surface and cannot function as an HIV-1 coreceptor.[170,315,439,620] Homozygotes for CCR5/Δ32 are only rarely infected with HIV-1 (and by X4 viruses), providing strong genetic evidence for the role of CCR5 in HIV-1 infection *in vivo*.

Membrane Fusion

The primary function of viral Env glycoproteins is to promote a membrane fusion reaction between viral and target-cell membranes. The fusion process proceeds in a series of steps: gp120 first interacts with CD4, which induces the formation of the coreceptor binding site; a ternary CD4–coreceptor–gp120 complex then forms; and finally, conformational changes take place in gp41 that ultimately trigger membrane fusion (Fig. 17.10).

Mutational analyses demonstrated that a hydrophobic region at the N-terminus of gp41, known as the "fusion peptide," plays a central role in membrane fusion mediated by HIV-1[112,233] (see Fig. 17.7). C-terminal to the gp41 fusion peptide are two amphipathic heptad repeat (HR) domains, HR1 and HR2 (see Fig. 17.7), that are also required for membrane fusion. Structures of the ectodomain of HIV-1 and SIV gp41, including HR1 and HR2, were determined by x-ray crystallography and nuclear magnetic resonance (NMR) spectroscopy.[93,107,692,731] These studies showed that HR1 and HR2 pack in an antiparallel fashion to generate a six-helix bundle (Fig. 17.10). The three HR1 domains of the Env trimer form a coiled-coil structure in the center of the bundle, with the HR2 domains packing into hydrophobic grooves on the outside of the HR1 trimer. The gp41 ectodomain structure resembles that of the fusion-competent (low-pH induced) form of influenza HA$_2$, indicating that HIV/SIV Env glycoproteins trigger membrane fusion by the same "spring-loaded" mechanism proposed for influenza virus,[87] likely an ancient mechanism for fusing membranes. Binding studies using native HIV-1 Env indicate that gp41 interacts with a soluble HR2-derived peptide only after CD4 binding, indicating that HR1 and HR2 undergo conformation changes after CD4 binding and that these rearrangements are required for formation of the six-helix bundle and membrane fusion.[242] Located between HR2 and the gp41 TMD is a Trp-rich region, known as the membrane-proximal external region (MPER), which plays a role in regulating Env conformation. Mutations in the MPER disrupt membrane fusion and infectivity,[619] and this region is the binding site for one class of broadly neutralizing antibodies. The cytoplasmic tail of gp41 also plays a role in modulating the fusion activity of Env, in part by regulating cell-surface expression levels of the gp120–gp41 complex and by influencing the conformation of gp120 and the ectodomain of gp41[115] (for review see Ref.[112]). The cytoplasmic tail contains several helical motifs often referred to as "lentiviral lytic peptides" (LLP1-LLP3) because of their ability to disrupt membranes (Fig. 17.7). Several NMR structures have been obtained for the cytoplasmic tail of HIV-1 gp41,[514,557] including a recent structure of the entire TMD and cytoplasmic tail embedded in a membrane bicell[557] (Fig. 17.9). While these structures differ in some important details, they confirm that the LLP regions interact intimately with the membrane and suggest that the cytoplasmic tail forms a trimeric baseplate around the trimeric TMD. The structure of the gp41 cytoplasmic tail in the context of a virus particle (i.e., in the presence of Gag) has not yet been solved.

A number of studies have shown that the HIV-1 membrane envelope is enriched in lipids (e.g., sphingolipids and cholesterol) that are concentrated within the cell plasma membrane in specialized microdomains known as lipid rafts.[13,505] This finding is consistent with evidence that HIV-1 assembly takes place in raft-like membrane microdomains (see below in Section on Virus Assembly and Release: The Gag Proteins). It has also been proposed that membrane fusion takes place in lipid rafts in the target cell plasma membrane, and depletion of cholesterol from either the virus particle or the target cell membrane disrupts fusion.[531] In addition to promoting cell-free HIV-1 infection, lipid rafts likely play an important role in HIV-1 transmission between T cells, as the VS is enriched in raft-like microdomains.[348]

Progress in understanding the molecular mechanism of membrane fusion has led to the development of inhibitors that block various aspects of virus fusion and entry (for review, see Ref.[752]). T-20 (enfuvirtide), approved for clinical use by the US

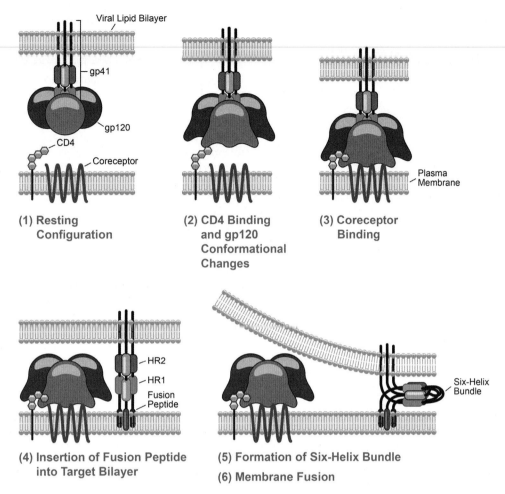

FIGURE 17.10 Schematic representation of the steps leading to membrane fusion. In the resting configuration, the Env glycoprotein complex is in its native state (*1*). CD4 binding (*2*) induces conformational changes in Env, which include opening up of the gp120 structure, which allow coreceptor binding (*3*). After the formation of a ternary gp120–CD4–coreceptor complex, gp41 adopts an extended conformation that allows the fusion peptide to insert into the target lipid bilayer (*4*). The formation of the gp41 six-helix bundle, which involves antiparallel interactions between the gp41 heptad repeats (HR1 and HR2) (*5*) brings the viral and cellular membranes together and membrane fusion takes place (*6*).

Food and Drug Administration (FDA) in 2003, is a 36-amino acid, gp41 HR2-derived peptide that interacts directly with HR1 during the conformational changes that take place after CD4 binding. The interaction of T-20 with gp41 prevents six-helix bundle formation, thereby blocking fusion. Resistance to T-20 arises both *in vitro* and in treated individuals, primarily through mutations in HR1.[598] T-20 is very costly and not orally bioavailable, reducing its current utility. A number of strategies have been employed to increase the potency of HR1/HR2 peptide-based inhibitors (reviewed in Ref.[752]). Given that it is straightforward to identify the HR1/HR2 repeats in the ectodomain of similar viral TM proteins, this type of therapeutic strategy could be rapidly developed for other enveloped viruses (such as SARS-CoV-2).

Additional approaches have been explored for inhibiting the fusion process. Ibalizumab, a CD4-targeting, humanized monoclonal antibody, was approved for clinical use in 2018. It binds the D1/D2 junction of CD4 and noncompetitively inhibits gp120 binding to the receptor.[205] A CCR5-based inhibitor, maraviroc, was approved in 2007 (for review, see Ref.[540]). Maraviroc functions by binding extracellular domains of CCR5 and inducing an allosteric change in the conformation of CCR5 that prevents gp120–CCR5 interaction.[212] Resistance to maraviroc can arise by acquisition of gp120 V3 loop mutations that allow HIV-1 to utilize the drug-bound coreceptor[733] or by the outgrowth of CXCR4-tropic strains.[494] Inhibitors that block gp120 binding to CD4 are also being developed. The first of these to be approved by the FDA is BMS-663068 (Fostemavir), approved in 2020. Other fusion and entry targets are being pursued, including small molecules that bind the MPER at docking sites for broadly neutralizing antibodies.[753]

Postentry Trafficking of the HIV Capsid

After membrane fusion deposits the viral core in the cytoplasm, it must traffic to the nuclear pore for eventual transit across the nuclear envelope (see Fig. 17.6). During the trafficking of the core particle to the nucleus, the surface of the core—known as the capsid, composed of an assembled lattice of CA protein—interacts with a series of host cell factors that either promote or interfere with core transport and stability. An early report showed that capsids associate with microtubules and use dynein to traffic toward the nucleus.[481] The dynein adapter protein bicaudal D2 (BICD2) helps promote trafficking on microtubules.[179,180] HIV-1 infection has been reported to stabilize microtubules[613] and proteins involved in microtubule stabilization are required for movement of capsids to the nucleus (for review, see Ref.[179]). The kinesin adapter fasciculation and elongation protein zeta-1 (FEZ1) directly engages incoming capsids[454] by binding to the highly basic pore at the center of the capsid hexamer[313] (see section below on CA). An additional protein, Sec24C, interacts with a pocket on the capsid that is the binding site for several other proteins involved in capsid nuclear import and viral DNA integration; this interaction involves Phe-Gly (FG) motifs on the host protein. Depletion of Sec24C destabilizes the capsid in the cytosol and thus interferes with the downstream events of nuclear import and DNA integration.[589]

Reverse Transcription

A defining characteristic of retroviruses is the ability to convert their single-stranded RNA genomes into double-stranded DNA during the early stages of infection.[28,697] The enzyme that catalyzes this reaction is RT, in conjunction with its associated ribonuclease H (RNase H) activity. Retroviral RTs have two enzymatic centers: (a) a DNA polymerase that can copy either RNA templates (for "minus-strand" DNA synthesis) or DNA templates (for second- or "plus-strand" DNA synthesis) and (b) RNase H (for the degradation of RNA present in DNA–RNA hybrid intermediates). RT was the first viral protein targeted by antiretroviral therapy, and RT inhibitors remain central to the treatment of people living with HIV (for reviews, see Refs.[307,659]).

The retroviral genome is packaged into the virion as a dimer of single-stranded RNA. As mentioned earlier, the two RNAs are held together in part by the DIS near their 5′ ends. Although each retroviral particle contains two copies of genomic RNA, only one provirus is formed per virion.[309] Retroviruses are, therefore, referred to as "pseudodiploid." As with most other DNA polymerases, RT is dependent on the 3′-OH group of an RNA or DNA primer to initiate polymerization. Retroviruses use specific tRNAs (tRNA^{Lys3} in the case of HIV-1) to initiate DNA synthesis. The mechanism of tRNA selection and placement on the template is complex, involving interactions with RT and NC as well as with the 18-nt PBS near the 5′ end of the viral genome.

Reverse transcription of the retroviral RNA genome to a double-stranded DNA copy is initiated after viral entry into the target cell and proceeds via a series of steps that are outlined briefly below (see E-Fig. 17.1). This is also described in Figure 8 of Chapter 15. (a) Minus-strand DNA synthesis is initiated from the 3′-OH of the tRNA bound to the PBS. DNA synthesis then proceeds a short distance to the 5′ end of the genome. (b) RNase H digests the RNA portion of the newly formed RNA–DNA hybrid, freeing the resulting short, single-stranded DNA fragment (known as the minus-strand strong-stop DNA). (c) The minus-strand strong-stop DNA is transferred to the 3′ end of the genome, where it hybridizes by virtue of a short region of homology (the "repeated" or R region) present at both 5′ and 3′ ends of the RNA genome (the first strand transfer). (d) Minus-strand synthesis, accompanied

by RNase H-mediated degradation of the RNA in the resulting RNA–DNA hybrid, continues along the length of the genome to the PBS that forms the 5′ end of the genome after the degradation of the early RNA/DNA hybrid of strong-stop DNA. (e) Fragments of RNA that were not removed by RNase H serve as primers for plus-strand synthesis. The major site of plus-strand priming is the polypurine tract (PPT) near the 3′ end of the genome (E-Fig. 17.1); however, residual RNA fragments that remain hybridized to regions outside the PPT can also be used for priming plus-strand synthesis. In the case of HIV-1, one such region, known as the central PPT, appears to be particularly important in this regard. (f) After plus-strand synthesis copies the initial minus-strand DNA product including a portion of the tRNA primer, RNase H removes that portion of tRNA in the RNA/DNA hybrid. This exposes the complement of the PBS (designated in lower case as pbs) at the 3′ end of the initial plus-strand DNA, allowing this short plus-strand DNA to anneal at its 3′ end with the complementary region at the 3′ end of the near full-length minus-strand DNA that paused after copying the PBS ("second-strand transfer"). (g) Plus- and minus-strand syntheses proceed to completion. Plus-strand synthesis terminates at the end of the minus strand and, for HIV-1, at a sequence known as the central termination signal (CTS). The position of the central PPT upstream of the CTS results in the displacement of approximately 100 nucleotides of plus-strand DNA and the formation of a triplex DNA structure. The final product of reverse transcription is a linear, double-stranded DNA molecule capable of serving as the substrate for integration.

In addition to providing an essential function in the virus replication cycle, the enzymatic activity of RT is routinely used in the laboratory to quantitatively monitor levels of progeny virions present in the supernatant of infected cultures and to elucidate the molecular details of virus replication. Also, the detection of viral DNA postinfection by real-time PCR provides one of the most reliable methods for monitoring entry and postentry steps in the virus replication cycle. Once inside the nucleus, some double-stranded viral DNA is ligated by nuclear enzymes to generate circular forms; although these circular DNA products do not integrate and are eventually lost, their formation is often used to monitor nuclear import.

The mature HIV-1 RT holoenzyme is a heterodimer of 66- and 51-kDa subunits. The 51-kDa subunit (p51) is derived from the 66-kDa (p66) subunit or some larger precursor by proteolytic removal of the C-terminal 15-kDa fragment of p66 by PR, cleaving at an internal site within a presumably partially unfolded RNase H domain (Figs. 17.4 and 17.11). Hundreds of structures of HIV-1 RT have been determined by x-ray crystallography in a number of studies.[307] Early studies crystallized RT in several contexts: (a) unliganded,[601] (b) bound to a short DNA duplex and the Fab portion of an anti-RT antibody,[330] (c) covalently linked to a complex of primer/template and dNTP,[310] and (d) bound to an RNA–DNA duplex.[621] A number of structures are also available for RT bound to nonnucleoside RT inhibitors (NNRTIs). The crystal structure of HIV-1 RT reveals that the p66 and p51 subunits are folded into similar subdomains, but these subdomains are arranged quite differently in the two subunits of the p66/p51 heterodimer. The p66 subunit can be visualized as a right hand, with the polymerase active site within the palm, and a deep, template-binding cleft formed by the palm, fingers, and thumb subdomains[331]

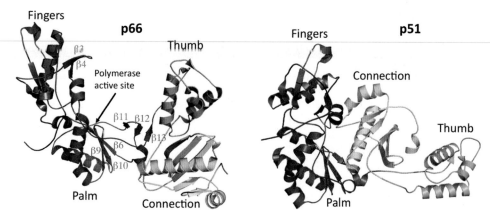

FIGURE 17.11 Ribbon diagrams of the p66 (*left*) and p51 (*right*) RT subunits. Polymerase active site and fingers, palm, thumb, and connection subdomains are shown. (Modified by Kalyas Das and Eddy Arnold from Jacobo-Molina A, Ding J, Nanni RG, et al. Crystal structure of human immunodeficiency virus type 1 reverse transcriptase complexed with double-stranded DNA at 3.0 Å resolution shows bent DNA. *Proc Natl Acad Sci USA* 1993;90(13):6320–6324. Copyright © 1993 National Academy of Sciences, USA.)

(Figs. 17.11 and 17.12). The polymerase domain is linked to RNase H by the connection subdomain. The active site, located in the palm, contains three critical Asp residues (Asp-110, Asp-185, and Asp-186) that are spacially in close proximity, and two Mg^{2+} ions that are coordinated by the negatively charged Asp side chains. Mutation of these Asp residues abolishes the polymerase activity of RT. The p51 subunit plays a structural role and does not form a polymerizing cleft; Asp-110, Asp-185, and Asp-186 of p51 are buried within the subunit. Approximately 18 bp of the primer/template duplex lie in the nucleic acid–binding cleft, stretching from the polymerase to the RNase H active sites. In the RT-primer/template-dNTP structure,[310] the presence of a dideoxynucleotide (ddNTP) at the 3′ end of the primer allows visualization of the catalytic complex blocked just prior to attack on the incoming dNTP. Comparison with previously obtained structures suggested a model whereby the fingers close in to trap the template and dNTP prior to nucleophilic

attack of the 3′-OH of the primer on the incoming dNTP. After the addition of the incoming dNTP to the growing chain, the fingers adopt a more open configuration, thereby releasing the pyrophosphate and enabling RT to bind the next dNTP. HIV-1 RNase H, the structure of which has been determined by x-ray crystallography, displays a global folding similar to that of *Escherichia coli* RNase H[163] and other nucleotide metabolizing enzymes, suggesting the ancestral enzyme appeared early in the evolution of life. The structure of human RNase H1 bound to an RNA/DNA hybrid has allowed the modeling of HIV-1 RNase H complexed with its substrate.[525] A structure of HIV-1 RNase H engaged in RNA cleavage has also been solved.[699]

As mentioned above, reverse transcription initiates from a tRNA^{Lys3} primer bound to the PBS. Initiation is known to proceed slowly relative to subsequent elongation and is characterized by frequent pausing events. Recent studies on the reverse transcription initiation complex indicate that the structure of

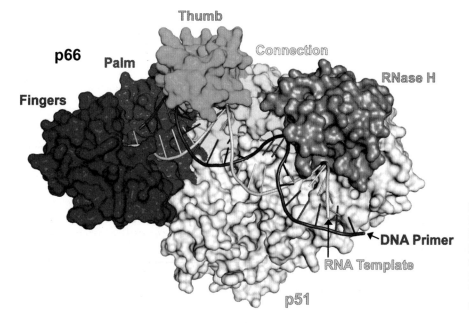

FIGURE 17.12 HIV-1 RT bound to an RNA/DNA template/primer. (Modified by Karen Kirby and Stefan Sarafianos from Singh K, Marchand B, Kirby KA, et al. Structural aspects of drug resistance and inhibition of HIV-1 reverse transcriptase. *Viruses* 2010;2(2):606–638. https://creativecommons.org/licenses/by/3.0/.)

the enzyme is regulated by the viral RNA and the primer, providing insights into the slow rate of initiation. The results of these studies also suggest that the initiation complex is particularly vulnerable to inhibition by NNRTIs.[407]

The high rate of variation among HIV-1 populations poses one of the fundamental challenges to effectively controlling this pathogen. Highly variable virus populations are largely a consequence of rapid virus replication rates, coupled with the error-prone nature of RT (which lacks a proof-reading function), and frequent template switching during reverse transcription[138] (for review, see Ref.[307]). Cell-free error rates for purified RTs have been determined,[35,574,599] as have *in vivo* retrovirus mutation rates.[1,192,464,543,544] Errors during retrovirus replication are also likely to be introduced by the cellular DNA-dependent RNA pol II during transcription of the viral RNA. The total HIV-1 *in vivo* mutation rate (a composite of substitutions, frameshifts, simple deletions, and deletions with insertions) was measured at approximately 1 to 3×10^{-5} per cycle of replication.[1,464]

As discussed earlier, retroviral particles contain two copies of single-stranded RNA, which are usually identical. During reverse transcription, RT frequently switches from one RNA template to the other in the dimer. RT also undergoes intramolecular jumps, that is, within the same RNA template.[542] Intramolecular jumps lead to mutations (e.g., deletions, insertions, and duplications), whereas intermolecular jumps generate recombinants if the two packaged RNAs are not genetically identical.[308] The intermolecular template switches that lead to recombination can occur when RT encounters a break in the RNA during polymerization—the so-called "forced copy choice" model.[137] Jumps during minus-strand synthesis can also occur in the absence of strand breaks,[355] and the stability of RT association with template is influenced by the balance between the enzyme's RNase H and polymerase activities—the "dynamic copy-choice" model.[319] Intermolecular strand transfers that lead to recombination are required for successful completion of reverse transcription, as blocking these events leads to large deletions in the viral genome and severe reductions in particle infectivity.[585] The impact of high rates of recombination and high replication rates on HIV-1 biology is substantial. As noted earlier, recombinants constitute the predominant strains currently circulating in certain parts of the world. Recombination also provides a mechanism for the rapid generation of multidrug-resistant HIV-1 variants by combining multiple drug-resistance mutations in one genome.

RT has long been a target for antiviral compounds, with AZT being the first antiretroviral approved for treatment of people living with HIV (in 1987). RT inhibitors are routinely prescribed, typically in combination with PR or IN inhibitors. There are two major classes of drugs that block reverse transcription: nucleoside RT inhibitors (NRTIs) and nonnucleoside RT inhibitors (NNRTIs). NRTIs are nucleotide mimics that lack the 3'-OH and thus act as chain terminators upon incorporation into DNA, whereas the NNRTIs inhibit DNA polymerization by binding a small hydrophobic pocket near the RT active site and inducing a change in the structure of RT that blocks DNA synthesis.[383] Resistance to RT inhibitors can develop in treated individuals; escape from NRTIs generally takes place by one of two mechanisms: (a) resistant RTs acquire the ability to selectively incorporate natural dNTPs but (at least partially) exclude the NRTI or (b) mutant RTs incorporate the NRTI but subsequently excise it from the terminated primer with the evolution of a rudimentary 3'-exonuclease activity. Resistance to NNRTIs occurs when mutations in RT interfere with the binding of the drug to the enzyme by disrupting key drug–enzyme interactions, changing the shape of the NNRTI binding pocket, or preventing entry of the drug into the binding pocket.[622] Finally, a significant effort has been directed toward developing inhibitors that target the RNaseH activity of RT, as this remains the only HIV enzymatic activity against which no drug is available.

Nuclear Import

Most retroviral genomes gain access to host cell chromosomal DNA during progression of the target cell through the cell cycle when the nuclear membrane dissolves. These retroviruses are, therefore, unable to efficiently infect noncycling cells. In contrast, as noted earlier, lentiviruses are able to productively infect nondividing cells (e.g., macrophages) and their genomes are competent to access the interphase nucleus of dividing cells. Although early studies proposed that the HIV-1 capsid uncoats (i.e., the CA subunits dissociate from the capsid) rapidly after membrane fusion, subsequent work demonstrated that at least some (and maybe most) CA subunits remain associated with the core particle, or RTC, as it traffics to the nucleus.[209] Analysis of chimeras between MLV (which is unable to infect nondividing cells) and HIV-1 revealed that the ability to infect nondividing cells maps to CA.[759] A C-terminally truncated, cytosolic form of cleavage and polyadenylation factor 6 (CPSF6, which is normally localized in the nucleus), referred to as CPSF6-358, was shown to block HIV-1 nuclear import but not to affect MLV infectivity.[413] Virus selection experiments in the presence of CPSF6-358 gave rise to a resistant mutant that contained a single amino acid change in CA (N74D). This CA-N74D mutant was not only resistant to inhibition by CPSF6-358 but also displayed an altered requirement for karyopherins and nuclear pore factors. These data supported a role for CA in nuclear import of the RTC and demonstrated that CA regulates HIV's utilization of nuclear transport and pore components.

Additional evidence accumulated in support of the model that not only is CA an integral part of the RTC but also that the capsid lattice must remain at least partially intact during trafficking to the nuclear envelope: (a) restriction factors such as tripartite motif-containing 5α (TRIM5α) and myxovirus resistance protein 2 (Mx2, also known as MxB), which block postentry and/or nuclear import events in the virus replication cycle (see below), recognize the assembled hexameric CA lattice on the capsid[235,245]; (b) nuclear pore components required for nuclear import (e.g., Nup153 and Nup358) bind to the capsid with much higher affinity than they bind nonassembled CA[54]; and (c) an intact capsid is likely required to shield the viral nucleic acid from detection by host innate immune sensors in the cytosol.[194] Recent studies have indeed provided compelling evidence that the HIV-1 capsid remains intact, or largely intact, until after import into the nucleus. Live-cell imaging of CA-labeled capsids revealed the import of intact capsids into the nucleus, with full uncoating taking place near the site of viral DNA integration.[89,420] This analysis used a system in which GFP, packaged into virions as an internal Gag–GFP fusion protein, becomes trapped within the capsid during Gag proteolysis and maturation and thus serves as a content marker for measuring the intactness of the capsid. GFP loss from the capsid took place in the nucleus almost simultaneously with loss of

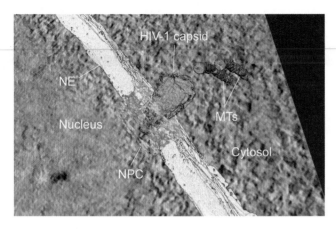

FIGURE 17.13 Cryoelectron tomographic reconstruction of an HIV-1 capsid entering a nuclear pore. Nuclear envelope (NE) is highlighted in *yellow*, HIV-1 capsid in *purple*, nuclear pore complex (NPC) in *light blue*, microtubules (MTs) in *red*. (Image provided by Vojtech Zila based on Zila V, Margiotta E, Turonova B, et al. Cone-shaped HIV-1 capsids are transported through intact nuclear pores. *Cell* 2021;184(4):1032–1046 e18.)

CA near the site of DNA integration.[420] Studies that examined the kinetics with which a nuclear pore-blocking agent inhibited HIV-1 infection[178] and sensitivity to the capsid-targeting small-molecule inhibitor PF-3450074 (PF74)[89,178] concluded that reverse transcription is likely completed in the nucleus and that intact CA hexamers survive nuclear import. One of the key arguments originally supporting the hypothesis that capsid uncoating must occur before nuclear entry was that the intact capsid is too large to traffic through the nuclear pore. However, a study that used a combination of light microscopy and cryoEM observed that whereas capsids in the nucleus appeared to be disrupted, apparently intact conical capsids could be visualized inside the central channel of the nuclear pore complex (Fig. 17.13). These observations indicated that the nuclear pore is large enough to accommodate an intact HIV-1 capsid.[789] The findings that reverse transcription is likely completed in the nucleus,[420] and that endogenous reverse transcription *in vitro* requires an intact capsid,[130] also support the hypothesis that uncoating takes place predominantly in the nucleus. Despite the evidence cited above, the topic of where uncoating occurs remains controversial, as some data support the hypothesis that uncoating occurs in the cytosol[461] or at the nuclear envelope.[226,227]

Postentry Blocks to Lentiviral Infection

A number of host cell restriction factors have been described that interfere with postentry steps in the HIV replication cycle. Several of these factors have likely imposed barriers to lentiviral transmission across primate species, and viruses that have crossed species have had to adapt to these factors in the new host. The best characterized of the factors that affect viral replication prior to integration include the cytidine deaminase apolipoprotein B mRNA-editing enzyme, catalytic polypeptide-like 3G (APOBEC3G) protein, and family members; TRIM5α; Mx2; and SAMHD1. APOBEC3G is counteracted by Vif, and SAMHD1 in antagonized by the HIV-2 Vpx protein; these restriction factors will, therefore, be discussed later in the context of the HIV-1 and HIV-2 accessory proteins.

TRIM5α and TRIMCyp

Decades ago, it was discovered that cells from mice of specific genetic backgrounds express dominant factors that block infection by certain subtypes of MLV. For example, the Friend virus susceptibility-1 (*Fv1*) allele[431,558] encodes resistance to distinct strains of MLV; *Fv1ⁿ* confers resistance to B-tropic MLV, whereas *Fv1ᵇ* cells cannot be efficiently infected by N-tropic MLV (N-MLV). The viral determinant of N- and B-tropism maps to a specific amino acid (residue 110) in the CA domain of Gag.[385] The *Fv1* block occurs early postentry, after reverse transcription but before integration.[345] It was demonstrated in the mid-1990s that *Fv1* encodes an endogenous Gag-like protein.[51]

Nonmurine cells do not harbor an *Fv1* gene.[51] However, seemingly analogous postentry restrictions have also been observed in a variety of mammalian cells. N-tropic MLV poorly infects cells from a number of mammalian species.[703] Similarly, HIV-1 infection is inefficient in cells derived from Old World (e.g., African green and rhesus) monkeys, whereas New World (e.g., owl and squirrel) monkey cells are poorly infected by SIV_mac.[298,302,653] The host factor responsible for postentry restriction of HIV-1 in rhesus macaque cells was demonstrated to be the IFN-inducible protein TRIM5α.[682] Expression of rhesus TRIM5α in human cells potently inhibits HIV-1 infection but has no effect on Moloney MLV infectivity. Conversely, knockdown of TRIM5α expression using small interfering RNA (siRNA) in rhesus cells markedly increases HIV-1 infectivity.[682] Subsequent studies indicated that, when expressed in human cells, TRIM5α derived from several New World monkey species restricts infection by SIV from African green monkeys (SIV_agm) and SIV adapted to replicate in macaques (SIV_mac).[669] Rhesus, African green monkey, and human TRIM5α can also diminish infection by the nonprimate lentivirus equine infectious anemia virus (EIAV).[286]

As their name implies, TRIM proteins contain three major domains: a RING domain that possesses ubiquitin ligase activity, a B-box 2 domain, and a coiled-coil domain (Fig. 17.14). The α isoform of TRIM5 (TRIM5α) also contains a C-terminal B30.2 or SPRY domain that is absent in other TRIM5 isoforms. This C-terminal B30.2/SPRY domain harbors the determinants responsible for the species specificity of TRIM5α-mediated restriction to retroviral infection[517,550,668,684,766]; a single amino acid change in the B30.2/SPRY domain of human TRIM5α converts it from a weak inhibitor of HIV-1 infection to one that behaves like rhesus TRIM5α in potently restricting HIV-1 infection.[766] This specificity is mediated through direct binding between the B30.2/SPRY domain and the CA protein on the incoming capsid.[405,427,642] Binding of TRIM5α to CA requires both TRIM5α dimerization and higher-order multimerization.[405,427] The higher-order multimers have been reported to be hexameric,[245,521] an observation that is relevant to the mechanism of TRIM5 restriction (see below). The importance of TRIM5α in combating retroviral infections is supported by the finding that the CA-binding B30.2/SPRY domain in TRIM5α has undergone positive selection during primate evolution.[344,627,668]

In owl monkey cells, HIV-1 infection is highly inefficient but is significantly enhanced by disrupting the interaction between CA and the cellular protein cyclophilin A (CypA) (see section on capsid). This observation suggested a link between CA–CypA binding and postentry restriction. The basis for this

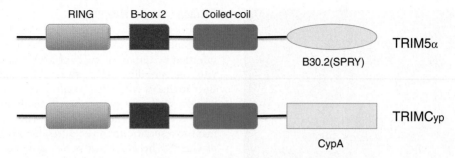

FIGURE 17.14 Domain organization of TRIM5α and TRIMCyp. The major domains—RING, B-box 2, coiled-coil, and B30.2 (SPRY), and cyclophilin A (CypA)—are shown. Gag-binding determinants of TRIM5α and TRIMCyp reside in the B30.2 (SPRY) and CypA domains, respectively.

link was revealed by the discovery that owl monkey cells express a form of TRIM5α in which the C-terminal B30.2/SPRY domain has been replaced by CypA[524,628] (Fig. 17.14). This unusual TRIM5 variant, designated TRIMCyp, restricts HIV-1 infection through a direct binding between the CypA portion of TRIMCyp and CA of the incoming particle. Thus, the ability of TRIMCyp to restrict HIV-1 infectivity in owl monkey cells is eliminated by mutations in the CypA-binding domain of CA or by treating the infected cells with drugs like cyclosporine A that block the CA–CypA interaction.[524,628] Given the short period of time HIV-1 has circulated in the human population, TRIM evolution in primates was not driven by selective pressure by HIV-1 but rather by SIVs. Nevertheless, TRIM-mediated restriction of HIV-1 provides useful information in understanding the antiviral activity of this family of restriction factors. In addition, human TRIM5α has been reported to potently block HIV-1 infection in primary T cells when the CA–CypA interaction is disrupted, suggesting that CypA binding to the incoming capsid protects it from TRIM5α restriction in human cells.[375]

TRIM family proteins, when overexpressed in cells, assemble into cytosolic complexes referred to as "cytoplasmic bodies".[594] Although preexisting TRIM5α or TRIMCyp cytoplasmic bodies are not required for restriction of retroviral infection,[550,667] microscopic examination of cells overexpressing rhesus TRIM5α early after HIV-1 infection revealed a colocalization between TRIM5α-induced cytoplasmic bodies and viral capsids.[99] These cytoplasmic bodies display features that suggest that they are associated with macroautophagy.[101]

Several lines of evidence support a model whereby binding of TRIM5α or TRIMCyp to CA on the incoming capsid contributes to a destabilization of the capsid and, consequently, a block to reverse transcription: (a) TRIM5α appears to accelerate CA uncoating early postinfection in the context of either HIV-1 or N-MLV.[683] (b) Incubation of in vitro-assembled capsid-like complexes with cell lysates containing TRIM5α or TRIMCyp disrupts the assembled structures.[61] (c) Treatment of infected cells with proteasome inhibitors reverses the ability of TRIM5α to prevent viral DNA synthesis, suggesting that TRIM5α induces the degradation of capsid in the proteasome.[745] It is important to note, however, that the mechanism of TRIM restriction in cells is still not fully understood, and although proteasome inhibitors rescue the TRIM-induced defect in DNA synthesis they do not rescue virus infectivity, suggesting that restriction is a multistep process.[745]

Structural studies have shed light on the mechanism of action of TRIM5α and TRIMCyp restriction.[246] In vitro, TRIM5α forms dimers, which assemble into a hexagonal lattice,[245] a feature of both TRIM5α and TRIMCyp.[428] Although TRIM lattice assembly occurs spontaneously, it is greatly facilitated by the presence of hexagonal arrays of in vitro-assembled CA. These findings suggest that restricting TRIM proteins assemble on top of incoming CA hexamers, thereby contributing to capsid disassembly and degradation (Fig. 17.15). Consistent with this model, a fragment of rhesus TRIM5α comprising the coiled-coil and B30.2/SPRY domain was shown to bind HIV-1 CA assemblies or virus-derived capsids in vitro and induce their disassembly from an extended CA hexameric lattice to individual hexamers.[780] Although binding of TRIM5α or TRIMCyp to the viral capsid induces capsid destabilization in vitro, the E3 ubiquitin ligase activity of the TRIM protein, which mediates TRIM autoubiquitylation, appears to contribute to restriction, presumably through recruitment of the proteasome. The immunoproteasome, a type of proteasome that is up-regulated by IFN, may promote capsid degradation.[341] TRIM5α binding to the CA lattice not only contributes to CA lattice disassembly and direct antiviral restriction but also triggers the innate immune response against retroviral infection. CA lattice recognition by TRIM5α reportedly leads to the generation of free polyubiquitin chains, which could in turn activate innate immune signaling.[551] In addition, the hexameric nature of the TRIM5α assemblies on the viral capsid leads to the formation of K63-linked polyubiquitin chains at the N-terminus of TRIM5α through RING domain–mediated autoubiquitylation; trivalent RING domain interactions at the vertices of the TRIM5α hexamer (Fig. 17.15) have been shown to be required for extension of K63-linked polyubiquitin chains. These chains are proposed to promote capsid disassembly and trigger immune signaling.[221]

Mx2

The Mx proteins are highly conserved across vertebrates and are IFN-inducible, dynamin-like GTPases. Humans encode Mx1 and Mx2 (also referred to as MxA and MxB, respectively). Mx1 interferes with the replication of a large number of viruses, but does not inhibit HIV. In 2013, it was reported independently by several groups that Mx2 exhibits anti-HIV activity.[265,359,440] Interestingly, the GTPase activity of Mx2 is not required for its antiviral activity. Mx2 is a dimeric protein that bears an N-terminal nuclear localization signal, and Mx1/Mx2 chimeras that

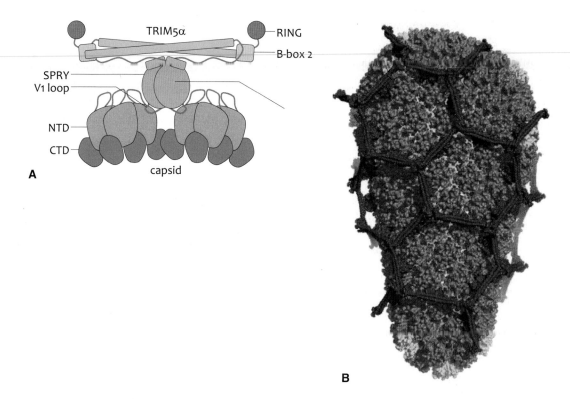

FIGURE 17.15 Capsid recognition by TRIM5α. A: Two SPRY domains bind the CA-NTD on the assembled capsid. **B:** TRIM5α (in *purple*) assembles on top of the capsid. CA hexamers are shown in *dark green*, pentamers in *light green/yellow*. The location of a trivalent RING domain interaction is indicated. (Adapted by permission from Nature: Ganser-Pornillos BK, Pornillos O. Restriction of HIV-1 and other retroviruses by TRIM5. *Nat Rev Microbiol* 2019;17(9):546–556. Copyright © 2019 Springer Nature.)

retain this region of Mx2 exhibit anti–HIV-1 activity.[265] This observation, coupled with the finding that Mx2 restriction is elicited not at the level of reverse transcription but at a nuclear import step,[265,359,440] suggests that Mx2 disrupts some aspect of capsid import into the nucleus. Indeed, Mx2 has been shown to interact with several nuclear pore components, potentially positioning the protein to disrupt the nuclear import of incoming HIV-1 capsids.[182]

Primate Mx2 proteins exhibit variable abilities to inhibit lentiviral infection; this species specificity maps to a single residue near the N-terminus of the protein that is under positive selection.[90] While the precise mechanism of Mx2 restriction is still uncertain, a number of studies have shown that mutations in CA can alleviate the antiviral activity of this host factor. Dimerization but not higher-order oligomerization of Mx2 is required for its antiviral activity and direct Mx2 binding to assembled CA has been demonstrated.[53,235]

Integration

Mutations that block retroviral DNA integration were first reported in avian and murine retroviral systems,[191,539,580,641] leading to the discovery of the essential viral enzyme IN, generated by PR-mediated cleavage of the C-terminal portion of the Gag–Pol polyprotein (see Fig. 17.6). The steps in the integration process were originally elucidated in studies using MLV,[81,241] but these findings apply to HIV as well. In all retroviral systems, integration proceeds in the same series of steps (Fig. 17.16): (a) 3′ processing: After its assembly with the viral DNA, IN cleaves immediately downstream from the invariant nucleotide sequence CA, typically removing two nucleotides from the 3′ termini of both strands of full-length, linear viral DNA, generating a preintegration substrate with 3′-recessed ends. (b) DNA strand transfer: In the nucleus, IN catalyzes a staggered cleavage in the cellular target DNA. The 3′-recessed ends of viral DNA are joined to the 5′ "overhanging" termini of the cleaved cellular DNA. (c) Gap repair: The cellular repair machinery fills the gap, thereby completing the integration process.[81,241,606] All integrated proviruses terminate with dinucleotides 5′-TG and CA-3′, whereas different genera yield different sized flanking duplications based on the spacing of the staggered chromosomal DNA cut; the lentiviral duplication of cellular DNA is 5 bp.

Our understanding of the chemistry of the retroviral integration reaction was greatly assisted by the development of *in vitro* integration assays. Purified IN can carry out 3′ processing and strand transfer reactions when combined with short synthetic oligonucleotides that mimic the viral DNA ends and a divalent metal ion (Mg^{2+} or Mn^{2+}).[152,365] Initial studies observed that the predominant product in *in vitro* assays using purified HIV-1 IN was a single end joined to one strand of the target, rather than the more physiologically relevant product in which both ends are integrated into the target ("concerted" or "full-site" integration).

Retroviral IN proteins are composed of three structurally and functionally distinct domains: an N-terminal, zinc-binding domain (NTD); a catalytic core domain (CCD); and a C-terminal domain (CTD) (Fig. 17.17). Problems with low solubility and propensity to aggregate initially hindered

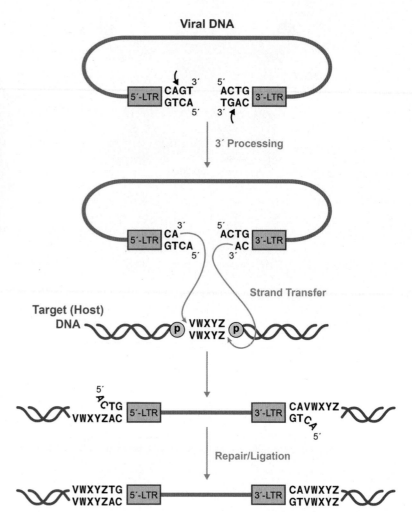

FIGURE 17.16 Schematic depiction of the HIV-1 integration process. During 3' processing, IN cleaves immediately downstream from the CA dinucleotide, removing two nucleotides from the 3' termini of both strands of full-length, linear viral DNA, generating a preintegration substrate with 3'-recessed ends. IN then catalyzes a staggered cleavage in the cellular target DNA. The 3'-recessed ends of viral DNA are joined to the 5' "overhanging" termini of the cleaved cellular DNA (strand transfer). The cellular repair machinery fills the gap, thereby completing the integration process (gap repair).

progress in defining the structure of the IN holoenzyme in its active state. However, the structures of all three domains independently and in various combinations were solved by x-ray crystallography or NMR methods. The NMR structure of the NTD[95] revealed three helical bundles with a zinc coordinated by invariant amino acids His-12, His-16, Cys-40, and Cys-43. Attempts at crystallography of the CCD were successful when a mutation was identified that greatly increased solubility without disrupting *in vitro* catalytic activity.[198] Each monomer of the core domain is composed of a five-stranded β-sheet flanked by helices; this structure bears striking resemblance to that of other polynucleotidyl transferases including RNase H and the bacteriophage MuA transposase.[198,596] Three highly conserved residues are found in analogous positions at the catalytic center of these enzymes; in HIV-1 IN, these residues are Asp-64, Asp-116, and Glu-152—often referred to as the D,D-35-E motif (Fig. 17.17). Mutations in this catalytic triad block HIV-1 IN function both *in vivo* and *in vitro*. The IN CTD, whose structure was initially solved by NMR,[201,442] adopts a five-stranded β-barrel folding topology reminiscent of Src homology 3 (SH3) domains. The crystal structure of an HIV-1 NTD-CCD IN fragment[726] revealed a dimer of dimers, with two inner monomers and two outer monomers, with an extensive intermolecular NTD–CTD interface that provided a preview of the interface evident in the structure of the full retroviral tetramer.

A breakthrough in IN structural biology was made possible by the realization that the IN of prototype foamy virus (PFV) is highly soluble and capable of concerted integration *in vitro* with short DNA substrates.[710] Although divergent at the overall amino acid sequence level, HIV-1 and PFV IN are structurally conserved. The IN tetramer bound to DNA oligonucleotides that mimic the viral DNA ends—which together form the active nucleoprotein complex referred to as the "intasome"—was crystallized and the structure solved.[277] This structure revealed that two monomers in the tetramer interact at a dimer interface and are responsible for all contacts with the DNA substrate; the other two monomers are on the outside of the complex and do not interact with each other or with DNA. The residues of the catalytic triad (D,D-35-E) of the inner mono-

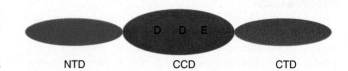

FIGURE 17.17 Schematic representation of an IN monomer. The three major structural domains—the N-terminal domain (NTD), catalytic core domain (CCD), and C-terminal domain (CTD)—are shown. The catalytic triad Asp-64, Asp-116, and Glu-152 is represented as D-D-E.

mers are oriented close to the 3'-OH of the viral DNA ends. Two metal ions are coordinated at the active site by the residues of the catalytic triad. The addition of model target DNA to the intasome allowed for crystallization of a complex containing both viral and target DNAs.[450] In the presence of Mg^{2+}, the strand transfer reaction took place during crystallization, whereas in the absence of divalent metal ions, strand transfer was blocked. This allowed capture of postcatalytic strand transfer and prestrand transfer complexes. These structures revealed that the target DNA, which binds in a cleft between the two halves of the intasome complex, adopts a highly bent conformation allowing the well-separated intasome active sites to access the scissile phosphodiester bonds in the target DNA. The viral (donor) DNA duplex is unpaired at the active site. Conformational changes that occur during catalysis are predicted to render the strand transfer reaction irreversible.[450] Following the original publication of the structures described above,[277,450] a number of additional PFV structures that contained potent inhibitors were solved (for review, see Ref.[476]).

Despite the utility of the PFV intasome structure, as mentioned, the sequences of the HIV-1 and PFV enzymes are highly divergent, sharing only approximately 20% amino acid sequence identity in the catalytic domain. Many of the mutations in HIV-1 IN that confer resistance to drugs targeting IN (see below) map to residues that are not conserved between the HIV-1 and PFV enzymes. These considerations led to efforts to solve the structure of the HIV-1 intasome by cryoEM methods.[541] These studies made use of the finding that fusion of the DNA-binding protein Sso7D to the N-terminus of HIV-1 IN increased enzyme activity and solubility, overcoming the propensity of HIV-1 IN to aggregate. Using this fusion protein, a cryoEM structure was solved for the HIV-1 IN tetramer in complex with joined viral and target DNA ends, referred to as the strand transfer complex (STC) (Fig. 17.18). The core tetrameric unit was observed to assemble into higher-order structures containing 12 or 16 IN protomers.[541] The biological relevance of these higher-order complexes remains to be fully explored, but it appears that the active complex contains multiple IN tetramers.

A number of host factors have been reported to bind directly to HIV-1 IN, including a 75-kDa, predominantly nuclear, chromatin-associated protein known as lens epithelium–derived

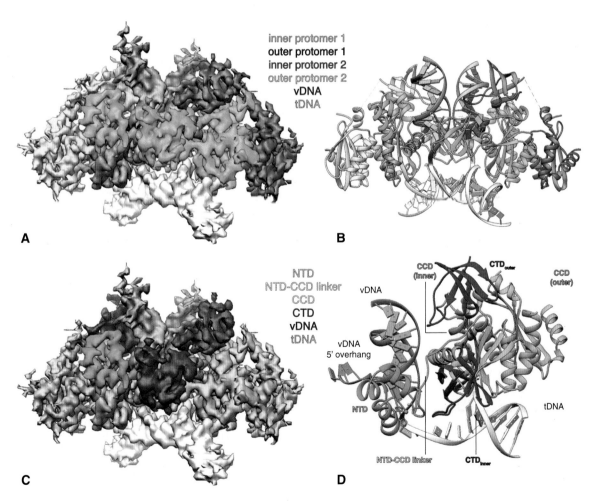

FIGURE 17.18 Structure of the HIV-1 strand transfer complex (STC). A: Cryo-EM reconstruction of the STC, with IN protomers indicated in *red, green, yellow,* and *blue*. Viral and target DNA are highlighted in *dark* and *light gray,* respectively. **B:** Atomic model derived from the cryo-EM density, colored as in **(A). C:** Segmented cryo-EM density and **(D)** asymmetric subunit of the atomic model, with IN N-terminal domain (NTD) in *green*, IN catalytic core domain (CCD) in *beige*, NTD-CCD linker in *blue*, and C-terminal domain (CTD) in *purple*.

growth factor (LEDGF/p75).[123,204] This protein was found to stimulate the strand transfer step of the integration reaction *in vitro*[123] and increase binding of IN to DNA.[91] Near-complete knock-down of LEDGF/p75 levels,[441] or use of a murine LEDGF/p75 knock-out cell line,[655] revealed markedly reduced HIV-1 infectivity in the absence of detectable LEDGF/p75 expression. Infectivity was also severely compromised by overexpression of the IN-binding domain (IBD) of LEDGF/p75.[168,441] In the case of both LEDGF/p75 depletion and LEDGF/p75-IBD overexpression, infectivity was disrupted at the integration step, and the effect was specific to lentiviruses, establishing LEDGF/p75 as a cellular cofactor for lentiviral integration. Studies in which siRNA-resistant LEDGF/p75 mutants were added back to LEDGF/p75-depleted cells identified domains of LEDGF/p75 required for its activity as an integration cofactor.[441,655,717] The observation that the LEDGF/p75-IBD and the chromatin-binding regions (the PWWP domain and AT-hook) (Fig. 17.19) are required for function supported the hypothesis that LEDGF/p75 functions to tether the PIC to target chromosomal DNA. Structural studies have provided further details of the IN–LEDGF/p75 interaction.[4,122,200]

Although the basic mechanism by which retroviruses integrate their DNAs into the host cell genome is highly conserved, different retroviruses differ in their target site selection.[488] For example, HIV-1 preferentially integrates within the bodies of actively transcribed genes in gene-rich regions; MLV favors transcription start sites but only weakly selects active genes. ASLV displays a strong preference for neither active genes nor transcription start sites. Target site selection, which impacts the development of retroviruses as vehicles for gene therapy, is influenced by interactions between components of the incoming viral complex—specifically CA and IN—and chromatin-associated host factors. CA–CPSF6 and IN–LEDGF/p75 interactions strongly influence, by different

mechanisms, HIV-1 integration into genes. The interaction between the incoming capsid and CPSF6 directs the viral complex to nuclear speckles in speckle-associated domains and the incoming capsid causes CPSF6 to cluster in these speckles.[644] Depletion of CPSF6, or mutation of the CPSF6 binding site in CA, in most cases does not substantially reduce the overall efficiency of virus infection but causes integration targeting to shift from gene-rich regions of the chromatin to gene-sparse regions.[2,225] Following CPSF6-mediated delivery of the PIC to gene-dense regions, IN–LEDGF/p75 binding tethers the viral DNA to chromatin (Fig. 17.19).

The function of LEDGF/p75 in promoting HIV-1 integration raises the possibility that the IN–LEDGF/p75 interaction could serve as a target for developing novel antiviral therapeutics. Small molecule "LEDGINs" (LEDGF/p75-IN inhibitors) were identified that block the IN–LEDGF/p75 interaction *in vitro* and inhibit HIV-1 infection at the integration step.[129] Although these molecules were originally identified based on their ability to block the IN–LEDGF/p75 interaction, it has become clear that their antiviral mechanism of action primarily results from their ability to induce IN aggregation and thus disrupt the role of IN in RNA condensation into the capsid during maturation (for review, see Ref.[379]) (also see section on Maturation). These compounds are now most often referred to as allosteric IN inhibitors (ALLINIs).

The IN protein is subject to extensive posttranscriptional modifications in the form of acetylation, SUMOylation, and phosphorylation. While the roles of these modifications in IN function are still under investigation, recent work has shown that mutation of Lys residues that are modified by acetylation, in particular IN residue Lys-258, has no effect on integration but markedly reduces viral gene expression from the integrated provirus.[735] Reduced viral RNA transcription is a result of misdirected integration into centromeric repeats. Polymorphisms in residue Lys-258 could thus lead to the formation of latent proviruses, suggesting a possible connection between altered integration site selection and latency.[734]

Diketo acid inhibitors have been developed that specifically and potently block the IN-mediated strand transfer reaction.[288] These IN strand transfer inhibitors (INSTIs) bind IN only in the presence of divalent metal and viral DNA and prevent the complex from associating with cellular (target) DNA. Although structurally diverse, INSTIs appear to have common features, including (a) a hydrophobic moiety composed of halobenzyl groups and (b) coplanar oxygen atoms that chelate the Mg^{+2} ions in the active site.[662] Work in the early 2000s showed that naphthyridine carboxamides inhibit the replication of a SHIV in rhesus macaques, setting the stage for *in vivo* use of INSTIs.[289] Further structure–activity relationship studies led to the development of raltegravir[687] and elvitegravir.[624] Raltegravir and elvitegravir were approved for clinical use in people living with HIV by the U.S. FDA in 2007 and 2014, respectively, and three other INSTIs, dolutegravir, bictegravir, and cabotegravir, are now approved for clinical use. The long-acting injectable Cabenuva combines cabotegravir with the NNRTI rilpivirine.

The observation that INSTIs are active against a wide range of retroviruses,[382] including PFV,[710] allowed structures to be determined for raltegravir and elvitegravir bound to the PFV IN active site.[277] These structural analyses showed that

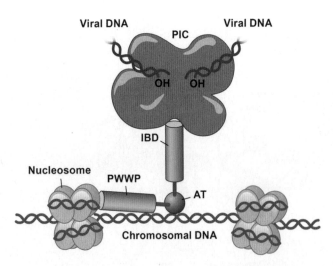

FIGURE 17.19 Model for the tethering of the preintegration complex to chromosomal DNA by LEDGF/p75. The preintegration complex (PIC), containing multimeric IN (*red*) and viral DNA (*blue*), is bound by the IN binding domain (IBD) of LEDGF. The AT hook (AT) domain of LEDGF is shown in complex with DNA; the PWWP domain is depicted bound to DNA and histone proteins in the nucleosome.

INSTIs chelate the metals in the enzyme active site and demonstrated that the halobenzyl moieties of the INSTI stack against the cytidine of the invariant CA dinucleotide and in doing so supplant the adenine ring and eject its associated DNA strand transfer 3′-OH nucleophile from the active site.[277,278,389] As with other HIV inhibitors, resistance develops both *in vitro* and *in vivo*. Several major pathways of resistance have been observed for raltegravir, and secondary mutations arise at a number of additional positions. The more recently developed INSTIs are more difficult for the virus to escape. The advances noted above in solving the structure of HIV-1 IN have provided a significant amount of structural information on the binding of INSTIs to HIV-1 IN.[354,662] This information will be useful in designing modified inhibitors that are active against INSTI-resistant HIV-1 mutants.

In addition to its primary role in viral DNA integration, a variety of studies have demonstrated a role for IN in RNA condensation in the viral core during maturation (see Maturation section).

Viral Gene Expression

The regulation of viral gene expression is rate limiting in the replication cycle. It occurs at the transcriptional and posttranscriptional levels and uses common cellular and unique viral mechanisms. Two viral proteins play a role in HIV gene expression, Tat and Rev, and both are RNA-binding proteins.

After viral integration, the HIV promoter, located within the 5′ LTR, is packaged into host chromatin and behaves in many ways like a highly signal-dependent human promoter. Viral transcription is executed by the cellular RNA polymerase II (Pol II), which forms a nonprocessive "paused" complex downstream of the start of transcription, generating short viral RNAs. RNA Pol II transitions to a processive state in elongation, allowing synthesis of full-length viral RNA, after

cellular activation or in the presence of Tat. The activity of the viral promoter is tightly connected to extracellular stimuli that induce cellular transcription factors (TFs) to translocate into the nuclear compartment and bind to various DNA elements that make up the promoter (Fig. 17.20). Distinct TF combinations drive transcription in different cell types (e.g., T cells and monocyte-derived macrophages), activated states (e.g., naive, effector and memory CD4+ T lymphocytes), and tissues (e.g., lymph nodes, gastrointestinal tract, and CNS) targeted by the virus. Posttranscriptionally, viral RNAs undergo distinct splicing steps that facilitate viral RNA export and translation; unspliced RNAs are effectively exported by the action of Rev.

Here we summarize the steps of basal and Tat-induced HIV transcription, and the roles of RNA splicing, nuclear export, and the Rev protein.

Basal HIV Transcription After Integration

Transcription of HIV, similar to eukaryotic genes comprises four key phases: initiation, promoter-proximal pausing, elongation, and termination.[647] Each phase involves dynamic, reversible, posttranslational modifications of Pol II.[780] Pol II contains 12 subunits, and the catalytic activity is encoded in the largest subunit, RPB1. RBP1 has a unique region called the C-terminal domain (CTD), which contains a heptad sequence (consensus Tyr1-Ser2-Pro3-Thr4-Ser5-Pro6-Ser7) that is repeated 52 times, making the CTD a highly repetitive, unstructured region of low sequence diversity.[570] This region is modified extensively posttranslationally; for example, serine residues, specifically Ser2 and Ser5, of the CTD are dynamically and reversibly phosphorylated.[88,199,335,556,773] Transcription also involves other features of gene regulation, such as nucleosome position, DNA sequence, DNA structure, and cotranscriptional processes.[15,42,349,569,616]

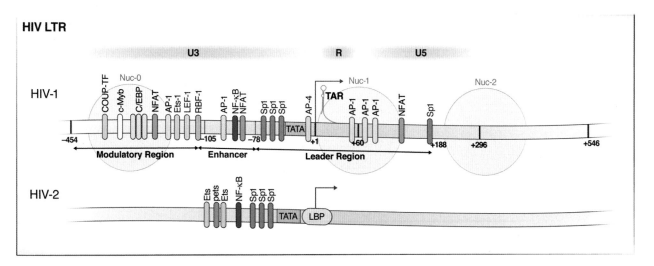

FIGURE 17.20 HIV-1 and HIV-2 long terminal repeat (LTR). The HIV-1 LTR is a duplicated 630+ base-pair (bp) element located at the termini of integrated proviral DNA. A blow-up of the 5′ LTR and adjacent cellular and Gag coding sequences is presented at the top. The HIV-1 LTR has been subdivided into three domains: the R (repeat) region is defined as a 96-nt repeat present at the 3′ and 5′ termini of HIV-1 genomic RNA; U5 is an 84-nt segment located immediately 3′ to the R region; and U3 is a 454-nt segment situated immediately 5′ to R. The 5′ LTR and adjacent gag leader sequence (GLS) are aligned with the subdivided LTR (*middle*) to indicate functionally important binding sites for transcriptional regulatory proteins. The positions of nucleosomes nuc 0, nuc 1, and nuc 2 are indicated. For HIV-2 (*bottom*), the unique binding sites for the peri-ets (pets) and E26 transforming specific (Ets) transcriptional factors are indicated.

HIV was one of the first systems in which promoter-proximal pausing of Pol II was described and intensely studied.[360] Multiple TF binding sites on the promoter recruit the Pol II preinitiation complex, a process observed even in latently infected cells. However, progression from promoter-proximal pausing into the elongation phase is prevented by the presence of negative elongation factors, suppressive placement of the first nucleosome (Nuc-1), and an absence of positive elongation factors, including the virally encoded Tat protein (Fig. 17.21). Without Tat, randomly and prematurely terminated HIV transcripts are produced. This Tat-deficient phenotype can be studied after transfection of LTR-driven reporter gene constructs in the absence of Tat and in cells harboring integrated HIV-1 proviruses with mutated Tat genes.[214,408,702] The presence or absence of Tat is also critical for the latent state of the virus.

LTR

The two LTRs flanking the HIV genome are assembled from different regions of the RNA genome representing the U3, R, and U5 regions (Fig. 17.20). The HIV-1 transcriptional promoter and multiple regulatory elements are located within the U3 region and function in the context of the 5′ LTR (Fig. 17.20). Their principal function is to recruit the Pol II holoenzyme to the start site (+1) of viral RNA synthesis (transcription start site/TSS), also defined as the first nucleotide in the LTR R region. In the presence of a functional 5′ LTR, transcription from the 3′ LTR is usually suppressed.[378]

The HIV-1 promoter can be divided into four main functional regions: a modulatory region (−455 to −104), the enhancer (−109 to −79), the core promoter (−78 to +1), and the leader region (+1 to +188) (Fig. 17.20). Both constitutive and inducible TFs recognize the *cis*-regulatory elements contained within these functional regions to enhance or repress HIV-1 transcription. Three TFs (nuclear factor-kappa B [NF-κB], activator protein 1 [AP-1], and nuclear factor of activated T cells [NFAT]) are important in regulating HIV-1 RNA synthesis in activated T cells after antigen-specific/MHC-restricted signaling through the T-cell receptor complex, whereas specificity protein 1 (Sp1) regulates basal transcription. These four TFs are further discussed below. In addition, there are binding sites for other TFs (e.g., COUP-TF, c-MyB, C/EBP, Ets-1, LEF-1, RBF-2, ATF4, and AP-4) that are involved in HIV transcription.

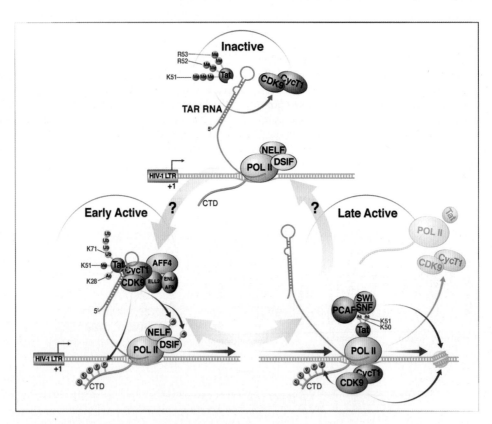

FIGURE 17.21 Regulation of HIV transcription. Tat-promoted phosphorylation of the C-terminal domain (CTD) of RNA polymerase II (Pol II) results in processive synthesis of human immunodeficiency virus 1 (HIV-1) messenger RNA (mRNA). In the absence of Tat binding to transactivation response region (TAR), the processivity of the RNA Pol II complex is impaired. When the activation domain of Tat interacts with the cyclin T (cycT1)–CDK9 complex, the conformation of Tat changes and its affinity and specificity for TAR RNA increase. By recruiting cycT1–CDK9 and the Super Elongation Complex (SEC, composed of AFF, ELL2, ENL/AF9) to a promoter-proximal location, Tat mediates the hyperphosphorylation of the CTD and promoter clearance (elongation) of the transcriptional complex. (Modified from Ott M, Geyer M, Zhou Q. The control of HIV transcription: keeping RNA polymerase II on track. *Cell Host Microbe* 2011;10(5):426–435. Copyright © 2011 Elsevier. With permission.)

Sp1

The LTRs of HIV and other primate lentiviruses contain three tandemly arranged binding sites for the constitutively expressed Sp1; these DNA elements are situated immediately upstream of a canonical Pol II TATA box (Fig. 17.20). The Sp1 and TATA elements constitute the HIV-1 core promoter and must all be present for basal levels of LTR-directed RNA synthesis.[281] Mutations that functionally inactivate all three Sp1 motifs eliminate detectable replication in Jurkat T cells and delay progeny virus production in CEM and H9 cells but have little effect on replication in activated PBMC.[417,605]

NF-κB

The two binding sites for the NF-κB/Rel family of TFs constitute the principal activatable enhancer elements in the HIV-1 LTR. The NF-κB sites (consensus sequence: GGGRNNYYCC) are located upstream and adjacent to the Sp1 binding motifs in all HIV-1 isolates.[516] In clade E strains, a single inactivating nucleotide deletion in the upstream NF-κB element converts it to a GA-binding protein (GABP) site, and clade C isolates carry three or four NF-κB sites.[25] *In vivo*, NF-κB is intimately involved in regulating inflammation, cell proliferation, and apoptosis. Because the various members of the NFκB family are present intracellularly as dimeric molecules, a heterogeneous population of homo- and heterodimers, with different functional specificities, bind to the two NF-κB sites in the HIV-1 LTR. For HIV-1 gene expression, the two most important forms of NF-κB are the p50/p50 homodimer, which functions as a repressor, and the p50/p65 heterodimer, which functions as an activator. In addition to its role in basal transcription, the Rel family member RelB interacts with Tat to further enhance HIV transcription.[727] Importantly, NF-κB synergizes with Sp1 and AP-1 family TFs in the activation of the HIV promoter. The LTRs of HIV-2 and SIV, while retaining the triplicated Sp1 motifs, each contain only a single NF-κB binding site (Fig. 17.20).

NFAT

Like NF-κB, members of the NFAT family of proteins are sequestered in the cytoplasm and transported into the nucleus after an increase in the levels of intracellular calcium.[700] Those increases activate the calcineurin serine/threonine phosphatase and result in the phosphorylation of NFAT, exposure of the NFAT nuclear localization sequence (NLS), and nuclear translocation of NFAT. This process is suppressed in resting T cells by the master regulator of cell quiescence, FOXO1. This protein acts by enhancing autophagy and reducing ER stress signals, which would otherwise activate HIV transcription by mobilizing NFAT and ATF4 TFs.[340,607,711]

AP-1

The rate of HIV-1 viral RNA synthesis can also be stimulated by AP1, which consists of Jun homodimers or Jun/Fos heterodimers. Depending on the HIV-1 subtype, AP1 binds to one or two DNA elements located immediately upstream of the two NF-κB sites in the HIV-1 LTR, or the three sites downstream of the TSS in the leader region. AP1 also cooperates with NF-κB and activates the viral promoter via the two NF-κB binding motifs. AP1 is activated by the c-Jun N-terminal kinase (JNK) and the extracellular signal-related kinase (ERK).[362]

Epigenetic Regulation of HIV

Eukaryotic gene expression is closely associated with nucleosome positioning.[631] Nucleosomes comprise 147 bp of DNA wrapped around an octamer of pairs of the four core histone proteins (i.e., H2A, H2B, H3, and H4). Promoter TF binding site accessibility is affected by the position of nucleosomes, and transcription machinery accesses DNA through the process of nucleosome remodeling. The positioning and stability of nucleosomes are regulated by their movement, deposition, or ejection by chromatin-remodeling complexes or posttranslational modification of the histone N-terminal tails.[71] These PTMs serve as a "histone code," allowing proteins with cognate recognition domains to interact with histones and then affect gene expression. The HIV epigenome is being targeted experimentally and clinically to manipulate the activity of the HIV provirus during latency.

When HIV-1 DNA becomes stably integrated into the host cell chromosomal DNA, it acquires precise nucleosomal positioning, independent from the integration site. Studies using DNA footprinting and restriction enzyme accessibility of integrated viral DNA revealed nucleosomes both upstream and downstream of the HIV-1 promoter (designated nuc-0, nuc-1, and nuc-2 in Fig. 17.20).[143] Nucleosome positioning defines two open chromatin regions encompassing (a) the promoter/enhancer sequences (−250 to +11 [relative to the transcription start site]) and (b) a downstream segment that begins within the 3′ portion of U5 and extends downstream of the PBS (+150 to +250). TFs are thought to bind to their cognate recognition motifs to maintain these open chromatin regions (Fig. 17.20). The effects of TFs on HIV-1 promoter activity depend on the function of coactivators and corepressors, which often induce chromatin remodeling by posttranslationally modifying histone tails on assembled nucleosomes.

Acetylation is one of the best studied histone modifications, and recruitment of histone acetyl transferases (HATs) and histone deacetyl transferases (HDACs) to the HIV LTR is mediated by TFs and other key transcriptional regulatory factors, such as BRD4, YY1, and the HUSH complex. Inhibitors of HDACs were the first epigenetic interventions experimentally and clinically tried to reverse HIV latency.[79,582,716] BRD4, a member of the bromodomain and ET domain (BET) protein family, binds acetylated histones through its double bromodomains. BRD4 exists in long and short isoforms; the long isoform recruits a critical cellular host factor, the positive transcription elongation factor (P-TEFb) to cellular promoters and is a transcriptional co-activator.[764] The short isoform, BRD4S, acts as a corepressor of HIV-1 transcription by binding to the catalytic subunit BRG1 of the SWI/SNF BAF complex, which promotes remodeling of nuc-1 in a repressive conformation downstream of the TSS.[60,146] Interestingly, other members of SWI/SNF activate HIV transcription in conjunction with the acetylated form of Tat (see below). Other bromodomain-containing proteins act on the HIV promoter: for example, the cellular factor P300/CBP-associated factor (PCAF) also interacts with the acetylated form of Tat through its bromodomain and coactivates the HIV LTR.[533,716]

The HIV promoter is also regulated by reversible methylation of lysines, arginines, and DNA. Proteins can be mono-, di-, or trimethylated, depending on the specificity of the methyltransferase. The histone lysine methyltransferase, SMYD2, represses HIV reactivation from latency by monomethylating lysine 20 of histone H4 at the HIV LTR. In addition, the reader protein L3MBTL1, which acts as a chromatin compactor, is recruited to the LTR in an SMYD2-dependent manner. The TF YY1 also represses HIV promoter activity by recruiting HDAC1.[47,151] Enhancer of Zeste 2 polycomb repressive complex 2 subunit (EZH2) associates with the promoter/enhancer region of HIV-1 proviruses in latently infected Jurkat T-cell lines and is found with the corresponding trimethylation mark at lysine27 in histone H3 (H3K27me3).[236] Knockdown of EZH2 with shRNA or treatment with an EZH2 inhibitor reactivates a significant portion of silenced proviruses.[522] Euchromatin histone methyltransferases (EHMTs) mono- and dimethylate histone 3 on lysine 9 (H3K9me1 and H3K9me2) in euchromatic regions of the genome[386] and both mammalian EHMTs, G9a and GLP, are responsible for transcriptional repression of the HIV-LTR by promoting repressive dimethylation at H3K9.[186,323] SUV39H1 specifically catalyzes trimethylation on histone H3 lysine 9 (H3K9me3) using monomethylated H3K9 as substrate.[588] H3K9me3 is a hallmark of facultative and constitutive heterochromatin and recruits heterochromatic protein 1α (HP1α), which binds H3K9me2/3 through its chromodomain.[237] Several studies link SUV39H1 to HIV-1 latency in microglial cells[465] and peripheral blood mononucleated cells (PBMCs) isolated from infected individuals.[196]

The human silencing hub (HUSH) complex is a key regulator of silencing endogenous retroviruses and transposable elements in mammalian genomes. The complex comprises three core proteins, TASOR, MPP8, and PPHLN1. Their exact functions are unknown, but by recruiting SETDB1, the complex is involved in reading and writing histone H3 lysine 9 trimethyl marks (H3K9me3) and spreads repressive chromatin marks. In several HIV latency models, inhibiting the HUSH complex reactivated the virus.[694]

DNA methylation involves the transfer of a methyl group onto cytosines to form 5-methylcytosine. DNA methylation of CpG (cytosine-proximal guanine) islands (CPGI) influences the chromatin environment and plays a role in epigenetic regulation of mammalian gene expression,[149] generally by recruiting repressors or blocking the binding of TFs.[495] The HIV-1 genome contains five CpGIs[111]: two surround the promoter region and flank the HIV-1 TSS and several TF binding sites at the 5′ LTR, two other CpGIs are located in the *env* gene, surrounding the HIV-1 antisense open reading frame, and the fifth CpGI is located in the 3′ LTR, where the antisense transcription start site is located.[104] In cultured HIV-1–infected cells, promoter DNA hypermethylation stabilizes HIV-1 latency and demethylating agents induce activation of HIV-1 transcription.[64,69,111,366,705] However, studies performed in infected individuals yielded controversial results.[63,300]

Tat

Tat is an indispensable viral protein that increases steady-state levels of viral RNA in a positive feedback loop by directing formation of a more processive Pol II transcription complex to produce itself and viral RNAs in virus-infected cells. When the *tat* gene is mutagenized, no detectable progeny virions are produced.[164] Tat is a small, pleiotropic protein that interacts with a set of critical host factors and links to TFs, the Pol II complex and the epigenetic machinery controlling HIV transcription.

Non–LTR-related functions of Tat include regulation of T-cell activity, apoptosis, oxidative stress, and inflammation.[7] Tat exerts its transactivator function by binding to the TAR RNA element. HIV-1 TAR encompasses the 5′-terminal 59 nt of all viral RNAs and folds into a stable stem-loop structure (Fig. 17.22). The minimal TAR element (mapping between bases +19 and +42) has three critical components: a base-paired stem, a trinucleotide bulge (with the sequence UCU at positions +23 to +25), and a hexanucleotide G-rich loop.[216] Sequences located in both the hexanucleotide loop and the bulge of HIV-1 TAR are required for Tat function. HIV-1 Tat binds to wild-type (WT) or "loop" mutants of TAR but not to TAR elements with alterations that affect the bulge region.[188,609] Interestingly, HIV-2 TAR forms a double stem-loop structure, each arm of which possesses a dinucleotide bulge and the hexanucleotide G-rich loop (Fig. 17.22).[202] The interaction between Tat and TAR is being explored as a drug target to block the interaction either to suppress HIV replication[202] or to enhance HIV latency by inducing a state of "deep latency."[421,485,503,504]

P-TEFb

The Tat/TAR complex activates HIV transcription both at the initiation and elongation steps. After initiation, Pol II pauses proximal to the promoter, at an average of 25 to 50 bp downstream of the TSS.[148] Establishment and maintenance of promoter-proximal pausing is performed by the interaction of the Pol II CTD with negative elongation factors NELF and DSIF.[121,758] This state is critical for HIV transcriptional regulation. Recruitment of P-TEFb catalyzes the transition of Pol II from a paused state to an actively elongating complex, called pause release.[148]

HIV research was critical in the discovery of P-TEFb. Reports describing the specific interaction of HIV-2 Tat with a cellular kinase provided the first mechanistic clues about Tat function.[294,295] The Tat-related kinase component in human P-TEFb was subsequently identified as CDK9, a 42-kDa CDC2-related kinase. However, the CDK9 catalytic subunit alone failed to bind to Tat in *in vitro* assays.[763] These unresolved issues were clarified with the isolation of an 87-kDa protein from nuclear extracts bound to Tat.[730] The new protein, named cyclin T (because it bound to Tat), is one of many cyclin regulatory subunits interacting with the CDK9 family of kinases (i.e., T1, T2a, T2b, or K).[548] Of these P-TEFb complexes, only those containing cyclin T1 directly bind to the HIV-1 Tat activation domain.[730]

P-TEFb is incorporated into a larger complex containing additional transcription elongation factors termed the superelongation complex (SEC). Besides P-TEFb, the SEC consists of the Pol II elongation factors eleven-nineteen Lys-rich leukemia (ELL) proteins and several frequent mixed lineage leukemia (MLL) translocation partners. ELL2 and P-TEFb act cooperatively to promote efficient Tat-mediated elongation.[290] AFF4, ENL, AF9, and elongation factor ELL2 are components of the Tat-P-TEFb complex, and Tat stabilizes ELL2.[290] P-TEFb phosphorylates Ser2 residues of the CTD to enhance polymerase processivity, but in the presence of Tat, it also phosphorylates serine 5.[469,552,575,636,785] P-TEFb also phosphorylates DSIF and NELF; phosphorylation of NELF leads to its dissociation from the Pol II complex, whereas phosphorylation of DSIF turns it into a positive elongation factor.[148]

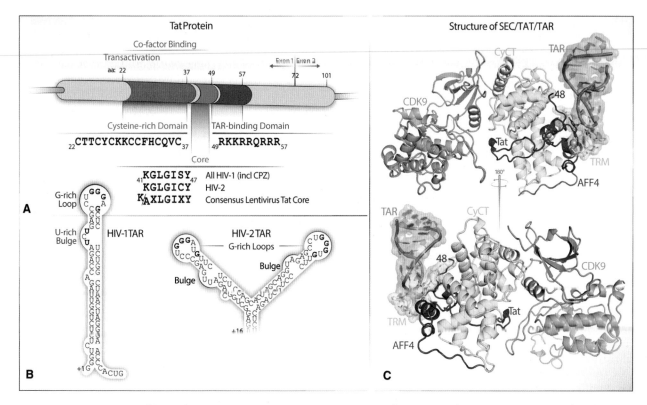

FIGURE 17.22 Structure of Tat and its transactivation response region (TAR) element. A: Schematic representation of the human immunodeficiency virus 1 (HIV-1) Tat protein with the cysteine-rich activation, core, and TAR-binding domains indicated. **B:** Structure of the stem-bulge-loop configurations of HIV-1 and HIV-2 TAR elements. **C:** Crystal structure of Tat/TAR binding in the presence of the super elongation complex.

In proliferating cells, P-TEFb is maintained in an inactive form in the cytoplasm through its reversible association with the 7SK small nuclear ribonucleoprotein (snRNP). The 7SK small nuclear RNA folds into a 3D scaffold that is stabilized by interactions with several proteins (Fig. 17.23). Of particular importance to HIV is the homodimer of the kinase inhibitor hexamethylene bisacetamide-inducible protein 1/2 (HEXIM). Several phosphorylation events, including especially Thr-186 on the CDK9 subunit, and acetylation of CDK9 and Cyclin T1, regulate activity and availability outside the 7SK snRNP.[125] In resting CD4+ T cells, P-TEFb regulation occurs through miRNA-mediated down-regulation of CycT1 and sequestration of inactive CDK9 in the cytoplasm.[124]

Tat expression during the early phase of productive infection results in the dissociation of 7SK snRNA from P-TEFb and formation of the Tat/P-TEFb complex.[643] This is facilitated, in part, by the fact that the Tat RNA-binding domain is highly homologous to the 7SK snRNP-interacting domain in the HEXIM1 inhibitor.[555,768] The interaction of Tat and the 7SKsnRNA releases HEXIM-1 from the 7SKsnRNA and relieves P-TEFb inhibition (Fig. 17.23). Moreover, subsequent P-TEFb inactivation is prevented by the interaction of Tat and the 7SKsnRNA, which prevents reassembly of the 7SKsnRNP complex.[29,509,555]

Structure

HIV-1 Tat contains 86 to 101 amino acid residues encoded by two exons (Fig. 17.22). A shorter, 72-amino acid "one-exon" HIV-1 Tat protein possesses all the transcriptional activating properties of full-length Tat, as measured in tissue culture infections or in LTR-driven reporter gene experiments. The termination codon after the first Tat exon is highly conserved among diverse HIV-1 isolates, suggesting that the one-exon and two-exon Tat proteins mediate different functions during productive viral infections *in vivo*. Immune modulatory effects of the second exon of Tat have been described.[532]

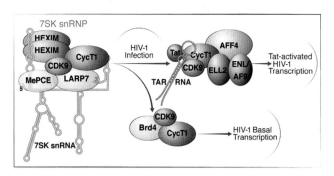

FIGURE 17.23 Differential Recruitment of P-TEFb from the 7SK snRNP during HIV Infection. The 7SK snRNP is a cellular reservoir of inactive P-TEFb that contains HEXIM1, an inhibitor of the CDK9 kinase activity. P-TEFb is recruited from the 7SK snRNP by Tat for transactivation of HIV-1 transcription or is released upon exposure of cells to hypertrophic or stress signals to associate with bromodomain-containing protein 4 (Brd4) to induce basal HIV transcription in the absence of Tat. (Modified from Ott M, Geyer M, Zhou Q. The control of HIV transcription: keeping RNA polymerase II on track. *Cell Host Microbe* 2011;10(5):426–435. Copyright © 2011 Elsevier. With permission. Ref.[5])

The functional organization of the HIV-1 Tat protein was deduced from TAR binding and transcriptional activation experiments with WT and mutagenized derivatives of Tat. The tripartite Tat activation (or effector) domain encompasses the N-terminal 48 residues, which include (a) a string of highly acidic amino acids (residues 1 to 21); (b) a Cys-rich region (seven invariant, six of which are required for function) at positions 22 to 37; and (c) a hydrophobic core segment (amino acids 38 to 48) that is highly conserved among HIV isolates (Fig. 17.22). The activation domain is critical for recruiting P-TEFb to TAR; mutations affecting this region drastically reduce or eliminate transactivation activity.[610] The TAR RNA binding domain of Tat was mapped to a Lys/Arg-rich region at residues 48 to 57 and is highly posttranslationally modified (Fig. 17.22). Peptides from this Tat segment bind to the TAR bulge region and a few base pairs surrounding the bulge, but with somewhat less affinity and specificity than does full-length Tat.[147]

While many structural studies have investigated Tat binding to TAR and P-TEFb binding to Tat, Tat binding to TAR is highly cooperative and involves formation of a trimolecular complex composed of Tat, TAR, and P-TEFb (including the SEC).[56,249,730,762,785] Upon binding of Tat/SEC, the TAR loop is stabilized by cross-loop hydrogen bonds. It makes structure-specific contacts with the side chains of the Tat–TAR recognition motif (TRM) of cyclin T1 and the zinc-coordinating region of Tat.[637] Despite limited resolution, it is clear that the TAR loop evolved to make high-affinity interactions with the cyclin T1 TRM, whereas Tat has three roles in the trimolecular complex: scaffolding and stabilizing the TRM, making specific interactions through its zinc-coordinating loop, and engaging in electrostatic interactions through its ARM (Fig. 17.22).

Besides P-TEFb, Tat has numerous other interacting partners in host cells as seen in proteomic screens[252,332] and described in functional studies.[56,249,730,785,788] These studies identified the SEC as a Tat/P-TEFb cofactor. Additional cofactors regulate the Tat/TAR/P-TEFb interaction, enhance HIV transcription elongation, link Tat to the cellular epigenetic machinery, or modify the host response to HIV infection.[120,290,535]

Posttranslational Modifications

Tat function is regulated by a series of PTMs, mainly in its RNA-binding domain. These modifications fine-tune Tat's function in transcription. For example, this function is inhibited by methylation of Arg52 and Arg53 by the arginine methyltransferase PRMT6 and methylation of Lys50 and Lys51 by the lysine methyltransferase SETDB1 as both inhibit the interaction with TAR and P-TEFb.[70,713]

Activating Tat modifications include phosphorylation, polyubiquitination, acetylation, and monomethylation. For example, Tat is acetylated on its lysine 28 residue by PCAF to mediate P-TEFb recruitment to the Tat–TAR complex.[156,374] Lys28 acetylation can be reversed by HDAC6.[316] Tat is also acetylated on Lys50 by the cellular proteins hGCN5 and p300/CBP to release the Tat–P-TEFb complex from TAR.[356,507] In addition, Tat is monomethylated by the lysine methyltransferase Set7/9 on lysine 51 and 71—both are needed for full Tat transactivation ability[11,535]—and Lys71 is also polyubiquitinated.[76] Demethylation of Tat on Lys51 by the demethylase LSD1 is important for Tat-mediated viral reactivation.[617] LSD1 also represses HIV transcription in microglial cells through its normal function as a histone demethylase.[410]

Function in Mice

Tat transactivation of HIV-1 LTR-driven gene expression is quite low in rodent cells but can be greatly augmented in rodent somatic cell hybrids containing human chromosome 12.[283] This defect can also be corrected by overexpressing human cyclin T in rodent cells, which results in enhanced Tat transactivation of the HIV-1 LTR to levels measured in human cells.[730] The murine homolog of human cyclin T binds to HIV-1 Tat, but the resulting Tat/murine cyclin T heterodimer is not efficiently recruited to TAR.[240,249] Substitution of Tyr260 in murine cyclin T with the Cys residue at that position in the human homolog also restores Tat activity in rodent cells.[56,249] Thus, the extremely weak activity of Tat in rodent cells is not due to a failure to form the Tat/cyclin T heterodimer; rather, the cross-species heterodimer that does form is unable to bind to TAR and deliver P-TEFb to a poorly processive transcription complex.

Latency

In addition to initiating productive virus infections, HIV-1 establishes latent infections in memory CD4[+] T cells and possibly other reservoir cells (e.g., macrophages) that persist in patients receiving ART.[132,217,741] The long half-life of memory T cells and their expansion after periodic restimulation prevent natural elimination of infected cells during the lifetime of infected individuals. Although most current latency studies are performed in the blood, the majority of reservoir cells reside in tissues, especially the gut and lymph nodes. Latency is maintained through homeostatic proliferation, antigenic stimulation and clonal expansion. In individuals on ART, lymph node CD4[+] T cells composed of about 65% T follicular helper cells, as defined by the expression of the cell-surface receptors CXCR5 and PD-1, were identified as the major sources of replication-competent HIV-1.[155]

Unlike other viruses such as herpes viruses, HIV lacks a dedicated latency program and encodes no proteins to actively regulate the establishment and maintenance of latency. In many ways, HIV latency can be defined as a lack of Tat; the HIV promoter becomes inactive and dependent on regulation through cellular TFs and extracellular stimuli. As such, HIV latency is a labile state of HIV with periodic low-level reactivation and homeostatic expansion of latent clones.[477] Importantly, latently infected lymphocytes carry replication-competent proviruses versus lymphocytes that contain defective proviruses that are not considered latent. As no or very few viral proteins are produced in latently infected cells, these latently infected cells are invisible to the immune system and persist during ART.

The size of the viral reservoir varies between individuals and depends on the onset of treatment, the viral set point, clade, and genetic diversity.[24,473,529] Approximately 1 in 10[6] CD4[+] T cells is latently infected in most patients.[657] The half-life of latently infected T cells was estimated to be 44 months, but predictions about whether the reservoir decays or increases over time are at odds.[24,473,529,549] The mechanisms responsible for establishing and maintaining latently infected CD4[+] T cells have only been partially elucidated. A prevailing model posits that latently infected cells arise from reversion of activated effector T cells to a quiescent memory T lymphocyte phenotype,[33,67,468,587] but they may also be the product of direct infection of resting CD4[+] T cells[97] or may arise in activated infected T cells before conversion to cellular quiescence.[110,587]

It is important to distinguish latent cells from the large number of cells with defective proviruses. The latter may outnumber truly latent cells by greater than a factor of greater than 10^{83} and obscure accurate detection of the active reservoir. While culturing T cells from ART-suppressed individuals in an *in vitro* viral outgrowth assay [such as the quantitative viral outgrowth assay (QVOA)] underestimates the size of the reservoir, analysis of integrated viral DNA overestimates it.[83] Recent advances in intact proviral DNA measurements either by droplet digital PCR or next generation sequencing aid in more accurately assessing the number of cells containing nondefective proviruses.[83,84,401]

There has been debate as to whether the very low levels of viremia (<50 copies of viral RNA/mL of plasma) in patients on ART[536,741] result from ongoing virus replication, perhaps in tissues not efficiently accessed by the antiretrovirals, or the release of small numbers of virus particles from the latent reservoir. The weight of the evidence points to an absence of ongoing low-level replication in the face of suppressive ART. Adding the integrase inhibitor raltegravir or other potent antiretroviral drugs on top of a suppressive ART regimen does not further reduce viral loads.[189,482] New drug-resistance mutations are typically not detected during fully suppressive antiretroviral therapy, as would be expected if even low-level virus replication were occurring.[189,293] In general, the maintenance of genetically uniform viral populations over time and the lack of emergence of genetic diversity during latency in patients on ART supports the concept that HIV persists in long-lived cells without ongoing cycles of viral replication.[368]

Role of Tat

The decision between latency and active infection is critically determined by Tat and the strength of the positive Tat feedback loop. Once the feedback loop is initiated, viral transcription appears to be largely independent of the cellular state.[587] Inhibition of Tat with the small-molecule didehydro-cortistatin A (dCA) suppressed viral reactivation in latency cell line models and primary CD4+ T cells explanted from virally suppressed individuals. Additionally, suppression was sustained beyond removal of antiretroviral and dCA treatment.[421,485,503,504] dCA binds the basic domain of Tat, blocking the Tat–TAR interaction and inhibiting Tat–P-TEFb–mediated viral transactivation.[485] Long-term treatment with dCA is associated with a tighter chromatin environment and a loss of Pol II occupancy on the HIV-1 genome.[421] These results support the critical role of Tat in driving active infection and the absence of Tat leading to latency.

Role of Cellular Factors

The balance between negative and positive cellular factors in the host cell influences the latency state of HIV (see Fig. 17.20). Significant effort is being invested to characterize existing cellular factors and to discover new ones involved in HIV latency as drug targets to overcome HIV latency and eradicate HIV. The principle is to inhibit repressors, to force the virus into reactivation (shock and kill), or to inhibit activators to force the virus into a deeper latency (block and lock). Current targets include modulators of T-cell quiescence (PKC activators and activators of the atypical NFκB),[339] epigenetic modulators (HDAC inhibitors, methyltransferase inhibitors, BET protein inhibitors),[60,65,69,146,190,466] metabolic regulators (mTOR pathway),[49] and long noncoding (lnc)RNAs involved in repression.[586] Multiple screens to identify new host factors

used shRNA or CRISPR knockouts to identify new host factors that, when inhibited, cause either HIV reactivation in latency models or prevent reactivation to induce more robust silencing.[49,75,311,387,429,438,583] These have identified a series of new host factors currently under investigation.

Role of Viral Integration Site

HIV-1 preferentially integrates into active cellular genes,[419,632] and proviruses in resting CD4+ T cells from patients on ART are integrated into the introns of transcriptionally active cellular genes.[275,754] Importantly, while the epigenetic organization of HIV is independent of the integration site, activity and regulation of neighboring genes or nuclear structures could affect HIV transcription in many ways. These mechanisms include transcriptional interference where gene expression activity of neighboring genes interferes with HIV transcription. A small fraction of integration sites are located in cellular heterochromatin—dense silenced regions of chromatin—that may directly affect HIV promoter activity.[33] In ELITE controllers—people living with HIV who maintain HIV viral loads below the level of detection even in the absence of ART—the latent reservoir is strongly silenced through heterochromatic mechanisms.[338] In addition, individuals on ART harbor a viral reservoir in T cells with the same integration sites.[142,453,723] This highlights the importance of clonal expansion in the persistence of the HIV reservoir during latency. Recent studies point to the importance of 3D chromatin spatial organization where latent integration sites line up with the nuclear periphery and are potentially silenced by the nuclear pore complex.[36,183,445]

Latency Models

Several *in vitro* cell systems have been used to determine how postintegration latency is maintained. The earliest studies involved monocyte-derived ACH2 or the T-cell–derived U1 cell lines.[135,223] However, these original cell lines contained defective HIV proviruses. Subsequently, clonal cell lines, called JLat cells, were developed using infected Jurkat cells, a T-cell lymphoblast-derived cell line.[350] Several JLat cell lines have proviruses at different integration sites and with varying reactivation abilities.[672] The viruses that have been used to generate these lines include viral genomes that express green fluorescent protein, GFP, in place of the viral structural proteins, which allows easy assessment of reactivated cells. Recently developed dual fluorescence models allow identification of the latently infected cell population from uninfected cells.[33,94,96]

Analogous models use infection of primary human CD4+ T cells. These systems include infection of resting CD4+ T cells, memory CD4+ T cells, or activated CD4+ T cells in conjunction with the rapid inclusion of ART to prevent virus spread, followed by the study of the small fraction of latently infected cells.[672] Some studies use additional molecular manipulations, such as the overexpression of the antiapoptotic protein Bcl-2 that allows the cells to better survive while re-entering a resting T-cell state.[366,468,615,761] The production of sufficient quantities of viable, latently infected cells and the diversity of integration sites remains problematic with primary CD4+ T-cell systems. None of these systems has so far proved to authentically replicate all natural aspects of HIV latency, although they have been a rich source of information about potential mechanisms of latency formation that is contributing to studies of latency *in vivo* and attempts to reverse it.

HIV RNA Splicing and Nuclear Export
Splicing
Retroviruses use the cellular posttranscriptional processing machinery. Like other primary RNA transcripts synthesized in eukaryotic cells, HIV pre-mRNAs undergo a series of modifications (e.g., capping, 3'-end cleavage, polyadenylation, and splicing) before their export to the cytoplasm. With few exceptions, introns in the nascent cellular mRNAs must be removed before export from the nucleus, presumably to prevent their translation into nonfunctional proteins. This requirement poses an obvious problem for retroviruses such as HIV, which must export a variety of intron-containing mRNAs into the cytoplasm (e.g., the unspliced 9.2-kb primary transcript for encapsidation into progeny virions and as mRNA for the Gag and Gag/Pol proteins, as well as several other partially spliced mRNAs such as those encoding the Env, Vif, and Vpr proteins).

HIV Splicing
A characteristic of HIV is that splicing has to be partially suppressed to produce the full range of mRNAs needed to encode the viral proteins.[203] In part, retroviruses solved the requirement for the removal of all intronic sequences from pre-mRNAs before nuclear export by incorporating suboptimal 3' splice acceptors into their genomes. These acceptors are functionally impaired due to short or interrupted polypyrimidine tracts, noncanonical branch points, and *cis*-acting inhibitory sequences, which dampen individual splice site usage. For example, purines within the polypyrimidine tracts associated with some HIV-1 3' splice sites impair splicing by reducing the affinity for the essential cellular splicing factor U2AF.[258,674] Most HIV-1 strains use four different splice donor or 5' splice sites and eight different acceptor or 3' splice sites to produce more than 40 different HIV-1 transcripts in virus-producing cells.[203,576,640] The frequency with which particular 5' and 3' splice sites are used depends on the relative strength of each site and the presence of adjacent *cis*-acting RNA elements. Probing of the structures of HIV-1 RNAs in cells revealed the presence of alternative RNA conformations at splice sites.[701]

All retroviruses must splice their primary RNA transcripts to generate *env* mRNAs, eliminating upstream *gag* and *pol* sequences in the process. For simple retroviruses (e.g., avian leukosis virus and murine leukemia virus), this is the only splicing reaction that the viral pre-mRNA undergoes (Fig. 17.24). In contrast, the splicing of HIV RNA is far more complex because of constitutive and alternatively used splice-donor and splice-acceptor motifs scattered through its genomic RNA. Three general classes of HIV-1 mRNAs have been identified in productively infected cells: (a) unspliced genomic RNA serves as the mRNA for synthesis of Gag and Pol; (b) partially spliced RNAs of 4.3 to 5.5 kb are translated into Vif, Vpr, Vpu, and Env; and (c) multiply or completely spliced viral mRNAs of 1.7 to 2.0 kb encode Tat, Rev, and Nef (Fig. 17.24). The first two classes of viral mRNA retain spliceable introns and yet are efficiently exported from the nucleus into the cytoplasm. Low levels of *tat* or *rev* mRNAs have been implicated in inducing viral latency.[276,500]

Different viral mRNA species occur at different relative abundances.[576,677] Interestingly, the strength of intrinsic splice sites and their observed abundances in mRNA are not correlated.[20] *Cis*-acting splicing elements direct splice site selection

in HIV-1 mRNA. These elements include exonic and intronic splicing silencers and exonic splicing enhancers. These enhancer and silencing sequences modulate alternative splicing of the HIV-1 primary RNA transcript by binding to SR proteins and hnRNPs (reviewed in Refs.[203,677]). hnRNP H1 has been reported to play a particularly key role in splicing regulation.[393] Variable usage of HIV 5' and 3' splice sites gives rise to several sets of distinct, closely related RNAs that serve as alternative templates for translation into the same protein. For example, 12 *rev*, five *nef*, eight *tat*, and 16 *env* mRNAs have been identified. This diversity of HIV-1 mRNA is due, in part, to the variable inclusion of two upstream 50- and 74-nt noncoding exons (Fig. 17.24) in many of the spliced RNA species; these two small exons are the result of splice donors downstream of the *vif* and *vpr* splice acceptors to provide exon definition to the splicing machinery allowing these acceptors to be recognized. The functional significance of multiply spliced mRNAs encoding the same viral protein, their relative abundance, and the hierarchy of HIV-1 splice site usage are not understood. However, mutations of splice sites and suppressive elements can have dramatic effects on HIV replication,[210,448,449,462] suggesting that maximum virus replication is balanced between the various species of HIV mRNA and the genome RNA.

RNA Polyadenylation
Normal metazoan 3' processing and polyadenylation of pre-mRNAs require recognition of the upstream AAUAAA and downstream GU-rich motifs surrounding the cleavage and poly(A) addition site. HIV-1 contains a duplicate set of AAUAAA and GU-rich core elements near the end of the R sequences found in the 5' and 3' LTRs. Similar to how HIV-1 prevents transcription initiation from the 3' LTR, it uses multiple regulatory elements to direct processing and polyadenylation specifically to the 3' R cleavage site. Many of the factors required for 3' processing and polyadenylation are directed to upstream enhancer elements (USE) in the 3' end of the viral genome.[158,255,709] Additionally, the splicing factor U1 snRNP acts to inhibit polyadenylation in the 5' R sequence by binding to the adjacent 5' splice site D1.[21,22]

Rev
Typically, transcripts from cellular genes that are unspliced and incompletely spliced are degraded in the nucleus. Complex retroviruses, such as HIV, deal with the restriction to the nuclear export of unspliced and incompletely spliced transcripts by encoding the Rev (Regulator of expression of viral proteins) protein. In the absence of Rev, the unspliced *gag/pol* and the partially spliced *vif*, *vpr*, and *vpu/env* mRNAs fail to be exported to the cytoplasm, thereby rendering the Rev-mutant viruses replication incompetent.[215,274]

Structure
HIV-1 Rev is a 19-kDa, predominantly nucleolar phosphoprotein containing 116 amino acid residues (Fig. 17.25). Like Tat, Rev is an RNA-binding protein encoded by two exons; it contains two functional regions: (a) an Arg-rich domain mediates RNA binding and nuclear localization (NLS), flanked by sequences that facilitate Rev multimerization, and (b) a hydrophobic segment, located between residues 73 and 84, contains several Leu residues within a region called the activation

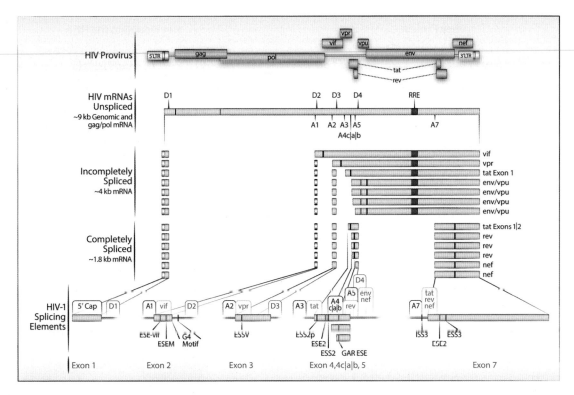

FIGURE 17.24 Locations of splice sites, exons, and splicing elements in the HIV-1 genome. *Top*: Schematic diagram of HIV-1 genome. The *dark blue* rectangles indicate open reading frames and are labeled with the gene names. The LTRs are shown at each edge of the genome. Full-length RNA transcripts begin at the 5′-end of the R region of the 5′-LTR (*left*) and 3′ processing and poly(A) addition takes place at the 3′-end of the R region in the 3′-LTR (*right*). *Middle*: Locations of 5′ss (*black bars*) and 3′ss (*red bars*) in the HIV-1 genome. The location of the RRE is shown by the *red rectangle*. The locations of the AUG codons used to initiate protein synthesis are shown as *purple bars* within the exons. *Bottom*: Locations of the known splicing regulatory elements in HIV-1. Splicing enhancers are designated by *green bars* and splicing silencers are designated by *red bars*. (Modified with permission of Eureka Science (FZC) from Stoltzfus CM, Madsen JM. Role of viral splicing elements and cellular RNA binding proteins in regulation of HIV-1 alternative RNA splicing. *Curr HIV Res* 2006;4(1):43–55; permission conveyed through Copyright Clearance Center, Inc.)

domain, which also promotes nuclear export (NES).[31,456] Mutation of any one of three critical leucines (residues 78, 81, or 83) within this domain eliminates Rev activity. Unlike *tat*, both *rev* exons are required for virus replication.[614]

RRE

Rev regulates the export of unspliced and partially spliced viral transcripts by binding to a *cis*-acting target, the Rev-responsive element (RRE) (Fig. 17.25). The RRE, located in a 250-nt segment spanning the junction between the gp120 and gp41 coding sequences of the *env* gene, is a complex RNA structure with a long stem terminating with multiple stem-loops branching from a large central bubble[215,456,604] (Fig. 17.25). This region of RNA has multiple possible conformations.[377,652] The RRE must be present within a Rev-responsive transcript and in the sense orientation to confer Rev responsiveness. Nuclease protection, chemical modification, and mutagenesis studies indicate that Rev specifically interacts with a 60+ nt portion of the RRE, designated stem-loop II (Fig. 17.25).[165,303,457]

Unlike the Tat–TAR interaction that requires multiple regions in Tat and TAR, this region of the RRE binds to Rev even when isolated from the complete RRE structure and mediates Rev responsiveness in functional assays.[314]

The determinants for high-affinity binding of Rev to RRE reside in the central purine-rich bubble of stem-loop II. This bubble contains unusual G:G and G:A base pairs that distort the duplex RNA structure and widen the major groove to accommodate the Rev protein.[31,304,457] An alpha-helical, Arg-rich, 17-residue peptide from the RNA-binding domain of Rev burrows deep into the major groove of a stem-loop II oligonucleotide to stabilize the non–Watson-Crick base pairs through specific interactions involving the Arg side chains.[32] The functionally complete RRE is approximately 350 nt in size, and an individual element may accommodate at least six Rev molecules, with multimerization being important for full Rev activity.[160,161,463]

Rev binds to the stem-loop IIB region of RRE as a monomer.[561] A crystal structure of truncated (N-terminal 70 aa) Rev bound to the RRE revealed that monomeric Rev folds into a helix-loop-helix structure, creating a hydrophobic core.[160,162] This core region becomes a dimerization interface for the cooperative binding of a second Rev monomer, which also interacts with a contiguous region of the RRE, thereby generating a "V"-shaped dimer structure. Similarly organized dimers cooperatively assemble into a tightly bound hexameric Rev-RRE RNP primed for nuclear export.

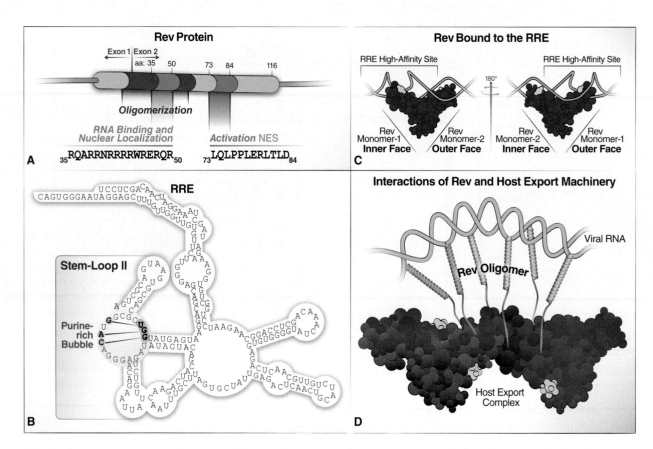

FIGURE 17.25 Rev and its response element, the RRE. A: A schematic representation of the human immunodeficiency virus 1 (HIV-1) Rev protein with its RNA-binding, activation, and oligomerization domains are shown at the top. The amino acid sequence of the leucine-rich nuclear export signal (NES) present in retroviral Rev/Rex proteins is also shown. The core tetramer motif, LxLy, where y is usually a charged residue and x is highly variable, is indicated. **B:** The structure of the RRE is presented at the bottom with the high-affinity target of HIV-1 Rev (stem-loop II) shown. The "bulged" G residues in stem-loop II able to form noncanonical purine–purine base pairs are *circled*. **C:** Rev binds to the RRE through its arginine-rich domain (ARD). In this model developed by Daugherty et al., the crystal structures of a Rev dimer are combined with the NMR structures of the Rev high affinity site. Notice the distortion of the RNA helix at the site of Rev binding. **D:** Model for the interactions between Rev and the nuclear export complex containing CRM-1 through the Rev nuclear export sequence (NES). The NES is an extended unstructured region emerging from one face of the Rev molecule. The core arginine-rich RNA binding domains interact with the RRE. (Adapted with permission from Daugherty MD, Booth DS, Jayaraman B, et al. HIV Rev response element (RRE) directs assembly of the Rev homooligomer into discrete asymmetric complexes. *Proc Natl Acad Sci U S A* 2010;107(28):12481–12486.)

Mutations affecting either the RNA-binding or the Leu-rich activation domains of Rev result in loss of function. For example, activation domain mutants bind to the RRE but are functionally inactive. They interfere with the transactivation mediated by WT Rev, exerting a *trans*-dominant effect in assays for Rev function.[455] Rev continuously shuttles between the nucleus and cytoplasm.[486] Mutations affecting the Rev activation domain abolish shuttling and restrict Rev to the nucleus. Multimerization-defective Rev mutants still bind to the high-affinity RRE site but are unable to form oligomeric complexes.[447]

The HIV-1 genome contains multiple sequence motifs, located in the *gag*, *pol*, and *env* genes, that contribute to a requirement for Rev. These *cis*-acting, AU-rich INS elements markedly impaired the expression of fused reporter genes by impeding RNA transport to the cytoplasm and/or decreasing RNA stability.[452,604] Cellular proteins likely bind to these inhibitory sequences, contributing to the nuclear retention and the intrinsic instability of intron-containing viral RNAs. Rev is able to reverse these effects, provided that an RRE is present in such transcripts.

Rev Cofactors

Rev engages key host factors to shuttle between the nucleus and cytoplasm.[486] Proteins bearing the basic-type NLS usually begin the nuclear import process by binding to a related transport protein, importin-α. Importin-α serves as a bridge, linking the NLS-containing substrate to importin-β. However, in contrast to most other proteins that carry a classic NLS, Rev appears to bind directly to importin-β. Furthermore, this heterodimeric complex is transported to the NPC, where the importin-β subunit successively binds to and dissociates from the resident nucleoporins, translocating the Rev substrate through the pore and into the nucleoplasm. The reverse process, nuclear export, uses transport receptors that are also members of the importin-β family. The best characterized of these is named Crm1 (for chromosome region maintenance 1), or exportin 1. The small GTPase molecule, Ran,[59] provides both the energy and directionality cues for nuclear import and export. Intracellularly, Ran cycles between two forms, RanGTP and RanGDP, which are concentrated primarily in the nucleus and cytoplasm, respectively.[328] Studies of HIV-1 Rev and related viral and cellular proteins bearing Leu-rich NES motifs (see below) led to the discovery and established the functions of many proteins involved in nuclear export.

Nuclear Export

The first unambiguous demonstration that Rev could promote the nuclear export of intron-containing viral RNA came from experiments in which purified Rev and RNA molecules containing the RRE were microinjected into cell nuclei.[218,732] These studies showed that the RRE-containing unspliced RNA substrates were transported from the nucleus into the cytoplasm only in the presence of Rev. Interestingly, the excised intron (containing the RRE), derived from those transcripts that did undergo splicing, was also detected in the cytoplasm, indicating that Rev-mediated nuclear export without inhibiting RNA splicing.[219]

The complete Rev nuclear transport cycle and its critical interacting partners are shown in Figure 17.26.[559] During the early, postintegration phase of the virus replication cycle, the HIV-1 mRNAs transported to the cytoplasm consist almost entirely of intronless, multiply spliced transcripts encoding Tat, Rev, and Nef. Rev uses its NLS to bind directly to importin-β in the cytoplasm and is translocated through the nuclear pore as a Rev/importin-β heterodimer. When the complex reaches the nucleus, the binding of RanGTP triggers the Rev/importin-β heterodimer to dissociate and release the Rev subunit. In the nucleoplasm, Rev initiates its role as a nuclear exporter by binding to RRE-containing HIV-1 pre-mRNAs and then multimerizes via cooperative protein–protein and protein–RNA interactions over the entire length of the RRE. When Rev oligomerizes on the RRE, its NES elements become aligned on the outside of an enlarging protein–RNA complex. Multimerized Rev/RRE then forms a functional complex with CRM1 in the presence of Ran in its GTP-bound form. The formation of this RNP is (a) sensitive to Rev NES mutations and (b) dissociated when RanGTP is hydrolyzed to its GDP-bound state.[23] The most likely scenario linking all available data is that the entry of RanGTP into a preexisting Rev/RRE/CRM1 RNP converts it into a functional export complex. Once the complex is formed, it is transported to the NPC, where the CRM1 subunit interacts with nucleoporins[224] and is then translocated into the cytoplasm. There, in the presence of Ran GAP1 and Ran BP1, the RanGTP component of the export complex is converted to the RanGDP form and the RNP disassembles.[263,523] Rev is released along with its unspliced and partially spliced HIV-1 RNA cargo, allowing the latter to be incorporated into progeny virions or translated into viral proteins. Rev, therefore, enables lentiviral intron-containing RNAs to elude in part or in total the cellular splicing machinery as well as the splicing quality control mechanisms and be transported to the cytoplasm via an export pathway not used by most cellular mRNAs.

Virus Assembly and Release: The Gag Proteins

The Gag proteins of HIV, like those of other retroviruses, are necessary and sufficient for the formation of noninfectious, virus-like particles (VLPs).[230,231] Orthoretroviral Gag proteins are synthesized as polyprotein precursors, Pr55^Gag in the case of HIV (Fig. 17.27).[27,229] As already noted, the mRNA for Pr55^Gag is the unspliced, full-length transcript that requires Rev for its transport to the cytoplasm. The HIV Pr55^Gag precursor

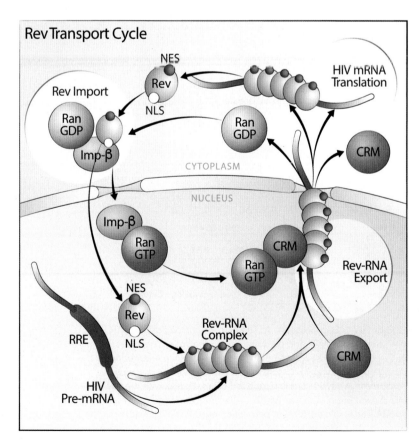

FIGURE 17.26 The Rev nuclear export cycle. Intronless, multiply spliced HIV-1 messenger RNAs (mRNAs) (tat, rev, and nef) use a Rev-independent pathway to exit the nucleus. Using its nuclear localization signal (NLS), newly synthesized Rev protein binds to importin β and the resulting heterodimer is translocated through the nuclear pore. In the nucleus, Rev/importin β dissociation is mediated by Ran(GTP) and the free Rev protein binds to Rev-responsive element (RRE)-containing viral pre-mRNA. The Rev–RRE RNA complex is converted to a functional export structure following the addition of CRM1 and Ran(GTP) and is transported through the nuclear pore. In the cytoplasm, RanBP1/RanGAP mediate the conversion of Ran(GTP) in the export complex to Ran(GDP), which then disassembles. After the release of Rev from intron-containing HIV-1 transcripts, the full-length viral RNA may be encapsidated into progeny virions or, as is the case for the partially spliced mRNA, may be translated into viral proteins. (Adapted with permission of Annual Reviews, Inc. from Pollard VW, Malim MH. The HIV-1 Rev protein. *Annu Rev Microbiol* 1998;52:491–532; permission conveyed through Copyright Clearance Center, Inc.)

is targeted to the plasma membrane rapidly after its synthesis where particles are assembled. The formation of noninfectious VLPs at the plasma membrane does not require the participation of viral genomic RNA, *pol*-encoded enzymes, or Env glycoproteins. However, the production of infectious virions requires the encapsidation of the viral RNA genome and the incorporation of the Env glycoproteins and the Gag–Pol polyprotein precursor Pr160[GagPol] into the virion. Retroviral Gag proteins perform several major functions during virus assembly, including (a) forming the structural framework of the virion, (b) encapsidating the viral genome, (c) targeting the nascent particle for export from the cell, and (d) acquiring a lipid bilayer, and associated Env glycoproteins during particle release (for reviews, see Ref.[231,689]). These processes require that Gag proteins participate in protein–protein, protein–RNA, and protein–lipid interactions. As described above, Gag proteins also play critical roles in the early, postentry stages of the virus replication cycle.

In the immature VLP, several thousand Gag monomers are aligned and packed radially, with the MA domain in association with the inner leaflet of the lipid bilayer and the NC domain,

bound to viral genomic RNA, facing the center of the virion (Fig. 17.28). Gag–Gag contacts are primarily mediated through the C-terminal domain of CA (CA-CTD) and SP1. Cryo-ET analyses have demonstrated that in immature VLPs Gag forms a hexameric lattice[77,167,744] (see below). The ability of the Gag lattice to curve into a sphere is afforded by gaps in the lattice. The CA N-terminal domain (CA-NTD) is arranged in a ring around a central pore in each hexamer; the CA-CTD is positioned just below the CA-NTD and links the hexamers together to form the lattice.[77] The region of the immature Gag lattice at the junction between the CA-CTD and adjoining SP1 folds into a six-helix bundle that plays key roles in virus assembly and subsequent maturation[639,722] (Fig. 17.29). This bundle is stabilized by the highly anionic cellular metabolite inositol hexakisphosphate (IP$_6$), which binds two electropositive rings formed by two Lys residues at the top of the six-helix bundle (Fig. 17.29).[181,458] Mutation of either of these Lys residues, or depleting cells of IP$_6$, interferes with virus particle assembly.[458,459]

When the *pol* ORF is expressed, the viral PR cleaves Pr55[Gag] during and/or shortly after virus particle release from the cell to

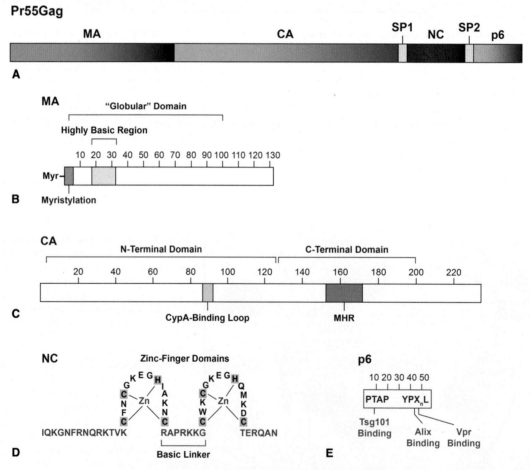

FIGURE 17.27 Linear organization of the major HIV-1 Gag proteins. A: The Gag precursor, Pr55[Gag], with the positions of the matrix (MA), capsid (CA), nucleocapsid (NC), and p6 domains and the spacer peptides, SP1 and SP2, indicated. **B:** MA, indicating the N-terminal myristic acid moiety and the sequence required for myristylation. The location of the highly basic region is also shown. **C:** CA, with N- and C-terminal domains, the major homology region (MHR), and the cyclophilin A (CypA)-binding loop indicated. **D:** NC, with the two zinc fingers and the zinc-coordinating residues shown. **E:** p6, with the Tsg101-, Alix-, and Vpr-binding regions/motifs indicated. Numbers indicate amino acid positions. (Adapted with permission of Annual Reviews, Inc. from Pollard VW, Malim MH. The HIV-1 Rev protein. *Annu Rev Microbiol* 1998;52:491–532; permission conveyed through Copyright Clearance Center, Inc.)

generate the mature Gag proteins MA, CA, NC, and p6, and spacer peptides SP1 and SP2 (Fig. 17.27A). Processing of the Gag and Gag–Pol precursor proteins by PR results in a major structural and morphological rearrangement, referred to as maturation, during which the cone-shaped core forms in the center of the virus particle (see section on Protease and Virus Maturation). In the mature virion, MA is localized immediately inside the lipid bilayer of the viral envelope, CA forms the cone-shaped outer shell of the core (the capsid) in the center of the particle, and NC is present in the core in a ribonucleoprotein complex with the viral genomic RNA and the viral enzymes IN and RT (see Fig. 17.28).

Matrix (MA): Membrane Binding, Gag Targeting, and Env Incorporation

The MA domain of Pr55[Gag] (Fig. 17.27b) performs several functions during the viral replication cycle. After Gag synthesis, it directs Pr55[Gag] to the plasma membrane via a multipartite membrane-binding signal. The affinity of the MA domain for membrane is provided in part by a myristic acid moiety covalently attached to the N-terminal Gly of MA after removal of the initiator Met by N-myristyl transferase. Mutation of the Gly myristate acceptor blocks binding of Gag to membrane and abolishes virus assembly in most systems. Sequences in MA downstream of the myristate also contribute to membrane binding; NMR and x-ray crystallographic analyses of HIV-1 MA (as well as the MA protein of a number of other retroviruses) demonstrate that a highly basic patch of amino acids (the highly basic region or HBR) clusters on the membrane-facing surface of MA (Fig. 17.27B).[297,474] The HBR interacts with negatively charged acidic phospholipids, in particular phosphatidylinositol (4,5) bisphosphate [PI(4,5)P$_2$], on the inner leaflet of the lipid bilayer, thereby stabilizing membrane interactions. As discussed in more detail below, mutations affecting the HBR can disrupt the targeting of Gag to the plasma membrane.[234,771,786]

MA adopts a primarily globular fold, containing five α-helices and a 3$_{10}$ helix.[297,474] MA crystallizes as a trimer[297] and assembles on PI(4,5)P$_2$-containing artificial membrane monolayers as a hexameric lattice of trimers.[10] Biochemical cross-linking studies have shown that in virions the MA domain of Gag, and the mature MA protein, also form trimers and that trimer formation is important for Env incorporation[695] (see below). Cryo-ET data confirm a trimeric arrangement of MA organized into a hexameric lattice in HIV-1 virions[579] (Fig. 17.30). Interestingly, the arrangement of MA within the lattice differs substantially between immature and mature particles, suggesting that MA undergoes a conformational rearrangement during particle maturation.[579] This rearrangement affects both the diameter of the central gap in the MA lattice and the charge of residues facing this gap (Fig. 17.30).[296] In addition, the results suggest that a lipid acyl chain, potentially that of PI(4,5)P$_2$, is extruded from the lipid bilayer during maturation and packs into a groove in MA.[579]

Although the cellular determinants that regulate the site of HIV-1 assembly remain to be fully defined, it is clear that PI(4,5)P$_2$ plays an important role in directing Gag to the plasma membrane[530] and anchoring it to the membrane.[506] An early study showed that depleting PI(4,5)P$_2$ from the plasma membrane leads to the retargeting of HIV-1 assembly to internal compartments and severely disrupts virus particle production.[530] Structural data indicate that PI(4,5)P$_2$ binds directly to MA via the HBR,[612,654] inducing the exposure of the N-terminal myristate[612] and allowing it to insert into the membrane. Although the NC domain of Gag is the primary determinant for Gag–RNA interaction, the MA HBR also binds RNA, particularly tRNA,[394] and this RNA binding inhibits MA association with PI(4,5)P$_2$-deficient, but not PI(4,5)P$_2$-containing, membranes. This mode of RNA regulation likely contributes to the selectivity of Gag for PI(4,5)P$_2$-enriched (i.e., plasma)

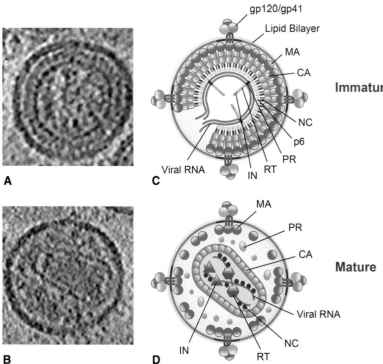

Immature

Mature

FIGURE 17.28 **Structural organization of immature and mature HIV-1 virions**. Cryoelectron micrographs of immature (**A**) and mature (**B**) virions. (Adapted from Keller PW, Adamson CS, Heymann JB, et al. HIV-1 maturation inhibitor bevirimat stabilizes the immature Gag lattice. *J Virol* 2011;85(4):1420–1428. Copyright © 2011 American Society for Microbiology.) Schematic representation of immature (**C**) and mature (**D**) HIV-1 particles, with labels indicating the gp120/gp41 subunits of the Env glycoprotein trimer, the lipid bilayer, and the viral RNA. **C:** The major domains in Gag [matrix (MA), capsid (CA), nucleocapsid (NC), and p6] and GagPol [protease (PR), reverse transcriptase (RT), and integrase (IN)] are labeled. In (**D**), locations of mature Gag and Pol products are indicated. (Modified with permission from Balasubramaniam M, Freed EO. New insights into HIV assembly and trafficking. *Physiology (Bethesda)* 2011;26(4):236–251. Copyright © 2011 The American Physiological Society.)

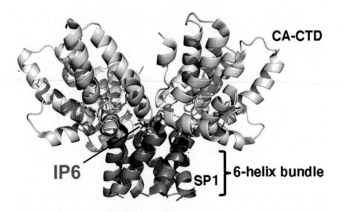

FIGURE 17.29 CA-SP1 six-helix bundle in the immature Gag lattice. The region of the immature Gag lattice spanning the junction between the CA-CTD and SP1 forms a six-helix bundle that helps stabilize the immature CA hexamer. The six-helix bundle, in turn, is stabilized by a molecule of IP$_6$, which is coordinated by two electropositive rings at the top of the bundle. Image constructed in PyMol from PDB accession 6BHR. (Image constructed in PyMol from PDB accession 6BHR723. Adapted from Wagner JM, Zadrozny KK, Chrustowicz J, et al. Crystal structure of an HIV assembly and maturation switch. *Elife* 2016;5:e17063. https://creativecommons.org/licenses/by/4.0/.)

membrane over more abundant, internal membranes that contain little PI(4,5)P$_2$.[10,131] Cross-linking immunoprecipitation (CLIP) sequencing data show minimal binding of MA to viral RNA, suggesting that MA does not play a major role in RNA packaging, and MA does not show preferential binding to the tRNA (tRNA[Lys3]) that serves as the primer for reverse transcription.[394] Structural analysis reveals a specific interaction between basic residues in MA and the elbow region of tRNA.[68]

Biochemical, microscopic, and pharmacological data indicate that HIV-1 assembly takes place in lipid rafts, the cholesterol- and glycosphingolipid-enriched microdomains discussed earlier in the context of virus entry. These specialized lipid microdomains may stabilize Gag–membrane binding and

facilitate assembly by serving as platforms for Gag–Gag interactions. Consistent with assembly taking place in lipid rafts, the lipid composition of HIV-1 particles is enriched in raft-like lipids such as cholesterol and sphingomyelin.[13,82]

The MA domain not only functions in regulating Gag trafficking but also plays an important role in the incorporation of the viral Env glycoproteins into virions (see below).

Capsid (CA): Gag Multimerization and Capsid Formation

The CA domain of Gag serves a central role in promoting virus assembly, and the mature CA protein forms the outer shell of the viral core (the capsid) after PR-mediated Gag processing. As already noted, CA contains two structural and functional domains, the CA-NTD and CA-CTD (Fig. 17.27C), which are connected by a short, flexible linker. This two-domain organization is a highly conserved feature among retroviral CA proteins. NMR and x-ray crystallographic data are available for both domains of HIV-1 CA[243,256,491] (Fig. 17.31A) and for CA in the assembled mature lattice.[267] In addition, structures of the CA domain of Gag in the immature lattice[638] and the mature CA protein in virion-derived viral capsids[476] have been solved by cryo-ET. The CA-NTD and CA-CTD both adopt highly helical conformations. The CA-NTD contains an exposed, CypA-binding loop and an N-terminal β-hairpin; the N-terminus of the CA-CTD contains the major homology region (MHR), which, apart from the zinc-finger motifs in NC, is the only sequence in Gag that displays significant amino acid sequence identity between divergent retroviral genera. Although CA assembles into a hexameric lattice in both the immature and mature particle, the arrangement of CA monomers is quite different in the immature and mature lattice, most strikingly in the CA-NTD.

Purified HIV-1 CA is capable of assembling into tubular or spherical particles *in vitro*. In the tubes assembled *in vitro*, CA is arranged in helical arrays in which the CA-NTD forms hexameric rings that are linked into a continuous lattice by the CA-CTD[425] (Fig. 17.31B and C). Similar CA hexamers are visualized in capsids obtained from purified HIV-1 virions,[78,767] indicating

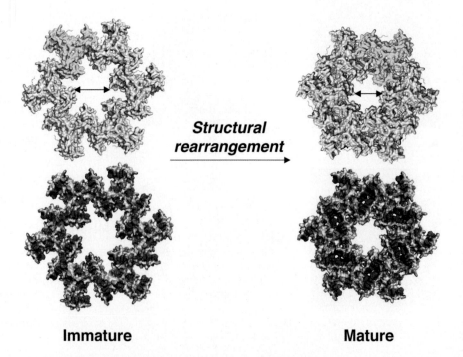

FIGURE 17.30 The MA lattice in HIV-1 virions reorganizes during virus maturation. *Left*, structure of the MA lattice in immature particles; right, its structure in the mature lattice. At the *top*, the hexamer-of-trimer arrangement of MA is shown, with one MA trimer highlighted in *yellow*. The difference in the diameter of the central gap in the MA lattice in immature and mature particles is illustrated by the *double-headed arrow*. At the *bottom* is shown the electrostatic surface potentials, with positive and negative surface potentials highlighted in *blue* and *red*, respectively. (Adapted from Hikichi Y, Freed EO. Maturation of HIV-1. *Science* 2021;373(6555):621–622. Reprinted with permission from AAAS. Structures made in PyMol with PDB accession numbers 7OVQ (immature) and 7OVR (mature).)

Immature   **Structural rearrangement** →   **Mature**

that the CA arrays assembled *in vitro* reflect the physiologically relevant higher-order CA organization. Indeed, these *in vitro* CA assemblies have provided a useful model for structural studies on the mature capsid lattice and have also been used extensively to identify and study host cell proteins that bind the capsid. As discussed above, in the immature particle, a large gap in the hexameric Gag lattice allows the lattice to curve and form a spherical structure. In contrast, the mature capsid is a closed structure; closure requires the introduction of 12 pentamers into the otherwise hexagonal lattice, with five pentamers at the narrow end and seven at the wide end (Fig. 17.31B).[567 and 568] This arrangement is reminiscent of the fullerene structures formed by elemental carbon.[244] Although the cores of other retroviruses can be cylindrical or spherical, they are also formed from similar hexagonal CA lattices; their different shapes arise through differences in the placement of the pentamers.[244] The hexameric lattice forms, and is stabilized by, several intermolecular CA–CA interfaces. At the center of both the capsid hexamer and pentamer is a positively charged pore, which includes Arg-18 and Lys-25 in the CA-NTD. This central pore is bound by two molecules of IP_6[181,460,593] (Fig. 17.31C) (note that, as mentioned above, IP_6 also binds and stabilizes the assembly of the immature Gag lattice by binding a distinct site located at the top of the six-helix bundle formed at the CA-SP1 junction of the immature lattice). Binding of IP_6 molecules to the Arg-18 pore stabilizes the mature capsid and may also play a role in regulating the import of dNTPs into the capsid after infection of the target cell.[130,460,593,755]

The peptidyl-prolyl *cis-trans* isomerase CypA is specifically incorporated into HIV-1 virions[444] as the result of an interaction between CypA and a Pro-rich loop in the CA-NTD that includes CA amino acid 90 (Figs. 17.27C and 17.31).[228,243,698] The relationship between CA–CypA binding and HIV-1 infectivity is complex; although CypA interacts with the CA domain of Pr55[Gag] during assembly, most biologically significant interactions between CA and CypA occur postentry. At least under some circumstances, CypA binding to CA in the target cell helps to counteract restriction mediated by TRIM5α and/or possibly other restriction factors and plays a role in modulating the interaction between the capsid and the nuclear import machinery.[34,285,665]

The critical roles that CA plays both early and late in the HIV-1 replication cycle make it a promising target for the development of antiretroviral agents. The ability of the small-molecule inhibitor PF74 to interfere with multiple steps in the HIV-1 replication has been studied extensively (for review, see Ref.[379]). PF74 binds a pocket at the interface between the CA-NTD of one CA subunit and the CA-CTD of the adjacent CA subunit in the mature capsid hexamer. The pocket at the CA-NTD/CA-CTD interface to which PF74 binds is also the docking site for two additional, structurally related CA inhibitors—GS-CA1 and GS-6207 (lenacapavir).[52,435,765] These latter compounds are highly potent (picomolar antiviral EC_{50}s in cell culture) and GS-6207/lenicapavir is currently undergoing clinical development as a long-acting antiretroviral.[435] Disruption of the CA-NTD/CA-CTD interface by these compounds inhibits virus assembly, perhaps by destabilizing Gag,[435] and interferes

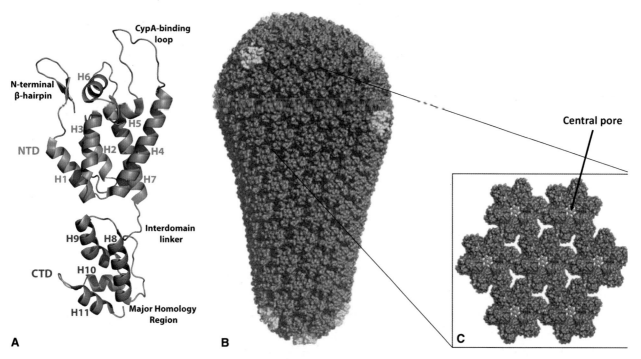

FIGURE 17.31 Structure of the capsid (CA) protein, the CA lattice, and the conical capsid. A: Structure of the CA monomer. N-terminal domain (NTD), C-terminal domain (CTD), linker region, and cyclophilin A-binding loop are indicated. Helices 1-11 (H1-H11) are labeled. Constructed in PyMol from PDB accession 2M8N.[177] **B:** Model of the HIV-1 capsid. CA-NTDs are highlighted in *orange*, CA-CTDs in *blue*. Pentamers, which close off the conical capsid at both wide and narrow ends, are highlighted in *greenish yellow*. (Adapted by permission from Nature: Pornillos O, Ganser-Pornillos BK, Yeager M. Atomic-level modelling of the HIV capsid. *Nature* 2011;469(7330):424–427. Copyright © 2011 Springer Nature.) **C:** Top view of a CA hexameric lattice. Note that hexamer-hexamer contacts are mediated by the CTDs. The central pore of the CA hexamer, which binds two molecules of IP_6, is indicated. (Adapted from Pornillos O, Ganser-Pornillos BK, Kelly BN, et al. X-ray structures of the hexameric building block of the HIV capsid. *Cell* 2009;137(7):1282–1292. Copyright © 2009 Elsevier. With permission.)

with the formation of the mature capsid lattice when used to treat virus-producer cells.[435] Treatment of target cells during HIV-1 infection causes a block in reverse transcription at high compound concentrations[765] and may stabilize viral capsids in the cytoplasm.[52] Although PF74, GS-CA1, and GS-6207/ lenacapavir display multiple inhibitory activities both early and late in the virus replication cycle, because the CA-NTD/CA-CTD interface is the docking site for host proteins involved in the stability and nuclear import of the capsid and subsequent viral DNA integration—for example, Sec24C in the cytoplasm, Nup153 at the nuclear pore, and CPSF6 at the nuclear pore and in the nucleus—these compounds appear to exert their strongest antiviral activity by blocking nuclear import of the capsid and DNA integration.[52,379] Mutations that confer resistance to these CA-NTD/CA-CTD interface-binding compounds cluster around the binding site.[379,765] Study of the complex, multimodal mechanism of action of these molecules will no doubt provide additional insights into the role of the CA-NTD/CA-CTD interface in HIV-1 replication and the value of this interface as an antiviral target.

Nucleocapsid (NC): RNA Encapsidation, Gag Multimerization, and Nucleic Acid Chaperone Activity

The third major domain synthesized as part of the Gag precursor is NC (see Fig. 17.27D). Like other Gag domains, NC—both as a domain of Gag and as a mature protein—serves multiple roles during the virus replication cycle. All orthoretroviral NC proteins contain one or two zinc-finger motifs; HIV-1 NC contains two zinc-finger motifs that bind zinc tightly both *in vitro* and in virions[50,671] and two clusters of basic residues flanking the first zinc finger. NMR data indicate that the two HIV-1 NC zinc fingers are brought together into a central globular domain by the highly basic and flexible linker domain (Fig. 17.32).[14,166,497,688,706] Mutations that abrogate zinc binding by retroviral NC abolish genome encapsidation and virus infectivity.[262]

A primary function of retroviral NC is to direct the packaging of the full-length, unspliced viral RNA into assembling virus particles. RNA packaging is driven by interactions between the NC domain of Gag and a packaging signal, historically referred to as ψ, in the full-length, unspliced viral RNA. Although one dimer of viral genomic RNA is usually packaged per virion,[116] monomeric RNA can be packaged if it contains two tandem packaging signals, presumably because it can fold into a structure that mimics that of a dimer.[618] These data suggest that the NC domain of Gag recognizes an RNA dimer. RNA dimerization is initiated by a short, palindromic sequence referred to as the dimerization initiation signal (DIS) (see Fig. 17.5).

The specificity of HIV-1 genome encapsidation results from an interaction between the NC domain of Gag and sequences within the approximately 400-nucleotide 5′ leader region of the viral RNA, which encompasses the 5′ untranslated region and a small portion of the 5′ end of the *gag* gene. Many different structures of various segments of the 5′ leader region have been proposed over the years, based on biochemical and structural data coupled with RNA folding algorithms (for review see Ref.[72]). The structure of the entire viral genomic RNA, purified from virus particles, has also been probed using SHAPE technology,[729] and it is possible that many regions

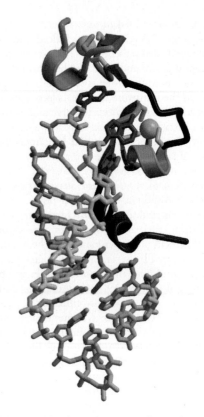

FIGURE 17.32 Complex between NC and stem-loop 3 (SL3) of the HIV-1 packaging signal. The two zinc ions coordinated by the zinc-finger domains are shown as *gray balls*. Color scheme: N-terminal 3₁₀ helix, *pink*; N-terminal zinc finger, *cyan*; linker, *red*; C-terminal zinc finger, *green*; cysteine and histidine side-chains, *yellow* and *cyan*, respectively. (Reprinted from Turner BG, Summers MF. Structural biology of HIV. *J Mol Biol* 1999;285(1):1–32. Copyright © 1999 Elsevier. With permission.)

of the RNA exist in multiple conformations.[701] While these approaches have generated a range of structural predictions, it is clear that the 5′ leader region folds into a series of stem-loops, which include TAR, the poly(A) stem-loop, PBS stem-loop, and four small stem-loops, SL1-SL4[72] (Fig. 17.5). SL1 contains the DIS, SL2 the major splice donor (SD), and SL4 the AUG translation initiation codon for *gag*. SL3 is often referred to as the ψ stem-loop, as it contains a high-affinity binding site for NC.[187] Early work suggested that alternative folding of these stem loops could regulate how a full-length viral RNA is utilized; that is, whether it is translated or packaged into virus particles.[318] This regulation was proposed to be in part determined by the availability of the DIS for intermolecular base pairing to form a dimeric RNA, and the accessibility of the *gag* AUG start codon for translation.

Advances in the use of NMR methods to solve RNA structures have resulted in novel insights into the folding of the 5′ leader region. Key studies focused on a 155-nucleotide portion of the 5′ leader region—referred to as the core encapsidation signal or ψᶜᴱˢ—containing deletions in TAR, poly(A), and PBS stem loops[292,367]; for review, see Ref.[72] An important observation from these studies was that the RNA forms a three-way junction structure in which bases in the SD stem-loop (SL2) engage in long-range base pairing. In this structure, the AUG start codon is sequestered, and NC binding sites are exposed, favoring packaging over translation. Because of heterogeneous start site usage during transcription, HIV-1 RNAs begin with 1, 2, or 3 guanosines (Gs). Interestingly, the 1G form of the RNA is favored for dimerization and is enriched in virions.[373,475] Structural analysis by NMR provides a model to explain the effect of the number of Gs at the 5′ end of the viral RNA on accessibility of the 5′ cap and the splice site recognition sequence[80] (Fig. 17.33). Our understanding of HIV-1 RNA structure and its role in packaging is still evolving; it is likely that a combination of NMR methods and other techniques, including biochemical approaches, small-angle X-ray scattering (SAXS), cryoEM, and atomic force microscopy (AFM), will provide additional insights into the structure and dynamics of the multifunctional 5′ leader region of full-length HIV-1 RNA.

A central challenge in elucidating the molecular mechanism of retroviral RNA packaging is that Gag must select the viral genomic RNA from a vast excess of cellular RNAs. CLIP sequencing data show that Gag exhibits only a several-fold preference for binding to viral over cellular RNAs in the cytosol,[394] and in the absence of viral genomic RNA retroviruses will package cellular RNAs to produce particles that are structurally similar to WT.[513,591] Under such conditions, 5′-capped, polyadenylated cellular mRNAs are packaged roughly in proportion to their level of expression in the cell.[611] However, the observation that nearly all HIV-1 virions contain two copies of genomic RNA[116] indicates that specific packaging of dimeric

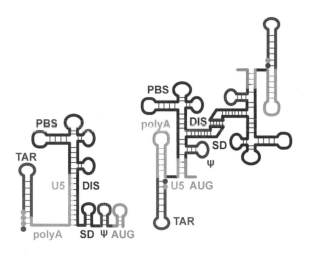

Cap3G (and Cap2G)
- monomeric
- retained in cells
- accessible cap
- functions as mRNA

Cap1G
- dimeric
- packaged in virions
- sequestered cap
- functions as gRNA

FIGURE 17.33 Model for two alternative structures of the capped HIV-1 leader RNA. RNAs with two or three 5′-guanosines fold into a monomeric structure with exposed cap. RNAs with one 5′ guanosine sequester the cap and form a dimer suitable for packaging. 5′ cap is indicated by the *red dot*; guanosines by *green dots*. (Adapted with permission of American Association for the Advancement of Science from Brown JD, Kharytonchyk S, Chaudry I, et al. Structural basis for transcriptional start site control of HIV-1 RNA fate. *Science* 2020;368(6489):413–417; permission conveyed through Copyright Clearance Center, Inc.)

viral genomic RNA is ultimately highly selective. NC engages in both sequence-specific and sequence-nonspecific interactions with nucleic acid, and NC is thought to coat the entire genomic RNA in the virion. In general, the sequence-specific interactions involve the zinc fingers in conjunction with the basic residues in NC, whereas nonspecific interactions are driven largely by the positive charge conferred by the basic residues. CLIP data showed that the nature of the contacts between viral RNA and NC (or the NC domain of Gag) shifts during virus assembly and maturation[394]; in cells, NC showed highly preferential binding to several regions within the genome, including the 5′ leader region and the RRE, whereas in immature virions, the NC domain of Gag bound to a large number of sites across the genome. In mature virions, NC–RNA contacts primarily involved the specific regions (e.g., the 5′ leader region and the RRE) that were preferred binding sites in the cell. A shift in nucleotide preference was also noted; in cells, NC bound preferentially to G-rich sequences whereas in virions it displayed an A-rich preference.[394] These data underscore the highly dynamic and context-dependent nature of NC–RNA binding.

Live-cell imaging experiments have demonstrated that HIV-1 genomic RNA localization at the plasma membrane is stabilized by initial interactions with a small number of Gag molecules.[352] In the absence of Gag expression, RNA associates with the plasma membrane only transiently and as a monomer. In the presence of Gag, stable dimers are visualized at the plasma membrane.[117] Although HIV-1 Gag can use cellular RNAs to assemble virus particles, both *in vitro* and cell-based studies have demonstrated that at low Gag concentrations, HIV-1 assembly is more efficient in the presence of packageable viral RNA than in its absence.[145,184] The ability of viral genomic RNA to promote assembly more efficiently than nonviral, cellular RNAs thus helps to explain the specificity and selectivity of viral RNA packaging.

In addition to its roles in RNA encapsidation and Gag assembly, NC plays other critical functions in HIV-1 replication. These are required for efficient reverse transcription and are attributed to the nucleic acid chaperone activity of NC.[418] This property enables NC to catalyze the refolding of nucleic acid molecules into structures with the most thermodynamically favorable conformation (i.e., the greatest number of base pairs). The nucleic acid chaperone activity of NC evidently requires that NC molecules coat nucleic acid at near-saturating levels of approximately one molecule of protein per five to eight nucleotides. NC, or the NC domain of Gag, contributes to placement of the tRNA^{Lys3} primer on the PBS, unwinding of the tRNA during the initiation of reverse transcription,[279] increased efficiency of minus-strand transfer by increasing the annealing of complementary R regions, removal of annealed RNA fragments during minus-strand strong stop DNA synthesis, destabilization of nucleic acid secondary structure during both minus- and plus-strand DNA synthesis, and stimulation of plus-strand transfer by promoting the removal of the tRNA primer and annealing of the PBS sequence in plus-strand strong-stop DNA to its minus-strand DNA complement.

The nucleic acid chaperone activity of NC has been demonstrated not only in *in vitro* assays but also by studying the effects of NC mutation on reverse transcription and virus infectivity in cells.[418] Mutations in HIV-1 NC impair infectivity by destabilizing newly reverse-transcribed viral DNA.[48] Studies performed with MLV demonstrated that changing the single CCHC zinc-finger motif to CCCC or CCHH had no effect on zinc binding, tRNA incorporation, RNA encapsidation, or RNA maturation but profoundly impaired virus infectivity.[260] Examination of viral DNA in mutant-infected cells revealed that full-length, circular DNA products were formed inefficiently and that a variety of mutations were present at the DNA ends.[260] Such aberrations, if present at the termini of linear DNAs, would render these DNAs unsuitable for integration. Analogous mutations in the zinc fingers of the HIV-1 NC have been reported[85,261,693]; these changes resulted in defects in reverse transcription, leading to a lack of circular DNA production, degradation of the viral DNA ends, and impaired virus infectivity.

Because NC participates in multiple steps in the virus replication cycle, it has been the target of drug development efforts. Although clinically effective NC inhibitors have not yet been identified, in part due to the lack of specificity of the inhibitors, this is a promising area for future research.

p6: Virus Release and Vpr/Vpx Incorporation

In addition to the MA, CA, and NC domains, HIV-1 encodes a Pro-rich, 6-kDa domain, known as p6, located at the C-terminus of Pr55[Gag] (see Fig. 17.27E). Deletion of p6 significantly disrupts HIV-1 particle production by blocking a late step in the budding process.[264] Particles assembled from p6 mutants display a release defect characterized by a striking accumulation of tethered virions at the plasma membrane (Fig. 17.34). The virus release function of p6 maps to a highly conserved Pro-Thr-Ala-Pro (PTAP) motif near the N-terminus of p6,[174,312] and to a lesser extent a Tyr-Pro-X_n-Leu (YPX$_n$L, where X is any amino acid and n = 1 to 3 residues) motif around amino acid residue 40 of p6.[679,720]

ESCRT Machinery and Virus Release

Mutational analyses of the Gag proteins of a number of retroviruses revealed the presence of motifs that, like PTAP of p6, promote the release of virions from the plasma membrane. These short sequences were termed "late" domains to reflect their role late in the budding process (for reviews, see Refs.[231,721]). Three general classes of retroviral late domains have been identified: PTAP (or PSAP), Pro-Pro-Pro-Tyr (PPPY), and YPX$_n$L. Analogous motifs function to promote the release of other families of enveloped viruses (e.g., the *Filoviridae*, *Paramyxoviridae*, *Rhabdoviridae*, and others), indicating a broadly conserved mechanism for enveloped virus release.

Retroviral late domains function by interacting directly with components of the cellular endosomal sorting complex required for transport (ESCRT) machinery,[436,478] which ultimately severs the membranous neck of the budding particle resulting in virus release. ESCRT machinery, which is functionally conserved from yeast to mammals, plays a key role in a number of cellular membrane scission events, for example, during the budding of cargo-laden vesicles into multivesicular bodies (MVBs) to generate intralumenal vesicles, and the abscission step of cytokinesis[100,498] (Fig. 17.35). These membrane scission events are topologically equivalent, that is, they are oriented away from the cytosol and are the topological inverse of endocytosis. Thus, retroviruses, and many other enveloped viruses, have evolved the ability to usurp cellular budding machinery to promote their release from the plasma membrane. The ESCRT machinery comprises a set of complexes that include ESCRT-0, I, II, III, Alix and the AAA ATPase Vps4, and associated factors (Fig. 17.35). ESCRT-0 first associates with endosomal membrane and cargo protein via phosphatidyl inositol-3-phosphate and ubiquitin binding, respectively, and subsequently recruits ESCRT-I to the membrane. *In vitro* reconstitution studies suggest that ESCRT-I and II provide the driving force for membrane budding, whereas ESCRT-III and Vps4 play the central role in the membrane scission event.[317,740] It has been reported that ESCRT-I forms helical assemblies that may help template ESCRT-III,[222] which in turn polymerizes to form spiral filaments that constrict membrane.[103] Vps4 assembles into a circular, hexameric structure that binds ESCRT-III subunits and, in a process driven by ATP hydrolysis, translocates the ESCRT-III subunits through a central pore, resulting in disassembly of the ESCRT-III lattice and membrane scission[492]; for review, see Ref.[478] HIV-1 release utilizes only a subset of the ESCRT machinery required for driving cellular processes; ESCRT-II appears to play only a relatively minor role, if any, in virus budding, and some ESCRT-III components are dispensable[404,499] (Fig. 17.35).

A link between the endosomal sorting pathway and HIV-1 budding was first suggested by the observation that the ESCRT-

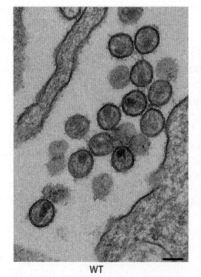
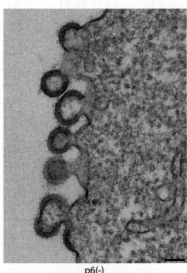

FIGURE 17.34 Morphology of WT versus p6-deleted HIV-1 visualized by thin-section transmission EM. Note the presence of released, mature particles in the WT micrograph (**left panel**) and tethered, immature particles in the p6-mutant micrograph (**right panel**). (Courtesy of Kunio Nagashima.)

WT   p6(-)

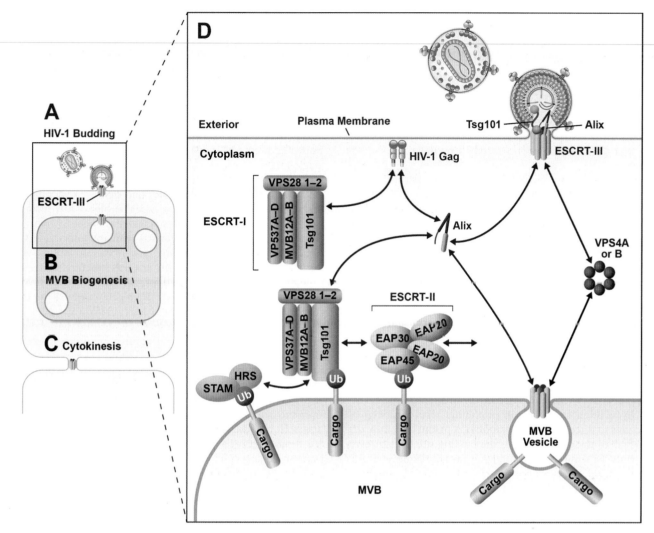

FIGURE 17.35 Role of endosomal sorting complex required for transport (ESCRT) machinery in membrane scission events. Virus budding **(A)**, multivesicular body (MVB) biogenesis **(B)**, and the abscission step of cytokinesis **(C)**. Panel **(D)** shows an enlarged view of MVB biogenesis (*bottom*) and HIV-1 budding (*top*). ESCRT-I, II, and III are labeled. While not explicitly labeled as such, the STAM/HRS complex is often referred to as ESCRT-0. Note that virus budding uses only a subset of ESCRT machinery, as described in the text. (Modified with permission from Balasubramaniam M, Freed EO. New insights into HIV assembly and trafficking. *Physiology* (*Bethesda*) 2011;26(4):236–251. Copyright © 2011 The American Physiological Society.)

I component Tsg101 interacts with p6, and that this interaction is dependent on the PTAP motif.[251,718] The functional significance of this interaction was supported by the finding that siRNA-mediated depletion of Tsg101 disrupts HIV-1 release,[251] as does overexpression of the N-terminal, Gag-binding domain of Tsg101 (TSG-5′).[173] Inhibition of release imposed by both Tsg101 depletion and overexpression of TSG-5′ is specific for PTAP-dependent budding, as the release of the PPPY-bearing MLV is unaffected.[173,251] The significance of p6–Tsg101 binding in HIV-1 release was also supported by the finding that fusing Tsg101 directly to the C-terminus of Gag rescued a p6 late-domain defect, indicating that the primary role of p6 in virus release is to bind Tsg101.[472] Broad disruption of the endosomal sorting pathway by overexpressing a dominant-negative mutant of Vps4 globally inhibits the budding of a number of retroviruses, suggesting that most, if not all, retroviruses depend on the ESCRT apparatus for their release. Whereas PTAP late domains function by interacting with the ESCRT-I

component Tsg101, the YPX$_n$L-type motif interacts with the ESCRT-associated factor Alix.[471,679,720] Alix can bridge ESCRT-I and ESCRT-III by interacting with both Tsg101 and one of the ESCRT-III subunits[471,679,720] (Fig. 17.35). PPPY-type late domains bind members of the Nedd4 family of E3 ubiquitin ligases.[231,678,721]

Although under most conditions PTAP serves as the dominant HIV-1 late domain, p6 also bears a conserved Alix-binding YPX$_n$L motif (Fig. 17.27E).[471,679,720] The presence of this alternative site for interaction between HIV-1 Gag and the ESCRT machinery suggests that under some circumstances, Alix plays a role in HIV-1 budding and release. Indeed, if the PTAP motif is eliminated by mutation, Alix overexpression partially rescues virus release.[707] Furthermore, mutation of the Alix binding site in p6 induces significant virus replication defects in T cells and macrophages. Simultaneous elimination of both Tsg101 and Alix binding sites in p6 abolishes virus replication.[239] These findings suggest some degree of functional redundancy between

PTAP and YPX$_n$L motifs in HIV-1 replication. In addition to binding the YPX$_n$L motif in HIV-1 p6, Alix has also been reported to interact with the NC domain of Gag.[197,563,564]

Live-cell imaging and superresolution microscopy have provided insights into the role of ESCRT machinery in HIV-1 release. Total internal reflection fluorescence (TIRF) microscopy and fluorescently tagged Gag and ESCRT components were used to follow the recruitment of ESCRT machinery during retrovirus assembly and release.[353] Gag assembly was typically completed within approximately 5 to 10 minutes of the initial appearance of an individual Gag punctum.[326,352] ESCRT-III components and Vps4 were transiently recruited late in this process, concomitant with the completion of assembly. As expected, late domain mutation largely ablated ESCRT-III recruitment but did not affect the kinetics of assembly.[326,353] Alternative models have been proposed regarding the timing of ESCRT-III recruitment and the topology and distribution of ESCRT components relative to the budding particle, with some data indicating that ESCRT-III leaves the site of assembly immediately prior to abscission (e.g., Ref.[343]) and an alternative model suggesting that some ESCRT-III components are located within the head of the assembling particle and help to drive membrane scission from the interior of the bud.[715] A consensus view of these topics has been presented.[436] Given the relatively limited role that ESCRT-II plays in HIV-1 release, and the secondary function served by Alix, precisely how ESCRT-I bridges to ESCRT-III in viral budding remains an open question.

In addition to its role in promoting virus budding, p6 functions to direct the incorporation of Vpr and Vpx into virions.[545,746] In the case of HIV-1, the binding site for Vpr overlaps with the sequence responsible for p6 association with Alix (Fig. 17.27E). The functions of Vpr and Vpx will be discussed in more detail in the section on Accessory Proteins.

Env Glycoprotein Incorporation Into Virions

As mentioned earlier, the cytoplasmic tail of most lentiviral Env glycoproteins is quite long (~150 amino acids, in the case of HIV-1) relative to those of other retroviruses. This long tail must be accommodated by the underlying Gag lattice during Env incorporation. Several models for HIV-1 Env incorporation can be postulated[112]: (a) passive incorporation, in which the Env glycoproteins are packaged into budding particles simply because they are present in the plasma membrane of the virus-producer cell; (b) direct Gag–Env interaction, in which contacts between the cytoplasmic tail of gp41 and the membrane-proximal portion of Gag (i.e., the MA domain) are required for the active recruitment of Env into virions; (c) Gag–Env co-targeting, whereby Gag and Env traffic to a common site on the plasma membrane (e.g., a lipid raft membrane microdomain), thereby concentrating Env at sites of Gag assembly; and (d) indirect Gag–Env interaction, according to which a host cell protein serves to link the gp41 cytoplasmic tail with the MA domain of Gag. Data in the literature can be invoked to support each of these models. The glycoproteins from heterologous viruses (e.g., MLV Env, VSV-G, SARS-CoV-2 spike), which contain short cytoplasmic tails, can be packaged into HIV-1 particles (a process known as pseudotyping), and some host cell membrane proteins are also present within the viral envelope. However, despite this apparently nonspecific incorporation, mutational analyses of MA and gp41 support the hypothesis that incorporation of HIV-1 Env glycoproteins is an active process that requires direct interactions between Env and MA, or at least an accommodation of the gp41 cytoplasmic tail by the Gag lattice. Although in some cell lines truncation of the gp41 cytoplasmic tail has little effect on Env incorporation, in most T-cell lines and in relevant primary cell types, for example, PBMCs and MDMs, gp41 truncations severely disrupt Env incorporation.[512]

Several studies have provided biochemical evidence in support of a direct MA–gp41 interaction.[8,9,150,750] High-resolution single-molecule tracking assays have demonstrated the trapping of Env at the sites of Gag assembly on the surface of infected cells. This trapping requires the long gp41 cytoplasmic tail and is ablated by a mutation in MA that blocks Env incorporation.[554] Together, such results support a model whereby the long gp41 cytoplasmic tail interacts with the underlying Gag lattice, leading to the retention Env in the assembling virus particle. HIV-1 MA was shown in early structural studies to crystallize as a trimer,[297] and both biochemical cross-linking data[695,696] and cryoET analysis[579] have demonstrated the existence of a trimeric arrangement of MA in HIV-1 particles.

As mentioned earlier, the gp41 cytoplasmic tail contains highly conserved endocytic and sorting motifs that regulate Env levels on the cell surface (Fig. 17.7). Low levels of surface Env likely contribute to the paucity of Env glycoproteins on HIV-1 virions (only ~12 Env trimers per virion[787]), reducing virus-induced cytopathicity and helping the virus avoid immune detection. These endocytosis and sorting motifs have also been proposed to direct the polarized sorting of Env to the VS to favor cell–cell transmission (e.g.,[176]) Based on this scenario, cellular factors involved in membrane protein recycling and sorting (e.g., Rab proteins and their adapters) could help to promote Env incorporation and viral spread. Rab11 family interacting protein 1C (FIP1C) has been proposed to play such a role.[578] A recent study of SIVmac infection of rhesus macaques demonstrated the importance of endocytosis/sorting motifs in lentiviral replication and pathogenesis *in vivo*.[409]

While some cellular proteins play a positive role in promoting Env trafficking and incorporation, others have been demonstrated to antagonize Env processing and transport, ultimately reducing Env incorporation into virions. These include the IFN-induced transmembrane (IFITM) proteins, ER mannosidase I, guanylate binding protein 5 (GBP5), galectin 3 binding protein (LGAL3SBP/90K), and the membrane-associated RING-CH (MARCH) E3 ubiquitin ligases (for review, see Ref.[38]). The roles that these proteins play in the biology of HIV-1 replication and spread remain to be characterized.

Protease (PR) and Virus Maturation

Early pulse-chase studies performed with avian retroviruses demonstrated that retroviral Gag proteins are initially synthesized as polyprotein precursors that are cleaved to generate smaller products.[719] Subsequent studies revealed that Gag precursor processing is mediated by the viral PR, and that proteolytic cleavage of the Gag and Gag–Pol precursors is essential for virus infectivity.[153,364] Sequence analysis of retroviral PRs indicated that they are related to cellular "aspartic" proteases such as pepsin and renin (for review, see Ref.[414]). Like these cellular enzymes, retroviral PRs use two apposed Asp residues in the active site to coordinate a water molecule that catalyzes the hydrolysis of a peptide bond in the target protein. However, unlike the cellular aspartic proteases, which function as pseudodimers (using two folds within the same molecule to generate the active site), retroviral PRs function as true dimers. Early X-ray crystallographic data from HIV-1 PR[406,519,738] indicated that the two monomers are held together in part by a four-stranded, antiparallel β-sheet derived from both N- and C-terminal ends of each monomer (Fig. 17.36).[737] The substrate-binding site is located within a cleft formed between the two monomers. Like their cellular homologs, the HIV-1 PR dimer contains flexible "flaps" that overhang the binding site and may stabilize the substrate within the cleft; the active-site Asp residues lie in the center of the dimer. Although some limited amino acid homology is observed surrounding active-site residues, the primary sequences of retroviral PRs are highly divergent, yet their structures are remarkably similar.

The first cleavage events catalyzed by retroviral PRs during or immediately after virion release from the cell are likely intramolecular[553] and serve to liberate PR from the Gag–Pol precursor. As mentioned earlier, after the release of PR from the Gag–Pol precursor, the dimeric enzyme cleaves a number of sites in both Gag and Gag–Pol (see Fig. 17.27). The efficiency with which PR cleaves the individual target sites in Gag and Gag–Pol varies widely and is influenced by the amino acid sequence at the site of cleavage and the context (i.e., degree of exposure or accessibility) of the cleavage site. The proteolytic processing of model proteins and substrate analogs by HIV-1 PR indicates that the binding cleft can accommodate a peptide of approximately seven residues in length, and synthetic peptides of this size are cleaved *in vitro*.[58] Although the primary amino acid sequence of each PR cleavage site is different, each target sequence must adopt a shape, or volume, that can fit into the "substrate envelope" of the enzyme.[573] As a consequence of the relatively divergent PR target sequences present in Gag, and the varying efficiencies with which these sites serve as substrates for PR activity, Gag cleavage takes place as an ordered, step-

wise cascade. Processing at the N-terminus of NC is the most rapid *in vitro*, whereas the cleavage converting CA-SP1 (p25) to CA (p24) is the slowest. Mutations in Gag that disrupt the ordered nature of PR-mediated processing severely disrupt virus assembly and/or subsequent maturation. Furthermore, HIV-1 mutants engineered to overexpress PR exhibit rapid, premature processing of Gag and Gag–Pol polyproteins and a block in virus production.[388] Thus, the activation of PR must be tightly controlled to prevent significant processing prior to the completion of assembly. A N-terminal Pro residue is a highly conserved feature of retroviral CA proteins[690]; while the viral PR prefers bulky hydrophobic residues adjacent to the scissile bond, it must be able to accommodate the steric effects imposed by the Pro to cleave the MA-CA junction.[571]

PR-mediated cleavage of the Gag and Gag–Pol precursors leads to maturation, which is characterized by a dramatic change in virion morphology[379,566] (Fig. 17.28). Maturation likely requires disassembly of the immature Gag lattice and reassembly of the mature capsid lattice post budding.[40] While CA adopts a predominantly hexameric arrangement in both the immature and the mature lattice, the sites of protein–protein interaction differ between the two lattices. As described earlier, formation of a fully closed capsid around the viral RNA during maturation is essential to protecting the viral genome during subsequent reverse transcription in the target cell, and preventing diffusional loss of RT from the RTC. The intact capsid also plays a central role in the trafficking of the core to, and across, the nuclear envelope and shields the viral nucleic acid from host innate sensing during the early events in the viral replication cycle.

Assembly of the conical capsid is the most readily apparent ultrastructural transition that the virus particle undergoes during maturation. However, several additional structural changes in the virion accompany Gag processing and capsid formation. The RNA dimer is more thermostable in mature than in immature virions,[238] and, as noted earlier, the contacts between NC,

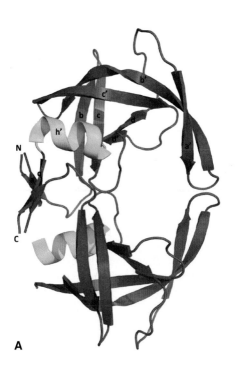
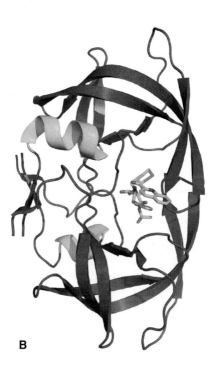

A   **B**

FIGURE 17.36 Structure of the HIV-1 PR dimer. Uncomplexed **(A)** or complexed **(B)** with the PR inhibitor Ro-31-8558. The following domains are indicated in the first half of the molecule: β-strands a (residues 1 to 4), b (residues 9 to 15), c, and d (residues 30 to 35). The active-site residues are at positions 25 to 27. The second half of the molecule is structurally related to the first half, with the following domains indicated: β-strands a' (residues 43 to 49), b' (residues 52 to 66), c' (residues 69 to 78), d' (residues 83 to 85), and helix h' (residues 86 to 94). The inner portion of the dimer interface is formed by β-strand q (residues 95 to 99). (Modified by Jerry Alexandratos with permission of Annual Reviews, Inc. from Wlodawer A, Erickson JW. Structure-based inhibitors of HIV-1 protease. *Annu Rev Biochem* 1993;62:543–585; permission conveyed through Copyright Clearance Center, Inc.)

and RNA change upon maturation.[394] The organization of the MA lattice appears to undergo a structural change following Gag processing[579] (Fig. 17.29), and, perhaps linked to changes in the MA lattice, the fusogenicity of Env is activated during maturation in a gp41 cytoplasmic tail-dependent manner.[511,749] Env has been shown to cluster in mature virions, again in a manner that is dependent on the gp41 cytoplasmic tail.[127] The cytoplasmic tail-dependent effect of particle maturation on Env function suggests that interactions between the gp41 cytoplasmic tail and the immature Gag lattice suppress fusion activity. Together, the diverse structural changes in the virion that are triggered by maturation could all be viewed as part of the process by which the virion is primed for infection of a new target cell.

When used in combination with other classes of antiretrovirals, competitive inhibitors of HIV-1 PR function have proven to be highly effective antiretroviral drugs, and nine such PR inhibitors are currently FDA approved. The earliest PR inhibitors were small oligopeptide derivatives that mimicked PR target sequences but contained nonhydrolyzable groups at the P1 and P1′ positions flanking the scissile bond that PR would normally cleave. The early, peptide-based inhibitors were subsequently modified to improve stability and bioavailability, and the structure of the PR active site was used to design novel inhibitory compounds.[738] Resistance to PR inhibitors arises as a result of changes throughout the enzyme. Some of these changes are directly responsible for conferring resistance, whereas others are adaptations to the fitness defects conferred by the primary resistance mutations. The substrate envelope concept, mentioned above, has been important in understanding resistance to PR inhibitors; amino acid residues in the enzyme that are contacted by portions of the inhibitor that protrude outside the substrate envelope are often the sites of resistance mutations.[392] As a result, PR inhibitors that fit within the substrate envelope are more difficult for the virus to evade and resistance requires a larger number of mutations. In addition to changes in PR itself, mutations that affect the targets of the enzyme (i.e., the cleavage sites in Gag), or the conformation or accessibility of those cleavage sites, can contribute to resistance.[195]

As described earlier, the primary function of IN is to catalyze the integration of the newly synthesized viral DNA into the genome of the target cell. However, it was noted in early studies that some IN mutations (referred to as "class II" IN mutations to distinguish them from mutations that blocked integration itself) exerted pleiotropic effects that included the formation of aberrant virions containing what appeared to be empty capsids and acentric electron density, presumed to contain the viral RNA, located outside of the capsid.[207] These results suggested that IN may play a role in the condensation of viral RNA into the capsid during particle maturation. Indeed, more recent studies (e.g.,[371]) demonstrated that IN binds specifically to viral RNA, resulting in the formation of RNP complexes in which IN plays a bridging role to condense the nucleic acid. IN-targeted inhibitors that induce IN multimerization (the ALLINIs, see section on Integration) produce a phenotype strikingly reminiscent of that exhibited by class II IN mutants (for review, see Ref.[208]); these compounds were shown to prevent IN–RNA binding.[371] Collectively, these findings demonstrate that in addition to catalyzing viral DNA integration, IN

plays a secondary role late in the virus replication cycle by promoting the condensation of viral genomic RNA into the assembling capsid core.

The highly ordered nature of Gag processing and the strict dependence on complete processing for proper virion maturation make the Gag processing cascade a potential target for drug development. The betulinic acid derivative dimethylsuccinyl betulinic acid (bevirimat) potently inhibits HIV-1 infectivity by targeting a late Gag processing event—the cleavage of the CA-SP1 processing intermediate to mature CA.[423,784] By specifically disrupting this step in Gag processing, treatment of virus-expressing cells with bevirimat leads to the formation of poorly infectious viral particles with aberrantly condensed cores. Selection in culture gives rise to bevirimat-resistant isolates that contain single amino acid substitutions flanking the CA/SP1 cleavage site.[3,423,784] In infected individuals, bevirimat can lead to significant reductions in viral loads,[597,661] providing proof-of-concept that compounds capable of disrupting specific steps in Gag processing can be clinically effective against HIV-1. In the case of bevirimat, however, polymorphisms in SP1 reduce susceptibility to the compound.[5,105,597] Efforts in recent years have focused on developing bevirimat analogs with increased potency that are capable of inhibiting a wide range of clinically relevant HIV-1 isolates (for review see Ref.[379]). A second, structurally distinct maturation inhibitor (known as PF-46396) that blocks CA-SP1 processing has been described.[62] Interestingly, mutations that confer resistance to PF-46396 map not only to residues surrounding the CA-SP1 cleavage site but also to the MHR in CA.[725] The study of these resistance mutations, and the mechanism by which they confer resistance, led to an increased understanding of the role of the CA-SP1 junction region in both assembly and maturation and helped to elucidate the mechanism of action of this class of inhibitors. In short, maturation inhibitors bind a central channel inside the CA-SP1 six-helix bundle (see section on Virus Assembly) and stabilize this highly dynamic structure.[370] Because some unfolding of the six-helix bundle is required for PR-mediated cleavage at the CA-SP1 junction, increased bundle stability prevents cleavage at that site, leading to a maturation defect[639,722] (for review, see Ref.[379]). In addition to compounds that block virus maturation by interfering with specific step(s) in Gag processing, condensation of a functional viral core can also be inhibited by molecules that bind the CA domain of Gag. Several compounds in this class are discussed in the CA section.

The Accessory Proteins

In addition to the viral structural proteins (Gag and Env), the *pol*-encoded enzymes (PR, RT, and IN), and the regulatory proteins (Rev and Tat), the HIV genome encodes several "accessory" proteins: Vif, Vpu, Vpr, Nef (and Vpx, in the case of HIV-2) (see Fig. 17.4). Although often dispensable for virus replication in immortalized cell lines, these gene products are required for efficient virus replication and disease induction *in vivo*. A primary function of these accessory proteins is to serve as adaptors to connect cellular substrates to the host cell proteasomal or lysosomal degradation machinery. The accessory proteins thus serve to counteract components of the cellular innate and adaptive immune responses that evolved to restrict retroviral infection.

Vif

As discussed earlier, the Vif protein derives its name (virus infectivity factor) from the observation that it plays a role in promoting virus infectivity. The presence of *vif* is a highly conserved feature among lentiviruses; a *vif* product is encoded by all lentiviruses except EIAV. Soon after the discovery of the *vif* gene,[220,664,680] it was noted that the requirement for Vif is strongly producer-cell dependent. Thus, certain cell lines are "permissive" for *vif*-defective mutants, whereas others, including primary lymphocytes, MDMs, and some T-cell lines, are "nonpermissive." A breakthrough came with the discovery that APOBEC3G is the primary host factor whose antiviral activity is neutralized by Vif.[651]

APOBEC3G is a member of a large family of DNA cytidine deaminases that are involved in mRNA editing and immunoglobulin gene diversification.[282] These enzymes contain one or two catalytic domains characterized by His/Cys-X-Glu-X$_{23-28}$-Pro-Cys-X$_2$-Cys motifs. In the absence of Vif, APOBEC3G is incorporated into HIV-1 virions in the producer cell. In the next round of infection, the virion-associated APOBEC3G converts cytidines to uridines during minus-strand DNA synthesis. Cytidine deamination during reverse transcription leads to G-to-A hypermutation of the viral plus-strand, introducing coding mutations and stop codons. In APOBEC3G-expressing

producer cells, Vif induces the degradation of APOBEC3G, thereby counteracting its antiviral activity[769] (Fig. 17.37). Some of the antiviral activity of APOBEC3G has been reported to be independent of cytidine deamination activity of the protein and involves suppression of reverse transcription via a direct interaction between RT and the restriction factor.[560]

Vif induces the degradation of APOBEC3G through the ubiquitin-proteasome pathway by interacting with the cellular proteins Cul5, elongins B and C, and ring-box-1 (Rbx1) to form an Skp1-cullin F-box (SCF)-like E3 ubiquitin ligase complex.[769] The transcription cofactor CBF-β is also recruited to this ubiquitin ligase complex[333] (Fig. 17.37). The formation of this complex leads to the ubiquitylation of APOBEC3G and its degradation in the 26S proteasome. The ability of Vif to induce the degradation of APOBEC3G is species specific; for example, HIV-1 Vif is inactive against simian APOBEC3G, and SIV$_{agm}$ Vif is unable to block the antiviral action of human APOBEC3G.

The ability of APOBEC3G to restrict HIV-1 replication is highly dependent on its incorporation into virions. APOBEC3G incorporation is rather promiscuous—the human protein can be packaged into, and inhibit, diverse retroviruses, including SIVs, EIAV, and MLV. Because these viruses are highly divergent at the protein sequence level, APOBEC3G

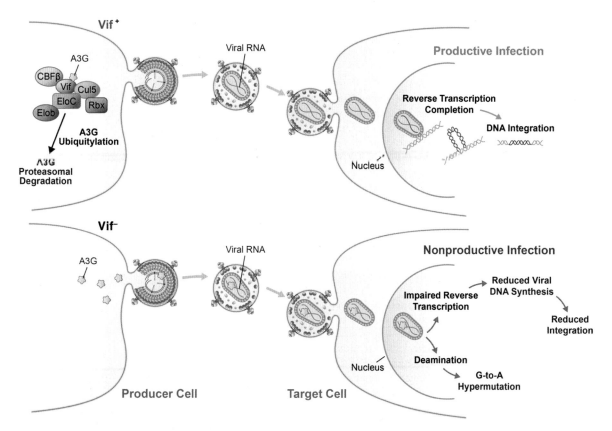

FIGURE 17.37 Proposed model for inactivation of APOBEC3G by Vif. *Top*: In APOBEC3G-expressing producer cells, Vif links APOBEC3G (A3G) to the cellular proteins Cul5, elongins B and C, and ring-box-1 (Rbx1) to form an Skp1-cullin F-box (SCF)-like E3 ubiquitin ligase complex, thereby inducing the proteasomal degradation of APOBEC3G and limiting its incorporation into virions. *Bottom*: In the absence of Vif, APOBEC3G is incorporated into virions. Its presence during reverse transcription in the target cell leads to impaired reverse transcription and integration, and deamination of cytidines to uridines, resulting in G-to-A hypermutation. (Adapted from Freed EO. HIV-1 and the host cell: an intimate association. *Trends Microbiol* 2004;12(4):170–177. Copyright © 2004 Elsevier. With permission.)

likely gains access to virions through a highly conserved structural element or by binding to molecules, for example RNA, present in all retroviral particles.[775] The antiviral potency of APOBEC3G is illustrated by the finding that fewer than 10 molecules of the protein are packaged per Vif(−) virion produced from primary T cells.[756]

Humans encode 11 APOBEC family members, with the APOBEC3 genes (APOBEC3A-H) being the most numerous.[282] Although APOBEC3G was originally identified as the cellular restriction factor that is inactivated by Vif,[651] other APOBECs, for example, APOBEC3D, F, and H, also display varying degrees of antiviral activity. The contribution of cytidine deamination–independent antiviral activity differs between APOBEC family members.[172] A number of structures of portions of the APOBEC proteins, in some cases in complex with Vif, CBF-β, Cul5, EloB/C or in complex with single-stranded DNA substrate, have been solved by NMR, x-ray crystallography, and cryoEM (for review, see Ref.[172]). The catalytic domains of APOBEC proteins share a common structural fold made up of six α-helices and five β-strands with a coordinated zinc ion at the catalytic site.

The interplay between Vif and APOBEC cytidine deaminases offers novel possibilities for antiretroviral therapy. For example, disrupting the binding between Vif and APOBECs with small-molecule inhibitors would unmask the antiviral activity of the cellular enzymes. Interfering with Vif-mediated APOBEC degradation could also theoretically be achieved by blocking the interaction of APOBECs with the SCF-like E3 ubiquitin ligase complex.[528]

Vpr

The *vpr* gene encodes a 14-kDa, 96-amino acid protein that is incorporated into virus particles.[140,770] Virion incorporation is mediated through an interaction with a (Leu-X-X)$_4$ motif in the p6 domain of Gag (Fig. 17.27E). The NMR structure of Vpr[496] reveals the presence of three α-helices folded around a hydrophobic core. The N- and C-termini of the protein are flexible. Although Vpr has little influence on HIV replication kinetics in proliferating PBMCs or T-cell lines in culture, in nondividing MDMs its effects are more pronounced. Several lines of evidence indicate that Vpr is also required for efficient replication and pathogenesis *in vivo*: Vpr mutations are observed in HIV-1 strains isolated from long-term nonprogressors,[666] and deletion of Vpr modestly decreases SIV pathogenicity in rhesus macaques.[403]

A number of Vpr activities have been reported. In particular, Vpr has been shown to (a) arrest infected cells in the G2/M phase of the cell cycle and induce apoptosis, (b) stimulate gene expression driven by the HIV-1 LTR, (c) promote HIV-1 replication in MDMs, and (d) activate the DNA damage response (DDR). Most activities described for Vpr can be linked to its ability to recruit target proteins to a ubiquitin ligase complex, resulting in their ubiquitylation and degradation in the proteasome. The challenges of deciphering Vpr function are highlighted by the observation that Vpr expression leads to the down-regulation of several dozen cellular proteins.[266] Notable cellular proteins that have been reported in multiple studies to be targeted for proteasomal degradation include uracil DNA glycosylase 2 (UNG2), the SLX4 complex, helicase-like transcription factor (HTLF), and the cell division cycle associated 2 (CDCA2) protein.[211] For the other primate lentiviral accessory proteins (Nef, Vif, Vpu,

and Vpx), there is consensus in the field regarding primary cellular targets; in contrast, it is not yet clearly established which of Vpr's many substrates are linked to the requirement for Vpr in HIV replication in physiological contexts.

An early report identified a Vpr-binding protein (VprBP)[781] that was later shown to bind damaged DNA specific binding protein 1 (DDB1), which in turn associates with cullin 4 (CUL4).[305,411,633] The interaction between Vpr and VprBP—subsequently renamed DCAF1 (DDB1- and CUL4-associated factor 1)—allows Vpr to recruit substrates into the E3 ubiquitin ligase complex, resulting in their ubiquitylation and proteasomal degradation. The effects of Vpr on the cellular proteome are almost entirely dependent upon the Vpr-DCAF1 interaction (e.g., Ref.[266]). While the biological consequences of Vpr-mediated UNG-2 degradation remain uncertain, the crystal structure of the DDB1-DCAF1-Vpr-UNG2 complex provides insights into the mechanism by which Vpr directs its substrate proteins for ubiquitylation and proteasomal degradation[747] (Fig. 17.38).

A number of studies have linked Vpr expression to the cellular DDR, which involves a network of factors involved in sensing and responding to DNA damage. Activation of the DDR triggers DNA repair, alters cell-cycle regulation, and can induce apoptosis. Several kinases play central roles in DDR, including ataxia telangiectasia Rad3-related (ATR), ataxia telangiectasia mutated (ATM), and DNA-dependent protein kinase (DNA-PK). Vpr expression leads to the degradation of a number of proteins involved in the DDR, including the DNA repair endonuclease Mus81 and HLTF.[211] Recent work has sug-

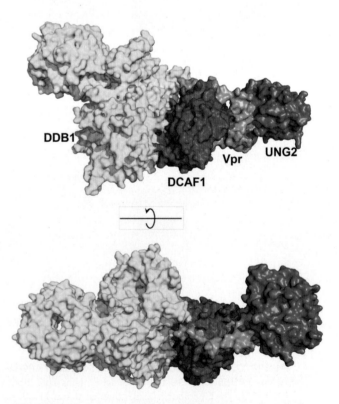

FIGURE 17.38 Structure of the complex between damaged DNA specific binding protein 1 (DDB1), and CUL4-associated factor 1 (DCAF1), Vpr, and uracil DNA glycosylase 2 (UNG2). Created in PyMol from PDB accession 5JK7.

gested that Vpr engages the DDR by two independent mechanisms: by inducing DNA damage and by blocking the repair of double-stranded DNA breaks.[422]

Another major and well-validated activity of Vpr, which is closely linked to its engagement of the DDR pathway, is the arrest of cells in the G2/M phase of the cell cycle (for review, see Ref.[211]). Cell-cycle arrest reportedly occurs within hours of infection and is not blocked by antiviral agents, suggesting that arrest can be initiated by virion-associated Vpr carried into the cell during infection.[562] A role for Vpr–DCAF1 binding in cell-cycle arrest is supported by the observation that this function of Vpr is abrogated by mutation of the DCAF1 binding site of Vpr or by DCAF1 depletion.[266,411,776] Vpr-induced cell cycle arrest is associated with the recruitment of the DDB1-CUL4 ubiquitin ligase complex to chromatin-associated nuclear foci, leading to proteasomal degradation of chromatin-bound cellular factor(s) and activation of ATR, which is involved in regulating the G2/M checkpoint.[39] Recent studies have identified the chromosome periphery protein coiled coil domain containing-137 (CCDC137) as a target for Vpr-mediated degradation.[266,776] As with many other Vpr substrates, the Vpr-CUL4 interaction is critical for CCDC137 degradation. Importantly, CRISPR/Cas9-mediated depletion of CCDC137 recapitulates several major Vpr activities—G2/M cell-cycle arrest, induction of DDR, and increased HIV-1 gene expression.[776] These results are consistent with CCDC137 being a key target for Vpr-mediated degradation.

Vpx

Members of the HIV-2/SIV$_{smm}$/SIV$_{mac}$ lineage of primate lentiviruses encode a *vpx* gene. The *vpx* and *vpr* genes are highly related, and it has been suggested that *vpx* arose by acquisition of the SIV$_{agm}$ *vpr* gene by recombination. Like Vpr, Vpx is incorporated into virus particles, also via an interaction with the C-terminal p6 domain of Gag. Although Vpr and Vpx share a common origin and both bind directly to DCAF1 to recruit target proteins to the DCAF1-DDB1-CUL4 E3 ubiquitin ligase complex, they diverge significantly in their functions.

The ability of Vpx to promote infection of nondividing cells (e.g., monocyte-derived macrophages, dendritic cells, and quiescent CD4+ T cells) is primarily a result of its ability to induce the degradation of the host cell restriction factor SAMHD1, a deoxynucleotide triphosphohydrolase that blocks reverse transcription in these cell types by reducing intracellular levels of dNTPs.[257,306,400] Treating macrophages and dendritic cells with Vpx-containing virions suppresses the block to subsequent infection by Vpx-deleted SIV$_{SM}$ or HIV-2. Likewise, HIV-1 infection of dendritic cells and monocytes can be enhanced by prior treatment of the cells with Vpx-containing SIVmac. Vpx-mediated degradation of SAMHD1 requires the engagement by Vpx of the DCAF1/DDB1/CUL4 E3 ubiquitin ligase complex discussed above in the context of Vpr activity.[648,673] SAMHD1 depletion in primary MDMs and MDDCs enhances infection by single-cycle reporter virus by increasing viral cDNA synthesis.[306,400] Some primate lentiviral Vpr proteins are able to induce the degradation of SAMHD1, but not that encoded by the HIV-1/SIVcpz lineage.[432]

SAMHD1 activity is regulated by phosphorylation and multimerization. Phosphorylation on residue Thr-592, which inactivates the enzyme's activity, is controlled by specific kinases

and phosphatases to achieve the appropriate concentrations of intracellular dNTPs during progression through the cell cycle.[154] SAMHD1 impairs the replication of several families of DNA viruses, which have evolved specific counter-measures against this cellular factor. For example, the β- and γ-herpesviruses encode a kinase that phosphorylates SAMHD1, thereby inhibiting its activity.[779] Binding of a combination of dGTP or GTP and dNTPs to allosteric sites on the enzyme induces the assembly of catalytically active SAMHD1 tetramers from two inactive dimers.[336] Phosphorylation of Thr-592 has been reported to reduce the stability of the SAMHD1 tetramer.[17]

SAMHD1 expression is IFN induced and this enzyme plays a diversity of roles in innate immunity.[119] The *SAMHD1* gene is defective in some patients with Aicardi-Goutiere syndrome (AGS), an autoimmune disorder that resembles congenital viral infection and is associated with inflammation and impaired breakdown of cytosolic nucleic acids.[595] Importantly, PBMCs from patients with AGS are highly susceptible to a spreading HIV-1 infection even in the absence of activation[43] consistent with the antiviral role of SAMHD1.

In addition to its primary role in directing the proteasomal degradation of SAMHD1, Vpx possesses other activities. Vpx and Vpr from some primate lentiviruses have been reported to target components of the human silencing hub (HUSH) complex, which represses retroviral gene expression. As with SAMHD1 degradation, this activity involves recruitment of DCAF1 and the associated E3 ubiquitin ligase complex. Vpx/Vpr-mediated degradation of the HUSH complex leads to activation of proviral gene expression.[128,772]

Vpu

A distinguishing feature of the HIV-1 lineage of primate lentiviruses is the presence of the *vpu* gene; it is absent from HIV-2 and from nearly all SIVs. Vpu is a multimeric, 81-amino acid, integral membrane phosphoprotein containing an N-terminal transmembrane anchor sequence and an approximately 50-amino acid cytoplasmic domain. Three α-helical domains have been predicted: one in the transmembrane sequence, the others in the cytoplasmic domain[743] (Fig 17.39). The sites of phosphorylation have been mapped to two Ser residues at positions 52 and 56.[635] Vpu is translated from a *vpu-env* bicistronic mRNA. Two principal functions for Vpu have been described: enhancement of virus release and degradation of CD4.

Early studies observed that HIV-1 clones lacking a functional *vpu* gene displayed a pronounced defect in virus particle production in some (Vpu-restrictive) but not in other (Vpu-permissive) cells.[681] The absence of Vpu had no discernible effect on the processing or transport of Gag proteins but caused

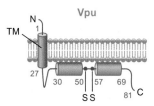

FIGURE 17.39 Schematic representation of the Vpu structure. The transmembrane (TM) and two predicted cytoplasmic helices are shown. The two phosphorylated Ser (S) residues are indicated. Numbers indicate amino acid positions.

apparently mature, fully budded virus particles to be retained at the plasma membrane and in intracellular vesicles.[380] In 2008, two groups independently reported that Vpu counteracts the IFN-inducible protein CD317 or BST-2 (bone marrow stromal cell antigen 2), renamed tetherin.[520,712] Vpu-permissive producer cells were shown to express low levels of tetherin, whereas Vpu-restrictive cells expressed high levels. Ectopic expression of tetherin in Vpu-permissive producer cells blocked the release of Vpu(−) but not Vpu(+) HIV-1. Conversely, siRNA-mediated depletion of tetherin from Vpu-restrictive cells converted these cells to a Vpu-permissive phenotype.

Tetherin is proposed to have an unusual topology in the plasma membrane, with an N-terminal cytoplasmic domain, a transmembrane region, an extracellular coiled-coil motif, and a C-terminal glycosylphosphatidylinositol (GPI) anchor that directs tetherin localization to lipid rafts[391] (Fig. 17.40). The extracellular domain of tetherin is glycosylated and includes three Cys residues that are involved in intermolecular disulfide cross-linking[527] (Fig. 17.40). X-ray crystallography studies demonstrate that the tetherin ectodomain forms an extended dimeric coiled coil.[634,760] Tetherin proteins from nonhuman species (e.g., rodents and nonhuman primates) retain the ability

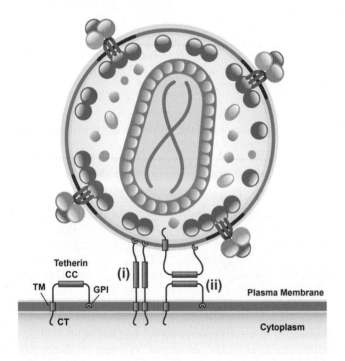

FIGURE 17.40 Hypothetical models for the tethering of HIV-1 virions to the cell surface by tetherin (CD317/BST-2). The tethered virion is at the top; tetherin is shown on the left anchored in the lipid bilayer of the plasma membrane, with the cytoplasmic tail (CT), transmembrane (TM), and coiled-coil (CC) domains and the GPI linkage indicated. In model (*i*), two molecules of tetherin are oriented in parallel, with the TM domains embedded in the plasma membrane and the GPI anchors in the viral membrane. In model (*ii*), one molecule is embedded in the viral membrane, the other in the plasma membrane, with the two molecules associating via their CC domains. (Adapted from Adamson CS, Freed EO. Novel approaches to inhibiting HIV-1 replication. *Antiviral Res* 2010;85(1):119–141. Copyright © 2010 Elsevier. With permission.)

to restrict HIV-1 release but are not counteracted by Vpu. The key amino acid differences that differentiate human from non-human tetherins in terms of their ability to be counteracted by Vpu map primarily to the transmembrane domain, and it has been demonstrated that the transmembrane domain of human tetherin interacts directly with Vpu.[327,602]

Tetherin has been shown to tether diverse enveloped viruses to the cell surface; these include viruses from many genera of *Retroviridae* (e.g., HIV-2, HTLV-1, MLV, EIAV, FIV, M-PMV, PFV) and nonretroviral enveloped viruses (e.g., filoviruses, arenaviruses, and herpesviruses). Several of these viruses have, in turn, evolved mechanisms to counteract tetherin restriction (for review see Ref.[193]). Whereas HIV-1 uses Vpu to neutralize tetherin, some strains of HIV-2 and SIV have evolved a mechanism whereby the Env glycoprotein induces the sequestration of tetherin in an intracellular, perinuclear compartment.[272] The glycoprotein of Ebola virus (a filovirus) has also been reported to possess antitetherin activity.[357] A number of SIVs use Nef to antagonize tetherin.[337,778] The ability of SIV Nef to counteract tetherin is primate species specific, with critical determinants for Nef antitetherin activity mapping to the N-terminal, cytoplasmic domain of tetherin. It is clear from the diverse strategies that enveloped viruses have evolved to counteract tetherin that this protein is a potent and broadly acting component of the host innate immune response. Although tetherin clearly restricts the release of enveloped viruses, the role of tetherin in cell–cell viral transfer remains to be defined. Some studies have reported that tetherin restricts cell–cell HIV-1 transfer,[102,390] whereas others concluded that tetherin actually promotes cell–cell transmission.[346] Nevertheless, the antitetherin activity of Vpu appears to be critical to HIV-1 replication and pathogenesis in a humanized mouse model.[757] By counteracting the tetherin-mediated accumulation of virus particles on the cell surface, Vpu reduces the susceptibility of infected cells to ADCC.[16] The ability of tetherin expression to sensitize infected cells to ADCC may help to explain the strong selective pressure on many different enveloped viruses to develop strategies to antagonize this restriction factor.

Sequence analysis of tetherin coding regions from across a number of primate species has revealed that it is undergoing rapid positive selection, likely in response to lentiviral infections.[484] Most notably, a motif in the cytoplasmic domain of tetherin that is required for Nef's antitetherin activity is deleted in humans,[433] rendering human tetherin resistant to antagonism by HIV-1 Nef. As discussed earlier in this chapter, HIV-1 infection in humans is thought to have originated from cross-species chimpanzee-to-human transmission of SIVcpz.[247] Although SIVcpz does encode Vpu, the SIVcpz protein does not possess antitetherin activity.[626] It therefore appears that Vpu acquired the ability to counteract tetherin after transmission of SIVcpz from chimps to humans.

The second main function of Vpu—CD4 degradation—has been characterized in some detail. Vpu binds directly to the cytoplasmic tail of CD4 in the ER; residues in the cytoplasmic domain of Vpu, and Vpu phosphorylation, are critical for CD4 down-regulation. Vpu is thought to mediate the degradation of CD4 by two distinct mechanisms: retention in the ER, and ER-associated degradation (ERAD).[451] Vpu simultaneously interacts with CD4 and the human β-transducin repeat-containing protein (h-βTrCP) subunit of the SCF (Skp–Cullin 1–F-box) ubiquitin ligase complex. CD4 is then targeted for ubiquitin-mediated proteasomal degradation.[467] The degradation of CD4 by Vpu prevents the Env glycoprotein precursor gp160 from interacting with CD4 intracellularly, thereby enabling Env to traffic to the cell surface. CD4 downmodulation also limits superinfection, and by preventing CD4-Env interactions at the cell surface, Vpu-mediated CD4 degradation may also prevent the exposure of CD4-induced Env epitopes that would, like the tetherin-induced accumulation of particles at the cell surface, render the infected cell susceptible to ADCC.[685]

In addition to counteracting tetherin and inducing the degradation of CD4, Vpu has also been reported to down-regulate a number of other cell-surface proteins.[581] While the consequences for HIV replication and pathogenesis are not entirely understood, these Vpu activities likely contribute to the evasion by HIV of both innate and adaptive arms of the host immune response.

Nef

The *nef* gene, present only in primate lentiviruses (see Figs. 17.3 and 17.4), encodes an approximately 25- to 34-kDa membrane-associated phosphoprotein that is incorporated into virions. Membrane binding, mediated by a covalently attached myristic acid moiety and a cluster of N-terminal basic residues, is critical for most Nef functions (Fig. 17.41). Nef is synthesized at high levels from the first multiply spliced mRNA transcript detected postinfection. Although Nef was originally labeled a "negative factor," it is now clear that in cultured cells Nef expression either has no effect on virus spread or modestly enhances replication kinetics. Positive effects of Nef on virus replication in culture are most pronounced when target cells are not highly activated. *In vivo*, Nef is a key contributor to sustained lentiviral replication and pathogenesis. Although numerous and complex functions for this viral protein have been described, the requirement for Nef in lentiviral pathogenesis, like that of the other accessory proteins, stems largely from its ability to hijack cellular trafficking pathways to antagonize host restriction factors and down-regulate the surface expression of proteins involved in innate and adaptive immunity (for review, see Ref.[86]).

Nef is composed of several structural domains: an N-terminal, flexible "anchor" domain, a "core" domain, and an internal loop (Fig. 17.41). The NMR structure of the core domain was determined in the mid-1990s,[269,270] and X-ray or NMR structures of the core domain were solved for the protein in a complex with Src homology 3 (SH3) domains[18,412] or with the cytoplasmic tail of CD4.[271] The internal loop and core domain contain acidic clusters and a dileucine motif important for the protein's interactions with cellular factors (Fig. 17.41).[86]

Deletion of the *nef* gene has a profound effect in the SIV/rhesus macaque animal model. Monkeys inoculated with *nef*-deleted mutants develop high-level antibody responses and are unable to sustain the infection.[372] Nef has also been proposed to play a major role in pathogenesis in HIV-1–infected humans. This hypothesis stems in part from the observation that individuals infected with virus isolates harboring Nef mutations progress to disease slowly.[169,376] Because of its pleiotropic properties and many dozens of reported interaction partners, the role of Nef in HIV/SIV pathogenesis has been difficult to decipher.

A number of functions for HIV-1, HIV-2, and SIV Nef have been reported: (a) down-regulation of a wide array of cell-surface molecules, including CD4, CD8, MHC I, the CD3 T-cell receptor complex, and the costimulatory molecule CD28; (b) enhancement of virus infectivity; (c) modulation of cellular activation and signaling pathways; and (d) the stimulation of extracellular vesicle production. Many of these functions are linked to a generalized disruption of endosomal trafficking induced by Nef.

Like the HIV-1 Env and Vpu proteins, Nef down-regulates cell-surface expression of CD4. Nef-induced CD4 down-regulation proceeds in a step-wise fashion: (a) Nef interacts with the cytoplasmic domain of CD4 and then associates with the clathrin adaptor protein complex 2 (AP-2) in clathrin-coated pits; this ternary CD4–Nef–AP-2 complex is then internalized.[109,434] The interaction between Nef and AP-2 involves an ExxxLL motif in Nef (Fig. 17.41)[396]; (b) Nef induces the ESCRT-dependent sorting of internalized CD4 to the MVB, and, ultimately, to the lysosome for degradation.[159] As discussed above in the context of Vpu, CD4 down-regulation helps limit superinfection and may reduce the exposure of CD4-induced epitopes in Env that would render infected cells susceptible to ADCC. Lentiviral Nef also down-regulates surface expression of CD3, CD8, and CD28 via the AP-2–dependent pathway (for review see Ref.[86]).

The mechanism by which Nef down-regulates MHC-I is distinct from that used to reduce CD4 expression and involves the formation of a Nef–MHC-I complex and AP-1–dependent redirection of MHC-I from the *trans*-Golgi network to lysosomes (review Ref.[86]). The binding of Nef to AP-1 involves an EEEE motif in Nef (Fig. 17.41). MHC-I down-regulation blocks proper antigen presentation—thereby limiting the ability of cytotoxic T lymphocytes to recognize and eliminate virus-infected cells—thus providing HIV and SIV with a mechanism for partially evading at least one component of the host immune response.[144] Nef also binds directly to β-COP, a component of the coatomer complex, via an EE motif (for review see Ref.[86]).

As mentioned earlier, HIV and SIV Nef contain a highly conserved consensus binding site (PxxP) for the Src homology 3 (SH3) domain of Src-family Tyr kinases (Fig 17.41). Nef has been reported to bind several of these kinases (e.g., Lyn, Hck, and Lck) and modulate their catalytic activities. Nef also reportedly binds and activates members of the Tec family kinases

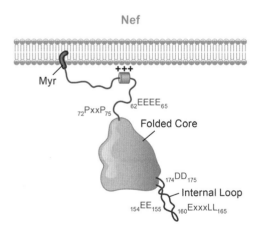

Nef

FIGURE 17.41 Schematic representation of the Nef structure. N-terminal myristic acid and polybasic sequence (+++) anchor Nef to the membrane. Amino acid numbering from the NL4-3 Nef strain of HIV-1 is indicated. The folded core with its internal loop are shown, as are several of the amino acid motifs responsible for Nef interactions with host cell proteins.

(e.g., Itk) (for review, see Ref.[675]). Because cellular kinases are intimately involved in signaling pathways, such interactions may stimulate HIV replication and gene expression. Nef also triggers the release of exosomes that contain factors including Nef itself.[483] It has been suggested that this Nef-induced exocytosis may play an important role in Nef function, although this remains an open question. An additional function of Nef is to induce the internalization of T-cell immunoglobulin and mucin domain (TIM) proteins, which retain virus particles on the plasma membrane by binding to phosphatidylserine in the viral lipid envelope.[424]

Many early studies showed that Nef enhances the infectivity of HIV-1 particles in single-cycle assays. In 2015, it was discovered that Nef expression leads to the down-regulation of members of the SERINC (for serine incorporator) family of proteins, and that SERINC5, and to a lesser extent SERINC3, is able to exert a potent antiviral activity in the absence of Nef.[603,708] The SERINC family of proteins, which comprise five members in humans (SERINC1-5), are multipass transmembrane proteins. In the absence of Nef expression, SERINC5 expressed in the virus-producer cell is incorporated into HIV-1 particles, causing a severe defect in virus particle infectivity. Nef expression leads to the endocytic uptake of SERINC5 from the cell surface in an AP-2–dependent manner, again using the ExxxLL motif of Nef for the interaction (Fig. 17.41). RNAi-mediated depletion of SERINC5 enhances the infectivity of Nef(−) virus, and ectopic expression of this host protein suppresses Nef(−) particle infectivity. The cryoEM structure of a *Drosophila* SERINC homolog reveals an unusual two-subdomain organization of the ten transmembrane domains.[577] Unlike many restriction factors, SERINC5 expression is not IFN inducible,[603,708] and this host factor does not show evidence of positive selection.[515] While primate lentiviruses use Nef to down-regulate SERINC proteins, MLV uses glycosylated Gag (GlycoGag)[603,708] and EIAV uses the S2 protein[108] for this purpose. That retroviruses encode multiple distinct genes to counteract SERINC proteins argues for the biological importance of these cellular inhibitory factors.

While the entry block imposed by SERINC5 incorporation into virus particles appears to be primarily at the step of fusion pore formation/expansion,[670,728] the precise mechanism by which SERINC proteins disrupt fusion remains enigmatic. The Env glycoproteins from different HIV-1 isolates differ in their sensitivity to restriction by SERINC5,[38,603,670,704,708] with the determinants of this sensitivity mapping to the variable loops of gp120.[37] The presence of SERINC5 in virus particles has been reported to alter the conformation of Env and render the virus more sensitive to neutralizing antibodies targeting gp41.[37,213,670] These results are consistent with a model whereby the presence of SERINC proteins in the viral membrane directly or indirectly force Env into a nonfusogenic state. Although an early report suggested that SERINC proteins alter cellular lipid biosynthesis[324] (hence the name Ser incorporator), SERINC5 expression was observed to not affect the lipid composition of HIV-1 particles.[704] However, recent data demonstrate that SERINC proteins are phosphatidylserine (PS) transporters that increase the concentration of PS on the extracellular leaflet of the lipid bilayer of infected cells and on HIV-1 particles.[268a,417a]

The Nef proteins of many SIVs and group O HIV-1 isolates possess the ability to antagonize the host restriction factor tetherin.[337,626,778] The capacity of Nef to counteract tetherin involves the removal of the host protein from sites of budding on the plasma membrane, and in the case of SIV Nef, requires Nef–AP-2 interaction.[777] In contrast, Nef from HIV-1 group O isolates induces the relocalization of tetherin to the *trans*-Golgi network by hijacking AP-1 complexes.[381,501]

Although it is well established that Nef is crucial to HIV and SIV pathogenesis, it remains to be determined which of the many functions attributed to Nef in culture are required for its ability to potentiate efficient replication and disease progression *in vivo*. Studies have been performed with SIV Nef mutants in an attempt to define which activities of Nef are required for the maintenance of high viral loads in infected animals. Results of these studies have suggested that mutations that interfere with the ability of Nef to down-regulate CD4, MHC-I, CD3, and CD28 attenuate virus replication *in vivo*.[320,508,629] Mutations that disrupt the ability of Nef to enhance virus infectivity *in vitro* are also detrimental to virus replication in monkeys.[320] Attempts to establish the *in vivo* significance of the many reported activities of HIV-1 Nef are complicated by the fact that individual mutations in key interaction motifs (Fig. 17.41) often disrupt multiple Nef activities, and by differences in the functional determinants of HIV-1 versus SIV Nef. This will remain an important area for future research.

PERSPECTIVES

Despite its relatively recent emergence as a major human pathogen, HIV-1 has become one of the most intensively studied and best understood viruses. As this chapter illustrates, an enormous amount of information has been obtained regarding the molecular, biochemical, biological, and structural details of all aspects of the HIV-1 replication cycle. Recent breakthroughs in our understanding of how lentiviruses parasitize host cell machinery to promote virus replication and, conversely, how the host cell has evolved to specifically restrict lentivirus infection have provided remarkable insights into the dynamic nature of this complex host–pathogen interaction. Although the wealth of information available on HIV-1 and related lentiviruses has led to the development of several classes of antiretroviral drugs that effectively suppress HIV-1 replication in infected patients, controlling the AIDS epidemic remains an elusive goal, particularly in resource-limited settings. In the absence of an effective vaccine or curative drug regimens, future progress in HIV research will be required to more effectively control this pathogen. HIV-1 research will also continue to drive advances in virology, immunology, and cellular, molecular, and structural biology.

ACKNOWLEDGMENTS

The authors would like to thank Danielle Lyons, Gary Howard, and John Carroll for assistance in the preparation of this chapter and Alex Kleinpeter, Yuta Hikichi, and Allen Kane for help with the figures.

REFERENCES

1. Abram ME, Ferris AL, Shao W, et al. Nature, position, and frequency of mutations made in a single cycle of HIV-1 replication. *J Virol* 2010;84(19):9864–9878.

2. Achuthan V, Perreira JM, Sowd GA, et al. Capsid-CPSF6 interaction licenses nuclear HIV-1 trafficking to sites of viral DNA integration. *Cell Host Microbe* 2018;24(3):392–404 e8.

3. Adamson CS, Ablan SD, Boeras I, et al. In vitro resistance to the human immunodeficiency virus type 1 maturation inhibitor PA-457 (Bevirimat). *J Virol* 2006;80(22):10957–10971.

4. Adamson CS, Freed EO. Novel approaches to inhibiting HIV-1 replication. *Antiviral Res* 2010;85(1):119–141.

5. Adamson CS, Sakalian M, Salzwedel K, et al. Polymorphisms in Gag spacer peptide 1 confer varying levels of resistance to the HIV-1 maturation inhibitor bevirimat. *Retrovirology* 2010;7:36.

6. Agosto LM, Uchil PD, Mothes W. HIV cell-to-cell transmission: effects on pathogenesis and antiretroviral therapy. *Trends Microbiol* 2015;23(5):289–295.

7. Ajasin D, Eugenin EA. HIV-1 Tat: role in bystander toxicity. *Front Cell Infect Microbiol* 2020;10:61.

8. Alfadhli A, Mack A, Ritchie C, et al. Trimer enhancement mutation effects on HIV-1 matrix protein binding activities. *J Virol* 2016;90(12):5657–5664.

9. Alfadhli A, Staubus AO, Tedbury PR, et al. Analysis of HIV-1 matrix-envelope cytoplasmic tail interactions. *J Virol* 2019;93(21):e01079-19.

10. Alfadhli A, Still A, Barklis E. Analysis of human immunodeficiency virus type 1 matrix binding to membranes and nucleic acids. *J Virol* 2009;83(23):12196–12203.

11. Ali I, Ramage H, Boehm D, et al. The HIV-1 Tat protein is monomethylated at lysine 71 by the lysine methyltransferase KMT7. *J Biol Chem* 2016;291(31):16240–16248.

12. Alkhatib G, Combadiere C, Broder CC, et al. CC CKR5: a RANTES, MIP-1a MIP-1b receptor as a fusion cofactor for macrophage-tropic HIV-1. *Science* 1996;272(5270):1955–1958.

13. Aloia RC, Tian H, Jensen FC. Lipid composition and fluidity of the human immunodeficiency virus envelope and host cell plasma membranes. *Proc Natl Acad Sci U S A* 1993;90(11):5181–5185.

14. Amarasinghe GK, De Guzman RN, Turner RB, et al. NMR structure of the HIV-1 nucleocapsid protein bound to stem-loop SL2 of the psi-RNA packaging signal. Implications for genome recognition. *J Mol Biol* 2000;301(2):491–511.

15. Aoi Y, Smith ER, Shah AP, et al. NELF regulates a promoter-proximal step distinct from RNA Pol II pause-release. *Mol Cell* 2020;78(2):261–274 e5.

16. Arias JF, Heyer LN, von Bredow B, et al. Tetherin antagonism by Vpu protects HIV-infected cells from antibody-dependent cell-mediated cytotoxicity. *Proc Natl Acad Sci U S A* 2014;111(17):6425–6430.

17. Arnold LH, Groom HC, Kunzelmann S, et al. Phospho-dependent regulation of SAMHD1 oligomerisation couples catalysis and restriction. *PLoS Pathog* 2015;11(10):e1005194.

18. Arold S, Franken P, Strub MP, et al. The crystal structure of HIV-1 Nef protein bound to the Fyn kinase SH3 domain suggests a role for this complex in altered T cell receptor signaling. *Structure* 1997;5(10):1361–1372.

19. Arthur LO, Bess JW Jr, Waters DJ, et al. Challenge of chimpanzees (Pan troglodytes) immunized with human immunodeficiency virus envelope glycoprotein gp120. *J Virol* 1989;63(12):5046–5053.

20. Asang C, Hauber I, Schaal H. Insights into the selective activation of alternatively used splice acceptors by the human immunodeficiency virus type 1 bidirectional splicing enhancer. *Nucleic Acids Res* 2008;36(5):1450–1463.

21. Ashe MP, Furger A, Proudfoot NJ. Stem-loop 1 of the U1 snRNP plays a critical role in the suppression of HIV-1 polyadenylation. *RNA* 2000;6(2):170–177.

22. Ashe MP, Griffin P, James W, et al. Poly(A) site selection in the HIV-1 provirus: inhibition of promoter-proximal polyadenylation by the downstream major splice donor site. *Genes Dev* 1995;9(23):3008–3025.

23. Askjaer P, Jensen TH, Nilsson J, et al. The specificity of the CRM1-Rev nuclear export signal interaction is mediated by RanGTP. *J Biol Chem* 1998;273(50):33414–33422.

24. Bachmann N, von Siebenthal C, Vongrad V, et al. Determinants of HIV-1 reservoir size and long-term dynamics during suppressive ART. *Nat Commun* 2019;10(1):3193.

25. Bachu M, Yalla S, Asokan M, et al. Multiple NF-kappaB sites in HIV-1 subtype C long terminal repeat confer superior magnitude of transcription and thereby the enhanced viral predominance. *J Biol Chem* 2012;287(53):44714–44735.

26. Baenziger S, Tussiwand R, Schlaepfer E, et al. Disseminated and sustained HIV infection in CD34+ cord blood cell-transplanted Rag2-/-gamma c-/- mice. *Proc Natl Acad Sci U S A* 2006;103(43):15951–15956.

27. Balasubramaniam M, Freed EO. New insights into HIV assembly and trafficking. *Physiology (Bethesda)* 2011;26(4):236–251.

28. Baltimore D. RNA-dependent DNA polymerase in virions of RNA tumour viruses. *Nature* 1970;226(252):1209–1211.

29. Barboric M, Yik JH, Czudnochowski N, et al. Tat competes with HEXIM1 to increase the active pool of P-TEFb for HIV-1 transcription. *Nucleic Acids Res* 2007;35(6):2003–2012.

30. Barre-Sinoussi F, Chermann JC, Rey F, et al. Isolation of a T-lymphotropic retrovirus from a patient at risk for acquired immune deficiency syndrome (AIDS). *Science* 1983;220(4599):868–871.

31. Bartel DP, Zapp ML, Green MR, et al. HIV-1 Rev regulation involves recognition of non-Watson-Crick base pairs in viral RNA. *Cell* 1991;67(3):529–536.

32. Battiste JL, Mao H, Rao NS, et al. Alpha helix-RNA major groove recognition in an HIV-1 rev peptide-RRE RNA complex. *Science* 1996;273(5281):1547–1551.

33. Battivelli E, Dahabieh MS, Abdel-Mohsen M, et al. Distinct chromatin functional states correlate with HIV latency reactivation in infected primary CD4(+) T cells. *Elife* 2018;7:e34655.

34. Battivelli E, Lecossier D, Matsuoka S, et al. Strain-specific differences in the impact of human TRIM5alpha, different TRIM5alpha alleles, and the inhibition of capsid-cyclophilin A interactions on the infectivity of HIV-1. *J Virol* 2010;84(21):11010–11019.

35. Bebenek K, Abbotts J, Roberts JD, et al. Specificity and mechanism of error-prone replication by human immunodeficiency virus-1 reverse transcriptase. *J Biol Chem* 1989;264(28):16948–16956.

36. Bedwell GJ, Engelman AN. Factors that mold the nuclear landscape of HIV-1 integration. *Nucleic Acids Res* 2021;49(2):621–635.

37. Beitari S, Ding S, Pan Q, et al. Effect of HIV-1 Env on SERINC5 antagonism. *J Virol* 2017;91(4):e02214-16.

38. Beitari S, Wang Y, Liu SL, et al. HIV-1 envelope glycoprotein at the interface of host restriction and virus evasion. *Viruses* 2019;11(4):311.

39. Belzile JP, Abrahamyan LG, Gerard FC, et al. Formation of mobile chromatin-associated nuclear foci containing HIV-1 Vpr and VPRBP is critical for the induction of G2 cell cycle arrest. *PLoS Pathog* 2010;6(9):e1001080.

40. Benjamin J, Ganser-Pornillos BK, Tivol WF, et al. Three-dimensional structure of HIV-1 virus-like particles by electron cryotomography. *J Mol Biol* 2005;346(2):577–588.

41. Benn S, Rutledge R, Folks T, et al. Genomic heterogeneity of AIDS retroviral isolates from North America and Zaire. *Science* 1985;230(4728):949–951.

42. Bentley DL. Coupling mRNA processing with transcription in time and space. *Nat Rev Genet* 2014;15(3):163–175.

43. Berger A, Sommer AF, Zwarg J, et al. SAMHD1-deficient CD14+ cells from individuals with Aicardi-Goutieres syndrome are highly susceptible to HIV-1 infection. *PLoS Pathog* 2012;7(12):e1002425.

44. Berges BK, Akkina SR, Folkvord JM, et al. Mucosal transmission of R5 and X4 tropic HIV-1 via vaginal and rectal routes in humanized Rag2-/- gammac -/- (RAG-hu) mice. *Virology* 2008;373(2):342–351.

45. Berkhout B, van Hemert FJ. The unusual nucleotide content of the HIV RNA genome results in a biased amino acid composition of HIV proteins. *Nucleic Acids Res* 1994;22(9):1705–1711.

46. Berlioz-Torrent C, Shacklett BL, Erdtmann L, et al. Interactions of the cytoplasmic domains of human and simian retroviral transmembrane proteins with components of the clathrin adaptor complexes modulate intracellular and cell surface expression of envelope glycoproteins. *J Virol* 1999;73(2):1350–1361.

47. Bernhard W, Barreto K, Raithatha S, et al. An upstream YY1 binding site on the HIV-1 LTR contributes to latent infection. *PLoS One* 2013;8(10):e77052.

48. Berthoux L, Pechoux C, Ottmann M, et al. Mutations in the N-terminal domain of human immunodeficiency virus type 1 nucleocapsid protein affect virion core structure and proviral DNA synthesis. *J Virol* 1997;71(9):6973–6981.

49. Besnard E, Hakre S, Kampmann M, et al. The mTOR Complex Controls HIV Latency. *Cell Host Microbe* 2016;20(6):785–797.

50. Bess JW Jr, Powell PJ, Issaq HJ, et al. Tightly bound zinc in human immunodeficiency virus type 1, human T-cell leukemia virus type I, and other retroviruses. *J Virol* 1992;66(2):840–847.

51. Best S, Le Tissier P, Towers G, et al. Positional cloning of the mouse retrovirus restriction gene Fv1. *Nature* 1996;382(6594):826–829.

52. Bester SM, Wei G, Zhao H, et al. Structural and mechanistic bases for a potent HIV-1 capsid inhibitor. *Science* 2020;370(6514):360–364.

53. Betancor G, Dicks MDJ, Jimenez-Guardeno JM, et al. The GTPase domain of MX2 interacts with the HIV-1 capsid, enabling its short isoform to moderate antiviral restriction. *Cell Rep* 2019;29(7):1923–1933 e3.

54. Bhattacharya A, Alam SL, Fricke T, et al. Structural basis of HIV-1 capsid recognition by PF74 and CPSF6. *Proc Natl Acad Sci U S A* 2014;111(52):18625–18630.

55. Bieniasz P, Telesnitsky A. Multiple, switchable protein: RNA interactions regulate human immunodeficiency virus type 1 assembly. *Annu Rev Virol* 2018;5(1):165–183.

56. Bieniasz PD, Grdina TA, Bogerd HP, et al. Recruitment of a protein complex containing Tat and cyclin T1 to TAR governs the species specificity of HIV-1 Tat. *EMBO J* 1998;17(23):7056–7065.

57. Bilbille Y, Vendeix FA, Guenther R, et al. The structure of the human tRNALys3 anticodon bound to the HIV genome is stabilized by modified nucleosides and adjacent mismatch base pairs. *Nucleic Acids Res* 2009;37(10):3342–3353.

58. Billich S, Knoop M-T, Hansen J, et al. Synthetic peptides as substrates and inhibitors of human immune deficiency virus-1 protease. *J Biol Chem* 1988;263(34):17905–17908.

59. Bischoff FR, Ponstingl H. Mitotic regulator protein RCC1 is complexed with a nuclear ras-related polypeptide. *Proc Natl Acad Sci U S A* 1991;88(23):10830–10834.

60. Bisgrove DA, Mahmoudi T, Henklein P, et al. Conserved P-TEFb-interacting domain of BRD4 inhibits HIV transcription. *Proc Natl Acad Sci U S A* 2007;104(34):13690–13695.

61. Black LR, Aiken C. TRIM5alpha disrupts the structure of assembled HIV-1 capsid complexes in vitro. *J Virol* 2010;84(13):6564–6569.

62. Blair WS, Cao J, Fok-Seang J, et al. New small-molecule inhibitor class targeting human immunodeficiency virus type 1 virion maturation. *Antimicrob Agents Chemother* 2009;53(12):5080–5087.

63. Blazkova J, Murray D, Justement JS, et al. Paucity of HIV DNA methylation in latently infected, resting CD4+ T cells from infected individuals receiving antiretroviral therapy. *J Virol* 2012;86(9):5390–5392.

64. Blazkova J, Trejbalova K, Gondois-Rey F, et al. CpG methylation controls reactivation of HIV from latency. *PLoS Pathog* 2009;5(8):e1000554.

65. Boehm D, Calvanese V, Dar RD, et al. BET bromodomain-targeting compounds reactivate HIV from latency via a Tat-independent mechanism. *Cell Cycle* 2013;12(3):452–462.

66. Boge M, Wyss S, Bonifacino JS, et al. A membrane-proximal tyrosine-based signal mediates internalization of the HIV-1 envelope glycoprotein via interaction with the AP-2 clathrin adaptor. *J Biol Chem* 1998;273(25):15773–15778.

67. Bosque A, Planelles V. Induction of HIV-1 latency and reactivation in primary memory CD4+ T cells. *Blood* 2009;113(1):58–65.

68. Bou-Nader C, Muecksch F, Brown JB, et al. HIV-1 matrix-tRNA complex structure reveals basis for host control of Gag localization. *Cell Host Microbe* 2021;29(9):1421–1436 e7.

69. Bouchat S, Delacourt N, Kula A, et al. Sequential treatment with 5-aza-2′-deoxycytidine and deacetylase inhibitors reactivates HIV-1. *EMBO Mol Med* 2016;8(2):117–138.

70. Boulanger MC, Liang C, Russell RS, et al. Methylation of Tat by PRMT6 regulates human immunodeficiency virus type 1 gene expression. *J Virol* 2005;79(1):124–131.

71. Bowman GD, Poirier MG. Post-translational modifications of histones that influence nucleosome dynamics. *Chem Rev* 2015;115(6):2274–2295.

72. Boyd PS, Brown JB, Brown JD, et al. NMR studies of retroviral genome packaging. *Viruses* 2020;12(10):1115.

73. Brainard DM, Seung E, Frahm N, et al. Induction of robust cellular and humoral virus-specific adaptive immune responses in human immunodeficiency virus-infected humanized BLT mice. *J Virol* 2009;83(14):7305–7321.

74. Brandariz-Nunez A, Valle-Casuso JC, White TE, et al. Role of SAMHD1 nuclear localization in restriction of HIV-1 and SIVmac. *Retrovirology* 2012;9:49.

75. Brass AL, Dykxhoorn DM, Benita Y, et al. Identification of host proteins required for HIV infection through a functional genomic screen. *Science* 2008;319(5865):921–926.

76. Bres V, Kiernan RE, Linares LK, et al. A non-proteolytic role for ubiquitin in Tat-mediated transactivation of the HIV-1 promoter. *Nat Cell Biol* 2003;5(8):754–761.

77. Briggs JA, Riches JD, Glass B, et al. Structure and assembly of immature HIV. *Proc Natl Acad Sci U S A* 2009;106(27):11090–11095.

78. Briggs JA, Wilk T, Welker R, et al. Structural organization of authentic, mature HIV-1 virions and cores. *EMBO J* 2003;22(7):1707–1715.

79. Brinkmann CR, Hojen JF, Rasmussen TA, et al. Treatment of HIV-infected individuals with the histone deacetylase inhibitor panobinostat results in increased numbers of regulatory T cells and limits ex vivo lipopolysaccharide-induced inflammatory responses. *mSphere* 2018;3(1):e00616-17.

80. Brown JD, Kharytonchyk S, Chaudry I, et al. Structural basis for transcriptional start site control of HIV-1 RNA fate. *Science* 2020;368(6489):413–417.

81. Brown PO, Bowerman B, Varmus HE, et al. Retroviral integration: structure of the initial covalent product and its precursor, and a role for the viral IN protein. *Proc Natl Acad Sci U S A* 1989;86(8):2525–2529.

82. Brugger B, Glass B, Haberkant P, et al. The HIV lipidome: a raft with an unusual composition. *Proc Natl Acad Sci U S A* 2006;103(8):2641–2646.

83. Bruner KM, Murray AJ, Pollack RA, et al. Defective proviruses rapidly accumulate during acute HIV-1 infection. *Nat Med* 2016;22(9):1043–1049.

84. Bruner KM, Wang Z, Simonetti FR, et al. A quantitative approach for measuring the reservoir of latent HIV-1 proviruses. *Nature* 2019;566(7742):120–125.

85. Buckman JS, Bosche WJ, Gorelick RJ. Human immunodeficiency virus type 1 nucleocapsid zn(2+) fingers are required for efficient reverse transcription, initial integration processes, and protection of newly synthesized viral DNA. *J Virol* 2003;77(2):1469–1480.

86. Buffalo CZ, Iwamoto Y, Hurley JH, et al. How HIV Nef proteins hijack membrane traffic to promote infection. *J Virol* 2019;93(24):e01322-19.

87. Bullough PA, Hughson FM, Skehel JJ, et al. Structure of influenza haemagglutinin at the pH of membrane fusion. *Nature* 1994;371(6492):37–43.

88. Buratowski S. Progression through the RNA polymerase II CTD cycle. *Mol Cell* 2009;36(4):541–546.

89. Burdick RC, Li C, Munshi M, et al. HIV-1 uncoats in the nucleus near sites of integration. *Proc Natl Acad Sci U S A* 2020;117(10):5486–5493.

90. Busnadiego I, Kane M, Rihn SJ, et al. Host and viral determinants of Mx2 antiretroviral activity. *J Virol* 2014;88(14):7738–7752.

91. Busschots K, Vercammen J, Emiliani S, et al. The interaction of LEDGF/p75 with integrase is lentivirus-specific and promotes DNA binding. *J Biol Chem* 2005;280(18):17841–17847.

92. Byland R, Vance PJ, Hoxie JA, et al. A conserved dileucine motif mediates clathrin and AP-2-dependent endocytosis of the HIV-1 envelope protein. *Mol Biol Cell* 2007;18(2):414–425.

93. Caffrey M, Cai M, Kaufman J, et al. Three-dimensional solution structure of the 44 kDa ectodomain of SIV gp41. *EMBO J* 1998;17(16):4572–4584.

94. Cai J, Gao H, Zhao J, et al. Infection with a newly designed dual fluorescent reporter HIV-1 effectively identifies latently infected CD4(+) T cells. *Elife* 2021;10:e63810.

95. Cai M, Zheng R, Caffrey M, et al. Solution structure of the N-terminal zinc binding domain of HIV-1 integrase. *Nat Struct Biol* 1997;4(7):567–577.

96. Calvanese V, Chavez L, Laurent T, et al. Dual-color HIV reporters trace a population of latently infected cells and enable their purification. *Virology* 2013;446(1–2):283–292.

97. Cameron PU, Saleh S, Sallmann G, et al. Establishment of HIV-1 latency in resting CD4+ T cells depends on chemokine-induced changes in the actin cytoskeleton. *Proc Natl Acad Sci U S A* 2010;107(39):16934–16939.

98. Campbell EM, Hope TJ. HIV-1 capsid: the multifaceted key player in HIV-1 infection. *Nat Rev Microbiol* 2015;13(8):471–483.

99. Campbell EM, Perez O, Anderson JL, et al. Visualization of a proteasome-independent intermediate during restriction of HIV-1 by rhesus TRIM5alpha. *J Cell Biol* 2008;180(3):549–561.

100. Carlton JG, Martin-Serrano J. Parallels between cytokinesis and retroviral budding: a role for the ESCRT machinery. *Science* 2007;316(5833):1908–1912.

101. Carter SD, Mamede JI, Hope TJ, et al. Correlated cryogenic fluorescence microscopy and electron cryo-tomography shows that exogenous TRIM5alpha can form hexagonal lattices or autophagy aggregates in vivo. *Proc Natl Acad Sci U S A* 2020;117(47):29702–29711.

102. Casartelli N, Sourisseau M, Feldmann J, et al. Tetherin restricts productive HIV-1 cell-to-cell transmission. *PLoS Pathog* 2010;6(6):e1000955.

103. Cashikar AG, Shim S, Roth R, et al. Structure of cellular ESCRT-III spirals and their relationship to HIV budding. *Elife* 2014;3:e02184.

104. Cassan E, Arigon-Chifolleau AM, Mesnard JM, et al. Concomitant emergence of the antisense protein gene of HIV-1 and of the pandemic. *Proc Natl Acad Sci U S A* 2016;113(41):11537–11542.

105. Castillo SA, Hernandez JE, Brothers CH. Long-term safety and tolerability of the lamivudine/abacavir combination as components of highly active antiretroviral therapy. *Drug Saf* 2006;29(9):811–826.

106. Chahroudi A, Bosinger SE, Vanderford TH, et al. Natural SIV hosts: showing AIDS the door. *Science* 2012;335(6073):1188–1193.

107. Chan DC, Fass D, Berger JM, et al. Core structure of gp41 from the HIV envelope glycoprotein. *Cell* 1997;89(2):263–273.

108. Chande A, Cuccurullo EC, Rosa A, et al. S2 from equine infectious anemia virus is an infectivity factor which counteracts the retroviral inhibitors SERINC5 and SERINC3. *Proc Natl Acad Sci U S A* 2016;113(46):13197–13202.

109. Chaudhuri R, Mattera R, Lindwasser OW, et al. A basic patch on alpha-adaptin is required for binding of human immunodeficiency virus type 1 Nef and cooperative assembly of a CD4-Nef-AP-2 complex. *J Virol* 2009;83(6):2518–2530.

110. Chavez L, Calvanese V, Verdin E. HIV latency is established directly and early in both resting and activated primary CD4 T cells. *PLoS Pathog* 2015;11(6):e1004955.

111. Chavez L, Kauder S, Verdin E. In vivo, in vitro, and in silico analysis of methylation of the HIV-1 provirus. *Methods* 2011;53(1):47–53.

112. Checkley MA, Luttge BG, Freed EO. HIV-1 envelope glycoprotein biosynthesis, trafficking, and incorporation. *J Mol Biol* 2011;410(4):582–608.

113. Chen B. Molecular mechanism of HIV-1 entry. *Trends Microbiol* 2019;27(10):878–891.

114. Chen B, Vogan EM, Gong H, et al. Structure of an unliganded simian immunodeficiency virus gp120 core. *Nature* 2005;433(7028):834–841.

115. Chen J, Kovacs JM, Peng H, et al. HIV-1 ENVELOPE. Effect of the cytoplasmic domain on antigenic characteristics of HIV-1 envelope glycoprotein. *Science* 2015;349(6244):191–195.

116. Chen J, Nikolaitchik O, Singh J, et al. High efficiency of HIV-1 genomic RNA packaging and heterozygote formation revealed by single virion analysis. *Proc Natl Acad Sci U S A* 2009;106(32):13535–13540.

117. Chen J, Rahman SA, Nikolaitchik OA, et al. HIV-1 RNA genome dimerizes on the plasma membrane in the presence of Gag protein. *Proc Natl Acad Sci U S A* 2016;113(2):E201–E208.

118. Chen P, Hubner W, Spinelli MA, et al. Predominant mode of human immunodeficiency virus transfer between T cells is mediated by sustained Env-dependent neutralization-resistant virological synapses. *J Virol* 2007;81(22):12582–12595.

119. Chen S, Bonifati S, Qin Z, et al. SAMHD1 suppression of antiviral immune responses. *Trends Microbiol* 2019;27(3):254–267.

120. Chen Y, Zhang L, Estaras C, et al. A gene-specific role for the Ssu72 RNAPII CTD phosphatase in HIV-1 Tat transactivation. *Genes Dev* 2014;28(20):2261–2275.

121. Cheng B, Price DH. Properties of RNA polymerase II elongation complexes before and after the P-TEFb-mediated transition into productive elongation. *J Biol Chem* 2007;282(30):21901–21912.

122. Cherepanov P, Ambrosio AL, Rahman S, et al. Structural basis for the recognition between HIV-1 integrase and transcriptional coactivator p75. *Proc Natl Acad Sci U S A* 2005;102(48):17308–17313.

123. Cherepanov P, Maertens G, Proost P, et al. HIV-1 integrase forms stable tetramers and associates with LEDGF/p75 protein in human cells. *J Biol Chem* 2003;278(1):372–381.

124. Chiang K, Sung TL, Rice AP. Regulation of cyclin T1 and HIV-1 replication by microRNAs in resting CD4+ T lymphocytes. *J Virol* 2012;86(6):3244–3252.

125. Cho S, Schroeder S, Ott M. CYCLINg through transcription: posttranslational modifications of P-TEFb regulate transcription elongation. *Cell Cycle* 2010;9(9):1697–1705.

126. Choe H, Farzan M, Sun Y, et al. The beta-chemokine receptors CCR3 and CCR5 facilitate infection by primary HIV-1 isolates. *Cell* 1996;85(7):1135–1148.

127. Chojnacki J, Staudt T, Glass B, et al. Maturation-dependent HIV-1 surface protein redistribution revealed by fluorescence nanoscopy. *Science* 2012;338(6106):524–528.

128. Chougui G, Munir-Matloob S, Matkovic R, et al. HIV-2/SIV viral protein X counteracts HUSH repressor complex. *Nat Microbiol* 2018;3(8):891–897.

129. Christ F, Voet A, Marchand A, et al. Rational design of small-molecule inhibitors of the LEDGF/p75-integrase interaction and HIV replication. *Nat Chem Biol* 2010;6(6):442–448.

130. Christensen DE, Ganser-Pornillos BK, Johnson JS, et al. Reconstitution and visualization of HIV-1 capsid-dependent replication and integration in vitro. *Science* 2020;370(6513):eabc8420.

131. Chukkapalli V, Oh SJ, Ono A. Opposing mechanisms involving RNA and lipids regulate HIV-1 Gag membrane binding through the highly basic region of the matrix domain. *Proc Natl Acad Sci U S A* 2010;107(4):1600–1605.

132. Chun TW, Finzi D, Margolick J, et al. In vivo fate of HIV-1-infected T cells: quantitative analysis of the transition to stable latency. *Nat Med* 1995;1(12):1284–1290.

133. Chun TW, Stuyver L, Mizell SB, et al. Presence of an inducible HIV-1 latent reservoir during highly active antiretroviral therapy. *Proc Natl Acad Sci U S A* 1997;94(24):13193–13197.

134. Clavel F, Guetard D, Brun-Vezinet F, et al. Isolation of a new human retrovirus from West African patients with AIDS. *Science* 1986;233(4761):343–346.

135. Clouse KA, Powell D, Washington I, et al. Monokine regulation of human immunodeficiency virus-1 expression in a chronically infected human T cell clone. *J Immunol* 1989;142(2):431–438.

136. Coffin J, Haase A, Levy JA, et al. Human immunodeficiency viruses. *Science* 1986;232(4751):697.

137. Coffin JM. Structure, replication, and recombination of retrovirus genomes: some unifying hypotheses. *J Gen Virol* 1979;42(1):1–26.

138. Coffin JM. HIV population dynamics in vivo: implications for genetic variation, pathogenesis, and therapy. *Science* 1995;267(5197):483–489.

139. Coffin JM, Bale MJ, Wells D, et al. Integration in oncogenes plays only a minor role in determining the in vivo distribution of HIV integration sites before or during suppressive antiretroviral therapy. *PLoS Pathog* 2021;17(4):e1009141.

140. Cohen EA, Terwilliger EF, Jalinoos Y, et al. Identification of HIV-1 vpr product and function. *J Acquir Immune Defic Syndr* 1990;3(1):11–18.

141. Cohen EA, Terwilliger EF, Sodroski JG, et al. Identification of a protein encoded by the vpu gene of HIV-1. *Nature* 1988;334(6182):532–534.

142. Cohn LB, Silva IT, Oliveira TY, et al. HIV-1 integration landscape during latent and active infection. *Cell* 2015;160(3):420–432.

143. Colin L, Van Lint C. Molecular control of HIV-1 postintegration latency: implications for the development of new therapeutic strategies. *Retrovirology* 2009;6:111.

144. Collins KL, Chen BK, Kalams SA, et al. HIV-1 Nef protein protects infected primary cells against killing by cytotoxic T lymphocytes. *Nature* 1998;391(6665):397–401.
145. Comas-Garcia M, Kroupa T, Datta SA, et al. Efficient support of virus-like particle assembly by the HIV-1 packaging signal. *Elife* 2018;7:e38438.
146. Conrad RJ, Fozouni P, Thomas S, et al. The short isoform of BRD4 promotes HIV-1 latency by engaging repressive SWI/SNF chromatin-remodeling complexes. *Mol Cell* 2017;67(6):1001–1012 e6.
147. Cordingley MG, LaFemina RL, Callahan PL, et al. Sequence-specific interaction of Tat protein and Tat peptides with the transactivation-responsive sequence element of human immunodeficiency virus type 1 in vitro. *Proc Natl Acad Sci U S A* 1990;87(22):8985–8989.
148. Core L, Adelman K. Promoter-proximal pausing of RNA polymerase II: a nexus of gene regulation. *Genes Dev* 2019;33(15–16):960–982.
149. Cortes-Rubio CN, Salgado-Montes de Oca G, Prado-Galbarro FJ, et al. Longitudinal variation in human immunodeficiency virus long terminal repeat methylation in individuals on suppressive antiretroviral therapy. *Clin Epigenetics* 2019;11(1):134.
150. Cosson P. Direct interaction between the envelope and matrix proteins of HIV-1. *EMBO J* 1996;15(21):5783–5788.
151. Coull JJ, Romerio F, Sun JM, et al. The human factors YY1 and LSF repress the human immunodeficiency virus type 1 long terminal repeat via recruitment of histone deacetylase 1. *J Virol* 2000;74(15):6790–6799.
152. Craigie R, Fujiwara T, Bushman F. The IN protein of Moloney murine leukemia virus processes the viral DNA ends and accomplishes their integration in vitro. *Cell* 1990;62(4):829–837.
153. Crawford S, Goff SP. A deletion mutation in the 5′ part of the *pol* gene of Moloney murine leukemia virus blocks proteolytic processing of the *gag* and *pol* polyproteins. *J Virol* 1985;53(3):899–907.
154. Cribier A, Descours B, Valadao AL, et al. Phosphorylation of SAMHD1 by cyclin A2/CDK1 regulates its restriction activity toward HIV-1. *Cell Rep* 2013;3(4):1036–1043.
155. Cubas RA, Mudd JC, Savoye AL, et al. Inadequate T follicular cell help impairs B cell immunity during HIV infection. *Nat Med* 2013;19(4):494–499.
156. D'Orso I, Frankel AD. Tat acetylation modulates assembly of a viral-host RNA-protein transcription complex. *Proc Natl Acad Sci U S A* 2009;106(9):3101–3106.
157. Daniel MD, Letvin NL, King NW, et al. Isolation of T-cell tropic HTLV-III-like retrovirus from macaques. *Science* 1985;228(4704):1201–1204.
158. Das AT, Klaver B, Berkhout B. A hairpin structure in the R region of the human immunodeficiency virus type 1 RNA genome is instrumental in polyadenylation site selection. *J Virol* 1999;73(1):81–91.
159. daSilva LL, Sougrat R, Burgos PV, et al. Human immunodeficiency virus type 1 Nef protein targets CD4 to the multivesicular body pathway. *J Virol* 2009;83(13):6578–6590.
160. Daugherty MD, Booth DS, Jayaraman B, et al. HIV Rev response element (RRE) directs assembly of the Rev homooligomer into discrete asymmetric complexes. *Proc Natl Acad Sci U S A* 2010;107(28):12481–12486.
161. Daugherty MD, D'Orso I, Frankel AD. A solution to limited genomic capacity: using adaptable binding surfaces to assemble the functional HIV Rev oligomer on RNA. *Mol Cell* 2008;31(6):824–834.
162. Daugherty MD, Liu B, Frankel AD. Structural basis for cooperative RNA binding and export complex assembly by HIV Rev. *Nat Struct Mol Biol* 2010;17(11):1337–1342.
163. Davies JF II, Hostomska Z, Hostomsky Z, et al. Crystal structure of the ribonuclease H domain of HIV-1 reverse transcriptase [see comments]. *Science* 1991;252(5002):88–95.
164. Dayton AI, Sodroski JG, Rosen CA, et al. The trans-activator gene of the human T cell lymphotropic virus type III is required for replication. *Cell* 1986;44(6):941–947.
165. Dayton ET, Powell DM, Dayton AI. Functional analysis of CAR, the target sequence for the Rev protein of HIV-1. *Science* 1989;246(4937):1625–1629.
166. De Guzman RN, Wu ZR, Stalling CC, et al. Structure of the HIV-1 nucleocapsid protein bound to the SL3 y-RNA recognition element. *Science* 1998;279(5349):384–388.
167. de Marco A, Muller B, Glass B, et al. Structural analysis of HIV-1 maturation using cryo-electron tomography. *PLoS Pathog* 2010;6(11):e1001215.
168. De Rijck J, Vandekerckhove L, Gijsbers R, et al. Overexpression of the lens epithelium-derived growth factor/p75 integrase binding domain inhibits human immunodeficiency virus replication. *J Virol* 2006;80(23):11498–11509.
169. Deacon NJ, Tsykin A, Solomon A, et al. Genomic structure of an attenuated quasi species of HIV-1 from a blood transfusion donor and recipients [see comments]. *Science* 1995;270(5238):988–991.
170. Dean M, Carrington M, Winkler C, et al. Genetic restriction of HIV-1 infection and progression to AIDS by a deletion allele of the *CKR5* structural gene. [see comments] [published erratum appears in *Science* 1996 Nov 15;274(5290):1069]. *Science* 1996;273(5283):1856–1862.
171. Debyser Z, De Vreese K, Pauwels R, et al. Differential inhibitory effects of TIBO derivatives on different strains of simian immunodeficiency virus. *J Gen Virol* 1992;73(Pt 7):1799–1804.
172. Delviks-Frankenberry KA, Desimmie BA, Pathak VK. Structural Insights into APOBEC3-mediated lentiviral restriction. *Viruses* 2020;12(6):587.
173. Demirov DG, Ono A, Orenstein JM, et al. Overexpression of the N-terminal domain of TSG101 inhibits HIV-1 budding by blocking late domain function. *Proc Natl Acad Sci U S A* 2002;99(2):955–960.
174. Demirov DG, Orenstein JM, Freed EO. The late domain of human immunodeficiency virus type 1 p6 promotes virus release in a cell type-dependent manner. *J Virol* 2002;76:105–117.
175. Deng H, Liu R, Ellmeier W, et al. Identification of a major co-receptor for primary isolates of HIV-1. *Nature* 1996;381(6584):661–666.
176. Deschambeault J, Lalonde JP, Cervantes-Acosta G, et al. Polarized human immunodeficiency virus budding in lymphocytes involves a tyrosine-based signal and favors cell-to-cell viral transmission. *J Virol* 1999;73(6):5010–5017.
177. Deshmukh L, Schwieters CD, Grishaev A, et al. Structure and dynamics of full-length HIV-1 capsid protein in solution. *J Am Chem Soc* 2013;135(43):16133–16147.
178. Dharan A, Bachmann N, Talley S, et al. Nuclear pore blockade reveals that HIV-1 completes reverse transcription and uncoating in the nucleus. *Nat Microbiol* 2020;5(9):1088–1095.
179. Dharan A, Campbell EM. Role of microtubules and microtubule-associated proteins in HIV-1 infection. *J Virol* 2018;92(16):e00085-18.
180. Dharan A, Opp S, Abdel-Rahim O, et al. Bicaudal D2 facilitates the cytoplasmic trafficking and nuclear import of HIV-1 genomes during infection. *Proc Natl Acad Sci U S A* 2017;114(50):E10707–E10716.
181. Dick RA, Zadrozny KK, Xu C, et al. Inositol phosphates are assembly co-factors for HIV-1. *Nature* 2018;560(7719):509–512.
182. Dicks MDJ, Betancor G, Jimenez-Guardeno JM, et al. Multiple components of the nuclear pore complex interact with the amino-terminus of MX2 to facilitate HIV-1 restriction. *PLoS Pathog* 2018;14(11):e1007408.
183. Dieudonne M, Maiuri P, Biancotto C, et al. Transcriptional competence of the integrated HIV-1 provirus at the nuclear periphery. *EMBO J* 2009;28(15):2231–2243.
184. Dilley KA, Nikolaitchik OA, Galli A, et al. Interactions between HIV-1 Gag and viral RNA genome enhance virion assembly. *J Virol* 2017;91(16):e02319-16.
185. Dimitrov DS, Willey RL, Sato H, et al. Quantitation of human immunodeficiency virus type 1 infection kinetics. *J Virol* 1993;67(4):2182–2190.
186. Ding D, Qu X, Li L, et al. Involvement of histone methyltransferase GLP in HIV-1 latency through catalysis of H3K9 dimethylation. *Virology* 2013;440(2):182–189.
187. Ding P, Kharytonchyk S, Waller A, et al. Identification of the initial nucleocapsid recognition element in the HIV-1 RNA packaging signal. *Proc Natl Acad Sci U S A* 2020;117(30):17737–17746.
188. Dingwall C, Ernberg I, Gait MJ, et al. HIV-1 tat protein stimulates transcription by binding to a U-rich bulge in the stem of the TAR RNA structure. *EMBO J* 1990;9(12):4145–4153.
189. Dinoso JB, Kim SY, Wiegand AM, et al. Treatment intensification does not reduce residual HIV-1 viremia in patients on highly active antiretroviral therapy. *Proc Natl Acad Sci U S A* 2009;106(23):9403–9408.
190. Divsalar DN, Simoben CV, Schonhofer C, et al. Novel histone deacetylase inhibitors and HIV-1 latency-reversing agents identified by large-scale virtual screening. *Front Pharmacol* 2020;11:905.
191. Donehower LA, Varmus HE. A mutant murine leukemia virus with a single missense codon in pol is defective in a function affecting integration. *Proc Natl Acad Sci U S A* 1984;81(20):6461–6465.
192. Dougherty JP, Temin HM. Determination of the rate of base-pair substitution and insertion mutations in retrovirus replication. *J Virol* 1988;62(8):2817–2822.
193. Douglas JL, Gustin JK, Viswanathan K, et al. The great escape: viral strategies to counter BST-2/tetherin. *PLoS Pathog* 2010;6(5):e1000913.
194. Doyle T, Goujon C, Malim MH. HIV-1 and interferons: who's interfering with whom? *Nat Rev Microbiol* 2015;13(7):403–413.
195. Doyon L, Croteau G, Thibeault D, et al. Second locus involved in human immunodeficiency virus type 1 resistance to protease inhibitors. *J Virol* 1996;70(6):3763–3769.
196. du Chene I, Basyuk E, Lin YL, et al. Suv39H1 and HP1gamma are responsible for chromatin-mediated HIV-1 transcriptional silencing and post-integration latency. *EMBO J* 2007;26(2):424–435.
197. Dussupt V, Javid MP, Abou-Jaoude G, et al. The nucleocapsid region of HIV-1 Gag cooperates with the PTAP and LYPXnL late domains to recruit the cellular machinery necessary for viral budding. *PLoS Pathog* 2009;5(3):e1000339.
198. Dyda F, Hickman AB, Jenkins TM, et al. Crystal structure of the catalytic domain of HIV-1 integrase: similarity to other polynucleotidyl transferases [see comments]. *Science* 1994;266(5193):1981–1986.
199. Eick D, Geyer M. The RNA polymerase II carboxy-terminal domain (CTD) code. *Chem Rev* 2013;113(11):8456–8490.
200. Eidahl JO, Crowe BL, North JA, et al. Structural basis for high-affinity binding of LEDGF PWWP to mononucleosomes. *Nucleic Acids Res* 2013;41(6):3924–3936.
201. Eijkelenboom AP, Lutzke RA, Boelens R, et al. The DNA-binding domain of HIV-1 integrase has an SH3-like fold. *Nat Struct Biol* 1995;2(9):807–810.
202. Emerman M, Guyader M, Montagnier L, et al. The specificity of the human immunodeficiency virus type 2 transactivator is different from that of human immunodeficiency virus type 1. *EMBO J* 1987;6(12):3755–3760.
203. Emery A, Swanstrom R. HIV-1: to splice or not to splice, that is the question. *Viruses* 2021;13(2):181.
204. Emiliani S, Mousnier A, Busschots K, et al. Integrase mutants defective for interaction with LEDGF/p75 are impaired in chromosome tethering and HIV-1 replication. *J Biol Chem* 2005;280(27):25517–25523.
205. Emu B, Fessel J, Schrader S, et al. Phase 3 study of ibalizumab for multidrug-resistant HIV-1. *N Engl J Med* 2018;379(7):645–654.
206. Endres MJ, Clapham PR, Marsh M, et al. CD4-independent infection by HIV-2 is mediated by fusin/CXCR4. *Cell* 1996;87(4):745–756.
207. Engelman A, Englund G, Orenstein JM, et al. Multiple effects of mutations in human immunodeficiency virus type 1 integrase on viral replication. *J Virol* 1995;69(5):2729–2736.
208. Engelman AN. Multifaceted HIV integrase functionalities and therapeutic strategies for their inhibition. *J Biol Chem* 2019;294(41):15137–15157.
209. Engelman AN. HIV capsid and integration targeting. *Viruses* 2021;13(1):125.
210. Exline CM, Feng Z, Stoltzfus CM. Negative and positive mRNA splicing elements act competitively to regulate human immunodeficiency virus type 1 vif gene expression. *J Virol* 2008;82(8):3921–3931.
211. Fabryova H, Strebel K. Vpr and its cellular interaction partners: R we there yet? *Cells* 2019;8(11):1310.
212. Fatkenheuer G, Pozniak AL, Johnson MA, et al. Efficacy of short-term monotherapy with maraviroc, a new CCR5 antagonist, in patients infected with HIV-1. *Nat Med* 2005;11(11):1170–1172.
213. Featherstone A, Aiken C. SERINC5 inhibits HIV-1 infectivity by altering the conformation of gp120 on HIV-1 particles. *J Virol* 2020;94(20)e00594-20.

214. Feinberg MB, Baltimore D, Frankel AD. The role of Tat in the human immunodeficiency virus life cycle indicates a primary effect on transcriptional elongation. *Proc Natl Acad Sci U S A* 1991;88(9):4045–4049.
215. Felber BK, Hadzopoulou-Cladaras M, Cladaras C, et al. rev protein of human immunodeficiency virus type 1 affects the stability and transport of the viral mRNA. *Proc Natl Acad Sci U S A* 1989;86(5):1495–1499.
216. Feng S, Holland EC. HIV-1 tat trans-activation requires the loop sequence within tar. *Nature* 1988;334(6178):165–167.
217. Finzi D, Hermankova M, Pierson T, et al. Identification of a reservoir for HIV-1 in patients on highly active antiretroviral therapy. *Science* 1997;278(5341):1295–1300.
218. Fischer U, Huber J, Boelens WC, et al. The HIV-1 Rev activation domain is a nuclear export signal that accesses an export pathway used by specific cellular RNAs. *Cell* 1995;82(3):475–483.
219. Fischer U, Meyer S, Teufel M, et al. Evidence that HIV-1 Rev directly promotes the nuclear export of unspliced RNA. *EMBO J* 1994;13(17):4105–4112.
220. Fisher AG, Ensoli B, Ivanoff L, et al. The *sor* gene of HIV-1 is required for efficient virus transmission in vitro. *Science* 1987;237(4817):888–893.
221. Fletcher AJ, Vaysburd M, Maslen S, et al. Trivalent RING assembly on retroviral capsids activates TRIM5 ubiquitination and innate immune signaling. *Cell Host Microbe* 2018;24(6):761–775 e6.
222. Flower TG, Takahashi Y, Hudait A, et al. A helical assembly of human ESCRT-I scaffolds reverse-topology membrane scission. *Nat Struct Mol Biol* 2020;27(6):570–580.
223. Folks TM, Justement J, Kinter A, et al. Cytokine-induced expression of HIV-1 in a chronically infected promonocyte cell line. *Science* 1987;238(4828):800–802.
224. Fornerod M, Ohno M, Yoshida M, et al. CRM1 is an export receptor for leucine-rich nuclear export signals. *Cell* 1997;90(6):1051–1060.
225. Francis AC, Marin M, Singh PK, et al. HIV-1 replication complexes accumulate in nuclear speckles and integrate into speckle-associated genomic domains. *Nat Commun* 2020;11(1):3505.
226. Francis AC, Melikyan GB. Live-cell imaging of early steps of single HIV-1 infection. *Viruses* 2018;10(5):275.
227. Francis AC, Melikyan GB. Single HIV-1 imaging reveals progression of infection through CA-dependent steps of docking at the nuclear pore, uncoating, and nuclear transport. *Cell Host Microbe* 2018;23(4):536–548 e6.
228. Franke EK, Yuan HE, Luban J. Specific incorporation of cyclophilin A into HIV-1 virions [see comments]. *Nature* 1994;372(6504):359–362.
229. Freed EO. HIV-1 Gag proteins: diverse functions in the virus life cycle. *Virology* 1998;251(1):1–15.
230. Freed EO. HIV-1 and the host cell: an intimate association. *Trends Microbiol* 2004;12(4):170–177.
231. Freed EO. HIV-1 assembly, release and maturation. *Nat Rev Microbiol* 2015;13(8):484–496.
232. Freed EO, Myers DJ, Risser R. Mutational analysis of the cleavage sequence of the human immunodeficiency virus type 1 envelope glycoprotein precursor gp160. *J Virol* 1989;63(11):4670–4675.
233. Freed EO, Myers DJ, Risser R. Characterization of the fusion domain of the human immunodeficiency virus type 1 envelope glycoprotein gp41. *Proc Natl Acad Sci U S A* 1990;87(12):4650–4654.
234. Freed EO, Orenstein JM, Buckler-White AJ, et al. Single amino acid changes in the human immunodeficiency virus type 1 matrix protein block virus particle production. *J Virol* 1994;68(8):5311–5320.
235. Fribourgh JL, Nguyen HC, Matreyek KA, et al. Structural insight into HIV-1 restriction by MxB. *Cell Host Microbe* 2014;16(5):627–638.
236. Friedman J, Cho WK, Chu CK, et al. Epigenetic silencing of HIV-1 by the histone H3 lysine 27 methyltransferase enhancer of Zeste 2. *J Virol* 2011;85(17):9078–9089.
237. Fritsch L, Robin P, Mathieu JR, et al. A subset of the histone H3 lysine 9 methyltransferases Suv39h1, G9a, GLP, and SETDB1 participate in a multimeric complex. *Mol Cell* 2010;37(1):46–56.
238. Fu W, Gorelick RJ, Rein A. Characterization of human immunodeficiency virus type 1 dimeric RNA from wild-type and protease-defective virions. *J Virol* 1994;68(8):5013–5018.
239. Fujii K, Munshi UM, Ablan SD, et al. Functional role of Alix in HIV-1 replication. *Virology* 2009;391(2):284–292.
240. Fujinaga K, Taube R, Wimmer J, et al. Interactions between human cyclin T, Tat, and the transactivation response element (TAR) are disrupted by a cysteine to tyrosine substitution found in mouse cyclin T. *Proc Natl Acad Sci U S A* 1999;96(4):1285–1290.
241. Fujiwara T, Mizuuchi K. Retroviral DNA integration: structure of an integration intermediate. *Cell* 1988;54(4):497–504.
242. Furuta RA, Wild CT, Weng Y, et al. Capture of an early fusion-active conformation of HIV-1 gp41 [published erratum appears in *Nat Struct Biol* 1998 Jul;5(7):612]. *Nat Struct Biol* 1998;5(4):276–279.
243. Gamble TR, Vajdos FF, Yoo S, et al. Crystal structure of human cyclophilin A bound to the amino-terminal domain of HIV-1 capsid. *Cell* 1996;87(7):1285–1294.
244. Ganser BK, Li S, Klishko VY, et al. Assembly and analysis of conical models for the HIV-1 core. *Science* 1999;283(5398):80–83.
245. Ganser-Pornillos BK, Chandrasekaran V, Pornillos O, et al. Hexagonal assembly of a restricting TRIM5alpha protein. *Proc Natl Acad Sci U S A* 2011;108(2):534–539.
246. Ganser-Pornillos BK, Pornillos O. Restriction of HIV-1 and other retroviruses by TRIM5. *Nat Rev Microbiol* 2019;17(9):546–556.
247. Gao F, Bailes E, Robertson DL, et al. Origin of HIV-1 in the chimpanzee *Pan troglodytes troglodytes*. *Nature* 1999;397(6718):436–441.
248. Gao F, Yue L, White AT, et al. Human infection by genetically diverse SIVSM-related HIV-2 in west Africa. *Nature* 1992;358(6386):495–499.
249. Garber ME, Wei P, KewalRamani VN, et al. The interaction between HIV-1 Tat and human cyclin T1 requires zinc and a critical cysteine residue that is not conserved in the murine CycT1 protein. *Genes Dev* 1998;12(22):3512–3527.
250. Garcia JV. In vivo platforms for analysis of HIV persistence and eradication. *J Clin Invest* 2016;126(2):424–431.
251. Garrus JE, von Schwedler UK, Pornillos OW, et al. Tsg101 and the vacuolar protein sorting pathway are essential for HIV-1 budding. *Cell* 2001;107(1):55–65.
252. Gautier VW, Gu L, O'Donoghue N, et al. In vitro nuclear interactome of the HIV-1 Tat protein. *Retrovirology* 2009;6:47.
253. Geijtenbeek TB, Kwon DS, Torensma R, et al. DC-SIGN, a dendritic cell-specific HIV-1-binding protein that enhances trans-infection of T cells. *Cell* 2000;100(5):587–597.
254. Gillgrass A, Wessels JM, Yang JX, et al. Advances in humanized mouse models to improve understanding of HIV-1 pathogenesis and immune responses. *Front Immunol* 2020;11:617516.
255. Gilmartin GM, Fleming ES, Oetjen J, et al. CPSF recognition of an HIV-1 mRNA 3′-processing enhancer: multiple sequence contacts involved in poly(A) site definition. *Genes Dev* 1995;9(1):72–83.
256. Gitti RK, Lee BM, Walker J, et al. Structure of the amino-terminal core domain of the HIV-1 capsid protein. *Science* 1996;273(5272):231–235.
257. Goldstone DC, Ennis-Adeniran V, Hedden JJ, et al. HIV-1 restriction factor SAMHD1 is a deoxynucleoside triphosphate triphosphohydrolase. *Nature* 2011;480(7377):379–382.
258. Goldstrohm AC, Greenleaf AL, Garcia-Blanco MA. Co-transcriptional splicing of pre-messenger RNAs: considerations for the mechanism of alternative splicing. *Gene* 2001;277(1–2):31–47.
259. Gonda MA, Wong-Staal F, Gallo RC, et al. Sequence homology and morphologic similarity of HTLV-III and visna virus, a pathogenic lentivirus. *Science* 1985;227(4683):173–177.
260. Gorelick RJ, Fu W, Gagliardi TD, et al. Characterization of the block in replication of nucleocapsid protein zinc finger mutants from moloney murine leukemia virus. *J Virol* 1999;73(10):8185–8195.
261. Gorelick RJ, Gagliardi TD, Bosche WJ, et al. Strict conservation of the retroviral nucleocapsid protein zinc finger is strongly influenced by its role in viral infection processes: characterization of HIV-1 particles containing mutant nucleocapsid zinc-coordinating sequences. *Virology* 1999;256(1):92–104.
262. Gorelick RJ, Henderson LE, Hanser JP, et al. Point mutants of Moloney murine leukemia virus that fail to package viral RNA: evidence for specific RNA recognition by a "zinc finger-like" protein sequence. *Proc Natl Acad Sci U S A* 1988;85(22):8420–8424.
263. Gorlich D, Mattaj IW. Nucleocytoplasmic transport. *Science* 1996;271(5255):1513–1518.
264. Gottlinger HG, Dorfman T, Sodroski JG, et al. Effect of mutations affecting the p6 gag protein on human immunodeficiency virus particle release. *Proc Natl Acad Sci U S A* 1991;88:3195–3199.
265. Goujon C, Moncorge O, Bauby H, et al. Human MX2 is an interferon-induced post-entry inhibitor of HIV-1 infection. *Nature* 2013;502(7472):559–562.
266. Greenwood EJD, Williamson JC, Sienkiewicz A, et al. Promiscuous targeting of cellular proteins by Vpr drives systems-level proteomic remodeling in HIV-1 infection. *Cell Rep* 2019;27(5):1579–1596 e7.
267. Gres AT, Kirby KA, KewalRamani VN, et al. STRUCTURAL VIROLOGY. X-ray crystal structures of native HIV-1 capsid protein reveal conformational variability. *Science* 2015;349(6243):99–103.
268. Gristick HB, von Boehmer L, West AP Jr, et al. Natively glycosylated HIV-1 Env structure reveals new mode for antibody recognition of the CD4-binding site. *Nat Struct Mol Biol* 2016;23(10):906–915.
268a. Grover JR, Yang Z, Leonhardt SA, et al. SERINC3 and SERINC5 inhibit HIV-1 infectivity by exposing phosphatidylserine on the viral surface. Cold Spring Harbor Retroviruses Meeting, abstract 10. 2021.
269. Grzesiek S, Bax A, Clore GM, et al. The solution structure of HIV-1 Nef reveals an unexpected fold and permits delineation of the binding surface for the SH3 domain of Hck tyrosine protein kinase. *Nat Struct Biol* 1996;3(4):340–345.
270. Grzesiek S, Bax A, Hu JS, et al. Refined solution structure and backbone dynamics of HIV-1 Nef. *Protein Sci* 1997;6(6):1248–1263.
271. Grzesiek S, Stahl SJ, Wingfield PT, et al. The CD4 determinant for downregulation by HIV-1 Nef directly binds to Nef. Mapping of the Nef binding surface by NMR. *Biochemistry* 1996;35(32):10256–10261.
272. Gupta RK, Mlcochova P, Pelchen-Matthews A, et al. Simian immunodeficiency virus envelope glycoprotein counteracts tetherin/BST-2/CD317 by intracellular sequestration. *Proc Natl Acad Sci U S A* 2009;106(49):20889–20894.
273. Haase AT. Early events in sexual transmission of HIV and SIV and opportunities for interventions. *Annu Rev Med* 2011;62:127–139.
274. Hammarskjold ML, Heimer J, Hammarskjold B, et al. Regulation of human immunodeficiency virus env expression by the rev gene product. *J Virol* 1989;63(5):1959–1966.
275. Han Y, Lassen K, Monie D, et al. Resting CD4+ T cells from human immunodeficiency virus type 1 (HIV-1)-infected individuals carry integrated HIV-1 genomes within actively transcribed host genes. *J Virol* 2004;78(12):6122–6133.
276. Hansen MMK, Wen WY, Ingerman E, et al. A post-transcriptional feedback mechanism for noise suppression and fate stabilization. *Cell* 2018;173(7):1609–1621 e15.
277. Hare S, Gupta SS, Valkov E, et al. Retroviral intasome assembly and inhibition of DNA strand transfer. *Nature* 2010;464(7286):232–236.
278. Hare S, Vos AM, Clayton RF, et al. Molecular mechanisms of retroviral integrase inhibition and the evolution of viral resistance. *Proc Natl Acad Sci U S A* 2010;107(46):20057–20062.
279. Hargittai MR, Gorelick RJ, Rouzina I, et al. Mechanistic insights into the kinetics of HIV-1 nucleocapsid protein-facilitated tRNA annealing to the primer binding site. *J Mol Biol* 2004;337(4):951–968.
280. Harlen KM, Trotta KL, Smith EE, et al. Comprehensive RNA polymerase II interactomes reveal distinct and varied roles for each phospho-CTD residue. *Cell Rep* 2016;15(10):2147–2158.
281. Harrich D, Garcia J, Wu F, et al. Role of SP1-binding domains in in vivo transcriptional regulation of the human immunodeficiency virus type 1 long terminal repeat. *J Virol* 1989;63(6):2585–2591.
282. Harris RS, Liddament MT. Retroviral restriction by APOBEC proteins. *Nat Rev Immunol* 2004;4(11):868–877.
283. Hart CE, Ou CY, Galphin JC, et al. Human chromosome 12 is required for elevated HIV-1 expression in human-hamster hybrid cells. *Science* 1989;246(4929):488–491.

284. Hatziioannou T, Evans DT. Animal models for HIV/AIDS research. *Nat Rev Microbiol* 2012;10(12):852–867.
285. Hatziioannou T, Perez-Caballero D, Cowan S, et al. Cyclophilin interactions with incoming human immunodeficiency virus type 1 capsids with opposing effects on infectivity in human cells. *J Virol* 2005;79(1):176–183.
286. Hatziioannou T, Perez-Caballero D, Yang A, et al. Retrovirus resistance factors Ref1 and Lv1 are species-specific variants of TRIM5alpha. *Proc Natl Acad Sci U S A* 2004;101(29):10774–10779.
287. Hayakawa J, Hsieh MM, Uchida N, et al. Busulfan produces efficient human cell engraftment in NOD/LtSz-Scid IL2Rgamma(null) mice. *Stem Cells* 2009;27(1):175–182.
288. Hazuda DJ, Felock P, Witmer M, et al. Inhibitors of strand transfer that prevent integration and inhibit HIV-1 replication in cells. *Science* 2000;287(5453):646–650.
289. Hazuda DJ, Young SD, Guare JP, et al. Integrase inhibitors and cellular immunity suppress retroviral replication in rhesus macaques. *Science* 2004;305(5683):528–532.
290. He N, Liu M, Hsu J, et al. HIV-1 Tat and host AFF4 recruit two transcription elongation factors into a bifunctional complex for coordinated activation of HIV-1 transcription. *Mol Cell* 2010;38(3):428–438.
291. Hemelaar J. The origin and diversity of the HIV-1 pandemic. *Trends Mol Med* 2012;18(3):182–192.
292. Heng X, Kharytonchyk S, Garcia EL, et al. Identification of a minimal region of the HIV-1 5′-leader required for RNA dimerization, NC binding, and packaging. *J Mol Biol* 2012;417(3):224–239.
293. Hermankova M, Ray SC, Ruff C, et al. HIV-1 drug resistance profiles in children and adults with viral load of <50 copies/ml receiving combination therapy. *JAMA* 2001;286(2):196–207.
294. Herrmann CH, Rice AP. Specific interaction of the human immunodeficiency virus Tat proteins with a cellular protein kinase. *Virology* 1993;197(2):601–608.
295. Herrmann CH, Rice AP. Lentivirus Tat proteins specifically associate with a cellular protein kinase, TAK, that hyperphosphorylates the carboxyl-terminal domain of the large subunit of RNA polymerase II: candidate for a Tat cofactor. *J Virol* 1995;69(3):1612–1620.
296. Hikichi Y, Freed EO. Maturation of HIV-1. *Science* 2021;373(6555):621–622.
297. Hill CP, Worthylake D, Bancroft DP, et al. Crystal structures of the trimeric human immunodeficiency virus type 1 matrix protein: implications for membrane association and assembly. *Proc Natl Acad Sci U S A* 1996;93(7):3099–3104.
298. Himathongkham S, Luciw PA. Restriction of HIV-1 (subtype B) replication at the entry step in rhesus macaque cells. *Virology* 1996;219(2):485–488.
299. Hirsch VM, Olmsted RA, Murphey-Corb M, et al. An African primate lentivirus (SIVsm) closely related to HIV-2. *Nature* 1989;339(6223):389–392.
300. Ho YC, Shan L, Hosmane NN, et al. Replication-competent noninduced proviruses in the latent reservoir increase barrier to HIV-1 cure. *Cell* 2013;155(3):540–551.
301. Hoffman TL, LaBranche CC, Zhang W, et al. Stable exposure of the coreceptor-binding site in a CD4-independent HIV- 1 envelope protein. *Proc Natl Acad Sci U S A* 1999;96(11):6359–6364.
302. Hofmann W, Schubert D, LaBonte J, et al. Species-specific, postentry barriers to primate immunodeficiency virus infection. *J Virol* 1999;73(12):10020–10028.
303. Holland SM, Ahmad N, Maitra RK, et al. Human immunodeficiency virus rev protein recognizes a target sequence in rev-responsive element RNA within the context of RNA secondary structure. *J Virol* 1990;64(12):5966–5975.
304. Holland SM, Chavez M, Gerstberger S, et al. A specific sequence with a bulged guanosine residue(s) in a stem-bulge-stem structure of Rev-responsive element RNA is required for trans activation by human immunodeficiency virus type 1 Rev. *J Virol* 1992;66(6):3699–3706.
305. Hrecka K, Gierszewska M, Srivastava S, et al. Lentiviral Vpr usurps Cul4-DDB1[VprBP] E3 ubiquitin ligase to modulate cell cycle. *Proc Natl Acad Sci U S A* 2007;104(28):11778–11783.
306. Hrecka K, Hao C, Gierszewska M, et al. Vpx relieves inhibition of HIV-1 infection of macrophages mediated by the SAMHD1 protein. *Nature* 2011;474(7353):658–661.
307. Hu WS, Hughes SH. HIV-1 reverse transcription. *Cold Spring Harb Perspect Med* 2012;2(10):a006882.
308. Hu WS, Rhodes T, Dang Q, et al. Retroviral recombination: review of genetic analyses. *Front Biosci* 2003;8:d143–d155.
309. Hu WS, Temin HM. Genetic consequences of packaging two RNA genomes in one retroviral particle: pseudodiploidy and high rate of genetic recombination. *Proc Natl Acad Sci U S A* 1990;87(4):1556–1560.
310. Huang H, Chopra R, Verdine GL, et al. Structure of a covalently trapped catalytic complex of HIV-1 reverse transcriptase: implications for drug resistance [see comments]. *Science* 1998;282(5394):1669–1675.
311. Huang H, Kong W, Jean M, et al. A CRISPR/Cas9 screen identifies the histone demethylase MINA53 as a novel HIV-1 latency-promoting gene (LPG). *Nucleic Acids Res* 2019;47(14):7333–7347.
312. Huang M, Orenstein JM, Martin MA, et al. p6^{Gag} is required for particle production from full-length human immunodeficiency virus type 1 molecular clones expressing protease. *J Virol* 1995;69(11):6810–6818.
313. Huang PT, Summers BJ, Xu C, et al. FEZ1 is recruited to a conserved cofactor site on capsid to promote HIV-1 trafficking. *Cell Rep* 2019;28(9):2373–2385 e7.
314. Huang XJ, Hope TJ, Bond BL, et al. Minimal Rev-response element for type 1 human immunodeficiency virus. *J Virol* 1991;65(4):2131–2134.
315. Huang Y, Paxton WA, Wolinsky SM, et al. The role of a mutant CCR5 allele in HIV-1 transmission and disease progression [see comments]. *Nat Med* 1996;2(11):1240–1243.
316. Huo L, Li D, Sun X, et al. Regulation of Tat acetylation and transactivation activity by the microtubule-associated deacetylase HDAC6. *J Biol Chem* 2011;286(11):9280–9286.
317. Hurley JH, Hanson PI. Membrane budding and scission by the ESCRT machinery: it's all in the neck. *Nat Rev Mol Cell Biol* 2010;11(8):556–566.
318. Huthoff H, Berkhout B. Two alternating structures of the HIV-1 leader RNA. *RNA* 2001;7(1):143–157.
319. Hwang CK, Svarovskaia ES, Pathak VK. Dynamic copy choice: steady state between murine leukemia virus polymerase and polymerase-dependent RNase H activity determines frequency of in vivo template switching. *Proc Natl Acad Sci U S A* 2001;98(21):12209–12214.
320. Iafrate AJ, Carl S, Bronson S, et al. Disrupting surfaces of nef required for downregulation of CD4 and for enhancement of virion infectivity attenuates simian immunodeficiency virus replication in vivo. *J Virol* 2000;74(21):9836–9844.
321. Igakura T, Stinchcombe JC, Goon PK, et al. Spread of HTLV-I between lymphocytes by virus-induced polarization of the cytoskeleton. *Science* 2003;299(5613):1713–1716.
322. Igarashi T, Endo Y, Englund G, et al. Emergence of a highly pathogenic simian/human immunodeficiency virus in a rhesus macaque treated with anti-CD8 mAb during a primary infection with a nonpathogenic virus. *Proc Natl Acad Sci U S A* 1999;96(24):14049–14054.
323. Imai K, Togami H, Okamoto T. Involvement of histone H3 lysine 9 (H3K9) methyltransferase G9a in the maintenance of HIV-1 latency and its reactivation by BIX01294. *J Biol Chem* 2010;285(22):16538–16545.
324. Inuzuka M, Hayakawa M, Ingi T. Serinc, an activity-regulated protein family, incorporates serine into membrane lipid synthesis. *J Biol Chem* 2005;280(42):35776–35783.
325. Ito M, Hiramatsu H, Kobayashi K, et al. NOD/SCID/gamma(c)(null) mouse: an excellent recipient mouse model for engraftment of human cells. *Blood* 2002;100(9):3175–3182.
326. Ivanchenko S, Godinez WJ, Lampe M, et al. Dynamics of HIV-1 assembly and release. *PLoS Pathog* 2009;5(11):e1000652.
327. Iwabu Y, Fujita H, Kinomoto M, et al. HIV-1 accessory protein Vpu internalizes cell-surface BST-2/tetherin through transmembrane interactions leading to lysosomes. *J Biol Chem* 2009;284(50):35060–35072.
328. Izaurralde E, Kutay U, von Kobbe C, et al. The asymmetric distribution of the constituents of the Ran system is essential for transport into and out of the nucleus. *EMBO J* 1997;16(21):6535–6547.
329. Jacks T, Power MD, Masiarz FR, et al. Characterization of ribosomal frameshifting in HIV-1 gag-pol expression. *Nature* 1988;331(6153):280–283.
330. Jacobo-Molina A, Clark AD Jr, Williams RL, et al. Crystals of a ternary complex of human immunodeficiency virus type 1 reverse transcriptase with a monoclonal antibody Fab fragment and double-stranded DNA diffract x-rays to 3.5-A resolution. *Proc Natl Acad Sci U S A* 1991;88(23):10895–10899.
331. Jacobo-Molina A, Ding J, Nanni RG, et al. Crystal structure of human immunodeficiency virus type 1 reverse transcriptase complexed with double-stranded DNA at 3.0 Å resolution shows bent DNA. *Proc Natl Acad Sci U S A* 1993;90(13):6320–6324.
332. Jager S, Cimermancic P, Gulbahce N, et al. Global landscape of HIV-human protein complexes. *Nature* 2011;481(7381):365–370.
333. Jager S, Kim DY, Hultquist JF, et al. Vif hijacks CBF-beta to degrade APOBEC3G and promote HIV-1 infection. *Nature* 2011;481(7381):371–375.
334. Javanbakht H, Halwani R, Cen S, et al. The interaction between HIV-1 Gag and human lysyl-tRNA synthetase during viral assembly. *J Biol Chem* 2003;278(30):27644–27651.
335. Jeronimo C, Collin P, Robert F. The RNA Polymerase II CTD: the increasing complexity of a low-complexity protein domain. *J Mol Biol* 2016;428(12):2607–2622.
336. Ji X, Tang C, Zhao Q, et al. Structural basis of cellular dNTP regulation by SAMHD1. *Proc Natl Acad Sci U S A* 2014;111(41):E4305–E4314.
337. Jia B, Serra-Moreno R, Neidermyer W, et al. Species-specific activity of SIV Nef and HIV-1 Vpu in overcoming restriction by tetherin/BST2. *PLoS Pathog* 2009;5(5):e1000429.
338. Jiang C, Lian X, Gao C, et al. Distinct viral reservoirs in individuals with spontaneous control of HIV-1. *Nature* 2020;585(7824):261–267.
339. Jiang G, Dandekar S. Targeting NF-kappaB signaling with protein kinase C agonists as an emerging strategy for combating HIV latency. *AIDS Res Hum Retroviruses* 2015;31(1):4–12.
340. Jiang G, Santos Rocha C, Hirao LA, et al. HIV exploits antiviral host innate GCN2-ATF4 signaling for establishing viral replication early in infection. *mBio* 2017;8(3):e01518-16.
341. Jimenez-Guardeno JM, Apolonia L, Betancor G, et al. Immunoproteasome activation enables human TRIM5alpha restriction of HIV-1. *Nat Microbiol* 2019;4(6):933–940.
342. Joag SV, Li Z, Foresman L, et al. Chimeric simian/human immunodeficiency virus that causes progressive loss of CD4+ T cells and AIDS in pig-tailed macaques. *J Virol* 1996;70(5):3189–3197.
343. Johnson DS, Bleck M, Simon SM. Timing of ESCRT-III protein recruitment and membrane scission during HIV-1 assembly. *Elife* 2018;7:e36221.
344. Johnson WE, Sawyer SL. Molecular evolution of the antiretroviral TRIM5 gene. *Immunogenetics* 2009;61(3):163–176.
345. Jolicoeur P, Baltimore D. Effect of Fv-1 gene product on proviral DNA formation and integration in cells infected with murine leukemia viruses. *Proc Natl Acad Sci U S A* 1976;73(7):2236–2240.
346. Jolly C, Booth NJ, Neil SJ. Cell-cell spread of human immunodeficiency virus type 1 overcomes tetherin/BST-2-mediated restriction in T cells. *J Virol* 2010;84(23):12185–12199.
347. Jolly C, Kashefi K, Hollinshead M, et al. HIV-1 cell to cell transfer across an Env-induced, actin-dependent synapse. *J Exp Med* 2004;199(2):283–293.
348. Jolly C, Sattentau QJ. Human immunodeficiency virus type 1 virological synapse formation in T cells requires lipid raft integrity. *J Virol* 2005;79(18):12088–12094.
349. Jonkers I, Lis JT. Getting up to speed with transcription elongation by RNA polymerase II. *Nat Rev Mol Cell Biol* 2015;16(3):167–177.
350. Jordan A, Bisgrove D, Verdin E. HIV reproducibly establishes a latent infection after acute infection of T cells in vitro. *EMBO J* 2003;22(8):1868–1877.
351. Joseph SB, Arrildt KT, Swanstrom AE, et al. Quantification of entry phenotypes of macrophage-tropic HIV-1 across a wide range of CD4 densities. *J Virol* 2014;88(4):1858–1869.
352. Jouvenet N, Simon SM, Bieniasz PD. Imaging the interaction of HIV-1 genomes and Gag during assembly of individual viral particles. *Proc Natl Acad Sci U S A* 2009;106(45):19114–19119.
353. Jouvenet N, Zhadina M, Bieniasz PD, et al. Dynamics of ESCRT protein recruitment during retroviral assembly. *Nat Cell Biol* 2011;13(4):394–401.

354. Jozwik IK, Passos DO, Lyumkis D. Structural biology of HIV integrase strand transfer inhibitors. *Trends Pharmacol Sci* 2020;41(9):611–626.

355. Julias JG, Hash D, Pathak VK. E⁻ vectors: development of novel self-inactivating and self-activating retroviral vectors for safer gene therapy. *J Virol* 1995;69(11):6839–6846.

356. Kaehlcke K, Dorr A, Hetzer-Egger C, et al. Acetylation of Tat defines a cyclinT1-independent step in HIV transactivation. *Mol Cell* 2003;12(1):167–176.

357. Kaletsky RL, Francica JR, Agrawal-Gamse C, et al. Tetherin-mediated restriction of filovirus budding is antagonized by the Ebola glycoprotein. *Proc Natl Acad Sci U S A* 2009;106(8):2886–2891.

358. Kalveram B, Lihoradova O, Ikegami T. NSs protein of rift valley fever virus promotes post-translational downregulation of the TFIIH subunit p62. *J Virol* 2011;85(13):6234–6243.

359. Kane M, Yadav SS, Bitzegeio J, et al. MX2 is an interferon-induced inhibitor of HIV-1 infection. *Nature* 2013;502(7472):563–566.

360. Kao SY, Calman AF, Luciw PA, et al. Anti-termination of transcription within the long terminal repeat of HIV-1 by tat gene product. *Nature* 1987;330(6147):489–493.

361. Kappes JC, Morrow CD, Lee SW, et al. Identification of a novel retroviral gene unique to human immunodeficiency virus type 2 and simian immunodeficiency virus SIVMAC. *J Virol* 1988;62(9):3501–3505.

362. Karin M. The regulation of AP-1 activity by mitogen-activated protein kinases. *J Biol Chem* 1995;270(28):16483–16486.

363. Karpel ME, Boutwell CL, Allen TM. BLT humanized mice as a small animal model of HIV infection. *Curr Opin Virol* 2015;13:75–80.

364. Katoh I, Yoshinaka Y, Rein A, et al. Murine leukemia virus maturation: protease region required for conversion from "immature" to "mature" core form and for virus infectivity. *Virology* 1985;145(2):280–292.

365. Katz RA, Merkel G, Kulkosky J, et al. The avian retroviral IN protein is both necessary and sufficient for integrative recombination in vitro. *Cell* 1990;63(1):87–95.

366. Kauder SE, Bosque A, Lindqvist A, et al. Epigenetic regulation of HIV-1 latency by cytosine methylation. *PLoS Pathog* 2009;5(6):e1000495.

367. Keane SC, Heng X, Lu K, et al. RNA structure. Structure of the HIV-1 RNA packaging signal. *Science* 2015;348(6237):917–921.

368. Kearney MF, Spindler J, Shao W, et al. Lack of detectable HIV-1 molecular evolution during suppressive antiretroviral therapy. *PLoS Pathog* 2014;10(3):e1004010.

369. Keele BF, Van Heuverswyn F, Li Y, et al. Chimpanzee reservoirs of pandemic and nonpandemic HIV-1. *Science* 2006;313(5786):523–526.

370. Keller PW, Adamson CS, Heymann JB, et al. HIV-1 maturation inhibitor bevirimat stabilizes the immature Gag lattice. *J Virol* 2011;85(4):1420–1428.

371. Kessl JJ, Kutluay SB, Townsend D, et al. HIV-1 integrase binds the viral RNA genome and is essential during virion morphogenesis. *Cell* 2016;166(5):1257–1268 e12.

372. Kestler HW, III, Ringler DJ, Mori K, et al. Importance of the *nef* gene for maintenance of high virus loads and for development of AIDS. *Cell* 1991;65(4):651–662.

373. Kharytonchyk S, Monti S, Smaldino PJ, et al. Transcriptional start site heterogeneity modulates the structure and function of the HIV-1 genome. *Proc Natl Acad Sci U S A* 2016;113(47):13378–13383.

374. Kiernan RE, Vanhulle C, Schiltz L, et al. HIV-1 tat transcriptional activity is regulated by acetylation. *EMBO J* 1999;18(21):6106–6118.

375. Kim K, Dauphin A, Komurlu S, et al. Cyclophilin A protects HIV-1 from restriction by human TRIM5alpha. *Nat Microbiol* 2019;4(12):2044–2051.

376. Kirchhoff F, Greenough TC, Brettler DB, et al. Brief report: absence of intact nef sequences in a long-term survivor with nonprogressive HIV-1 infection. *N Engl J Med* 1995;332(4):228–232.

377. Kjems J, Sharp PA. The basic domain of Rev from human immunodeficiency virus type 1 specifically blocks the entry of U4/U6.U5 small nuclear ribonucleoprotein in spliceosome assembly. *J Virol* 1993;67(8):4769–4776.

378. Klaver B, Berkhout B. Comparison of 5′ and 3′ long terminal repeat promoter function in human immunodeficiency virus. *J Virol* 1994;68(6):3830–3840.

379. Kleinpeter AB, Freed EO. HIV-1 maturation: lessons learned from inhibitors. *Viruses* 2020;12(9):940.

380. Klimkait T, Strebel K, Hoggan MD, et al. The human immunodeficiency virus type 1-specific protein *vpu* is required for efficient virus maturation and release. *J Virol* 1990;64(2):621–629.

381. Kluge SF, Mack K, Iyer SS, et al. Nef proteins of epidemic HIV-1 group O strains antagonize human tetherin. *Cell Host Microbe* 2014;16(5):639–650.

382. Koh Y, Matreyek KA, Engelman A. Differential sensitivities of retroviruses to integrase strand transfer inhibitors. *J Virol* 2011;85(7):3677–3682.

383. Kohlstaedt LA, Wang J, Friedman JM, et al. Crystal structure at 3.5 Å resolution of HIV-1 reverse transcriptase complexed with an inhibitor. *Science* 1992;256(5065):1783–1790.

384. Kolchinsky P, Mirzabekov T, Farzan M, et al. Adaptation of a CCR5-using, primary human immunodeficiency virus type 1 isolate for CD4-independent replication. *J Virol* 1999;73(10):8120–8126.

385. Kozak CA, Chakraborti A. Single amino acid changes in the murine leukemia virus capsid protein gene define the target of Fv1 resistance. *Virology* 1996;225(2):300–305.

386. Kramer JM. Regulation of cell differentiation and function by the euchromatin histone methyltransferases G9a and GLP. *Biochem Cell Biol* 2016;94(1):26–32.

387. Krasnopolsky S, Kuzmina A, Taube R. Genome-wide CRISPR knockout screen identifies ZNF304 as a silencer of HIV transcription that promotes viral latency. *PLoS Pathog* 2020;16(9):e1008834.

388. Kräusslich H-G. Human immunodeficiency virus proteinase dimer as component of the viral polyprotein prevents particle assembly and viral infectivity. *Proc Natl Acad Sci U S A* 1991;88(8):3213–3217.

389. Krishnan L, Li X, Naraharisetty HL, et al. Structure-based modeling of the functional HIV-1 intasome and its inhibition. *Proc Natl Acad Sci U S A* 2010;107(36):15910–15915.

390. Kuhl BD, Sloan RD, Donahue DA, et al. Tetherin restricts direct cell-to-cell infection of HIV-1. *Retrovirology* 2010;7:115.

391. Kupzig S, Korolchuk V, Rollason R, et al. Bst-2/HM1.24 is a raft-associated apical membrane protein with an unusual topology. *Traffic* 2003;4(10):694–709.

392. Kurt Yilmaz N, Swanstrom R, Schiffer CA. Improving viral protease inhibitors to counter drug resistance. *Trends Microbiol* 2016;24(7):547–557.

393. Kutluay SB, Emery A, Penumutchu SR, et al. Genome-wide analysis of heterogeneous nuclear ribonucleoprotein (hnRNP) binding to HIV-1 RNA reveals a key role for hnRNP H1 in alternative viral mRNA splicing. *J Virol* 2019;93(21):e01048-19.

394. Kutluay SB, Zang T, Blanco-Melo D, et al. Global changes in the RNA binding specificity of HIV-1 gag regulate virion genesis. *Cell* 2014;159(5):1096–1109.

395. Kwon DS, Gregorio G, Bitton N, et al. DC-SIGN-mediated internalization of HIV is required for trans-enhancement of T cell infection. *Immunity* 2002;16(1):135–144.

396. Kwon Y, Kaake RM, Echeverria I, et al. Structural basis of CD4 downregulation by HIV-1 Nef. *Nat Struct Mol Biol* 2020;27(9):822–828.

397. Kwong PD, Wyatt R, Robinson J, et al. Structure of an HIV gp120 envelope glycoprotein in complex with the CD4 receptor and a neutralizing human antibody [In Process Citation]. *Nature* 1998;393(6686):648–659.

398. LaBranche CC, Sauter MM, Haggarty BS, et al. A single amino acid change in the cytoplasmic domain of the simian immunodeficiency virus transmembrane molecule increases envelope glycoprotein expression on infected cells. *J Virol* 1995;69(9):5217–5227.

399. Lackner AA, Veazey RS. Current concepts in AIDS pathogenesis: insights from the SIV/macaque model. *Annu Rev Med* 2007;58:461–476.

400. Laguette N, Sobhian B, Casartelli N, et al. SAMHD1 is the dendritic- and myeloid-cell-specific HIV-1 restriction factor counteracted by Vpx. *Nature* 2011;474(7353):654–657.

401. Laird GM, Eisele EE, Rabi SA, et al. Rapid quantification of the latent reservoir for HIV-1 using a viral outgrowth assay. *PLoS Pathog* 2013;9(5):e1003398.

402. Lan P, Tonomura N, Shimizu A, et al. Reconstitution of a functional human immune system in immunodeficient mice through combined human fetal thymus/liver and CD34+ cell transplantation. *Blood* 2006;108(2):487–492.

403. Lang SM, Weeger M, Stahl-Hennig C, et al. Importance of vpr for infection of rhesus monkeys with simian immunodeficiency virus. *J Virol* 1993;67(2):902–912.

404. Langelier C, von Schwedler UK, Fisher RD, et al. Human ESCRT-II complex and its role in human immunodeficiency virus type 1 release. *J Virol* 2006;80(19):9465–9480.

405. Langelier CR, Sandrin V, Eckert DM, et al. Biochemical characterization of a recombinant TRIM5alpha protein that restricts human immunodeficiency virus type 1 replication. *J Virol* 2008;82(23):11682–11694.

406. Lapatto R, Blundell T, Hemmings A, et al. X-ray analysis of HIV-1 proteinase at 2.7 Å resolution confirms structural homology among retroviral enzymes. *Nature* 1989;342(6247):299–302.

407. Larsen KP, Mathiharan YK, Kappel K, et al. Architecture of an HIV-1 reverse transcriptase initiation complex. *Nature* 2018;557(7703):118-122.

408. Laspia MF, Rice AP, Mathews MB. HIV-1 Tat protein increases transcriptional initiation and stabilizes elongation. *Cell* 1989;59(2):283–292.

409. Lawrence SP, Elser SE, Torben W, et al. A tyrosine-based trafficking signal in the simian immunodeficiency virus envelope cytoplasmic domain is strongly selected for pathogenic SIV infection. *bioRxiv* 2021. doi: 10.1101/2021.03.31.437834.

410. Le Douce V, Colin L, Redel L, et al. LSD1 cooperates with CTIP2 to promote HIV-1 transcriptional silencing. *Nucleic Acids Res* 2012;40(5):1904–1915.

411. Le Rouzic E, Belaidouni N, Estrabaud E, et al. HIV1 Vpr arrests the cell cycle by recruiting DCAF1/VprBP, a receptor of the Cul4-DDB1 ubiquitin ligase. *Cell Cycle* 2007;6(2):182–188.

412. Lee CH, Saksela K, Mirza UA, et al. Crystal structure of the conserved core of HIV-1 Nef complexed with a Src family SH3 domain. *Cell* 1996;85(6):931–942.

413. Lee K, Ambrose Z, Martin TD, et al. Flexible use of nuclear import pathways by HIV-1. *Cell Host Microbe* 2010;7(3):221–233.

414. Lee SK, Potempa M, Swanstrom R. The choreography of HIV-1 proteolytic processing and virion assembly. *J Biol Chem* 2012;287(49):40867–40874.

415. Lemey P, Pybus OG, Wang B, et al. Tracing the origin and history of the HIV-2 epidemic. *Proc Natl Acad Sci U S A* 2003;100(11):6588–6592.

416. Leonard CK, Spellman MW, Riddle L, et al. Assignment of intrachain disulfide bonds and characterization of potential glycosylation sites of the type 1 recombinant human immunodeficiency virus envelope glycoprotein (gp120) expressed in Chinese hamster ovary cells. *J Biol Chem* 1990;265(18):10373–10382.

417. Leonard J, Parrott C, Buckler-White AJ, et al. The NF-kappa B binding sites in the human immunodeficiency virus type 1 long terminal repeat are not required for virus infectivity. *J Virol* 1989;63(11):4919–4924.

417a. Leonhardt SA, Purdy MD, Grover J, et al. Cryo-EM structures of the human HIV-1 restriction factor SERINC3 and function as a lipid flippase. Cold Spring Harbor Retroviruses Meeting, abstract 9. 2021.

418. Levin JG, Guo J, Rouzina I, et al. Nucleic acid chaperone activity of HIV-1 nucleocapsid protein: critical role in reverse transcription and molecular mechanism. *Prog Nucleic Acid Res Mol Biol* 2005;80:217–286.

419. Lewinski MK, Bisgrove D, Shinn P, et al. Genome-wide analysis of chromosomal features repressing human immunodeficiency virus transcription. *J Virol* 2005;79(11):6610–6619.

420. Li C, Burdick RC, Nagashima K, et al. HIV-1 cores retain their integrity until minutes before uncoating in the nucleus. *Proc Natl Acad Sci U S A* 2021;118(10):e2019467118.

421. Li C, Mousseau G, Valente ST. Tat inhibition by didehydro-Cortistatin A promotes heterochromatin formation at the HIV-1 long terminal repeat. *Epigenetics Chromatin* 2019;12(1):23.

422. Li D, Lopez A, Sandoval C, et al. HIV Vpr modulates the host DNA damage response at two independent steps to damage DNA and repress double-strand DNA break repair. *mBio* 2020;11(4):e00940-20.

423. Li F, Goila-Gaur R, Salzwedel K, et al. PA-457: a potent HIV inhibitor that disrupts core condensation by targeting a late step in Gag processing. *Proc Natl Acad Sci U S A* 2003;100(23):13555–13560.

424. Li M, Waheed AA, Yu J, et al. TIM-mediated inhibition of HIV-1 release is antagonized by Nef but potentiated by SERINC proteins. *Proc Natl Acad Sci U S A* 2019;116(12):5705–5714.

425. Li S, Hill CP, Sundquist WI, et al. Image reconstructions of helical assemblies of the HIV-1 CA protein. *Nature* 2000;407(6802):409–413.

426. Li X, Krishnan L, Cherepanov P, et al. Structural biology of retroviral DNA integration. *Virology* 2011;411(2):194–205.

427. Li X, Sodroski J. The TRIM5alpha B-box 2 domain promotes cooperative binding to the retroviral capsid by mediating higher-order self-association. *J Virol* 2008;82(23):11495–11502.

428. Li YL, Chandrasekaran V, Carter SD, et al. Primate TRIM5 proteins form hexagonal nets on HIV-1 capsids. *Elife* 2016;5:e16269.

429. Li Z, Hajian C, Greene WC. Identification of unrecognized host factors promoting HIV-1 latency. *PLoS Pathog* 2020;16(12):e1009055.

430. Li Z, Li W, Lu M, et al. Subnanometer structures of HIV-1 envelope trimers on aldrithiol-2-inactivated virus particles. *Nat Struct Mol Biol* 2020;27(8):726–734.

431. Lilly F. Susceptibility to two strains of Friend leukemia virus in mice. *Science* 1967;155(761):461–462.

432. Lim ES, Fregoso OI, McCoy CO, et al. The ability of primate lentiviruses to degrade the monocyte restriction factor SAMHD1 preceded the birth of the viral accessory protein Vpx. *Cell Host Microbe* 2012;11(2):194–204.

433. Lim ES, Malik HS, Emerman M. Ancient adaptive evolution of tetherin shaped the functions of Vpu and Nef in human immunodeficiency virus and primate lentiviruses. *J Virol* 2010;84(14):7124–7134.

434. Lindwasser OW, Smith WJ, Chaudhuri R, et al. A diacidic motif in human immunodeficiency virus type 1 Nef is a novel determinant of binding to AP-2. *J Virol* 2008;82(3):1166–1174.

435. Link JO, Rhee MS, Tse WC, et al. Clinical targeting of HIV capsid protein with a long-acting small molecule. *Nature* 2020;584(7822):614–618.

436. Lippincott-Schwartz J, Freed EO, van Engelenburg SB. A consensus view of ESCRT-mediated human immunodeficiency virus type 1 abscission. *Annu Rev Virol* 2017;4(1):309–325.

437. Liu J, Bartesaghi A, Borgnia MJ, et al. Molecular architecture of native HIV-1 gp120 trimers. *Nature* 2008;455(7209):109–113.

438. Liu L, Oliveira NM, Cheney KM, et al. A whole genome screen for HIV restriction factors. *Retrovirology* 2011;8:94.

439. Liu R, Paxton WA, Choe S, et al. Homozygous defect in HIV-1 coreceptor accounts for resistance of some multiply-exposed individuals to HIV-1 infection. *Cell* 1996;86(3):367–377.

440. Liu Z, Pan Q, Ding S, et al. The interferon-inducible MxB protein inhibits HIV-1 infection. *Cell Host Microbe* 2013;14(4):398–410.

441. Llano M, Saenz DT, Meehan A, et al. An essential role for LEDGF/p75 in HIV integration. *Science* 2006;314(5798):461–464.

442. Lodi PJ, Ernst JA, Kuszewski J, et al. Solution structure of the DNA binding domain of HIV-1 integrase. *Biochemistry* 1995;34(31):9826–9833.

443. Los Alamos National Lab (LANL). HIV circulating recombinant forms (CRFs) HIV sequence data base Web site. Published 2011. Updated Feb 3, 2011. http://www.hiv.lanl.gov/content/sequence/HIV/CRFs/CRFs.html. Accessed 2011.

444. Luban J, Bossolt KL, Franke EK, et al. Human immunodeficiency virus type 1 Gag protein binds to cyclophilins A and B. *Cell* 1993;73(6):1067–1078. https://www.hiv.lanl.gov/content/index

445. Lucic B, Chen HC, Kuzman M, et al. Spatially clustered loci with multiple enhancers are frequent targets of HIV-1 integration. *Nat Commun* 2019;10(1):4059.

446. Maddon PJ, Dalgleish AG, McDougal JS, et al. The T4 gene encodes the AIDS virus receptor and is expressed in the immune system and the brain. *Cell* 1986;47(3):333–348.

447. Madore SJ, Tiley LS, Malim MH, et al. Sequence requirements for Rev multimerization in vivo. *Virology* 1994;202(1):186–194.

448. Madsen JM, Stoltzfus CM. An exonic splicing silencer downstream of the 3′ splice site A2 is required for efficient human immunodeficiency virus type 1 replication. *J Virol* 2005;79(16):10478–10486.

449. Madsen JM, Stoltzfus CM. A suboptimal 5′ splice site downstream of HIV-1 splice site A1 is required for unspliced viral mRNA accumulation and efficient virus replication. *Retrovirology* 2006;3:10.

450. Maertens GN, Hare S, Cherepanov P. The mechanism of retroviral integration from X-ray structures of its key intermediates. *Nature* 2010;468(7321):326–329.

451. Magadan JG, Perez-Victoria FJ, Sougrat R, et al. Multilayered mechanism of CD4 downregulation by HIV-1 Vpu involving distinct ER retention and ERAD targeting steps. *PLoS Pathog* 2010;6(4):e1000869.

452. Maldarelli F, Martin MA, Strebel K. Identification of posttranscriptionally active inhibitory sequences in human immunodeficiency virus type 1 RNA: novel level of gene regulation. *J Virol* 1991;65(11):5732–5743.

453. Maldarelli F, Wu X, Su L, et al. HIV latency. Specific HIV integration sites are linked to clonal expansion and persistence of infected cells. *Science* 2014;345(6193):179–183.

454. Malikov V, da Silva ES, Jovasevic V, et al. HIV-1 capsids bind and exploit the kinesin-1 adaptor FEZ1 for inward movement to the nucleus. *Nat Commun* 2015;6:6660.

455. Malim MH, Bohnlein S, Hauber J, et al. Functional dissection of the HIV-1 Rev trans-activator—derivation of a trans-dominant repressor of Rev function. *Cell* 1989;58(1):205–214.

456. Malim MH, Hauber J, Le SY, et al. The HIV-1 rev trans-activator acts through a structured target sequence to activate nuclear export of unspliced viral mRNA. *Nature* 1989;338(6212):254–257.

457. Malim MH, Tiley LS, McCarn DF, et al. HIV-1 structural gene expression requires binding of the Rev trans-activator to its RNA target sequence. *Cell* 1990;60(4):675–683.

458. Mallery DL, Faysal KMR, Kleinpeter A, et al. Cellular IP6 levels limit HIV production while viruses that cannot efficiently package IP6 are attenuated for infection and replication. *Cell Rep* 2019;29(12):3983–3996 e4.

459. Mallery DL, Kleinpeter AB, Renner N, et al. A stable immature lattice packages IP6 for HIV capsid maturation. *Sci Adv* 2021;7(11):eabe4716.

460. Mallery DL, Marquez CL, McEwan WA, et al. IP6 is an HIV pocket factor that prevents capsid collapse and promotes DNA synthesis. *Elife* 2018;7:e35335.

461. Mamede JI, Cianci GC, Anderson MR, et al. Early cytoplasmic uncoating is associated with infectivity of HIV-1. *Proc Natl Acad Sci U S A* 2017;114(34):E7169–E7178.

462. Mandal D, Feng Z, Stoltzfus CM. Gag-processing defect of human immunodeficiency virus type 1 integrase E246 and G247 mutants is caused by activation of an overlapping 5′ splice site. *J Virol* 2008;82(3):1600–1604.

463. Mann DA, Mikaelian I, Zemmel RW, et al. A molecular rheostat. Co-operative rev binding to stem I of the rev response element modulates human immunodeficiency virus type 1 late gene expression. *J Mol Biol* 1994;241(2):193–207.

464. Mansky LM, Temin HM. Lower in vivo mutation rate of human immunodeficiency virus type 1 than that predicted from the fidelity of purified reverse transcriptase. *J Virol* 1995;69(8):5087–5094.

465. Marban C, Suzanne S, Dequiedt F, et al. Recruitment of chromatin-modifying enzymes by CTIP2 promotes HIV-1 transcriptional silencing. *EMBO J* 2007;26(2):412–423.

466. Margolis DM. Histone deacetylase inhibitors and HIV latency. *Curr Opin HIV AIDS* 2011;6(1):25–29.

467. Margottin F, Bour SP, Durand H, et al. A novel human WD protein, h-bTrCP, that interacts with HIV-1 Vpu connects CD4 to the ER degradation pathway through an F-box motif. *Mol Cell* 1998;1(4):565–574.

468. Marini A, Harper JM, Romerio F. An in vitro system to model the establishment and reactivation of HIV-1 latency. *J Immunol* 2008;181(11):7713–7720.

469. Marshall NF, Price DH. Purification of P-TEFb, a transcription factor required for the transition into productive elongation. *J Biol Chem* 1995;270(21):12335–12338.

470. Martin KA, Wyatt R, Farzan M, et al. CD4-independent binding of SIV gp120 to rhesus CCR5. *Science* 1997;278(5342):1470–1473.

471. Martin-Serrano J, Yaravoy A, Perez-Caballero D, et al. Divergent retroviral late-budding domains recruit vacuolar protein sorting factors by using alternative adaptor proteins. *Proc Natl Acad Sci U S A* 2003;100:12414–12419.

472. Martin-Serrano J, Zang T, Bieniasz PD. HIV-1 and Ebola virus encode small peptide motifs that recruit Tsg101 to sites of particle assembly to facilitate egress. *Nat Med* 2001;7:1313–1319.

473. Massanella M, Puthanakit T, Leyre L, et al. Continuous prophylactic antiretrovirals/antiretroviral therapy since birth reduces seeding and persistence of the viral reservoir in children vertically infected with human immunodeficiency virus. *Clin Infect Dis* 2021;73(3):427–438.

474. Massiah MA, Starich MR, Paschall C, et al. Three-dimensional structure of the human immunodeficiency virus type 1 matrix protein. *J Mol Biol* 1994;244(2):198–223.

475. Masuda T, Sato Y, Huang YL, et al. Fate of HIV-1 cDNA intermediates during reverse transcription is dictated by transcription initiation site of virus genomic RNA. *Sci Rep* 2015;5:17680.

476. Mattei S, Glass B, Hagen WJ, et al. The structure and flexibility of conical HIV-1 capsids determined within intact virions. *Science* 2016;354(6318):1434–1437.

477. Mbonye U, Karn J. The molecular basis for human immunodeficiency virus latency. *Annu Rev Virol* 2017;4(1):261–285.

478. McCullough J, Frost A, Sundquist WI. Structures, functions, and dynamics of ESCRT-III/Vps4 membrane remodeling and fission complexes. *Annu Rev Cell Dev Biol* 2018;34:85–109.

479. McCune JM, Rabin LB, Feinberg MB, et al. Endoproteolytic cleavage of gp160 is required for the activation of human immunodeficiency virus. *Cell* 1988;53(1):55–67.

480. McCutchan FE. Understanding the genetic diversity of HIV-1. *AIDS* 2000;14 (Suppl 3):S31–S44.

481. McDonald D, Vodicka MA, Lucero G, et al. Visualization of the intracellular behavior of HIV in living cells. *J Cell Biol* 2002;159(3):441–452.

482. McMahon D, Jones J, Wiegand A, et al. Short-course raltegravir intensification does not reduce persistent low-level viremia in patients with HIV-1 suppression during receipt of combination antiretroviral therapy. *Clin Infect Dis* 2010;50(6):912–919.

483. McNamara RP, Costantini LM, Myers TA, et al. Nef secretion into extracellular vesicles or exosomes is conserved across human and simian immunodeficiency viruses. *mBio* 2018;9(1):e02344-17.

484. McNatt MW, Zang T, Hatziioannou T, et al. Species-specific activity of HIV-1 Vpu and positive selection of tetherin transmembrane domain variants. *PLoS Pathog* 2009;5(2):e1000300.

485. Mediouni S, Chinthalapudi K, Ekka MK, et al. Didehydro-Cortistatin A inhibits HIV-1 by specifically binding to the unstructured basic region of Tat. *MBio* 2019;10(1):e02662-18.

486. Meyer BE, Malim MH. The HIV-1 Rev trans-activator shuttles between the nucleus and the cytoplasm. *Genes Dev* 1994;8(13):1538–1547.

487. Meyerhans A, Cheynier R, Albert J, et al. Temporal fluctuations in HIV quasispecies in vivo are not reflected by sequential HIV isolations. *Cell* 1989;58(5):901–910.

488. Mitchell RS, Beitzel BF, Schroder AR, et al. Retroviral DNA integration: ASLV, HIV, and MLV show distinct target site preferences. *PLoS Biol* 2004;2(8):E234.

489. Centers for Disease Control (CDC). Pneumocystis pneumonia—Los Angeles. *Morb Mortal Wkly Rep* 1981;30(21):250–252.

490. Moeser M, Nielsen JR, Joseph SB. Macrophage tropism in pathogenic HIV-1 and SIV infections. *Viruses* 2020;12(10):1077.

491. Momany C, Kovari LC, Prongay AJ, et al. Crystal structure of dimeric HIV-1 capsid protein. *Nat Struct Biol* 1996;3(9):763–770.

492. Monroe N, Han H, Shen PS, et al. Structural basis of protein translocation by the Vps4-Vta1 AAA ATPase. *Elife* 2017;6:e24487.

493. Montagnier L, Chermann JC, Barré-Sinoussi F, et al. A new human T-lymphotropic retrovirus: characterization and possible role in lymphadenopathy and acquired immune deficiency syndromes. In: Gallo RC, Essex ME, Gross L, eds. *Human T-Cell Leukemia/Lymphoma Virus The Family of Human T-Lymphotropic Retroviruses: Their Role in Malignancies and Association with AIDS.* Cold Spring Harbor, NY: Cold Spring Harbor Laboratory; 1984:363–379.

494. Moore JP, Kuritzkes DR. A piece de resistance: how HIV-1 escapes small molecule CCR5 inhibitors. *Curr Opin HIV AIDS* 2009;4(2):118–124.

495. Moore LD, Le T, Fan G. DNA methylation and its basic function. *Neuropsychopharmacology* 2013;38(1):23–38.

496. Morellet N, Bouaziz S, Petitjean P, et al. NMR structure of the HIV-1 regulatory protein VPR. *J Mol Biol* 2003;327(1):215–227.

497. Morellet N, Jullian N, De Rocquigny H, et al. Determination of the structure of the nucleocapsid protein NCp7 from the human immunodeficiency virus type 1 by 1H NMR. *EMBO J* 1992;11(8):3059–3065.

498. Morita E, Sandrin V, Chung HY, et al. Human ESCRT and ALIX proteins interact with proteins of the midbody and function in cytokinesis. *EMBO J* 2007;26(19):4215–4227.

499. Morita E, Sandrin V, McCullough J, et al. ESCRT-III protein requirements for HIV-1 budding. *Cell Host Microbe* 2011;9(3):235–242.

500. Moron-Lopez S, Telwatte S, Sarabia I, et al. Human splice factors contribute to latent HIV infection in primary cell models and blood CD4+ T cells from ART-treated individuals. *PLoS Pathog* 2020;16(11):e1009060.

501. Morris KL, Buffalo CZ, Sturzel CM, et al. HIV-1 Nefs are cargo-sensitive AP-1 trimerization switches in tetherin downregulation. *Cell* 2018;174(3):659–671 e14.

502. Mosier DE, Gulizia RJ, Baird SM, et al. Human immunodeficiency virus infection of human-PBL-SCID mice. *Science* 1991;251(4995):791–794.

503. Mousseau G, Clementz MA, Bakeman WN, et al. An analog of the natural steroidal alkaloid cortistatin A potently suppresses Tat-dependent HIV transcription. *Cell Host Microbe* 2012;12(1):97–108.

504. Mousseau G, Kessing CF, Fromentin R, et al. The Tat inhibitor didehydro-cortistatin A prevents HIV-1 reactivation from latency. *MBio* 2015;6(4):e00465.

505. Mucksch F, Citir M, Luchtenborg C, et al. Quantification of phosphoinositides reveals strong enrichment of PIP2 in HIV-1 compared to producer cell membranes. *Sci Rep* 2019;9(1):17661.

506. Mucksch F, Laketa V, Muller B, et al. Synchronized HIV assembly by tunable PIP2 changes reveals PIP2 requirement for stable Gag anchoring. *Elife* 2017;6:e25287.

507. Mujtaba S, He Y, Zeng L, et al. Structural basis of lysine-acetylated HIV-1 Tat recognition by PCAF bromodomain. *Mol Cell* 2002;9(3):575–586.

508. Munch J, Stolte N, Fuchs D, et al. Efficient class I major histocompatibility complex down-regulation by simian immunodeficiency virus Nef is associated with a strong selective advantage in infected rhesus macaques. *J Virol* 2001;75(21):10532–10536.

509. Muniz L, Egloff S, Ughy B, et al. Controlling cellular P-TEFb activity by the HIV-1 transcriptional transactivator Tat. *PLoS Pathog* 2010;6(10):e1001152.

510. Munro JB, Gorman J, Ma X, et al. Conformational dynamics of single HIV-1 envelope trimers on the surface of native virions. *Science* 2014;346(6210):759–763.

511. Murakami T, Ablan S, Freed EO, et al. Regulation of human immunodeficiency virus type 1 Env-mediated membrane fusion by viral protease activity. *J Virol* 2004;78(2):1026–1031.

512. Murakami T, Freed EO. The long cytoplasmic tail of gp41 is required in a cell type-dependent manner for HIV-1 envelope glycoprotein incorporation into virions. *Proc Natl Acad Sci U S A* 2000;97(1):343–348.

513. Muriaux D, Mirro J, Harvin D, et al. RNA is a structural element in retrovirus particles. *Proc Natl Acad Sci U S A* 2001;98(9):5246–5251.

514. Murphy RE, Samal AB, Vlach J, et al. Solution structure and membrane interaction of the cytoplasmic tail of HIV-1 gp41 protein. *Structure* 2017;25(11):1708–1718 e5.

515. Murrell B, Vollbrecht T, Guatelli J, et al. The evolutionary histories of antiretroviral proteins SERINC3 and SERINC5 do not support an evolutionary arms race in primates. *J Virol* 2016;90(18):8085–8089.

516. Nabel G, Baltimore D. An inducible transcription factor activates expression of human immunodeficiency virus in T cells. *Nature* 1987;326(6114):711–713.

517. Nakayama EE, Miyoshi H, Nagai Y, et al. A specific region of 37 amino acid residues in the SPRY (B30.2) domain of African green monkey TRIM5alpha determines species-specific restriction of simian immunodeficiency virus SIVmac infection. *J Virol* 2005;79(14):8870–8877.

518. Namikawa R, Kaneshima H, Lieberman M, et al. Infection of the SCID-hu mouse by HIV-1. *Science* 1988;242(4886):1684–1686.

519. Navia MA, Fitzgerald PMD, McKeever BM, et al. Three-dimensional structure of aspartyl protease from human immunodeficiency virus HIV-1. *Nature* 1989;337(6208):615–620.

520. Neil SJ, Zang T, Bieniasz PD. Tetherin inhibits retrovirus release and is antagonized by HIV-1 Vpu. *Nature* 2008;451(7177):425–430.

521. Nepveu-Traversy ME, Berube J, Berthoux L. TRIM5alpha and TRIMCyp form apparent hexamers and their multimeric state is not affected by exposure to restriction-sensitive viruses or by treatment with pharmacological inhibitors. *Retrovirology* 2009;6:100.

522. Nguyen K, Das B, Dobrowolski C, et al. Multiple histone lysine methyltransferases are required for the establishment and maintenance of HIV-1 latency. *MBio* 2017;8(1):e00133-17.

523. Nigg EA. Nucleocytoplasmic transport: signals, mechanisms and regulation. *Nature* 1997;386(6627):779–787.

524. Nisole S, Lynch C, Stoye JP, et al. A Trim5-cyclophilin A fusion protein found in owl monkey kidney cells can restrict HIV-1. *Proc Natl Acad Sci U S A* 2004;101(36):13324–13328.

525. Nowotny M, Gaidamakov SA, Ghirlando R, et al. Structure of human RNase H1 complexed with an RNA/DNA hybrid: insight into HIV reverse transcription. *Mol Cell* 2007;28(2):264–276.

526. Ohno H, Aguilar RC, Fournier MC, et al. Interaction of endocytic signals from the HIV-1 envelope glycoprotein complex with members of the adaptor medium chain family. *Virology* 1997;238(2):305–315.

527. Ohtomo T, Sugamata Y, Ozaki Y, et al. Molecular cloning and characterization of a surface antigen preferentially overexpressed on multiple myeloma cells. *Biochem Biophys Res Commun* 1999;258(3):583–591.

528. Olson ME, Harris RS, Harki DA. APOBEC enzymes as targets for virus and cancer therapy. *Cell Chem Biol* 2018;25(1):36–49.

529. Omondi FH, Chandrarathna S, Mujib S, et al. HIV subtype and Nef-mediated immune evasion function correlate with viral reservoir size in early-treated individuals. *J Virol* 2019;93(6):e01832-18.

530. Ono A, Ablan SD, Lockett SJ, et al. Phosphatidylinositol (4,5) bisphosphate regulates HIV-1 Gag targeting to the plasma membrane. *Proc Natl Acad Sci U S A* 2004;101(41):14889–14894.

531. Ono A, Freed EO. Role of lipid rafts in virus replication. *Adv Virus Res* 2005;64:311–358.

532. Ott M, Emiliani S, Van Lint C, et al. Immune hyperactivation of HIV-1-infected T cells mediated by Tat and the CD28 pathway. *Science* 1997;275(5305):1481–1485.

533. Ott M, Geyer M, Zhou Q. The control of HIV transcription: keeping RNA polymerase II on track. *Cell Host Microbe* 2011;10(5):426–435.

534. Ozorowski G, Pallesen J, de Val N, et al. Open and closed structures reveal allostery and pliability in the HIV-1 envelope spike. *Nature* 2017;547(7663):360–363.

535. Pagans S, Kauder SE, Kaehlcke K, et al. The cellular lysine methyltransferase Set7/9-KMT7 binds HIV-1 TAR RNA, monomethylates the viral transactivator Tat, and enhances HIV transcription. *Cell Host Microbe* 2010;7(3):234–244.

536. Palmer S, Maldarelli F, Wiegand A, et al. Low-level viremia persists for at least 7 years in patients on suppressive antiretroviral therapy. *Proc Natl Acad Sci U S A* 2008;105(10):3879–3884.

537. Pancera M, Zhou T, Druz A, et al. Structure and immune recognition of trimeric prefusion HIV-1 Env. *Nature* 2014;514(7523):455–461.

538. Pandrea I, Apetrei C. Where the wild things are: pathogenesis of SIV infection in African nonhuman primate hosts. *Curr HIV/AIDS Rep* 2010;7(1):28–36.

539. Panganiban AT, Temin HM. The retrovirus pol gene encodes a product required for DNA integration: identification of a retrovirus int locus. *Proc Natl Acad Sci U S A* 1984;81(24):7885–7889.

540. Parra J, Portilla J, Pulido F, et al. Clinical utility of maraviroc. *Clin Drug Investig* 2011;31(8):527–542.

541. Passos DO, Li M, Yang R, et al. Cryo-EM structures and atomic model of the HIV-1 strand transfer complex intasome. *Science* 2017;355(6320):89–92.

542. Pathak VK, Hu W-S. "Might as Well Jump!" Template switching by retroviral reverse transcriptase, defective genome formation, and recombination. *Semin Virol* 1997;8:141–150.

543. Pathak VK, Temin HM. Broad spectrum of in vivo forward mutations, hypermutations, and mutational hotspots in a retroviral shuttle vector after a single replication cycle: deletions and deletions with insertions. *Proc Natl Acad Sci U S A* 1990;87(16):6024–6028.

544. Pathak VK, Temin HM. Broad spectrum of in vivo forward mutations, hypermutations, and mutational hotspots in a retroviral shuttle vector after a single replication cycle: substitutions, frameshifts, and hypermutations. *Proc Natl Acad Sci U S A* 1990;87(16):6019–6023.

545. Paxton W, Connor RI, Landau NR. Incorporation of Vpr into human immunodeficiency virus type 1 virions: requirement for the p6 region of gag and mutational analysis. *J Virol* 1993;67:7229–7237.

546. Pearson T, Greiner DL, Shultz LD. Creation of "humanized" mice to study human immunity. *Curr Protoc Immunol* 2008;Chapter 15:Unit 15.21.

547. Peeters M. Recombinant HIV sequences: their role in the global epidemic. In: Kuiken C, Foley B, Hahn B, et al., eds. *HIV Sequence Compendium 2000*. Los Alamos, New Mexico: Los Alamos National Laboratory; 2000:39–54.

548. Peng J, Zhu Y, Milton JT, et al. Identification of multiple cyclin subunits of human P-TEFb. *Genes Dev* 1998;12(5):755–762.

549. Perelson AS, Neumann AU, Markowitz M, et al. HIV-1 dynamics in vivo: virion clearance rate, infected cell life-span, and viral generation time. *Science* 1996;271(5255):1582–1586.

550. Perez-Caballero D, Hatziioannou T, Yang A, et al. Human tripartite motif 5alpha domains responsible for retrovirus restriction activity and specificity. *J Virol* 2005;79(14):8969–8978.

551. Pertel T, Hausmann S, Morger D, et al. TRIM5 is an innate immune sensor for the retrovirus capsid lattice. *Nature* 2011;472(7343):361–365.

552. Peterlin BM, Price DH. Controlling the elongation phase of transcription with P-TEFb. *Mol Cell* 2006;23(3):297–305.

553. Pettit SC, Everitt LE, Choudhury S, et al. Initial cleavage of the human immunodeficiency virus type 1 GagPol precursor by its activated protease occurs by an intramolecular mechanism. *J Virol* 2004;78(16):8477–8485.

554. Pezeshkian N, Groves NS, van Engelenburg SB. Single-molecule imaging of HIV-1 envelope glycoprotein dynamics and Gag lattice association exposes determinants responsible for virus incorporation. *Proc Natl Acad Sci U S A* 2019;116(50):25269–25277.

555. Pham VV, Salguero C, Khan SN, et al. HIV-1 Tat interactions with cellular 7SK and viral TAR RNAs identifies dual structural mimicry. *Nat Commun* 2018;9(1):4266.

556. Phatnani HP, Greenleaf AL. Phosphorylation and functions of the RNA polymerase II CTD. *Genes Dev* 2006;20(21):2922–2936.

557. Piai A, Fu Q, Sharp AK, et al. NMR model of the entire membrane-interacting region of the HIV-1 fusion protein and its perturbation of membrane morphology. *J Am Chem Soc* 2021;143(17):6609–6615.

558. Pincus T, Hartley JW, Rowe WP. A major genetic locus affecting resistance to infection with murine leukemia viruses. I. Tissue culture studies of naturally occurring viruses. *J Exp Med* 1971;133(6):1219–1233.

559. Pollard VW, Malim MH. The HIV-1 Rev protein. *Annu Rev Microbiol* 1998;52:491–532.

560. Pollpeter D, Parsons M, Sobala AE, et al. Deep sequencing of HIV-1 reverse transcripts reveals the multifaceted antiviral functions of APOBEC3G. *Nat Microbiol* 2018;3(2):220–233.

561. Pond SJ, Ridgeway WK, Robertson R, et al. HIV-1 Rev protein assembles on viral RNA one molecule at a time. *Proc Natl Acad Sci U S A* 2009;106(5):1404–1408.

562. Poon B, Grovit-Ferbas K, Stewart SA, et al. Cell cycle arrest by Vpr in HIV-1 virions and insensitivity to antiretroviral agents. *Science* 1998;281(5374):266–269.

563. Popov S, Popova E, Inoue M, et al. Human immunodeficiency virus type 1 Gag engages the Bro1 domain of ALIX/AIP1 through the nucleocapsid. *J Virol* 2008;82(3):1389–1398.

564. Popov S, Popova E, Inoue M, et al. Divergent Bro1 domains share the capacity to bind human immunodeficiency virus type 1 nucleocapsid and to enhance virus-like particle production. *J Virol* 2009;83(14):7185–7193.

565. Popovic M, Sarngadharan MG, Read E, et al. Detection, isolation, and continuous production of cytopathic retroviruses (HTLV-III) from patients with AIDS and pre-AIDS. *Science* 1984;224(4648):497–500.

566. Pornillos O, Ganser-Pornillos BK. Maturation of retroviruses. *Curr Opin Virol* 2019;36:47–55.

567. Pornillos O, Ganser-Pornillos BK, Kelly BN, et al. X-ray structures of the hexameric building block of the HIV capsid. *Cell* 2009;137(7):1282–1292.

568. Pornillos O, Ganser-Pornillos BK, Yeager M. Atomic-level modelling of the HIV capsid. *Nature* 2011;469(7330):424–427.

569. Porrua O, Libri D. Transcription termination and the control of the transcriptome: why, where and how to stop. *Nat Rev Mol Cell Biol* 2015;16(3):190–202.

570. Portz B, Lu F, Gibbs EB, et al. Structural heterogeneity in the intrinsically disordered RNA polymerase II C-terminal domain. *Nat Commun* 2017;8:15231.

571. Potempa M, Lee SK, Kurt Yilmaz N, et al. HIV-1 protease uses bi-specific S2/S2′ subsites to optimize cleavage of two classes of target sites. *J Mol Biol* 2018;430(24):5182–5195.

572. Potempa S, Picard L, Reeves JD, et al. CD4-independent infection by human immunodeficiency virus type 2 strain ROD/B: the role of the N-terminal domain of CXCR-4 in fusion and entry. *J Virol* 1997;71(6):4419–4424.

573. Prabu-Jeyabalan M, Nalivaika E, Schiffer CA. Substrate shape determines specificity of recognition for HIV-1 protease: analysis of crystal structures of six substrate complexes. *Structure* 2002;10(3):369–381.

574. Preston BD, Poiesz BJ, Loeb LA. Fidelity of HIV-1 reverse transcriptase. *Science* 1988;242(4882):1168–1171.

575. Price DH. P-TEFb, a cyclin-dependent kinase controlling elongation by RNA polymerase II. *Mol Cell Biol* 2000;20(8):2629–2634.

576. Purcell DF, Martin MA. Alternative splicing of human immunodeficiency virus type 1 mRNA modulates viral protein expression, replication, and infectivity. *J Virol* 1993;67(11):6365–6378.

577. Pye VE, Rosa A, Bertelli C, et al. A bipartite structural organization defines the SERINC family of HIV-1 restriction factors. *Nat Struct Mol Biol* 2020;27(1):78–83.

578. Qi M, Williams JA, Chu H, et al. Rab11-FIP1C and Rab14 direct plasma membrane sorting and particle incorporation of the HIV-1 envelope glycoprotein complex. *PLoS Pathog* 2013;9(4):e1003278.

579. Qu K, Ke Z, Zila V, et al. Maturation of the matrix and viral membrane of HIV-1. *Science* 2021;373(6555):700–704.

580. Quinn TP, Grandgenett DP. Genetic evidence that the avian retrovirus DNA endonuclease domain of pol is necessary for viral integration. *J Virol* 1988;62(7):2307–2312.

581. Ramirez PW, Sharma S, Singh R, et al. Plasma membrane-associated restriction factors and their counteraction by HIV-1 accessory proteins. *Cells* 2019;8(9):1020.

582. Rasmussen TA, Lewin SR. Shocking HIV out of hiding: where are we with clinical trials of latency reversing agents? *Curr Opin HIV AIDS* 2016;11(4):394–401.

583. Rathore A, Iketani S, Wang P, et al. CRISPR-based gene knockout screens reveal deubiquitinases involved in HIV-1 latency in two Jurkat cell models. *Sci Rep* 2020;10(1):5350.

584. Ratner L, Haseltine W, Patarca R, et al. Complete nucleotide sequence of the AIDS virus, HTLV-III. *Nature* 1985;313(6000):277–284.

585. Rawson JMO, Nikolaitchik OA, Keele BF, et al. Recombination is required for efficient HIV-1 replication and the maintenance of viral genome integrity. *Nucleic Acids Res* 2018;46(20):10535–10545.

586. Ray RM, Morris KV. Long non-coding RNAs mechanisms of action in HIV-1 modulation and the identification of novel therapeutic targets. *Noncoding RNA* 2020;6(1):12.

587. Razooky BS, Pai A, Aull K, et al. A hardwired HIV latency program. *Cell* 2015;160(5):990–1001.

588. Rea S, Eisenhaber F, O'Carroll D, et al. Regulation of chromatin structure by site-specific histone H3 methyltransferases. *Nature* 2000;406(6796):593–599.

589. Rebensburg SV, Wei G, Larue RC, et al. Sec24C is an HIV-1 host dependency factor crucial for virus replication. *Nat Microbiol* 2021;6(4):435–444.

590. Reimann KA, Li JT, Veazey R, et al. A chimeric simian/human immunodeficiency virus expressing a primary patient human immunodeficiency virus type 1 isolate env causes an AIDS-like disease after in vivo passage in rhesus monkeys. *J Virol* 1996;70(10):6922–6928.

591. Rein A. RNA packaging in HIV. *Trends Microbiol* 2019;27(8):715–723.

592. Ren J, Bird LE, Chamberlain PP, et al. Structure of HIV-2 reverse transcriptase at 2.35-A resolution and the mechanism of resistance to non-nucleoside inhibitors. *Proc Natl Acad Sci U S A* 2002;99(22):14410–14415.

593. Renner N, Mallery DL, Faysal KMR, et al. A lysine ring in HIV capsid pores coordinates IP6 to drive mature capsid assembly. *PLoS Pathog* 2021;17(2):e1009164.

594. Reymond A, Meroni G, Fantozzi A, et al. The tripartite motif family identifies cell compartments. *EMBO J* 2001;20(9):2140–2151.

595. Rice GI, Bond J, Asipu A, et al. Mutations involved in Aicardi-Goutieres syndrome implicate SAMHD1 as regulator of the innate immune response. *Nat Genet* 2009;41(7):829–832.

596. Rice P, Mizuuchi K. Structure of the bacteriophage Mu transposase core: a common structural motif for DNA transposition and retroviral integration. *Cell* 1995;82(2):209–220.

597. Richards J, McCallister S. Maturation inhibitors as new antiretroviral agents. *J HIV Ther* 2008;13(4):79–82.

598. Rimsky LT, Shugars DC, Matthews TJ. Determinants of human immunodeficiency virus type 1 resistance to gp41-derived inhibitory peptides. *J Virol* 1998;72(2):986–993.

599. Roberts JD, Bebenek K, Kunkel TA. The accuracy of reverse transcriptase from HIV-1. *Science* 1988;242(4882):1171–1173.

600. Robertson DL, Anderson JP, Bradac JA, et al. HIV-1 nomenclature proposal. In: Kuiken C, Foley B, Hahn BH, et al., eds. *Human Retroviruses and AIDS 1999*. Los Alamos, NM: Los Alamos National Laboratory; 1999:492–505.

601. Rodgers DW, Gamblin SJ, Harris BA, et al. The structure of unliganded reverse transcriptase from the human immunodeficiency virus type 1. *Proc Natl Acad Sci U S A* 1995;92(4):1222–1226.

602. Rong L, Zhang J, Lu J, et al. The transmembrane domain of BST-2 determines its sensitivity to down-modulation by human immunodeficiency virus type 1 Vpu. *J Virol* 2009;83(15):7536–7546.

603. Rosa A, Chande A, Ziglio S, et al. HIV-1 Nef promotes infection by excluding SERINC5 from virion incorporation. *Nature* 2015;526(7572):212–217.

604. Rosen CA, Terwilliger E, Dayton A, et al. Intragenic cis-acting art gene-responsive sequences of the human immunodeficiency virus. *Proc Natl Acad Sci U S A* 1988;85(7):2071–2075.

605. Ross EK, Buckler-White AJ, Rabson AB, et al. Contribution of NF-kappa B and Sp1 binding motifs to the replicative capacity of human immunodeficiency virus type 1: distinct patterns of viral growth are determined by T-cell types. *J Virol* 1991;65(8):4350–4358.

606. Roth MJ, Schwartzberg PL, Goff SP. Structure of the termini of DNA intermediates in the integration of retroviral DNA: dependence on IN function and terminal DNA sequence. *Cell* 1989;58(1):47–54.

607. Roux A, Leroy H, De Muylder B, et al. FOXO1 transcription factor plays a key role in T cell-HIV-1 interaction. *PLoS Pathog* 2019;15(5):e1007669.

608. Rowell JF, Stanhope PE, Siliciano RF. Endocytosis of endogenously synthesized HIV-1 envelope protein. Mechanism and role in processing for association with class II MHC. *J Immunol* 1995;155(1):473–488.

609. Roy S, Delling U, Chen CH, et al. A bulge structure in HIV-1 TAR RNA is required for Tat binding and Tat-mediated trans-activation. *Genes Dev* 1990;4(8):1365–1373.

610. Ruben S, Perkins A, Purcell R, et al. Structural and functional characterization of human immunodeficiency virus tat protein. *J Virol* 1989;63(1):1–8.

611. Rulli SJ Jr, Hibbert CS, Mirro J, et al. Selective and nonselective packaging of cellular RNAs in retrovirus particles. *J Virol* 2007;81(12):6623–6631.

612. Saad JS, Miller J, Tai J, et al. Structural basis for targeting HIV-1 Gag proteins to the plasma membrane for virus assembly. *Proc Natl Acad Sci U S A* 2006;103(30):11364–11369.

613. Sabo Y, Walsh D, Barry DS, et al. HIV-1 induces the formation of stable microtubules to enhance early infection. *Cell Host Microbe* 2013;14(5):535–546.

614. Sadaie MR, Rappaport J, Benter T, et al. Missense mutations in an infectious human immunodeficiency viral genome: functional mapping of tat and identification of the rev splice acceptor. *Proc Natl Acad Sci U S A* 1988;85(23):9224–9228.

615. Sahu GK, Lee K, Ji J, et al. A novel in vitro system to generate and study latently HIV-infected long-lived normal CD4+ T-lymphocytes. *Virology* 2006;355(2):127–137.

616. Sainsbury S, Bernecky C, Cramer P. Structural basis of transcription initiation by RNA polymerase II. *Nat Rev Mol Cell Biol* 2015;16(3):129–143.

617. Sakane N, Kwon HS, Pagans S, et al. Activation of HIV transcription by the viral Tat protein requires a demethylation step mediated by lysine-specific demethylase 1 (LSD1/KDM1). *PLoS Pathog* 2011;7(8):e1002184.

618. Sakuragi J, Shioda T, Panganiban AT. Duplication of the primary encapsidation and dimer linkage region of human immunodeficiency virus type 1 RNA results in the appearance of monomeric RNA in virions. *J Virol* 2001;75(6):2557–2565.

619. Salzwedel K, West JT, Hunter E. A conserved tryptophan-rich motif in the membrane-proximal region of the human immunodeficiency virus type 1 gp41 ectodomain is important for Env-mediated fusion and virus infectivity. *J Virol* 1999;73(3):2469–2480.

620. Samson M, Libert F, Doranz BJ, et al. Resistance to HIV-1 infection in caucasian individuals bearing mutant alleles of the CCR-5 chemokine receptor gene [see comments]. *Nature* 1996;382(6593):722–725.

621. Sarafianos SG, Das K, Tantillo C, et al. Crystal structure of HIV-1 reverse transcriptase in complex with a polypurine tract RNA:DNA. *EMBO J* 2001;20(6):1449–1461.

622. Sarafianos SG, Marchand B, Das K, et al. Structure and function of HIV-1 reverse transcriptase: molecular mechanisms of polymerization and inhibition. *J Mol Biol* 2009;385(3):693–713.

623. Sarngadharan MG, Popovic M, Bruch L, et al. Antibodies reactive with human T-lymphotropic retroviruses (HTLV-III) in the serum of patients with AIDS. *Science* 1984;224(4648):506–508.

624. Sato M, Motomura T, Aramaki H, et al. Novel HIV-1 integrase inhibitors derived from quinolone antibiotics. *J Med Chem* 2006;49(5):1506–1508.

625. Sattentau QJ. Cell-to-cell spread of retroviruses. *Viruses* 2010;2:1306–1321.

626. Sauter D, Schindler M, Specht A, et al. Tetherin-driven adaptation of Vpu and Nef function and the evolution of pandemic and nonpandemic HIV-1 strains. *Cell Host Microbe* 2009;6(5):409–421.

627. Sawyer SL, Wu LI, Emerman M, et al. Positive selection of primate TRIM5alpha identifies a critical species-specific retroviral restriction domain. *Proc Natl Acad Sci U S A* 2005;102(8):2832–2837.

628. Sayah DM, Sokolskaja E, Berthoux L, et al. Cyclophilin A retrotransposition into TRIM5 explains owl monkey resistance to HIV-1. *Nature* 2004;430(6999):569–573.

629. Schindler M, Munch J, Brenner M, et al. Comprehensive analysis of nef functions selected in simian immunodeficiency virus-infected macaques. *J Virol* 2004;78(19):10588–10597.

630. Schmidt F, Keele BF, Del Prete GQ, et al. Derivation of simian tropic HIV-1 infectious clone reveals virus adaptation to a new host. *Proc Natl Acad Sci U S A* 2019;116(21):10504–10509.

631. Schones DE, Cui K, Cuddapah S, et al. Dynamic regulation of nucleosome positioning in the human genome. *Cell* 2008;132(5):887–898.

632. Schroder AR, Shinn P, Chen H, et al. HIV-1 integration in the human genome favors active genes and local hotspots. *Cell* 2002;110(4):521–529.

633. Schrofelbauer B, Hakata Y, Landau NR. HIV-1 Vpr function is mediated by interaction with the damage-specific DNA-binding protein DDB1. *Proc Natl Acad Sci U S A* 2007;104(10):4130–4135.

634. Schubert HL, Zhai Q, Sandrin V, et al. Structural and functional studies on the extracellular domain of BST2/tetherin in reduced and oxidized conformations. *Proc Natl Acad Sci U S A* 2010;107(42):17951–17956.

635. Schubert U, Henklein P, Boldyreff B, et al. The human immunodeficiency virus type 1 encoded Vpu protein is phosphorylated by casein kinase-2 (CK-2) at positions Ser52 and Ser56 within a predicted alpha-helix-turn-alpha-helix-motif. *J Mol Biol* 1994;236(1):16–25.

636. Schuller R, Forne I, Straub T, et al. Heptad-Specific Phosphorylation of RNA Polymerase II CTD. *Mol Cell* 2016;61(2):305–314.

637. Schulze-Gahmen U, Hurley JH. Structural mechanism for HIV-1 TAR loop recognition by Tat and the super elongation complex. *Proc Natl Acad Sci U S A* 2018;115(51):12973–12978.

638. Schur FK, Hagen WJ, Rumlova M, et al. Structure of the immature HIV-1 capsid in intact virus particles at 8.8 A resolution. *Nature* 2015;517(7535):505–508.

639. Schur FK, Obr M, Hagen WJ, et al. An atomic model of HIV-1 capsid-SP1 reveals structures regulating assembly and maturation. *Science* 2016;353(6298):506–508.

640. Schwartz S, Felber BK, Benko DM, et al. Cloning and functional analysis of multiply spliced mRNA species of human immunodeficiency virus type 1. *J Virol* 1990;64(6):2519–2529.

641. Schwartzberg P, Colicelli J, Goff SP. Construction and analysis of deletion mutations in the pol gene of Moloney murine leukemia virus: a new viral function required for productive infection. *Cell* 1984;37(3):1043–1052.

642. Sebastian S, Luban J. TRIM5alpha selectively binds a restriction-sensitive retroviral capsid. *Retrovirology* 2005;2:40.
643. Sedore SC, Byers SA, Biglione S, et al. Manipulation of P-TEFb control machinery by HIV: recruitment of P-TEFb from the large form by Tat and binding of HEXIM1 to TAR. *Nucleic Acids Res* 2007;35(13):4347–4358.
644. Selyutina A, Persaud M, Lee K, et al. Nuclear import of the HIV-1 core precedes reverse transcription and uncoating. *Cell Rep* 2020;32(13):108201.
645. Sengupta S, Siliciano RF. Targeting the latent reservoir for HIV-1. *Immunity* 2018;48(5):872–895.
646. Shaik MM, Peng H, Lu J, et al. Structural basis of coreceptor recognition by HIV-1 envelope spike. *Nature* 2019;565(7739):318–323.
647. Shandilya J, Roberts SG. The transcription cycle in eukaryotes: from productive initiation to RNA polymerase II recycling. *Biochim Biophys Acta* 2012;1819(5):391–400.
648. Sharova N, Wu Y, Zhu X, et al. Primate lentiviral Vpx commandeers DDB1 to counteract a macrophage restriction. *PLoS Pathog* 2008;4(5):e1000057.
649. Sharp PM, Hahn BH. Origins of HIV and the AIDS pandemic. *Cold Spring Harb Perspect Med* 2011;1(1):a006841.
650. Sharp PM, Shaw GM, Hahn BH. Simian immunodeficiency virus infection of chimpanzees. *J Virol* 2005;79(7):3891–3902.
651. Sheehy AM, Gaddis NC, Choi JD, et al. Isolation of a human gene that inhibits HIV-1 infection and is suppressed by the viral Vif protein. *Nature* 2002;418(6898):646–650.
652. Sherpa C, Rausch JW, Le Grice SF, et al. The HIV-1 Rev response element (RRE) adopts alternative conformations that promote different rates of virus replication. *Nucleic Acids Res* 2015;43(9):4676–4686.
653. Shibata R, Kawamura M, Sakai H, et al. Generation of a chimeric human and simian immunodeficiency virus infectious to monkey peripheral blood mononuclear cells. *J Virol* 1991;65(7):3514–3520.
654. Shkriabai N, Datta SA, Zhao Z, et al. Interactions of HIV-1 Gag with assembly cofactors. *Biochemistry* 2006;45(13):4077–4083.
655. Shun MC, Raghavendra NK, Vandegraaff N, et al. LEDGF/p75 functions downstream from preintegration complex formation to effect gene-specific HIV-1 integration. *Genes Dev* 2007;21(14):1767–1778.
656. Shytaj IL, Norelli S, Chirullo B, et al. A highly intensified ART regimen induces long-term viral suppression and restriction of the viral reservoir in a simian AIDS model. *PLoS Pathog* 2012;8(6):e1002774.
657. Simonetti FR, White JA, Tumiotto C, et al. Intact proviral DNA assay analysis of large cohorts of people with HIV provides a benchmark for the frequency and composition of persistent proviral DNA. *Proc Natl Acad Sci U S A* 2020;117(31):18692–18700.
658. Simonetti FR, Zhang H, Soroosh GP, et al. Antigen-driven clonal selection shapes the persistence of HIV-1-infected CD4+ T cells in vivo. *J Clin Invest* 2021;131(3):e145254.
659. Singh K, Marchand B, Kirby KA, et al. Structural aspects of drug resistance and inhibition of HIV-1 reverse transcriptase. *Viruses* 2010;2(2):606–638.
660. Smith DJ, Lin LJ, Moon H, et al. Propagating humanized BLT mice for the study of human immunology and immunotherapy. *Stem Cells Dev* 2016;25(24):1863–1873.
661. Smith PF, Ogundele A, Forrest A, et al. Phase I and II study of the safety, virologic effect, and pharmacokinetics/pharmacodynamics of single-dose 3-o-(3′,3′-dimethylsuccinyl)betulinic acid (bevirimat) against human immunodeficiency virus infection. *Antimicrob Agents Chemother* 2007;51(10):3574–3581.
662. Smith SJ, Zhao XZ, Passos DO, et al. Integrase strand transfer inhibitors are effective anti-HIV drugs. *Viruses* 2021;13(2):205.
663. Sodora DL, Allan JS, Apetrei C, et al. Toward an AIDS vaccine: lessons from natural simian immunodeficiency virus infections of African nonhuman primate hosts. *Nat Med* 2009;15(8):861–865.
664. Sodroski J, Goh WC, Rosen C, et al. Replicative and cytopathic potential of HTLV-III/LAV with *sor* gene deletions. *Science* 1986;231(4745):1549–1553.
665. Sokolskaja E, Sayah DM, Luban J. Target cell cyclophilin A modulates human immunodeficiency virus type 1 infectivity. *J Virol* 2004;78(23):12800–12808.
666. Somasundaran M, Sharkey M, Brichacek B, et al. Evidence for a cytopathogenicity determinant in HIV-1 Vpr. *Proc Natl Acad Sci U S A* 2002;99(14):9503–9508.
667. Song B, Diaz-Griffero F, Park DH, et al. TRIM5alpha association with cytoplasmic bodies is not required for antiretroviral activity. *Virology* 2005;343(2):201–211.
668. Song B, Gold B, O'Huigin C, et al. The B30.2(SPRY) domain of the retroviral restriction factor TRIM5alpha exhibits lineage-specific length and sequence variation in primates. *J Virol* 2005;79(10):6111–6121.
669. Song B, Javanbakht H, Perron M, et al. Retrovirus restriction by TRIM5alpha variants from Old World and New World primates. *J Virol* 2005;79(7):3930–3937.
670. Sood C, Marin M, Chande A, et al. SERINC5 protein inhibits HIV-1 fusion pore formation by promoting functional inactivation of envelope glycoproteins. *J Biol Chem* 2017;292(14):6014–6026.
671. South TL, Blake PR, Sowder RC III, et al. The nucleocapsid protein isolated from HIV-1 particles binds zinc and forms retroviral-type zinc fingers. *Biochemistry* 1990;29(34):7786–7789.
672. Spina CA, Anderson J, Archin NM, et al. An in-depth comparison of latent HIV-1 reactivation in multiple cell model systems and resting CD4+ T cells from aviremic patients. *PLoS Pathog* 2013;9(12):e1003834.
673. Srivastava S, Swanson SK, Manel N, et al. Lentiviral Vpx accessory factor targets VprBP/DCAF1 substrate adaptor for cullin 4 E3 ubiquitin ligase to enable macrophage infection. *PLoS Pathog* 2008;4(5):e1000059.
674. Staffa A, Cochrane A. The tat/rev intron of human immunodeficiency virus type 1 is inefficiently spliced because of suboptimal signals in the 3′ splice site. *J Virol* 1994;68(5):3071–3079.
675. Staudt RP, Alvarado JJ, Emert-Sedlak LA, et al. Structure, function, and inhibitor targeting of HIV-1 Nef-effector kinase complexes. *J Biol Chem* 2020;295(44):15158–15171.
676. Stevenson M, Stanwick TL, Dempsey MP, et al. HIV-1 replication is controlled at the level of T cell activation and proviral integration. *EMBO J* 1990;9(5):1551–1560.
677. Stoltzfus CM, Madsen JM. Role of viral splicing elements and cellular RNA binding proteins in regulation of HIV-1 alternative RNA splicing. *Curr HIV Res* 2006;4(1):43–55.
678. Strack B, Calistri A, Accola MA, et al. A role for ubiquitin ligase recruitment in retrovirus release. *Proc Natl Acad Sci U S A* 2000;97(24):13063–13068.
679. Strack B, Calistri A, Craig S, et al. AIP1/ALIX is a binding partner for HIV-1 p6 and EIAV p9 functioning in virus budding. *Cell* 2003;114:689–699.
680. Strebel K, Daugherty D, Clouse K, et al. The HIV 'A' (sor) gene product is essential for virus infectivity. *Nature* 1987;328(6132):728–730.
681. Strebel K, Klimkait T, Martin MA. A novel gene of HIV-1, vpu, and its 16-kilodalton product. *Science* 1988;241(4870):1221–1223.
682. Stremlau M, Owens CM, Perron MJ, et al. The cytoplasmic body component TRIM5alpha restricts HIV-1 infection in Old World monkeys. *Nature* 2004;427(6977):848–853.
683. Stremlau M, Perron M, Lee M, et al. Specific recognition and accelerated uncoating of retroviral capsids by the TRIM5alpha restriction factor. *Proc Natl Acad Sci U S A* 2006;103(14):5514–5519.
684. Stremlau M, Perron M, Welikala S, et al. Species-specific variation in the B30.2(SPRY) domain of TRIM5alpha determines the potency of human immunodeficiency virus restriction. *J Virol* 2005;79(5):3139–3145.
685. Sugden SM, Bego MG, Pham TN, et al. Remodeling of the host cell plasma membrane by HIV-1 Nef and Vpu: a strategy to ensure viral fitness and persistence. *Viruses* 2016;8(3):67.
686. Sui Y, Gordon S, Franchini G, et al. Nonhuman primate models for HIV/AIDS vaccine development. *Curr Protoc Immunol* 2013;102:12.14.1–12.14.30.
687. Summa V, Petrocchi A, Bonelli F, et al. Discovery of raltegravir, a potent, selective orally bioavailable HIV-integrase inhibitor for the treatment of HIV-AIDS infection. *J Med Chem* 2008;51(18):5843–5855.
688. Summers MF, Henderson LE, Chance MR, et al. Nucleocapsid zinc fingers detected in retroviruses: EXAFS studies of intact viruses and the solution-state structure of the nucleocapsid protein from HIV-1. *Protein Sci* 1992;1(5):563–574.
689. Sundquist WI, Krausslich HG. HIV-1 assembly, budding, and maturation. *Cold Spring Harb Perspect Med* 2012;2(7):a006924.
690. Swanstrom, R, Sundquist WI. Stephan Oroszlan and the proteolytic processing of retroviral proteins: following A Pro. *Viruses* 2021;13(11):2218.
691. Takehisa J, Zekeng L, Ido E, et al. Human immunodeficiency virus type 1 intergroup (M/O) recombination in cameroon. *J Virol* 1999;73(8):6810–6820.
692. Tan K, Liu J, Wang J, et al. Atomic structure of a thermostable subdomain of HIV-1 gp41. *Proc Natl Acad Sci U S A* 1997;94(23):12303–12308.
693. Tanchou V, Decimo D, Pechoux C, et al. Role of the N-terminal zinc finger of human immunodeficiency virus type 1 nucleocapsid protein in virus structure and replication. *J Virol* 1998;72(5):4442–4447.
694. Tchasovnikarova IA, Timms RT, Matheson NJ, et al. GENE SILENCING. Epigenetic silencing by the HUSH complex mediates position-effect variegation in human cells. *Science* 2015;348(6242):1481–1485.
695. Tedbury PR, Novikova M, Ablan SD, et al. Biochemical evidence of a role for matrix trimerization in HIV-1 envelope glycoprotein incorporation. *Proc Natl Acad Sci U S A* 2016;113(2):E182–E190.
696. Tedbury PR, Novikova M, Alfadhli A, et al. HIV-1 matrix trimerization-impaired mutants are rescued by matrix substitutions that enhance envelope glycoprotein incorporation. *J Virol* 2019;94(1):e01526-19.
697. Temin HM, Mizutani S. RNA-dependent DNA polymerase in virions of Rous sarcoma virus. *Nature* 1970;226(252):1211–1213.
698. Thali M, Bukovsky A, Kondo E, et al. Functional association of cyclophilin A with HIV-1 virions [see comments]. *Nature* 1994;372(6504):363–365.
699. Tian L, Kim MS, Li H, et al. Structure of HIV-1 reverse transcriptase cleaving RNA in an RNA/DNA hybrid. *Proc Natl Acad Sci U S A* 2018;115(3):507–512.
700. Timmerman LA, Clipstone NA, Ho SN, et al. Rapid shuttling of NF-AT in discrimination of Ca2+ signals and immunosuppression. *Nature* 1996;383(6603):837–840.
701. Tomezsko PJ, Corbin VDA, Gupta P, et al. Determination of RNA structural diversity and its role in HIV-1 RNA splicing. *Nature* 2020;582(7812):438–442.
702. Toohey MG, Jones KA. In vitro formation of short RNA polymerase II transcripts that terminate within the HIV-1 and HIV-2 promoter-proximal downstream regions. *Genes Dev* 1989;3(3):265–282.
703. Towers G, Bock M, Martin S, et al. A conserved mechanism of retrovirus restriction in mammals. *Proc Natl Acad Sci U S A* 2000;97(22):12295–12299.
704. Trautz B, Wiedemann H, Luchtenborg C, et al. The host-cell restriction factor SERINC5 restricts HIV-1 infectivity without altering the lipid composition and organization of viral particles. *J Biol Chem* 2017;292(33):13702–13713.
705. Trejbalova K, Kovarova D, Blazkova J, et al. Development of 5′ LTR DNA methylation of latent HIV-1 provirus in cell line models and in long-term-infected individuals. *Clin Epigenetics* 2016;8:19.
706. Turner BG, Summers MF. Structural biology of HIV. *J Mol Biol* 1999;285(1):1–32.
707. Usami Y, Popov S, Gottlinger HG. Potent rescue of human immunodeficiency virus type 1 late domain mutants by ALIX/AIP1 depends on its CHMP4 binding site. *J Virol* 2007;81(12):6614–6622.
708. Usami Y, Wu Y, Gottlinger HG. SERINC3 and SERINC5 restrict HIV-1 infectivity and are counteracted by Nef. *Nature* 2015;526(7572):218–223.
709. Valente ST, Gilmartin GM, Venkatarama K, et al. HIV-1 mRNA 3′ end processing is distinctively regulated by eIF3f, CDK11, and splice factor 9G8. *Mol Cell* 2009;36(2):279–289.
710. Valkov E, Gupta SS, Hare S, et al. Functional and structural characterization of the integrase from the prototype foamy virus. *Nucleic Acids Res* 2009;37(1):243–255.
711. Vallejo-Gracia A, Chen IP, Perrone R, et al. FOXO1 promotes HIV latency by suppressing ER stress in T cells. *Nat Microbiol* 2020;5(9):1144–1157.
712. Van Damme N, Goff D, Katsura C, et al. The interferon-induced protein BST-2 restricts HIV-1 release and is downregulated from the cell surface by the viral Vpu protein. *Cell Host Microbe* 2008;3(4):245–252.
713. Van Duyne R, Easley R, Wu W, et al. Lysine methylation of HIV-1 Tat regulates transcriptional activity of the viral LTR. *Retrovirology* 2008;5:40.
714. Van Duyne R, Kuo LS, Pham P, et al. Mutations in the HIV-1 envelope glycoprotein can broadly rescue blocks at multiple steps in the virus replication cycle. *Proc Natl Acad Sci U S A* 2019;116(18):9040–9049.

715. Van Engelenburg SB, Shtengel G, Sengupta P, et al. Distribution of ESCRT machinery at HIV assembly sites reveals virus scaffolding of ESCRT subunits. *Science* 2014;343(6171):653–656.

716. Van Lint C, Emiliani S, Ott M, et al. Transcriptional activation and chromatin remodeling of the HIV-1 promoter in response to histone acetylation. *EMBO J* 1996;15(5):1112–1120.

717. Vandekerckhove L, Christ F, Van Maele B, et al. Transient and stable knockdown of the integrase cofactor LEDGF/p75 reveals its role in the replication cycle of human immunodeficiency virus. *J Virol* 2006;80(4):1886–1896.

718. VerPlank L, Bouamr F, LaGrassa TJ, et al. Tsg101, a homologue of ubiquitin-conjugating (E2) enzymes, binds the L domain in HIV type 1 Pr55Gag. *Proc Natl Acad Sci U S A* 2001;98:7724–7729.

719. Vogt VM, Eisenman R, Diggelmann H. Generation of avian myeloblastosis virus structural proteins by proteolytic cleavage of a precursor polypeptide. *J Mol Biol* 1975;96(3):471–493.

720. von Schwedler UK, Stuchell M, Muller B, et al. The protein network of HIV budding. *Cell* 2003;114(6):701–713.

721. Votteler J, Sundquist WI. Virus budding and the ESCRT pathway. *Cell Host Microbe* 2013;14(3):232–241.

722. Wagner JM, Zadrozny KK, Chrustowicz J, et al. Crystal structure of an HIV assembly and maturation switch. *Elife* 2016;5:e17063.

723. Wagner TA, McLaughlin S, Garg K, et al. HIV latency. Proliferation of cells with HIV integrated into cancer genes contributes to persistent infection. *Science* 2014;345(6196):570–573.

724. Wain-Hobson S, Sonigo P, Danos O, et al. Nucleotide sequence of the AIDS virus, LAV. *Cell* 1985;40(1):9–17.

725. Waki K, Durell SR, Soheilian F, et al. Structural and functional insights into the HIV-1 maturation inhibitor binding pocket. *PLoS Pathog* 2012;8(11):e1002997.

726. Wang JY, Ling H, Yang W, et al. Structure of a two-domain fragment of HIV-1 integrase: implications for domain organization in the intact protein. *EMBO J* 2001;20(24):7333–7343.

727. Wang M, Yang W, Chen Y, et al. Cellular RelB interacts with the transactivator Tat and enhance HIV-1 expression. *Retrovirology* 2018;15(1):65.

728. Ward AE, Kiessling V, Pornillos O, et al. HIV-cell membrane fusion intermediates are restricted by Serincs as revealed by cryo-electron and TIRF microscopy. *J Biol Chem* 2020;295(45):15183–15195.

729. Watts JM, Dang KK, Gorelick RJ, et al. Architecture and secondary structure of an entire HIV-1 RNA genome. *Nature* 2009;460(7256):711–716.

730. Wei P, Garber ME, Fang SM, et al. A novel CDK9-associated C-type cyclin interacts directly with HIV-1 Tat and mediates its high-affinity, loop-specific binding to TAR RNA. *Cell* 1998;92(4):451–462.

731. Weissenhorn W, Dessen A, Harrison SC, et al. Atomic structure of the ectodomain from HIV-1 gp41. *Nature* 1997;387(6631):426–430.

732. Wen W, Meinkoth JL, Tsien RY, et al. Identification of a signal for rapid export of proteins from the nucleus. *Cell* 1995;82(3):463–473.

733. Westby M, Smith-Burchnell C, Mori J, et al. Reduced maximal inhibition in phenotypic susceptibility assays indicates that viral strains resistant to the CCR5 antagonist maraviroc utilize inhibitor-bound receptor for entry. *J Virol* 2007;81(5):2359–2371.

734. Winans S, Yu HJ, de Los Santos K, et al. A point mutation in HIV-1 integrase redirects proviral integration into centromeric repeats. *Nat Comm* 2022;13(1):1474.

735. Winans S, Goff SP. Mutations altering acetylated residues in the CTD of HIV-1 integrase cause defects in proviral transcription at early times after integration of viral DNA. *PLoS Pathog* 2020;16(12):e1009147.

736. Witvrouw M, Pannecouque C, Van Laethem K, et al. Activity of non-nucleoside reverse transcriptase inhibitors against HIV-2 and SIV. *AIDS* 1999;13(12):1477–1483.

737. Wlodawer A, Erickson JW. Structure based inhibitors of HIV-1 protease. *Annu Rev Biochem* 1993;62:543–585.

738. Wlodawer A, Miller M, Jaskólski M, et al. Conserved folding in retroviral proteases: crystal structure of a synthetic HIV-1 protease. *Science* 1989;245(4918):616–621.

739. Wolfs TF, Zwart G, Bakker M, et al. HIV-1 genomic RNA diversification following sexual and parenteral virus transmission. *Virology* 1992;189(1):103–110.

740. Wollert T, Wunder C, Lippincott-Schwartz J, et al. Membrane scission by the ESCRT-III complex. *Nature* 2009;458(7235):172–177.

741. Wong JK, Hezareh M, Gunthard HF, et al. Recovery of replication-competent HIV despite prolonged suppression of plasma viremia. *Science* 1997;278(5341):1291–1295.

742. Worobey M, Gemmel M, Teuwen DE, et al. Direct evidence of extensive diversity of HIV-1 in Kinshasa by 1960. *Nature* 2008;455(7213):661–664.

743. Wray V, Kinder R, Federau T, et al. Solution structure and orientation of the transmembrane anchor domain of the HIV-1-encoded virus protein U by high-resolution and solid-state NMR spectroscopy. *Biochemistry* 1999;38(16):5272–5282.

744. Wright ER, Schooler JB, Ding HJ, et al. Electron cryotomography of immature HIV-1 virions reveals the structure of the CA and SP1 Gag shells. *EMBO J* 2007;26(8):2218–2226.

745. Wu X, Anderson JL, Campbell EM, et al. Proteasome inhibitors uncouple rhesus TRIM5alpha restriction of HIV-1 reverse transcription and infection. *Proc Natl Acad Sci U S A* 2006;103(19):7465–7470.

746. Wu X, Conway JA, Kim J, et al. Localization of the Vpx packaging signal within the C terminus of the human immunodeficiency virus type 2 Gag precursor protein. *J Virol* 1994;68:6161–6169.

747. Wu Y, Zhou X, Barnes CO, et al. The DDB1-DCAF1-Vpr-UNG2 crystal structure reveals how HIV-1 Vpr steers human UNG2 toward destruction. *Nat Struct Mol Biol* 2016;23(10):933–940.

748. Wyatt R, Kwong PD, Desjardins E, et al. The antigenic structure of the HIV gp120 envelope glycoprotein [In Process Citation]. *Nature* 1998;393(6686):705–711.

749. Wyma DJ, Jiang J, Shi J, et al. Coupling of human immunodeficiency virus type 1 fusion to virion maturation: a novel role of the gp41 cytoplasmic tail. *J Virol* 2004;78(7):3429–3435.

750. Wyma DJ, Kotov A, Aiken C. Evidence for a stable interaction of gp41 with Pr55(Gag) in immature human immunodeficiency virus type 1 particles. *J Virol* 2000;74(20):9381–9387.

751. Wyss S, Berlioz-Torrent C, Boge M, et al. The highly conserved C-terminal dileucine motif in the cytosolic domain of the human immunodeficiency virus type 1 envelope glycoprotein is critical for its association with the AP-1 clathrin adaptor [correction of adapter]. *J Virol* 2001;75(6):2982–2992.

752. Xiao T, Cai Y, Chen B. HIV-1 entry and membrane fusion inhibitors. *Viruses* 2021;13(5):735.

753. Xiao T, Frey G, Fu Q, et al. HIV-1 fusion inhibitors targeting the membrane-proximal external region of Env spikes. *Nat Chem Biol* 2020;16(5):529–537.

754. Xing S, Bullen CK, Shroff NS, et al. Disulfiram reactivates latent HIV-1 in a Bcl-2-transduced primary CD4+ T cell model without inducing global T cell activation. *J Virol* 2011;85(12):6060–6064.

755. Xu C, Fischer DK, Rankovic S, et al. Permeability of the HIV-1 capsid to metabolites modulates viral DNA synthesis. *PLoS Biol* 2020;18(12):e3001015.

756. Xu H, Chertova E, Chen J, et al. Stoichiometry of the antiviral protein APOBEC3G in HIV-1 virions. *Virology* 2007;360(2):247–256.

757. Yamada E, Nakaoka S, Klein L, et al. Human-specific adaptations in Vpu conferring anti-tetherin activity are critical for efficient early HIV-1 replication in vivo. *Cell Host Microbe* 2018;23(1):110–120 e7.

758. Yamaguchi Y, Takagi T, Wada T, et al. NELF, a multisubunit complex containing RD, cooperates with DSIF to repress RNA polymerase II elongation. *Cell* 1999;97(1):41–51.

759. Yamashita M, Emerman M. Capsid is a dominant determinant of retrovirus infectivity in nondividing cells. *J Virol* 2004;78(11):5670–5678.

760. Yang H, Wang J, Jia X, et al. Structural insight into the mechanisms of enveloped virus tethering by tetherin. *Proc Natl Acad Sci U S A* 2010;107(43):18428–18432.

761. Yang HC, Xing S, Shan L, et al. Small-molecule screening using a human primary cell model of HIV latency identifies compounds that reverse latency without cellular activation. *J Clin Invest* 2009;119(11):3473–3486.

762. Yang X, Gold MO, Tang DN, et al. TAK, an HIV Tat-associated kinase, is a member of the cyclin-dependent family of protein kinases and is induced by activation of peripheral blood lymphocytes and differentiation of promonocytic cell lines. *Proc Natl Acad Sci U S A* 1997;94(23):12331–12336.

763. Yang X, Herrmann CH, Rice AP. The human immunodeficiency virus Tat proteins specifically associate with TAK in vivo and require the carboxyl-terminal domain of RNA polymerase II for function. *J Virol* 1996;70(7):4576–4584.

764. Yang Z, Yik JH, Chen R, et al. Recruitment of P-TEFb for stimulation of transcriptional elongation by the bromodomain protein Brd4. *Mol Cell* 2005;19(4):535–545.

765. Yant SR, Mulato A, Hansen D, et al. A highly potent long-acting small-molecule HIV-1 capsid inhibitor with efficacy in a humanized mouse model. *Nat Med* 2019;25(9):1377–1384.

766. Yap MW, Nisole S, Stoye JP. A single amino acid change in the SPRY domain of human Trim5alpha leads to HIV-1 restriction. *Curr Biol* 2005;15(1):73–78.

767. Yeager M. Design of in vitro symmetric complexes and analysis by hybrid methods reveal mechanisms of HIV capsid assembly. *J Mol Biol* 2011;410(4):534–552.

768. Yik JH, Chen R, Pezda AC, et al. A human immunodeficiency virus type 1 Tat-like arginine-rich RNA-binding domain is essential for HEXIM1 to inhibit RNA polymerase II transcription through 7SK snRNA-mediated inactivation of P-TEFb. *Mol Cell Biol* 2004;24(12):5094–5105.

769. Yu X, Yu Y, Liu B, et al. Induction of APOBEC3G ubiquitination and degradation by an HIV-1 Vif-Cul5-SCF complex. *Science* 2003;302(5647):1056–1060.

770. Yuan X, Matsuda Z, Matsuda M, et al. Human immunodeficiency virus *vpr* gene encodes a virion-associated protein. *AIDS Res Hum Retroviruses* 1990;6(11):1265–1271.

771. Yuan X, Yu X, Lee TH, et al. Mutations in the N-terminal region of human immunodeficiency virus type 1 matrix protein block intracellular transport of the Gag precursor. *J Virol* 1993;67(11):6387–6394.

772. Yurkovetskiy L, Guney MH, Kim K, et al. Primate immunodeficiency virus proteins Vpx and Vpr counteract transcriptional repression of proviruses by the HUSH complex. *Nat Microbiol* 2018;3(12):1354–1361.

773. Zaborowska J, Egloff S, Murphy S. The pol II CTD: new twists in the tail. *Nat Struct Mol Biol* 2016;23(9):771–777.

774. Zack JA, Arrigo SJ, Weitsman SR, et al. HIV-1 entry into quiescent primary lymphocytes: molecular analysis reveals a labile, latent viral structure. *Cell* 1990;61(2):213–222.

775. Zennou V, Perez-Caballero D, Gottlinger H, et al. APOBEC3G incorporation into human immunodeficiency virus type 1 particles. *J Virol* 2004;78(21):12058–12061.

776. Zhang F, Bieniasz PD. HIV-1 Vpr induces cell cycle arrest and enhances viral gene expression by depleting CCDC137. *Elife* 2020;9:e55806.

777. Zhang F, Landford WN, Ng M, et al. SIV Nef proteins recruit the AP-2 complex to antagonize Tetherin and facilitate virion release. *PLoS Pathog* 2011;7(5):e1002039.

778. Zhang F, Wilson SJ, Landford WC, et al. Nef proteins from simian immunodeficiency viruses are tetherin antagonists. *Cell Host Microbe* 2009;6(1):54–67.

779. Zhang K, Lv DW, Li R. Conserved herpesvirus protein kinases target SAMHD1 to facilitate virus replication. *Cell Rep* 2019;28(2):449–459 e5.

780. Zhao G, Ke D, Vu T, et al. Rhesus TRIM5alpha disrupts the HIV-1 capsid at the inter-hexamer interfaces. *PLoS Pathog* 2011;7(3):e1002009.

781. Zhao LJ, Mukherjee S, Narayan O. Biochemical mechanism of HIV-I Vpr function. Specific interaction with a cellular protein. *J Biol Chem* 1994;269(22):15577–15582.

782. Zhong P, Agosto LM, Ilinskaya A, et al. Cell-to-cell transmission can overcome multiple donor and target cell barriers imposed on cell-free HIV. *PLoS One* 2013;8(1):e53138.

783. Zhong P, Agosto LM, Munro JB, et al. Cell-to-cell transmission of viruses. *Curr Opin Virol* 2013;3(1):44–50.

784. Zhou J, Yuan X, Dismuke D, et al. Small-molecule inhibition of human immunodeficiency virus type 1 replication by specific targeting of the final step of virion maturation. *J Virol* 2004;78(2):922–929.

785. Zhou Q, Chen D, Pierstorff E, et al. Transcription elongation factor P-TEFb mediates Tat activation of HIV-1 transcription at multiple stages. *EMBO J* 1998;17(13):3681–3691.

786. Zhou W, Resh MD. Differential membrane binding of the human immunodeficiency virus type 1 matrix protein. *J Virol* 1996;70(12):8540–8548.

787. Zhu P, Chertova E, Bess J Jr, et al. Electron tomography analysis of envelope glycoprotein trimers on HIV and simian immunodeficiency virus virions. *Proc Natl Acad Sci U S A* 2003;100(26):15812–15817.

788. Zhu Y, Pe'ery T, Peng J, et al. Transcription elongation factor P-TEFb is required for HIV-1 tat transactivation in vitro. *Genes Dev* 1997;11(20):2622–2632.

789. Zila V, Margiotta E, Turonova B, et al. Cone-shaped HIV-1 capsids are transported through intact nuclear pores. *Cell* 2021;184(4):1032–1046 e18.

HIV-1: Pathogenesis, Clinical Manifestations, and Treatment

Eileen P. Scully • Daniel R. Kuritzkes

History
Infectious agent
Epidemiology
  Origin of HIV
  Current global distribution
  Mechanisms of transmission
Pathogenesis and pathology
  Acute infection and CD4 cell depletion
  Establishment of a latent viral reservoir
  Host immunity
  Innate immune responses
  Adaptive humoral immune responses
  Adaptive cellular immune responses
  Virus-specific CD4 T cells
  Host genetics and viral control
  Reasons for immune failure
Clinical features
  Primary infection
  Chronic infection
  Advanced disease
  Non-AIDS complications of HIV infection
  Determinants of disease progression
Diagnosis
  Differential diagnosis
  Laboratory diagnosis
Prevention and control
  Treatment
  Treatment as prevention
  Postexposure prophylaxis
  Preexposure prophylaxis
  Prospects for HIV eradication
  HIV vaccines
Perspective

HISTORY

Human immunodeficiency virus (HIV) infection is fundamentally a direct infection of the immune system. The main clinical manifestation of infection is a progressive and ultimately profound defect in cell-mediated immune responses essential for protection against a variety of normally innocuous agents. These opportunistic infections are the major sources of morbidity and mortality in patients with advanced disease. Over the 40 years since the original identification of a new immunodeficiency syndrome that was ultimately shown to be caused by HIV,[74] the infection has become a grave humanitarian crisis with far ranging impact on international political and economic stability and contributes greatly to global health inequalities in terms of access to life-saving therapies and prevention.

INFECTIOUS AGENT

The clinical syndrome is primarily caused by infection with HIV-1, a pathogenic retrovirus in the lentiviral genus. A similar although somewhat attenuated clinical syndrome is associated with infection with HIV-2, but with distinct origin and a geographically restricted region of endemicity. A defining feature of these viruses is their interaction with the cellular receptor CD4 found on both T cells and macrophages. Please refer to Chapter 15 for detailed discussion of the structure, genetic, and functional details of these viruses.

EPIDEMIOLOGY

Initial clues to the emerging HIV epidemic came from two linked observations in 1980–1981. One was from front-line physicians, predominantly in New York and California, who were confronted with previously healthy young men presenting with symptoms of profound unexplained immune deficiency. The other was at the Centers for Disease Control and Prevention (CDC) in Atlanta, which noted a marked increase in the number of requests for pentamidine, a drug used to treat an infection associated with severe immunodeficiency. The link between these observations was the sudden upsurge in cases of *Pneumocystis jirovecii* (formerly *P. carinii*) pneumonia being diagnosed in young men who have sex with men (MSM), an opportunistic infection previously seen in the setting of immune suppression accompanying cancer chemotherapy, but now, for the first time, appearing in persons with no obvious disposition to develop immune deficiency. Thus, a new clinical entity—acquired immune deficiency syndrome (AIDS)—was defined.

By 1984, the viral etiology of AIDS was established through the isolation of a lymphotropic retrovirus, HIV type 1 (HIV-1), from affected persons along with the detection of HIV-1 antibodies in persons at risk.[28,171,396,431] It was clear that certain groups were particularly at risk, including MSM, persons using injection drugs, recipients of blood transfusions, and people with hemophilia, and the mechanisms bloodborne and sexual transmission began to be defined.[111,243] By April 1985, a blood test for detection of antibodies was licensed, and the extent of the epidemic began to unfold. Since the initial detection of the epidemic in the United States and Europe, the World Health Organization (WHO) estimates that 76 million people have been infected with the virus, and as of 2020, approximately 38 million people were living with HIV/AIDS (Fig. 18.1). Globally there are some regions in which transmission is concentrated in specific risk groups, and other areas where the epidemic is generalized meaning that transmission will persist in the general population even with focused prevention efforts in higher risk populations.[478] The WHO African region has the highest burden of infection, accounting for almost two-thirds of all global infections and with an estimated prevalence of 3.7% and a disproportionate infection rate among young girls and women. Expansion of access to testing and to antiretroviral therapy (ART) are key pillars of the strategy to interrupt the epidemic. The 2014 United Nations Programme on HIV and AIDS (UNAIDS) goals center around identifying 90% of infections, insuring 90% of people living with HIV have access to ART and that 90% achieve full viral suppression (so-called "90-90-90" goal).[192] Progress toward these goals has been uneven.[288] Whereas in 2019 new infections had decreased by more than 20% compared to 2010, there were still 1.7 million new infections and an estimated 690,000 AIDS-related deaths.

Origin of HIV

HIV is a zoonotic pathogen. The global epidemic of HIV-1 is the result of cross-species infection of humans by a chimpanzee lentivirus, simian immunodeficiency virus (SIV_{cpz}), which occurred in west central Africa.[175] Chimpanzees, in turn, appear to have acquired SIV_{cpz} sometime after their divergence into multiple subspecies. *Pan troglodytes* and *P.t. schweinfurthii* are naturally infected, whereas other closely related species are not, suggesting that SIV_{cpz} is unlikely to have coevolved with its natural host.[445] How SIV initially arose as a new virus in chimpanzees remains unclear. There is evidence of transmission of two other ancestral SIV species from monkeys to chimpanzees,[445] and diversity within SIV is likely the result of multiple cross-species transmission and recombination events.[33] The timing of the origin of primate lentiviruses more broadly is not clear,[432] although data indicating evolutionary pressure on primate genes suggest that these viruses have been present in the primate population for a prolonged period of time.[101,326] The other causative agent of AIDS, HIV-2 arose from cross-species transmissions of SIV_{smm} to humans in West Africa.[430] There is evidence of at least 9 cross-species transmission events for HIV-2 although the distribution of HIV-2 continues to be restricted.[20] Of note, while some SIVs cause minimal pathology and no immunodeficiency in their natural hosts (i.e., SIV_{smm} in sooty mangabeys),[82] epidemiologic evidence documents decreased survival in chimpanzee troops infected by SIV_{cpz}.[263] Experimental transmission of SIV to susceptible non-natural hosts can result in progressive and profound immunodeficiency and AIDS.[430] Although the reasons for differences in transmissibility and pathogenicity resulting from cross-species transmission are not fully understood, it is clear that immune defenses and viral accessory proteins that mediate immune evasion play an important role. Host restriction factors including apolipoprotein B messenger RNA (mRNA)–editing enzyme, catalytic polypeptide-like 3G (APOBEC3G), tetherin, and tripartite motif 5 alpha (TRIM-5α) create barriers that viruses must overcome in order to become established and survive within a new host species (see Chapter 17).

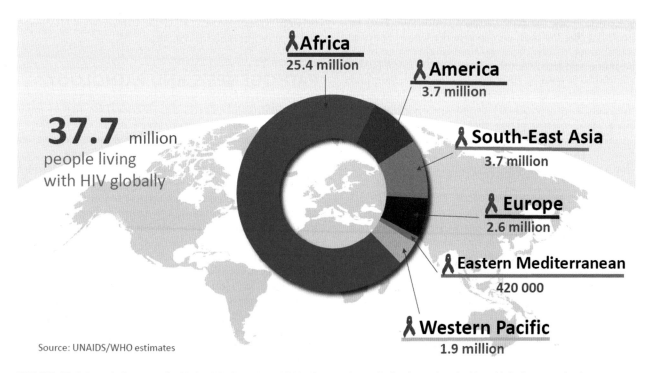

FIGURE 18.1 People living with HIV by WHO region, 2020. (Source: https://cdn.who.int/media/docs/default-source/hq-hiv-hepatitis-and-stis-library/2021_global_summary_web_v32.pdf?sfvrsn=4b8815ad_30. Accessed November 9, 2021.)

For HIV-1, at least four distinct cross-species transmissions are thought to have occurred, giving rise to four highly divergent genetic lineages of infection, termed groups M, N, O, and P.[206,379,392,453] Groups M (major) and N both emerged as the result of a cross-species transmission event from chimpanzees to humans. Groups O and P were likely transmitted from gorillas to chimpanzees and subsequently to humans[432,444] and constitute a very small minority of infections, with some indication that P may represent a lineage that will extinguish.[4] Group M is by far the most widespread, accounting for more than 95% of global cases. The greatest genetic diversity in group M is found in the area near Kinshasa in central Africa, suggesting that the pandemic strain likely emerged in this region of Africa. Multiple studies have attempted to date the emergence of group M in the human population using a variety of approaches, HIV sequence datasets, and assumptions about rates of sequence evolution, with all centering around the turn of the 20th century as the timing of introduction of HIV-1 group M.[150,272,426,522,530] Inclusion of a near-full length HIV-1 genome extracted from an archived, fixed tissue specimen from Kinshasa in 1966 yielded a similar estimate of the origin of the HIV-1 epidemic, providing additional empirical support for this understanding of the evolution of pandemic group M HIV-1.[202]

Current Global Distribution

The most heavily affected global region is Africa, with an estimated 26 million persons currently infected with HIV, approximately two-thirds of the global population of people living with HIV. In the decade between 2010 and 2019, diagnoses and deaths from HIV decreased in both the African region and in Southeast Asia where 3.7 million people are estimated to be living with HIV. In the Americas, which also have approximately 3.7 million people living with HIV, diagnoses increased modestly by 7%, although deaths declined by 20%. The viruses fueling these epidemics vary according to geographic region, with clade C virus being the most prevalent worldwide and clade B currently being the most prevalent in the United States and Western Europe. Clades differ one from another by up to 35% at the amino acid level; within a single clade variation between isolates can be as great as 20%. Errors in reverse transcription, which occur because the viral reverse transcriptase lacks an editing function, lead to variability of individual virus sequences within a single infected person that can exceed what is seen with other viruses (e.g., influenza) over the course of a global epidemic.[179] This variation remains a challenge for efforts to develop a preventative vaccine.

Mechanisms of Transmission

Most cases of HIV infection worldwide are the result of sexual transmission, but important alternative modes of transmission also include parenteral transmission (e.g., through injection drug use) and transmission from mother to infant (vertical transmission). In most global regions, key populations (MSM, people who inject drugs, transgender women, and sex workers) and their sexual partners account for the vast majority of new infections (78% to 99%). Africa is a notable exception: in 2019, key populations accounted for only 28% of new infections, with the vast majority of transmissions occurring through heterosexual exposure. The actual risk of transmission per exposure varies widely (Table 18.1). For sexual transmission, the risk of male to male transmission is greater than the

TABLE 18.1 Risk of transmission of HIV-1	
Sexual transmission	
Receptive penile–vaginal intercourse	8 in 10,000
Insertive penile–vaginal intercourse	4 in 10,000
Receptive anal intercourse	138 in 100,000
Insertive anal intercourse	11 in 100,000
Oral intercourse	Low
Parenteral transmission	
Transfusion of infected blood	250 in 10,000
Needle sharing	63 in 10,000
Needle stick	23 in 10,000
Transmission from mother to infant	
Without ART	2,260 in 10,000[120]
With ART	4 in 1,000

ART, antiretroviral therapy.
Adapted with permission from Patel P, Borkowf CB, Brooks JT, et al. Estimating per-act HIV transmission risk: a systematic review. *AIDS* 2014;28(10):1509–1519.

risk of heterosexual transmission and is highest in persons practicing receptive anal intercourse.[377,421] Overall, the greatest risk of transmission is from contaminated blood transfusions, with greater than 90 of 100 persons becoming infected, although transfusion-related infections are rare now that blood is routinely screened for this pathogen.[377,438] The rate of transmission depends on the inoculum size delivered, but local defense mechanisms in the vaginal and rectal mucosa also likely modulate the risk of infection after a sexual exposure. Initial population studies performed in Africa suggest that there is a threshold viral load (~1,500 RNA copies/mL plasma) below which the likelihood of sexual transmission is greatly reduced.[197,397] These studies were subsequently validated with clinical trials demonstrating that there is no risk of linked viral transmissions between sexual partners when the partner with HIV has had full viral suppression for 6 months.[31,98,415]

PATHOGENESIS AND PATHOLOGY

HIV-1 infects and kills cells that are critical for effective immune responses. Through interactions between the viral envelope and its cellular receptor, CD4 and a chemokine coreceptor, either CCR5 or CXCR4 (see Chapter 17), the virus infects key cells of the adaptive immune response, the CD4 T cell. Depletion of these cells correlates with the clinical manifestations of disease associated with profound immune suppression. The course of disease varies enormously among infected persons. The time from acute infection to the development of AIDS, defined by a CD4 cell count of less than 200 cells/μL or the appearance of AIDS-defining opportunistic infections or cancers, can be as rapid as 6 months.[385] Other persons have been known to be infected for more than 25 years and to maintain normal CD4 cell counts and exhibit no evidence of CD4 cell decline or immune deficiency, despite never having received ART.[338] Initial modeling estimates from the pre-ART era conducted in all male populations suggested a median time to developing AIDS of 9.8 years.[22] This estimate is supported by a retrospective analysis of vaccine trial participants found to have HIV that yielded an estimated survival time of 12.1 years.[268]

A precise explanation for these differences in disease development remains elusive, but there is evidence for contributions from host and viral genetic factors, as well as events early around the time of seroconversion.

Acute Infection and CD4 Cell Depletion

The median viral load in plasma at the time of peak viremia during acute infection is approximately 10^6 to 10^7 RNA copies/mL, which drops to a mean set point of 30,000 copies/mL within the first 6 to 12 months of infection. Longitudinal studies from the Multicenter AIDS Cohort Study (MACS), which were initiated before the availability of effective antiviral therapy, revealed the interquartile ranges of viral load and their relationship to risk of disease progression (Fig. 18.2). Analyses from these data sets indicate that HIV viral load and the initial slope of virus decay after seroconversion are highly associated with disease progression.[305] After the initial seroconversion period, HIV viral load remains linked to risk of AIDS progression in MACS participants followed for more than 10 years.[335] The determinants of initial peak viremia and set point viral load include both intrinsic viral characteristics and host determinants. In one study of subtype B virus using phylogenetic analysis, viral sequence accounted for a substantial proportion of variation in set point viral load.[5] Multiple cohort analyses identify viral load of the transmitting partner as a key determinant in viral load in the newly infected individual; in general, this association is strong but explains a minority of the variance in set point viral load. Incorporation into the analysis of features including HLA haplotype of both partners and the gender of the newly infected person further explains the variance in set point viral load.[218,293,529] The majority of the initial studies were conducted in MSM, with subsequent studies confirming a relationship between set point viral load and progression in women as well.[283] However, women tend to have lower HIV viral loads,[172] although this does not protect against disease progression.[471] The impact of HLA haplotype likely reflects the constriction of viral evolution associated with specific protective immune responses to HIV, as discussed below.[190]

During the period of acute infection, CD4 depletion occurs both in the peripheral blood and from the gastrointestinal (GI) tract.[494] Studies in humans infected with HIV[53,332] and in the SIV macaque model[289,323] describe the profound impact of early infection on the gut. Infection and depletion of large numbers of both resting and activated memory CD4 cells in the gut during primary infection may contribute to initial peak viremia and limit the diversity of subsequent adaptive responses[53,332] (Fig. 18.3). Acute SIV infection is characterized by infection of the gut-associated lymphoid tissue, with between 30% and 60% of all gut-associated CD4 cells becoming productively infected, leading to massive depletion of these cells in only 4 days.[323] The memory cell population including activated and resting memory cells is particularly vulnerable; a substantial portion of this population is lost early during infection.[289] Early initiation of ART is not sufficient to block initial depletion of these cells in the nonhuman primate (NHP) model but appears to enhance restoration of these populations.[103,497] Notably, many pathologic manifestations of HIV occur at mucosal surfaces including esophageal candidiasis, CMV enteritis, and HIV enteropathy. These findings are consistent with the emerging understanding that mucosal T cells play an important role in balancing local immune responses and serve an effective barrier function.[493] Specifically, CD4 T cells that produce IL-17 and/or IL-22 are implicated in maintaining the homeostasis and integrity of the intestinal mucosa. These cells are susceptible to infection with HIV *in vitro* and are depleted in the NHP SIV model and in humans with HIV.[51,340,422,525] This loss of epithelial integrity within the gut mucosa allows translocation of gut-associated microbial products into the systemic

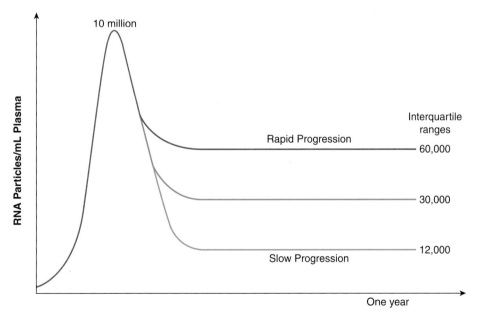

FIGURE 18.2 Interquartile ranges of viral load within 1 year of acute human immunodeficiency virus (HIV) infection. (Adapted from Lyles RH, Munoz A, Yamashita TE, et al. Natural history of human immunodeficiency virus type 1 viremia after seroconversion and proximal to AIDS in a large cohort of homosexual men. *J Infect Dis* 2000;181:872–880.)

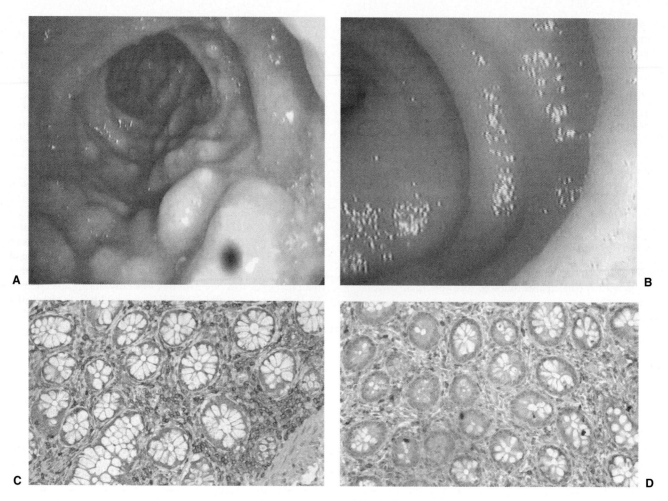

FIGURE 18.3 Appearance of the terminal ileum in human immunodeficiency virus (HIV) infection. A: Uninfected. **B:** HIV infected, showing dramatic loss of lymphoid tissue. **C:** Uninfected, showing numerous CD4 T cells in the lamina propria by immunohistochemical staining. **D:** HIV infected, showing depletion of CD4 T cells in the lamina propria.

circulation.[148] These products are a major driver of the systemic immune activation that is a predominant feature of pathogenic HIV and SIV infections.[51,52] The loss of CD4 T cells from the gut during acute infection, therefore, has two effects on the immune system: depletion of a substantial number of memory CD4 T cells and microbial translocation, which establishes a state of chronic immune activation that further promotes systemic HIV infection and replication.

The impact of HIV-associated CD4 depletion on T-cell receptor (TCR) diversity has been studied in multiple settings based on analyses of TCR Vβ gene usage and TCR sequence diversity. Initial studies demonstrated skewing of the TCR repertoire.[104] Follow-up studies showed a drop in TCR diversity overall but more comparable levels of diversity within T cell subsets.[30] The precise consequences of this substantial early loss of T cells in the context of limited thymic function and potential for repopulation are unknown. It is notable that the profound initial depletion typically is not associated with increased susceptibility to opportunistic infections, suggesting some recovery in immune function. Another key question centers around the decline from peak viremia to set point viral load at steady state. Potential factors responsible for this transition include the depletion of mucosal cells that support high levels of replication

and the rise of a virus-specific adaptive immune response; modeling studies highlight the potential contributions of these different mechanisms to limiting viral replication.[386]

Establishment of a Latent Viral Reservoir

During the period of acute infection, a stable reservoir of HIV-infected resting memory CD4 cells is established that harbors replication-competent, integrated provirus.[91,158] Evidence for the very early establishment of a latent reservoir comes from the observation that even in persons treated immediately after infection subsequent treatment interruption results in viral rebound.[99,219] Studies with SIV in NHPs confirm the early establishment of the reservoir; latently infected cells can be identified in the gastrointestinal tract and spleen and mesenteric lymph nodes in animals treated 3 to 4 days after infection, even in some animals treated within 1 day after inoculation with SIV.[398,509,510] Because proviruses that form this latent reservoir are not transcriptionally active, no viral proteins or enzymes are produced. These infected cells, therefore, are protected from the effects of antiviral drug therapy that depend on active replication and from immune recognition and elimination. This latent reservoir is present whether the viral load is high or low, and it persists even after prolonged ART.[157] Current estimates suggest that in persons on suppressive ART, the number of CD4+ T cells that harbor intact proviral DNA averages around 800 per 10^6, the vast majority of which are defective, carrying deletions, truncations, or hypermutations.[228,454] A little more than 50 in 10^6 CD4 cells harbor genetically intact proviruses, but only approximately 1 in 10^6 CD4 cells harbor replication-competent HIV proviruses that can be induced by a single round of maximal *in vitro* stimulation.[454] These defective proviruses accumulate early during HIV infection[58] and make it challenging to quantify the replication competent reservoir, which is the only source of rebound virus. Although previously considered the gold standard for assessing reservoir size, it is now understood that quantitative viral outgrowth assays provide only a minimal estimate of the size of the latent reservoir because not all replication-competent proviruses are induced by a single round of stimulation. These assays nevertheless established that the half-life for decline of the replication-competent HIV reservoir is at least 44 months, suggesting that it would take more than 70 years to achieve viral eradication by gradual senescence of these cells.[110,450] Consequently, persistence of this latent reservoir is the principal barrier to cure of HIV infection.

It is now generally accepted that homeostatic proliferation and antigen-driven expansion of CD4+ T cells harboring HIV proviruses, rather than ongoing viral replication, are the mechanisms responsible for persistence of the latent reservoir. Integration site analysis provides evidence for clonal expansion of cells harboring defective and intact, replication-competent proviral sequences.[60,232,303,308,454] The presence of identical proviral integrants in clonally amplified CD4 T cells provides evidence that latently infected T cells can undergo proliferative expansion without necessarily inducing viral expression that leads to cell death.[455] In most cases, clonal expansion cannot be explained by insertional mutagenesis but is due to antigen-specific stimulation.[306,455] Episodic exposure to cognate antigen may lead to fluctuations over time in the size of a particular proviral clone, explaining the dynamic nature of the viral reservoir.

Host Immunity

Whereas HIV infection is associated with immune depletion in the vast majority of individuals, there is substantial variability in the course of disease progression. In rare cases, nonprogressive infection (i.e., with preservation of CD4 count) can occur with or without natural suppression of viremia. Although in rare cases defective viruses have been associated with an attenuated clinical course,[124,266] the majority of data indicate that innate and adaptive immune responses as well as host genetic factors are the primary determinants of outcomes.

Innate Immune Responses

The initial immune response to HIV involves innate immune mechanisms. Nonhuman primates infected with SIV demonstrate activation of interferon signaling as early as 1 day after infection. Notably, these initial responses do not include antiviral restriction factors but are inflammatory, with expression of inflammasome components and chemokines that may recruit additional cells susceptible to infection.[27] Days later, there is rise of antiviral interferon signaling that corresponds to higher levels of local SIV RNA production.[27,304] Studies of the hyperacute phase of HIV infection in humans have delineated features of the early immune response in the peripheral blood.[262] Plasmacytoid dendritic cells (pDCs) respond to HIV

viral sequences with IFN α production[32]; pDCs also are important early sources of IFN-α in NHP models of SIV infection. Work from hyperacute infection in human cohorts suggests that pDCs may recruit immune cells through IFN-independent mechanisms. Specific phenotypes of dendritic cell function may be responsible for priming optimized T-cell responses in elite controllers.[320]

Inflammatory cytokines including CXCL10 are rapidly up-regulated in response to plasma viremia; monocytes and macrophages are key regulators of this process.[255,452] With plasma viremia, monocytes expand and up-regulate pathogen recognition and antiviral genes.[261,262,349] Continued expression of HLA-DR by monocytes and macrophages during acute and early infection may contribute to expansion of suppressive Treg cells[298] and may be linked to induction of an exhaustion phenotype in T cell populations. Inflammatory cytokines contribute to the environment of immune activation that is a signature of HIV pathogenesis; early studies identified the close relationship between T-cell activation markers and disease progression.[186,187] In addition to classical innate immune cells and T cells, HIV has a direct impact on the innate-like cytotoxic lymphocyte population (ILC) including natural killer (NK) cells, mucosal-associated invariant T (MAIT) cells, and ILC helper cell populations.[140,262] NK cells expand and express cytolytic gene programs in acute HIV infection, although they show dysregulated phenotypes in chronic infection.[8,261] Genomic determinants of NK cell function including KIR and HLA suggest a direct role for NK cells in the response to HIV.[7,16,318] The identification of HIV antigen-specific NK cells with recall responses has opened questions about the potential to direct NK cells responses with vaccination. The precise roles of innate lymphoid cells in the immune response to HIV and the pathogenesis incurred by their depletion or dysfunction are areas of active research.

Adaptive Humoral Immune Responses

Antibodies to HIV appear within weeks of initial infection. The viral envelope glycoprotein is heavily glycosylated by sugar residues that prevent antibody binding to the underlying peptidic structure without disrupting receptor binding.[504] A subset of these antibodies nevertheless have neutralizing function and select rapidly for escape mutants characterized by alterations in glycosylation sites that constitute the glycan shield.[411] This selection is an iterative process: new antibody responses develop to neutralize the mutant virus, which then escapes again. A minority of individuals develop broadly neutralizing antibodies (bNAbs) capable of neutralizing multiple strains of HIV-1.[37,132,233,291,451,468,501] Specific regions of HIV Env targeted by bNAbs include the CD4 biding site, the V1V2 loop apex, glycan targets on the V2 loop, and the membrane proximal external region (MPER). Binding to the envelope glycoprotein trimer on the surface of free virions or following CD4-gp120 binding prevents the fusion of the viral and cell membranes that is essential for viral entry.[61] There is little evidence to suggest that antibodies contribute to immune control in chronic infection.[393] However, the therapeutic use of bNAbs isolated from patients is a strategy under evaluation for both prevention of HIV and for targeting of the reservoir in cure strategies.[72,470] Current vaccine efforts seek to leverage the understanding of naturally emerging bNAbs to inform immunogen design.[62]

Adaptive Cellular Immune Responses

CD8 T-Cell Responses

Expansion of CD8 T cells that recognize specific viral proteins presented by HLA class I molecules on the infected cell surface is a key feature of adaptive cellular immunity. Recognition via the TCR of a viral (foreign/nonself) protein presented as a short 8 to 10 amino acid peptide in the groove of a class I molecule can result in the directed lysis of that cell by CD8 T cells. In a successful response to infection, the kinetics of virus production, peptide presentation via class I, CD8 T-cell recognition, and the activation state of the CD8 T cell allow the elimination of virus-infected cells, thereby interrupting the production of progeny virus. The importance of these CD8 responses can be inferred from the genetic footprints in HIV sequences that result from evolution to escape directed T-cell control (discussed below).

In the early weeks following HIV infection, viral load rises to a peak averaging 1×10^6 copies/mL and then drops to a viral set point that averages 30,000 copies/mL.[305,418] As discussed above, the decline occurs in the context of depletion of gut CD4 cells that support replication and a rise in innate immune responses. Also coincident with this drop in viremia is the appearance of HIV-specific CD8 T cells, suggesting that these cells have an active antiviral effect.[45,275] Studies in the NHP model of SIV infection support a role for CD8 cells. Although transient depletion of CD8 cells with a monoclonal antibody during primary infection does not significantly change viral kinetics or peak viremia, viral set points are higher.[436] In chronic infection, depletion of CD8 cells is associated with a rise in virus levels followed by a decline with reemergence of CD8 populations.[247] Studies of acute HIV infection demonstrate that HIV-specific CD8 T cells are activated and expand early during infection, with progressive functional dysregulation that may partially be ameliorated by early initiation of ART.[129,356,477] Thus, there is evidence of effective immune recognition of HIV, although these responses are inadequate to achieve full control of viral replication.

The efficacy of the CD8 T-cell response depends on a number of host and viral determinants. Dysfunctional responses and susceptibility to apoptosis are cell-intrinsic limitations of CD8 T-cell effectiveness in controlling HIV infection. Additional factors include immune evasion through variations in specific viral epitopes targeted by the adaptive immune response, as well as the breadth and magnitude of that response. Responses have been observed to all nine HIV viral proteins, and, in most persons, an average of more than a dozen viral peptides are simultaneously targeted.[3,35] The precise drivers of which epitopes are targeted (immunodominance of antigens) in viral infections in general are incompletely understood, but host genetics (HLA haplotype) and viral factors both contribute.[87] The immunodominance of responses to nonprotective epitopes is one feature of inefficient immune responses to HIV.[163] Escape from CTL control influences HIV diversity and, when escape mutations occur in appropriate viral proteins, can affect the viral replication capacity.[6,10,48] The *in vitro* reduction in replication capacity is consistent with *in vivo* association of Gag-dominant responses with lower HIV viral load, highlighting the importance of appropriately targeted responses.[400,535]

Evasion of CD8 T-cell recognition by viral mutation can be mediated at several different levels: mutations may interfere with antigen processing or presentation or may alter epitope residues required for TCR recognition.[46] Certain viral proteins are more constrained than others in the mutational burden that can be tolerated, and efforts to identify optimal targets of CD8 T-cell recognition have used both quantitative modeling of fitness costs[29,116,155] and novel approaches assessing structural topology of viral epitopes.[167] These considerations are critical for designing preventive vaccines that elicit a CD8 T-cell response and for therapeutic vaccine strategies to boost endogenous immune recognition and eliminate the viral reservoir.[331] The only CD8 T-cell response with substantial protective efficacy in preventive vaccine studies in NHP models is notable for its atypical restriction by major histocompatibility complex E, which may also provide insight into the potential for epitope targeting.[208,209] Therapeutic vaccines focused on HIV cure will have to contend with the substantial burden of escape mutations in the latent reservoir highlighting the importance of identifying specific conserved and vulnerable antigenic targets.[131]

Virus-Specific CD4 T Cells

The optimal coordination of antibody and CD8 CTL responses depends on the presence of virus-specific CD4 T cells. These cells are also the primary target of infection by HIV, however, and asymmetric depletion of specific functional subsets may influence their helper function. Whereas data suggest that HIV-specific CD4 T cells are enriched for HIV proviral DNA, the majority of HIV-specific T cells are not infected.[137] The antigenic targets of CD4 T-cell recognition are less well defined as compared to CD8 T-cell epitopes, although data have indicated that a greater breadth in the overall CD4 T-cell response and responses targeting the HIV Gag protein are associated with lower levels of viremia.[402] Although less clear than for CD8 T cells, there is evidence in NHP SIV models for mutations that allow escape from CD4 T-cell recognition and correlative data linking HIV sequence polymorphisms and HLA II genotypes, suggesting selective pressure.[63,145] CD4 T helper cell function can support CD8 T-cell proliferation, although attempts to augment this CD4 T-cell support through vaccination or cytokine support (IL-2) have not led to improvement in clinical or virologic outcomes.[2,240,257,412,418,419]

CD4 T cells are classified into multiple functional lineages including T helper 1, T helper 2, T helper 17, follicular T helper, and T regulatory subsets. As discussed above, depletion of Th17 and Th1 CD4 cells at mucosal sites is a feature of acute HIV infection.[304] The HIV-specific CD4 response detected in the periphery includes production of both IFN-γ and IL-17, which may signal a dysfunctional polarization.[89,528] Despite secretion of IFN-γ, overall function of these CD4 cells appears to be impaired.[210,240] Atypical CD4 T-cell activity including cytolytic function has been documented.[462] A role for CD4 T-cell responses despite evidence for functional compromise is supported by the association of CD4 T-cell activation during later acute infection and subsequent preservation of CD4 cell counts.[524]

CD4 T cells responding to coinfecting pathogens may have specific features that affect their susceptibility to infection with HIV. Initial studies suggested that CD4 T cells that express β chemokines (which bind to CCR5 and block HIV entry) may be more resistant to HIV infection and depletion than those that do not.[71,182] However, as HIV most efficiently infects activated CD4 cells, it is likely that infection events occur with higher frequency in pathogen-specific, activated and expanded CD4 T cells. This concept is supported by the identification of enrichment of proviral DNA in CD4 cells responding to Epstein-Barr virus (EBV)/CMV antigens and implicating antigen-driven clonal expansion in the maintenance of the HIV-1 reservoir.[220,455]

Host Genetics and Viral Control

The course of HIV disease is moderated by a variety of host genetic factors. Among the most important are polymorphisms in the genes encoding the chemokine coreceptors and their ligands, and in the HLA genes. HIV-1 uses one of two chemokine receptors as coreceptor for virus entry into CD4 cells: CCR5 or CXCR4.[130,138,153] Approximately 10% of Caucasians carry a defective allele that has a 32-base pair (bp) deletion in the CCR5 gene (ccr5Δ32); 1% are homozygous for this deletion and resist infection by CCR5-using (R5) viruses.[297,428] Infected individuals who are heterozygous for the ccr5Δ32 allele have a slower rate of disease progression than do those who are homozygous for the wild-type allele.[125] This effect is limited to patients with R5 strains of HIV-1, presumably because other viruses use the CXCR4 receptor (X4 virus).[50,337] A mutation in the CCR2 gene, CCR2–64I, likewise reduces the rate of disease progression,[273,459] possibly by delaying emergence of X4 virus.[490] By contrast, mutations in the promoter region of CCR5 (CCR5 P1) are associated with accelerated disease progression.[317] Other analyses have failed, however, to show a significant effect of

CCR5 and CCR2 genotype after controlling for CD4 cell count, plasma HIV-1 RNA level, and viral tropism.[184,239]

Copy number of the gene encoding the natural ligand for CCR5 (CCL3L1, previously known as MIP-1α) also influences the rate of disease progression. Higher CCL3L1 copy number is associated with a lower risk of progression, which is most pronounced in patients with polymorphisms that reduce the level of functional CCR5 on the cell surface.[189] Variable effects on progression have been noted for the SDF1-3′A polymorphism, which affects the untranslated region of the mRNA encoding stromal-derived factor (SDF-1, also known as CXCL12), the natural ligand of CXCR4.[115,189,513]

Several studies have related host HLA haplotype to the rate of HIV disease progression (Fig. 18.4).[70] For example, presence of the HLA-B27 and B57 alleles is associated with slow progression.[9,152,383] Conversely, persons carrying class I alleles B*35 or Cw*04 progress to AIDS significantly more rapidly than do those lacking these alleles.[69,176] Maximal heterozygosity at HLA class I loci A, B, and C is associated with delayed onset of AIDS.[253] Polymorphisms resulting in increased surface expression of HLA-A are associated with poor control of HIV due to enhanced expression of HLA-E, the ligand for the inhibitory NKG2A natural killer cell receptor.[401] By contrast, polymorphisms that increase surface expression of HLA-C are associated with lower virus load.[16] Given that HLA antigen class I molecules play an essential role in antigen presentation to CD8+ CTL, these findings provide strong, albeit indirect, evidence for the importance of CTL in moderating the rate of HIV disease progression.

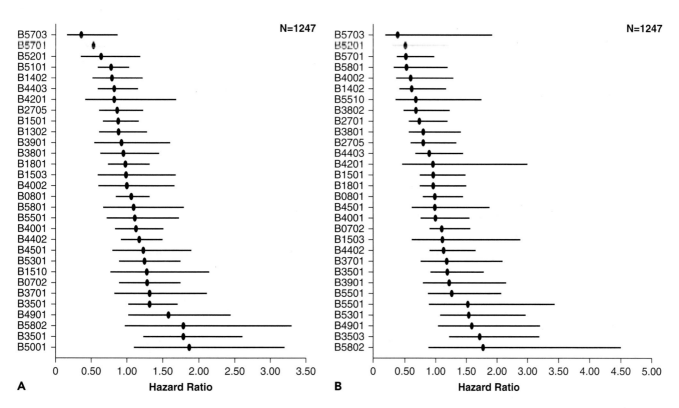

FIGURE 18.4 Relative hazard of disease progression by human leukocyte antigen (HLA) class I type. A: Relative hazard of progression to a CD4 count of less than 200/mm³. **B:** Relative hazard of progression to acquired immunodeficiency disease syndrome (AIDS) by the 1987 AIDS defining criteria.

Variation in the killer immunoglobulin-like receptor (KIR) genes also affects the course of disease. These receptors are found on NK cells and regulate NK activity by recognition of certain HLA class I molecules on the surface of target cells.[498] The effect of KIR alleles appears to be related to the presence or absence of specific HLA-B or HLA-C alleles.[181] For example, when present together with the HLA-B *Bw4-80Ile* allele, the activating KIR allele *KIR3DS1* is associated with delayed disease progression.[318] By contrast, in the absence of HLA-B *Bw4-80Ile*, the presence of *KIR3DS1* is associated with more rapid disease progression. Similarly, presence of the inhibitory KIR allele *KIR3DL1* together with HLA-B*57S is highly protective against disease progression.[301] The *KIR2DS2* allele appears to be associated with more rapid CD4 decline over time, but has no effect on viral load, whereas HLA-B*5701* and B*2705* alleles are associated with significantly lower levels of viremia.[180] A more detailed understanding of the interactions between HLA and KIR genotypes and the balance between CD8 and NK responses that lead to favorable outcomes will provide opportunities for vaccine targeting.

Reasons for Immune Failure

Functional Defects

Given the multiplicity of immune responses generated in response to HIV, including production of broadly neutralizing antibodies, virus-specific CD4 and CD8 T-cell responses, and activation of innate immune responses, why is the immune system unable to contain HIV replication in the vast majority of persons with HIV? Immune escape due to viral variation limits the ability of antibodies to neutralize autologous virus. Aberrant differentiation of CD4 T-cell populations likely also contributes to the ineffectiveness of the immune response. Viremic infection results in an overrepresentation of T-follicular helper cell (T_{fh}) phenotypes; this skewing is not observed in individuals with spontaneous control of viral replication, who show patterns of gene expression consistent with Th1, Th17, and Th22 CD4 T-cell differentiation programs.[347] Functional CD8 T-cell responses associated with lower viral load and spontaneous control of HIV replication include polyfunctionality (simultaneous expression of multiple cytokines, cytolytic function, proliferation, and maturation).[36,122,221,222,339] Which of these aspects of the CD8 T-cell response in chronic HIV infection is a cause as opposed to an effect of ongoing viral replication is often unclear. What is clear, however, is that chronic antigenic stimulation by persistent viruses can lead to exhaustion of CD8 T cells by preventing them from completing the normal progression to renewable memory cells.[507,508] Surface expression on CD8 T cells of molecules associated with T-cell regulation (i.e., programmed death 1 [PD-1], 2B4, CD160, lymphocyte activation gene 3 [LAG-3]) is associated with chronic antigen exposure and ineffective viral clearance by CD8 T cells.[26,38] HIV-specific T cells show aberrant expression of coregulatory molecules and specific epigenetic programs that favor PD-1 expression and can adversely affect HIV-specific CD8 T-cell function and longevity.[121,384,484,526,527] Coregulatory molecule expression can also be aberrant on CD4 T cells, thereby imparting indirect effects on the CD8 T-cell response.[256,261] In addition, myeloid DCs can be infected with HIV, which may contribute to impaired DC function in infected persons.[302,311,435] Efforts to ameliorate this antigen-specific dysfunction are a focus of curative strategies.[154]

Immune Escape and Evasion

As discussed in the section on CD8 T-cell responses above, there is substantial evidence of CTL-mediated escape mutations in HIV linked to specific HLA alleles, highlighting the balance between the immune response and virus evolution. On a population level, clear evidence indicates viral imprinting by host CD8 T-cell responses: persons with certain HLA alleles have a significantly increased prevalence of certain viral polymorphisms that appear to be driven by immune escape.[260] HIV also evades immune recognition through down-regulation of HLA class I molecules mediated by the viral Nef protein, limiting the capacity for CD8 T-cell recognition of productively infected cells.[100,284,441] Likewise, viral latency contributes to immune evasion as latently infected cells do not express viral proteins and remain invisible to the immune system. Taken together, the immune response to HIV infection demonstrates the impact of host genetics on pathogen recognition, the interplay between viral evolutionary constraints and immune evasion in individuals and populations, and the consequences of dysfunctional immune responses for pathogen control.

CLINICAL FEATURES

Advancing immunodeficiency caused by the progressive loss of CD4+ T lymphocytes underlies the cardinal clinical manifestations of HIV-1 infection. The myriad opportunistic infections and malignancies characteristic of AIDS are a consequence of the resulting profound defect in cellular immunity. In addition, a number of clinical syndromes are attributable directly to infection of specific organs by HIV-1. The course of HIV-1 disease can be divided into three stages: primary (or acute) infection, chronic (asymptomatic) infection, and advanced disease (AIDS) (Fig. 18.5). The duration of each stage is highly variable and can be altered by ART. Several systems for classifying the different stages of HIV-1 disease have been developed, the most widely used of which include those developed by the CDC (Table 18.2) and the WHO.[76,518] Although these classification systems are valuable epidemiologic tools, their role in the assessment and clinical management of individual patients has been more limited.

Primary Infection

Acquisition of HIV-1 infection is accompanied by relatively nonspecific symptoms of an acute viral illness in approximately 50% to 70% of infected individuals.[250] Symptoms, which usually begin 2 weeks after exposure, frequently include fever, pharyngitis, headache, arthralgias, myalgias, malaise, and weight loss.[114,217] A nonpruritic, maculopapular rash on the face and trunk occurs in up to 70% of cases.[483] In addition, generalized lymphadenopathy is a frequent finding. Mucocutaneous ulceration and weight loss help distinguish primary HIV-1 infection from other viral syndromes.[168,217] Aseptic meningoencephalitis is the most common neurologic manifestation of primary HIV-1 infection.[483] Symptoms of primary infection resolve within 3 to 4 weeks in most patients. Persistence of symptoms beyond 8 to 12 weeks along with a severely depressed CD4+ T-lymphocyte count and high plasma HIV-1 RNA levels may predict more rapid progression of disease.

Laboratory characteristics of primary HIV-1 infection include lymphopenia and a decrease in the absolute CD4+

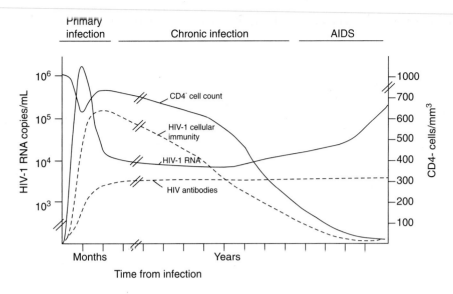

FIGURE 18.5 Changes in plasma human immunodeficiency virus type 1 (HIV-1) RNA level, CD4+ cell count, HIV-1-specific antibody titers, and HIV-1-specific cellular immune responses over the course of HIV-1 infection.

T-lymphocyte count, usually accompanied by an increase in circulating activated CD8+ T cells.[106] Other hematologic abnormalities are unusual, except for mild thrombocytosis. Modest elevations in serum aspartate transaminase and alkaline phosphate may be present, but clinically significant hepatitis is uncommon.[483] Plasma HIV-1 RNA titers generally peak 1 week following the onset of symptoms, averaging 10^6 to 10^7 copies/mL and decline to steady-state levels (between 10^3 and 10^5 copies/mL) by 2 months after infection.[292,305]

Chronic Infection

Following resolution of primary infection and establishment of a virologic *quasi-steady state*,[226] a prolonged period of asymptomatic chronic infection ensues. Although most patients remain asymptomatic during much of this phase, ongoing viral replication and CD4 lymphocyte depletion make the term *clinical latency* inappropriate. The loss of CD4 T cells proceeds at

an average rate of 30 to 60 cells/mm³/year, although CD4 cell counts can remain stable for several years before a period of rapid decline.[334] A small proportion of patients (<1%) experience progression to AIDS within 1 to 2 years.[351,385] Rapid progression may be associated with transmission of syncytium-inducing (SI) variants of HIV-1 (i.e., viruses that use the CXCR4 coreceptor, also known as *X4 viruses*).[92,279,360]

Fatigue and lymphadenopathy are noted by many patients during this otherwise asymptomatic phase of HIV-1 infection. Minor clinical events, such as oral hairy leukoplakia (caused by EBV infection of oral epithelial cells), oral and vaginal candidiasis, herpes zoster, and a variety of other dermatologic conditions, may be early signs of clinical progression. With advancing disease, night sweats and weight loss become more common.

A variety of systemic manifestations of HIV-1 infection involving nearly every organ system can occur during the chronic phase of disease. Remission in response to ART

TABLE 18.2   CDC classification system for HIV infection

	Clinical Categories		
CD4 Cell Categories	**A** Asymptomatic, Lymphadenopathy, or Acute Infection	**B** Symptomatic,[a] not Category A or C	**C** Clinical AIDS[b]
>500/mm³ (>29%)	A1	B1	C1
200–499/mm³ (14%–28%)	A2	B2	C2
<200/mm³ (<14%)	A3	B3	C3

[a]Examples of these symptoms include bacillary angiomatosis; thrush; vulvovaginal candidiasis; cervical dysplasia or carcinoma *in situ*; constitutional symptoms such as fever or diarrhea of greater than 1 month duration; oral hairy leukoplakia; multidermatomal or recurrent herpes zoster; immune thrombocytopenic purpura; listeriosis; pelvic inflammatory disease; and peripheral neuropathy.
[b]Candidiasis of the esophagus or respiratory tract; invasive cervical cancer; extrapulmonary coccidioidomycosis; cryptosporidiosis; extralymphatic cytomegalovirus infection; herpes simplex with mucocutaneous ulcer greater than 1 month duration, or bronchitis, pneumonitis, or esophagitis; extrapulmonary histoplasmosis; HIV-associated dementia; CNS lymphoma; non-Hodgkin lymphoma; pulmonary tuberculosis; disseminated *M. tuberculosis*, *M. avium* complex, or *M. kansasii* infection; nocardiosis; *Pneumocystis jirovecii* pneumonia; recurrent bacterial pneumonia; progressive multifocal leukoencephalopathy; recurrent *Salmonella* septicemia; extraintestinal strongyloidiasis; toxoplasmosis.

Adapted from the Centers for Disease Control and Prevention. 1993 revised classification system for HIV infection and expanded surveillance case definition for AIDS among adolescents and adults. *MMWR Morbid Mortal Wkly Rep* 1992;41(RR-17):1–19.

suggests a direct role for HIV-1 in the pathogenesis of these disorders. Dermatologic conditions are particularly common among persons with HIV-1, including seborrheic dermatitis, papular pruritic eruption, and eosinophilic folliculitis.[107] Neurologic manifestations include disorders of both the central nervous system (CNS) and peripheral nervous system, in addition to opportunistic infections and malignancies of the CNS. HIV-associated neurological dysfunction (HAND, previously known as AIDS dementia complex) and distal symmetric polyneuropathy, which occur in up to 27% and 35% of patients, respectively, are among the most frequently encountered HIV-related neurologic complications.[456,461] Wasting associated with HIV infection remains highly prevalent in resource-limited settings and is an independent predictor of mortality.[312] Anorexia, malabsorption, and inappropriate nutrient utilization all contribute to the loss of lean body mass in patients with AIDS.[201,274]

Other organ system–specific complications of HIV infection include nonspecific interstitial pneumonitis and lymphocytic interstitial pneumonitis, disorders of the gastrointestinal tract, endocrine dysfunction, anemia and neutropenia, immune-mediated thrombocytopenia, and a variety of rheumatologic syndromes.[368] In addition, HIV-associated nephropathy leading to renal insufficiency is particularly common among African Americans and injection drug users.[476,514]

Advanced Disease

Opportunistic infections and malignancies are rare in HIV-infected persons with CD4 counts above 500 cells/mm^3 but increase as the CD4 count declines below this benchmark. Oral candidiasis, pneumococcal infections, tuberculosis, and reactivation of herpes simplex and varicella zoster viruses become more common. The risk of life-threatening complications, including *Pneumocystis jirovecii* (formerly, *P. carinii*) pneumonia, candida esophagitis, disseminated histoplasmosis and other systemic fungal infections, toxoplasma encephalitis, and cryptococcal meningitis increases substantially once the CD4 lymphocyte count drops below 200 cells/mm^3.[321] Opportunistic infections, such as disseminated *Mycobacterium avium* complex infection; reactivation of cytomegalovirus (CMV) infection, cryptosporidiosis, and microsporidiosis; and progressive multifocal leukoencephalopathy caused by JC virus reactivation, are all indicative of a profound defect in cellular immunity and usually occur at CD4 counts below 50 cells/mm^3. Malignancies associated with AIDS generally are related to underlying viral infection, including Kaposi's sarcoma (KS) caused by infection with human herpes virus 8; lymphomas associated with EBV infection; and cervical and anal carcinoma associated with human papilloma virus infection. Although potent ART has clearly reduced the risk of KS and non-Hodgkin lymphoma, the effect on Hodgkin lymphoma is less clear.[41,42,449] Whereas the incidence of lung cancer is also increased in persons with HIV infection, age-adjusted rates of other malignancies (e.g., breast and prostate cancer) are comparable to those found in the general population.[199,448]

Non-AIDS Complications of HIV Infection

A number of end-organ complications not traditionally considered "AIDS-defining" events have been recognized to occur more frequently in HIV-1–infected patients.[314,359] These include an increased risk of cardiovascular disease, non-AIDS defining malignancies, HAND, and HIV-associated nephropathy

(HIVAN) and may also include loss of bone mineral density (BMD) and other changes typically associated with increasing age, suggesting that HIV-1 infection may accelerate the aging process more generally. Moreover, as the population with HIV ages, the proportion of people with HIV (PWH) with one or more significant medical comorbidities increases.[515]

With respect to cardiovascular risk, a number of studies suggest increased risk of myocardial infarction in HIV-1–infected patients as compared to control populations matched for traditional cardiovascular risk factors such as age, family history, hyperlipidemia, hypertension, diabetes, and smoking.[225,359,486] More striking is the finding that interrupting ART significantly increases the risk of cardiovascular events, independent of CD4 cell count.[142,388] This increased risk was correlated with an increase in plasma levels of inflammatory markers such as IL-6 and high-specificity C-reactive protein (hsCRP).[278,420] In addition, a number of studies have shown adverse changes in surrogate markers associated with cardiovascular risk such as flow-mediated vasodilatation, carotid intima-media thickness, and coronary artery calcification in patients with HIV-1 infection.[112,200] The extent to which these changes can be prevented or reversed by ART is an active area of current research.

Patients with HIV-1 infection also show lower BMD and an increased risk of fractures compared to age-matched, uninfected controls.[485] The causes of HIV-associated loss of BMD are poorly understood and most likely are multifactorial, including increased immune activation and inflammation, renal tubular dysfunction, low vitamin D levels, and other endocrine abnormalities.[11] Paradoxically, initiation of ART may be associated with a decrease in BMD, which subsequently stabilizes.[56] This effect is most pronounced in patients starting ART regimens containing tenofovir disoproxil fumarate (TDF; see "Drug Toxicity" under Section Treatment and Control, below).

Determinants of Disease Progression

Numerous viral and host factors contribute to determining the rate of HIV disease progression. The plasma HIV-1 RNA level, or viral load, reflects the rate of virus replication and is a powerful independent prognostic factor for the risk of disease progression.[335,382] Data from the MACS show that in the absence of ART individuals with plasma HIV-1 RNA levels greater than 100,000 copies/mL 6 months after seroconversion are 10 times more likely to progress to AIDS within 5 years than are those with lower steady-state levels of viremia.[333] Similarly, for patients with established HIV-1 infection, a steady-state viral load of more than 30,000 copies/mL is associated with a more than fivefold greater risk of disease progression within 3 years as compared with patients with viral loads of 3,000 to 10,000 copies/mL.[334]

According to a Poisson regression model based on data from the Concerted Action on Seroconversion to AIDS and Death in Europe (CASCADE) collaboration of 22 cohorts from Europe, Canada, and Australia, in the absence of combination ART, the 6-month risk of AIDS for a 25-year-old patient with a CD4 cell count of 350/mm^3 ranges from 0.6% at a viral load of 3,000 copies/mL to 2.5% at a viral load of 300,000 copies/mL.[387] At a CD4 count of 100 cells/mm^3, the AIDS risk at the same viral loads increases to 3.7% and 14.5%, respectively. The risk of disease progression has been reduced substantially since the introduction of potent combination ART.[141] Progression to AIDS among persons infected with HIV-2 proceeds at a significantly slower rate as compared with infection with HIV 1.[242,322] Epidemiologic and cohort studies show that HIV-2 infection generally results in lower steady-state levels of viremia (10^3 copies/mL) and a more gradual decline in CD4 cell counts.[17,34,242]

Age at the time of infection is an independent risk factor for disease progression, with older persons being at significantly greater risk, perhaps as a consequence of diminished thymic reserve.[14,119] The role of gender in determining disease progression is less clear. Most studies show that HIV-1–infected men and women progress to AIDS at similar rates.[123,341] Early in the course of infection, however, women tend to have significantly lower plasma HIV-1 RNA levels than men.[12,13,151] This difference disappears as disease progresses. Because overall progression rates are comparable between the sexes, these observations imply that compared with men, women experience HIV-1 disease progression at lower viral loads.

Although virus replication, and consequently viral load, is the engine that drives progression to AIDS, the CD4 cell count is the most useful marker for predicting the immediate risk of developing particular opportunistic infections.[141] Moreover, differences in viral load explain only a small fraction of the variability in rates of CD4 cell decline in patients not receiving ART,[417] suggesting that other factors such as immune activation drive CD4 cell loss in HIV infection (see "Pathogenesis"). Indeed, the proportion of activated CD8+ T cells, measured as the percentage of cells expressing CD38, predicts the risk of disease progression independently of viral load and CD4 count.[40,186,187,296] Levels of IL-6 and hsCRP are elevated in patients with HIV infection and independently predict the development of opportunistic diseases.[416] Moreover, increases in soluble markers of inflammation and coagulation including IL-6, soluble TNF receptor (sTNFR)-I, sTNFR-II, kynurenine-to-tryptophan ratio and D-dimer 1 year after initiation of ART were associated with increases in non-AIDS defining events defined as myocardial infarction, stroke, non–AIDS-defining cancer, non–AIDS-defining serious bacterial infection, or death.[481]

The role of chemokine receptor tropism in determining the rate of disease progression remains unresolved. The prevalence of X4 variants increases with decreasing CD4 cell count, and several studies show a significantly increased risk of disease progression among patients with X4 (SI) virus.[57,270,348,439] Macaques infected with a simian-HIV (SHIV) (SIV/HIV chimera) that expresses an X4 HIV-1 envelope show rapid depletion of CD4 cells, suggesting a causal role of X4 viruses in rapid disease progression.[229,362] X4 variants, however, emerge in only half of patients who progress to AIDS.[49,409] The long interval between infection and emergence of X4 viruses in most patients argues for strong selection against X4 viruses early in the course of HIV disease. Therefore, the possibility that emergence of X4 variants is a consequence, rather than a cause, of advancing immunodeficiency remains a plausible alternative explanation for the apparent association of X4 virus with disease progression.

Coinfecting viral pathogens have varied effects on the rate of disease progression. Patients with CMV viremia were twice as likely to experience disease progression and four times more likely to die.[464] Asymptomatic CMV replication may also contribute to ongoing immune activation.[235] Similarly, higher levels of EBV DNA are associated with an increased risk of non-AIDS events.[185] Although the course of both hepatitis B (HBV) and hepatitis C virus (HCV) infection is worse in patients with HIV-1 infection, the effect of hepatitis coinfection on AIDS progression is less clear, with some studies suggesting accelerated progression of HIV-1 infection among coinfected patients and other studies showing no effect[88,424,474,482]; overall, the evidence suggests no significant effect of either HBV or HCV coinfection on the course HIV-1 infection.[413]

DIAGNOSIS

Differential Diagnosis

The occurrence of opportunistic infections such as *P. jirovecii* pneumonia, candida esophagitis, cryptococcal meningitis, toxoplasmosis, or chronic ulcerative herpes simplex in the absence of a known cause of immunodeficiency should raise the possibility of HIV-1 infection. Recurrent or disseminated varicella zoster infection, pneumococcal infection in a young adult, oral or recurrent vulvovaginal candidiasis, disseminated papillomavirus infection, persistent fever, night sweats, lymphadenopathy, weight loss, and chronic diarrhea all may be evidence of infection with HIV-1. A diagnosis of HIV-1 infection also should be considered in patients with unexplained lymphopenia, anemia, or neutropenia, and in cases of idiopathic thrombocytopenia.

The differential diagnosis of acute HIV-1 infection is broad and includes other viral syndromes, such as acute EBV, CMV, adenovirus, influenza, SARS-CoV-2 and enterovirus infection that can be associated with fever, myalgias, rash, lymphadenopathy, pharyngitis, aseptic meningitis, or lymphopenia. Acute Lyme disease, secondary syphilis, rickettsial infection, anaplasmosis, and babesiosis all have features in common with primary HIV-1 infection but are readily excluded by appropriate laboratory tests.

Laboratory Diagnosis

The laboratory diagnosis of HIV infection usually is made by an antigen/antibody immunoassay that detects antibodies to HIV-1 and HIV-2.[79] The mean time to seroconversion during acute HIV infection is 25 days.[64] Antibodies to HIV become detectable within 6 to 12 weeks of infection in most infected individuals and in virtually all patients within 6 months (Fig. 18.6).[169,227] The time to serologic detection of HIV after initial infection can be reduced by 7 days through the use of "4th generation" diagnostic tests, which combine detection of HIV antibodies and core (p24) antigen.[146,373] In addition to the standard HIV immunoassay, rapid diagnostic tests have been developed.[216,364,457] The simplicity and wide range of operating temperature for certain of these assays make them particularly well suited for use in point-of-care testing (e.g., a hospital emergency department or physician office) and in resource-limited settings,[254,492] but specificity of these rapid tests may be lower than expected when applied to populations with a low prevalence of HIV infection.[499]

Previously, sera that gave a positive reaction by an initial antibody screening assay (EIA, chemiluminometric, or rapid immunoassay) were retested to exclude the possibility of clerical or laboratory error, and repeatedly reactive sera were then tested by a confirmatory assay such as a western blot to verify that reactive antibodies were directed against HIV antigens. The availability of combination HIV-1/2 antibody/antigen detection assays has streamlined testing algorithms (Fig. 18.7). The sensitivity of

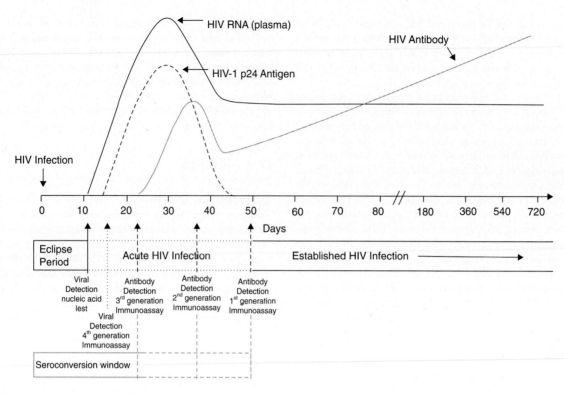

FIGURE 18.6 Sequence of appearance of laboratory markers of HIV-1 infection. (Centers for Disease Control and Prevention and Association of Public Health Laboratories. Laboratory Testing for the Diagnosis of HIV Infection: Updated Recommendations. http://dx.doi.org/10.15620/cdc.23447. Published June 27, 2014.)

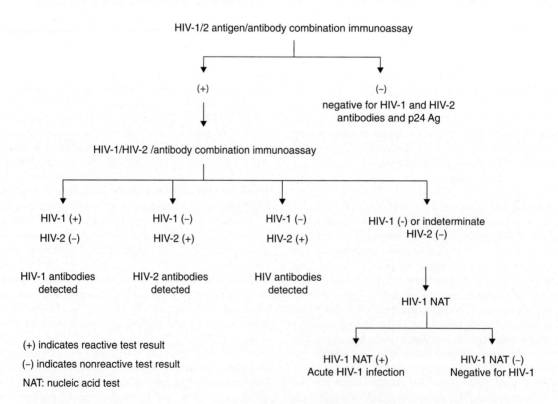

FIGURE 18.7 Recommended algorithm for laboratory testing of serum or plasma specimens for HIV.
(Centers for Disease Control and Prevention and Association of Public Health Laboratories. Laboratory Testing for the Diagnosis of HIV Infection: Updated Recommendations. http://dx.doi.org/10.15620/cdc.23447. Published June 27, 2014.)

FDA-approved tests for the diagnosis of established HIV-1 infection range from 99.76% to 100.0%, with specificities of 99.50% to 100%.[79] In settings where HIV prevalence exceeds 5%, confirmation of an initial rapid HIV antibody test by a second test that uses different antigens can serve to make a diagnosis of HIV infection.[81] Combination HIV-1–HIV-2 assays are reported to have a sensitivity of 100% for detection of HIV-2.[21]

The diagnosis of primary HIV-1 infection before seroconversion depends on detection of HIV-1 capsid (p24) antigen or HIV-1 RNA in plasma. The sensitivity and specificity of the p24 antigen assay for diagnosis of acute HIV-1 infection range from 79% to 89% and 99% to 100%, respectively.[114,217] Quantitative HIV-1 RNA assays are highly sensitive (100%), but because of occasional false-positive findings, tests have a specificity of only 95% to 97%.[114,217] Plasma HIV-1 RNA levels generally exceed 10,000 copies/mL during acute infection, and most false-positive findings generally have values below 3,000 copies/mL.[217] Therefore, accuracy of quantitative plasma HIV-1 RNA assays for diagnosing primary HIV-1 infection can be improved if only values that exceed 5,000 copies/mL are considered true positives.[217]

Serologic testing of infants born of mothers infected with HIV-1 is complicated by the presence of maternal anti-HIV antibodies that decay over 12 to 15 months. Persistence of antibody beyond 15 months of age is evidence of HIV-1 infection in the infant.[75] Two negative antibody tests obtained at least 1 month apart in infants older than 6 months of age effectively exclude HIV-1 infection. Earlier diagnosis depends on detection of HIV-1 RNA in plasma or HIV-1 proviral DNA in peripheral blood mononuclear cells. A DNA polymerase chain reaction (PCR) test is positive in approximately 40% of infected children by age 48 hours, and in 93% of infected children by age 14 days.[139] A qualitative HIV-1 RNA test based on transcription-mediated amplification showed 100% sensitivity and greater than 99% specificity as compared to DNA PCR for infant diagnosis of HIV-1 infection using whole blood or dried blood spots, respectively.[472]

PREVENTION AND CONTROL

Treatment

The advent of combination ART for the treatment of HIV infection has resulted in a dramatic reduction in morbidity and mortality from this disease worldwide. In the United States, AIDS-related mortality has decreased by more than 80% since the introduction of combination ART in the mid-1990s[370] (Fig. 18.8). With prompt initiation of ART, people with HIV may live near-normal lifespans.[491] The rollout of ART in South Africa resulted in a 10-year increase in life expectancy.[13] More than thirty antiretroviral drugs and drug combinations are approved for the treatment of HIV-1 infection (Table 18.3), with more in clinical development. The experience with ART has served as a model for the feasibility of treating chronic viral infections and established important paradigms that have been applied successfully to the treatment of other chronic infections such as HBV and HCV.

Targets for Antiretroviral Drugs

The replication cycle of HIV-1 involves multiple steps, many of which have been successfully exploited as targets for

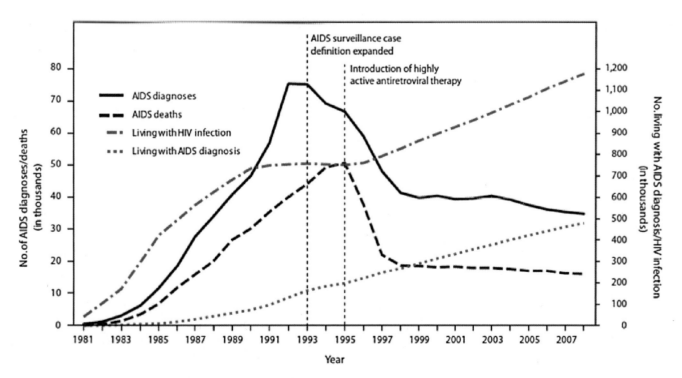

FIGURE 18.8 Estimated number of acquired immunodeficiency disease syndrome (AIDS) diagnoses and deaths and estimated number of persons living with AIDS diagnosis and living with diagnosed or undiagnosed human immunodeficiency virus (HIV) infection among persons aged 13 years or older in the United States, 1981–2008. (From Centers for Disease Control and Prevention. HIV surveillance–United States, 1981–2008. *MMWR Morbid Mortal Wkly Rep* 2011;60:689–693.)

TABLE 18.3 Generic names and common abbreviations for FDA-approved antiretrovirals (2021)

Nucleoside reverse transcriptase inhibitors (NRTIs)		Protease inhibitors (PIs)	
Abacavir	ABC	Amprenavir[a]	APV
Emtricitabine	FTC	fos-Amprenavir	fAPV
Didanosine[a]	ddI	Atazanavir	ATV
Lamivudine	3TC	Darunavir	DRV
Stavudine[a]	d4T	Indinavir	IDV
Zalcitabine[a]	ddC	Lopinavir[b]	LPV
Zidovudine	ZDV	Nelfinavir	NFV
		Saquinavir	SQV
		Ritonavir[c]	RTV
		Tipranavir	TPV
Nucleotide RT inhibitor (NtRTI)		**Attachment inhibitor**	
Tenofovir alafenamide	TAF	Fostemsavir	FTV
Tenofovir disoproxil fumarate	TDF		
Nonnucleoside RT inhibitors (NNRTIs)		**Postattachment inhibitor**	
Delavirdine[d]	DLV	Ibalizumab	
Doravirine	DOR		
Efavirenz	EFV	**CCR5 antagonist**	
Etravirine	ETV	Maraviroc	MVC
Nevirapine	NVP		
Rilpivirine	RPV		
Integrase strand transfer inhibitor (INSTI)		**Fusion inhibitor**	
Bictegravir[e]	BIC	Enfuvirtide	ENF
Cabotegravir	CAB		
Dolutegravir	DTG		
Elvitegravir	EVG		
Raltegravir	RAL		

[a]Withdrawn from market by manufacturer.
[b]Available only as coformulation with ritonavir.
[c]Used principally for pharmacologic enhancement of other antiretroviral agents.
[d]Not recommended and rarely used.
[e]Available only as coformulation with FTC plus TAF.

antiretroviral drug development (Fig. 18.9). The first step in the virus life cycle is virus entry, a multistep process that involves attachment, coreceptor binding, and fusion of the cell and virus membranes. Temsavir, administered as the prodrug fostemsavir, binds to gp120 and blocks the binding of gp120 to the primary viral receptor, CD4.[207,276] The humanized monoclonal antibody (ibalizumab) binds to domain 2 of the extracellular portion of CD4 and acts as a postattachment inhibitor of virus entry.[144,241,280] Potent inhibition of HIV-1 replication has been demonstrated in randomized clinical trials by

maraviroc, a small-molecule chemokine receptor antagonist that prevents binding of gp120 to CCR5.[105,203] The efficacy of the fusion inhibitor enfuvirtide (T-20), a synthetic 36-amino acid oligopeptide, was demonstrated in a series of randomized clinical trials.[281] This drug blocks virus fusion by preventing the formation of a six-helix bundle by two heptad repeats (HR-1 and HR-2) in the trimeric gp41 ectodomain.[511,512] In addition to these specific entry inhibitors, bNAbs that target a variety of epitopes on gp120 or gp41 may neutralize HIV.[267] Several bNAbs have been shown to reduce plasma viremia in early phase clinical trials and are now in development for treatment and prevention of HIV.[73,306]

Inhibition of reverse transcriptase (RT) by substrate analogs (nucleoside and nucleotide RT inhibitors [NRTIs]) and by noncompetitive inhibitors (nonnucleoside RT inhibitors [NNRTIs]) constitutes the mainstay of most antiretroviral regimens. Because the NRTIs lack a 3′-OH group, once incorporated into the growing complementary DNA (cDNA) strand, they act as chain terminators, bringing reverse transcription to a halt.[376] Another feature of the NRTIs is their need for phosphorylation by intracellular nucleoside and nucleotide kinases to generate the active deoxynucleotide triphosphate (dNTP) forms of these drugs. Activity of these kinases can differ between cell types (lymphocyte vs. monocyte or macrophage) and their activation state, accounting for variations in drug activity.[177] The NRTIs have formed the backbone of ART since the introduction of zidovudine in 1987. A novel class of nucleoside analog that functions as both chain terminator and inhibits translocation of RT along the genomic viral RNA, known as nucleoside RT translocation inhibitors (NRTTIs), is currently in clinical development.[315,427]

The NNRTIs are a chemically diverse class of drugs that occupy a potential drug-binding pocket in RT distinct from the dNTP binding site. Binding induces conformational changes that essentially inactivate RT[147]; in this respect, the NNRTIs can be considered allosteric inhibitors of RT function.[465] Currently approved NNRTIs generally are inactive against HIV-2, which lacks tyrosine residues at positions 181 and 188 that are essential for drug binding.[404]

Following reverse transcription, the resulting linear double-stranded DNA (dsDNA) molecule must be integrated into the host chromosome. The process of integration, which is catalyzed by the virally encoded integrase, is a multistep process that involves formation of a preintegration complex, nuclear importation, endonucleolytic processing of the 3′ ends of the DNA molecule, and a strand-transfer reaction that results in covalent attachment of the viral and cellular DNA (see Chapter 17). The development of appropriate high-throughput screening assays allowed identification of specific inhibitors of the strand-transfer reaction.[215] Regimens that include the integrase inhibitors bictegravir and dolutegravir are now considered preferred first-line regimens.[374,423]

Inhibition of HIV-1 protease prevents processing of the Gag and Gag-Pol polyprotein precursors into their mature substituents, which comprise the structural proteins of the virus core particle (capsid, matrix, and nucleoprotein) as well as the three virally encoded enzymes (protease, reverse transcriptase, and integrase) required for virus replication. In contrast to inhibitors of virus entry, reverse transcription and integration, which act at early (preintegration) steps in the virus life

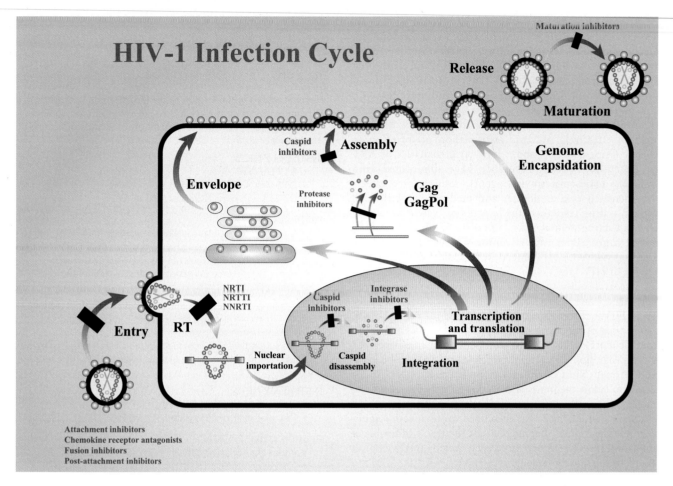

FIGURE 18.9 Points of attack in the human immunodeficiency virus type 1 (HIV-1) virus lifecycle for antiretroviral drugs.

cycle, protease inhibitors act at late (postintegration) stages of the life cycle, resulting in the release of noninfectious virions.[160,249,378] Most protease inhibitors are peptidic or peptidomimetic compounds designed as analogs of the cleavage sites found within the Gag and Gag-Pol precursor proteins. Because of their relatively poor oral bioavailability, most protease inhibitors are coadministered with a low dose of ritonavir or cobicistat, potent inhibitors of the 3A4 isozyme of cytochrome P450 (CYP 3A4)[264]; CYP 3A4 is responsible for metabolism of most of these drugs.

Maturation inhibitors block proteolytic processing the Gag-Pol polyprotein at the capsid (CA)-spacer peptide 1 (SP1) cleavage site. In contrast to HIV protease inhibitors, which bind to the substrate binding site on the enzyme, maturation inhibitors bind directly to the polyprotein, thereby hindering access of the protease to its substrate. Polymorphisms at or near the CA-SP1 cleavage site limited activity of the first-generation maturation inhibitor bevirimat,[460] but next-generation candidates have potent activity against a broader range of viral isolates and are now in clinical development.[467] Drugs targeting the HIV-1 capsid (p24 protein) inhibit multiple capsid-dependent steps in the virus life cycle, including proper CA assembly and disassembly. Proper capsid assembly is essential for formation of mature, infectious virions, whereas disassembly is necessary for the completion of reverse transcription and viral

integration. The investigational capsid inhibitor lenacapavir has potent *in vitro* and *in vivo* antiviral activity and can be formulated for once-monthly oral or twice yearly subcutaneous administration.[294] A phase 2 to 3 study of lenacapavir in highly treatment-experienced patients with multidrug resistance HIV demonstrated high rates of viral suppression when combined with other active agents.[442]

Principles of Antiretroviral Therapeutics

The demonstration in 1987 that zidovudine increases survival of individuals with advanced HIV-1 disease[159] ushered in the era of ART. Subsequent development of additional NRTIs created possibilities for combination therapy.[336,437] The NNRTIs had even greater potency as antiretroviral agents, but rapid emergence of resistance initially hindered their development.[86,117,211] The discovery of protease inhibitors with a higher genetic barrier to resistance provided sufficiently potent regimens that could achieve durable suppression of virus replication.[204] At the same time, viral dynamics studies demonstrated high rates of HIV-1 replication and turnover of the HIV-1 quasi-species and suggested the inevitable emergence of drug resistance when ART does not completely inhibit replication.[226,382,505] These observations provided the theoretic basis for use of potent drug combinations with the goal of suppressing plasma HIV-1 RNA levels to below the limits of detection of the most sensitive assays available.[212]

After years of debate, the benefits of ART for all patients with HIV infection are well established. Three randomized, placebo-controlled trials including START (Strategic Timing of Antiretroviral Therapy), TEMPRANO, and HIV Prevention Trials Network (HPTN) protocol 052 document a significant decrease in morbidity and mortality with immediate initiation of ART even at CD4 cell count ≥500 cells/mm[3],[97],[238],[479] In addition, ART for persons with HIV infection effectively prevents transmission of infection to others.[97] Prior concerns about long-term toxicities of ART and potential for drug resistance have diminished with newer less-toxic antiretroviral agents, coformulated tablets with increased ease of dosing, and medications with high barriers to drug resistance; the benefits of early ART clearly outweigh any potential risks. Since 2016, the WHO HIV treatment guidelines have recommended initiation of ART for all persons with HIV infection regardless of CD4 count or stage of HIV infection.

The availability of potent, once-daily single-tablet regimens that are safe and well tolerated has made durable suppression of HIV-1 replication an achievable goal for most patients. A large body of data from randomized control trials and longitudinal cohort studies informs treatment guidelines developed by various groups. The general principles are clear: to be effective, treatment must be sufficiently potent to suppress plasma viremia to below the limits of detection of sensitive assays and must be sufficiently simple and well tolerated that patients will be capable of adhering to the prescribed regimen with a minimum of missed doses. Because current therapy is incapable of eradicating HIV-1 infection, once such therapy is started most patients will require it lifelong.

Preferred regimens include an integrase strand transfer inhibitor (INSTI), either bictegravir or dolutegravir, in combination with tenofovir (TFV) plus emtricitabine (FTC) or lamivudine (3TC) (Table 18.4).[149],[374],[423],[520] Randomized trials have shown the efficacy and long-term durability of such regimens.[366],[399] For many patients, a two-drug regimen containing dolutegravir plus 3TC is sufficient to achieve and maintain durable virologic suppression.[65],[66] Various two- and three-drug combinations of NRTIs, NNRTIs, PIs, and/or INSTIs are suitable alternative or second-line regimens for patients who do not tolerate or have experienced treatment failure on a preferred first-line regimen.[374],[423] In addition, long-acting injectable formulations of the INSTI cabotegravir plus the NNRTI rilpivirine offer an alternative to daily oral therapy for appropriate patients.[365],[367],[475] Because recommendations change as new data become available, readers should consult the *Department of Health and Human Services Guidelines for Use of Antiretroviral Agents in Adults and Adolescents with HIV*, which is updated regularly and may be found at http://aidsinfo.nih.gov.

Pharmacologic interactions between different antiretroviral drugs, or between antiretroviral drugs and drugs used to treat common coinfections, significantly complicate the use of ART in many settings. Most troublesome are the interactions of NNRTIs, PIs, and INSTIs with the cytochrome P450 (CYP) system. Perhaps the greatest challenge is the difficulty of combining standard antituberculosis regimens with first-line ART because of the profound induction of CYP by rifampin, an essential component of antituberculosis regimens.[135],[136]

TABLE 18.4 Recommended antiretroviral regimens for initial therapy (updated June 3, 2021)

Recommended Initial Regimens for Most People with HIV
Recommended regimens are those with demonstrated durable virologic efficacy, favorable tolerability and toxicity profiles, and ease of use.

INSTI plus 2 NRTIs:
- BIC/TAF/FTC
- DTG/ABC/3TC—if HLA-B*5701 negative
- DTG plus (TAF or TDF) plus (FTC or 3TC)

INSTI plus 1 NRTI:
- DTG/3TC, except for individuals with HIV RNA >500,000 copies/mL, HBV coinfection, or in whom ART is to be started before the results of HIV genotypic resistance testing for reverse transcriptase or HBV testing are available.

Recommended Initial Regimens in Certain Clinical Situations
These regimens are effective and tolerable but have some disadvantages when compared with the regimens listed above or have less supporting data from randomized clinical trials. However, in certain clinical situations, one of these regimens may be preferred.

INSTI plus 2 NRTIs:
- EVG/c/(TAF or TDF)a/FTC
- RAL plus (FAT or TDF) plus (FTC or 3TC)

Boosted PI plus 2 NRTIs:
- In general, boosted DRV is preferred over boosted ATV
- (DRV/c or DRV/r) plus (TAF or TDF)a plus (FTC or 3TC)
- (ATV/c or ATV/r) plus (TAF or TDF)a plus (FTC or 3TC)
- (DRV/c or DRV/r) plus ABC/3TC —if HLA-B*5701 negative

NNRTI plus 2 NRTIs:
- DOR/TDF/3TC or DOR plus TAF/FTC
- EFV plus (TAF or TDF) plus (FTC or 3TC)
  - EFV 600 mg plus TDF plus (FTC or 3TC)
  - EFV 400 mg/TDF/3TC
  - EFV 600 mg plus TAF/FTC
- RPV/(TAF or TDF)/FTC—if HIV RNA <100,000 copies/mL and CD4 count >200 cells/mm³

Regimens to Consider When ABC, TAF, and TDF Cannot Be Used or Are Not Optimal:
- DTG/3TC except for individuals with HIV RNA >500,000 copies/mL, HBV coinfection, or in whom ART is to be started before the results of HIV genotypic resistance testing for reverse transcriptase or HBV testing are available
- DRV/r plus RAL twice a day—if HIV RNA <100,000 copies/mL and CD4 count >200 cells/mm³
- DRV/r once daily plus 3TC

aFTC and 3TC may be used interchangeably in each of the regimens listed in the table.
bATV/c, ATV/r, DRV/c, and DRV/r denote dosing of the indicated protease inhibitor together with pharmacologic enhancement by cobicistat or low-dose ritonavir, respectively.

Abbreviations of drug names are given in Table 18.3.

Adapted from DHHS Guidelines for the Use of Antiretroviral Agents in HIV-1-Infected Adults and Adolescents (http://www.aidsinfo.nih.gov/ContentFiles/AdultandAdolescentGL.pdf).

Virologic and Immunologic Effects of Antiretroviral Therapy

A brisk decrease in plasma HIV-1 RNA levels should be expected following treatment initiation, with at least a 1-$\log_{10}$ reduction within 14 days. In most patients, plasma HIV-1 RNA should fall to less than 50 copies/mL by week 16 to 24, depending on the starting viral load. Failure to achieve the expected drop in plasma viremia raises concerns regarding the degree of treatment adherence or presence of drug-resistant virus. The initial rapid decay in plasma viremia reflects the half-life of productively infected, activated cells.[382] By contrast, the decay in latently infected resting memory (CD45RA−RO+) CD4 cells is almost imperceptible.[157] Replication-competent HIV-1 can be recovered from these latently infected cells by the use of sensitive culture techniques.[91,158,516] As noted above in Pathogenesis and Pathology, the half-life of this replication competent HIV reservoir is at least 44 months, limiting prospects for viral eradication by ART alone.[110,450]

Although patients with plasma HIV-1 RNA levels below the limit of detection by routine clinical tests are considered to have "undetectable" viral loads, residual viremia (1 to 50 copies/mL) can be detected in nearly all patients when sufficiently sensitive methods are applied.[371] The absence of viral evolution over time in subjects with detectable residual viremia and the inability to suppress residual viremia through intensification of ART by additional antiretroviral drugs argues against ongoing replication as a source of this virus.[25,134,174,330] Some patients experience transient episodes of detectable plasma viremia (*blips*). In most studies, the occurrence of blips has not been associated with emergence of drug resistance or an increased risk of treatment failure.[357,358] Mathematic modeling of the frequency of these blips suggests that they represent stochastic bursts of replication, perhaps caused by intercurrent episodes of immune activation.[133,380]

The rapid decline in plasma HIV-1 RNA is accompanied by a similarly brisk increase in CD4 T lymphocytes in most patients. On average, the CD4 cell count increases by 50 to 100 cells/mm^3 in the first 4 weeks of therapy, followed by a more gradual, but steady, increase thereafter.[286] Most of this initial increase in CD4 cell counts is thought to be the result of redistribution of memory CD4 T cells from lymphoid tissues into the peripheral blood.[369] The subsequent slower increase is attributed, in turn, to the gradual increase in naïve CD4 T cells that is thought to represent production of naïve CD4 T cells.[18,102,533] By the end of the first year of therapy, total CD4 cell counts increase by an average of 175 cells/mm^3.[173,299,503] Patients remaining on ART over 7 years experience a CD4 count increase of 300 to 600 cells/mm^3, depending on the CD4 count at the time of ART initiation.[299] Patients with incomplete suppression of plasma viremia also show significant increases in CD4 cell counts, but the magnitude of this increase is blunted compared with patients with complete viral suppression.[258,259,480]

Viral suppression reduces generalized immune activation, as judged by the number or percentage of CD38+DR+ CD4 and CD8 cells.[286] The proportion of activated cells remains greater, however, than that found in seronegative controls.[246,458] Higher levels of immune activation are associated with lower levels of CD4 cell restoration on ART.[246] Reconstitution of the follicular DC network in lymphoid tissues can occur over time,[534] but central memory T cells (Tcm) do not appear to be reconstituted by successful ART.[143]

The numeric increase in CD4 T cells is accompanied by laboratory and clinical evidence of reconstitution in pathogen-specific immunity. Proliferative responses to recall antigens such as *Candida albicans* and CMV can be demonstrated after 12 to 48 weeks of therapy.[18,102,286,363,395] Prophylactic therapy to prevent new or recurrent episodes of *P. jirovecii* pneumonia,[165,166,269] disseminated *Mycobacterium avium* complex infection,[1,113] histoplasmosis,[188] and CMV retinitis[307,488] can be discontinued safely in patients who have shown a satisfactory virologic and immunologic response to therapy. By contrast, lymphocyte proliferative responses to HIV antigens remain limited,[18,102] although some studies have shown improvements in HIV-specific immunity by enzyme-linked immunospot (ELISPOT) assay or intracellular cytokine staining.[44,395]

Immune reconstitution can be accompanied by a pathologic inflammatory response to previously treated or subclinical opportunistic infections. The immune reconstitution inflammatory syndrome (IRIS) occurs in up to one third of patients beginning ART and is best described in association with CMV retinitis, disseminated *Mycobacterium tuberculosis*, or *M. avium* complex infection, and cryptococcal meningitis.[54,403,446,447] Patients with IRIS are more likely to have started an initial ART regimen soon after diagnosis of an opportunistic infection, a low CD4 count below 50 cells/mm^3, and to have a more rapid decrease in plasma HIV-1 RNA levels.[350,447] Management includes continuation of ART, treatment of the associated opportunistic infection, and a brief course of steroids if the extent of inflammation risks significant end-organ damage or is life threatening.[224]

Drug Toxicity

A wide range of toxicities of varying severity has been described. In the case of the NRTIs, the more serious include anemia and neutropenia,[410] peripheral neuropathy (stavudine [d4T], didanosine [ddI], zalcitabine [ddC]),[39,156,345] pancreatitis (ddI and ddC),[194] and life-threatening lactic acidosis.[85,300] Severe peripheral lipoatrophy has been associated with use of d4T, ddI, and zidovudine (ZDV), most likely caused by inhibition of mitochondrial DNA polymerase γ.[67,251] As a result, these drugs are no longer recommended, and ddC, ddI and d4T have been withdrawn from the market. Fatal hypersensitivity reactions can occur with abacavir in patients carrying the HLA B*5701 allele.[223,309,319,390] Abacavir may also contribute to an increased risk of cardiovascular disease.[109,407,425,521] Although TDF generally is well tolerated, concerns have been raised regarding loss of BMD.[327,469] Reductions in BMD associated with TDF appear to be exacerbated when the drug is combined with a boosted protease inhibitor.[55,346] Similarly, concerns over potential nephrotoxicity have limited TDF use in patients with impaired renal function.[252,265] An alternative formulation, tenofovir alafenamide (TAF), results in much higher intracellular concentrations of the active moiety tenofovir diphosphate in lymphocytes and hepatocytes at much lower plasma concentrations of tenofovir, resulting in reduced loss of BMD and less impact on markers of renal tubular injury.[170,434]

Use of nevirapine and efavirenz can be complicated by rash and hepatotoxicity. In the case of nevirapine, rash may be severe (Stevens-Johnson syndrome).[394] Life-threatening hypersensitivity hepatitis can occur with nevirapine, particularly in women with CD4+ T-cell counts greater than 250/mm^3.[429] CNS side effects are a common cause of treatment discontinuation with efavirenz.[93]

Gastrointestinal intolerance, hepatoxicity, and hyperlipidemia are the most frequent dose-limiting toxicities associated with the protease inhibitors. The incidence of hepatotoxicity may be significantly increased among HCV coinfected patients.[473] In addition, several drugs in this class significantly impair insulin sensitivity, possibly by an inhibitory effect on the glucose transporter GLUT4.[352] The combination of insulin resistance and hyperlipidemia can increase the risk of cardiovascular disease among patients receiving certain protease inhibitors.[164] Hyperbilirubinemia, nephrolithiasis, and rash are additional concerns with certain members of this class.[83,342,361,408,414]

Integrase strand transfer inhibitors are generally well tolerated. Infrequent side effects including neuropsychiatric adverse events such as insomnia, depression, and suicidal ideation have been reported in patients receiving raltegravir and dolutegravir, but the incidence of CNS side effects with INSTIs is far less common than observed with efavirenz.[230,287,502] Unintentional and sometimes excessive weight gain has emerged as a potential side effect of INSTI-based ART.[495,496] This effect has been observed in treatment-naïve patients initiating an INSTI-based regimen as well as in treatment-experienced patients switching to an INSTI regimen.[310] The magnitude of weight gain varies by gender and race/ethnicity, being greatest among black African women.[495] Weight gain appears greatest with dolutegravir and bictegravir, particularly when these INSTIs are used together with TAF (Fig. 18.10).[433,495] The mechanism of this weight gain remains unclear. Some weight gain occurs in all persons with HIV upon initiation of ART and is attributed to a "return to health." Whether the greater weight gain observed with certain INSTIs and TAF is due to a direct effect of these drugs is the subject of active investigation.

Initial results of an observational study in Botswana raised concerns that dolutegravir increased the risk of neural tube defects in infants born to women exposed to this drug at the time of conception.[532] With expanded surveillance, the incidence of neural tube defects in exposed and unexposed infants was no longer statistically significant.[531] In addition, a retrospective cohort study of pregnancy outcomes in Brazil of women with possible dolutegravir exposure within 8 weeks of the estimated time of conception found no increased risk of neural tube defects.[381] Consequently, current treatment guidelines recommend dolutegravir as a preferred drug for women with HIV who are trying to conceive and in all trimesters of pregnancy.[375]

When a change in therapy is prompted by drug toxicity, an alternative agent should be substituted for the offending drug without interrupting treatment. When toxicity is sufficiently severe to require suspension of dosing, all drugs in a regimen should be discontinued to avoid exposure of the virus to a partially suppressive regimen, which can result in selection of drug resistance (see Drug Resistance).

Treatment Failure

Numerous factors contribute to the failure of highly active antiretroviral therapy (HAART), including poor adherence (because of the complexity or poor tolerability of certain regimens)[237,517]; pharmacologic factors, including drug–drug interactions that impair absorption or accelerate clearance[353]; host factors (e.g., low CD4 cell count at the start of treatment and HLA haplotype)[231,271,389]; drug resistance acquired by transmission of a resistant isolate or selected by previous suboptimal therapy[295]; and preexisting drug-resistant minority variants.[290] Each of these factors leads to incomplete suppression of viral replication, which in turn leads to selection of drug-resistant variants.

The definition of treatment failure depends on where in the course of treatment an individual patient stands. For patients on a first or second regimen, treatment failure usually is defined as confirmed evidence of detectable viremia after an initial virologic response, or failure to achieve a response. Prompt switching to a new potent regimen is advised to reestablish virologic suppression, prevent emergence of drug resistance, and preserve future treatment options.[245,354] Although many clinicians do not alter therapy unless the level of viremia exceeds 1,000 to 5,000 copies/mL, persistent low levels of detectable viremia can be associated with accumulation of drug resistance mutations.[354]

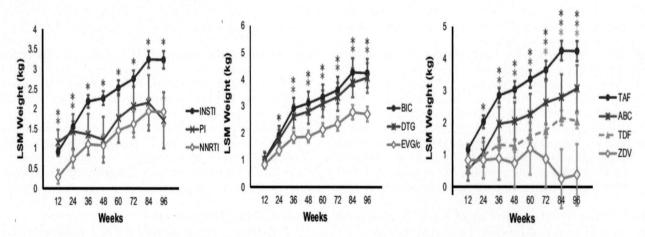

FIGURE 18.10 Weight change in trials participants initiating antiretroviral therapy. Data shown are least squares mean weight change (kg). INSTI, integrase strand transfer inhibitor; PI, protease inhibitor; NNRTI, nonnucleoside reverse transcriptase inhibitor; BIC, bictegravir; DTG, dolutegravir; EVG/c, elvitegravir/cobicistat; TAF, tenofovir alafenamide; ABC, abacavir; TDF, tenofovir disoproxil fumarate; ZDV, zidovudine. (Modified from Sax PE, Erlandson KM, Lake JE, et al. Weight gain following initiation of antiretroviral therapy: risk factors in randomized comparative clinical trials. *Clin Infect Dis* 2020;71(6):1379–1389. Reproduced by permission of Oxford University Press.)

For patients with more extensive treatment histories, the situation is more complex. By this point, most patients already will have been exposed to more classes of antiretroviral agents and may have developed resistance to at least one agent within each drug class. Therefore, the presence of detectable plasma HIV-1 RNA is less useful as a marker of treatment failure. In this situation, symptomatic evidence of treatment failure can include increasing fatigue, malaise, and night sweats; objective evidence includes weight loss, a rising viral load, falling CD4 cell count, and occurrence of new, recurrent, or worsening AIDS-related opportunistic infections.

Even when complete virologic suppression cannot be achieved, ART continues to provide clinical benefits. Studies show that mean CD4 cell counts remain above pretherapy levels through 96 weeks of follow-up in patients experiencing virologic failure of a protease inhibitor regimen.[126] Maintenance of stable CD4 cell counts depends on continued administration of ART, even in patients with apparent virologic failure of their regimen.[127] An analysis of data pooled from 13 cohorts in Europe, North America, and Australia showed the continuing immunologic and clinical benefits of ART despite virologic failure.[285] Those with plasma HIV-1 RNA levels above 10,000 copies/mL and CD4 cell counts below 200 cells/µL were at greatest risk of disease progression. Within each viral load and CD4 count stratum, the risk of disease progression was significantly lower for those who continued on ART despite virologic failure, confirming the persistent benefit of treatment in the setting of ongoing virus replication and presumed drug resistance.

Drug Resistance

As discussed above, the high error rate of HIV-1 RT and rapid turnover of the virus population contribute to the generation of extensive genetic variation in the HIV-1 quasi-species. These factors provide a mechanism for rapid emergence of drug resistance in the setting of partially effective ART. Resistance emerges at a rate proportional to the frequency of preexisting variants and their relative growth advantage in the presence of drug.[95] Support for this model is provided by observations from monotherapy studies with different classes of antiretroviral drugs. For example, resistance to lamivudine emerges within weeks of initiating monotherapy because of point mutations that result in a thousand-fold reduction in drug activity.[440] By contrast, resistance to tenofovir emerges slowly.[313] In the case of most PIs and INSTIs, high-level resistance occurs as a consequence of the accumulation of multiple mutations over time.[84,234,344] Given the extensive array of mutations implicated in resistance to various classes of antiretroviral drugs, a detailed discussion of resistance to individual drugs is beyond the scope of this chapter. The reader is referred instead to excellent reviews of this subject[47,94,506] and to the several websites that maintain a comprehensive listing of HIV-1 drug resistance data (www.hiv.lanl.gov; http://hivdb.stanford.edu; www.iasusa.org).

The clinical significance of antiretroviral drug resistance was demonstrated not long after the introduction of ZDV and ddI by studies that showed accelerated immunologic decline and disease progression in patients receiving nucleoside analogs to which their viruses had become resistant.[118,244,277] The relationship between resistance to PI-based ART regimens and clinical progression is more complex.[126,127] Drug resistance comes at a cost to the virus in terms of replication capacity. Diminished replication capacity and residual activity of some drugs against resistant viruses may account for persisting reductions in disease progression and AIDS-related mortality in the developed world despite the increasing prevalence of antiretroviral drug resistance. Whereas the prevalence of antiretroviral (ARV) drug resistance and transmitted drug resistance appears to be stable or decreasing in high-income countries, increasing ARV resistance in specific populations and in lower and middle-income countries is cause for concern.

Resistance to antiretroviral agents can be assessed by genotypic and phenotypic assays. These tests are an important tool for management decisions related to therapy initiation or regimen modification. Properly used, they can lead to improved virologic outcomes for patients infected with HIV-1.

Treatment as Prevention

Evidence that the risk of HIV-1 transmission correlates with viral load in the source patient leads naturally to the hypothesis that decreasing circulating levels of HIV-1 by effective ART will reduce transmission.[191,248,397,480] This hypothesis is supported by the successful use of ART to prevent perinatal and breast-milk transmission of HIV-1 from infected mothers to their infants.[103,443] Prevention of mother-to-child transmission has evolved to consist of combination ART during pregnancy with a goal of virologic suppression by the time of delivery and perinatal prophylaxis with ART for the newborn. These advances in perinatal care have reduced the risk of HIV transmission from mother to child to less than 1%.[78,120] Comprehensive guidelines for the use of antiretroviral drugs in pregnant women with HIV infection and interventions to reduce perinatal HIV transmission in the United States have been developed.[375] Observational studies among HIV-1 discordant couples show a substantially reduced risk of HIV transmission when the infected partner is receiving ART.[15,406] These data have been confirmed in a randomized trial showing a 96% reduction in the risk of sexual transmission of HIV in the group randomized to receive ART.[97] As a result, the CDC and WHO now include treatment as prevention as a major component of their HIV prevention programs.[80,519] Additional studies have confirmed the efficacy of successful ART with virologic suppression to prevent HIV transmission in other settings and patient populations.[415] Moreover, rollout of ART is associated with decreased community HIV viral load, which has also been associated with a reduction in HIV incidence.[463]

Postexposure Prophylaxis

Administration of ART immediately after HIV exposure can prevent acquisition of HIV. A single case–control study in 1997 demonstrated that postexposure prophylaxis (PEP) with zidovudine reduced acquisition of HIV after percutaneous workplace exposure by approximately 80%.[68] Additional observational studies have examined the availability, uptake, use, and tolerability of various PEP regimens in a variety of settings, including both occupational and nonoccupational (e.g., sexual) exposures.[162,324] HIV incidence is so low in these studies that efficacy is difficult to confirm, but the absence of new infections is reassuring. The CDC now recommends a three-drug regimen of TDF, emtricitabine (FTC), and either dolutegravir or raltegravir, initiated within 72 hours (ideally within 24 hours) after potential exposure and continued for 28 days, as the preferred regimen for PEP for HIV-negative individuals after both occupational and nonoccupational exposures.

Preexposure Prophylaxis

Studies in NHPs showing that administration of antiretroviral drugs could prevent infection by SIV or SHIV[178,487] led to the Preexposure Prophylaxis Initiative (iPrEx) study in MSM, which demonstrated a 44% reduction in HIV acquisition in participants who received fixed-dose TDF plus FTC as compared to placebo; the effect was even greater (92% protection) when among participants in whom adherence was documented by detectable levels of study drug.[193] The Partners PrEP study subsequently confirmed the efficacy of TDF-FTC for prevention of HIV acquisition in serodiscordant heterosexual couples in Kenya and Uganda.[23] Although subsequent studies have confirmed the efficacy of TDF plus FTC as PrEP in MSM and injection drug users (IDU),[90,328,343] trials of oral PrEP in women have been disappointing, largely because of low levels of adherence.[316,489] The combination of TAF plus FTC has also demonstrated efficacy in preventing HIV in MSM and transgender women but has not yet been studied in cisgender women.[325] Two large randomized clinical trials have demonstrated the superiority of the long-acting injectable INSTI cabotegravir administered by intramuscular injection every 2 months as compared to daily oral TDF plus FTC in men and women.[128,282] By contrast, the Antibody-Mediated Prevention (AMP) trials found that the bNAb VRC01 did not significantly protect against HIV in men or women.[108] This result was explained by the high prevalence of VRC01 resistance among HIV strains circulating in the study population; significant protection was found against infection by viruses susceptible to this bNAb.[108] These results establish proof of concept that bNAbs can protect against infection by susceptible HIV but suggest that combinations of bNAbs or bNAbs engineered to have multiple specificities will be needed to offer broad protection. Prevention Guidelines published by the CDC recommend PrEP as a prevention option for sexually active MSM, heterosexually active men and women at substantial risk of HIV acquisition, and adult IDUs.[77]

Prospects for HIV Eradication

As discussed earlier in this chapter, the establishment of a reservoir of latently infected, resting CD4 lymphocytes results in the lifelong persistence of HIV-1 infection. To date, long-term remission or cure has been reported in two individuals with HIV who underwent allogeneic stem cell transplants with a donor homozygous for *CCR5Δ32*.[205,236] These unique cases have spurred a global effort aimed at discovering feasible, scalable approaches for an HIV cure. While the fruits of these efforts remain uncertain, it is likely that a combination of approaches that stimulate latently infected cells to produce viral antigens, enhance HIV-specific immunity, and enhance access of HIV-specific cytotoxic cells to cells harboring this reservoir will be needed.

HIV Vaccines

Vaccines are arguably the most powerful medical intervention for preventing virus infections. Despite the obvious need, and years of intense research, the development of an effective vaccine against HIV has been elusive. Many approaches have been tried, but only four basic vaccine platforms have shown adequate promise to warrant large scale efficacy testing. Initial efforts were directed at using recombinant envelope proteins to stimulate antibodies to block infection. Although these vaccines did stimulate envelope binding antibodies, they failed to induce antibodies capable of neutralizing strains of HIV other than easy to neutralize laboratory-grown viruses, and the trials failed to demonstrate protection against HIV infection.[161,391] The inability to induce bNAbs through vaccination has continued to be a vexing problem and is related to a number of factors, including sequence variability, especially within exterior loops of Env that are highly immunogenic but that can easily mutate to avoid recognition, and the heavy glycosylation of Env.[468] The isolation of bNAbs from HIV-infected subjects, and the identification of the antigenic target of these antibodies on the HIV Env, have raised hopes that an immunogen can be developed that targets conserved sites of vulnerability on the HIV Env.[372,500,501,523] The autoreactivity of some bNAb lineages, however, suggests that immune tolerance mechanisms may limit vaccine-induced elicitation of these responses and will need to be considered in immunogen design.[214]

Because of the failure of early vaccines to protect against HIV acquisition, a subsequent approach was to stimulate broad HIV-specific CD8 T-cell responses in the hope that these responses would at least control viral replication in those who became infected with HIV, thereby limiting the impact of the infection upon the vaccinated individual, and potentially influencing the subsequent transmission of HIV to other individuals. A trial of a recombinant adenovirus type 5 vaccine was performed, and although it did stimulate strong CD8 T-cell responses, it failed to protect vaccinees from infection or affect their viral loads, and actually increased HIV acquisition within subjects with preexisting immunity to the vaccine vector (adenovirus type 5).[59,329] Although the mechanism underlying the increase in acquisition remains uncertain, the failure of this trial has severely dampened enthusiasm for T-cell–based vaccine strategies.

A vaccine that combined priming with a canary pox-based vector and boosting with recombinant envelope protein (gp120) showed modest (31%) protection against HIV acquisition in a low-risk predominantly heterosexual population[405]; neither neutralizing antibody responses nor virus-specific CD8 T-cell responses correlated with protection.[213] Failure of a second phase 3 trial based conducted in South Africa with immunogens adapted to subtype C virus has significantly dampened enthusiasm for this approach.[195] An alternative prime-boost strategy using adenovirus 26 recombinants expressing a mosaic of HIV antigens from different clades followed by boosting with subtype C envelope glycoprotein likewise failed to show protection in a phase 2b trial conducted in women in sub-Saharan Africa.[355]

Other Prevention Strategies

Sexual behavioral change can clearly diminish the risk of becoming infected, as has been shown in Zimbabwe with a reduction in casual sex and a delay in sexual debut accounting for the greatest differences.[198] In addition, knowledge of the mechanisms of transmission (discussed previously) has led to other nonvaccine interventions aimed at reducing transmission. It was long assumed that the mucosa of the male foreskin was a site of HIV acquisition in men, a contention supported by epidemiologic data. This was confirmed when an initial trial of more than 3,000 uncircumcised men who were randomized to be offered immediate circumcision or circumcision after a 21-month period of follow-up was stopped after an interim analysis at 18 months revealed that circumcision conferred 60% protection from HIV infection.[19] These findings have been confirmed in two subsequent randomized clinical trials,[24,196] and efforts are ongoing to deploy circumcision to high-risk male populations.

PERSPECTIVE

Since AIDS was first described 40 years ago, extraordinary advances in understanding the pathogenesis of HIV infection have led to unprecedented advances in therapeutics and prevention of this pandemic retroviral infection. Whereas the basic principles are clear, implementation of policies that would provide global access to proven interventions for treatment and prevention of HIV has encountered significant political and financial obstacles over the years. Persisting stigmatization of people with HIV and criminalization of behaviors associated with acquisition of HIV infection continue to fuel the spread of HIV and create barriers to equitable access to care. We possess the tools to bring an end to the HIV pandemic—all that is needed is the social, political, and economic will to employ them.

Despite the wealth of knowledge accumulated since its discovery, important scientific questions remain regarding HIV. Chief among these is the ongoing quest for an effective preventive vaccine suitable for global deployment. How to induce protective immunity against the ever increasing diversity of HIV-1 subtypes and circulating recombinant forms continues to challenge vaccine developers. Similarly, advances in our understanding of mechanisms of viral latency and the factors that contribute to persistence of the latent reservoir have yet to yield feasible, scalable approaches to HIV-1 remission or cure. In their absence, how to counteract inappropriate immune activation that persists in people on ART with fully suppressed viral replication in order to prevent the end-organ damage associated with that inflammation requires continued basic and clinical investigation.

REFERENCES

1. Aberg JA, Williams PL, Liu T, et al. A study of discontinuing maintenance therapy in human immunodeficiency virus-infected subjects with disseminated Mycobacterium avium complex: AIDS Clinical Trial Group 393 Study Team. *J Infect Dis* 2003;187:1046–1052.
2. Abrams D, Levy Y, Losso MH, et al. Interleukin-2 therapy in patients with HIV infection. *N Engl J Med* 2009;361:1548–1559.
3. Addo MM, Yu XG, Rathod A, et al. Comprehensive epitope analysis of human immunodeficiency virus type 1 (HIV-1)-specific T-cell responses directed against the entire expressed HIV-1 genome demonstrate broadly directed responses, but no correlation to viral load. *J Virol* 2003;77:2081–2092.
4. Alessandri-Gradt E, De Oliveira F, Leoz M, et al. HIV-1 group P infection: towards a dead-end infection? *AIDS* 2018;32:1317–1322.
5. Alizon S, von Wyl V, Stadler T, et al. Phylogenetic approach reveals that virus genotype largely determines HIV set-point viral load. *PLoS Pathog* 2010;6:e1001123.
6. Allen TM, Altfeld M, Geer SC, et al. Selective escape from CD8+ T-cell responses represents a major driving force of human immunodeficiency virus type 1 (HIV-1) sequence diversity and reveals constraints on HIV-1 evolution. *J Virol* 2005;79:13239–13249.
7. Alter G, Heckerman D, Schneidewind A, et al. HIV-1 adaptation to NK-cell-mediated immune pressure. *Nature* 2011;476:96–100.
8. Alter G, Teigen N, Davis BT, et al. Sequential deregulation of NK cell subset distribution and function starting in acute HIV-1 infection. *Blood* 2005;106:3366–3369.
9. Altfeld M, Addo MM, Rosenberg ES, et al. Influence of HLA-B57 on clinical presentation and viral control during acute HIV-1 infection. *AIDS* 2003;17:2581–2591.
10. Altfeld M, Rosenberg ES, Shankarappa R, et al. Cellular immune responses and viral diversity in individuals treated during acute and early HIV-1 infection. *J Exp Med* 2001;193:169–180.
11. Amorosa V, Tebas P. Bone disease and HIV infection. *Clin Infect Dis* 2006;42:108–114.
12. Anastos K, Gange SJ, Lau B, et al. Association of race and gender with HIV-1 RNA levels and immunologic progression. *J Acquir Immune Defic Syndr* 2000;24:218–226.
13. Anastos K, Kalish LA, Hessol NA, et al. The relative value of CD4 cell count and quantitative HIV-1 RNA in predicting survival in HIV-1 infected women: results of the women's interagency HIV study. *AIDS* 1999;13:1717–1726.
14. Pezzotti P, Phillips AN, Dorrucci M, et al. Category of exposure to HIV and age in the progression to AIDS: longitudinal study of 1199 people with known dates of seroconversion. HIV Italian Seroconversion Study Group. *BMJ* 1996;313:583–586.
15. Anglemyer A, Rutherford GW, Egger M, et al. Antiretroviral therapy for prevention of HIV transmission in HIV-discordant couples. *Cochrane Database Syst Rev* 2011;(5):CD009153.
16. Apps R, Qi Y, Carlson JM, et al. Influence of HLA-C expression level on HIV control. *Science* 2013;340:87–91.
17. Ariyoshi K, Jaffar S, Alabi AS, et al. Plasma RNA viral load predicts the rate of CD4 T cell decline and death in HIV-2-infected patients in West Africa. *AIDS* 2000;14:339–344.
18. Autran B, Carcelain G, Li TS, et al. Positive effects of combined antiretroviral therapy on CD4+ T cell homeostasis and function in advanced HIV disease. *Science* 1997;277:112–116.
19. Auvert B, Taljaard D, Lagarde E, et al. Randomized, controlled intervention trial of male circumcision for reduction of HIV infection risk: the ANRS 1265 Trial. *PLoS Med* 2005;2:e298.
20. Ayouba A, Akoua-Koffi C, Calvignac-Spencer S, et al. Evidence for continuing cross-species transmission of SIVsmm to humans: characterization of a new HIV-2 lineage in rural Cote d'Ivoire. *AIDS* 2013;27:2488–2491.
21. Ayres L, Avillez F, Garcia-Benito A, et al. Multicenter evaluation of a new recombinant enzyme immunoassay for the combined detection of antibody to HIV-1 and HIV-2. *AIDS* 1990;4:131–138.
22. Bacchetti P, Moss AR. Incubation period of AIDS in San Francisco. *Nature* 1989;338:251–253.
23. Baeten JM, Donnell D, Ndase P, et al. Antiretroviral prophylaxis for HIV prevention in heterosexual men and women. *N Engl J Med* 2012;367:399–410.
24. Bailey RC, Moses S, Parker CB, et al. Male circumcision for HIV prevention in young men in Kisumu, Kenya: a randomised controlled trial. *Lancet* 2007;369:643–656.
25. Bailey JR, Sedaghat AR, Kieffer T, et al. Residual human immunodeficiency virus type 1 viremia in some patients on antiretroviral therapy is dominated by a small number of invariant clones rarely found in circulating CD4+ T cells. *J Virol* 2006;80:6441–6457.
26. Barber DL, Wherry EJ, Masopust D, et al. Restoring function in exhausted CD8 T cells during chronic viral infection. *Nature* 2006;439:682–687.
27. Barouch DH, Ghneim K, Bosche WJ, et al. Rapid inflammasome activation following mucosal SIV infection of rhesus monkeys. *Cell* 2016;165:656–667.
28. Barre-Sinoussi F, Chermann JC, Rey F, et al. Isolation of a T-lymphotropic retrovirus from a patient at risk for acquired immune deficiency syndrome (AIDS). *Science* 1983;220:868–871.
29. Barton JP, Goonetilleke N, Butler TC, et al. Relative rate and location of intra-host HIV evolution to evade cellular immunity are predictable. *Nat Commun* 2016;7:11660.
30. Baum PD, Young JJ, Schmidt D, et al. Blood T-cell receptor diversity decreases during the course of HIV infection, but the potential for a diverse repertoire persists. *Blood* 2012;119:3469–3477.
31. Bavinton BR, Pinto AN, Phanuphak N, et al. Viral suppression and HIV transmission in serodiscordant male couples: an international, prospective, observational, cohort study. *Lancet HIV* 2018;5:e438–e447.
32. Beignon AS, McKenna K, Skoberne M, et al. Endocytosis of HIV-1 activates plasmacytoid dendritic cells via Toll-like receptor-viral RNA interactions. *J Clin Invest* 2005;115:3265–3275.
33. Bell SM, Bedford T. Modern-day SIV viral diversity generated by extensive recombination and cross-species transmission. *PLoS Pathog* 2017;13:e1006466.
34. Berry N, Ariyoshi K, Jaffar S, et al. Low peripheral blood viral HIV-2 RNA in individuals with high CD4 percentage differentiates HIV-2 from HIV-1 infection. *J Hum Virol* 1998;1:457–468.
35. Betts MR, Ambrozak DR, Douek DC, et al. Analysis of total human immunodeficiency virus (HIV)-specific CD4(+) and CD8(+) T-cell responses: relationship to viral load in untreated HIV infection. *J Virol* 2001;75:11983–11991.
36. Betts MR, Nason MC, West SM, et al. HIV nonprogressors preferentially maintain highly functional HIV-specific CD8+ T cells. *Blood* 2006;107:4781–4789.
37. Binley JM, Lybarger EA, Crooks ET, et al. Profiling the specificity of neutralizing antibodies in a large panel of plasmas from patients chronically infected with human immunodeficiency virus type 1 subtypes B and C. *J Virol* 2008;82:11651–11668.
38. Blackburn SD, Shin H, Haining WN, et al. Coregulation of CD8+ T cell exhaustion by multiple inhibitory receptors during chronic viral infection. *Nat Immunol* 2009;10:29–37.
39. Blum AS, Dal Pan GJ, Feinberg J, et al. Low-dose zalcitabine-related toxic neuropathy: frequency, natural history, and risk factors. *Neurology* 1996;46:999–1003.
40. Bofill M, Mocroft A, Lipman M, et al. Increased numbers of primed activated CD8+CD38+CD45RO+ T cells predict the decline of CD4+ T cells in HIV-1-infected patients. *AIDS* 1996;10:827–834.
41. Bohlius J, Schmidlin K, Boue F, et al. HIV-1-related Hodgkin lymphoma in the era of combination antiretroviral therapy: incidence and evolution of CD4+ T-cell lymphocytes. *Blood* 2011;117:6100–6108.
42. Bonnet F, Lewden C, May T, et al. Malignancy-related causes of death in human immunodeficiency virus-infected patients in the era of highly active antiretroviral therapy. *Cancer* 2004;101:317–324.
43. Bor J, Herbst AJ, Newell ML, et al. Increases in adult life expectancy in rural South Africa: valuing the scale-up of HIV treatment. *Science* 2013;339:961–965.
44. Boritz E, Palmer BE, Livingston B, et al. Diverse repertoire of HIV-1 p24-specific, IFN-gamma-producing CD4+ T cell clones following immune reconstitution on highly active antiretroviral therapy. *J Immunol* 2003;170:1106–1116.
45. Borrow P, Lewicki H, Hahn BH, et al. Virus-specific CD8+ cytotoxic T-lymphocyte activity associated with control of viremia in primary human immunodeficiency virus type 1 infection. *J Virol* 1994;68:6103–6110.

46. Boucau J, Le Gall S. Antigen processing and presentation in HIV infection. *Mol Immunol* 2019;113:67–74.
47. Boucher CA, Bobkova MR, Geretti AM, et al. State of the art in HIV drug resistance: science and technology knowledge gap. *AIDS Rev* 2018;20:27–42.
48. Boutwell CL, Carlson JM, Lin TH, et al. Frequent and variable cytotoxic-T-lymphocyte escape-associated fitness costs in the human immunodeficiency virus type 1 subtype B Gag proteins. *J Virol* 2013;87:3952–3965.
49. Bozzette SA, McCutchan JA, Spector SA, et al. A cross-sectional comparison of persons with syncytium- and non-syncytium-inducing human immunodeficiency virus. *J Infect Dis* 1993;168:1374–1379.
50. Bratt G, Sandstrom E, Albert J, et al. The influence of MT-2 tropism on the prognostic implications of the 32 deletion in the CCR-5 gene. *AIDS* 1997;11:1415–1419.
51. Brenchley JM, Paiardini M, Knox KS, et al. Differential Th17 CD4 T-cell depletion in pathogenic and nonpathogenic lentiviral infections. *Blood* 2008;112:2826–2835.
52. Brenchley JM, Price DA, Schacker TW, et al. Microbial translocation is a cause of systemic immune activation in chronic HIV infection. *Nat Med* 2006;12:1365–1371.
53. Brenchley JM, Schacker TW, Ruff LE, et al. CD4+ T cell depletion during all stages of HIV disease occurs predominantly in the gastrointestinal tract. *J Exp Med* 2004;200:749–759.
54. Breton G, Adle-Biassette H, Therby A, et al. Immune reconstitution inflammatory syndrome in HIV-infected patients with disseminated histoplasmosis. *AIDS* 2006;20:119–121.
55. Brown TT, Moser C, Currier JS, et al. Changes in bone mineral density after initiation of antiretroviral treatment with tenofovir disoproxil fumarate/emtricitabine plus atazanavir/ritonavir, darunavir/ritonavir, or raltegravir. *J Infect Dis* 2015;212:1241–1249.
56. Brown TT, Qaqish RB. Antiretroviral therapy and the prevalence of osteopenia and osteoporosis: a meta-analytic review. *AIDS* 2006;20:2165–2174.
57. Brumme ZL, Goodrich J, Mayer HB, et al. Molecular and clinical epidemiology of CXCR4-using HIV-1 in a large population of antiretroviral-naive individuals. *J Infect Dis* 2005;192:466–474.
58. Bruner KM, Murray AJ, Pollack RA, et al. Defective proviruses rapidly accumulate during acute HIV-1 infection. *Nat Med* 2016;22:1043–1049.
59. Buchbinder SP, Mehrotra DV, Duerr A, et al. Efficacy assessment of a cell-mediated immunity HIV-1 vaccine (the Step Study): a double-blind, randomised, placebo-controlled, test-of-concept trial. *Lancet* 2008;372:1881–1893.
60. Bui JK, Sobolewski MD, Keele BF, et al. Proviruses with identical sequences comprise a large fraction of the replication-competent HIV reservoir. *PLoS Pathog* 2017;13:e1006283.
61. Burton DR, Desrosiers RC, Doms RW, et al. HIV vaccine design and the neutralizing antibody problem. *Nat Immunol* 2004;5:233–236.
62. Burton DR, Hangartner L. Broadly neutralizing antibodies to HIV and their role in vaccine design. *Annu Rev Immunol* 2016;34:635–659.
63. Burwitz BJ, Giraldo-Vela JP, Reed J, et al. CD8+ and CD4+ cytotoxic T cell escape mutations precede breakthrough SIVmac239 viremia in an elite controller. *Retrovirology* 2012;9:91.
64. Busch MP, Lee LL, Satten GA, et al. Time course of detection of viral and serologic markers preceding human immunodeficiency virus type 1 seroconversion: implications for screening of blood and tissue donors. *Transfusion* 1995;35:91–97.
65. Cahn P, Madero JS, Arribas JR, et al. Dolutegravir plus lamivudine versus dolutegravir plus tenofovir disoproxil fumarate and emtricitabine in antiretroviral-naive adults with HIV-1 infection (GEMINI-1 and GEMINI-2): week 48 results from two multicentre, double-blind, randomised, non-inferiority, phase 3 trials. *Lancet* 2019;393:143–155.
66. Cahn P, Madero JS, Arribas JR, et al. Durable efficacy of dolutegravir plus lamivudine in antiretroviral treatment-naive adults with HIV-1 infection: 96-week results from the GEMINI-1 and GEMINI-2 randomized clinical trials. *J Acquir Immune Defic Syndr* 2020;83:310–318.
67. Carr A, Samars K, Burton S, et al. A syndrome of peripheral lipodystrophy, hyperlipidaemia and insulin resistance in patients receiving HIV protease inhibitors. *AIDS* 1998;12:F51–F58.
68. Cardo DM, Culver DH, Ciesielski CA, et al. A case-control study of HIV seroconversion in health care workers after percutaneous exposure. *N Engl J Med* 1997;337:1485–1490.
69. Carrington M, Nelson GW, Martin MP, et al. HLA and HIV-1: heterozygote advantage and B*35-Cw*04 disadvantage. *Science* 1999;283:1753.
70. Carrington M, Walker BD. Immunogenetics of spontaneous control of HIV. *Annu Rev Med* 2012;63:131–145.
71. Casazza JP, Brenchley JM, Hill BJ, et al. Autocrine production of beta-chemokines protects CMV-Specific CD4 T cells from HIV infection. *PLoS Pathog* 2009;5:e1000646.
72. Caskey M. Broadly neutralizing antibodies for the treatment and prevention of HIV infection. *Curr Opin HIV AIDS* 2020;15:49–55.
73. Caskey M, Klein F, Lorenzi JC, et al. Viraemia suppressed in HIV-1-infected humans by broadly neutralizing antibody 3BNC117. *Nature* 2015;522:487–491.
74. Centers for Disease Control. Kaposi's sarcoma and Pneumocystis pneumonia among homosexual men—New York City and California. *MMWR Morb Mortal Wkly Rep* 1981;30:305–308.
75. Centers for Disease Control. Classification system for human immunodeficiency virus (HIV) in children under 13 years of age. *MMWR Morb Mortal Wkly Rep* 1987;36:225–236.
76. Centers for Disease Control and Prevention. 1993 revised classification system for HIV infection and expanded surveillance case definition for AIDS among adolescents and adults. *MMWR Recomm Rep* 1992;41(RR-17):1–19.
77. Centers for Disease Control and Prevention. Preexposure prophylaxis for the prevention of HIV infection in the United States—2017 Update: a clinical practice guideline. https://www.cdc.gov/hiv/pdf/risk/prep/cdc-hiv-prep-guidelines-2017.pdf. Accessed April 29, 2021.
78. Centers for Disease Control and Prevention. HIV and Pregnant Women, Infants, and Children. https://www.cdc.gov/hiv/group/gender/pregnantwomen/. Accessed April 30, 2021.
79. Centers for Disease Control and Prevention, Association of Public Health Laboratories. 2014 (updated 2018). http://dx.doi.org/10.15620/cdc.23447. Accessed April 30, 2021.
80. Centers for Disease Control and Prevention, Health Resources and Services Administration, National Institutes of Health, American Academy of HIV Medicine, Association of Nurses in AIDS Care, International Association of Providers of AIDS Care, et al. Recommendations for HIV prevention with adults and adolescents with HIV in the United States, 2014 (ammended December 30, 2016). https://stacks.cdc.gov/view/cdc/44064. Accessed April 30, 2021.
81. Centers for Disease Control and Prevention/World Health Organization. *Guidelines for Assuring the Accuracy and Reliability of HIV Rapid Testing*. Geneva: World Health Organization; 2005.
82. Chahroudi A, Bosinger SE, Vanderford TH, et al. Natural SIV hosts: showing AIDS the door. *Science* 2012;335:1188–1193.
83. Chan-Tack KM, Truffa MM, Struble KA, et al. Atazanavir-associated nephrolithiasis: cases from the US Food and Drug Administration's Adverse Event Reporting System. *AIDS* 2007;21:1215–1218.
84. Charpentier C, Karmochkine M, Laureillard D, et al. Drug resistance profiles for the HIV integrase gene in patients failing raltegravir salvage therapy. *HIV Med* 2008;9:765–770.
85. Chattha G, Arieff AI, Cummings C, et al. Lactic acidosis complicating the acquired immunodeficiency syndrome. *Ann Intern Med* 1993;118:37–39.
86. Cheeseman SH, Havlir D, McLaughlin MM, et al. Phase I/II evaluation of nevirapine alone and in combination with zidovudine for infection with human immunodeficiency virus. *J Acquir Immune Defic Syndr Hum Retrovirol* 1995;8:141–151.
87. Chen W, Anton LC, Bennink JR, et al. Dissecting the multifactorial causes of immunodominance in class I-restricted T cell responses to viruses. *Immunity* 2000;12:83–93.
88. Chen TY, Ding EL, Seage III GR, et al. Meta-analysis: increased mortality associated with hepatitis C in HIV-infected persons is unrelated to HIV disease progression. *Clin Infect Dis* 2009;49:1605–1615.
89. Chevalier MF, Julg B, Pyo A, et al. HIV-1-specific interleukin-21+ CD4+ T cell responses contribute to durable viral control through the modulation of HIV-specific CD8+ T cell function. *J Virol* 2011;85:733–741.
90. Choopanya K, Martin M, Suntharasamai P, et al. Antiretroviral prophylaxis for HIV infection in injecting drug users in Bangkok, Thailand (the Bangkok Tenofovir Study): a randomised, double-blind, placebo-controlled phase 3 trial. *Lancet* 2013;381:2083–2090.
91. Chun T, Carruth L, Finzi D, et al. Quantification of latent tissue reservoirs and total body viral load in HIV-1 infection. *Nature* 1997;387:183–188.
92. Clark SJ, Saag MS, Decker WD, et al. High titers of cytopathic virus in plasma of patients with symptomatic primary HIV-1 infection. *N Engl J Med* 1991;324:954–960.
93. Clifford DB, Evans S, Yang Y, et al. Impact of efavirenz on neuropsychological performance and symptoms in HIV-infected individuals. *Ann Intern Med* 2005;143:714–721.
94. Clutter DS, Jordan MR, Bertagnolio S, et al. HIV-1 drug resistance and resistance testing. *Infect Genet Evol* 2016;46:292–307.
95. Coffin JM. HIV population dynamics in vivo: implications for genetic variation, pathogenesis, and therapy. *Science* 1995;267:483–489.
96. Coffin JM, Bale MJ, Wells D, et al. Integration in oncogenes plays only a minor role in determining the in vivo distribution of HIV integration sites before or during suppressive antiretroviral therapy. *PLoS Pathog* 2021;17:e1009141.
97. Cohen MS, Chen YQ, McCauley M, et al. Prevention of HIV-1 infection with early antiretroviral therapy. *N Engl J Med* 2011;365:493–505.
98. Cohen MS, Chen YQ, McCauley M, et al. Antiretroviral therapy for the prevention of HIV-1 transmission. *N Engl J Med* 2016;375:830–839.
99. Colby DJ, Trautmann L, Pinyakorn S, et al. Rapid HIV RNA rebound after antiretroviral treatment interruption in persons durably suppressed in Fiebig I acute HIV infection. *Nat Med* 2018;24:923–926.
100. Collins KL, Chen BK, Kalams SA, et al. HIV-1 Nef protein protects infected primary cells against killing by cytotoxic T lymphocytes. *Nature* 1998;391:397–401.
101. Compton AA, Emerman M. Convergence and divergence in the evolution of the APOBEC3G-Vif interaction reveal ancient origins of simian immunodeficiency viruses. *PLoS Pathog* 2013;9:e1003135.
102. Connick E, Lederman MM, Kotzin B, et al. Immune reconstitution in the first year of potent antiretroviral therapy and its relationship to virologic response. *J Infect Dis* 2000;181:358–363.
103. Connor EM, Sperling RS, Gelber R, et al. Reduction of maternal-infant transmission of human immunodeficiency virus type 1 with zidovudine treatment. *N Engl J Med* 1994;331:1173–1180.
104. Connors M, Kovacs JA, Krevat S, et al. HIV infection induces changes in CD4+ T-cell phenotype and depletions within the CD4+ T-cell repertoire that are not immediately restored by antiviral or immune-based therapies. *Nat Med* 1997;3:533–540.
105. Cooper DA, Heera J, Goodrich J, et al. Maraviroc versus efavirenz, both in combination with zidovudine-lamivudine, for the treatment of antiretroviral-naive subjects with CCR5-tropic HIV-1 infection. *J Infect Dis* 2010;201:803–813.
106. Cooper DA, Tindall B, Wilson EJ, et al. Characterization of T lymphocyte responses during primary infection with human immunodeficiency virus. *J Infect Dis* 1988;157:889–896.
107. Coopman SA, Johnson RA, Platt R, et al. Cutaneous disease and drug reactions in HIV infection. *N Engl J Med* 1993;328:1670–1674.
108. Corey L, Gilbert PB, Juraska M, et al. Two randomized trials of neutralizing antibodies to prevent HIV-1 acquisition. *N Engl J Med* 2021;384:1003–1014.
109. Costagliola D, Lang S, Mary-Krause M, et al. Abacavir and cardiovascular risk: reviewing the evidence. *Curr HIV/AIDS Rep* 2010;7:127–133.
110. Crooks AM, Bateson R, Cope AB, et al. Precise quantitation of the latent HIV-1 reservoir: implications for eradication strategies. *J Infect Dis* 2015;212:1361–1365.
111. Curran JW, Lawrence DN, Jaffe H, et al. Acquired immunodeficiency syndrome (AIDS) associated with transfusions. *N Engl J Med* 1984;310:69–75.
112. Currier JS, Kendall MA, Henry WK, et al. Progression of carotid artery intima-media thickening in HIV-infected and uninfected adults. *AIDS* 2007;21:1137–1145.
113. Currier JS, Williams PL, Koletar SL, et al. Discontinuation of Mycobacterium avium complex prophylaxis in patients with antiretroviral therapy-induced increases in CD4+ cell count. A randomized, double-blind, placebo-controlled trial. AIDS Clinical Trials Group 362 Study Team. *Ann Intern Med* 2000;133:493–503.

114. Daar ES, Little S, Pitt J, et al. Diagnosis of primary HIV-1 infection. Los angeles county primary HIV infection recruitment network. *Ann Intern Med* 2001;134:25–29.
115. Daar ES, Lynn HS, Donfield SM, et al. Stromal cell-derived factor-1 genotype, coreceptor tropism, and HIV type 1 disease progression. *J Infect Dis* 2005;192:1597–1605.
116. Dahirel V, Shekhar K, Pereyra F, et al. Coordinate linkage of HIV evolution reveals regions of immunological vulnerability. *Proc Natl Acad Sci U S A* 2011;108:11530–11535.
117. D'Aquila RT, Hughes MD, Johnson VA, et al. Nevirapine, zidovudine, and didanosine compared with zidovudine and didanosine in patients with HIV-1 infection. A randomized, double-blind, placebo-controlled trial. National Institute of Allergy and Infectious Diseases AIDS Clinical Trials Group Protocol 241 Investigators. *Ann Intern Med* 1996;124:1019–1030.
118. D'Aquila RT, Johnson VA, Welles SL, et al. Zidovudine resistance and HIV-1 disease progression during antiretroviral therapy. AIDS Clinical Trials Group Protocol 116B/117 Team and the Virology Committee Resistance Working Group. *Ann Intern Med* 1995;122:401–408.
119. Darby SC, Ewart DW, Giangrande PL, et al. Importance of age at infection with HIV-1 for survival and development of AIDS in UK haemophilia population. UK Haemophilia Centre Directors' Organisation. *Lancet* 1996;347:1573–1579.
120. Davey S, Ajibola G, Maswabi K, et al. Mother-to-child HIV transmission with in utero dolutegravir vs. efavirenz in Botswana. *J Acquir Immune Defic Syndr* 2020;84:235–241.
121. Day CL, Kaufmann DE, Kiepiela P, et al. PD-1 expression on HIV-specific T cells is associated with T-cell exhaustion and disease progression. *Nature* 2006;443:350–354.
122. Day CL, Kiepiela P, Leslie AJ, et al. Proliferative capacity of epitope-specific CD8 T-cell responses is inversely related to viral load in chronic human immunodeficiency virus type 1 infection. *J Virol* 2007;81:434–438.
123. de la Hera GM, Ferreros I, del Amo J, et al. Gender differences in progression to AIDS and death from HIV seroconversion in a cohort of injecting drug users from 1986 to 2001. *J Epidemiol Community Health*. 2004;58:944–950.
124. Deacon NJ, Tsykin A, Solomon A, et al. Genomic structure of an attenuated quasi species of HIV-1 from a blood transfusion donor and recipients. *Science* 1995;270:988–991.
125. Dean M, Carrington M, Winkler C, et al. Genetic restriction of HIV-1 infection and progression to AIDS by a deletion allele of the CKR5 structural gene. *Science* 1996;273:1856–1862.
126. Deeks S, Barbour JD, Martin JN, et al. Sustained CD4+ T cell response after virologic failure of protease inhibitor-based regimens in patients with human immunodeficiency virus infection. *J Infect Dis* 2000;181:946–953.
127. Deeks SG, Wrin T, Liegler T, et al. Virologic and immunologic consequences of discontinuing combination antiretroviral-drug therapy in HIV-infected patients with detectable viremia. *N Engl J Med* 2001;344:472–480.
128. Delany-Moretlwe S, Hughes J, Bock P, et al. Long acting injectable cabotegravir is safe and effective in preventing HIV infection in cisgender women: interim results from HPTN 084. HIV R4P Virtual; 27 January 2021. Abstract HY01.02LB.
129. Demers KR, Makedonas G, Buggert M, et al. Temporal dynamics of CD8+ T cell effector responses during primary HIV infection. *PLoS Pathog* 2016;12:e1005805.
130. Deng HK, Liu R, Ellmeier W, et al. Identification of a major co-receptor for primary isolates of HIV-1. *Nature* 1996;381:661–666.
131. Deng K, Pertea M, Rongvaux A, et al. Broad CTL response is required to clear latent HIV-1 due to dominance of escape mutations. *Nature* 2015;517:381–385.
132. Dhillon AK, Donners H, Pantophlet R, et al. Dissecting the neutralizing antibody specificities of broadly neutralizing sera from human immunodeficiency virus type 1-infected donors. *J Virol* 2007;81:6548–6562.
133. Di Mascio M, Markowitz M, Louie M, et al. Viral blip dynamics during highly active antiretroviral therapy. *J Virol* 2003;77:12165–12172.
134. Dinoso JB, Kim SY, Wiegand AM, et al. Treatment intensification does not reduce residual HIV-1 viremia in patients on highly active antiretroviral therapy. *Proc Natl Acad Sci U S A* 2009;106:9403–9408.
135. Dooley KE, Kaplan R, Mwelase N, et al. Dolutegravir-based antiretroviral therapy for patients coinfected with tuberculosis and human immunodeficiency virus: a multicenter, noncomparative, open-label, randomized trial. *Clin Infect Dis* 2020;70:549–556.
136. Dooley KE, Sayre P, Borland J, et al. Safety, tolerability, and pharmacokinetics of the HIV integrase inhibitor dolutegravir given twice daily with rifampin or once daily with rifabutin: results of a phase 1 study among healthy subjects. *J Acquir Immune Defic Syndr* 2013;62:21–27.
137. Douek DC, Brenchley JM, Betts MR, et al. HIV preferentially infects HIV-specific CD4+ T cells. *Nature* 2002;417:95–98.
138. Dragic T, Litwin V, Allaway GP, et al. HIV-1 entry into CD4+ cells is mediated by the chemokine receptor CC-CKR-5. *Nature* 1996;381:667–673.
139. Dunn DT, Brandt CD, Krivine A, et al. The sensitivity of HIV-1 DNA polymerase chain reaction in the neonatal period and the relative contributions of intra-uterine and intra-partum transmission. *AIDS* 1995;9:F7–F11.
140. Eberl G, Colonna M, Di Santo JP, et al. Innate lymphoid cells. Innate lymphoid cells: a new paradigm in immunology. *Science* 2015;348:aaa6566.
141. Egger M, May M, Chene G, et al. Prognosis of HIV-1-infected patients starting highly active antiretroviral therapy: a collaborative analysis of prospective studies. *Lancet* 2002;360:119–129.
142. El Sadr WM, Lundgren JD, Neaton JD, et al. CD4+ count-guided interruption of antiretroviral treatment. *N Engl J Med* 2006;355:2283–2296.
143. Elrefaei M, McElroy MD, Preas CP, et al. Central memory CD4+ T cell responses in chronic HIV infection are not restored by antiretroviral therapy. *J Immunol* 2004;173:2184–2189.
144. Emu B, Fessel J, Schrader S, et al. Phase 3 study of ibalizumab for multidrug-resistant HIV-1. *N Engl J Med* 2018;379:645–654.
145. Erdmann N, Du VY, Carlson J, et al. HLA Class-II associated HIV polymorphisms predict escape from CD4+ T Cell responses. *PLoS Pathog* 2015;11:e1005111.
146. Eshleman SH, Khaki L, Laeyendecker O, et al. Detection of individuals with acute HIV-1 infection using the ARCHITECT HIV Ag/Ab Combo assay. *J Acquir Immune Defic Syndr* 2009;52:121–124.
147. Esnouf R, Ren J, Ross C, et al. Mechanism of inhibition of HIV-1 reverse transcriptase by non-nucleoside inhibitors. *Nat Struct Biol* 1995;2:303–308.
148. Estes JD, Harris LD, Klatt NR, et al. Damaged intestinal epithelial integrity linked to microbial translocation in pathogenic simian immunodeficiency virus infections. *PLoS Pathog* 2010;6:e1001052.
149. European AIDS Clinical Society. Guidelines Version 10.1. 2020. https://www.eacsociety.org/files/guidelines-10.1_30032021_1.pdf. Accessed April 29, 2021.
150. Faria NR, Rambaut A, Suchard MA, et al. HIV epidemiology. The early spread and epidemic ignition of HIV-1 in human populations. *Science* 2014;346:56–61.
151. Farzadegan H, Hoover DR, Astemborski J, et al. Sex differences in HIV-1 viral load and progression to AIDS. *Lancet* 1998;352:1510–1514.
152. Fellay J, Shianna KV, Ge D, et al. A whole-genome association study of major determinants for host control of HIV-1. *Science* 2007;317:944–947.
153. Feng Y, Broder CC, Kennedy PE, et al. HIV-1 entry cofactor: functional cDNA cloning of a seven-transmembrane G protein-coupled receptor. *Science* 1996;272:872–877.
154. Fenwick C, Joo V, Jacquier P, et al. T-cell exhaustion in HIV infection. *Immunol Rev* 2019;292:149–163.
155. Ferguson AL, Mann JK, Omarjee S, et al. Translating HIV sequences into quantitative fitness landscapes predicts viral vulnerabilities for rational immunogen design. *Immunity* 2013;38:606–617.
156. Fichtenbaum CJ, Clifford DB, Powderly WG. Risk factors for dideoxynucleoside-induced toxic neuropathy in patients with the human immunodeficiency virus infection. *J Acquir Immune Defic Syndr Hum Retrovirol* 1995;10:169–174.
157. Finzi D, Blankson J, Siliciano JD, et al. Latent infection of CD4+ T cells provides a mechanism for lifelong persistence of HIV-1, even in patients on effective combination therapy. *Nat Med* 1999;5:512–525.
158. Finzi D, Hermankova M, Pierson T, et al. Identification of a reservoir for HIV-1 in patients on highly active antiretroviral therapy. *Science* 1997;278:1295–1300.
159. Fischl MA, Richman DD, Grieco MH, et al. The efficacy of azidothymidine (AZT) in the treatment of patients with AIDS and AIDS-related complex. A double-blind, placebo-controlled trial. *N Engl J Med* 1987;317:185–191.
160. Flexner C. HIV-protease inhibitors. *N Engl J Med* 1998;338:1281–1292.
161. Flynn NM, Forthal DN, Harro CD. Placebo-controlled phase 3 trial of a recombinant glycoprotein 120 vaccine to prevent HIV-1 infection. *J Infect Dis* 2005;191:654–665.
162. Ford N, Shubber Z, Calmy A, et al. Choice of antiretroviral drugs for postexposure prophylaxis for adults and adolescents: a systematic review. *Clin Infect Dis* 2015;60(Suppl 3):S170–S176.
163. Frahm N, Kiepiela P, Adams S, et al. Control of human immunodeficiency virus replication by cytotoxic T lymphocytes targeting subdominant epitopes. *Nat Immunol* 2006;7:173–178.
164. Friis-Moller N, Sabin CA, Weber R, et al. Combination antiretroviral therapy and the risk of myocardial infarction. *N Engl J Med* 2003;349:1993–2003.
165. Furrer H, Opravil M, Rossi M, et al. Discontinuation of primary prophylaxis in HIV-infected patients at high risk of Pneumocystis carinii pneumonia: prospective multicentre study. *AIDS* 2001;15:501–507.
166. Furrer H, Telenti A, Rossi M, et al. Discontinuing or withholding primary prophylaxis against Mycobacterium avium in patients on successful antiretroviral combination therapy. The Swiss HIV Cohort Study. *AIDS* 2000;14:1409–1412.
167. Gaiha GD, Rossin EJ, Urbach J, et al. Structural topology defines protective CD8(+) T cell epitopes in the HIV proteome. *Science* 2019;364:480–484.
168. Gaines H, von Sydow M, Pehrson PO, et al. Clinical picture of primary HIV infection presenting as a glandular fever-like illness. *Br Med J* 1988;297:1363–1368.
169. Gaines H, von Sydow M, Sonnerborg A, et al. Antibody response in primary human immunodeficiency virus infection. *Lancet* 1987;i:1249–1253.
170. Gallant JE, Daar ES, Raffi F, et al. Efficacy and safety of tenofovir alafenamide versus tenofovir disoproxil fumarate given as fixed-dose combinations containing emtricitabine as backbones for treatment of HIV-1 infection in virologically suppressed adults: a randomised, double-blind, active-controlled phase 3 trial. *Lancet HIV* 2016;3:e158–e165.
171. Gallo RC, Sarin PS, Gelmann EP, et al. Isolation of human T-cell leukemia virus in acquired immune deficiency syndrome (AIDS). *Science* 1983;220:865–867.
172. Gandhi M, Bacchetti P, Miotti P, et al. Does patient sex affect human immunodeficiency virus levels? *Clin Infect Dis* 2002;35(3):313–322.
173. Gandhi RT, Spritzler J, Chan E, et al. Effect of baseline- and treatment-related factors on immunologic recovery after initiation of antiretroviral therapy in HIV-1-positive subjects: results from ACTG 384. *J Acquir Immune Defic Syndr* 2006;42:426–434.
174. Gandhi RT, Zheng L, Bosch RJ, et al. The effect of raltegravir intensification on low-level residual viremia in HIV-infected patients on antiretroviral therapy: a randomized controlled trial. *PLoS Med* 2010;7:e1000321.
175. Gao F, Bailes E, Robertson DL, et al. Origin of HIV-1 in the chimpanzee Pan troglodytes troglodytes. *Nature* 1999;397:436–442.
176. Gao X, Nelson GW, Karacki P, et al. Effects of a single amino acid change in NHC class I molecules on the rate of progression to AIDS. *N Engl J Med* 2001;344:1668–1675.
177. Gao WY, Shirasaka T, Johns DG, et al. Differential phosphorylation of dideoxynucleotides in resting and activated peripheral blood mononuclear cells. *J Clin Invest* 1993;91:2326–2333.
178. Garcia-Lerma JG, Otten RA, Qari SH, et al. Prevention of rectal SHIV transmission in macaques by daily or intermittent prophylaxis with emtricitabine and tenofovir. *PLoS Med* 2008;5:e28.
179. Gaschen B, Taylor J, Yusim K, et al. Diversity considerations in HIV-1 vaccine selection. *Science* 2002;296:2354–2360.
180. Gaudieri S, DeSantis D, McKinnon E, et al. Killer immunoglobulin-like receptors and HLA act both independently and synergistically to modify HIV disease progression. *Genes Immun* 2005;6:683–690.
181. Gaudieri S, Nolan D, McKinnon E, et al. Associations between KIR epitope combinations expressed by HLA-B/-C haplotypes found in an HIV-1 infected study population may influence NK mediated immune responses. *Mol Immunol* 2005;42:557–560.

182. Geldmacher C, Ngwenyama N, Schuetz A, et al. Preferential infection and depletion of Mycobacterium tuberculosis-specific CD4 T cells after HIV-1 infection. *J Exp Med* 2010;207:2869–2881.
183. George MD, Reay E, Sankaran S, et al. Early antiretroviral therapy for simian immunodeficiency virus infection leads to mucosal CD4+ T-cell restoration and enhanced gene expression regulating mucosal repair and regeneration. *J Virol* 2005;79:2709–2719.
184. Geskus RB, Meyer L, Hubert JB, et al. Causal pathways of the effects of age and the CCR5-Delta32, CCR2-64I, and SDF-1 3'A alleles on AIDS development. *J Acquir Immune Defic Syndr* 2005;39:321–326.
185. Gianella S, Moser C, Vitomirov A, et al. Presence of asymptomatic cytomegalovirus and Epstein—Barr virus DNA in blood of persons with HIV starting antiretroviral therapy is associated with non-AIDS clinical events. *AIDS* 2020;34:849–857.
186. Giorgi JV, Hultin LE, McKeating JA, et al. Shorter survival in advanced human immunodeficiency virus type 1 infection is more closely associated with T lymphocyte activation than with plasma virus burden or virus chemokine coreceptor usage. *J Infect Dis* 1999;179:859–870.
187. Giorgi JV, Liu Z, Hultin LE, et al. Elevated levels of CD38+ CD8+ T cells in HIV infection add to the prognostic value of low CD4+ T cell levels results of 6 years of follow-up. *J Acquir Immune Defic Syndr* 1997;6:904–912.
188. Goldman M, Zackin R, Fichtenbaum CJ, et al. Safety of discontinuation of maintenance therapy for disseminated histoplasmosis after immunologic response to antiretroviral therapy. *Clin Infect Dis* 2004;38:1485–1489.
189. Gonzalez E, Kulkarni H, Bolivar H, et al. The influence of CCL3L1 gene-containing segmental duplications on HIV-1/AIDS susceptibility. *Science* 2005;307:1434–1440.
190. Goulder PJ, Walker BD. HIV and HLA class I: an evolving relationship. *Immunity* 2012;37:426–440.
191. Granich RM, Gilks CF, Dye C, et al. Universal voluntary HIV testing with immediate antiretroviral therapy as a strategy for elimination of HIV transmission: a mathematical model. *Lancet* 2009;373:48–57.
192. Granich R, Williams B, Montaner J, et al. 90-90-90 and ending AIDS: necessary and feasible. *Lancet* 2017;390:341–343.
193. Grant RM, Lama JR, Anderson PL, et al. Preexposure chemoprophylaxis for HIV prevention in men who have sex with men. *N Engl J Med* 2010;363:2587–2599.
194. Grasela TH, Walawander CA, Beltangady M, et al. Analysis of potential risk factors associated withthe development of pancreatitis in Phase I patients with AIDS or AIDS-related complex receiving didanosine. *J Infect Dis* 1994;169:1250–1255.
195. Gray GE, Bekker LG, Laher F, et al. Vaccine efficacy of ALVAC-HIV and bivalent subtype C gp120-MF59 in adults. *N Engl J Med* 2021;384:1089–1100.
196. Gray RH, Kigozi G, Serwadda D, et al. Male circumcision for HIV prevention in men in Rakai, Uganda: a randomised trial. *Lancet* 2007;369:657–666.
197. Gray RH, Wawer MH, Brokmeyer R, et al. Probability of HIV-1 transmission per coital act in monogamous, heterosexual, HIV-1-discordant couples in Rakai, Uganda. *Lancet* 2001;357:1149–1153.
198. Gregson S, Garnett GP, Nyamukapa CA, et al. HIV decline associated with behavior change in eastern Zimbabwe. *Science* 2006;311:664–666.
199. Grulich AE, van Leeuwen MT, Falster MO. Incidence of cancers in people with HIV/AIDS compared with immunosuppressed transplant recipients: a meta-analysis. *Lancet* 2007;370:59–67.
200. Grunfeld C, Delaney JA, Wanke C, et al. Preclinical atherosclerosis due to HIV infection: carotid intima-medial thickness measurements from the FRAM study. *AIDS* 2009;23:1841–1849.
201. Grunfeld C, Feingold KR. Metabolic disturbances and wasting in the acquired immunodeficiency syndrome. *N Engl J Med* 1992;327:329–337.
202. Gryseels S, Watts TD, Kabongo Mpolesha JM, et al. A near full-length HIV-1 genome from 1966 recovered from formalin-fixed paraffin-embedded tissue. *Proc Natl Acad Sci U S A* 2020;117:12222–12229.
203. Gulick RM, Lalezari J, Goodrich J, et al. Maraviroc for previously treated patients with R5 HIV-1 infection. *N Engl J Med* 2008;359:1429–1441.
204. Gulick RM, Mellors JW, Havlir D, et al. Treatment with indinavir, zidovudine and lamivudine in adults with human immunodeficiency virus infection and prior antiretroviral therapy. *N Engl J Med* 1997;337:734–740.
205. Gupta RK, Abdul-Jawad S, McCoy LE, et al. HIV-1 remission following CCR5Delta32/Delta32 haematopoietic stem-cell transplantation. *Nature* 2019;568:244–248.
206. Gurtler LG, Hauser PH, Eberle J, et al. A new subtype of human immunodeficiency virus type 1 (MVP-5180) from Cameroon. *J Virol* 1994;68:1581–1585.
207. Hanna GJ, Lalezari J, Hellinger JA, et al. Antiviral activity, pharmacokinetics, and safety of BMS-488043, a novel oral small-molecule HIV-1 attachment inhibitor, in HIV-1-infected subjects. *Antimicrob Agents Chemother* 2011;55:722–728.
208. Hansen SG, Sacha JB, Hughes CM, et al. Cytomegalovirus vectors violate CD8+ T cell epitope recognition paradigms. *Science* 2013;340:1237874.
209. Hansen SG, Wu HL, Burwitz BJ, et al. Broadly targeted CD8(+) T cell responses restricted by major histocompatibility complex E. *Science* 2016;351:714–720.
210. Harari A, Petitpierre S, Vallelian F, et al. Skewed representation of functionally distinct populations of virus-specific CD4 T cells in HIV-1-infected subjects with progressive disease: changes after antiretroviral therapy. *Blood* 2004;103:966–972.
211. Havlir D, Cheeseman SH, McLaughlin M, et al. High-dose nevirapine: safety, pharmacokinetics, and antiviral effect in patients with human immunodeficiency virus infection. *J Infect Dis* 1995;171:537–545.
212. Havlir DV, Richman DD. Viral dynamics of HIV: implications for drug development and therapeutic strategies. *Ann Intern Med* 1996;124:984–994.
213. Haynes BF, Gilbert PB, McElrath MJ, et al. Immune-correlates analysis of an HIV-1 vaccine efficacy trial. *N Engl J Med* 2012;366:1275–1286.
214. Haynes BF, Mascola JR. The quest for an antibody-based HIV vaccine. *Immunol Rev* 2017;275(1):5–10.
215. Hazuda DJ, Felock P, Witmer M, et al. Inhibitors of strand transfer that prevent integration and inhibit HIV-1 replication in cells. *Science* 2000;287:646–650.
216. Heberling RL, Kalter SS, Marx PA, et al. Dot immunobinding assay compared with enzyme-linked immunosorbent assay for rapid and specific detection of retrovirus antibody induced by human or simian acquired immunodeficiency syndrome. *J Clin Microbiol* 1988;26:765–767.
217. Hecht FM, Busch MP, Rawal B, et al. Use of laboratory tests and clinical symptoms for identification of primary HIV infection. *AIDS* 2002;16:1119–1129.
218. Hecht FM, Hartogensis W, Bragg L, et al. HIV RNA level in early infection is predicted by viral load in the transmission source. *AIDS* 2010;24:941–945.
219. Henrich TJ, Hatano H, Bacon O, et al. HIV-1 persistence following extremely early initiation of antiretroviral therapy (ART) during acute HIV-1 infection: an observational study. *PLoS Med* 2017;14:e1002417.
220. Henrich TJ, Hobbs KS, Hanhauser E, et al. Human immunodeficiency virus type 1 persistence following systemic chemotherapy for malignancy. *J Infect Dis* 2017;216:254–262.
221. Hersperger AR, Pereyra F, Nason M, et al. Perforin expression directly ex vivo by HIV-specific CD8 T-cells is a correlate of HIV elite control. *PLoS Pathog* 2010;6:e1000917.
222. Hess C, Altfeld M, Thomas SY, et al. HIV-1 specific CD8+ T cells with an effector phenotype and control of viral replication. *Lancet* 2004;363:863–866.
223. Hetherington S, McGuirk S, Powell G, et al. Hypersensitivity reactions during therapy with the nucleoside reverse transcriptase inhibitor abacavir. *Clin Ther* 2001;23:1603–1614.
224. Hirsch HH, Kaufmann G, Sendi P, et al. Immune reconstitution in HIV-infected patients. *Clin Infect Dis* 2004;38:1159–1166.
225. Ho JE, Hsue PY. Cardiovascular manifestations of HIV infection. *Heart* 2009;95: 1193–1202.
226. Ho DD, Neumann AU, Perelson AS. Rapid turnover of plasma virions and CD4 lymphocytes in HIV-1 infection. *Nature* 1995;373:123–126.
227. Ho DD, Sarngadharan MG, Resnick L, et al. Primary human T-lymphotropic virus type III infection. *Ann Intern Med* 1985;103:880–883.
228. Ho YC, Shan L, Hosmane NN, et al. Replication-competent noninduced proviruses in the latent reservoir increase barrier to HIV-1 cure. *Cell* 2013;155:540–551.
229. Ho SH, Shek L, Gettie A, et al. V3 loop-determined coreceptor preference dictates the dynamics of CD4+-T-cell loss in simian-human immunodeficiency virus-infected macaques. *J Virol* 2005;79:12296–12303.
230. Hoffmann C, Llibre JM. Neuropsychiatric adverse events with dolutegravir and other integrase strand transfer inhibitors. *AIDS Rev* 2019;21:4–10.
231. Hogg RS, Yip B, Chan KJ, et al. Rates of disease progression by baseline CD4 count and viral load after initiating triple-drug therapy. *JAMA* 2001;286:2568–2577.
232. Hosmane NN, Kwon KJ, Bruner KM, et al. Proliferation of latently infected CD4(+) T cells carrying replication-competent HIV-1: potential role in latent reservoir dynamics. *J Exp Med* 2017;214:959–972.
233. Hraber P, Seaman MS, Bailer RT, et al. Prevalence of broadly neutralizing antibody responses during chronic HIV-1 infection. *AIDS* 2014;28:163–169.
234. Hu Z, Kuritzkes DR. Effect of raltegravir resistance mutations in HIV-1 integrase on viral fitness. *J Acquir Immune Defic Syndr* 2010;55:148–155.
235. Hunt PW, Martin JN, Sinclair E, et al. Valganciclovir reduces T Cell activation in HIV-infected individuals with incomplete CD4+ T Cell recovery on antiretroviral therapy. *J Infect Dis* 2011;203:1474–1483.
236. Hutter G, Nowak D, Mossner M, et al. Long-term control of HIV by CCR5 Delta32/Delta32 stem-cell transplantation. *N Engl J Med* 2009;360:692–698.
237. Ickovics JR, Cameron A, Zackin R, et al. Consequences and determinants of adherence to antiretroviral medication: results from adult AIDS Clinical Trials Group Protocol 370. *Antivir Ther* 2002;7:185–193.
238. INSIGHT START Study Group. Initiation of antiretroviral therapy in early asymptomatic HIV infection. *N Engl J Med* 2015;373:795–807.
239. Ioannidis JP, Rosenberg PS, Goedert JJ, et al. Effects of CCR5-Delta32, CCR2-64I, and SDF-1 3'A alleles on HIV-1 disease progression: an international meta-analysis of individual-patient data. *Ann Intern Med* 2001;135:782–795.
240. Iyasere C, Tilton JC, Johnson AJ, et al. Diminished proliferation of human immunodeficiency virus-specific CD4+ T cells is associated with diminished interleukin-2 (IL-2) production and is recovered by exogenous IL-2. *J Virol* 2003;77:10900–10909.
241. Jacobson JM, Kuritzkes DR, Godofsky E, et al. Safety, pharmacokinetics, and antiretroviral activity of multiple doses of ibalizumab (formerly TNX-355), an anti-CD4 monoclonal antibody, in human immunodeficiency virus type 1-infected adults. *Antimicrob Agents Chemother* 2009;53:450–457.
242. Jaffar S, Grant AD, Whitworth J, et al. The natural history of HIV-1 and HIV-2 infections in adults in Africa: a literature review. *Bull World Health Organ* 2004;82: 462–469.
243. Jaffe HW, Francis DP, McLane MF, et al. Transfusion-associated AIDS: serologic evidence of human T-cell leukemia virus infection of donors. *Science* 1984;223:1309–1312.
244. Japour AJ, Welles S, D'Aquila RT, et al. Prevalence and clinical significance of zidovudine resistance mutations in human immunodeficiency virus isolated from patients after long-term zidovudine treatment. AIDS Clinical Trials Group 116B/117 Study Team and the Virology Committee Resistance Working Group. *J Infect Dis* 1995;171:1172–1179.
245. Jiang H, Deeks SG, Kuritzkes DR, et al. Assessing resistance costs of antiretroviral therapies via measures of future drug options. *J Infect Dis* 2003;188:1001–1008.
246. Jiang W, Lederman MM, Hunt P, et al. Plasma levels of bacterial DNA correlate with immune activation and the magnitude of immune restoration in persons with antiretroviral-treated HIV infection. *J Infect Dis* 2009;199:1177–1185.
247. Jin X, Bauer DE, Tuttleton SE, et al. Dramatic rise in plasma ciremia after CD8+ T cell depletion in simian immunodeficiency virus-infected macaques. *J Exp Med* 1999;189 991–998.
248. John GC, Nduati RW, Mbori-Ngacha DA, et al. Correlates of mother-to-child human immunodeficiency virus type 1 (HIV-1) transmission: association with maternal plasma HIV-1 RNA load, genital HIV-1 DNA shedding, and breast infections. *J Infect Dis* 2001;183:206–212.
249. Johnson M, Grinsztejn B, Rodriguez C, et al. 96-week comparison of once-daily atazanavir/ritonavir and twice-daily lopinavir/ritonavir in patients with multiple virologic failures. *AIDS* 2006;20:711–718.

250. Kahn JO, Walker BD. Acute human immunodeficiency virus type 1 infection. *N Engl J Med* 1998;339:33–39.

251. Kakuda TN. Pharmacology of nucleoside and nucleotide reverse transcriptase inhibitor-induced mitochondrial toxicity. *Clin Ther* 2000;22:685–708.

252. Karras A, Lafaurie M, Furco A, et al. Tenofovir-related nephrotoxicity in human immunodeficiency virus-infected patients: three cases of renal failure, Fanconi syndrome, and nephrogenic diabetes insipidus. *Clin Infect Dis* 2003;36:1070–1073.

253. Kaslow RA, Carrington M, Apple R, et al. Influence of combinations of human major histocompatibility complex genes on the course of HIV-1 infection. *Nat Med* 1996;2: 405–411.

254. Kassler WJ, Haley C, Jones WK, et al. Performance of a rapid, on-site human immunodeficiency virus antibody assay in a public health setting. *J Clin Microbiol* 1995;33: 2899–2902.

255. Katsikis PD, Mueller YM, Villinger F. The cytokine network of acute HIV infection: a promising target for vaccines and therapy to reduce viral set-point? *PLoS Pathog* 2011;7:e1002055.

256. Kaufmann DE, Kavanagh DG, Pereyra F, et al. Upregulation of CTLA-4 by HIV-specific CD4+ T cells correlates with disease progression and defines a reversible immune dysfunction. *Nat Immunol* 2007;8:1246–1254.

257. Kaufmann DE, Lichterfeld M, Altfeld M, et al. Limited durability of viral control following treated acute HIV infection. *PLoS Med* 2004;1:e36.

258. Kaufmann D, Munoz M, Bleiber G, et al. Virological and immunological characteristics of HIV treatment failure. *AIDS* 2000;14:1767–1774.

259. Kaufmann D, Pantaleo G, Sudre P, et al. CD4-cell count in HIV-1-infected individuals remaining viraemic with highly active antiretroviral therapy (HAART). Swiss HIV cohort study [letter]. *Lancet* 1998;351:723–724.

260. Kawashima Y, Pfafferott K, Frater J, et al. Adaptation of HIV-1 to human leukocyte antigen class I. *Nature* 2009;458:641–645.

261. Kazer SW, Aicher TP, Muema DM, et al. Integrated single-cell analysis of multicellular immune dynamics during hyperacute HIV-1 infection. *Nat Med* 2020;26:511–518.

262. Kazer SW, Walker BD, Shalek AK. Evolution and diversity of immune responses during acute HIV infection. *Immunity* 2020;53:908–924.

263. Keele BF, Jones JH, Terio KA, et al. Increased mortality and AIDS-like immunopathology in wild chimpanzees infected with SIVcpz. *Nature* 2009;460:515–519.

264. Kempf DJ, Marsh KC, Kumar G, et al. Pharmacokinetic enhancement of inhibitors of the human immunodeficiency virus protease by coadministration with ritonavir. *Antimicrob Agents Chemother* 1997;41:654–660.

265. Kinai E, Hanabusa H. Renal tubular toxicity associated with tenofovir assessed using urine-beta 2 microglobulin, percentage of tubular reabsorption of phosphate and alkaline phosphatase levels. *AIDS* 2005;19:2031–2033.

266. Kirchhoff F, Greenough TC, Brettler DB, et al. Brief report: absence of intact nef sequences in a long-term survivor with nonprogressive HIV-1 infection. *N Engl J Med* 1995;332:228–232.

267. Klein F, Mouquet H, Dosenovic P, et al. Antibodies in HIV-1 vaccine development and therapy. *Science* 2013;341:1199–1204.

268. Koblin BA, van Benthem BH, Buchbinder SP, et al. Long-term survival after infection with human immunodeficiency virus type 1 (HIV-1) among homosexual men in hepatitis B vaccine trial cohorts in Amsterdam, New York City, and San Francisco, 1978–1995. *Am J Epidemiol* 1999;150:1026–1030.

269. Koletar SL, Heald AE, Finkelstein D, et al. A prospective study of discontinuing primary and secondary Pneumocystis carinii pneumonia prophylaxis after CD4 cell count increase to > 200 x 10⁶/l. *AIDS* 2001;15:1509–1515.

270. Koot M, Keet IPM, Vos AHV, et al. Prognostic value of HIV-1 syncytium-inducing phenotype for rate of CD4+ cell depletion and progression to AIDS. *Ann Intern Med* 1993;118:681–688.

271. Kopp JB, Smith MW, Nelson GW, et al. MYH9 is a major-effect risk gene for focal segmental glomerulosclerosis. *Nat Genet* 2008;40:1175–1184.

272. Korber B, Muldoon M, Theiler J, et al. Timing the ancestor of the HIV-1 pandemic strains. *Science* 2000;288:1789–1796.

273. Kostrikis LG, Huang Y, Moore JP, et al. A chemokine receptor CCR2 allele delays HIV-1 disease progression and is associated with a CCR5 promoter mutation. *Nat Med* 1998;4:350–353.

274. Kotler DP, Grunfeld C. Pathophysiology and treatment of the AIDS wasting syndrome. In: Volberding P, Jacobson MA, eds. *AIDS Clinical Review 1995/1996*. New York: Marcel Dekker, Inc.; 1995:229–275.

275. Koup RA, Safrit JT, Cao Y, et al. Temporal association of cellular immune responses with the initial control of viremia in primary human immunodeficiency virus type 1 syndrome. *J Virol* 1994;68:4650–4655.

276. Kozal M, Aberg J, Pialoux G, et al. Fostemsavir in adults with multidrug-resistant HIV-1 infection. *N Engl J Med* 2020;382:1232–1243.

277. Kozal MJ, Kroodsma K, Winters MA, et al. Didanosine resistance in HIV-infected patients switched from zidovudine to didanosine monotherapy. *Ann Intern Med* 1994;121:263–268.

278. Kuller LH, Tracy R, Belloso W, et al. Inflammatory and coagulation biomarkers and mortality in patients with HIV infection. *PLoS Med* 2008;5:e203.

279. Kuritzkes DR, Bell S, Bakhtiari M. Rapid CD4+ cell decline after sexual transmission of a zidovudine-resistant syncytium-forming isolate of HIV-1. *AIDS* 1994;8:1017–1019.

280. Kuritzkes DR, Jacobson J, Powderly WG, et al. Antiretroviral activity of the anti-CD4 monoclonal antibody TNX-355 in patients infected with human immunodeficiency virus type 1. *J Infect Dis* 2004;189:286–291.

281. Lalezari JP, Henry K, O'Hearn M, et al. Enfuvirtide, an HIV-1 fusion inhibitor, for drug-resistant HIV infection in North and South America. *N Engl J Med* 2003;348:2175–2185.

282. Landovitz RJ, Donnell D, Clement ME, et al. Cabotegravir for HIV prevention in cisgender men and transgender women. *N Engl J Med* 2021;385:595–608.

283. Lavreys L, Baeten JM, Chohan V, et al. Higher set point plasma viral load and more-severe acute HIV type 1 (HIV-1) illness predict mortality among high-risk HIV-1-infected African women. *Clin Infect Dis* 2006;42:1333–1339.

284. Le Gall S, Erdtmann L, Benichou S, et al. Nef interacts with the mu subunit of clathrin adaptor complexes and reveals a cryptic sorting signal in MHC I molecules. *Immunity* 1998;8:483–495.

285. Ledergerber B, Lundgren JD, Walker AS, et al. Predictors of trend in CD4-positive T-cell count and mortality among HIV-1-infected individuals with virological failure to all three antiretroviral-drug classes. *Lancet* 2004;364:51–62.

286. Lederman M, Connick E, Landay A, et al. Immunologic responses associated with 12 weeks of combination antiretroviral therapy consisting of zidovudine, lamivudine, and ritonavir: results of AIDS clinical trials group protocol 315. *J Infect Dis* 1998;178:70–79.

287. Lennox JL, DeJesus E, Lazzarin A, et al. Safety and efficacy of raltegravir-based versus efavirenz-based combination therapy in treatment-naive patients with HIV-1 infection: a multicentre, double-blind randomised controlled trial. *Lancet* 2009;374:796–806.

288. Levi J, Raymond A, Pozniak A, et al. Can the UNAIDS 90-90-90 target be achieved? A systematic analysis of national HIV treatment cascades. *BMJ Glob Health* 2016;1:e000010.

289. Li Q, Duan L, Estes JD, et al. Peak SIV replication in resting memory CD4+ T cells depletes gut lamina propria CD4+ T cells. *Nature* 2005;434:1148–1152.

290. Li JZ, Paredes R, Ribaudo HJ, et al. Low-frequency HIV-1 drug resistance mutations and risk of NNRTI-based antiretroviral treatment failure: a systematic review and pooled analysis. *JAMA* 2011;305:1327–1335.

291. Li Y, Svehla K, Louder MK, et al. Analysis of neutralization specificities in polyclonal sera derived from human immunodeficiency virus type 1-infected individuals. *J Virol* 2009;83:1045–1059.

292. Lindback S, Karlsson AC, Mittler J, et al. Viral dynamics in primary HIV-1 infection. Karolinska Institutet Primary HIV Infection Study Group. *AIDS.* 2000;14:2283–2291.

293. Lingappa JR, Thomas KK, Hughes JP, et al. Partner characteristics predicting HIV-1 set point in sexually acquired HIV-1 among African seroconverters. *AIDS Res Hum Retroviruses* 2013;29:164–171.

294. Link JO, Rhee MS, Tse WC, et al. Clinical targeting of HIV capsid protein with a long-acting small molecule. *Nature* 2020;584:614–618.

295. Little SJ, Holte S, Routy JP, et al. Antiretroviral-drug resistance among patients recently infected with HIV. *N Engl J Med* 2002;347:385–394.

296. Liu Z, Cumberland WG, Hultin LE, et al. Elevated CD38 antigen expression on CD8+ T cells is a stronger marker for the risk of chronic HIV disease progression to AIDS and death in the Multicenter AIDS Cohort Study than CD4+ cell count, soluble immune activation markers, or combinations of HLA-DR and CD38 expression. *J Acquir Immune Defic Syndr Hum Retrovirol* 1997;16:83–92.

297. Liu R, Paxton WA, Choe S, et al. Homozygous defect in HIV-1 coreceptor accounts for resistance of some multiply-exposed individuals to HIV-1 infection. *Cell* 1996;86:367–377.

298. Liu L, Zhang Q, Chen P, et al. Foxp3(+)Helios(+) regulatory T cells are associated with monocyte subsets and their PD-1 expression during acute HIV-1 infection. *BMC Immunol* 2019;20:38.

299. Lok JJ, Bosch RJ, Benson CA, et al. Long-term increase in CD4+ T-cell counts during combination antiretroviral therapy for HIV-1 infection. *AIDS* 2010;24:1867–1876.

300. Lonergan JT, Behling C, Pfander H, et al. Hyperlactatemia and hepatic abnormalities in 10 human immunodeficiency virus-infected patients receiving nucleoside analogue combination regimens. *Clin Infect Dis* 2000;31:162–166.

301. Lopez-Vazquez A, Mina-Blanco A, Martinez-Borra J, et al. Interaction between KIR3DL1 and HLA-B*57 supertype alleles influences the progression of HIV-1 infection in a Zambian population. *Hum Immunol* 2005;66:285–289.

302. Lore K, Sonnerborg A, Brostrom C, et al. Accumulation of DC-SIGN+CD40+ dendritic cells with reduced CD80 and CD86 expression in lymphoid tissue during acute HIV-1 infection. *AIDS* 2002;16:683–692.

303. Lorenzi JC, Cohen YZ, Cohn LB, et al. Paired quantitative and qualitative assessment of the replication-competent HIV-1 reservoir and comparison with integrated proviral DNA. *Proc Natl Acad Sci U S A* 2016;113:E7908–E7916.

304. Lu W, Ma F, Churbanov A, et al. Virus-host mucosal interactions during early SIV rectal transmission. *Virology* 2014;464-465:406–414.

305. Lyles RH, Munoz A, Yamashita TE, et al. Natural history of human immunodeficiency virus type 1 viremia after seroconversion and proximal to AIDS in a large cohort of homosexual men. *J Infect Dis* 2000;181:872–880.

306. Lynch RM, Boritz E, Coates EE, et al. Virologic effects of broadly neutralizing antibody VRC01 administration during chronic HIV-1 infection. *Sci Transl Med* 2015;7:319ra206.

307. Macdonald JC, Torriani FJ, Morse LS, et al. Lack of reactivation of cytomegalovirus (CMV) retinitis after stopping CMV maintenance therapy in AIDS patients with sustained elevations in CD4 T cells in response to highly active antiretroviral therapy. *J Infect Dis* 1998;177:1182–1187.

308. Maldarelli F, Wu X, Su L, et al. HIV latency. Specific HIV integration sites are linked to clonal expansion and persistence of infected cells. *Science* 2014;345:179–183.

309. Mallal S, Nolan D, Witt C, et al. Association between presence of HLA-B*5701, HLA-DR7, and HLA-DQ3 and hypersensitivity to HIV-1 reverse-transcriptase inhibitor abacavir. *Lancet* 2002;359:727–732.

310. Mallon PW, Brunet L, Hsu RK, et al. Weight gain before and after switch from TDF to TAF in a U.S. cohort study. *J Int AIDS Soc* 2021;24:e25702.

311. Manches O, Frleta D, Bhardwaj N. Dendritic cells in progression and pathology of HIV infection. *Trends Immunol* 2014;35:114–122.

312. Mangili A, Murman DH, Zampini AM, et al. Nutrition and HIV infection: review of weight loss and wasting in the era of highly active antiretroviral therapy from the nutrition for healthy living cohort. *Clin Infect Dis* 2006;42:836–842.

313. Margot NA, Lu B, Cheng A, et al. Resistance development over 144 weeks in treatment-naive patients receiving tenofovir disoproxil fumarate or stavudine with lamivudine and efavirenz in Study 903. *HIV Med* 2006;7:442–450.

314. Marin B, Thiebaut R, Bucher HC, et al. Non-AIDS-defining deaths and immunodeficiency in the era of combination antiretroviral therapy. *AIDS* 2009;23:1743–1753.
315. Markowitz M, Grobler JA. Islatravir for the treatment and prevention of infection with the human immunodeficiency virus type 1. *Curr Opin HIV AIDS* 2020;15:27–32.
316. Marrazzo JM, Ramjee G, Richardson BA, et al. Tenofovir-based preexposure prophylaxis for HIV infection among African women. *N Engl J Med* 2015;372:509–518.
317. Martin MP, Dean M, Smith MW, et al. Genetic acceleration of AIDS progression by a promoter variant of CCR5. *Science* 1998;282:1907–1911.
318. Martin MP, Gao X, Lee JH, et al. Epistatic interaction between KIR3DS1 and HLA-B delays the progression to AIDS. *Nat Genet* 2002;31:429–434.
319. Martin AM, Nolan D, Gaudieri S, et al. Predisposition to abacavir hypersensitivity conferred by HLA-B*5701 and a haplotypic Hsp70-Hom variant. *Proc Natl Acad Sci U S A* 2004;101:4180–4185.
320. Martin-Gayo E, Buzon MJ, Ouyang Z, et al. Potent cell-intrinsic immune responses in dendritic cells facilitate HIV-1-specific T cell immunity in HIV-1 elite controllers. *PLoS Pathog* 2015;11:e1004930.
321. Masur H, Ognibene FP, Yarchoan R, et al. CD4 counts as predictors of opprotunistic pneumonia in human immunodeficiency virus (HIV) infection. *Ann Intern Med* 1989;111:223–231.
322. Matheron S, Pueyo S, Damond F, et al. Factors associated with clinical progression in HIV-2 infected-patients: the French ANRS cohort. *AIDS* 2003;17:2593–2601.
323. Mattapallil JJ, Douek DC, Hill B, et al. Massive infection and loss of memory CD4+ T cells in multiple tissues during acute SIV infection. *Nature* 2005;434:1093–1097.
324. Mayer KH, Mimiaga MJ, Gelman M, et al. Raltegravir, tenofovir DF, and emtricitabine for postexposure prophylaxis to prevent the sexual transmission of HIV: safety, tolerability, and adherence. *J Acquir Immune Defic Syndr* 2012;59:354–359.
325. Mayer KH, Molina JM, Thompson MA, et al. Emtricitabine and tenofovir alafenamide vs emtricitabine and tenofovir disoproxil fumarate for HIV pre-exposure prophylaxis (DISCOVER): primary results from a randomised, double-blind, multicentre, active-controlled, phase 3, non-inferiority trial. *Lancet* 2020;396:239–254.
326. McCarthy KR, Kirmaier A, Autissier P, et al. Evolutionary and functional analysis of old world primate TRIM5 reveals the ancient emergence of primate lentiviruses and convergent evolution targeting a conserved capsid interface. *PLoS Pathog* 2015;11:e1005085.
327. McComsey GA, Kitch D, Daar ES, et al. Bone mineral density and fractures in antiretroviral-naive persons randomized to receive abacavir-lamivudine or tenofovir disoproxil fumarate-emtricitabine along with efavirenz or atazanavir-ritonavir: AIDS Clinical Trials Group A5224s, a substudy of ACTG A5202. *J Infect Dis* 2011;203:1791–1801.
328. McCormack S, Dunn DT, Desai M, et al. Pre-exposure prophylaxis to prevent the acquisition of HIV-1 infection (PROUD): effectiveness results from the pilot phase of a pragmatic open-label randomised trial. *Lancet* 2016;387:53–60.
329. McElrath MJ, De Rosa SC, Moodie Z, et al. HIV-1 vaccine-induced immunity in the test-of-concept Step Study: a case-cohort analysis. *Lancet* 2008;372:1894–1905.
330. McMahon D, Jones J, Wiegand A, et al. Short-course raltegravir intensification does not reduce persistent low-level viremia in patients with HIV-1 suppression during receipt of combination antiretroviral therapy. *Clin Infect Dis.* 2010;50:912–919.
331. McMichael AJ, Carrington M. Topological perspective on HIV escape. *Science* 2019;364:438–439.
332. Mehandru S, Poles MA, Tenner-Racz K, et al. Primary HIV-1 infection is associated with preferential depletion of CD4+ T lymphocytes from effector sites in the gastrointestinal tract. *J Exp Med* 2004;200:761–770.
333. Mellors JW, Kingsley LA, Rinaldo CR, et al. Quantitation of HIV-1 RNA in plasma predicts outcome after seroconversion. *Ann Intern Med* 1995;122:573–579.
334. Mellors JW, Munoz A, Giorgi JV, et al. Plasma viral load and CD4 + lymphocytes as prognostic markers of HIV-1 infection. *Ann Intern Med* 1997;126:946–954.
335. Mellors JW, Rinaldo CR, Gupta P, et al. Prognosis of HIV-1 infection predicted by quantity of virus in plasma. *Science* 1996;272:1167–1170.
336. Meng TC, Fischl MA, Boota AM, et al. Combination therapy with zidovudine and dideoxycytidine in patients with advanced human immunodeficiency virus infection. A phase I/II study. *Ann Intern Med* 1992;116:13–20.
337. Michael NL, Louie LG, Rohrbaugh AL, et al. The role of CCR5 and CCR2 polymorphisms in HIV-1 transmission and disease progression. *Nat Med* 1997;3:1160–1162.
338. Migueles SA, Connors M. Long-term nonprogressive disease among untreated HIV-infected individuals: clinical implications of understanding immune control of HIV. *JAMA* 2010;304:194–201.
339. Migueles SA, Osborne CM, Royce C, et al. Lytic granule loading of CD8+ T cells is required for HIV-infected cell elimination associated with immune control. *Immunity* 2008;29:1009–1021.
340. Mitsuki YY, Tuen M, Hioe CE. Differential effects of HIV transmission from monocyte-derived dendritic cells vs. monocytes to IL-17+CD4+ T cells. *J Leukoc Biol* 2017;101:339–350.
341. Mocroft A, Gill MJ, Davidson W, et al. Are there gender differences in starting protease inhibitors, HAART, and disease progression despite equal access to care? *J Acquir Immune Defic Syndr* 2000;24:475–482.
342. Molina JM, Andrade-Villanueva J, Echevarria J, et al. Once-daily atazanavir/ritonavir versus twice-daily lopinavir/ritonavir, each in combination with tenofovir and emtricitabine, for management of antiretroviral-naive HIV-1-infected patients: 48 week efficacy and safety results of the CASTLE study. *Lancet* 2008;372:646–655.
343. Molina JM, Capitant C, Spire B, et al. On-demand preexposure prophylaxis in men at high risk for HIV-1 infection. *N Engl J Med* 2015;373:2237–2246.
344. Molla A, Korneyeva M, Gao Q, et al. Ordered accumulation of mutations in HIV protease confers resistance to ritonavir. *Nat Med* 1996;2:760–766.
345. Moore RD, Wong WME, Keruly JC, et al. Incidence of neuropathy in HIV-infected patients on monotherapy versus those on combination therapy with didanosine, stavudine and hydroxyurea. *AIDS* 2000;14:273–278.
346. Moran CA, Weitzmann MN, Ofotokun I. The protease inhibitors and HIV-associated bone loss. *Curr Opin HIV AIDS* 2016;11:333–342.
347. Morou A, Brunet-Ratnasingham E, Dube M, et al. Altered differentiation is central to HIV-specific CD4(+) T cell dysfunction in progressive disease. *Nat Immunol* 2019;20:1059–1070.
348. Moyle GJ, Wildfire A, Mandalia S, et al. Epidemiology and predictive factors for chemokine receptor use in HIV-1 infection. *J Infect Dis* 2005;191:866–872.
349. Muema DM, Akilimali NA, Ndumnego OC, et al. Association between the cytokine storm, immune cell dynamics, and viral replicative capacity in hyperacute HIV infection. *BMC Med* 2020;18:81.
350. Muller M, Wandel S, Colebunders R, et al. Immune reconstitution inflammatory syndrome in patients starting antiretroviral therapy for HIV infection: a systematic review and meta-analysis. *Lancet Infect Dis* 2010;10:251–261.
351. Munoz A, Sabin CA, Phillips AN. The incubation period of AIDS. *AIDS* 1997;11(Suppl A):S69–S76.
352. Murata H, Hruz PW, Mueckler M. Indinavir inhibits the glucose transporter isoform Glut4 at physiologic concentrations. *AIDS* 2002;16:859–863.
353. Murphy RL, Sommadossi JP, Lamson M, et al. Antiviral effect and pharmacokinetic interaction between nevirapine and indinavir in persons infected with HIV-1. *J Infect Dis* 1999;179:1116–1123.
354. Napravnik S, Edwards D, Stewart P, et al. HIV-1 drug resistance evolution among patients on potent combination antiretroviral therapy with detectable viremia. *J Acquir Immune Defic Syndr* 2005;40:34–40.
355. National Institutes of Health. News Releases. https://www.nih.gov/news-events/news-releases/hiv-vaccine-candidate-does-not-sufficiently-protect-women-against-hiv-infection. Accessed November 9, 2021.
356. Ndhlovu ZM, Kamya P, Mewalal N, et al. Magnitude and kinetics of CD8+ T cell activation during hyperacute HIV infection impact viral set point. *Immunity* 2015;43:591–604.
357. Nettles RE, Kieffer TL. Update on HIV-1 viral load blips. *Curr Opin HIV AIDS* 2006;1:157–161.
358. Nettles RE, Kieffer TL, Kwon P, et al. Intermittent HIV-1 viremia (blips) and drug resistance in patients receiving HAART. *JAMA* 2005;293:817–829.
359. Neuhaus J, Angus B, Kowalska JD, et al. Risk of all-cause mortality associated with nonfatal AIDS and serious non-AIDS events among adults infected with HIV. *AIDS* 2010;24:697–706.
360. Nielsen C, Pedersen C, Lundgren JD, et al. Biological properties of HIV isolates in primary HIV infection: consequences for the subsequent course of infection. *AIDS* 1993;7:1035–1040.
361. Nishijima T, Gatanaga H, Teruya K, et al. Skin rash induced by ritonavir-boosted darunavir is common, but generally tolerable in an observational setting. *J Infect Chemother* 2014;20:285–287.
362. Nishimura Y, Brown CR, Mattapallil JJ, et al. Resting naive CD4+ T cells are massively infected and eliminated by X4-tropic simian-human immunodeficiency viruses in macaques. *Proc Natl Acad Sci U S A* 2005;102:8000–8005.
363. Notermans DW, Pakker NG, Hamann D, et al. Immune reconstitution after 2 years of successful potent antiretroviral therapy in previously untreated human immunodeficiency virus type 1-infected adults. *J Infect Dis* 1999;180:1050–1056.
364. O'Connell RJ, Merritt TM, Malia JA, et al. Performance of the OraQuick rapid antibody test for diagnosis of human immunodeficiency virus type 1 infection in patients with various levels of exposure to highly active antiretroviral therapy. *J Clin Microbiol* 2003;41:2153–2155.
365. Orkin C, Arasteh K, Gorgolas Hernandez-Mora M, et al. Long-acting cabotegravir and rilpivirine after oral induction for HIV-1 infection. *N Engl J Med* 2020;382:1124–1135.
366. Orkin C, DeJesus E, Sax PE, et al. Fixed-dose combination bictegravir, emtricitabine, and tenofovir alafenamide versus dolutegravir-containing regimens for initial treatment of HIV-1 infection: week 144 results from two randomised, double-blind, multicentre, phase 3, non-inferiority trials. *Lancet HIV* 2020;7:e389–e400.
367. Overton ET, Richmond G, Rizzardini G, et al. Long-acting cabotegravir and rilpivirine dosed every 2 months in adults with HIV-1 infection (ATLAS-2M), 48-week results: a randomised, multicentre, open-label, phase 3b, non-inferiority study. *Lancet* 2021;396:1994–2005.
368. Pacheco D, Ballesteros F, Gonzalez M, et al. [Acute polyarthritis in a patient with AIDS. Clinical report]. *Rev Med Chil* 1989;117:910–913.
369. Pakker NG, Notermans DW, de Boer RJ, et al. Biphasic kinetics of peripheral blood T cells after triple combination therapy in HIV-1 infection: a composite of redistribution and proliferation. *Nat Med* 1998;4:208–214.
370. Palella FJ, Delaney KM, Moorman AC, et al. Declining morbidity and mortality among patients with advanced human immunodeficiency virus infection. HIV outpatient study investigators. *N Engl J Med* 1998;338:853–860.
371. Palmer S, Maldarelli F, Wiegand A, et al. Low-level viremia persists for at least 7 years in patients on suppressive antiretroviral therapy. *Proc Natl Acad Sci U S A* 2008;105:3879–3884.
372. Pancera M, McLellan JS, Wu X, et al. Crystal structure of PG16 and chimeric dissection with somatically related PG9: structure-function analysis of two quaternary-specific antibodies that effectively neutralize HIV-1. *J Virol* 2010;84:8098–8110.
373. Pandori MW, Hackett J Jr, Louie B, et al. Assessment of the ability of a fourth-generation immunoassay for human immunodeficiency virus (HIV) antibody and p24 antigen to detect both acute and recent HIV infections in a high-risk setting. *J Clin Microbiol* 2009;47:2639–2642.
374. Panel on Antiretroviral Guidelines for Adults and Adolescents. Guidelines for the use of antiretroviral agents in adults and adolescents with HIV. Department of Health and Human Services. http://www.aidsinfo.nih.gov/ContentFiles/AdultandAdolescentGL.pdf. Accessed May 3, 2021.
375. Panel on Treatment of Pregnant Women with HIV Infection and Prevention of Perinatal Transmission. Recommendations for use of antiretroviral drugs in pregnant HIV-1-infected women for maternal health and interventions to reduce perinatal HIV transmission in the United States. 2020:1–470. https://clinicalinfo.hiv.gov/en/guidelines/perinatal/. Accessed April 30, 2021.

376. Parker WB, White EL, Shaddix SC, et al. Mechanism of inhibition of human immunodeficiency virus type 1 reverse transcriptase and human DNA polymerases alpha, beta, and gamma by the 5′-triphosphates of carbovir, 3′-azido-3′-deoxythymidine, 2′,3′-dideoxyguanosine and 3′-deoxythymidine. A novel RNA template for the evaluation of antiretroviral drugs. *J Biol Chem* 1991;266:1754–1762.
377. Patel P, Borkowf CB, Brooks JT, et al. Estimating per-act HIV transmission risk: a systematic review. *AIDS* 2014;28:1509–1519.
378. Patick AK, Potts KE. Protease inhibitors as antiviral agents. *Clin Microbiol Rev* 1998;11:614–627.
379. Peeters M, Gueye A, Mboup S, et al. Geographical distribution of HIV-1 group O viruses in Africa. *AIDS* 1997;11:493–498.
380. Percus JK, Percus OE, Markowitz M, et al. The distribution of viral blips observed in HIV-1 infected patients treated with combination antiretroviral therapy. *Bull Math Biol* 2003;65:263–277.
381. Pereira GFM, Kim A, Jalil EM, et al. Dolutegravir and pregnancy outcomes in women on antiretroviral therapy in Brazil: a retrospective national cohort study. *Lancet HIV* 2021;8:e33–e41.
382. Perelson AS, Neumann AU, Markowitz M, et al. HIV-1 dynamics in vivo: virion clearance rate, infected cell life-span, and viral generation time. *Science* 1996;271:1582–1586.
383. Pereyra F, Jia X, McLaren PJ, et al. The major genetic determinants of HIV-1 control affect HLA class I peptide presentation. *Science* 2010;330:1551–1557.
384. Petrovas C, Casazza JP, Brenchley JM, et al. PD-1 is a regulator of virus-specific CD8+ T cell survival in HIV infection. *J Exp Med* 2006;203:2281–2292.
385. Phair J, Jacobson L, Detels R, et al. Acquired immune deficiency syndrome occurring within 5 years of infection with human immunodeficiency virus type-1: the Multicenter AIDS Cohort Study. *J Acquir Immune Defic Syndr* 1992;5:490–496.
386. Phillips AN. Reduction of HIV concentration during acute infection: independence from a specific immune response. *Science* 1996;271:497–499.
387. Phillips A. Short-term risk of AIDS according to current CD4 cell count and viral load in antiretroviral drug-naive individuals and those treated in the monotherapy era. *AIDS* 2004;18:51–58.
388. Phillips AN, Carr A, Neuhaus J, et al. Interruption of antiretroviral therapy and risk of cardiovascular disease in persons with HIV-1 infection: exploratory analyses from the SMART trial. *Antivir Ther* 2008;13:177–187.
389. Phillips AN, Staszewski S, Weber R, et al. HIV viral load response to antiretroviral therapy according to the baseline CD4 cell count and viral load. *JAMA* 2001;286:2560–2567.
390. Phillips EJ, Wong GA, Kaul R, et al. Clinical and immunogenetic correlates of abacavir hypersensitivity. *AIDS* 2005;19:979–981.
391. Pitisuttithum P, Gilbert P, Gurwith M, et al. Randomized, double-blind, placebo-controlled efficacy trial of a bivalent recombinant glycoprotein 120 HIV-1 vaccine among injection drug users in Bangkok, Thailand. *J Infect Dis* 2006;194:1661–1671.
392. Plantier JC, Leoz M, Dickerson JE, et al. A new human immunodeficiency virus derived from gorillas. *Nat Med* 2009;15:871–872.
393. Poignard P, Sabbe R, Picchio GR, et al. Neutralizing antibodies have limited effects on the control of established HIV-1 infection in vivo. *Immunity* 1999;10:431–438.
394. Pollard RB, Robinson P, Dransfield K. Safety profile of nevirapine, a nonnucleoside reverse transcriptase inhibitor for the treatment of human immunodeficiency virus infection. *Clin Ther* 1998;20:1071–1092.
395. Pontesilli O, Kerkhof-Garde S, Noterman DW, et al. Functional T cell Reconstitution and HIV-1-specific cell-mediated immunity during highly active antiretroviral therapy. *J Infect Dis* 1999;180:76–86.
396. Popovic M, Sarngadharan MG, Read E, et al. Detection, isolation, and continuous production of cytopathic retroviruses (HTLV-III) from patients with AIDS and pre-AIDS. *Science* 1984;224:497–500.
397. Quinn TC, Wawer MJ, Sewankambo N, et al. Viral load and heterosexual transmission of human immunodeficiency virus type 1. *N Engl J Med* 2000;342:921–928.
398. Rabezanahary H, Moukambi F, Palesch D, et al. Despite early antiretroviral therapy effector memory and follicular helper CD4 T cells are major reservoirs in visceral lymphoid tissues of SIV-infected macaques. *Mucosal Immunol* 2020;13:149–160.
399. Raffi F, Rachlis A, Stellbrink HJ, et al. Once-daily dolutegravir versus raltegravir in antiretroviral-naive adults with HIV-1 infection: 48 week results from the randomised, double-blind, non-inferiority SPRING-2 study. *Lancet* 2013;381:735–743.
400. Ramduth D, Chetty P, Mngquandaniso NC, et al. Differential immunogenicity of HIV-1 clade C proteins in eliciting CD8+ and CD4+ cell responses. *J Infect Dis* 2005;192:1588–1596.
401. Ramsuran V, Naranbhai V, Horowitz A, et al. Elevated HLA-A expression impairs HIV control through inhibition of NKG2A-expressing cells. *Science* 2018;359:86–90.
402. Ranasinghe S, Flanders M, Cutler S, et al. HIV-specific CD4 T cell responses to different viral proteins have discordant associations with viral load and clinical outcome. *J Virol* 2012;86:277–283.
403. Ratnam I, Chiu C, Kandala NB, et al. Incidence and risk factors for immune reconstitution inflammatory syndrome in an ethnically diverse HIV type 1-infected cohort. *Clin Infect Dis* 2006;42:418–427.
404. Ren J, Nichols C, Bird L, et al. Structural mechanisms of drug resistance for mutations at codons 181 and 188 in HIV-1 reverse transcriptase and the improved resilience of second generation non-nucleoside inhibitors. *J Mol Biol* 2001;312:795–805.
405. Rerks-Ngarm S, Pitisuttithum P, Nitayaphan S, et al. Vaccination with ALVAC and AIDSVAX to prevent HIV-1 infection in Thailand. *N Engl J Med* 2009;361:2209–2220.
406. Reynolds SJ, Makumbi F, Nakigozi G, et al. HIV-1 transmission among HIV-1 discordant couples before and after the introduction of antiretroviral therapy. *AIDS* 2011;25:473–477.
407. Ribaudo HJ, Benson CA, Zheng Y, et al. No risk of myocardial infarction associated with initial antiretroviral treatment containing abacavir: short and long-term results from ACTG A5001/ALLRT. *Clin Infect Dis* 2011;52:929–940.
408. Ribaudo HJ, Daar ES, Tierney C, et al. Impact of UGT1A1 Gilbert variant on discontinuation of ritonavir-boosted atazanavir in AIDS Clinical Trials Group Study A5202. *J Infect Dis* 2013;207:420–425.
409. Richman DD, Bozzette SA. The impact of the syncytium-inducing phenotype of human immunodeficiency virus on disease progression. *J Infect Dis* 1994;169:968–974.
410. Richman DD, Fischl MA, Grieco MH, et al. The toxicitiy of azidothymidine (AZT) in the treatment of patients with AIDS and AIDS-related complex. A double-blind, placebo-controlled trial. *N Engl J Med* 1987;317:192–197.
411. Richman DD, Wrin T, Little SJ, et al. Rapid evolution of the neutralizing antibody response to HIV type 1 infection. *Proc Natl Acad Sci U S A* 2003;100:4144–4149.
412. Robbins GK, Addo MM, Troung H, et al. Augmentation of HIV-1-specific T helper cell responses in chronic HIV-1 infection by therapeutic immunization. *AIDS* 2003;17:1121–1126.
413. Rockstroh JK. Influence of viral hepatitis on HIV infection. *J Hepatol* 2006;44(1 Suppl):S25–S27.
414. Rockwood N, Mandalia S, Bower M, et al. Ritonavir-boosted atazanavir exposure is associated with an increased rate of renal stones compared with efavirenz, ritonavir-boosted lopinavir and ritonavir-boosted darunavir. *AIDS* 2011;25:1671–1673.
415. Rodger AJ, Cambiano V, Bruun T, et al. Sexual activity without condoms and risk of HIV transmission in serodifferent couples when the HIV-positive partner is using suppressive antiretroviral therapy. *JAMA* 2016;316:171–181.
416. Rodger AJ, Fox Z, Lundgren JD, et al. Activation and coagulation biomarkers are independent predictors of the development of opportunistic disease in patients with HIV infection. *J Infect Dis* 2009;200:973–983.
417. Rodriguez B, Sethi AK, Cheruvu VK, et al. Predictive value of plasma HIV RNA level on rate of CD4 T-cell decline in untreated HIV infection. *JAMA* 2006;296:1498–1506.
418. Rosenberg E, Altfeld M, Poon SH, et al. Immune control of HIV-1 after early treatment of acute infection. *Nature* 2000;407:523–526.
419. Rosenberg ES, Graham BS, Chan ES, et al. Safety and immunogenicity of therapeutic DNA vaccination in individuals treated with antiretroviral therapy during acute/early HIV-1 infection. *PLoS One* 2010;5:e10555.
420. Ross AC, Rizk N, O'Riordan MA, et al. Relationship between inflammatory markers, endothelial activation markers, and carotid intima-media thickness in HIV-infected patients receiving antiretroviral therapy. *Clin Infect Dis* 2009;49:1119–1127.
421. Royce RA, Sena A, Cates W, et al. Sexual transmission of HIV. *N Engl J Med* 1997;336:1072–1078.
422. Ryan ES, Micci L, Fromentin R, et al. Loss of function of intestinal IL-17 and IL-22 producing cells contributes to inflammation and viral persistence in SIV-infected rhesus macaques. *PLoS Pathog* 2016;12:e1005412.
423. Saag MS, Gandhi RT, Hoy JF, et al. Antiretroviral drugs for treatment and prevention of HIV infection in adults: 2020 recommendations of the international antiviral society-USA panel. *JAMA* 2020;324:1651–1669.
424. Sabin CA, Telfer P, Phillips AN, et al. The association between hepatitis C virus genotype and human immunodeficiency virus disease progression in a cohort of hemophilic men. *J Infect Dis* 1997;175:164–168.
425. Sabin CA, Worm SW, Weber R, et al. Use of nucleoside reverse transcriptase inhibitors and risk of myocardial infarction in HIV-infected patients enrolled in the D:A:D study: a multi-cohort collaboration. *Lancet* 2008;371:1417–1426.
426. Salemi M, Strimmer K, Hall WW, et al. Dating the common ancestor of SIVcpz and HIV-1 group M and the origin of HIV-1 subtypes using a new method to uncover clock-like molecular evolution. *FASEB J* 2001;15:276–278.
427. Salie ZL, Kirby KA, Michailidis E, et al. Structural basis of HIV inhibition by translocation-defective RT inhibitor 4′-ethynyl-2-fluoro-2′-deoxyadenosine (EFdA). *Proc Natl Acad Sci U S A* 2016;113:9274–9279.
428. Samson M, Libert F, Doranz BJ, et al. Resistance to HIV-1 infection in caucasian individuals bearing mutant alleles of th eCCR-5 chemokine receptor gene. *Nature* 1996;382:722–725.
429. Sanne I, Mommeja-Marin H, Hinkle J, et al. Severe hepatotoxicity associated with nevirapine use in HIV-infected subjects. *J Infect Dis* 2005;191:825–829.
430. Santiago ML, Range F, Keele BF, et al. Simian immunodeficiency virus infection in free-ranging sooty mangabeys (Cercocebus atys atys) from the Tai Forest, Cote d'Ivoire: implications for the origin of epidemic human immunodeficiency virus type 2. *J Virol* 2005;79:12515–12527.
431. Sarngadharan MG, Popovic M, Bruch L, et al. Antibodies reactive with human T-lymphotropic retroviruses (HTLV-III) in the serum of patients with AIDS. *Science* 1984;224:506–508.
432. Sauter D, Kirchhoff F. Key viral adaptations preceding the AIDS pandemic. *Cell Host Microbe* 2019;25:27–38.
433. Sax PE, Erlandson KM, Lake JE, et al. Weight gain following initiation of antiretroviral therapy: risk factors in randomized comparative clinical trials. *Clin Infect Dis* 2020;71:1379–1389.
434. Sax PE, Pozniak A, Montes ML, et al. Coformulated bictegravir, emtricitabine, and tenofovir alafenamide versus dolutegravir with emtricitabine and tenofovir alafenamide, for initial treatment of HIV-1 infection (GS-US-380-1490): a randomised, double-blind, multicentre, phase 3, non-inferiority trial. *Lancet* 2017;390:2073–2082.
435. Schmitt N, Nugeyre MT, Scott-Algara D, et al. Differential susceptibility of human thymic dendritic cell subsets to X4 and R5 HIV-1 infection. *AIDS* 2006;20:533–542.
436. Schmitz JE, Kuroda MJ, Santra S, et al. Control of viremia in simian immunodeficiency virus infection by CD8+ lymphocytes. *Science* 1999;283:857–860.
437. Schooley RT, Ramirez-Ronda C, Lange JMA, et al. Virologic and immunologic benefits of initial combination therapy with zidovudine and zalcitabine or didanosine compared to zidovudine monotherapy. *J Infect Dis* 1996;173:1354–1366.
438. Schreiber GB, Busch MP, Kleinman SH, et al. The risk of transfusion-transmitted viral infections. The Retrovirus Epidemiology Donor Study. *N Engl J Med* 1996;334:1685–1690.
439. Schuitemaker H, Koot M, Kootstra NA, et al. Biological phenotype of human immunodeficiency virus type 1 clones at different stages of infection: progression of disease is associated with a shift from monocytotropic to T-cell-tropic virus populations. *J Virol* 1992;66:1354–1360.

440. Schuurman R, Nijhuis M, van Leeuwen R, et al. Rapid changes in human immunodeficiency virus type 1 RNA load and appearance of drug-resistant virus populations in persons treated with lamivudine (3TC). *J Infect Dis* 1995;171:1411–1419.

441. Schwartz O, Marechal V, Le Gall S, et al. Endocytosis of major histocompatibility complex class I molecules is induced by the HIV-1 Nef protein. *Nat Med* 1996;2:338–342.

442. Segal-Maurer S, Castagna A, Berhe M, et al. Potent antiviral activity of lenacapavir in phase 2/3 in heavily ART-experienced PWH. Virtual CROI 2021. (held virtually): International Antiviral Society-USA; 2021 [Abstract 127].

443. Shapiro RL, Hughes MD, Ogwu A, et al. Antiretroviral regimens in pregnancy and breast-feeding in Botswana. *N Engl J Med* 2010;362:2282–2294.

444. Sharp PM, Hahn BH. Origins of HIV and the AIDS pandemic. *Cold Spring Harb Perspect Med* 2011;1:a006841.

445. Sharp PM, Shaw GM, Hahn BH. Simian immunodeficiency virus infection of chimpanzees. *J Virol* 2005;79:3891–3902.

446. Shelburne SA III, Darcourt J, White AC Jr, et al. The role of immune reconstitution inflammatory syndrome in AIDS-related Cryptococcus neoformans disease in the era of highly active antiretroviral therapy. *Clin Infect Dis* 2005;40:1049–1052.

447. Shelburne SA, Visnegarwala F, Darcourt J, et al. Incidence and risk factors for immune reconstitution inflammatory syndrome during highly active antiretroviral therapy. *AIDS* 2005;19:399–406.

448. Shiels MS, Pfeiffer RM, Engels EA. Age at cancer diagnosis among persons with AIDS in the United States. *Ann Intern Med* 2010;153:452–460.

449. Shiels MS, Pfeiffer RM, Hall HI, et al. Proportions of Kaposi sarcoma, selected non-Hodgkin lymphomas, and cervical cancer in the United States occurring in persons with AIDS, 1980-2007. *JAMA* 2011;305:1450–1459.

450. Siliciano JD, Kajdas J, Finzi D, et al. Long-term follow-up studies confirm the stability of the latent reservoir for HIV-1 in resting CD4+ T cells. *Nat Med* 2003;9:727–728.

451. Simek MD, Rida W, Priddy FH, et al. Human immunodeficiency virus type 1 elite neutralizers: individuals with broad and potent neutralizing activity identified by using a high-throughput neutralization assay together with an analytical selection algorithm. *J Virol* 2009;83:7337–7348.

452. Simmons RP, Scully EP, Groden EE, et al. HIV-1 infection induces strong production of IP-10 through TLR7/9-dependent pathways. *AIDS* 2013;27:2505–2517.

453. Simon F, Mauclere P, Roques P, et al. Identification of a new human immunodeficiency virus type 1 distinct from group M and group O. *Nat Med* 1998;4:1032–1037.

454. Simonetti FR, White JA, Tumiotto C, et al. Intact proviral DNA assay analysis of large cohorts of people with HIV provides a benchmark for the frequency and composition of persistent proviral DNA. *Proc Natl Acad Sci U S A* 2020;117:18692–18700.

455. Simonetti FR, Zhang H, Soroosh GP, et al. Antigen-driven clonal selection shapes the persistence of HIV-1-infected CD4+ T cells in vivo. *J Clin Invest* 2021;131:e145254.

456. Simpson DM, Tagliati M. Neurologic manifestations of HIV infection. *Ann Intern Med* 1994;121:769–785.

457. Sirivichayakul S, Phanuphak P, Tanprasert S, et al. Evaluation of a 2-minute anti-human immunodeficiency virus (HIV) test using the autologous erythrocyte agglutination technique with populations differing in HIV prevalence. *J Clin Microbiol* 1993;31:1373–1375.

458. Smith K, Aga E, Bosch RJ, et al. Long-term changes in circulating CD4 T lymphocytes in virologically suppressed patients after 6 years of highly active antiretroviral therapy. *AIDS* 2004;18:1953–1956.

459. Smith MW, Dean M, Carrington M, et al. Contrasting genetic influence of CCR2 and CCR5 variants on HIV-1 infection and disease progression. *Science* 1997;277:959–965.

460. Smith PF, Ogundele A, Forrest A, et al. Phase I and II study of the safety, virologic effect, and pharmacokinetics/pharmacodynamics of single-dose 3-o-(3′,3′-dimethylsuccinyl)betulinic acid (bevirimat) against human immunodeficiency virus infection. *Antimicrob Agents Chemother* 2007;51:3574–3581.

461. So YT, Holtzman DM, Abrams DI, et al. Peripheral neuropathy associated with acquired immunodeficiency syndrome. Prevalence and clinical features from a population-based survey. *Arch Neurol* 1988;45:945–948.

462. Soghoian DZ, Jessen H, Flanders M, et al. HIV-specific cytolytic CD4 T cell responses during acute HIV infection predict disease outcome. *Sci Transl Med* 2012;4:123ra25.

463. Solomon SS, Mehta SH, McFall AM, et al. Community viral load, antiretroviral therapy coverage, and HIV incidence in India: a cross-sectional, comparative study. *Lancet HIV* 2016;3:e183–e190.

464. Spector SA, Wong R, Hsia K, et al. Plasma cytomegalovirus (CMV) DNA load predicts CMV disease and survival in AIDS patients. *J Clin Invest* 1998;101:497–502.

465. Spence RA, Kati WM, Anderson KS, et al. Mechanism of inhibition of HIV-1 reverse transcriptase nonnucleoside inhibitors. *Science* 1995;267:988–993.

466. Sperling RS, Shapiro DE, Coombs RW, et al. Maternal viral load, zidovudine treatment, and the risk of transmission of human immunodeficiency virus type 1 from mother to infant. *N Engl J Med* 1996;335:1621–1629.

467. Spinner C, Felizarta FB, Rizzardini G, et al. Phase IIA proof-of-concept trial of next-generation maturation inhibitor GSK3630254. Virtual CROI 2021. (held virtually): International Antiviral Society-USA; 2021 [Abstract 126].

468. Stamatatos L, Morris L, Burton DR, et al. Neutralizing antibodies generated during natural HIV-1 infection: good news for an HIV-1 vaccine? *Nat Med* 2009;15:866–870.

469. Stellbrink HJ, Orkin C, Arribas JR, et al. Comparison of changes in bone density and turnover with abacavir-lamivudine versus tenofovir-emtricitabine in HIV-infected adults: 48-week results from the ASSERT study. *Clin Infect Dis* 2010;51:963–972.

470. Stephenson KE, Wagh K, Korber B, et al. Vaccines and broadly neutralizing antibodies for HIV-1 prevention. *Annu Rev Immunol* 2020;38:673–703.

471. Sterling TR, Vlahov D, Astemborski J, et al. Initial plasma HIV-1 RNA levels and progression to AIDS in women and men. *N Engl J Med* 2001;344:720–725.

472. Stevens WS, Noble L, Berrie L, et al. Ultra-high-throughput, automated nucleic acid detection of human immunodeficiency virus (HIV) for infant infection diagnosis using the Gen-Probe Aptima HIV-1 screening assay. *J Clin Microbiol* 2009;47:2465–2469.

473. Sulkowski MS, Mehta SH, Chaisson RE, et al. Hepatotoxicity associated with protease inhibitor-based antiretroviral regimens with or without concurrent ritonavir. *AIDS* 2004;18:2277–2284.

474. Sullivan PS, Hanson DL, Teshale EH, et al. Effect of hepatitis C infection on progression of HIV disease and early response to initial antiretroviral therapy. *AIDS* 2006;20:1171–1179.

475. Swindells S, Andrade-Villanueva JF, Richmond GJ, et al. Long-acting cabotegravir and rilpivirine for maintenance of HIV-1 suppression. *N Engl J Med* 2020;382:1112–1123.

476. Szczech LA, Gupta SK, Habash R, et al. The clinical epidemiology and course of the spectrum of renal diseases associated with HIV infection. *Kidney Int* 2004;66:1145–1152.

477. Takata H, Buranapraditkun S, Kessing C, et al. Delayed differentiation of potent effector CD8(+) T cells reducing viremia and reservoir seeding in acute HIV infection. *Sci Transl Med* 2017;9:eaag1809.

478. Tanser F, de Oliveira T, Maheu-Giroux M, et al. Concentrated HIV subepidemics in generalized epidemic settings. *Curr Opin HIV AIDS* 2014;9:115–125.

479. TEMPRANO ANRS Study Group. A trial of early antiretrovirals and isoniazid preventive therapy in Africa. *N Engl J Med* 2015;373:808–822.

480. Tenorio A, Smith KY, Kuritzkes DR, et al. HIV-1-infected antiretroviral-treated patients with prolonged partial viral suppression: clinical, virologic, and immunologic course. *J Acquir Immune Defic Syndr* 2003;34:491–496.

481. Tenorio AR, Zheng Y, Bosch RJ, et al. Soluble markers of inflammation and coagulation but not T-cell activation predict non-AIDS-defining morbid events during suppressive antiretroviral treatment. *J Infect Dis* 2014;210:1248–1259.

482. Thein HH, Yi Q, Dore GJ, et al. Natural history of hepatitis C virus infection in HIV-infected individuals and the impact of HIV in the era of highly active antiretroviral therapy: a meta-analysis. *AIDS* 2008;22:1979–1991.

483. Tindall B, Barker S, Donovan B, et al. Characterization of the acute clinical illness associated with human immunodeficiency virus infection. *Arch Intern Med* 1988;148:945–949.

484. Trautmann L, Janbazian L, Chomont N, et al. Upregulation of PD-1 expression on HIV-specific CD8+ T cells leads to reversible immune dysfunction. *Nat Med* 2006;12:1198–1202.

485. Triant VA, Brown TT, Lee H, et al. Fracture prevalence among human immunodeficiency virus (HIV)-infected versus non-HIV-infected patients in a large U.S. healthcare system. *J Clin Endocrinol Metab* 2008;93:3499–3504.

486. Triant VA, Lee H, Hadigan C, et al. Increased acute myocardial infarction rates and cardiovascular risk factors among patients with human immunodeficiency virus disease. *J Clin Endocrinol Metab* 2007;92:2506–2512.

487. Tsai CC, Follis KE, Sabo A, et al. Prevention of SIV infection in macaques by (R)-9-(2-phosphonylmethoxypropyl)adenine. *Science* 1995;270:1197–1199.

488. Tural C, Romeu J, Sirera G, et al. Long-lasting remission of cytomegalovirus retinitis without maintenance therapy in human immunodeficiency virus-infected patients. *J Infect Dis* 1998;177:1080–1083.

489. Van Damme L, Corneli A, Ahmed K, et al. Preexposure prophylaxis for HIV infection among African women. *N Engl J Med* 2012;367:411–422.

490. van Rij RP, de Roda Husman AM, Brouwer M, et al. Role of CCR2 genotype in the clinical course of syncytium-inducing (SI) or non-SI HIV-1 infection and in the time to conversion to SI virus variants. *J Infect Dis* 1998;178:1806–1811.

491. van Sighem A, Gras L, Reiss P. Life expectancy of recently diagnosed asymptomatic HIV-infected patients approaches that of uninfected individuals. *AIDS* 2010;24:1527–1535.

492. Van de Perre P, Nzaramba D, Allen S, et al. Comparison of six serological assays for human immunodeficiency virus antibody detection in developing countries. *J Clin Microbiol* 1988;26:552–556.

493. Veazey RS. Intestinal CD4 depletion in HIV/SIV infection. *Curr Immunol Rev* 2019;15:76–91.

494. Veazey RS, DeMaria M, Chalifoux LV, et al. Gastrointestinal tract as a major site of CD4+ T cell depletion and viral replication in SIV infection. *Science* 1998;280:427–431.

495. Venter WDF, Moorhouse M, Sokhela S, et al. Dolutegravir plus two different prodrugs of tenofovir to treat HIV. *N Engl J Med* 2019;381:803–815.

496. Venter WDF, Sokhela S, Simmons B, et al. Dolutegravir with emtricitabine and tenofovir alafenamide or tenofovir disoproxil fumarate versus efavirenz, emtricitabine, and tenofovir disoproxil fumarate for initial treatment of HIV-1 infection (ADVANCE): week 96 results from a randomised, phase 3, non-inferiority trial. *Lancet HIV* 2020;7:e666–e676.

497. Verhoeven D, Sankaran S, Silvey M, et al. Antiviral therapy during primary simian immunodeficiency virus infection fails to prevent acute loss of CD4+ T cells in gut mucosa but enhances their rapid restoration through central memory T cells. *J Virol* 2008;82:4016–4027.

498. Vilches C, Parham P. KIR: diverse, rapidly evolving receptors of innate and adaptive immunity. *Annu Rev Immunol* 2002;20:217–251.

499. Walensky RP, Arbelaez C, Reichmann WM, et al. Revising expectations from rapid HIV tests in the emergency department. *Ann Intern Med* 2008;149:153–160.

500. Walker LM, Phogat SK, Chan-Hui PY, et al. Broad and potent neutralizing antibodies from an African donor reveal a new HIV-1 vaccine target. *Science* 2009;326:285–289.

501. Walker LM, Simek MD, Priddy F, et al. A limited number of antibody specificities mediate broad and potent serum neutralization in selected HIV-1 infected individuals. *PLoS Pathog* 2010;6:e1001028.

502. Walmsley SL, Antela A, Clumeck N, et al. Dolutegravir plus abacavir-lamivudine for the treatment of HIV-1 infection. *N Engl J Med* 2013;369:1807–1818.

503. Walmsley S, Bernstein B, King M, et al. Lopinavir-Ritonavir versus nelfinavir for the initial treatment of HIV infection. *N Engl J Med* 2002;346:2039–2046.

504. Wei X, Decker JM, Wang S, et al. Antibody neutralization and escape by HIV-1. *Nature* 2003;422:307–312.

505. Wei X, Ghosh SK, Taylor ME, et al. Viral dynamics in human immunodeficiency virus type 1 infection. *Nature* 1995;373:117–122.

506. Wensing AM, Calvez V, Ceccherini-Silberstein F, et al. 2019 update of the drug resistance mutations in HIV-1. *Top Antivir Med* 2019;27:111–121.

507. Wherry EJ, Blattman JN, Murali-Krishna K, et al. Viral persistence alters CD8 T-cell immunodominance and tissue distribution and results in distinct stages of functional impairment. *J Virol* 2003;77:4911–4927.

508. Wherry EJ, Teichgraber V, Becker TC, et al. Lineage relationship and protective immunity of memory CD8 T cell subsets. *Nat Immunol* 2003;4:225–234.

509. Whitney JB, Hill AL, Sanisetty S, et al. Rapid seeding of the viral reservoir prior to SIV viraemia in rhesus monkeys. *Nature* 2014;512:74–77.

510. Whitney JB, Lim SY, Osuna CE, et al. Prevention of SIVmac251 reservoir seeding in rhesus monkeys by early antiretroviral therapy. *Nat Commun* 2018;9:5429.

511. Wild C, Greenwell T, Shugars D, et al. The inhibitory activity of an HIV type 1 peptide correlates with its ability to interact with a leucine zipper structure. *AIDS Res Hum Retroviruses* 1995;11:323–325.

512. Wild CT, Shugars DC, Greenwell TK, et al. Peptides corresponding to a predictive alpha-helical domain of human immunodeficiency virus type 1 gp41 are potent inhibitors of virus infection. *Proc Natl Acad Sci U S A* 1994;91:9770–9774.

513. Winkler C, Modi W, Smith MW, et al. Genetic restriction of AIDS pathogenesis by an SDF-1 chemokine gene variant. ALIVE Study, Hemophilia Growth and Development Study (HGDS), Multicenter AIDS Cohort Study (MACS), Multicenter Hemophilia Cohort Study (MHCS), San Francisco City Cohort (SFCC). *Science* 1998;279:389–393.

514. Winston JA, Bruggeman LA, Ross MD, et al. Nephropathy and establishment of a renal reservoir of HIV type 1 during primary infection. *N Engl J Med* 2001;344:1979–1984.

515. Winston A, De Francesco D, Post F, et al. Comorbidity indices in people with HIV and considerations for coronavirus disease 2019 outcomes. *AIDS* 2020;34:1795–1800.

516. Wong JK, Hezareh M, Gunthard HF, et al. Recovery of replication-competent HIV despite prolonged suppression of plasma viremia. *Science* 1997;278:1291–1295.

517. Wood E, Hogg RS, Yip B, et al. Effect of medication adherence on survival of HIV-infected adults who start highly active antiretroviral therapy when the CD4+ cell count is 0.200 to 0.350 x 10⁹ cells/L. *Ann Intern Med* 2003;139:810–816.

518. World Health Organization. *WHO Case Definitions of HIV for Surveillance and Revised Clinical Staging and Immunological Classification of HIV-Related Disease in Adults and Children*. Geneva: WHO Press; 2007.

519. World Health Organization. *Programmatic Update: Antiretroviral Treatment as Prevention (TASP) of HIV and TB*. Geneva: World Health Organization; 2012.

520. World Health Organization. *Update of Recommendations on First- and Second-line Antiretroviral Regimens*. Geneva, Switzerland: World Health Organization; 2019:1–16.

521. Worm SW, Sabin C, Weber R, et al. Risk of myocardial infarction in patients with HIV infection exposed to specific individual antiretroviral drugs from the 3 major drug classes: the data collection on adverse events of anti-HIV drugs (D:A:D) study. *J Infect Dis* 2010;201:318–330.

522. Worobey M, Gemmel M, Teuwen DE, et al. Direct evidence of extensive diversity of HIV-1 in Kinshasa by 1960. *Nature* 2008;455:661–664.

523. Wu X, Yang ZY, Li Y, et al. Rational design of envelope identifies broadly neutralizing human monoclonal antibodies to HIV-1. *Science* 2010;329:856–861.

524. Xia H, Jiang W, Zhang X, et al. Elevated level of CD4(+) T Cell immune activation in acutely HIV-1-infected stage associates with increased IL-2 production and cycling expression, and subsequent CD4(+) T Cell preservation. *Front Immunol* 2018;9:616.

525. Xu H, Wang X, Liu DX, et al. IL-17-producing innate lymphoid cells are restricted to mucosal tissues and are depleted in SIV-infected macaques. *Mucosal Immunol* 2012;5:658–669.

526. Yamamoto T, Price DA, Casazza JP, et al. Surface expression patterns of negative regulatory molecules identify determinants of virus-specific CD8+ T-cell exhaustion in HIV infection. *Blood* 2011;117:4805–4815.

527. Youngblood B, Noto A, Porichis F, et al. Cutting edge: prolonged exposure to HIV reinforces a poised epigenetic program for PD-1 expression in virus-specific CD8 T cells. *J Immunol* 2013;191:540–544.

528. Yue FY, Merchant A, Kovacs CM, et al. Virus-specific interleukin-17-producing CD4+ T cells are detectable in early human immunodeficiency virus type 1 infection. *J Virol* 2008;82:6767–6771.

529. Yue L, Prentice HA, Farmer P, et al. Cumulative impact of host and viral factors on HIV-1 viral-load control during early infection. *J Virol* 2013;87:708–715.

530. Yusim K, Peeters M, Pybus OG, et al. Using human immunodeficiency virus type 1 sequences to infer historical features of the acquired immune deficiency syndrome epidemic and human immunodeficiency virus evolution. *Philos Trans R Soc Lond B Biol Sci* 2001;356:855–866.

531. Zash R, Holmes L, Diseko M, et al. Update on neural tube defects with antiretroviral exposure in the Tsepamo study, Botswana. 23rd International AIDS Conference (conducted virtually), 6-10 July, 2020. International AIDS Society. Abstract OAXLB0102.

532. Zash R, Makhema J, Shapiro RL. Neural-tube defects with dolutegravir treatment from the time of conception. *N Engl J Med* 2018;379:979–981.

533. Zhang ZQ, Notermans DW, Sedgewick G, et al. Kinetics of CD4+ T cell repopulation of lymphoid tissues after treatment of HIV-1 infection. *Proc Natl Acad Sci U S A* 1998;95:1154–1159.

534. Zhang ZQ, Schuler T, Cavert W, et al. Reversibility of the pathological changes in the follicular dendritic cell network with treatment of HIV-1 infection. *Proc Natl Acad Sci U S A* 1999;96:5169–5172.

535. Zuniga R, Lucchetti A, Galvan P, et al. Relative dominance of Gag p24-specific cytotoxic T lymphocytes is associated with human immunodeficiency virus control. *J Virol* 2006;80:3122–3125.

Nonhuman Lentiviruses

Ronald C. Desrosiers • David T. Evans

History
Infectious agent
Genome organization and composition
Propagation
    Propagation and cell culture
    Host range
    Restriction
    Receptor use
    Germline integration
Pathogenesis and pathology
    Portals of entry
    Cell and tissue tropism
    Immune responses and persistence
    Virulence
    Clinical and pathologic features
    Contributions of individual genes and genetic elements
    Genetic resistance
Diagnosis
Prevention and control
Research on vaccine development
Research on therapeutic regimens
Perspective

HISTORY

Use of the term "slow virus infections" and identification of the first lentivirus is generally credited to Sigurdsson et al.[321–323] Twenty karakul sheep imported into Iceland from Germany in 1933 resulted in the transmission of a chronic disease that led to the death of more than 100,000 sheep in the decades that followed. Sigurdsson et al. not only described the disease but also demonstrated that it was due to a transmissible agent[321–323] and used the term "slow virus infections" to refer to this disease.[320] In 1960, Sigurdsson et al. described the cultivation of the transmissible agent in tissue culture,[324] and Gudnadottir and Palsson were able to reproduce the disease with the culture-grown virus.[126] The diseases in the sheep were called *maedi* (Icelandic for dyspnea; i.e., a lung disease resulting in difficulty breathing) and *visna* (Icelandic for a state of progressive apathy, a "fading away" resulting from brain disease). Both disease states result from the same virus, now referred to as maedi/visna virus (MVV). MVV and related viruses are called lentiviruses, which is derived from the Latin *lentus* for slow. Approximately 600,000 sheep were slaughtered in Iceland in 1965 to eradicate MVV from the island.

The maedi/visna disease in Icelandic sheep, although the first specifically shown to be caused by a lentivirus, is probably not, however, the first description of a lentiviral disease. Vallée and Carré described in 1904 the infectious nature of a chronic disease in horses,[354] which is now known to be caused by the lentivirus equine infectious anemia virus (EIAV). A chronic, progressive interstitial pneumonia had also been described in South African sheep in 1915 and in Montana sheep in 1923 before the identification of MVV.[222] Work with EIAV was largely on a parallel track with that of MVV, and the first description of EIAV cultivation appeared in 1961.[180] Only subsequently were EIAV and MVV shown to belong to the lentivirus genus on the basis of morphologic criteria.[118,258,375]

The scenario of disease outbreak leading to the identification of a new lentivirus has repeated itself dramatically on several occasions in more recent history. In 1964, an emerging infectious disease was first detected in Bali cattle in the Jembrana district of Bali.[282,328] Bali cattle are the domesticated form of the wild banteng (*Bos javanicus*). Within 12 months, 26,000 of the 300,000 cattle on the island died of the disease. The cause of the disease was subsequently traced to a bovine lentivirus, now called Jembrana disease virus (JDV), which is a distinct variant of bovine immunodeficiency virus (BIV).[43,170] Bali cattle are particularly sensitive to disease caused by this virus.[329,330,380] Outbreaks of immunodeficiency disease and lymphoma in captive colonies of macaques were subsequently traced to the introduction of a simian lentivirus from African monkeys.[23,68,214,219] Simian immunodeficiency viruses (SIVs) naturally infect African apes and Old World monkeys but are not found in macaques or other Asian nonhuman primate species. The origins of the human immunodeficiency viruses have followed a similar pattern. HIV-2 in western Africa quite clearly originated from SIVsmm in sooty mangabey monkeys.[49,79,104,142,197,225] Sooty mangabeys are naturally infected with SIVsmm at high frequency, and the habitat of sooty mangabeys coincides with the same geographic region of western Africa where HIV-2 is most prevalent. SIVsmm also groups phylogenetically with HIV-2. The origins of HIV-1 have similarly been traced to SIVs of great apes in West Central Africa.[313]

The earliest descriptions of the isolation of HIV and its association with acquired immunodeficiency syndrome (AIDS) did not appreciate that the virus was a lentivirus.[18,275] Only subsequently, through more careful examination of electron micrographs and sequence analysis, did this become clear.[119,235] At the time, study of lentiviruses was an obscure discipline with which many scientists were not familiar.

From a historical perspective, MVV and EIAV were discovered, isolated, and characterized long before the discovery of HIV.[180,324] Lentiviruses identified after the discovery of HIV-1 have used a nomenclature similar to that for HIV-1 (i.e., "immunodeficiency virus"). BIV, originally isolated from a cow with a chronic disease by Van Der Maaten et al. in 1972,[356] received little attention until after the discovery of HIV. Subsequent to the discovery of HIV-1, lentiviruses were isolated from monkeys and cats (Table 19.1). Although the discovery of MVV, EIAV, and BIV predates that of HIV-1, HIV-1 has received such intense scrutiny that much more is known about it than any of the other lentiviruses. New information about the nonhuman lentiviruses is thus usually compared with what is known for HIV-1.

INFECTIOUS AGENT

Lentiviruses have been isolated from sheep, goats, horses, cattle, cats, monkeys, and humans (Table 19.1). Genetic analysis of a lentivirus from goats, caprine arthritis–encephalitis

TABLE 19.1	Known lentiviruses	
Species	Virus	Year That Cultivation Was First Published
Sheep/goats	Maedi/visna virus; caprine arthritis encephalitis virus	1960[324]
Horses	Equine infectious anemia virus	1961[180]
Cattle	Bovine immunodeficiency virus; Jembrana disease virus	1972[356]
Humans	Human immunodeficiency virus	1983[18]
Monkeys	Simian immunodeficiency virus	1985[356]
Cats	Feline immunodeficiency virus	1987[260]

virus (CAEV) revealed that it clusters closely with MVV[353] and belongs in a single group with MVV. Therefore, based on host species and viral genetics, five distinct groups of lentiviruses are recognized (Fig. 19.1). It is important to note that even within

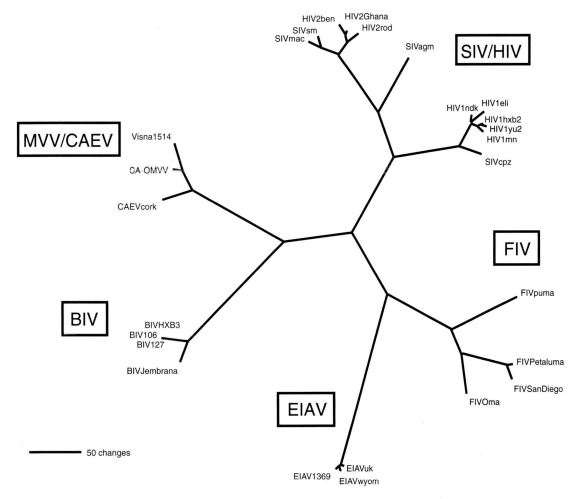

FIGURE 19.1 Phylogeny of the lentiviruses. Five distinct phylogenetic groups of lentiviruses. The unrooted tree depicts the phylogenetic relationships among the five recognized groups of lentiviruses. The tree is based on an amino acid alignment of 470 residues of reverse transcriptase from representative members of each group, including bovine immunodeficiency virus (BIV), equine infectious anemia virus (EIAV), feline immunodeficiency virus (FIV), maedi/visna virus, caprine arthritis–encephalitis virus (MVV/CAEV), and the simian and human immunodeficiency viruses (SIV/HIV). Maximum parsimony (shown) and neighbor-joining (not shown) analyses give trees of nearly identical topology. Branch lengths are proportional to the number of amino acid substitutions.

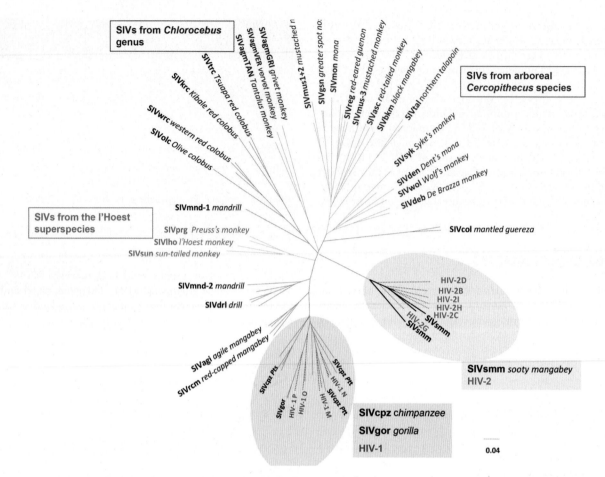

FIGURE 19.2 Phylogeny of primate lentiviruses. The tree depicts the phylogenetic relationships among the human and simian immunodeficiency viruses and is based on neighbor-joining analysis of a 294 bp sequence in *pol*. Branch lengths that are drawn to scale indicate the number of nucleotide substitutions per site. (Courtesy of Martine Peeters. Redrawn from Peeters M, Ma D, Liegeois F, et al. Simian immunodeficiency virus infections in the wild. In: Ansari AA, Silvestri G, eds. *Natural Hosts of SIV: Implication in AIDS.* Amsterdam, The Netherlands: Elsevier; 2014:37–67. Copyright © 2014 Elsevier. With permission.)

a single group, discrete subgroups can be defined based on host species, geography, and genetic distance. For example, among the nonhuman primate lentiviruses, different subgroups exist for the SIVs from African green monkeys, sooty mangabeys, Sykes' monkeys, and L'Hoest's monkeys (Fig. 19.2 and Table 19.2).

All lentiviruses have a common morphology that distinguishes them from other retroviruses (see Chapter 17). Lentiviruses bud from the plasma membrane without a preformed nucleoid, and mature particles typically have a conical or rod-shaped nucleoid core (Fig. 19.3). Classification into the lentivirus subgroup by morphologic criteria alone is entirely consistent with phylogenetic analysis of *pol* gene sequences. Viruses classified as lentiviruses have *pol* gene sequences more closely related to one another than to other retroviruses, and all have the same characteristic morphology. All lentiviruses have a propensity to replicate in macrophages, all exhibit long-term persistent viral replication in their natural host, and all are associated with a chronic progressive disease course in susceptible hosts. The primate lentiviruses have acquired use of CD4 as one of two receptors used sequentially by virus for entry into cells (Table 19.3). FIV has also been shown to use a similar two receptor mechanism for entry. However, nonprimate lentiviruses, including FIV, do not use CD4 as an entry receptor. The chronic disease induced by primate lentiviruses has

an immunodeficiency component because of the infection of CD4+ lymphocytes. All lentiviruses have a number of auxiliary (or accessory) genes in addition to the *gag*, *pol*, and *env* genes found in all retroviruses.

GENOME ORGANIZATION AND COMPOSITION

Widespread use of DNA sequencing has greatly enhanced our understanding of the phylogenetic relationships and the gene products of lentiviruses. Based on sequence analysis, five discrete groups of lentiviruses are now recognized (Fig. 19.1). Extensive diversity exists even within a group. For example, among the SIVs, distinct subgroups have been defined from the African green monkey, sooty mangabey monkey, L'Hoest's monkey, Sykes' monkey, and other genera (Table 19.2 and Fig. 19.2). Of the 69 nonhuman primate species known to inhabit sub-Saharan Africa, SIV infection has been demonstrated in at least 45 of them, and partial or complete viral sequence information is available for 39 of them.[262] Since some species have not yet been surveyed, additional SIV lineages may still be discovered. Extensive diversity has also been observed for FIV in wild and captive cat species.[42,346] Among the four subspecies of African

TABLE 19.2 Partial listing of primate lentiviruses[a]

Virus Designation	Primate Lentivirus Group	Species (Common)	Species (Formal)	Subspecies Isolates	References
HIV-1	HIV-1/SIVcpz/SIVgor	Humans	Homo sapiens		18
SIVcpzPtt	HIV-1/SIVcpz/SIVgor	Central African chimpanzee	Pan troglodytes	P. t. troglodytes	168,295
SIVcpzPtt	HIV-1/SIVcpz/SIVgor	Eastern chimpanzee	Pan troglodytes	P. t. schweinfurthii	293
SIVgor	HIV-1/SIVcpz/SIVgor	Western lowland gorillas	Gorilla gorilla	G. g. gorilla	358
SIVsmm	HIV-2/SIVsmm/SIVmac	Sooty mangabeys	Cercocebus atys		100,142,242
SIVmac	HIV-2/SIVsmm/SIVmac	Macaques	Macaca mulatta M. nemestrina M. nemestrina M. arctoides		23,68,248
HIV-2	HIV-2/SIVsmm/SIVmac	Humans	Homo sapiens		52,189
SIVagmGri	SIVagm	African green monkeys	Chlorocebus aethiops	C. a. grivet	3,97,183,239,251
SIVagmVer	SIVagm	African green monkeys	Chlorocebus aethiops	C. a. vervet	3,97,183,239,251
SIVagmTan	SIVagm	African green monkeys	Chlorocebus aethiops	C. a. tantalus	3,97,183,239,251
SIVagmSab	SIVagm	African green monkeys	Chlorocebus aethiops	C. a. sabeus	3,97,183,239,251
SIVsyk	SIVsyk	Sykes' monkeys	Cercopithecus mitis	C. a. alboqularis	91,141
SIVgsn	SIVgsn/SIVmon/SIVmus	Greater spot-nosed monkey	Cercopithecus nictitans		62
SIVmon	SIVgsn/SIVmon/SIVmus	Mona monkey	Cercopithecus mona		59
SIVmus	SIVgsn/SIVmon/SIVmus	Mustached monkey	Cercopithecus cephus		59
SIVlho	SIVsun/SIVlho	L'Hoest monkey	Cercopithecus lhoesti	C. l. lhoesti	139
SIVsun	SIVsun/SIVlho	Sun-tailed monkey	Cercopithecus lhoesti	C. l. solatus	20
SIVdeb	SIVdeb	DeBrazza monkey	Cercopithecus neglectus		27
SIVden	SIVdeb	Dent's mona monkey	Cercopithecus	C. m. denti	70
SIVrcm	SIVrcm	Red-capped mangabey	Cercocebus torquatus	C. t. torquatus	21,48
SIVmnd	SIVmnd-1	Mandrill	Mandrillus sphinx		334,349
SIVmnd	SIVmnd-2	Mandrill	Mandrillus Sphinx		261,334
SIVdrl	SIVmnd-2	Drill	Mandrillus leucophaeus		53,150
SIVcol	SIVcol	Querza colobus	Colobus querza		61
SIVolc	SIVolc	Olive colobus	Procolobus badius		60
SIVwrc	SIVwrc	Western red colobus	Piliocolobus badius		60
SIVtal	SIVtal	Angolian talapoin monkey	Miopithecus talapoin		255
SIVtal	SIVtal	Gabon talapoin monkey	Miopithecus ogouensis		261

[a]In addition to the primate lentiviruses listed, serologic surveys for the detection of antibodies to SIV have suggested SIV infection of a variety of other species.[215,251,344]

green monkeys (vervet, grivet, tantalus, and sabeus), discrete sub-subgroups of SIVagm have been defined (Table 19.2). These four subspecies naturally inhabit distinct or sometimes partially overlapping habitats that cover almost all of sub-Saharan Africa. The JDV also represents a distinct subgroup relative to the original BIV isolate.[43]

The *pol* gene generally exhibits the greatest degree of sequence conservation. *Pol* sequences are therefore often used for the comparison of lentiviruses from different groups, subgroups, or sub-subgroups. Sequences from one subgroup of SIV (e.g., SIVsmm) will typically exhibit only 55% to 60%

amino acid identity in Pol when compared with sequences from another SIV subgroup (e.g., SIVagm). Diverse members within a subgroup may exhibit as little as 75% to 80% amino acid identity in Pol, but the number is typically higher. When different groups of lentiviruses are compared, for example, MVV with SIV, amino acid identity in Pol is typically 35% or less. Similarity in other genes is even lower. Nonetheless, lentiviral sequences are clearly more closely related to one another than to other retroviruses.

All known lentiviruses have at least three genes in addition to *gag*, *pol*, and *env* that are present in all replication-competent

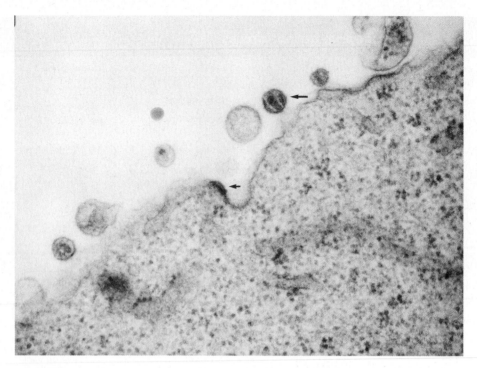

FIGURE 19.3 Lentivirus morphogenesis and morphology. This electron micrograph of a cell infected with simian immunodeficiency virus shows virus budding from the cell in the absence of preformed particles (*lower arrow*) and a mature particle with a cylindrical or rod-shaped nucleoid (*upper arrow*). (Courtesy of John MacKey.)

retroviruses (Fig. 19.4 and Tables 19.4 and 19.5). These additional genes contribute to the more complex biology of lentiviruses, which includes persistent virus replication and immune evasion as discussed in more detail later in this chapter. A *rev* gene that encodes a protein responsible for the nuclear export of unspliced viral RNA transcripts through interactions with a region of RNA secondary structure, referred to as the Rev response element (RRE), is present in all lentiviruses.[274] Interestingly, although neither the sequence nor the location of the RRE is conserved, its function appears to be the same in all lentiviruses.[274] A *vif* gene, whose primary function is to counteract restriction by members of the APOBEC3 family of cytosine deaminases, is consistently present in five of the six lentivirus groups; EIAV stands alone in lacking a *vif* gene.

TABLE 19.3	Properties of lentiviruses		
Property	**HIV-1**	**SIV**	**MVV, EIAV, BIV, FIV**
Morphogenesis/morphology	Lenti	Lenti	Lenti
Macrophage tropism	Yes	Yes	Yes
CD4 lymphocyte tropism	Yes	Yes	No
Use of CD4 as receptor for virus entry	Yes	Yes	No
Use of chemokine receptors as receptor for virus entry	Yes	Yes	Yes (FIV)
Natural modes of transmission	Sex, blood, vertical	Sex, blood, vertical	Insects, saliva/aerosols, blood, sex, vertical
Genes in addition to *gag, pol, env, tat,* and *rev* activities	6	5 or 6	3 or more
	Yes	Yes	Yes
dUTPase	No	No	Yes
Persistent viral replication	Yes	Yes	Yes
Chronic, debilitating disease[a]	Yes	Yes	Yes
Immunodeficiency[a]	Yes	Yes	No (MVV, EIAV, BIV), Yes (FIV)

[a]In susceptible hosts. Not all hosts are susceptible to disease.

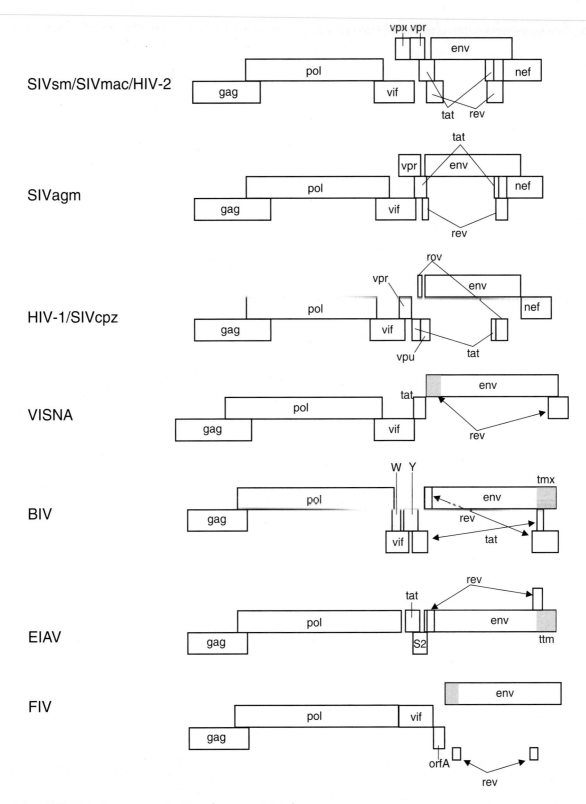

FIGURE 19.4 Genome organization of representative lentiviruses.

A *nef* gene is found at the 3′ end of all primate lentiviruses (Table 19.5). The nonprimate lentiviruses do not have a *nef* gene. However, cells infected with EIAV and BIV make spliced mRNAs that encode the Ttm and Tmx proteins, which correspond to the carboxy-terminal portion of Env.[22,117] It is possible that these viral proteins represent evolutionary precursors of Nef. All lentiviruses except FIV contain an unusually long (>120 amino acids) Env cytoplasmic domain.[277] In the intergenic region between *vif* and *env*, a number of other genes are present, particularly in the primate lentiviruses. A *vpr* gene is present in all known primate lentiviruses. The HIV-2/SIVsmm, SIVmnd-2, and SIVrcm lineages also have a *vpx* gene in this

TABLE 19.4 Accessory genes in nonprimate lentiviruses

MVV[a]	EIAV[b]	BIV[c]	FIV[d]
vif	tat (S1)	vif	vif
tat	rev (S3)	tat	rev
rev	S2	rev	tat (orfA)
	ttm	tmx	
		vpw?	
		vpy?	

[a]Valas S, Benoit C, Guionaud C, et al. North American and French caprine arthritis-encephalitis viruses emerge from ovine maedi-visna viruses. *Virology* 1997;237:307–318. Ref.[353]

[b]Maury W. Regulation of equine infectious anemia virus expression. *J Biomed Sci* 1998:11–23. Ref.[228]

[c]Gonda M. The lentiviruses of cattle. In: Levy JA, ed. *Retroviridae*. New York: Plenum Press; 1994. Ref.[116]

[d]Olmsted RA, Barnes AK, Yamamoto JK, et al. Molecular cloning of feline immunodeficiency virus. *Proc Natl Acad Sci U S A* 1989;86:2448–2452. Ref.[252]

region that is a paralog of *vpr*. The nonprimate lentiviruses have genes between *vif* and *env* with varied roles. BIV encodes a Tat protein from this location that acts on a trans-activation response element similar to the primate lentiviruses.[210] In other ruminant lentiviruses, a small protein encoded from this region was originally thought to be transcriptional trans-activator but may actually have activity more similar to Vpr.[365] Likewise, a small protein encoded in a similar region of FIV, termed OrfA, down-regulates the CD134 receptor for this virus from the surface of infected cells, similar to CD4 down-regulation by primate lentiviral Nef proteins.[144] Only two groups of primate lentiviruses have consistently been found to have a *vpu* gene: HIV-1/SIVcpz/gor and SIVgsn/mon/mus (Table 19.5). SIVden from a pet Dent's Mona monkey (*Cercopithecus mona denti*) was also found to contain a *vpu* gene, although this virus clusters phylogenetically with SIVdeb from DeBrazza monkeys.[70]

All nonprimate lentiviruses except BIV encode deoxyuridine triphosphatase (dUTPase) from a distinct open reading frame within the *pol* gene.[89] dUTPase converts dUTP to a precursor of dTTP, which reduces dUTP concentrations in infected cells. By doing so, dUTPase prevents mis-incorporation of uracil into viral DNA, thereby reducing the accumulation of G-to-A transitions in the viral genome. dUTPase is particularly important for lentiviral replication in nondividing cells such as macrophages where cellular dUTPase levels are

especially low. Curiously, dUTPase coding sequences are absent from the primate lentiviruses. The explanation for this is not entirely clear, but may be related to the evolution of Vpr and Vpx to facilitate virus replication in nondividing cells. This is consistent with the transitional genomic structure of an endogenous lentivirus found in a prosimian species, the gray mouse lemur (*Microcebus murinus*), which encodes dUTPase but lacks a *vpr* gene.[111] Thus, dUTPase may have been lost during the course of primate lentiviral evolution as a result of the acquisition of Vpr.

PROPAGATION

Propagation and Cell Culture

Primary isolates from all lentivirus groups can be grown in macrophage cultures of their respective host species. Other types of cells may also be used depending on the virus (Table 19.6), and virus isolates may be adapted to replicate in particular cell types. Examples include FIV replication in Crandell feline kidney cells and the replication of SIV and HIV-1 in immortalized T-cell lines (Table 19.6). However, it is important to note that lentiviral replication in cell culture can select for phenotypic changes that do not represent natural replication in infected hosts.

Host Range

SIVs naturally infect a variety of African apes and Old World monkeys, but natural infection of Asian nonhuman primates has never been documented. The SIVs from sooty mangabeys and African green monkeys when introduced into macaque species (Asian monkeys) can cause an AIDS-like disease.[100,140,242] In fact, SIVsmm from sooty mangabeys was accidentally introduced into captive macaque colonies in the United States and disseminated unknowingly for more than a decade before it was discovered and eliminated.[7,66,219] At least one case of laboratory-acquired human infection with SIVmac has been documented.[173,333]

Baboons do not appear to naturally harbor their own SIV. However, cross-species transmission of SIV to baboons in the wild has been documented. Of 279 baboon sera taken from native habitats in Tanzania and Ethiopia, 2 animals had strong reactivity to SIVagm antigens and 1 of these animals was later shown to harbor SIVagm in plasma.[181] The virus sequences from this baboon clustered with the vervet subtype of SIVagm, consistent with the overlapping habitat of vervet monkeys in the region where the baboon samples were taken.[158] An SIVagm variant has similarly been detected in a chacma baboon of southern Africa.[359] There is additional evidence for

TABLE 19.5 Accessory genes of primate lentiviruses

Primate Lentiviruses	Vif	Vpx	Vpr	Vpu	Tat	Rev	Nef
SIVagm, SIVsyk, SIVmnd-1, SIVlho, SIVsun, SIVcol, SIVtal, SIVdeb, SIVwrc, SIVolc, SIVkrc, and SIVkrtg	+	–	+	–	+	+	+
HIV-1[a], SIVcpz[a], SIVgor[a], SIVgsn, SIVmus, SIVmon, and SIVden[b]	+	–	+	+	+	+	+
HIV-2, SIVmac, SIVsmm, SIVrcm, SIVmnd-2, SIVdrl, and SIVagi	+	+	+	–	+	+	+

[a]Unlike the other viruses in this group, the *env* and *nef* genes of HIV-1, SIVcpz, and SIVgor do not overlap.
[b]Although SIVden has a *vpu* gene, it is more closely to SIVdeb and SIVsyk than to the other viruses in this group.

TABLE 19.6   Cell substrates for growing lentiviruses

Lentivirus Group	Growth on Macrophages	Other Cell Types	Adaptation to Growth
HIV-1	Yes	Stimulated, primary, human CD4⁺ lymphocytes	Human tumor T-cell lines
SIV	Yes	Stimulated, primary, monkey CD4⁺ lymphocytes	Human tumor T-cell lines
MVV/CAEV	Yes	Choroid plexus cells; primary synovial cells; endothelial cells	—
FIV	Yes	Primary, stimulated feline lymphocytes	Crandell feline kidney cells
EIAV	Yes	—	Fetal equine kidney; equine dermal
BIV	Yes	—	Bovine, rabbit, canine fibroblasts

the cross-species transmission of SIVagm from West African green monkeys (*Cercopithecus aethiops sabeus*) to patas monkeys (*Erythrocebus patas*).[28] Baboons can also be infected experimentally with HIV-2.[211]

It is generally accepted that HIV-2 arose from the zoonotic transmission of SIVsmm from sooty mangabeys to humans. HIV-2 is primarily found in western Africa and has only slowly made its way to other parts of the world. The native habitat of the sooty mangabey is the coastal forest region of western Africa, which corresponds to regions where HIV-2 is most prevalent. SIVsmm also has the same genomic organization and groups phylogenetically with HIV-2 (Figs. 19.2 and 19.4).[104,142] Of the nine distinct groups of HIV-2 thought to represent independent cross-species transmission events, most are limited to a few cases in West Africa.[313] The two groups of HIV-2 that account for the majority of spread (groups A and B) are closely related to SIVsmm isolates that have been identified in wild sooty mangabeys of the Taï forest in Côte d'Ivoire.[294]

Noninvasive fecal sampling techniques for great apes in the wild have provided a wealth of data on the origins of HIV-1. Molecular epidemiological studies of thousands of samples collected from wild chimpanzee and gorilla populations across Africa have identified SIV strains related to each of the four groups of HIV-1 (groups M, N, O, and P). SIVcpz has been found in only two of the four subspecies of the common chimpanzee; *Pan troglodytes troglodytes* in West Central Africa and *P. t. schweinfurthii* in East Africa.[168,357] These subspecies harbor their own lineages (SIVcpzPtt and SIVcpzPts), and while SIVcpzPtt sequences are closely related to HIV-1, viruses similar to SIVcpzPts have not been found in humans.[262] Detailed phylogenetic analyses indicate that HIV-1 group M, which is responsible for the global AIDS pandemic, and HIV-1 group N, which has only been found in a few individuals, originated from SIVcpzPtt in geographically distinct populations of chimpanzees in southern Cameroon.[168,203,291,357] Extensive fecal sampling and sequencing have similarly shown that western lowland gorillas (*Gorilla gorilla gorilla*) are naturally infected with their own SIV and that SIVgor probably originated from the transmission of SIVcpzPtt from chimpanzees to gorillas.[358] HIV-1 groups O and P are more closely related to SIVgor than to SIVcpzPtt, and phylogeographic analyses have traced the ancestors of these viruses to distinct populations of gorillas in southern Cameroon.[69,262] Whereas HIV-1 group O has been found in approximately 100,000 individuals in West Central Africa, HIV-1 group P has only been identified in a handful of patients.

The absence of SIVcpz in two of the four chimpanzee subspecies (*P. t. ellioti* and *P. t. vellerosus*) and the genetic composition of the virus in the subspecies that do harbor SIVcpz suggest that chimpanzees may have acquired SIV relatively recently. A recent origin for SIVcpz is also consistent with the finding that at least some chimpanzees develop an AIDS-like disease from SIVcpz infection.[92,290,342] SIVcpz is more closely related to SIVrcm in Pol and to SIVgsn in Env than it is to the corresponding sequences of other SIVs.[14] Furthermore, the range of the chimpanzees (*P. t. troglodytes*) in West Central Africa overlaps with the ranges of both red-capped mangabeys and greater spot-nosed monkeys, and chimpanzees have been known to prey on monkeys for food (Fig. 19.5). Thus, SIVcpz may have recently emerged from an ancestral recombination between viruses similar to SIVrcm and SIVgsn.

Attempts to infect species other than great apes with HIV-1 have failed. HIV-1 is infectious for chimpanzees and chimpanzee-passaged HIV-1 has shown pathogenic potential[249,253]; however, HIV-1 does not replicate in Old World monkeys. The two strongest blocks to HIV-1 replication in monkeys are the restriction factors TRIM5 and APOBEC3.[315,337] Simian-tropic strains of HIV-1 have now been engineered with defined sequence changes that overcome each of these restriction factors to allow persistent virus replication in macaques.[134,305]

The nonprimate lentiviruses are also restricted in their host range, as reflected by their replication only in the same or in closely related genera. BIV is a notable exception in that it has been reported to infect New Zealand white rabbits.[270] However, cross-species transmission does occur. The transmission of CAEV from goats to sheep has been observed,[271] although CAEV is genetically similar enough to MVV to qualify as a quasi-species of this lentivirus. Studies have also shown that domestic cats can be infected by puma FIV (FIVpco) and lion FIV (FIVple).[360,361] Although no overt disease symptoms have been documented for the latter, long-term studies have not been performed.

Restriction

Mammals express a number of gene products termed "restriction factors" that interfere with specific stages of virus replication at the cellular level. The best characterized of these are the APOBEC3, TRIM5, tetherin, SAMHD1, MX2, SERINC5, and ZAP proteins.[123,148,165,189,243,315,337,355] To replicate efficiently in their respective hosts, lentiviruses have evolved mechanisms to overcome each of these factors. Resistance to restriction can occur by the expression of a viral protein (usually an accessory

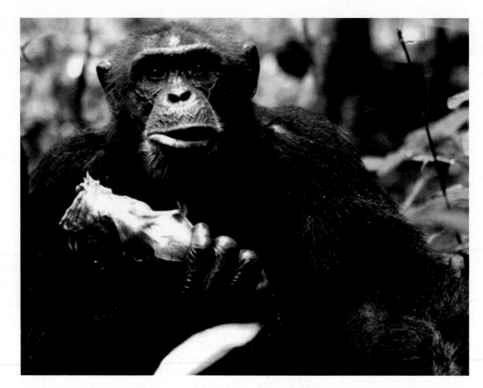

FIGURE 19.5 Chimpanzee "Sagu" eating a spine and rib cage of a red colobus monkey. Photo by Cristina Gomes, Max-Planck-Institute for Evolutionary Anthropology. (Photo by Cristina Gomes, Max-Plank Institute for Evolutionary Anthropology. Reprinted from Leendertz SA, Locatelli S, Boesch C, et al. No evidence for transmission of SIVwrc from western red colobus monkeys (Piliocolobus badius badius) to wild West African chimpanzees (Photo by Cristina Gomes, Max-Planck-Institute for Evolutionary Anthropology; Tropical Conservation Institute, Florida International University. Reprinted from Leendertz SA, Locatelli S, Boesch C, et al. No evidence for transmission of SIVwrc from western red colobus monkeys (Piliocolobus badius badius) to wild West African chimpanzees (Pan troglodytes verus) despite high exposure through hunting. *BMC Microbiol* 2011;11(1):24. Ref.[196])

protein) that directly antagonizes the restriction factor or by changes in the viral target sequence that reduce sensitivity to restriction. Viral pathogens have in turn caused selection for sequence variation in restriction factors among different species and in some cases within the same species. As a consequence, a few of these species-specific differences represent important barriers to the cross-species transmission of lentiviruses.[232,234,299,301] Key properties of each of the restriction factors discussed below are summarized in Table 19.7.

APOBEC3

The apolipoprotein B mRNA editing enzyme, catalytic polypeptide-like 3 (APOBEC3 or A3) proteins are a family of mammalian cytosine deaminases that inhibit the replication of lentiviruses as well as other retroviruses and retroelements. Humans and other primate species express seven distinct A3 genes (A3A, A3B, A3C, A3D, A3F, A3G, and A3H),[190] of which A3D, A3F, A3G, and A3H are able to restrict HIV-1 and SIV.[151] If unopposed, A3 proteins become incorporated

TABLE 19.7   Lentiviral restriction factors

Restriction Factor	Antilentiviral Isoforms	Viral Resistance	Interferon-Inducible	Positive Selection	Barrier to Cross-Species Transmission
APOBEC3	A3D, A3F, A3G, and A3H	Vif[a]	Some isoforms	Yes	Strong
TRIM5	TRIM5α and TRIM-Cyp	Capsid[b]	Yes	Yes	Strong
Tetherin	L-tetherin and S-tetherin	Nef[a], Vpu[a], Env[a]	Yes	Yes	Weak
SAMHD1	SAMHD1	Vpx[a], Vpr[a]	Yes	Yes	Weak
MX2	MX2	Capsid[b]	Yes	Yes	Possibly
SERINC5	SERINC3 and SERINC5	Nef[a], S2[a]	No	No	Unlikely
ZAP	ZAP-L and ZAP-S	Viral RNA[b]	Yes	Yes	Unlikely

[a]Viral antagonist.
[b]Viral target of restriction.

into virions where they catalyze the conversion of cytosines into uracils during the minus-strand cDNA synthesis step of reverse transcription. These uracils then template the insertion of adenines during plus-strand cDNA synthesis, resulting in guanine-to-adenine (G-to-A) transitions in the proviral DNA.[132,396] Lentiviruses overcome this restriction by expressing Vif, which mediates A3 degradation in productively infected cells thereby preventing A3 incorporation into virions. In the absence of antagonism by Vif, the accumulation of extensive G-to-A substitutions results in catastrophic hypermutation of the viral genome, which prevents further virus replication.[133,194]

A3 antagonism by Vif is often species-dependent. HIV-1 Vif can degrade the A3G proteins of humans and chimpanzees but not those of African green monkeys or rhesus macaques.[325] Conversely, SIVagm Vif can degrade African green monkey A3G but not human A3G.[325] This specificity is governed by a single amino acid difference between human and monkey A3G that is critical for binding to Vif.[30,307] The failure of HIV-1 Vif to counteract the A3 proteins of Old World monkeys represents a major barrier to HIV-1 replication in these species. Likewise, the inability of SIVagm Vif to counteract human APOBEC3G is a significant barrier to the zoonotic transmission of this group of viruses to humans. As an illustration of the evolutionary dynamics driving A3G variation and viral adaptation, amino acid differences were identified in the A3G proteins of four different subspecies of African green monkeys that confer resistance to antagonism by the Vif proteins of SIVagm strains from other subspecies but not from the same subspecies.[56]

TRIM5

Isoforms of the tripartite motif-containing protein 5 (TRIM5), most notably the alpha isoform (TRIM5α), impose a postentry block to virus infection that represents a major host range determinant for lentiviruses and other types of retroviruses.[337] Evolutionary analyses indicate that TRIM5 has been coevolving with retroviral pathogens for tens of millions of years, perhaps since the radiation of eutherian mammals.[300] Homologs of the TRIM5 gene have been found in the genomes of primates, cows, pigs, dogs, rabbits, rats, and mice,[300] and antiviral activity has been demonstrated for the TRIM5 proteins of various species of Old and New World primates[136,292,331] as well as for the TRIM5 proteins of rabbits and cows.[303,395] TRIM5 typically does not block infection by retroviruses adapted to a particular host but exhibits variable patterns of restriction against the retroviruses of other species.[136] Differences in sensitivity to restriction reflect sequence variation in the viral capsid protein and in the domains of TRIM5 predicted to interact with capsid.[246,383,394] The mechanism of restriction remains to be fully defined but appears to involve TRIM5 recognition of the hexagonal capsid symmetry of intact retroviral core particles and the formation of a higher-order lattice around the core that destabilizes it before the completion of reverse transcription.[103]

One of the more peculiar twists in TRIM5 evolution is the independent emergence of a TRIM5-cyclophilin A (TRIM5-Cyp) isoform in at least two different primate lineages. Owl monkey cells exhibit a potent postentry block to HIV-1 infection due to a TRIM5-Cyp fusion resulting from the retrotransposition of an open reading frame for CypA into an intron of TRIM5.[302] A similar TRIM5-Cyp fusion occurred in macaques as a result the insertion of CypA into the 3′ UTR of TRIM5.[366,384] In this case,

macaque TRIM5 Cyp poorly restricts HIV-1 but does block infection by other lentiviruses such as HIV-2, SIVagm, and FIV.[366,384]

TRIM5 polymorphisms may also result in variable courses of infection within a single species. In contrast to SIV strains such as SIVmac239 that are well-adapted to rhesus macaques and consistently result in high viral loads, rhesus macaques infected with SIVsmE543-3 exhibit considerable animal-to-animal variation in plasma viremia. Kirmaier et al. found that this variation reflects differences in TRIM5 genotype and that the adaptation of SIVsmE543-3 for efficient replication in rhesus macaques is associated with amino acid changes in the viral capsid that confer resistance to restrictive variants of TRIM5α.[176] The susceptibility of SIVsmE543-3 to certain allotypes of rhesus macaque TRIM5α appears to be a result of the incomplete adaptation of the virus to this species, since SIVsmE543-3 was derived after the sequential passage of SIVsmm in only two rhesus macaques.[135,130]

Tetherin

Tetherin (BST-2 or CD317) is an interferon-inducible transmembrane protein that inhibits the detachment of enveloped viruses from infected cells. Although initially identified as the cellular factor that accounts for a defect in the release of vpu-deleted HIV-1 from restrictive cells,[243,355] tetherin has since been shown to have broad antiviral activity against diverse families of enveloped viruses.[244] The antiviral activity of tetherin is a function of its unique topology, which includes an N-terminal cytoplasmic domain, a membrane-spanning domain, an extracellular coiled-coil domain, and a C-terminal glycosylphosphatidylinositol anchor.[184,265] These features allow opposite ends of tetherin dimers to become incorporated into viral and cellular membranes, physically linking budding virions to the surface of infected cells.[95,127,265] Tetherin may also amplify other immune responses. Virion-induced cross-linking of tetherin stimulates NK-κB signaling and the release of proinflammatory cytokines,[102] and the accumulation of captured virions on the cell surface increases the susceptibility of infected cells to antibody-dependent cellular cytotoxicity.[10] Thus, tetherin may serve as a link between innate and adaptive immunity to enhance the elimination of virus-infected cells by antibodies.

Among the primate lentiviruses, at least three different viral proteins have evolved to counteract tetherin. Most SIVs, including phylogenetically diverse viruses such as SIVcpz, SIVagm, and SIVsmm, use Nef to counteract the tetherin proteins of their simian hosts.[156,298,402] However, the SIVs of Old World monkeys that have a vpu gene (SIVgsn, SIVmon, and SIVmus) use Vpu as a tetherin antagonist.[298] HIV-1 group M and HIV-2 evolved to use Vpu and Env, respectively, to counteract human tetherin because of the loss of a five amino acid sequence from the cytoplasmic domain of human tetherin that confers susceptibility to Nef.[156,192,243,355] Thus, even though the SIVs that gave rise to HIV-1 and HIV-2 (SIVcpz and SIVsmm) use Nef to antagonize tetherin in their natural hosts, the absence of sequences from the N-terminus of human tetherin that confer sensitivity to Nef explains why HIV-1 group M evolved to use Vpu and why HIV-2, which lacks a vpu gene, evolved to use Env to counteract human tetherin. The resistance of human tetherin to Nef does not appear to be absolute, however, since the Nef proteins of HIV-1 group O and certain HIV-1 group M isolates are able to counteract human tetherin.[9,178]

Species-specific differences in tetherin represent a potential barrier to cross-species transmission. HIV-1 Vpu counteracts human, chimpanzee, and gorilla tetherin but is ineffective against the tetherin orthologs of Old World monkeys.[156,232,298] Conversely, the Nef proteins of SIVcpz, SIVsmm, and SIVagm counteract the tetherin proteins of their respective hosts but are generally ineffective against human tetherin.[156,298,402] Differences in the susceptibility of tetherin to antagonism by Vpu and Nef map to amino acid residues at sites of contact with these viral proteins. Whereas variation in the membrane-spanning domain accounts for differences in susceptibility to Vpu, it is the cytoplasmic domain of tetherin that accounts for differences in susceptibility to Nef. This is consistent with the rapid evolution of sequences coding for the cytoplasmic and transmembrane domains of tetherin in response to the selective pressure of viral pathogens.[232]

Several instances of lentiviral adaptation to tetherin in primates have been documented. These include compensatory changes in the Env cytoplasmic domain of a *nef*-deleted strain of SIV that regained a pathogenic phenotype in rhesus macaques,[311] changes in Nef that restore the ability to counteract tetherin in HIV-1–infected chimpanzees,[122] adaptation of the Vpu protein of a simian-tropic HIV-1 to antagonize macaque tetherin,[134] and compensatory changes in Nef that restore tetherin antagonism during the replication of a tetherin-sensitive SIV *nef* mutant in rhesus macaques.[340] Together, these observations indicate that the primate lentiviruses are under strong selective pressure to overcome restriction by tetherin.

SAMHD1

Sterile alpha motif and histidine–aspartic acid domain–containing protein 1 (SAMHD1) is a GTP/dGTP-activated triphosphohydrolase that cleaves deoxynucleotide triphosphates (dNTPs) into their deoxynucleoside and inorganic triphosphate components.[115] In nondividing cells, SAMHD1 forms catalytically active tetramers that maintain intracellular dNTP pools below concentrations needed to complete reverse transcription.[11,115] The Vpx proteins of HIV-2 and SIVsmm/mac alleviate this barrier to infection of differentiated myeloid cells (macrophages and dendritic cells) and resting CD4+ T cells by targeting SAMHD1 for proteasomal degradation.[15,148,189] However, Vpx is only expressed by the HIV-2/SIVsmm, SIVmnd-2, and SIVrcm lineages of primate lentiviruses (Table 19.5).

An evolutionary analysis of SAMHD1 antagonism revealed that the Vpr proteins of some SIVs, including SIVagm, SIVdeb, and SIVmus, acquired the ability to degrade their host's SAMHD1 proteins.[208] Vpr and Vpx are related by gene duplication; however, unlike Vpx, Vpr is expressed by all primate lentiviruses. Phylogenetic analyses suggest that the functionalization of Vpr to counteract SAMHD1 occurred prior to the gene duplication that gave rise to Vpx in SIVs of the *Cercopithecinae* subfamily of Old World monkeys.[208] Comparisons of the SAMHD1-coding sequences among Old and New World primates also revealed evidence of positive selection among *Cercopithecinae* species, including at sites essential for interactions with Vpx.[208] Lentiviral antagonism may therefore have driven SAMHD1 evolution in these species, and species-specific differences in SAMHD1 represent a potential barrier to cross-species transmission.

MX2

The myxovirus resistance (MX) proteins are a family of dynamin-like GTPases found in vertebrates that are strongly inducible by type I interferons. Mammals typically express two paralogous MX proteins, MX1 and MX2 (also known as MXA and MXB), which differ in their spectrum of antiviral activity. Whereas MX1 has broad activity against diverse families of RNA viruses, including orthomyxoviruses, paramyxoviruses, and rhabdoviruses (but not retroviruses), MX2 was thought to lack antiviral activity until it was identified as an interferon-stimulated gene product responsible for differences in resistance to HIV-1 infection.[123,165] Although its mechanism of antiviral activity is not fully understood, MX2 is thought to impede nuclear import of pre-integration complexes. This is consistent with the inhibition of HIV-1 replication at a step after reverse transcription but before proviral integration, the localization of MX2 to nuclear pores, and the physical interactions of MX2 with multiple components of the nuclear import machinery.[84,123,165]

Similar to TRIM5, MX2 binds to surfaces of the HIV-1 capsid, and it is differences in capsid protein sequences that differentially affect virus restriction by MX2.[25,39,326] However, MX2 does not impose as stringent of a block to HIV-1 infection as TRIM5, and sensitivity to MX2 is dependent on cyclophilin A as well as cell type and cell cycle variation in the expression of nucleoporins.[164] Sequence variation and signatures of positive selection among the MX2 orthologs of different species indicate evolutionary conflict with viral pathogens.[39] Serial passage of HIV-1 in cell lines that overexpress MX2[39] and the adaptation of simian-tropic HIV-1 to macaques[305] can also select for amino acid changes in capsid that confer resistance to MX2. However, the sensitivity of primary HIV-1 isolates to human MX2, including interferon-resistant transmitted/founder viruses, as well as the general sensitivity of other primate lentiviruses to the MX2 proteins of their simian hosts,[39] suggests that MX2 is not a significant barrier to the cross-species transmission of the primate lentiviruses.

SERINC5

Serine incorporator 3 and 5 (SERINC3 and SERINC5) were identified as the cellular factors that account for producer cell-dependent impairment of the infectivity of *nef*-deleted HIV-1.[287,352] In the absence of Nef, these multipass transmembrane proteins become incorporated into budding virions and potently inhibit HIV-1 infectivity.[287,352] SERINC homologs are found in all eukaryotes, including five paralogous gene products in humans (SERINC1-5), that are distinguished by a unique bipartite domain structure composed of 10 membrane-spanning alpha helices.[279] Although SERINC3 and SERINC5 both impair HIV-1 infectivity and are expressed in primary lymphocytes, the majority of antiretroviral activity can be attributed to SERINC5.[287,352]

There is a general consensus that SERINC5 inhibits the formation and expansion of fusion pores between viral and cellular membranes,[287,352,372] thereby impairing the delivery of the viral nucleocapsid to the cytoplasm. How this occurs is less clear. SERINC5 does not appear to alter the lipid composition of viral membranes as its name might suggest.[345] Instead, differences in the sensitivity of HIV-1 to SERINC5 map to Env.[352] The ability of SERINC5 to increase the sensitivity of HIV-1 to certain neutralizing antibodies[337] suggests that SERINC5 directly modifies Env conformation. There is also evidence that SERINC5 prevents the clustering of Env trimers on the surface of virions,[47] which may inhibit fusion by reducing the number of Env–receptor contacts that can mediate entry.

SERINC5 antagonism is broadly conserved among the Nef proteins of phylogenetically diverse primate lentiviruses.[137] Accessory proteins of other retroviruses have also evolved to counteract SERINC5, including the glycoGag protein of murine leukemia virus (MLV) and the S2 protein of EIAV.[45,287,352] Thus, the SERINC proteins appear to have broad antiviral activity that has impacted the course of retroviral evolution. However, unlike other restriction factors discussed thus far, the SERINCs do not appear to be evolving under positive selection. SERINC proteins are generally well conserved with few amino acid differences between species (e.g., human and macaque SERINC5 share 99% amino acid identity). As a consequence, the Nef proteins of HIV-1, HIV-2, and diverse SIVs are able to counteract human, simian, and even murine orthologs of SERINC3 and SERINC5.[137] Likewise, EIAV S2 and MLV glycoGag counteract human, rodent, and lagomorph SERINC3/5.[75] Thus, the SERINC proteins are unlikely to represent a significant barrier to lentiviral transmission between species.

ZAP

The zinc finger antiviral protein (ZAP, also known as PARP13) was initially identified as a cellular gene product that specifically depletes viral mRNAs in the cytoplasm of MLV-infected cells.[105] This factor was subsequently shown to have broad antiviral activity against diverse families of RNA viruses.[121,404] The specificity of ZAP is dependent on the CG dinucleotide content of viral RNAs; increasing the frequency of GCs in HIV-1 increases the depletion of viral transcripts in the cytoplasm.[339] Because vertebrate genomes contain a lower than expected frequency of CG dinucleotides, ZAP can differentiate viral RNAs from host cellular mRNAs based on their CG content.[339]

The antiviral activity of ZAP is not fully understood but is dependent on binding to RNA GC dinucleotides[233] and the formation of a complex with at least two cofactors, TRIM25 and KHNYN.[94,202] TRIM25 regulates ZAP by a poorly understood mechanism,[403] and KHNYN contains an endonuclease domain that is essential for the cytoplasmic depletion of HIV-1 RNAs.[94] ZAP and TRIM25 are both interferon-inducible,[314] and the *ZAP* gene encodes long and short protein isoforms (ZAP-L and ZAP-S) that are products of alternative splicing.[169] Although both isoforms have antiviral activity, ZAP-L is reported to have greater activity against retroviruses. Signatures of recurrent positive selection are also localized to the PARP-like domain that is present in ZAP-L but not ZAP-S.[169] Lentiviruses are unlikely, however, to account for this selective pressure; since like many RNA viruses, they have evolved to evade ZAP by maintaining low CG frequencies. Thus, ZAP is unlikely to represent a significant barrier to the cross-species transmission of lentiviruses.

Receptor Use

HIV-1 uses a sequential two-receptor system that includes CD4 as a primary receptor and a seven transmembrane chemokine receptor as a secondary receptor for entry into target cells (see Chapter 17). The overwhelming majority of naturally transmitted HIV-1 field isolates use CCR5 as a second receptor, although variants that are able to use CXCR4 as an alternative co-receptor may arise at later stages of infection.[162] A 32 base pair deletion in the *CCR5* gene (*CCR5Δ32*) occurs with an allelic frequency of approximately 10% in people of European descent. *CCR5Δ32* homozygotes are extremely resistant to HIV-1 infection. However, among the few documented cases of HIV-1 infection of *CCR5Δ32* homozygotes, CCR5 inactivation does not protect against high viral loads and disease progression because of the utilization of CXCR4 by HIV-1 in these individuals.[327] The SIVs that have been examined to date are similar to HIV-1 in their use of CD4 and CCR5 as primary and secondary receptors, but rarely use CXCR4. However, many SIVs are also able to use additional chemokine receptors that are not utilized by HIV-1. Depending on the SIV strain, these receptors may include CXCR6 (STRL33 or Bonzo), GPR15 (BOB), CCR2b, CCR3, and GPR1.

The use of alternative co-receptors may help to explain high levels of persistent SIV replication without progressive CD4+ T-cell depletion in natural hosts. Early studies revealed that SIVrcm can use CXCR6 and CCR2b rather than CCR5 for entry,[21,48] which probably accounts for the replication of this virus in red-capped mangabeys (*Cercocebus torquatus torquatus*) with homozygous deletions in *CCR5*. More recently, SIVsmm and SIVagm were also found to use CXCR6 for infection of primary CD4+ T cells from their natural hosts, the sooty mangabey (*Cercocebus atys*) and the African green monkey (*Chlorocebus* spp.).[90,286,377] This is consistent with exceedingly low or absent CCR5 expression on CD4+ lymphocytes of these species,[256] and possibly also with the downmodulation of CD4 on a subset of memory T cells in African green monkeys.[19] On the other hand, SIVcpz and SIVmac, which are pathogenic in chimpanzees and rhesus macaques, respectively, are unable to use their hosts' CXCR6 for entry—which appears to be a property of Env in the case of SIVcpz and an amino acid difference in rhesus macaque CXCR6 in the case of SIVmac.[378] Hence, these viruses depend on high levels of CCR5 for efficient replication in their respective hosts. The observation that CXCR6 is expressed on a subset of effector memory CD4+ T cells in sooty mangabeys distinct from the central memory population that expresses CCR5 raises the intriguing possibility that some natural hosts may be able to sustain high levels of SIV replication without CD4+ T-cell depletion because the virus is replicating in a cell population that is more easily replaced.[378]

FIV also uses a two-receptor mechanism and shares with HIV the use of CXCR4 as a co-receptor for cell entry.[272,381] FIV infection is modulated by soluble stromal cell–derived factor-1 (SDF-1), the natural ligand for CXCR4,[145] and is inhibited by the CXCR4 antagonist AMD3100. However, FIV uses the T-cell activation marker CD134 as the initial binding receptor rather than CD4.[72,318] CD134 is a member of the TNF receptor superfamily and has the typical four-domain structure. The outermost domain is responsible for receptor activity and as few as five amino acid changes can make human CD134 a viable receptor for FIV.[71] Certain lion FIVs also use CD134 and CXCR4 sequentially for entry.[230] This two-receptor mechanism used by the primate lentiviruses and by FIV conceals critical surfaces of the envelope glycoprotein from host antibody responses prior to conformational changes that mediate entry.

EIAV also uses a member of the TNF receptor superfamily for entry, a protein called ELR1, which is expressed on macrophages that are the primary target cells for this virus.[399,400] Little information is currently available about the receptors used by other nonprimate lentiviruses, leaving a number of fundamental questions central to lentiviral evolution and receptor biology unanswered. Do all lentiviruses use a two-receptor system for entry into target cells? Is the second receptor always a seven membrane-spanning chemokine receptor? Did evolutionary changes result in a switch from a one-receptor system to a two-receptor system or a switch from one two-receptor system to another two-receptor system?

Germline Integration

Many retroviruses not only infect their hosts exogenously but may also be inherited in a mendelian fashion, either as highly defective genomes, solo long terminal repeats (LTRs), or in the case of the murine and feline gammaretroviruses as inducible infectious agents. However, endogenous lentiviruses have not been found in the vast majority of species examined, suggesting that germline integration for lentiviruses is much rarer than for other types of retroviruses. The absence of endogenous lentiviruses was thought to reflect the recent evolutionary origin of lentiviruses, the lack of lentiviral receptors on germ cells, and the cytopathic nature of lentiviral infection. Nevertheless, there are now four examples of germline transmission of nonreplicating lentiviral elements. Since entering the germline, these elements have been expanded and shuffled by host genetic mechanisms and are now inherited as multiple copies of various defective forms by all individuals of their respective host species. These elements no longer express functional viral proteins due to the accumulation of numerous in-frame stop codons and frameshift mutations in coding regions.

The first endogenous lentivirus to be identified was in the European rabbit (*Oryctolagus cuniculus*). Rabbit endogenous lentivirus type K (RELIK) as it was termed has unmistakable lentiviral sequences, including *gag*, *pol*, *env*, *tat*, and *rev* genes.[166] The *pol* gene of RELIK encodes dUTPase similar to the nonprimate lentiviruses and like EIAV lacks an open reading frame for *vif*.[166] Subsequent to the identification of RELIK, endogenous lentiviruses were also identified in two different genera of Malagasy lemurs (*Microcebus* and *Cheirog*aleus),[111,112] mustelids (weasels and ferrets),[65,128] and a colugo (*Galeopterus variegatus*).[129] These lentiviral elements are phylogenetically distinct from one another in accordance with independent introductions into the germlines of these species. Estimates of the time since these lentiviral sequences entered the germline vary between 1.9 and 14.3 million years (Table 19.8). These findings therefore indicate that lentiviruses are much older than previously appreciated.

Inspection of the endogenous lentiviruses found in the gray mouse lemur (*M. murinus*) and the fat-tailed dwarf lemur

(*C. medius*) revealed that they represent distinct germline insertions and are phylogenetically basal to all extant lineages of exogenous primate lentiviruses.[111,112] In addition to *gag*, *pol*, and *env*, these prosimian immunodeficiency viruses (pSIVgml and pSIVfdl) contain a *vif* gene and a putative open reading frame in a similar position as *nef*, albeit with no discernible similarity to the *nef* genes of known SIVs.[111] However, similar to the nonprimate lentiviruses, pSIVgml and pSIVfdl have a dUTPase coding region in *pol* and lack orthologs of the primate lentiviral *vpr* and *vpx* genes. Hence, the endogenous lentiviruses of lemurs exhibit transitional features intermediate to the nonprimate and primate lentiviruses.

PATHOGENESIS AND PATHOLOGY

Portals of Entry

The primary mode of natural transmission of the nonhuman lentiviruses varies considerably with the virus. EIAV may be the most interesting because it is the only lentivirus for which there is good evidence for vector-borne transmission. During disease episodes, levels of infectious virus in the plasma of horses can exceed 10^4/mL. The horse fly appears to be more efficient than mosquitoes, fleas, or other insects for being able to transmit EIAV. Transmission has been documented by following a single horse fly that took a blood meal on an infected pony during an acute clinical period.[155] Transmission via blood can also be mediated by inappropriate veterinary practices involving needles or scalpels.

Work on natural modes of infection has demonstrated the capability of both vertical and horizontal transmission of FIV, MVV/CAEV, and EIAV.[40] Vertical transmission can occur *in utero*, during parturition, and postnatally via milk. Vertical transmission by these viruses parallels that observed with HIV in humans. Contact transmission is also common, particularly for MVV/CAEV and EIAV, when animals are herded closely together in barns or stables. These viruses can be found in semen, lung excretions, and saliva. For cats, bite wounds are believed to be the most important route of transmission in adult animals.[390] Transmission via grooming/licking has also been observed,[74] and experimental infection of cats can be achieved via oronasal administration. FIV infection is much more prevalent in free-roaming males than in females, consistent with increased fighting and biting among male cats. Cats allowed to roam free in areas with high cat density are at the greatest risk of becoming infected.

Information about natural modes of SIV transmission has been harder to come by. One study of wild grivet monkeys in

TABLE 19.8 Summary of known endogenous lentiviruses

Host	Geographic Location	Estimated Time of Endogenization	Genes Present
Rabbit	Europe	5.7–7 M years	*gag, pol, env, tat, rev*
Lemur	Madagascar	1.9–4.2 M years	*gag, pol, env, tat, rev, vif*
Weasel (Ferret)	Widespread	8.8–11.8 M years	*gag, pol, env, tat, rev, vif*
Colugo	Southeast Asia	~14.3 M years	*gag, pol, env, tat, orf1*[a], *orf2*[a]

[a]The proteins encoded by *orf1* and *orf2* do not share any significant similarity with other known lentiviral accessory elements.

Awash National Park in Ethiopia analyzed SIVagm serologic status with age, sex, and risk.[267] Infection was nearly universal in females of reproductive age and nearly absent in younger females. In males, infection was observed in only those that were fully adult. The findings support a predominantly sexual mode of SIV transmission among grivets. Male-to-male transmission by aggressive contacts may also be a prominent mode by which SIV is spread.[245] Maternal–infant transmission of SIV has been documented in captive animals.[179] Experimental SIV infection of laboratory animals is routinely achieved by intravenous injection or by mucosal inoculation.

Cell and Tissue Tropism

Despite the varied modes of transmission, all lentiviruses are disseminated to an assortment of tissue sites by the blood. Dissemination can occur as cell-free virus or by virus-infected monocytes or lymphocytes. Differences in the cellular tropism of primate versus nonprimate lentiviruses relate largely to receptor use as discussed earlier. Infection by the primate lentiviruses SIV and HIV is seen in CD4+ lymphocytes and macrophages, with CD4+ lymphocytes vastly predominating in terms of numbers of infected cells. For the nonprimate lentiviruses, infection of macrophages typically predominates, but infection can also be seen in other cell types. Replication in tissue macrophages is a unifying feature of all lentiviruses.

The principal anatomical sites of MVV and CAEV infection have varied with the study and with the strain of virus used. Because many studies have used experimental infection, the origin of the virus and the cell type on which it was grown must be considered when interpreting the results. Various reports have localized MVV principally to the lungs, mammary glands, joints, lymph nodes, the spleen, and the brain. Tissue macrophages are the principal target cell in which MVV and CAEV sequences are consistently found. However, in keeping with the broad range of cell types that can support replication in culture, evidence has been presented for MVV/CAEV infection of other cell types, including epithelial and fibroblast cells of the choroid plexus, intestine, and kidneys. An important observation first made with MVV is that although the virus may reside in relatively undifferentiated monocytes in peripheral blood, MVV expression is greatest in differentiated tissue macrophages.[109,263] This led to the "Trojan horse" concept for MVV and for other lentiviruses whereby undifferentiated monocytes in peripheral blood may carry the proviral genome with little or no viral protein expression until they reach tissues where they differentiate into macrophages and begin to produce virus.

A variety of studies have also shown tissue macrophages to be the predominant cell type for productive infection with EIAV.[231,250,310] Virus replication has been noted in the spleen, liver, kidney, lymph nodes, lung, heart, brain, stomach, bone marrow, thymus, adrenals, and intestine. Although EIAV can be adapted to replicate on fibroblasts, the virus that comes out of horses during viremic episodes is derived principally from macrophages. The anemia caused by EIAV is hemolytic and results from the formation of antigen–antibody complexes that can associate with the surface of erythrocytes. The kidneys are also affected by antigen–antibody complex formation.

FIV appears to be unusual among the nonprimate lentiviruses in that it has been found more consistently in a broader range of cell types, particularly lymphocytes, in addition to macrophages. Analyses of tissue and cellular tropism have primarily depended on experimentally infected cats and FIV grown in activated peripheral blood mononuclear cell (PBMC) cultures. However, studies with naturally infected cats have yielded similar findings. FIV has been found in a variety of cell types including CD4+ T lymphocytes, B cells, CD8+ T cells, macrophages, bone marrow–derived cells, and cells of the central nervous system (CNS). Macrophages, microglia, and astrocytes, but not neurons, in the brains of infected cats have been identified as targets of FIV infection.[86] The propensity of FIV to replicate in and deplete CD4+ T lymphocytes is consistent with use of the activated T-cell marker CD134 (OX40) as the initial receptor and CXCR4 as a co-receptor for cell entry.[71,72,318]

The major sites of SIV replication in macaques at early stage of infection are the gastrointestinal tract, thymus, spleen, and other lymphoid tissues.[187,362] SIV is found at early time points within periarteriolar lymphoid sheaths in the spleen, paracortex of lymph nodes, and the medulla of the thymus. The gastrointestinal tract contains most of the lymphoid tissue in the body, and activated T lymphocytes of the gastrointestinal mucosa express CCR5 in great abundance. SIV infection of rhesus monkeys results in profound and selective depletion of CD4+ T cells in the intestine within days of infection, before such changes are evident in peripheral lymphoid tissues. Thus, the gastrointestinal tract appears to be a major site of SIV replication and CD4+ T-cell depletion.[362,363] Subsequent to these pioneering studies in SIV-infected macaques, the gut-associated lymphoid tissues were shown to be the major site of HIV-1 replication during acute infection.[35] The predominate replication of HIV-1 in the human gut is again associated with a preference for activated CD4+CCR5+ memory T cells.[227] Within the thymus, marked depletion of thymic progenitors occurs by 21 days after infection of macaques with pathogenic SIV; this depletion is followed temporally by increased cell proliferation in the thymus and a rebound in thymocyte progenitors.[389] The distribution of virus within lymphoid organs varies with the inoculum. In some animals, SIV can be found in the CNS early after infection. The infected cells in the brain, whether at early or later stages of SIV-induced encephalitis (SIVE), are primarily cells of the monocyte/macrophage lineage[296] and may include perivascular macrophages that have migrated from the blood or resident microglial cells.[382] A neurovirulent infectious molecular clone of SIV that results in SIVE in approximately 50% of rhesus macaques after about a year of infection was recently described as a more physiological model for HIV-associated neuropathology than earlier systems that depend on immunomodulation of SIV infection to induce rapid progression to SIVE.[195,226]

Immune Responses and Persistence

Monkeys infected with SIV and animals infected with other lentiviruses typically develop strong antibody and CD8+ T-cell responses to the virus. These immune responses persist at high levels for the lifetime of the infected host, regardless of whether infection occurs by natural or experimental means. Approximately 20% to 30% of macaques infected with some AIDS-causing strains of SIV develop a more rapid disease course, make few or no antibodies to the virus, and develop AIDS within 3 to 7 months. The magnitude of the SIV-specific antibody response varies with the extent of virus replication. SIV deletion mutants that are progressively more attenuated and result in lower viral loads elicit weaker antibody responses (Fig. 19.6).[80]

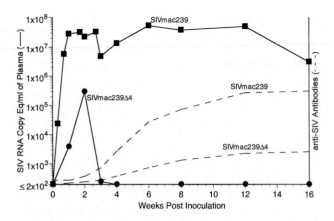

FIGURE 19.6 Attenuation by accessory gene deletion lowers viral load and reduces the strength of the antiviral antibody response. SIVmac239Δ4 has inactivating deletions in *vpr*, *vpx*, and two in *nef*.

CD8[+] T cells recognize and kill virus-infected cells presenting viral peptides on their cell surface in complex with MHC class I molecules. The importance of CD8[+] lymphocytes in limiting the extent of SIV replication was demonstrated by depleting CD8[+] T cells with anti-CD8 antibodies.[306] When CD8[+] cells are depleted during primary infection, virus replication proceeds unabated after peak viremia; this contrasts with non-depleted animals, in which immune responses typically reduce viral loads after 14 days of infection.[306] Depletion of CD8[+] lymphocytes during chronic SIV infection results in an immediate increase in viral loads that is suppressed again by the reappearance of virus-specific CD8[+] T cells.[306]

In macaques infected with wild-type, pathogenic strains of SIV, CD4[+] T-cell responses to viral antigens are typically weak or absent. However, infection with *nef*-deleted, live attenuated strains of SIV results in strong CD4[+] helper T-cell responses.[107] This situation may be analogous to HIV-1 infection in which virus-specific CD4[+] T-cell responses are weak or absent in most individuals but are often strong in nonprogressors that are able to control virus replication.[288] These observations suggest a struggle during early stages of infection, where CD4[+] helper T cells respond to sites of virus replication only to become targets of virus infection. In most cases, the virus wins resulting in progressive CD4[+] T-cell depletion, immunodeficiency, and ultimately progression to AIDS. However, under certain circumstances virus-specific CD4[+] T cells are preserved and are able to support the development of antibody and CD8[+] T-cell responses needed to contain virus replication.

Lentiviral persistence is achieved primarily through continuous virus replication. In HIV-1–infected individuals and SIV-infected animals, millions of CD4[+] T lymphocytes are infected and turned over every day throughout months and years of ongoing virus replication.[143,374] This does not mean that latent infection does not occur. Latent infection of quiescent cells with transcriptionally silent proviruses is a key component of the viral reservoir, which persists indefinitely even under conditions of complete suppression of virus replication with antiretroviral drugs. However, in the absence of antiretroviral therapy, virus replication continues unabated in most HIV-infected individuals and SIV-infected animals. This is also true of nonpathogenic SIV infection of natural hosts, which exhibit ongoing virus replication, high viral loads in plasma, CD4[+] T-cell turnover, and sustained antibody and CD8[+] T-cell responses.[44]

EIAV is unusual among the lentiviruses for the episodic nature of its persistent viral replication. Infection of horses with EIAV is associated with recurring episodes of fever, anemia, and thrombocytopenia. These episodes of clinical disease coincide with bursts of virus replication, which may be weeks or months apart. While the virus replicating in an infected horse during these periods is resistant to neutralization by contemporaneous serum, EIAV variants from earlier episodes can be neutralized by the same serum.[236]

Lentiviruses have evolved multiple mechanisms of immune evasion that allow them to replicate persistently in the face of vigorous host immune responses. In addition to overcoming innate immunity as discussed in the context of restriction factors, these include mechanisms of resistance to adaptive immunity. A few of the features that confer resistance to antibody and T-cell responses are summarized below and depicted in Figure 19.7.

Resistance to Antibodies

Structural studies have confirmed that the envelope glycoproteins of HIV-1 and SIV form trimers consisting of three noncovalently bound gp120 and gp41 subunits.[163,379] Outer domain surfaces of Env trimers are covered by extensive N-linked glycosylation that creates a "glycan shield" to prevent antibody binding to underlying polypeptides.[283] SIV strains lacking N-linked glycosylation sites in Env are more sensitive to antibody-mediated neutralization and are able to elicit higher neutralizing antibody titers in infected macaques.[283] Surfaces of Env that must be conserved to interact with cellular receptors are concealed by "conformational masking."[186] The CD4-binding site in gp120 is a deeply recessed pocket that is not accessible to most antibodies, and the co-receptor binding site is not even formed prior to CD4 engagement. Some of the most antigenic surfaces of Env (those that elicit the strongest binding antibody responses) are occluded by oligomerization via gp120-gp120 and gp120-gp41 contacts. Other Env surfaces that are readily accessible to antibodies, such as the variable loops, rapidly acquire amino acid changes to escape antibody binding.[38,373,387] On average, there are also only 8 to 14 Env trimers per virion,[50,398] which prevents antibodies from cross-linking Env trimers on virions, thereby preventing neutralization by all but the highest affinity antibodies that are capable of binding to Env using a single Fab arm.

Many of the structural features of Env that provide resistance to neutralization also protect virus-infected cells from elimination by antibodies. With a few notable exceptions,[96,367] antibodies that mediate antibody-dependent cellular cytotoxicity (ADCC) also neutralize virus infectivity,[368] which is consistent with the idea that antibodies that can bind to functional Env trimers on virions can also bind to Env trimers on the surface of virus-infected cells. Additional mechanisms of resistance to ADCC include CD4 downmodulation by Vpu and Nef,[364] which prevents exposure of CD4-inducible epitopes on the inner domain of gp120 that are normally occluded in "closed" Env trimers, and tetherin downmodulation by Vpu,[10] which prevents the accumulation of captured virions on the plasma membrane.

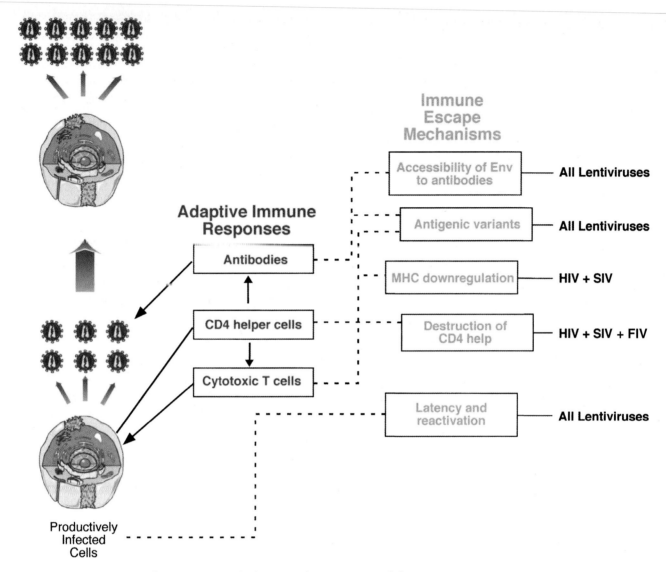

FIGURE 19.7 Mechanisms of immune evasion by human and simian immunodeficiency viruses.

MHC Class I Down-regulation

The Nef proteins of HIV-1 and SIV downmodulate HLA A and B molecules from the surface of virus-infected cells, reducing their sensitivity to lysis by cytotoxic CD8⁺ T cells.[55,309,338] More recently, the Vpu proteins of certain primary HIV-1 isolates were also found to downmodulate HLA C,[8] providing additional resistance to HLA C–restricted CD8⁺ T cells.

Destruction of CD4⁺ Helper T Cells

The primate lentiviruses preferentially replicate in virus-specific CD4⁺ lymphocytes,[85] which are activated by ongoing virus replication. As a result, CD4⁺ helper T cells needed to support antibody and CD8⁺ T-cell responses are depleted. A similar mechanism may apply to FIV, which uses CD134 to infect CD4⁺ lymphocytes in cats.

Escape Variants

The error-prone nature of reverse transcription coupled with high levels of persistent virus replication generates an enormous pool of genetic diversity within a single infected host for the selection of immunological escape variants. The emergence of lentiviral variants that escape neutralizing antibodies was first described for EIAV, MVV, and CAEV. Subsequent work has provided exquisite detail on the emergence of SIV and HIV-1 variants that escape both antibody and CD8⁺ T-cell responses.[32,38,93,285,373]

Virulence

Not all lentiviral infections are uniformly pathogenic. Although a few instances of AIDS-like disease have been reported in African monkeys naturally infected with SIV,[209,229,257] the primate lentiviruses are generally not associated with disease in their natural hosts. Lifelong subclinical infections have also been documented for EIAV and MVV. Breeds of horses and sheep vary in their susceptibility to EIAV and MVV and may even vary in the degree of susceptibility to specific disease manifestations. For example, the classic CNS form of MVV infection originally observed in Iceland is only rarely seen elsewhere. Some strains of SIV are also much less pathogenic than others in susceptible macaque monkeys, and certain strains attenuated by deletion mutations appear to be nonpathogenic.

The diseases associated with lentiviral infections are typically chronic and manifest over a prolonged period. However, there are some prominent exceptions. SIVsmPbj14 is acutely lethal in rhesus monkeys. Monkeys infected with SIVsmPBj14 typically die within 14 days with very high viral loads, severe gastrointestinal disease, cytokine dysregulation, lymphoproliferative disease, and organ system failure.[82,99,101] The unusual properties of this strain have been attributed in large part to the presence of a tyrosine residue at position 17 of the Nef protein.[87] This tyrosine creates an immunoreceptor tyrosine-based activation motif (ITAM) that imparts on the virus the ability to cause lymphocyte activation and to replicate to high titers in unstimulated PBMC cultures.[87] The BIV variant that is the cause of Jembrana disease in Bali cattle also can be acutely pathogenic. About 17% of Bali cattle infected either naturally or experimentally with JDV die with an acute disease within the first few weeks.[83,380] During acute disease, infectious titers reach 10^8/mL of plasma. JDV has remarkable similarities to the disease induced by SIVsmPBj14. There is marked enlargement of lymph nodes and spleen, which feature proliferating lymphoblastoid cells. Proliferating lymphoid infiltrates are also found in many other tissues. The disease in horses induced by EIAV is often considered more acute than that occurring with other lentiviruses. The first episode of anemia usually occurs 2 to 6 weeks after EIAV infection. Subsequent disease cycles are irregular, appearing weeks to months apart, and usually last 3 to 5 days. The frequency and severity of disease episodes usually declines with time, and usually ends within the first year after an average of six to eight episodes.

Everything that we know about the pathogenesis of SIV in macaques and HIV-1 in humans points to the importance of viral loads. Whereas high viral loads bode poorly, low viral loads are indicative of a better prognosis. Because sooty mangabeys and African green monkeys do not get sick from their SIVs, most scientists assumed that the viral loads in these species would be low. Quite unexpectedly, they are not.[36,114,284] Naturally infected sooty mangabeys and African green monkeys live normal lifespans with plasma viral loads of 10^5 to 10^6 RNA copies/mL, levels at which disease progression usually occurs with HIV-1 in humans and SIV in macaques.[36,114,167,284] The SIVs infecting these species are fully capable of inducing AIDS when passaged in macaques. Distinguishing features of SIV infection of natural hosts include the absence of chronic immune activation, preservation of mucosal integrity, lack of microbial translocation, maintenance of healthy CD4+ T-cell counts, and preservation of normal lymph node architecture.[44] A strong case has been made that chronic immune activation as a consequence of the loss of mucosal integrity and translocation of microbial antigens (e.g., bacterial lipopolysaccharide, peptidoglycans, and nucleic acids) is a major factor contributing to pathogenic HIV-1 and SIV infection.[34]

Clinical and Pathologic Features

Good reviews are available on the clinical and pathologic features of nonhuman lentiviral infections.[26,40,161,218,254,264] Some of the most prominent findings are highlighted here.

EIAV

Only equine species are susceptible to natural or experimental infection with EIAV. In contrast to infections with HIV, SIV, and FIV, immunosuppression is not a feature of EIAV. Clinical disease is usually divided into acute, subacute, and chronic phases. Acute disease typically results in a fever as high as 108°F 1 to 4 weeks after infection. Anemia is not a prominent feature at the outset. Excessive thirst, loss of appetite, weakness, depression, and hemorrhage are seen in the acute phase. Acute disease may result in death. The subacute form is characterized by relapsing fever and recurrence of other signs. Recurrent episodes may be brought on by hard work or malnutrition. In its chronic form, animals may remain thin despite adequate availability of food, and red cell counts are typically well below normal. Clinical signs in late disease appear to result principally from hemolytic anemia. Erythrocytes of infected horses are coated with antibodies and complement factor 3, and destruction of red cells is immunologically mediated. Osmotic fragility, shortened half-life, and phagocytosis contribute to erythrocyte destruction. Bone marrow may also be depressed, but this seems less important than immune-mediated destruction. Hemorrhage, jaundice, and edema are commonly found at necropsy. The nature and severity of lesions vary with disease course and duration of illness.

MVV and CAEV

Although maedi (pneumonia) and visna (wasting, depression, paralysis) were once thought to be separate diseases, it is now clear that they are both caused by the same virus. In contrast to infections with HIV, SIV, and FIV, immunosuppression is not a feature of maedi/visna. Polyarthritis and mastitis are also seen as a result of viral infection. Disease is usually seen only in adult sheep because of the lengthy incubation period, typically 3 to 8 years. The lungs of affected sheep may be two to five times their normal weight and exhibit a rubbery loss of elasticity.[161] These abnormalities result from a gross thickening of the alveolar walls caused by infiltration and proliferation of reticuloendothelial or mesenchymal cells that invade the septa (Fig. 19.8A and B). Lymph nodules occur along the bronchi and bronchioles. There is progressive weight loss. Dyspnea is initially apparent only after exercise, but it progresses. Severely dyspneic sheep spend much time lying down. Lesions in the brain consist of demyelination and lymphocytic infiltration (Fig. 19.8C and D). Trembling of facial muscles and lips may occur. Clinical signs of visna usually begin with weakness of the hind legs, and this eventually leads to paraplegia. Diseases caused by CAEV in goats are similar to those of MVV in sheep, except arthritis is usually most prominent and pneumonia is usually of lesser severity. Joints are swollen and painful, and this is exacerbated by cold weather. The basic lesion is a proliferative synovitis of joints, tendon sheaths, and bursae.

FIV

Primary infection by FIV may lead to low-grade fever, generalized lymphadenopathy, and sometimes diarrhea. During the ensuing months and years, progressing disease is associated with lymphopenia, recurrent fever, lymphadenopathy, anemia, diarrhea, and weight loss of protracted duration. CD4 T-cell counts and other cell subsets may be depressed. The final stages of disease are associated with chronic secondary infections, particularly gingivitis, dermatitis, and infections of the upper respiratory tract. Opportunistic infections that have been observed include calicivirus, herpesviruses, toxoplasma, and

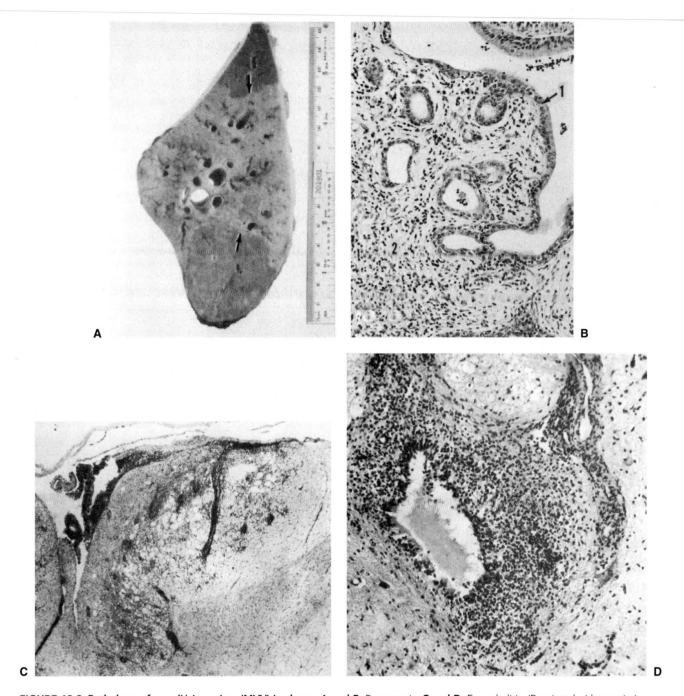

FIGURE 19.8 Pathology of maedi/visna virus (MVV) in sheep. A and B: Pneumonia. **C and D:** Encephalitis. (Reprinted with permission from Jones TC, Hunt RD, King NW. Diseases caused by viruses. In: Cann C, ed. *Veterinary Pathology.* 6th ed. Baltimore, MD: Lippincott Williams & Wilkins; 1997:197–370.)

cryptococcus. Neurologic abnormalities also have been noted, including dementia, twitching tremors, and convulsions. Pathologic lesions primarily reflect those of opportunistic infection.

SIV

SIV infection of rhesus monkeys is generally considered the closest model of HIV-1 infection of humans. SIV infection of natural hosts (e.g., SIVagm in African green monkeys or SIVsmm in sooty mangabeys) is in general not associated with disease, although there may be occasional exceptions.[209,229,257]

When SIVsmm was inadvertently introduced into macaque species (Asian Old World primates) in captivity, AIDS-like disease and lymphomas ensued.[7,68,219] AIDS-like disease is generally induced experimentally in macaque monkeys with SIVmac, SIVsmm, or less frequently with SIVagm. As with other lentiviruses, SIV establishes a chronic active infection with a prodromal period of months to years before clinical signs appear. Immunodeficiency is usually, but not always, associated with marked declines in CD4+ lymphocyte counts. Macrophages are also infected. Generalized lymphadenopathy typically occurs and is characterized by hyperplasia followed by lymphoid depletion in terminal stages (Fig. 19.9A and B). The gastrointestinal tract, where activated T lymphocytes predominate, appears to be the major site of early viral replication and loss of CD4+ T cells (Fig. 19.9C).[362] However, CXCR4-using viruses may cause a profound loss of CD4+ T cells in the periphery that is not paralleled in the intestine.[269] Marked depletion of progenitor cells occurs in the thymus by 21 days postinfection; although a rebound occurs subsequently, thymic dysinvolution is typically seen at terminal stages (Fig. 19.9D and E).[389] Nodular lymphocytic infiltrates in a variety of tissues (Fig. 19.9C), interstitial pneumonia with syncytial cells ("giant cell pneumonia") (Fig. 19.9H and I), and granulomatous encephalitis (Fig. 19.9F and G) are variably present. Opportunistic infections usually occur, and these can influence the specific nature of the clinical signs. Common opportunistic infections include *Pneumocystis carinii* pneumonia, generalized cytomegalovirus infection, cryptosporidiosis, and *Mycobacterium avium*.

A significant number of AIDS research studies in macaques now utilize recombinant forms of SIVmac with HIV-1 *env*, *tat*, and *rev* genes, referred to as simian-human immunodeficiency viruses (SHIVs). First-generation SHIVs, such as SHIV89.6P, were X4-tropic (use CXCR4 as co-receptor) and acutely pathogenic. However, these SHIVs proved to be paradoxically easy to protect against by vaccination and are no longer considered rigorous challenge viruses for vaccine studies.[135] Several pathogenic SHIVs that use CCR5 as a co-receptor have now been developed. A few of these SHIVs result in high viral loads during chronic infection and progressive CD4+ T-cell turnover that resembles the pathogenesis of the SIVmac strains from which they were derived.[201,319] These SHIVs have become especially useful for the preclinical evaluation of HIV-1 Env-specific antibodies in macaque models.

Contributions of Individual Genes and Genetic Elements

Lentiviruses, like other retroviruses, replicate through a proviral DNA intermediate. Proviral DNA clones that contain a full-length lentiviral genome are therefore sufficient to initiate a spreading infection after physical or chemical delivery into permissive cells. Infectious molecular clones (IMCs) of lentiviruses have been used to study the functions of open reading frames not found in other retroviruses and to gauge their relative importance in the context of experimental animal infection. The first molecular clone of a lentivirus that was not only shown to be infectious but also pathogenic was for SIVmac.[171] Pathogenic IMCs were subsequently obtained for EIAV, CAEV, FIV, and other SIV isolates.[58,74,138,259]

Deoxyuridine Triphosphatase

A dUTPase reading frame is located within the *pol* gene of the nonprimate lentiviruses and in the transition region between *gag* and *pol* of type D retroviruses. dUTPase catalyzes the conversion of dUTP to dUMP and inorganic pyrophosphate. dUMP is a key precursor of dTTP, which is required for cDNA synthesis during reverse transcription. dUTPase activity also minimizes the mutagenic effects of misincorporation of dUTP into viral DNA. The impact of eliminating the dUTPase open reading frame (DU) has been studied for EIAV, FIV, CAEV, and

MVV. In all cases, DU− viruses still replicate in cultured cells. However, the loss of DU dramatically impairs virus replication in nondividing macrophages with low dNTP pools.[343,369] Compared to wild-type EIAV, DU− EIAV exhibited 5- to 10-fold lower peak viral loads in plasma, and the pathogenicity of both DU− EIAV and DU− CAEV was attenuated.[204,369] Moreover, DU− FIV and DU− CAEV were found to accumulate increased levels of mutations, particularly G-to-A transitions.[198,350] Visna viruses lacking DU also showed decreased viral loads in experimentally infected sheep but still produced neuropathogenic effects upon direct intracerebral inoculation.[266]

Tat

Lentiviral Tat proteins can be divided into two groups depending on whether their transactivating activities involve binding to an RNA secondary structure at the 5' end of nascent viral transcripts known as the transactivation response (TAR) element.[31,73,237] Whereas the efficiency of transcription is strongly enhanced for HIV-1, SIV, EIAV, and BIV by their respective Tat proteins in a cyclin T1– and viral RNA–dependent manner, transcription is fully active for MVV and FIV in the absence of any viral proteins. The products of MVV *tat* and FIV *orfA* may therefore have functions more similar to those of other accessory proteins.[46,108,365] Similar to CD4 downmodulation by Nef, FIV OrfA downmodulates the CD134 receptor of the virus from the surface of infected cells.[144] BIV Tat is unusual in that it is able to bind to an RNA sequence element independent of cyclin T1, but transactivation is nonetheless dependent on cyclin T1.[31]

Rev

The lentiviral Rev protein mediates the nuclear export of unspliced viral genomic RNA (gRNA) and a subset of partially spliced, intron-containing mRNAs that encode the Vif, Vpr, Vpx, Vpu, and Env proteins.[274] Rev multimerizes on an RNA secondary structure at the 3' end of the viral genome known as the Rev-responsive element (RRE).[274] Interactions between Rev and the chromosomal region maintenance 1 (CRM1) protein (also known as exportin-1) shuttle viral transcripts from the nucleus to the cytoplasm, where Rev and CRM1 disengage to allow protein translation or packaging of gRNA.[274] Importantly, Rev and Tat are translated from multiply spliced transcripts and therefore are not dependent on Rev for nuclear export. Although Rev and RRE sequences vary, this mechanism is used by all lentiviruses and is essential for replication.[274]

S2

The *S2* gene is unique to EIAV and encodes a 7-kDa protein that bears no homology to other known retroviral proteins. The S2 protein was found to counteract the effects of SERINC3 and SERINC5 on viral infectivity by excluding these factors from virions.[45] Similar to Nef, this activity is dependent on N-terminal myristoylation and a dileucine motif in S2 required for the recruitment of AP-2 for clathrin-mediated endocytosis of SERINC3/5.[45] The phenotype of *S2*-deleted EIAV also resembles the phenotype of *nef*-deleted SIV. An EIAV derivative lacking S2 replicated normally in fetal equine kidney cells, monocyte-derived macrophages, and differentiated macrophages[200] but exhibited lower viral loads and decreased pathogenesis compared to wild-type EIAV in infected horses.[199]

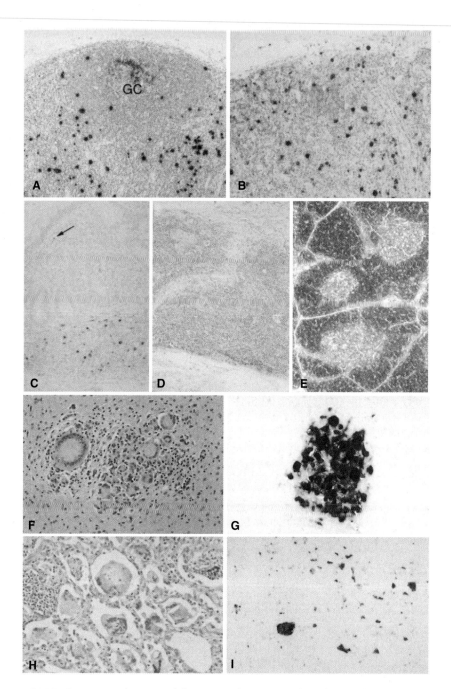

FIGURE 19.9 Acquired immunodeficiency syndrome in monkeys: histopathologic lesions and simian immunodeficiency virus localization. A–C: *In situ* hybridization for SIV RNA in lymph nodes (**A, B**) and intestine (**C**). In (**A**), numerous individual positive cells can be seen in the paracortex of the lymph node of an animal 8 weeks after infection. In addition, diffuse staining of the germinal center (*GC*) of a lymphoid follicle consistent with trapping of virus on follicular dendritic cells can be seen. Note that the lymphoid architecture is relatively intact at this early time point, in contrast to a lymph node from an animal with terminal AIDS in (**B**). Although the lymph node in (**B**) shows severe lymphoid depletion with no evidence of lymphoid follicles, numerous SIV-infected cells can be seen. In (**C**), numerous infected cells in the intestine can be seen in a submucosal lymphoid nodule with a rare positive cell (*arrow*) in the overlying lamina propria of this animal 2 months after infection. **D and E:** Thymic atrophy. Infection with SIV is associated with profound dysinvolution of the thymus (**D**), as opposed to a normal thymus (**E**) with discrete cortex and medulla. **F and G:** SIV encephalitis. Infection with SIV results in inflammation of the brain in 25% to 50% of the animals that are infected. The brain lesions are characterized by aggregates of mononuclear cells and multinucleated giant cells (**F**). Cells in the lesions contain abundant SIV nucleic acid by *in situ* hybridization (**G**). **H and I:** Giant cell pneumonia. Multinucleated giant cells in this pneumonia (**H**) as well as numerous mononuclear cells contain abundant SIV nucleic acid by *in situ* hybridization (**I**). (Figure and legend courtesy of Andrew Lackner.)

Vif

With the exception of EIAV, all lentiviruses have a *vif* gene (Fig. 19.4 and Tables 19.4 and 19.5). Vif is required to overcome a producer-cell block to virus infectivity imposed by members of the APOBEC3 family of cytidine deaminases.[29,205,315] Accordingly, Vif is critical for virus replication *in vivo* and in cells expressing A3G, A3F, and A3H.[80,312] In the absence of Vif, A3G, A3F, and in some cases, A3H become incorporated into virus particles and catalyze cytidine deamination of minus strand DNA during reverse transcription.[132,194] This leads to the accumulation of G-to-A transitions in the plus strand that inactivate the viral genome (see "Restriction" section of this chapter). Vif counteracts this restriction by recruiting the cullin-5-elongin B/C-Rbx ubiquitin ligase complex, which mediates the polyubiquitylation and proteasomal degradation of A3 proteins.[220,316] By depleting intracellular A3 levels, Vif prevents the incorporation of these proteins into virions.

Nef

A *nef* gene is present in all of the primate lentiviruses but is not found in the nonprimate lentiviruses (Fig. 19.4 and Tables 19.4 and 19.5). The Nef sequences of HIV-1 and SIVsmm/mac correspond in most regions. However, SIVsmm/mac Nef is approximately 40 to 50 amino acids longer due to additional N-terminal sequences that are not found in HIV-1 Nef. A multitude of functional activities have been attributed to Nef. Most of these functions, including CD4 and MHC class I downmodulation, lymphocyte activation, and infectivity enhancement, are shared by the Nef proteins of HIV-1 and SIV. CD4 downmodulation prevents CD4 binding to Env and the exposure of CD4-inducible epitopes that render virus-infected cells susceptible to elimination by antibodies.[364] Selective downmodulation of certain MHC class I molecules, but not others, enables HIV- and SIV-infected cells to evade recognition and destruction by virus-specific CD8+ T cells, while simultaneously inhibiting NK cell responses.[54,77,338] Infectivity enhancement reflects the downmodulation of SERINC5, and to a lesser extent SERINC3, which prevents the incorporation of these factors into virions.[287,352]

Additional functions of the Nef proteins of SIV and HIV-2 have been identified that are not shared by HIV-1 Nef. The Nef proteins of HIV-2 and diverse SIVs down-regulate the T-cell receptor (TCR) through interactions with the CD3ζ chain.[146,304] TCR downmodulation reduces the sensitivity of infected CD4+ T cells to activation and has been proposed to contribute to the nonpathogenic nature of SIV infection in natural hosts.[304] The Nef proteins of most SIVs, with the exception of SIVgsn/mon/mus, also counteract restriction by the tetherin proteins of their simian hosts by downmodulating tetherin from the surface of infected cells.[156,298,402] This activity is dependent on a five-amino acid sequence that is present in the cytoplasmic domain of the tetherin orthologs of apes and Old World monkeys but is missing from human tetherin.[156,402] Recent structural studies have revealed that Nef acts as a cargo adaptor for clathrin-mediated endocytosis of cellular transmembrane proteins.[37,157,185] By using different surfaces and conformations to form multimeric complexes with the cytoplasmic domains of specific cargo proteins and AP-1 or AP-2 subunits,[37,157,185] Nef is able to selectively downmodulate several different transmembrane proteins from the cell surface, which helps to explain how Nef is able to serve so many functions.

Nef also plays a role in lymphocyte activation. The Nef proteins of HIV-1 and SIV potentiate NF-κB activation, which enhances virus replication by stimulating viral gene transcription from the LTR promoter.[297] Nef additionally increases IL-2 production from infected cells, and *nef*-deleted viruses are accordingly more dependent on exogenous IL-2 for replication.[1,113] Polymorphisms in Nef can also impact cellular activation, as illustrated by the identification of an ITAM in SIVpbj14 Nef that accounts for the unusual ability of SIVpbj14 to replicate in unstimulated CD4+ T cells and for the highly pathogenic phenotype of this virus in macaques.[87]

Nef is not essential for virus replication *in vitro* but is important for efficient virus replication and pathogenesis in infected hosts. SIV strains with deletions in *nef* are highly attenuated compared with wild-type virus.[172] Peak viral loads are typically two to three logs lower during acute infection, and set-point viral loads are frequently undetectable during chronic infection with *nef*-deleted SIV. Most monkeys infected with SIVmac239Δ*nef* have survived without disease and with undetectable viral loads for as long as they have been studied. However, despite marked attenuation, SIVmac239Δ*nef* infection is clearly persistent. Approximately 10% to 20% of monkeys infected with SIVmac239Δ*nef* develop moderate viral loads and eventually progress to AIDS as a result of the accumulation of genetic changes by the virus that restore a pathogenic phenotype.[2] Among these changes, substitutions in the gp41 cytoplasmic domain of serially passaged, *nef*-deleted SIV have been shown to restore the ability to counteract tetherin.[311] The phenotype of *nef*-deleted HIV-1 in humans appears to be similar to *nef*-deleted SIV in monkeys. Although infection with *nef*-deleted HIV-1 is clearly attenuated,[76,174] some individuals have developed signs of disease progression.[125,193]

Vpr

A *vpr* gene is present in all primate lentiviruses and encodes a protein of approximately 14-kDa that is specifically incorporated into virions through binding interactions with the p6 domain of Gag. Vpr directs a number of cellular proteins for proteasomal degradation by recruiting the cullin-4A–containing E3 ubiquitin ligase complex (CRL4) through binding interactions with VprBP (DCAF1).[147,191,308] Several DNA repair enzymes have been identified as targets of Vpr-mediated degradation, including the nuclear isoform of uracil–DNA glycosylase (UNG2),[33,149] helicase-like transcription factor (HTLF),[149] exonuclease 1 (EXO1),[391] the structure-specific endonuclease regulator complex (SLX4),[188] and the methylcytosine dioxygenase TET2.[216] Degradation of the base excision repair enzymes UNG2 and TET2 may prevent cDNA products of reverse transcription from triggering DNA repair mechanisms as a consequence of high levels of uracil incorporation owing to elevated dUTP pools in macrophages.[149] Vpr-mediated degradation of HTLF and EXO1 also affords an advantage to HIV-1 replication in T cells,[392] consistent with the idea that the turnover of these enzymes prevents the processing of branched cDNA intermediates of reverse transcription.

Vpr additionally targets the coiled-coil domain–containing-137 (CCDC137) protein for proteasomal degradation.[401] Although the cellular function of CCDC137 is poorly understood, the degradation of this chromosome periphery protein is sufficient to account for the long-standing observation that Vpr induces G2/M cell cycle arrest.[401] Whereas CCDC137 depletion increases HIV-1 gene expression by approximately 10-fold in macrophages, it only increases viral gene expression by approximately twofold in CD4+ lymphocytes.[401] These observations are consistent with a greater effect of *vpr* deletion on virus replication in macrophages than in CD4+ lymphocytes[16,57] and the modest attenuation of SIVmac239Δ*vpr* replication in rhesus macaques.[110] Interestingly, HIV-2 Vpr does not degrade human HTLF or UNG2,[149] only partially depletes CCDC137,[401] and SIVmac Vpr does not degrade human CCDC137,[401] which suggests species-specific differences in these activities.

Vpx

Vpx and *vpr* are related by gene duplication. However, in contrast to *vpr*, which is present in all of the primate lentiviruses, the *vpx* gene is only found in a subset of primate lentiviruses (Table 19.5). Like Vpr, Vpx is packaged into virions through interactions with the p6 domain of Gag and mediates the proteasomal degradation of cellular proteins by binding to DCAF1 and recruiting CRL4.[335] Vpx is required for efficient SIVsmm/mac replication in terminally differentiated, nondividing myeloid cells (macrophages and dendritic cells) and in resting CD4+ lymphocytes. Vpx can also enhance HIV-1 infection of these cell types. This phenotype reflects the degradation of SAMHD1,[15,148,189] a triphosphohydrolase that maintains dNTP concentrations in nondividing cells below the threshold required to complete reverse transcription.[115] Accordingly, deletion of *vpx* has a greater effect than deletion of *vpr* on the attenuation of SIV replication in macaques. Nevertheless, more than half of the animals infected with SIVmac239Δ*vpx* progress to AIDS.[110] An analysis of necropsy tissue from animals infected with *vpx*-deleted SIV revealed little or no infected macrophages at the time of death indicating that AIDS can occur without significant macrophage infection.[376]

In addition to SAMHD1, the Vpx proteins of SIVsmm/mac and HIV-2 degrade the transgene activation suppressor (TASOR) subunit of the human silencing hub (HUSH).[51] The HUSH complex recruits an H3K9me3 methyltransferase implicated in the epigenetic repression of retroelements. Vpx-mediated depletion of HUSH reduces H3K9me3 chromosomal marks and reactivates transcription from latent HIV-1 proviruses.[51] The effects of Vpx are stronger for SIVmac LTR–driven gene expression, suggesting that this activity is especially important for the replication of SIVsmm/mac and HIV-2.[51] However, whereas the Vpx proteins of SIVrcm and SIVmnd2 are unable to degrade human TASOR, the Vpr proteins of two phylogenetically distinct SIVs (SIVagm and SIVlst) can degrade human TASOR and activate HIV-1 transcription.[51] These observations suggest species specificity in the antagonism of HUSH and that this function also preceded evolution of the of *vpx* gene.

Env

Env encodes an extensively glycosylated viral protein that is cleaved into surface (SU) and transmembrane (TM) subunits by furin proteases in the Golgi. Three SU and three TM subunits (which correspond to gp120 and gp41 for the primate lentiviruses) associate noncovalently to form Env trimers on the surface of virions. Env binding to receptor(s) on the surface of susceptible cells induces conformational changes that mediate membrane fusion and virus entry. As the only viral protein exposed on the surface of infected cells and virions, it is the only viral-encoded target of antibodies that can neutralize viral infectivity and eliminate virus-infected cells by Fc-mediated mechanisms.

A distinguishing feature of lentiviral envelope glycoproteins is the unusual length of their cytoplasmic tails. These sequences range in length from approximately 50 amino acids for FIV to over 200 amino acids for EIAV and are typically 150 and 164 amino acids for HIV-1 and SIVsmm/mac, respectively. The cytoplasmic domains (CDs) of the primate lentiviral Env proteins have been studied most extensively and are known to participate in the trafficking and incorporation of Env into virions.[277] Both HIV-1 and SIV Env contain a highly conserved, membrane-proximal, tyrosine-based motif in their CDs that serves as an AP-2–binding site for clathrin-mediated endocytosis.[24,398] The HIV-1 CD also contains a motif implicated in Rab11-family interacting protein 1C (FIP1C)- and Rab14-dependent sorting of Env to sites of virus assembly.[280,281] The incorporation of SIV Env into virions is not dependent on FIP1C, however,[177] and SIV replication in human CD4+ T cells selects for CD truncations,[182] suggesting species-specific differences in Env trafficking. Although a direct physical interaction between the Env CD and the viral matrix (MA) protein has been difficult to confirm biochemically, genetic evidence supports an interaction between the HIV-1 Env CD and MA.[240,341] The CDs of HIV-1 and SIV Env may also enhance virus replication in minimally activated CD4+ T cells by stimulating NF-κB activation.[276]

U3

The U3 regions of the primate lentiviruses are unusually long compared with their counterparts in the nonprimate lentiviruses.[153] Most of this length can be accounted for by the overlap of *nef* coding sequences with the U3 region of the LTR. This is supported by several observations. In monkeys infected with *nef*-deleted SIV missing 182 bp in the region that is unique to *nef*, the virus consistently loses approximately 300 bp of sequence in the *nef*-U3 overlap.[175] However, the 12 terminal nucleotides of U3 required for integration and an approximately 50 bp sequence at the 3′ end of *nef* immediately upstream of the NF-κB binding site are retained.[152,221,273] In one case of human infection with a *nef*-deleted HIV-1 variant, sequences in the region of *nef*-U3 overlap were also progressively lost over time, while terminal U3 nucleotides and an approximately 50 bp sequence upstream of the NF-κB site were retained.[174]

NF-κB and Sp1

Sequence elements in the U3 region of the LTR for binding NF-κB and Sp1 transcription factors have been defined as major promoter elements for HIV-1, HIV-2, and SIV. Nevertheless, the removal of NF-κB or Sp1 binding sites from both LTRs surprisingly did not detectably attenuate SIVmac239 replication in rhesus monkeys.[152] The removal of both NF-κB and Sp1 binding sites did attenuate SIVmac239 but not markedly so.[154] This is likely to be predominantly or exclusively due to an enhancer element present within the 50 bp sequence immediately upstream of the NF-κB binding region that coincides with the *nef* coding region.[152,221,273] Although HIV-1 replication appears more heavily dependent on the presence of the NF-κB and Sp1 sites,[289] there is also evidence for an enhancer element upstream of the NF-κB binding sequence of this virus.[88,174]

Genetic Resistance

Host genetic determinants that influence resistance to disease occur for all lentiviruses. The best documented examples come from studies of HIV-1 in humans because of the availability of large, well-characterized patient cohorts. Differences in susceptibility to HIV-1 infection and progression to disease are associated with polymorphisms in many genes, but particularly in the *CCR5*, *HLA*, and *KIR* genes (see Chapter 17). Among the nonhuman lentiviruses, genetic resistance is best characterized for SIV infection of the rhesus macaque because of the extensive use of this species as an animal model.

Certain *MHC class I* alleles have been associated with the control of SIV replication in rhesus macaques. *Mamu* (*Macaca mulatta*)-*A*01*, a common *MHC class I* allele present in 22% of Indian origin rhesus macaques, is associated with a fivefold reduction in chronic phase viral loads.[238] *Mamu-B*08* and *Mamu-B*17*, which are present in 6% and 11% of Indian origin rhesus macaques, respectively, are significantly overrepresented among elite controllers (animals that contain plasma viremia below 1,000 copies/mL).[212,393] The protective effect of *Mamu-B*08* is particularly strong and is associated on average with more than a sevenfold reduction in chronic phase viral loads.[212] The protective effect of *Mamu-B*17* is less consistent, since viral loads in *Mamu-B*17*–positive animals vary considerably.[385] Interestingly, Mamu-B*08 binds a similar set of peptides as HLA-B*2705, which is associated with the control of HIV-1 replication in humans.[213] CD8 depletion studies and studies of CD8+ T-cell escape suggest that these MHC class I associations primarily reflect virus-specific CD8+ T-cell responses.

TRIM5 polymorphisms are also associated with differences in the ability of macaques to contain the replication of some SIV strains. SIVsmE543-3 and SIVsmE660 were derived by experimental infection of rhesus macaques with SIVsmm isolated from sooty mangabeys, and as a consequence of the incomplete adaptation to rhesus macaques, they exhibit considerable animal-to-animal variation in both acute and chronic phase viral loads. This variation in viral loads reflects differences in susceptibility to restriction by TRIM5.[176] Thus, the sensitivity of SIVsmE543-3 and SIVsmE660 to restrictive variants of rhesus macaque TRIM5 is an important consideration for the interpretation and design of animal studies using these viruses. SIVsmm replication in rhesus macaques expressing restrictive variants of TRIM5 nevertheless selects for amino acid changes in capsid that confer resistance to these variants at later stages of infection. These capsid changes can be engineered back into SIVsmm to generate infectious molecular clones that bypass the confounding effects of TRIM5 genotype in animal studies.[386]

DIAGNOSIS

Because lentiviral infections are persistent, antiviral antibodies are present throughout the lifetime of the infected host. Detection of antibodies to viral antigens is thus the most widely used method for diagnosing viral infection. A variety of methods are commonly used for antibody detection. These include enzyme-linked immunosorbent assay (ELISA), Western blot, gel diffusion, indirect immunofluorescence, hemagglutination, complement fixation, and neutralization assays. The commonly used Coggins test for the detection of EIAV infection is a gel diffusion assay for the detection of antiviral antibodies. ELISA methods for the detection of antibodies to FIV are available. It is estimated that 2% to 3% of cats in the United States are FIV positive. ELISA and Western blots are most commonly used for the detection of antibodies to SIV; detection by ELISA is usually routine but can be complicated by the history of the monkey, whether the antibodies are to the same or a different type of SIV (i.e., cross-reactive), and in an experimental setting, the presence of antibodies at low levels due to attenuation or intervention. Positivity can be confirmed by virus isolation or by identification of viral antigens or viral RNA in plasma or cells. The presence of specific clinical signs and clear demonstration of the presence of virus-specific antibodies is usually sufficient for a definitive diagnosis.

PREVENTION AND CONTROL

MVV was eradicated from Iceland by a drastic slaughter policy before the availability of diagnostic tests. Test and removal programs, either voluntary or mandated, continue to be used as an effective means of control. Buyers of horses have increasingly sought negative test certification for EIAV, and negative test certification is required as a condition for entry to many racetracks, sales yards, and shows. Horses imported into the United States and some other countries are required to have a negative test certificate. Testing within a state is not always compulsory, nor is it compulsory for an owner to destroy a positive horse. For FIV, testing is routinely available for cats under veterinary care, and animals in shelters are also routinely screened. However, test and removal programs and certification at the point of sale have been sparingly applied to FIV.

Two vaccines have been used in the field for the prevention of lentivirus infections. A live attenuated EIAV strain was developed by researchers by repeated passage of the virus in donkey cells.[317] This EIAV vaccine has been extensively used in China and in Cuba, where it has been administered to millions of horses with apparent safety and efficacy. An accumulation of nucleotide substitutions rather than deletions appears to be the basis for the attenuation of EIAV.[370] An EIAV vaccine virus derived from a single proviral clone did not fare as well in vaccine challenge experiments as the actual vaccine, which contains extensive sequence diversity.[217] The live attenuated EIAV vaccine was administered to 61 million horses and mules in China from 1975 to the 1990s, and this nationwide vaccination program ended the incidence of equine infectious anemia in the country.[371] A vaccine against FIV consisting of two inactivated virus subtypes was available in the United States and Canada from 2002 to 2017[278] but has been discontinued because of questionable efficacy.[336]

RESEARCH ON VACCINE DEVELOPMENT

One important application of nonhuman lentiviruses is in the area of vaccine research. The development of a safe and effective AIDS vaccine is certainly one of the greatest challenges of our time. Yet, after more than three decades of research, we still lack the basic scientific knowledge needed to achieve this goal. While vaccines designed to stimulate virus-specific T cell responses can reduce viral loads in nonhuman primate models, at least under conditions where protection is assessed against viruses closely matched to the vaccine and the time of challenge is only a few weeks after the last vaccine dose, conventional T-cell responses alone are not sufficient to prevent infection. On the other hand, passive antibody transfer experiments have shown that potent broadly neutralizing antibodies that are able to bind with high affinity to conserved, conformational features of the HIV-1 envelope glycoprotein can afford complete protection. However, it is presently unclear how to elicit these types of antibodies by vaccination.

A myriad of vaccine approaches have been evaluated in macaque models, including many prime and boost vaccine regimens with different combinations of recombinant DNA, poxviral, or adenoviral vectors. While pathogenic strains of SIV have been used most commonly as challenge viruses, SHIVs have also been extensively used to assess protection by vaccines designed to elicit antibodies to the HIV-1 envelope glycoprotein. Rather than attempting to cover the multitude of vectors and prime-boost vaccine regimens that have been tested over the years, we will focus on a few approaches that highlight key concepts or promising advances.

Early expectations were raised when inactivated whole SIV was found to provide protection against pathogenic strains of SIV.[81,241] Hope was quickly dashed, however, when it was found that protection occurred only when the vaccine and challenge stocks were grown in human cells.[63,64] When the vaccine was prepared in human cells and the challenge virus was grown in monkey cells, protection was not observed. Human cellular antigens present in virus preparations appear to have conferred protection when the challenge virus was grown in the same human cells. MHC class II antigens were present in greater abundance in virus particles than the viral envelope glycoprotein and may have been among the xenoantigens that contributed to protection.[12,13]

There are good reasons for believing that development of an effective vaccine against HIV is going to be a very difficult task. First and foremost, despite enormous antibody and cellular responses to HIV-1, these immune responses do not stop continuous virus replication and CD4+ T-cell destruction. Not only do these immune responses not control virus replication in an already infected individual, they are routinely unable to protect against superinfection by a different strain of the virus.[268] HIV-1 field isolates have extraordinary genetic variability, and neutralizing antibody responses are typically strain specific[285]; methods by which a vaccine could deal with this diversity have yet to be devised. These difficulties have been borne out through seven large-scale efficacy trials in humans, the most recent of which was another disappointing failure.[124]

Vaccine studies in animal models can provide useful information in several ways. Head-to-head comparisons of different vaccine approaches can shed light on which approaches perform more effectively, at least under defined experimental conditions. In-depth analyses of individual vaccine approaches also may provide fundamental insights into immunologic control and what is needed for protective immunity. With these goals in mind, vaccine approaches that have been tried in monkey models include a variety of Env subunit approaches, replication-competent and replication-defective recombinant viruses, single-cycle SIV, recombinant DNA and RNA, and prime-boost protocols that use combinations of these approaches. A few themes arising from these studies are worth noting.

The particular virus that is used for challenge is one of the most important factors that determine whether or not a vaccine/challenge study will be successful. Easy-to-neutralize, nonpathogenic challenge viruses have proven relatively easy to protect against. Difficult-to-neutralize, pathogenic viruses, which are considered representative of naturally transmitted HIV-1 field isolates, have proven very difficult to protect against. A homologous cloned virus challenge is less stringent than a closely matched, uncloned virus challenge, which in turn is much less stringent than a challenge with a virus with natural levels of sequence divergence. The timing of the challenge is also a factor. Many of the vaccine approaches mentioned above induce transient immune responses that decline dramatically after peaking a few weeks after the last vaccine boost. Other important considerations are the dose and route of challenge. High doses of challenge virus are more difficult to protect against than low challenge doses and it is more difficult to protect against intravenous challenge than mucosal challenge. For these reasons, the use of repeated, low-dose mucosal inoculation, usually via the rectal mucosa, is now widely used as a challenge model to better approximate sexual transmission of HIV-1.

Live attenuated strains of SIV have performed most impressively as vaccines in experimental monkey studies.[67,98] Single and combinations of mutations in *nef*, *vpr*, *vpx*, and LTR sequences have been used. In general, the ability to achieve protection has varied inversely with the degree of attenuation.[160] While protection against homologous challenge with SIVmac239 has been impressive, only minimal protection has been observed against challenge with a heterologous strain of SIV.[388] Nevertheless, because of the potential for live attenuated viruses to regain a pathogenic phenotype as a result of the accumulation of genetic changes,[2] this approach is not under serious consideration for clinical use in people.

Interesting results have also been obtained with recombinant herpesviruses. Herpesviruses persist for life, and immune responses to their antigens are maintained in an active state. Herpesviruses have large genomes and can accommodate large amounts of genetic information. A lab-adapted strain of rhesus macaque cytomegalovirus (rhCMV) called 68-1 has been used as a vaccine vector to express SIV antigens in monkeys. These recombinants stimulate unconventional CD8+ T-cell responses with extraordinary breadth and unusual restriction characteristics. More than half of the monkeys immunized with such rhCMV recombinants have exhibited early and complete virologic control following SIVmac239 challenge.[130,131] A gamma-2 herpesvirus of rhesus monkeys, rhesus rhadinovirus (RRV), has also been used to deliver a near-full-length SIV genome that expresses all nine SIV gene products and assembles non-infectious virus particles. Protection against SIVmac239 acquisition has been observed with this vaccine strain following challenge by both mucosal and intravenous routes.[120,224]

The use of adeno-associated virus (AAV) as a vector to achieve long-term delivery of potent broadly neutralizing monoclonal antibodies is another promising approach being intensively studied in rhesus monkey models. When delivered to muscle, the muscle cells can become factories for long-term antibody production. Protection against SIV and SHIV challenges has been observed with this approach.[96,106,159] However, antidrug antibody (ADA) responses to vectored antibodies or antibody-like molecules can severely impair antibody delivery. ADA responses remain a major challenge to realizing the potential of this approach.[223]

RESEARCH ON THERAPEUTIC REGIMENS

Antiviral drugs used against HIV-1 in people have been developed with little or no input from animal models of lentiviral infection. However, animal models can provide valuable information for investigation of certain types of therapeutic intervention. For example, there is currently great interest in the idea of using so-called latency reversing agents (LRAs) in combination with antiretroviral therapy (ART) to reactivate viral gene expression in latently infected cells so that these cells can be targeted and eliminated by antiviral responses. LRAs are highly exploratory, and monkey models are quite reasonably being used to examine their feasibility.[247] A number of companies are also exploring approaches to long-acting ART formulations in an attempt to reduce the frequency with which these drugs must be taken, and monkey models are being used to address their feasibility.[6]

Many of the antiretroviral drugs developed for use against HIV-1 in humans are less potent against SIV, and the bioavailability of some of these drugs can also differ between humans and macaques.[5] After extensive testing, the current "gold standard" ART regimen for suppressing SIV replication in monkeys is a daily subcutaneous injection of tenofovir, emtricitabine, and dolutegravir.[78] Reverse transcriptase (RT)-SHIVs, in which the RT reading frame of SIV has been replaced with that of HIV-1, have been developed.[4,351] Macaques infected with these RT-SHIVs have been used to study the emergence of drug resistance mutations.[5,351] A minimally modified simian-tropic HIV-1 that replicates in pigtail macaques may also be useful for therapeutic studies in primate models.[305]

Early studies showed that treatment of SIV-infected monkeys with tenofovir (PMPA; R-9-2-phosphonylmethoxypropyl adenine) for 4 weeks starting at 24 hours after experimental SIV infection resulted in impressive virological control after discontinuing drug treatment.[206,348] Delaying the initiation of therapy to 48 or 72 hours, or shortening the duration of treatment, significantly reduced efficacy.[347] Interestingly, when three such animals off therapy for 6 weeks were subsequently challenged intravenously with SIVsmE660, one animal was completely protected, and the other two showed dramatic reductions in viral load.[207] What is most startling and difficult to understand is that protection was achieved in these animals in the absence of readily measurable SIV-specific antibody or cellular immune responses at the time of challenge. Continuation of this line of investigation could provide important insights into immune-mediated control outside the bounds of our current level of understanding.

A variety of gene therapy strategies for inhibiting lentiviral replication and depleting viral reservoirs are also being tested in nonhuman primate models. Recent approaches include editing of the *CCR5* gene in hematopoietic stem cells (HSCs)

and transduction of HSCs with chimeric antigen receptors (CARs).[17,41,397] These approaches rely on either the differentiation of HSCs into *CCR5*-deleted T cells that are resistant to HIV-1 and SHIV infection or into cytotoxic T lymphocytes expressing CARs that allow them to recognize and kill HIV-infected cells. Another promising gene therapy approach that is currently under investigation in macaque models is the use of AAV vectors for long-term delivery of potent broadly neutralizing antibodies.[223]

PERSPECTIVE

The global AIDS crisis brought on by HIV-1 has focused attention on nonhuman lentiviruses as a source of information that will shed light on the human condition. Lentiviral infections of domesticated animals are economically important in their own right and have been studied historically in this context. The lack of a practical animal model for infection with HIV-1 that recapitulates features of human infection has led to the extensive investigation of nonhuman lentiviruses in naturally or experimentally infected hosts as analog model systems. Critical areas for future progress include a better understanding of lentiviral pathogenesis, improvements in therapy, and perhaps most importantly, the development of a safe, effective, long-acting, and affordable vaccine or other preventative measure. The most remarkable feature of lentiviruses, and perhaps the most important for the eventual control of HIV-1, is their ability to replicate continuously and unrelentingly in the presence of strong immune responses. The advancement of therapeutic regimens and the development of effective vaccines against HIV-1 will ultimately need to deal with the propensity of this group of viruses to generate and tolerate genetic changes that enable the evasion of host immune responses.

REFERENCES

1. Alexander L, Du Z, Rosenzweig M, et al. A role for natural simian immunodeficiency virus and human immunodeficiency virus type 1 nef alleles in lymphocyte activation. *J Virol* 1997;71:6094–6099.
2. Alexander L, Illyinskii PO, Lang SM, et al. Determinants of increased replicative capacity of serially passaged simian immunodeficiency virus with nef deleted in rhesus monkeys. *J Virol* 2003;77:6823–6835.
3. Allan JS, Kanda P, Kennedy RC, et al. Isolation and characterization of simian immunodeficiency viruses from two subspecies of African green monkeys. *AIDS Res Hum Retroviruses* 1990;6:275–285.
4. Ambrose Z, Boltz V, Palmer S, et al. In vitro characterization of a simian immunodeficiency virus-human immunodeficiency virus (HIV) chimera expressing HIV type 1 reverse transcriptase to study antiviral resistance in pigtail macaques. *J Virol* 2004;78:13553–13561.
5. Ambrose Z, Palmer S, Boltz VF, et al. Suppression of viremia and evolution of human immunodeficiency virus type 1 drug resistance in a macaque model for antiretroviral therapy. *J Virol* 2007;81:12145–12155.
6. Andrews CD, Bernard LS, Poon AY, et al. Cabotegravir long acting injection protects macaques against intravenous challenge with SIVmac251. *AIDS* 2017;31:461–467.
7. Apetrei C, Kaur A, Lerche NW, et al. Molecular epidemiology of simian immunodeficiency virus SIVsm in U.S. primate centers unravels the origin of SIVmac and SIVstm. *J Virol* 2005;79:8991–9005.
8. Apps R, Del Prete GQ, Chatterjee P, et al. HIV-1 Vpu mediates HLA-C downregulation. *Cell Host Microbe* 2016;19:686–695.
9. Arias JF, Colomer-Lluch M, von Bredow B, et al. Tetherin Antagonism by HIV-1 Group M Nef Proteins. *J Virol* 2016;90:10701–10714.
10. Arias JF, Heyer LN, von Bredow B, et al. Tetherin antagonism by Vpu protects HIV-infected cells from antibody-dependent cell-mediated cytotoxicity. *Proc Natl Acad Sci U S A* 2014;111:6425–6430.
11. Arnold LH, Groom HC, Kunzelmann S, et al. Phospho-dependent Regulation of SAMHD1 Oligomerisation Couples Catalysis and Restriction. *PLoS Pathog* 2015;11:e1005194.
12. Arthur LO, Bess JW Jr, Sowder RC II, et al. Cellular proteins bound to immunodeficiency viruses: implications for pathogenesis and vaccines. *Science* 1992;258:1935–1938.
13. Arthur LO, Bess JW Jr, Urban RG, et al. Macaques immunized with HLA-DR are protected from SIV challenge. *J Virol* 1995;69:3117–3124.

14. Bailes E, Gao F, Bibollet-Ruche F, et al. Hybrid origin of SIV in chimpanzees. *Science* 2003;300:1713.
15. Baldauf HM, Pan X, Erikson E, et al. SAMHD1 restricts HIV-1 infection in resting CD4(+) T cells. *Nat Med* 2012;18:1682–1687.
16. Balliet JW, Kolson DL, Eiger G, et al. Distinct effects in primary macrophages and lymphocytes of the human immunodeficiency virus type 1 accessory genes vpr, vpu, and nef: mutational analysis of a primary HIV-1 isolate. *Virology* 1994;200:623–631.
17. Barber-Axthelm IM, Barber-Axthelm V, Sze KY, et al. Stem cell-derived CAR T cells traffic to HIV reservoirs in macaques. *JCI Insight* 2021;6(1):e141502.
18. Barre-Sinoussi F, Chermann JC, Rey F, et al. Isolation of a T-lymphotropic retrovirus from a patient at risk for acquired immune deficiency syndrome (AIDS). *Science* 1983;220:868–871.
19. Beaumier CM, Harris LD, Goldstein S, et al. CD4 downregulation by memory CD4+ T cells in vivo renders African green monkeys resistant to progressive SIVagm infection. *Nat Med* 2009;15:879–885.
20. Beer BE, Bailes E, Goeken R, et al. Simian immunodeficiency virus (SIV) from sun-tailed monkeys (Cercopithecus solatus): evidence for host-dependent evolution of SIV within the C. lhoesti superspecies. *J Virol* 1999;73:7734–7744.
21. Beer BE, Foley BT, Kuiken CL, et al. Characterization of novel simian immunodeficiency viruses from red-capped mangabeys from Nigeria (SIVrcmNG409 and -NG411). *J Virol* 2001;75:12014–12027.
22. Beisel CE, Edwards JF, Dunn LL, et al. Analysis of multiple mRNAs from pathogenic equine infectious anemia virus (EIAV) in an acutely infected horse reveals a novel protein, Ttm, derived from the carboxy terminus of the EIAV transmembrane protein. *J Virol* 1993;67:832–842.
23. Benveniste RE, Arthur LO, Tsai C-C, et al. Isolation of a lentivirus from a macaque with lymphoma: comparison with HTLV-III/LAV and other lentiviruses. *J Virol* 1986;60:483–490.
24. Berlioz-Torrent C, Shacklett BL, Erdtmann L, et al. Interactions of the cytoplasmic domains of human and simian retroviral transmembrane proteins with components of the clathrin adaptor complexes modulate intracellular and cell surface expression of envelope glycoproteins. *J Virol* 1999;73:1350–1361.
25. Betancor G, Dicks MDJ, Jimenez-Guardeno JM, et al. The GTPase domain of MX2 interacts with the HIV-1 capsid, enabling its short isoform to moderate antiviral restriction. *Cell Rep* 2019;29:1923–1933 e3.
26. Bhatia S, Sood R. Bovine immunodeficiency virus. In: Bayry J, ed. *Emerging and Re-emerging Infectious Diseases of Livestock*. Switzerland, Cham: Springer; 2017:301–308.
27. Bibollet-Ruche F, Bailes E, Gao F, et al. New simian immunodeficiency virus infecting De Brazza's monkeys (Cercopithecus neglectus): evidence for a cercopithecus monkey virus clade. *J Virol* 2004;78:7748–7762.
28. Bibollet-Ruche F, Galat-Luong A, Cuny G, et al. Simian immunodeficiency virus infection in a patas monkey (Erythrocebus patas): evidence for cross-species transmission from African green monkeys (Cercopithecus aethiops sabaeus) in the wild. *J Gen Virol* 1996;77:773–781.
29. Bishop KN, Holmes RK, Sheehy AM, et al. Cytidine deamination of retroviral DNA by diverse APOBEC proteins. *Curr Biol* 2004;14:1392–1396.
30. Bogerd HP, Doehle BP, Wiegand HL, et al. A single amino acid difference in the host APOBEC3G protein controls the primate species specificity of HIV type 1 virion infectivity factor. *Proc Natl Acad Sci U S A* 2004;101:3770–3774.
31. Bogerd HP, Wiegand HL, Bieniasz PD, et al. Functional differences between human and bovine immunodeficiency virus tat transcription factors. *J Virol* 2000;74:4666–4671.
32. Borrow P, Lewicki H, Wei X, et al. Antiviral pressure exerted by HIV-1-specific cytotoxic T lymphocytes (CTLs) during primary infection demonstrated by rapid selection of CTL escape virus. *Nat Med* 1997;3:205–211.
33. Bouhamdan M, Benichou S, Rey F, et al. Human immunodeficiency virus type 1 Vpr protein binds to the uracil DNA glycosylase DNA repair enzyme. *J Virol* 1996;70:697–704.
34. Brenchley JM, Price DA, Schacker TW, et al. Microbial translocation is a cause of systemic immune activation in chronic HIV infection. *Nat Med* 2006;12:1365–1371.
35. Brenchley JM, Schacker TW, Ruff LE, et al. CD4+ T cell depletion during all stages of HIV disease occurs predominantly in the gastrointestinal tract. *J Exp Med* 2004;200:749–759.
36. Broussard SR, Staprans SI, White R, et al. Simian immunodeficiency virus replicates to high levels in naturally infected African green monkeys without inducing immunologic or neurologic disease. *J Virol* 2001;75:2262–2275.
37. Buffalo CZ, Sturzel CM, Heusinger E, et al. Structural basis for tetherin antagonism as a barrier to zoonotic lentiviral transmission. *Cell Host Microbe* 2019;26:359–368 e8.
38. Burns D, Collignon, C, Desrosiers, RC. Simian immunodeficiency virus mutants resistant to serum neutralization arise during persistent infection of rhesus monkeys. *J Virol* 1993;67:4104–4113.
39. Busnadiego I, Kane M, Rihn SJ, et al. Host and viral determinants of Mx2 antiretroviral activity. *J Virol* 2014;88:7738–7752.
40. Campbell R, Robinson, WF. The comparative pathology of the lentiviruses. *J Comp Pathol* 1998;119:333–395.
41. Cardozo-Ojeda EF, Duke ER, Peterson CW, et al. Thresholds for post-rebound SHIV control after CCR5 gene-edited autologous hematopoietic cell transplantation. *Elife* 2021;10:e57646.
42. Carpenter MA, Brown EW, Culver M, et al. Genetic and phylogenetic divergence of feline immunodeficiency virus in the puma (Puma concolor). *J Virol* 1996;70:6682–6693.
43. Chadwick BJ, Coelen RJ, Wilcox GE, et al. Nucleotide sequence analysis of Jembrana disease virus: a bovine lentivirus associated with an acute disease syndrome. *J Gen Virol* 1995;76:1637–1650.
44. Chahroudi A, Bosinger SE, Vanderford TH, et al. Natural SIV hosts: showing AIDS the door. *Science* 2012;335:1188–1193.
45. Chande A, Cuccurullo EC, Rosa A, et al. S2 from equine infectious anemia virus is an infectivity factor which counteracts the retroviral inhibitors SERINC5 and SERINC3. *Proc Natl Acad Sci U S A* 2016;113:13197–13202.
46. Chatterji U, de Parseval A, Elder JH. Feline immunodeficiency virus OrfA is distinct from other lentivirus transactivators. *J Virol* 2002;76:9624–9634.
47. Chen YC, Sood C, Marin M, et al. Super-resolution fluorescence imaging reveals that serine incorporator protein 5 inhibits human immunodeficiency virus fusion by disrupting envelope glycoprotein clusters. *ACS Nano* 2020;14:10929–10943.
48. Chen Z, Kwon D, Jin Z, et al. Natural infection of a homozygous delta24 CCR5 red-capped mangabey with an R2b tropic simian immunodeficiency virus. *J Exp Med* 1998;188:2057–2065.
49. Chen Z, Luckay A, Sodora DL, et al. Human immunodeficiency virus type 2 (HIV-2) seroprevalence and characterization of a distinct HIV-2 genetic subtype from the natural range of simian immunodeficiency virus-infected sooty mangabeys. *J Virol* 1997;71:3953–3960.
50. Chertova E, Bess JW Jr, Crise BJ, et al. Envelope glycoprotein incorporation, not shedding of surface envelope glycoprotein (gp120/SU), is the primary determinant of SU content of purified human immunodeficiency virus type 1 and simian immunodeficiency virus. *J Virol* 2002;76:5315–5325.
51. Chougui G, Munir-Matloob S, Matkovic R, et al. HIV-2/SIV viral protein X counteracts HUSH repressor complex. *Nat Microbiol* 2018;3:891–897.
52. Clavel F, Guetaro D, Brun-Vezinet F, et al. Isolation of a new human retrovirus from West African patients with AIDS. *Science* 1986;233:343–346.
53. Clewley JP, Lewis JC, Brown DW, et al. A novel simian immunodeficiency virus (SIVdrl) pol sequence from the drill monkey, Mandrillus leucophaeus. *J Virol* 1998;72:10305–10309.
54. Cohen GB, Gandhi RT, Davis DM, et al. The selective downregulation of class I major histocompatibility complex proteins by HIV-1 protects HIV-infected cells from NK cells. *Immunity* 1999;10:661–671.
55. Collins KL, Chen BK, Kalams SA, et al. HIV-1 Nef protein protects infected primary cells against killing by cytotoxic T lymphocytes. *Nature* 1998;391:397–401.
56. Compton AA, Hirsch VM, Emerman M. The host restriction factor APOBEC3G and retroviral Vif protein coevolve due to ongoing genetic conflict. *Cell Host Microbe* 2012;11:91–98.
57. Connor RI, Chen BK, Choe S, et al. Vpr is required for efficient replication of human immunodeficiency virus type-1 in mononuclear phagocytes. *Virology* 1995;206:935–944.
58. Cook RF, Leroux C, Cook SJ, et al. Development and characterization of an in vivo pathogenic molecular clone of equine infectious anemia virus. *J Virol* 1998;72:1383–1393.
59. Courgnaud V, Abela B, Pourrut X, et al. Identification of a new simian immunodeficiency virus lineage with a vpu gene present among different cercopithecus monkeys (C. mona, C. cephus, and C. nictitans) from Cameroon. *J Virol* 2003;77:12523–12534.
60. Courgnaud V, Formenty P, Akoua-Koffi C, et al. Partial molecular characterization of two simian immunodeficiency viruses (SIV) from African colobids: SIVwrc from Western red colobus (Piliocolobus badius) and SIVolc from olive colobus (Procolobus verus). *J Virol* 2003;77:744–748.
61. Courgnaud V, Pourrut X, Bibollet-Ruche F, et al. Characterization of a novel simian immunodeficiency virus from guereza colobus monkeys (Colobus guereza) in Cameroon: a new lineage in the nonhuman primate lentivirus family. *J Virol* 2001;75:857–866.
62. Courgnaud V, Salemi M, Pourrut X, et al. Characterization of a novel simian immunodeficiency virus with a vpu gene from greater spot-nosed monkeys (Cercopithecus nictitans) provides new insights into simian/human immunodeficiency virus phylogeny. *J Virol* 2002;76:8298–8309.
63. Cranage MP, Ashworth LAE, Greenaway PJ, et al. AIDS vaccine developments. *Nature* 1992;355:684–686.
64. Cranage MP, Polyanskaya N, McBride B, et al. Studies on the specificity of the vaccine effect elicited by inactivated simian immunodeficiency virus. *AIDS Res Hum Retroviruses* 1993;9:13–22.
65. Cui J, Holmes EC. Endogenous lentiviruses in the ferret genome. *J Virol* 2012;86:3383–3385.
66. Daniel M, Letvin N, Sehgal P, et al. Prevalence of antibodies to 3 retroviruses in a captive colony of macaque monkeys. *Int J Cancer* 1988;41:601–608.
67. Daniel MD, Kirchhoff F, Czajak SC, et al. Protective effects of a live-attenuated SIV vaccine with a deletion in the *nef* gene. *Science* 1992;258:1938–1941.
68. Daniel MD, Letvin NL, King NW, et al. Isolation of T-cell tropic HTLV-III-like retrovirus from macaques. *Science* 1985;228:1201–1204.
69. D'Arc M, Ayouba A, Esteban A, et al. Origin of the HIV-1 group O epidemic in western lowland gorillas. *Proc Natl Acad Sci U S A* 2015;112:E1343–E1352.
70. Dazza MC, Ekwalanga M, Nende M, et al. Characterization of a novel vpu-harboring simian immunodeficiency virus from a Dent's Mona monkey (Cercopithecus mona denti). *J Virol* 2005;79:8560–8571.
71. de Parseval A, Chatterji U, Morris G, et al. Structural mapping of CD134 residues critical for interaction with feline immunodeficiency virus. *Nat Struct Mol Biol* 2005;12:60–66.
72. de Parseval A, Chatterji U, Sun P, et al. Feline immunodeficiency virus targets activated CD4+ T cells by using CD134 as a binding receptor. *Proc Natl Acad Sci U S A* 2004;101:13044–13049.
73. de Parseval A, Elder, JH. Demonstration that orf2 encodes the feline immunodeficiency virus transactivating (Tat) protein and characterization of a unique gene product with partial rev activity. *J Virol* 1999;73:608–617.
74. de Rozieres S, Mathiason CK, Rolston MR, et al. Characterization of a highly pathogenic molecular clone of feline immunodeficiency virus clade C. *J Virol* 2004;78:8971–8982.
75. de Sousa-Pereira P, Abrantes J, Bauernfried S, et al. The antiviral activity of rodent and lagomorph SERINC3 and SERINC5 is counteracted by known viral antagonists. *J Gen Virol* 2019;100:278–288.
76. Deacon NJ, Tsykin A, Solomon A, et al. Genomic structure of an attenuated quasi species of HIV-1 from a blood transfusion donor and recipients. *Science* 1995;270:988–991.
77. DeGottardi MQ, Specht A, Metcalf B, et al. Selective downregulation of rhesus macaque and sooty mangabey major histocompatibility complex class I molecules by Nef alleles of simian immunodeficiency virus and human immunodeficiency virus type 2. *J Virol* 2008;82:3139–3146.
78. Del Prete GQ, Smedley J, Macallister R, et al. Short communication: comparative evaluation of coformulated injectable combination antiretroviral therapy regimens in simian immunodeficiency virus-infected rhesus Macaques. *AIDS Res Hum Retroviruses* 2016;32:163–168.
79. Desrosiers RC. HIV-1 origins: A finger on the missing link. *Nature* 1990;345:288–289.
80. Desrosiers RC, Lifson JD, Gibbs JS, et al. Identification of highly attenuated mutants of simian immunodeficiency virus. *J Virol* 1998;72:1431–1437.
81. Desrosiers RC, Wyand MS, Kodama T, et al. Vaccine protection against simian immunodeficiency virus infection. *Proc Natl Acad Sci U S A* 1989;86:6353–6357.

82. Dewhurst S, Embretson JE, Anderson DC, et al. Sequence analysis and acute pathogenicity of molecularly cloned SIV$_{smmPBj14}$. *Nature* 1990;345:636–640.

83. Dharma DM, Budiantono A, Campbell RS, et al. Studies on experimental Jembrana disease in Bali cattle. III. Pathology. *J Comp Pathol* 1991;105:397–414.

84. Dicks MDJ, Betancor G, Jimenez-Guardeno JM, et al. Multiple components of the nuclear pore complex interact with the amino-terminus of MX2 to facilitate HIV-1 restriction. *PLoS Pathog* 2018;14:e1007408.

85. Douek DC, Brenchley JM, Betts MR, et al. HIV preferentially infects HIV-specific CD4+ T cells. *Nature* 2002;417:95–98.

86. Dow SW, Poss ML, Hoover EA. Feline immunodeficiency virus: a neurotropic lentivirus. *J Acquir Immune Defic Syndr* 1990;3:658–668.

87. Du Z, Lang SM, Sasseville VG, et al. Identification of a *nef* allele that causes lymphocyte activation and acute disease in macaque monkeys. *Cell* 1995;82:665–674.

88. Duverger A, Wolschendorf F, Zhang M, et al. An AP-1 binding site in the enhancer/core element of the HIV-1 promoter controls the ability of HIV-1 to establish latent infection. *J Virol* 2013;87:2264–2277.

89. Elder JH, Lerner DL, Hasselkus-Light CS, et al. Distinct subsets of retroviruses encode dUTPase. *J Virol* 1992;66:1791–1794.

90. Elliott ST, Wetzel KS, Francella N, et al. Dualtropic CXCR6/CCR5 simian immunodeficiency virus (SIV) infection of sooty mangabey primary lymphocytes: distinct coreceptor use in natural versus pathogenic hosts of SIV. *J Virol* 2015;89:9252–9261.

91. Emau P, McClure HM, Isahakia M, et al. Isolation from African Sykes' monkeys (Cercopithecus mitis) of a lentivirus related to human and simian immunodeficiency viruses. *J Virol* 1991;65:2135–2140.

92. Etienne L, Nerrienet E, LeBreton M, et al. Characterization of a new simian immunodeficiency virus strain in a naturally infected Pan troglodytes troglodytes chimpanzee with AIDS related symptoms. *Retrovirology* 2011;8:4.

93. Evans DT, O'Connor DH, Jing P, et al. Virus-specific cytotoxic T-lymphocyte responses select for amino acid variation in simian immunodeficiency virus Env and Nef. *Nat Med* 1999;5:1270–1276.

94. Ficarelli M, Wilson H, Pedro Galao R, et al. KHNYN is essential for the zinc finger antiviral protein (ZAP) to restrict HIV-1 containing clustered CpG dinucleotides. *Elife* 2019;8:e46767.

95. Fitzpatrick K, Skasko M, Deerinck TJ, et al. Direct restriction of virus release and incorporation of the interferon-induced protein BST-2 into HIV-1 particles. *PLoS Pathog* 2010;6:e1000701.

96. Fuchs SP, Martinez-Navio JM, Piatak M Jr, et al. AAV-delivered antibody mediates significant protective effects against SIVmac239 challenge in the absence of neutralizing activity. *PLoS Pathog* 2015;11:e1005090.

97. Fukasawa M, Muira T, Hasegawa A, et al. Sequence of simian immunodeficiency virus from African green monkey, a new member of the HIV/SIV group. *Nature* 1988;333:457–461.

98. Fukazawa Y, Park H, Cameron MJ, et al. Lymph node T cell responses predict the efficacy of live attenuated SIV vaccines. *Nat Med* 2012;18:1673–1681.

99. Fultz PN. Replication of an acutely lethal simian immunodeficiency virus activates and induces proliferation of lymphocytes. *J Virol* 1991;65:4902–4909.

100. Fultz PN, McClure HM, Anderson DC, et al. Isolation of a T-lymphotropic retrovirus from naturally infected sooty mangabey monkeys (Cercocebus atys). *Proc Natl Acad Sci U S A* 1986;83:5286–5290.

101. Fultz PN, McClure HM, Anderson DC, et al. Identification and biologic characterization of an acutely lethal variant of simian immunodeficiency virus from sooty mangabeys (SIV/SMM). *AIDS Res Hum Retroviruses* 1989;5:397–409.

102. Galao RP, Pickering S, Curnock R, et al. Retroviral retention activates a Syk-dependent HemITAM in human tetherin. *Cell Host Microbe* 2014;16:291–303.

103. Ganser-Pornillos BK, Pornillos O. Restriction of HIV-1 and other retroviruses by TRIM5. *Nat Rev Microbiol* 2019;17:546–556.

104. Gao F, Yue L, White AT, et al. Human infection by genetically diverse SIVsm-related HIV-2 in west Africa. *Nature* 1992;358:495–499.

105. Gao G, Guo X, Goff SP. Inhibition of retroviral RNA production by ZAP, a CCCH-type zinc finger protein. *Science* 2002;297:1703–1706.

106. Gardner MR, Kattenhorn LM, Kondur HR, et al. AAV-expressed eCD4-Ig provides durable protection from multiple SHIV challenges. *Nature* 2015;519:87–91.

107. Gauduin MC, Yu Y, Barabasz A, et al. Induction of a virus-specific effector-memory CD4+ T cell response by attenuated SIV infection. *J Exp Med* 2006;203:2661–2672.

108. Gemeniano MC, Sawai ET, Sparger EE. Feline immunodeficiency virus Orf-A localizes to the nucleus and induces cell cycle arrest. *Virology* 2004;325:167–174.

109. Gendelman HE, Narayan O, Kennedy-Stoskopf S, et al. Tropism of sheep lentiviruses for monocytes: susceptibility to infection and virus gene expression increase during maturation of monocytes to macrophages. *J Virol* 1986;58:67–74.

110. Gibbs JS, Lackner AA, Lang SM, et al. Progression to AIDS in the absence of genes for vpr or vpx. *J Virol* 1995;69:2378–2383.

111. Gifford RJ, Katzourakis A, Tristem M, et al. A transitional endogenous lentivirus from the genome of a basal primate and implications for lentivirus evolution. *Proc Natl Acad Sci U S A* 2008;105:20362–20367.

112. Gilbert C, Maxfield DG, Goodman SM, et al. Parallel germline infiltration of a lentivirus in two Malagasy lemurs. *PLoS Genet* 2009;5:e1000425.

113. Glushakova S, Grivel JC, Suryanarayana K, et al. Nef enhances human immunodeficiency virus replication and responsiveness to interleukin-2 in human lymphoid tissue ex vivo. *J Virol* 1999;73:3968–3974.

114. Goldstein S, Ourmanov I, Brown CR, et al. Wide range of viral load in healthy African green monkeys naturally infected with simian immunodeficiency virus. *J Virol* 2000;74:11744–11753.

115. Goldstone DC, Ennis-Adeniran V, Hedden JJ, et al. HIV-1 restriction factor SAMHD1 is a deoxynucleoside triphosphate triphosphohydrolase. *Nature* 2011;480:379–382.

116. Gonda M. The lentiviruses of cattle. In: Levy JA, ed. *Retroviridae*. New York: Plenum Press; 1994.

117. Gonda MA, Braun MJ, Carter SG, et al. Characterization and molecular cloning of a bovine lentivirus related to human immunodeficiency virus. *Nature* 1987;330:388–391.

118. Gonda MA, Charman HP, Walker JL, et al. Scanning and transmission electron microscopic study of equine infectious anemia virus. *Am J Vet Res* 1978;39:731–740.

119. Gonda MA, Wong-Staal F, Gallo RC, et al. Sequence homology and morphologic similarity of HTLV-III and visna virus, a pathogenic lentivirus. *Science* 1985;227:173–177.

120. Gonzalez-Nieto L, Castro IM, Bischof GF, et al. Vaccine protection against rectal acquisition of SIVmac239 in rhesus macaques. *PLoS Pathog* 2019;15:e1008015.

121. Goodier JL, Pereira GC, Cheung LE, et al. The broad-spectrum antiviral protein ZAP restricts human retrotransposition. *PLoS Genet* 2015;11:e1005252.

122. Gotz N, Sauter D, Usmani SM, et al. Reacquisition of Nef-mediated tetherin antagonism in a single in vivo passage of HIV-1 through its original chimpanzee host. *Cell Host Microbe* 2012;12:373–380.

123. Goujon C, Moncorge O, Bauby H, et al. Human MX2 is an interferon-induced post-entry inhibitor of HIV-1 infection. *Nature* 2013;502:559–562.

124. Gray GE, Bekker LG, Laher F, et al. Vaccine efficacy of ALVAC-HIV and bivalent subtype C gp120-MF59 in adults. *N Engl J Med* 2021;384:1089–1100.

125. Greenough T, Sullivan JL, Desrosiers RC. Declining CD4 T-cell counts in a person infected with *nef*-deleted HIV-1. *N Engl J Med* 1999;340:236–237.

126. Gudnadottir M, Palsson PA. Transmission of maedi by inoculation of a virus grown in tissue culture from maedi-affected lungs. *J Infect Dis* 1967;117:1–6.

127. Hammonds J, Wang JJ, Yi H, et al. Immunoelectron microscopic evidence for Tetherin/BST2 as the physical bridge between HIV-1 virions and the plasma membrane. *PLoS Pathog* 2010;6:e1000749.

128. Han GZ, Worobey M. Endogenous lentiviral elements in the weasel family (Mustelidae). *Mol Biol Evol* 2012;29:2905–2908.

129. Han GZ, Worobey M. A primitive endogenous lentivirus in a colugo: insights into the early evolution of lentiviruses. *Mol Biol Evol* 2015;32:211–215.

130. Hansen SG, Ford JC, Lewis MS, et al. Profound early control of highly pathogenic SIV by an effector memory T-cell vaccine. *Nature* 2011;473:523–527.

131. Hansen SG, Marshall EE, Malouli D, et al. A live-attenuated RhCMV/SIV vaccine shows long-term efficacy against heterologous SIV challenge. *Sci Transl Med* 2019;11(501):eaaw2607.

132. Harris RS, Bishop KN, Sheehy AM, et al. DNA deamination mediates innate immunity to retroviral infection. *Cell* 2003;113:803–809.

133. Harris RS, Sheehy AM, Craig HM, et al. DNA deamination: not just a trigger for antibody diversification but also a mechanism for defense against retroviruses. *Nat Immunol* 2003;4:641–643.

134. Hatziioannou T, Del Prete GQ, Keele BF, et al. HIV-1-induced AIDS in monkeys. *Science* 2014;344:1401–1405.

135. Hatziioannou T, Evans DT. Animal models for HIV/AIDS research. *Nat Rev Microbiol* 2012;10:852–867.

136. Hatziioannou T, Perez-Caballero D, Yang A, et al. Retrovirus resistance factors Ref1 and Lv1 are species-specific variants of TRIM5alpha. *Proc Natl Acad Sci U S A* 2004;101:10774–10779.

137. Heigele A, Kmiec D, Regensburger K, et al. The potency of Nef-mediated SERINC5 antagonism correlates with the prevalence of primate lentiviruses in the wild. *Cell Host Microbe* 2016;20:381–391.

138. Hirsch V, Adger-Johnson D, Campbell B, et al. A molecularly cloned, pathogenic, neutralization-resistant simian immunodeficiency virus, SIVsmE543-3. *J Virol* 1997;71:1608–1620.

139. Hirsch VM, Campbell BJ, Bailes E, et al. Characterization of a novel simian immunodeficiency virus (SIV) from L'Hoest monkeys (Cercopithecus l'hoesti): implications for the origins of SIVmnd and other primate lentiviruses. *J Virol* 1999;73:1036–1045.

140. Hirsch VM, Dapolito G, Johnson PR, et al. Induction of AIDS by simian immunodeficiency virus from an African green monkey: species-specific variation in pathogenicity correlates with the extent of in vivo replication. *J Virol* 1995;69:955–967.

141. Hirsch VM, Dapolito GA, Goldstein S, et al. A distinct African lentivirus from Sykes' monkeys. *J Virol* 1993;67:1517–1528.

142. Hirsch VM, Olmsted RA, Murphey-Corb M, et al. An African primate lentivirus (SIVsm) closely related to HIV-2. *Nature* 1989;339:389–392.

143. Ho DD, Neuman AU, Perelson AS, et al. Rapid turnover of plasma virions and CD4 lymphocytes in HIV-1 infection. *Nature* 1995;373:123–126.

144. Hong Y, Fink E, Hu QY, et al. OrfA downregulates feline immunodeficiency virus primary receptor CD134 on the host cell surface and is important in viral infection. *J Virol* 2010;84:7225–7232.

145. Hosie MJ, Broere N, Hesselgesser J, et al. Modulation of feline immunodeficiency virus infection by stromal cell-derived factor. *J Virol* 1998;72:2097–2104.

146. Howe AY, Jung JU, Desrosiers RC. Zeta chain of the T-cell receptor interacts with nef of simian immunodeficiency virus and human Immunodeficiency virus type 2. *J Virol* 1998;72:9827–9834.

147. Hrecka K, Gierszewska M, Srivastava S, et al. Lentiviral Vpr usurps Cul4-DDB1[VprBP] E3 ubiquitin ligase to modulate cell cycle. *Proc Natl Acad Sci U S A* 2007;104:11778–11783.

148. Hrecka K, Hao C, Gierszewska M, et al. Vpx relieves inhibition of HIV-1 infection of macrophages mediated by the SAMHD1 protein. *Nature* 2011;474:658–661.

149. Hrecka K, Hao C, Shun MC, et al. HIV-1 and HIV-2 exhibit divergent interactions with HLTF and UNG2 DNA repair proteins. *Proc Natl Acad Sci U S A* 2016;113:E3921–E3930.

150. Hu J, Switzer WM, Foley BT, et al. Characterization and comparison of recombinant simian immunodeficiency virus from drill (Mandrillus leucophaeus) and mandrill (Mandrillus sphinx) isolates. *J Virol* 2003;77:4867–4880.

151. Hultquist JF, Lengyel JA, Refsland EW, et al. Human and rhesus APOBEC3D, APOBEC3F, APOBEC3G, and APOBEC3H demonstrate a conserved capacity to restrict Vif-deficient HIV-1. *J Virol* 2011;85:11220–11234.

152. Ilyinskii PO, Desrosiers RC. Efficient transcription and replication of simian immunodeficiency virus in the absence of NF-kB and Sp1 binding elements. *J Virol* 1996;70:3118–3126.

153. Ilyinskii PO, Daniel MD, Simon MA, et al. The role of upstream U3 sequences in the pathogenesis of simian immunodeficiency virus-induced AIDS in rhesus monkeys. *J Virol* 1994;68:5933–5944.

154. Ilyinskii PO, Simon MA, Czajak SC, et al. Induction of AIDS by simian immunodeficiency virus lacking NF-kB and SP1 binding elements. *J Virol* 1997;71:1880–1887.

155. Issel C, Foil, LD. Studies on equine infectious anemia virus transmission by insects. *J Am Vet Med Assoc* 1984;184:293–297.

156. Jia B, Serra-Moreno R, Neidermyer W, et al. Species-specific activity of SIV Nef and HIV-1 Vpu in overcoming restriction by tetherin/BST2. *PLoS Pathog* 2009;5:e1000429.

157. Jia X, Singh R, Homann S, et al. Structural basis of evasion of cellular adaptive immunity by HIV-1 Nef. *Nat Struct Mol Biol* 2012;19:701–706.

158. Jin MJ, Rogers J, Phillips-Conroy JE, et al. Infection of a yellow baboon with simian immunodeficiency virus from African green monkeys: evidence for cross-species transmission in the wild. *J Virol* 1994;68:8454–8460.

159. Johnson PR, Schnepp BC, Zhang J, et al. Vector-mediated gene transfer engenders long-lived neutralizing activity and protection against SIV infection in monkeys. *Nat Med* 2009;15:901–906.

160. Johnson RP, Lifson JD, Czajak SC, et al. Highly attenuated vaccine strains of simian immunodeficiency virus protect against vaginal challenge: inverse relation of degree of protection with level of attenuation. *J Virol* 1999;73:4952–4961.

161. Jones T, Hunt RD, King NW. Diseases caused by viruses. In: Cann C, ed. *Veterinary Pathology*. Baltimore, MD: Lippincott Williams & Wilkins; 1997:197–370.

162. Joseph SB, Swanstrom R. The evolution of HIV-1 entry phenotypes as a guide to changing target cells. *J Leukoc Biol* 2018;103:421–431.

163. Julien JP, Cupo A, Sok D, et al. Crystal structure of a soluble cleaved HIV-1 envelope trimer. *Science* 2013;342:1477–1483.

164. Kane M, Rebensburg SV, Takata MA, et al. Nuclear pore heterogeneity influences HIV-1 infection and the antiviral activity of MX2. *Elife* 2018;7:e35738.

165. Kane M, Yadav SS, Bitzegeio J, et al. MX2 is an interferon-induced inhibitor of HIV-1 infection. *Nature* 2013;502:563–566.

166. Katzourakis A, Tristem M, Pybus OG, et al. Discovery and analysis of the first endogenous lentivirus. *Proc Natl Acad Sci U S A* 2007;104:6261–6265.

167. Kaur A, Grant RM, Means RE, et al. Diverse host responses and outcomes following simian immunodeficiency virus SIVmac239 infection in sooty mangabeys and rhesus macaques. *J Virol* 1998;72:9597–9611.

168. Keele BF, Van Heuverswyn F, Li Y, et al. Chimpanzee reservoirs of pandemic and nonpandemic HIV-1. *Science* 2006;313:523–526.

169. Kerns JA, Emerman M, Malik HS. Positive selection and increased antiviral activity associated with the PARP-containing isoform of human zinc-finger antiviral protein. *PLoS Genet* 2008;4:e21.

170. Kertayadnya G, Wilcox GE, Soeharsono S, et al. Characteristics of a retrovirus associated with Jembrana disease in Bali cattle. *J Gen Virol* 1993;74:1765–1778.

171. Kestler H, Kodama T, Ringler D, et al. Induction of AIDS in rhesus monkeys by molecularly cloned simian immunodeficiency virus. *Science* 1990;248:1109–1112.

172. Kestler HW III, Ringler DJ, Mori K, et al. Importance of the *nef* gene for maintenance of high virus loads and for the development of AIDS. *Cell* 1991;65:651–662.

173. Khabbaz RF, Heneine W, George JR, et al. Brief report: infection of a laboratory worker with simian immunodeficiency virus. *N Engl J Med* 1994;330:172–177.

174. Kirchhoff F, Greenough TC, Brettler DB, et al. Absence of intact *nef* sequences in a long-term survivor with nonprogressive HIV-1 infection. *N Engl J Med* 1995;332:228–232.

175. Kirchhoff F, Kestler HW III, Desrosiers RC. Upstream U3 sequences in simian immunodeficiency virus are selectively deleted in vivo in the absence of an intact *nef* gene. *J Virol* 1994;68:2031–2037.

176. Kirmaier A, Wu F, Newman RM, et al. TRIM5 suppresses cross-species transmission of a primate immunodeficiency virus and selects for emergence of resistant variants in the new species. *PLoS Biol* 2010;8(8):e1000462.

177. Kirschman J, Qi M, Ding L, et al. HIV-1 envelope glycoprotein trafficking through the endosomal recycling compartment is required for particle incorporation. *J Virol* 2018;92(5):e01893-17.

178. Kluge SF, Mack K, Iyer SS, et al. Nef proteins of epidemic HIV-1 group O strains antagonize human tetherin. *Cell Host Microbe* 2014;16:639–650.

179. Klumpp SA, Novembre FJ, Anderson DC, et al. Clinical and pathologic findings in infant rhesus macaques infected with SIVsmm by maternal transmission. *J Med Primatol* 1993;22:169–176.

180. Kobayashi K. Studies on the cultivation of equine infectious anemia virus *in vitro*. I. Serial cultivation of the virus in the culture of various horse tissues. *Virus* 1961;11:177–189.

181. Kodama T, Silva DP, Daniel MD, et al. Prevalence of antibodies to SIV in baboons in their native habitat. *AIDS Res Hum Retroviruses* 1989;5(3):337–343.

182. Kodama T, Wooley DP, Naidu YM, et al. Significance of premature stop codons in env of simian immunodeficiency virus. *J Virol* 1989;63:4709–4714.

183. Kraus G, Werner A, Baier M, et al. Isolation of human immunodeficiency virus-related simian immunodeficiency viruses from African green monkeys. *Proc Natl Acad Sci U S A* 1989;86:2892–2896.

184. Kupzig S, Korolchuk V, Rollason R, et al. Bst-2/HM1.24 is a raft-associated apical membrane protein with an unusual topology. *Traffic* 2003;4:694–709.

185. Kwon Y, Kaake RM, Echeverria I, et al. Structural basis of CD4 downregulation by HIV-1 Nef. *Nat Struct Mol Biol* 2020;27:822–828.

186. Kwong PD, Doyle ML, Casper DJ, et al. HIV-1 evades antibody-mediated neutralization through conformational masking of receptor-binding sites. *Nature* 2002;420:678–682.

187. Lackner A, Vogel P, Ramos R, et al. Early events in tissues during infection with pathogenic (SIVmac239) and nonpathogenic (SIVmac1A11) molecular clones of SIV. *Am J Pathol* 1994;145:428–439.

188. Laguette N, Bregnard C, Hue P, et al. Premature activation of the SLX4 complex by Vpr promotes G2/M arrest and escape from innate immune sensing. *Cell* 2014;156:134–145.

189. Laguette N, Sobhian B, Casartelli N, et al. SAMHD1 is the dendritic- and myeloid-cell-specific HIV-1 restriction factor counteracted by Vpx. *Nature* 2011;474:654–657.

190. LaRue RS, Jonsson SR, Silverstein KA, et al. The artiodactyl APOBEC3 innate immune repertoire shows evidence for a multi-functional domain organization that existed in the ancestor of placental mammals. *BMC Mol Biol* 2008;9:104.

191. Le Rouzic E, Belaidouni N, Estrabaud E, et al. HIV1 Vpr arrests the cell cycle by recruiting DCAF1/VprBP, a receptor of the Cul4-DDB1 ubiquitin ligase. *Cell Cycle* 2007;6:182–188.

192. Le Tortorec A, Neil SJ. Antagonism to and intracellular sequestration of human tetherin by the human immunodeficiency virus type 2 envelope glycoprotein. *J Virol* 2009;83:11966–11978.

193. Learmont JC, Geczy AF, Mills J, et al. Immunologic and virologic status after 14 to 18 years of infection with an attenuated strain of HIV-1. A report from the Sydney Blood Bank Cohort. *N Engl J Med* 1999;340:1715–1722.

194. Lecossier D, Bouchonnet F, Clavel F, et al. Hypermutation of HIV-1 DNA in the absence of the Vif protein. *Science* 2003;300:1112.

195. Lee CA, Beasley E, Sundar K, et al. Simian immunodeficiency virus-infected memory CD4(+) T cells infiltrate to the site of infected macrophages in the neuroparenchyma of a chronic macaque model of neurological complications of AIDS. *mBio* 2020;11:e00602-20.

196. Leendertz SA, Locatelli S, Boesch C, et al. No evidence for transmission of SIVwrc from western red colobus monkeys (Piliocolobus badius badius) to wild West African chimpanzees (Pan troglodytes verus) despite high exposure through hunting. *BMC Microbiol* 2011;11:24.

197. Lemey P, Pybus OG, Wang B, et al. Tracing the origin and history of the HIV-2 epidemic. *Proc Natl Acad Sci U S A* 2003;100:6588–6592.

198. Lerner DL, Wagaman PC, Phillips TR, et al. Increased mutation frequency of feline immunodeficiency virus lacking functional deoxyuridine-triphosphatase. *Proc Natl Acad Sci U S A* 1995;92:7480–7484.

199. Li F, Leroux C, Craigo JK, et al. The S2 gene of equine infectious anemia virus is a highly conserved determinant of viral replication and virulence properties in experimentally infected ponies. *J Virol* 2000;74:573–579.

200. Li F, Puffer BA, Montelaro RC. The S2 gene of equine infectious anemia virus is dispensable for viral replication in vitro. *J Virol* 1998;72:8344–8348.

201. Li H, Wang S, Kong R, et al. Envelope residue 375 substitutions in simian-human immunodeficiency viruses enhance CD4 binding and replication in rhesus macaques. *Proc Natl Acad Sci U S A* 2016;113:E3413–E3422.

202. Li MM, Lau Z, Cheung P, et al. TRIM25 enhances the antiviral action of Zinc-Finger Antiviral Protein (ZAP). *PLoS Pathog* 2017;13:e1006145.

203. Li Y, Ndjango JB, Learn GH, et al. Eastern chimpanzees, but not bonobos, represent a simian immunodeficiency virus reservoir. *J Virol* 2012;86:10776–10791.

204. Lichtenstein DL, Rushlow KE, Cook RF, et al. Replication in vitro and in vivo of an equine infectious anemia virus mutant deficient in dUTPase activity. *J Virol* 1995;69:2881–2888.

205. Liddament MT, Brown WL, Schumacher AJ, et al. APOBEC3F properties and hypermutation preferences indicate activity against HIV-1 in vivo. *Curr Biol* 2004;14:1385–1391.

206. Lifson JD, Rossio JL, Arnaout R, et al. Containment of simian immunodeficiency virus infection: cellular immune responses and protection from rechallenge following transient postinoculation antiretroviral treatment. *J Virol* 2000;74:2584–2593.

207. Lifson JD, Rossio JL, Piatak M Jr, et al. Role of CD8(+) lymphocytes in control of simian immunodeficiency virus infection and resistance to rechallenge after transient early antiretroviral treatment. *J Virol* 2001;75:10187–10199.

208. Lim ES, Fregoso OI, McCoy CO, et al. The ability of primate lentiviruses to degrade the monocyte restriction factor SAMHD1 preceded the birth of the viral accessory protein Vpx. *Cell Host Microbe* 2012;11:194–204.

209. Ling B, Apetrei C, Pandrea I, et al. Classic AIDS in a sooty mangabey after an 18-year natural infection. *J Virol* 2004;78:8902–8908.

210. Liu ZQ, Sheridan D, Wood C. Identification and characterization of the bovine immunodeficiency-like virus tat gene. *J Virol* 1992;66:5137–5140.

211. Locher CP, Barnett SW, Herndier BG, et al. Human immunodeficiency virus-2 infection in baboons is an animal model for human immunodeficiency virus pathogenesis in humans. *Arch Pathol Lab Med* 1998;122:523–533.

212. Loffredo JT, Maxwell J, Qi Y, et al. Mamu-b*08-positive macaques control simian immunodeficiency virus replication. *J Virol* 2007;81:8827–8832.

213. Loffredo JT, Sidney J, Bean AT, et al. Two MHC class I molecules associated with elite control of immunodeficiency virus replication, Mamu-B*08 and HLA-B*2705, bind peptides with sequence similarity. *J Immunol* 2009;182:7763–7775.

214. Lowenstine LJ, Lerche NW, Yee JL, et al. Evidence for a lentiviral etiology in an epizootic of immune deficiency and lymphoma in stump-tailed macaques (Macaca arctoides). *J Med Primatol* 1992;21:1–14.

215. Lowenstine LJ, Pedersen NC, Higgins J, et al. Seroepidemiologic survey of captive Old-World primates for antibodies to human and simian retroviruses, and isolation of a lentivirus from sooty mangabeys (Cercocebus atys). *Int J Cancer* 1986;38:563–574.

216. Lv L, Wang Q, Xu Y, et al. Vpr targets TET2 for degradation by CRL4(VprBP) E3 ligase to sustain IL-6 expression and enhance HIV-1 replication. *Mol Cell* 2018;70:961–970 e5.

217. Ma J, Shi N, Jiang CG, et al. A proviral derivative from a reference attenuated EIAV vaccine strain failed to elicit protective immunity. *Virology* 2011;410:96–106.

218. Malik P, Singha H, Sarkar S. Equine infectious anemia. In: Bayry J, ed. *Emerging and Re-emerging Infectious Diseases of Livestock*. 2017:215–336.

219. Mansfield KG, Lerch NW, Gardner MB, et al. Origins of simian immunodeficiency virus infection in macaques at the New England Regional Primate Research Center. *J Med Primatol* 1995;24:116–122.

220. Marin M, Rose KM, Kozak SL, et al. HIV-1 Vif protein binds the editing enzyme APOBEC3G and induces its degradation. *Nat Med* 2003;9:1398–1403.

221. Markovitz DM, Smith MJ, Hilfinger J, et al. Activation of the human immunodeficiency virus type 2 enhancer is dependent on purine box and kB regulatory elements. *J Virol* 1992;66:5479–5484.

222. Marsh H. Progressive pneumonia in sheep. *J Am Vet Med Assoc* 1923;62:458–473.

223. Martinez-Navio JM, Fuchs SP, Pantry SN, et al. Adeno-associated virus delivery of anti-HIV monoclonal antibodies can drive long-term virologic suppression. *Immunity* 2019;50:567–575 e5.

224. Martins MA, Bischof GF, Shin YC, et al. Vaccine protection against SIVmac239 acquisition. *Proc Natl Acad Sci U S A* 2019;116:1739–1744.

225. Marx P. Unsolved questions over the origin of HIV and AIDS. *ASM News* 2005;71:15–17.
226. Matsuda K, Riddick NE, Lee CA, et al. A SIV molecular clone that targets the CNS and induces neuroAIDS in rhesus macaques. *PLoS Pathog* 2017;13:e1006538.
227. Mattapallil JJ, Douek DC, Hill B, et al. Massive infection and loss of memory CD4+ T cells in multiple tissues during acute SIV infection. *Nature* 2005;434:1093–1097.
228. Maury W. Regulation of equine infectious anemia virus expression. *J Biomed Sci* 1998;5(1):11–23.
229. McClure HM, Anderson DC, Gordon TP, et al. Natural simian immunodeficiency virus infection in nonhuman primates. *Top Primatol* 1992;3:425–438.
230. McEwan WA, McMonagle EL, Logan N, et al. Genetically divergent strains of feline immunodeficiency virus from the domestic cat (Felis catus) and the African lion (Panthera leo) share usage of CD134 and CXCR4 as entry receptors. *J Virol* 2008;82:10953–10958.
231. McGuire TC, Crawford TB, Henson JB. Immunofluorescent localization of equine infectious anemia virus in tissue. *Am J Pathol* 1971;62:283–294.
232. McNatt MW, Zang T, Hatziioannou T, et al. Species-specific activity of HIV-1 Vpu and positive selection of tetherin transmembrane domain variants. *PLoS Pathog* 2009;5:e1000300.
233. Meagher JL, Takata M, Goncalves-Carneiro D, et al. Structure of the zinc-finger antiviral protein in complex with RNA reveals a mechanism for selective targeting of CG-rich viral sequences. *Proc Natl Acad Sci U S A* 2019;116:24303–24309.
234. Monit C, Morris ER, Ruis C, et al. Positive selection in dNTPase SAMHD1 throughout mammalian evolution. *Proc Natl Acad Sci U S A* 2019;116:18647–18654.
235. Montagnier L, Dauguet C, Axler C, et al. A new type of retrovirus isolated from patients presenting with lymphadenopathy and acquired immune deficiency syndrome: structural and antigenic relatedness with equine infectious anemia virus. *Ann Virol* 1984;135 E:119–134.
236. Montelaro RC, Ball JM, Rushlow KE. Equine retroviruses. In: Levy JA, ed. *The Retroviridae*. New York: Plenum Press; 1993:257.
237. Morse BA, Carruth LM, Clements JE. Targeting of the visna virus tat protein to AP-1 sites: interactions with the bZIP domains of fos and jun in vitro and in vivo. *J Virol* 1999;73:37–45.
238. Mothe BR, Weinfurter J, Wang C, et al. Expression of the major histocompatibility complex class I molecule Mamu-A*01 is associated with control of simian immunodeficiency virus SIVmac239 replication. *J Virol* 2003;77:2736–2740.
239. Muller MC, Saksena NK, Nerrienet E, et al. Simian immunodeficiency viruses from central and western Africa: evidence for a new species-specific lentivirus in tantalus monkeys. *J Virol* 1993;67:1227–1235.
240. Murakami T, Freed EO. Genetic evidence for an interaction between human immunodeficiency virus type 1 matrix and alpha-helix 2 of the gp41 cytoplasmic tail. *J Virol* 2000;74:3548–3554.
241. Murphey-Corb M, Martin LN, Davison-Fairburn B, et al. A formalin-inactivated whole SIV vaccine confers protection in macaques. *Science* 1989;246:1293–1297.
242. Murphey-Corb M, Martin LN, Rangan SRS, et al. Isolation of an HTLV-III-related retrovirus from macaques with simian AIDS and its possible origin in asymptomatic mangabeys. *Nature* 1986;321:435–437.
243. Neil SJ, Zang T, Bieniasz PD. Tetherin inhibits retrovirus release and is antagonized by HIV-1 Vpu. *Nature* 2008;451:425–430.
244. Neil SJ. The antiviral activities of tetherin. *Curr Top Microbiol Immunol* 2013;371:67–104.
245. Nerrienet E, Amouretti X, Muller-Trutwin MC, et al. Phylogenetic analysis of SIV and STLV type I in mandrills (Mandrillus sphinx): indications that intracolony transmissions are predominantly the result of male-to-male aggressive contacts. *AIDS Res Hum Retroviruses* 1998;14:785–796.
246. Newman RM, Hall L, Connole M, et al. Balancing selection and the evolution of functional polymorphism in Old World monkey TRIM5alpha. *Proc Natl Acad Sci U S A* 2006;103:19134–19139.
247. Nixon CC, Mavigner M, Sampey GC, et al. Systemic HIV and SIV latency reversal via non-canonical NF-kappaB signalling in vivo. *Nature* 2020;578:160–165.
248. Novembre FJ, Hirsch VM, McClure HM, et al. SIV from stump-tailed macaques: molecular characterization of a highly transmissible primate lentivirus. *Virology* 1992;186:783–787.
249. Novembre FJ, Saucier M, Anderson DC, et al. Development of AIDS in a chimpanzees infected with human immunodeficiency virus type. *J Virol* 1997;71:4086–4091.
250. Oaks JL, McGuire TC, Ulibarri C, et al. Equine infectious anemia virus is found in tissue macrophages during subclinical infection. *J Virol* 1998;72:7263–7269.
251. Ohta Y, Masuda T, Tsujimoto H, et al. Isolation of simian immunodeficiency virus from African green monkeys and seroepidemiologic survey of the virus in various non-human primates. *Int J Cancer* 1988;41:115–122.
252. Olmsted RA, Barnes AK, Yamamoto JK, et al. Molecular cloning of feline immunodeficiency virus. *Proc Natl Acad Sci U S A* 1989;86:2448–2452.
253. O'Neil SP, Novembre FJ, Hill AB, et al. Progressive infection in a subset of HIV-1-positive chimpanzees. *J Infect Dis* 2000;182:1051–1062.
254. Orandle MS, Baldwin CJ. Clinical and pathological features associated with feline immunodeficiency virus infection in cats. *Iowa State Univ Vet.* 1995;7(2):61–65.
255. Osterhaus AD, Pedersen N, van Amerongen G, et al. Isolation and partial characterization of a lentivirus from talapoin monkeys (Myopithecus talapoin). *Virology* 1999;260:116–124.
256. Pandrea I, Apetrei C, Gordon S, et al. Paucity of CD4+CCR5+ T cells is a typical feature of natural SIV hosts. *Blood* 2007;109:1069–1076.
257. Pandrea I, Onanga R, Rouquet P, et al. Chronic SIV infection ultimately causes immunodeficiency in African non-human primates. *AIDS* 2001;15:2461–2462.
258. Parekh B, Issel CJ, Montelaro RC. Equine infectious anemia virus, a putative lentivirus, contains polypeptides analogous to prototype-C oncornaviruses. *Virology* 1980;107:520–525.
259. Payne SL, Qi XM, Shao H, et al. Disease induction by virus derived from molecular clones of equine infectious anemia virus. *J Virol* 1998;72:483–487.
260. Pedersen NC, Ho EW, Brown ML, et al. Isolation of a T-lymphotropic virus from domestic cats with an immunodeficiency-like syndrome. *Science* 1987;235:790–793.
261. Peeters M, Courgnaud V, Abela B, et al. Risk to human health from a plethora of simian immunodeficiency viruses in primate bushmeat. *Emerg Infect Dis* 2002;8:451–457.
262. Peeters M, Ma D, Liegeois F, et al. Simian immunodeficiency virus infections in the wild. In: Ansari AA, Silvestri G, eds. *Natural Hosts of SIV*. Elsevier; 2014:37–67.
263. Peluso R, Haase A, Stowring L, et al. A Trojan horse mechanism for the spread of visna virus in monocytes. *Virology* 1985;147:231–236.
264. Pepin M, Vitu C, Russo P, et al. Maedi-visna virus infection in sheep: a review. *Vet Res* 1998;29:341–367.
265. Perez-Caballero D, Zang T, Ebrahimi A, et al. Tetherin inhibits HIV-1 release by directly tethering virions to cells. *Cell* 2009;139:499–511.
266. Petursson G, Turelli P, Matthiasdottir S, et al. Visna virus dUTPase is dispensable for neuropathogenicity. *J Virol* 1998;72:1657–1661.
267. Phillips-Conroy JE, Jolly CJ, Petros B, et al. Sexual transmission of SIVagm in wild grivet monkeys. *J Med Primatol* 1994;23:1–7.
268. Piantadosi A, Chohan B, Chohan V, et al. Chronic HIV-1 infection frequently fails to protect against superinfection. *PLoS Pathog* 2007;3:e177.
269. Picker LJ, Hagen SI, Lum R, et al. Insufficient production and tissue delivery of CD4+ memory T cells in rapidly progressive simian immunodeficiency virus infection. *J Exp Med* 2004;200:1299–1314.
270. Pifat DY, Ennis WH, Ward JM, et al. Persistent infection of rabbits with bovine immunodeficiency-like virus. *J Virol* 1992;66:4518–4524.
271. Pisoni G, Quasso A, Moroni P. Phylogenetic analysis of small-ruminant lentivirus subtype B1 in mixed flocks: evidence for natural transmission from goats to sheep. *Virology* 2005;339:147–152.
272. Poeschla EM, Looney DJ. CXCR4 is required by a nonprimate lentivirus: heterologous expression of feline immunodeficiency virus in human, rodent, and feline cells. *J Virol* 1998;72:6858–6866.
273. Pohlmann S, Floos S, Ilyinskii PO, et al. Sequences just upstream of the simian immunodeficiency virus core enhancer allow efficient replication in the absence of NF-kappaB and Sp1 binding elements. *J Virol* 1998;72:5589–5598.
274. Pollard VW, Malim MH. The HIV-1 Rev protein. *Annu Rev Microbiol* 1998;52:491–532.
275. Popovic M, Sarngadharan MG, Read E, et al. Detection, isolation, and continuous production of cytopathic retroviruses (HTLV-III) from patients with AIDS and pre-AIDS. *Science* 1984;224:497–500.
276. Postler TS, Desrosiers RC. The cytoplasmic domain of the HIV-1 glycoprotein gp41 induces NF-kappaB activation through TGF-beta-activated kinase 1. *Cell Host Microbe* 2012;11:181–193.
277. Postler TS, Desrosiers RC. The tale of the long tail: the cytoplasmic domain of HIV-1 gp41. *J Virol* 2013;87:2–15.
278. Pu R, Coleman J, Omori M, et al. Dual-subtype FIV vaccine protects cats against in vivo swarms of both homologous and heterologous subtype FIV isolates. *AIDS* 2001;15:1225–1237.
279. Pye VE, Rosa A, Bertelli C, et al. A bipartite structural organization defines the SERINC family of HIV-1 restriction factors. *Nat Struct Mol Biol* 2020;27:78–83.
280. Qi M, Chu H, Chen X, et al. A tyrosine-based motif in the HIV-1 envelope glycoprotein tail mediates cell-type- and Rab11-FIP1C-dependent incorporation into virions. *Proc Natl Acad Sci U S A* 2015;112:7575–7580.
281. Qi M, Williams JA, Chu H, et al. Rab11-FIP1C and Rab14 direct plasma membrane sorting and particle incorporation of the HIV-1 envelope glycoprotein complex. *PLoS Pathog* 2013;9:e1003278.
282. Ramachandran S. Early observations and research of Jembrana disease in Bali and other Indonesian islands. In: *Jembrana Disease and The Bovine Lentiviruses*. Canberra, Australia: ACIAR Proceedings; 1997.
283. Reitter J, Means RE, Desrosiers RC. A role for carbohydrates in immune evasion in AIDS. *Nat Med* 1998;4:679–684.
284. Rey-Cuille MA, Berthier JL, Bomsel-Demontoy MC, et al. Simian immunodeficiency virus replicates to high levels in sooty mangabeys without inducing disease. *J Virol* 1998;72:3872–3886.
285. Richman DD, Wrin T, Little SJ, et al. Rapid evolution of the neutralizing antibody response to HIV type 1 infection. *Proc Natl Acad Sci U S A* 2003;100:4144–4149.
286. Riddick NE, Wu F, Matsuda K, et al. Simian immunodeficiency virus SIVagm efficiently utilizes non-CCR5 entry pathways in African Green Monkey lymphocytes: potential role for GPR15 and CXCR6 as viral coreceptors. *J Virol* 2015;90:2316–2331.
287. Rosa A, Chande A, Ziglio S, et al. HIV-1 Nef promotes infection by excluding SERINC5 from virion incorporation. *Nature* 2015;526:212–217.
288. Rosenberg ES, Billingsley JM, Caliendo AM, et al. Vigorous HIV-1-specific $CD4^+$ T cell responses associated with control of viremia. *Science* 1997;278:1447–1450.
289. Ross EK, Buckler-White AJ, Rabson AB, et al. Contribution of NF-kB and Sp1 binding motifs to the replicative capacity of human immunodeficiency virus type 1: distinct patterns of viral growth are determined by T-cell types. *J Virol* 1991;65:4350–4358.
290. Rudicell RS, Holland Jones J, Wroblewski EE, et al. Impact of simian immunodeficiency virus infection on chimpanzee population dynamics. *PLoS Pathog* 2010;6:e1001116.
291. Rudicell RS, Piel AK, Stewart F, et al. High prevalence of simian immunodeficiency virus infection in a community of savanna chimpanzees. *J Virol* 2011;85:9918–9928.
292. Saenz DT, Teo W, Olsen JC, et al. Restriction of feline immunodeficiency virus by Ref1, Lv1, and primate TRIM5alpha proteins. *J Virol* 2005;79:15175–15188.
293. Santiago ML, Lukasik M, Kamenya S, et al. Foci of endemic simian immunodeficiency virus infection in wild-living eastern chimpanzees (Pan troglodytes schweinfurthii). *J Virol* 2003;77:7545–7562.
294. Santiago ML, Range F, Keele BF, et al. Simian immunodeficiency virus infection in free-ranging sooty mangabeys (Cercocebus atys atys) from the Tai Forest, Cote d'Ivoire: implications for the origin of epidemic human immunodeficiency virus type 2. *J Virol* 2005;79:12515–12527.
295. Santiago ML, Rodenburg CM, Kamenya S, et al. SIVcpz in wild chimpanzees. *Science* 2002;295:465.
296. Sasseville V, Lackner A A. Neuropathogenesis of simian immunodeficiency virus infection in macaque monkeys. *J Neurovirol* 1997;3:1–9.
297. Sauter D, Hotter D, Van Driessche B, et al. Differential regulation of NF-kappaB-mediated proviral and antiviral host gene expression by primate lentiviral Nef and Vpu proteins. *Cell Rep* 2015;10:586–599.

298. Sauter D, Schindler M, Specht A, et al. Tetherin-driven adaptation of Vpu and Nef function and the evolution of pandemic and nonpandemic HIV-1 strains. *Cell Host Microbe* 2009;6:409–421.
299. Sawyer SL, Emerman M, Malik HS. Ancient adaptive evolution of the primate antiviral DNA-editing enzyme APOBEC3G. *PLoS Biol* 2004;2:E275.
300. Sawyer SL, Emerman M, Malik HS. Discordant evolution of the adjacent antiretroviral genes TRIM22 and TRIM5 in mammals. *PLoS Pathog* 2007;3:e197.
301. Sawyer SL, Wu LI, Emerman M, et al. Positive selection of primate TRIM5alpha identifies a critical species-specific retroviral restriction domain. *Proc Natl Acad Sci U S A* 2005;102:2832–2837.
302. Sayah DM, Sokolskaja E, Berthoux L, et al. Cyclophilin A retrotransposition into TRIM5 explains owl monkey resistance to HIV-1. *Nature* 2004;430:569–573.
303. Schaller T, Hue S, Towers GJ. An active TRIM5 protein in rabbits indicates a common antiviral ancestor for mammalian TRIM5 proteins. *J Virol* 2007;81:11713–11721.
304. Schindler M, Munch J, Kutsch O, et al. Nef-mediated suppression of T cell activation was lost in a lentiviral lineage that gave rise to HIV-1. *Cell* 2006;125:1055–1067.
305. Schmidt F, Keele BF, Del Prete GQ, et al. Derivation of simian tropic HIV-1 infectious clone reveals virus adaptation to a new host. *Proc Natl Acad Sci U S A* 2019;116: 10504–10509.
306. Schmitz JE, Kuroda MJ, Santra S, et al. Control of viremia in simian immunodeficiency virus infection by CD8+ lymphocytes. *Science* 1999;283:857–860.
307. Schrofelbauer B, Chen D, Landau NR. A single amino acid of APOBEC3G controls its species-specific interaction with virion infectivity factor (Vif). *Proc Natl Acad Sci U S A* 2004;101:3927–3932.
308. Schrofelbauer B, Hakata Y, Landau NR. HIV-1 Vpr function is mediated by interaction with the damage-specific DNA-binding protein DDB1. *Proc Natl Acad Sci U S A* 2007;104:4130–4135.
309. Schwartz O, Marechal V, LeGall S, et al. Endocytosis of major histocompatibility complex class I molecules is induced by the HIV-1 nef protein. *Nat Med* 1996;2:338–342.
310. Sellon DC, Perry ST, Coggins L, et al. Wild-type equine infectious anemia virus replicates in vivo predominantly in tissue macrophages, not in peripheral blood monocytes. *J Virol* 1992;66:5906–5913.
311. Serra-Moreno R, Jia B, Breed M, et al. Compensatory changes in the cytoplasmic tail of gp41 confer resistance to tetherin/BST-2 in a pathogenic nef-deleted SIV. *Cell Host Microbe* 2011;9:46–57.
312. Shacklett BL, Luciw PA. Analysis of the vif gene of feline immunodeficiency virus. *Virology* 1994;204:860–867.
313. Sharp PM, Hahn BH. Origins of HIV and the AIDS pandemic. *Cold Spring Harb Perspect Med* 2011;1:a006841.
314. Shaw AE, Hughes J, Gu Q, et al. Fundamental properties of the mammalian innate immune system revealed by multispecies comparison of type I interferon responses. *PLoS Biol* 2017;15:e2004086.
315. Sheehy AM, Gaddis NC, Choi JD, et al. Isolation of a human gene that inhibits HIV-1 infection and is suppressed by the viral Vif protein. *Nature* 2002;418:646–650.
316. Sheehy AM, Gaddis NC, Malim MH. The antiretroviral enzyme APOBEC3G is degraded by the proteasome in response to HIV-1 Vif. *Nat Med* 2003;9:1404–1407.
317. Shen R, Wang Z. Development and use of an equine infectious anemia donkey leukocyte attenuated vaccine. In: Tashjian R, ed. *Equine Infectious Anemia. A National Review of Policies, Programs, and Future Objections*. Amarillo, TX: American Quarter Horse Association; 1985:135–248.
318. Shimojima M, Miyazawa T, Ikeda Y, et al. Use of CD134 as a primary receptor by the feline immunodeficiency virus. *Science* 2004;303:1192–1195.
319. Shingai M, Donau OK, Schmidt SD, et al. Most rhesus macaques infected with the CCR5-tropic SHIV(AD8) generate cross-reactive antibodies that neutralize multiple HIV-1 strains. *Proc Natl Acad Sci U S A* 2012;109:19769–19774.
320. Sigurdsson B. RIDA; a chronic encephalitis of sheep. With general remarks on infections which develop slowly and some of their special characteristics. *Br Vet J* 1954;110:354–358.
321. Sigurdsson B, Grimsson H, Palsson PA. Maedi, a chronic progressive infection of sheep's lungs. *J Infect Dis* 1952;90:23–241.
322. Sigurdsson B, Pálsson PA. Visna of sheep. A slow, demyelinating infection. *Br J Exp Pathol* 1958;39:519.
323. Sigurdsson B, Palsson PA, Grimsson H. Visna, a demyelinating transmissible disease of sheep. *J Neuropathol Exp Neurol* 1957;16:389–403.
324. Sigurdsson B, Thormar H, Pálsson PA. Cultivation of visna virus in tissue culture. *Arch Gesamte Virusforsch* 1960;10:368.
325. Simon JH, Miller DL, Fouchier RA, et al. The regulation of primate immunodeficiency virus infectivity by Vif is cell species restricted: a role for Vif in determining virus host range and cross-species transmission. *EMBO J* 1998;17:1259–1267.
326. Smaga SS, Xu C, Summers BJ, et al. MxB restricts HIV-1 by targeting the Tri-hexamer interface of the viral capsid. *Structure* 2019;27:1234–1245 e5.
327. Smolen-Dzirba J, Rosinska M, Janiec J, et al. HIV-1 infection in persons homozygous for CCR5-Delta32 allele: the next case and the review. *AIDS Rev* 2017;19:219–230.
328. Soeharsono S. Current information on Jembrana disease distribution in Indonesia. In: *Jembrana Disease and the Bovine Lentiviruses. ACIAR Proceedings*. Canberra, Australia: ACIAR; 1997.
329. Soeharsono S, Wilcox GE, Dharma DM, et al. Species differences in the reaction of cattle to Jembrana disease virus infection. *J Comp Pathol* 1995;112:391–402.
330. Soeharsono S, Wilcox GE, Putra AA, et al. The transmission of Jembrana disease, a lentivirus disease of Bos javanicus cattle. *Epidemiol Infect* 1995;115:367–374.
331. Song B, Javanbakht H, Perron M, et al. Retrovirus restriction by TRIM5alpha variants from Old World and New World primates. *J Virol* 2005;79:3930–3937.
332. Sood C, Marin M, Chande A, et al. SERINC5 protein inhibits HIV-1 fusion pore formation by promoting functional inactivation of envelope glycoproteins. *J Biol Chem* 2017;292:6014–6026.
333. Sotir M, Switzer W, Schable C, et al. Risk of occupational exposure to potentially infectious nonhuman primate materials and to simian immunodeficiency virus. *J Med Primatol* 1997;26:233–240.
334. Souquiere S, Bibollet-Ruche F, Robertson DL, et al. Wild Mandrillus sphinx are carriers of two types of lentivirus. *J Virol* 2001;75:7086–7096.
335. Srivastava S, Swanson SK, Manel N, et al. Lentiviral Vpx accessory factor targets VprBP/DCAF1 substrate adaptor for cullin 4 E3 ubiquitin ligase to enable macrophage infection. *PLoS Pathog* 2008;4:e1000059.
336. Stickney A, Ghosh S, Cave NJ, et al. Lack of protection against feline immunodeficiency virus infection among domestic cats in New Zealand vaccinated with the Fel-O-Vax(R) FIV vaccine. *Vet Microbiol* 2020;250:108865.
337. Stremlau M, Owens CM, Perron MJ, et al. The cytoplasmic body component TRIM5alpha restricts HIV-1 infection in Old World monkeys. *Nature* 2004;427:848–853.
338. Swigut T, Alexander L, Morgan J, et al. Impact of Nef-mediated downregulation of major histocompatibility complex class I on immune response to simian immunodeficiency virus. *J Virol* 2004;78:13335–13344.
339. Takata MA, Goncalves-Carneiro D, Zang TM, et al. CG dinucleotide suppression enables antiviral defence targeting non-self RNA. *Nature* 2017;550:124–127.
340. Tavakoli-Tameh A, Janaka SK, Zarbock K, et al. Loss of tetherin antagonism by Nef impairs SIV replication during acute infection of rhesus macaques. *PLoS Pathog* 2020;16:e1008487.
341. Tedbury PR, Ablan SD, Freed EO. Global rescue of defects in HIV-1 envelope glycoprotein incorporation: implications for matrix structure. *PLoS Pathog* 2013;9:e1003739.
342. Terio KA, Kinsel MJ, Raphael J, et al. Pathologic lesions in chimpanzees (Pan trogylodytes schweinfurthii) from Gombe National Park, Tanzania, 2004-2010. *J Zoo Wildl Med* 2011;42:597–607.
343. Threadgill DS, Steagall WK, Flaherty MT, et al. Characterization of equine infectious anemia virus dUTPase: growth properties of a dUTPase-deficient mutant. *J Virol* 1993;67:2592–2600.
344. Tomonaga K, Katahira J, Fukasawa M, et al. Isolation and characterization of simian immunodeficiency virus from African white-crowned mangabey monkeys (Cercocebus torquatus lunulatus). *Arch Virol* 1993;129:77–92.
345. Trautz B, Wiedemann H, Luchtenborg C, et al. The host-cell restriction factor SERINC5 restricts HIV-1 infectivity without altering the lipid composition and organization of viral particles. *J Biol Chem* 2017;292:13702–13713.
346. Troyer JL, Pecon-Slattery J, Roelke ME, et al. Patterns of feline immunodeficiency virus multiple infection and genome divergence in a free-ranging population of African lions. *J Virol* 2004;78:3777–3791.
347. Tsai CC, Emau P, Follis KE, et al. Effectiveness of postinoculation (R)-9-(2-phosphonylmethoxypropyl) adenine treatment for prevention of persistent simian immunodeficiency virus SIVmne infection depends critically on timing of initiation and duration of treatment. *J Virol* 1998;72:4265–4273.
348. Tsai CC, Follis KE, Sabo A, et al. Prevention of SIV infection in macaques by (R)-9-(2-phosphonylmethoxypropyl)adenine. *Science* 1995;270:1197–1199.
349. Tsujimoto H, Hasegawa A, Maki N, et al. Sequence of a novel simian immunodeficiency virus from a wild-caught African mandrill. *Nature* 1989;341:539–541.
350. Turelli P, Guiguen F, Mornex JF, et al. dUTPase-minus caprine arthritis-encephalitis virus is attenuated for pathogenesis and accumulates G-to-A substitutions. *J Virol* 1997;71: 4522–4530.
351. Überla K, Stahl Hennig C, Böttiger D, et al. Animal model for the therapy of acquired immunodeficiency syndrome with reverse transcriptase inhibitors. *Proc Natl Acad Sci U S A* 1995;92:8210–8214.
352. Usami Y, Wu Y, Gottlinger HG. SERINC3 and SERINC5 restrict HIV-1 infectivity and are counteracted by Nef. *Nature* 2015;526:218–223.
353. Valas S, Benoit C, Guionaud C, et al. North American and French caprine arthritis-encephalitis viruses emerge from ovine maedi-visna viruses. *Virology* 1997;237:307–318.
354. Vallée H, Carré H. Sur la nature infectieuse de l'anaemie du cheval. *C R Hebd Seances Acad Sci* 1904;139:331–333.
355. Van Damme N, Goff D, Katsura C, et al. The interferon-induced protein BST-2 restricts HIV-1 release and is downregulated from the cell surface by the viral Vpu protein. *Cell Host Microbe* 2008;3:245–252.
356. Van Der Maaten MJ, Boothe AD, Seger CL. Isolation of a virus from cattle with persistent lymphocytosis. *J Natl Cancer Inst* 1972;49:1649.
357. Van Heuverswyn F, Li Y, Bailes E, et al. Genetic diversity and phylogeographic clustering of SIVcpzPtt in wild chimpanzees in Cameroon. *Virology* 2007;368:155–171.
358. Van Heuverswyn F, Li Y, Neel C, et al. Human immunodeficiency viruses: SIV infection in wild gorillas. *Nature* 2006;444:164.
359. van Rensburg EJ, Engelbrecht S, Mwenda J, et al. Simian immunodeficiency viruses (SIVs) from eastern and southern Africa: detection of a SIVagm variant from a chacma baboon. *J Gen Virol* 1998;79:1809–1814.
360. VandeWoude S, O'Brien SJ, Hoover EA. Infectivity of lion and puma lentiviruses for domestic cats. *J Gen Virol* 1997;78(Pt 4):795–800.
361. VandeWoude S, Troyer J, Poss M. Restrictions to cross-species transmission of lentiviral infection gleaned from studies of FIV. *Vet Immunol Immunopathol* 2010;134:25–32.
362. Veazey RS, DeMaria M, Chalifoux LV, et al. Gastrointestinal tract as a major site of CD4+ T cell depletion and viral replication in SIV infection. *Science* 1998;280:427–431.
363. Veazey RS, Tham IC, Mansfield KG, et al. Identifying the target cell in primary simian immunodeficiency virus (SIV) infection: highly activated memory CD4(+) T cells are rapidly eliminated in early SIV infection in vivo. *J Virol* 2000;74:57–64.
364. Veillette M, Desormeaux A, Medjahed H, et al. Interaction with cellular CD4 exposes HIV-1 envelope epitopes targeted by antibody-dependent cell-mediated cytotoxicity. *J Virol* 2014;88:2633–2644.
365. Villet S, Bouzar BA, Morin T, et al. Maedi-visna virus and caprine arthritis encephalitis virus genomes encode a Vpr-like but no Tat protein. *J Virol* 2003;77:9632–9638.
366. Virgen CA, Kratovac Z, Bieniasz PD, et al. Independent genesis of chimeric TRIM5-cyclophilin proteins in two primate species. *Proc Natl Acad Sci U S A* 2008;105: 3563–3568.
367. von Bredow B, Andrabi R, Grunst M, et al. Differences in the binding affinity of an HIV-1 V2 apex-specific antibody for the SIVsmm/mac envelope glycoprotein uncouple antibody-dependent cellular cytotoxicity from neutralization. *MBio* 2019;10(4):e01255-19.

368. von Bredow B, Arias JF, Heyer LN, et al. Comparison of antibody-dependent cell-mediated cytotoxicity and virus neutralization by HIV-1 Env-specific monoclonal antibodies. *J Virol* 2016;90:6127–6139.

369. Wagaman PC, Hasselkus-Light CS, Henson M, et al. Molecular cloning and characterization of deoxyuridine triphosphatase from feline immunodeficiency virus (FIV). *Virology* 1993;196:451–457.

370. Wang X, Wang S, Lin Y, et al. Genomic comparison between attenuated Chinese equine infectious anemia virus vaccine strains and their parental virulent strains. *Arch Virol* 2011;156:353–357.

371. Wang XF, Lin YZ, Li Q, et al. Genetic evolution during the development of an attenuated EIAV vaccine. *Retrovirology* 2016;13:9.

372. Ward AE, Kiessling V, Pornillos O, et al. HIV-cell membrane fusion intermediates are restricted by Serincs as revealed by cryo-electron and TIRF microscopy. *J Biol Chem* 2020;295:15183–15195.

373. Wei X, Decker JM, Wang S, et al. Antibody neutralization and escape by HIV-1. *Nature* 2003;422:307–312.

374. Wei X, Ghosh SK, Taylor ME, et al. Viral dynamics in human immunodeficiency virus type 1 infection. *Nature* 1995;373:117–122.

375. Weiland F, Matheka HD, Coggins L, et al. Electron microscopic studies on equine infectious anemia virus (EIAV). Brief report. *Arch Virol* 1977;55:335–340.

376. Westmoreland SV, Converse AP, Hrecka K, et al. SIV vpx is essential for macrophage infection but not for development of AIDS. *PLoS One* 2014;9:e84463.

377. Wetzel KS, Yi Y, Elliott STC, et al. CXCR6-mediated simian immunodeficiency virus SIVagmSab entry into Sabaeus African Green Monkey lymphocytes implicates widespread use of non-CCR5 pathways in natural host infections. *J Virol* 2017;91(4):e01626-16.

378. Wetzel KS, Yi Y, Yadav A, et al. Loss of CXCR6 coreceptor usage characterizes pathogenic lentiviruses. *PLoS Pathog* 2018;14:e1007003.

379. White TA, Bartesaghi A, Borgnia MJ, et al. Three-dimensional structures of soluble CD4-bound states of trimeric simian immunodeficiency virus envelope glycoproteins determined by using cryo-electron tomography. *J Virol* 2011;85:12114–12123.

380. Wilcox GE. Jembrana disease. *Aust Vet J* 1997;75:492–493.

381. Willett BJ, Hosie MJ, Neil JC, et al. Common mechanisms of infection by lentiviruses. *Nature* 1997;385:587.

382. Williams KC, Corey S, Westmoreland SV, et al. Perivascular macrophages are the primary cell type productively infected by simian immunodeficiency virus in the brains of macaques: implications for the neuropathogenesis of AIDS. *J Exp Med* 2001;193:905–915.

383. Wilson SJ, Webb BL, Maplanka C, et al. Rhesus macaque TRIM5 alleles have divergent antiretroviral specificities. *J Virol* 2008;82:7243–7247.

384. Wilson SJ, Webb BL, Ylinen LM, et al. Independent evolution of an antiviral TRIMCyp in rhesus macaques. *Proc Natl Acad Sci U S A* 2008;105:3557–3562.

385. Wojcechowskyj JA, Yant LJ, Wiseman RW, et al. Control of simian immunodeficiency virus SIVmac239 is not predicted by inheritance of Mamu-B*17-containing haplotypes. *J Virol* 2007;81:406–410.

386. Wu F, Kirmaier A, Goeken R, et al. TRIM5 alpha drives SIVsmm evolution in rhesus macaques. *PLoS Pathog* 2013;9:e1003577.

387. Wu F, Ourmanov I, Kuwata T, et al. Sequential evolution and escape from neutralization of simian immunodeficiency virus SIVsmE660 clones in rhesus macaques. *J Virol* 2012;86:8835–8847.

388. Wyand MS, Manson K, Montefiori DC, et al. Protection by live, attenuated simian immunodeficiency virus against heterologous challenge. *J Virol* 1999;73:8356–8363.

389. Wykrzykowska JJ, Rosenzweig M, Veazey RS, et al. Early regeneration of thymic progenitors in rhesus macaques infected with simian immunodeficiency virus. *J Exp Med* 1998;187:1767–1778.

390. Yamamoto JK, Sparger E, Ho EW, et al. Epidemiologic and clinical aspects of feline immunodeficiency virus infection in cats from the continental United States and Canada and possible mode of transmission. *J Am Vet Med Assoc* 1989;194:213–220.

391. Yan J, Shun MC, Hao C, et al. HIV-1 Vpr reprograms CLR4(DCAF1) E3 ubiquitin ligase to antagonize exonuclease 1-mediated restriction of HIV-1 infection. *mBio* 2018;9(5):e01732-18.

392. Yan J, Shun MC, Zhang Y, et al. HIV-1 Vpr counteracts HLTF-mediated restriction of HIV-1 infection in T cells. *Proc Natl Acad Sci U S A* 2019;116:9568–9577.

393. Yant LJ, Friedrich TC, Johnson RC, et al. The high-frequency major histocompatibility complex class I allele Mamu-B*17 is associated with control of simian immunodeficiency virus SIVmac239 replication. *J Virol* 2006;80:5074–5077.

394. Yap MW, Nisole S, Stoye JP. A single amino acid change in the SPRY domain of human Trim5alpha leads to HIV-1 restriction. *Curr Biol* 2005;15:73–78.

395. Ylinen LM, Keckesova Z, Webb BL, et al. Isolation of an active Lv1 gene from cattle indicates that tripartite motif protein-mediated innate immunity to retroviral infection is widespread among mammals. *J Virol* 2006;80:7332–7338.

396. Yu Q, Konig R, Pillai S, et al. Single-strand specificity of APOBEC3G accounts for minus-strand deamination of the HIV genome. *Nat Struct Mol Biol* 2004;11:435–442.

397. Yu S, Ou Y, Xiao H, et al. Experimental treatment of SIV-infected Macaques via autograft of CCR5-disrupted hematopoietic stem and progenitor cells. *Mol Ther Methods Clin Dev* 2020;17:520–531.

398. Yuste E, Reeves JD, Doms RW, et al. Modulation of Env content in virions of simian immunodeficiency virus: correlation with cell surface expression and virion infectivity. *J Virol* 2004;78:6775–6785.

399. Zhang B, Jin S, Jin J, et al. A tumor necrosis factor receptor family protein serves as a cellular receptor for the macrophage-tropic equine lentivirus. *Proc Natl Acad Sci U S A* 2005;102:9918–9923.

400. Zhang B, Montelaro RC. Replication of equine infectious anemia virus in engineered mouse NIH 3T3 cells. *J Virol* 2009;83:2034–2037.

401. Zhang F, Bieniasz PD. HIV-1 Vpr induces cell cycle arrest and enhances viral gene expression by depleting CCDC137. *Elife* 2020;9:e55806.

402. Zhang F, Wilson SJ, Landford WC, et al. Nef proteins from simian immunodeficiency viruses are tetherin antagonists. *Cell Host Microbe* 2009;6:54–67.

403. Zheng X, Wang X, Tu F, et al. TRIM25 is required for the antiviral activity of zinc finger antiviral protein. *J Virol* 2017;91(9):e00088-17.

404. Zhu Y, Chen G, Lv F, et al. Zinc-finger antiviral protein inhibits HIV-1 infection by selectively targeting multiply spliced viral mRNAs for degradation. *Proc Natl Acad Sci U S A* 2011;108:15834–15839.

Foamy Viruses

Dirk Lindemann • Ottmar Herchenröder

Overview
Foamy virus isolation and diagnosis of infection
Natural history and trans-species transmissions
Evolution of foamy viruses
Replication *in vitro*
Replication in the natural host *in vivo*
Apathogenicity of foamy viruses
Virion structure
Genome structure and organization
Virion-associated proteins
  Gag
  Pol
  Env
Nonstructural proteins
  Tas
  Bet
Stages of replication
  The early phase: establishing the provirus (Fig. 20.14)
  The late phase: generation of progeny viruses (Fig. 20.15)

OVERVIEW

Foamy viruses (FVs) are found in numerous mammalian species. Basically all simian and prosimian species investigated to date harbor exogenous FVs. Otherwise, FVs were found for instance in cattle, horses, and felines. Human beings are no natural hosts for FV, although transmissions from apes or monkeys to man do occur since these viruses exhibit a broad tropism with respect to both, cell and species type. Like all other retroviruses, FVs establish lifelong persistent infections but according to current knowledge do not cause any obvious disease, be it within the species of origin or after zoonotic transmission. Although the FV genomes are typical for complex retroviruses, their polymerases are phylogenetically related to those of other retroviruses, and their reverse transcription mechanism employs a tRNA primer. Consequently, FVs were classified as a separate subfamily in the *Retroviridae* family, the Spumaretrovirinae, because their replication cycle deviates from that observed in all other retroviruses. Therefore, and with respect to their potential use as vectors systems and to gain valuable insights into zoonotic virus transmissions, this "Cinderella" group of viruses is worth to be thoroughly investigated.[283,284]

The term "foamy virus" was coined in the 1950s to acknowledge the spontaneous formation of a typical foamy cytopathic effect (CPE) observed in FV infected cell cultures (Fig. 20.1; Video 20.1). This CPE is characterized by multinucleated syncytia and vacuolization in primary monkey kidney cell cultures causing a "foamy" appearance.[53,174,214,230] The CPE observed before destruction of the cell cultures was later attributed to the fact that the donor monkeys were latently infected with a transmittable agent, and it became the light microscopy hallmark of *in vitro* FV propagation. Following the discovery of reverse transcriptase, FVs were identified to be retroviruses.[193] The first 30 years of FV research dealt mainly with the identification of infected monkeys, prior to sacrifice, as sources of primary cell cultures used to diagnose human transmissible diseases.[41] Molecular cloning of the first FV—at that time believed to be a human isolate—permitted initial functional studies on their replication.[216] FV research gained momentum following the discovery that these viruses replicate differently from all other retroviruses.[151,298] These studies culminated in the finding that the FV infectious genome consists of DNA rather than RNA.[180,225,303] In brief, the FV replication strategy combines those of retroviruses with some characteristics of hepadnaviruses, such as hepatitis B virus (HBV), with other properties unique to FVs.[133,212,214] Consequently, retroviral taxonomy was updated into two retroviral subfamilies, the Orthoretrovirinae, which encompass all other retrovirus genera, and the Spumaretrovirinae, which currently contain five genera of spumaviruses (*spuma*, latin for foam).[125,152] This chapter will summarize our knowledge of FV epidemiology and biology. We shall focus on FVs of nonhuman primates (NHPs) and mention the nonprimate viruses only when they become relevant depending on the scientific context. For particular aspects such as FV vectors, the reader is referred to more specialized reviews.[148,149,204,206,252]

FOAMY VIRUS ISOLATION AND DIAGNOSIS OF INFECTION

FV isolation is easiest by cocultivating fibroblasts obtained from throat or buccal swabs with a stable cell line, although many other tissues as virus sources can be used.[104,174,187,235] FVs are also shed in feces. With refined isolation techniques, noninvasive FV nucleic acids detection from fecal samples or saliva remnants on food leftovers have become feasible in native habitats.[154,243,253] FV replication *in vitro* is strongly inhibited by different types of interferon (IFN), and virus recovery from

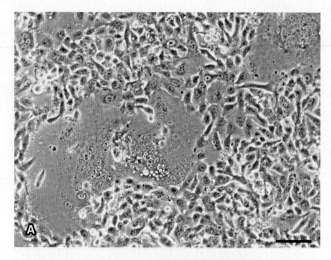

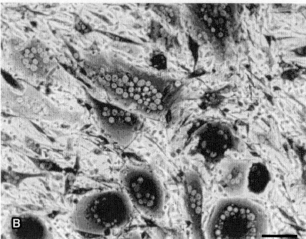

FIGURE 20.1 Cytopathic effect induced by foamy viruses in adherent cells. A: Formation of multinucleated and vacuolated syncytia after transfecting BHK-LTR-lacZ indicator cells with a full-length infectious clone of Western chimpanzee simian foamy virus (SFVpve). **B:** The indicator cells bear the β-galactosidase gene under control of the PFV-LTR. Staining of SFVpve-infected cells with X-gal. Since both prototype foamy virus (PFV) and SFVpve originated from chimpanzees, their transactivators coactivate each other's promoters. Scale bar: 100 μm.

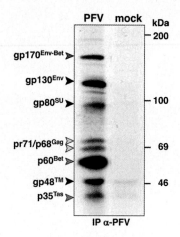

FIGURE 20.2 Radioimmunoprecipitation analysis of prototype foamy virus infected cells. 293T cells metabolically labeled with [35]SMet/Cys were transfected with a prototype foamy virus (PFV) proviral expression construct (lane 1, PFV) or an empty expression vector (lane 2, mock), lysed, and precipitated with a foamy virus–positive chimpanzee serum. Immunodominant proteins are indicated by *arrowheads (left)* and molecular weight markers are shown on the *right*.

NATURAL HISTORY AND TRANS-SPECIES TRANSMISSIONS

Various vertebrate species are naturally infected with FVs. Figure 20.3 gives an overview of the currently known exogenous spumavirus genera and FV species. Extensively studied are simian foamy viruses (SFVs) of Great Apes, Old and New World monkeys, and prosimians.[104,105,174,214,235] Probably all monkey species harbor a FV.[113,154] Otherwise, FV infections appear to occur worldwide in bovines and other *Artiodactyla*, equines, and felidae, and one report shows FVs in a bat species.[66,125,134,167,174,214,218,271] The prevalence in the natural hosts in the wild is usually over 30% and may reach 100%.[104,154,174,214] It is generally assumed that FVs are transmitted among NHPs through saliva via social contacts, including aggressive activities such as biting among young animals.[32,154] These contacts and lactation are also suspected to be the main transmission route of the feline foamy virus (FFV), whereas bovine foamy virus (BFV) probably is mainly transmitted via milk from infected cows to their offspring.[220,291] It is, therefore, not unlikely that FVs are, in terms of prevalence, the most successful of all retroviruses. Although host restriction factors show some species restriction (see later discussion), FVs have been reported to cross the species barrier between monkeys and apes in captivity or in the wild.[104,139,154] In their hosts, FVs cause lifelong persistent infections of benign nature, often in the presence of neutralizing antibodies.[104,174,214] Laboratory animals, such as mice and rabbits, have also been infected in the absence of overt disease.[28,232,240] However, none of these reports yielded a suitable animal model that mimics replication in the natural host.

Humans are not a natural host of FVs.[214] Indeed, the most intensely studied FV isolate was once believed to be of human origin but is meanwhile designated as the prototype foamy virus (PFV).[1,161,213] Initial reports on naturally occurring human infections[162,166] were not confirmed

peripheral blood lymphocytes is greatly enhanced by the addition of anti–γ-interferon (γ-IFN) antibodies.[8,64,171] A virus isolate displaying the typical CPE (Fig. 20.1) should be confirmed by detection of reverse transcriptase activity, by immunofluorescence assay (IFA) demonstrating a predominantly nuclear antigen, or via polymerase chain reaction (PCR).[104,174,214,247] FV infection in the host can be diagnosed serologically by demonstrating antibodies against the main structural proteins, typically the Gag doublet as well as the accessory protein Bet.[79] The choice of antigen in immunoblots or radioimmunoprecipitation (Fig. 20.2) is crucial, because the reactions are, at least in part, virus type specific.[107,115,126] Seropositivity has to be verified by nucleic acid detection. PCR amplification of a conserved fragment of approximately 420 bp from the integrase (IN) domain within the *pol* gene is most expedient.[243] The tools of choice for basic research on FV are molecular clones carrying a full proviral genome of a virus isolate.[100,216]

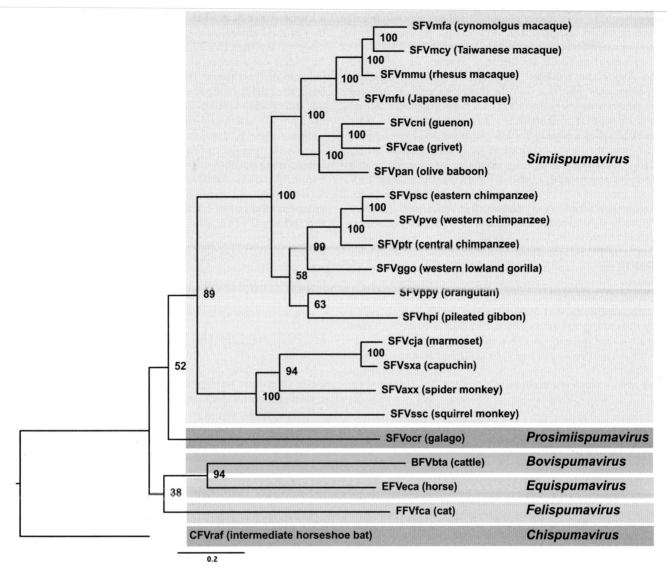

FIGURE 20.3 Spumaretrovirus phylogeny. The tree was generated using aligned nucleotide sequences beginning approximately in the middle of the *pol* gene and extending to approximately the middle of the *env* gene, corresponding to positions 5089–7927 of SFVpsc. Unrooted tree is depicted as rooted for ease of visualization. Branches are labeled with virus names; corresponding host names are given in parentheses. Branches corresponding to viruses within the same genus are indicated with *colored boxes* and genus names. Percent bootstrap support (100 replicates) is indicated for each node. Sequences were aligned using MUSCLE 3.8.425 and phylogeny inferred using PhyML 3.2.2 (HKY85 substitution model and the NNI search option) as implemented in Geneious Prime 2020.2.3. Image was created using FigTree 1.4.4 and Adobe Illustrator CC. Virus genome accession numbers are SFVcni (JQ867466); SFVcae (NC_010820); SFVpan (MK241969); SFVmfa (LC094267); SFVmcy (MN585198.1); SFVmmu (MF280817); SFVmfu (AB923518); SFVpve (NC_001364); SFVpsc (KX087159); SFVptr (JQ867463); SFVggo (HM245790); SFVppy (AJ544579); SFVhpi (MF621235); SFVsxa (KP143760); SFVcja (GU356395); SFVaxx (EU010385); SFVssc (GU356394); SFVocr (KM233624); FFVfca (Y08851); EFVeca (AF201902); BFVbta (NC_001831); and CFVraf (JQ814855). (Courtesy of A.S. Khan, Silver Spring, USA and W.E. Johnson, Chestnut Hill, USA.)

after large-scale screening of more than 5,000 samples using sophisticated methodological combinations of serology and PCR.[3,247] Formerly postulated associations of FVs with human diseases such as autoimmune disorders or neurologic conditions of unknown origin could never be validated.[45,97,223,248] Because of the close nucleotide sequence homology to FVs from the *Pan troglodytes verus* chimpanzee subspecies, initially called SFVcpz and now designated SFVpve,[99,154] the first documented human isolate from a Kenyan patient is believed to have resulted from a zoonotic transmission.[58] Primate FVs

are not circulating in the human population, but humans are susceptible to zoonotic transmissions of NHP FVs.[204,244,261] Worldwide, over a hundred human infections with NHP FVs have been thoroughly confirmed. In a survey, the Centers for Disease Control and Prevention identified approximately 2% seropositives and virus DNA positives among several hundred samples from persons occupationally exposed to NHPs, and virus could be isolated in several instances. Some of these infections dated back to severe monkey bites decades before.[24,98] FV infections were also identified in African bushmeat hunters.[31,71,292] Other persons at risk are those living in close proximity to quasi-wild NHPs (e.g., at Asian temple sites) or individuals possessing NHP as pets.[114]

Human infections are lifelong; however, none induced any disease and remained unrecognized prior to respective investigations. The viral load in buffy-coat cells of infected humans revealed very low FV DNA copy numbers.[31] Moreover, in contrast to lentiviruses, *in vivo* adaptation to what could be called a human FV has not occurred. Even decades after infection, FV nucleotide sequences in humans barely change, and the transmitting donor species can be readily identified as over time, a baboon FV will remain a baboon FV in a human host.[24,98,250] There is no indication of human-to-human transmission even between close contacts.[204] But since FV can be transmitted by transfusion,[27,124] infected persons are advised not to donate blood to avoid virus spreading.[96] Special cases were FV transmissions to end-stage diseased recipients of NHP xenotransplants.[5] For reasons not fully understood, humans appear to be "dead-end" hosts for primate FVs. Concerning infections in humans with other than NHP FVs, it is worth mentioning that antibody screening of more than 200 veterinarians at risk of acquiring FFV did not reveal a single positive case.[29] Based on this result, it appears also unlikely that bovine or equine foamy virus can infect humans.[204] Why throughout the evolution of humans FVs have not adapted to this species remains a mystery.

EVOLUTION OF FOAMY VIRUSES

Exogenous FVs are ancient retroviruses. While the prominent pathogenic retroviruses like simian immunodeficiency viruses (SIVs) and simian T-lymphotropic viruses (STLVs), or the D-type retroviruses including Mason-Pfizer monkey virus (MPMV) are only inherent in African or Asian monkeys, respectively, the higher evolutionary age of primate FV is reflected in that they are the only known exogenous primate retroviruses also found in the Neotropis, precisely in South and Central America.[235] Over the last decade, researchers have uncovered a number of endogenous foamy viral sequences in several species testifying that exogenous FVs were around before the advent of mammals. First, Katzourakis et al.[122] reported the detection of endogenous FVs in the South American sloths genome (*Choloepus hoffmanni*). Han and Worobey described endogenous FVs in a lemur species, the Madagascan aye-aye (*Daubentonia madagascariensis*), in the Coelacanth genome (*Latimeria chalumnae*), and the Cape golden mole (*Chrysochloris asiatica*), suggesting that endogenous FVs existed more than 400 million years ago.[82] An evolutionary gap was filled after detecting endogenous FV in the reptile species tuatara (*Sphenodon punctatus*).[281] Currently, and on the basis of additional foamy-like endogenous sequences in fish and amphibians, it is believed that this retroviral lineage and probably retroviruses as a whole originated in ancient marine life.[2]

Apparently, when an exogenous FV has adapted to its host, it mutates only slightly faster than the host mitochondrial DNA. The substitution rate of SFVs has been estimated to be around 1.7×10^{-8} per site and year.[263] This makes FVs the most genetically stable of viruses with an RNA phase in their replication. For instance, the FV mutation rate is approximately

10 times lower than STLV-1, a virus that replicates primarily by a proviral expansion mechanism, that is, through DNA (see Chapter 16). Therefore, FVs are of extraordinary genetic stability and, if not acquired by trans-species transmissions, always point to the host species from which they were derived. Curiously, the fidelity of the reverse transcriptase enzyme (RT) does not reflect this enormous genetic stability. If analyzed *in vitro*, the PFV RT was found to be of exceptional high processivity but of low fidelity.[25,26,219] The mutation rate of PFV RT ($\sim 1.7 \times 10^{-4}$ per site and replication round) is similar to that of human immunodeficiency virus (HIV). Most mutations found were small deletions and insertions.[26] If analyzed in cell culture, such deletions and insertions were not found. However, a point mutation error rate of 1.1×10^{-5} per site and round of replication remained.[68] Thus, the genetic stability of FVs at the molecular level is not currently understood, and the involvement of yet unidentified specific cellular factor(s) or the very limited replication in specific tissues in persistently infected hosts may play a role in this process.

REPLICATION *IN VITRO*

The host cell range for FVs is quite broad and includes species-independent primary cells or cell lines of fibroblastoid, epithelial, and lymphoblastoid origin, such as various B and T lymphocytes, and cells of erythroid and of myeloid lineages.[104,174,214,302] Upon replication in adherent cell cultures, FVs induce massive multinucleated giant cell CPE (Fig. 20.1; Video 20.1), and apoptosis is thought to be the ultimate cause of cell death.[178] Vacuolization of cells is often only observed using primary isolates. The paucity of cell lines resistant to FV infections or FV glycoprotein complex (GPC)-mediated membrane fusion has hindered the identification of the cellular receptor(s) required for entry by classical approaches. It is now appreciated that all FVs use the same cellular receptor, including those present on bird, reptile, and fish cells.[13,101,258] Two cell lines reported to be refractory to infection, Pac-2 zebrafish embryonic fibroblasts and the G1E-ER4 human erythroid precursors,[258] were later found to block virus replication intracellularly. Thus, systematic screenings of complementary DNA (cDNA) libraries for FV receptor-related genes are still pending.

Whereas the characteristic CPE develops in adherent cells, this hallmark of FVs is often absent in cells of lymphoblastoid origin, in which FVs appear to become latent but intermittently capable of being reactivated. Latently infected cells do not undergo syncytium formation and death but proliferate with normal kinetics and produce low amounts of virus.[302] Interestingly, chemical treatment of lymphocytes, for example, with phorbol esters may induce the latent virus and cause cell death owing to activated viral replication.[177,302] Although this is reminiscent of the lymphotropic herpesviruses, the molecular basis for FV reactivation has not been investigated nor have sites within the cellular or FV DNA genome responsive to the drug-mediated reactivation been mapped. Whether the methylation of FV DNA that has been observed in a cell culture model[245] contributes to *in vivo* latency remains unresolved, because there is no evidence of transcriptional down-regulation of FV vectors by methylation following their introduction *in vivo*.[102,190]

REPLICATION IN THE NATURAL HOST IN VIVO

Liu et al.[154] used methods similar to those employed to demonstrate that HIV-1 was derived from SIV from chimpanzees (SIVcpz; i.e., the authors collected and analyzed fecal samples from wild chimpanzees; see Chapter 19). It was found that SFVs are widely distributed among chimpanzees in the wild with a phylogeographic distribution. In these animals, FVs are transmitted horizontally, because babies younger than 2 years were free from FVs and infection rates increased with age. Moreover, superinfection of chimpanzees by SFVs from lower primates and subsequently recombination events occur. The most interesting finding by these authors has been the detection of viral RNA (vRNA) but not viral DNA (vDNA) in the fecal samples.[154] This issue directly relates to the FV replication pathway (see later discussion). However, Liu et al.[154] did not investigate whether the RNA-containing virus transmits the infection, and it is not known in which cell type these viruses were produced. It is possible that the DNA content in the fecal samples may have been too low to be detected even with very sensitive methods.

The tissue distribution of SFV and sites of in vivo replication have been investigated using another approach. As expected from the broad host cell range of FVs seen in vitro, vDNA was detected at a frequency of one genome copy per 10^2 to 10^3 cells in every organ examined.[62] Because animals in this study were perfused prior to the analysis of nucleic acids, infected lymphocytes were not detected, although these cells were the probable vehicles of virus dissemination in vivo.[62,63] As judged from in situ hybridization experiments, vRNA, indicative of active virus replication, was confined to superficial cells of the oral mucosa.[62,185] Thus, it appears that only cells, which are destined to be shed, are productively infected and undergo lytic replication in vivo. Differential expression of yet undisclosed host factors restricting viral replication in other tissues is a likely explanation for this observation.

It was subsequently found that in severely immunosuppressed, dually SFV- and SIV-infected macaques, the predominant site of FV replication changed from the oral mucosa to the small intestine.[184] However, diseases attributable to SFV did not occur. This was also observed in cats dually infected with feline immunodeficiency virus (FIV) and FFV.[11,306] One case of a human coinfected by HIV-1 and SFV from mandrills has also been reported, without clinical consequences that could be attributed to the SFV infection.[262]

APATHOGENICITY OF FOAMY VIRUSES

For decades in the last century, several pathogenic conditions in humans were attributed to PFV, formerly called human foamy virus (HFV) or in some earlier publications human spumaretrovirus (HSRV). Prompted by a gathering in the mid-1990s of all laboratories involved in FV research and subsequent cross-examinations on sera, two essential perceptions were agreed upon: humans do not naturally harbor FV and neither in the natural hosts nor after zoonotic transmission to man do FV cause any disease.[284] After it was proven that PFV, originally isolated from an African patient,[1] had originated from a chimpanzee, and thorough analyses of samples from patients with diseases once attributed to FV infections, this consensus was sustained.[99,243] This notion seems strange, since to the layperson, a virus infection and a disease seem to belong together. Instead, the pathogenicity of an infectious agent may require an explanation, not the apathogenicity of what has been called a "perfect parasite" whose "interest" is to multiply its genome without doing harm, with the FVs as a prominent example.[276] It appears that FVs have coevolved with their hosts over millions of years to do exactly this.[2]

Certainly, some arguments can be made in favor of this hypothesis. The site of active replication in vivo determines to a large extent the pathogenicity of an infectious agent. FVs appear to mainly replicate in cells of the oral and occasionally the intestinal mucosa, both tissues, that are destined to be desquamated.[62,63] However, during the establishment of persistence, it is likely that lymphocytes become infected and shed low amounts of virus that disseminate throughout the body. Once persistence is established, FV genes may no longer be expressed in lymphocytes. A second factor contributing to the benign character of FV infections is that the Tas transactivator appears to be specific for its autologous cognate viral promoters.[100,155] The off-target activation of gene expression upon zoonotic transmission may probably be a rare event, although Tas has been demonstrated to activate transcription of some cellular genes in vitro.[128,278] Furthermore, the integration of FVs does not induce the activation of cellular oncogenes because they lack strong enhancer elements and their LTRs were recently reported to harbor insulator sequences.[61,78] In addition, a strong polyadenylation signal in the LTR seems to prevent a read-through of viral transcripts into cellular genes for activation.[95,242]

Meanwhile, newer reports challenge to some extent the fully innocent nature of FVs, however, just as a cofactor in conjunction with other conditions. Cameroonian and French researchers thoroughly examined hunters residing in the Cameroonian rain forest of whom numerous contracted zoonotic transmissible agents and among those NHP FV. Gorilla FV for instance seems to alter hematological parameters inversely correlated to the presence of strong neutralizing antibodies.[132] A case–control study revealed that the cases had numerous deviations in their immune parameters compared to the controls.[71] In such FV-positive individuals, coinfections with other retroviruses do occur and the viruses may influence each other.[226] After experimental infection of two rhesus monkey cohorts with the pathogenic SIVmac239 strain, the naturally FV-positive animals developed higher SIV plasma loads, their CD4-positive T cells decay was steeper, and they died earlier than the FV-negative monkeys.[40] Appreciating the latter reports and during the continuous inventory of the planet's virome, FVs should, therefore, not be released from the watch list.

VIRION STRUCTURE

By ultrastructural analysis, FVs appear as immature-looking core particles surrounded by a lipid bilayer with embedded prominent Env proteins[104,174,214,287] (Fig. 20.4; Video 20.2). Investigations using electron microscopy (EM) or electron tomography (ET) techniques suggest that the FV virions have a diameter of approximately 110 nm and contain a core of about 60 nm

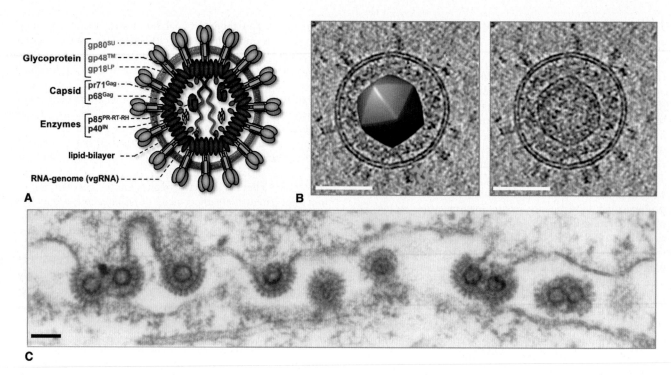

FIGURE 20.4 Structure of foamy virus (FV) virions. A: Schematic representation of the prototype foamy virus (PFV) particle structure prior to reverse transcription initiation. pr, precursor protein; p, protein; gp, glycoprotein. **B:** Cryo-electron tomography of a wild-type PFV virion. The *left* image has the central, polyhedral capsid structure highlighted in *red* and two oligomeric glycoprotein spike structures in *green*. Scale bar: 50 nm. (Courtesy of P. Rosenthal and T. Calcraft, London, UK.) **C:** Electron micrograph of negative stained PFV budding structures at cellular membranes of 293T cells transfected with proviral expression constructs. Scale bar: 100 nm. (**Panel A** adapted from Lindemann D, Rethwilm A. Foamy virus biology and its application for vector development. *Viruses* 2011;3(5):561–585.)

diameter.[52,104,174,214,287] The core has an isometric, angular, and immature morphology owing to the very limited cleavage of the Gag precursor protein by the viral protease (PR) (see later discussion). The cores of infectious FV virions are made up of the Gag precursor (pr71[Gag] for PFV) and its large processing product (p68[Gag] for PFV) at a ratio of 1:1 up to 1:4[35] (Fig. 20.2). This Gag doublet is inherent in all FVs,[79] although the nonprimate FV capsid proteins are considerably smaller than their primate relatives.[103,134,221,271] Whether the FV core is made up of a hexameric lattice as observed for mature orthoretroviral capsids is currently unknown. However, the recently determined 3D structure of the central, capsid-like Gag domain, which share the same core fold as the N- (NtD$_{CA}$) and C-terminal domains (CtD$_{CA}$) of archetypal orthoretroviral CAs, may suggest so. In addition, the FV core is characterized by being surrounded by an unusual, less ordered shell of density, termed matrix (MA) layer or intermediate shell (Fig. 20.4B and C). It follows the virus membrane at budding, subsequently relocates to the capsid's edges in released virions, and displays different width characteristics for individual FV genera.[287] The intermediate shell is likely formed by the Gag N-terminal domain (NtD) for which a subdomain structure is available,[77] which points outward to the cytoplasmic domains (CyDs) of the FV GPC.[52,287]

The prominent surface spikes are characteristic for FV virions and average 15 nm in length (Fig. 20.4). The mature FV GPCs are organized as tripartite oligomeric protrusions that are frequently arranged in elaborate lattice structures on the virion surface[52,287] (Fig. 20.11). A feature that PFV shares with HBV is the formation of subviral particles (SVPs) consisting only of membranous Env-containing vesicles devoid of cores.[251,256]

It appears that FV particles contain fewer Pol molecules than orthoretroviruses, which is consistent with the high processive activity of its RT.[25,219] The interpretation of other studies demonstrating equal amounts of Pol in foamy- and orthoretroviruses[35] have been complicated by the detection of significant amounts of extraparticular Pol protein present in FV particle preparations of different origin as reported by Swiersy et al.[260] This study and others also revealed that in sharp contrast to orthoretroviruses, FV replication tolerates a great imbalance in the intracellular amounts of Gag and Pol molecules.[137,260] This is owing to the unusual Pol encapsidation strategy of FVs (see later discussion), in which vgRNA is the limiting factor at conditions of high cellular levels of Pol.

Extracellular FV virions obtained after transient transfection of proviral expression constructs into packaging cells or upon virus propagation in tumor cells *in vitro* harbor viral and cellular RNAs.[80] Viral nucleic acid present within the FV core appears to be a mixture of RNA and DNA. vRNA dominates at a ratio of approximately 1:1 to 7:1, depending on the genomic region analyzed long terminal repeat (LTR) versus *gag*.[225,303,304] Consistent with this, both forms of nucleic acid were detected in plasma and saliva of an experimentally infected cynomolgus macaque by PCR and RT-PCR.[27] However, in feces samples collected from chimpanzee in the wild, only vRNA but not vDNA was detectable,[154] as mentioned above. Full-length double-stranded viral genomic DNA (vgDNA) was shown to be present in roughly 5% to 20% of FV virions produced by *in vitro* propagation,[225,303,304] and functional studies using the RT-inhibiting drug AZT indicated vgDNA to be the relevant genome for infection, at least at the high multiplicity of infection (MOI) studied.[171,180,304] Because vgDNA was found in both, PFV and FFV virions, the idea that FVs are facultative DNA viruses may be generalized.[225]

However, it has not been investigated in much detail to what extent reverse transcription (RTr) is taking place late in the replication cycle. For instance, it is likely that there are genomic regions, such as the gap in the plus strand cDNA (see later discussion), that still remain single stranded. The finding of more LTR than *gag* region reverse transcripts in virions clearly indicates this.[225,303] In addition, because more vRNA than vDNA is found in virions, it would be interesting to know whether infectious, purely RNA-containing viruses are generated from specific cell types in natural or zoonotic hosts *in vivo*, as the detection of only vRNA in feces samples of FV infected wild chimpanzees may suggest,[154] or whether other tissues like the oral mucosa that support active replication of FVs *in vivo* release a mixture viruses containing one or the other form of viral nucleic acid as indicated by another study.[27]

It is with respect to RTr taking place at a late step in viral replication that FVs diverge at most from orthoretroviruses, which display a vRNA to DNA ratio of approximately 10^5:1 in extracellular virions.[225] The most compelling evidence for this are experiments in which the infectivity of virion-extracted FV DNA has been demonstrated.[171,225,303] Thus, FV replication functionally combines features of orthoretroviruses and hepad-naviruses (Fig. 20.5). Because of this analogy to the hepadnaviral replication cycle (see Chapter 18, Volume 2 DNA Viruses), the full-length FV RNA packaged into the virion should be viewed as the pregenome or viral genomic RNA (vgRNA).

In addition to RTr in late phases of FV particle morphogenesis, it has been shown that, similar to orthoretroviruses, RTr also occurs during the early phases of FV replication upon target cell entry *in vitro*.[46,304] Given the aforementioned ratios of RNA to DNA in extracellular viruses generated by *in vitro* propagation, RTr during the early phase of FV replication *in vitro* may only become relevant at a very low MOI, when the amount of virion DNA may be too low to sustain a productive infection.[304] Furthermore, the discrepant results reported about the relevance of the differentially timed RTr events for FV infectivity may reflect the inherent differences in the cell types used for virus production.[46,171,180,225,303,304] In essence, the generally accepted view that virions contain either an RNA or DNA genome, but not both, may not apply to FVs.

The physical stability of FVs has not been directly compared with that of orthoretroviruses. However, owing to their immature core and a particular Env topology (see later discussion), these virions are probably quite stable. This is illustrated by the fact that vector particles can be concentrated more than 100-fold (i.e., by ultracentrifugation) without significant loss of infectivity.[72,101]

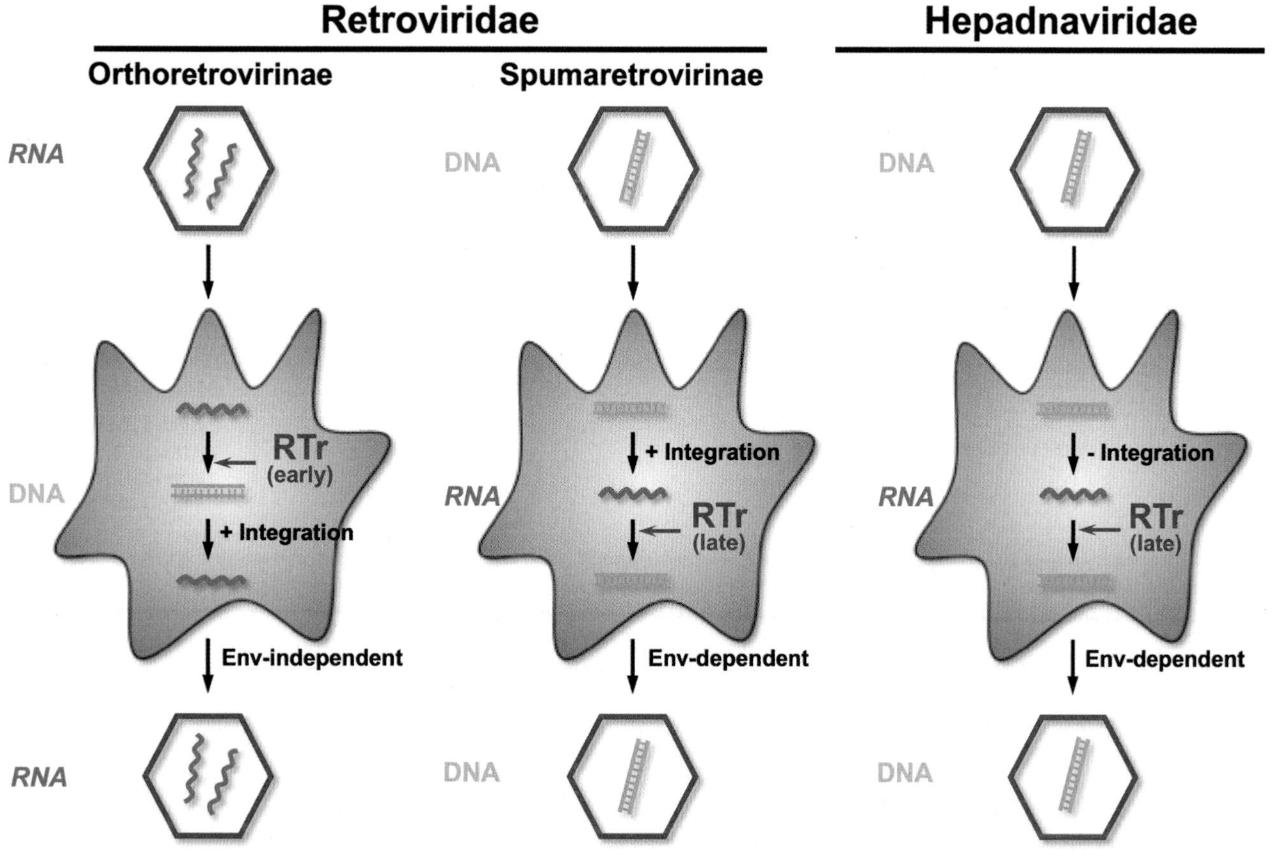

FIGURE 20.5 Principle replication strategies of reverse transcribing viruses. Orthoretroviruses (*left panel*) are RNA viruses that reverse transcribe early in replication, replicate through a DNA intermediate, and exhibit obligate virus-mediated integration into the cellular genome. Hepadnaviruses (*right panel*) are essentially DNA viruses, replicate through an RNA intermediate, and do not integrate. The retroviral subfamily of spumaretroviruses (*middle panel*) functionally combines both pathways by being DNA viruses that reverse transcribe late in replication like hepadnaviruses and integrate like orthoretroviruses.

GENOME STRUCTURE AND ORGANIZATION

All FV genomes share common genome structures.[215] The schematic representation of the PFV genome is shown in Figure 20.6. The general organization of the canonical *gag*, *pol*, and *env* genes and accessory open reading frames (ORFs) downstream of *env* reaching into the 3′ LTR resembles other complex retroviruses. FVs encode two such ORFs, which in older litera-

ture were designated bel1 and bel2. The first ORF *(tas)* encodes the transcriptional transactivator Tas, and *orf-2* is partially used to express a fusion protein designated Bet. In PFV, Bet consists of the first 88 amino acids of Tas fused to the bulk of the coding capacity of *orf-2*. It is noteworthy that no independent protein is expressed from *orf-2* alone in any of the known FVs.

Unique for all FVs is a second, internal promoter (IP) near the 3′ end of the *env* gene, which mainly drives expression of the accessory ORFs[155,158] (Fig. 20.6). FV proviruses are

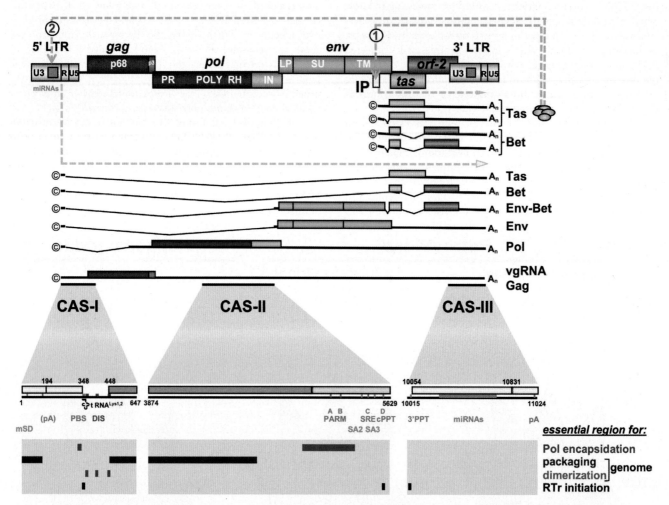

FIGURE 20.6 Foamy virus provirus organization, genomic and structural gene transcripts, and essential cis-acting viral RNA sequence elements. Top: Schematic illustration of the prototype foamy virus (PFV) proviral DNA genome structure with long terminal repeats (LTRs) and ORFs indicated as *boxes*. For ORFs encoding Gag, Pol, and Env precursor proteins, the regions encompassing the mature subunits generated by proteolytic processing are indicated in differential *colors* and labeled accordingly. Underneath, unspliced and spliced transcripts originating at the LTR or internal promoter (IP) including the full-length viral RNA genome (vgRNA) or giving rise to the viral structural (Gag, Pol, Env) and accessory (Tas, Bet) proteins are indicated. The respective coding capacities of individual transcripts are indicated to the *right*. The bimodal transcriptional stimulation of FV transcription by Tas at both, the IP and the LTR promoter, is indicated by *dashed yellow arrows*. **Bottom:** Cis-acting sequence (CAS) elements localized within the full-length vgRNA, which are essential for viral replication, are indicated by *black bars* underneath. Functionally important or essential RNA sequence motifs are marked in each enlarged CAS element below. *Numbers* represent nucleotide positions of the PFV vgRNA (HSRV2 isolate). Individual regions within the vgRNA essential for specific functions in viral replication as indicated to the *right* are marked as differentially *colored bars*. U3, unique 3′ LTR region; R, repeat LTR region; U5, unique 5′ LTR region; miRNAs, microRNA Pol III expression cassettes; p68, Gag p68 subunit; p3, Gag p3 subunit; PR, Pol protease domain; POLY, Pol polymerase domain; RH, Pol RNase H domain; IN, Pol integrase subunit; LP, Env leader peptide subunit; SU, Env surface subunit; TM, Env transmembrane subunit; ©, cap structure; An, poly-A tail; mSD, major splice donor; PBS, primer binding site; DIS, dimerization sites; PARM, protease activating RNA motif; SRE, splicing regulatory element; cPPT, central poly-purine tract; 3′ PPT, 3′ poly-purine tract; pA, polyadenylation signal; A–D, purine-rich (PuR) sequence motifs A through D; RTr, reverse transcription. (Adapted from Lindemann D, Rethwilm A. Foamy virus biology and its application for vector development. *Viruses* 2011;3:561–585.)

12 to 13 kb long and thereby larger than those of most other retroviruses. Their size is partially attributed to the extraordinary long U3 regions of the LTR, which can be explained in part by the overlapping *orf-2* (Fig. 20.6). However, in the case of PFV, the accessory *orf-2* reaches only 300 bp into the 5′ end of the more than 1.4 kb long U3 region. In addition, very few enhancer elements, such as those for AP-1 and Ets-1,[173,239] and the short sequence motifs responsive to the viral transactivator (see later discussion), are present at the 3′ end of U3. The enhancer elements are involved in regulating LTR-derived expression of the structural genes. For many years, several hundred bases in the U3 region remained devoid of known functions until the discovery of one or more RNA Pol III-directed microRNA (miRNA) cassettes[129,285] (Fig. 20.6). For BFV and SFVcae, miRNA expression was experimentally confirmed and a first study examining the possible functions of BFV miRNAs suggest a role in modulating cellular antiviral defense mechanisms.[33] Bioinformatic analysis suggests that nearly all FV genomes contain at least one miRNA cassette.[129,170]

There are length differences in the *gag* genes in different FVs, with those in FVs from cats, bovines, and equines being shorter than those from primates.[103,172,271,290] In sharp contrast to their orthoretroviral cousins, the FV Gag proteins are more variable than the Env proteins. Primate lentiviruses for instance have an amino acid conservation of roughly 60% in Gag and 40% in Env compared to 45% in Gag and 65% in Env among primate FVs.[214,267] It is likely that this curiosity of FV biology is a consequence of the process of adaptation to and coevolution with their natural hosts. Furthermore, this finding is consistent with the use of the same cellular receptor(s) by all FVs.

Like orthoretroviruses, FV genomes contain elements, designated as cis-active sequences (CAS) that harbor secondary and tertiary structures essential for various aspects of viral replication (Fig. 20.6). The first region, CAS-1, is located in the 5′ untranslated leader of the vgRNA and extends into the *gag* gene. It includes the R-U5 region of the LTR, the primer binding site (PBS), which is complementary to the cellular transfer RNA(Lys1,2) and conserved among all FVs and elements conferring dimerization of the vgRNA.[30,60,172] CAS-I has functions in RTr and splice regulation as well as in vgRNA and Pol encapsidation.[92–94,153,293]

However, FVs require another cis-acting genomic RNA element, CAS-II, for viral infectivity and FV vector function[59,91,93,153,293] (Fig. 20.6). CAS-II is reported to harbor additional RNA packaging elements in its 5′ part, while its 3′ portion contains the major Pol encapsidation signal (PES) and four purine-rich sequence elements (PuR-A to -D).[197,198,286] PuR-A and -B appear to be essential elements of the PES element of CAS-II and have been reported to promote FV PR-RT dimerization (protease-activating RNA motif, PARM) and thereby probably Pol precursor encapsidation.[86] PuR-C was shown to represent a splicing regulatory element (SRE) preventing further processing of full-length Gag and single-spliced *Pol* mRNA.[181] PuR-D, found in all sequenced FV genomes, has been demonstrated to serve as a second internal or central poly-purine tract (PPT), similarly to what has been reported for HIV, as an initiation site for plus-strand DNA synthesis during RTr, in addition to the 3′ PPT upstream of the 3′ LTR.[7,197,246,272,286] Finally, a third element, CAS-III, is located far downstream on the vgRNA. It contains the 3′ PPT and the LTR (U3-R) sequences needed for RTr and integration as well

as transcription initiation and polyadenylation upon proviral integration[148] (Fig. 20.6).

VIRION-ASSOCIATED PROTEINS

Gag

The FV capsid proteins have several unusual characteristics compared to orthoretroviral Gag proteins. They are neither cleaved into the canonical matrix (MA), capsid (CA), and nucleocapsid (NC) subunits nor are several sequence motifs present, which are conserved in all orthoretroviral Gag proteins (Fig. 20.7). These include the N-terminal myristoylation signal of the MA domain, the major homology region in the CA domain, or the cysteine-histidine (CH) boxes in the NC domain. Instead of Gag subunit processing observed with orthoretroviruses, at least half of the particle-associated FV Gag molecules are truncated approximately 3 to 4 kD C-terminally by pol-encoded PR processing at a singular cleavage site. In the case of PFV, this generates a large p68^{Gag} and a small p3^{Gag} product from the pr71^{Gag} precursor molecule[67] (Fig. 20.7A). Whereas the p68^{Gag} cleavage product together with the pr71^{Gag} precursor forms the capsid of free PFV virions, the smaller p3^{Gag} so far could not be detected in extracellular virus particles (Figs. 20.2 and 20.4A). Whether this is due to limitations in the sensitivity of the detection methods employed, or may indicate that Gag precursor processing starts before the PFV capsid is fully assembled and this small processing product thereby evades encapsidation, is unclear. The p3^{Gag} postprocessing cellular localization, fate, function, and possible functions remain to be elucidated.[55] FV Gag cleavage is required for infectivity, as FVs expressing only the pr71^{Gag} precursor are not infectious and often produce aberrantly formed capsids.[55,130,305] Mutants expressing only the large p68^{Gag} cleavage product are infectious albeit at 10- to 50-fold lower titers.[55,108,257,305] Secondary protease cleavage sites, located in the central part of FV Gag, have been identified *in vitro*, using recombinant proteins and peptides[200] (Fig. 20.7A). They are proposed to be utilized for a viral disassembly process involving proteolytic processing of Gag by the FV PR and cellular proteases following entry into target cells.[73,140,200] However, the essential requirement of the Gag processing by FV PR at the secondary cleavage sites for viral replication is a matter of debate.[108,140] Thus, FV capsid disassembly appears to be a unique process that involves viral and cellular protease-mediated processing.

In the FV Gag precursors, currently five major regions or domains can be structurally and functionally distinguished (Fig. 20.7A): an NtD; a proline-rich (P-rich) region of variable length mainly responsible for the size variation among Gag precursor proteins of different FV genera (52 to 71 kDa); a central capsid (CA) domain; a glycine–arginine–rich (GR-rich) region; and the C-terminal p3^{Gag} domain, with the first four located in the p68^{Gag} subunit. For PFV, of two of those, 3D structures were recently solved, namely the 180 aa NtD and the 178 aa central CA[10,77] (Fig. 20.7B and C).

Various peptide and structural motifs have been identified and characterized to variable extent in FV Gag proteins (Fig. 20.7). Four coiled-coil domains (CC1-4) are predicted to be present in PFV Gag,[199,269] and functions have been assigned to the first three located in the NtD (Fig. 20.7A and B). The N-terminal CC1 (aa 14–24) has been suggested to interact with

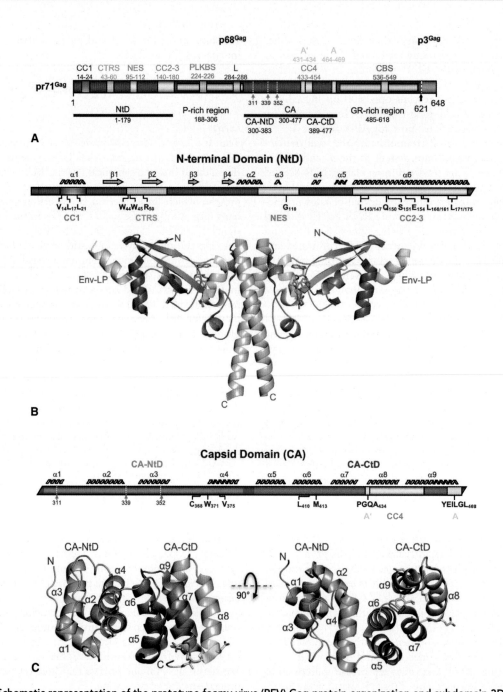

FIGURE 20.7 Schematic representation of the prototype foamy virus (PFV) Gag protein organization and subdomain 3D structures.
A: PFV Gag protein organization and selected functional motifs highlighted by the *colored boxes*. The organization of the N-terminal domain (NtD) and the central capsid-like (CA) domain are shown in the enlargements in **B** and **C**. Numbers indicate amino acid (aa) sequence positions of PFV Gag. The *black arrow* indicates the viral protease cleavage site of pr71^{Gag} for processing into p68^{Gag} and p3^{Gag} utilized during virus morphogenesis, *gray arrows* mark secondary cleavage sites of potential processing upon virus entry. *Gray boxes* represent the proline-rich (P-rich) and glycine–arginine–rich (GR-rich) regions, respectively. CC1 to CC4, coiled-coil domains 1 to 4; CTRS, cytoplasmic targeting and retention signal; NES, nuclear export sequence; PLKBS, polo-like kinase binding site; L, late budding domain motif; A, assembly motif YxxLGL; A', assembly motif PGQA; CBS, chromatin binding sequence. **B:** Crystal structure of PFV Gag NtD-Env LP complex (PDB ID: 4JMR). *Upper*, PFV Gag enlargement showing just the PFV Gag NtD, secondary structure elements indicated above. *Lower*, cartoon representation of the crystal structure of the PFV Gag NtD homodimer. The functional sequence motifs, CC1 Env-binding region (*blue*), CTRS (*orange*), NES (*green*) and CC2-3 dimer interface coiled-coil (*cyan*) are color coded as in the schematic. Residue side chains in the GWWGQ core of the CTRS are shown in stick representation. The helical regions of the Env-LP bound at the periphery of the Gag-NtD head domain are colored *gold*. **C:** 3D solution NMR structure of the central PFV Gag capsid (CA) domains (PDB ID: 5M1H). *Upper*, PFV Gag CA enlargement with secondary structure elements indicated above. *Lower*, cartoon representation of the PFV Gag CA structure. The backbone of the N-terminal capsid domain (CA-NtD) and C-terminal capsid domain (CA-CtD) are shown in *pink* and *brown*. Helices in the structure are numbered sequentially from N- to C-terminus in the left- and right-hand views. The CC4, PGQA, and YxxLGL sequence motifs are color coded as in the schematic. Residue side chains in the PGQA and YxxLGL sequence motifs in the α7-α8 connecting loop and C-terminal of α9 are shown in stick representation. (**Panel A** adapted from Lindemann D, Rethwilm A. Foamy virus biology and its application for vector development. *Viruses* 2011;3(5):561–585. https://creativecommons.org/licenses/by/3.0/. **panels B and C** 3D-ribbon structure cartoons of panels B and C courtesy of Ian A. Taylor, London, UK)

the CyD of the Env leader peptide (LP) according to initial biochemical analyses.[34,146,207,288] A direct interaction was confirmed later by 3D structural data of Gag NtD-Env LP peptide cocrystals[77] (Fig. 20.7B). CC2 (aa 130–146) has been reported to harbor a domain necessary for Gag multimerization,[269] and CC3 (aa 161–180) is believed to be required for incoming capsids to interact with the dynein light chain 8 for retrograde movement along the cellular microtubule network to the microtubule organizing center (MTOC).[199] The Gag NtD 3D structure revealed an extended, single coiled-coil structure comprised by CC2 and CC3 essential for dimerization of the NtD.[77] The function of CC4 (aa 436–453), which is located at the C-terminus of the PFV Gag CA domain (Fig. 20.7C), whose 3D structure was recently determined,[10] remains unknown.

C-terminally of CC4 the PFV Gag CA domain also harbors an evolutionary conserved YxxLGL sequence termed assembly motif (A-motif; aa 464–469) (Fig. 20.7A and C) shown to be essential for both, capsid assembly and RTr.[168] The PFV Gag CA structure revealed the presence of two all α-helical domains (CA-NtD) and (CA-CtD) that, although having no sequence similarity, both share the same core fold as the N-(NtD$_{CA}$) and C-terminal domains (CtD$_{CA}$) of archetypal orthoretroviral CAs (Fig. 20.7C). The tyrosine residue of the A-motif at the C-terminus of an α-helix 9 in the PFV CA-CtD appears to be involved in hydrophobic interactions forming part of the core of the CA-CtD bundle. In contrast, the LGL portion of the A-motif is exposed and forms a continuous hydrophobic surface patch together with a second, A′-motif (aa 431–434, PGQA) in an α-helix 8 (Fig. 20.7C). It is speculated that it is involved in interactions that give rise to hexameric assemblies analogous to those formed in orthoretrovirus capsids.[10] This study has also identified a previously unknown hydrophobic interface between PFV CA-NtD α-helices 2 and 4 and CA-CtD α-helices 5 and 6 (Fig. 20.7C). The relevance of this interface for correct capsid assembly and generation of infectious virions has been demonstrated by cryo-electron tomography and infectivity analysis of viral mutants with alterations in key residues of this hydrophobic interface.[10]

In primate FVs, the GR-rich region is organized in three 11 to 13 aa-long clusters, termed GR boxes I to III, which is not the case in other FVs including the ancient endogenous FVs[103,237,271,290] (Fig. 20.7A). Initial studies assigned various functions to individual PFV Gag GR boxes, like vgRNA or Pol protein encapsidation, RTr, capsid assembly, viral infectivity, or nuclear localization of PFV Gag.[182,237,270,300] However, in respect to vgRNA packaging, a more recent report suggests that encapsidation of the PFV vgRNA and cellular RNAs are mediated by the cooperative action of arginine residues in the GR-rich domain.[80]

Nuclear localization of the Gag protein is a common feature of most FVs proven by a strong nuclear fluorescence using homologous serum in IFA. Intracellular distribution and/or trafficking of FV Gag proteins is affected by several peptide motifs. The NtD harbors a nuclear export signal (NES) at aa 95–112 (Fig. 20.7A and B). It is proposed to be responsible for the active nuclear export of Gag after its nuclear interaction with vgRNA[208] and to antagonize another trafficking signal located in the GR-rich region, the chromatin binding signal (CBS) at aa 536–549.[145,182,270] Furthermore, GR-I and GR-III sequences were reported to promote nucleolar targeting of

PFV Gag, a function that appears to be naturally antagonized by the CBS located in GR-II.[192] By this regulatory circuit, a putative temporal nuclear trafficking of Gag is achieved, which may be involved in selective encapsidation of vgRNA during assembly of the virion.[208] However, this proposed function of PFV Gag is challenged by other studies. Either, involvement of Gag in nuclear vgRNA export was not observed,[23] or Gag nuclear localization was seen as a passive process achieved only by CBS-mediated chromatin tethering upon nuclear membrane breakdown during host cell mitosis, rather than its active nuclear import into interphase cell nuclei.[145,182] These studies rather suggest a primary role of the CBS during virus entry by enabling Gag association with cellular chromosomes through direct CBS–nucleosome interaction and appears to be important for tethering the FV preintegration complex to cellular chromatin, thereby determining the integration site profile of FVs.[145]

Similar to MPMV, a cytoplasmic targeting and retention signal (CTRS, aa 43–60) is also located at the NtD of PFV Gag[34,51,249] (Fig. 20.7A and B). However, unlike MPMV, mutation of a conserved arginine in the CTRS did not lead to a switch from a B/D to a C-type capsid assembly strategy. Instead, mutation of the analogous arginine in PFV Gag completely abolished particle release.[51,146] This suggests that the CTRS of MPMV and FV Gag are functionally different.

A late assembly (L) domain specified by the motif PSAP (aa 284–287 of PFV Gag) and located at the C-terminus of the P-rich region (Fig. 20.7A) interacts with the cellular export machinery vacuolar protein sorting (VPS) via TSG101 to mediate release of virus particles from the plasma membrane.[195,255] However, PSAP motifs are absent in nonprimate FV Gag proteins, and their functional L-domains remain to be identified.[255] Interestingly, ubiquitination of PFV Gag—a common feature of orthoretroviral capsids upon interaction with the VPS machinery—has not been observed as discussed below.[256] This suggests that ubiquitin conjugation to transacting cellular factors, not the Gag protein itself, may be critical for ubiquitin-dependent particle release of enveloped viruses.[307,308]

In addition to the proteolytic processing of the FV Gag precursor, several additional posttranslational modifications of PFV Gag were reported. The latter is phosphorylated at unspecified serine residues with unknown functional consequences.[55] Furthermore, particle-associated PFV Gag was found to be phosphorylated at threonine 225 (T$_{225}$), which is located in a polo-like kinase (PLK) S-T/S-P consensus binding sequence[310] (Fig. 20.7A). Upon host cell entry, Gag phosphorylated at T$_{225}$ interacts with PLK1 and/or PLK2 and relocalizes the PLKs to mitotic condensed chromatin, a process which is dependent on a functional Gag CBS. PFV mutants deficient in PLK interaction displayed reduced infectivity due to a delayed and decreased integration efficiency and an increased preference for heterochromatin integration sites. This demonstrates that PFV Gag–PLK interactions are important for early viral replication steps and may be involved in the mitosis-dependent disassembly and integration process of FVs. Furthermore, PFV Gag was reported to interact with cellular protein arginine methyltransferases (PMRTs) 1 and 5, which results in Gag methylation at several arginine residues.[192] Methylation of PFV Gag arginine 540 (R$_{540}$), which is a key residue of the CBS (Fig. 20.7A), was reported to mask its chromatin tethering function and result in a GR-I and GR-III dependent nucleolar relocalization of Gag in interphase nuclei. Other posttranslational modifications, like N-terminal myristoylation or ubiquitination, reported for orthoretroviral Gag proteins, could not be detected for FV Gag proteins. The absence of ubiquitination is not surprising since an unusual and distinguishing feature of FV Gag proteins is their paucity of lysine residues.[171,256,308] PFV Gag contains only a single lysine residue essential for replication in primary cells.[171] This notable feature may be the reason for the FVs ability to remain biologically active for a quite prolonged time after infecting resting cells.

In summary, FV capsids share various features with the cores of hepadnaviruses (i.e., glycoprotein dependence for budding, nuclear localization, and the presence of arginine-rich motifs) as well as with orthoretroviruses (i.e., presence of an L-domain and a CTRS). There are also Gag characteristics that are unique to FVs, particularly their unusual cleavage pattern. Furthermore, alterations of conserved FV Gag motifs result in morphologic defects that affect the ability of capsids to support intraparticle RTr and render such mutants noninfectious.

Pol

Unlike orthoretroviruses, FV Pol is translated from its own spliced mRNA, using the major splice donor (mSD) in the R region of the LTR and a suboptimal splice acceptor in the *gag* ORF, instead from the full-length vgRNA (Fig. 20.6). The latter prevents *pol* mRNA from becoming too abundant.[22,56,116,136,156,298] Historically, the discovery of a spliced pol mRNA and large amounts of vgDNA in extracellular virions represent a landmark in retrovirus research.[298] PFV Pol is translated separately from Gag as a large, approximately 127-kD polyprotein harboring the four enzymatic domains of PR, polymerase (POLY), RNase H (RH), and IN from N- to C-terminus (Fig. 20.8A). Deviating from other retroviruses, the PFV pr127[Pol] precursor is processed by the viral PR during or following capsid assembly into only two mature subunits: p85[PR-RT] and p40[IN].[67] FV PR does not exist as a separate subunit and instead remains covalently attached to the N-terminus of the RT POLY domain through a peptide linker (Fig. 20.8A). This unique element (aa 93–120) is not present in other RTs and consists of an unstructured region followed by an alpha-helix.[188] Studies with deletion variants indicated that it is an integral part of the RT domain, which is important for activity and solubility.[241] Both PR-RT and IN localize to the nucleus in infected cells.[110] FV Pol precursor processing is required for virus replication.[130,224] For the PFV IN subunit, NLS sequence motifs have been characterized.[6,109]

On the other hand, FV mutants have been reported to be replication competent when Pol was expressed in-frame with the preceding *gag* ORF or by an orthoretroviral-like frameshift mechanism.[137,260] From orthoretroviruses, it is known that expression of a Gag-Pol fusion protein alone is incompatible with viral replication owing to severe particle assembly or release defects.[280] Furthermore, these defects often involved the orthoretroviral PR that was either found to be inactive or hyperactive. The finding that FV replication tolerates expression of an in-frame Gag-Pol fusion protein indicates a mode of Pol encapsidation and regulation of PR domain activity that is unique to these viruses and different from that observed for orthoretrovi-

ruses (see later discussion). In the BFV system, equal amounts of *gag* and *pol* mRNAs have been reported.[103] Whether this also leads to similar amounts of intracellular Gag and Pol proteins has not been investigated.

All retroviral PRs including the FV PR belong to the family of aspartic PRs and are active as dimers. Each subunit of the homodimer provides one catalytic aspartate residue situated in the conserved motif Asp-Thr-Ser-Gly in order to create the active site. So the question arises, how FV Pol dimerization is accomplished. In orthoretroviruses, this is facilitated by Gag oligomerization of the Gag-Pol fusion protein, which is not possible in FVs. Biochemical and biophysical evidence point to transient dimer formation of FV Pol, as the enzyme is always purified as a monomer, except under nonphysiologic conditions of high salt.[87] A role of RNA in PR activation was proposed by Hartl et al.[86] by identifying a *pol* ORF-located RNA PARM present on vgRNA (Fig. 20.6). By binding to PARM, the full-length p85[PR-RT] subunit including its C-terminal RH domain dimerizes and PR is activated.[86,241] Although the entire process has not yet been elucidated, this mechanism could explain the replication competence of viral mutants expressing an in-frame Gag-Pol protein,[137,260] because they can also rely on activation of PR by PARM, which would be the rate-limiting step for PR dimerization. The mechanism of PR activation by binding to RNA is unique among retroviruses and explains the necessity of a PR-RT fusion protein. Thus, premature PR activity before virus assembly can be avoided.[86]

FV RTs bear the motif YxDD in the active center and are sensitive to nucleoside analog RT inhibitors, such as AZT[131,138,219,222] (Fig. 20.8B). Both, the RH domain and the connection subdomain of RT substantially contribute to polymerase integrity and stability as well as polymerase activity and substrate binding[241] (Fig. 20.8B–D). RH is an endonuclease covalently coupled to the POLY domain of Pol and hydrolyzes the RNA template strand in RNA/DNA hybrids during RTr. This activity is essential for virus replication.[210,268] Like the murine leukemia virus (MLV) enzyme, but unlike HIV RT, FV RH possesses a protruding basic loop and the so-called C-helix[25,142] (Fig. 20.8E). This has been validated in the solution structure of the PFV RH domain alone[143] and in the complete White-tufted-ear marmoset SFV (SFVcja) PR-RT subunit crystal structure,[188] indicating a function of the basic loop in substrate binding. Strikingly, PFV RH is inhibited by HIV-1 RH inhibitors, suggesting a similar inhibitor binding pocket of the two proteins.[42]

Only very recently, the first 3D structures of complete, mature PR-RT subunits from SFVcja in complex with different substrates were solved by X-ray crystallography and cryo-electron microscopy reconstruction[188] (Fig. 20.8C and D). Surprisingly, differential oligomeric states were observed depending on the type of nucleic acid substrate used. Full-length SFVcja PR-RT monomers bound to RNA/DNA hybrid substrates (Fig. 20.8C), whereas dsDNA substrates were found in complex with asymmetric homodimers of either RH-deleted or full-length SFVcja PR-RT (Fig. 20.8D), resembling HIV-1 p66/p51 RT heterodimers. This not only is the first report of a retroviral RT to adopt different oligomeric configurations but may suggest that FV −strand and +strand DNA synthesis may be executed by different enzyme configurations. Perhaps the monomeric or dimeric state of this enzymatic complex may also be attributed to the sequential order of FV polyprotein

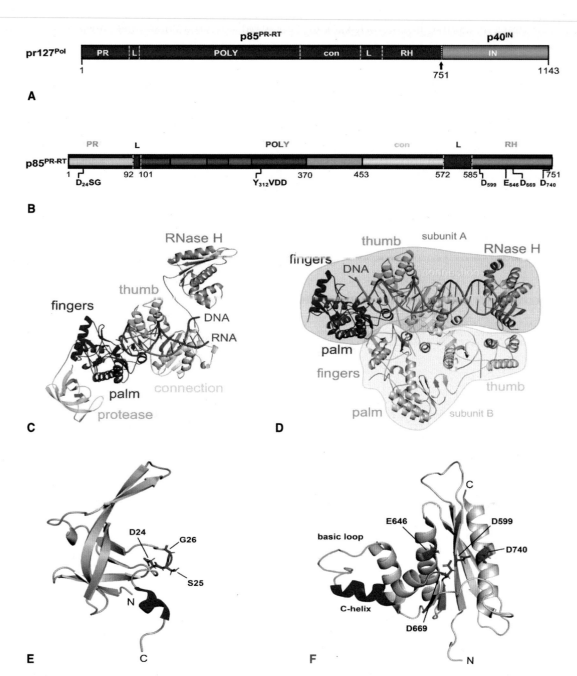

FIGURE 20.8 Schematic representation of the foamy virus Pol protein organization and PR-RT subunit/subdomain 3D structures. A: Schematic of the prototype foamy virus (PFV) Pol precursor protein. *Numbers* indicate amino acid positions of PFV Pol. The *black arrow* marks the cleavage site of pr127^{Pol} for processing into p85^{PR-RT} and p40^{IN}. (Subdomains of PR-RT: PR, protease; L, linker; POLY, polymerase; con, connection; RH, RNase H; IN: integrase subunit.) **B:** Schematic representation of the PFV Pol p85^{PR-RT} subunit organization. Individual subdomains are indicated by differently *colored boxes*. PR (*light blue*); POLY palm (*dark red*); POLY fingers (*dark blue*); POLY thumb (*green*); con (*yellow*); RH (*orange*). Active site residues of PR, POLY, and RH are marked. **C:** Cartoon representation of monomeric White-tufted-ear marmoset simian foamy virus (SFVcja) PR-RT in complex with an RNA/DNA hybrid substrate (pdb:7O0G). **D:** Cryo-EM reconstruction of dimeric SFVcja PR-RT in complex with a 22 bp/2 nt overhang dsDNA substrate. Lighter shades of colors are used for domains/subdomains of subunit B (pdb:7O24). **E:** Cartoon representation of the solution structure of the Taiwanese macaque simian foamy virus (SFVmcy) protease (PR) monomer. The flap region (*red*) and the C-terminal α-helix (*blue*) are highlighted. The conserved amino acids D24, S25, and G26 forming the active site in the dimer are depicted in red as sticks (pdb:2JYS). **F:** Ribbon diagram of the solution structure of the PFV RNase H. The C-helix is highlighted in *blue*; the basic loop in *green*. The active site residues D599, E646, D669, and D740 are depicted in *red* as sticks (pdb:2LSN). (**Panel A** adapted from Lindemann D, Rethwilm A. Foamy virus biology and its application for vector development. *Viruses* 2011;3(5):561–585; **panels C and D** courtesy of Marcin Nowotny, Warsaw, Poland; **panels E and F** courtesy of Birgitta M. Wöhrl, University of Bayreuth, Germany.)

processing by the viral PR, of which we unfortunately know so little until now.

FV replication depends on integration mediated by the active IN. A 4-bp duplication of staggered chromosomal nucleotides occurs at the site of integration.[57,176] Orthoretroviruses utilize 3′ end processing as the initial step of the integration reaction. This involves the removal of two nucleotides from each terminus of the blunt-ended linear vDNA. During FV integration, only the 3′ terminus (within the U5 region) of the vDNA undergoes processing, whereas the 5′ end (the U3 region of the LTR) remains unprocessed, possibly because it is already suitable for integration.[57,118] In 2010, a seminal study was published that described the crystal structure of full-length PFV IN bound to its cognate DNA as a tight complex, termed the intasome[83] (Fig. 20.9). This achievement was possible because, unlike orthoretroviral IN proteins, the recombinant PFV IN is uniquely soluble and catalytically active *in vitro*.[275] These properties contrast with the aggregation and poor enzymatic activity

observed with other retroviral INs, regardless of the expression system.

Classically, retroviral INs are subdivided into three domains (Fig. 20.9A): an N-terminal Zn²⁺ binding domain (NTD), characterized by pairs of His and Cys residues (HHCC motif), that is expanded by an approximately 40 aa residue NTD extension domain (NED) in FV-, γ-, and ε-retrovirus INs; a catalytic core domain (CCD), harboring the Asp, Asp-35-Glu (DD35E) motif; and a nucleic acid–binding Arg/Lys-rich C-terminal domain (CTD).[144] These domains are connected by nonconserved flexible linkers. Early studies reported unspecific DNA-binding activity by the CTD, and it was assumed that retroviral INs would adopt a dimeric or tetrameric structure when engaged with the vDNA ends.[144] It was also hypothesized that multimers were highly flexible, and several contrasting structures of the retroviral intasome had been proposed. Crystallization of the PFV intasome has revealed the definitive answer to a long-standing

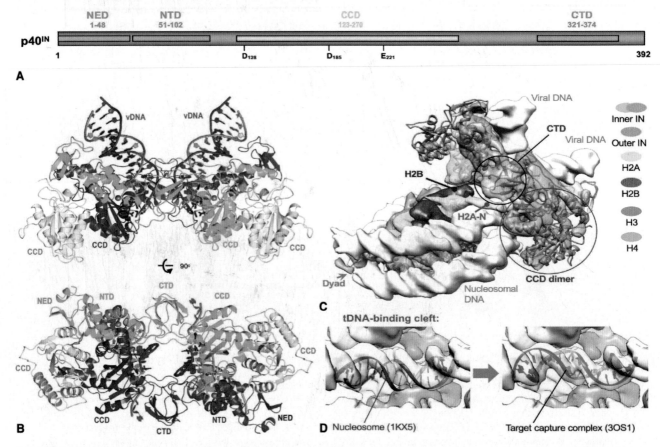

FIGURE 20.9 The architecture of the prototype foamy virus (PFV) intasome. A: Schematic representation of the PFV Pol p40^IN subunit organization. Individual subdomains are indicated by differentially *colored boxes*. Amino-terminal domain (NTD, *green*); NTD extension domain (NED, *green*); catalytic core domain (CCD, *yellow*); carboxyterminal domain (CTD, *green*). Active site residues of the D,D-35-E motif of the CCD are marked. **B:** The crystal structure (PDB ID 3OY9) is shown as viewed along (*bottom panel*) or perpendicular (*top panel*) to its twofold axis. Viral DNA (vDNA) chains are shown as cartoons and colored by chain (*magenta*: reactive strand; *orange*: nontransferred strand); vDNA bases and active site IN residues are shown as sticks. *Gray spheres* are metal cations. Locations of IN domains (NTD, CTD, and CCD) are indicated. **C:** Segmented electron density map as semitransparent surface with docked PFV intasome and nucleosome structures shown as ribbons. H2B, the N-terminal tail of H2A (H2A-N), the CTD and one of the CCD dimers are indicated. **D:** Nucleosomal DNA within the tDNA-binding cleft of the intasome. DNA conformations as in available nucleosome structures (*left*) and as in the crystals of the PFV target capture complex (*right*) produce local electron density cross-correlation scores of 0.36 and 0.70, respectively. Protein Data Bank accessions are indicated in *brackets*. (**Panel B** courtesy of Peter Cherepanov, Francis Crick Institute, London, UK; **panels C and D** reprinted by permission from Nature: Maskell DP, Renault L, Serrao E, et al. Structural basis for retroviral integration into nucleosomes. *Nature* 2015;523(7560):366–369. Copyright © 2015 Springer Nature.)

puzzle. The foamyviral integration apparatus contains a tetramer of IN, assembled on a pair of vDNA ends, in which all three IN domains and interdomain linkers are involved in intimate protein–protein and protein–DNA interactions cross-linking the complex in a rigid structure[83] (Fig. 20.9B). Further cocrystallization of the PFV intasome with target DNA to mimic of the host cell chromosomal DNA revealed the assembly of the entire retroviral synaptic integration complex prior to and following strand transfer.[165] Structures of the PFV intasome–nucleosome complex revealed a multivalent intasome–nucleosome interface involving both gyres of nucleosomal DNA and one H2A-H2B histone heterodimer[169] (Fig. 20.9C and D; Video 20.3). Without altering the histone octamer, the cellular target DNA is lifted from the surface of the H2A-H2B heterodimer by a looping-and-sliding mechanism to allow integration at preferred locations.[169,289] Moreover, because of the structural and functional similarity of

PFV and HIV-1 INs, the mechanism of action of several HIV IN strand transfer inhibitors in clinical use (raltegravir, elvitegravir, and dolutegravir) was elucidated.[84,85] Using the PFV intasome as a surrogate for its HIV counterpart, it was shown that these small molecule inhibitors bind to the active site of IN and displace the reactive 3′ hydroxyl group of the vDNA, thereby preventing strand transfer.[144] After solving the PFV intasome structure, it was believed that retroviral integrases generally function as a tetrameric complex. However, subsequent elucidation of other retroviral intasome structures revealed that α- and β-retroviruses require eight, and lentiviruses up to sixteen integrase subunits, to assemble the intasome core structure.[54]

Env

The Env glycoprotein of FVs has an unusual primary structure and topology[70,150] (Figs. 20.10 and 20.11). It is synthesized as

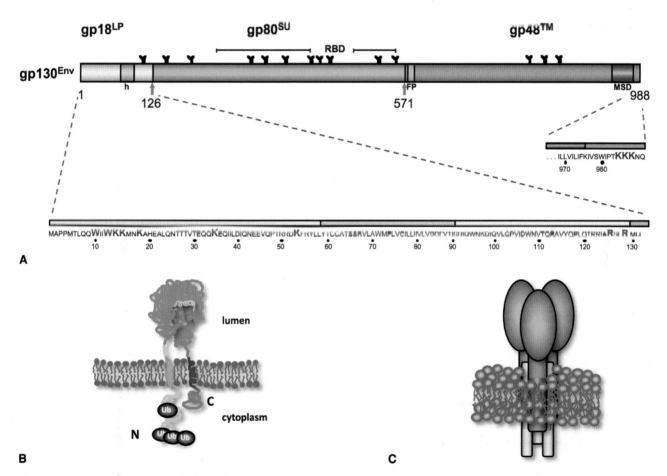

FIGURE 20.10 Schematic representation of the prototype foamy virus (PFV) Env protein domain organization and membrane topology. A: Schematic representation of the prototype foamy virus (PFV) Env protein organization. The furin cleavage sites within the gp130[Env] precursor used to generate the mature gp18[LP], gp80[SU], and gp48[TM] subunits are indicated by *gray arrows*. The individual subunits are shown as boxes in different shades of *green*. Hydrophobic sequences spanning the membrane in the gp18[LP] (h) and the gp48[TM] (membrane-spanning domain, MSD) subunit as well as the fusion peptide (FP) are indicated. The amino acid sequence of the PFV Env gp18[LP] subunit and the cytoplasmic domain of the gp48[TM] subunit are shown in the enlargements below. The conserved WxxW and RxxR motif in LP are highlighted in *red* and the lysine residues potentially ubiquitinated in *blue*. The KKxx ER retrieval signal at the C-terminus is highlighted. The approximate positions of PFV Env N-glycosylation sites are marked by *Y-shaped symbols*. **B:** Schematic membrane topology of the monomeric unprocessed Env precursor protein with ubiquitination (Ub) sites in the leader peptide regulating subviral particle release. The N- and C-termini of the protein are indicated. **C:** Schematic view of the trimeric PFV glycoprotein complex assembled from mature LP, SU, and TM subunits. Color coding of subunits and hydrophobic h, MSD, and FP peptides in **B** and **C** is identical to **A**. (**Panels A to C** adapted from Lindemann D, Rethwilm A. Foamy virus biology and its application for vector development. *Viruses* 2011;3(5):561–585. https://creativecommons.org/licenses/by/3.0/.)

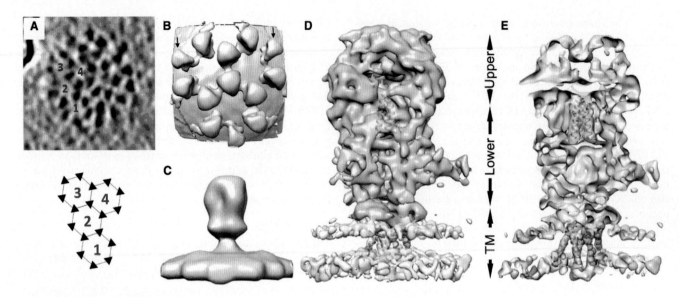

FIGURE 20.11 Prototype foamy virus (PFV) glycoprotein structures on cell-free virions. A and B: 0.8-nm-thick tomographic slice perpendicular to the glycoprotein long axis and its corresponding schematic of interlocked hexagonal assemblies of trimers. *Numbers* are indicated at the center of each hexagon, and *triangles* represent the positions of each trimer of Env in the hexagonal network. **B:** Top view of intertwined hexagonal assemblies. **C:** Side view of a single trimer. **D and E:** *In situ* single particle 3D reconstruction of PFV glycoprotein by cryo-EM. Full **(D)** and cut-away **(E)** side views of a single PFV Env trimer (sharpened map) after threefold symmetry application (~9 Å resolution at FSC = 0.143). The densities corresponding to the extracellular domains and the viral membrane are colored *salmon* and *gray*, respectively in **(D)**. The three central helices attributed to gp48 fusion peptide are represented by three *green* α-helices each being 22 residues long. The transmembrane helices (TMHs) are represented by three inner (colored *blue*) and three outer (colored *orange*) α-helices. In **(E)**, the densities surrounding the three central helices and the three inner and outer TMHs are colored *green, blue,* and *orange,* respectively, while the remaining of the spike is *gray* colored. **(Panels A to E** adapted from Effantin G, Estrozi LF, Aschman N, et al. Cryo-electron microscopy structure of the native prototype foamy virus glycoprotein and virus architecture. *PLoS Pathog* 2016;12(7):e1005721. https://creativecommons.org/licenses/by/4.0/.)

a large precursor protein, in case of PFV comprising 988 aa (gp130[Env]), from spliced subgenomic mRNAs (Fig. 20.6). FV Env is tripartite, consisting of gp18[LP] (LP), gp80[SU] surface (SU), and gp48[TM] transmembrane (TM) subunits[150] (Figs. 20.4A and 20.10B and C). The Env precursor is not cotranslationally processed by the cellular signal peptidase complex, which naturally removes N-terminal signal peptides required for targeting glycoproteins to the secretory pathway. Therefore, unlike orthoretroviruses, which have their glycoprotein anchored in the cellular lipid membrane only via the TM domain, the FV Env precursor spans the membrane twice with the N- and C-terminal regions of the precursor located in the cytoplasm[150] (Figs. 20.10B and 20.11D and E). The peptide backbone of the PFV Env precursor protein is cleaved between LP and SU (after aa 126) and between SU and TM (after aa 571), during transport to the cell surface in the late Golgi complex, by furin-like cellular proteases.[49,69] The SU-TM cleavage is required for infectivity, whereas the LP-SU cleavage is not.[49] Furthermore, PFV and FFV Env precursors, and possibly their mature LP as well, are substrates for SPase and signal peptide peptidase-like (SPPL) proteases.[69,70,277] Whether SPase- and SPPL-mediated cleavage of FV Env is of functional relevance for viral replication or just involved in cellular degradation of Elp/LP has not been investigated.

As a consequence, the mature LP subunit is an integral component of the mature tripartite and trimeric Env GPC present on released FV particles[52,287] (Figs. 20.4A; 20.10B and C; 20.11). It transverses the viral membrane at the N-terminus (a type II transmembrane protein), as does the TM subunit at the C-terminus of

Env (a type I transmembrane protein)[150,288] (Figs. 20.10B and C, 20.11D and E). All three Env subunits are heavily glycosylated. Fourteen N-linked glycosylation sites have been mapped, only two of which, N8 and N13 located in PFV SU and PFV TM, respectively, are essential for viral infectivity[163] (Fig. 20.10A).

The C-terminal CyD of the TM subunit comprising 16 aa is rather short, and its presence is not required for particle egress[202] (Fig. 20.10A). In contrast, the N-terminal CyD of the LP subunit, comprising approximately 68 aa, is considerably longer. Alteration of conserved tryptophan residues herein, at aa positions 10 and 13 of the PFV LP, abolished interaction with the Gag protein.[77,150,288] Not only is FV Env required for export of capsids, but Gag expression is also necessary for the transport of Env to the cell surface.[203] This observation implied that highly specific interactions influence the intracellular distribution and trafficking of both proteins.[34,65,202] Coimmunoprecipitation analyses and surface plasmon resonance to define an N-terminal LP "budding domain" suggested and demonstrated that a direct interaction of LP and Gag with both tryptophan residues is critical and essential.[150,207,288] Indeed, this has been confirmed by solving the crystal structure of an N-terminal MA-like domain of PFV Gag comprising aa 1–179 and variants thereof cocrystallized with peptides representing the first 20 aa of the PFV LP N-terminus[77] (Fig. 20.7B).

Aside from its interaction with Gag, additional factors appear to regulate Env intracellular trafficking and transport to the cell surface. First, a dilysine motif, known to be responsible for retrieval of glycoproteins to the endoplasmic reticulum (ER), is present near the C-terminus of the TM of most FV Env proteins[75] (Fig. 20.10A). Although this signal can sort Env to the ER, it is not required for efficient virus replication of PFV[76] and, in comparison to the other factors, has only a weak effect on Env intracellular distribution. Second, posttranslational ubiquitination of four of five lysine residues located within the LP subunit N-terminal CyD also appears to mediate efficient Env removal from the cell surface as observed for PFV as well as for SFVmcy, a monkey FV formerly designated SFVmac[254,256] (Fig. 20.10A). In contrast, FFV Env LP appears not to be ubiquitinated.[69] Whether this type of posttranslational modification occurs in nonprimate FVs like BFV or EFV and has a crucial function in their intracellular GP trafficking has not been investigated. Third, BFV Env lacking the dilysine ER retrieval signal was recently shown to be palmitoylated at two conserved cysteine residues located close to the lipid membrane in the N-terminal CyD of the LP subunit.[36] BFV Env mutants with inactivated palmitoylation sites showed an impaired Env cell surface expression and membrane fusion activity.[36]

The PFV Env has been shown to support not only viral particle release from cells but also release of SVP from other cellular membranes harboring the viral glycoprotein.[251] This is again analogous to a similar process observed in hepadnaviruses, which secrete vast amounts of SVPs, the so-called Australia antigen (see Chapter 18, Volume 2 DNA Viruses). Ubiquitination appears to suppress the intrinsic activity of the primate FV glycoprotein to induce SVP release, and mutants of the lysine-specifying codons in the LP CyD release large amounts of SVP.[256] These PFV Env mutants appear to be particularly well suited to pseudotype orthoretroviral capsids, in contrast to wild-type PFV Env, probably owing to its low level of cell surface expression.[81]

Surprisingly, the gp130[Env] is not the only FV glycoprotein synthesized. Using conserved splice sites within *env* ORF of the FV genome (Fig. 20.6), alternatively spliced *env* transcripts are generated. In case of PFV, this leads to translation of proteins consisting of Env lacking the membrane-spanning domain (MSD) and CyD of TM fused in-frame with the Bet protein (Env-Bet)[74,147] or, as in the case of FFV, Env lacking only the MSD of TM fused to the orf-2 encoded peptide sequence (Env-Bel2).[21] The Env-Bet fusion protein and its processing products LP, SU, and ΔTM-Bet are secreted into the supernatant of PFV-infected cells but are not associated with the viral particle.[147] This fusion protein is synthesized at about 50% of the level of particle-associated gp130[Env], suggesting that it may have a useful function *in vivo*. In cell culture, however, replication-competent PFV mutants deficient in Env-Bet synthesis do not exhibit a distinctive phenotype, and no revertants with restored Env-Bet expression have been observed.[147]

In summary, the biosynthesis and membrane topology of the FV Env are highly unusual for retroviral GPs. The Env LP subunit is an integral component of the particle-associated Env complex and harbors in its CyD the major interaction domain with FV capsid essential for viral particle budding. The interaction of Env with Gag and ubiquitination of the CyD of the Env LP subunit seem to be the main determinants of its intracellular transport and are probably dominant over the C-terminal dilysine motif. Furthermore, some properties of orthoretroviral Gag proteins, such as ubiquitination and budding functions, have been delegated to Env in FVs. In addition, the function of the unusual Env-Bet/Bel-2 fusion proteins is unknown.

NONSTRUCTURAL PROTEINS

Tas

Tas is the transactivator of spumaviruses and essential for replication.[160,217] PFV Tas is a 35-kD nuclear protein that binds to upstream DNA elements in, and augments gene expression from, both the IP and the U3 LTR promoter[37,123,157] (Fig. 20.6). Most Tas protein is translated from a spliced mRNA initiated at the IP.[12,21,155,183] Among the FVs, Tas is variable in size with 209 aa in FFV and 300 aa in PFV and has a modular organization[155,179,209,211] (Fig. 20.12). Its N-terminus contains a region of variable length that is shared with Bet (SR) and harbors several multimerization domains (MMDs). Unique to Tas are a DNA-binding central domain (CD) of approximately 100 aa, a basic NLS, and a C-terminal acidic activation domain (AD) of around 30 aa.

Except for the AD, Tas shows no homology to known cellular proteins, and there is little or no cross-transactivation between different FVs.[100,155] The reason for this is the species specificity of the Tas DNA-binding CD, which is highly variable in aa sequence among different FV Tas proteins. This is consistent with the highly divergent DNA targets that mediate Tas function among different FVs. In contrast, the Tas AD shares key amino acids with other viral and cellular transcription activators and is also active in yeast.[16] For transcriptional activation, the Tas protein has to multimerize. This process that is apparently facilitated by residues of the MMDs mainly located within the N-terminal SR. This property has been demonstrated experimentally for BFV Tas and can probably be generalized to all FV Tas proteins.[266] Little is known about likely cellular factors that might interact with Tas.[127] Phosphorylation by DNA-PK is required for full Tas activity, and only acetylated Tas protein has full DNA-binding capacity.[20,38] In addition, the yeast ADA2 adaptor molecule is required for Tas AD-mediated activation in yeast.[16]

Research carried out on cellular factors engaged with BFV Tas has led to the identification of RelB as its interaction partner to activate the nuclear factor κB (NF-κB) pathway.[279]

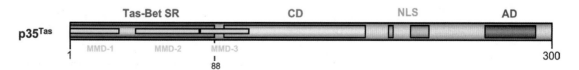

FIGURE 20.12 Schematic outline of prototype foamy virus (PFV) Tas protein. Functional domains are indicated as differentially *colored boxes*. SR, Tas-Bet shared N-terminal region; MMD-1 to 3, multimerization domains 1 to 3; CD, conserved domain; NLS, nuclear localization signal; AD, activation domain.

However, whether these results also apply to Tas proteins other than BFV Tas is not known. Furthermore, the NF-κB–mediated transcriptional enhancement seen is unlikely to explain the full activity of Tas. It can also activate cellular genes if they happen to harbor Tas responsive DNA elements. This has been investigated for various human genes activated by PFV Tas.[155,278]

Bet

Bet is the least conserved of all FV proteins (Fig. 20.13). It is translated predominantly from multiply spliced mRNAs originating at the IP and to a minor extent from mRNA variants initiating at the LTR promoter[12,183] (Fig. 20.6). The splice sites located within the *tas* ORF utilized for generation of the bet mRNA are highly efficient, resulting in Bet to be always made in vast excess over Tas. In transfected or infected cells, Bet is found in the cytoplasm and the nucleus. The nuclear localization is mediated by a C-terminal NLS (Fig. 20.13). Because SR at the N-terminus contains the MMD of Tas, it is likely that Bet also multimerizes via this domain. 3D structures of Bet are not available. A recent bioinformatic protein structure modeling of PFV Bet consisting of 482 aa predicts an organization in two domains. The protein consists of a smaller NtD with 164 aa, which includes the N-terminal 88 aa shared region, and a larger C-terminal domain (CtD) with 318 aa.[111]

For a long time, no clear function could be attributed to Bet. For PFV, Bet was shown to be dispensable for *in vitro* replication in most cell types, with only a minimal decrease in viral titers.[12,297] The first generation of FV vectors actually had the *orf-2* region encoding for most of Bet replaced by sequences of interest putting them under Tas-dependent transcriptional control of the IP or of an inserted heterologous promoter.[238] For FFV, a more drastic reduction in viral titers was observed for Bet-deficient viruses when grown on feline CRFK, but not on human 293T cells.[4] This observation eventually led to the identification of Bet being an antagonist of APOBEC3 (A3) proteins, similar to HIV Vif.[159,196] Whereas SR of FFV Bet was shown to be dispensable, conserved motifs (CMs) within its C-terminus are essential for A3 antagonization[164] (Fig. 20.13).

The splice sites that lead to generation of the Bet protein appear to be so efficient that they are used also in vgRNA. An integrated FV has been described that carries the characteristic deletion leading to the generation of Bet (ΔTas)[233] (Fig. 20.6). As the vgRNA leading to ΔTas carries all features necessary for successful packaging and RTr, ΔTas infects new cells where it integrates. ΔTas has been found *in vitro* and also *in vivo* in a rabbit infection model and in the monkey to a considerable extent.[21,62,232,233] ΔTas provirus is replication incompetent because of its *tas* gene deletion; however, it is not transcriptionally silent. Owing to the basal activity of the IP (see later

discussion), there is still some residual bet gene expression. The magnitude of viral transcription depends on the number of integrated copies of ΔTas and probably also depends on the site of integration where cellular promoter/enhancer elements could augment levels of Bet mRNA.[233] Cells expressing Bet become resistant to superinfection by homologous virus, a feature that has so far not been further investigated.[17,233] Furthermore, a role in promoting viral persistence has been discussed for Bet in general and ΔTas in particular.[175,233] Functionally, ΔTas behaves like a defective interfering genome. However, whether the typical oscillating frequency of DI viruses occurs with ΔTas has not been investigated. Because only either Bet or Tas can be made, and since FV gene expression starts with the translation of Tas (see later discussion), it has been speculated that Bet synthesis represents the molecular switch, which determines viral latency.[175]

STAGES OF REPLICATION

The Early Phase: Establishing the Provirus (Fig. 20.14)

Attachment

FVs bind via a receptor-binding domain located in the Env SU subunit[48] (Fig. 20.10), to yet unknown, probably ubiquitously expressed and evolutionary conserved cellular receptor molecules. Overexpression of FV Env in target cells results in superinfection resistance toward the parental virus as well as FVs derived from other species. This suggests that all FVs use same entry receptor(s).[13] Proteoglycans contribute significantly to FV entry but do not appear to be the major cellular receptor.[186,205,258]

Entry and Intracellular Trafficking

Uptake of most FVs predominantly seems to involve endocytosis and a pH-dependent FV Env-mediated fusion process.[50,201,259] Only PFV Env displays a significant fusion activity at neutral pH and enables fusion to take place at the plasma membrane as well. Single particle tracing of FVs entering the target cells revealed a unique intermediate fusion step characterized by tethering of glycoprotein and capsid but separation of up to 400 nm before final separation of both viral components.[50] After release into the cytoplasm, intact FV capsids migrate along the microtubular network to the centrosome, where they accumulate.[50,234,259] Retrograde movement of FV capsids appears to utilize dynein motor complexes and involves an interaction of its dynein light chain 8 component with the CC3 domain of FV Gag.[199]

A few other host cell factors interacting with FV components during the early replication phases have been identified.

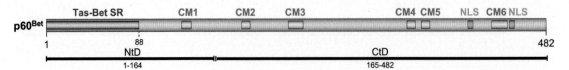

FIGURE 20.13 Schematic outline of prototype foamy virus (PFV) Bet protein. Functional domains are indicated as differentially *colored boxes*. SR, Tas-Bet shared N-terminal region; CM1 to 6, conserved motifs 1 to 6; NLS, bipartite nuclear localization signal.

TRIM5a, a well-known restriction factor for various retro-viruses, was shown to restrict FVs in a species-specific manner.[191,296] The specificity of TRIM5a has been mapped to variable residues of the B30.2 domain, which are important for neutralization of lentiviruses, and to the N-terminal half of FV Gag.[296] The activity of TRIM5a against several retroviral capsid proteins, including those of FVs, which do not mature into the canonical orthoretrovial MA, CA, and NC subunits, implies an even wider structural recognition pattern than previously assumed.

Uncoating

Intact FV capsids that accumulate at the centrosome in G_0-resting cells can remain functionally active for weeks, allowing productive infection to proceed upon their re-entry into the cell cycle.[141] It is generally agreed upon that mitosis is required for FV replication and that the latency period from cell entry to integration and gene expression, owing to the facultative vDNA genome, can be very long.[15,47,141,194,273] Most productive infections are attributed to FV particles that have their vgRNA reverse transcribed into vgDNA prior to target cell infection.[171,180] However, some genome RTr takes place upon FV host cell entry and seems to add to viral infectivity predominantly under conditions of a low MOI.[46,304] The trigger that initiates RTr during FV entry has not been identified.

Disassembly of FV capsids accumulated at the centrosome is reported to involve Gag cleavage by yet uncharacterized cellular protease(s), and potentially the viral protease, in a cell cycle–dependent manner.[73,108,140,259] Upon mitotic breakdown of the nuclear membrane, the vDNA and fragments of Gag gain access to the chromosome, whereas active nuclear import of Gag into interphase nuclei is not observed.[182,259]

Capsid disassembly is essential for further steps in FV replication but also makes the virus vulnerable to cellular defense mechanisms. It leads to exposure of a key pathogen-associated molecular pattern, the viral nucleic acids, recognized by the innate immune system and triggering antiviral responses in different immune cell types. Toll-like receptor 7 (TLR7) expressed in plasmacytoid dendritic cells was shown to be the likely factor in endosomal sensing of FV RNA resulting in the induction of type I IFN.[227] Replicating virus was not found to be required for this type of IFN induction. Furthermore, FV RTr products already present in FV particles taken up by various myeloid immune cells induced an efficient innate immune response.[14] It required FV particles with an active RT, was largely unaffected by RTr inhibition during viral entry, and was dependent on RTr products to be derived from full-length vgRNA. RTr products were sensed in the cytoplasm in a cGAS and STING-dependent manner by the innate immune system in host cells of the myeloid lineage.

Integration

Productive viral replication requires insertion of the provirus into the host genome mediated by the viral integrase,[57,176] although unintegrated vDNA appears to be transcriptionally active, similarly as reported for orthoretroviruses.[47] Like other retroviruses, there are no preferred sites of FV integration. Analyses of PFV integration site patterns have revealed that in sharp contrast to HIV-1 and MLV, PFV disfavors integration into genes.[145,169,189,274] Recent studies using Gag mutants of PFV, SFVmcy,[145] or FFV[282] demonstrated a functional role for the CBS in proviral integration and integration site distribution. PFV and SFVmcy Gag CBS mutant viruses are characterized by a wild-type–like integration efficiency but a massive redistribution of integration sites toward centromeres in different cell lines,[145] whereas FFV Gag CBS mutants display a strongly reduced integration efficiency.[282] Lesbats and colleagues[145] showed that the PFV Gag CBS is essential and sufficient for a direct interaction with nucleosomes. By determining a crystal structure of the PFV Gag CBS bound to mononucleosomes, they found that this viral entity directly interacts with the histone octamer, engaging the H2A-H2B acidic patch in a manner similar to other acid patch–binding proteins such as herpesvirus latency-associated nuclear antigen. How PFV Gag is embedded within the extensive PFV intasome–nucleosome interface,[169] which involves a lift off of cellular DNA from the H2A-H2B heterodimer during the integration process, remains to be determined.

Unlike other retroviruses, the contribution of cellular proteins to FV integration and integration site distribution is largely unknown. Only cellular PLK, and PLK-2 in particular, was shown to interact with PFV Gag during virus entry.[310] The PLK–Gag interaction is dependent on the phosphorylation of a PLKBS in Gag (Fig. 20.7A) by a yet uncharacterized cellular kinase. Thereby cellular PLKs are relocalized to mitotic chromatin in a PFV Gag CBS-dependent manner. PFV Gag PLKBS mutants display a delayed and reduced integration, which is accompanied with an enhanced preference to integrate into heterochromatin.

The Late Phase: Generation of Progeny Viruses (Fig. 20.15)

Transcription

Like orthoretroviruses, FVs exploit the cellular transcription machinery to initiate virus propagation. FV transcription is special, as a cascade of events is launched by the action of two viral promoters and one transcriptional transactivator. FV gene expression (Fig. 20.6) begins with the production of the *tas* and *bet* genes' transcripts directed by and initiated at the IP located in the *env* ORF.[158] This is mediated by the weak basal transcriptional activity of the IP, whereas the U3 promoter in the LTR of the provirus has no, or almost no, basal activity.[123,157]

In FFV, enhancer elements upstream of the IP that are implicated in its basal transcriptional activity include sites for SP-1[18,290]; however, their biological function has not been characterized in any depth. In BFV, AP-1 sites in this location have been partially characterized[294] and may control the basal gene expression that it directs.

As a consequence of the IP's low basal activity, some Tas protein is made, which subsequently binds with high affinity to specific DNA elements—namely, Tas-binding sites (TBS) upstream of the IP—resulting in a positive feedback loop of *tas* gene expression (Fig. 20.6). Once sufficient amounts of Tas have been synthesized by this mechanism, the transactivator also binds with lower affinity but higher avidity to upstream promoter elements in the 5′ LTR U3 region. At this step, the expression of all structural genes and, to some extent, additional LTR-directed Tas and Bet expression set on and virus production is initiated.[18,155]

The IP and LTR U3 TBSs are essential for Tas-mediated transactivation and have been determined and characterized in detail, for example, by electromobility shift assays for PFV,

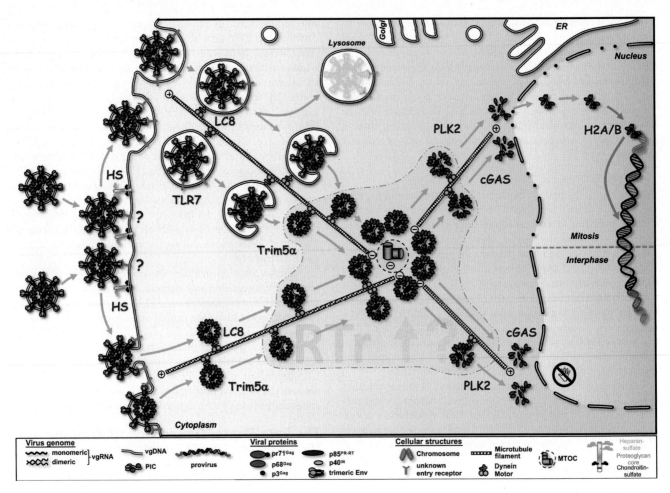

FIGURE 20.14 Early steps of FV replication. Pathways of FV particle attachment, uptake, intracellular trafficking, virion disassembly, and proviral integration are illustrated. Putative early steps of FV replication that may include RTr in vgRNA bearing capsids are marked in a *dashed area* as follows: RTr ↑?. Known cellular cofactors involved in early steps of FV replication are mentioned at the respective subcellular locations. Further details can be found in the inserted legend and throughout the main text.

SFVmcy, FFV, and BFV.[19,88,121,264,309] However, no real TBS consensus sequence has been pinpointed. Furthermore, even within each specific FV species, the IP and U3 TBS show only very weak homology. In general, it can be noted that the finer details of Tas-mediated regulation of FV gene expression, in particular the involvement of cellular proteins, remain to be elucidated. The IFN-induced leucine zipper protein human IFN-induced 35 kDa protein (IFP35) has been previously reported to down-regulate BFV and PFV transcription and replication by interacting with the respective transactivators.[265] Furthermore, N-Myc interactor (Nmi) of man and cattle, an IFN-stimulated gene (ISG), was found to bind the respective Tas proteins of PFV and BFV. Binding interferes with viral replication by sequestering the protein in the cytoplasm.[106] More recently, PHD finger domain protein-11 (PHF11), another ISG identified in a screen as an antiviral factor of PFV replication, was reported to inhibit the basal expression from the IP, thereby preventing Tas expression.[119,120]

The LTR structure of FVs is unique with respect to the location of the mSD, which is located upstream of the polyadenylation signal (pA) (Fig. 20.6). For the expression of full-length genomic transcripts, the vgRNA, FVs suppress premature polyadenylation at the 5′ LTR pA site by U1 small nuclear ribo-

nucleoprotein (U1snRNP) binding to the 5′ LTR mSD.[242] At their 3′ LTR, FV transcripts fold in a different secondary structure that presumably blocks access of U1snRNP and thereby activates polyadenylation at the 3′ end of the RNAs.

Nuclear RNA Export

FV nuclear RNA export also appears to be unique. Similar to other complex retroviruses, the foamyviral regulatory protein Tas acts at the transcriptional level. A posttranscriptional regulator, such as Rev of HIV or Rex of T-lymphotropic retroviruses, has never been identified in FVs. The peculiarities of FV gene regulation—one transcriptional activator and two active promoters—allow a biphasic mode of FV gene expression analogous to other complex retroviruses.[43] However, this does not circumvent a central problem of all retroviruses: regulation of nuclear export of intron-bearing mRNAs containing functional splice sites.[44] As detailed elsewhere in this book (see Chapters 15, 16, and 17), complex retroviruses solve this problem by interacting with the karyopherin CRM1 by using a viral regulatory protein, which binds to an RNA secondary structure embedded in viral mRNAs. In contrast, some simple retroviruses utilize the NXF1/NXT1-mediated cellular mRNA export pathway by means of a constitutive transport element

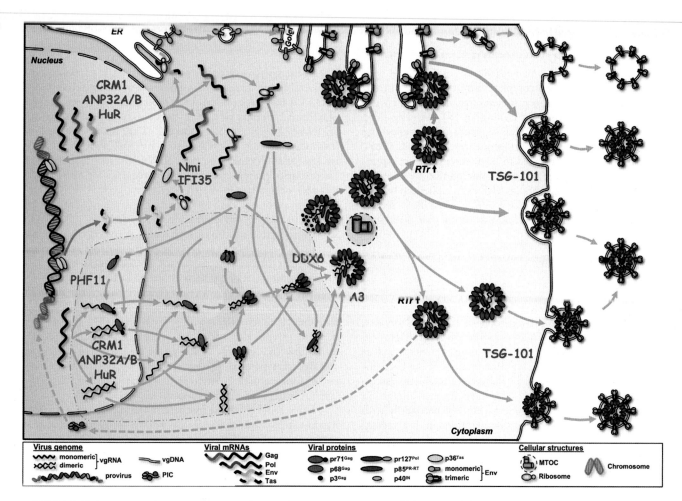

FIGURE 20.15 Late steps of FV replication. Pathways of FV RNA and protein trafficking resulting in capsid assembly and particle release are illustrated. Known and putative trafficking pathways (marked by the *dashed area* with the question mark in the center) of viral RNAs from the nucleus into the cytoplasm to the capsid assembly site at the microtubule organizing center (MTOC) are shown. Putative RNA–protein interactions and assembly intermediates are depicted. Four different variants of vgRNA dimerization throughout the transport pathway to the assembly site are illustrated. Known cellular cofactors involved in late steps of FV replication are mentioned at the respective subcellular locations. *Dashed arrows* indicate the potential pathway leading to reintegration of vgDNA originating from preassembled capsids, which underwent reverse transcription prior to particle release. Further details can be found in the inserted legend and throughout the main text.

(CTE) located within their genomic mRNAs.[44] PFV vgRNA and Gag-ecoding mRNA appears to make use of yet another, so far undisclosed pathway.[23] Nuclear export of FV RNA is, on one hand, CRM1 dependent and, on the other, relies on the presence of additional cellular proteins. The host cell HuR protein binds to the unspliced PFV vgRNA, and two cellular adapter molecules, ANP32A and ANP32B, mediate the interaction between the RNA-bound complex and CRM1.[18,23] The FV RNA elements in question have not yet been characterized. The consequences of this viral nuclear RNA export mechanism on the synthesis of early response cellular proteins, whose mRNAs normally use this export pathway, are unknown. It is tempting to speculate that FVs, by making use of a nuclear mRNA export pathway involving cellular proteins also required for the synthesis of early response proteins, may outcompete the latter.

Translation

The Gag and Pol proteins, as well as the accessory gene products Tas and Bet, are translated on free ribosomes in the cyto-plasm. It should be remembered that *pol* translation of FVs as a separate protein from a spliced mRNA is unique among retroviruses (see above). The Env protein is targeted to the secretory pathway by ribosomal translation in the rough ER and displays a highly unusual biosynthesis and membrane topology[150,288] (see above).

Translation of pr71[Gag], encoded in the vgRNA containing the authentic *gag* 5′ UTR, appears to use a ribosomal shunting mechanism[236] (Fig. 20.6). This is a mechanism that is used by plant pararetroviruses to translate their Gag homolog and involves the selective jumping of ribosomes to the translation initiation site.[231] In addition, FV Gag translation is regulated at different levels. At least three genetic elements were reported to influence expression of Gag, in context of its natural environment of the full-length vgRNA (Fig. 20.6). The first one is the mSD found in the *gag* 5′ UTR sequences, which regulates 5′ LTR pA site suppression[242] (see above). Its presence appears to be crucial for the translation of the Gag protein from vgRNA or from expression constructs harboring the authentic 5′ UTR sequences and FV *gag* ORF.[91–93,153,229,242] The second element, although poorly characterized, appears to be located within the *gag* ORF itself and inhibits expression of authentic *gag* ORFs in the absence of its 5′ UTR.[92,93,153,229] Its inhibitory effect can be neutralized by replacing the authentic FV *gag* 5′ UTR with a heterologous SD site or a complete intron sequence but not by adding such sequences downstream of an authentic PFV *gag* ORF with 5′ UTR sequences lacking an SD site. The third element is found in the 3′ UTR sequence of Gag-encoding mRNAs. It is one of the four PuR sequences, element C (PuR-C), which was initially reported to be essential for Gag expression, without knowing the underlying mechanism.[197] Recently, PuR-C was shown to represent an SRE overlapping the branch point of a strong env-specific 3′ ss (SA3).[181] Most likely, serine-rich protein binding the PuR-C results in suboptimal recognition of the major *env* 3′ ss BP by SF1/mBBP, thereby permitting retention of the *env* intron and formation of unspliced *gag* and singly spliced *pol* transcripts.

Capsid Assembly

FV capsid assembly follows a retrovirus type B/D morphotype strategy. Gag is the driving force of FV in this process, since neither Pol nor vgRNA are essential for intracellular capsid assembly. C-terminal FV Gag truncation mutants as well as full-length PFV Gag with 23 arginine residues of the C-terminal GR-rich domain changed to alanine are unable to assemble normal shaped capsids.[34,80] This suggests that interaction of Gag with nucleic acids in general, but not necessarily with vgRNA, through its C-terminal GR-rich domain, is a prerequisite for the assembly of FV capsids with normal morphology or virus-like structures. FV morphogenesis includes the microtubule-dependent transport of Gag proteins to the centrosome involving the CTRS within Gag[51,299] (Fig. 20.7). The Gag CC2 domain mediates FV capsid preassembly at the centrosome.[269]

An important question concerning assembly deals with the mechanism of Pol protein encapsidation. Pol packaging via protein–protein interaction of the fused Gag precursor, as it occurs with orthoretroviruses, cannot apply to FVs since Pol is separately expressed from its own spliced mRNA[56,116,136,156,298] (Fig. 20.6). FV Pol precursor, but not its mature cleavage products PR-RT and IN, are packaged into assembling capsids after provirus-derived expression.[108,198,224] Two competing views on this mechanism exist for the initial step of Pol incorporation. One favors Gag-Pol protein–protein interactions when proviral mutants were analyzed. Another concept arose from subgenomic vector analyses, where Gag and Pol seem to interact in that the viral vgRNA serves as a bridging molecule.[94,108,135,198] Currently, it cannot be excluded that both mechanisms are involved in packaging the Pol precursor. However, details of the temporal and spatial regulation of FV vgRNA and Pol encapsidation as well as the contribution of cellular factors have not been well characterized. Only a cellular DEAD-box RNA helicase, DDX6, was described to promote vgRNA encapsidation by a yet unclear mechanism independent of a direct interaction with FV Gag.[301] Furthermore, it is yet unclear whether all three viral components, vgRNA, Gag, and Pol, are transported separately to the centrosome and capsid assembly initiates and proceeds at this key organelle in the FV replication cycle, or if assembly intermediates encompassing two or all components are formed before or during transport to the centrosome. The order of protein–nucleic acid interactions is also still unknown. Whether Gag or Pol first interact with vgRNA, or whether both

bind simultaneously, perhaps enhanced by additional viral and/or cellular protein–protein interactions, remains to be elucidated.

Although the exact time point of RTr with respect to capsid assembly and maturation is unknown, preassembled intracellular FV capsids, generated upon propagation *in vitro*, contain significant amounts of already reverse transcribed, infectious vgDNA.[171,180,225,303] In this respect, FVs are unique among retroviruses but show a similarity to HBV replication (see Chapter 18, Fields Virology Volume 2, DNA Viruses). Gag, but not Pol precursor protein cleavage, is a prerequisite for intraparticle RTr that occurs late in the FV replication cycle.[55,108,224] Therefore, Gag precursor cleavage appears to be the initiating event for intraparticle RTr in assembling FV capsids.[108]

Orthoretroviruses can occasionally behave like retrotransposons and reshuttle their genome to the nucleus without an extracellular phase. The frequency of such intracellular retrotransposition (IRT) has been estimated to be 1 per 10^6 proviruses and is thought to reflect the frequency at which the RNA genome is prematurely reverse transcribed.[89,225] For PFV, this frequency is much higher with approximately 5% and thereby concordant with late RTr of the vgRNA.[89] It was subsequently found that IRT strongly depended on the particular FV isolate and the cell type used for analysis.[90,225] Thus, IRT is not a general phenomenon of FVs. However, the late phase of RTr of the vgRNA is required for this process.

Some cellular defense mechanisms tackle viruses at late replication steps. One of few factors known to interfere with FV replication are members of a family of evolutionarily conserved cytidine deaminases, the apolipoprotein B mRNA editing enzyme, catalytic polypeptide-like 3 (APOBEC3; A3) proteins.[111] As observed for other retroviruses, the A3s are encapsidated into the nascent virus particle due to specific Gag-A3 interactions. The antiviral activity is mediated by cytidine deamination of the viral reverse transcript during RTr that results in G-to-A hypermutations of the viral genome. FVs encode the accessory Bet protein (Fig. 20.13) to preserve genome stability and counteract A3s.[159,228] Unlike the HIV-1 Vif protein, which prevents A3 particle incorporation by routing it to the proteasomal degradation pathway, Bet prevents A3 encapsidation by binding, inhibiting its dimerization, and quantitatively trapping the deaminase.[39,112,196] The Bet-specific orf-2–encoded domain of FFV Bet, but not the shared N-terminal Tas domain, was found to be essential for feline A3 binding and inactivation.[164] The PFV and FFV Bet function was found to be broadly active against various primate or feline A3s.[196] However, some species specificity was also observed, as PFV Bet was found to be inactive against all or some mouse, feline, and rhesus monkey A3 proteins, as well as against human A3DE and A3H.[196] Because RTr of FV RNA takes place to a significant degree in virus-producing cells, A3 restriction of FVs occurs at a different point in the replication cycle than that reported for orthoretroviruses.[159]

Membrane Envelopment and Release

One of the most distinctive features of FVs is the failure of their capsids to spontaneously bud from cellular membranes and generate virus-like particles. This is owing to the absence of a membrane-targeting signal in Gag[9,65,202] (Fig. 20.7A). For cellular egress, FVs require the cognate envelope protein, with which their own capsids specifically interact. Coexpression of FV Gag and FV Env is required to detect capsids secreted into the cell culture supernatant. Biochemical and biophysical investigations with PFV and FFV[70,207,288] suggested that a direct interaction between Gag and Env occurs (Fig. 20.7B). This aspect was later confirmed by determination of 3D structures derived from of Gag and Env subdomain cocrystals.[77] This interaction is mediated by the N-terminal Gag CC1 of capsids preassembled at the centrosome, and the connection with the N-terminus of the envelope LP subunit CyD[34,150,288] presumably takes place at the trans-Golgi network.[299]

Budding of FVs occurs at intracellular membranes and the plasma membrane with differences in the relative contribution of the sites depending on the FV species studied.[134,150,299] Primate FVs, like other retroviruses, have been shown to exploit the cellular VPS machinery, through a TSG101-Gag L-domain interaction, for this process[195,255] (Fig. 20.7A). It appears likely that also nonprimate FVs make use of the same mechanism, though they lack the classical PSAP L domain motif conserved in primate FV Gag proteins. Only recently, in BFV Gag, nonclassical PLPI and YGPL motifs with L-domain function were identified and shown to promote BFV budding in a TSG101- and ALIX-dependent manner.[279a] Whether release of FFV that depends on the host cell VPS machinery has yet to be demonstrated.

CD317/tetherin is an integral membrane protein with an N-terminal MSD and a C-terminal glycosyl-phosphatidylinositol anchor. It interacts directly with the actin cytoskeleton and blocks the release of various enveloped viruses, including orthoretroviruses, from infected cells. CD317 is also active against FVs.[117,295] Unlike in HIV-1 and HIV-2, a FV protein antagonizing tetherin has not yet been identified. The activity of tetherin against PFV shows some mechanistic differences in comparison to HIV-1, because dimerization-deficient tetherin inhibits PFV replication with the same efficiency as the wild-type factor.[295]

Perspectives

Above we learned, that foamy viruses are "the other complex retroviruses" since they are apparently apathogenic and follow a different replication strategy as their cousins. The latter issue justified their classification as an own subfamily within the family of retroviruses. For the future, there remain many questions to be addressed, both in the field and in the laboratory.

Certainly, more exogenous FVs await their discovery, possibly in species beyond those known so far in simians, prosimians, and probably, other classes of mammalia. Researchers in the field and in primate facilities should investigate possible impacts of coinfections with FV and other viruses. It will be interesting to elucidate further in how the immune system maintains the constant replication for instance in the oral mucosa without harming the host. An animal model with well-characterized tools for immunologic studies and smaller than primates or cats would be very helpful for these studies. Will we ever understand why mouse and man are apparently spared from foamy viruses?

This question leads to whether more endogenous FV remnant sequence stretches will be identified in the genome of vertebrates. Could such new discoveries find a mutualistic contribution of ancient FVs to modern life?

On the molecular side, the yet unknown receptor(s) still await discovery. Certainly, the intracellular fate of both, the incoming FVs and the assembly and release of virus offspring, may hold further surprises in comparison to other more extensively studied retroviruses. FVs are characterized by accumulation of intact capsids at the centrosome of nondividing cells that can remain biologically active for weeks. What triggers uncoating of these latent capsids upon host cell entry into mitosis? In orthoretroviruses, genome packaging is quite well understood. How do FVs selectively package their vgRNA upon capsid assembly? Another peculiar aspect of the FV replication cycle is the formation of a truncated provirus lacking the bulk part of the transactivator gene only allowing low expression levels of Bet. Does the shortened provirus play any role in FV persistence?

Aside from basic research on their replication, FVs have been exploited as useful tools for gene transfer purposes. It will be interesting to see a first gene therapy clinical trial being initiated using FV-derived vectors or components thereof for treatment of patients.

Ultimately, foamy viruses, like Cinderella, may surprise scientists once more at second glance. Further research will show.

ACKNOWLEDGMENTS

We like to express our thanks to all the scientists who permitted us to use their figures or parts thereof for this edition. Also, we apologize to those in the yet limited foamy virus researcher's community whose contributions did not find their way into this chapter. We shall reconvene in person, once the other virus That-Must-Not-Be-Named, which restricted our freedom, including ours while assembling this chapter, will be under tight control!

REFERENCES

1. Achong BG, Mansell PW, Epstein MA, et al. An unusual virus in cultures from a human nasopharyngeal carcinoma. *J Natl Cancer Inst* 1971;46:299–307.
2. Aiewsakun P, Katzourakis A. Marine origin of retroviruses in the early Palaeozoic Era. *Nat Commun* 2017;8:13954.
3. Ali M, Taylor GP, Pitman RJ, et al. No evidence of antibody to human foamy virus in widespread human populations. *AIDS Res Hum Retroviruses* 1996;12:1473–1483.
4. Alke A, Schwantes A, Kido K, et al. The bet gene of feline foamy virus is required for virus replication. *Virology* 2001;287:310–320.
5. Allan JS, Broussard SR, Michaels MG, et al. Amplification of simian retroviral sequences from human recipients of baboon liver transplants. *AIDS Res Hum Retroviruses* 1998;14:821–824.
6. An DG, Hyun U, Shin CG. Characterization of nuclear localization signals of the prototype foamy virus integrase. *J Gen Virol* 2008;89:1680–1684.
7. Arhel N, Munier S, Souque P, et al. Nuclear import defect of human immunodeficiency virus type 1 DNA flap mutants is not dependent on the viral strain or target cell type. *J Virol* 2006;80:10262–10269.
8. Bähr A, Singer A, Hain A, et al. Interferon but not MxB inhibits foamy retroviruses. *Virology* 2016;488:51–60.
9. Baldwin DN, Linial ML. The roles of Pol and Env in the assembly pathway of human foamy virus. *J Virol* 1998;72:3658–3665.
10. Ball NJ, Nicastro G, Dutta M, et al. Structure of a spumaretrovirus Gag central domain reveals an ancient retroviral capsid. *PLoS Pathog* 2016;12:e1005981.
11. Bandecchi P, Matteucci D, Baldinotti F, et al. Prevalence of feline immunodeficiency virus and other retroviral infections in sick cats in Italy. *Vet Immunol Immunopathol* 1992;31:337–345.
12. Baunach G, Maurer B, Hahn H, et al. Functional analysis of human foamy virus accessory reading frames. *J Virol* 1993;67:5411–5418.
13. Berg A, Pietschmann T, Rethwilm A, et al. Determinants of foamy virus envelope glycoprotein mediated resistance to superinfection. *Virology* 2003;314:243–252.
14. Bergez M, Weber J, Riess M, et al. Insights into innate sensing of prototype foamy viruses in myeloid cells. *Viruses* 2019;11:1095.
15. Bieniasz PD, Weiss RA, McClure MO. Cell cycle dependence of foamy retrovirus infection. *J Virol* 1995;69:7295–7299.
16. Blair WS, Bogerd H, Cullen BR. Genetic analysis indicates that the human foamy virus Bel-1 protein contains a transcription activation domain of the acidic class. *J Virol* 1994;68:3803–3808.
17. Bock M, Heinkelein M, Lindemann D, et al. Cells expressing the human foamy virus (HFV) accessory Bet protein are resistant to productive HFV superinfection. *Virology* 1998;250:194–204.

18. Bodem J. Regulation of foamy viral transcription and RNA export. *Adv Virus Res* 2011;81:1–31.
19. Bodem J, Kang Y, Flügel RM. Comparative functional characterization of the feline foamy virus transactivator reveals its species specificity. *Virology* 2004;318:32–36.
20. Bodem J, Kräusslich HG, Rethwilm A. Acetylation of the foamy virus transactivator Tas by PCAF augments promoter-binding affinity and virus transcription. *J Gen Virol* 2007;88:259–263.
21. Bodem J, Löchelt M, Delius H, et al. Detection of subgenomic cDNAs and mapping of feline foamy virus mRNAs reveals complex patterns of transcription. *Virology* 1998;244:417–426.
22. Bodem J, Löchelt M, Winkler I, et al. Characterization of the spliced *pol* transcript of feline foamy virus: the splice acceptor site of the *pol* transcript is located in *gag* of foamy viruses. *J Virol* 1996;70:9024–9027.
23. Bodem J, Schied T, Gabriel R, et al. Foamy virus nuclear RNA export is distinct from that of other retroviruses. *J Virol* 2011;85:2333–2341.
24. Boneva RS, Switzer WM, Spira TJ, et al. Clinical and virological characterization of persistent human infection with simian foamy viruses. *AIDS Res Hum Retroviruses* 2007;23:1330–1337.
25. Boyer PL, Stenbak CR, Clark PK, et al. Characterization of the polymerase and RNase H activities of human foamy virus reverse transcriptase. *J Virol* 2004;78:6112–6121.
26. Boyer PL, Stenbak CR, Hoberman D, et al. In vitro fidelity of the prototype primate foamy virus (PFV) RT compared to HIV-1 RT. *Virology* 2007;367:253–264.
27. Brooks JI, Merks HW, Fournier J, et al. Characterization of blood-borne transmission of simian foamy virus. *Transfusion* 2007;47:162–170.
28. Brown P, Moreau-Dubois MC, Gajdusek DC. Persistent asymptomatic infection of the laboratory mouse by simian foamy virus type 6: a new model of retrovirus latency. *Arch Virol* 1982;71:229–234.
29. Butera ST, Brown J, Callahan ME, et al. Survey of veterinary conference attendees for evidence of zoonotic infection by feline retroviruses. *J Am Vet Med Assoc* 2000;217:1475–1479.
30. Cain D, Erlwein O, Grigg A, et al. Palindromic sequence plays a critical role in human foamy virus dimerization. *J Virol* 2001;75:3731–3739.
31. Calattini S, Betsem EBA, Froment A, et al. Simian foamy virus transmission from apes to humans, rural Cameroon. *Emerg Infect Dis* 2007;13:1314–1320.
32. Calattini S, Wanert F, Thierry B, et al. Modes of transmission and genetic diversity of foamy viruses in a Macaca tonkeana colony. *Retrovirology* 2006;3:23.
33. Cao W, Stricker E, Hotz-Wagenblatt A, et al. Functional analyses of bovine foamy virus-encoded miRNAs reveal the importance of a defined miRNA for virus replication and host-virus interaction. *Viruses* 2020;12:1250.
34. Cartellieri M, Herchenröder O, Rudolph W, et al. N-terminal Gag domain required for foamy virus particle assembly and export. *J Virol* 2005;79:12464–12476.
35. Cartellieri M, Rudolph W, Herchenröder O, et al. Determination of the relative amounts of Gag and Pol proteins in foamy virus particles. *Retrovirology* 2005;2:44.
36. Chai K, Wang Z, Xu Y, et al. Palmitoylation of the bovine foamy virus envelope glycoprotein is required for viral replication. *Viruses* 2020;13:31.
37. Chang J, Lee KJ, Jang KL, et al. Human foamy virus Bel1 transactivator contains a bipartite nuclear localization determinant which is sensitive to protein context and triple multimerization domains. *J Virol* 1995;69:801–808.
38. Chang R, Tan J, Xu F, et al. Lysine acetylation sites in bovine foamy virus transactivator BTas are important for its DNA binding activity. *Virology* 2011;418:21–26.
39. Chareza S, Slavkovic Lukic D, Liu Y, et al. Molecular and functional interactions of cat APOBEC3 and feline foamy and immunodeficiency virus proteins: different ways to counteract host-encoded restriction. *Virology* 2012;424:138–146.
40. Choudhary A, Galvin TA, Williams DK, et al. Influence of naturally occurring simian foamy viruses (SFVs) on SIV disease progression in the rhesus macaque (*Macaca mulatta*) model. *Viruses* 2013;5:1414–1430.
41. Clarke JK, Attridge JT, Gay FW. The morphogenesis of simian foamy agents. *J Gen Virol* 1969;4:183–188.
42. Corona A, Schneider A, Schweimer K, et al. Inhibition of foamy virus reverse transcriptase by human immunodeficiency virus type 1 RNase H inhibitors. *Antimicrob Agents Chemother* 2014;58:4086–4093.
43. Cullen BR. Retroviruses as model systems for the study of nuclear RNA export pathways. *Virology* 1998;249:203–210.
44. Cullen BR. Nuclear RNA export. *J Cell Sci* 2003;116:587–597.
45. Debons-Guillemin MC, Valla J, Gazeau J, et al. No evidence of spumaretrovirus infection markers in 19 cases of De Quervain's thyroiditis [letter]. *AIDS Res Hum Retroviruses* 1992;8:1547.
46. Delelis O, Saïb A, Sonigo P. Biphasic DNA synthesis in spumaviruses. *J Virol* 2003;77:8141–8146.
47. Deyle DR, Li Y, Olson EM, et al. Nonintegrating foamy virus vectors. *J Virol* 2010;84:9341–9349.
48. Duda A, Lüftenegger D, Pietschmann T, et al. Characterization of the prototype foamy virus envelope glycoprotein receptor-binding domain. *J Virol* 2006;80:8158–8167.
49. Duda A, Stange A, Lüftenegger D, et al. Prototype foamy virus envelope glycoprotein leader peptide processing is mediated by a furin-like cellular protease, but cleavage is not essential for viral infectivity. *J Virol* 2004;78:13865–13870.
50. Dupont A, Glück IM, Ponti D, et al. Identification of an intermediate step in foamy virus fusion. *Viruses* 2020;12:1472.
51. Eastman SW, Linial ML. Identification of a conserved residue of foamy virus Gag required for intracellular capsid assembly. *J Virol* 2001;75:6857–6864.
52. Effantin G, Estrozi LF, Aschman N, et al. Cryo-electron microscopy structure of the native prototype foamy virus glycoprotein and virus architecture. *PLoS Pathog* 2016;12:e1005721.
53. Enders JF, Peebles TC. Propagation in tissue cultures of cytopathogenic agents from patients with measles. *Proc Soc Exp Biol Med* 1954;86:277–286.
54. Engelman AN, Cherepanov P. Retroviral intasomes arising. *Curr Opin Struct Biol* 2017;47:23–29.
55. Enssle J, Fischer N, Moebes A, et al. Carboxy-terminal cleavage of the human foamy virus Gag precursor molecule is an essential step in the viral life cycle. *J Virol* 1997;71:7312–7317.
56. Enssle J, Jordan I, Mauer B, et al. Foamy virus reverse transcriptase is expressed independently from the Gag protein. *Proc Natl Acad Sci USA* 1996;93:4137–4141.
57. Enssle J, Moebes A, Heinkelein M, et al. An active foamy virus integrase is required for virus replication. *J Gen Virol* 1999;80(Pt 6):1445–1452.
58. Epstein MA. Simian retroviral infections in human beings. *Lancet* 2004;364:138–139; author reply 139–140.
59. Erlwein O, Bieniasz PD, McClure MO. Sequences in pol are required for transfer of human foamy virus-based vectors. *J Virol* 1998;72:5510–5516.
60. Erlwein O, Cain D, Fischer N, et al. Identification of sites that act together to direct dimerization of human foamy virus RNA in vitro. *Virology* 1997;229:251–258.
61. Everson EM, Olzsko ME, Leap DJ, et al. A comparison of foamy and lentiviral vector genotoxicity in SCID-repopulating cells shows foamy vectors are less prone to clonal dominance. *Mol Ther Methods Clin Dev* 2016;3:16048.
62. Falcone V, Leupold J, Clotten J, et al. Sites of simian foamy virus persistence in naturally infected African green monkeys: latent provirus is ubiquitous, whereas viral replication is restricted to the oral mucosa. *Virology* 1999;257:7–14.
63. Falcone V, Schweizer M, Neumann-Haefelin D. Replication of primate foamy viruses in natural and experimental hosts. *Curr Top Microbiol Immunol* 2003;277:161–180.
64. Falcone V, Schweizer M, Toniolo A, et al. Gamma interferon is a major suppressive factor produced by activated human peripheral blood lymphocytes that is able to inhibit foamy virus-induced cytopathic effects. *J Virol* 1999;73:1724–1728.
65. Fischer N, Heinkelein M, Lindemann D, et al. Foamy virus particle formation. *J Virol* 1998;72:1610–1615.
66. Flanagan M. Isolation of a spumavirus from a sheep. *Aust Vet J* 1992;69:112–113.
67. Flügel RM, Pfrepper KI. Proteolytic processing of foamy virus Gag and Pol proteins. *Curr Top Microbiol Immunol* 2003;277:63–88.
68. Gärtner K, Wiktorowicz T, Park J, et al. Accuracy estimation of foamy virus genome copying. *Retrovirology* 2009;6:32.
69. Geiselhart V, Bastone P, Kempf T, et al. Furin-mediated cleavage of the feline foamy virus Env leader protein. *J Virol* 2004;78:13573–13581.
70. Geiselhart V, Schwantes A, Bastone P, et al. Features of the Env leader protein and the N-terminal Gag domain of feline foamy virus important for virus morphogenesis. *Virology* 2003;310:235–244.
71. Gessain A, Montange T, Betsem E, et al. Case–control study of the immune status of humans infected with zoonotic gorilla simian foamy viruses. *J Infect Dis* 2020;221:1724–1733.
72. Gharwan H, Hirata RK, Wang P, et al. Transduction of human embryonic stem cells by foamy virus vectors. *Mol Ther* 2007;15:1827–1833.
73. Giron ML, Colas S, Wybier J, et al. Expression and maturation of human foamy virus Gag precursor polypeptides. *J Virol* 1997;71:1635–1639.
74. Giron ML, Rozain F, Debons-Guillemin MC, et al. Human foamy virus polypeptides: identification of env and bel gene products. *J Virol* 1993;67:3596–3600.
75. Goepfert PA, Shaw KL, Ritter GD Jr, et al. A sorting motif localizes the foamy virus glycoprotein to the endoplasmic reticulum. *J Virol* 1997;71:778–784.
76. Goepfert PA, Shaw K, Wang G, et al. An endoplasmic reticulum retrieval signal partitions human foamy virus maturation to intracytoplasmic membranes. *J Virol* 1999;73:7210–7217.
77. Goldstone DC, Flower TG, Ball NJ, et al. A unique spumavirus Gag N-terminal domain with functional properties of orthoretroviral matrix and capsid. *PLoS Pathog* 2013;9:e1003376.
78. Goodman MA, Arumugam P, Pillis DM, et al. Foamy virus vector carries a strong insulator in its long terminal repeat which reduces its genotoxic potential. *J Virol* 2018;92:e01639-17.
79. Hahn H, Baunach G, Bräutigam S, et al. Reactivity of primate sera to foamy virus Gag and Bet proteins. *J Gen Virol* 1994;75(Pt 10):2635–2644.
80. Hamann MV, Müllers E, Reh J, et al. The cooperative function of arginine residues in the Prototype Foamy Virus Gag C-terminus mediates viral and cellular RNA encapsidation. *Retrovirology* 2014;11:87.
81. Hamann MV, Stanke N, Müllers E, et al. Efficient transient genetic manipulation in vitro and in vivo by prototype foamy virus-mediated nonviral RNA transfer. *Mol Ther* 2014;22:1460–1471.
82. Han GZ, Worobey M. Endogenous viral sequences from the Cape golden mole (*Chrysochloris asiatica*) reveal the presence of foamy viruses in all major placental mammal clades. *PLoS One* 2014;9:e97931.
83. Hare S, Gupta SS, Valkov E, et al. Retroviral intasome assembly and inhibition of DNA strand transfer. *Nature* 2010;464:232–236.
84. Hare S, Smith SJ, Metifiot M, et al. Structural and functional analyses of the second-generation integrase strand transfer inhibitor dolutegravir (S/GSK1349572). *Mol Pharmacol* 2011;80:565–572.
85. Hare S, Vos AM, Clayton RF, et al. Molecular mechanisms of retroviral integrase inhibition and the evolution of viral resistance. *Proc Natl Acad Sci USA* 2010;107:20057–20062.
86. Hartl MJ, Bodem J, Jochheim F, et al. Regulation of foamy virus protease activity by viral RNA: a novel and unique mechanism among retroviruses. *J Virol* 2011;85:4462–4469.
87. Hartl MJ, Schweimer K, Reger MH, et al. Formation of transient dimers by a retroviral protease. *Biochem J* 2010;427:197–203.
88. He F, Blair WS, Fukushima J, et al. The human foamy virus Bel-1 transcription factor is a sequence-specific DNA binding protein. *J Virol* 1996;70:3902–3908.
89. Heinkelein M, Pietschmann T, Jarmy G, et al. Efficient intracellular retrotransposition of an exogenous primate retrovirus genome. *EMBO J* 2000;19:3436–3445.
90. Heinkelein M, Rammling M, Juretzek T, et al. Retrotransposition and cell-to-cell transfer of foamy viruses. *J Virol* 2003;77:11855–11858.
91. Heinkelein M, Schmidt M, Fischer N, et al. Characterization of a cis-acting sequence in the Pol region required to transfer human foamy virus vectors. *J Virol* 1998;72:6307–6314.
92. Heinkelein M, Thurow J, Dressler M, et al. Complex effects of deletions in the 5' untranslated region of primate foamy virus on viral gene expression and RNA packaging. *J Virol* 2000;74:3141–3148.
93. Heinkelein M, Dressler M, Jarmy G, et al. Improved primate foamy virus vectors and packaging constructs. *J Virol* 2002;76:3774–3783.

94. Heinkelein M, Leurs C, Rammling M, et al. Pregenomic RNA is required for efficient incorporation of pol polyprotein into foamy virus capsids. *J Virol* 2002;76:10069–10073.

95. Hendrie PC, Huo Y, Stolitenko RB, et al. A rapid and quantitative assay for measuring neighboring gene activation by vector proviruses. *Mol Ther* 2008;16:534–540.

96. Heneine W, Kuehnert MJ. Preserving blood safety against emerging retroviruses. *Transfusion* 2006;46:1276–1278.

97. Heneine W, Musey VC, Sinha SD, et al. Absence of evidence for human spumaretrovirus sequences in patients with Graves' disease [letter]. *J Acquir Immune Defic Syndr Hum Retrovirol* 1995;9:99–101.

98. Heneine W, Switzer WM, Sandstrom P, et al. Identification of a human population infected with simian foamy viruses [see comments]. *Nat Med* 1998;4:403–407.

99. Herchenröder O, Renne R, Loncar D, et al. Isolation, cloning, and sequencing of simian foamy viruses from chimpanzees (SFVcpz): high homology to human foamy virus (HFV). *Virology* 1994;201:187–199.

100. Herchenröder O, Turek R, Neumann-Haefelin D, et al. Infectious proviral clones of chimpanzee foamy virus (SFVcpz) generated by long PCR reveal close functional relatedness to human foamy virus. *Virology* 1995;214:685–689.

101. Hill CL, Bieniasz PD, McClure MO. Properties of human foamy virus relevant to its development as a vector for gene therapy. *J Gen Virol* 1999;80:2003–2009.

102. Hirata RK, Miller AD, Andrews RG, et al. Transduction of hematopoietic cells by foamy virus vectors. *Blood* 1996;88:3654–3661.

103. Holzschu DL, Delaney MA, Renshaw RW, et al. The nucleotide sequence and spliced pol mRNA levels of the nonprimate spumavirus bovine foamy virus. *J Virol* 1998;72:2177–2182.

104. Hooks JJ, Gibbs CJ Jr. The foamy viruses. *Bacteriol Rev* 1975;39:169–185.

105. Hooks JJ, Gibbs CJ Jr, Cutchins EC, et al. Characterization and distribution of two new foamy viruses isolated from chimpanzees. *Arch Gesamte Virusforsch* 1972;38:38–55.

106. Hu X, Yang W, Liu R, et al. N-Myc interactor inhibits prototype foamy virus by sequestering viral Tas protein in the cytoplasm. *J Virol* 2014;88:7036–7044.

107. Hussain AI, Shanmugam V, Bhullar VB, et al. Screening for simian foamy virus infection by using a combined antigen Western blot assay: evidence for a wide distribution among Old World primates and identification of four new divergent viruses. *Virology* 2003;309:248–257.

108. Hütter S, Müllers E, Stanke N, et al. Prototype foamy virus protease activity is essential for intraparticle reverse transcription initiation but not absolutely required for uncoating upon host cell entry. *J Virol* 2013;87:3163–3176.

109. Hyun U, Lee DH, Shin CG. Minimal size of prototype foamy virus integrase for nuclear localization. *Acta Virol* 2011;55:169–174.

110. Imrich H, Heinkelein M, Herchenröder O, et al. Primate foamy virus Pol proteins are imported into the nucleus. *J Gen Virol* 2000;81:2941–2947.

111. Jaguva Vasudevan AA, Becker D, Luedde T, et al. Foamy viruses, bet, and APOBEC3 restriction. *Viruses* 2021;13:504.

112. Jaguva Vasudevan AA, Perkovic M, Bulliard Y, et al. Prototype foamy virus bet impairs the dimerization and cytosolic solubility of human APOBEC3G. *J Virol* 2013;87:9030–9040.

113. Johnston PB. Taxonomic features of seven serotypes of simian and ape foamy viruses. *Infect Immun* 1971;3:793–799.

114. Jones-Engel L, May CC, Engel GA, et al. Diverse contexts of zoonotic transmission of simian foamy viruses in Asia. *Emerg Infect Dis* 2008;14:1200–1208.

115. Jones-Engel L, Steinkraus KA, Murray SM, et al. Sensitive assays for simian foamy viruses reveal a high prevalence of infection in commensal, free-ranging Asian monkeys. *J Virol* 2007;81:7330–7337.

116. Jordan I, Enssle J, Güttler E, et al. Expression of human foamy virus reverse transcriptase involves a spliced pol mRNA. *Virology* 1996;224:314–319.

117. Jouvenet N, Neil SJ, Zhadina M, et al. Broad-spectrum inhibition of retroviral and filoviral particle release by tetherin. *J Virol* 2009;83:1837–1844.

118. Juretzek T, Holm T, Gärtner K, et al. Foamy virus integration. *J Virol* 2004;78:2472–2477.

119. Kane M, Mele V, Liberatore RA, et al. Inhibition of spumavirus gene expression by PHF11. *PLoS Pathog* 2020;16:e1008644.

120. Kane M, Zang TM, Rihn SJ, et al. Identification of interferon-stimulated genes with antiretroviral activity. *Cell Host Microbe* 2016;20:392–405.

121. Kang Y, Blair WS, Cullen BR. Identification and functional characterization of a high-affinity Bel-1 DNA binding site located in the human foamy virus internal promoter. *J Virol* 1998;72:504–511.

122. Katzourakis A, Gifford RJ, Tristem M, et al. Macroevolution of complex retroviruses. *Science* 2009;325:1512.

123. Keller A, Partin KM, Löchelt M, et al. Characterization of the transcriptional trans activator of human foamy retrovirus. *J Virol* 1991;65:2589–2594.

124. Khan AS, Kumar D. Simian foamy virus infection by whole-blood transfer in rhesus macaques: potential for transfusion transmission in humans. *Transfusion* 2006;46:1352–1359.

125. Khan AS, Bodem J, Buseyne F, et al. Spumaretroviruses: updated taxonomy and nomenclature. *Virology* 2018;516:158–164.

126. Khan IH, Mendoza S, Yee J, et al. Simultaneous detection of antibodies to six nonhuman-primate viruses by multiplex microbead immunoassay. *Clin Vaccine Immunol* 2006;13:45–52.

127. Kido K, Bannert H, Gronostajski RM, et al. Bel1-mediated transactivation of the spumaretroviral internal promoter is repressed by nuclear factor I. *J Biol Chem* 2003;278:11836–11842.

128. Kido K, Doerks A, Löchelt M, et al. Identification and functional characterization of an intragenic DNA binding site for the spumaretroviral trans-activator in the human p57Kip2 gene. *J Biol Chem* 2002;277:12032–12039.

129. Kincaid RP, Chen Y, Cox JE, et al. Noncanonical microRNA (miRNA) biogenesis gives rise to retroviral mimics of lymphoproliferative and immunosuppressive host miRNAs. *mBio* 2014;5:e00074.

130. Konvalinka J, Löchelt M, Zentgraf H, et al. Active foamy virus proteinase is essential for virus infectivity but not for formation of a Pol polyprotein. *J Virol* 1995;69:7264–7268.

131. Kretzschmar B, Nowrouzi A, Hartl MJ, et al. AZT-resistant foamy virus. *Virology* 2008;370:151–157.

132. Lambert C, Couteaudier M, Gouzil J, et al. Potent neutralizing antibodies in humans infected with zoonotic simian foamy viruses target conserved epitopes located in the dimorphic domain of the surface envelope protein. *PLoS Pathog* 2018;14:e1007293.

133. Lecellier CH, Saïb A. Foamy viruses: between retroviruses and pararetroviruses. *Virology* 2000;271:1–8.

134. Lecellier CH, Neves M, Giron ML, et al. Further characterization of equine foamy virus reveals unusual features among the foamy viruses. *J Virol* 2002;76:7220–7227.

135. Lee EG, Linial ML. The C terminus of foamy retrovirus Gag contains determinants for encapsidation of Pol protein into virions. *J Virol* 2008;82:10803–10810.

136. Lee EG, Kuppers D, Horn M, et al. A premature termination codon mutation at the C terminus of foamy virus Gag downregulates the levels of spliced pol mRNA. *J Virol* 2008;82:1656–1664.

137. Lee EG, Sinicrope A, Jackson DL, et al. Foamy virus Pol protein expressed as a Gag-Pol fusion retains enzymatic activities, allowing for infectious virus production. *J Virol* 2012;86:5992–6001.

138. Lee CC, Ye F, Tarantal AF. Comparison of growth and differentiation of fetal and adult rhesus monkey mesenchymal stem cells. *Stem Cells Dev* 2006;15:209–220.

139. Leendertz FH, Zirkel F, Couacy-Hymann E, et al. Interspecies transmission of simian foamy virus in a natural predator–prey system. *J Virol* 2008;82:7741–7744.

140. Lehmann-Che J, Giron ML, Delelis O, et al. Protease-dependent uncoating of a complex retrovirus. *J Virol* 2005;79:9244–9253.

141. Lehmann-Che J, Renault N, Giron ML, et al. Centrosomal latency of incoming foamy viruses in resting cells. *PLoS Pathog* 2007;3:e74.

142. Leo B, Hartl MJ, Schweimer K, et al. Insights into the structure and activity of prototype foamy virus RNase H. *Retrovirology* 2012;9:14.

143. Leo B, Schweimer K, Rösch P, et al. The solution structure of the prototype foamy virus RNase H domain indicates an important role of the basic loop in substrate binding. *Retrovirology* 2012;9:73.

144. Lesbats P, Engelman AN, Cherepanov P. Retroviral DNA integration. *Chem Rev* 2016;116:12730–12757.

145. Lesbats P, Serrao E, Maskell DP, et al. Structural basis for spumavirus GAG tethering to chromatin. *Proc Natl Acad Sci USA* 2017;114:5509–5514.

146. Life RB, Lee EG, Eastman SW, et al. Mutations in the amino terminus of foamy virus Gag disrupt morphology and infectivity but do not target assembly. *J Virol* 2008;82:6109–6119.

147. Lindemann D, Rethwilm A. Characterization of a human foamy virus 170-kilodalton Env-Bet fusion protein generated by alternative splicing. *J Virol* 1998;72:4088–4094.

148. Lindemann D, Rethwilm A. Foamy virus biology and its application for vector development. *Viruses* 2011;3:561–585.

149. Lindemann D, Hütter S, Wei G, et al. The unique, the known, and the unknown of spumaretrovirus assembly. *Viruses* 2021;13:105.

150. Lindemann D, Pietschmann T, Picard-Maureau M, et al. A particle-associated glycoprotein signal peptide essential for virus maturation and infectivity. *J Virol* 2001;75:5762–5771.

151. Linial ML. Foamy viruses are unconventional retroviruses. *J Virol* 1999;73:1747–1755.

152. Linial M, Fan H, Hahn B, et al. Retroviridae. In: Fauquet C, Mayo M, Maniloff J, et al., eds. *Virus Taxonomy*. 2nd ed. Elsevier Inc.; 2005:421–440.

153. Liu W, Backes P, Löchelt M. Importance of the major splice donor and redefinition of cis-acting sequences of gutless feline foamy virus vectors. *Virology* 2009;394:208–217.

154. Liu W, Worobey M, Li Y, et al. Molecular ecology and natural history of simian foamy virus infection in wild-living chimpanzees. *PLoS Pathog* 2008;4:e1000097.

155. Löchelt M. Foamy virus transactivation and gene expression. *Curr Top Microbiol Immunol* 2003;277:27–61.

156. Löchelt M, Flügel RM. The human foamy virus pol gene is expressed as a Pro-Pol polyprotein and not as a Gag-Pol fusion protein. *J Virol* 1996;70:1033–1040.

157. Löchelt M, Flügel RM, Aboud M. The human foamy virus internal promoter directs the expression of the functional Bel 1 transactivator and Bet protein early after infection. *J Virol* 1994;68:638–645.

158. Löchelt M, Muranyi W, Flügel RM. Human foamy virus genome possesses an internal, Bel-1-dependent and functional promoter. *Proc Natl Acad Sci USA* 1993;90:7317–7321.

159. Löchelt M, Romen F, Bastone P, et al. The antiretroviral activity of APOBEC3 is inhibited by the foamy virus accessory Bet protein. *Proc Natl Acad Sci USA* 2005;102:7982–7987.

160. Löchelt M, Zentgraf H, Flügel RM. Construction of an infectious DNA clone of the full-length human spumaretrovirus genome and mutagenesis of the bel 1 gene. *Virology* 1991;184:43–54.

161. Loh PC, Achong BC, Epstein MA. Further biological properties of the human syncytial virus. *Intervirology* 1977;8:204–217.

162. Loh PC, Matsuura F, Mizumoto C. Seroepidemiology of human syncytial virus: antibody prevalence in the Pacific. *Intervirology* 1980;13:87–90.

163. Lüftenegger D, Picard-Maureau M, Stanke N, et al. Analysis and function of prototype foamy virus envelope N glycosylation. *J Virol* 2005;79:7664–7672.

164. Lukic DS, Hotz-Wagenblatt A, Lei J, et al. Identification of the feline foamy virus Bet domain essential for APOBEC3 counteraction. *Retrovirology* 2013;10:76.

165. Maertens GN, Hare S, Cherepanov P. The mechanism of retroviral integration from X-ray structures of its key intermediates. *Nature* 2010;468:326–329.

166. Mahnke C, Kashaiya P, Rössler J, et al. Human spumavirus antibodies in sera from African patients. *Arch Virol* 1992;123:243–253.

167. Malmquist WA, Van der Maaten MJ, Boothe AD. Isolation, immunodiffusion, immunofluorescence, and electron microscopy of a syncytial virus of lymphosarcomatous and apparently normal cattle. *Cancer Res* 1969;29:188–200.

168. Mannigel I, Stange A, Zentgraf H, et al. Correct capsid assembly mediated by a conserved YXXLGL motif in prototype foamy virus Gag is essential for infectivity and reverse transcription of the viral genome. *J Virol* 2007;81:3317–3326.

169. Maskell DP, Renault L, Serrao E, et al. Structural basis for retroviral integration into nucleosomes. *Nature* 2015;523:366–369.

170. Materniak-Kornas M, Tan J, Heit-Mondrzyk A, et al. Bovine foamy virus: shared and unique molecular features in vitro and in vivo. *Viruses* 2019;11:1084.

171. Matthes D, Wiktorowicz T, Zahn J, et al. Basic residues in the foamy virus Gag protein. *J Virol* 2011;85:3986–3995.
172. Maurer B, Bannert H, Darai G, et al. Analysis of the primary structure of the long terminal repeat and the *gag* and *pol* genes of the human spumaretrovirus. *J Virol* 1988;62:1590–1597.
173. Maurer B, Serfling E, ter Meulen V, et al. Transcription factor AP-1 modulates the activity of the human foamy virus long terminal repeat. *J Virol* 1991;65:6353–6357.
174. Meiering CD, Linial ML. Historical perspective of foamy virus epidemiology and infection. *Clin Microbiol Rev* 2001;14:165–176.
175. Meiering CD, Linial ML. Reactivation of a complex retrovirus is controlled by a molecular switch and is inhibited by a viral protein. *Proc Natl Acad Sci USA* 2002;99:15130–15135.
176. Meiering CD, Comstock KE, Linial ML. Multiple integrations of human foamy virus in persistently infected human erythroleukemia cells. *J Virol* 2000;74:1718–1726.
177. Meiering CD, Rubio C, May C, et al. Cell-type-specific regulation of the two foamy virus promoters. *J Virol* 2001;75:6547–6557.
178. Mergia A, Blackwell J, Papadi G, et al. Simian foamy virus type 1 (SFV-1) induces apoptosis. *Virus Res* 1997;50:129–137.
179. Mergia A, Renshaw-Gegg LW, Stout MW, et al. Functional domains of the simian foamy virus type 1 transcriptional transactivator (Taf). *J Virol* 1993;67:4598–4604.
180. Moebes A, Enssle J, Bieniasz PD, et al. Human foamy virus reverse transcription that occurs late in the viral replication cycle. *J Virol* 1997;71:7305–7311.
181. Moschall R, Denk S, Erkelenz S, et al. A purine-rich element in foamy virus pol regulates env splicing and gag/pol expression. *Retrovirology* 2017;14:10.
182. Müllers E, Stirnnagel K, Kaulfuss S, et al. Prototype foamy virus gag nuclear localization: a novel pathway among retroviruses. *J Virol* 2011;85:9276–9285.
183. Muranyi W, Flügel RM. Analysis of splicing patterns of human spumaretrovirus by polymerase chain reaction reveals complex RNA structures. *J Virol* 1991;65:727–735.
184. Murray SM, Picker LJ, Axthelm MK, et al. Expanded tissue targets for foamy virus replication with simian immunodeficiency virus-induced immunosuppression. *J Virol* 2006;80:663–670.
185. Murray SM, Picker LJ, Axthelm MK, et al. Replication in a superficial epithelial cell niche explains the lack of pathogenicity of primate foamy virus infections. *J Virol* 2008;82:5981–5985.
186. Nasimuzzaman M, Persons DA. Cell Membrane-associated heparan sulfate is a receptor for prototype foamy virus in human, monkey, and rodent cells. *Mol Ther* 2012;20:1158–1166.
187. Neumann-Haefelin D, Rethwilm A, Bauer G, et al. Characterization of a foamy virus isolated from *Cercopithecus aethiops* lymphoblastoid cells. *Med Microbiol Immunol* 1983;172:75–86.
188. Nowacka M, Nowak E, Czarnocki-Cieciura M, et al. Structures of substrate complexes of foamy viral protease-reverse transcriptase. *J Virol* 2021;95:e0084821.
189. Nowrouzi A, Dittrich M, Klanke C, et al. Genome-wide mapping of foamy virus vector integrations into a human cell line. *J Gen Virol* 2006;87:1339–1347.
190. Ohmine K, Li Y, Bauer TR Jr, et al. Tracking of specific integrant clones in dogs treated with foamy virus vectors. *Hum Gene Ther* 2011;22:217–224.
191. Pacheco B, Finzi A, McGee-Estrada K, et al. Species-specific inhibition of foamy viruses from South American monkeys by New World Monkey TRIM5{alpha} proteins. *J Virol* 2010;84:4095–4099.
192. Paris J, Tobaly-Tapiero J, Giron ML, et al. The invariant arginine within the chromatin-binding motif regulates both nucleolar localization and chromatin binding of Foamy virus Gag. *Retrovirology* 2018;15:48.
193. Parks WD, Todaro GJ, Scolnick EM, et al. RNA dependent DNA polymerase in primate syncytium-forming (foamy) viruses. *Nature* 1971;229:258–260.
194. Patton GS, Erlwein O, McClure MO. Cell-cycle dependence of foamy virus vectors. *J Gen Virol* 2004;85:2925–2930.
195. Patton GS, Morris SA, Chung W, et al. Identification of domains in gag important for prototypic foamy virus egress. *J Virol* 2005;79:6392–6399.
196. Perkovic M, Schmidt S, Marino D, et al. Species-specific inhibition of APOBEC3C by the prototype foamy virus protein bet. *J Biol Chem* 2009;284:5819–5826.
197. Peters K, Barg N, Gärtner K, et al. Complex effects of foamy virus central purine-rich regions on viral replication. *Virology* 2008;373:51–60.
198. Peters K, Wiktorowicz T, Heinkelein M, et al. RNA and protein requirements for incorporation of the Pol protein into foamy virus particles. *J Virol* 2005;79:7005–7013.
199. Petit C, Giron ML, Tobaly-Tapiero J, et al. Targeting of incoming retroviral Gag to the centrosome involves a direct interaction with the dynein light chain 8. *J Cell Sci* 2003;116:3433–3442.
200. Pfrepper KI, Löchelt M, Rackwitz HR, et al. Molecular characterization of proteolytic processing of the Gag proteins of human spumavirus. *J Virol* 1999;73:7907–7911.
201. Picard-Maureau M, Jarmy G, Berg A, et al. Foamy virus envelope glycoprotein-mediated entry involves a pH-dependent fusion process. *J Virol* 2003;77:4722–4730.
202. Pietschmann T, Heinkelein M, Heldmann M, et al. Foamy virus capsids require the cognate envelope protein for particle export. *J Virol* 1999;73:2613–2621.
203. Pietschmann T, Zentgraf H, Rethwilm A, et al. An evolutionarily conserved positively charged amino acid in the putative membrane-spanning domain of the foamy virus envelope protein controls fusion activity. *J Virol* 2000;74:4474–4482.
204. Pinto-Santini DM, Stenbak CR, Linial ML. Foamy virus zoonotic infections. *Retrovirology* 2017;14:55.
205. Plochmann K, Horn A, Gschmack E, et al. Heparan sulfate is an attachment factor for foamy virus entry. *J Virol* 2012;86:10028–10035.
206. Rajawat YS, Humbert O, Kiem HP. In-vivo gene therapy with foamy virus vectors. *Viruses* 2019;11:1091.
207. Reh J, Stange A, Götz A, et al. An N-terminal domain helical motif of Prototype Foamy Virus Gag with dual functions essential for particle egress and viral infectivity. *Retrovirology* 2013;10:45.
208. Renault N, Tobaly-Tapiero J, Paris J, et al. A nuclear export signal within the structural Gag protein is required for prototype foamy virus replication. *Retrovirology* 2011;8:6.
209. Renne R, Friedl E, Schweizer M, et al. Genomic organization and expression of simian foamy virus type 3 (SFV-3). *Virology* 1992;186:597–608.
210. Repaske R, Hartley JW, Kavlick MF, et al. Inhibition of RNase H activity and viral replication by single mutations in the 3′ region of Moloney murine leukemia virus reverse transcriptase. *J Virol* 1989;63:1460–1464.
211. Rethwilm A. Regulation of foamy virus gene expression. *Curr Top Microbiol Immunol* 1995;193:1–24.
212. Rethwilm A. Unexpected replication pathways of foamy viruses. *J Acquir Immune Defic Syndr Hum Retrovirol* 1996;13(Suppl 1):S248–253.
213. Rethwilm A. The replication strategy of foamy viruses. *Curr Top Microbiol Immunol* 2003;277:1–26.
214. Rethwilm A. Foamy viruses. In: Mahy BWJ, ter Meulen V, eds. *Topley & Wilson's Microbiology Virology*. Edward Arnold; 2005:1304–1321.
215. Rethwilm A, Baunach G, Netzer KO, et al. Infectious DNA of the human spumaretrovirus. *Nucleic Acids Res* 1990;18:733–738.
216. Rethwilm A, Darai G, Rösen A, et al. Molecular cloning of the genome of human spumaretrovirus. *Gene* 1987;59:19–28.
217. Rethwilm A, Erlwein O, Baunach G, et al. The transcriptional transactivator of human foamy virus maps to the bel 1 genomic region. *Proc Natl Acad Sci USA* 1991;88:941–945.
218. Riggs JL, Oshirls, Taylor DO, et al. Syncytium-forming agent isolated from domestic cats. *Nature* 1969;222:1190–1191.
219. Rinke CS, Boyer PL, Sullivan MD, et al. Mutation of the catalytic domain of the foamy virus reverse transcriptase leads to loss of processivity and infectivity. *J Virol* 2002;76:7560–7570.
220. Romen F, Backes P, Materniak M, et al. Serological detection systems for identification of cows shedding bovine foamy virus via milk. *Virology* 2007;364:123–131.
221. Romen F, Pawlita M, Sehr P, et al. Antibodies against Gag are diagnostic markers for feline foamy virus infections while Env and Bet reactivity is undetectable in a substantial fraction of infected cats. *Virology* 2006;345:502–508.
222. Rosenblum LL, Patton G, Grigg AR, et al. Differential susceptibility of retroviruses to nucleoside analogues. *Antivir Chem Chemother* 2001;12:91–97.
223. Rösener M, Hahn H, Kranz M, et al. Absence of serological evidence for foamy virus infection in patients with amyotrophic lateral sclerosis. *J Med Virol* 1996;48:222–226.
224. Roy J, Linial ML. Role of the foamy virus Pol cleavage site in viral replication. *J Virol* 2007;81:4956–4962.
225. Roy J, Rudolph W, Juretzek T, et al. Feline foamy virus genome and replication strategy. *J Virol* 2003;77:11324–11331.
226. Rua R, Betsem E, Montange T, et al. In vivo cellular tropism of gorilla simian foamy virus in blood of infected humans. *J Virol* 2014;88:13429–13435.
227. Rua R, Lepelley A, Gessain A, et al. Innate sensing of foamy viruses by human hematopoietic cells. *J Virol* 2012;86:909–918.
228. Russell RA, Wiegand HL, Moore MD, et al. Foamy virus Bet proteins function as novel inhibitors of the APOBEC3 family of innate antiretroviral defense factors. *J Virol* 2005;79:8724–8731.
229. Russell RA, Zeng Y, Erlwein O, et al. The R region found in the human foamy virus long terminal repeat is critical for both Gag and Pol protein expression. *J Virol* 2001;75:6817–6824.
230. Rustigian R, Johnston P, Reihart H. Infection of monkey kidney tissue cultures with virus-like agents. *Proc Soc Exp Biol Med* 1955;88:8–16.
231. Ryabova LA, Hohn T. Ribosome shunting in the cauliflower mosaic virus 35S RNA leader is a special case of reinitiation of translation functioning in plant and animal systems. *Genes Dev* 2000;14:817–829.
232. Saïb A, Neves M, Giron ML, et al. Long-term persistent infection of domestic rabbits by the human foamy virus. *Virology* 1997;228:263–268.
233. Saïb A, Peries J, de The H. A defective human foamy provirus generated by pregenome splicing. *EMBO J* 1993;12:4439–4444.
234. Saïb A, Puvion-Dutilleul F, Schmid M, et al. Nuclear targeting of incoming human foamy virus Gag proteins involves a centriolar step. *J Virol* 1997;71:1155–1161.
235. Santos AF, Cavalcante LTF, Muniz CP, et al. Simian foamy viruses in Central and South America: a new world of discovery. *Viruses* 2019;11:967.
236. Schepetilnikov M, Schott G, Katsarou K, et al. Molecular dissection of the prototype foamy virus (PFV) RNA 5′-UTR identifies essential elements of a ribosomal shunt. *Nucleic Acids Res* 2009;37:5838–5847.
237. Schliephake AW, Rethwilm A. Nuclear localization of foamy virus Gag precursor protein. *J Virol* 1994;68:4946–4954.
238. Schmidt M, Rethwilm A. Replicating foamy virus-based vectors directing high level expression of foreign genes. *Virology* 1995;210:167–178.
239. Schmidt M, Herchenröder O, Heeney J, et al. Long terminal repeat U3 length polymorphism of human foamy virus. *Virology* 1997;230:167–178.
240. Schmidt M, Niewiesk S, Heeney J, et al. Mouse model to study the replication of primate foamy viruses. *J Gen Virol* 1997;78(Pt 8):1929–1933.
241. Schneider A, Peter D, Schmitt J, et al. Structural requirements for enzymatic activities of foamy virus protease-reverse transcriptase. *Proteins* 2014;82:375–385.
242. Schrom EM, Moschall R, Hartl MJ, et al. U1snRNP-mediated suppression of polyadenylation in conjunction with the RNA structure controls poly (A) site selection in foamy viruses. *Retrovirology* 2013;10:55.
243. Schweizer M, Neumann-Haefelin D. Phylogenetic analysis of primate foamy viruses by comparison of pol sequences. *Virology* 1995;207:577–582.
244. Schweizer M, Falcone V, Gänge J, et al. Simian foamy virus isolated from an accidentally infected human individual. *J Virol* 1997;71:4821–4824.
245. Schweizer M, Fleps U, Jäckle A, et al. Simian foamy virus type 3 (SFV-3) in latently infected Vero cells: reactivation by demethylation of proviral DNA. *Virology* 1993;192:663–666.
246. Schweizer M, Renne R, Neumann-Haefelin D. Structural analysis of proviral DNA in simian foamy virus (LK-3)-infected cells. *Arch Virol* 1989;109:103–114.
247. Schweizer M, Turek R, Hahn H, et al. Markers of foamy virus infections in monkeys, apes, and accidentally infected humans: appropriate testing fails to confirm suspected foamy virus prevalence in humans. *AIDS Res Hum Retroviruses* 1995;11:161–170.
248. Schweizer M, Turek R, Reinhardt M, et al. Absence of foamy virus DNA in Graves' disease. *AIDS Res Hum Retroviruses* 1994;10:601–605.
249. Sfakianos JN, LaCasse RA, Hunter E. The M-PMV cytoplasmic targeting-retention signal directs nascent Gag polypeptides to a pericentriolar region of the cell. *Traffic* 2003;4:660–670.
250. Shankar A, Shanmugam V, Switzer WM. Complete genome sequence of a baboon simian foamy virus isolated from an infected human. *Microbiol Resour Announc* 2020;9:e00522-20.

251. Shaw KL, Lindemann D, Mulligan MJ, et al. Foamy virus envelope glycoprotein is sufficient for particle budding and release. *J Virol* 2003;77:2338–2348.

252. Simantirakis E, Tsironis I, Vassilopoulos G. FV vectors as alternative gene vehicles for gene transfer in HSCs. *Viruses* 2020;12:332.

253. Smiley Evans T, Gilardi KV, Barry PA, et al. Detection of viruses using discarded plants from wild mountain gorillas and golden monkeys. *Am J Primatol* 2016;78:1222–1234.

254. Stange A, Lüftenegger D, Reh J, et al. Subviral particle release determinants of prototype foamy virus. *J Virol* 2008;82:9858–9869.

255. Stange A, Mannigel I, Peters K, et al. Characterization of prototype foamy virus gag late assembly domain motifs and their role in particle egress and infectivity. *J Virol* 2005;79:5466–5476.

256. Stanke N, Stange A, Lüftenegger D, et al. Ubiquitination of the prototype foamy virus envelope glycoprotein leader peptide regulates subviral particle release. *J Virol* 2005;79:15074–15083.

257. Stenbak CR, Linial ML. Role of the C terminus of foamy virus Gag in RNA packaging and Pol expression. *J Virol* 2004;78:9423–9430.

258. Stirnnagel K, Lüftenegger D, Stange A, et al. Analysis of prototype foamy virus particle-host cell interaction with autofluorescent retroviral particles. *Retrovirology* 2010;7:45.

259. Stirnnagel K, Schupp D, Dupont A, et al. Differential pH-dependent cellular uptake pathways among foamy viruses elucidated using dual-colored fluorescent particles. *Retrovirology* 2012;9:71.

260. Swiersy A, Wiek C, Reh J, et al. Orthoretroviral-like prototype foamy virus Gag-Pol expression is compatible with viral replication. *Retrovirology* 2011;8:66.

261. Switzer WM, Bhullar V, Shanmugam V, et al. Frequent simian foamy virus infection in persons occupationally exposed to nonhuman primates. *J Virol* 2004;78:2780–2789.

262. Switzer WM, Garcia AD, Yang C, et al. Coinfection with HIV-1 and simian foamy virus in West Central Africans. *J Infect Dis* 2008;197:1389–1393.

263. Switzer WM, Salemi M, Shanmugam V, et al. Ancient co-speciation of simian foamy viruses and primates. *Nature* 2005;434:376–380.

264. Tan J, Hao P, Jia R, et al. Identification and functional characterization of BTas transactivator as a DNA-binding protein. *Virology* 2010;405:408–413.

265. Tan J, Qiao W, Wang J, et al. IFP35 is involved in the antiviral function of interferon by association with the viral tas transactivator of bovine foamy virus. *J Virol* 2008;82:4275–4283.

266. Tan J, Qiao W, Xu F, et al. Dimerization of BTas is required for the transactivational activity of bovine foamy virus. *Virology* 2008;376:236–241.

267. Thümer L, Rethwilm A, Holmes EC, et al. The complete nucleotide sequence of a New World simian foamy virus. *Virology* 2007;369:191–197.

268. Tisdale M, Schulze T, Larder BA, et al. Mutations within the RNase H domain of human immunodeficiency virus type 1 reverse transcriptase abolish virus infectivity. *J Gen Virol* 1991;72(Pt 1):59–66.

269. Tobaly-Tapiero J, Bittoun P, Giron ML, et al. Human foamy virus capsid formation requires an interaction domain in the N terminus of Gag. *J Virol* 2001;75:4367–4375.

270. Tobaly-Tapiero J, Bittoun P, Lehmann-Che J, et al. Chromatin tethering of incoming foamy virus by the structural Gag protein. *Traffic* 2008;9:1717–1727.

271. Tobaly-Tapiero J, Bittoun P, Neves M, et al. Isolation and characterization of an equine foamy virus. *J Virol* 2000;74:4064–4073.

272. Tobaly-Tapiero J, Kupiec JJ, Santillana-Hayat M, et al. Further characterization of the gapped DNA intermediates of human spumavirus: evidence for a dual initiation of plus-strand DNA synthesis. *J Gen Virol* 1991;72(Pt 3):605–608.

273. Trobridge G, Russell DW. Cell cycle requirements for transduction by foamy virus vectors compared to those of oncovirus and lentivirus vectors. *J Virol* 2004;78:2327–2335.

274. Trobridge GD, Miller DG, Jacobs MA, et al. Foamy virus vector integration sites in normal human cells. *Proc Natl Acad Sci USA* 2006;103:1498–1503.

275. Valkov E, Gupta SS, Hare S, et al. Functional and structural characterization of the integrase from the prototype foamy virus. *Nucleic Acids Res* 2009;37:243–255.

276. Vassilopoulos G, Rethwilm A. The usefulness of a perfect parasite. *Gene Ther* 2008;15:1299–1301.

277. Voss M, Fukumori A, Kuhn PH, et al. Foamy virus envelope protein is a substrate for signal peptide peptidase-like 3 (SPPL3). *J Biol Chem* 2012;287:43401–43409.

278. Wagner A, Doerks A, Aboud M, et al. Induction of cellular genes is mediated by the Bel1 transactivator in foamy virus-infected human cells. *J Virol* 2000;74:4441–4447.

279. Wang J, Tan J, Guo H, et al. Bovine foamy virus transactivator BTas interacts with cellular RelB to enhance viral transcription. *J Virol* 2010;84:11888–11897.

279a. Wang Z, Li R, Liu C, et al. Characterization of bovine foamy virus gag late assembly domain motifs and their role in recruiting ESCRT for budding. *Viruses* 2022;13:522.

280. Weaver TA, Talbot KJ, Panganiban AT. Spleen necrosis virus gag polyprotein is necessary for particle assembly and release but not for proteolytic processing. *J Virol* 1990;64:2642–2652.

281. Wei X, Chen Y, Duan G, et al. A reptilian endogenous foamy virus sheds light on the early evolution of retroviruses. *Virus Evol* 2019;5:vez001.

282. Wei G, Kehl T, Bao Q, et al. The chromatin binding domain, including the QPQRYG motif, of feline foamy virus Gag is required for viral DNA integration and nuclear accumulation of Gag and the viral genome. *Virology* 2018;524:56–68.

283. Weiss RA. Foamy retroviruses. A virus in search of a disease [news]. *Nature* 1988;333:497–498.

284. Weiss RA. Reverse transcription. Foamy viruses bubble on [news]. *Nature* 1996;380:201.

285. Whisnant AW, Kehl T, Bao Q, et al. Identification of novel, highly expressed retroviral microRNAs in cells infected by bovine foamy virus. *J Virol* 2014;88:4679–4686.

286. Wiktorowicz T, Peters K, Armbruster N, et al. Generation of an improved foamy virus vector by dissection of cis-acting sequences. *J Gen Virol* 2009;90:481–487.

287. Wilk T, de Haas F, Wagner A, et al. The intact retroviral Env glycoprotein of human foamy virus is a trimer. *J Virol* 2000;74:2885–2887.

288. Wilk T, Geiselhart V, Frech M, et al. Specific interaction of a novel foamy virus Env leader protein with the N-terminal Gag domain. *J Virol* 2001;75:7995–8007.

289. Wilson MD, Renault L, Maskell DP, et al. Retroviral integration into nucleosomes through DNA looping and sliding along the histone octamer. *Nat Commun* 2019;10:4189.

290. Winkler I, Bodem J, Haas L, et al. Characterization of the genome of feline foamy virus and its proteins shows distinct features different from those of primate spumaviruses. *J Virol* 1997;71:6727–6741.

291. Winkler IG, Löchelt M, Flower RL. Epidemiology of feline foamy virus and feline immunodeficiency virus infections in domestic and feral cats: a seroepidemiological study. *J Clin Microbiol* 1999;37:2848–2851.

292. Wolfe ND, Switzer WM, Carr JK, et al. Naturally acquired simian retrovirus infections in central African hunters. *Lancet* 2004;363:932–937.

293. Wu M, Chari S, Yanchis T, et al. cis-Acting sequences required for simian foamy virus type 1 vectors. *J Virol* 1998;72:3451–3454.

294. Wu Y, Tan J, Su Y, et al. Transcription factor AP1 modulates the internal promoter activity of bovine foamy virus. *Virus Res* 2010;147:139–144.

295. Xu F, Tan J, Liu R, et al. Tetherin inhibits prototypic foamy virus release. *Virol J* 2011;8:198.

296. Yap MW, Lindemann D, Stanke N, et al. Restriction of foamy viruses by primate Trim5alpha. *J Virol* 2008;82:5429–5439.

297. Yu SF, Linial ML. Analysis of the role of the bel and bet open reading frames of human foamy virus by using a new quantitative assay. *J Virol* 1993;67:6618–6624.

298. Yu SF, Baldwin DN, Gwynn SR, et al. Human foamy virus replication: a pathway distinct from that of retroviruses and hepadnaviruses. *Science* 1996;271:1579–1582.

299. Yu SF, Eastman SW, Linial ML. Foamy virus capsid assembly occurs at a pericentriolar region through a cytoplasmic targeting/retention signal in Gag. *Traffic* 2006;7:966–977.

300. Yu SF, Edelmann K, Strong RK, et al. The carboxyl terminus of the human foamy virus Gag protein contains separable nucleic acid binding and nuclear transport domains. *J Virol* 1996;70:8255–8262.

301. Yu SF, Lujan P, Jackson DL, et al. The DEAD-box RNA helicase DDX6 is required for efficient encapsidation of a retroviral genome. *PLoS Pathog* 2011;7:e1002303.

302. Yu SF, Stone J, Linial ML. Productive persistent infection of hematopoietic cells by human foamy virus. *J Virol* 1996;70:1250–1254.

303. Yu SF, Sullivan MD, Linial ML. Evidence that the human foamy virus genome is DNA. *J Virol* 1999;73:1565–1572.

304. Zamborlini A, Renault N, Saïb A, et al. Early reverse transcription is essential for productive foamy virus infection. *PLoS One* 2010;5:e11023.

305. Zemba M, Wilk T, Rutten T, et al. The carboxy-terminal p3Gag domain of the human foamy virus Gag precursor is required for efficient virus infectivity. *Virology* 1998;247:7–13.

306. Zenger E, Brown WC, Song W, et al. Evaluation of cofactor effect of feline syncytium-forming virus on feline immunodeficiency virus infection. *Am J Vet Res* 1993;54:713–718.

307. Zhadina M, Bieniasz PD. Functional interchangeability of late domains, late domain cofactors and ubiquitin in viral budding. *PLoS Pathog* 2010;6:e1001153.

308. Zhadina M, McClure MO, Johnson MC, et al. Ubiquitin-dependent virus particle budding without viral protein ubiquitination. *Proc Natl Acad Sci USA* 2007;104:20031–20036.

309. Zou JX, Luciw PA. The transcriptional transactivator of simian foamy virus 1 binds to a DNA target element in the viral internal promoter. *Proc Natl Acad Sci USA* 1996;93:326–330.

310. Zurnic I, Hütter S, Rzeha U, et al. Interactions of prototype foamy virus capsids with host cell polo-like kinases are important for efficient viral DNA integration. *PLoS Pathog* 2016;12:e1005860.

Severe Acute Respiratory Syndrome Coronavirus 2 (SARS-CoV-2)

Stephen A. Goldstein • Brenda G. Hogue • Julian L. Leibowitz • Susan R. Weiss

History of human coronaviruses
Evolution of SARS-CoV-2–related viruses
  Phylogenetic structure of SARS-related coronaviruses
    (SARSr-CoV)
Origin and evolution of SARS-CoV
  Evolutionary history of SARS-CoV-2
  Evolution of ACE2 usage by SARS-related coronaviruses
    (SARSr-CoVs)
  Recombination drives diversification of SARS-CoV-2 lineage
    viruses
SARS-CoV-2 replication and structural proteins (Fig. 21.5)
  Spike (S) protein
  Membrane (M) protein
  Envelope (E) protein
  Nucleocapsid (N) protein
  SARS-CoV-2 assembly and release
Nonstructural proteins (Table 21.1)
  Nsp1
  Nsp2
  Nsp3
  Nsp4 and Nsp6
  Nsp5
  The replicase complex: Nsp7-Nsp16
SARS-CoV-2 accessory proteins
  ORF3a
  ORF3b
  ORF6
  ORF7a
  ORF7b
  ORF8
  ORF9b
  Recombinant viruses
SARS-CoV-2 variants—transmission and immune evasion
SARS-CoV-2: secondary transmission to wild and domestic
  animals

HISTORY OF HUMAN CORONAVIRUSES

While the first highly lethal human coronavirus (HCoV), severe acute respiratory syndrome coronavirus (SARS-CoV), was identified in late 2002, human respiratory coronaviruses were isolated more than 50 years before that. HCoV-229E and related strains were isolated in human embryonic intestine cell cultures. HCoV-OC43 and related viruses were isolated human tracheal from organ cultures and later adapted to grow in suckling mice. Early literature suggested that HCoVes may be associated with enteric disease[104,172] and also multiple sclerosis,[104,260] but neither has been confirmed.

From that time forward, there was extensive research performed on the basic mechanisms of coronavirus replication, including cell entry, cell to cell fusion, mRNA synthesis, protein expression, and host–virus interactions including innate and adaptive immune responses. Most of these studies were performed on the model murine coronavirus mouse hepatitis virus (MHV), the avian infectious bronchitis virus (IBV), and bovine coronavirus (BCV). All of these systems were more amenable to molecular biology studies than the human viruses since these were more difficult to work with in cell culture and there were no useful animal models for the human viruses.

In late 2002, severe acute respiratory syndrome (SARS)-CoV emerged in southern China, causing an epidemic, shocking coronavirologists to the reality that members of this virus family could be etiologic agents of highly lethal respiratory disease in humans and furthermore making coronaviruses known to the general public (Fig. 21.1A). SARS-CoV disappeared after 6 or 7 months, but during that time caused 8,069 infections and 774 deaths. In the years after the SARS epidemic, it was discovered that bats were the hosts for many SARS-like coronaviruses[197,210] and that SARS-CoV was likely transmitted to humans through an intermediate host, the palm civet.

Following the SARS epidemic, two other HCoVes were identified, NL63[299] and HKU1,[198] causing respiratory symptoms (Fig. 21.1A). Approximately 10 years later in 2012, the deadlier Middle East respiratory syndrome (MERS)-CoV emerged in Saudi Arabia. MERS-CoV was found also to have its origin in bats, and to have a reservoir in the intermediate animal, the camel, and continues to spread from camel to human (Fig. 21.1A). While less transmissible among humans, MERS-CoV has a higher mortality rate and continues to cause infections in humans (https://Orf.who.int/emergencies/disease-outbreak-news/item/2021-DON317). In late 2019, a SARS-CoV–like virus emerged in Wuhan China, far from the site of the first SARS-CoV infections (Fig. 21.1A). SARS-CoV-2, the cause of coronavirus disease 2019 (COVID-19), causes severe respiratory disease with a lower fatality rate than SARS-CoV, even though it spreads more quickly, sometimes from asymptomatic individuals around the world. Since its emergence, SARS-CoV-2 has caused the largest and most serious global pandemic since the 1918 influenza. It is still not completely understood why this virus, which is similar to SARS-CoV, was able to spread more readily to cause the global pandemic.

Coronaviruses are divided into four genera designated as alpha, beta, gamma, and delta. All genera have similar genome organizations (structural proteins and nonstructural proteins including replicase proteins) but differ in their nonessential accessory proteins that are often involved in evading or antagonizing host cell responses. The less pathogenic, HCoVes are grouped in the *Alphacoronavirus* genus (229E, NL63, and related viruses) or the *Betacoronavirus* genus (Fig. 21.1B). The latter genus is further divided into subgroups and lineages based on the phylogenetic relatedness. These include the nonhighly pathogenic embeco or lineage a (OC43, HKU-1) and the highly pathogenic sarbeco or lineage b (SARS-CoV, SARS-CoV-2 and related bat CoVs) and merbeco or lineage c (MERS-CoV and related bat CoVs) (Fig. 21.1B).

EVOLUTION OF SARS-CoV-2–RELATED VIRUSES

The discovery of SARS-CoV-2 and ensuing pandemic[439] has focused attention on the evolution and origins of this viral lineage. SARS-CoV-2 and the 2002–2003 epidemic SARS-CoV fall within the *SARSr(elated)-CoV* species in the *Sarbecovirus*

subgenus of *Betacoronavirus*[62] (Fig. 21.1B). This group of *SARSr-CoVs* was unknown prior to the SARS-CoV epidemic but is now known to comprise at least several hundred viruses[143,196] present not only throughout China but also in southeast Asia,[383] Japan,[259] South Korea,[201] Europe,[81] and sub-Saharan Africa.[291,396] SARSr-CoVs are evidently not narrowly restricted from a geographic standpoint, though the degree of public health concern emanating from different viral reservoirs remains unclear. Both 21st century spillovers of SARSr-CoVs have occurred in mainland China.

Phylogenetic Structure of SARS-Related Coronaviruses (SARSr-CoV)

In the period since the emergence of SARS-CoV (detailed below), dozens of related full-length genomes and additional partial genomes have been described, largely through metagenomic analyses. SARSr-CoV sequences have been identified primarily in East Asia spanning Japan, South Korea, China, Thailand, and Cambodia. Based on geographic distribution of the reservoir species, primarily *Rhinolophus* bats, such viruses surely circulate elsewhere in southeast Asia. In addition, distantly related SARSr-CoVs have been identified in Europe and Africa. The wide distribution suggests an ancient origin of this group of viruses. A 2021 study by Wells et al.[396] conducted a phylogenetic analysis of the RNA-dependent RNA polymerase (RdRp)-encoding region of ORF1ab (described in detail below) and identified five distinct lineages within *SARSr-CoV* (Fig. 21.2). Four of these are distributed throughout East Asia while the

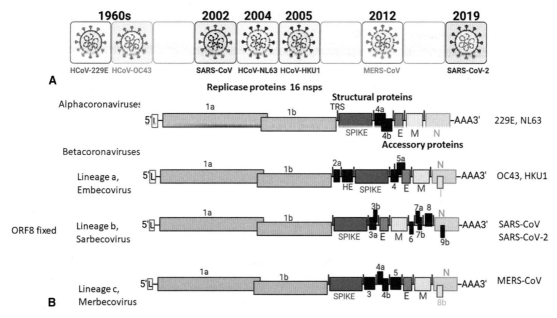

FIGURE 21.1 A: Timeline of detection of human coronaviruses. Common cold human coronaviruses HCoV-OC43 and HCoV-229E have been known since the 1960s; HCoV-NL63 and HCoV-HKU-1 were identified in 2004–2005. The first highly pathogenic human SARS-CoV coronavirus was identified in 2002, MERS-CoV in 2012, and SARS-CoV-2 in 2019. **B:** Human coronavirus genome structure. Human coronaviruses are found in the alphavirus genus and in three lineages of betacoronaviruses, embeco (lineage a), sarbeco (lineage b), and merbeco (lineage c). The genomes have 5' capped ends and leader (L) sequences. The intergenic short *light brown bars* are transcription regulatory sequence, which mark the initiation site of transcription of each subgenomic mRNA. All coronaviruses encode 16 nonstructural proteins (nsps) in 5' open reading frames 1a and 1b. Genes encoding structural proteins are arrayed in the 3' portion of the genome in the order spike (S), small membrane (E), membrane (M), and nucleocapsid (N). Lineage specific accessory genes are found interspersed among the structural genes (*dark brown bars*). ORF8 of SARS-CoV evolved into ORF8a and ORFb but remains as an intact ORF8 in SARS-CoV-2 (as shown in the figure). (Created by Alejandra Fausto using Biorender.com.)

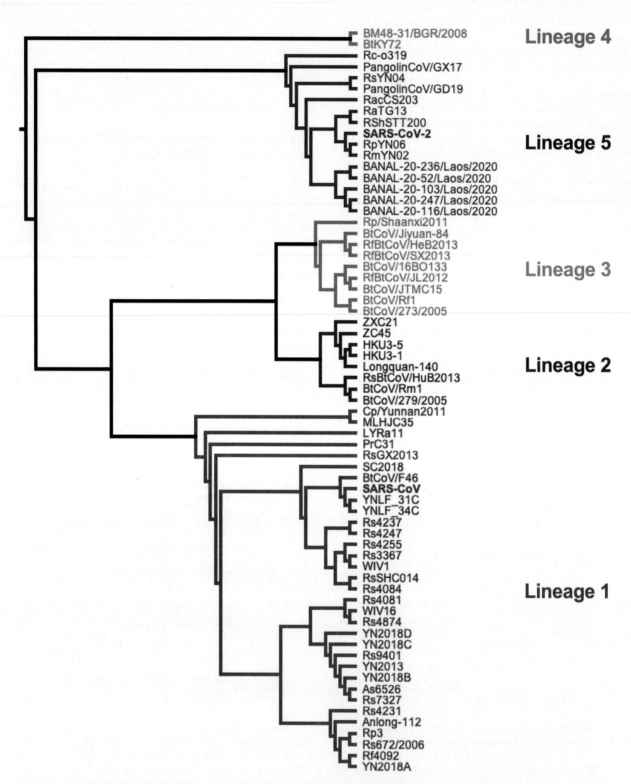

FIGURE 21.2 RdRp phylogenetic tree. Maximum-likelihood phylogenetic tree of the RdRp-encoding region of ORF1ab. This tree demonstrated the segregation of *SARSrelated(r)-CoV* into 5 RdRp lineages with SARS-CoV and SARS-CoV-2 each defining two widely divergent lineages. Viruses shown able to use human ACE-2 are bolded. To construct the tree, representative *SARSr-CoV* sequences were obtained from GenBank or GISAID and aligned to the RdRp-encoding region of SARS-CoV-2 using MAFFT. A tree was then inferred using FastTree.

fifth comprises the African and European SARSr-CoVs. Notably, three of the Asian lineages fall onto sub-branches within a single branch, including SARS-CoV and related viruses. The SARS-CoV-2–like viruses are on a distant branch and exhibit greater than 10% genetic distance in RdRp from SARS-CoV–like viruses; they are comparably distant as the European and African viruses and the relative phylogenetic positions of the Africa/Europe and SARS-CoV-2–like viruses remain somewhat uncertain. This suggests that the split between the SARS-CoV and SARS-CoV-2 branches was quite ancient despite their common receptor [angiotensin converting enzyme −2 (ACE2)] usage, possibly approaching 1,000 years ago.[396] SARS-CoV and SARS-CoV-2 are much more closely related to different non–ACE2-utilizing viruses than they are to each other, suggesting a complex evolutionary history of ACE2-binding spike proteins. Interestingly NL63, an alphacoronavirus also uses ACE2 as its receptor[251] indicating receptor utilization is not always useful for determining relatedness of viruses.

ORIGIN AND EVOLUTION OF SARS-CoV

Though the definitive origin of SARS-CoV-2 remains unknown, the historical example of SARS-CoV provides valuable context and guidance given the likely similar ecological niche occupied by the two viruses. The SARS-CoV epidemic began as a cluster of unusual pneumonia cases in spring 2003 in Hong Kong[200,369] and retrospectively was determined to have begun the preceding fall in Guangdong in mainland China.[434] Via both electron microscopy and genomic analyses, a coronavirus was identified as the etiological agent of these outbreaks.[82,285] Ultimately, greater than 8,000 cases and nearly 800 deaths due to SARS-CoV were recorded globally (https://Orf.who.int/publications/m/item/summary-of-probable-sars-cases-with-onset-of-illness-from-1-november-2002-to-31-july-2003).

Field investigators quickly determined that small mammals in live animal markets but not on rural farms were infected, suggesting they were an intermediate rather than reservoir host.[123] By 2005, viruses related to SARS-CoV had been identified in *Rhinolophus* (horseshoe) bats in mainland China,[210] establishing them as the reservoir host for these viruses. Although numerous viruses were quickly identified with greater than 90% nucleotide identity to SARS-CoV, only in 2013 was a bat virus, BtCoV/WIV1, isolated that is able to infect human cells via the SARS-CoV receptor ACE2.[102,209] Over the next several years, additional such viruses were isolated and shown able to replicate in primary human airway epithelial (HAE) cells.[244,246,418,427,437] Most recently, dozens of novel members of the species *SARSr-CoV* have been identified in Chinese horseshoe bats[196] though many are characterized based only on partial sequences of the ORF1ab region encoding the RdRp. Although SARSr-CoVs have been found throughout China, the closest related viruses to SARS-CoV have been identified in the southern Chinese province of Yunnan.

The discovery and genome analysis of diverse SARSr-CoVs in bats have revealed a critical role for recombination in the evolution of SARS-CoV. Despite the isolation of BtCoV/WIV1 in 2013, several genomic mysteries remained regarding the evolutionary history of SARS-CoV. Although BtCoV/WIV1 infects human cells via ACE2, the receptor binding domain (RBD) of its spike protein is distinct from

SARS-CoV,[102,418] and the ORF3b and ORF8 accessory proteins (putative functions described below) of SARS-CoV are highly divergent from the orthologs encoded by its otherwise closest relatives, indicative of recombination. The ORF8 of SARS-CoV famously experienced a 29 nucleotide deletion, splitting it into two open-reading frames, early in the human epidemic.[261] A comprehensive 2017 report from a bat sampling study conducted by the Wuhan Institute of Virology reported bat SARSr-CoVs with nearly identical ORF8 genes to SARS-CoV, whereas other viruses such as BtCoV/WIV1 were most closely related to SARS-CoV in other regions of the genome.[143] The same study identified the first close relative of SARS-CoV ORF3b in a bat SARSr-CoV in a different genome from the SARS-CoV–like ORF8, indicating multiple recombination events produced the immediate progenitor virus to SARS-CoV, which has nevertheless not been identified in a natural reservoir.

Evolutionary History of SARS-CoV-2

Despite intense sampling of bat populations for SARSr-CoVs between 2003 and 2019, the SARS-CoV-2 lineage remained largely undiscovered prior to early 2020. The genome of SARS-CoV-2 was first published on Virological.org on January 10, 2020 and characterized in greater detail the following month.[440] This study also provided the first insight into the evolutionary origins of the pandemic virus, describing a virus, BtCoV/RaTG13, with approximately 96% nucleotide identity to SARS-CoV-2, a comparable similarity to SARS-CoV and its closest known relative. A partial RdRp sequence of BtCoV/RaTG13 was previously reported in 2016 as a possibly new lineage within *SARSr-CoV*.[103] The sample containing this viral sequence was collected from a *Rhinolophus affinis* bat in an abandoned mineshaft in Yunnan province in southern China, the same region of China from which the closest relatives of SARS-CoV have been identified, though farther south. These viruses exhibit only 79% to 80% nucleotide identity to SARS-CoV across the entire genome and qualify as a novel lineage of *SARSr-CoV*.

Since the initial discovery of SARS-CoV-2, several other viral genome sequences in this lineage have been identified in previously collected samples (Fig. 21.2). Shortly after the full genomic characterization of SARS-CoV-2 in February 2020, related viral sequences were identified in pangolins seized in antitrafficking operations in the southern Chinese provinces of Guangxi and Guangdong. In particular, a sequence from a pangolin seized in Guangdong province yielded a complete genome sequence exhibiting high (>90%) identity to SARS-CoV-2 and an even higher identity to SARS-CoV-2 in the spike RBD than BtCoV/RaTG13, with all six critical residues for ACE2 binding conserved.[192,384,408] Despite the apparent association of SARS-CoV-2–like viruses with pangolins, whether they are a reservoir host or incidentally infected during wildlife trafficking remains unclear. A 2009–2019 study in Malaysia sampled greater than 300 pangolins entering the wildlife trade and found no evidence of coronavirus infection.[202] In contrast, pangolins with evidence of coronavirus infection have been seized "downstream" in trafficking networks in Thailand and southern China and in some cases shown evidence of severe lung disease,[408] suggesting that at least under stress conditions pangolins are susceptible to disease caused by these viruses.

Discoveries of additional related viruses reported later in 2020 and early in 2021 have further populated the SARS-CoV-2–like branch of the *Sarbecovirus* phylogenetic tree (Fig. 21.2). Whereas most viruses on the SARS-CoV branch have been identified in *Rhinolophus sinicus*, the SARS-CoV-2 branch

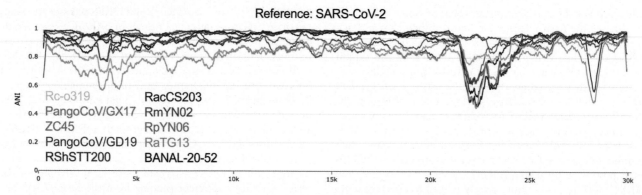

FIGURE 21.3 Average nucleotide identity analysis of SARS-CoV-2–related virus genomes using SARS-CoV-2 as the reference genome. Sliding window analysis showing nucleotide identity (ANI) of related viruses to SARS-CoV-2 generated in IDPlot. Large decreases in ANI are often indicative of genomic recombination with divergent SARSr-CoVs. Putative recombination hotspots at approximately 22 kb and 28 kb correspond to the spike and ORF8 genes, respectively. Numbers on the y axis correspond to nucleotides of the coronavirus genome.

exhibits an apparently more diverse host range. BtCoV/RmYN02 was sequenced from a *R. malayanus* sample taken in southern Yunnan and exhibits even higher nucleotide identity to SARS-CoV-2 in ORF1ab than does BtCoV/RaTG13,[440] with recombination apparently accounting for lower genome-wide identity (Fig. 21.3). Based on the relatedness of SARS-CoV-2 with closely related viruses in ORF1ab, it is estimated to have had a common ancestor with BtCoV/RaTG13 approximately 52 years ago and with BtCoV/RmYN02 approximately 37 years ago,[389] though the confidence intervals for these estimates overlap, producing considerable uncertainty as to the exact evolutionary relationships. In March 2021, a new virus sequence was reported from Yunnan province with high identity to SARS-CoV-2. BtCoV/RpYN06 exhibits 94.5% genome-scale nucleotide identity to SARS-CoV-2 and 97.2% identity in the entirety of ORF1ab, making it equivalently close to SARS-CoV-2 as BtCoV/RmYN02 (Fig. 21.3).[441] Although all of these viruses are too distantly related to SARS-CoV-2 to have been the progenitor of the pandemic virus, the

discovery of these viruses within a limited geographic area raises the possibility that the SARS-CoV-2 progenitor naturally circulates in southern Yunnan province. However, sampling bias and the recently expanded known range of SARS-CoV-2–related virus lends considerable uncertainty to this hypothesis.

While most interest on the origins of SARS-CoV-2 has focused on Yunnan province, the early 2021 report of a closely related virus in Thai *Rhinopholus* bats[383] expands the known geographic range of this viral lineage. BtCoV/RacCS203 exhibits similar identity to SARS-CoV-2 as BtCoV/RmYN02 and is the most closely related virus to the latter. Another southeast Asian SARS-CoV-2–like virus was identified retrospectively from *Rhinolophus shameli* samples collected in 2010 in Cambodia. This virus exhibits 92.6% genome-wide identity to SARS-CoV-2 and contains a SARS-CoV-2–like RBD, including conservation of five out of six critical ACE2 contact residues (Fig. 21.4).[148] Continued efforts to identify the origin of SARS-CoV-2 are likely to include wildlife sampling in southern

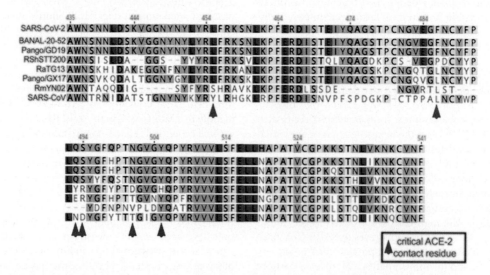

FIGURE 21.4 Receptor binding motif (RBM) alignment. Multiple sequence alignment of SARS-CoV-2–like virus (plus SARS-CoV) receptor binding motifs within the receptor binding domain. Six critical residues for interaction with ACE-2 are indicated by *red arrows*. RmYN02, which is not predicted to use ACE-2, contains deletions, one of which removes two of the critical residues. All 6 residues are conserved in BANAL-20-52 and PangolinCoV/GD19 and 5 in RShSTT200. The lack of conservation with SARS-CoV demonstrates the tolerance of ACE-2 binding to mutations in this region.

China and in southeast Asia, which has seen extremely limited virus surveillance previously. At the time of this writing, the progenitor of SARS-CoV-2 has not been discovered, but the best estimates are that the virus emerged from a genetic pool of viruses circulating widely across southern China and southeast Asia. To this point, recently a group of viruses were isolated in Laos with very high identity to SARS-CoV-2; BANAL-52 has 96.8 % genome wide identity and conservation of all six critical ACE2 binding residues (Figs. 21.3 and 21.4).[361]

Evolution of ACE2 Usage by SARS-Related Coronaviruses (SARSr-CoVs)

The emergence in humans of SARS-CoV and SARS-CoV-2 owes principally to their ability to utilize the human cell surface protease ACE2 as a receptor for cell attachment and entry. ACE2 binding is mediated by the RBD (Fig. 21.4), located in the C-terminal portion of the spike protein S1 subunit. ACE2 usage is far from ubiquitous among SARSr-CoVs. A 2020 study by Letko et al. that demonstrated ACE2 utilization by the SARS-CoV-2 spike[207] segregated SARSr-CoV spike proteins into three groups based on ACE2 usage. Non–ACE2-utilizing viruses, in comparison, contain one or two deletions that encompass some of the ACE2 contact residues[207,305] and the receptor used by these viruses for entry is currently unknown.

The phylogenetic distance between SARS-CoV-2 and SARS-CoV is in contrast to the similarity of their RBDs and use of a common receptor. Wells et al. found that although SARS-CoV was discovered first and this lineage is best represented in currently sampled diverse viruses, ACE2 binding is ancestral in the SARS-CoV-2 lineage and introgressed via recombination into the SARS-CoV lineage where it is widespread but not ubiquitous. Similarly, in the SARS-CoV-2 lineage, the ancestral RBD has been lost by multiple viruses via recombination.[23]

Notably with respect to the potential for human transmission, the binding affinity of numerous bat SARSr-CoV spikes is higher for human than *R. sinicus* ACE2,[125] reflecting rapid evolution of the gene due to selective pressure imposed by SARSr-CoVs. Further evidence supports a generalist evolutionary trajectory of ACE2 binding SARSr-CoV spikes, calling into question the need for adaptation of the RBD to facilitate cross-species transmission. BtCoV/WIV1 readily mediates infectivity in a range of mammalian species.[437] Additionally, a 2021 study by MacLean et al. found evidence for powerful diversifying selection in the SARS-CoV-2 lineage RBDs, suggesting that rather than converging on an ACE2 binding solution highly specific to particular hosts, evolutionary pressures diversify their sequences resulting in generalist viruses.[232]

Indeed, analysis of the ACE2-interaction region of the RBD of these viruses (Fig. 21.4) suggests high tolerability to amino acid diversity of ACE2 binding. Six residues in the SARS-CoV spike, Y442, L472, N479, D480, T487, and Y491, were previously identified as critical for binding to ACE2[11,387] corresponding to amino acids L455, F486, Q493, S494, N501, and Y505 in SARS-CoV-2; only the final tyrosine is conserved. Despite this sequence variation, affinity for human ACE2 is sufficiently high for both spike proteins to effectively mediate infection. In the SARS-CoV-2 lineage, only Y505 is conserved in BtCoV/RaTG13, whereas in PangolinCoV/GD19, all six residues are conserved (Fig. 21.4), confirming that the SARS-CoV-2 RBD is highly conserved with that of viruses circulating in wildlife.

It has recently been discovered that viruses with RBD containing all six critical human ACE2 binding residues are also found in bats, as illustrated by the recently identified BtCoV BANAL-50 isolates (Fig. 21.4).[361] Other related viruses, such as BtCoV/RmYN02, contain deletions that eliminate some of these residues and presumably must use an alternative receptor. Their potential for human infection is unknown.

Recombination Drives Diversification of SARS-CoV-2 Lineage Viruses

Genomic recombination is a common feature in coronavirus evolution and clear signatures are evident among SARSr-CoVs. Given the apparent recombinant nature of SARS-CoV,[143,199] immediate interest arose in whether SARS-CoV-2 similarly arose via recombination in a reservoir or intermediate host. Recombination is most frequent in the 3′ end of the genome[121] and particularly in the spike gene,[107,116] which may produce differences in tropism, receptor usage, and host range. This is easily observed on a large scale in the incongruence between RdRp and spike phylogenies[396] as well as in large changes in average nucleotide identity within the RdRp-defined SARS-CoV-2 lineage of *SARSr-CoV* (Fig. 21.2).

Although a flurry of preliminary studies suggested a recent recombinant origin of SARS-CoV-2, studies by Boni et al.[23] and Nielsen et al.[389] found no evidence supporting this hypothesis. The consistently high genome-wide nucleotide identity with RaTG13 (Fig. 21.3) suggests little change in genome composition since the last common ancestor of these viruses but does not preclude recombination in deeper evolutionary history. However, evidence of recombination is striking in other viruses on the SARS-CoV-2 branch of *SARSr-CoV*, including in RpYN06 and RmYN02, which are more closely related to SARS-CoV-2 than RaTG13 in large regions of their genome (Fig. 21.3). The considerable genomic distance between these viruses and SARS-CoV-2 in the spike gene (and ORF8 in the case of RmYN02) is clear evidence that SARS-CoV-2–like viruses circulate alongside and coinfect host animals with more distantly related SARSr-CoVs. Therefore, viruses outside the SARS-CoV-2 branch may contribute genetic material to viruses within it, expanding the genetic diversity with the potential to contribute to future pandemics.

SARS-CoV-2 REPLICATION AND STRUCTURAL PROTEINS (FIG. 21.5)

SARS-CoV-2, like other coronaviruses, has a positive-sense, single-stranded RNA genome consisting of almost 30,000 nucleotides.[109,112,227] The genome is capped and also has a leader sequence at the 5′ end of the RNA (Fig. 21.1B). The original SARS-CoV-2 isolates exhibit 79.6% identity to the SARS-CoV genome at the nucleotide level.[404,439] Approximately two-thirds of the 5′ end of the genome contains open reading frames (ORFs) 1a and 1b that encode primarily proteins involved in replication. The 3′ one-third of the genome encodes the structural proteins and eight accessory genes (Fig. 21.1B).[404,439] SARS-CoV-2 virions have four structural proteins, the spike (S), envelope (E), membrane (M) anchored in the viral envelope, and the nucleocapsid (N), which encapsidates the single-stranded RNA genome (Fig. 21.6). Spike trimers prominently

Model of coronavirus life cycle

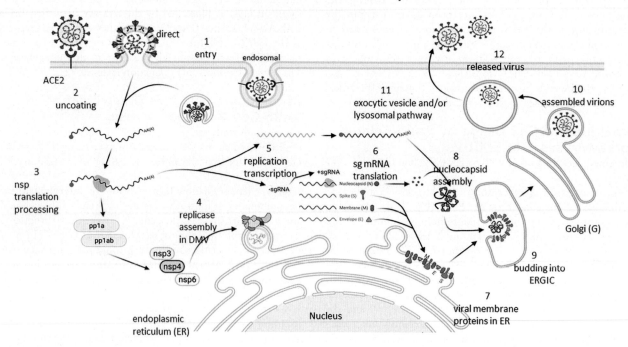

FIGURE 21.5 Model of coronavirus life cycle. *1.* Virus enters the cell by both direct fusion of the viral membrane with the cellular plasma membrane or is endocytosed and enters the cell by fusion between the viral and endosomal membranes, both processes mediated by spike that has been activated by proteolytic cleavage. *2.* Viral genome RNA is uncoated. *3.* Genome RNA is translated from ORFs1a and 1b into polyproteins pp1a and pp1ab, which are processed into replicase proteins. *4.* The replicase complex is assembled on double membrane vesicles (DMV) at the endoplasmic reticulum (ER). *5.* Genome RNA is replicated through a negative strand intermediate and subgenomic negative strand RNAs are transcribed from genome and then copied into subgenomic mRNAs. *6.* Subgenomic (sg) mRNAs are translated into viral structural and accessory proteins. *7.* Viral membrane proteins spike (S), membrane (M), and envelope (E) are inserted into ER membranes. *8.* Viral nucleocapsid protein (N) complexes with genome RNA to form nucleocapsids. *9.* Nucleocapsids bud into the ER–Golgi intermediate compartment (ERGIC) in regions containing viral membrane proteins to form progeny virions. *10.* Spike protein on virions is cleaved by furin in the Golgi. *11.* Virus is transported to the cell surface in exocytic vesicles and/or through the lysosomal pathway. *12.* Progeny virus is released into the extracellular space. (Created by Alejandra Fausto using Biorender.com.)

extend from the envelope and the helical nucleocapsid consisting of the viral genome and N protein form a dense core when viewed by EM (Fig. 21.6B and C). Coronavirus entry into cells is receptor mediated through interactions of the S protein with host cell ACE2. Virus replication and assembly takes place in the cytoplasm (Fig. 21.5).

Spike (S) Protein

Spike (S) proteins extend from the viral envelope as trimers to give coronaviruses their characteristic crown-like appearance. The proteins play important roles in infectivity, host range, and pathogenesis.[208,287] SARS-CoV-2 S protein is the host receptor binding protein that, like SARS-CoV and HCoV-NL63 S proteins, mediates entry into host cells by binding to hACE2.[137,207,386] The S protein exhibits significant structural and sequence homology with SARS-CoV S. Initial SARS-CoV-2 S isolates shared approximately 76% amino acid identity with SARS-CoV S.[227,404] Like other coronaviruses, SARS-CoV-2 S proteins are the major target for neutralizing antibodies, therapeutic monoclonal antibodies, and vaccine development.

SARS-CoV-2 S exhibits the same overall structural features as other coronavirus S proteins. The proteins are type I transmembrane proteins that form homotrimers. S protein monomers consist of two subunits, the N-terminal S1 extracellular amino end head region and the S2 carboxy end stalk, transmembrane domain (TMD) and short viral endo-domain tail (Fig. 21.7). The S1 subunit consists of the N-terminal domain (NTD) and the C-terminal domain (CTD), which contains the RBD.[137,207,386,402,439] The S2 subunit contains two heptad-repeat (HR) domains and a hydrophobic fusion peptide that mediates membrane fusion.[207,208,367,386,402] The proteins are class I fusion glycoproteins.[208] SARS-CoV-2 S protein is highly glycosylated at 66 N-linked sites on each trimeric S, which shields the RBD in its prefusion conformation.[394,435]

Coronavirus S proteins are cleaved sequentially by host cellular proteases at the S1/S2 junction and S2′ sites (Fig. 21.7) to promote viral virus–host membrane fusion and entry,[134] although cleavage at the S1/S2 junction may not be required for activation of all coronavirus S proteins, for example in alphacoronaviruses.[398] The S2′ cleavage site is located in the

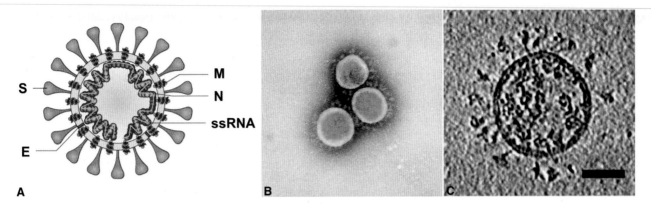

FIGURE 21.6 SARS-CoV-2 virions contain four structural proteins, spike (S), envelope (E), membrane (M), and nucleocapsid (N). **A:** Schematic of the virion shows the S trimers, M and E proteins anchored in the viral lipid envelope. The positive-sense, single-strand RNA genome (ssRNA) encapsidated by the N protein is packaged inside the particle. **B:** SARS-CoV-2 transmission electron micrograph of virus particles that is color-enhanced (NIAID). **C:** EM tomographic slice of a SARS-CoV-2 virion showing granular density of the ssRNA encapsidated by the N protein and S trimers extending from the viral envelope. (**Panel A** adapted by permission from Nature: V'kovski P, Kratzel A, Steiner S, et al. Coronavirus biology and replication: implications for SARS-CoV-2. *Nat Rev Microbiol* 2021;19(3):155–170. Copyright © 2020 Springer Nature, Ref.[379]. **Panel C** adapted by permission from Nature: Ke Z, Oton J, Qu K, et al. Structures and distributions of SARS-CoV-2 spike proteins on intact virions. *Nature* 2020;588(7838):498–502. Copyright © 2020 Springer Nature.)

S2 subunit between the amino end helix region and the fusion peptide (Fig. 21.7). SARS-CoV-2 S differs from SARS-CoV S in that it has a multibasic furin cleavage site ($R_{682}RAR\downarrow S_{686}$) at the S1/S2 junction.[136,386,402] MERS-CoV S is also cleaved by furin in producer cells.[136,325] Less pathogenic hCoV-HKU1 and hCoV-OC43, also have furin cleavage sites at the S1/S2 junction.[63,252] Furin is a Golgi-associated protease that cleaves the S1/S2 junction during virus assembly or transport through the secretory pathway.[252] The SARS-CoV-2 S1/S2 multibasic cleavage site with the additional arginine residues is presented in an exposed loop.[386,402]

Cleavage at the S2' site primes the protein by revealing the fusion peptide in the S2 domain that is necessary for fusion of viral and cellular membranes during entry. SARS-CoV S2' site is cleaved by either cell surface protease TMPRSS2, a member of the type II transmembrane serine protease 2 family

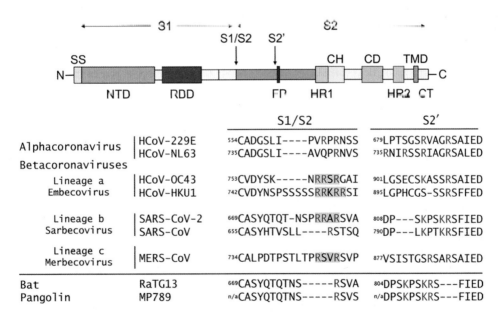

FIGURE 21.7 Summary of the functions and domain organization of full-length (1,273 amino acids) SARS-CoV-2 spike (S) protein. Amino acid sequence alignments of the S1/S2 and S2' cleavage sites of human alphacoronavirus (HCoV-229E, HCoV-NL63), betacoronavirus embeco (a, HCoV-OC43, HCoV-HKU1), sarbeco (b, SARS-CoV-2, SARS-CoV) and merbeco (c, MERS-CoV) lineages, and bat RaTG13 and pangolin MP789 are shown. Basic residues are highlighted in *red*. Multibasic S1/S2 cleavage sites are highlighted with *gray boxes*. SS, signal sequence; NTD, N-terminal domain; RBD, receptor binding domain; CTD; carboxy-terminal domains 1 and 2; S1/S2, furin cleavage site; S2', protease cleavage site; FP, fusion peptide; HR, heptad repeats 1 and 2; CH, central helix; CD, connector domain; TMD, transmembrane domain; CT, cytoplasmic tail (intravirion domain).

of enzymes, or endosomal cysteine protease cathepsin B or L.[106,239,336] SARS-CoV-2 S is primed by TMPRSS2 cleavage at S2′ and the TMPRSS2 inhibitor camostat mesylate blocks infection in Calu-3 and primary human lung cells.[137] Cleavage at the S2′ site is necessary for fusion and entry into human lung cells.[136] SARS-CoV-2 S, like MERS-CoV, requires cleavage by furin at the S1/S2 site for downstream activation by membrane-associated transmembrane serine protease 2 (TMPRSS2) cleavage at S2′ in lung cells.[22,136]

Aside from the furin cleavage site at the S1/S2 junction that is not present in SARS-CoV S, SARS-CoV-2 S protein exhibits other distinctive characteristics compared with that other sarbecoviruses.[136,325] The S proteins have NTD loops that are divergent from other sarbecoviruses.[386] The S1 RBD is structurally divergent and has been reported to bind hACE2 receptor with higher affinity than SARS-CoV S RBD.[386,402] The RBD consists of a core structure and a receptor-binding motif (RBM) located in an extended loop, flanked by alpha-helices[193,326]

Coronavirus S proteins are very dynamic structures during entry and infection. Prefusion S exists in a metastable state, which transitions between conformations with all three RBDs in the down conformation where the RBM is not in a position to bind to its cognate ACE2 receptor, to conformations in which one or more of the trimers adopt a conformation with the RBD in up position with their RBM positioned to engage with ACE2.[402] S undergoes changes during entry and infection as the viral envelope membrane fuses with host cell membranes.[208] In the postfusion state, the trimers have all three RBDs in the up conformation.[34,90,181,386] S1 binding to the receptor results in conformational changes that trigger S2 extension to reveal the hydrophobic fusion peptide that promotes virus and cell membrane fusion during entry.[208,238] The protein assumes a postfusion stabilization of helical bundles as the protein refolds.[34,386]

Most coronavirus S proteins, including SARS-CoV-2, transport to some extent to the cell surface in infected cells. This promotes cell-to-cell fusion that results in multinucleated syncytia that provides a mechanism for virus spread.[370,442] This is seen in infected Calu-3 or A549 cells derived from the respiratory tract.[136,262]

Coronaviruses can enter cells by two different routes (Fig. 21.5).[157,338] Following binding of virus to a cellular receptor, virion can be endocytosed or alternatively, the viral envelope fuses directly with the host cell surface membrane. Previous studies with other coronavirus that use similar entry mechanism provided significant insight that helped inform how SARS-CoV-2 enters cells. In the direct plasma membrane route, the SARS-CoV-2 S protein, as well as MERS-CoV S, has already been cleaved at the S1/S2 site by furin during synthesis in infected host producer cells.[136,325] Following attachment to the receptor, S cleavage at the S2′ site by membrane-associated TMPRSS2 initiates fusion between the viral and host cell membranes. Cleavage allows the fusion peptide to insert into the host cell membrane to promote fusion between the viral and cell membrane. Fusion between the membranes results in release of the viral nucleocapsid (viral genome coated by nucleocapsid (N) protein) into the cytoplasm to initiate replication.

In the case of entry by the endosomal route, virus attaches to its receptor and is then endocytosed. The low pH environment of the endosome activates cleavage by the protease cathepsin L, resulting in fusion of viral and endosomal membranes and release of the nucleocapsid into the cytoplasm to initi-

ate infection.[21] The pathway(s) used depends on the proteases available, which can vary among cell types and the sequence of the S protein.[252,338] Some cell types may favor one pathway or the other. In lung-derived cells, SARS-CoV-2 entry is dependent on both furin for S1/S2 junction cleavage and TMRPSS2 for the second S2′ cleavage.[22] It is possible that in other cell types different proteases and one or the other pathways is primarily utilized or alternatively both pathways can be used by the same virus in a particular cell type.

Spike cleavage is important for entry but can also play a role in virus spread. Following synthesis at endoplasmic reticulum membranes, coronavirus S proteins traffics through the exocytic pathway and for those with a furin cleavage site, such as SARS-CoV-2, cleavage occurs in the Golgi. In the endoplasmic reticulum Golgi intermediate compartment (ERGIC)/ Golgi region, some S molecules are retained through interaction with the membrane (M) protein where virions are assembled (see additional details in the assembly section). The S protein that is not retained is transported to the plasma membrane where it can mediate fusion with receptor bearing neighboring cells, thus allowing cell to cell spread of virus shielded from the extracellular immune responses. This promotes cell-to-cell fusion that results in multinucleated syncytia that provides a mechanism for virus spread.[370,442] This is seen in infected Calu-3 or A549 cells derived from the respiratory tract.[136,213,262] However, it is not known to what extent, if at all, this promotes viral spread *in vivo*. While no obvious cell to cell fusion was observed in induced pluripotent stem cell (iPSC)-derived AT2 cells, robust cell fusion was observed in iPSC-derived cardiomyocytes.[213] The dynamics of this spread are determined at least in part by the levels of ACE2, TMPRSS2, and furin in each cell line.

Significant progress toward understanding the structural biology of SARS-CoV-2 S was made quickly after the virus emerged. Multiple cryo-EM structures have been determined using X-ray crystallography or cryo-electron microscopy (cryoEM) for SARS-CoV-2 S protein in prefusion and postfusion conformations. SARS-CoV-2 S bound to ACE2 has been determined at the atomic level.[193,243,326,386,410] The ectodomain of SARS-CoV-2 S was determined by cryo-EM at 3.5-angstrom resolution of a prefusion trimer.[402] The crystal structure of SARS-CoV-2 RBD complexed with ACE2 shows that the binding ridge is more compact than the SARS-CoV binding ridge and that residue differences stabilize two binding hotspots compared to SARS-CoV RBD, which results in higher receptor binding affinity than previously measured for SARS-CoV RBD.[326] S trimers exists in both down and up conformations on virions when examined by cryo-EM tomography.[174,218,371,419] Trimers were observed to tilt relative to the viral membrane due to flexibility of the membrane-proximal stalk region that functions like a hinge.[174]

Coronaviruses evolution is slowed as a result of 3′-5′ exonuclease proofreading activity of nonstructural protein 14 (nsp14). Nonetheless, mutations in SARS-CoV-2 S have emerged during the COVID-19 pandemic, referred to as "variants of concern." Changes in the spike protein are particularly important since these can affect both receptor and antibody binding, resulting in changes in infectivity, transmission, antibody binding, and vaccine escape. The strongest spike neutralizing epitopes are located in the RBD. SARS-CoV-2 RBD has three nonoverlapping antigenic sites.[365] A major change during evolution of S since the emergence of COVID-19 is a D614G (Asp614 to Gly) change in S1. Multiple studies suggest that the change increases infectivity and transmission.[54,187,429,432]

Membrane (M) Protein

Coronavirus membrane (M) proteins play a major role in assembly of virus particles. The proteins are highly conserved in their overall architecture. SARS-CoV-2 M consists of 222 amino acids with a theoretical molecular weight of approximately 25 kDa, which aligns with the overall characteristics of other coronavirus M proteins. The protein is 91% identical to SARS-CoV M protein at the amino acid level. M proteins are type III membrane proteins, consisting of three TMDs, a short N-terminal ectodomain and a long, approximately 100 amino acid C-terminal intravirion tail.[140,310] Coronavirus M proteins are glycosylated on the NTD with either N-linked or O-linked glycans.[140,264,286] SARS-CoV-2 M has a predicted N-glycosylation site in the N-terminal ectodomain. Prior to incorporation into assembled virions, the C-terminal tail is located in the cytoplasm and where it plays a role in trafficking to and localization in the Golgi.[69,214,223,264,288] The tail associates with the inner leaflet of the plasma membrane where it interacts with the viral nucleocapsid during budding.[68] M proteins can homo-oligomerize and interact with other virion components, including S, N, and E.[68,69,242] For all coronaviruses, virus-like particles (VLPs) can be efficiently assembled with protein M, S, and E.[372,376] Recent studies indicate that SARS-CoV-2 M protein is also required for VLP formation and plays a role in retention of the S protein for incorporation into the particles.[26,295]

Envelope (E) Protein

Coronavirus E proteins are small, 8.4 to 12 kDa (74 to 109 amino acids), multifunctional membrane proteins that play roles in virus assembly, egress, inflammation, and pathogenesis.[140,318] The proteins localize at the site of assembly in the ERGIC.[270,376] SARS-CoV-2 E consists of 75 amino acids that share 96% identity with SARS-CoV E protein but exhibit very low identity with other coronavirus E proteins. Nonetheless, SARS-CoV-2 E exhibits the same overall structure and key conserved amino acids characteristic of the proteins across the virus family. All E proteins consist of an NTD, a long alpha helical TMD and a C-terminal hydrophilic domain, including conservation of cysteine and proline residues in the C-terminus.[140,311] Structural data and *in vitro* measurement have shown that E proteins multimerize to form a pentamer in the membrane bilayer and form ion channels that are known as viroporins.[18,283,289] SARS-CoV-2 E, like SARS-CoV E, also assembles into pentameric ion channels in membranes.[237,318] Structural models based on NMR studies in either micelles or liposomes have been produced for SARS-CoV and SARS-CoV-2 E proteins.[237,353] Comparison of the models suggest that SARS-CoV-2 ion channels exhibit a more simple architecture, but it was suggested that based on the high sequence homology between the two E proteins that the structural difference may be due to experimental differences in the NMR studies.[18] This indicates that understanding of the proteins will benefit from additional structural and functional studies that directly compare the E proteins from multiple coronaviruses. E proteins are posttranslationally modified by palmitoylation at conserved cysteine residues located on the C-terminal side of the third TMD, which affects its interactions with the membrane

bilayer.[25,225] The proteins are expressed at a high level in infected cells, but only a few molecules are assembled into virus particles.[140,311]

Of the four coronavirus structural proteins, the E viroporin protein and its functions are the least understood. Studies have shown that E proteins play diverse roles, including modulating virion assembly/membrane budding, trafficking, and release by exocytosis, as well as virion stability and pathogenesis.[140,212,311,318,319] It is well established that E proteins colocalize and interact with M proteins during virus assembly.[286,318] Mechanistically how E proteins contribute to virus assembly is still not fully understood since the requirement for E during the process varies among coronaviruses.[72,278] The roles of E may be associated with the viroporin activity and/or contributions to membrane curvature or scission during assembly and budding.[271,311,318]

SARS-CoV-2 E protein and SARS-CoV E both contain PDZ-domain binding motifs (PBMs) in the C-terminus. The E PBMs interact with PALS1, a PDZ containing protein that is important for epithelial polarity in mammalian cells.[44,162,362] The C-terminal PBMs have four residues (DLLV) that are conserved between SARS-CoV and SARS-CoV-2. C-terminal peptides containing the conserved residues show that the SARS-CoV-2 peptide exhibits enhanced binding to the PALS1 PDZ domain.[368] A cryo-EM structure of PALS1 with SARS-CoV-2 E CTD containing the PBM shows that conserved residues DLLV bind a pocket formed by PALS1 PDZ and SH3 domains.[44] A crystal structure of SARS-CoV and SARS-CoV-2 E protein PBMs with PALS1 PDZ has also shown binding to a pocket in the latter domain.[159] These structural studies suggest that the E protein C-terminal PMD interactions with PALS1 may play a role in pathogenesis by interference with lung epithelial cell junction integrity.[73,362] E protein is expressed at high levels in SARS-CoV-2 infected lung epithelial cells.[401] Previously, it was suggested that SARS-CoV E localizes at the site of virus assembly where recruitment of PALS1 may disrupt lung cell polarity and vascular structure.[362] SARS and SARS-CoV-2 E proteins also interact with other cellular junction proteins, including PDZ-containing syntenin adhesion junction protein, and tight junction ZO-1 protein.[35,42,162] Thus, E protein interactions with these proteins and its viroporin activity likely contribute to significant inflammation, tight junction breakdown, vascular leakage, and immune-mediated damage that results in acute respiratory distress syndrome (ARDS). Indeed, a recent study suggests that SARS-CoV-2 E contributes to pathological damage that resembles ARDS.[406]

Nucleocapsid (N) Protein

Coronavirus nucleocapsid (N) proteins are multifunctional phosphoproteins that encapsidate the viral RNA to form a ribonucleoprotein complex (vRNP) that mediates packaging into virus particles.[188] N protein is recruited to replication–transcription complexes where it participates in RNA synthesis and is thought to promote RNA template switching to facilitate addition of the 5′ leader sequence during subgenomic mRNA synthesis.[60,243,377,444] Full-length SARS-CoV-2 N protein consists of 419 amino acids that has a theoretical molecular weight of 45.6 kDa. SARS-CoV-2 N protein shares 90.52% identify at the amino acid level with SARS-CoV N. The protein exhibits the same overall modular architecture as other CoV N proteins with conserved, folded N-terminal

(NTD) and C-terminal (CTD) domains. The NTD interacts with the viral RNA genome packaging signal and the CTD associates to form dimers that are thought to facilitate vRNP assembly.[145,282,352,420] The ordered NTD and CTD are flanked by intrinsically disordered regions (IRDs) and separated by a conserved central IDR that contains a serine/arginine-rich (SR) region that is phosphorylated in infected cells. A high-resolution structure of SARS-CoV-2 N dimerization domain shows a compact structure similar to other betacoronaviruses, whereas extension to include the CTD results in homotetramer formation.[420] SARS-CoV N crystal structures previously showed a helical assembly of dimer domains that was proposed to form the basis for helical nucleocapsid filaments in virions.[49] SARS-CoV-2 N dimer–dimer packing modes, revealed in the crystal structures, shows that the N protein would not assemble into helical filaments. This suggests that CTD dimers may not form the basis for interaction with the viral RNA and assembly of N protein helical filaments or globular vRNPs that were recently also described using cryoEM tomography.[182,420]

SARS-CoV-2 Assembly and Release

Coronaviruses assemble at the endoplasmic reticulum Golgi intermediate compartment (ERGIC) and Golgi where virions bud into to the lumen (Fig. 21.5).[184,349,366] *In situ* cryo-EM tomography studies have shown that SARS-CoV-2 virions bud into high vesicle density areas in close proximity to ER and Golgi-like membranes.[182] As with other coronaviruses, SARS-CoV-2 structural proteins (S, M, N, E) interact to drive budding at ERGIC membranes. The M protein plays a significant role in virus assembly through its interactions with the other structural proteins.[140] Coexpression of the E and M proteins is sufficient in many cases for the production of noninfectious VLPs, which forms the basic structure for the viral envelope.[30,311] SARS-CoV-2 and SARS-CoV E and M proteins are required for formation of VLPs, but coexpression with the N protein enhances particle production.[26,30,295] SARS-CoV-2 E and M proteins are required for retention and maturation of S proteins at the site of assembly, as has been shown for other coronaviruses.[26,30,295] SARS-CoV-2 S trimers localized in ERGIC members do not alone drive membrane curvature but appear to laterally reorganize in the envelope during virion assembly.[182] Viral ribonucleoprotein complexes consisting of the genomic RNA and N protein accumulate at the curved membranes where budding takes place, possibly recruited by bending of the membranes to help drive the budding process.[182]

SARS-CoV-2 efficiently infects differentiated HAE cells.[442] Peak SARS-CoV-2 release from the apical surface of HAE cells occurs 48 to 72 hours postinfection, whereas HCoV-NL63 and SARS-CoV exhibit slower kinetics with peak virus production occurring 72 to 96 hours pi.[340]

Less is known about how coronaviruses are released, or egress, from cells. After coronavirus particles are assembled, these traffic through the Golgi where glycosylation and other posttranslational processing occur.[241,274] Previous studies have supported that virus particles are released through the exocytic secretory pathway.[30,231,366] New information has emerged with SARS-CoV-2 that describe the use a lysosomal, Arl8b-dependent pathway for egress and release.[105] In this study, SARS-CoV-2 and MHV particles were observed to bud into ERGIC membranes, transport to the Golgi, as previously seen, but to diverge by trafficking to lysosomes for egress and release from

cells. Additionally, lysosomal deacidification was observed that resulted in disruption of antigen presentation pathways.[105] SARS-CoV-2 ORF3a protein has been implicated to promote lysosomal exocytosis, but the mechanism is not understood.[53] Further studies are warranted to fully understand coronavirus egress and release from infected cells.

NONSTRUCTURAL PROTEINS (TABLE 21.1)

SARS-CoV-2 and other betacoronaviruses encode 16 nonstructural proteins, nsp1-nsp16 within ORF1a and ORF1b (Fig. 21.1B). They are synthesized similarly to other coronaviruses; as two long overlapping polyproteins that are cotranslationally processed to individual nsps by either a papain-like protease domain contained within nsp3 (nsp1, nsp2, and nsp3) or by the 3C-like protease domain contained in nsp5 (nsp4-16).

Nsp1

SARS-CoV-2 Nsp1 is the first protein encoded in the ORF1a/ORF1ab polyproteins. It is proteolytically cleaved from the ORF1a precursor polyprotein by the papain-like protease domain in nsp3, as is the nsp1 of other coronaviruses. This results in a protein that is 180 amino acids long and is 84.4% sequence identical with SARS-CoV nsp1. This high degree of sequence conservation between SARS-CoV and SARS-CoV-2 nsp1 proteins (Table 21.1) results in a high degree of functional and structural similarity. The nsp1 proteins of both viruses interfere with host gene expression (reviewed in Ref.[263]) and consequently antagonize the development of an interferon response in infected cells.[158,168,206,263,265,395,405]

The molecular basis for the inhibition of host protein synthesis by nsp1 has been extensively investigated for SARS-CoV. Studies utilizing ectopic overexpression of nsp1 and purified bacterially expressed SARS-CoV nsp1 demonstrated that nsp1 promotes degradation of host mRNAs, binds to the 40S ribosomal subunit, inhibits formation of the 80S ribosome, and inhibits translation of capped RNAs during the initiation process.[167,168,224] Binding of nsp1 to the 40S ribosome preinitiation complex results in endonucleolytic cleavage of 5′ capped host mRNAs near their 5′ end during translation elongation.[146,167,168,356] Nsp1 does not contain a recognized nuclease motif and a direct ribonuclease activity has not been shown with purified protein, suggesting that nsp1 recruits a host nuclease.[146,411] SARS-CoV nsp1 does not induce cleavage of SARS-CoV viral mRNAs, and protection from endonucleolytic cleavage was conferred on reporter mRNAs by adding the SARS-CoV 5′ leader sequence to their 5′ ends.[146,356] However, when purified recombinant nsp1 protein was added to *in vitro* translation reactions programmed with a viral mRNA or a host mRNA carrying the 5′leader sequence and thus resistant to nsp1-mediated cleavage, protein synthesis was still inhibited, suggesting that nsp1 directly inhibited protein synthesis independently of its cleavage at the 5′ termini of host mRNAs.[147] However, cotransfection of a nsp1 expression plasmid and a SARS-CoV-5′UTR-luciferase construct failed to significantly inhibit luciferase expression.[356] Additional studies demonstrated that the first stem-loop in the 5′UTR bound to nsp1 and was sufficient to protect mRNAs from nucleolytic degradation.[356] NMR analysis of the SARS-CoV nsp1 protein

TABLE 21.1　Nonstructural proteins (NSPs) of SARS-CoV-2

Protein	Size (AA)	Sequence Identity With SARS-CoV	Functional Roles
Nsp1	180	84.4%	Immune evasion, inhibitor of translation
Nsp2	638	68.3%	Unknown
Nsp3	1945	76.0%	Papain-like protease releases nsp1-nsp4 from pp1a, immune evasion, DMV formation
Nsp4	500	80%	DMV formation
Nsp5	306	96.1%	Main protease (Mpro) releases nsp5-nsp16 from pp1a
Nsp6	290	88.2%	DMV formation
Nsp7	83	98.8%	Component of core replication/transcription complex
Nsp8	198	97.5%	Component of core replication/transcription complex
Nsp9	113	97.3%	Acceptor for nsp12 NiRAN nucleotide transferase activity; component of extended replication/transcription complex
Nsp10	139	99.3%	Cofactor for nsp14 exonuclease activity; cofactor for nsp16 2-2'-O-methyl transferase activity
Nsp11	13	84.6%	Unknown if functional, also contained in nsp12 N-terminal NiRAN domain due to programmed ribosomal frameshifting
Nsp12	932	96.4%	RNA-dependent RNA polymerase; nucleotidyl transferase
Nsp13	601	99.8%	Helicase, nucleotide triphosphatase
Nsp14	527	99.1%	3' exonuclease with RNA proofreading activity; 5'Cap synthesis, N-methyl transferase activity
Nsp15	346	88.7%	Endonuclease, immune evasion
Nsp16	298	93.3%	5' cap synthesis, 2'-O-methyl transferase activity

SARS-CoV-2 and other betacoronaviruses contain 16 nonstructural proteins, nsp1-nsp16. They are synthesized similarly in other coronaviruses as two long overlapping polyproteins, which are cotranslationally processed to individual nsps by either a papain-like protease domain contained within nsp3 (nsp1, nsp2, and nsp3) or by the 3C-like protease domain contained in nsp5 (nsp4-16). DMV, double membrane vesicles.

indicated that the N-terminal 12 amino acids are unstructured, that amino acids 13 to 128 form a well-folded globular domain, followed by a second C-terminal unstructured domain.[8] The globular domain is made up of a 6-stranded beta-barrel with a long alpha helical segment, residues 36 to 49, across one barrel opening, and a second short alpha helical segment, residues 62 to 64 positioned next to the barrel. Additionally, there are two locally disordered regions at residues 77 to 86 and 121 to 128. Reverse genetic studies by Narayanan[265] implicated the CTD in the inhibition of translation. Viruses carrying K164A/H165A mutations in this CTD inhibited host protein synthesis and degraded host mRNAs much less efficiently than wild type virus and allowed greater expression of interferon-β, ISG15 and ISG56, implying lesser inhibition of innate immune responses to infection.[265] A deletion mutant within this region of the CTD was attenuated in a mouse model of SARS.[163] In addition to inhibiting host protein synthesis, Wathelet et al.[395] showed that overexpression of SARS-CoV nsp1 interferes with induction of interferon-β synthesis by Sendai virus infection by inhibiting activation of the transcription factors IRF-3, IRF-7. NF-KB and c-Jun that are required for induction of interferon-β mRNA synthesis.[395] In the same work, these authors also showed that overexpression of nsp1 inhibited downstream signaling by interferons by decreasing phosphorylation of STAT1 after exposure of cells to interferon. Additionally, overexpression of nsp1 inhibited progression of cells through the cell cycle.[395] Introduction of mutations in two basic surface exposed residues, R124 and

K125, greatly attenuated these effects of nsp1.[395] SARS-CoV carrying these nsp1 mutations are more sensitive to the antiviral effect of interferon than wild-type virus and replicate less well than wild-type in interferon competent cells. SARS-CoV nsp1 has also been shown to bind to Nup93 and thus disrupt the nucleocytoplasmic transport of host cell proteins.[108]

Similarly, to SARS-CoV nsp1, SARS-CoV-2 nsp1 inhibits the translation of host mRNAs in both cell-free and cell-based assays.[17,194,320,363,364,423] Studies of SARS-CoV-2 nsp1 interactions with the ribosome and the 5'UTR of the virus have advanced our understanding of the mechanism by which nsp1 inhibits protein synthesis while allowing translation of viral mRNAs.[17,194,320,333,363,364,423] Cryoelectron microscopy (cryo-EM) revealed that nsp1 bound to 40S ribosomal subunits with two alpha helices of the previously structurally uncharacterized CTD positioned in the mRNA entry channel, obstructing it.[320,363,423] The conserved residues K164 and H165 essential for nsp1 inhibition of protein synthesis and induction of an interferon response are located in a loop flanked by two alpha helices.[17,363] These amino acids interact with 18S rRNA helix h18 and the two nsp1 helices interact with ribosomal proteins uS5 of the ribosomal body and with uS3 of the ribosomal head.[17,320,363,423] These interactions do not block binding of the mRNA to the ribosome, but rather prevent the physiologic conformation of the 48S preinitiation complex by restricting rotation of the 40S ribosomal head and the loading of the mRNA into the entry channel.[423] SL1, the first stem loop of the

5'UTR, when present at the 5'end of an mRNA, interacts with the globular NTD of nsp1, allowing entry of mRNA into the entry channel and subsequent translation.[17,194,333,364] The structure of the NTD (amino acids 10 to 127) has been determined by X-ray crystallography[57,321] and is similar overall to the structure of the SARS-CoV nsp1 NTD, with some alterations in surface exposed loops. A previously unreported activity of nsp1 is its inhibition of mRNA export from the nucleus. Zhang et al.[433] have shown that nsp1 interacts with the nuclear mRNA export machinery by binding to the nuclear export receptor NFX1, and that infection with SARS-CoV2 inhibits the translocation of polyadenylated RNAs from the nucleus to the cytoplasm, a similar effect to that observed with NFX depletion. This effect could be replicated by nsp1 overexpression and the inhibition of mRNA nuclear export could be overcome by overexpressing NFX1 in SARS-CoV-2–infected cells. Furthermore, nsp1 overexpression was shown to displace NFX1 from its binding partners at the nucleopore complex, providing a functional basis for these observations.

Nsp2

A relatively limited number of studies have been done on coronavirus nsp2, including SARS and SARS-CoV-2 nsp2, making it one of the poorly understood coronavirus proteins. The 638 amino acid nsp2 protein is proteolytically cleaved from the ORF1a precursor polyprotein by the papain-like protease domain in nsp3.[297] Nsp2 proteins of SARS-CoV and SARS-CoV-2 are not as well conserved as many of the other nonstructural proteins, with only 68.3% sequence identity. The protein is not essential for SARS-CoV, and presumably SARS-CoV-2, or for MHV replication in cell cultures as viable mutants of SARS-CoV and MHV in which the entire nsp2 coding sequence has been deleted have been recovered using reverse genetics.[117] These mutants were attenuated for viral replication in permissive cell cultures reaching titers 1 to 1.5 logs lower than the corresponding isogenic wild-type virus. There have been few functional studies of this protein, but Prentice et al.[297] showed that SARS-CoV nsp2 colocalizes with nsp3 and nsp8 in double membrane vesicular structures (DMVs) associated with viral RNA synthesis. Using the MHV system, Hagemeijer et al.[128] demonstrated that fluorescently tagged nsp2 expressed by transient transfection was diffusely located in the cytoplasmic in uninfected cells but was recruited to DMVs, the site of coronavirus RNA synthesis, in MHV-infected cells. The association of nsp2 with DMVs was confirmed by immune-cryo-EM. Experiments expressing overlapping truncations of nsp2 fused with a fluorescent reporter revealed that the C-terminal fragment spanning amino acids 247 to 585 was sufficient for this localization to DMVs. Photobleaching experiments demonstrated that once recruited to DMVs nsp2 was not freely exchangeable after photobleaching. A yeast two-hybrid screen followed by confirmatory coprecipitation assays of overexpressed proteins in mammalian cells to identify binding partners among SARS-CoV proteins identified nsp4 and nsp6, two proteins associated with DMVs, nsp8, nsp11, and nsp16, associated with viral RNA synthesis and capping, and the SARS-CoV ORF3a protein, a virion associated accessory protein,[154,330] as binding partners for nsp2.[380]

A study to identify potential SARS-CoV nsp2 host binding partners by an overexpression pull-down mass spectroscopy strategy identified 11 proteins, and the binding of two of these

protein PHB1 and PHB2 were verified by western blotting assays.[61] These two proteins have been associated with a variety of cellular processes: cell cycle progression, mitochondrial biogenesis, cell differentiation, and apoptosis.[61] A comparative study using a similar affinity purification mass spectroscopy strategy to probe host protein interactions with nsp2 identified 4 proteins, ERLIN1, ERLIN2, RNF170, and TMEM, that interacted with both SARS-CoV and SARS-CoV-2 nsp2 proteins and 16 proteins that bound uniquely to each one.[66] This study also confirmed the binding of SARS-CoV nsp2 to PHB2. Immunofluorescence colocalization indicated that considerable nsp2 localized to ER membranes in uninfected cell.[66] Protein binding network and gene enrichment analyses suggest a role for nsp2 in interacting with the mitochondrial ER interface.[66] As yet, there have been no studies to confirm these interactions with host proteins in infected cells nor to assess the functional importance of any of the nsp2–host protein interactions in virus infected cells.

Two studies of genetic variation in isolates of SARS-CoV-2 have identified an interesting pattern of sequence variation involving nsp2.[296,426] Zeng et al.[426] identified two epistatic linkages of a nsp2 T85I mutation to both a Q57H mutation in the ORF3a protein and to a noncoding sequence change in nsp14. Pohl et al.[296] examined 14 low passage isolates for differences in their ability to replicate in Vero cells or bronchial epithelial cells. The three isolates that replicated well in the bronchial epithelial cells but relatively poorly in Vero cells all contained the linked nsp2 T85I and ORF3a Q57H mutations. The frequency of these changes reflected the frequency with which this linkage is found in SARS-CoV-2 and they were not further selected in culture by passage of the 14 viruses studied. The mechanism(s) underlying this linkage are unknown.

Nsp3

Nsp3 is the largest and most structurally complex of the ORF1a encoded nonstructural proteins (Fig. 21.8). It is proteolytically cleaved from the primary OF1a translation product, by the papain-like protease domain contained within nsp3 itself.[443] It is a multidomain protein of 1945 amino acids in SARS-CoV-2, a 1922 amino acid protein in SARS-CoV, and contains 15 recognized domains.[206] The difference in size between the SARS-CoV and SARS-CoV-2 nsp3 proteins is largely due to a 19 amino acid deletion in the hypervariable domain in the N-terminal region plus two smaller, two and three amino acid deletions in this same region. The functional significance, if any, of these deletions is unknown. The domain organization and functions of SARS-CoV nsp3 are summarized in Figure 21.8. The various domains are discussed below moving from the N-terminus to the C-terminus of nsp3.

Structural and functional characterizations for many these domains have been performed for SARS-CoV and for the more distantly related betacoronavirus, MHV, and will be briefly summarized.

The nsp3 most N-terminal domain contains a ubiquitin-like fold and is designated Ubl1 since it is the first of two ubiquitin-like domains in coronavirus nsp3 proteins. The structure of the SARS-CoV Ubl1 domain has been determined by NMR spectroscopy.[322] Two functions have been assigned to this domain: a ssRNA binding activity[323] and, for the MHV nsp3 Ubl1 domain, a nucleocapsid (N) protein binding activity, which plays an important role in the initial stages of viral

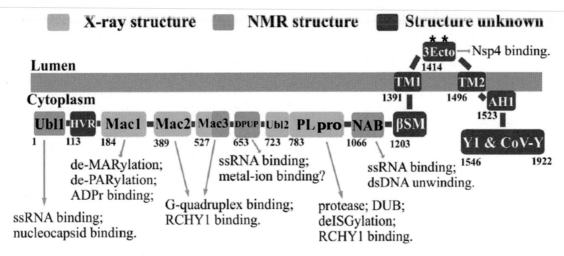

FIGURE 21.8 Summary of the functions and domain organization of SARS-CoV Nsp3. Nsp3 is bound to double-membrane vesicles recruited from the endoplasmic reticulum membrane. The protein passes through this membrane twice, via two transmembrane regions, TM1 and TM2. AH1 is possibly an amphipathic helix attached to the ER membrane, next to TM2. Except for the 3Ecto domain, all other Nsp3 domains are located in the cytosol. All domains with known three-dimensional structures are indicated in *light green* (X-ray structures) or *orange* (NMR structures), whereas parts with unknown structure are in *red*. The best-characterized functions of each domain of Nsp3 are shown. *Asterisks* indicate the Asn1431 and Asn1434 glycosylation sites in the 3Ecto domain. Ubl, ubiquitin-like fold; HVR, hypervariable region; Mac, macrodomain; DPUP, domain preceding Ubl; NAB, nucleic acid binding domain; betaSM, betacoronavirus-specific marker. (Adapted from Lei J, Kusov Y, Hilgenfeld R. Nsp3 of coronaviruses: Structures and functions of a large multi-domain protein. *Antiviral Res* 2018;149:58–74. Copyright © 2017 Elsevier. With permission.)

replication and is postulated to tether the viral genome to newly translated replicase–transcriptase complex.[60,150] The hypervariable domain is an intrinsically disordered, glutamic acid rich region of unknown function which is poorly conserved among coronaviruses.[???] It is dispensable for MHV in that recombinant viruses containing deletions in this region could be generated by reverse genetics and had no discernable phenotype.[150]

Following the hypervariable region is a conserved macro domain, initially named the X domain. It was bioinformatically predicted to have an ADP-ribose-1″-phosphate (ADPR) phosphatase activity,[345] and this activity was subsequently demonstrated for the SARS macro domain by Saikatendu et al. and a structure determined by X-ray crystallography.[314] The enzyme contains a deep cleft in its surface containing the substrate binding pocket. Asparagine 41 is essential for macro domain phosphatase activity[88]; however, recombinant SARS-CoV containing the same asparagine 41 alanine mutation is viable and replicates to the same titer as wild-type virus in Vero cells, albeit slightly more slowly.[189] In addition to its rather weak ADPR phosphatase activity, coronavirus macro domains have been reported to have hydrolase activity removing mono- and poly-ADP-ribose conjugated to proteins (deMARylation and dePARylation, respectively), posttranslational modifications that regulate innate immune responses.[92] Recently, the SARS-CoV, SARS-CoV-2 and MERS-CoV macrodomains were all determined to have a deMARylation activity rather than a dePARylation activity.[7] Recombinant mouse adapted SARS-CoV carrying mutations inactivating ADPR enzymatic activity were attenuated in mice and induced a greater interferon response than the parental mouse adapted virus.[92]

Following the macro domain is a region of nsp3 that was originally designated as the SARS unique domain or SUD.[345]

This region contains 3 subdomains, SUD-N, SUD-M, and SUD-C. SUD-N and SUD-M are macro domains, designated Mac2 and Mac3, and have been structurally characterized, are devoid of enzymatic activity, but bind RNAs containing G-quadraplexes.[???] This binding activity is essential for viral RNA replication and transcription.[190] Mac2Mac3 also binds to and stabilizes the RCHY1 protein, an E3-ubiquitin ligase targeting p53, an inhibitor of SARS-CoV replication.[235] The SUD-C subdomain, also known as DPUP, is not required for replication of a SARS-replicon, but its deletion leads to greatly decreased replication.[190] The functional role of the Ubl2 domain in virus replication and pathogenesis is unclear as it does not appear to affect the catalytic activity of the adjacent papain-like protease domain, and there are conflicting results in the literature regarding its role in antagonizing innate immune responses.[59,98]

Adjacent to the Ubl2 domain is the papain-like protease (PLpro) domain. The single SARS-CoV PLpro domain proteolytically cleaves the ORF1a encoded precursor polypeptide (pp1a) at LXGG sites found at the boundaries between nsp1, nsp2, nsp3, and nsp4, an activity required for viral replication. The structure of the SARS-CoV PLpro protease domain has been determined by X-ray crystallography and contains four Cys residues that coordinate zinc and the Cys-His-Asp catalytic triad of papain-like proteases.[19,303] In addition to its role in generating nsps1-4 from its polyprotein precursor, PLpro also cleaves ubiquitin and ISG15 (an antiviral protein induced by interferon and containing two ubiquitin-like domains) at their C-terminal LXGG motifs and this cleavage event removes them from proteins to which they have been conjugated.[19,216] Both ubiquitination and ISG15ylation play important roles in innate immune signaling pathways, thus deubiquitination (DUB) and deISGylation by overexpressed SARS-CoV PLpro unsurprisingly inhibited innate immune signaling.[302] The PLpro domain contains two binding pockets for ubiquitin and the structurally related ISG15 that are separate from the 4 substrate binding pockets for their coronavirus substrates.[302,303] Devaraj et al. have reported that interference with IRF3 by overexpressed SARS-CoV PLpro does not require it to be enzymatically active.[78] In contrast, Deng et al.[75] created recombinant MHV strains with mutations, which decreased binding of ubiquitin and ISG15 to the MHV PLpro2 domain, greatly decreasing DUB and deISGylation activities, yet still allowing MHV polyprotein processing by PLpro2 and thus recovery of infectious virus. These viruses activated an interferon response more quickly than the parental wild-type virus in macrophages and significantly decreased virus titer in the livers of infected mice. The SARS PLpro has been a target for the development of antivirals blocking its proteolytic activity and several compounds with IC_{50}s in the low micromolar range with good selectivity in biochemical assays have been developed (reviewed in Refs.[15,205]).

The next two domains, the nucleic acid binding (NAB) domain and betacoronavirus specific domain (βSM), have not been extensively studied. The NAB domain binds to ssRNA and its structure has been determined by NMR.[268,323] Even less is known about the betacoronavirus specific domain. Nsp3 contains two TMDs[277] separated by a 3Ecto domain, which is situated on the luminal side of the ER membrane.[277] When Nsp3 is coexpressed with nsp4, they induce curvature of ER-derived membranes,[130] and when coexpressed with nsp4 and nsp6, they induce the formation of double membrane vesicles (DMVs) similar to the coronavirus replication organelle.[13,101] The nsp3 3Ecto domain interacts with the luminal loops of nsp4 driving membrane curvature necessary for DMV formation.[129,130] The second nsp3 TMD is followed by a hydrophobic amphipathic helical domain (AH1) that is located on the cytosolic side of the ER membrane. The C-terminal region contains two domains designated as the Y1 and Y-CoV domains. Their function is unknown.

The SARS-CoV-2 nsp3 protein has largely been studied in the context of inhibitors of its two enzymatic activities, the macro domain's deMARylation activity and the PLpro domain's proteinase activity. The structure of the SARS-CoV-2 PLpro domain has been determined by X-ray crystallography and is quite similar to the previously determined structure of the SARS-CoV PLpro domain.[101] Both enzymes cleave a model peptide substrate mimicking the cleavage site between nsp2 and nsp3 with similar efficiencies.[101] However, the two enzymes differ in their preferences toward ubiquitinated and ISGylated substrates with the SARS-CoV enzyme preferring ubiquitinated substrates and the SARS-CoV-2 enzyme preferring ISGylated substrates.[101,334] The basis for this difference has been determined by cocrystallization of these enzymes with ubiquitin or ISG15 and solving the structures of PLpro complexed with these molecules.[334] Additionally, it has been reported that purified SARS-CoV-2 PLpro cleaves IRF3 at an LGGG motif *in vitro*,[256] correlating with the observation that decreased levels of IRF3 are observed in SARS-CoV-2 infected cells in tissue culture. Several SARS-CoV protease inhibitors, including the noncovalent inhibitor GRL-0617,[15,304] are also effective against SARS-CoV-2[183,334] inhibiting both viral replication and the PLpro deubiquitinating and deISGylase activities. Additionally, GRL0167 treatment of SARS-CoV-2 infected cells increased

the level of ISG15ylated IRF3 and increased the levels of interferon stimulated proteins over that detected in infected but untreated cells, suggesting that the inhibitor was effective in reversing the SARS-CoV-2 inhibition of the antiviral interferon response.[334]

The second enzymatically active domain in SARS-CoV-2 nsp3, the Mac1 ADP-ribosylhydrolase, has also been studied as a potential drug target. It has been suggested that the deMARylation of STAT1 may contribute to the cytokine storm associated with severe COVID-19[58] making the Mac1 domain a possible therapeutic target. Its three-dimensional structure has been determined by four different groups[7,31,248,300] and its interaction with various substrates characterized. As mentioned above, the SARS-CoV-2 macrodomain has deMARylating activity but not dePARylating activity, with the SARS-CoV-2 enzyme being somewhat more active than the SARS-CoV Mac1 domain. Potential binding pockets for both the adenosyl and ribose moieties of substrates were identified[7,31,248,300] and potential inhibitors identified by virtual screening and optimization of inhibitors of a structurally related human poly(ADP-ribose) glycohydrolase.[31] Screening against various nucleotides and nucleotide analogues demonstrated considerable flexibility of the adenosyl binding pocket and a surprising interaction with active metabolites of remdesivir suggesting another possible approach to developing inhibitors.[269]

Nsp4 and Nsp6

The nsp4 and nsp6 proteins are 500 and 290 amino acids long, respectively. At its N-terminus, nsp4 is cleaved from nsp3 by PLpro, and at its C-terminus, it is cleaved from nsp5 by Mpro, the protease contained within nsp5. Nsp6 is released from the coronavirus pp1a polyprotein by Mpro. Nsp4 contains four TMDs with both the N- and CTDs exposed to the cytoplasm, an approximately 100 amino acid CTD, and a relatively large luminal loop between the first and second TMDs.[276] The luminal loop of nsp3 and the first large luminal loop of nsp4 are necessary for DMV formation.[130,347] Nsp3, nsp4, and nsp6 all localize to the endoplasmic reticulum when expressed separately; coexpression of nsp3, nsp4, and nsp6 result in relocalization of these proteins to perinuclear foci.[12,129,130,276] Electron tomography studies of cells coexpressing nsp3 and nsp4 in the absence of nsp6 demonstrated that these two proteins are sufficient to form structures, which resemble the DMV replication organelle found in infected cells.[279] This is supported by the earlier colocalization of these proteins in perinuclear foci containing nsp8,[297] a component of the RNA replication machinery (see below) in infected cells.

There have been a limited number of studies of the SARS-CoV-2 nsp4 and nsp6 proteins. An overexpression screen for proteins that antagonize the interferon response has shown that nsp6 suppresses type I interferon secretion in response to poly(I:C).[405] Further examination of the effect of nsp6 overexpression on interferon induction and responses to interferon showed that this inhibited phosphorylation of TBK1 and its downstream target, IRF3, two events necessary for the induction of interferon-β, and down-regulated interferon receptor signaling by inhibiting phosphorylation of STAT1 and STAT2. As yet, the mechanism by which nsp6 produces these effects is unknown; nor have these effects of nsp6 on the interferon response been verified in infected cells. A screen for host binding partners with individually overexpressed SARS-CoV-2 proteins identified the ER receptor protein sigma-1 as an interaction partner with nsp6 and several mitochondrial proteins that are part of the TIM complex were identified as binding partners for nsp4.[113] Small molecule ligands (inhibitors) of sigma-1, including a number of compounds in clinical use such as haloperidol and hydroxychloroquine, inhibited viral replication in Vero cells, as did inhibitors of the sigma-2 receptor.[113] Genome sequencing of SARS-CoV-2 isolates have shown that a nsp6 L37F mutation is epistatically linked to a mutation in the accessory ORF3a gene.[426] This mutation has recurred in different countries on multiple occasions and an association with milder disease has been suggested.[373,388]

Nsp5

Nsp5 is a highly conserved 306 amino acid protein in SARS-CoV and SARS-CoV-2, with 96.1% amino acid identity between the two proteins. This protein contains the main protease (Mpro), also referred to as the 3C-like protease (3CLpro), due to its similar substrate specificity and some structural similarities to the picornavirus 3C protease. Mpro is responsible for the majority of the processing of the pp1a and pp1b polyproteins, releasing nsp4-nsp16 from these polyproteins.[9,345] Its enzymatic activity is essential for coronavirus replication. The structures of the SARS-CoV and SARS-CoV-2 Mpro have been solved by X-ray crystallography[9,414,430] and reveal a protein with a chymotrypsin like beta barrel domain (domain I, amino acids 10 to 99) and an adjacent picornavirus 3C-like beta-barrel domain (domain II, residues 100 to 182), which together make up a chymotrypsin-like fold but contain a catalytic dyad of His41 and Cys145 in the active site, rather than the serine–histidine–aspartate catalytic triad of chymotrypsin (Fig. 21.9). A substrate binding cleft separates domains I and II, and there are three substrate binding pockets that provide substrate specificity. A third domain consists of 5 alpha helices and mediates dimerization, which is required for enzymatic activity.[331] Mpro has strong sequence specificity requiring a glutamine in the P1 position (just N-terminal of the cleavage site), a strong preference for leucine immediately upstream (P2 position) of the glutamine, although other bulky hydrophobic amino acids can be recognized, no real amino acid preference in the P3 position, a preference for small neutral amino acids (valine, serine, threonine, proline) in the P4 position, and a strong preference for serine or alanine just C-terminal to the cleavage site (P1′ position). Substrate binding pockets (termed S1-S4, and S1′) have been identified for each of these positions. In addition to its essential role in viral replication, SARS-CoV and SARS-CoV-2 Mpro have been suggested to have a role in pathogenesis. Proteins that are components of the innate immune response expressed *in vitro* and incubated with purified recombinant SARS-CoV-2 Mpro identified NLRP12, a negative regulator of

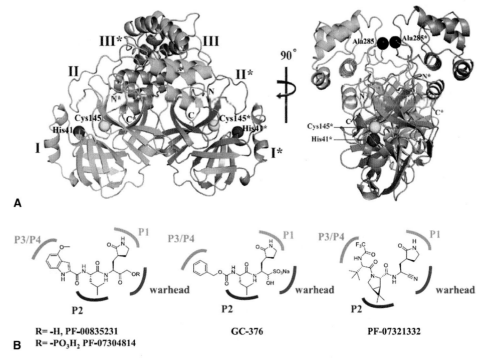

FIGURE 21.9 The structure of the SARS-CoV-2 Mpro, the protease contained within nsp5, and Mpro inhibitors. A: The three-dimensional structure of a dimer of SARS-CoV-2 Mpro. The protomers of the dimeric molecule are shown in *light blue* (protomer A) and *orange* (protomer B). Domains are labeled by Roman numerals and those in protomer B are marked with *asterisks*. The N- and C-terminals are labeled and the positions of the catalytic His41 and Cys145 are indicated by *blue* and *yellow spheres*, respectively. (From Zhang L, Lin D, Sun X, et al. Crystal structure of SARS-CoV-2 main protease provides a basis for design of improved α-ketoamide inhibitors. *Science* 2020;368(6489):409–412. Reprinted with permission from AAAS.) **B:** The structures of the most advanced Mpro inhibitors. (Reprinted from Vandyck K, Deval J. Considerations for the discovery and development of 3-chymotrypsin-like cysteine protease inhibitors targeting SARS-CoV-2 infection. *Curr Opin Virol* 2021;49:36–40. Copyright © 2021 Elsevier. With permission.)

the release of inflammatory cytokines, and TAB1, another regulator of the inflammatory response, NRP, as potential targets for cleavage by Mpro.[256] Levels of both proteins were decreased in SARS-CoV-2–infected ACE2-expressing 293 cells, consistent with these proteins being targeted by Mpro, although specific Mpro cleavage products were not reported.[256]

Because of its essential role in viral replication and the structural information that is available, Mpro has been a therapeutic target for SARS, MERS, and SARS-CoV-2 (reviewed in Ref.[219]). Coronavirus Mpro is well conserved and some broadly active compounds inhibiting Mpro from multiple coronaviruses have been developed. Inhibitors can generally be classified as being peptidomimetic, which bind in the S1, S2, S3, and S1' substrate binding pockets or allosteric inhibitors binding elsewhere and altering the substrate binding interface sites.[219] Peptidomimentic compounds may contain ketones, ketoamide, aldehyde, or Michael receptors as reactive moieties, which covalently link to the active site cysteine or be noncovalent reversible inhibitors. Prior to the COVID-19 pandemic, a number of inhibitors of Mpro were developed and inhibit viral replication in cell cultures; several had broad anticoronavirus activity as well.[9,24,175,176,415] The compound GC376, a bisufite adduct of a dipepityl-aldehyde Mpro inhibitor (GC373), has been shown to be an effective inhibitor of replication for multiple coronaviruses[175,176] and has been used to successfully treat an otherwise fatal infection of cats with the feline coronavirus, infectious peritonitis virus.[177] A derivative of GC376 has also been used to protect mice expressing the human MERS-CoV receptor from otherwise lethal infection with MERS-CoV and inhibit the replication of SARS-CoV-2 in cultured primary human airway cells[301] and in Vero cells.[382] PF-07321332[374,436] is an oral Mpro inhibitor containing a nitrile warhead (Fig. 21.9B), which when combined with ritonavir, was shown to reduce hospitalization in SARS-CoV-2 infected persons in the interim analysis of the EPIC-HR phase 2/3 clinical trial (NCT04960202).[280] A third peptidomimetic Mpro inhibitor developed against SARS-CoV, N3,[415] contains a Michael receptor warhead, and is also active against SARS-CoV-2.[164] An X-ray crystallographic screen of a library of drugs and drug-like compounds identified two allosteric inhibitors, which bound at or near the Mpro dimer interface resulting in a narrowing of the substrate binding cleft and altering the substrate binding site.[124] Computational and biochemical screens of libraries of approved or investigational drugs and natural products identified a number of additional inhibitors of SARS-CoV-2 Mpro, which also inhibited SARS-CoV-2 replication.[164] Among these are cinanserin, a serotonin antagonist, disulfiram, an inhibitor of aldehyde dehydrogenase used to treat alcoholism, and ebselem, a selenorganic compound, and carmofur, a 5-fluorouracil derivative used as a chemotherapeutic agent. Cinanserin[48] had previously been identified as an inhibitor of the SARS enzyme and was an effective antiviral in tissue culture. Inhibitors of other viral proteases such as boceprevir, a ketoaminde inhibitor of hepatitis C virus ns3 protease, is also effective against SARS-CoV-2 Mpro.[100] Lopinavir, a drug targeting the HIV protease, also inhibited SARS-CoV Mpro, SARS-CoV replication *in vitro*, and had modest effectiveness in an open label clinical trial during the 2002–2003 SARS outbreak.[56,403] However, a clinical trial during the COVID-19 outbreak indicated that this drug was not effective in hospitalized patients.[39] Clinical trials of ebselem (NCT04484025 and NCT04483973) and disulfiram (NCT04485130) have been registered at ClinicalTrials.gov.

The Replicase Complex: Nsp7-Nsp16
Overview

Coronavirus RNA replication and transcription is a complex process that requires enzymatic machinery able to carry out the discontinuous coronavirus transcription process and replicate the very large coronavirus genome. The nine proteins that carry out these processes, nsp7-nsp10 and nsp12-16, carry a number of enzymatic and nonenzymatic functions (summarized in Table 21.1) and they have been colocalized to the DMVs that are the site of coronavirus RNA synthesis in the cell.[27,77,115,127] During the 2002–2003 SARS outbreak, many of the enzymatic activities were predicted by a comparative bioinformatic analysis prior to being demonstrated biochemically.[345] Nsp12 contains the typical seven sequence motifs (A-G) of an RNA-dependent RNA polymerase (RdRp)[110,409] and has been reported to have primer-dependent[358] and primer-independent RdRp activity.[6] Bioinformatic analyses of nsp12 suggested that it lacked priming loops needed for positioning NTPs for initiating RNA synthesis and sequence comparison grouped it with primer-dependent RdRps such as the picornavirus 3Dpol based on the presence or absence of a motif implicated in primer recognition.[409] Additional nsps with identified enzymatic activities in coronavirus RNA synthesis and modification are nsp13, which has 5'-3' helicase and nucleotide triphosphatase activities[155]; nsp14, which has a N7-methyltransferase activity that methylates the N7 position of guanosine in the 5' cap of viral positive-sense RNAs producing a Cap-0 structure[50] and a 3' 5' exoribonuclease activity which carries out a proof-reading function during coronavirus RNA synthesis[84,254]; and nsp16, which has a 2'-O-methyl transferase activity which methylates the 2'-O position of the ribose of the first nucleotide of the 5' end of coronavirus mRNAs to form a Cap-1 structure.[70] Nsp15 has an endoribonuclease activity, which when expressed cleaves dsRNA with a strong preference for U residues.[156] Mutants with catalytically inactive nsp15 promote increased accumulation of dsRNA and consequent activation of innate immune antiviral pathways including IFN production and signaling, OAS/RNase L and PKR pathways; such mutants are reported to have modest[170] to severe[179] defects in viral replication.[170] While the exact mechanisms underlying how nsp15 functions in the evasion of the host innate immune response are unknown, it is proposed to act by either degrading poly (U) on minus strand RNA[126] or by degrading positive sense genome RNA.[10] Nsp8 has been reported to have an RdRp activity that synthesizes, in a primer-independent manner, short oligoribonucleotides and thus was speculated to function as primase for nsp12 RNA synthesis.[151] Subsequent work with a complex of nsp7, nsp8, and nsp12 has called this conclusion into question (see below).[351] Nsps 7, 9, and 10 are devoid of enzymatic activities but form a number of different complexes with nsp8, nsp12, nsp13, nsp14, and nsp16 and have important regulatory roles in coronavirus RNA synthesis and modification.[344]

Core Replicase/Transcriptase Complex Proteins (Nsp12, Nsp8, and Nsp7)
Nsp12

The SARS-CoV and SARS-CoV-2 nsp12 proteins are 932 amino acids in length and are proteolytically cleaved from their pp1ab precursor by the nsp5 Mpro.[345] The two proteins are 96.4% identical in amino acid sequence. Nsp12 contains two domains, an N-terminal domain of approximately 300 amino acids, the NiRAN (nidovirus RdRp associated nucleotidyltransferase) domain found in all nidovirus RdRp proteins, a roughly 500 amino acid C-terminal RdRp domain, with these two domains being joined by a linker region.[204] The coronavirus RdRp domain has a similar architecture to other viral RdRps and can be described as resembling a cupped right hand with a thumb region, fingers and a palm, and contains a conserved SDD motif as part of the polymerase active site rather than the GDD motif found in most other RdRps, as well as the other seven (A-G) motifs associated with RdRp activity.[110,180,409] Purified recombinant SARS-CoV nsp12 has a very modest level of *in vitro* polymerase activity with low processivity when presented with a template RNA that has been annealed to an RNA primer.[358] A complex of nsp12 with nsp8 and nsp7 greatly increased polymerase activity and processivity.[351] This tetrameric complex consists of one molecule of nsp12 bound to an nsp7-nsp8 heterodimer and a single molecule of nsp8. The complex exhibits both primer-independent *de novo* initiation of RNA synthesis and primer-dependent RdRp activity, and both these activities depend on the presence of an intact catalytic site in the RdRp domain of nsp12.[351] The SARS-CoV nsp12 was refractory to crystallization but its structure was determined in 2019 by cryo-EM of the complex of nsp12 bound to nsp7 and nsp8 (Fig. 21.10).[180] In this structure, the N-terminal NiRAN domain and the linker (interface) domain contact the RdRp domain at the outer surface of the fingers and the base of the palm subdomains. RNA entry and exit channels were identified in the RdRp domain as was the NTP binding channel. In addition, two previously unsuspected metal-binding sites were identified, one in the linker domain (H295-C301-C306-C310) and the second in the RdRp fingers subdomain (C487-H642-C645-C646). Although zinc was found ligated at these metal binding sites in the cryo-EM generated structure, subsequent work[133] showed that these metal binding sites were occupied by Fe-S clusters in infected cells, that binding of the Fe-S clusters to RdRp is essential for polymerase activity, and that treatment of infected cells with a compound that oxidizes and disassem-

bles FeS clusters strongly inhibited SARS-CoV-2 replication in infected cells. The nsp7-nsp8 heterodimer is bound above the RdRp thumb subdomain and the second molecule of nsp8 contacts nsp12 at the outside surface near the top of the finger subdomain of the RdRp domain and at the linker domain, which is adjacent to the to the RdRp fingers subdomain. The complex of nsp12 with nsp7 and nsp8 is the core structure of the coronavirus replication machinery. It provides a platform for larger complexes containing additional nsps involved in RNA synthesis and modification and has been used in assays of potential RdRp inhibitors (see below).

The nsp12 NiRAN domain is unique to nidoviruses and was first characterized by Lehmann et al.[204] This domain is conserved in all nidoviruses and a bioinformatic analysis identified three conserved motifs designated A_N, B_N, and C_N. The NiRAN domain has a nucleotidyl transferase activity with a preference for UTP over other nucleotide triphosphates.[204,342] When the SARS nsp12 was incubated with a UTP or GTP substrate, this activity transfers a UMP or GMP to the epsilon amino group of a conserved lysine residue at amino acid 73 in SARS-CoV nsp12 by formation of a phosphoramidate bond. In this assay, there was a strong preference for UTP over GTP and other nucleotide triphosphates were not utilized. The transferase activity was shown to be essential for nidovirus replication by a series of reverse genetic experiments with SARS-CoV and for the related arterivirus, equine arteritis virus, in which infectious viruses carrying mutations in the conserved residues in motifs A_N, B_N, and C_N required for the transferase activity could not be recovered. Three possible functions for this transferase activity were put forward: it could function as an RNA ligase, it could provide the as yet unidentified guanylyltransferase activity needed for 5′ cap formation, or by transferring a UMP to a protein target it could have a protein priming function for minus-strand RNA synthesis. A subsequent set of experiments using HCoV-229E and SARS-CoV-2 nsp12 demonstrated that the NiRAN domain nucleotidyltransferase activity was much more active when it was provided with nsp9 as a substrate, that the N-terminal asparagine of nsp9 was the target of the nucleotide

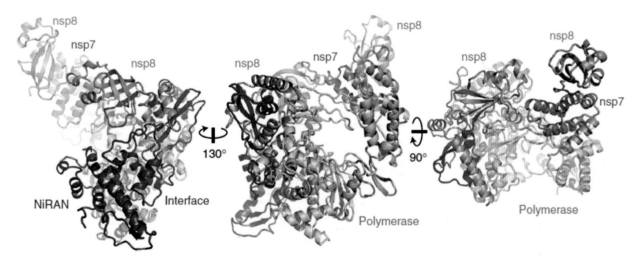

FIGURE 21.10 The structure of the SARS-CoV nsp12-nsp7-(nsp8)2 complex. SARS-CoV nsp12 contains a large N-terminal extension composed of the NiRAN domain (*dark red*) and an interface domain (*purple*) adjacent to the polymerase domain (*orange*). nsp12 binds to a heterodimer of nsp7 (*blue*) and nsp8 (*green*) as well as to a second subunit of nsp8. (Adapted from Kirchdoerfer RN, Ward AB. Structure of the SARS-CoV nsp12 polymerase bound to nsp7 and nsp8 co-factors. *Nat Commun* 2019;10(1):2342. https://creativecommons.org/licenses/by/4.0/.)

transfer reaction, and that this was vital for virus replication.[342] Recent studies with the SARS-CoV-2 nsp12 demonstrated that in the presence of nsp13, a protein that binds to nsp12 (see discussion of replication/transcription complexes below) and contains both helicase and NTPase activity, the NiRAN domain was capable of transferring GMP to ppA-RNA. Thus the nsp12 NiRAN domain appears to be able to function as a guanylyl transferase, carrying out one of the early steps in the synthesis of a 5′ cap.[412] This activity was diminished by the addition of nsp9 to the complex.

The RdRp and nucleotidyl transferase activities exhibited by nsp12 are attractive targets for antivirals. Prior to the COVID-19 outbreak, remdesivir (GS-5734), a prodrug of a nucleoside analogue of adenine (GS-441524) and a broad-spectrum inhibitor of viral RdRps, was shown to be an effective inhibitor of coronavirus replication in cell culture and protective in a mouse model of SARS.[328] Its activity against coronaviruses is notable as most other nucleoside analogues are relatively ineffective because of the coronavirus nsp14 exonuclease proofreading activity (see section on nsp14 below).[3] With the advent of the COVID-19 pandemic, remdesivir or its biochemically active triphosphate form was rapidly shown to be an effective inhibitor of the SARS-CoV-2 RdRp in biochemical assays,[114] of SARS-CoV-2 replication in cell culture,[298,391] and showed efficacy in mouse[298] and macaque[400] models of COVID-19. Incorporation of remdesivir into an elongating RNA by the SARS-CoV-2 RdRp results in delayed chain termination of RNA synthesis at the +3 position, three nucleotides after the site of remdesivir incorporation,[114] similar to the mechanism observed in SARS and MERS coronaviruses.[111] The cryo-EM structure of the RdRp domain in complex with an elongating RNA in the presence of remdesivir demonstrated a steric clash with nsp12 serine-861 that prevented the incorporation of a fourth nucleotide after the incorporated remdesivir monophosphate.[185,421] Mutation of serine 861 to a less bulky glycine eliminates chain termination.[357] A second mechanism of action has been proposed in which remdesivir that has been incorporated into a successfully elongated RNA acts as a poor template for subsequent rounds of RNA synthesis due to mispositioning of the incorporated remdesivir monophosphate in the RdRp active site.[357] Passage of SARS-CoV and MHV in cell culture in the presence of remdesivir resulted in the accumulation of mutant viruses that had acquired resistance to the drug. These mutations were F480L and V557L in the SARS-CoV RdRp.[3] Both mutations are in the fingers subdomain of the RdRp, and V557L is in RdRp motif F, which forms a channel for incoming NTPs, suggesting that the mutation may affect RdRp fidelity.

The COVID-19 pandemic spurred a series of computational and high throughput screens to identify potential inhibitors of SARS-CoV-2 replication. Multiple nucleoside analogues currently used as antivirals for other RNA viruses were tested as their triphosphate derivatives as inhibitors of primer elongation by the SARS-CoV-2 core polymerase complex.[55] The triphosphate derivatives of sofosbuvir, tenofovir, alovudine, and abacavir are incorporated in the elongating RNA by the RdRp and terminate further elongation. Sofosbuvir has been shown to have activity in inhibiting SARS-CoV-2 replication in cell culture, as was daclatasvir, a second nucleoside inhibitor of HCV replication.[312] A meta-analysis of a number of small clinical trials of sofosbuvir in combination daclatasvir in COVID-19 patients suggested that this combination improved survival and

shortened the time to clinical recovery,[339] although the modest number of patients enrolled in the trials and differences in trial design precluded definitive conclusions on efficacy. Three additional nucleoside analogs, favipiravir, β-D-N⁴-hydroxycytidine (EIDD-1931), and a prodrug of EIDD-1931, EIDD-2801, inhibit coronavirus replication by a different mechanism, inducing an increase in the rate of transition mutations in replicating genomes resulting in error catastrophe.[4,327,329] EIDD-2801 (molnupiravir) was developed to address the rapid catabolism of EIDD-1931 in the intestine of nonhuman primates.[281] EIDD-2081 improved pulmonary function, decreased viral titer in the lungs, and decreased weight loss in mouse models of SARS, MERS, and in mouse and hamster models of COVID-19.[308,329,385] EIDD-2801 can be given orally, was effective in preclinical studies, and reduced hospitalization in SARS-CoV-2–infected persons.[281]

Nsp7 and Nsp8

These two relatively small (83 to 198 amino acids) proteins are part of the coronavirus RNA replication/transcription machinery and are localized to the DMV RNA replication compartment in coronavirus infected cells.[27] They are released from the pp1a and pp1ab precursor polypeptides by the nsp5 Mpro domain.[74,345] Nsp7 and nsp8 are highly conserved with 98.8% and 97.5% sequence identity between the respective SARS-CoV and SARS-CoV-2 proteins. Structures of the SARS-CoV nsp7 have been determined by NMR[290] and by X-ray crystallography,[428] with the latter structure being determined in an in vitro assembled hexadecameric ring-like complex consisting of 8 molecules of nsp7 complexed with 8 molecules of nsp8. Nsp7 contains four alpha helices in both structures, although the helices are oriented somewhat differently in space in the two structures. The nsp8 molecules in the hexameric complex take on two conformations, one which generally has been described as a golf club with the N-terminal shaft (residues 6 to 104) consisting of three helices and the C-terminal head consisting of a beta-barrel and three helical segments folded into a tight hydrophobic domain. In the second nsp8 conformation, described as a bent golf club, the longest helix in the shaft domain contains a bend and thus is divided into two shorter helical segments.[428] In the ring-like complex, the inner surface of this ring is positively charged and provides a surface for binding dsRNA with the long helices of nsp8 interacting with the RNA. As mentioned earlier, purified recombinant SARS nsp8 was shown to have a template-dependent RNA polymerase activity producing short, 6 nucleotides long, RNA products and has been suggested to act as primase for the nsp12 RNA-dependent RNA polymerase (RdRp), nsp12.[151] Formation of the complex of nsp8 with nsp7 stimulates this polymerase activity and also allowed nsp8 to perform primer extension RNA synthesis as well as the de novo RNA synthesis described earlier although it was still about 20-fold less active than the nsp12 RdRp.[359] Mutations of basic residues in the helical shaft of nsp8 abolished RNA binding and polymerase activity and mutagenesis of conserved D/ExD/E motifs identified residues in the nsp8 N-terminal helical domain required for polymerase activity of the complex.[359,428] It should be kept in mind that the physiological relevance of the hexadecameric ring-like structure in viral replication is unclear since complexes with nsp12 have nsp7:nsp8:nsp12 ratios of 1:2:1 and polymerase activity is dependent on the nsp12 catalytic center.[351]

Nsp9

Nsp9 is a 113 amino acid protein that is a component of extended transcription/replication complexes.[412] The protein is released from the pp1a and pp1ab precursor polypeptides by the nsp5 Mpro domain.[74,345] In MHV-infected cells, nsp9 was localized to the DMV along with other components of the replicative machinery.[27] The sequences of the SARS-CoV and SARS-CoV-2 proteins are 97.3% identical and bacterially overexpressed SARS-CoV protein was crystallized and its three-dimensional structure determined.[88,354] Nsp9 was dimerized in the crystal structure with each molecule of nsp9 having the overall conformation of a six-stranded conical-shaped β-barrel with projecting loops flanked by a C-terminal α-helix bound to the β-barrel through hydrophobic interactions. The outward facing side of the helix is the dimerization interface between two molecules of nsp9. Dynamic light scattering measurements suggested that nsp9 was dimeric in solution while gel permeation chromatography suggested that nsp9 was monomeric in solution. Equilibrium sedimentation analysis suggested that the dimer and the monomeric forms of nsp9 were in equilibrium with each other.[354] Further experiments employing site-directed mutagenesis demonstrated that a conserved GXXXG protein interaction motif spanning residues 100 to 104 was critical for dimerization and crucial for successful virus replication.[250] Dimerization positions a patch of basic amino acids in each monomer adjacent to each other providing an area of high electrostatic potential to serve as binding region for RNA. Surface plasma resonance and electrophoretic mobility shift studies demonstrated that nsp9 was a ssRNA binding protein.[88,354]

With the advent of the COVID-19 pandemic, the SARS-CoV-2 nsp9 was overexpressed, purified, crystallized, and its structure determined by X-ray crystallography fairly early in the course of the pandemic.[217] Gel permeation chromatography demonstrated that the purified protein was a dimer in solution and that its affinity for short polyU or polyT oligonucleotides was very low. The structure of the SARS-CoV-2 nsp9 was very similar to that of the SARS molecule as could be expected from their high degree of sequence identity. As noted above, nsp9 is a target for the nsp12 NiRAN domain catalyzed nucleotide transferase activity resulting in NMPylation of the nsp9 N-terminal asparagine residue, which is vital for virus replication.[342] Cryo-EM of an extended replicase/transcriptase complex consisting of nsp7-nsp8$_2$-nsp9-nsp12-nsp13$_2$ showed that nsp9 was positioned with its N-terminus near the catalytic center of the nsp12 NiRAN domain.[412]

Nsp13

Nsp13 is a 601 amino acid protein that is a component of extended transcription/replication complexes.[412] The SARS-CoV-2 nsp13 is 99.8% identical with the SARS-CoV nsp13, only differing from SARS-CoV nsp13 at residue 570 where a valine is substituted for an isoleucine. It is released from the pp1ab precursor polypeptide by the nsp5 Mpro domain[74,345] and localizes to the DMV, along with other components of the replicative machinery.[77,155] Nsp13 contains C-terminal helicase and N-terminal zinc finger (ZF) domains identified by bioinformatics analyses of the IBV and SARS-CoV genomes.[110,345] The helicase domain contains 11 motifs associated with the SF1 family of helicases, with motifs I and II, also known as Walker A and B boxes, being required for NTP binding and hydrolysis.[324] It most closely resembles helicases of the Upf1

family.[703] Biochemical analyses of purified recombinant nsp13 from several coronaviruses, including SARS-CoV, were shown to have both NTPase and helicase activities.[135,155,324] Studies with the HCoV-229E[324] and the SARS-CoV nsp13[155] established that the helicase was capable of unwinding both DNA and RNA duplexes with protruding 5′ ends in a 5′ to 3′ direction. The presence of a substrate for the helicase greatly stimulated its NTPase activity and a K288A mutation in motif I that interfered with NTP binding abolished both helicase NTPase and helicase activity, providing evidence that the NTPase activity provided the energy for NSP13 unwinding RNA duplexes. Further investigation of the NTPase activity demonstrated that it was able to hydrolyze the 5′ triphosphate of a single-stranded RNA molecule to produce an RNA with a 5′ diphosphate. This 5′ NTPase activity was hypothesized to carry out the first step in synthesizing the 5′cap found on coronavirus mRNAs and the genome. A K288A mutation abolished this triphosphatase activity as well the NTPase and helicase activities. A kinetic analysis of nsp13 helicase activity demonstrated that unwinding a nucleic acid duplex took place in discrete steps of 9.3 nucleotides at a rate of 30 steps per second, and the addition of nsp12 to the reaction doubled the step size thus increasing the rate of unwinding two-fold, suggesting an association between the two proteins.[1] Structures were determined for the MERS-CoV and SARS-CoV nsp13 molecules in 2017 and 2019, respectively.[133,160] Both molecules were dimers in the crystallographic asymmetric unit, although the dimers were packed differently in the two structures. The structures of the two enzymes were very similar with both structures containing five domains: an N-terminal Cys-His rich domain binding 3 zinc atoms (designated ZBD or CH domains) and corresponding to the ZF domain identified bioinformatically,[110,345] an α-helical stalk domain, a β-barrel domain (designated the 1B domain) followed by two RecA-like domains designated RecA1 (residues 241 to 443) and RecA2 (residues 444 to 596). These domains are arranged to form a pyramidal shaped molecule with the two RecA-like domains containing the first seven core SF1 family helicase motifs plus the 1B domain forming the base of the pyramid, the α-helical stalk domain lying atop the RecA1 and 1B domains with the zinc binding domain sitting above the α-helical stalk. The seven conserved SF1 family helicase motifs are located in a cleft between the two RecA-like domains, and this cleft contains the nucleotide binding pocket. A comparison of the nsp13 structure with the related arterivirus helicase and the Upf1 helicase suggested that the 3′ end of a bound ssRNA is located in a 6 to 12 angstrom wide tunnel formed by the 1B, stalk and RecA1 domains, with the 5′end of the RNA sitting atop the RecA2 domain. A binding site for nsp12 on the adjacent surfaces of the nsp13 ZBD and 1B domains was identified in 2019.[133] Mutagenesis studies with the HCoV-229E nsp13 and a related arterivirus nsp10 indicated that an intact and functional ZBD was essential for ATPase and helicase activity and thus for viral replication.[324] Unsurprisingly, a compound that inhibited the unwinding activity of the SARS-CoV helicase also inhibited the replication of a SARS-CoV RNA replicon.[2]

Studies of the SARS-CoV-2 nsp13 have either focused on identifying inhibitors of the NTPase and helicase activities[424] or have been cryo-EM studies of nsp13 in complex with the replication/transcription complex (nsp7-nsp8$_2$-nsp12-nsp13$_2$) or in a extended replication complex additionally containing nsp9.[52,236,411,412] Although there have been multiple computational and enzymatic screens for inhibitors of the NTPase and helicase activities, there have been relatively few which investigated viral replication in infected cells and SARS-CoV-2 infection of animals. Prior to the COVID-19 pandemic, bismuth compounds had been identified as inhibitors of the SARS-CoV nsp13 helicase and viral replication in infected cells.[416] The compound ranitidine bismuth citrate is a potent inhibitor of purified nsp13 SARS-CoV-2 helicase and NTPase activities and inhibited virus replication in both infected cells and in SARS-CoV-2–infected Syrian hamsters while also decreasing the severity of pneumonitis in these animals.[424] Treatment of purified nsp13 with bismuth compounds displaces zinc ions from the nsp13 zinc binding domain suggesting that this alters the interaction of this domain with the enzymatically active helicase. Cryo-EM studies[52,417] of a replication/transcription complex (nsp7-nsp8$_2$-nsp12-nsp13$_2$) with a partially double-stranded RNA template-primer demonstrated that the two nsp13 molecules interacted through their 1B domains. The 1B domain of one molecule of nsp13, designated nsp13-1, bound to the nsp12 interface domain (links the RdrRp and NiRAN domains) while its ZBD domain bound to nsp8-1. The ZBD of the second molecule of nsp13, designated nsp13-2, bound to the nsp8-2 helical domain and the RdRp thumb domain, while its 1B domain made additional contacts with nsp8-2. The unpaired 5′ extension of the template RNA protrudes from the nsp12 catalytic site into the nsp13-2 RNA binding channel.[52,236,411] It should be noted that as nsp12 RdRp progresses along the template RNA in a 3′ to 5′ direction and the nsp13 helicase unwinds RNA in the 5′ to 3′ direction, these two molecules' movements along the template RNA oppose each other. If the helicase prevails, the RdRp will move backward on the template,[52,236] a process called backtracking. Molecular dynamic simulations suggested that one or more misincorporated nucleotides at the elongating 3′end of the newly synthesized RNA will spontaneously fray away from the template and enter the nucleotide binding tunnel of the RdRp, a result supported by RNA-protein cross-linking experiments.[236] Structural studies support a model where the RdRp motif F provides a strand-separating structure directing the frayed end of the elongating RNA to the nucleotide binding tunnel during backtracking. Backtracking has been suggested to play a role in the template switching event that is central to leader-body joining, an essential step in coronavirus transcription.[236] It has also been suggested that this provides a mechanism to extrude an elongating RNA with a misincorporated nucleotide or nucleotide analogue through the nucleotide entry tunnel, providing access to the nsp14 exonuclease that provides a proof-reading function for coronavirus RNA synthesis (see below for a discussion of nsp14).

Coronavirus Capping Machinery Proteins (Nsp10, Nsp14, and Nsp16)

The capping reactions

There are five coronavirus proteins involved in the addition of a 5′ cap to positive sense virus-specific RNAs that are synthesized by the replication/transcription complex: nsp13, nsp12, nsp14, nsp16, and nsp10. The NTPase activity of nsp13 removes the gamma-phosphate from the 5′-triphosphate of nascent RNA

transcripts and the nsp12 NiRAN domain appears to provide a guanylyltransferase activity to produce a GpppN at the 5′end of the newly synthesized RNAs (see sections on nsp12 and nsp13 above). The next two steps in producing a 5′ cap are the addition of a methyl group at the N7 position of the guanine by nsp14's N7-methyl transferase activity to produce a Cap-0 structure, followed by a second methyl transferase reaction mediated by nsp16, adding methyl groups to the 2′-O position of the first RNA nucleotide (produces a Cap-1 structure) or to the first and second RNA nucleotides to produce a Cap-2 structure. The presence of a 5′ cap structure is essential for mRNA recognition by translation initiation factor eIF4E and thus translation of viral RNA and for replication,[93,95] and it also plays a role in avoiding recognition by the innate immune system.[445] Both nsp14 and nsp16 form heterodimers with nsp10, and these interactions and their functional effects are described in more detail below.

Nsp10

The SARS-CoV and SARS-CoV-2 nsp10 proteins are 139 amino acids in length and are proteolytically cleaved from their pp1ab precursor by the nsp5 Mpro.[345] The two proteins are 99.3% identical in amino acid sequence, with the two differences being a nonconservative change from a proline (SARS-CoV) to an alanine (SARS-CoV-2) at position 23 and a conservative arginine (SARS-CoV) to lysine change (SARS-CoV-2) at amino acid 113. Nsp10 has an important role in viral replication and RNA synthesis, as demonstrated by a biochemical analysis of a MHV temperature sensitive mutant, tsLA6, that was mapped to nsp10 by sequencing the mutant and spontaneous revertants[315] and by reverse genetic experiments with MHV and SARS-CoV.[29,79] A yeast two-hybrid screen of the 16 SARS-CoV ORF1ab encoded proteins demonstrated that nsp10 could self-associate and strongly interacted with both nsp14 and nsp16.[152] X-ray crystallography of purified SARS-CoV nsp10 provided a single domain structure composed of two N-terminal antiparallel alpha-helices stacked against a beta-sheet core and three additional alpha-helical regions followed by a coiled C-terminus.[165] The protein contains two conserved zinc fingers and in MHV these were shown to play an essential role in RNA synthesis.[79] A cluster of basic amino acids on its surface is thought to mediate its modest single- and double-stranded NAB activity.[165] Structures of the SARS-CoV nsp10-nsp16[71] and nsp10-nsp14[230] heterodimers have been determined and interaction surfaces mapped for both by their X-ray crystallographic structures. The interaction of nsp10 with nsp14 is exclusively with the nsp14 exonuclease domain and significantly activates nsp14 exonuclease activity.[230] The nsp10 interaction surfaces for these two proteins partially overlap, thus excluding a single nsp10 molecule simultaneously interacting with both nsp14 and nsp16. The functional role of these interactions will be discussed in more detail under nsp14 and nsp16 below.

The SARS-CoV-2 nsp10 structure has been resolved by X-ray crystallography and was virtually identical to the structures determined for SARS-CoV nsp10.[306] The nsp10 structure in complexes with nsp14,[215,220] with nsp16,[307,378] and with an extended replication/transcription complex have been determined by either cryo-EM or X-ray crystallography studies and will be discussed below.

Nsp14

The SARS-CoV and SARS-CoV-2 nsp14 proteins are 527 amino acids in length and are proteolytically cleaved from their pp1ab precursor by the nsp5 Mpro.[345] Nsp14 contains two domains each with a different enzymatic activity, an N-terminal exonuclease activity, designated as ExoN,[254,345] and an N7-methyl transferase activity.[50] The ExoN domain was predicted to be a 3-to-5′ exonuclease belonging to the DEDD super family of DNA and RNA exonucleases, so named because of the conserved amino acids in three motifs (motifs I, II, and III)[345] essential for nsp14's nuclease activity.[254] A fifth residue, a histidine, is conserved 4 amino acids upstream of the last conserved aspartate in motif III, making ExoN a member of the DEDDh subfamily of the DEDD superfamily. The four acidic residues are part of the catalytic site and form two metal binding sites needed for catalytic activity.[344] The ExoN domain also contains a zinc finger-like domain inserted between motifs I and II of the DEDDh helicases.[345] Based on the role of some members of the DEDD family of exonucleases in DNA proofreading and the conservation of this domain in coronaviruses, toroviruses, and roniviruses, viruses with very large genomes in the Nidovirus family, and its absence in the smaller arteriviruses, it was speculated that this nsp14 domain might have a role in RNA proofreading or template switching during subgenomic RNA synthesis.[345]

Biochemical characterization of overexpressed and purified SARS-CoV ExoN demonstrated that the enzyme digested both single- and double-stranded RNA substrates in the predicted 3′-to- 5′ direction, but not DNA.[254] The pattern of cleavage products obtained suggested that the target of this enzyme might be partially single-stranded RNAs. As noted under nsp10, binding of nsp10 to nsp14 greatly stimulated nsp14 ExoN nuclease activity.[230] This complex is able to efficiently carry out the excision of mismatches at the 3′ end of a dsRNA, an activity consistent with a role in RNA proofreading. Additionally, the complex was shown to be able to excise remdesivir-MP from the 3′end of a synthetic dsRNA substrate, suggesting a role in resistance of coronaviruses to nucleoside analogues.[94] Coexpression of nsp10 and nsp14 allowed the purification of nsp10-nsp14 complexes and determination of their structure by X-ray crystallography.[230] Nsp14 contained two domains, an N-terminal ExoN domain encompassing amino acids 1 to 287 and a C-terminal N7-methyltransferase domain of amino acids 288 to 527. The structure defined the nsp10-nsp14 interaction surface showing that nsp10 interacts exclusively with the ExoN domain. The structure revealed that the ExoN catalytic residues are D (aspartic acid) 90, E (glutamic acid) 92, E191 rather than the conserved D at position 243 in SARS-CoV nsp14 that was thought to be part of the ExoN active site, H (histidine) 268, and D273. The structure also revealed two zinc fingers with the first zinc finger positioned between motifs I and II with the second zinc finger overlapping domain III. Both are required for nuclease activity. The interaction of nsp14 with nsp10 produced a change in nsp14 conformation that stabilized the ExoN active site with a concomitant increase in ExoN enzymatic activity.[94] In addition to interacting with nsp10, nsp14 interacts with nsp12 and the core RdRp complex consisting of nsp7-nsp8₂-nsp12, suggesting that a super-molecular replication/transcriptase complex might exist to carry out both RNA synthesis, RNA proof-reading, and the enzymatic reactions necessary for cap formation on mRNAs.[94,351] In this complex, nsp12 interacts with both the ExoN and N7-methyltransferase domains of nsp14.

Reverse genetic experiments with the alphacoronavirus HCoV-229E demonstrated that replacing any of the four conserved DDED residues in the exonuclease catalytic site was lethal for virus replication due to greatly reduced viral RNA synthesis, suggesting that the exonuclease activity was a potential therapeutic target.[254] Mutations in the MHV and SARS-CoV nsp14 ExoN active site were not lethal but resulted in viruses with impaired viral RNA synthesis and modest growth deficits[84,85] while significantly increasing mutation rates, supporting the idea that the ExoN domain had a functional role in RNA proofreading. Interestingly, similar mutations in the MERS-CoV nsp14 ExoN domain severely impaired enzymatic activity and markedly reduced viral RNA synthesis and were lethal to MERS-CoV, suggesting a possible role in replication beyond proofreading.[273] This was confirmed in a study of recombination in three betacoronaviruses, MHV, MERS-CoV, and SARS-CoV-2, which demonstrated that recombination events were extensive during RNA synthesis, and that inactivating mutations in the ExoN domain decreased the frequency and altered the spectrum of recombination products.[121] Importantly, the ExoN nuclease activity plays a key role in the relative resistance of coronaviruses to some nucleoside analogues. Recombinant MHV and SARS-CoV carrying catalytically inactivating mutations in the ExoN domain had a 300-fold decrease in growth in response to 5-fluorouracil (5-FU) compared to the more modest effect of the drug on wild-type viruses.[343] The increased response to 5-FU is accompanied by a 24-fold increase in the mutation rate over that observed during infections with wild-type viruses treated with an equivalent dose of 5-FU. The majority of the increased number of mutations were the A-to-G and U-to-C transitions that are expected from incorporation of 5-FU into replicating genomes followed by mispairing of the incorporated 5-FUMP during subsequent rounds of RNA synthesis. Additionally, recombinant MHV strains with a catalytically inactive ExoN were more than 5-fold more sensitive to remdesivir than wild-type virus.[3] These observations support the idea that at least one function of the nsp14 ExoN domain is RNA proofreading, and it may mediate relative resistance of coronaviruses to nucleoside analogues.[3,343] In addition to its proofreading function, mutations rendering ExoN catalytically inactive increase MHV's sensitivity to interferon; the nsp14 ExoN activity is necessary for MHV to replicate in macrophages and overcome the cell's innate immune response,[41] suggesting a role for this domain in immune evasion by coronaviruses. This is consistent with the observation that SARS-CoV carrying a catalytically inactive ExoN domain is attenuated in an aged mouse model of SARS.[118]

With the onset of COVID-19 pandemic, the role of the ExoN domain in SARS-CoV-2 replication and potential resistance to nucleoside analogues was investigated. Inactivating mutations in the catalytic site of ExoN were lethal, similarly to this effect in MERS-CoV.[273] This contrasts with the effect of similar mutations in the SARS-CoV enzyme where infectious virus could be recovered in reverse genetic experiments[84,85] and is surprising considering the much closer similarity of the SARS-CoV-2 ExoN domain to the SARS-CoV enzyme (99.7% identity) than to the MERS-CoV sequence (63% identity).

Similar to findings for other coronaviruses, binding of SARS-CoV-2 nsp10 to nsp14 activates its ExoN activity.[229] The substrate specificity of the SARS-CoV-2 ExoN domain is similar to that of the SARS-CoV nsp14 in that it removes mismatched nucleotides at the 3′ end of a dsRNA, with the exception that it is also able to hydrolyze RNAs in the context of a 3′ mismatched RNA:DNA hybrid.[229] The structural basis of mismatch recognition has been investigated by cryo-EM studies of synthetic templates bound to SARS-CoV-2 nsp10-nsp14 heterodimers (Fig. 21.11).[220] Binding of a partially double-stranded RNA with a 5′ single-stranded extension and a mismatched 3′-terminal base pair to the nsp10-nsp14 heterodimer resulted in local conformational changes of the ExoN domain, slightly narrowing the RNA binding site and shifting the position of the catalytic residues stabilizing an active conformation of the enzyme. The binding of ExoN to the substrate RNA encompasses the last 2 residues of the fully base-paired nucleotides, flipping the template strand unpaired nucleotide out of the RNA helix, leaving the template mis-incorporated nucleotide as a 3′ single strand extension in the active site. This same study demonstrated that ExoN was capable of removing remdesivir-MP that had been incorporated into substrate

RNA, consistent with earlier work showing that sensitivity to remdesivir is increased in coronaviruses carrying mutations in the ExoN catalytic site.[3] Another cryo-EM study of a complex with the stoichiometry of nsp7-nsp8$_2$-nsp9-nsp12-nsp13$_2$-nsp10-nsp14 and a partially base-paired template RNA with a 5′ unpaired extension revealed that the nsp10-nsp14 complex bound to the extended replication complex (nsp7-nsp8$_2$-nsp9-nsp12-nsp13$_2$) in a shallow valley present between nsp9 and the nsp12 NiRAN domain with both of those domains contacting the nsp14 ExoN domain and nsp10 being in contact with the NiRAN domain (Fig. 21.11A and B).[413] In the images captured by cryo-EM, a greater proportion of the molecules of this complex were side by side antiparallel dimers rather than monomers (Fig. 21.11C). In this dimer, the catalytic site of the ExoN domain is in relative proximity to the RdRp NTP entry tunnel suggesting that backtracking of the RdRp could allow extrusion of the 3′ end of a mis-paired backtracked primer strand RNA where it would be accessible to the ExoN bound to the opposite nsp12 molecule. The cryo-EM data does not exclude the possibility that RNA proofreading is carried out by a nsp10-nsp14 heterodimer acting on a monomeric replication/transcription complex composed of nsp7-nsp8$_2$-nsp9-

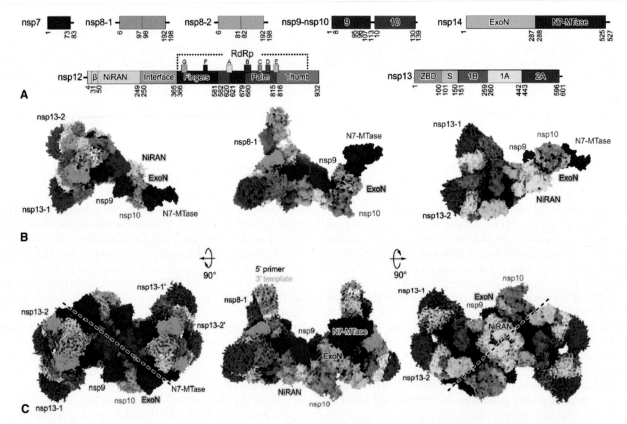

FIGURE 21.11 The cryoelectron microscopy structures of monomeric and dimeric SARS-CoV-2 extended replication/transcription complexes containing nsp10-nsp14 heterodimer. A: A schematic diagram of the domain structure of each component of the complex. Nsp7, *deep purple*; nsp8-1, *gray*; nsp8-2, *green cyan*; nsp9, *purple blue*; nsp10, *slate*; nsp12 NiRAN, *yellow*; nsp12 Interface, *orange*; nsp12 fingers, *blue*; nsp12 palm, *red*; nsp12 thumb, *forest green*; nsp13 ZBD, *light green*; nsp13 S, *salmon*; nsp13 1B, *violet*; nsp13 1A, *sand*; nsp13 2A, *hot pink*; nsp14 ExoN, *pale green*; nsp14 N7-MTase, *brown*. **B:** Three perpendicular views of the cryoelectron microscopy densities of the monomeric complex. **C:** Three perpendicular views of the cryoelectron microscopy densities of the dimeric complex. The *dashed lines* roughly indicate the boundary between the two complexes making up the dimer. (Adapted from Yan L, Ge J, Zheng L, et al. Cryo-EM Structure of an extended SARS-CoV-2 replication and transcription complex reveals an intermediate state in cap synthesis. *Cell* 2021;184(1):184–193.e10. Copyright © 2020 Elsevier. With permission.)

nsp12-nsp13₂ or nsp8₂-nsp9-nsp12-nsp13₂-nsp10-nsp14. The data demonstrating that ExoN activity was necessary for SARS-CoV-2 viability and that other coronaviruses that were able to tolerate mutational inactivation of ExoN were more sensitive to antivirals such as remdesivir has led to computational and biochemical screens for inhibitors of ExoN activity. One screen has identified two compounds, patulin and aurintricarboxylic acid, that inhibit SARS-CoV-2 nsp10-nsp14 ExoN activity in a concentration-dependent manner and inhibited SARS-CoV-2 replication at low micromolar concentration[37] and synergized with remdesivir in inhibiting virus replication.

Chen et al.[50] first identified SARS-CoV nsp14 as having a guanine N7-methyltransferase (N7-MTase) activity by a functional genetic screen in yeast seeking enzymes needed for 5'cap formation. N7-MTase catalyzes the reaction that is the third step in cap formation. Biochemical analyses with purified nsp14 confirmed that the protein transferred a methyl group from S-adenosyl methionine (SAM) to the guanine N7 position of a GpppRNA substrate to synthesize a Cap-0 structure. They further mapped the activity to the CTD of nsp14 by mutagenesis. Alignment with other N7-MTases and an analysis of predicted secondary structure allowed the identification of a conserved DxG motif that is part of the SAM binding site in other methyl transferases. Mutations in this site abolished nsp14 N7-MTase activity in the yeast trans-complementation assay without affecting its ExoN activity. Similarly, mutations in the nsp14 ExoN catalytic site did not inactivate N7-MTase activity. Further experiments using a SARS-CoV replicon demonstrated that RNA replication and transcription were significantly impaired in replicons carrying inactivating mutations in the DxG motif, demonstrating the importance of the N7-MTase activity in viral replication. Biochemical characterization of purified bacterially expressed nsp14 confirmed the previous results of the yeast complementation assay and demonstrated the requirement for SAM as a the methyl donor.[28] Binding of nsp10 to nsp14 failed to augment N7-MTase activity.[28] The crystal structure of the nsp14-nsp10 heterodimer[230] showed that the N7-MTase domain contained an atypical MTase fold. It contains a beta-sheet containing five beta-strands rather than the usual seven strands, with the first four strands oriented parallel to one another with the last strand in an antiparallel orientation. Additionally, there is a small three-stranded antiparallel beta-sheet that is inserted perpendicularly to the central beta-sheet between the last two strands of the central sheet, which together with an N-terminal alpha-helix forms a pocket that tightly accommodates GpppA with the guanine N7 proximal to the methyl group of SAM in a position to effect the methyl transfer reaction. Mutation of residues making up the GpppA binding pocket confirmed their role in positioning the guanine in the appropriate position and orientation to accept the methyl group. There is also a zinc finger located distil to the N7-MTase active site.

The structural studies of the SARS-CoV-2 extended replication complex (nsp7-nsp8₂-nsp9-nsp12-nsp13₂) have shed some additional understanding of how the 5′ ends of the coronavirus mRNAs are generated.[413] In this complex, the catalytic site of the nsp12 NiRAN domain responsible for the guanylyl transfer reaction to the dephosphorylated 5′ end of the of elongating RNA is opposite the catalytic site of the nsp14 N7-MTase. The N7-MTase zinc finger of unknown function

is positioned on a potential transfer path of the GpppRNA to the N7-MTase active site and is hypothesized to play a role in this transfer. The outbreak of the COVID-19 pandemic triggered a search for inhibitors of the SARS-CoV-2 N7-MTase. Two biochemical screens of chemical libraries using purified nsp14 identified a number of inhibitors of the N7-MTase.[20,173] The most potent inhibitors without toxicity inhibited viral replication at low micromolar concentrations. A study on the role of SARS-CoV-2 nsps1-16 as inhibitors of protein synthesis and the interferon response identified ectopically overexpressed nsp14 as potential inhibitor of these processes.[142] Mutational inactivation of either the SARS-CoV-2 nsp14 ExoN endonuclease or the N7-MTase activities abrogated nsp14's ability to inhibit translation, and the inhibition of translation was augmented by coexpression of nsp10, suggesting that nsp14 enzymatic activities are important in this effect. It has not yet been shown that nsp14 mediates an inhibitory effect on translation during virus infection, nor is the mechanism understood.

Nsp16

Nsp16 is a 298 amino acid protein and is released from the pp1ab precursor polypeptide by the nsp5 Mpro domain.[74,345] The sequences of the SARS-CoV and SARS-CoV-2 proteins are 93.3% identical. Nsp16 was predicted to have a 2′O-methyltransferase (2′O-MTase) activity based on comparative sequence analysis.[345,381] It contains the four conserved catalytic amino acids, K-D-K-E, and a conserved SAM binding site that is characteristic of this family of enzymes. Biochemical assays of bacterially expressed and purified feline coronavirus (FeCoV) nsp16 demonstrated that it was able to bind to a Cap-0 (⁷ᵐᵉGpppRNA) containing short RNA substrate and transfer a methyl group from SAM to the 2′-O position of the first transcribed nucleotide, the last step in the synthesis of a fully functional 5′ cap (Cap-1). The enzyme had a requirement for the guanine N7-methyl group to be present for nsp16 to bind the RNA substrate, positioning it downstream of the N7-methyltransferase reaction catalyzed by nsp14 in 5′cap synthesis.[70] Mutational analysis confirmed that the K-D-K-E residues were essential for enzyme activity. Although the FeCoV nsp16 is able to carry out this reaction in the absence of other viral proteins, the 2′O-MTase activity of SARS-CoV nsp16 is absolutely dependent on nsp10 binding.[28,228] Binding of nsp10 to nsp16 enabled SARS-CoV nsp16 to bind both its substrates, ⁷ᵐᵉGpppRNA and SAM.[51] The structure of the SARS-CoV nsp16 complexed with nsp10 was determined by X-ray crystallography and contains a canonical seven-stranded beta-sheet methyltransferase fold.[51,71] Mutations of the SARS-CoV nsp10-nsp16 binding interface that abolish their interaction also abolish nsp16 2′O-methyltransferase activity.[51,71,228] S-adenosylhomocysteine (SAH), a product of the methyltransferase reaction after the methyl group has been transferred from SAM to the RNA, was visualized and identified in the SAM binding pocket. The residues making up the SAM binding pocket are conserved among coronaviruses nsp16s. Binding of SAM in its nsp16 binding pocket increased the formation of enzymatically active nsp10-nsp16 complexes through an allosteric effect.[14] Conversely, dissociation of SAH, a product of the methyl transferase reaction, from the SAM binding pocket promoted the dissociation of the nsp10-nsp16 complex. Mutation of the K-D-K-E residues to alanine abolished SARS-CoV nsp16 methyltransferase activity; similarly, mutation of the amino acids lining the SAM binding pocket severely compromised activity.[71] A hydrophobic putative RNA binding groove leading to the catalytic site was identified using the vaccinia virus VP39 methyltransferase bound to RNA as a template.

The function of 2′-O methylation on mammalian and viral mRNAs was uncertain for many years as it is not required for mRNA translation.[65] A role for this RNA modification in distinguishing host from nonhost mRNAs was first described in West Nile virus, a flavivirus, vaccinia virus, a poxvirus, and the coronavirus MHV, where mutational inactivation of these viruses' 2′O-MTase activities made these viruses more sensitive to interferon and the interferon-stimulated IFIT proteins.[65] This implicated the coronavirus nsp16 in immune evasion. Mutational inactivation of nsp16 in MHV or HCoV-229E resulted in increased interferon production in infected macrophages accompanied by decreased viral replication compared to recombinant viruses with a wild-type nsp16 gene.[445] The induction of interferon upon infection with a 2′O-MTase deficient recombinant mutant MHV was dependent upon the macrophage having a functioning MDA5 protein. The role of nsp16 in immune evasion *in vivo* was demonstrated by the failure of a recombinant 2′-OMT mutant of MHV-A59 to productively infect the liver and spleen of mice challenged by intraperitoneal inoculation.[445] These observations were extended to SARS-CoV using the MA15 mouse adapted SARS-CoV model, where mutational inactivation of the SARS-CoV nsp16 2′OMTase activity resulted in an attenuated infection both *in vitro* and *in vivo* and the attenuated viruses were more sensitive to interferon.[245] As was the case for MHV, the attenuation of nsp16 mutants was dependent on intact MDA5 and IFIT proteins. The ability of attenuated 2′OMTase negative nsp16 mutants to serve as an attenuated live virus vaccine platform was also examined. Immunization of mice with mouse adapted SARS-CoV with an enzymatically inactive nsp16 elicited protective immunity to challenge with wild-type MA15. Similar results were obtained with MERS-CoV carrying a 2′OMTase mutation in nsp16[247] suggesting that this approach to the development of live-attenuated vaccines might be applicable to a wide range of coronaviruses. Because the enzyme activity of nsp16 is dependent upon its allosteric activation by binding to nsp10, short peptides or peptidomimetic compounds targeting the interaction interface of these two proteins is a potential approach to an antiviral therapy. This approach was tested experimentally by the development of a short peptide targeting the nsp10-nsp16 interaction and demonstrated that it inhibited 2′-OMTase activity of a number of coronaviruses *in vitro* and inhibited MHV replication in cell cultures and attenuated infection and pathogenesis *in vivo*.[390]

With the onset of the COVID-19 pandemic, four groups determined the structure of SARS-CoV-2 nsp10-nsp16 complexes by X-ray crystallography.[253,307,378,399] The structures were similar to that determined for the SARS-CoV nsp16. Structures in the presence and absence of a cap analogue, [7me]GpppA, SAM, SAH, or the SAH analogue sinefungin, were also determined and allowed identification of the Cap-0 binding and SAM binding pockets.[253,307,378,399] Nsp16 undergoes a conformational change upon binding SAM and its RNA substrate bringing the nsp16 catalytic residues and its substrates into closer proximity.[378] The presence of divalent cations stabilizes interactions between nsp16 and its RNA substrate enhancing the alignment of the RNA in the active site.[253] A comparison of the SARS-CoV-2 nsp16 structure to mammalian methyltransferases revealed a four amino acid insertion, which is unique to coronaviruses and promotes nsp16's catalytic activity by altering the conformation of the RNA backbone in its binding groove.[253] This four residue insertion was suggested as a promising target for the design of coronavirus-specific inhibitors of the nsp16 2′OMTase activity. In addition to the well-described role of nsp16's 2′OMTase activity in immune evasion described earlier, it has been reported that overexpressed nsp16 binds to U1/U2 snRNAs and thus inhibits splicing.[16] The observation that nsp16 can be identified in the nucleus of SARS-CoV-2–infected cells by immunofluorescent staining supports the idea that nsp16 may suppress the interferon response by interfering with the proper splicing of interferon and interferon responsive transcripts. Identification of the structural basis for binding to U1/U2 snRNAs followed up by reverse genetic experiments is needed to provide confirmation of the effect of nsp16 on splicing during SARS-CoV-2 infection.

SARS-CoV-2 ACCESSORY PROTEINS

Coronavirus accessory proteins differ among the lineages of human viruses. The proteins encoded by these genes often function to antagonize the host cell innate immune responses.

Like other RNA viruses, coronaviruses produce double-stranded (ds)RNA early during the infection cycle as an intermediate in genome replication and messenger mRNA transcription.[346] Host cell pattern recognition receptors (PRRs) sense viral dsRNA as pathogenic nonself and respond by activating several antiviral pathways critical for early defense against viral invasion. DsRNA sensing by cytosolic PRRs leads to activation of three key pathways, interferon (IFN) production and signaling, oligoadenylate-ribonuclease L (OAS-RNase L), and protein kinase R (PKR).[149] Detection of dsRNA by MDA5 during coronavirus infection[309] leads to signaling through mitochondrial antiviral signaling (MAVS) protein leading to activation and nuclear translocation of transcription factor IRF3 and production of type I (α/β) and type III (λ) interferon (IFN). Upon binding to its specific cell surface receptor, IFN promotes phosphorylation by Janus kinase (JAK) and translocation to the nucleus of signal transducers and activators of transcription (STAT)1 and STAT2, which induce expression of IFN stimulated genes (ISGs) with antiviral activities.[226,294] In parallel, dsRNA is also sensed by oligoadenylate synthetases (OASs), primarily OAS3, which synthesize 2′,5′-linked oligoadenylates (2-5A),[211,397] which induce dimerization and activation of RNase L, leading to degradation of viral and host single-stranded sRNA and protein synthesis inhibition.[80] Finally, also in parallel, dsRNA sensing by PKR induces PKR autophosphorylation, permitting PKR to phosphorylate the translation initiation factor eIF2α leading to protein synthesis inhibition.[313] While RNase L and PKR antiviral activities are not dependent on IFN production,[397] OASs and PKR are encoded by ISGs; therefore, these pathways can be activated and/or further up-regulated by IFNs. Similarly, RNase L and PKR activation can promote cellular stress, inflammation, and/or apoptotic death.[16,43,45,169,234,438] Thus, these antiviral pathways

TABLE 21.2 Accessory proteins of SARS-CoV-2 compared to SARS-CoV

Accessory Proteins	SARS-CoV-2 Amino Acid Number	SARS-CoV Amino Acid Number	% Identity to SARS-CoV	Function
ORF3a	275	274	72.4	Viroporin, viral assembly
ORF3b	22	154	61.1	IFN antagonist when overexpressed
ORF6	61	63	68.9	Inhibits nuclear import pathway
ORF7a	121	122	85.2	IFN antagonist when overexpressed
ORF7b	43	44	85.4	Unknown
ORF8	121	122	29.5 (40 aa)	Reported to degrade MHC class 1; induce ER stress response when overexpressed; viruses with deletions found in humans
ORF8a	N/A	39	31.7% (in overlap)	Unknown
ORF8b	N/A	84	40.5% (overlap)	Unknown
ORF9b	97	98	72.4	IFN antagonist when overexpressed

IFN, interferon.
ORF8 of SARS-CoV evolved into ORF8a and ORF8b but remains intact in SARS-CoV-2.

are also destructive to the cell, thus further reducing host cell viability.

Coronaviruses utilize a large portion of their genomes to encode proteins that antagonize host defenses by many diverse mechanisms. These include some of the ORF1a/1b encoded proteins conserved among all coronaviruses (discussed above). In addition, each lineage of CoV encodes a unique set of accessory genes encoding proteins that promote evasion and/or antagonism of dsRNA-induced pathways described above (Fig. 21.1B; Table 21.2). These proteins are named by the ORFs encoding them. CoV proteins are usually translated from the 5′ ORF of each individual mRNA. However, there are less often two CoV proteins translated from separate ORFs encoded by the same RNA and in those cases the downstream ORFs are designated "b," for example, ORF3a,b and ORFs7a,7b. The ORFs for accessory proteins in the SARS-CoV-2 genome are named with the same numbers as their homologues in SARS-CoV.[166,249] These accessory proteins will be described below and summarized in Table 21.2.

ORF3a

The SARS-CoV-2 ORF3a protein is similar to that of SARS-CoV, containing three transmembrane domains (TMDs),[153] potassium ion channel activity, and a role in virion assembly and budding. The SARS-CoV ORF3a encoded protein accumulates and localizes to vesicles containing markers for late endosomes and is necessary for SARS-CoV–induced Golgi fragmentation.[97] Consistent with this, a recombinant mutant SARS-CoV-2 with a knockout of ORF3a was attenuated for weight loss and mortality of K18 mice expressing the human ACE2 receptor.[337]

ORF3b

The very short (22 amino acid) ORF3b encoded protein of SARS-CoV-2, when overexpressed, was found to antagonize transcription from an IFNβ promoter construct and to prevent IRF3 localization to the nucleus, while the corresponding SARS-CoV 153 amino acid proteins does not have this activity.[186] IFN antagonism was associated with the cytoplasmic

localization noted for SARS-CoV-2 ORF3b but not that of SARS-CoV. Paradoxically, longer versions of ORF3b were isolated from two COVID-19 patients with severe disease and were associated with stronger antagonism of transcription from an IFNβ promoter in an *in vitro* assay. Interestingly, short forms of ORF3b are found in bat viruses related to both SARS-CoV and SARS-CoV-2. Confirmation of the role of this protein in the virus life cycle is needed.

ORF6

The ORF6 encoded protein was initially described for SARS-CoV and shown to prevent translocation of STAT1 to the nucleus, by sequestering nuclear import factors on the membranes of the rough endoplasmic reticulum and Golgi.[99] Subsequently, the SARS-CoV ORF6 encoded protein was shown to more generally antagonize karyopherin-dependent nuclear import of additional transcription factors needed for an effective host response to viral infections.[341] Interestingly, a similar mechanism is utilized by MERS-CoV in that the NS4b protein was shown to antagonize the translocation of NF-κB, a transcription factor important for induction of inflammatory cytokines by competing for binding to karyopherins.[38] The SARS-CoV-2 ORF6 encoded protein localizes to the nuclear pore complex (NPC) where it binds directly to the Nup98-Rae1 complex via its carboxyterminal end, to target the nuclear import pathway and in doing so reduces docking of karyopherin/importin and the attached transcription factors.[255] The SARS-CoV protein also binds to this complex; however, SARS-CoV-2 more strongly disrupts nucleocytoplasmic transport than its SARS-CoV homolog. Not surprisingly a recombinant SARS-CoV-2 ORF6 knockout virus was attenuated inducing less weight loss and mortality during infection of K18 mice expressing the human ACE2 receptor.[337]

ORF7a

The SARS-CoV ORF7a encodes a protein of 122 amino acids containing a TMD and cytoplasmic tail, which is localized to the Golgi complex and in lesser amounts to the endoplasmic reticulum (ER) and ER–Golgi intermediate compartment.[317]

Its luminal portion is similar in topology to members of the immunoglobulin superfamily.[266] The ORF7a encoded protein has been reported to be incorporated into SARS-CoV particles by interacting with viral structural proteins E and M[144] and in addition to contribute to apoptosis.[317,375]

The SARS-CoV-2 ORF7a encoded protein, when over-expressed, antagonizes type 1 IFN signaling as evidenced by inhibition of expression from an interferon-sensitive response element containing promoter (ISRE) driving expression of luciferase. This occurs by preventing phosphorylation of STAT2, a transcription factor required for IFN signaling and this depends on ubiquitination the ORF7a protein.[40] Interestingly, mutations in the carboxy terminal portion of ORF7a protein were identified in clinical isolates of SARS-CoV-2 and shown to have a replication defect as well reduce the antagonism of IFN.[267]

Since the ORF7a encoded proteins of SARS-CoV and SARS-Cov2 are 85.2% identical and 95.9% similar, it is very likely that they have similar functions. However, studies of each protein, usually by overexpression, as described above, have revealed different activities. Thus, further studies utilizing infectious virus are needed to determine the actual function of the ORF7a encoded protein during the life cycle.

ORF7b

The 44 amino acid SARS-CoV ORF7b encoded protein is an integral membrane protein that is localized to the Golgi and has been shown, like the ORF7a protein, to participate in inducing apoptosis.[292,316] The SARS-CoV-2 ORF7b encoded protein, like the ORF7a protein, is very similar to that of SARS-CoV and likely to have similar functions.

ORF8

ORF8 encodes a protein of 121 amino acids with a signal sequence. As such it is found ER membrane associated and also secreted into the extracellular space and in serum in humans. Antibodies to the ORF8 encoded protein were detected early in patients before the detection of antinucleocapsid antibodies and proposed to be an early marker for infection and perhaps have diagnostic value.[392] The ORF8 of SARS-CoV evolved into two smaller ORFs, 8a and 8b, following a 29 nucleotide deletion early in the SARS epidemic,[275] suggesting the protein encoded in ORF8 was not required for viral replication in humans. SARS-CoV-2 has thus far retained ORF8, which is conserved among related bat coronaviruses. However, interestingly, isolates with deletions or mutations have been reported in different parts of the world. As early as January 2020, a variant with a 382 nucleotide deletion encompassing part of ORF7b and ORF8, including its transcriptional regulatory sequence (TRS), was reported in Singapore, accounting for 23.6% (45/191) of the sequenced viruses.[350] These viruses replicated to a similar extent in cell culture and produced similar viral loads in people. However, infection with this variant was associated with milder disease[422] and this variant died out due to control of viral spread in Singapore. Variants with deletions in parts of ORFs7b and 8 from 62 to 345 nucleotides were also identified in Taiwan, Australia, Bangladesh, and Spain,[350] and the genome of the alpha variant (B.1.1.7) also contains a stop codon in ORF8 (C27972T; Q27stop) producing a truncated protein.

While it is clear that SARS-CoV-2 ORF8 encoded protein is not required for replication in cell culture or humans, there are several studies addressing its function. The ORF8 encoded protein when overexpressed bound to MHC class I and directed its degradation resulting in less antigen presentation on the cell surface, a type of immune evasion.[431] ORF8 overexpression, but not the overexpression of other SARS-CoV-2 accessory proteins, has also been reported to induce ER stress responses within transfected cells; however, the consequences of such activation have not yet been characterized using viral mutants with deletion of ORF8 n.[83] This finding is derived from data in cell culture and the relevance to infection of humans needs to be validated . However, a recombinant virus in which ORF8 was deleted replicated in cell culture with similar kinetics to wild-type virus and demonstrated similar pathogenesis in K18 human ACE2 expressing mice indicating ORF8 expression is not required for pathogenesis in this mouse model.[337]

ORF9b

The ORF9b encoded protein of SARS-CoV-2 is quite similar in sequence and structure to that of SARS-CoV.[332] The ORF9b encoded protein is localized to the membrane of mitochondria where it associates with TOM70, an outer membrane mitochondrial protein that serves as receptor of the mitochondrial antiviral-signaling (MAVS) protein. When overexpressed, the ORF9b encoded protein suppresses type I interferon responses.[161] As with many other accessory gene products, this has yet to be confirmed in the context of infection.

Recombinant Viruses

As described above, often initial investigations with a new pathogen identify host antagonists by overexpression of each individual protein and assessment of effects on IFN production or signaling. While this is a good first step, the most definitive way to prove this function is to produce a recombinant virus and identify the steps in virus–host interactions that are altered. Several groups have developed reverse genetics systems needed to construct mutant viruses. Using a Bacterial Artificial Chromosome (BAC) cloning system, a group of mutant recombinant viruses were constructed in which ORF3a, ORF6, ORF7a, ORF7b, or ORF8 were deleted.[337] Most of these viruses demonstrated smaller plaque morphology compared to parental virus, suggesting they may have defects in viral spread, and mutants with deletions of ORF7a and ORF8 showed lower levels of replication in several cell lines. When K18 mice bearing human ACE2 receptor were infected with each of these mutant viruses, those deleted for ORF3a, ORF7a, ORF7b, or ORF6 were attenuated in morbidity and mortality with the most striking attenuation exhibited by viruses lacking expression of the ORF3a or ORF6 encoded proteins. These data suggest that these proteins most likely contribute to SARS-CoV-2 virulence.

SARS-CoV-2 VARIANTS— TRANSMISSION AND IMMUNE EVASION

From the earliest time of detection in December 2019, SARS-CoV-2 has efficiently been transmitted between people. Without genome sequences and/or isolates from the earliest period of human transmission, it is impossible to know definitively whether adaptation in an intermediate host before transmission to humans modified the transmissibility. One line of evidence suggests a single spike mutation, threonine to alanine at amino acid in position 372 (T372A) occurred during this period and may confer a significant fitness benefit during infection of human cells.[171] In the subsequent first several months of the pandemic phase of SARS-CoV-2, emergence of an additional mutation occurred, with viruses bearing G614D (glycine at position 614 rather than aspartic acid) rising to dominance worldwide.[187] Functional studies in cell culture and animals have confirmed that this amino acid change alters spike protein functionality[425,432] and enhances upper respiratory tract replication in animal models, conferring increased transmissibility.[293]

In the several months following the emergence of D614G, SARS-CoV-2 exhibited a remarkable degree of genetic stability, with variation due solely to genetic drift and an apparent absence of further adaptation to humans. In late 2020, coincident with a global acceleration in the number of cases, several variants of suspected altered biological properties emerged—some have been formally classified as variants of concern (VOC).

The first of these to be identified was initially detected by robust genomic sequencing in the United Kingdom and classified as lineage B.1.1.7 (alpha), defined by 14 amino acid changes and 3 deletions, including an N501Y substitution in the spike RBD.[67] Early studies identified a 30% to 70% transmission advantage for the alpha variant,[67] which has been replicated in settings other than the United Kingdom including during spread of this lineage in the United States.[393] Two other significant VOCs containing N501Y have emerged: B.1.351 (beta) first identified in South Africa[360] and P.1 (gamma)[64,91] identified in Brazil. Both of these lineages, like the alpha variant, contain an unusually large number of mutations overall, suggesting they may have evolved during prolonged infection of an immunocompromised individual, and both share a concerning suite of RBD mutations.

Beta and gamma variants contain substitutions at spike positions 417 (K417N/T), 484 (E484K), and 501 (N501Y) in addition to unique, lineage-defining mutations. Of these, E484K is of particular concern due to its potential to mediate immune escape, increasing the possibility of reinfection and potentially the frequency of breakthrough infections of vaccinated individuals. Substantial research earlier in the pandemic included deep mutational scanning of the spike RBD to identify changes that alter affinity for ACE2[348] and reduce serum neutralization.[119] In these assays, changes at position 484, specifically to K, P, or Q, produced the most substantial reductions in neutralization potency by human convalescent serum, though the effect was highly variable between individuals. In contrast, N501Y increases affinity for ACE2, possibly contributing to its higher transmissibility but does not appear to mediate any notable antibody escape.

Laboratory studies to determine how these variants might impact vaccine efficacy suggest that the alpha variant is fully susceptible to sera from vaccines,[86] whereas beta and gamma variants are neutralized less potently by serum from vaccinated individuals.[87,138] Most vaccines are expected to retain substantial efficacy against these established variants, although whether efficacy is retained at the maximal possible level remains unclear. Data from Israel reported in April 2021 suggest the beta variant may produce an increased likelihood of breakthrough infection in vaccinated individuals, but there are no data to support increased severity or transmission of such infections.[191] Finally, as of spring 2021, the potential for booster vaccines matched to VOCs has already been contemplated and appears promising. Serum from individuals infected with the beta variant potently neutralizes gamma and wild-type spike proteins, suggesting a vaccine encoding the beta spike may produce broad efficacy[257] against a variety of SARS-CoV-2 variants.

In addition to these three VOCs identified in fall and winter 2020, a fourth variant of concern was identified in early 2021 in California, identified as lineage B.1.427/429 (epsilon) containing RBD mutation L452R. This lineage appears to exhibit approximately 20% enhance transmissibility compared to variants previously circulating in the United States[76] but does not appear to pose a significant threat to vaccine efficacy[120] and in June 2021 was downgraded to a variant of interest as its frequency declined in competition of alpha and delta variants. As SARS-CoV-2 continues to circulate at high levels globally, additional variants continue to emerge. Amino acid changes at spike positions 484 and 681, most commonly E484K and P681H/R, respectively, repeatedly emerge in various lineages. This signal of convergent evolution is consistent with experimental support for E484K conferring a fitness advantage in the face of individual and population immunity, so as global vaccine coverage increases, viruses containing K484 may rise to dominance globally. Continued surveillance activities will be required to ensure vaccine formulations are optimized for dominant circulating viruses, and infrastructure put in place to deliver updated vaccines as warranted.

In late spring 2021, an additional variant of concern, B.1.617.2 (delta), was identified associated with the catastrophic SARS-CoV-2 epidemic in India. The delta variant contains RBD amino acid changes L452R and T478K, as well as a P681R substitution preceding the S1/S2 furin cleavage site. Following introduction to the United Kingdom, this variant rapidly displaced the alpha variant as the dominant lineage.[36,46] Compared to other VOC, delta is estimated to have the largest increase in reproductive number over nonvariant of concern lineages, explaining its displacement of the alpha variant where the two lineages have circulated in the same populations.[36] However, as with other variants, the role of specific amino acid changes in spike and other genes in enhancing transmission remains unclear. The P681R change in the delta variant enhances spike protein cleavage at S1/S2[284] and the furin cleavage site plays an important role in transmission and pathogenesis in ferrets. However, the significance of this with respect to transmission in humans is unknown. Finally, the delta variant exhibits enhanced neutralization resistance to convalescent and vaccine sera, but of a lower magnitude than the beta variant[221,222] and estimates of the impact on vaccine effectiveness are ongoing at the time of writing but expected to be modest in fully vaccinated individuals.

SARS-CoV-2: SECONDARY TRANSMISSION TO WILD AND DOMESTIC ANIMALS

In addition to its high infectivity in humans, SARS-CoV-2 exhibits a broad documented and predicted host range. Experimental infections of nonhuman primates,[258] hamsters,[308] ferrets,[178] and raccoon dogs[96] result in robust viral replication and, in some cases, disease. Although most of these represent experimental animal models, the susceptibility of raccoon dogs bears on their potential role as intermediate hosts, and they were widely solid in Wuhan markets in the fall of 2019.[407]

In silico structural modeling combined with functional binding studies have further expanded our understanding of the potential SARS-CoV-2 host range. Generally, in silico modeling has been informative but not perfectly correlated with functional binding assays. One comprehensive study, for example, predicted high binding affinity for human ACE-2 and very low affinity to Chinese pangolin (*M. pentadactyla*) ACE-2, a species closely related to the Malayan pangolin (*Manis javanica*), which is susceptible to viruses closely related to SARS-CoV-2.[192,384,407] The ACE-2 proteins of the two species share 99% amino acid identity. A more recent study, however, found that SARS-CoV-2 spike binds to Malayan pangolin ACE-2 with equivalent high identity as to human ACE-2, suggesting in silico studies may not be perfectly predictive of *in vivo* susceptibility.[272]

In numerous instances, humans have transmitted ACE-2 to domestic animals or captive wildlife, highlighting the potential for SARS-CoV-2 to establish new reservoirs outside its presumed natural range of southeast Asia and/or southern China. During the current period of continued epidemic transmission in humans, flare-ups from secondary reservoirs is not a major concern, but in a possible low endemicity future new outbreaks could be sparked from animal reservoirs worldwide, should they become established. Multiple diverse species factor in these potential concerns. While domestic rodents appear not susceptible to SARS-CoV-2, deer mice, a widely distributed wild rodent, are highly susceptible[89,122] and are a reservoir for other viruses that infect humans. Thus, the potential infection of wild deer mice represents a potential "spill-back" scenario for the permanent circulation of SARS-CoV-2 in wildlife, with the potential to seed future human outbreaks.[47] Additionally, widespread SARS-CoV-2 infection of white-tailed deer has been documented in North America.[47,131] Transmission from deer back to humans has not yet been identified, but the potential clearly exists given close contact between humans and these animals. Although the additional public health risk posed by such transmission may be limited while circulation remains high in the human population, as circulation ebbs spillback events may pose a greater risk of sparking local outbreaks.

Among domestic animals, felines and mink represent the most frequent animals infected via contact with infected humans. The most notorious instance of feline SARS-CoV-2 infection has been the infection of captive lions and tigers at the Bronx Zoo in 2020.[240] Other studies have found that infected humans routinely transmit SARS-CoV-2 to domestic cats.[33,132,141] Mink have proved particularly susceptible, and mink farms a fertile ground for large outbreaks and the emergence of potentially significant amino acid substitutions in the spike RBD. Mink outbreaks have occurred on farms in both North America[33,335] and Europe.[5,32,195] On multiple occasions, mink-derived viruses have spilled back into the human population resulting in community spread of these variants. This is of particular concern because mink-associated mutations such as spike Y453F are associated with reduced susceptibility to neutralization by some monoclonal antibodies,[139] raising the possibility that mink-derived outbreaks may produce infections

resistant to some therapeutics and increasing the need for the mink farming industry to implement rigorous biosecurity practices. Mink may also represent a potential spillback reservoir as wild and feral minks have repeatedly found to be infected with SARS-CoV-2, though whether such a reservoir would pose significant risk to humans remains unclear.

The broad potential host range of SARS-CoV-2 highlights its generalist properties as described by MacLean et al.[232] produced during its evolution in bats. In addition to secondary infections among domestic animals, captive and feral animals such as cats and mink may prove able to sustain SARS-CoV-2 transmission as new reservoir hosts. Given that these animals, in addition to susceptible wild rodents, come into frequent contact with other animals as well as humans the potential exists to spark human outbreaks with variants marked in some cases by altered neutralization susceptibility. This warrants continued surveillance, improved biosecurity in farming industries, and the necessity to suppress human transmission to minimize the risk of spillback.

REFERENCES

1. Adedeji AO, et al. Mechanism of nucleic acid unwinding by SARS-CoV helicase. *PLoS One* 2012;7:e36521.
2. Adedeji AO, et al. Severe acute respiratory syndrome coronavirus replication inhibitor that interferes with the nucleic acid unwinding of the viral helicase. *Antimicrob Agents Chemother* 2012;56:4718–4728.
3. Agostini ML, et al. Coronavirus susceptibility to the antiviral remdesivir (GS-5734) is mediated by the viral polymerase and the proofreading exoribonuclease. *MBio* 2018;9.
4. Agostini ML, et al. Small-molecule antiviral β-d-N (4)-hydroxycytidine inhibits a proofreading-intact coronavirus with a high genetic barrier to resistance. *J Virol* 2019;93.
5. Aguilo-Gisbert J, et al. First description of SARS-CoV-2 infection in two Feral American Mink (Neovison vison) caught in the wild. *Animals (Basel)* 2021;11.
6. Ahn DG, Choi JK, Taylor DR, et al. Biochemical characterization of a recombinant SARS coronavirus nsp12 RNA-dependent RNA polymerase capable of copying viral RNA templates. *Arch Virol* 2012;157:2095–2104.
7. Alhammad YMO, et al. The SARS-CoV-2 conserved macrodomain is a Mono-ADP-ribosylhydrolase. *J Virol* 2021;95.
8. Almeida MS, Johnson MA, Herrmann T, et al. Novel beta-barrel fold in the nuclear magnetic resonance structure of the replicase nonstructural protein 1 from the severe acute respiratory syndrome coronavirus. *J Virol* 2007;81:3151–3161.
9. Anand K, Ziebuhr J, Wadhwani P, et al. Coronavirus main proteinase (3CLpro) structure: basis for design of anti-SARS drugs. *Science* 2003;300:1763–1767.
10. Ancar R, et al. Physiologic RNA targets and refined sequence specificity of coronavirus EndoU. *RNA* 2020;26:1976–1999.
11. Andersen KG, Rambaut A, Lipkin WI, et al. The proximal origin of SARS-CoV-2. *Nat Med* 2020;26:450–452.
12. Angeletti S, et al. COVID-2019: the role of the nsp2 and nsp3 in its pathogenesis. *J Med Virol* 2020;92:584–588.
13. Angelini MM, Akhlaghpour M, Neuman BW, et al. Severe acute respiratory syndrome coronavirus nonstructural proteins 3, 4, and 6 induce double-membrane vesicles. *MBio* 2013;4.
14. Aouadi W, et al. Binding of the Methyl Donor S-Adenosyl-l-Methionine to Middle East respiratory syndrome coronavirus 2'-O-Methyltransferase nsp16 promotes recruitment of the allosteric activator nsp10. *J Virol* 2017;91.
15. Báez-Santos YM, St John SE, Mesecar AD. The SARS-coronavirus papain-like protease: structure, function and inhibition by designed antiviral compounds. *Antiviral Res* 2015;115:21–38.
16. Banerjee S, Chakrabarti A, Jha BK, et al. Cell-type-specific effects of RNase L on viral induction of beta interferon. *MBio* 2014;5:e00856.
17. Banerjee AK, et al. SARS-CoV-2 disrupts splicing, translation, and protein trafficking to suppress host defenses. *Cell* 2020;183:1325–1339.e1321.
18. Barrantes FJ. Structural biology of coronavirus ion channels. *Acta Crystallogr D Struct Biol* 2021;77:391–402.
19. Barretto N, et al. The papain-like protease of severe acute respiratory syndrome coronavirus has deubiquitinating activity. *J Virol* 2005;79:15189–15198.
20. Basu S, et al. Identifying SARS-CoV-2 antiviral compounds by screening for small molecule inhibitors of Nsp14 RNA cap methyltransferase. *Biochem J* 2021;478:2481–2497.
21. Bayati A, Kumar R, Francis V, et al. SARS-CoV-2 infects cells after viral entry via clathrin-mediated endocytosis. *J Biol Chem* 2021;296:100306.
22. Bestle D, et al. TMPRSS2 and furin are both essential for proteolytic activation of SARS-CoV-2 in human airway cells. *Life Sci Alliance* 2020;3.
23. Boni MF, et al. Evolutionary origins of the SARS-CoV-2 sarbecovirus lineage responsible for the COVID-19 pandemic. *Nat Microbiol* 2020;5:1408–1417. doi: 10.1038/s41564-020-0771-4.
24. Boras B, et al. Preclinical characterization of an intravenous coronavirus 3CL protease inhibitor for the potential treatment of COVID19. *Nat Commun* 2021;12:6055.

25. Boscarino JA, Logan HL, Lacny JJ, et al. Envelope protein palmitoylations are crucial for murine coronavirus assembly. *J Virol* 2008;82:2989–2999.
26. Boson B, et al. The SARS-CoV-2 envelope and membrane proteins modulate maturation and retention of the spike protein, allowing assembly of virus-like particles. *J Biol Chem* 2021;296:100111.
27. Bost AG, Carnahan RH, Lu XT, et al. Four proteins processed from the replicase gene polyprotein of mouse hepatitis virus colocalize in the cell periphery and adjacent to sites of virion assembly. *J Virol* 2000;74:3379–3387.
28. Bouvet M, et al. In vitro reconstitution of SARS-coronavirus mRNA cap methylation. *PLoS Pathog* 2010;6:e1000863.
29. Bouvet M, et al. Coronavirus Nsp10, a critical co-factor for activation of multiple replicative enzymes. *J Biol Chem* 2014;289:25783–25796.
30. Bracquemond D, Muriaux D. Betacoronavirus assembly: clues and perspectives for elucidating SARS-CoV-2 particle formation and egress. *mBio* 2021;12:e0237121.
31. Brosey CA, et al. Targeting SARS-CoV-2 Nsp3 macrodomain structure with insights from human poly(ADP-ribose) glycohydrolase (PARG) structures with inhibitors. *Prog Biophys Mol Biol* 2021;163:171–186. doi: 10.1016/j.pbiomolbio.2021.02.002.
32. Burkholz S, et al. Paired SARS-CoV-2 spike protein mutations observed during ongoing SARS-CoV-2 viral transfer from humans to minks and back to humans. *Infect Genet Evol* 2021;93:104897.
33. Cai Y, et al. CD26/DPP4 cell-surface expression in bat cells correlates with bat cell susceptibility to Middle East respiratory syndrome coronavirus (MERS-CoV) infection and evolution of persistent infection. *PLoS One* 2014;9:e112060.
34. Cai Y, et al. Distinct conformational states of SARS-CoV-2 spike protein. *Science* 2020;369:1586–1592.
35. Caillet-Saguy C, et al. Host PDZ-containing proteins targeted by SARS-CoV-2. *FEBS J* 2021;288:5148–5162.
36. Campbell F, et al. Increased transmissibility and global spread of SARS-CoV-2 variants of concern as at June 2021. *Euro Surveill* 2021;26.
37. Canal B, et al. Identifying SARS-CoV-2 antiviral compounds by screening for small molecule inhibitors of nsp14/nsp10 exoribonuclease. *Biochem J* 2021;478:2445–2464.
38. Canton J, et al. MERS-CoV 4b protein interferes with the NF-kappaB-dependent innate immune response during infection. *PLoS Pathog* 2018;14:e1006838.
39. Cao B, et al. A trial of lopinavir-ritonavir in adults hospitalized with severe Covid-19. *N Engl J Med* 2020;382:1787–1799.
40. Cao Z, et al. Ubiquitination of SARS-CoV-2 ORF7a promotes antagonism of interferon response. *Cell Mol Immunol* 2021;18:746–748.
41. Case JB, et al. Murine hepatitis virus nsp14 exoribonuclease activity is required for resistance to innate immunity. *J Virol* 2018;92.
42. Castaño-Rodriguez C, et al. Role of severe acute respiratory syndrome coronavirus viroporins E, 3a, and 8a in replication and pathogenesis. *MBio* 2018;9.
43. Castelli JC, et al. A study of the interferon antiviral mechanism: apoptosis activation by the 2-5A system. *J Exp Med* 1997;186:967–972.
44. Chai J, et al. Structural basis for SARS-CoV-2 envelope protein recognition of human cell junction protein PALS1. *Nat Commun* 2021;12:3433.
45. Chakrabarti A, et al. RNase L activates the NLRP3 inflammasome during viral infections. *Cell Host Microbe* 2015;17:466–477.
46. Challen R, et al. Early epidemiological signatures of novel SARS-CoV-2 variants: establishment of B.1.617.2 in England. *medRxiv* 2021. doi: https://doi.org/10.1101/2021.06.05.21258365.
47. Chandler JC, et al. SARS-CoV-2 exposure in wild white-tailed deer (Odocoileus virginianus). *Proc Natl Acad Sci U S A* 2021;118.
48. Chen L, et al. Cinanserin is an inhibitor of the 3C-like proteinase of severe acute respiratory syndrome coronavirus and strongly reduces virus replication in vitro. *J Virol* 2005;79:7095–7103.
49. Chen CY, et al. Structure of the SARS coronavirus nucleocapsid protein RNA-binding dimerization domain suggests a mechanism for helical packaging of viral RNA. *J Mol Biol* 2007;368:1075–1086.
50. Chen Y, et al. Functional screen reveals SARS coronavirus nonstructural protein nsp14 as a novel cap N7 methyltransferase. *Proc Natl Acad Sci U S A* 2009;106:3484–3489.
51. Chen Y, et al. Biochemical and structural insights into the mechanisms of SARS coronavirus RNA ribose 2′-O-methylation by nsp16/nsp10 protein complex. *PLoS Pathog* 2011;7:e1002294.
52. Chen J, et al. Structural basis for helicase-polymerase coupling in the SARS-CoV-2 replication-transcription complex. *Cell* 2020;182:1560–1573.e1513.
53. Chen D, et al. ORF3a of SARS-CoV-2 promotes lysosomal exocytosis-mediated viral egress. *Dev Cell* 2021;56:3250–3263.e5. doi: 10.1016/j.devcel.2021.10.006.
54. Cheng YW, et al. D614G substitution of SARS-CoV-2 spike protein increases syncytium formation and virus titer via enhanced furin-mediated spike cleavage. *MBio* 2021;12:e0058721.
55. Chien M, et al. Nucleotide analogues as inhibitors of SARS-CoV-2 polymerase, a key drug target for COVID-19. *J Proteome Res* 2020;19:4690–4697.
56. Chu CM, et al. Role of lopinavir/ritonavir in the treatment of SARS: initial virological and clinical findings. *Thorax* 2004;59:252–256.
57. Clark LK, Green TJ, Petit CM. Structure of nonstructural protein 1 from SARS-CoV-2. *J Virol* 2021;95.
58. Claverie JM. A putative role of de-Mono-ADP-Ribosylation of STAT1 by the SARS-CoV-2 Nsp3 protein in the cytokine storm syndrome of COVID-19. *Viruses* 2020;12.
59. Clementz MA, et al. Deubiquitinating and interferon antagonism activities of coronavirus papain-like proteases. *J Virol* 2010;84:4619–4629.
60. Cong Y, et al. Nucleocapsid protein recruitment to replication-transcription complexes plays a crucial role in coronaviral life cycle. *J Virol* 2020;94.
61. Cornillez-Ty CT, Liao L, Yates JR III, et al. Severe acute respiratory syndrome coronavirus nonstructural protein 2 interacts with a host protein complex involved in mitochondrial biogenesis and intracellular signaling. *J Virol* 2009;83:10314–10318.
62. Coronaviridae Study Group of the International Committee on Taxonomy of Viruses. The species Severe acute respiratory syndrome-related coronavirus: classifying 2019-nCoV and naming it SARS-CoV-2. *Nat Microbiol* 2020;5:536–544.
63. Coutard B, et al. The spike glycoprotein of the new coronavirus 2019-nCoV contains a furin-like cleavage site absent in CoV of the same clade. *Antiviral Res* 2020;176:104742.
64. Coutinho RM, et al. Model-based estimation of transmissibility and reinfection of SARS-CoV-2 P.1 variant. *Commun Med* 2021;1(48).
65. Daffis S, et al. 2′-O methylation of the viral mRNA cap evades host restriction by IFIT family members. *Nature* 2010;468:452–456.
66. Davies JP, Almasy KM, McDonald EF, et al. Comparative multiplexed interactomics of SARS-CoV-2 and homologous coronavirus nonstructural proteins identifies unique and shared host-cell dependencies. *ACS Infect Dis* 2020;6:3174–3189.
67. Davies NG, et al. Estimated transmissibility and impact of SARS-CoV-2 lineage B.1.1.7 in England. *Science* 2021;372:eabg3055.
68. de Haan CA, Kuo L, Masters PS, et al. Coronavirus particle assembly: primary structure requirements of the membrane protein. *J Virol* 1998;72:6838–6850.
69. de Haan CA, Rottier PJ. Molecular interactions in the assembly of coronaviruses. *Adv Virus Res* 2005;64:165–230.
70. Decroly E, et al. Coronavirus nonstructural protein 16 is a cap-0 binding enzyme possessing (nucleoside-2′O)-methyltransferase activity. *J Virol* 2008;82:8071–8084.
71. Decroly E, et al. Crystal structure and functional analysis of the SARS-coronavirus RNA cap 2′-O-methyltransferase nsp10/nsp16 complex. *PLoS Pathog* 2011;7:e1002059.
72. DeDiego ML, et al. A severe acute respiratory syndrome coronavirus that lacks the E gene is attenuated in vitro and in vivo. *J Virol* 2007;81:1701–1713.
73. DeDiego ML, et al. Coronavirus virulence genes with main focus on SARS-CoV envelope gene. *Virus Res* 2014;194:124–137.
74. Deming DJ, Graham RL, Denison MR, et al. Processing of open reading frame 1a replicase proteins nsp7 to nsp10 in murine hepatitis virus strain A59 replication. *J Virol* 2007;81:10280–10291.
75. Deng X, et al. Structure-guided mutagenesis alters deubiquitinating activity and attenuates pathogenesis of a murine coronavirus. *J Virol* 2020;94:e01734.
76. Deng X, et al. Transmission, infectivity, and antibody neutralization of an emerging SARS-CoV-2 variant in California carrying a L452R spike protein mutation. *medRxiv* 2021;2021.03.07.21252647. doi: 10.1101/2021.03.07.21252647.
77. Denison MR, et al. The putative helicase of the coronavirus mouse hepatitis virus is processed from the replicase gene polyprotein and localizes in complexes that are active in viral RNA synthesis. *J Virol* 1999;73:6862–6871.
78. Devaraj SG, et al. Regulation of IRF-3-dependent innate immunity by the papain-like protease domain of the severe acute respiratory syndrome coronavirus. *J Biol Chem* 2007;282:32208–32221.
79. Donaldson EF, Sims AC, Graham RL, et al. Murine hepatitis virus replicase protein nsp10 is a critical regulator of viral RNA synthesis. *J Virol* 2007;81:6356–6368.
80. Dong B, Silverman RH. 2-5A-dependent RNase molecules dimerize during activation by 2-5A. *J Biol Chem* 1995;270:4133–4137.
81. Drexler JF, et al. Genomic characterization of severe acute respiratory syndrome-related coronavirus in european bats and classification of coronaviruses based on partial RNA-dependent RNA polymerase gene sequences. *J Virol* 2010;84:11336–11349.
82. Drosten C, et al. Identification of a novel coronavirus in patients with severe acute respiratory syndrome. *N Engl J Med* 2003;348:1967–1976.
83. Echavarria-Consuegra L, et al. Manipulation of the unfolded protein response: a pharmacological strategy against coronavirus infection. *PLoS Pathog* 2021;17:e1009644.
84. Eckerle LD, Lu X, Sperry SM, et al. High fidelity of murine hepatitis virus replication is decreased in nsp14 exoribonuclease mutants. *J Virol* 2007;81:12135–12144.
85. Eckerle LD, et al. Infidelity of SARS-CoV Nsp14-exonuclease mutant virus replication is revealed by complete genome sequencing. *PLoS Pathog* 2010;6:e1000896.
86. Edara VV, et al. Infection and mRNA-1273 vaccine antibodies neutralize SARS-CoV-2 UK variant. *medRxiv* 2021;2021.02.02.21250799.
87. Edara VV, et al. Infection- and vaccine-induced antibody binding and neutralization of the B.1.351 SARS-CoV-2 variant. *Cell Host Microbe* 2021;29:516–521.e513.
88. Egloff MP, et al. Structural and functional basis for ADP-ribose and poly(ADP-ribose) binding by viral macro domains. *J Virol* 2006;80:8493–8502.
89. Fagre A, et al. SARS-CoV-2 infection, neuropathogenesis and transmission among deer mice: implications for spillback to New World rodents. *PLoS Pathog* 2021;17:e1009585.
90. Fan X, Cao D, Kong L, et al. Cryo-EM analysis of the post-fusion structure of the SARS-CoV spike glycoprotein. *Nat Commun* 2020;11:3618.
91. Faria NR, et al. Genomics and epidemiology of the P.1 SARS-CoV-2 lineage in Manaus, Brazil. *Science* 2021;372:815–821. doi: 10.1126/science.abh2644, eabh2644.
92. Fehr AR, et al. The conserved coronavirus macrodomain promotes virulence and suppresses the innate immune response during severe acute respiratory syndrome coronavirus infection. *MBio* 2016;7.
93. Ferron F, Decroly E, Selisko B, et al. The viral RNA capping machinery as a target for antiviral drugs. *Antiviral Res* 2012;96:21–31.
94. Ferron F, et al. Structural and molecular basis of mismatch correction and ribavirin excision from coronavirus RNA. *Proc Natl Acad Sci U S A* 2018;115:E162–E171.
95. Filipowicz W, et al. A protein binding the methylated 5′-terminal sequence, m7GpppN, of eukaryotic messenger RNA. *Proc Natl Acad Sci U S A* 1976;73:1559–1563.
96. Freuling CM, et al. Susceptibility of raccoon dogs for experimental SARS-CoV-2 infection. *Emerg Infect Dis* 2020;26:2982–2985.
97. Freundt EC, et al. The open reading frame 3a protein of severe acute respiratory syndrome-associated coronavirus promotes membrane rearrangement and cell death. *J Virol* 2010;84:1097–1109.
98. Frieman M, Ratia K, Johnston RE, et al. Severe acute respiratory syndrome coronavirus papain-like protease ubiquitin-like domain and catalytic domain regulate antagonism of IRF3 and NF-kappaB signaling. *J Virol* 2009;83:6689–6705.
99. Frieman M, et al. Severe acute respiratory syndrome coronavirus ORF6 antagonizes STAT1 function by sequestering nuclear import factors on the rough endoplasmic reticulum/Golgi membrane. *J Virol* 2007;81:9812–9824.
100. Fu L, et al. Both boceprevir and GC376 efficaciously inhibit SARS-CoV-2 by targeting its main protease. *Nat Commun* 2020;11:4417.
101. Gao X, et al. Crystal structure of SARS-CoV-2 papain-like protease. *Acta Pharm Sin B* 2021;11:237–245.

102. Ge XY, et al. Isolation and characterization of a bat SARS-like coronavirus that uses the ACE2 receptor. *Nature* 2013;503:535–538.
103. Ge XY, et al. Coexistence of multiple coronaviruses in several bat colonies in an abandoned mineshaft. *Virol Sin* 2016;31:31–40.
104. Gerna G, et al. Coronaviruses and gastroenteritis: evidence of antigenic relatedness between human enteric coronavirus strains and human coronavirus OC43. *Microbiologica* 1984;7:315–322.
105. Ghosh S, et al. β-Coronaviruses use lysosomes for egress instead of the biosynthetic secretory pathway. *Cell* 2020;183:1520–1535.e1514.
106. Glowacka I, et al. Evidence that TMPRSS2 activates the severe acute respiratory syndrome coronavirus spike protein for membrane fusion and reduces viral control by the humoral immune response. *J Virol* 2011;85:4122–4134.
107. Goldstein SA, Brown J, Pedersen BS, et al. Extensive recombination-driven coronavirus diversification expands the pool of potential pandemic pathogens. *bioRxiv* 2021;10.1101/2021.02.03.429646.
108. Gomez GN, Abrar F, Dodhia MP, et al. SARS coronavirus protein nsp1 disrupts localization of Nup93 from the nuclear pore complex. *Biochem Cell Biol* 2019;97:758–766.
109. Gorbalenya AB, Baric S, de Groot R, et al. The species severe acute respiratory syndrome-related coronavirus: classifying 2019-nCoV and naming it SARS-CoV-2. *Nat Microbiol* 2020;5:536–544.
110. Gorbalenya AE, Koonin EV, Donchenko AP, et al. Coronavirus genome: prediction of putative functional domains in the non-structural polyprotein by comparative amino acid sequence analysis. *Nucleic Acids Res* 1989;17:4847–4861.
111. Gordon CJ, Tchesnokov EP, Feng JY, et al. The antiviral compound remdesivir potently inhibits RNA-dependent RNA polymerase from Middle East respiratory syndrome coronavirus. *J Biol Chem* 2020;295:4773–4779.
112. Gordon DE, et al. Comparative host-coronavirus protein interaction networks reveal pan-viral disease mechanisms. *Science* 2020;370.
113. Gordon DE, et al. A SARS-CoV-2 protein interaction map reveals targets for drug repurposing. *Nature* 2020;583:459–468.
114. Gordon CJ, et al. Remdesivir is a direct-acting antiviral that inhibits RNA-dependent RNA polymerase from severe acute respiratory syndrome coronavirus 2 with high potency. *J Biol Chem* 2020;295:6785–6797.
115. Gosert R, Kanjanahaluethai A, Egger D, et al. RNA replication of mouse hepatitis virus takes place at double-membrane vesicles. *J Virol* 2002;76:3697–3708.
116. Graham RL, Baric RS. Recombination, reservoirs, and the modular spike: mechanisms of coronavirus cross-species transmission. *J Virol* 2010;84:3134–3146.
117. Graham RL, Sims AC, Brockway SM, et al. The nsp2 replicase proteins of murine hepatitis virus and severe acute respiratory syndrome coronavirus are dispensable for viral replication. *J Virol* 2005;79:13399–13411.
118. Graham RL, et al. A live, impaired-fidelity coronavirus vaccine protects in an aged, immunocompromised mouse model of lethal disease. *Nat Med* 2012;18:1820–1826.
119. Greaney AJ, et al. The SARS-CoV-2 mRNA-1273 vaccine elicits more RBD-focused neutralization, but with broader antibody binding within the RBD. *bioRxiv* 2021;2021.04.14.439844.
120. Greaney AJ, et al. Comprehensive mapping of mutations in the SARS-CoV-2 receptor-binding domain that affect recognition by polyclonal human plasma antibodies. *Cell Host Microbe* 2021;29:463–476.e466.
121. Gribble J, et al. The coronavirus proofreading exoribonuclease mediates extensive viral recombination. *PLoS Pathog* 2021;17:e1009226.
122. Griffin BD, et al. SARS-CoV-2 infection and transmission in the North American deer mouse. *Nat Commun* 2021;12:3612.
123. Guan Y, et al. Isolation and characterization of viruses related to the SARS coronavirus from animals in Southern China. *Science* 2003;302:276–278.
124. Günther S, et al. X-ray screening identifies active site and allosteric inhibitors of SARS-CoV-2 main protease. *Science* 2021;372:642–646.
125. Guo H, et al. Evolutionary arms race between virus and host drives genetic diversity in bat severe acute respiratory syndrome-related coronavirus spike genes. *J Virol* 2020;94.
126. Hackbart M, Deng X, Baker SC. Coronavirus endoribonuclease targets viral polyuridine sequences to evade activating host sensors. *Proc Natl Acad Sci U S A* 2020;117:8094–8103.
127. Hagemeijer MC, Vonk AM, Monastyrska I, et al. Visualizing coronavirus RNA synthesis in time by using click chemistry. *J Virol* 2012;86:5808–5816.
128. Hagemeijer MC, et al. Dynamics of coronavirus replication-transcription complexes. *J Virol* 2010;84:2134–2149.
129. Hagemeijer MC, et al. Mobility and interactions of coronavirus nonstructural protein 4. *J Virol* 2011;85:4572–4577.
130. Hagemeijer MC, et al. Membrane rearrangements mediated by coronavirus nonstructural proteins 3 and 4. *Virology* 2014;458-459:125–135.
131. Hale VL, et al. SARS-CoV-2 infection in free-ranging white-tailed deer (Odocoileus virginianus). *bioRxiv* 2021. Nature volume 602, pages 481–486 (2022).
132. Hamer SA, et al. SARS-CoV-2 infections and viral isolations among serially tested cats and dogs in households with infected owners in Texas, USA. *Viruses* 2021;13.
133. Hao W, et al. Crystal structure of Middle East respiratory syndrome coronavirus helicase. *PLoS Pathog* 2017;13:e1006474.
134. Heald-Sargent T, Gallagher T. Ready, set, fuse! The coronavirus spike protein and acquisition of fusion competence. *Viruses* 2012;4:557–580.
135. Heusipp G, Harms U, Siddell SG, et al. Identification of an ATPase activity associated with a 71-kilodalton polypeptide encoded in gene 1 of the human coronavirus 229E. *J Virol* 1997;71:5631–5634.
136. Hoffmann M, Kleine-Weber H, Pöhlmann S. A multibasic cleavage site in the spike protein of SARS-CoV-2 is essential for infection of human lung cells. *Mol Cell* 2020;78:779–784.e5. doi: 10.1016/j.molcel.2020.04.022.
137. Hoffmann M, et al. SARS-CoV-2 cell entry depends on ACE2 and TMPRSS2 and is blocked by a clinically proven protease inhibitor. *Cell* 2020;181:271–280.e278.
138. Hoffmann M, et al. SARS-CoV-2 variants B.1.351 and P.1 escape from neutralizing antibodies. *Cell* 2021;184:2384–2393.e23. doi: 10.1016/j.cell.2021.03.036.
139. Hoffmann M, et al. SARS-CoV-2 mutations acquired in mink reduce antibody-mediated neutralization. *Cell Rep* 2021;35:109017.
140. Hogue BG, Machamer CM. Coronavirus structural proteins and assembly. In: Perlman SG, ed. *The Nidoviruses*. Washington, DC: American Society for Microbiology Press; 2008:179–200.
141. Hosie MJ, et al. Anthropogenic infection of cats during the 2020 COVID-19 pandemic. *Viruses* 2021;13.
142. Hsu JC, Laurent-Rolle M, Pawlak JB, et al. Translational shutdown and evasion of the innate immune response by SARS-CoV-2 NSP14 protein. *Proc Natl Acad Sci U S A* 2021;118.
143. Hu B, et al. Discovery of a rich gene pool of bat SARS-related coronaviruses provides new insights into the origin of SARS coronavirus. *PLoS Pathog* 2017;13:e1006698.
144. Huang C, Ito N, Tseng CT, et al. Severe acute respiratory syndrome coronavirus 7a accessory protein is a viral structural protein. *J Virol* 2006;80:7287–7294.
145. Huang Q, et al. Structure of the N-terminal RNA-binding domain of the SARS CoV nucleocapsid protein. *Biochemistry* 2004;43:6059–6063.
146. Huang C, et al. SARS coronavirus nsp1 protein induces template-dependent endonucleolytic cleavage of mRNAs: viral mRNAs are resistant to nsp1-induced RNA cleavage. *PLoS Pathog* 2011;7:e1002433.
147. Huang C, et al. Alphacoronavirus transmissible gastroenteritis virus nsp1 protein suppresses protein translation in mammalian cells and in cell-free HeLa cell extracts but not in rabbit reticulocyte lysate. *J Virol* 2011;85:638–643.
148. Hul V, et al. A novel SARS-CoV-2 related coronavirus in bats from Cambodia. *Nat Commun* 2021;12(6563).
149. Hur S. Double-stranded RNA sensors and modulators in innate immunity. *Annu Rev Immunol* 2019;37:349–375.
150. Hurst KR, Koetzner CA, Masters PS. Characterization of a critical interaction between the coronavirus nucleocapsid protein and nonstructural protein 3 of the viral replicase-transcriptase complex. *J Virol* 2013;87:9159–9172.
151. Imbert I, et al. A second, non-canonical RNA-dependent RNA polymerase in SARS coronavirus. *Embo J* 2006;25:4933–4942.
152. Imbert I, et al. The SARS-Coronavirus PLnc domain of nsp3 as a replication/transcription scaffolding protein. *Virus Res* 2008;133:136–148.
153. Issa E, Merhi G, Panossian B, et al. SARS-CoV-2 and ORF3a: nonsynonymous mutations, functional domains, and viral pathogenesis. *mSystems* 2020;5.
154. Ito N, et al. Severe acute respiratory syndrome coronavirus 3a protein is a viral structural protein. *J Virol* 2005;79:3182–3186.
155. Ivanov KA, et al. Multiple enzymatic activities associated with severe acute respiratory syndrome coronavirus helicase. *J Virol* 2004;78:5619–5632.
156. Ivanov KA, et al. Major genetic marker of nidoviruses encodes a replicative endoribonuclease. *Proc Natl Acad Sci U S A* 2004;101:12694–12699.
157. Jackson CB, Farzan M, Chen B, et al. Mechanisms of SARS-CoV-2 entry into cells. *Nat Rev Mol Cell Biol* 2022;23:3–20. doi: 10.1038/s41580-021-00418-x, 1–18.
158. Jauregui AR, Savalia D, Lowry VK, et al. Identification of residues of SARS-CoV nsp1 that differentially affect inhibition of gene expression and antiviral signaling. *PLoS One* 2013;8:e62416.
159. Javorsky A, Humbert PO, Kvansakul M. Structural basis of coronavirus E protein interactions with human PALS1 PDZ domain. *Commun Biol* 2021;4:724.
160. Jia Z, et al. Delicate structural coordination of the severe acute respiratory syndrome coronavirus Nsp13 upon ATP hydrolysis. *Nucleic Acids Res* 2019;47:6538–6550.
161. Jiang HW, et al. SARS-CoV-2 Orf9b suppresses type I interferon responses by targeting TOM70. *Cell Mol Immunol* 2020;17:998–1000.
162. Jimenez-Guardeno JM, et al. The PDZ-binding motif of severe acute respiratory syndrome coronavirus envelope protein is a determinant of viral pathogenesis. *PLoS Pathog* 2014;10:e1004320.
163. Jimenez-Guardeno JM, et al. Identification of the mechanisms causing reversion to virulence in an attenuated SARS-CoV for the design of a genetically stable vaccine. *PLoS Pathog* 2015;11:e1005215.
164. Jin Z, et al. Structure of M^{pro} from SARS-CoV-2 and discovery of its inhibitors. *Nature* 2020;582:289–293.
165. Joseph JS, et al. Crystal structure of nonstructural protein 10 from the severe acute respiratory syndrome coronavirus reveals a novel fold with two zinc-binding motifs. *J Virol* 2006;80:7894–7901.
166. Jungreis I, et al. Conflicting and ambiguous names of overlapping ORFs in the SARS-CoV-2 genome: a homology-based resolution. *Virology* 2021;558:145–151.
167. Kamitani W, Huang C, Narayanan K, et al. A two-pronged strategy to suppress host protein synthesis by SARS coronavirus Nsp1 protein. *Nat Struct Mol Biol* 2009;16:1134–1140.
168. Kamitani W, et al. Severe acute respiratory syndrome coronavirus nsp1 protein suppresses host gene expression by promoting host mRNA degradation. *Proc Natl Acad Sci U S A* 2006;103:12885–12890.
169. Kang R, Tang D. PKR-dependent inflammatory signals. *Sci Signal* 2012;5:pe47.
170. Kang H, et al. Biochemical and genetic analyses of murine hepatitis virus Nsp15 endoribonuclease. *J Virol* 2007;81:13587–13597.
171. Kang L, et al. A selective sweep in the Spike gene has driven SARS-CoV-2 human adaptation. *Cell* 2021;184:4392–4400.e4.
172. Kapikian AZ. The coronaviruses. *Dev Biol Stand* 1975;28:42–64.
173. Kasprzyk R, et al. Identification and evaluation of potential SARS-CoV-2 antiviral agents targeting mRNA cap guanine N7-Methyltransferase. *Antiviral Res* 2021;193:105142.
174. Ke Z, et al. Structures and distributions of SARS-CoV-2 spike proteins on intact virions. *Nature* 2020;588:498–502.
175. Kim Y, et al. Broad-spectrum antivirals against 3C or 3C-like proteases of picornaviruses, noroviruses, and coronaviruses. *J Virol* 2012;86:11754–11762.
176. Kim Y, et al. Broad-spectrum inhibitors against 3C-like proteases of feline coronaviruses and feline caliciviruses. *J Virol* 2015;89:4942–4950.
177. Kim Y, et al. Reversal of the progression of fatal coronavirus infection in cats by a broad-spectrum coronavirus protease inhibitor. *PLoS Pathog* 2016;12:e1005531.

178. Kim YI, et al. Infection and rapid transmission of SARS-CoV-2 in ferrets. *Cell Host Microbe* 2020;27:704–709.
179. Kindler E, et al. Early endonuclease-mediated evasion of RNA sensing ensures efficient coronavirus replication. *PLoS Pathog* 2017;13:e1006195.
180. Kirchdoerfer RN, Ward AB. Structure of the SARS-CoV nsp12 polymerase bound to nsp7 and nsp8 co-factors. *Nat Commun* 2019;10:2342.
181. Kirchdoerfer RN, et al. Pre-fusion structure of a human coronavirus spike protein. *Nature* 2016;531:118–121.
182. Klein S, et al. SARS-CoV-2 structure and replication characterized by in situ cryo-electron tomography. *Nat Commun* 2020;11:5885.
183. Klemm T, et al. Mechanism and inhibition of the papain-like protease, PLpro, of SARS-CoV-2. *EMBO J* 2020;39:e106275.
184. Klumperman J, et al. Coronavirus M proteins accumulate in the Golgi complex beyond the site of virion budding. *J Virol* 1994;68:6523–6534.
185. Kokic G, et al. Mechanism of SARS-CoV-2 polymerase stalling by remdesivir. *Nat Commun* 2021;12:279.
186. Konno Y, et al. SARS-CoV-2 ORF3b is a potent interferon antagonist whose activity is increased by a naturally occurring elongation variant. *Cell Rep* 2020;32:108185.
187. Korber B, et al. Tracking changes in SARS-CoV-2 spike: evidence that D614G increases infectivity of the COVID-19 virus. *Cell* 2020;182:812–827.e819.
188. Krupovic M, Koonin EV. Multiple origins of viral capsid proteins from cellular ancestors. *Proc Natl Acad Sci U S A* 2017;114:E2401–E2410.
189. Kuri T, et al. The ADP-ribose-1''-monophosphatase domains of severe acute respiratory syndrome coronavirus and human coronavirus 229E mediate resistance to antiviral interferon responses. *J Gen Virol* 2011;92:1899–1905.
190. Kusov Y, Tan J, Alvarez E, et al. A G-quadruplex-binding macrodomain within the "SARS-unique domain" is essential for the activity of the SARS-coronavirus replication-transcription complex. *Virology* 2015;484:313–322.
191. Kustin T, et al. Evidence for increased breakthrough rates of SARS-CoV-2 variants of concern in BNT162b2 mRNA vaccinated individuals. *Nat Med* 2021;27:1379–1384.
192. Lam TTY, et al. Identifying SARS-CoV-2-related coronaviruses in Malayan pangolins. *Nature* 2020;583:282–285.
193. Lan J, et al. Structure of the SARS-CoV-2 spike receptor-binding domain bound to the ACE2 receptor. *Nature* 2020;581:215–220.
194. Lapointe CP, et al. Dynamic competition between SARS-CoV-2 NSP1 and mRNA on the human ribosome inhibits translation initiation. *Proc Natl Acad Sci U S A* 2021;118.
195. Larsen HD, et al. Preliminary report of an outbreak of SARS-CoV-2 in mink and mink farmers associated with community spread, Denmark, June to November 2020. *Euro Surveill* 2021;26.
196. Latinne A, et al. Origin and cross-species transmission of bat coronaviruses in China. *Nat Commun* 2020;11:4235.
197. Lau SK, et al. Severe acute respiratory syndrome coronavirus-like virus in Chinese horseshoe bats. *Proc Natl Acad Sci U S A* 2005;102:14040–14045.
198. Lau SK, et al. Coronavirus HKU1 and other coronavirus infections in Hong Kong. *J Clin Microbiol* 2006;44:2063–2071.
199. Lau SKP, et al. Severe acute respiratory syndrome (SARS) coronavirus ORF8 protein is acquired from SARS-related coronavirus from greater horseshoe bats through recombination. *J Virol* 2015;89:10532–10547.
200. Lee N, et al. A major outbreak of severe acute respiratory syndrome in Hong Kong. *N Engl J Med* 2003;348:1986–1994.
201. Lee S, et al. Genetic characteristics of coronaviruses from Korean bats in 2016. *Microb Ecol* 2018;75:174–182.
202. Lee J, et al. No evidence of coronaviruses or other potentially zoonotic viruses in sunda pangolins (Manis javanica) entering the wildlife trade via Malaysia. *Ecohealth* 2020;17:406–418.
203. Lehmann KC, Snijder EJ, Posthuma CC, et al. What we know but do not understand about nidovirus helicases. *Virus Res* 2015;202:12–32.
204. Lehmann KC, et al. Discovery of an essential nucleotidylating activity associated with a newly delineated conserved domain in the RNA polymerase-containing protein of all nidoviruses. *Nucleic Acids Res* 2015;43:8416–8434.
205. Lei J, Kusov Y, Hilgenfeld R. Nsp3 of coronaviruses: structures and functions of a large multi-domain protein. *Antiviral Res* 2018;149:58–74.
206. Lei X, et al. Activation and evasion of type I interferon responses by SARS-CoV-2. *Nat Commun* 2020;11:3810.
207. Letko M, Marzi A, Munster V. Functional assessment of cell entry and receptor usage for SARS-CoV-2 and other lineage B betacoronaviruses. *Nat Microbiol* 2020;5:562–569.
208. Li F. Structure, function, and evolution of coronavirus spike proteins. *Annu Rev Virol* 2016;3:237–261.
209. Li W, et al. Angiotensin-converting enzyme 2 is a functional receptor for the SARS coronavirus. *Nature* 2003;426:450–454.
210. Li W, et al. Bats are natural reservoirs of SARS-like coronaviruses. *Science* 2005;310:676–679.
211. Li Y, et al. Activation of RNase L is dependent on OAS3 expression during infection with diverse human viruses. *Proc Natl Acad Sci U S A* 2016;113:2241–2246.
212. Li S, et al. Regulation of the ER stress response by the ion channel activity of the infectious bronchitis coronavirus envelope protein modulates virion release, apoptosis, viral fitness, and pathogenesis. *Front Microbiol* 2019;10:3022.
213. Li Y, et al. SARS-CoV-2 induces double-stranded RNA-mediated innate immune responses in respiratory epithelial-derived cells and cardiomyocytes. *Proc Natl Acad Sci U S A* 2021;118.
214. Lim KP, Liu DX. The missing link in coronavirus assembly. Retention of the avian coronavirus infectious bronchitis virus envelope protein in the pre-Golgi compartments and physical interaction between the envelope and membrane proteins. *J Biol Chem* 2001;276:17515–17523.
215. Lin S, et al. Crystal structure of SARS-CoV-2 nsp10 bound to nsp14-ExoN domain reveals an exoribonuclease with both structural and functional integrity. *Nucleic Acids Res* 2021;49:5382–5392.
216. Lindner HA, et al. The papain-like protease from the severe acute respiratory syndrome coronavirus is a deubiquitinating enzyme. *J Virol* 2005;79:15199–15208.
217. Littler DR, Gully BS, Colson RN, et al. Crystal structure of the SARS-CoV-2 non-structural protein 9, Nsp9. *iScience* 2020;23:101258.
218. Liu C, et al. The architecture of inactivated SARS-CoV-2 with postfusion spikes revealed by Cryo-EM and Cryo-ET. *Structure* 2020;28:1218–1224.e1214.
219. Liu Y, et al. The development of Coronavirus 3C-Like protease (3CL(pro)) inhibitors from 2010 to 2020. *Eur J Med Chem* 2020;206:112711.
220. Liu C, et al. Structural basis of mismatch recognition by a SARS-CoV-2 proofreading enzyme. *Science* 2021;373:1142–1146.
221. Liu C, et al. Reduced neutralization of SARS-CoV-2 B.1.617 by vaccine and convalescent serum. *Cell* 2021;184:4220–4236.e13. doi: 10.1016/j.cell.2021.06.020.
222. Liu J, et al. BNT162b2-elicited neutralization of B.1.617 and other SARS-CoV-2 variants. *Nature* 2021;596:273–275. doi: 10.1038/s41586-021-03693-y.
223. Locker JK, et al. The cytoplasmic tail of mouse hepatitis virus M protein is essential but not sufficient for its retention in the Golgi complex. *J Biol Chem* 1994;269:28263–28269.
224. Lokugamage KG, Narayanan K, Huang C, et al. Severe acute respiratory syndrome coronavirus protein nsp1 is a novel eukaryotic translation inhibitor that represses multiple steps of translation initiation. *J Virol* 2012;86:13598–13608.
225. Lopez LA, Riffle AJ, Pike SL, et al. Importance of conserved cysteine residues in the coronavirus envelope protein. *J Virol* 2008;82:3000–3010.
226. Lopusna K, et al. Interferons lambda, new cytokines with antiviral activity. *Acta Virol* 2013;57:171–179.
227. Lu R, et al. Genomic characterisation and epidemiology of 2019 novel coronavirus: implications for virus origins and receptor binding. *Lancet* 2020;395:565–574. doi: 10.1016/s0140-6736(20)30251-8.
228. Lugari A, et al. Molecular mapping of the RNA Cap 2′-O-methyltransferase activation interface between severe acute respiratory syndrome coronavirus nsp10 and nsp16. *J Biol Chem* 2010;285:33230–33241.
229. Ma Z, Pourfarjam Y, Kim IK. Reconstitution and functional characterization of SARS-CoV-2 proofreading complex. *Protein Expr Purif* 2021;185:105894.
230. Ma Y, et al. Structural basis and functional analysis of the SARS coronavirus nsp14-nsp10 complex. *Proc Natl Acad Sci U S A* 2015;112:9436–9441.
231. Machamer CE. Accommodation of large cargo within Golgi cisternae. *Histochem Cell Biol* 2013;140:261–269.
232. MacLean OA, et al. Natural selection in the evolution of SARS-CoV-2 in bats created a generalist virus and highly capable human pathogen. *PLoS Biol* 2021;19:e3001115.
233. Maio N, et al. Fe-S cofactors in the SARS-CoV-2 RNA-dependent RNA polymerase are potential antiviral targets. *Science* 2021;373:236–241.
234. Malathi K, Dong B, Gale M Jr, et al. Small self-RNA generated by RNase L amplifies antiviral innate immunity. *Nature* 2007;448:816–819.
235. Ma-Lauer Y, et al. p53 down-regulates SARS coronavirus replication and is targeted by the SARS-unique domain and PLpro via E3 ubiquitin ligase RCHY1. *Proc Natl Acad Sci U S A* 2016;113:E5192–E5201.
236. Malone B, et al. Structural basis for backtracking by the SARS-CoV-2 replication-transcription complex. *Proc Natl Acad Sci U S A* 2021;118.
237. Mandala VS, et al. Structure and drug binding of the SARS-CoV-2 envelope protein transmembrane domain in lipid bilayers. *Nat Struct Mol Biol* 2020;27:1202–1208.
238. Matsuyama S, Taguchi F. Two-step conformational changes in a coronavirus envelope glycoprotein mediated by receptor binding and proteolysis. *J Virol* 2009;83:11133–11141.
239. Matsuyama S, et al. Efficient activation of the severe acute respiratory syndrome coronavirus spike protein by the transmembrane protease TMPRSS2. *J Virol* 2010;84:12658–12664.
240. McAloose D, et al. From people to panthera: natural SARS-CoV-2 infection in tigers and lions at the bronx zoo. *MBio* 2020;11.
241. McBride CE, Li J, Machamer CE. The cytoplasmic tail of the severe acute respiratory syndrome coronavirus spike protein contains a novel endoplasmic reticulum retrieval signal that binds COPI and promotes interaction with membrane protein. *J Virol* 2007;81:2418–2428.
242. McBride CE, Machamer CE. A single tyrosine in the severe acute respiratory syndrome coronavirus membrane protein cytoplasmic tail is important for efficient interaction with spike protein. *J Virol* 2010;84:1891–1901.
243. McBride R, van Zyl M, Fielding BC. The coronavirus nucleocapsid is a multifunctional protein. *Viruses* 2014;6:2991–3018.
244. Menachery VD. MERS vaccine candidate offers promise, but questions remain. *EBioMedicine* 2015;2:1292–1293.
245. Menachery VD, et al. Attenuation and restoration of severe acute respiratory syndrome coronavirus mutant lacking 2′-o-methyltransferase activity. *J Virol* 2014;88:4251–4264.
246. Menachery VD, et al. Corrigendum: a SARS-like cluster of circulating bat coronaviruses shows potential for human emergence. *Nat Med* 2016;22:446.
247. Menachery VD, et al. Middle East respiratory syndrome coronavirus nonstructural protein 16 is necessary for interferon resistance and viral pathogenesis. *mSphere* 2017;2.
248. Michalska K, et al. Crystal structures of SARS-CoV-2 ADP-ribose phosphatase: from the apo form to ligand complexes. *IUCrJ* 2020;7:814–824.
249. Michel CJ, Mayer C, Poch O, et al. Characterization of accessory genes in coronavirus genomes. *Virol J* 2020;17:131.
250. Miknis ZJ, et al. Severe acute respiratory syndrome coronavirus nsp9 dimerization is essential for efficient viral growth. *J Virol* 2009;83:3007–3018.
251. Milewska A, et al. Entry of human coronavirus NL63 into the Cell. *J Virol* 2018;92.
252. Millet JK, Whittaker GR. Host cell proteases: critical determinants of coronavirus tropism and pathogenesis. *Virus Res* 2015;202:120–134.
253. Minasov G, et al. Mn(2+) coordinates Cap-0-RNA to align substrates for efficient 2′-O-methyl transfer by SARS-CoV-2 nsp16. *Sci Signal* 2021;14.
254. Minskaia E, et al. Discovery of an RNA virus 3′->5′ exoribonuclease that is critically involved in coronavirus RNA synthesis. *Proc Natl Acad Sci U S A* 2006;103:5108–5113.
255. Miorin L, et al. SARS-CoV-2 Orf6 hijacks Nup98 to block STAT nuclear import and antagonize interferon signaling. *Proc Natl Acad Sci* 2020;117:28344–28354. doi: 10.1073/pnas.2016650117, 202016650.

256. Moustaqil M, et al. SARS-CoV-2 proteases PLpro and 3CLpro cleave IRF3 and critical modulators of inflammatory pathways (NLRP12 and TAB1): implications for disease presentation across species. *Emerg Microbes Infect* 2021;10:178–195.

257. Moyo-Gwete T, et al. Cross-reactive neutralizing antibody responses elicited by SARS-CoV-2 501Y.V2 (B.1.351). *N Engl J Med* 2021;384:2161–2163. doi: 10.1056/nejmc2104192.

258. Munster VJ, et al. Respiratory disease in rhesus macaques inoculated with SARS-CoV-2. *Nature* 2020;585:268–272.

259. Murakami S, et al. Detection and characterization of bat sarbecovirus phylogenetically related to SARS-CoV-2, Japan. *Emerg Infect Dis* 2020;26:3025–3029.

260. Murray RS, MacMillan B, Cabirac G, et al. Detection of coronavirus RNA in CNS tissue of multiple sclerosis and control patients. *Adv Exp Med Biol* 1990;276:505–510 .

261. Muth D, et al. Attenuation of replication by a 29 nucleotide deletion in SARS-coronavirus acquired during the early stages of human-to-human transmission. *Sci Rep* 2018;8:15177.

262. Mykytyn AZ, et al. SARS-CoV-2 entry into human airway organoids is serine protease-mediated and facilitated by the multibasic cleavage site. *Elife* 2021;10.

263. Nakagawa K, Makino S. Mechanisms of coronavirus Nsp1-mediated control of host and viral gene expression. *Cells* 2021;10:300.

264. Nal B, et al. Differential maturation and subcellular localization of severe acute respiratory syndrome coronavirus surface proteins S, M and E. *J Gen Virol* 2005;86:1423–1434.

265. Narayanan K, et al. Severe acute respiratory syndrome coronavirus nsp1 suppresses host gene expression, including that of type I interferon, in infected cells. *J Virol* 2008;82:4471–4479.

266. Nelson CA, Pekosz A, Lee CA, et al. Structure and intracellular targeting of the SARS-coronavirus Orf7a accessory protein. *Structure* 2005;13:75–85.

267. Nemudryi A, et al. SARS-CoV-2 genomic surveillance identifies naturally occurring truncation of ORF7a that limits immune suppression. *Cell Rep* 2021;35:109197.

268. Neuman BW, et al. Proteomics analysis unravels the functional repertoire of coronavirus nonstructural protein 3. *J Virol* 2008;82:5279–5294.

269. Ni X, et al. Structural insights into plasticity and discovery of remdesivir metabolite GS-441524 binding in SARS-CoV-2 macrodomain. *ACS Med Chem Lett* 2021;12:603–609.

270. Nieto-Torres JL, et al. Subcellular location and topology of severe acute respiratory syndrome coronavirus envelope protein. *Virology* 2011;415:69–82.

271. Nieva JL, Madan V, Carrasco L. Viroporins: structure and biological functions. *Nat Rev Microbiol* 2012;10:563–574.

272. Niu S, et al. Molecular basis of cross-species ACE2 interactions with SARS-CoV-2-like viruses of pangolin origin. *EMBO J* 2021;40:e107786. doi: 10.15252/embj.2021107786, e107786.

273. Ogando NS, et al. The enzymatic activity of the nsp14 exoribonuclease is critical for replication of MERS-CoV and SARS-CoV-2. *J Virol* 2020;94.

274. Oostra M, de Haan CA, de Groot RJ, et al. Glycosylation of the severe acute respiratory syndrome coronavirus triple-spanning membrane proteins 3a and M. *J Virol* 2006;80:2326–2336.

275. Oostra M, de Haan CA, Rottier PJ. The 29-nucleotide deletion present in human but not in animal severe acute respiratory syndrome coronaviruses disrupts the functional expression of open reading frame 8. *J Virol* 2007;81:13876–13888.

276. Oostra M, et al. Localization and membrane topology of coronavirus nonstructural protein 4: involvement of the early secretory pathway in replication. *J Virol* 2007;81:12323–12336.

277. Oostra M, et al. Topology and membrane anchoring of the coronavirus replication complex: not all hydrophobic domains of nsp3 and nsp6 are membrane spanning. *J Virol* 2008;82:12392–12405.

278. Ortego J, Escors D, Laude H, et al. Generation of a replication-competent, propagation-deficient virus vector based on the transmissible gastroenteritis coronavirus genome. *J Virol* 2002;76:11518–11529.

279. Oudshoorn D, et al. Expression and cleavage of middle east respiratory syndrome coronavirus nsp3-4 polyprotein induce the formation of double-membrane vesicles that mimic those associated with coronaviral RNA replication. *MBio* 2017;8.

280. Owen DR, et al. An oral SARS-CoV-2 M^pro inhibitor clinical candidate for the treatment of COVID-19. *Science* 2021;374:1586–1593. doi: 10.1126/science.abl4784.

281. Painter GR, Natchus MG, Cohen O, et al. Developing a direct acting, orally available antiviral agent in a pandemic: the evolution of molnupiravir as a potential treatment for COVID-19. *Curr Opin Virol* 2021;50:17–22.

282. Parker MM, Masters PS. Sequence comparison of the N genes of five strains of the coronavirus mouse hepatitis virus suggests a three domain structure for the nucleocapsid protein. *Virology* 1990;179:463–468.

283. Parthasarathy K, et al. Structural flexibility of the pentameric SARS coronavirus envelope protein ion channel. *Biophys J* 2008;95:L39–L41.

284. Peacock TP, et al. The furin cleavage site in the SARS-CoV-2 spike protein is required for transmission in ferrets. *Nat Microbiol* 2021;6:899–909. doi: 10.1038/s41564-021-00908-w.

285. Peiris JS, et al. Coronavirus as a possible cause of severe acute respiratory syndrome. *Lancet* 2003;361:1319–1325.

286. Perlman SM. Coronaviridae: the viruses and their replication. In: Howley PMK, Whelan DM, eds. *Fields Virology.* Vol. 1, Chap. 10. Philadelphia, PA: Wolters Kluwer; 2020:410–421.

287. Perlman S, Netland J. Coronaviruses post-SARS: update on replication and pathogenesis. *Nat Rev Microbiol* 2009;7:439–450.

288. Perrier A, et al. The C-terminal domain of the MERS coronavirus M protein contains a trans-Golgi network localization signal. *J Biol Chem* 2019;294:14406–14421.

289. Pervushin K, et al. Structure and inhibition of the SARS coronavirus envelope protein ion channel. *PLoS Pathog* 2009;5:e1000511.

290. Peti W, et al. Structural genomics of the severe acute respiratory syndrome coronavirus: nuclear magnetic resonance structure of the protein nsp7. *J Virol* 2005;79:12905–12913.

291. Pfefferle S, et al. Distant relatives of severe acute respiratory syndrome coronavirus and close relatives of human coronavirus 229E in bats, Ghana. *Emerg Infect Dis* 2009;15:1377–1384.

292. Pfefferle S, et al. Reverse genetic characterization of the natural genomic deletion in SARS-Coronavirus strain Frankfurt-1 open reading frame 7b reveals an attenuating function of the 7b protein in-vitro and in-vivo. *Virol J* 2009;6:131.

293. Plante JA, et al. Spike mutation D614G alters SARS-CoV-2 fitness. *Nature* 2021;592:116–121.

294. Platanias LC. Mechanisms of type-I and type-II-interferon-mediated signalling. *Nat Rev Immunol* 2005;5:375–386.

295. Plescia CB, et al. SARS-CoV-2 viral budding and entry can be modeled using BSL-2 level virus-like particles. *J Biol Chem* 2021;296:100103.

296. Pohl MO, et al. SARS-CoV-2 variants reveal features critical for replication in primary human cells. *PLoS Biol* 2021;19:e3001006.

297. Prentice E, McAuliffe J, Lu X, et al. Identification and characterization of severe acute respiratory syndrome coronavirus replicase proteins. *J Virol* 2004;78:9977–9986.

298. Pruijssers AJ, et al. Remdesivir inhibits SARS-CoV-2 in human lung cells and chimeric SARS-CoV expressing the SARS-CoV-2 RNA polymerase in mice. *Cell Rep* 2020;32:107940.

299. Pyrc K, Jebbink MF, Berkhout B, et al. Genome structure and transcriptional regulation of human coronavirus NL63. *Virol J* 2004;1:7.

300. Rack JGM, et al. Viral macrodomains: a structural and evolutionary assessment of the pharmacological potential. *Open Biol* 2020;10:200237.

301. Rathnayake AD, et al. 3C-like protease inhibitors block coronavirus replication in vitro and improve survival in MERS-CoV-infected mice. *Sci Transl Med* 2020;12.

302. Ratia K, Kilianski A, Baez-Santos YM, et al. Structural basis for the ubiquitin-linkage specificity and deISGylating activity of SARS-CoV papain-like protease. *PLoS Pathog* 2014;10:e1004113.

303. Ratia K, et al. Severe acute respiratory syndrome coronavirus papain-like protease: structure of a viral deubiquitinating enzyme. *Proc Natl Acad Sci U S A* 2006;103:5717–5722.

304. Ratia K, et al. A noncovalent class of papain like protease/deubiquitinase inhibitors blocks SARS virus replication. *Proc Natl Acad Sci U S A* 2008;105:16119–16124.

305. Ren W, et al. Difference in receptor usage between severe acute respiratory syndrome (SARS) coronavirus and SARS-like coronavirus of bat origin. *J Virol* 2008;82:1899–1907.

306. Rogstam A, et al. Crystal structure of non-structural protein 10 from severe acute respiratory syndrome coronavirus-2. *Int J Mol Sci* 2020;21.

307. Rosas-Lemus M, et al. High-resolution structures of the SARS-CoV-2 2'-O-methyltransferase reveal strategies for structure-based inhibitor design. *Sci Signal* 2020;13.

308. Rosenke K, et al. Defining the Syrian hamster as a highly susceptible preclinical model for SARS-CoV-2 infection. *Emerg Microbes Infect* 2020;9:2673–2684.

309. Roth-Cross JK, Bender SJ, Weiss SR. Murine coronavirus mouse hepatitis virus is recognized by MDA5 and induces type I interferon in brain macrophages/microglia. *J Virol* 2008;82:9829–9838.

310. Rottier PJ. The coronavirus membrane glycoprotein. In: Siddell SG, ed. *The Coronaviridae.* New York: Plenum Press; 1995:115–139.

311. Ruch TR, Machamer CE. The coronavirus e protein: assembly and beyond. *Viruses* 2012;4:363–382.

312. Sacramento CQ, et al. In vitro antiviral activity of the anti-HCV drugs daclatasvir and sofosbuvir against SARS-CoV-2, the aetiological agent of COVID-19. *J Antimicrob Chemother* 2021;76:1874–1885.

313. Sadler AJ, Williams BR. Interferon-inducible antiviral effectors. *Nat Rev Immunol* 2008;8:559–568.

314. Saikatendu KS, et al. Structural basis of severe acute respiratory syndrome coronavirus ADP-ribose-1''-phosphate dephosphorylation by a conserved domain of nsP3. *Structure* 2005;13:1665–1675.

315. Sawicki SG, et al. Functional and genetic analysis of coronavirus replicase-transcriptase proteins. *PLoS Pathog* 2005;1:e39.

316. Schaecher SR, Diamond MS, Pekosz A. The transmembrane domain of the severe acute respiratory syndrome coronavirus ORF7b protein is necessary and sufficient for its retention in the Golgi complex. *J Virol* 2008;82:9477–9491.

317. Schaecher SR, Touchette E, Schriewer J, et al. Severe acute respiratory syndrome coronavirus gene 7 products contribute to virus-induced apoptosis. *J Virol* 2007;81:11054–11068.

318. Schoeman D, Fielding BC. Coronavirus envelope protein: current knowledge. *Virol J* 2019;16:69.

319. Schoeman D, Fielding BC. Is there a link between the pathogenic human coronavirus envelope protein and immunopathology? A review of the literature. *Front Microbiol* 2020;11:2086.

320. Schubert K, et al. SARS-CoV-2 Nsp1 binds the ribosomal mRNA channel to inhibit translation. *Nat Struct Mol Biol* 2020;27:959–966. doi: 10.1038/s41594-020-0511-8.

321. Semper C, Watanabe N, Savchenko A. Structural characterization of nonstructural protein 1 from SARS-CoV-2. *iScience* 2021;24:101903.

322. Serrano P, et al. Nuclear magnetic resonance structure of the N-terminal domain of nonstructural protein 3 from the severe acute respiratory syndrome coronavirus. *J Virol* 2007;81:12049–12060.

323. Serrano P, et al. Nuclear magnetic resonance structure of the nucleic acid-binding domain of severe acute respiratory syndrome coronavirus nonstructural protein 3. *J Virol* 2009;83:12998–13008.

324. Seybert A, Hegyi A, Siddell SG, et al. The human coronavirus 229E superfamily 1 helicase has RNA and DNA duplex-unwinding activities with 5'-to-3' polarity. *RNA* 2000;6:1056–1068.

325. Shang J, et al. Cell entry mechanisms of SARS-CoV-2. *Proc Natl Acad Sci U S A* 2020;117:11727–11734.

326. Shang J, et al. Structural basis of receptor recognition by SARS-CoV-2. *Nature* 2020;581:221–224.

327. Shannon A, et al. Rapid incorporation of Favipiravir by the fast and permissive viral RNA polymerase complex results in SARS-CoV-2 lethal mutagenesis. *Nat Commun* 2020;11:4682.

328. Sheahan TP, et al. Broad-spectrum antiviral GS-5734 inhibits both epidemic and zoonotic coronaviruses. *Sci Transl Med* 2017;9.

329. Sheahan TP, et al. An orally bioavailable broad-spectrum antiviral inhibits SARS-CoV-2 in human airway epithelial cell cultures and multiple coronaviruses in mice. *Sci Transl Med* 2020;12:eabb5883.
330. Shen S, et al. The severe acute respiratory syndrome coronavirus 3a is a novel structural protein. *Biochem Biophys Res Commun* 2005;330:286–292.
331. Shi J, Sivaraman J, Song J. Mechanism for controlling the dimer-monomer switch and coupling dimerization to catalysis of the severe acute respiratory syndrome coronavirus 3C-like protease. *J Virol* 2008;82:4620–4629.
332. Shi CS, et al. SARS-coronavirus open reading frame-9b suppresses innate immunity by targeting mitochondria and the MAVS/TRAF3/TRAF6 signalosome. *J Immunol* 2014;193:3080–3089.
333. Shi M, et al. SARS-CoV-2 Nsp1 suppresses host but not viral translation through a bipartite mechanism. *bioRxiv* 2020;2020.09.18.302901. doi: 10.1101/2020.09.18.302901.
334. Shin D, et al. Papain-like protease regulates SARS-CoV-2 viral spread and innate immunity. *Nature* 2020;587:657–662.
335. Shriner SA, et al. SARS-CoV-2 exposure in escaped mink, Utah, USA. *Emerg Infect Dis* 2021;27:988–990.
336. Shulla A, et al. A transmembrane serine protease is linked to the severe acute respiratory syndrome coronavirus receptor and activates virus entry. *J Virol* 2011;85:873–882.
337. Silvas J, et al. Contribution of SARS-CoV-2 accessory proteins to viral pathogenicity in K18 hACE2 transgenic mice. *bioRxiv* 2021. doi: 10.1101/2021.03.09.434696, 2021.2003.2009.434696 .
338. Simmons G, Zmora P, Gierer S, et al. Proteolytic activation of the SARS-coronavirus spike protein: cutting enzymes at the cutting edge of antiviral research. *Antiviral Res* 2013;100:605–614.
339. Simmons B, et al. Sofosbuvir/daclatasvir regimens for the treatment of COVID-19: an individual patient data meta-analysis. *J Antimicrob Chemother* 2021;76:286–291.
340. Sims AC, Burkett SE, Yount B, et al. SARS-CoV replication and pathogenesis in an in vitro model of the human conducting airway epithelium. *Virus Res* 2008;133:33–44.
341. Sims AC, et al. Release of severe acute respiratory syndrome coronavirus nuclear import block enhances host transcription in human lung cells. *J Virol* 2013;87:3885–3902.
342. Slanina H, et al. Coronavirus replication-transcription complex: vital and selective NMPylation of a conserved site in nsp9 by the NiRAN-RdRp subunit. *Proc Natl Acad Sci U S A* 2021;118.
343. Smith EC, Blanc H, Surdel MC, et al. Coronaviruses lacking exoribonuclease activity are susceptible to lethal mutagenesis: evidence for proofreading and potential therapeutics. *PLoS Pathog* 2013;9:e1003565.
344. Snijder EJ, Decroly E, Ziebuhr J. The nonstructural proteins directing coronavirus RNA synthesis and processing. *Adv Virus Res* 2016;96:59–126.
345. Snijder EJ, et al. Unique and conserved features of genome and proteome of SARS-coronavirus, an early split-off from the coronavirus group 2 lineage. *J Mol Biol* 2003;331: 991–1004.
346. Sola I, Almazan F, Zuniga S, et al. Continuous and discontinuous RNA synthesis in coronaviruses. *Annu Rev Virol* 2015;2:265–288.
347. Sparks JS, Lu X, Denison MR. Genetic analysis of murine hepatitis virus nsp4 in virus replication. *J Virol* 2007;81:12554–12563.
348. Starr TN, et al. Deep mutational scanning of SARS-CoV-2 receptor binding domain reveals constraints on folding and ACE2 binding. *Cell* 2020;182:1295–1310.
349. Stertz S, et al. The intracellular sites of early replication and budding of SARS-coronavirus. *Virology* 2007;361:304–315.
350. Su YAO, et al. Discovery and genomic characterization of a 382-nucleotide deletion in ORF7b and ORF8 during the early evolution of SARS-CoV-2. *MBio* 2020;114:e01610. doi: 10.1128/mBio.01610-20.
351. Subissi L, et al. One severe acute respiratory syndrome coronavirus protein complex integrates processive RNA polymerase and exonuclease activities. *Proc Natl Acad Sci U S A* 2014;111:E3900–E3909.
352. Surjit M, Liu B, Kumar P, et al. The nucleocapsid protein of the SARS coronavirus is capable of self-association through a C-terminal 209 amino acid interaction domain. *Biochem Biophys Res Commun* 2004;317:1030–1036.
353. Surya W, Li Y, Torres J. Structural model of the SARS coronavirus E channel in LMPG micelles. *Biochim Biophys Acta Biomembr* 2018;1860:1309–1317.
354. Sutton G, et al. The nsp9 replicase protein of SARS-coronavirus, structure and functional insights. *Structure* 2004;12:341–353.
355. Tan J, et al. The SARS-unique domain (SUD) of SARS coronavirus contains two macrodomains that bind G-quadruplexes. *PLoS Pathog* 2009;5:e1000428.
356. Tanaka T, Kamitani W, DeDiego ML, et al. Severe acute respiratory syndrome coronavirus nsp1 facilitates efficient propagation in cells through a specific translational shutoff of host mRNA. *J Virol* 2012;86:11128–11137.
357. Tchesnokov EP, et al. Template-dependent inhibition of coronavirus RNA-dependent RNA polymerase by remdesivir reveals a second mechanism of action. *J Biol Chem* 2020;295:16156–16165.
358. te Velthuis AJ, Arnold JJ, Cameron CE, et al. The RNA polymerase activity of SARS-coronavirus nsp12 is primer dependent. *Nucleic Acids Res* 2010;38:203–214.
359. te Velthuis AJ, van den Worm SH, Snijder EJ. The SARS-coronavirus nsp7+nsp8 complex is a unique multimeric RNA polymerase capable of both de novo initiation and primer extension. *Nucleic Acids Res* 2012;40:1737–1747.
360. Tegally H, et al. Emergence and rapid spread of a new severe acute respiratory syndrome-related coronavirus 2 (SARS-CoV-2) lineage with multiple spike mutations in South Africa. *medRxiv* 2020. https://doi.org/10.1101/2020.12.21.20248640.
361. Temmam S, et al. Bat coronaviruses related to SARS-CoV-2 and infectious for human cells. *Nature* 2021. doi: 10.21203/rs.3.rs-871965/v1. https://doi.org/10.1038/s41586-022-04532-4.
362. Teoh KT, et al. The SARS coronavirus E protein interacts with PALS1 and alters tight junction formation and epithelial morphogenesis. *Mol Biol Cell* 2010;21:3838–3852.
363. Thoms M, et al. Structural basis for translational shutdown and immune evasion by the Nsp1 protein of SARS-CoV-2. *Science* 2020;369:1249–1255.
364. Tidu A, et al. The viral protein NSP1 acts as a ribosome gatekeeper for shutting down host translation and fostering SARS-CoV-2 translation. *RNA* 2020;27:253–264.
365. Tong P, et al. Memory B cell repertoire for recognition of evolving SARS-CoV-2 spike. *Cell* 2021;184:4969–4980.e4915.
366. Tooze J, Tooze SA, Fuller SD. Sorting of progeny coronavirus from condensed secretory proteins at the exit from the trans-Golgi network of AtT20 cells. *J Cell Biol* 1987;105:1215–1226.
367. Tortorici MA, Veesler D. Structural insights into coronavirus entry. *Adv Virus Res* 2019;105:93–116.
368. Toto A, et al. Comparing the binding properties of peptides mimicking the envelope protein of SARS-CoV and SARS-CoV-2 to the PDZ domain of the tight junction-associated PALS1 protein. *Protein Sci* 2020;29:2038–2042.
369. Tsang KW, et al. A cluster of cases of severe acute respiratory syndrome in Hong Kong. *N Engl J Med* 2003;348:1977–1985.
370. Tseng CT, et al. Apical entry and release of severe acute respiratory syndrome-associated coronavirus in polarized Calu-3 lung epithelial cells. *J Virol* 2005;79:9470–9479.
371. Turoňová B, et al. In situ structural analysis of SARS-CoV-2 spike reveals flexibility mediated by three hinges. *Science* 2020;370:203–208.
372. Ujike M, Taguchi F. Incorporation of spike and membrane glycoproteins into coronavirus virions. *Viruses* 2015;7:1700–1725.
373. van Dorp L, et al. Emergence of genomic diversity and recurrent mutations in SARS-CoV-2. *Infect Genet Evol* 2020;83:104351.
374. Vandyck K, Deval J. Considerations for the discovery and development of 3-chymotrypsin-like cysteine protease inhibitors targeting SARS-CoV-2 infection. *Curr Opin Virol* 2021;49:36–40.
375. Vasilenko N, Moshynskyy I, Zakhartchouk A. SARS coronavirus protein 7a interacts with human Ap4A-hydrolase. *Virol J* 2010;7:31.
376. Venkatagopalan P, Daskalova SM, Lopez LA, et al. Coronavirus envelope (E) protein remains at the site of assembly. *Virology* 2015;478:75–85.
377. Verheije MH, et al. The coronavirus nucleocapsid protein is dynamically associated with the replication-transcription complexes. *J Virol* 2010;84:11575–11579.
378. Viswanathan T, et al. Structural basis of RNA cap modification by SARS-CoV-2. *Nat Commun* 2020;11:3718.
379. V'Kovski P, Kratzel A, Steiner S, et al. Coronavirus biology and replication: implications for SARS-CoV-2. *Nat Rev Microbiol* 2021;19:155–170.
380. von Brunn A, et al. Analysis of intraviral protein-protein interactions of the SARS coronavirus ORFeome. *PLoS One* 2007;2:e459.
381. von Grotthuss M, Wyrwicz LS, Rychlewski L. mRNA cap-1 methyltransferase in the SARS genome. *Cell* 2003;113:701–702.
382. Vuong W, et al. Feline coronavirus drug inhibits the main protease of SARS-CoV-2 and blocks virus replication. *Nat Commun* 2020;11:4282.
383. Wacharapluesadee S, et al. Evidence for SARS-CoV-2 related coronaviruses circulating in bats and pangolins in Southeast Asia. *Nat Commun* 2021;12:972.
384. Wahba L, et al. An extensive meta-metagenomic search identifies SARS-CoV-2-homologous sequences in pangolin lung viromes. *mSphere* 2020;5.
385. Wahl A, et al. SARS-CoV-2 infection is effectively treated and prevented by EIDD-2801. *Nature* 2021;591:451–457.
386. Walls AC, et al. Structure, function, and antigenicity of the SARS-CoV-2 spike glycoprotein. *Cell* 2020;181:281–292.e286.
387. Wan Y, Shang J, Graham R, et al. Receptor recognition by the novel coronavirus from Wuhan: an analysis based on decade-long structural studies of SARS Coronavirus. *J Virol* 2020;94.
388. Wang R, Chen J, Hozumi Y, et al. Decoding asymptomatic COVID-19 infection and transmission. *J Phys Chem Lett* 2020;11:10007–10015.
389. Wang H, Pipes L, Nielsen R. Synonymous mutations and the molecular evolution of SARS-CoV-2 origins. *Virus Evol* 2021;7.
390. Wang Y, et al. Coronavirus nsp10/nsp16 methyltransferase can be targeted by nsp10-derived peptide in vitro and in vivo to reduce replication and pathogenesis. *J Virol* 2015;89:8416–8427.
391. Wang M, et al. Remdesivir and chloroquine effectively inhibit the recently emerged novel coronavirus (2019-nCoV) in vitro. *Cell Res* 2020;30:269–271.
392. Wang X, et al. Accurate diagnosis of COVID-19 by a novel immunogenic secreted SARS-CoV-2 orf8 Protein. *MBio* 2020;11.
393. Washington NL, et al. Emergence and rapid transmission of SARS-CoV-2 B.1.1.7 in the United States. *Cell* 2021;184:2587–2594.e7. doi: 10.1016/j.cell.2021.03.052.
394. Watanabe Y, Allen JD, Wrapp D, et al. Site-specific glycan analysis of the SARS-CoV-2 spike. *Science* 2020;369:330–333.
395. Wathelet MG, Orr M, Frieman MB, et al. Severe acute respiratory syndrome coronavirus evades antiviral signaling: role of nsp1 and rational design of an attenuated strain. *J Virol* 2007;81:11620–11633.
396. Wells HL, et al. The evolutionary history of ACE2 usage within the coronavirus subgenus Sarbecovirus. *Virus Evol* 2021;7:veab007.
397. Whelan JN, Li Y, Silverman RH, et al. Zika virus production is resistant to RNase L antiviral activity. *J Virol* 2019;93.
398. Whittaker GR, Daniel S, Millet JK. Coronavirus entry: how we arrived at SARS-CoV-2. *Curr Opin Virol* 2021;47:113–120.
399. Wilamowski M, et al. 2′-O methylation of RNA cap in SARS-CoV-2 captured by serial crystallography. *Proc Natl Acad Sci U S A* 2021;118.
400. Williamson BN, et al. Clinical benefit of remdesivir in rhesus macaques infected with SARS-CoV-2. *Nature* 2020;585:273–276.
401. Wong NA, Saier MH Jr. The SARS-Coronavirus infection cycle: a survey of viral membrane proteins, their functional interactions and pathogenesis. *Int J Mol Sci* 2021;22.
402. Wrapp D, et al. Cryo-EM structure of the 2019-nCoV spike in the prefusion conformation. *Science* 2020;367:1260–1263.
403. Wu CY, et al. Small molecules targeting severe acute respiratory syndrome human coronavirus. *Proc Natl Acad Sci U S A* 2004;101:10012–10017.

404. Wu F, et al. A new coronavirus associated with human respiratory disease in China. *Nature* 2020;579:265–269.

405. Xia H, et al. Evasion of type-I interferon by SARS-CoV-2. *Cell Rep* 2020;10:8234.

406. Xia B, et al. SARS-CoV-2 envelope protein causes acute respiratory distress syndrome (ARDS)-like pathological damages and constitutes an antiviral target. *Cell Res* 2021;31:847–860.

407. Xiao X, Newman C, Buesching CD, et al. Animal sales from Wuhan wet markets immediately prior to the COVID-19 pandemic. *Sci Rep* 2021;11:11898.

408. Xiao K, et al. Isolation of SARS-CoV-2-related coronavirus from Malayan pangolins. *Nature* 2020;583:286–289.

409. Xu X, et al. Molecular model of SARS coronavirus polymerase: implications for biochemical functions and drug design. *Nucleic Acids Res* 2003;31:7117–7130.

410. Yan R, et al. Structural basis for the recognition of SARS-CoV-2 by full-length human ACE2. *Science* 2020;367:1444–1448.

411. Yan L, et al. Architecture of a SARS-CoV-2 mini replication and transcription complex. *Nat Commun* 2020;11:5874.

412. Yan L, et al. Cryo-EM structure of an extended SARS-CoV-2 replication and transcription complex reveals an intermediate state in cap synthesis. *Cell* 2021;184:184–193.e110.

413. Yan L, et al. Coupling of N7-methyltransferase and 3'-5' exoribonuclease with SARS-CoV-2 polymerase reveals mechanisms for capping and proofreading. *Cell* 2021;184:3474–3485.e3411.

414. Yang H, et al. The crystal structures of severe acute respiratory syndrome virus main protease and its complex with an inhibitor. *Proc Natl Acad Sci U S A* 2003;100:13190–13195.

415. Yang H, et al. Design of wide-spectrum inhibitors targeting coronavirus main proteases. *PLoS Biol* 2005;3:e324.

416. Yang N, et al. Bismuth complexes inhibit the SARS coronavirus. *Angew Chem Int Ed Engl* 2007;46:6464–6468.

417. Yang Y, et al. The structural and accessory proteins M, ORF 4a, ORF 4b, and ORF 5 of Middle East respiratory syndrome coronavirus (MERS-CoV) are potent interferon antagonists. *Protein Cell* 2013;4:951–961.

418. Yang XL, et al. Isolation and characterization of a novel bat coronavirus closely related to the direct progenitor of severe acute respiratory syndrome coronavirus. *J Virol* 2016;90:3253–3256.

419. Yao H, et al. Molecular architecture of the SARS-CoV-2 virus. *Cell* 2020;183:730–738.e713.

420. Ye Q, West AMV, Silletti S, et al. Architecture and self-assembly of the SARS-CoV-2 nucleocapsid protein. *Protein Sci* 2020;29:1890–1901.

421. Yin W, et al. Structural basis for inhibition of the RNA-dependent RNA polymerase from SARS-CoV-2 by remdesivir. *Science* 2020;368:1499–1504.

422. Young BE, et al. Effects of a major deletion in the SARS-CoV-2 genome on the severity of infection and the inflammatory response: an observational cohort study. *Lancet* 2020;396:603–611.

423. Yuan S, et al. Nonstructural protein 1 of SARS-CoV-2 is a potent pathogenicity factor redirecting host protein synthesis machinery toward viral RNA. *Mol Cell* 2020;80:1055–1066.e1056.

424. Yuan S, et al. Metallodrug ranitidine bismuth citrate suppresses SARS-CoV-2 replication and relieves virus-associated pneumonia in Syrian hamsters. *Nat Microbiol* 2020;5:1439–1448.

425. Yurkovetskiy L, et al. Structural and functional analysis of the D614G SARS-CoV-2 spike protein variant. *Cell* 2020;183:739–751.e738.

426. Zeng HL, Dichio V, Rodríguez Horta E, et al. Global analysis of more than 50,000 SARS-CoV-2 genomes reveals epistasis between eight viral genes. *Proc Natl Acad Sci U S A* 2020;117:31519–31526.

427. Zeng LP, et al. Bat severe acute respiratory syndrome-like coronavirus WIV1 encodes an extra accessory protein, ORFX, involved in modulation of the host immune response. *J Virol* 2016;90:6573–6582.

428. Zhai Y, et al. Insights into SARS-CoV transcription and replication from the structure of the nsp7-nsp8 hexadecamer. *Nat Struct Mol Biol* 2005;12:980–986.

429. Zhang L, et al. SARS-CoV-2 spike-protein D614G mutation increases virion spike density and infectivity. *Nat Commun* 2020;11:6013.

430. Zhang L, et al. Crystal structure of SARS-CoV-2 main protease provides a basis for design of improved α-ketoamide inhibitors. *Science* 2020;368:409–412.

431. Zhang Y, et al. The ORF8 protein of SARS-CoV-2 mediates immune evasion through potently downregulating MHC-I. *PNAS* 2021;118(23):e2024202118.

432. Zhang J, et al. Structural impact on SARS-CoV-2 spike protein by D614G substitution. *Science* 2021;372:525–530.

433. Zhang K, et al. Nsp1 protein of SARS-CoV-2 disrupts the mRNA export machinery to inhibit host gene expression. *Sci Adv* 2021;7.

434. Zhao Z, et al. Description and clinical treatment of an early outbreak of severe acute respiratory syndrome (SARS) in Guangzhou, PR China. *J Med Microbiol* 2003;52:715–720.

435. Zhao P, et al. Virus-receptor interactions of glycosylated SARS-CoV-2 spike and human ACE2 receptor. *Cell Host Microbe* 2020;28:586–601.e586.

436. Zhao Y, et al. Crystal structure of SARS-CoV-2 main protease in complex with protease inhibitor PF-07321332. *Protein Cell* 2021. doi: 10.1007/s13238-021-00883-2.

437. Zheng M, et al. Bat SARS-Like WIV1 coronavirus uses the ACE2 of multiple animal species as receptor and evades IFITM3 restriction via TMPRSS2 activation of membrane fusion. *Emerg Microbes Infect* 2020;9:1567–1579.

438. Zhou A, et al. Interferon action and apoptosis are defective in mice devoid of 2',5'-oligoadenylate-dependent RNase L. *EMBO J* 1997;16:6355–6363.

439. Zhou P, et al. A pneumonia outbreak associated with a new coronavirus of probable bat origin. *Nature* 2020;579:270–273.

440. Zhou H, et al. A novel bat coronavirus closely related to SARS-CoV-2 contains natural insertions at the S1/S2 cleavage site of the spike protein. *Curr Biol* 2020;30:2196–2203.e2193.

441. Zhou H, et al. Identification of novel bat coronaviruses sheds light on the evolutionary origins of SARS-CoV-2 and related viruses. *Cell* 2021;184:4380–4391.

442. Zhu N, et al. Morphogenesis and cytopathic effect of SARS-CoV-2 infection in human airway epithelial cells. *Nat Commun* 2020;11:3910.

443. Ziebuhr J, Snijder EJ, Gorbalenya AE. Virus-encoded proteinases and proteolytic processing in the Nidovirales. *J Gen Virol* 2000;81:853–879.

444. Zúñiga S, et al. Coronavirus nucleocapsid protein facilitates template switching and is required for efficient transcription. *J Virol* 2010;84:2169–2175.

445. Zust R, et al. Ribose 2'-O-methylation provides a molecular signature for the distinction of self and non-self mRNA dependent on the RNA sensor Mda5. *Nat Immunol* 2011;12:137–143.

SARS-CoV-2/COVID-19: Clinical Characteristics, Prevention, and Treatment

John H. Beigel • Timothy M. Uyeki

Introduction
Pathogenesis
  Pathophysiology
  Pathology
  Immune responses to SARS-CoV-2
SARS-CoV-2 variant viruses
Epidemiologic parameters
  Transmission dynamics
  Transmission modes
  Duration of infectiousness
Clinical disease
  Severity of disease
  Spectrum of disease
Clinical complications
  Respiratory complications
  Extrapulmonary complications
  Coinfections
  Laboratory findings
  Radiographic and imaging findings
Risk factors for severe disease
Special populations
  Children
  Pregnancy
  Vertical transmission
Clinical issues after infection
  SARS-CoV-2 reinfection
  Post-COVID conditions
  Multisystem inflammatory syndrome
Diagnostic testing
  Viral tests
  Serology
Clinical management
  General
Monoclonal antibodies
Bamlanivimab/etesevimab
  Casirivimab/imdevimab
  Sotrovimab
  Regdanvimab
  Variants and monoclonal antibodies
Antiviral agents
  Remdesivir
  Other antiviral agents
Anti-inflammatory
  Dexamethasone
  Baricitinib
  IL-6 pathway inhibitors
  Other anti-inflammatory agents

Convalescent plasma
Antithrombotic prophylaxis
  Ineffective therapies
Treatment of COVID-19
  Outpatients
  Hospitalized patients
Infection prevention and control
Vaccine
  Adverse events
  Myocarditis/pericarditis
  Thrombosis with thrombocytopenia
  Guillain-Barré syndrome
  Variant viruses
  Additional vaccine dose in immunocompromised
  Vaccine booster
Perspective
Addendum, April 2022
  Epidemiology
  COVID-19 Vaccines
  Therapeutics

INTRODUCTION

In late 2019, the emergence of a novel respiratory virus caused an unprecedented threat to public health and became a global pandemic. The causative virus was rapidly identified[764] (later named severe acute respiratory syndrome coronavirus 2, or SARS-CoV-2) and descriptions of the clinical characteristics of the disease (referred to as COVID-19) and complications were quickly published.[137,263,301,690] Within weeks, trials of candidate vaccines and investigational therapeutics began. Within months, there were emergency use authorizations issued in the United States for therapeutics and early approvals in other countries of accurate diagnostics, several efficacious therapeutics were identified in clinical trials, and increased understanding of the pathogenesis and sequelae of the disease were recognized. Within a year, there was authorization or initial approvals of highly effective vaccines worldwide. The emergence of viral variants could reduce the effectiveness of the vaccines and may impact some of the advances noted above in the future. This chapter summarizes the current understanding of clinical characteristics, prevention, and treatment of COVID-19, as of late 2021, primarily based upon findings that preceded emergence of the SARS-CoV-2 Delta (B.1.617.2) variant of concern, while noting the pandemic continues to evolve and the field continues to advance.

PATHOGENESIS

Pathophysiology

Following host cell binding, the viral and cell membranes fuse, enabling virus entry into the cell[444] followed by RNA genome replication and translation.[79] SARS-CoV-2 infection induces cellular death via pyroptosis, a highly inflammatory form of programmed cell death commonly seen with cytopathic viruses.[217] This process also causes the release of various damage-associated molecular patterns (DAMPs) and pathogen-associated molecular patterns (PAMPs). Pattern Recognition Receptors such as toll-like receptors (TLRs) recognize PAMPs and DAMPs triggering induction of proinflammatory cytokine transcription factors such as NF-κβ, as well as activating interferon regulatory factors that mediate the type I interferon–dependent antiviral response.[391] In some patients, SARS-CoV-2 suppresses the early type I and III interferon responses, an immune evasion strategy employed by the virus, leading to early failure to control the virus.[74]

After SARS-CoV-2 infection, two waves of cellular responses occur. First, a rapid recruitment of monocytes and macrophages into the lungs occurs early after infection.[344,373] Then T cells infiltrate into the lungs where they initiate a specific response to clear the virus.[135] This results in an increase in proinflammatory cytokines and chemokines and the recruitment of immune cells into affected sites. Several cohort studies

in SARS-CoV-2 have observed increased levels of interleukin-6 (IL-6), IL-2, granulocyte colony-stimulating factor (G-CSF), IL-7, IL-10, interferon (IFN)-inducible protein-10 (IP-10), monocyte chemoattractant protein-1 (MCP1), IFN-γ, macrophage inflammatory protein 1α (MIP1α), and tumor necrosis factor (TNF-α).[301,650]

In most individuals with SARS-CoV-2 infection, the cytokine release and activation of an antiviral interferon response followed by immune cell recruitment result in successful SARS-CoV-2 clearance. In a subset of patients, there is progression to a hyperinflammatory state that may manifest by organ dysfunction (Fig. 22.1). This hyperinflammatory state is sometimes called a cytokine storm, which is generally described as a collection of clinical manifestations resulting from an overactivated and dysregulated immune response. Cytokine storms are associated with various disorders, such as uncontrolled infectious diseases associated with certain acquired or inherited immunodeficiencies, autoinflammatory diseases, or following therapeutic interventions.[135] Distinguishing an appropriate innate immune response triggered by viral infection from a dysregulated abnormal inflammatory response can be difficult, though the clinical benefit in modifying this innate immune response (described below in Treatment) suggests that the cytokine activation may contribute to pathogenesis.

Coagulation abnormalities and a high incidence of thrombotic events occur in COVID-19 patients. Early reports demonstrated prolonged activated partial thromboplastin time (aPTT), prothrombin time, and elevated D-dimer.[137,690] A meta-analysis reported that the frequency of disseminated intravascular coagulation (DIC) was 3% in hospitalized COVID-19

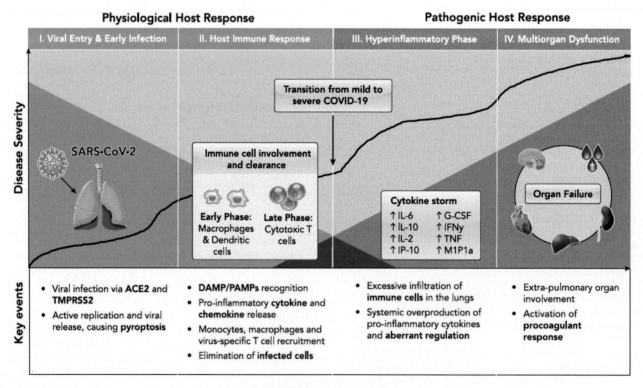

FIGURE 22.1 Characterization of COVID-19 disease progression. The *dark blue* shading indicates physiological viral host response over time, and the *dark red* shading indicates a pathogenic hyperinflammatory host. (Reprinted with permission from Bohn MK, Hall A, Sepiashvili L, et al. Pathophysiology of COVID-19: mechanisms underlying disease severity and progression. *Physiology (Bethesda).* 2020;35(5):288–301. Copyright © 2020 The American Physiological Society.)

patients, DIC was associated with greater severity of illness, and deaths.[762] One study reported that 71.4% of nonsurvivors and 0.6% of recovered cases met the criteria for DIC during hospitalization.[645] Autopsy data observed fibrin thrombi in pulmonary small arterial vessels in 87% of fatal cases.[109] Complement-mediated pulmonary tissue damage and microvascular injury have been observed in severe COVID-19.[433] Together, these data suggest that hypercoagulability in addition to hyperinflammation may contribute to the pathogenesis of severe COVID-19.

Pathology

The primary pathology of COVID-19 in the lungs is diffuse alveolar damage (DAD), organizing pneumonia, reactive type II pneumocytes, and chronic interstitial pneumonia (Fig. 22.2A).[103] There are additional reports of diffuse proteinaceous edema and hyaline membranes.[363] Macroscopically, this can appear as very heavy wet lungs[593] (Fig. 22.2B). There is also massive capillary congestion often accompanied by microthrombi despite anticoagulation.[455] In the proliferative phase of DAD, there is an interstitial infiltrate of lymphocytes and florid, atypical type 2 pneumocyte hyperplasia (within the cytoplasm of which some authors have demonstrated viral inclusions/protein/RNA), sometimes associated with squamous metaplasia.[593] Occasionally, the lung consolidation consists of intra-alveolar neutrophilic infiltration, consistent with superimposed bacterial bronchopneumonia,[662] though only directly visualized or detected by culture or PCR in 8%.[159] Severe tracheobronchitis including aphthous ulcers[81] and mononuclear inflammation[455] have been described.

Angiotensin converting enzyme 2 (ACE2) is abundantly present in human epithelial cells of the lung, as well as in endothelial cells of the arterial and venous vessels,[266] suggesting direct viral infection and injury of the vascular endothelium is possible. Postmortem studies have confirmed venous thromboembolic disease in the majority of patients that died (Fig. 22.2C).[709] This has been attributed to increased levels of von Willebrand factor, Toll-like receptor activation, complement deposition, and tissue factor pathway activation.[242,640]

Histology demonstrated inflammation of the myocardium with predominance of macrophages, and myocyte necrosis has occasionally been reported on endomyocardial biopsy, generally performed after patients present with symptoms of myocarditis or heart failure.[588] Autopsy series have demonstrated accumulation of inflammatory cells in the endocardium[662] and myocardium.[662] The early clinical hypothesis that atherosclerotic plaque rupture results in coronary artery thrombosis has not been supported by postmortem studies.[593]

The primary pathology findings in the liver are those reflective of underlying diseases such as obesity.[593] While elevated liver function tests are seen in many patients, most autopsy series demonstrate nonspecific passive congestion with centrilobular necrosis and collapse. Kupffer cell activation and proliferation has rarely been reported,[376] and it is unknown if this is responsible for liver dysfunction or simply reflective of the viremia. The primary findings in the kidneys are also reflective of preexisting diseases: diabetic and hypertensive nephropathy. Acute tubular injury and myoglobin casts have also been commonly reported.[630] Noteworthy for its absence in most of the published studies has been glomerular capillary thrombi/evidence of thrombotic microangiopathy (TMA), diverging from the findings in typical DIC.[593]

In the few published case series examining whole brains, there are infrequent reports of widespread microthrombi, microinfarcts and microhemorrhages, global or watershed anoxic injury, and rarely a focal infiltrate of T lymphocytes and microglia.[90,593] White pulp atrophy of the spleen has been commonly described.[87,463] Lymphoid depletion has also been documented in lymph nodes, with some studies finding reactive plasmablastic proliferation[463] and hemophagocytosis.[90] Rarely, skeletal muscle may have mononuclear myositis associated with myocyte necrosis.[463]

Immune Responses to SARS-CoV-2

T-Cell Immunity

Both T- and B-cell responses against SARS-CoV-2 are detected approximately 1 week after the onset of symptoms. The notion that activated T cells are key determinants of protection may explain the increased susceptibility of older individuals to severe COVID-19.[282] Aging is associated with thymic involution, which depletes the potential to generate new T-cell repertoires. In contrast, T-cell repertoires are abundant in children which may explain their resistance to severe disease.[366]

CD8+ T cells are important for directly attacking and killing virus-infected cells, whereas CD4+ T cells are crucial to prime both CD8+ T cells and B cells.[650] CD4+ T cells are also responsible for cytokine production to drive immune cell

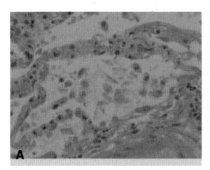
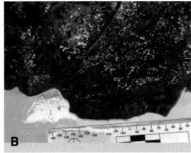
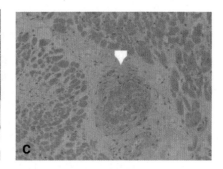

FIGURE 22.2 Typical autopsy findings in severe COVID-19. A: Diffuse alveolar damage—congestion/proliferation phases, with lymphocytic infiltration of alveolar septa. **B:** Typical macroscopic appearance of COVID-19 lung. **C:** Thrombus in intramyocardial arteriole (*arrowhead*), with surrounding subacute microinfarct. (Reprinted from Sekhawat V, Green A, Mahadeva U. COVID-19 autopsies: conclusions from international studies. *Diagn Histopathol (Oxf)*. 2021;27(3):103–107. Copyright © 2020 Elsevier. With permission.)

recruitment. After SARS-CoV-1 infection, the CD4+ T-cell response includes production of IFN-γ, TNF, and IL-2, suggesting a T_H1 cell response to control the infection.[318,610] Spike-reactive CD4+ T cells not only were detected in most infected individuals but also have been detected in up to 1/3 of uninfected unvaccinated controls.[88] The SARS-CoV-2-reactive CD4+ T cells from healthy controls also responded to the spike proteins of human endemic coronaviruses 229E and OC43 suggesting a cross reactive response to the seasonal coronaviruses. These findings support the importance of CD4+ T cells in creating effective cross-reactive immune responses. It has been suggested that frequent exposure to endemic coronaviruses in children are part of the reason of decreased severity of disease in this population.

In patients with COVID-19, CD8+ T cells exhibiting activated phenotypes are commonly observed, although the absolute number of CD8+ T cells is decreased.[561] SARS-CoV-2–specific CD8+ T-cell responses have been identified in most individuals after recovery from COVID-19.[258] These responses are specific to a wide range of SARS-CoV-2 antigens, including spike, nucleocapsid, and membrane proteins, as well as other nonstructural proteins.[258,377] In the acute phase of COVID-19, SARS-CoV-2–specific CD8+ T cells express activation markers (CD38 and HLA-DR), Ki-67, inhibitor checkpoint receptors (PD-1, TIM-3, and LAG-3), and cytotoxic proteins (perforin and granzyme B), indicating that these cells are activated and proliferate with a high cytotoxic capacity.[594] However, an exhausted CD8+ T-cell phenotype with an up-regulation of inhibitory receptors such as PD-1, TIM-3, LAG-3, CTLA-4, NKG2A, and CD39, has been described in patients with COVID-19, particularly in those with severe disease.[561,618] After recovery from the acute illness, SARS-CoV-2–specific T-cell responses are maintained in convalescent individuals up to 10 months postinfection, indicating that SARS-CoV-2–specific T-cell memory develops successfully and is long lasting.[561] Depletion of CD8+ T cells in convalescent macaques partially abrogated the protective efficacy of natural immunity against rechallenge with SARS-CoV-2 suggesting cellular immunity is important for long-term protection.[452]

B-Cell Immunity

B-cell activation and rapid production of antigen-specific antibodies are critical for the control of viral infections. B-cell responses occur concomitantly with T-cell responses, starting around 1 week after symptom onset.[650] The seroconversion rate and antibody levels increased rapidly during the first 2 weeks after symptom onset with the cumulative seropositive rate reaching 50% by day 11 and 100% by day 39.[282,485,653] Moreover, the median seroconversion time of total antibody, IgM, and IgG were observed at day 11, 12, and 14, respectively.[751] Poor antibody responses are associated with ineffective SARS-CoV-2 clearance in some patients.[733] Adoptive transfer of purified IgG from convalescent rhesus macaques protects naive recipient macaques against challenge with SARS-CoV-2 in a dose-dependent fashion.[452]

After infection, there are high-level IgG, IgM, and IgA reactivity to the structural proteins—spike (S), matrix (M), and nucleocapsid (N) of SARS-CoV-2, as well as accessory proteins such as ORF3a and ORF7a.[106] Antibodies against the N protein typically arise first.[643,719] Uninfected unvaccinated individuals can have antibodies that cross-react to SARS-CoV-2, likely from prior seasonal coronavirus, and are mainly targeted to N and the carboxy portion of the S (S2) proteins.[222] Antibodies to the amino portion of S (S1) and the receptor binding domain (RBD) are more specific to SARS-CoV-2 infections. With acute infection, substantial populations of endemic human coronavirus reactive antibody-secreting cells expand signifying preexisting immunity though these antibodies were generally nonneutralizing and nonprotective *in vivo*.[199] In a vaccinated population, the risk of symptomatic COVID-19 decreased with increasing levels of anti-spike IgG, anti-RBD IgG, pseudovirus neutralization, and live-virus neutralization titers.[213] Correlates of protection have not been established after infection, but likely entail similar immunologic parameters.

Antibody responses tend to be higher in more severe cases, although there is considerable heterogeneity.[429] Memory B cells persist or increase even as antibody levels wane.[583] There have also been reports of B cells undergoing somatic hypermutation over the course of 6 months, consistent with persistent antigen.[228] It is unknown if protection against COVID-19 is durable over years, given that protection against other circulating coronaviruses tends to be short lived, as seen by increased reinfection after 1 year.[203,429] Modeling suggests that a loss in protection from SARS-CoV-2 infection may occur, while protection from severe disease including hospitalization and death should be largely retained.[349]

SARS-CoV-2 VARIANT VIRUSES

Genetic variants of SARS-CoV-2 have been emerging and circulating around the world throughout the COVID-19 pandemic. Variants of interest are those strains with specific genetic markers that have been associated with changes to receptor binding, reduced neutralization by antibodies generated against previous infection or vaccination, reduced efficacy of treatments, potential diagnostic impact, or predicted increase in transmissibility or disease severity.[123] Variants being monitored include variants for which there are data indicating a potential or clear impact on approved or authorized medical countermeasures or that have been associated with more severe disease or increased transmission, but the variant viruses are no longer detected or are circulating at very low levels in the United States. Variants of Concern are those strains with evidence of an increase in transmissibility, more severe disease (e.g., increased hospitalizations or deaths), significant reduction in neutralization by antibodies generated during previous infection or vaccination, reduced effectiveness of treatments or vaccines, or diagnostic detection failures.[123] The Delta (B.1.617.2) and Omicron (B.1.1.529) variants are currently classified as Variants of Concern. Alpha (B.1.1.7), Beta (B.1.351), Gamma (P.1), and others are currently considered variants being monitored.

Alpha (B.1.1.7)
- First identified in September 2020 in the United Kingdom. Includes sublineage with E484K mutation. Most recently has become a minority of isolates.[245]

- Associated with higher viral concentrations in nasopharyngeal swabs compared to the original (wild-type) virus.[178]
- Approximately 30% increased transmission relative to non-variants.[107]
- In postvaccination sera, exhibited a 1.7-fold reduction in pseudovirus neutralization and 1.3-fold reduction in live virus neutralization compared to wild-type (D614G).[518]
- Risk of death was reported as 55% to 64% higher when compared to other strains.[128,178]

Beta (B.1.351)
- First identified in September 2020 in South Africa, but declined in 2021.[245]
- Approximately 25% increased transmission relative to the original wild-type strain.[107]
- In postvaccination sera, exhibited a 6.9-fold reduction in pseudovirus neutralization and 4.6-fold reduction in live virus neutralization compared to wild-type (D614G).[518]

Gamma (P.1)
- First identified in October 2020 in Brazil. Most recently has decreased in prevalence in much of the world but continues to widely circulate in South America.[245]
- Approximately 40% increased transmission relative to the original wild-type strain.[107]
- In postvaccination sera, exhibited a 3.2-fold reduction in pseudovirus neutralization compared to wild-type (D614G).[518]

Delta (B.1.617.2)
- First identified in September 2020 in India. Includes sublineages AY.1 to AY.12. This strain became widespread and the most common isolate in many countries during 2021.[245]
- Approximately 100% increased transmission relative to the original wild-type strain.[107]
- In postvaccination sera, exhibited a 2.4-fold reduction in pseudovirus neutralization compared to wild-type (D614G).[518]

Omicron (B.1.1.529)
- First identified in November 2021 in Botswana and reported to WHO on November 24, 2021. Contains mutations associated with reduced neutralization to some anti-SARS-CoV-2 monoclonal antibodies, increased transmissibility, and immune escape.[104,715]

Other variants being monitored, but have not widely circulated, include the following:

• Epsilon	B.1.427 and B.1.429
• Eta	B.1.525
• Iota	B.1.526
• Kappa	B.1.617.1
• Zeta	P.2
• Mu	B.1.621, B.1.621.1

As variant viruses have the potential to significantly evolve, the data in this chapter including epidemiology, transmission, pathogenesis, and efficacy of vaccines and therapeutics may change; thus, awareness of the circulating variants and their impact on the parameters above is critical to understanding and managing COVID-19.

EPIDEMIOLOGIC PARAMETERS

Transmission Dynamics

Based upon data from studies conducted when the original Wuhan SARS-CoV-2 strain was predominant, the incubation period for COVID-19 was estimated to be a median of 5.1 days (95% CI 4.5 to 5.8)[374] and a mean of 5.2 days after SARS-CoV-2 infection (95% CI 4.1 to 7)[399,744] with a range estimated in different populations and countries to be 4 to 7 days.[17,205,345,447,700,748] A pooled analysis estimated that 97.5% of symptomatic illness occurs within 11.5 days (CI 8.2 to 15.6) of SARS-CoV-2 infection.[374] Meta-analyses have estimated the serial interval (time from illness onset in an index case to illness onset in a secondary case) to be 5.2 to 5.4 days suggesting transmission occurs early after symptom onset.[17,541,748] The pooled mean serial interval in China was 4.9 days (range 1.9 to 6.5) after the pandemic peak compared to 6.2 days (range 5.1 to 7.8) before the pandemic peak and may have been affected by differences in time to the isolation of index cases.[19] The SARS-CoV-2 incubation period might vary in different variants. For example, an investigation of an outbreak of COVID-19 due to the Delta variant in mid-2021 in southern China reported a median incubation period of 4 days and a median serial interval of 3 days, both shorter than what has been reported for non-Delta SARS-CoV-2 infections.[747]

Secondary attack rates can vary by transmission settings (e.g., households, workplaces, social settings, health care facilities)[660] and extent of prevention and control measures; secondary transmission is highest in households.[427,660] One study estimated that susceptibility to SARS-CoV-2 infection increased with older age and that most secondary and tertiary transmission occurred in households.[299] A meta-analysis reported that the overall estimated secondary household attack rate for SARS-CoV-2 infection was 18.9% but was 24.5% for the Delta variant.[427] In one study of SARS-CoV-2–infected index cases aged 7 to 19 years old, of whom 88% were symptomatic, transmission occurred in 18% of households with a secondary attack rate of 45%.[157] The basic reproduction number (R_0, the average number of secondary cases resulting from exposure to an index case) is typically greater than 2 but has been estimated to vary from 0.48 to 14.8 on a large cruise ship.[231]

Some SARS-CoV-2 variants, such as those comprising the Alpha lineage, are estimated to have a substantially higher estimated basic reproduction number and are associated with greater transmissibility in community settings than earlier circulating SARS-CoV-2 viruses.[177] The Delta variant was estimated to have 55% higher transmissibility than the Alpha variant.[107]

SARS-CoV-2 can be transmitted by infected persons before they are symptomatic,[288,539,720] and by those who never develop symptoms,[720] but secondary attack rates are likely lower than from symptomatic individuals. One study estimated that the latent period (time from infection to becoming infectious) was 5.5 days.[726] Estimates of secondary attack rates can vary depending on the definition of asymptomatic versus symptomatic or pauci-symptomatic and whether the data were based upon cross-sectional or longitudinal assessments. Two meta-analyses reported that the secondary attack rate was substantially lower in contacts of asymptomatic-infected persons compared with contacts of symptomatic SARS-CoV-2–

infected persons.[92,428] One meta-analysis estimated that the secondary attack rate for asymptomatic index cases was 1.9% but was 9.3% for presymptomatic and 13.6% for symptomatic index cases.[660] Another meta-analysis reported that the relative risk for transmission from asymptomatically infected persons was 42% lower than from symptomatic persons,[99] indicating that most transmission of SARS-CoV-2 is from symptomatic persons or infected persons just before symptom onset. A prospective study of U.S. households reported that the incidence of SARS-CoV-2 infections was similar among children and adults, but a greater proportion of infections among children were asymptomatic compared with adults.[181]

However, depending on the population and the number of asymptomatic individuals, asymptomatic SARS-CoV-2 infections may contribute substantially to transmission. One study that analyzed detailed contact tracing data from China found no difference in transmissibility between symptomatic and asymptomatically infected persons or between age groups and estimated that presymptomatic infected persons accounted for 59% of transmission events.[299] A study in university residence halls reported that transmission from SARS-CoV-2–infected persons, most of whom were asymptomatic, to their roommates was more likely to occur from index cases with higher estimated viral RNA levels compared to index cases with lower estimated viral RNA levels.[72] One study of a large SARS-CoV-2 outbreak among cruise ship passengers estimated that asymptomatic persons were the source for 69% of SARS-CoV-2 infections.[206]

Transmission Modes

Respiratory transmission through expelled large droplets and small particle droplet nuclei generated through aerosols is the primary mode of SARS-CoV-2 spread. SARS-CoV-2 has been isolated from nasopharyngeal,[105,280,302,394,737] oropharyngeal,[280,302] saliva,[320] sputum,[302] and bronchoalveolar lavage fluid[764] specimens of COVID-19 patients, indicating the potential for respiratory transmission. SARS-CoV-2 can be isolated from upper respiratory tract specimens of asymptomatic and presymptomatic individuals.[35,101,475,477] SARS-CoV-2 RNA is detectable in exhaled breath condensate from patients[423,578,760] and experimentally infected rhesus macaques,[204] suggesting potential for transmission through breathing or speech to close contacts. However, SARS-CoV-2 RNA may be more frequently detectable in aerosols produced by talking and singing, especially early in the clinical course, than in exhaled breath specimens.[162] Experimentally infected ferrets can transmit infectious SARS-CoV-2 through droplets to ferrets in an adjacent cage.[562] Air sampling from COVID-19 patients in hospital rooms has occasionally detected SARS-CoV-2 RNA, but the isolation of infectious virus is uncommon.[200,381,497,587] Superspreading events have occurred in nightclubs and bars,[133,331,472,633] on an aircraft carrier,[337] and aboard a cruise ship.[208] Epidemiological investigations have documented SARS-CoV-2 transmission in other closed settings including planes,[150,347] restaurants,[362,401,418,419] fitness centers and exercise facilities,[48,155,261,317,389] church services,[338] and church choir practice.[275] Air sampling has detected SARS-CoV-2 RNA after Cesarean and vaginal deliveries from asymptomatic pregnant women.[291] These events suggest that droplet spread facilitated by airflow or airborne transmission of aerosolized small particle SARS-CoV-2 more than 2 m is possible. Generally, these exposures are for periods of time of 30 minutes or more, but transmission can occur with exposures as short as 5 minutes.[362]

Infectious SARS-CoV-2 has rarely been isolated from non-respiratory specimens such as urine[320,635] or feces.[175,192,320,725] Viral RNA has been detected more frequently in feces than other nonrespiratory specimens.[140,143,509,571,711] SARS-CoV-2 RNA has been identified by sampling air in toilets and bathrooms of COVID-19 patients,[70,410] although infectious virus was not recovered.[70] One study suggested that fecal aerosol transmission of SARS-CoV-2 may have contributed to an outbreak of COVID-19 in a high-rise building in southern China.[332] Although SARS-CoV-2 RNA is detectable in plasma[65,136,210] and serum,[27,139] particularly in critically ill COVID-19 patients,[65,136,652] and is suggestive of viremia, infectious SARS-CoV-2 virus has not been isolated from blood.[27]

Extrapulmonary dissemination through viremia could explain the detection of viral RNA in cardiac tissues and recovery of infectious virus in urine. Some autopsy studies have reported extrapulmonary SARS-CoV-2 infection of multiple organ tissues based upon electron microscopy findings, but one comprehensive study noted that many of these reported results are based upon a misidentification of nonviral subcellular structures.[94] SARS-CoV-2 RNA was detected in the cerebrospinal fluid of an adolescent diagnosed with Guillain-Barré syndrome.[33] Detection of SARS-CoV-2 RNA has been reported infrequently in semen in patients with acute illness and recovered COVID-19 patients.[227,249,397] Detection of SARS-CoV-2 RNA has very rarely been reported in vaginal fluid[40,540,591,621,736] or amniotic fluid.[359,537,686] SARS-CoV-2 RNA has been detected infrequently in breast milk samples, but replication-competent virus has not been identified.[129,165,260] While respiratory droplets and secretions pose the highest potential of containing infectious SARS-CoV-2, and virus has been isolated sporadically from urine and feces during the acute phase of COVID-19, given the paucity of available data in which viral culture was performed on extrapulmonary specimens that tested positive for SARS-CoV-2 RNA, all extrapulmonary specimens should be considered potentially infectious during the acute phase of COVID-19, especially in patients with severe illness.

One experimental study demonstrated that SARS-CoV-2 can remain viable on different surfaces up to 72 hours and that aerosols may be viable for several hours.[677] Although SARS-CoV-2 RNA has been detected on various surfaces for prolonged periods, suggesting potential for fomite transmission, viral culture of patient fomites, and surfaces in households and health care settings and a quarantine hotel has only yielded recovery of infectious virus from one surface sample.[64,439,461]

Reverse zoonosis of SARS-CoV-2 transmission from people to animals has been reported in domesticated dogs and cats, farmed mink, captive tigers, and lions.[273,274,435] Experimental infection models are established in mice, Syrian golden hamsters, Chinese hamsters, cats, dogs, ferrets, raccoon dogs, cattle, tree shrews, and nonhuman primates (cynomolgus and rhesus macaques, and common marmosets),[83,435] However, animal-to-human SARS-CoV-2 transmission has only been reported from farmed mink, an event that also had evidence of reverse zoonosis and viral evolution in mink.[372,502]

Duration of Infectiousness

Peak SARS-CoV-2 RNA levels in the upper respiratory tract are typically observed during the first week after symptom onset and in the lower respiratory tract of persons with severe COVID-19 during the 2nd week of illness.[126] Reverse transcription polymerase chain reaction (RT-PCR) detection of SARS-CoV-2 RNA was most frequent in nasopharyngeal swab specimens collected within 4 days of symptoms onset in one systematic review.[437] SARS-CoV-2 RNA levels may be higher in respiratory specimens infected with the Alpha or Delta variants than viruses not considered variants of concern or interest.[326,395] In hospitalized COVID-19 patients, infection with the Delta variant was associated with significantly lower cycle threshold values and longer duration of SARS-CoV-2 RNA detection compared with wild-type SARS-CoV-2 from the first pandemic wave in Singapore.[495] Unvaccinated and fully vaccinated persons infected with the SARS-CoV-2 Delta variant may have similar viral RNA levels in respiratory specimens.[89,145] One meta-analysis of studies on wild-type Wuhan SARS-CoV-2 infections reported that the mean duration of SARS-CoV-2 RNA detection was 17 days (maximum 83 days) in the upper respiratory tract, 14.6 days in the lower respiratory tract (maximum 59 days), 17.2 days in stool (maximum 126 days), and 16.6 days in serum specimens (maximum 60 days).[126] Longer duration of SARS-CoV-2 RNA detection is associated with older age.[126,731,758] While SARS-CoV-2 RNA can be detected for prolonged periods in different clinical specimens from persons with asymptomatic infection, mild-to-moderate disease, and severe COVID-19, the presence of viral RNA does not necessarily indicate that infectious virus is present. Therefore, studies to assess evidence of replication–competent SARS-CoV-2, such as isolation in viral culture, are needed to inform the duration of infectiousness.

The duration of detection of infectious virus is shorter than detection of viral RNA. SARS-CoV-2 infectious virus has been isolated from upper respiratory tract specimens of asymptomatic[35,294,614] and presymptomatic persons.[35,486] In persons with mild-to-moderate COVID-19, SARS-CoV-2 RNA can be detected for prolonged periods, but infectious virus identified by viral culture is unlikely to be present in upper respiratory tract specimens beyond 8 to 10 days after illness onset.[35,93,504,521,711] However, one case report described isolation of SARS-CoV-2 infectious virus from sputum up to 18 days from illness onset in a patient with mild COVID-19 who had evidence of an endogenous antibody response[409] and an asymptomatic, previously healthy immunocompetent adolescent hospitalized for injuries sustained in a motor vehicle accident had SARS-CoV-2 isolated from a throat swab and tracheal aspirate specimens 54 days after hospital admission.[582] One study estimated that isolation of infectious virus was highest 2 days before symptom onset to 1 day after onset and declined within 7 days after onset.[288] Patients with severe disease may have a longer duration of infectiousness compared to patients with mild-to-moderate COVID-19. In hospitalized patients with severe COVID-19, SARS-CoV-2 has been isolated from respiratory specimens up to 20 days from illness onset, but infectious virus is unlikely to be recovered after 15 days from illness onset or when a neutralizing antibody titer of 1:80 was present.[679]

Some severely immunocompromised persons can have infectious SARS-CoV-2 detected in the upper respiratory tract for prolonged periods and pose a transmission risk to close contacts. Prolonged detection of the replication–competent infectious virus has been reported in case reports of patients with chronic lymphocytic leukemia and acquired hypogammaglobulinemia, lymphoma, hematopoietic stem cell transplant, kidney transplant, heart transplant, chimeric antigen receptor T-cell therapy, or AIDS, and with shedding often beyond 20 days and as long as 143 days after an initial positive SARS-CoV-2 test results.[42,44,46,62,149,188,478,648] During prolonged SARS-CoV-2 replication in immunocompromised patients, especially those who are severely immunocompromised, viral evolution with emergence of mutations can occur with potential implications for treatment.[42,46,149,413]

CLINICAL DISEASE

Severity of Disease

Patients with SARS-CoV-2 infection can have clinical manifestations ranging from no symptoms to critical illness (Fig. 22.3). Discussions of severity of disease and treatment require a common understanding on how to define severity of disease. The US National Institutes of Health (NIH) COVID-19 Treatment guidelines define the following groups[289]:

- *Asymptomatic Infection:* Individuals who test positive for SARS-CoV-2 using a virologic test but who have no symptoms consistent with COVID-19.
- *Mild Illness:* Individuals who have any of the various signs and symptoms of COVID-19 but do not have shortness of breath, dyspnea, or abnormal chest imaging.
- *Moderate Illness:* Individuals with evidence of lower respiratory disease during clinical assessment or imaging and oxygen saturation (SpO_2) $\geq$94% on room air at sea level.
- *Severe Illness:* Individuals who have SpO_2 <94% on room air at sea level, a ratio of arterial partial pressure of oxygen to fraction of inspired oxygen (PaO_2/FiO_2) less than 300 mm Hg, respiratory frequency greater than 30 breaths/min, or lung infiltrates greater than 50%.
- *Critical Illness:* Individuals who have respiratory failure, septic shock, or multiple organ dysfunction.

The World Health Organization (WHO) defines the criteria for severity of illness slightly differently[716]:

- Nonsevere COVID-19: Absence of any criteria for severe or critical COVID-19.
  - Nonsevere is further divided into moderate (evidence of pneumonia), or mild (no evidence of pneumonia).
- Severe COVID-19: Any of the following:
  - Oxygen saturation less than 90% on room air.
  - Respiratory rate greater than 30 breaths/min in adults and children greater than 5 years old; $\geq$60 breaths/min in children less than 2 months old; $\geq$50 in children 2 to 11 months old; and $\geq$40 in children 1 to 5 years old.
  - Signs of severe respiratory distress including accessory muscle use and inability to complete full sentences. In children, this may include chest wall indrawing, grunting, central cyanosis, or the presence of any other general danger signs.
- Critical COVID-19: acute respiratory distress syndrome (ARDS), sepsis, septic shock, or other conditions that would require the provision of life-sustaining therapies such as mechanical ventilation (invasive or noninvasive) or vasopressor therapy.

The definitions used by the U.S. Food and Drug Administration (FDA) for descriptions for COVID-19 therapeutics generally align with the NIH COVID-19 Treatment Guidelines,[308,672] but sponsors of FDA-regulated trials are permitted to develop study-specific criteria. Clinical trials will use established criteria,[567] develop their own severity of illness criteria,[60] or not use any categorizations.[551,558]

Spectrum of Disease

The clinical spectrum of SARS-CoV-2 infection ranges from asymptomatic to critical illness with fatal outcomes. Meta-analyses have estimated that 17% (95% CI 14 to 20)[99] to 20% (95% CI 17 to 25)[92] of persons with SARS-CoV-2 infection remain asymptomatic, although the asymptomatic proportion of infected persons has been estimated to be as high as 65%.[451] One study of more than 44,000 laboratory-confirmed COVID-19 patients in China reported that 81% had a mild-to-moderate illness, 14% had severe disease requiring hospitalization, and an additional 5% were critically ill and required admission to an intensive care unit.[722]

For symptomatic COVID-19, signs and symptoms can vary by age and underlying medical conditions, are nonspecific and highly variable, and may overlap with symptoms of other respiratory viral infections. In nonhospitalized adult patients, COVID-19 often begins as cough, fever, fatigue or weakness, and headache.[73,538] Among adults with laboratory-confirmed COVID-19, the most common systemic signs and symptoms were fever, fatigue, myalgia, and rigors, and the most common respiratory symptoms are cough, typically nonproductive, dyspnea, wheezing, and chest pain.[254] Other symptoms may be chills, hyposmia or anosmia, headache, and less commonly nausea, vomiting, diarrhea, abdominal pain, sore throat, hypogeusia or ageusia, nasal congestion, rhinorrhea, or conjunctivitis.[254] Olfactory dysfunction, predominantly presenting as anosmia, may precede, accompany, or follow other COVID-19 symptoms in persons with a mild-to-moderate illness.[380] Gastrointestinal symptoms (nausea, vomiting, diarrhea, or abdominal pain) can occur without respiratory symptoms or may precede or occur concurrently with respiratory symptoms.[323,422,508,555] A wide range of focal and diffuse central nervous system and peripheral nervous system signs and symptoms occur in patients with COVID-19.[264,564] Delirium with impaired consciousness, disorientation, and hypoactive symptoms or agitation can occur in older adults.[341]

Dermatologic findings occur with variable frequency in COVID-19 patients. One meta-analysis reported that the prevalence of skin manifestations was 1%,[586] but some studies of COVID-19 patients have reported higher frequencies of cutaneous lesions.[182,586] Skin lesions most commonly reported include erythematous rash (macular, papular, morbilliform), less frequently pruritic plaques, urticaria, painful chilblain-like lesions of the hands and toes, vesicles, livedoid vasculitis, and necrotic lesions.[182,246,321,522,586] Limb lesions are more common than truncal and facial lesions.[522] Chilblain-like acral lesions (painful inflammation of small blood vessels in the skin) are associated with younger and nonsevere illnesses and last longer than other cutaneous findings.[443] Urticaria, exanthems, and livedoid lesions may occur during the 2 weeks after COVID-19 symptom onset, whereas chilblain-like lesions are observed after the first 2 weeks; purpuric and petechial lesions can occur anytime during the 4 weeks after onset of other COVID-19 symptoms.[246]

In adults with uncomplicated mild-to-moderate COVID-19 not requiring hospital admission, approximately half improve and return to their baseline health by 2 to 3 weeks after illness onset, but impaired recovery is more common with increasing age and comorbidities.[647,654] In persons who have progressive disease, dyspnea may occur in the 2nd week of illness during the inflammatory phase of COVID-19. The median time from illness onset to hospital presentation was 4 days in the United Kingdom[194] and 5 to 7 days in the United States.[169,170] Among patients reported in early studies from Wuhan, China, who had

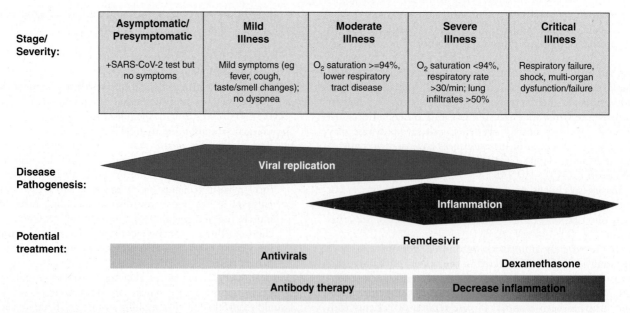

FIGURE 22.3 Characteristics, diagnosis, and pathogenesis of COVID-19 according to disease stage or severity. (From Gandhi RT. The multidimensional challenge of treating coronavirus disease 2019 (COVID-19): remdesivir is a foot in the door. *Clin Infect Dis* 2021;73(11):e4175–e4178. Reproduced by permission of Oxford University Press.)

severe COVID-19, the median time from illness onset to experiencing dyspnea was 5 to 8 days[301,690,759] and the median time from onset to hospitalization was 7 to 11 days.[301,690,759]

Acute respiratory distress syndrome (ARDS), a syndrome of progressive pulmonary infiltrates and hypoxia, generally occurs 8 to 12 days after illness and often requires admission to an intensive care unit and either high oxygen requirements or mechanical ventilation.[301,690,759] A meta-analysis of critically ill COVID-19 patients in 17 countries reported that the median time from illness onset to ICU admission was 9 days, with a median ICU duration of 10.8 days.[642] U.S. studies of hospitalized adults during the early months of the first pandemic wave reported that 19% to 32% of COVID-19 patients required ICU admission.[169,350,570] Duration of hospitalization for COVID-19 patients has changed over time as clinical management has evolved, infection prevention and control criteria for requiring in-hospital isolation have changed, and some patients with pneumonia and hypoxia are discharged on supplemental oxygen.[52] One study in two U.S. states reported that the estimated median duration of hospitalization in survivors was 9 days versus nearly 13 days for COVID-19 patients that died, and the median duration of ICU stay was nearly 11 days.[393] Among studies of hospitalized COVID-19 patients in New York City from the early spring pandemic wave, one study reported that the median length of stay was 7 days, but it was 36 days for critically ill patients.[523]

In the United States, overall in-hospital mortality during the first pandemic wave was 20%[570] but declined over the first 6 months.[37] A large U.S. study reported that in-hospital mortality decreased from 16.4% during March to April 2020 to 8.6% during September to October 2020.[61] In contrast, the ages of hospitalized patients and in-hospital mortality increased during the second pandemic wave in South Africa.[319] One meta-analysis estimated an overall pooled mortality of 39% (95% CI 23% to 56%) for COVID-19 patients with ARDS during the first pandemic wave.[283] While overall 90-day mortality in critically ill adults in France, Belgium, and Switzerland during the initial pandemic wave was 31%, 90-day mortality ranged from 30% in patients diagnosed with mild ARDS at ICU admission to 50% in those with severe ARDS. However, overall mortality declined significantly from 42% to 25% from February to May 2020.[167] In Brazil, overall in-hospital mortality from February to August 2020 was 38% but was 59% in ICU patients and 80% in mechanically ventilated patients.[542] One meta-analysis of COVID-19 patients admitted to ICUs in 17 countries during the first pandemic wave reported overall 28.1% ICU mortality.[642] One meta-analysis estimated overall in-hospital mortality in mechanically ventilated patients to be 45% during the first 6 months of the pandemic and ranged from 48% in patients aged ≤40 years to 84% in those aged greater than 80 years.[402]

High levels of hospital strain from the patient surge are associated with a greater risk of death in critically ill COVID-19 patients.[665] One large U.S. study of data from 558 hospitals reported that surge in COVID-19 patient caseload was associated with an increased risk of in-hospital mortality across wards, ICUs, and intubated COVID-19 patients.[329] The association was stronger during the summer 2020 pandemic wave than the first wave despite wider use of corticosteroids as the standard of care and less frequent intubation at hospital admission. While COVID-19–related mortality declined after the early months of the first pandemic wave,[216,234,386,573,629] including in critically ill patients,[29] and was likely due to multiple factors, including improvements in clinical management, over-

all mortality due to COVID-19 was substantially higher when excess deaths not initially attributed to COVID-19 were considered and analyzed.[626]

Patients who survive hospitalization for COVID-19 are at risk of related complications that may require readmission. One U.S. study of COVID-19 patients hospitalized during the first pandemic wave reported that readmission within 60 days of hospital discharge was more common among those discharged to a skilled nursing facility or those needing home health care than for those discharged home for self-care.[375] The risk of hospital readmission increased with age ≥65 years, presence of certain chronic medical conditions, and hospitalization within 3 months preceding COVID-19 hospitalization. A U.K. study of the first pandemic wave reported that 28% of COVID-19 patients discharged from the hospital were readmitted or died within 60 days.[312] Among elderly predominantly male veterans with COVID-19 who survived hospitalization during the first pandemic wave in the United States, 27% were readmitted or died within 60 days of discharge.[195] However, in a younger population (median 51 years) discharged on supplemental oxygen from an emergency department or after hospitalization, the 30-day hospital readmission rate was 8.5%.[52]

CLINICAL COMPLICATIONS

Respiratory Complications

The most common pulmonary complication of COVID-19 is pneumonia, typically bilateral and manifested by dyspnea and shortness of breath with hypoxemia that may progress to respiratory failure and ARDS,[464,529,642] pulmonary emboli,[230,566] and coinfections (see "Coinfections"). Hypoxemia (oxygen saturation <92%) or respiratory rate greater than 22/minute at hospital admission was associated with an increased risk of in-hospital death.[132] However, hypoxemia can be clinically inapparent without dyspnea, including in critically ill COVID-19 patients. One study reported that occult hypoxemia was not detected by pulse oximetry nearly three times more frequently in Black patients than White patients.[615] Progression of pneumonia to hypoxemic respiratory failure and acute respiratory distress syndrome (ARDS) is common.[690,759]

Extrapulmonary Complications

A broad spectrum of extrapulmonary complications occurs in COVID-19, with differences in clinical phenotypes, complications, and involvement of different organ systems, including sepsis, septic shock, and multiorgan dysfunction or failure resulting in severe to critical illness.[500] Cardiac complications include acute cardiac injury, myocarditis, acute coronary syndrome, heart failure, arrhythmias, thromboembolic events, and sudden cardiac death.[404,754] One study reported that while myocarditis is rare, COVID-19 was associated with 15.7 times the risk for myocarditis compared with patients without COVID-19, and the risk was highest for persons aged less than 16 years or ≥75 years.[77] Uncommonly, myocarditis associated with recent SARS-CoV-2 infection in college athletes can be detected by laboratory and imaging studies and may be subclinical.[174] Acute myocardial injury with elevated troponin levels is associated with cardiovascular and noncardiovascular complications and death.[267,367,414,608]

Acute kidney injury is prevalent in 8% to 10% of hospitalized COVID-19 patients and approximately 20% of critically ill patients and is associated with in-hospital death.[141,355,410,730] Among critically ill COVID-19 patients with acute kidney injury requiring renal replacement therapy, mortality is high, and a high proportion of survivors require renal replacement therapy at hospital discharge.[270] Gastrointestinal complications reported in critically ill COVID-19 patients include pancreatitis, acute hepatic injury (transaminitis), gastrointestinal bleeding, severe ileus, acute megacolon, and intestinal ischemia.[328]

Neurologic complications of COVID-19 include encephalopathy, meningoencephalitis, impaired consciousness, syncope, seizures, Guillain-Barré syndrome, myelitis, ischemic stroke, cardioembolic stroke, intracerebral hemorrhage, cranial nerve impairment, visual deficits and oculomotor impairment, neuroinflammatory disorders, peripheral neuropathies, and altered mental status with neuropsychiatric disorders.[264,279,490,681,732] Altered mental status during hospitalization is associated with prolonged hospitalization, ICU admission, intubation, and in-hospital mortality.[127,340] Musculoskeletal complications include myositis, myopathy, and uncommonly rhabdomyolysis; rhabdomyolysis is associated with in-hospital death.[239,343] In one U.K. study, neurologic complications had the strongest associations with worsened ability to self-care than before COVID-19.[197]

SARS-CoV-2 infection of the respiratory tract can induce a hypercoagulable state.[1,290,307,333,353,498,645] Coagulopathy with microvascular and macrovascular venous thromboembolism and arterial thrombi occur in COVID-19 patients.[237,498] The prevalence of venous thromboembolism, including pulmonary embolism and deep venous thrombosis, has been reported in more than 25% of critically ill COVID-19 patients, with a higher risk of death compared with COVID-19 patients without venous thromboembolism,[356] and can occur despite prophylactic anticoagulation.[144,322,743] Autopsy studies have shown that deep venous thromboembolism is often unrecognized before death.[664,709] Cerebral venous sinus thrombosis is an uncommon complication of COVID-19 but is associated with high mortality in critically ill children and adults, with or without concurrent venous thromboembolism.[51,173,293,311,599,670] Pulmonary and systemic arterial thrombi and coronary arterial thrombi leading to myocardial infarction, with high mortality, can occur despite anticoagulation.[154,342,458] In survivors of hospitalization, venous thromboembolism requiring rehospitalization can occur within 90 days after initial discharge.[241]

Coinfections

Community-acquired invasive bacterial or fungal coinfection with SARS-CoV-2 causing secondary bacterial or fungal pneumonia is uncommon at hospital admission,[9,235,305,334,335,369,370,388,574,577,666,682] including admission to the intensive care unit.[575] While bacteremia at hospital admission is uncommon,[371,596,658,739] the prevalence of bacterial bloodstream infections in COVID-19 patients at admission is higher in long-term care facility residents than in noninstitutionalized persons.[13] Limited data are available on SARS-CoV-2 and *Mycobacterium tuberculosis* coinfection, but tuberculosis may contribute to higher disease severity and mortality of COVID-19 regardless of HIV status.[459,641,707] Community-acquired coinfections with respiratory syncytial virus, influenza viruses, rhinoviruses, enteroviruses, human coronaviruses, adenoviruses, parainfluenza viruses, or human metapneumovirus in hospitalized COVID-19 patients are infrequent.[23,96,235,379,590,702] Data on SARS-CoV-2 and influenza virus coinfection are limited, but severe to fatal illness has occurred.[166,168,284,628,724,757] People with HIV who develop

COVID-19 may have a higher risk of death than those without HIV.[68,634,707] SARS-CoV-2 and dengue virus coinfections have been described in critically ill patients.[580]

Critically ill COVID-19 patients are at risk for hospital-acquired multidrug resistant bacterial and fungal infections (e.g., *Aspergillus* sp., *Candida* sp.) and ventilator-associated pneumonia, contributing to high mortality.[76,368,430,531,546,708] Gram-negative bacteria and *Staphylococcus aureus* were identified in nearly all cases of ventilator-associated pneumonia in critically ill COVID-19 patients in a multicenter cohort study in Italy.[256] Hospital-acquired infections were significantly associated with prolonged duration of mechanical ventilation, ICU admission, and hospital admission; septic shock nearly doubled in-hospital mortality compared to patients without hospital-acquired infections.[256] However, a U.K. study reported that bacterial coinfection or hospital-acquired infection was not associated with in-hospital mortality in critically ill COVID-19 patients.[577] A study in India reported that the development of mucormycosis more than 1 week after onset of COVID-19 symptoms was associated with hypoxemia due to COVID-19 and inappropriate use of corticosteroids at high doses or when not clinically indicated.[511]

Laboratory Findings

In hospitalized patients with COVID-19, several laboratory biomarkers are associated with poor outcomes (e.g., intensive care admission, invasive mechanical ventilation, in-hospital death), including lymphopenia, thrombocytopenia, and elevated white blood cell count; neutrophil count; C-reactive protein (CRP); procalcitonin; D-dimer; N-terminal pronatriuretic peptide; creatine kinase; aspartate aminotransferase (AST); alanine aminotransferase (ALT); creatinine; and lactate dehydrogenase (LDH).[436,501,718,746,761] An elevated neutrophil to lymphocyte ratio and an elevated LDH level were associated with severe COVID-19, and elevated CRP and B-type natriuretic peptide (BNP) were associated with disease progression in severe and critical illness.[407] The neutrophil-to-lymphocyte ratio was significantly higher in moderately ill and severely ill COVID-19 patients than in mild illnesses and significantly higher in fatal cases than in nonfatal cases.[20]

Compared with nonseverely ill patients, a meta-analysis showed that severely ill COVID-19 patients had significantly higher levels of CRP, erythrocyte sedimentation rate (ESR), procalcitonin (PCT), interleukin-6 (IL-6), IL-10, IL-2R, serum amyloid A (SAA), and neutrophil-to-lymphocyte ratio (NLR), and fatal cases had significantly higher levels of CRP, IL-6, procalcitonin, ferritin, and NLR compared with survivors.[434] One study reported that elevated levels of cardiac troponin I, D-dimer, CRP, and LDH at hospital admission were associated with an increased risk of 30-day all-cause death.[519]

Although many COVID-19 prognostic models that rely partly or entirely upon biomarkers attempted to predict mortality or progression to severe disease, a systematic review and critical appraisal concluded that these models were poorly reported and at high risk of bias and that one promising model needs further validation.[675] A prognostic tool based upon detailed clinical and biomarker data was developed to calculate the risk of disease progression in hospitalized adult COVID-19 patients using readily available clinical data, but further validation is also needed.[713]

Higher SARS-CoV-2 RNA levels or lower RT-PCR cycle threshold values in respiratory tract specimens have been associated with increased disease severity in most but not all studies,[22,34,86,184,268,378,432,438,474,536,543] and prolonged SARS-CoV-2

RNA detection is associated with severe or critical COVID-19.[225,462,728] SARS-CoV-2 RNA levels in the lower respiratory tract may be associated with mortality.[91] Observational studies have reported that qualitative and quantitative detection of SARS-CoV-2 RNA in plasma or serum is associated with ICU admission, mechanical ventilation, and death.[65,210,295,533,727] Detection of SARS-CoV-2 RNA in fecal specimens during hospitalization was associated with increased risk of death, and stool specimens from patients who subsequently died had higher SARS-CoV-2 RNA levels compared with survivors.[175] Higher plasma SARS-CoV-2 RNA levels are associated with biomarkers of disease severity and inflammation, such as lower absolute lymphocyte counts; higher levels of CRP, ferritin, IL-6, and chemokines (CXCL10, CCL2); and elevated markers of endothelial dysfunction (VCAM-1, angiopoietin-2, ICAM-1), coagulation activation (D-dimer, INR), tissue damage (LDH, ALT), neutrophil count and activation (myeloperoxidase, GM-CSF), and antiinflammatory molecules (PD-L1, IL-10).[65,210]

Radiographic and Imaging Findings

Chest radiographic and computerized tomography (CT) findings in COVID-19 patients with pneumonia are nonspecific and overlap with other respiratory viral infections.[160] CT is more sensitive than a chest x-ray, but portable chest x-ray is often used to assess pneumonia in the emergency department and hospitalized patients because of infection control requirements and time needed for disinfection of the CT scanner and equipment.[314,576] Chest radiographs of patients with COVID-19 pneumonia typically demonstrate multifocal bilateral peripheral air-space confluent or patchy opacities and consolidation, although unilateral abnormalities may be observed.[335,406] As pneumonia progresses to respiratory failure, chest radiographs demonstrate diffuse opacities and consolidation.[314] Chest CT may reveal evidence of pneumonia with ground glass opacities in asymptomatic persons with SARS-CoV-2 infection or before symptom onset.[18,454,742] Chest CT images from patients with COVID-19 pneumonia frequently demonstrate bilateral, peripheral ground-glass opacities, more commonly in the lower lobes than upper lobes.[53,66,493,606,613,696,729,734,753] (Fig. 22.4). A cross-sectional study reported that the extent of total lung segment involvement observed by chest CT scan was positively correlated with peripheral neutrophil count and negatively correlated with peripheral lymphocyte count.[695] Pleural effusion is infrequent but is more common in critically ill COVID-19 patients than non-ICU patients.[734] One study of serial chest CT scans from adult COVID-19 patients with mild-to-moderate illness showed maximum lung involvement peaks at 9 to 13 days after illness onset.[506] Lung ultrasound has also been used in emergency department settings to diagnose COVID-19 pneumonia.[306]

RISK FACTORS FOR SEVERE DISEASE

The risk of ICU admission, in-hospital death, and overall death with COVID-19 increase with increasing age.[67,255,350,525] One study estimated that 82% of unrecognized deaths attributable to COVID-19 in the United States were among persons aged ≥65 years.[313] People with multiple chronic medical conditions are at higher risk for severe disease, ICU admission, and death with COVID-19 than persons with few or no comorbid conditions.[262,350,570,749]

The COVID-19 pandemic has highlighted racial and ethnic disparities and health inequities. Most studies have reported that Black and Hispanic persons have

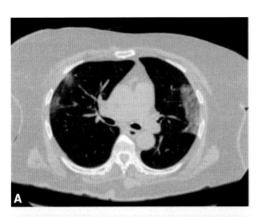

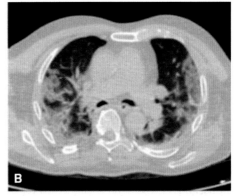

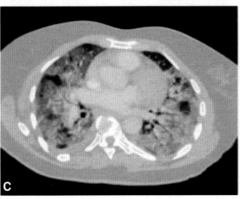

FIGURE 22.4 Chest computed tomography in three patients with COVID-19. A: Noncontrast examination with rounded, bilateral ground glass opacities (*dashed arrow*) and interlobular septal thickening giving appearance of crazy paving (*solid arrow*). **B:** Noncontrast examination with rounded, bilateral ground glass opacities and areas of surrounding consolidation giving appearance of reverse halo sign (*solid arrow*). **C:** Contrast-enhanced examination with ground glass and dense consolidation bilaterally and air bronchogram (*solid arrow*). (From Kaufman AE, Naidu S, Ramachandran S, et al. Review of radiographic findings in COVID-19. *World J Radiol* 2020;12(8):142–155. Reprinted by permission of Baishideng Publishing Group Inc.)

experienced disproportionately higher morbidity and mortality from COVID-19 than other racial groups in the United States[45,425,534] CDC population-based COVID-19 hospital surveillance during March 2020 to February 2021 indicated that American Indian or Alaska Native, Latino, Black, and Asian or Pacific Islander persons had higher cumulative age-adjusted rates of hospitalization, ICU admission, and death compared with White persons.[7,117] One U.S. study reported that Black patients hospitalized with COVID-19 were more likely to die or be discharged to hospice care than White patients, possibly due to differences in the hospitals to which Black and White patients were admitted.[36] A study in Mexico City highlighted socioeconomic disparities and reported that unemployed persons, persons without specific occupations, those who worked at home, and retired persons had increased risks of adverse outcomes from COVID-19, including death.[31] Higher COVID-19–related mortality was reported in United States nursing homes with higher proportions of minority residents than in nursing homes with low proportions of minority residents.[400] Viral factors, such as infection with a SARS-CoV-2 variant virus of concern, may also increase the risk of severe COVID-19 disease. Infection with the Alpha (B.1.1.7) variant or Delta (B.1.617.2) variant is associated with increased risk of hospitalization, critical illness, and death.[49,178,259,491,513,604] Infection with the Delta variant was associated with 1.88 times higher odds of pneumonia compared with non-Delta wild-type virus infection in Singapore,[495] and the Delta variant was associated with a significantly higher risk of emergency care visit or hospital admission compared with the Alpha variant in England.[671] A Canadian study reported that infection with the Delta variant was associated with a significantly increased risk of ICU admission and death compared to infection with other SARS-CoV-2 variants.[219] A U.S. study that was restricted to hospitalized COVID-19 patients did not find any significant increases in the proportion of adult patients with severe outcomes before and during the predominance of the Delta variant.[651,671]

A U.S. study reported that a history of metastatic cancer, myocardial infarction, cerebrovascular disease, heart failure, hemiplegia, dementia, diabetes, chronic pulmonary disease, and hyperlipidemia were all significantly associated with increased risk of in-hospital COVID-19–related death.[570] A U.K. study reported that solid organ transplant; hematologic malignancy; neurologic disease other than stroke or dementia; diabetes; liver disease; nonhematologic cancer; respiratory disease excluding asthma, asplenia, rheumatoid arthritis, lupus, or psoriasis; cardiac disease; and asthma with recent corticosteroid use were associated with a higher risk of COVID-19–related death.[710] A study of COVID-19 patients in China reported that although persons with Type 2 diabetes were at increased risk of 28-day mortality, those with well-controlled blood glucose levels had a significantly lower risk of in-hospital death.[763] Obesity, defined as body mass index (BMI) $\geq$30 kg/m^2 is associated with an increased risk of severe COVID-19, including ICU admission, invasive mechanical ventilation, and death, with the risk of severe outcomes increasing with higher BMI.[26,233,358,530,649] Overweight (BMI $\geq$25 and <30 kg/m^2) is also associated with an increased risk of hospitalization, ICU admission, and death.[233,358] Being underweight (BMI <18.5 kg/m^2) is associated with an increased risk for COVID-19 hospitalization and death.[233,358]

The CDC considers available evidence indicating that the following conditions are associated with increased risk of severe COVID-19: (a) comorbidities supported by at least one meta-analysis or systematic review or other review method including cancer, cerebrovascular disease, chronic kidney disease, chronic lung diseases (limited to interstitial lung disease, pulmonary embolism, pulmonary hypertension, bronchopulmonary dysplasia, bronchiectasis, chronic obstructive pulmonary disease), chronic liver diseases (limited to cirrhosis, nonalcoholic fatty liver disease, alcoholic liver disease, autoimmune hepatitis), diabetes mellitus type 1 and type 2, heart conditions (such as heart failure, coronary artery disease, or cardiomyopathies), obesity (BMI $\geq$30 kg/m^2), pregnancy and recent pregnancy, smoking (current and former), tuberculosis; (b) comorbidities supported by at least one observational study including children with certain underlying conditions, Down syndrome, HIV, neurologic conditions including dementia, overweight (BMI $\geq$25 kg/m^2, but <30 kg/m^2), sickle cell disease, solid organ or blood stem cell transplantation, substance use disorders, use of corticosteroids or other immunosuppressive medications; (c) comorbidities supported mostly by case series, case reports or other study design with small sample size including cystic fibrosis, and thalassemia; and (d) comorbidities supported by mixed evidence including asthma, hypertension, and, possibly, immune deficiencies (except people with moderate to severe immune compromise due to a medical condition or receipt of immunosuppressive medications or treatments).[125]

SPECIAL POPULATIONS

Children

Signs and symptoms of SARS-CoV-2 infection in children are similar to those in adults, with most children experiencing mild to moderate illness.[442] A U.K. study reported that headache and fatigue were the most common symptoms of COVID-19 among schoolchildren, and approximately 75% experienced fever, cough, anosmia, or a combination of these symptoms.[460] Although upper respiratory tract symptoms are common in children with SARS-CoV-2 infection, many symptoms involving multiple organ systems have been described.[63] A systematic review of neonatal SARS-CoV-2 infections reported that 45% were asymptomatic while symptomatic infants manifested signs of respiratory distress and pneumonia, feeding difficulties, diarrhea, vomiting, hypertonia or hypotonia, irritability, lethargy, apnea, hypotension, tachycardia, conjunctivitis, hypothermia, and rash.[545] A systematic review of COVID-19 in predominantly hospitalized children and adolescents reported that fever and cough were the most common signs and symptoms and that rhinorrhea, sore throat, headache, fatigue, myalgia, diarrhea, and vomiting occurred in less than 10% to 20% of patients.[685] A multinational retrospective study reported that dyspnea, bronchiolitis, anosmia, and gastrointestinal symptoms were more common in hospitalized children with COVID-19 than with influenza.[198] A higher proportion of asymptomatic SARS-CoV-2 infections has been reported in children, particularly in young children, than in adults.[69,638]

Hospitalization rates in children with COVID-19 are typically highest in young children[351] but may also be high in adolescents.[287] While overall hospitalization rates and in-hospital mortality are substantially lower in children than in adults with COVID-19, more than 30% of hospitalized adolescent patients with COVID-19 required intensive care admission in a U.S. study.[287] During March 2020 to mid-August 2021, based on the CDC population-based surveillance, cumulative COVID-19–associated hospitalization rates in U.S. children were highest in children aged less than 5 years, followed closely by adolescents aged 12 to 17 years, and were lowest in those aged 5 to 11 years.[190,287] Hospitalization rates in children and adolescents with COVID-19 during 2020–2021 were higher than for seasonal influenza and increased with spread of the Delta variant,[287] but severity among hospitalized children was similar to that during pre-Delta circulation.[190,616] Median duration of hospitalization of children aged less than 18 years with COVID-19 in the United States ranged from 2 to 3 days.[611] A multinational study reported a higher proportion of pneumonia and hypoxemia among children hospitalized with COVID-19 compared with influenza.[198]

Risk factors for severe respiratory disease with SARS-CoV-2–associated deaths in children include obesity and hypoxia on admission.[214] A U.S. study reported that among hospitalized children aged less than 2 years, underlying medical conditions associated with severe COVID-19 (ICU admission, mechanical ventilation, or in-hospital death) were chronic lung disease, neurologic disorders, cardiovascular disease, prematurity, and airway abnormality.[714] Among hospitalized children aged 2 to 17 years, feeding tube dependence, diabetes mellitus, and obesity were associated with severe COVID-19.[714] A cross-sectional analysis of a large administrative database of COVID-19 patients aged ≤18 years reported that the strongest risk factors for hospitalization were type 1 diabetes and obesity, and the strongest risk factors for severe COVID-19 (intensive care unit admission, invasive mechanical ventilation, or death) were type 1 diabetes, and cardiac and circulatory anomalies.[357] A systematic review and meta-analysis reported that risk factors for progression to severe or critical COVID-19 in children were chronic neurological diseases, obesity, presence of gastrointestinal symptoms, ARDS, and age less than 6 months.[607] Among 112 U.S. children who died from COVID-19–related conditions, including 16 (14%) with multisystem-inflammatory syndrome in children (MIS-C, discussed below), 86% had at least one chronic medical condition, most commonly obesity, asthma or reactive airway disease, and developmental disorders, and 52% had ≥3 underlying medical conditions.[450] In a large cross-sectional study in the United States, type 1 diabetes, cardiac and circulatory congenital anomalies, epilepsy or convulsions, obesity, hypertension, and sleep/wake disorders including sleep apnea were associated with ICU admission, invasive mechanical ventilation, or death among patients aged ≤18 years, and prematurity was associated with severe COVID-19 among children aged ≤1 year.[357] A study in Brazil reported that hospitalized children aged less than 2 years or 12 to 19 years had a higher risk of death than those aged 2 to 11 years.[494]

Health inequities are also apparent in children—those living in more impoverished regions or of indigenous ethnicity were at higher risk of death compared with white patients.[494] CDC population-based surveillance indicated that COVID-19-associated hospitalization rates among persons aged less than 18 years were highest in non-Hispanic American Indian or Alaska Native, non-Hispanic Black, and Hispanic or Latino children during March 2020 to October 2021.[116] A study of children admitted to children's hospitals in the United States during April to September 2020 reported that greater disease severity was associated with Black or other non-White race.[32] A study of participating family practitioners in England reported that Asian children were more likely to be hospitalized for COVID-19 and to be admitted to an intensive care unit compared with White children, and that Black children and children of mixed or other races had significantly greater hospitalizations of ≥36 hours than White children.[579]

Pregnancy

Clinical characteristics of pregnant women with SARS-CoV-2 infection are similar to those in nonpregnant persons.[21,445] Although the risk of severe COVID-19 among pregnant women is low, one U.S. study reported that symptomatic pregnant women with laboratory-confirmed SARS-CoV-2 infection were at increased risk for critical illness requiring intensive care admission, invasive mechanical ventilation, extracorporeal membrane oxygenation (ECMO), and death compared with symptomatic nonpregnant women of reproductive age with SARS-CoV-2 infection.[740] A meta-analysis reported that pregnant women and those recently pregnant with SARS-CoV-2 infection were at increased risk of ICU admission, invasive mechanical ventilation, and ECMO compared with nonpregnant women of reproductive age with SARS-CoV-2 infection.[21] In one U.S. study, severe COVID-19 among pregnant women was associated with underlying prepregnancy medical conditions such as obesity, chronic lung disease, hypertension, and diabetes.[229] The risk of severe complications increased with the increasing prevalence of chronic medical or pregnancy-related conditions. Among pregnant and postpartum women with COVID-19 and ARDS in Brazil, postpartum women had an increased risk of ICU admission, mechanical ventilation, and death.[433] A meta-analysis reported that SARS-CoV-2 infection increases the risk of complications such as preeclampsia and adverse pregnancy outcomes such as preterm birth and stillbirth compared with pregnant women without SARS-CoV-2 infection.[704] Babies born to mothers with SARS-CoV-2 infection have a higher risk of admission to a neonatal intensive care unit than babies born to mothers without SARS-CoV-2 infection.[21]

SARS-CoV-2 can rarely infect placental tissues and is not associated with specific placental injury.[315] Some studies have reported that histologic features of maternal vascular malperfusion were significantly higher in placentas from women with SARS-CoV-2 infection compared with placentas from women without SARS-CoV-2 infection.[315,510]

Vertical Transmission

In two combined large pregnancy cohorts from the United States and United Kingdom, SARS-CoV-2 infection was reported in 1.8% and 2% of babies born to mothers with SARS-CoV-2 infection.[473] An international cohort study reported that among women who tested positive for SARS-CoV-2, 13% of their neonates tested positive for SARS-CoV-2 and that Cesarean delivery, but not breastfeeding, was associated with increased risk of a neonatal SARS-CoV-2–positive test result.[684] A meta-analysis of reported neonatal SARS-CoV-2 infections reported that most infections were due to postpartum transmission, and approximately 30% were likely due to vertical transmission.[545] A systematic review of Chinese studies reported that rooming of mothers and newborn infants together did not increase the risk of SARS-CoV-2 transmission compared with isolation of newborns from their mothers.[545,689] A systematic review reported that detection of SARS-CoV-2 RNA in the breast milk of mothers with confirmed COVID-19 is very uncommon,[361] and there is no evidence to date of SARS-CoV-2 transmission through breast milk.[113] One study reported detection of SARS-CoV-2 RNA in a small percentage of breast milk specimens tested from women with SARS-CoV-2 infection, but subgenomic RNA was not detected, suggesting that infectious virus was not present.[360] Breast milk of mothers with SARS-CoV-2 infection can contain antibodies to SARS-CoV-2.[56,201,360]

CLINICAL ISSUES AFTER INFECTION

SARS-CoV-2 Reinfection

Reinfection with SARS-CoV-2 appears to be relatively uncommon, has been described primarily in immunocompetent persons, and typically does not occur until several months after the initial infection.[153,272,277,492] One systematic review reported that the median interval of reinfection after initial SARS-CoV-2 infection was 113.5 days (range 1.5 to more than 8 months) after initial SARS-CoV-2 infection, with reinfections resulting in a wide range of disease severity.[153] Reinfections with SARS-CoV-2 from the same virus clade as the initial infection or with variant viruses are possible but do not necessarily result in different symptoms or duration of illness.[153,253,488,560,623] Overall, the frequency of reinfection, the correlates of immune protection from reinfection, and the duration of immune protection from reinfection with an antigenically similar virus or variant after initial SARS-CoV-2 infection are under investigation. Data from Qatar and England indicate that prior SARS-CoV-2 infection confers substantial protection against reinfection and significantly reduces the risk of severe COVID-19.[4,5,272]

Post-COVID Conditions

Following COVID-19 illness, most persons recover and return to baseline health. However, some persons, including those initially asymptomatic or with clinically mild illness, may experience a wide range of new or persistent symptoms, lasting more than 4 weeks after SARS-CoV-2 infection.[12,122,632] Post-COVID conditions (previously referred to as long-COVID or postacute sequelae of SARS-CoV-2 infection [PASC]) include any new or chronic symptoms from COVID-19.[479] Challenges to characterizing post-COVID conditions include variability among studies in symptoms that were captured, differences in study design (cross-sectional vs. prospective longitudinal follow-up at defined periods), follow-up periods after SARS-CoV-2 infection, and whether a comparison group was included without SARS-CoV-2 infection.[479]

Persistent signs and symptoms reported in adults include fever, fatigue, headache, cough, difficulty breathing, chest pain, palpitations, joint pain, myalgia, hair loss, ageusia, anosmia, dizziness with standing, and neuropsychiatric symptoms such as depression and anxiety.[100,122,252,300,467,484,517] Neurocognitive deficits affecting short-term memory and difficulties in thinking or ability to concentrate have been reported in adults, including after mild COVID-19.[24,122,224,252,276,563,619] The overall frequency of post-COVID-19 symptoms in either nonhospitalized or hospitalized persons with SARS-CoV-2 infection is not well understood but appears to be substantially higher among adults who experienced more severe illness requiring hospitalization. A wide prevalence of abnormalities has been reported in cross-sectional and longitudinal studies with differences in intervals since illness onset or hospital discharge.[100] A large U.S. study reported that after the first 30 days of illness, persons with COVID-19 who were not hospitalized had a significantly higher risk of death, greater need for outpatient care, and higher burden of respiratory and nonrespiratory conditions compared to persons without COVID-19.[100] A small prospective study in Norway reported that more than half of young adults who experienced mild COVID-19 had persistent symptoms, including ageusia, anosmia, fatigue, dyspnea, impaired concentration, and memory problems.[75] Another U.S. study reported that the risk of continuing to experience symptoms 2 months after a positive SARS-CoV-2 test result was significantly higher in women, persons with at least one preexisting condition, and persons aged 40 to 54 years.[735]

In a prospective 1-year follow-up study among Italian adults who experienced mild-to-moderate COVID-19 with an altered sense of smell and taste, the majority had recovered function, and more than 20% had improvement, but 8.6% reported worse or unchanged smell or taste impairment.[75,84] A German study reported that only 22.9% of patients had fully recovered symptoms by 1 year, fatigue and dyspnea increased in adults between 5 and 12 months after COVID-19, and the most frequently reported persistent symptoms at 1 year include reduced exercise capacity, fatigue, dyspnea, and difficulty with concentrating, word-finding, and sleeping.[592]

Adult patients who survived hospitalization for severe or critical COVID-19 illness may experience persistent symptoms related to respiratory (e.g., acute respiratory distress syndrome) or extrapulmonary complications of COVID-19 (e.g., myocarditis, thrombosis, prolonged invasive mechanical ventilation). A large U.S. study reported that after the first 30 days of illness, persons with COVID-19 who were hospitalized had a significantly increased risk of death, higher risk of outpatient care, and greater burden of pulmonary and extrapulmonary disorders compared with persons who were hospitalized for seasonal influenza or other causes.[14] Specific symptoms include fatigue, muscle weakness, anxiety, depression, difficulty sleeping, breathlessness, ageusia, and anosmia and may persist for 4 to 6 months or as long as 1 year.[215,224,300,431,467,517] A single center cross-sectional study of cognitive functioning in adults who were assessed a mean of 7.6 months after COVID-19 diagnosis reported that hospitalized patients were significantly more likely to have impairments in attention, executive functioning, memory encoding, and memory recall than patients who received outpatient care.[57]

Data are more limited on post-COVID conditions in children than for adults. A small follow-up study in Italy of children who had been hospitalized primarily for mild-to-moderate COVID-19 reported that clinical recovery with normalization of laboratory and pulmonary abnormalities identified on lung ultrasound had resolved within 5 weeks after discharge.[191] A large study of children with COVID-19 in the United Kingdom reported that 4.4% experienced symptoms of ≥28 days and only 1.8% had symptoms for at least 56 days.[460] A small study among persons isolated at home for COVID-19 in Norway and followed up at 6 months reported that 6% of children aged less than 16 years reported symptoms compared with 18% to 27% of those aged ≥16 years.[75] After hospitalization for COVID-19, a study in Russia reported that some children may experience persistent fatigue, sleep disturbance, and altered sense of smell for at least 6 to 7 months.[499] Older children may have a higher frequency of persistent symptoms 4 to 7 months after initial COVID-19 illness than younger children.[95,499]

At 6 months follow-up of a cohort of adults in Singapore with a wide range of disease severity ranging from asymptomatic SARS-CoV-2 infection to severe COVID-19, all individuals had higher levels of multiple growth factors, cytokines, and chemokines compared with healthy controls.[496] Although most inflammatory biomarkers declined over time, recovered COVID-19 patients had evidence of ongoing chronic inflammation (high levels of IL-17A, IL-12p70, stem cell factor, IL-1β) and high levels of biomarkers associated with endothelial repair and angiogenesis (BDNF, MIP-1β, VEGF) that did not differ by acute COVID-19 disease severity.[300]

A large study of hospitalized COVID-19 patients in China reported that those who required respiratory support with high-flow oxygen, noninvasive or invasive mechanical ventilation had a higher risk of diffusion impairment measured by pulmonary function testing.[300] They also had a higher risk of anxiety, depression, fatigue, and muscle weakness than patients not requiring supplemental oxygen at 6 months after hospital discharge. Notably, 13% of discharged COVID-19 patients without evidence of kidney injury during hospitalization had decreased glomerular filtration rate 6 months after discharge.[300] At 1-year of follow-up of the same cohort, the proportion of patients reporting at least one persistent symptom decreased significantly compared to 6 months after hospital discharge, although 49% still reported symptoms.[303] Furthermore, the proportion of patients with dyspnea and either anxiety or depression increased significantly at 1-year of follow-up compared to 6 months after hospital discharge.[303] A prospective study of hospitalized COVID-19 patients in China without chronic cardiopulmonary disease or history of cigarette smoking and who did not require invasive mechanical ventilation, followed every 3 months for 1 year, reported that although dyspnea declined and pulmonary function improved over time, impaired lung diffusion capacity for carbon dioxide and abnormal chest CT findings persisted at 12 months in some patients.[721]

A small Chinese study of COVID-19 patients after hospital discharge for severe or critical illness reported that age greater than 48 years, receipt of corticosteroid treatment during hospitalization, evidence of bronchiectasis, and greater than 75% of lung opacification at hospital discharge were independently associated with pulmonary fibrosis at 7 months after discharge.[408] Cardiopulmonary testing revealed that patients with pulmonary fibrosis 7 months after hospital discharge had significantly decreased maximum oxygen consumption, decreased metabolic equivalents, and increased ventilation to carbon dioxide production than patients without fibrosis, suggesting cardiopulmonary insufficiency.[408] Data to inform clinical management of patients with post COVID-19 conditions are very limited, and clinical management is mainly supportive depending upon the persistence and severity of specific symptoms and clinically significant abnormalities.[479] Clinical algorithms for follow-up evaluation of respiratory disease in discharged patients have been proposed in the United Kingdom.[240]

Multisystem-Inflammatory Syndrome

Multisystem-inflammatory syndrome in children (MIS-C) is a rare, severe complication of SARS-CoV-2 infection with higher incidence among Black, Hispanic, and Asian or Pacific Islander persons than White persons, and in those aged less than 5 years or 6 to 10 years.[211,516] The CDC MIS-C case definition is an individual aged less than 21 years presenting with fever greater than 38.0°C or subjective fever for ≥24 hours, laboratory evidence of inflammation (including, but not limited to, one or more of the following: an elevated CRP, ESR, fibrinogen, procalcitonin, D-dimer, ferritin, lactic acid dehydrogenase [LDH], or IL-6, elevated neutrophils, reduced lymphocytes, and low albumin), and evidence of clinically severe illness requiring hospitalization, with multisystem (>2) organ involvement (cardiac, renal, respiratory, hematologic, gastrointestinal, dermatologic or neurological).[118] There must be no plausible alternative diagnoses and either evidence of current or recent SARS-CoV-2 infection by RT-PCR, serology, or antigen test, or exposure to a suspected or confirmed COVID-19 case within the 4 weeks before the onset of symptoms.

While MIS-C generally occurs 2 to 6 weeks after COVID-19 illness, one report described an adolescent with MIS-C that occurred 16 weeks after COVID-19 illness onset.[158] Admission to an intensive care unit for MIS-C is more likely for children aged ≥6 years compared with those aged less than 5 years,[2] while young infants may experience a relatively milder clinical course with MIS-C than older children.[247] U.S. studies reported that compared with persons in the general population aged less than 20 years, MIS-C was more frequent among Hispanic and non-Hispanic Black children,[625] and non-Hispanic Black patients were more likely to be admitted to an ICU compared with non-Hispanic White patients.[2] Compared to persons aged less than 21 years with COVID-19 in the United States, MIS-C was more frequent in non-Hispanic Black children.[625] A study from Turkey reported that the risk of ICU admission for MIS-C patients increased significantly with older age and decreased serum albumin levels.[285] In one well-characterized U.S. cohort, cardiac complications (e.g., systolic myocardial dysfunction and valvular regurgitation) were significantly more frequent in MIS-C patients who required critical care support than in MIS-C patients who did not require ICU admission.[187] Another U.S. study reported that 65% of MIS-C patients had abnormal left ventricular function.[130] Confirmed and probable MIS-C patients had significantly elevated levels of soluble interleukin 2 receptor (sIL2R), IL-10, and IL-6 compared with non-MIS-C control patients.[187] ICU admission for MIS-C patients was associated with increased D-dimer, troponin, brain natriuretic peptide (BNP), proBNP, CRP, and IL-6, and decreased counts of platelets and lymphocytes.[2]

Clinical care of MIS-C patients is supportive care of complications and the use immunomodulator therapy. Although data from controlled clinical trials of treatment of MIS-C patients are not available, observational studies assessed the clinical benefit of immunomodulatory treatment. A U.S. observational cohort study reported that the combination of intravenous immune globulin (IVIG) and glucocorticoid treatment was associated with a significantly lower risk of cardiovascular dysfunction (left ventricular ejection fraction <55% or refractory shock) on or after day 2 from treatment initiation.[617] The relative benefit of IVIG versus glucocorticoid therapy is not known. An international observational cohort study compared IVIG alone, IVIG plus glucocorticoids, and glucocorticoids alone and reported no significant differences in the use of inotropes or invasive mechanical ventilation or death occurring on or after 2 days of treatment, and no significant differences in reduction in disease severity by day 2.[448] A small longitudinal study of MIS-C patients, nearly all of whom were treated with immunomodulators, reported that left ventricular dysfunction or coronary abnormalities resolved between 8 weeks and 6 months after admission.[108] Another small longitudinal study of MIS-C patients reported that by 1-year after hospitalization, the majority had resolved cardiac abnormalities and abnormal laboratory markers, but 25% still had persistently elevated D-dimer levels.[179]

Multisystem inflammatory syndrome in adults (MIS-A) is a very rare and severe complication of SARS-CoV-2 infection in adults and has similar findings to MIS-C with a wide range of severity and organ system involvement.[180,468] The CDC MIS-A case definition specifies that both clinical and laboratory criteria must be met in a patient without a more likely alternative diagnosis aged ≥21 years who is hospitalized for ≥24 hours or with an illness resulting in death, with a subjective or documented fever of ≥ 38.0°C for ≥24 hours before hospitalization or within the first 3 days of hospitalization, and at least three clinical criteria with at least one being a primary clinical criteria[121]:

- Primary clinical criteria
  - Severe cardiac illness, or
  - Rash and nonpurulent conjunctivitis
- Secondary clinical criteria
  - New-onset neurologic signs and symptoms
  - Shock or hypotension not attributable to medical therapy
  - Abdominal pain, vomiting, or diarrhea, or
  - Thrombocytopenia
- Laboratory evidence of inflammation
  - Elevated levels of two or more: CRP, ferritin, IL-6, ESR, procalcitonin, and
  - Positive SARS-CoV-2 test during the current illness by RT-PCR, serology, or antigen detection.

For patients who experienced typical COVID-19 symptoms before MIS-A, the interval after onset of COVID-19 symptoms to development of MIS-A was approximately 2 to 5 weeks.[468] Similar to MIS-C, no randomized controlled trials are available to inform clinical management of patients with MIS-A, and data on optimal treatment are limited. Therefore, clinical management of patients with MIS-A is supportive care of complications and immunomodulator therapy.

DIAGNOSTIC TESTING

Viral Tests

The U.S. Food and Drug Administration issued emergency use authorizations for more than 300 SARS-CoV-2 diagnostic tests.[674] Commercially available viral tests for diagnosis of acute SARS-CoV-2 infection detect either SARS-CoV-2 antigens or nucleic acids in respiratory or saliva specimens. Most of the available SARS-CoV-2 diagnostic tests are singleplex assays, while multiplex assays that detect other respiratory pathogens

such as influenza A and B viruses or bacterial pathogens are also available. Both rapid antigen and rapid molecular point-of-care assays that produce results within 30 minutes are available for use in health care settings, and some have received emergency use authorization for home use. Some kits are available for self-collection of respiratory or saliva specimens and testing at home or to send for testing at a designated laboratory. Supervised self-collection of mid-turbinate nasal swab or saliva specimens has a similar yield for detection of SARS-CoV-2 compared with clinician-collected nasopharyngeal swabs.[354]

Nucleic acid amplification tests (NAATs) are molecular assays with high sensitivity and very high specificity to detect SARS-CoV-2 in respiratory specimens or saliva of persons with SARS-CoV-2 infection. Laboratory-based NAATs such as RT-PCR assays have higher sensitivity and specificity than point-of-care molecular assays. Most NAATs such as RT-PCR assays detect one or more RNA target genes such as the envelope (env), nucleocapsid (N), spike (S), RNA-dependent RNA polymerase (RdRp), and ORF1 genes.[597] Rapid molecular assays have higher sensitivity than rapid antigen tests to detect SARS-CoV-2, but both typically have high specificity in persons with COVID-19.[758] One meta-analysis reported that NAATs had a pooled sensitivity of 90.4% and specificity of 98.1%.[476] Rapid antigen tests have much lower sensitivity than molecular assays to detect asymptomatic SARS-CoV-2 infection.[532,535]

Commercially available SARS-CoV-2 assays differ by the specific kinds of clinical specimens recommended for testing. Although nasopharyngeal swab specimens have higher sensitivity than other upper respiratory specimens for detecting SARS-CoV-2, meta-analyses have reported that saliva specimens have similar or slightly lower sensitivity than nasopharyngeal swabs for detecting SARS-CoV-2 by RT-PCR.[55,97,383] Combined nasal and oropharyngeal swabs have similar sensitivity to nasopharyngeal swabs to detect SARS-CoV-2 RNA by NAATs.[383,668] SARS-CoV-2 RNA may be detected in saliva specimens more frequently than in deep throat saliva/posterior oropharyngeal saliva specimens.[466] Midturbinate nasal swabs have similar frequency of detection of SARS-CoV-2 antigen as nasopharyngeal swabs.[403] Provider-collected nasopharyngeal swabs and self-collected saliva specimens have higher frequency of detection of SARS-CoV-2 by NAAT than self-collected anterior nasal swabs.[278] SARS-CoV-2 RNA can be detected for a longer duration in sputum specimens than in nasopharyngeal swab specimens.[692] In hospitalized patients with COVID-19, SARS-CoV-2 RNA may be detected in lower respiratory tract specimens (bronchoalveolar lavage fluid) when SARS-CoV-2 RNA is not detected in sputum or upper respiratory tract specimens[98,694] and SARS-CoV-2 RNA can be detected for a longer duration in respiratory specimens of patients with severe disease than in those with mild disease.[474,728,756]

Interpretation of SARS-CoV-2 testing results in a person with suspected COVID-19 should consider the prevalence of SARS-CoV-2 in the patient population, the individual's pretest probability of SARS-CoV-2 infection based upon exposures, signs and symptoms, and time from illness onset, the type of the clinical specimen, and the characteristics of the test used (e.g., sensitivity and specificity) to inform the posttest probability of testing positive or negative.[701] Negative test results in persons suspected of having COVID-19 (e.g., high pretest probability) should be considered as potentially false-negative results, particularly when SARS-CoV-2 prevalence is high in the community[712] If a rapid antigen test is negative in a person with a high pretest probability of SARS-CoV-2 infection, confirmation with a NAAT should be considered. Positive test results in persons with low pretest probability during periods of low SARS-CoV-2 circulation could be potentially false-positive results, and additional SARS-CoV-2 testing can confirm results.

Serology

Serological assays differ in methodologies (e.g., lateral flow immunoassay, chemiluminescent immunoassay, enzyme-linked immunosorbent assay, microneutralization assay) and the kinds of antibodies detected (i.e., pan Ig, total Ig, IgG, IgA, IgM, and neutralizing antibodies). Commercially available serological tests can help establish recent or history of SARS-CoV-2 infection but generally lack sensitivity to identify acute infection. Serological testing may be useful in establishing a diagnosis of recent SARS-CoV-2 infection in pediatric patients with MIS-C who have negative SARS-CoV-2 NAAT results.[572] Virus-specific IgM antibodies begin to increase during the first week after illness onset, peak after 2 weeks, and decline after that, while virus-specific IgG antibodies are detectable after 1 week, increase until peaking at approximately 25 days after onset, declining gradually after 1 month, and may remain elevated for many weeks or months.[364,424] Virus-specific IgA antibodies follow a similar pattern to virus-specific IgM antibodies.[364] One meta-analysis reported that pooled percentages of IgM and IgG seroconversion were 37.5% by day 7 and 73.3% by day 14 after illness onset.[745] Estimated sensitivities and specificities at day 21 after onset were 87.2% and 97.3% for IgM and 91.3% and 96% for IgG, respectively.[745] Detection of IgM and IgG at day 14 after onset by enzyme-linked immunosorbent assay (ELISA) was more accurate than other serological methods.[745] Point of care lateral flow immunoassays have lower sensitivity than other serological testing methods.[405]

The dynamics of the neutralizing antibody response, such as peak antibody levels, the kinetics of antibody decline, and duration of antibodies, are highly variable among COVID-19 patients.[146] Neutralizing antibodies typically increase in the 2nd and 3rd weeks after illness onset, peak at about 1 month, and gradually decline over 3 to 4 months.[691] Some patients with mild disease may have little or no neutralizing antibody response.[387] Patients with severe disease may develop neutralizing antibodies later than patients with mild disease.[667] Hospitalized patients with COVID-19 who survive develop higher neutralizing antibody levels than persons with mild disease or asymptomatic SARS-CoV-2 infection.[667] Hospitalized COVID-19 patients who are immunocompromised may have lower IgG levels than immunocompetent persons[183] and may not have evidence of an antibody response by commercial serological assays.[281] One study reported that patients with persistence of neutralizing antibodies continued to have high systemic concentrations of proinflammatory cytokines, including when assessed at 6 months after illness onset.[146] In another study conducted 6 months after SARS-CoV-2 infection, anti-SARS-CoV-2 nucleocapsid IgG antibodies were detected in 66.7%, and neutralizing antibodies were detected in 86.9% of patients who had experienced a wide range of disease severity.[487] A follow-up study showed that neutralizing activity against wild-type SARS-CoV-2 remained stable 6 to 12 months after SARS-CoV-2 infection.[698] Another longitudinal study reported

that while antibody titers to the virus specific receptor-binding domain, spike IgG, and neutralizing antibody titers all declined over the first 6 months after recovery from COVID-19, these titers remained stable from 6 to 12 months after recovery.[212]

A small follow-up study of patients with asymptomatic or symptomatic SARS-CoV-2 infection reported that although neutralizing antibody titers decreased during the first 6 months after infection, these titers declined slowly between 6 and 12 months after infection, and all patients had detectable neutralizing antibody titers at 12 months.[148] A 1-year follow-up study of patients who had SARS-CoV-2 infection early in the first pandemic wave in China reported that although 90% had detectable SARS-CoV-2–specific IgG antibodies against the nucleocapsid protein and the receptor-binding domain of the spike protein, low titers of neutralizing antibodies against the homologous virus were detected in 42.5%.[723] However, only 22.6% had low neutralizing antibody titers against the B.1.351 (Beta) variant.

CLINICAL MANAGEMENT

General

With the urgency of the pandemic and the time required for the discovery of new drugs, most early approaches to therapy involved repurposing available agents.[683] Anti-SARS-CoV-2 monoclonal antibodies are the exception, with rapid isolation of monoclonal antibodies, most often from the B cells of patients who have recently recovered from SARS-CoV-2, and in some cases from individuals who were infected with SARS-CoV-1 in 2003.[441] Over 400 drugs have undergone trials in COVID-19.[683] Of these, several therapeutics have demonstrated efficacy in clinical trials for treatment of patients with COVID-19: Four anti-SARS-CoV-2 monoclonal antibody products (bamlanivimab/etesevimab, casirivimab/imdevimab, sotrovimab, regdanvimab), one antiviral (remdesivir), and three anti-inflammatory agents (dexamethasone, baricitinib, tocilizumab). Convalescent plasma was made available under emergency use authorization and used widely initially but lacked rigorous trials to inform efficacy and safety. The clinical utility and effectiveness of these treatments varies by specific susceptibility and resistance characteristics of SARS-CoV-2 infection, time from onset to clinical presentation (Fig. 22.2), complications, severity of illness, and risk factors. Evidence-based recommendations for clinical management of hospitalized patients with COVID-19 are available from the NIH COVID-19 Treatment Guidelines Panel,[483] WHO,[716] and other organizations.

MONOCLONAL ANTIBODIES

Monoclonal antibodies historically have had mixed success in the treatment of severe viral diseases. Late initiation of therapy has not shown success in influenza, with most monoclonal antibodies failing to show any clinical benefit.[58] While a monoclonal antibody is approved for prevention of respiratory syncytial virus (RSV) disease, it has not been effective for treatment.[15] Monoclonal antibodies did show benefit in the treatment of Ebola, with ansuvimab (mAb114) and atoltivimab/maftivimab/odesivimab (REGN-EB3) demonstrating superior efficacy over other treatments,[471] and by extension to prior studies over standard of care.[176]

Anti-SARS-CoV-2 monoclonal antibodies, directed against the spike glycoprotein, are likely to be most effective when used for treatment early in the course of COVID-19 disease, before patients develop an innate and adaptive immune response, viral replication is increasing, and marked inflammation has occurred (Fig. 22.5).

BAMLANIVIMAB/ETESEVIMAB

Bamlanivimab (LY-CoV555) was the first monoclonal antibody that received emergency use authorization. The BLAZE-1 trial was a randomized, double-blind, placebo-controlled clinical trial studying bamlanivimab to treat outpatients with mild to moderate COVID-19 and given bamlanivimab or placebo within 3 days of diagnosis. Interim results suggested that treatment with bamlanivimab reduced COVID-19–related hospitalizations or emergency room visits within 28 days after treatment.[138] As the study was ongoing, the active arm was modified to add a second monoclonal etesevimab (LY-CoV016, also known as JS016). The final analysis demonstrated that treatment with bamlanivimab/etesevimab was associated with a 4.8% absolute decrease (70% relative decrease) in COVID-19–related hospitalizations or emergency room visits and a dose-dependent change in viral load at day 11 (log viral load reduction of −0.57 at the highest dose).[196,250] In February 2021, the FDA granted an Emergency Use Authorization (EUA) for the combination of bamlanivimab/etesevimab for treatment of mild-to-moderate non-hospitalized COVID-19 in at-risk patients. Clinical benefit of bamlanivimab was not demonstrated for those already hospitalized, and the trial was halted due to the lack of efficacy.[421] Additional analysis

demonstrated possible benefit for those that were seronegative at study entry (relative risk [RR] = 1.24) but harm if seropositive (RR = 0.74).[6]

Monoclonal antibodies may be even more effective for prophylaxis. Prophylactic efficacy of bamlanivimab was evaluated among residents and staff of skilled nursing and assisted living facilities after a reported confirmed SARS-CoV-2 case at a facility. Bamlanivimab reduced the incidence of COVID-19 in the prevention population compared with placebo (8.5% vs. 15.2%, $p < 0.001$).[161] This benefit was mainly seen in the residents (8.8% vs. 22.5%, $p < 0.001$) and less pronounced in the staff (8.4% vs. 12.2%). The efficacy of bamlanivimab/etesevimab (and all monoclonal antibody products) can be affected by variant strains of the virus (see "Variants and Monoclonal Antibodies"). Current circulating variants have variable susceptibilities to the available anti-SARS-CoV-2 monoclonal antibodies.

Casirivimab/Imdevimab

In outpatients with COVID-19, the monoclonal combination casirivimab/imdevimab reduced hospitalization or all-cause death by half (6% in treated compared to 3% control in the phase 2, and 4.6% in treated compared to 1.3% control in the phase 3).[705,706] This treatment effect was largest among patients that were serum antibody negative at baseline (15% and 6%, respectively).[706] Casirivimab/imdevimab is effective in prophylaxis in household contacts of those with SARS-CoV-2, with an 81% reduction in symptomatic SARS-CoV-2 infection. In a treatment study of hospitalized patients with COVID-19, there was no difference in mortality when casirivimab/imdevimab was added to standard care (mortality 20% vs. 21%, $p = 0.17$).[553] In an analysis of seronegative patients (as determined later, not at the time of study entry), mortality was decreased by 6% (24% vs. 30%, $p = 0.0010$).

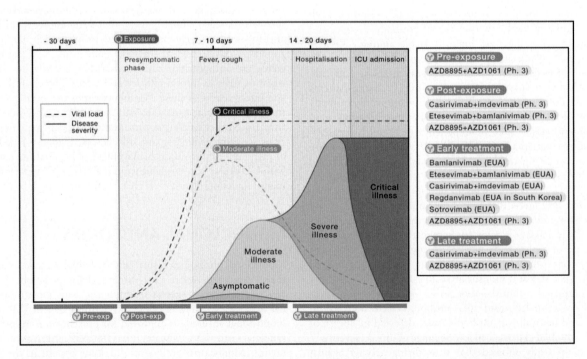

FIGURE 22.5 Viral load and disease severity in SARS-CoV-2 infections. Adapted from Corti D, Purcell LA, Snell G, et al. Tackling COVID-19 with neutralizing monoclonal antibodies. *Cell* 2021;184(12):3086–3108. Copyright © 2021 Elsevier. With permission.

Casirivimab/imdevimab can also be used for prophylaxis. The COV-2069 trial evaluated casirivimab/imdevimab in household contacts after one member was diagnosed with SARS-CoV-2 infection. Casirivimab/imdevimab was associated with 72% protection against symptomatic infections in the first week and 93% in subsequent weeks.[556] In July 2021, the EUA was revised to allow treatment with casirivimab/imdevimab in outpatients at risk for progressing to severe disease and in post-exposure prophylaxis (e.g., household contacts).

Sotrovimab

Sotrovimab (VIR-7831) was evaluated in a phase 3 trial in nonhospitalized patients with symptomatic COVID-19 and at least one risk factor for disease progression. In an interim analysis, sotrovimab reduced the risk of COVID-19 progression to hospitalization or death by 85% ($p = 0.002$).[269] A trial in a hospitalized population that was stopped after treatment with sotrovimab in addition to standard care showed no improvement over usual care alone.[482] Sotrovimab is available for treatment of outpatients infected with SARS-CoV-2 and who are at high risk for progression to severe COVID-19.

Regdanvimab

Regdanvimab (CT-P59) received conditional marketing authorization from South Korea's drug safety agency. In a phase 3 trial in nonhospitalized patients with symptomatic COVID-19 and at least one risk factor for disease progression, regdanvimab significantly reduced the risk of hospitalization or death by 72% ($p < 0.0001$).[112]

Variants and Monoclonal Antibodies

All available monoclonal antibodies are sensitive to one or more of the mutations found in receptor-binding domain (RBD) residues at positions 417, 452, or 484 that are carried by multiple circulating variants including the Delta variant (B.1.617).[164,449,553,622,693] These variants may decrease the ability of the monoclonal antibodies to bind the virus and could impact effectiveness.

Alpha (B.1.1.7)
• No impact on susceptibility to available monoclonal antibody treatments.[123]

Beta (B.1.351)
• Significantly reduced susceptibility to the combination of bamlanivimab/etesevimab monoclonal antibody treatment.[123]
• Other monoclonal antibody treatments are not significantly affected.

Gamma (P.1)
• Significantly reduced susceptibility to the combination of bamlanivimab/etesevimab monoclonal antibody treatment.[123]
• Other monoclonal antibody treatments are not significantly affected.

Delta (B.1.617.2)
• No impact on susceptibility to EUA monoclonal antibody treatments.[123]

ANTIVIRAL AGENTS

Remdesivir

Shortly after the emergence of SARS-CoV-2 in China, case reports described the empiric use of remdesivir to treat COVID-19.[296] RNA-dependent RNA polymerase is a nonstructural protein that is highly conserved, making it an attractive antiviral target.[16] Remdesivir (GS-5734) is a prodrug of a cyano-adenosine nucleoside analog. Remdesivir undergoes rapid intracellular conversion to an alanine metabolite (GS-704277), then to the nucleoside analog (GS-441524), and then the pharmacologically active nucleoside triphosphate form (GS-443902) (Fig. 22.6).[202] GS-443902 acts as an analog of ATP and competes with the endogenous ATP substrate for incorporation into SARS-CoV-2 RNA via RNA-dependent RNA polymerase (RdRp), leading to chain termination and inhibition of viral replication.

Remdesivir was discovered in research programs looking for treatments of hepatitis C (HCV) and respiratory syncytial virus (RSV).[244] It inhibits the RNA-dependent RNA polymerase in many RNA viruses, including filoviruses (e.g., Ebola, Sudan, Marburg), paramyxoviruses (e.g., RSV, Nipah, Hendra), and pathogenic coronaviruses.[411,412,699] Studies in human airway epithelial cell assays demonstrated that remdesivir inhibits replication of coronaviruses, including MERS-CoV.[602] In mouse infection models, remdesivir had therapeutic efficacy against SARS-CoV-1 and MERS-CoV.[602,603] In a nonhuman primate study, therapeutic remdesivir treatment initiated 12 hours postinoculation with MERS-CoV provided clinical benefit with a reduction in clinical signs, reduced virus replication in the lungs, and decreased presence and severity of lung lesions.[185,186]

Four randomized efficacy trials evaluated the efficacy of remdesivir, and one compared two treatment durations (Table 22.1). The first trial implemented in response to the SARS-CoV-2 outbreak was in Hubei, China. Wang et al. conducted a randomized, double-blind, multicenter, placebo-controlled trial of 237 hospitalized adults at 10 hospitals with laboratory-confirmed SARS-CoV-2 infection, with severe disease (oxygen saturation ≤94% and radiologically confirmed pneumonia).[697] The primary end point was time to clinical improvement, defined as decline of two levels on a six-point ordinal scale (from 1 = discharged to 6 = death) or hospital discharge. In the 237 participants enrolled, the time to clinical improvement was 21 days in the remdesivir group compared to 23 days in the placebo group (HR 1.23, 95% CI 0.87 to 1.75). The Adaptive COVID-19 Treatment Trial (ACTT) was the second trial implemented for evaluating remdesivir for treatment of COVID-19. ACTT was also a randomized, blinded placebo-controlled trial. In 1,062 hospitalized adults with COVID-19, the median time to recovery (defined as being discharged or still hospitalized but no longer requiring medical care) was shorter with remdesivir than with placebo (10 vs. 15 days; RR 1.29, 95% CI 1.12 to 1.49).[60] Those with more moderate disease (no oxygen or low flow oxygen) had better outcomes (HR 1.29 and 1.45 respectively) than those with severe or critical disease (high-flow oxygen HR 1.09; mechanical ventilation, HR 0.98).

The SIMPLE-Moderate trial was an open-label trial of 584 hospitalized adults with moderate COVID-19 (pneumonia and

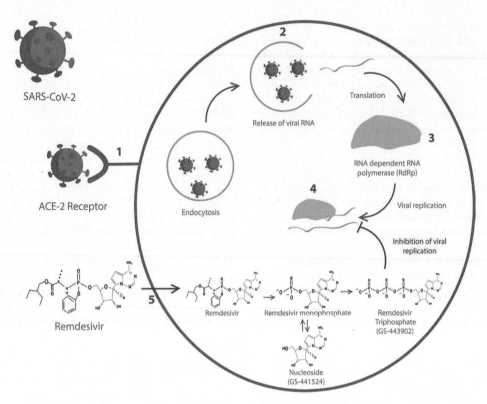

FIGURE 22.6 Mechanism of remdesivir. Entry of SARS-CoV-2 into the target cell (*1*) by binding to the ACE-2 receptor on the cell surface. Once SARS-CoV-2 enters the cell, it releases its viral RNA (*2*). SARS-CoV-2 uses the host machinery to translate RNA (*3*) into RNA-dependent RNA polymerase (RdRp). RdRp is then used to facilitate viral replication (*4*). Once remdesivir enters the cell (*5*), it is converted into remdesivir triphosphate, which competes with endogenous ATP, which is used as a source of nucleotide, for incorporation into RdRp, leading to chain termination. Courtesy of Lama Al-Abdi. From Aleissa MM, Silverman EA, Paredes Acosta LM, et al. New perspectives on antimicrobial agents: remdesivir treatment for COVID-19. *Antimicrob Agents Chemother* 2020;65(1):e01814–20. Ref.[16])

room air oxygen saturation >94%) who were randomized to receive remdesivir for either 5 or 10 days or standard treatment (no remdesivir). Patients who received remdesivir for 5 days, but not those who received it for 10 days, were more likely to improve their clinical status on day 11 than those who received standard treatment (odds ratio 1.65; 95% CI 1.09–2.48).[620] This trial only enrolled those not requiring any supplemen-

tal oxygen at baseline. The Solidarity trial, sponsored by the WHO, enrolled 11,330 hospitalized adults with COVID-19 randomized to receive one of four treatments: remdesivir, hydroxychloroquine, lopinavir/ritonavir, or interferon beta. Controls received the local standard of care. An interim analysis found that none of the drugs including remdesivir affected in-hospital mortality.[688]

TABLE 22.1 Summary of pivotal trials of remdesivir

Trial	Study Size	Randomized	Blinded	Control	Primary End Point
Wang et al.[697]	237	Yes	Yes	Placebo + SOC	Time to 2-point improvement in ordinal score
ACTT[60]	1062	Yes	Yes	Placebo + SOC	Time to recovery (hospital discharge or resolution of active medical issues)
Spinner et al.[620]	584	Yes	No	SOC	Clinical Status on Day 11
Solidarity[688]	2,750 (remdesivir arm)	Yes, to acceptable arms	No	SOC	Mortality
Goldman et al.[248]	397	Yes	No	Remdesivir 10 days	Clinical improvement of 2 points or more

ACTT, Adaptive COVID-19 Treatment Trial; SOC, Standard of care.

SIMPLE-Severe was an open-label trial of 397 hospitalized adults with severe COVID-19 (pneumonia and oxygen saturation of ≤94% or requiring supplemental oxygen) randomized to receive remdesivir for either 5 or 10 days (the trial did not have a nontreated group). Clinical improvement of ≥2 points on a 7-point ordinal scale on day 14, the primary end point, occurred in 65% of patients treated with remdesivir for 5 days compared to 54% of those treated for 10 days ($p = 0.14$).[248] All-cause mortality at day 14 was 8% in the 5-day treatment group versus 11% in the 10-day treatment group.[248]

Observational studies are helpful to frame real-world data compared to the randomized trials above. Using a U.S. nationwide database, survival for adults hospitalized with COVID-19 from August to November 2020 on high-flow/noninvasive or low-flow oxygen treated with remdesivir ($N = 19,589$) was compared to those who did not receive remdesivir ($N = 8,703$). After adjusting for baseline and clinical covariates, those treated with remdesivir had a significantly lower risk of 14-day mortality (low flow oxygen HR 0.68 (0.60 to 0.77), high flow oxygen 0.81 (0.70 to 0.93)).[470] A separate analysis assessed mortality after COVID-19 using U.S.–based claims data. Those treated with remdesivir ($N = 9,271$) had a reduced risk of death (HR = 0.79) compared to matched controls ($N = 9,271$). Those treated also had a significantly greater likelihood of discharge by day 28, compared with controls. These findings were most pronounced in patients with lower oxygen requirements at baseline, but the benefit was across all groups, including those on mechanical ventilation.[151]

The totality of the data suggests that remdesivir is effective in the treatment of COVID-19. Some subgroups may benefit more than others, though no trials were designed and adequately powered to answer this question. There appears to be a consistent benefit in hospitalized patients receiving no oxygen, low-flow, or high-flow oxygen, but not requiring mechanical ventilation. Those on mechanical ventilation (invasive or noninvasive) may not benefit from remdesivir alone. It is unclear if remdesivir improves mortality. None of the randomized studies demonstrated an improvement in mortality, though observational studies with a much larger sample size did. However, decreased time in the hospital and decreased utilization of other hospital resources are meaningful to an individual and essential to health care systems that are often stretched thin during the pandemic. Remdesivir has been approved or authorized for temporary use in the treatment of COVID-19 in at least 48 countries, and as of October 2021 is the only antiviral for COVID-19 approved in most countries.[309]

Other Antiviral Agents

Favipiravir is currently licensed in several countries for the treatment of influenza. Favipiravir (T-705) is an inhibitor of RNA-dependent RNA polymerase and has been evaluated for multiple viral diseases. Multiple groups have reported benefit from favipiravir in case series or small clinical trials. The largest randomized placebo-controlled trial involved 156 Japanese patients with COVID-19 with nonsevere pneumonia. The time to nondetectable SARS-CoV-2 viral RNA was 11.9 days for the favipiravir group and 14.7 days for the placebo group ($p = 0.0136$).[226] Other studies have reported no benefit from favipiravir.[82] The PRESCO study is a larger blinded trial with results anticipated in late 2021.

Molnupiravir (MK-4482, EIDD-2801) is an orally bioavailable prodrug of the ribonucleoside analog N^4-hydroxycytidine, which also inhibits RNA-dependent RNA polymerase.[663] In a phase 2 trial in an outpatient population, treatment with molnupiravir significantly decreased virus isolation at day 3 compared to placebo (1.9% and 16.7%, respectively, $p = 0.02$).[218] Molnupiravir reduced the risk of hospitalization or death in outpatients with mild-to-moderate COVID-19 by approximately 30% when treatment was initiated within 5 days of illness onset.[457] A study in a hospitalized population (Move-In) was stopped for lack of efficacy.[457]

Nirmatrelvir (PF-07321332) is an inhibitor of the SARS-CoV-2 main protease (Mpro, also referred to as 3CL).[503] It is metabolized via cytochrome p450 CYP3A4 and is coadministered with ritonavir, a potent CYP3A4 inhibitor, to extend the serum half-life. Pfizer announced results of a phase 2/3 trial that randomized nonhospitalized adult COVID-19 patients who were at high risk of progressing to severe illness to receive placebo or nirmatrelvir/ritonavir. The rates of hospitalization or death in the nirmatrelvir/ritonavir and control arms were 1% and 6.7%, respectively, resulting in a risk reduction of 85%.[524]

ANTI-INFLAMMATORY

Early in the pandemic, it was recognized that COVID-19 was associated with an acute hyperinflammatory syndrome. The hypercytokinemia was thought to be contributing to the respiratory syndrome by injury of alveolar epithelial cells and vascular endothelial cells.[520] Higher levels of inflammation, especially IL-6, IL-8, and TNF-α, were strong predictors of worse outcomes.[189] As a result, more than 100 antiinflammatory agents have been tried in the treatment of COVID-19. Only three drugs have been proven in multiple studies to improve outcomes: dexamethasone, baricitinib, tocilizumab.[110] Two of these (baricitinib and tocilizumab) have been FDA authorized for emergency use. Dexamethasone has become the standard of care despite never having the scrutiny of an FDA or European Medicines Agency (EMA) review.

Anti-inflammatory strategies are not appropriate for all patients. Dexamethasone, baricitinib, and tocilizumab all have data suggestive of a lack of benefit or even potential harm in some patients with mild (outpatient) or moderate (not requiring oxygen) disease. Understanding the limitations of the data and defining populations most likely to benefit are critical to optimal use of these agents.

Dexamethasone

Dexamethasone is a glucocorticoid that can modify the immune response through the activation of transcription factors belonging to the superfamily of nuclear receptors.[589] Dexamethasone can decrease pro-inflammatory cytokines such as IL-6 and TNF-α by down-regulating transcription. Early in the COVID-19 pandemic, there was hesitancy to use dexamethasone given a lack of benefit seen in SARS-CoV-1.[80,220,382] The majority of the efficacy data on dexamethasone comes from the RECOVERY trial, a large, randomized, open-label trial in the United Kingdom.[297] This trial included hospitalized patients with confirmed or suspected COVID-19 who had no specific contraindications to dexamethasone. The 28-day mortality for the entire population decreased from 25.7% in the control arm to 22.9% with dexamethasone (rate ratio [RR] 0.83, 95% CI 0.75 to 0.93). Patients on invasive mechanical ventilation at baseline had a 36% relative reduction in mortality (29.3 vs. 41.4%, RR 0.64, 95% CI 0.51 to 0.81), while patients on oxygen therapy at baseline had an 18% relative reduction in mortality (23.3% vs. 26.2%, RR 0.82, 95% CI 0.72 to 0.94). In contrast, a benefit was not seen among patients who did not require either oxygen or ventilatory support; there was a non-statistically significant trend toward higher mortality (17.8% vs. 14%, RR 1.19, 95% CI 0.91 to 1.55). These findings have generally held up in meta-analyses across 10 randomized trials (overall RR 0.88).[398]

It is not clear if all glucocorticoids are equally effective. A meta-analysis that pooled data from seven randomized clinical trials that evaluated the efficacy of different corticosteroids in 1,703 critically ill patients with COVID-19 demonstrated less mortality (OR 0.70; 95% CI 0.48 to 1.01, $p = 0.053$) based on the random-effects meta-analysis. The OR was smallest (largest benefit) for dexamethasone (OR 0.64; 95% CI 0.50 to 0.82; $p < 0.001$).[624] Methylprednisolone had fairly limited benefit (OR was 0.91 (95% CI 0.29 to 2.87; $p = 0.87$)). The benefit of dexamethasone depends on the severity of disease and mortality in each population. When control mortality was less than 10% to 20%, there was increased risk of death from glucocorticoids.[398] In a low-risk population with a control mortality of less than 5%, glucocorticoids increased the risk of death three- to fivefold.[398] Dexamethasone is the primary anti-inflammatory agent for those in a hyperinflammatory state from COVID-19, as clinically evident by increasing oxygen requirement, or advancement to requiring more respiratory support including high flow oxygen, noninvasive mechanical ventilation, or invasive mechanical ventilation.[483]

Baricitinib

Baricitinib is a Janus kinase inhibitor approved for the treatment of rheumatoid arthritis. The cytokine receptor family responsible for amplification of the inflammatory cascade in response to TNF-α, IL-6, IFN, and other cytokines require the Janus kinase-signal transduction and activation of transcription (JAK–STAT) pathway to effect signal transduction.[390] Targeting this pathway is critical in other inflammatory mediated diseases and thus an early target for reducing inflammation from COVID-19. In a randomized trial of 1,033 hospitalized adults with COVID-19, baricitinib plus remdesivir reduced time to recovery (defined as hospital discharge or continued hospitalization without need for oxygen or medical care) compared with placebo plus remdesivir (7 vs. 8 days, rate ratio for recovery 1.16, 95% CI 1.01 to 1.32).[330] Among the 216 patients on high-flow oxygen or noninvasive ventilation at baseline, the median recovery time with baricitinib was 10 days versus 18 days with placebo (RR 1.51, 95% CI 1.10 to 2.08). In those patients not on oxygen, there was a slight increase in time to recovery (5 vs. 4 days, rate ratio 0.88). Overall, there was also a trend toward lower 29-day mortality with the addition of baricitinib to remdesivir (5.1% vs. 7.8%; HR 0.65, 95% CI 0.39 to 10.9), but this was not statistically significant.

A second placebo-controlled, randomized trial of 1,525 hospitalized adults with COVID-19 evaluated baricitinib in addition to standard of care, which could include glucocorticoids and did not require remdesivir. Twenty-eight-day mortality was reduced (8.1% vs. 13.1% with placebo; HR 0.57, 95% CI 0.41 to 0.78).[440] Among the subgroup of patients on high-flow oxygen or noninvasive ventilation at baseline, the mortality with baricitinib was 17.5% versus 29.4% with placebo (HR 0.52, 95% CI 0.33 to 0.80). This is also supported by efficacy studies of other JAK inhibitors such as tofacitinib,[265] though currently only baricitinib is available under a EUA.

IL-6 Pathway Inhibitors

Given the pathogenesis and increased IL-6 demonstrated in severe disease, the IL-6 receptor blockers tocilizumab and sarilumab were evaluated for the treatment of COVID-19. In an open-label trial in the United Kingdom that included 4,116 patients with suspected or confirmed COVID-19, hypoxia, and a CRP level ≥75 mg/L, adding tocilizumab to usual care reduced the 28-day mortality rate compared with standard care alone (31% vs. 35%, relative risk 0.85, 95% CI 0.76 to 0.94).[550] A subgroup analysis suggested that those on glucocorticoids were more likely to benefit from tocilizumab than were individuals not on glucocorticoids, but this may reflect benefit in those with most severe disease rather than a requirement of dual therapy. Another open label study of tocilizumab or sarilumab demonstrated an improvement in organ support–free days (median 10 [IQR −1 to 16] in the tocilizumab group, 11 [0 to 16] in the sarilumab group, and 0 [IQR −1 to 15] in the control group).[558] 90-day survival was also improved (combined HR 1.61 (95% CI 1.25 to 2.08)). In the EMPACTA trial, tocilizumab reduced the percentage of patients progressing to mechanical ventilation or death by day 28 (12.0% vs. 19.3%).[584] Two other smaller studies support the benefit of tocilizumab.[584,750]

Several trials, however, gave conflicting results and failed to identify a mortality benefit or other clear clinical benefit with these agents.[292,567,585,627] In the COVACTA trial, in 452 hospitalized patients with severe COVID-19 pneumonia, the median value for clinical status on the ordinal scale at day 28 was 1.0 (discharged or ready for discharge) in the tocilizumab group and 2.0 (non-ICU hospitalization without supplemental oxygen) in the placebo group.[440] This was considered not statistically different ($p = 0.31$). In the REMDACTA trial, in 649 hospitalized patients with severe COVID-19 pneumonia, tocilizumab had no statistically significant differences observed between treatment groups for time to hospital discharge or ready for discharge through 28 days of follow-up.

The reasons for the different findings among trials are uncertain. In meta-analyses, tocilizumab does not have benefit in the general hospitalized COVID-19 population.[703] The most benefit was seen in those most critically ill. Many of the beneficial studies had a higher proportion of participants who were receiving steroids suggesting IL-6 blockade may only provide benefit when combined with steroids.[38] Additionally, the discrepant results may be related to the endpoint chosen—positive studies generally evaluated prevention of deterioration (death or mechanical ventilation), while negative studies generally evaluated improvement in recovery (hospital discharge or clinical status by ordinal score).

Sarilumab was evaluated with tocilizumab in an open label study that demonstrated the benefit of either drug in addition to standard care.[558] The study was stopped early with only 48 participants treated with sarilumab in the trial. A meta-analysis of other small trials with sarilumab failed to show benefit.[657]

No other published trials that compared tocilizumab with sarilumab are available at the time of this writing. While sarilumab might be expected to have similar benefits to tocilizumab given the same mechanism of action, the available data are insufficient to make definitive recommendations for sarilumab.[289]

Other Anti-Inflammatory Agents

At least 300 trials with at least 30 unique anti-inflammatory or immunomodulatory effects are being evaluated.[396] It is likely that additional anti-inflammatory agents will be proven to have benefit, and some may receive emergency use authorization or formal approval. However, lacking well powered definitive studies and regulatory review, no conclusive statements can be made about the clinical utility of these agents.

CONVALESCENT PLASMA

Plasma from persons who have recovered from an infection is often tried for severe infectious diseases for which few therapeutic options exist, such as severe acute respiratory syndrome (SARS-CoV-1) in 2003,[142] pandemic influenza in 2009,[420] and Ebola in 2016.[678] Unfortunately, most of these reports have failed to show efficacy in definitive clinical trials.[59] Early in the pandemic, convalescent plasma was used for treatment of COVID-19. Early case series suggested benefit.[605] Unfortunately, most studies with convalescent plasma have remained as case series or retrospective cohorts, and no adequately powered randomized trials have been performed.[223] The largest randomized control trials showed no reduction in disease progression or reduction of mortality.[10,549,612]

Other analyses such as case series and reviews of expanded access programs have reported much more encouraging results. Following transfusion of plasma, most patients improved, most notably in mild to moderately ill patients.[327] Critically ill/end-stage patients on ventilators showed worsening of disease status after treatment with convalescent plasma. In analysis of those treated with plasma, the risk of death within 30 days was lower in those that received plasma with high titers of antibody to SARS-CoV-2 compared to those that received medium or low titer plasma (22.3%, 27.4%, and 29.6%, respectively) potentially representing a dose (titer) effect. Given the potential for benefit and the known safety profile of plasma, the FDA authorized high titer COVID-19 convalescent plasma to be used in the treatment of hospitalized patients with COVID-19 early in the disease course and for those who have impaired humoral immunity and cannot produce an adequate antibody response. Given these mixed results, most guidelines have not endorsed treatment with convalescent plasma.

ANTITHROMBOTIC PROPHYLAXIS

Several studies suggest a high rate of thromboembolic complications among hospitalized patients with COVID-19, particularly those who are critically ill. Pharmacologic prophylaxis of venous thromboembolism is generally indicated for all hospitalized patients with COVID-19. A recent meta-analysis identified 66 relevant studies in patients with COVID-19 and showed an estimated overall prevalence of venous thromboembolism of 14·1%.[385,489] A variety of antithrombotic agents, doses, and

durations of therapy are being assessed in more than 75 randomized controlled trials spanning outpatients, hospitalized patients in medical wards, and critically ill patients with COVID-19.[639]

Therapeutic heparin was studied in critically ill patients with COVID-19. Based on interim data, an open-label, multiplatform randomized study discontinued enrollment for ICU patients when the futility boundary for the primary end point was reached and a potential for harm could not be excluded. There was no improvement in in-hospital survival (64.3% vs. 65.3%), and those treated with heparin potentially had higher major bleeding (3.1% vs. 2.4%).[559] The INSPIRATION trial evaluated intermediate dose low molecular weight heparin versus the standard dose. There was no difference in the primary outcome, a composite of venous or arterial thrombosis, treatment with extracorporeal membrane oxygenation, or mortality (45.7% vs. 44.1%).[310] Again, major bleeding was slightly higher in the intermediate dose arm (2.5% vs. 1.4%). One multiplatform trial in patients with COVID-19 admitted to hospital wards treated with therapeutic heparin decreased the need for oxygen support from approximately 25% to 18%.[385] However, given the potential that therapeutic doses of heparin can cause harm if patients progress to high flow oxygen, most guidelines committees still recommend only routine thromboprophylaxis dosed heparin in COVID-19.[385]

Ineffective Therapies

While the field of therapeutics is dynamic and there are likely to be more effective therapeutics advanced through clinical development, there are several therapeutics that have been shown to be ineffective and should not be used. These include the following:

- Aspirin (in hospitalized population)[554]
- Azithromycin (in hospitalized population)[548]
- Colchicine (in hospitalized population)[443]
- High dose zinc and vitamin C (outpatient and hospitalized populations)[316,659]
- Hydroxychloroquine (postexposure prophylaxis, outpatient, and hospitalized populations)[8,43,85,298,507,598]
- Interferon beta (in hospitalized population)[8,507]
- Lopinavir/ritonavir (in hospitalized population)[8,507,547,598]
- Ivermectin[565]

TREATMENT OF COVID-19

The treatment of COVID-19 depends on clinical symptoms and severity of disease at presentation. Clinical management has changed throughout the COVID-19 pandemic and continues to evolve, as evidence from clinical trials and observational studies inform clinical practice. While there are multiple therapeutic options and the general framework of when these agents should be used are known (Fig. 22.7), there is much that is not known about the optimal combinations, timing, and populations. Evidence-based guidelines such as those from the National Institutes of Health COVID-19 Treatment Guidelines Panel[483] are invaluable when determining optimal treatments.

Outpatients

Clinical care of outpatients is mainly supportive and includes close monitoring for complications, hypoxia, and clinical deterioration. For outpatients, as of mid-2021, the only

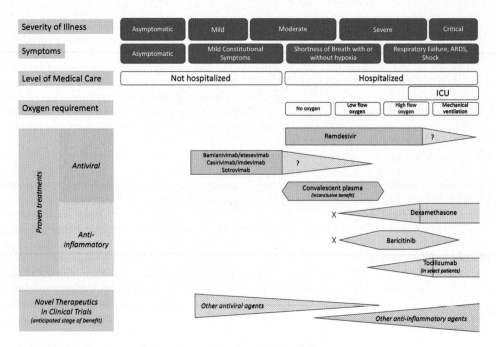

FIGURE 22.7 Summary of treatment options by severity of disease.

SARS-CoV-2–specific treatments with proven clinical benefit in randomized placebo-control clinical trials are the anti-SARS-CoV-2 monoclonal antibodies that target the SARS-CoV-2 spike protein.[138,250,706] The clinical benefit of anti-SARS-CoV-2 monoclonal antibodies is greatest in persons without baseline immunity against SARS-CoV-2 infection[706] and when administered before endogenous antibodies are present. The selection of antibody must be guided by knowledge of circulating variants and the ability of the available monoclonal antibodies to neutralize the likely infecting virus. There is no evidence that treatment with glucocorticoids or other immunosuppressants benefit this population, and some evidence to suggest harm. The oral antivirals molnupiravir and PF-07321332, if approved or authorized for early use, could revolutionize the treatment of COVID-19 prior to hospitalization.

Hospitalized Patients

Clinical care of hospitalized patients generally is a combination of an antiviral (remdesivir) and an anti-inflammatory agent (generally dexamethasone, but also baricitinib and tocilizumab) plus supportive care including oxygen therapy and routine dosed thromboprophylaxis. Remdesivir has the most benefit in those on low flow oxygen or not yet on oxygen. Those not on oxygen will typically do well regardless of treatment. In resource-limited situations, remdesivir may not be given.

The decision of when to treat with an anti-inflammatory agent and what agent(s) to use is more challenging. In general, those not on oxygen do not need treatment with an anti-inflammatory, and several trials suggest harm in this population. Those with a rapidly deteriorating respiratory status, on high flow oxygen, or on mechanical ventilation benefit most from anti-inflammatory agents. Dexamethasone is currently the standard of care, but baricitinib and tocilizumab may represent effective alternatives. Defining the timing, dose, combination, and populations for each still requires additional research.

INFECTION PREVENTION AND CONTROL

During the early months of the COVID-19 pandemic, nosocomial SARS-CoV-2 infections in health care personnel highlighted the importance of the availability of recommended personal protective equipment and strict compliance with recommended infection prevention and control measures.[78,152,755] Health care personnel (HCP) should be educated and trained on proper use, donning, and doffing of recommended personal protective equipment. CDC recommends that for care of patients with suspected or confirmed COVID-19 in ambulatory care settings, source control for both HCP and patients should be applied with a properly fitted cloth mask, facemask, or respirator except for children aged less than 2 years, and patients should be isolated by placement in an examination room with the door closed.[120] In general, health care personnel should follow standard and transmission-based precautions and wear a fit-tested N95 respirator (or similar respirator approved under standards used in other countries similar to National Institute for Occupational Safety and Health (NIOSH)–approved N95 filtering facepiece respirators), or a well-fitting facemask, gown, gloves, and eye protection.[120] HCP working in facilities located in areas with moderate to substantial community SARS-CoV-2 transmission should wear a properly fitted cloth mask, facemask, or respirator for source control while in the facility and for protection during all patient care encounters. Health care facilities should optimize the use of engineering controls to improve indoor air quality and reduce or eliminate exposures by shielding HCP and other patients from infected individuals. Patients hospitalized with suspected or confirmed COVID-19 should be placed in a single room (with the door closed) with a dedicated bathroom. Sharing of rooms can result in the transmission of SARS-CoV-2 from persons with unrecognized infection to their unvaccinated roommates.[336] Negative pressure Airborne Infection Isolation Rooms (AIIRs) should be prioritized for patients who are undergoing aerosol-generating procedures.

VACCINE

The S protein of coronaviruses plays essential roles in cell receptor binding, tissue tropism, and pathogenesis and is the primary target of neutralizing antibodies elicited by natural infections.[243] S protein consists of an S1 subunit that determines receptor recognition via its receptor-binding domain (RBD) and an S2 subunit responsible for membrane fusion.[172] Vaccine-induced neutralizing antibodies (nAbs) correlate with protection and reduction of viral loads in nonhuman primates (NHPs) after SARS-CoV-2 infection.[456,738] In humans, the risk of symptomatic COVID-19 decreased with increasing levels of anti-spike IgG, anti-RBD IgG, pseudovirus neutralization titer, and live-virus neutralization titer.[213] In contrast, there were no significant associations between any of the assays and protection against asymptomatic infection. Depletion of T cells in mice impairs virus clearance in SARS-CoV-1 and SARS-CoV-2 infections[636,752], and the development of robust virus–specific CD4+ and CD8+ responses are associated with milder disease, suggesting T-cell responses are also protective against severe COVID-19.[172,446]

Any SARS-CoV-2 vaccine must avoid enhancing the viral replication and clinical disease, a phenomenon known as enhanced respiratory disease (ERD). ERD is a broad category that includes antibody-dependent enhancement (ADE) and non–antibody-based mechanisms.[384] ADE occurs through two distinct mechanisms: enhanced antibody-mediated virus uptake by Fc gamma receptor IIa (FcγRIIa)-expressing phagocytic cells leading to increased viral replication, or excessive antibody Fc-mediated effector functions or immune complex formation causing enhanced inflammation and immunopathology.[384] For nonmacrophage tropic respiratory viruses, non-neutralizing antibodies can induce ERD by forming immune complexes that deposit into airway tissues and activate cytokine and complement pathways.[251,384,527] ERD and ADE have been well documented in vitro for several viruses, including human immunodeficiency virus (HIV), Ebola, influenza, and flaviviruses.[384] Studies of mice vaccinated with SARS-CoV-1 showed enhanced immunopathology in animals following viral challenge when the T-cell response was Th2 biased.[669] Passive transfer studies have illustrated that anti-S antibody confers protection from SARS-CoV-1 replication in the mouse model without potentiating disease.[631]

Coronavirus S protein can readily transition from an unstable prefusion state to a stable postfusion state during cellular binding or spontaneously independent of target cells.[102] The prefusion antibody epitopes are most likely to lead to neutralizing responses.[352] The prefusion coronavirus S proteins can be stabilized with two proline mutations.[505] Stabilization of the S protein in the prefusion conformation significantly increases expression, conformational homogeneity, and increased elicitation of antibody responses.[505] Therefore, an ideal vaccine would target the SARS-CoV-2 S protein (preferably a stabilized S), evoke both the humoral and cellular arms of the immune system, induce primarily a Th1 cell–biased response, and not have evidence of ERD. As of October 2021, there are 128 COVID-19 vaccines in clinical development (including those licensed and in development for other age groups) and an additional 194 in preclinical development.[717] These can be divided into eight different types of vaccines[680,717] including the following:

- DNA
- Inactivated virus
- Live attenuated virus
- Protein subunit
- RNA
- Virus-like particle
- Viral vector (nonreplicating and replicating)
- Antigen-presenting cell + viral vector (nonreplicating and replicating)

Protein subunit vaccines are the most common platform in clinical development (35%), followed by RNA (17%), non-replicating viral vector, and inactivated virus.[717] Three COVID-19 vaccines are currently approved or authorized by the U.S. Food and Drug Administration (FDA) for emergency use: two mRNA vaccines (Pfizer-BioNTech and Moderna) and one viral vector vaccine (Johnson & Johnson/Janssen). Other vaccines that have received approvals or authorizations in other countries and are widely available include two viral vector vaccines (AstraZeneca and CanSino Biologics), and two inactivated SARS-CoV-2 vaccines (Sinovac and Sinopharm), and one protein subunit vaccine (Medigen).[717]

Vaccine efficacy refers to how well a vaccine performs in a carefully controlled clinical trial. All currently available (approved or emergency use authorized) COVID-19 vaccines demonstrated efficacy against symptomatic, laboratory-confirmed COVID-19 in adults ≥18 years.[124] The Pfizer-BioNTech COVID-19 vaccine also demonstrated high efficacy against symptomatic, laboratory-confirmed COVID-19 in adolescents aged 12 to 17 years and children aged 5 to 11 years. All authorized COVID-19 vaccines have also demonstrated high effectiveness against severe disease (generally defined as requiring hospitalization) and high effectiveness against death from COVID-19[124] (Table 22.2). No trials have compared efficacy between any of the authorized vaccines in the same study population at the same time. One observational study reported that persons with prior SARS-CoV-2 infection ≥6 months before receiving their first dose of COVID-19 mRNA vaccine had a significantly lower risk of breakthrough infection compared with those infected less than 6 months before receiving their first dose.[3] To date, there has been no evidence of vaccine-associated ERD in any COVID-19 vaccine studies.

Vaccine effectiveness describes a vaccine's performance in real-world observational studies. Multiple studies (Table 22.3) from the United States and other countries demonstrate that the currently approved or authorized COVID-19 vaccines are highly effective against SARS-CoV-2 infection (including both symptomatic and asymptomatic infections) and sequelae, including severe disease, hospitalization, and death.

Data from the clinical trials among adults suggest that COVID-19 vaccines may also protect against asymptomatic infection.[124] In the Moderna trial, among people who had received a first dose, the number of asymptomatic people who tested positive for SARS-CoV-2 at their second-dose appointment was approximately 67% lower among vaccines than among placebo. Efficacy of the Janssen COVID-19 vaccine against asymptomatic infection was 74% in a subset of trial participants. Additionally, COVID-19 vaccines can reduce asymptomatic SARS-CoV-2 infection and transmission.

TABLE 22.2	Characteristics and initial reported efficacy of select SARS-CoV-2 vaccines			
Manufacturer	Pfizer/BioNTech[528]	Moderna[47]	Janssen[581]	AstraZeneca[687]
Name	BNT162b2	mRNA-1273	Ad26.COV2.S	ChAdOx1 nCoV-19
Vaccine type	mRNA	mRNA	Adenovirus vector	Adenovirus vector
Stabilized prefusion S	Yes	Yes	Yes	No
Age	≥5 years old	≥18 years old	≥18 years old	≥18 years old
Schedule	Two doses 21 days apart	Two doses 28 days apart	One dose	Two doses 4–12 weeks apart
Initial efficacy[a] 95% CI	95% (90.3–97.6)	94.1% (89.3–96.8)	66.1% (55.0–74.8)	70.4% (54.8–80.6)

[a]Vaccine efficacy (VE) based on initial assessments and studies conducted when the Delta variant was not predominant; VE is less certain and may be reduced against Delta and other variants.

Adverse Events

Postvaccination reactogenicity events commonly occur in the first 24 to 48 hours and include injection site pain and erythema and systemic symptoms such as fever, myalgias, fatigue, and headache.[131,238,286,601] For vaccines requiring two doses, the frequency and severity of the systemic events generally increased after the second dose.[47,528] Injection site and systemic adverse events were more common among younger participants (18 to <65 years of age) than among older participants (≥65 years of age).[47] SARS-CoV-2 vaccines approved or authorized for emergency use in the United States are recommended for pregnant women, and accumulating evidence supports their safety when administered during any stage of pregnancy.[119,348,609,741]

Less common but more severe reactions include hypersensitivity reactions. Anaphylaxis, a life-threatening allergic reaction that rarely occurs after vaccination, can occur with these vaccines. The incidence is approximately 5 in 1,000,000 vaccinations.[257]

Myocarditis/Pericarditis

Myocarditis is an inflammation of the heart muscle, and pericarditis is an inflammation of the pericardium, the lining that surrounds the heart, and has been associated with the mRNA vaccines (Pfizer-BioNTech and Moderna).[569] Myocarditis may be suggested by one or more of the following clinical symptoms: chest pain, pressure, or discomfort; dyspnea, shortness of breath, or pain with breathing; palpitations; or syncope.[236] It occurs most commonly within 4 days after the second vaccine, more commonly in men, and typically in those under 30 years of age (median 26 years).[236] Other diagnostic signs include elevated troponin, abnormal imaging such as cardiac magnetic resonance imaging (MRI), and ST or T wave changes on electrocardiogram (ECG).[193,465] The current risk benefit is still thought to favor vaccination in all age groups (currently age 5 years or older).

Thrombosis With Thrombocytopenia

Thrombosis with thrombocytopenia syndrome (TTS) is a rare syndrome associated with the adenovirus-based COVID-19 vaccines (ChAdOx1 nCoV-19 and Ad26.COV2.S COVID-19). TTS is manifested by acute venous or arterial thrombosis and new-onset thrombocytopenia in patients with no recent known exposure to heparin.[426] Thrombosis typically involves atypical locations, including cerebral venous thrombosis and splanchnic

vein thrombosis.[514] TTS should be suspected in patients with severe persistent (lasting over 3 days) headache, abdominal pain, vomiting, dyspnea, chest pain, leg pain, or leg swelling, which are present 4 to 30 days after receiving either the ChAdOx1 nCoV-19 or AD26.COV2.S vaccine.[415] TTS mimics autoimmune heparin-induced thrombocytopenia and can be mediated by platelet-activating antibodies against platelet factor 4.[365] Diagnostic criteria have been established (must meet all five criteria): COVID vaccine 4 to 42 days prior to symptom onset, any venous or arterial thrombosis (often cerebral or abdominal), thrombocytopenia (platelet count <150 × 10^9/L), positive PF4 "HIT" (heparin-induced thrombocytopenia) ELISA, and a markedly elevated D-dimer (>4 times upper limit of normal).[25,365] Treatment may include intravenous immunoglobulin and anticoagulation while avoiding both heparin-based agents and platelet transfusions.

Guillain-Barré Syndrome

Rare cases of the neurological disorder, Guillain-Barré syndrome, have been reported following vaccination with the Janssen COVID-19 and AstraZeneca vaccines and generally occur within 42 days of vaccination.[207,324] Guillain-Barré syndrome generally presents as progressive ascending limb weakness associated with reduced or absent reflexes.[600] This syndrome has been associated with infections such as Campylobacter jejuni and Zika virus, and other vaccines including the 1976 H1N1 influenza vaccine.[512,600] The incidence is not known but appears to be approximately 6.2 to 9 per 1,000,000 vaccinations. Guillain-Barré does rarely occur after SARS-CoV-2 infection[11] but not enough is known about vaccine-associated and post-SARS-CoV-2 infection Guillain-Barré to know if their pathophysiology is related. Plasma exchange and intravenous immunoglobulin are the primary treatments for Guillain-Barré syndrome.[304,544]

Variant Viruses

COVID-19 vaccines have been demonstrated to reduce the risk of severe disease and death from circulating variants (Tables 22.4 and 22.5).

Additional Vaccine Dose in Immunocompromised

Vaccination is particularly important for people with immunocompromising conditions, who are at increased risk of

TABLE 22.3   Effectiveness against SARS-CoV-2 infection, symptomatic disease, and hospitalization

Country	Population	Vaccine	Outcome	Effectiveness for Symptomatic Disease[a]
United States[515]	Adults (≥18 years old)	Pfizer-BioNTech or Moderna	SARS-CoV-2 infection	89%
United States[676]	Adults (≥18 years old)	Pfizer-BioNTech or Moderna	Hospitalization	96%
United States[163]	Adults (≥18 years old)	Johnson & Johnson/Janssen	SARS-CoV-2 infection	77%
Israel[271]	General population ≥16 years	Pfizer-BioNTech	Symptomatic disease	>97%
			Hospitalization	97%
			Death	97%
Sweden[71]	Adults (≥18 years old)	Pfizer-BioNTech	SARS-CoV-2 infection	86%
Norway[595]	Adults (>18 years old)	Pfizer-BioNTech or Moderna	SARS-CoV-2 infection	54.5% (Alpha)
				64.6% (Delta)
United Kingdom[416]	Adults (≥16 years old)	Pfizer-BioNTech	SARS-CoV-2 infection	93.7% (Alpha)
				88.0% (Delta)
United States[655]	Adults ≥ 65 years old	Pfizer-BioNTech or Moderna	Hospitalization	94%
United Kingdom[417]	Adults aged ≥80 years, including those with multiple underlying conditions	Pfizer-BioNTech	Symptomatic disease	85%
United States[111]	Residents in a skilled nursing facility	Pfizer-BioNTech	Symptomatic disease	87%
			Hospitalization	94%
United States[480]		Pfizer-BioNTech or Moderna	SARS-CoV-2 infection	74.7% (pre-Delta)
				53.1% (Delta)
Denmark[469]	Long-term care facility residents	Pfizer-BioNTech	SARS-CoV-2 infection	64%
United States[637]	Health care workers	Pfizer-BioNTech	SARS-CoV-2 infection	97%
		Moderna	SARS-CoV-2 infection	99%
United States[661]	Health care workers, first responders, and other essential and frontline workers	Pfizer-BioNTech or Moderna	SARS-CoV-2 infection	90%
United States[526]	Health care workers	Pfizer-BioNTech or Moderna	Symptomatic disease	94%
Israel[30]	Health care workers	Pfizer-BioNTech	Symptomatic disease	>97%
Italy[209]	Health care workers	Pfizer-BioNTech	Symptomatic disease	>95%
United States[221]	Health care workers	Pfizer-BioNTech, Moderna or Janssen	SARS-CoV-2 infection	91% (before Delta)
				66% (Delta)

[a]Vaccine effectiveness (VE) based on studies conducted when the Delta variant was not predominant; VE is less certain and may be reduced against Delta and other variants.
Adapted from Centers for Disease Control and Prevention. COVID-19 Vaccines and Vaccination. https://www.ncbi.nlm.nih.gov/pubmed/34009769. Ref.[114]

severe COVID-19 illness. Recent studies in several countries found significantly lower vaccine effectiveness among immunocompromised adults compared to those without immunocompromising conditions (vaccine effectiveness 47% to 81% in immunocompromised compared to 90% to 94% if not immunocompromised).[39,134,147,346,656] People with moderately to severely compromised immune systems should receive an additional dose of mRNA COVID-19 vaccine at least 28 days after a second dose of Pfizer-BioNTech COVID-19 vaccine or Moderna COVID-19 vaccine.[115] This includes people who have

TABLE 22.4 Effectiveness of COVID-19 vaccination against SARS-CoV-2 infection and symptomatic disease (including severe disease and hospitalization) caused by the delta variant

Country	Population	Vaccine	Outcome	Vaccine Effectiveness
United Kingdom[417]	General population ≥16 years	Pfizer-BioNTech	Symptomatic disease	88%
Canada[481]	General population ≥16 years	Pfizer-BioNTech	Symptomatic disease	85%
United Kingdom (Scotland)[481]	General population	Pfizer-BioNTech	SARS-CoV-2 infection	79%
United Kingdom[416]	General population	Pfizer-BioNTech	SARS-CoV-2 infection	80%
United States[221]	Health care workers, first responders, and other essential and frontline workers	Pfizer-BioNTech, Moderna, or Janssen	SARS-CoV-2 infection	66%
Qatar[646]	General population ≥12 years	Moderna	SARS-CoV-2 infection	85%
		Pfizer-BioNTech	SARS-CoV-2 infection	54%
		Moderna	Symptomatic disease	86%
		Pfizer-BioNTech	Symptomatic disease	56%
		Moderna	Severe, critical, or fatal disease	100%
		Pfizer-BioNTech	Severe, critical, or fatal disease	90%

From Centers for Disease Control and Prevention. COVID-19 Vaccines and Vaccination. https://www.ncbi.nlm.nih.gov/pubmed/34009769. Ref.[114]

- Been receiving active cancer treatment for tumors or cancers of the blood
- Received an organ transplant and are taking medicine to suppress the immune system
- Received a stem cell transplant within the last 2 years or are taking medicine to suppress the immune system
- Moderate or severe primary immunodeficiency (such as DiGeorge syndrome, Wiskott-Aldrich syndrome)
- Advanced or untreated HIV infection
- Active treatment with high-dose corticosteroids or other drugs that may suppress the immune response

This additional dose of an mRNA COVID-19 vaccine is intended to improve the initial response to the vaccine series and is different than a booster (described below).

Vaccine Booster

Emerging evidence also shows that vaccine effectiveness against SARS-CoV-2 infections is decreasing over time. Six months after a primary vaccination series, neutralizing antibodies have been found to decrease at least 0.5 log.[518] Additionally, there is a 2.4-fold decrease in pseudovirus neutralization of Delta compared to D614G.[518]

TABLE 22.5 Effectiveness of COVID-19 vaccination against asymptomatic SARS-CoV-2 infection when different variants predominated

Country	Population	Vaccine	Dominant Variant(s)	Vaccine Effectiveness
Israel[557]	Health care workers	Pfizer-BioNTech	Alpha	65%
United States (California)[28]	General population ≥18 years	Pfizer-BioNTech or Moderna	Epsilon, Alpha	68%
United States[644]	Preprocedural adult patients	Pfizer-BioNTech or Moderna	Ancestral strain	80%
Qatar[644]	General population ≥12 years	Moderna	Delta	80%
		Pfizer-BioNTech	Delta	36%
Israel[30]	Health care workers	Pfizer-BioNTech	Alpha	86%
Israel[271]	General population ≥16 years	Pfizer-BioNTech	Alpha	92%
Israel[171]	General population ≥16 years	Pfizer-BioNTech	Ancestral strain, Alpha	90%

Adapted from Centers for Disease Control and Prevention. COVID-19 Vaccines and Vaccination. https://www.ncbi.nlm.nih.gov/pubmed/34009769. Ref.[114]

In a high-risk population of nursing home residents, two doses of mRNA vaccines were 74.7% effective against infection early in the vaccination program (March to May 2021) and declined to 53.1% effective at preventing infection later (June to July 2021) when the Delta variant predominated.[480] In a population at high risk of SARS-CoV-2 exposure (health care personnel, first responders, and other essential and frontline workers), estimates of effectiveness declined from 91% before predominance of the Delta variant to 66%.[221] In a general adult population, the overall age-adjusted vaccine effectiveness declined from 91.7% to 79.8% in a similar period of time.[568] Effectiveness against COVID-19–associated hospitalization has not declined as much, though this differs based on age: vaccine was 79.8% effective among adults aged ≥65 years and 95.1% among those aged 18 to 64 years.[50] Taken together, these data suggest waning vaccine effectiveness, likely due to both waning antibodies and a more infectious delta variant.

Persons receiving a homologous booster dose of vaccine 6 to 8 months after a primary series of two doses of 50 or 100 µg of mRNA-1273 had a 1.7-fold increase in neutralizing titer compared to 28 days after the second injection of the primary series.[156] A homologous booster with the Ad26.COV2.S vaccine given 2 months after the primary vaccination resulted in a 4-fold increase in antibodies when given at 2 months and a 12-fold increase in antibodies when the booster was given at 6 months.[325] By 2 weeks after the booster dose, the rate of confirmed SARS-CoV-2 infection was lower in the booster group than in the nonboosted group by a factor of 11.3, and the rate of severe illness was lower by a factor of 19.5.[54] In persons with breakthrough infections after a booster dose of vaccine, there was a viral load reduction suggesting restored vaccine-associated decrease in transmissibility.[392]

Limiting vaccine recipients to a homologous booster would pose logistical challenges. Heterologous boosts have been evaluated using the three vaccines available in the United States. In all nine combinations, booster vaccines increased the neutralizing activity against a D614G pseudovirus (4.2- to 76-fold) and binding antibody titers (4.6- to 56-fold) for all combinations; homologous booster vaccines increased neutralizing antibody titers 4.2- to 20-fold, whereas heterologous boost increased titers 6.2- to 76-fold.[41] While some differences in reactogenicity following the booster dose were present, no new safety concerns were identified as compared with the characterized safety profiles of the vaccines when used for primary vaccination.

On November 19, 2021, the FDA authorized COVID-19 booster vaccines for all individuals 18 years of age and older.[673]

- A single booster dose of the Moderna or Pfizer COVID-19 vaccine can be administered at least 6 months after completion of the primary series.
- A single booster dose of the Janssen (Johnson and Johnson) COVID-19 vaccine may be given at least 2 months after completion of the single-dose primary regimen to individuals 18 years of age and older.

PERSPECTIVE

The COVID-19 pandemic is an unparalleled public health crisis. In under 2 years since its emergence, there have been over 250 million confirmed COVID-19 cases and more than 5 million deaths reported to the WHO, and this will likely continue to increase until there is widespread availability and acceptance of vaccines. This pandemic has been associated with remarkable scientific advances in a short period of time, including:

- Rapid isolation of the causative organism.
- Extensive characterization of the clinical spectrum of SARS-CoV-2 infection, complications, and persistence of symptoms.
- The development of over 300 diagnostic assays to detect infection.
- Unparalleled pace for developing highly effective vaccines, leading to at least 10 vaccines being approved or authorized by regulatory authorities and over 5 billion doses of vaccine administered worldwide.
- At least five monoclonal antibodies have received early authorization use for the prevention and early treatment of disease.
- Clinical trials have demonstrated conclusive efficacy of four therapeutics including one novel antiviral (remdesivir, now approved in about 50 countries), and three repurposed agents (dexamethasone, baricitinib, and tocilizumab).

It is challenging to write a chapter for such a quick moving field with important new developments reported daily. Much of the data cited were from studies conducted during the COVID-19 pandemic before Delta and Omicron variants were predominant. SARS-CoV-2 will continue to evolve in unpredictable ways with unknown effects upon transmission dynamics, disease severity, response to therapeutics, and clinical management. Vaccines will continue to advance, with additional constructs receiving authorization for early use and additional vaccines likely receiving full approval. Future vaccines might be given intranasally to enhance local immune responses, may be modified in response to variants, or may have activity against multiple different coronaviruses. Data will become available on the durability of immunity acquired from SARS-CoV-2 infection and/or vaccination, including against evolving SARS-CoV-2 variants. These data, along with understanding of breakthroughs and risk factors, will inform recommendations on additional vaccines. Therapeutics will continue to advance, and additional agents are likely to be approved, both for early treatment of outpatients and for hospitalized patients. The therapeutics field will also likely continue to be refined, with better understanding of which agents in which combination should be used in each specific population affording a more tailored precision medicine approach. There will be better understanding of the long-term effects of SARS-CoV-2 infection, including complications, and how to best treat post-COVID conditions, MIS-C, and MIS-A. While this chapter attempts to document current understanding of the field and highlights some common themes, it will need to be supplemented with contemporaneous data and guidelines to ensure that researchers and clinicians are aware of current best practices to optimize clinical management of this evolving viral disease. Clinicians should refer to updated evidence-based guidelines such as from the NIH COVID-19 Treatment Guidelines Panel for the latest recommendations on clinical management of patients with COVID-19.[483]

ADDENDUM, APRIL 2022

Given the rapidly changing COVID-19 pandemic, continued unpredictable evolution of SARS-CoV-2, and rapid advancement of science and product development in response to the pandemic, this addendum was added as close to publishing as possible. By necessity, it is abbreviated but conveys the latest developments as well as sources of additional information.

Epidemiology

A comprehensive analysis estimated that 3.39 billion people, or 43% of the global population, had been infected with SARS-CoV-2 as of mid-November 2021, up to the beginning of circulation of the Omicron variant.[162a] The Omicron variant caused a higher incidence of SARS-CoV-2 infections and COVID-19 cases per period of time, but less severe overall disease compared to other variants to date.[312a,428a] The Omicron variant was associated with a shorter incubation period (median 3 days) compared with the Delta variant (median 4 days).[87a,254a] The risks of hospitalization, critical illness, and death in infected adults with the Omicron variant were substantially lower compared to the Delta variant,[490a,651a] but hospitalization rates in children aged <5 years were much higher.[651a] Sera from patients previously infected with SARS-CoV-2 (6 to 12 months prior) had low or no neutralizing activity against the Omicron variant,[526a] and sera from those given the mRNA-1273 vaccine showed a 6.3 times lower peak titers for the Omicron variant compared to D164G.[504a] Epidemiological data suggest that the Omicron variant is associated with an increase in reinfection compared with prior variants, and a higher frequency of asymptomatic infections has been reported.[236a]

COVID-19 Vaccines

The FDA authorized Pfizer-BioNTech COVID-19 vaccine and Moderna COVID-19 vaccine as a single booster dose for persons aged ≥18 years after completing a primary series with a different vaccine (based on data discussed earlier in the chapter). The FDA fully approved the two-dose Moderna COVID-19 vaccine (Spikevax) for the primary prevention of COVID-19 in persons aged ≥18 years.[9h] The FDA extended the prior approval of the two-dose Pfizer-BioNTech COVID-19 vaccine to children aged ≥5 years, as a third primary series dose for immunocompromised persons aged ≥5 years, and as a booster dose for persons aged ≥12 years at least 5 months after completing a primary vaccine series. The ACIP recommended preferential use of mRNA COVID-19 vaccines over Johnson & Johnson COVID-19 vaccine due to increased risk of thrombosis with thrombocytopenia syndrome (TTS).[119a]

Vaccine effectiveness (VE) against SARS-CoV-2 infection and symptomatic illness declines over time for two doses, and the VE is largely restored after three doses.[211a,221a,661a] Protection against severe disease remains high without the booster.[210a] VE against hospitalization for COVID-19 mRNA vaccines was 85% for two doses against the Alpha and Delta variants, 94% for three doses against Delta variant, 65% for two doses against Omicron variant, and 86% for three doses against Omicron variant.[374a] During March 2021-January 2022, VE for COVID-19 mRNA vaccines against invasive mechanical ventilation or in-hospital death in adults was 90% and was higher for three doses (94%) than two doses (88%).[655a] Among children aged 12 to 18 years, effectiveness of a two-dose BNT162B2 mRNA vaccine against hospitalization was 92% to 93% up to 44 weeks after vaccination when Delta variant predominated but was 40% a median of 23 weeks after vaccination when Omicron variant predominated.[533a] However, VE was 79% against critical illness during the Omicron variant period.[533a] A second booster dose of BNT162B2 mRNA vaccine in persons aged ≥60 years had higher protection against severe COVID-19 than a single booster dose in Israel during the Omicron period.[54a] Given these data, the FDA also authorized a second booster dose with either Pfizer-BioNTech or the Moderna COVID-19 vaccines at least 4 months after an initial booster dose for persons aged ≥50 years and for people aged ≥12 years with immunocompromising conditions.[9c]

For the latest COVID-19 vaccine emergency use instructions, see: https://www.cdc.gov/vaccines/covid-19/eui/index.html. For the latest COVID-19 vaccine recommendations, see: https://www.cdc.gov/vaccines/covid-19/clinical-considerations/covid-19-vaccines-us.html.

Therapeutics

Treatment of nonhospitalized patients at high risk for severe COVID-19 with remdesivir (intravenously daily for 3 days) within 7 days of symptom onset was associated with a 87% lower risk of hospitalization or death as compared to placebo.[250a] Based on these data, the FDA approved IV remdesivir for treatment of nonhospitalized adults and children aged ≥12 years weighing ≥40 kg with mild-to-moderate COVID-19 and authorized IV remdesivir for children aged <12 years weighing ≥3.5 kg within 7 days of symptom onset.[9g] FDA authorized oral nirmatrelvir–ritonavir (twice daily for 5 days) for treatment of nonhospitalized patients aged ≥12 years and weighing ≥40 kg at high risk for severe disease within 5 days of symptom onset[9b] based on an randomized trial that showed nirmatrelvir–ritonavir reduced risk of hospitalization or death by 89% versus placebo in high-risk adult outpatients.[274a] The FDA also authorized oral molnupiravir (twice daily for 5 days) for treatment of nonhospitalized patients aged ≥18 years with mild-to-moderate COVID-19 and high risk of disease progression within 5 days of symptom onset,[9a] based on a trial that reported treatment with molnupiravir-reduced hospitalization or death by 30% compared to placebo in high-risk outpatients.[319a] Molnupiravir is not recommended in children, pregnant, or lactating persons.

The FDA authorized the long-acting anti-SARS-CoV-2 monoclonal antibodies tixagevimab–cilgavimab for preexposure prophylaxis of persons aged ≥12 years weighing at least 40 kg with moderate to severe immunocompromise who are not expected to respond to COVID-19 vaccination.[9d] Tixagevimab–cilgavimab has a half-life of approximately 85 days making it a good option for those who may need prophylaxis for a prolonged period of time. The FDA authorization was updated to recommend an additional dose in prior recipients and a higher dose in persons not previously administered tixagevimab–cilgavimab due to reduced activity against circulating Omicron subvariants.[9f] The FDA also authorized bebtelovimab as another monoclonal antibody for the treatment of mild-to-moderate COVID-19 in adults and pediatric patients (12 years of age and older weighing at least 40 kg) with SARS-CoV-2 who are at high risk for progressing to severe COVID-19.[9e] Bebtelovimab is notable for retaining activity against the Omicron variant and subvariants.

With the emergence of SARS-CoV-2 variants and subvariants with reduced susceptibility to some anti-SARS-CoV-2 monoclonal antibodies, the FDA also limited authorization of some products for treatment or postprophylaxis (i.e., bamlanivimab–etesevimab, casirivimab–imdevimab, and sotrovimab). For the latest information on authorized anti-SARS-CoV-2 monoclonal antibodies, see: https://www.fda.gov/emergency-preparedness-and-response/mcm-legal-regulatory-and-policy-framework/emergency-use-authorization#coviddrugs. For the latest treatment recommendations for COVID-19 patients, see: https://www.covid19treatmentguidelines.nih.gov/management/clinical-management/.

REFERENCES

1. Abou-Ismail MY, Diamond A, Kapoor S, et al. The hypercoagulable state in COVID-19: incidence, pathophysiology, and management. *Thromb Res* 2020;194:101–115. doi: 10.1016/j.thromres.2020.06.029.
2. Abrams JY, Oster ME, Godfred-Cato SE, et al. Factors linked to severe outcomes in multisystem inflammatory syndrome in children (MIS-C) in the USA: a retrospective surveillance study. *Lancet Child Adolesc Health* 2021;5(5):323–331. doi: 10.1016/s2352-4642(21)00050-x.
3. Abu-Raddad LJ, Chemaitelly H, Ayoub HH, et al. Association of prior SARS-CoV-2 infection with risk of breakthrough infection following mRNA vaccination in Qatar. *JAMA* 2021;326(19):1930–1939. doi: 10.1001/jama.2021.19623.
4. Abu-Raddad LJ, Chemaitelly H, Bertollini R. Severity of SARS-CoV-2 reinfections as compared with primary infections. *N Engl J Med* 2021;385(26):2487–2489. doi: 10.1056/NEJMc2108120.
5. Abu-Raddad LJ, Chemaitelly H, Coyle P, et al. SARS-CoV-2 antibody-positivity protects against reinfection for at least seven months with 95% efficacy. *EClinicalMedicine* 2021;35:100861. doi: 10.1016/j.eclinm.2021.100861.
6. ACTIV-3/TICO Bamlanivimab Study Group, Lundgren JD, Grund B, et al. Clinical and virological response to a neutralizing monoclonal antibody for hospitalized patients with COVID-19. *medRxiv* 2021:2021.07.19.21260559. doi: 10.1101/2021.07.19.21260559.
7. Acosta AM, Garg S, Pham H, et al. Racial and ethnic disparities in rates of COVID-19-associated hospitalization, intensive care unit admission, and in-hospital death in the United States From March 2020 to February 2021. *JAMA Netw Open* 2021;4(10):e2130479. doi: 10.1001/jamanetworkopen.2021.30479.
8. Ader F, Peiffer-Smadja N, Poissy J, et al. An open-label randomized controlled trial of the effect of lopinavir/ritonavir, lopinavir/ritonavir plus IFN-β-1a and hydroxychloroquine in hospitalized patients with COVID-19. *Clin Microbiol Infect* 2021;27(12):1826–1837. doi: 10.1016/j.cmi.2021.05.020.
9. Adler H, Ball R, Fisher M, et al. Low rate of bacterial co-infection in patients with COVID-19. *Lancet Microbe* 2020;1(2):e62. doi: 10.1016/s2666-5247(20)30036-7

9a. Administration USFDA. Coronavirus (COVID-19) Update: FDA Authorizes Additional Oral Antiviral for Treatment of COVID-19 in Certain Adults. https://www.fda.gov/news-events/press-announcements/coronavirus-covid-19-update-fda-authorizes-additional-oral-antiviral-treatment-covid-19-certain

9b. Administration USFDA. Coronavirus (COVID-19) Update: FDA Authorizes First Oral Antiviral for Treatment of COVID-19. https://www.fda.gov/news-events/press-announcements/coronavirus-covid-19-update-fda-authorizes-first-oral-antiviral-treatment-covid-19

9c. Administration USFDA. Coronavirus (COVID-19) Update: FDA Authorizes Second Booster Dose of Two COVID-19 Vaccines for Older and Immunocompromised Individuals. https://www.fda.gov/news-events/press-announcements/coronavirus-covid-19-update-fda-authorizes-second-booster-dose-two-covid-19-vaccines-older-and

9d. Administration USFDA. Coronavirus (COVID-19) Update: FDA Authorizes New Long-Acting Monoclonal Antibodies for Pre-exposure Prevention of COVID-19 in Certain Individuals. https://www.fda.gov/news-events/press-announcements/coronavirus-covid-19-update-fda-authorizes-new-long-acting-monoclonal-antibodies-pre-exposure

9e. Administration USFDA. Coronavirus (COVID-19) Update: FDA Authorizes New Monoclonal Antibody for Treatment of COVID-19 that Retains Activity Against Omicron Variant. https://www.fda.gov/news-events/press-announcements/coronavirus-covid-19-update-fda-authorizes-new-monoclonal-antibody-treatment-covid-19-retains

9f. Administration USFDA. FDA authorizes revisions to Evusheld dosing. https://www.fda.gov/drugs/drug-safety-and-availability/fda-authorizes-revisions-evusheld-dosing

9g. Administration USFDA. FDA Takes Actions to Expand Use of Treatment for Outpatients with Mild-to-Moderate COVID-19. https://www.fda.gov/news-events/press-announcements/fda-takes-actions-expand-use-treatment-outpatients-mild-moderate-covid-19

9h. Administration USFDA. Spikevax and Moderna COVID-19 Vaccine. https://www.fda.gov/emergency-preparedness-and-response/coronavirus-disease-2019-covid-19/spikevax-and-moderna-covid-19-vaccine

10. Agarwal A, Mukherjee A, Kumar G, et al. Convalescent plasma in the management of moderate covid-19 in adults in India: open label phase II multicentre randomised controlled trial (PLACID Trial). *BMJ* 2020;371:m3939. doi: 10.1136/bmj.m3939.
11. Ahmad I, Rathore FA. Guillain-Barré syndrome in COVID-19: a scoping review. *medRxiv* 2020:2020.06.13.20130062. doi: 10.1101/2020.06.13.20130062.
12. Aiyegbusi OL, Hughes SE, Turner G, et al. Symptoms, complications and management of long COVID: a review. *J R Soc Med* 2021;114(9):428–442. doi: 10.1177/01410768211032850.
13. Akagi EF, Sharma M, Johnson LB, et al. Clinical features and risk factors for community-onset bloodstream infections among coronavirus disease 2019 (COVID-19) patients. *Infect Control Hosp Epidemiol* 2021;42(7):899–901. doi: 10.1017/ice.2021.88.
14. Al-Aly Z, Xie Y, Bowe B. High-dimensional characterization of post-acute sequelae of COVID-19. *Nature* 2021;594(7862):259–264. doi: 10.1038/s41586-021-03553-9.
15. Alansari K, Toaimah FH, Almatar DH, et al. Monoclonal antibody treatment of RSV bronchiolitis in young infants: a randomized trial. *Pediatrics* 2019;143(3):e20182308. doi: 10.1542/peds.2018-2308.
16. Aleissa MM, Silverman EA, Paredes Acosta LM, et al. New perspectives on antimicrobial agents: remdesivir treatment for COVID-19. *Antimicrob Agents Chemother* 2020;65(1):e01814-20. doi: 10.1128/AAC.01814-20.
17. Alene M, Yismaw L, Assemie MA, et al. Serial interval and incubation period of COVID-19: a systematic review and meta-analysis. *BMC Infect Dis* 2021;21(1):257. doi: 10.1186/s12879-021-05950-x.
18. Ali RMM, Ghonimy MBI. Radiological findings spectrum of asymptomatic coronavirus (COVID-19) patients. *Egypt J Radiol Nucl Med* 2020;51(1):156. doi: 10.1186/s43055-020-00266-3.
19. Ali ST, Yeung A, Shan S, et al. Serial intervals and case isolation delays for COVID-19: a systematic review and meta-analysis. *Clin Infect Dis* 2021;ciab491. doi: 10.1093/cid/ciab491.
20. Alkhatip A, Kamel MG, Hamza MK, et al. The diagnostic and prognostic role of neutrophil-to-lymphocyte ratio in COVID-19: a systematic review and meta-analysis. *Expert Rev Mol Diagn* 2021;21(5):505–514. doi: 10.1080/14737159.2021.1915773.
21. Allotey J, Stallings E, Bonet M, et al. Clinical manifestations, risk factors, and maternal and perinatal outcomes of coronavirus disease 2019 in pregnancy: living systematic review and meta-analysis. *BMJ* 2020;370:m3320. doi: 10.1136/bmj.m3320.
22. Alteri C, Cento V, Vecchi M, et al. Nasopharyngeal SARS-CoV-2 load at hospital admission as predictor of mortality. *Clin Infect Dis* 2021;72(10):1868–1869. doi: 10.1093/cid/ciaa956.
23. Alvares PA. SARS-CoV-2 and respiratory syncytial virus coinfection in hospitalized pediatric patients. *Pediatr Infect Dis J* 2021;40(4):e164–e166. doi: 10.1097/inf.0000000000003057.
24. Amdal CD, Pe M, Falk RS, et al. Health-related quality of life issues, including symptoms, in patients with active COVID-19 or post COVID-19; a systematic literature review. *Qual Life Res* 2021:1–15. doi: 10.1007/s11136-021-02908-z.
25. American Society of Hematology. Thrombosis with Thrombocytopenia Syndrome (also termed Vaccine-induced Immune Thrombotic Thrombocytopenia). https://www.hematology.org/covid-19/vaccine-induced-immune-thrombotic-thrombocytopenia#:~:text=1%20If%20TTS%20is%20suspected%2C%20perform%20immediate%20CBC,prior%20to%20any%20therapies%207%20Fibrinogen%20and%20D-dimer. Accessed October 30, 2021.
26. Anderson MR, Geleris J, Anderson DR, et al. Body mass index and risk for intubation or death in SARS-CoV-2 infection: a retrospective cohort study. *Ann Intern Med* 2020;173(10):782–790. doi: 10.7326/m20-3214.
27. Andersson MI, Arancibia-Carcamo CV, Auckland K, et al. SARS-CoV-2 RNA detected in blood products from patients with COVID-19 is not associated with infectious virus. *Wellcome Open Res* 2020;5:181. doi: 10.12688/wellcomeopenres.16002.2.
28. Andrejko K, Pry J, Myers JF, et al. Early evidence of COVID-19 vaccine effectiveness within the general population of California. *medRxiv* 2021:2021.04.08.21255135. doi: 10.1101/2021.04.08.21255135.
29. Anesi GL, Jablonski J, Harhay MO, et al. Characteristics, outcomes, and trends of patients with COVID-19-related critical illness at a learning health system in the United States. *Ann Intern Med* 2021;174(5):613–621. doi: 10.7326/m20-5327.
30. Angel Y, Spitzer A, Henig O, et al. Association between vaccination with BNT162b2 and incidence of symptomatic and asymptomatic SARS-CoV-2 infections among health care workers. *JAMA* 2021;325(24):2457–2465. doi: 10.1001/jama.2021.7152.
31. Antonio-Villa NE, Fernandez-Chirino L, Pisanty-Alatorre J, et al. Comprehensive evaluation of the impact of sociodemographic inequalities on adverse outcomes and excess mortality during the COVID-19 pandemic in Mexico City. *Clin Infect Dis* 2021:ciab577. doi: 10.1093/cid/ciab577.
32. Antoon JW, Grijalva CG, Thurm C, et al. Factors associated with COVID-19 disease severity in US children and adolescents. *J Hosp Med* 2021;16(10):603–610. doi: 10.12788/jhm.3689.
33. Araújo NM, Ferreira LC, Dantas DP, et al. First report of SARS-CoV-2 detection in cerebrospinal fluid in a child with Guillain-Barré syndrome. *Pediatr Infect Dis J* 2021;40(7):e274–e276. doi: 10.1097/inf.0000000000003146.
34. Argyropoulos KV, Serrano A, Hu J, et al. Association of initial viral load in severe acute respiratory syndrome coronavirus 2 (SARS-CoV-2) patients with outcome and symptoms. *Am J Pathol* 2020;190(9):1881–1887. doi: 10.1016/j.ajpath.2020.07.001.
35. Arons MM, Hatfield KM, Reddy SC, et al. Presymptomatic SARS-CoV-2 infections and transmission in a skilled nursing facility. *N Engl J Med* 2020;382(22):2081–2090. doi: 10.1056/NEJMoa2008457.
36. Asch DA, Islam MN, Sheils NE, et al. Patient and hospital factors associated with differences in mortality rates among black and white US medicare beneficiaries hospitalized with COVID-19 infection. *JAMA Netw Open* 2021;4(6):e2112842. doi: 10.1001/jamanetworkopen.2021.12842.
37. Asch DA, Sheils NE, Islam MN, et al. Variation in US hospital mortality rates for patients admitted with COVID-19 during the first 6 months of the pandemic. *JAMA Intern Med* 2021;181(4):471–478. doi: 10.1001/jamainternmed.2020.8193.
38. Ascierto PA, Fu B, Wei H. IL-6 modulation for COVID-19: the right patients at the right time? *J Immunother Cancer* 2021;9(4):e002285. doi: 10.1136/jitc-2020-002285.
39. Aslam S, Adler E, Mekeel K, et al. Clinical effectiveness of COVID-19 vaccination in solid organ transplant recipients. *Transpl Infect Dis* 2021;23(5):e13705. doi: 10.1111/tid.13705.
40. Aslan MM, Uslu Yuvacı H, Köse O, et al. SARS-CoV-2 is not present in the vaginal fluid of pregnant women with COVID-19. *J Matern Fetal Neonatal Med* 2020:1–3. doi: 10.1080/14767058.2020.1793318.
41. Atmar RL, Lyke KE, Deming ME, et al. Heterologous SARS-CoV-2 booster vaccinations—preliminary report. *medRxiv* 2021:2021.10.10.21264827. doi: 10.1101/2021.10.10.21264827.
42. Avanzato VA, Matson MJ, Seifert SN, et al. Case study: prolonged infectious SARS-CoV-2 Shedding from an asymptomatic immunocompromised individual with cancer. *Cell* 2020;183(7):1901–1912.e9. doi: 10.1016/j.cell.2020.10.049.
43. Axfors C, Schmitt AM, Janiaud P, et al. Mortality outcomes with hydroxychloroquine and chloroquine in COVID-19 from an international collaborative meta-analysis of randomized trials. *Nat Commun* 2021;12(1):2349. doi: 10.1038/s41467-021-22446-z.

44. Aydillo T, Gonzalez-Reiche AS, Aslam S, et al. Shedding of viable SARS-CoV-2 after immunosuppressive therapy for cancer. *N Engl J Med* 2020;383(26):2586–2588. doi: 10.1056/NEJMc2031670.

45. Azar KMJ, Shen Z, Romanelli RJ, et al. Disparities in outcomes among COVID-19 patients in a large health care system in California. *Health Aff (Millwood)* 2020;39(7):1253–1262. doi: 10.1377/hlthaff.2020.00598.

46. Baang JH, Smith C, Mirabelli C, et al. Prolonged severe acute respiratory syndrome coronavirus 2 replication in an immunocompromised patient. *J Infect Dis* 2021;223(1):23–27. doi: 10.1093/infdis/jiaa666.

47. Baden LR, El Sahly HM, Essink B, et al. Efficacy and safety of the mRNA-1273 SARS-CoV-2 vaccine. *N Engl J Med* 2021;384(5):403–416. doi: 10.1056/NEJMoa2035389.

48. Bae S, Kim H, Jung TY, et al. Epidemiological characteristics of COVID-19 outbreak at fitness centers in Cheonan, Korea. *J Korean Med Sci* 2020;35(31):e288. doi: 10.3346/jkms.2020.35.e288.

49. Bager P, Wohlfahrt J, Fonager J, et al. Risk of hospitalisation associated with infection with SARS-CoV-2 lineage B.1.1.7 in Denmark: an observational cohort study. *Lancet Infect Dis* 2021;21(11):1507–1517. doi: 10.1016/s1473-3099(21)00290-5.

50. Bajema KL, Dahl RM, Prill MM, et al. Effectiveness of COVID-19 mRNA vaccines against COVID-19-associated hospitalization—Five Veterans Affairs Medical Centers, United States, February 1-August 6, 2021. *MMWR Morb Mortal Wkly Rep* 2021;70(37):1294–1299. doi: 10.15585/mmwr.mm7037e3.

51. Baldini T, Asioli GM, Romoli M, et al. Cerebral venous thrombosis and severe acute respiratory syndrome coronavirus-2 infection: a systematic review and meta-analysis. *Eur J Neurol* 2021;28(10):3478–3490. doi: 10.1111/ene.14727.

52. Banerjee J, Canamar CP, Voyageur C, et al. Mortality and readmission rates among patients with COVID-19 after discharge from acute care setting with supplemental oxygen. *JAMA Netw Open* 2021;4(4):e213990. doi: 10.1001/jamanetworkopen.2021.3990.

53. Bao C, Liu X, Zhang H, et al. Coronavirus disease 2019 (COVID-19) CT findings: a systematic review and meta-analysis. *J Am Coll Radiol* 2020;17(6):701–709. doi: 10.1016/j.jacr.2020.03.006.

54. Bar-On YM, Goldberg Y, Mandel M, et al. Protection of BNT162b2 Vaccine Booster against Covid-19 in Israel. *N Engl J Med* 2021;385(15):1393–1400. doi: 10.1056/NEJMoa2114255.

54a. Bar-On YM, Goldberg Y, Mandel M, et al. Protection by a fourth dose of BNT162b2 against Omicron in Israel. *N Engl J Med* 2022. doi: 10.1056/NEJMoa2201570.

55. Bastos ML, Perlman-Arrow S, Menzies D, et al. The sensitivity and costs of testing for SARS-CoV-2 infection with saliva versus nasopharyngeal swabs: a systematic review and meta-analysis. *Ann Intern Med* 2021;174(4):501–510. doi: 10.7326/m20-6569.

56. Bauerl C, Randazzo W, Sanchez G, et al. SARS-CoV-2 RNA and antibody detection in breast milk from a prospective multicentre study in Spain. *Arch Dis Child Fetal Neonatal Ed* 2021:fetalneonatal-2021-322463. doi: 10.1136/archdischild-2021-322463.

57. Becker JH, Lin JJ, Doernberg M, et al. Assessment of Cognitive Function in Patients After COVID-19 Infection. *JAMA Netw Open* 2021;4(10):e2130645. doi: 10.1001/jamanetworkopen.2021.30645.

58. Beigel JH. Polyclonal and monoclonal antibodies for the treatment of influenza. *Curr Opin Infect Dis* 2018;31(6):527–534. doi: 10.1097/qco.0000000000000499.

59. Beigel JH, Tebas P, Elie-Turenne MC, et al. Immune plasma for the treatment of severe influenza: an open-label, multicentre, phase 2 randomised study. *Lancet Respir Med* 2017;5(6):500–511. doi: 10.1016/s2213-2600(17)30174-1.

60. Beigel JH, Tomashek KM, Dodd LE, et al. Remdesivir for the treatment of Covid-19 - final report. *N Engl J Med* 2020;383(19):1813–1826. doi: 10.1056/NEJMoa2007764.

61. Bennett TD, Moffitt RA, Hajagos JG, et al. Clinical Characterization and Prediction of Clinical Severity of SARS-CoV-2 Infection Among US Adults Using Data From the US National COVID Cohort Collaborative. *JAMA Netw Open* 2021;4(7):e2116901. doi: 10.1001/jamanetworkopen.2021.16901.

62. Benotmane I, Risch S, Doderer-Lang C, et al. Long-term shedding of viable SARS-CoV-2 in kidney transplant recipients with COVID-19. *Am J Transplant* 2021;21(8):2871–2875. doi: 10.1111/ajt.16636.

63. Benou S, Ladhani S, Dimitriou G, et al. Atypical manifestations of severe acute respiratory syndrome coronavirus 2 infection in children: a systematic review. *Curr Pediatr Rev* 2021;17(3):162–171. doi: 10.2174/1573396317666210406153302.

64. Ben-Shmuel A, Brosh-Nissimov T, Glinert I, et al. Detection and infectivity potential of severe acute respiratory syndrome coronavirus 2 (SARS-CoV-2) environmental contamination in isolation units and quarantine facilities. *Clin Microbiol Infect* 2020;26(12):1658–1662. doi: 10.1016/j.cmi.2020.09.004.

65. Bermejo-Martin JF, González-Rivera M, Almansa R, et al. Viral RNA load in plasma is associated with critical illness and a dysregulated host response in COVID-19. *Crit Care* 2020;24(1):691. doi: 10.1186/s13054-020-03398-0.

66. Bernheim A, Mei X, Huang M, et al. Chest CT findings in coronavirus disease-19 (COVID-19): relationship to duration of infection. *Radiology* 2020;295(3):200463. doi: 10.1148/radiol.2020200463.

67. Bhaskaran K, Bacon S, Evans SJ, et al. Factors associated with deaths due to COVID-19 versus other causes: population-based cohort analysis of UK primary care data and linked national death registrations within the OpenSAFELY platform. *Lancet Reg Health Eur* 2021;6:100109. doi: 10.1016/j.lanepe.2021.100109.

68. Bhaskaran K, Rentsch CT, MacKenna B, et al. HIV infection and COVID-19 death: a population-based cohort analysis of UK primary care data and linked national death registrations within the OpenSAFELY platform. *Lancet HIV* 2021;8(1):e24–e32. doi: 10.1016/s2352-3018(20)30305-2.

69. Bhuiyan MU, Stiboy E, Hassan MZ, et al. Epidemiology of COVID-19 infection in young children under five years: a systematic review and meta-analysis. *Vaccine* 2021;39(4):667–677. doi: 10.1016/j.vaccine.2020.11.078.

70. Birgand G, Peiffer-Smadja N, Fournier S, et al. Assessment of air contamination by SARS-CoV-2 in hospital settings. *JAMA Netw Open* 2020;3(12):e2033232. doi: 10.1001/jamanetworkopen.2020.33232.

71. Björk J, Inghammar M, Moghaddassi M, et al. Effectiveness of the BNT162b2 vaccine in preventing COVID-19 in the working age population – first results from a cohort study in Southern Sweden. *medRxiv* 2021:2021.04.20.21254636. doi: 10.1101/2021.04.20.21254636.

72. Bjorkman KK, Saldi TK, Lasda E, et al. Higher viral load drives infrequent SARS-CoV-2 transmission between asymptomatic residence hall roommates. *J Infect Dis* 2021;224(8):1316–1324. doi: 10.1093/infdis/jiab386.

73. Blair PW, Brown DM, Jang M, et al. The clinical course of COVID-19 in the outpatient setting: a prospective cohort study. *Open Forum Infect Dis* 2021;8(2):ofab007. doi: 10.1093/ofid/ofab007.

74. Blanco-Melo D, Nilsson-Payant BE, Liu WC, et al. Imbalanced host response to SARS-CoV-2 drives development of COVID-19. *Cell* 2020;181(5):1036–1045 e9. doi: 10.1016/j.cell.2020.04.026.

75. Blomberg B, Mohn KG, Brokstad KA, et al. Long COVID in a prospective cohort of home-isolated patients. *Nat Med* 2021;27(9):1607–1613. doi: 10.1038/s41591-021-01433-3.

76. Blonz G, Kouatchet A, Chudeau N, et al. Epidemiology and microbiology of ventilator-associated pneumonia in COVID-19 patients: a multicenter retrospective study in 188 patients in an un-inundated French region. *Crit Care* 2021;25(1):72. doi: 10.1186/s13054-021-03493-w.

77. Boehmer TK, Kompaniyets L, Lavery AM, et al. Association between COVID-19 and myocarditis using hospital-based administrative data—United States, March 2020-January 2021. *MMWR Morb Mortal Wkly Rep* 2021;70(35):1228–1232. doi: 10.15585/mmwr.mm7035e5.

78. Boffetta P, Violante F, Durando P, et al. Determinants of SARS-CoV-2 infection in Italian healthcare workers: a multicenter study. *Sci Rep* 2021;11(1):5788. doi: 10.1038/s41598-021-85215-4.

79. Bohn MK, Hall A, Sepiashvili L, et al. Pathophysiology of COVID-19: mechanisms underlying disease severity and progression. *Physiology (Bethesda)* 2020;35(5):288–301. doi: 10.1152/physiol.00019.2020.

80. Booth CM, Matukas LM, Tomlinson GA, et al. Clinical features and short-term outcomes of 144 patients with SARS in the greater Toronto area. *JAMA* 2003;289(21):2801–2809. doi: 10.1001/jama.289.21.JOC30885.

81. Borczuk AC, Salvatore SP, Seshan SV, et al. COVID-19 pulmonary pathology: a multi-institutional autopsy cohort from Italy and New York City. *Mod Pathol* 2020;33(11):2156–2168. doi: 10.1038/s41379-020-00661-1.

82. Bosaeed M, Mahmoud E, Alharbi A, et al. Favipiravir and hydroxychloroquine combination therapy in patients with moderate to severe COVID-19 (FACCT Trial): an open-label, multicenter, randomized, controlled trial. *Infect Dis Ther* 2021;10(4):2291–2307. doi: 10.1007/s40121-021-00496-6.

83. Bosco-Lauth AM, Hartwig AE, Porter SM, et al. Experimental infection of domestic dogs and cats with SARS-CoV-2: pathogenesis, transmission, and response to reexposure in cats. *Proc Natl Acad Sci U S A* 2020;117(42):26382–26388. doi: 10.1073/pnas.2013102117.

84. Boscolo-Rizzo P, Guida F, Polesel J, et al. Self-reported smell and taste recovery in coronavirus disease 2019 patients: a one-year prospective study. *Eur Arch Otorhinolaryngol* 2021:1–6. doi: 10.1007/s00405-021-06839-w.

85. Boulware DR, Pullen MF, Bangdiwala AS, et al. A randomized trial of hydroxychloroquine as postexposure prophylaxis for Covid-19. *N Engl J Med* 2020;383(6):517–525. doi: 10.1056/NEJMoa2016638.

86. Boyapati A, Wipperman MF, Ehmann PJ, et al. Baseline SARS-CoV-2 viral load is associated with COVID-19 disease severity and clinical outcomes: post-hoc analyses of a phase 2/3 trial. *J Infect Dis* 2021;224(11):1830–1838. doi: 10.1093/infdis/jiab445.

87. Bradley BT, Maioli H, Johnston R, et al. Histopathology and ultrastructural findings of fatal COVID-19 infections in Washington State: a case series. *Lancet* 2020;396(10247):320–332. doi: 10.1016/s0140-6736(20)31305-2.

87a. Brandal LT, MacDonald E, Veneti L, et al. Outbreak caused by the SARS-CoV-2 Omicron variant in Norway, November to December 2021. *Eurosurveillance* 2021;26(50):2101147. doi: doi:https://doi.org/10.2807/1560-7917.ES.2021.26.50.2101147.

88. Braun J, Loyal L, Frentsch M, et al. SARS-CoV-2-reactive T cells in healthy donors and patients with COVID-19. *Nature* 2020;587(7833):270–274. doi: 10.1038/s41586-020-2598-9.

89. Brown CM, Vostok J, Johnson H, et al. Outbreak of SARS-CoV-2 infections, including COVID-19 vaccine breakthrough infections, associated with large public gatherings—Barnstable County, Massachusetts, July 2021. *MMWR Morb Mortal Wkly Rep* 2021;70(31):1059–1062. doi: 10.15585/mmwr.mm7031e2.

90. Bryce C, Grimes Z, Pujadas E, et al. Pathophysiology of SARS-CoV-2: targeting of endothelial cells renders a complex disease with thrombotic microangiopathy and aberrant immune response. The Mount Sinai COVID-19 autopsy experience. *medRxiv* 2020:2020.05.18.20099960. doi: 10.1101/2020.05.18.20099960.

91. Buetti N, Wicky PH, Le Hingrat Q, et al. SARS-CoV-2 detection in the lower respiratory tract of invasively ventilated ARDS patients. *Crit Care* 2020;24(1):610. doi: 10.1186/s13054-020-03323-5.

92. Buitrago-Garcia D, Egli-Gany D, Counotte MJ, et al. Occurrence and transmission potential of asymptomatic and presymptomatic SARS-CoV-2 infections: a living systematic review and meta-analysis. *PLoS Med* 2020;17(9):e1003346. doi: 10.1371/journal.pmed.1003346.

93. Bullard J, Dust K, Funk D, et al. Predicting infectious severe acute respiratory syndrome coronavirus 2 from diagnostic samples. *Clin Infect Dis* 2020;71(10):2663–2666. doi: 10.1093/cid/ciaa638.

94. Bullock HA, Goldsmith CS, Zaki SR, et al. Difficulties in differentiating coronaviruses from subcellular structures in human tissues by electron microscopy. *Emerg Infect Dis* 2021;27(4):1023–1031. doi: 10.3201/eid2704.204337.

95. Buonsenso D, Munblit D, De Rose C, et al. Preliminary evidence on long COVID in children. *Acta Paediatr* 2021;110(7):2208–2211. doi: 10.1111/apa.15870.

96. Burrel S, Hausfater P, Dres M, et al. Co-infection of SARS-CoV-2 with other respiratory viruses and performance of lower respiratory tract samples for the diagnosis of COVID-19. *Int J Infect Dis* 2021;102:10–13. doi: 10.1016/j.ijid.2020.10.040.

97. Butler-Laporte G, Lawandi A, Schiller I, et al. Comparison of saliva and nasopharyngeal swab nucleic acid amplification testing for detection of SARS-CoV-2: a systematic review and meta-analysis. *JAMA Intern Med* 2021;181(3):353–360. doi: 10.1001/jamainternmed.2020.8876.

98. Bwire GM, Majigo MV, Njiro BJ, et al. Detection profile of SARS-CoV-2 using RT-PCR in different types of clinical specimens: a systematic review and meta-analysis. *J Med Virol* 2021;93(2):719–725. doi: 10.1002/jmv.26349.
99. Byambasuren Oea. Estimating the extent of true asymptomatic COVID-19 and its potential for community transmission: systematic review and meta-analysis. *J Assoc Med Microbiol Infect Dis Canada* 2020;5.
100. Cabrera Martimbianco AL, Pacheco RL, Bagattini ÂM, et al. Frequency, signs and symptoms, and criteria adopted for long COVID-19: a systematic review. *Int J Clin Pract* 2021;75(10):e14357. doi: 10.1111/ijcp.14357.
101. Caccuri F, Zani A, Messali S, et al. A persistently replicating SARS-CoV-2 variant derived from an asymptomatic individual. *J Transl Med* 2020;18(1):362. doi: 10.1186/s12967-020-02535-1.
102. Cai Y, Zhang J, Xiao T, et al. Distinct conformational states of SARS-CoV-2 spike protein. *Science* 2020;369(6511):1586–1592. doi: 10.1126/science.abd4251.
103. Calabrese F, Pezzuto F, Fortarezza F, et al. Pulmonary pathology and COVID-19: lessons from autopsy. The experience of European Pulmonary Pathologists. *Virchows Arch* 2020;477(3):359–372. doi: 10.1007/s00428-020-02886-6.
104. Callaway E. Heavily mutated Omicron variant puts scientists on alert. *Nature* 2021;600(7887):21. doi: 10.1038/d41586-021-03552-w.
105. Caly L, Druce J, Roberts J, et al. Isolation and rapid sharing of the 2019 novel coronavirus (SARS-CoV-2) from the first patient diagnosed with COVID-19 in Australia. *Med J Aust* 2020;212(10):459–462. doi: 10.5694/mja2.50569.
106. Camerini D, Randall AZ, Trappl-Kimmons K, et al. Mapping SARS-CoV-2 antibody epitopes in COVID-19 patients with a multi-coronavirus protein microarray. *Microbiol Spectr* 2021;9(2):e0141621. doi: 10.1128/Spectrum.01416-21.
107. Campbell F, Archer B, Laurenson-Schafer H, et al. Increased transmissibility and global spread of SARS-CoV-2 variants of concern as at June 2021. *Euro Surveill* 2021;26(24):2100509. doi: 10.2807/1560-7917.Es.2021.26.24.2100509.
108. Capone CA, Misra N, Ganigara M, et al. Six month follow-up of patients with multisystem inflammatory syndrome in children. *Pediatrics* 2021;148(4):e2021050973. doi: 10.1542/peds.2021-050973.
109. Carsana L, Sonzogni A, Nasr A, et al. Pulmonary post-mortem findings in a series of COVID-19 cases from northern Italy: a two-centre descriptive study. *Lancet Infect Dis* 2020;20(10):1135–1140. doi: 10.1016/S1473-3099(20)30434-5.
110. Castleman Disease Collaborative Network. CORONA Data Viewer. https://cdcn.org/corona-data-viewer/Accessed July 31, 2021.
111. Cavanaugh AM, Fortier S, Lewis P, et al. COVID-19 outbreak associated with a SARS-CoV-2 R.1 lineage variant in a skilled nursing facility after vaccination program - Kentucky, March 2021. *MMWR Morb Mortal Wkly Rep* 2021;70(17):639–643. doi: 10.15585/mmwr.mm7017e2.
112. Celltrion Healthcare. Celltrion announces positive top-line results from global Phase III trial of regdanvimab (CT-P59), an anti-COVID-19 monoclonal antibody treatment. Updated June 6, 2021. https://www.celltrionhealthcare.com/en-us/board/newsdetail?modify_key=498&pagenumber=1&keyword=&keyword_type=
113. Centeno-Tablante E, Medina-Rivera M, Finkelstein JL, et al. Transmission of SARS-CoV-2 through breast milk and breastfeeding: a living systematic review. *Ann N Y Acad Sci* 2021;1484(1):32–54. doi: 10.1111/nyas.14477.
114. Centers for Disease Control and Prevention. COVID-19 Vaccines and Vaccination. https://www.ncbi.nlm.nih.gov/pubmed/34009769.
115. Centers for Disease Control and Prevention. COVID-19 Vaccines for Moderately to Severely Immunocompromised People. https://www.cdc.gov/coronavirus/2019-ncov/vaccines/recommendations/immuno.html. Accessed October 30, 2021.
116. Centers for Disease Control and Prevention. Disparities in COVID-19-Associated Hospitalizations: Racial and Ethnic Health Disparities. https://www.cdc.gov/coronavirus/2019-ncov/community/health-equity/racial-ethnic-disparities/disparities-hospitalization.html. Accessed October 30, 2021.
117. Centers for Disease Control and Prevention. Health Disparities Provisional Death Counts for Coronavirus Disease 2019 (COVID-19). https://www.cdc.gov/nchs/nvss/vsrr/covid19/health_disparities.htm. Accessed June 6, 2021.
118. Centers for Disease Control and Prevention. Information for Healthcare Providers about Multisystem Inflammatory Syndrome in Children (MIS-C) Case Definition for MIS-C. Centers for Disease Control and Prevention. 2021. https://www.cdc.gov/mis-c/hcp/. Accessed June 20, 2021.
119. Centers for Disease Control and Prevention. Interim Clinical Considerations for Use of COVID-19 Vaccines Currently Approved or Authorized in the United States. Considerations involving pregnancy, lactation, and fertility. https://www.cdc.gov/vaccines/covid-19/clinical-considerations/covid-19-vaccines-us.html#pregnant. Accessed September 7, 2021.
119a. Centers for Disease Control and Prevention. Use of COVID-19 Vaccines in the United States. https://www.cdc.gov/vaccines/covid-19/clinical-considerations/covid-19-vaccines-us.html
120. Centers for Disease Control and Prevention. Interim Infection Prevention and Control Recommendations for Healthcare Personnel During the Coronavirus Disease 2019 (COVID-19) Pandemic. https://www.cdc.gov/coronavirus/2019-ncov/hcp/infection-control-recommendations.html. Accessed May 31, 2021.
121. Centers for Disease Control and Prevention. Multisystem Inflammatory Syndrome in Adults (MIS-A) – Case Definition. 2021. https://www.cdc.gov/mis-c/mis-a/hcp.html. Accessed June 20, 2021.
122. Centers for Disease Control and Prevention. Post-COVID Conditions: Information for Healthcare Providers. 2021. https://www.cdc.gov/coronavirus/2019-ncov/hcp/clinical-care/post-covid-conditions.html. Accessed July 4, 2021.
123. Centers for Disease Control and Prevention. SARS-CoV-2 Variant Classifications and Definitions. Updated July 27, 2021. https://www.cdc.gov/coronavirus/2019-ncov/variants/variant-info.html#ConcernAccessed July 31, 2021.
124. Centers for Disease Control and Prevention. Science Brief: COVID-19 Vaccines and Vaccination. Updated September 15, 2021. https://www.cdc.gov/coronavirus/2019-ncov/science/science-briefs/fully-vaccinated-people.html. Accessed October 30, 2021.
125. Centers for Disease Control and Prevention. Underlying Medical Conditions Associated with Higher Risk for Severe COVID-19: Information for Healthcare Providers. Updated October 14, 2021. Accessed October 16, 2021.
126. Cevik M, Tate M, Lloyd O, et al. SARS-CoV-2, SARS-CoV, and MERS-CoV viral load dynamics, duration of viral shedding, and infectiousness: a systematic review and meta-analysis. *Lancet Microbe* 2021;2(1):e13–e22. doi: 10.1016/s2666-5247(20)30172-5.
127. Chachkhiani D, Soliman MY, Barua D, et al. Neurological complications in a predominantly African American sample of COVID-19 predict worse outcomes during hospitalization. *Clin Neurol Neurosurg* 2020;197:106173. doi: 10.1016/j.clineuro.2020.106173.
128. Challen R, Brooks-Pollock E, Read JM, et al. Risk of mortality in patients infected with SARS-CoV-2 variant of concern 202012/1: matched cohort study. *BMJ* 2021;372:n579. doi: 10.1136/bmj.n579.
129. Chambers C, Krogstad P, Bertrand K, et al. Evaluation for SARS-CoV-2 in breast milk from 18 infected women. *JAMA* 2020;324(13):1347–1348. doi: 10.1001/jama.2020.15580.
130. Chang JC, Matsubara D, Morgan RW, et al. Skewed cytokine responses rather than the magnitude of the cytokine storm may drive cardiac dysfunction in multisystem inflammatory syndrome in children. *J Am Heart Assoc* 2021;10(16):e021428. doi: 10.1161/jaha.121.021428.
131. Chapin-Bardales J, Gee J, Myers T. Reactogenicity following receipt of mRNA-Based COVID-19 vaccines. *JAMA* 2021;325(21):2201–2202. doi: 10.1001/jama.2021.5374.
132. Chatterjee NA, Jensen PN, Harris AW, et al. Admission respiratory status predicts mortality in COVID-19. *Influenza Other Respir Viruses* 2021;15(5):569–572. doi: 10.1111/irv.12869.
133. Chau NVV, Hong NTT, Ngoc NM, et al. Superspreading event of SARS-CoV-2 infection at a bar, Ho Chi Minh City, Vietnam. *Emerg Infect Dis* 2021;27(1):310–314. doi: 10.3201/eid2701.203480.
134. Chemaitelly H, AlMukdad S, Joy JP, et al. SARS-CoV-2 vaccine effectiveness in immunosuppressed kidney transplant recipients. *medRxiv* 2021:2021.08.07.21261578. doi: 10.1101/2021.08.07.21261578.
135. Chen J, Lau YF, Lamirande EW, et al. Cellular immune responses to severe acute respiratory syndrome coronavirus (SARS-CoV) infection in senescent BALB/c mice: CD4+ T cells are important in control of SARS-CoV infection. *J Virol* 2010;84(3):1289–1301. doi: 10.1128/jvi.01281-09.
136. Chen L, Wang G, Long X, et al. Dynamics of blood viral load is strongly associated with clinical outcomes in coronavirus disease 2019 (COVID-19) patients: a prospective cohort study. *J Mol Diagn* 2021;23(1):10–18. doi: 10.1016/j.jmoldx.2020.10.007.
137. Chen N, Zhou M, Dong X, et al. Epidemiological and clinical characteristics of 99 cases of 2019 novel coronavirus pneumonia in Wuhan, China: a descriptive study. *Lancet* 2020;395(10223):507–513. doi: 10.1016/S0140-6736(20)30211-7.
138. Chen P, Nirula A, Heller B, et al. SARS-CoV-2 neutralizing antibody LY-CoV555 in outpatients with Covid-19. *N Engl J Med* 2021;384(3):229–237. doi: 10.1056/NEJMoa2029849.
139. Chen X, Zhao B, Qu Y, et al. Detectable serum severe acute respiratory syndrome coronavirus 2 viral load (RNAemia) is closely correlated with drastically elevated interleukin 6 level in critically ill patients with coronavirus disease 2019. *Clin Infect Dis* 2020;71(8):1937–1942. doi: 10.1093/cid/ciaa449.
140. Chen Y, Chen L, Deng Q, et al. The presence of SARS-CoV-2 RNA in the feces of COVID-19 patients. *J Med Virol* 2020;92(7):833–840. doi: 10.1002/jmv.25825.
141. Cheng Y, Luo R, Wang K, et al. Kidney disease is associated with in-hospital death of patients with COVID-19. *Kidney Int* 2020;97(5):829–838. doi: 10.1016/j.kint.2020.03.005.
142. Cheng Y, Wong R, Soo YO, et al. Use of convalescent plasma therapy in SARS patients in Hong Kong. *Eur J Clin Microbiol Infect Dis* 2005;24(1):44–46. doi: 10.1007/s10096-004-1271-9.
143. Cheung KS, Hung IFN, Chan PPY, et al. Gastrointestinal manifestations of SARS-CoV-2 infection and virus load in fecal samples from a Hong Kong cohort: systematic review and meta-analysis. *Gastroenterology* 2020;159(1):81–95. doi: 10.1053/j.gastro.2020.03.065.
144. Chi G, Lee JJ, Jamil A, et al. Venous thromboembolism among hospitalized patients with COVID-19 undergoing thromboprophylaxis: a systematic review and meta-analysis. *J Clin Med* 2020;9(8):2489. doi: 10.3390/jcm9082489.
145. Chia PY, Xiang Ong SW, Chiew CJ, et al. Virological and serological kinetics of SARS-CoV-2 Delta variant vaccine-breakthrough infections: a multi-center cohort study. *medRxiv* 2021:2021.07.28.21261295. doi: 10.1101/2021.07.28.21261295.
146. Chia WN, Zhu F, Ong SWX, et al. Dynamics of SARS-CoV-2 neutralising antibody responses and duration of immunity: a longitudinal study. *Lancet Microbe* 2021;2(6):e240–e249. doi: 10.1016/s2666-5247(21)00025-2.
147. Chodick G, Tene L, Rotem RS, et al. The effectiveness of the TWO-DOSE BNT162b2 vaccine: analysis of real-world data. *Clin Infect Dis* 2022;74(3):472–478. doi: 10.1093/cid/ciab438.
148. Choe PG, Kang CK, Kim KH, et al. Persistence of neutralizing antibody response up to one year after asymptomatic or symptomatic SARS-CoV-2 infection. *J Infect Dis* 2021;224(6):1097–1099. doi: 10.1093/infdis/jiab339.
149. Choi B, Choudhary MC, Regan J, et al. Persistence and evolution of SARS-CoV-2 in an immunocompromised host. *N Engl J Med* 2020;383(23):2291–2293. doi: 10.1056/NEJMc2031364.
150. Choi EM, Chu DKW, Cheng PKC, et al. In-flight transmission of SARS-CoV-2. *Emerg Infect Dis* 2020;26(11):2713–2716. doi: 10.3201/eid2611.203254.
151. Chokkalingam AP, Li H, Asubonteng J, et al. Comparative Effectiveness Of Remdesivir Treatment In Patients Hospitalized With Covid-19. Presented at: World Microbe Forum; 2021; Session CIVP103. https://www.abstractsonline.com/pp8/#!/9286/presentation/10403.
152. Chou R, Dana T, Buckley DI, et al. Epidemiology of and risk factors for coronavirus infection in health care workers: a living rapid review. *Ann Intern Med* 2020;173(2):120–136. doi: 10.7326/m20-1632.
153. Choudhary MC, Crain CR, Qiu X, et al. SARS-CoV-2 sequence characteristics of COVID-19 persistence and reinfection. *Clin Infect Dis* 2022;74(2):237–245. doi: 10.1093/cid/ciab380.
154. Choudry FA, Hamshere SM, Rathod KS, et al. High thrombus burden in patients with COVID-19 presenting with ST-segment elevation myocardial infarction. *J Am Coll Cardiol* 2020;76(10):1168–1176. doi: 10.1016/j.jacc.2020.07.022.

155. Chu DKW, Gu H, Chang LDJ, et al. SARS-CoV-2 superspread in fitness center, Hong Kong, China, March 2021. *Emerg Infect Dis* 2021;27(8):2230–2232. doi: 10.3201/eid2708.210833.

156. Chu L, Montefiori D, Huang W, et al. Immune memory response after a booster injection of mRNA-1273 for severe acute respiratory syndrome coronavirus-2 (SARS-CoV-2). *medRxiv* 2021:2021.09.29.21264089. doi: 10.1101/2021.09.29.21264089.

157. Chu VT, Yousaf AR, Chang K, et al. Household transmission of SARS-CoV-2 from children and adolescents. *N Engl J Med* 2021;385(10):954–956. doi: 10.1056/NEJMc2031915.

158. Cirks BT, Rowe SJ, Jiang SY, et al. Sixteen weeks later: expanding the risk period for multisystem inflammatory syndrome in children. *J Pediatric Infect Dis Soc* 2021;10(5):686–690. doi: 10.1093/jpids/piab007.

159. Clancy CJ, Schwartz IS, Kula B, et al. Bacterial superinfections among persons with coronavirus disease 2019: a comprehensive review of data from postmortem studies. *Open Forum Infect Dis* 2021;8(3). doi: 10.1093/ofid/ofab065.

160. Cleverley J, Piper J, Jones MM. The role of chest radiography in confirming covid-19 pneumonia. *BMJ* 2020;370:m2426. doi: 10.1136/bmj.m2426.

161. Cohen MS, Nirula A, Mulligan MJ, et al. Effect of bamlanivimab vs placebo on incidence of COVID-19 among residents and staff of skilled nursing and assisted living facilities: a randomized clinical trial. *JAMA* 2021;326(1):46–55. doi: 10.1001/jama.2021.8828.

162. Coleman KK, Tay DJW, Sen Tan K, et al. Viral load of SARS-CoV-2 in respiratory aerosols emitted by COVID-19 patients while breathing, talking, and singing. *Clin Infect Dis* 2021;ciab691. doi: 10.1093/cid/ciab691.

162a. Collaborators C-CI. Estimating global, regional, and national daily and cumulative infections with SARS-CoV-2 through Nov 14, 2021: a statistical analysis. *Lancet* 2022. doi: 10.1016/s0140-6736(22)00484-6.

163. Corchado-Garcia J, Puyraimond-Zemmour D, Hughes T, et al. Real-world effectiveness of Ad26.COV2.S adenoviral vector vaccine for COVID-19. *medRxiv* 2021:2021.04.27.21256193. doi: 10.1101/2021.04.27.21256193.

164. Corti D, Purcell LA, Snell G, et al. Tackling COVID-19 with neutralizing monoclonal antibodies. *Cell* 2021;184(12):3086–3108. doi: 10.1016/j.cell.2021.05.005.

165. Costa S, Posteraro B, Marchetti S, et al. Excretion of SARS-CoV-2 in human breast milk. *Clin Microbiol Infect* 2020;26(10):1430–1432. doi: 10.1016/j.cmi.2020.05.027.

166. Coutinho A, Riaz A, Makan A, et al. Lessons of the month: co-infection with SARS-CoV-2 and influenza B virus in a patient with community-acquired pneumonia. *Clin Med (Lond)* 2020;20(6):e262–e263. doi: 10.7861/clinmed.2020-0598.

167. COVID-ICU Group on behalf of the REVA Network and the COVID-ICU Investigators. Clinical characteristics and day-90 outcomes of 4244 critically ill adults with COVID-19: a prospective cohort study. *Intensive Care Med* 2021;47(1):60–73. doi: 10.1007/s00134-020-06294-x.

168. Cuadrado-Payán E, Montagud-Marrahi E, Torres-Elorza M, et al. SARS-CoV-2 and influenza virus co-infection. *Lancet* 2020;395(10236):e84. doi: 10.1016/s0140-6736(20)31052-7.

169. Cummings MJ, Baldwin MR, Abrams D, et al. Epidemiology, clinical course, and outcomes of critically ill adults with COVID-19 in New York City: a prospective cohort study. *Lancet* 2020;395(10239):1763–1770. doi: 10.1016/s0140-6736(20)31189-2.

170. da Silva JF, Hernandez-Romieu AC, Browning SD, et al. COVID-19 clinical phenotypes: presentation and temporal progression of disease in a cohort of hospitalized adults in Georgia, United States. *Open Forum Infect Dis* 2021;8(1):ofaa596. doi: 10.1093/ofid/ofaa596.

171. Dagan N, Barda N, Kepten E, et al. BNT162b2 mRNA Covid-19 vaccine in a nationwide mass vaccination setting. *N Engl J Med* 2021;384(15):1412–1423. doi: 10.1056/NEJMoa2101765.

172. Dai L, Gao GF. Viral targets for vaccines against COVID-19. *Nat Rev Immunol* 2021;21(2):73–82. doi: 10.1038/s41577-020-00480-0.

173. Dakay K, Cooper J, Bloomfield J, et al. Cerebral venous sinus thrombosis in COVID-19 infection: a case series and review of the literature. *J Stroke Cerebrovasc Dis* 2021;30(1):105434. doi: 10.1016/j.jstrokecerebrovasdis.2020.105434.

174. Daniels CJ, Rajpal S, Greenshields JT, et al. Prevalence of clinical and subclinical myocarditis in competitive athletes with recent SARS-CoV-2 infection: results from the big ten COVID-19 cardiac registry. *JAMA Cardiol* 2021;6(9):1078–1087.doi: 10.1001/jamacardio.2021.2065.

175. Das Adhikari U, Eng G, Farcasanu M, et al. Fecal SARS-CoV-2 RNA is associated with decreased COVID-19 survival. *Clin Infect Dis* 2021:ciab623. doi: 10.1093/cid/ciab623.

176. Davey RT, Jr., Dodd L, Proschan MA, et al. A randomized, controlled trial of ZMapp for Ebola virus infection. *N Engl J Med* 2016;375(15):1448–1456. doi: 10.1056/NEJMoa1604330.

177. Davies NG, Abbott S, Barnard RC, et al. Estimated transmissibility and impact of SARS-CoV-2 lineage B.1.1.7 in England. *Science* 2021;372(6538):eabg3055. doi: 10.1126/science.abg3055.

178. Davies NG, Jarvis CI, Edmunds WJ, et al. Increased mortality in community-tested cases of SARS-CoV-2 lineage B.1.1.7. *Nature* 2021;593(7858):270–274. doi: 10.1038/s41586-021-03426-1.

179. Davies P, du Pré P, Lillie J, et al. One-year outcomes of critical care patients post-COVID-19 multisystem inflammatory syndrome in children. *JAMA Pediatr* 2021;175(12):1281–1283. doi: 10.1001/jamapediatrics.2021.2993.

180. Davogustto GE, Clark DE, Hardison E, et al. Characteristics associated with multisystem inflammatory syndrome among adults with SARS-CoV-2 infection. *JAMA Netw Open* 2021;4(5):e2110323. doi: 10.1001/jamanetworkopen.2021.10323.

181. Dawood FS, Porucznik CA, Veguilla V, et al. Incidence rates, household infection risk, and clinical characteristics of SARS-CoV-2 infection among children and adults in Utah and New York City, New York. *JAMA Pediatr* 2021;176(1):59–67.doi: 10.1001/jamapediatrics.2021.4217.

182. De Giorgi V, Recalcati S, Jia Z, et al. Cutaneous manifestations related to coronavirus disease 2019 (COVID-19): a prospective study from China and Italy. *J Am Acad Dermatol* 2020;83(2):674–675. doi: 10.1016/j.jaad.2020.05.073.

183. De Greef J, Scohy A, Zech F, et al. Determinants of IgG antibodies kinetics after severe and critical COVID-19. *J Med Virol* 2021;93(9):5416–5424. doi: 10.1002/jmv.27059.

184. de la Calle C, Lalueza A, Mancheño-Losa M, et al. Impact of viral load at admission on the development of respiratory failure in hospitalized patients with SARS-CoV-2 infection. *Eur J Clin Microbiol Infect Dis* 2021:1–8. doi: 10.1007/s10096-020-04150-w.

185. de Wit E, Feldmann F, Cronin J, et al. Prophylactic and therapeutic remdesivir (GS-5734) treatment in the rhesus macaque model of MERS-CoV infection. *Proc Natl Acad Sci* 2020;117(12):6771–6776. doi: 10.1073/pnas.1922083117.

186. de Wit E, Rasmussen AL, Falzarano D, et al. Middle East respiratory syndrome coronavirus (MERS-CoV) causes transient lower respiratory tract infection in rhesus macaques. *Proc Natl Acad Sci U S A* 2013;110(41):16598–16603. doi: 10.1073/pnas.1310744110.

187. DeBiasi RL, Harahsheh AS, Srinivasalu H, et al. Multisystem inflammatory syndrome of children: subphenotypes, risk factors, biomarkers, cytokine profiles, and viral sequencing. *J Pediatr* 2021;237:125–135.e18. doi: 10.1016/j.jpeds.2021.06.002.

188. Decker A, Welzel M, Laubner K, et al. Prolonged SARS-CoV-2 shedding and mild course of COVID-19 in a patient after recent heart transplantation. *Am J Transplant* 2020;20(11):3239–3245. doi: 10.1111/ajt.16133.

189. Del Valle DM, Kim-Schulze S, Hsin-Hui H, et al. An inflammatory cytokine signature helps predict COVID-19 severity and death. *medRxiv* 2020:2020.05.28.20115758. doi: 10.1101/2020.05.28.20115758.

190. Delahoy MJ, Ujamaa D, Whitaker M, et al. Hospitalizations Associated with COVID-19 Among Children and Adolescents - COVID-NET, 14 States, March 1, 2020-August 14, 2021. *MMWR Morb Mortal Wkly Rep* 2021;70(36):1255–1260. doi: 10.15585/mmwr.mm7036e2.

191. Denina M, Pruccoli G, Scolfaro C, et al. Sequelae of COVID-19 in Hospitalized Children: a 4-Months Follow-Up. *Pediatr Infect Dis J* 2020;39(12):e458–e459. doi: 10.1097/inf.0000000000002937.

192. Dergham J, Delerce J, Bedotto M, et al. Isolation of viable SARS-CoV-2 virus from feces of an immunocompromised patient suggesting a possible fecal mode of transmission. *J Clin Med* 2021;10(12):2696. doi: 10.3390/jcm10122696.

193. Dionne A, Sperotto F, Chamberlain S, et al. Association of myocarditis with BNT162b2 messenger RNA COVID-19 vaccine in a case series of children. *JAMA Cardiol* 2021;6(12):1446–1450. doi: 10.1001/jamacardio.2021.3471.

194. Docherty AB, Harrison EM, Green CA, et al. Features of 20 133 UK patients in hospital with covid-19 using the ISARIC WHO Clinical Characterisation Protocol: prospective observational cohort study. *BMJ* 2020;369:m1985. doi: 10.1136/bmj.m1985.

195. Donnelly JP, Wang XQ, Iwashyna TJ, et al. Readmission and death after initial hospital discharge among patients with COVID-19 in a large multihospital system. *JAMA* 2021;325(3):304–306. doi: 10.1001/jama.2020.21465.

196. Dougan M, Nirula A, Azizad M, et al. Bamlanivimab plus etesevimab in mild or moderate Covid-19. *N Engl J Med* 2021;385(15):1382–1392. doi: 10.1056/NEJMoa2102685.

197. Drake TM, Riad AM, Fairfield CJ, et al. Characterisation of in-hospital complications associated with COVID-19 using the ISARIC WHO clinical characterisation protocol UK: a prospective, multicentre cohort study. *Lancet* 2021;398(10296):223–237. doi: 10.1016/s0140-6736(21)00799-6.

198. Duarte-Salles T, Vizcaya D, Pistillo A, et al. Thirty-day outcomes of children and adolescents with COVID-19: an international experience. *Pediatrics* 2021;148(3):e2020042929. doi: 10.1542/peds.2020-042929.

199. Dugan HL, Stamper CT, Li L, et al. Profiling B cell immunodominance after SARS-CoV-2 infection reveals antibody evolution to non-neutralizing viral targets. *Immunity* 2021;54(6):1290–1303.e7. doi: 10.1016/j.immuni.2021.05.001.

200. Dumont-Leblond N, Veillette M, Mubareka S, et al. Low incidence of airborne SARS-CoV-2 in acute care hospital rooms with optimized ventilation. *Emerg Microbes Infect* 2020;9(1):2597–2605. doi: 10.1080/22221751.2020.1850184.

201. Duncombe CJ, McCulloch DJ, Shuey KD, et al. Dynamics of breast milk antibody titer in the six months following SARS-CoV-2 infection. *J Clin Virol* 2021;142:104916. doi: 10.1016/j.jcv.2021.104916.

202. Eastman RT, Roth JS, Brimacombe KR, et al. Remdesivir: a review of its discovery and development leading to emergency use authorization for treatment of COVID-19. *ACS Cent Sci* 2020;6(5):672–683.

203. Edridge AWD, Kaczorowska J, Hoste ACR, et al. Seasonal coronavirus protective immunity is short-lasting. *Nat Med* 2020;26(11):1691–1693. doi: 10.1038/s41591-020-1083-1.

204. Edwards DA, Ausiello D, Salzman J, et al. Exhaled aerosol increases with COVID-19 infection, age, and obesity. *Proc Natl Acad Sci U S A* 2021;118(8):e2021830118. doi: 10.1073/pnas.2021830118.

205. Elias C, Sekri A, Leblanc P, et al. Incubation period of COVID-19: a meta-analysis. *Int J Infect Dis* 2021;104:708–710. doi: 10.1016/j.ijid.2021.01.069.

206. Emery JC, Russell TW, Liu Y, et al. The contribution of asymptomatic SARS-CoV-2 infections to transmission on the Diamond Princess cruise ship. *Elife* 2020;9.doi: 10.7554/eLife.58699.

207. European Medicines Agency. COVID-19 Vaccine Janssen: Guillain-Barré syndrome listed as a very rare side effect. Updated July 22, 2021. https://www.ema.europa.eu/en/news/covid-19-vaccine-janssen-guillain-barre-syndrome-listed-very-rare-side-effect. Accessed July 25, 2021.

208. Expert Taskforce for the COVID-19 Cruise Ship Outbreak. Epidemiology of COVID-19 outbreak on cruise ship quarantined at Yokohama, Japan, February 2020. *Emerg Infect Dis* 2020;26(11):2591–2597. doi: 10.3201/eid2611.201165.

209. Fabiani M, Ramigni M, Gobbetto V, et al. Effectiveness of the Comirnaty (BNT162b2, BioNTech/Pfizer) vaccine in preventing SARS-CoV-2 infection among healthcare workers, Treviso province, Veneto region, Italy, 27 December 2020 to 24 March 2021. *Euro Surveill* 2021;26(17):2100420. doi: 10.2807/1560-7917.ES.2021.26.17.2100420.

210. Fajnzylber J, Regan J, Coxen K, et al. SARS-CoV-2 viral load is associated with increased disease severity and mortality. *Nat Commun* 2020;11(1):5493. doi: 10.1038/s41467-020-19057-5.

210a. Feikin DR, Higdon MM, Abu-Raddad LJ, et al. Duration of effectiveness of vaccines against SARS-CoV-2 infection and COVID-19 disease: results of a systematic review and meta-regression. *Lancet* 2022;399(10328):924–944. doi: 10.1016/s0140-6736(22)00152-0.

211. Feldstein LR, Rose EB, Horwitz SM, et al. Multisystem inflammatory syndrome in U.S. children and adolescents. *N Engl J Med* 2020;383(4):334–346. doi: 10.1056/NEJMoa2021680.

211a. Ferdinands JM, Rao S, Dixon BE, et al. Waning 2-dose and 3-dose effectiveness of mRNA vaccines against COVID-19-associated emergency department and urgent care encounters and hospitalizations among adults during periods of Delta and Omicron variant predominance - VISION network, 10 states, August 2021-January 2022. *MMWR Morb Mortal Wkly Rep* 2022;71(7):255–263. doi: 10.15585/mmwr.mm7107e2.

212. Feng C, Shi J, Fan Q, et al. Protective humoral and cellular immune responses to SARS-CoV-2 persist up to 1 year after recovery. *Nat Commun* 2021;12(1):4984. doi: 10.1038/s41467-021-25312-0.

213. Feng S, Phillips DJ, White T, et al. Correlates of protection against symptomatic and asymptomatic SARS-CoV-2 infection. *Nat Med* 2021;27(11):2032–2040. doi: 10.1038/s41591-021-01540-1.

214. Fernandes DM, Oliveira CR, Guerguis S, et al. Severe acute respiratory syndrome coronavirus 2 clinical syndromes and predictors of disease severity in hospitalized children and youth. *J Pediatr* 2021;230:23–31.e10. doi: 10.1016/j.jpeds.2020.11.016.

215. Fernández-de-Las-Peñas DC. Anxiety, depression and poor sleep quality as long-term post-COVID sequelae in previously hospitalized patients: a multicenter study. *J Infect* 2021;83(4):496–522. doi: 10.1016/j.jinf.2021.06.022.

216. Finelli L, Gupta V, Petigara T, et al. Mortality among US patients hospitalized with SARS-CoV-2 infection in 2020. *JAMA Netw Open* 2021;4(4):e216556. doi: 10.1001/jamanetworkopen.2021.6556

217. Fink SL, Cookson BT. Apoptosis, pyroptosis, and necrosis: mechanistic description of dead and dying eukaryotic cells. *Infect Immun* 2005;73(4):1907–1916. doi: 10.1128/IAI.73.4.1907-1916.2005.

218. Fischer W, Eron JJ, Holman W, et al. Molnupiravir, an oral antiviral treatment for COVID-19. *medRxiv* 2021:2021.06.17.21258639. doi: 10.1101/2021.06.17.21258639.

219. Fisman DN, Tuite AR. Evaluation of the relative virulence of novel SARS-CoV-2 variants: a retrospective cohort study in Ontario, Canada. *CMAJ* 2021;193(42):E1619–E1625. doi: 10.1503/cmaj.211248.

220. Fowler RA, Lapinsky SE, Hallett D, et al. Critically ill patients with severe acute respiratory syndrome. *JAMA* 2003;290(3):367–373. doi: 10.1001/jama.290.3.367.

221. Fowlkes A, Gaglani M, Groover K, et al. Effectiveness of COVID-19 vaccines in preventing SARS-CoV-2 infection among frontline workers before and during B.1.617.2 (Delta) variant predominance - eight U.S. locations, December 2020-August 2021. *MMWR Morb Mortal Wkly Rep* 2021;70(34):1167–1169. doi: 10.15585/mmwr.mm7034e4.

221a. Fowlkes AL, Yoon SK, Lutrick K, et al. Effectiveness of 2-dose BNT162b2 (Pfizer BioNTech) mRNA vaccine in preventing SARS-CoV-2 infection among children aged 5–11 years and adolescents aged 12–15 years - PROTECT cohort, July 2021-February 2022. *MMWR Morb Mortal Wkly Rep* 2022;71(11):422–428. doi: 10.15585/mmwr.mm7111e1.

222. Fraley E, LeMaster C, Banerjee D, et al. Cross-reactive antibody immunity against SARS-CoV-2 in children and adults. *Cell Mol Immunol* 2021;18(7):1826–1828. doi: 10.1038/s41423-021-00700-0.

223. Franchini M, Liumbruno GM. Convalescent plasma for the treatment of severe COVID-19. *Biologics* 2021;15:31–38. doi: 10.2147/btt.S272063.

224. Frontera JA, Yang D, Lewis A, et al. A prospective study of long-term outcomes among hospitalized COVID-19 patients with and without neurological complications. *J Neurol Sci* 2021;426:117486. doi: 10.1016/j.jns.2021.117486.

225. Fu Y, Li Y, Guo E, et al. Dynamics and correlation among viral positivity, seroconversion, and disease severity in COVID-19: a retrospective study. *Ann Intern Med* 2021;174(4):453–461. doi: 10.7326/m20-3337.

226. Fujifilm Japan. Anti-influenza drug Avigan® Tablet Meets Primary Endpoint in Phase III Clinical Trial in Japan for COVID-19 patients. Updated September 23, 2020. https://www.fujifilm.com/jp/en/news/hq/5451?_ga=2.102248257.1948831102.1612073055-48278478.1612073055. Accessed July 31, 2021.

227. Gacci M, Coppi M, Baldi E, et al. Semen impairment and occurrence of SARS-CoV-2 virus in semen after recovery from COVID-19. *Hum Reprod* 2021;36(6):1520–1529. doi: 10.1093/humrep/deab026.

228. Gaebler C, Wang Z, Lorenzi JCC, et al. Evolution of antibody immunity to SARS-CoV-2. *Nature* 2021;591(7851):639–644. doi: 10.1038/s41586-021-03207-w.

229. Galang RR, Newton SM, Woodworth KR, et al. Risk factors for illness severity among pregnant women with confirmed severe acute respiratory syndrome coronavirus 2 infection-surveillance for emerging threats to mothers and babies network, 22 state, local, and territorial health departments, 29 March 2020-5 March 2021. *Clin Infect Dis* 2021;73(Suppl 1):S17–S23. doi: 10.1093/cid/ciab432.

230. Gallastegui N, Zhou JY, Drygalski AV, et al. Pulmonary embolism does not have an unusually high incidence among hospitalized COVID19 patients. *Clin Appl Thromb Hemost* 2021;27:1076029621996471. doi: 10.1177/1076029621996471.

231. Gallo LG, Oliveira AFM, Abrahão AA, et al. Ten epidemiological parameters of COVID-19: use of rapid literature review to inform predictive models during the pandemic. *Front Public Health* 2020;8:598547. doi: 10.3389/fpubh.2020.598547.

232. Gandhi RT, Lynch JB, del Rio C. Mild or moderate Covid-19. *N Engl J Med* 2020;383(18):1757–1766. doi: 10.1056/NEJMcp2009249.

233. Gao M, Piernas C, Astbury NM, et al. Associations between body-mass index and COVID-19 severity in 6·9 million people in England: a prospective, community-based, cohort study. *Lancet Diabetes Endocrinol* 2021;9(6):350–359. doi: 10.1016/s2213-8587(21)00089-9.

234. Garcia-Vidal C, Cózar-Llistó A, Meira F, et al. Trends in mortality of hospitalised COVID-19 patients: a single centre observational cohort study from Spain. *Lancet Reg Health Eur* 2021;3:100041. doi: 10.1016/j.lanepe.2021.100041.

235. Garcia-Vidal C, Sanjuan G, Moreno-García E, et al. Incidence of co-infections and superinfections in hospitalized patients with COVID-19: a retrospective cohort study. *Clin Microbiol Infect* 2021;27(1):83–88. doi: 10.1016/j.cmi.2020.07.041.

236. Gargano JW, Wallace M, Hadler SC, et al. Use of mRNA COVID-19 vaccine after reports of myocarditis among vaccine recipients: update from the Advisory Committee on Immunization Practices - United States, June 2021. *MMWR Morb Mortal Wkly Rep* 2021;70(27):977–982. doi: 10.15585/mmwr.mm7027e2.

236a. Garrett N, Tapley A, Andriesen J, et al. High asymptomatic carriage with the Omicron variant in South Africa. *Clin Infect Dis* 2022. doi: 10.1093/cid/ciac237.

237. Gąsecka A, Borovac JA, Guerreiro RA, et al. Thrombotic complications in patients with COVID-19: pathophysiological mechanisms, diagnosis, and treatment. *Cardiovasc Drugs Ther* 2021;35(2):215–229. doi: 10.1007/s10557-020-07084-9.

238. Gee J, Marquez P, Su J, et al. First month of COVID-19 vaccine safety monitoring - United States, December 14, 2020-January 13, 2021. *MMWR Morb Mortal Wkly Rep* 2021;70(8):283–288. doi: 10.15585/mmwr.mm7008e3.

239. Geng Y, Ma Q, Du YS, et al. Rhabdomyolysis is associated with in-hospital mortality in patients with COVID-19. *Shock* 2021;56(3):360–367. doi: 10.1097/shk.0000000000001725.

240. George PM, Barratt SL, Condliffe R, et al. Respiratory follow-up of patients with COVID-19 pneumonia. *Thorax* 2020;75(11):1009–1016. doi: 10.1136/thoraxjnl-2020-215314.

241. Giannis D, Allen S, Tsang J, et al. Post-discharge thromboembolic outcomes and mortality of hospitalized COVID-19 patients: the CORE-19 registry. *Blood* 2021;137(20):2838–2847. doi: 10.1182/blood.2020010529.

242. Giannis D, Ziogas IA, Gianni P. Coagulation disorders in coronavirus infected patients: COVID-19, SARS-CoV-1, MERS-CoV and lessons from the past. *J Clin Virol* 2020;127:104362. doi: 10.1016/j.jcv.2020.104362.

243. Gierer S, Bertram S, Kaup F, et al. The spike protein of the emerging betacoronavirus EMC uses a novel coronavirus receptor for entry, can be activated by TMPRSS2, and is targeted by neutralizing antibodies. *J Virol* 2013;87(10):5502–5511. doi: 10.1128/JVI.00128-13.

244. Gilead Sciences I. Development of Remdesivir. https://www.gilead.com/-/media/gilead-corporate/files/pdfs/covid-19/gilead_rdv-development-fact-sheet-2020.pdf. Accessed June 12, 2021.

245. GISAID. Tracking of Variants. https://www.gisaid.org/hcov19-variants/. Accessed Aug 7, 2021.

246. Gisondi P, Di Leo S, Bellinato F, et al. Time of onset of selected skin lesions associated with COVID-19: a systematic review. *Dermatol Ther (Heidelb)* 2021;11(3):695–705. doi: 10.1007/s13555-021-00526-8.

247. Godfred-Cato S, Tsang CA, Giovanni J, et al. Multisystem inflammatory syndrome in infants <12 months of age, United States, May 2020-January 2021. *Pediatr Infect Dis J* 2021;40(7):601–605. doi: 10.1097/inf.0000000000003149.

248. Goldman JD, Lye DCB, Hui DS, et al. Remdesivir for 5 or 10 days in patients with severe Covid-19. *N Engl J Med* 2020;383(19):1827–1837. doi: 10.1056/NEJMoa2015301.

249. Gonzalez DC, Khodamoradi K, Pai R, et al. A systematic review on the investigation of SARS-CoV-2 in semen. *Res Rep Urol* 2020;12:615–621. doi: 10.2147/rru.S277679.

250. Gottlieb RL, Nirula A, Chen P, et al. Effect of bamlanivimab as monotherapy or in combination with etesevimab on viral load in patients with mild to moderate COVID-19: a randomized clinical trial. *JAMA* 2021;325(7):632–644. doi: 10.1001/jama.2021.0202.

250a. Gottlieb RL, Vaca CE, Paredes R, et al. Early remdesivir to prevent progression to severe Covid-19 in outpatients. *N Engl J Med* 2022;386(4):305–315. doi: 10.1056/NEJMoa2116846.

251. Graham BS. Vaccines against respiratory syncytial virus: the time has finally come. *Vaccine* 2016;34(30):3535–3541. doi: 10.1016/j.vaccine.2016.04.083.

252. Graham EL, Clark JR, Orban ZS, et al. Persistent neurologic symptoms and cognitive dysfunction in non-hospitalized Covid-19 "long haulers". *Ann Clin Transl Neurol* 2021;8(5):1073–1085. doi: 10.1002/acn3.51350.

253. Graham MS, Sudre CH, May A, et al. Changes in symptomatology, reinfection, and transmissibility associated with the SARS-CoV-2 variant B.1.1.7: an ecological study. *Lancet Public Health* 2021;6(5):e335–e345. doi: 10.1016/s2468-2667(21)00055-4.

254. Grant MC, Geoghegan L, Arbyn M, et al. The prevalence of symptoms in 24,410 adults infected by the novel coronavirus (SARS-CoV-2; COVID-19): a systematic review and meta-analysis of 148 studies from 9 countries. *PLoS One* 2020;15(6):e0234765. doi: 10.1371/journal.pone.0234765.

254a. Grant R, Charmet T, Schaeffer L, et al. Impact of SARS-CoV-2 Delta variant on incubation, transmission settings and vaccine effectiveness: results from a nationwide case-control study in France. *Lancet Reg Health Eur* 2022;13:100278. doi: 10.1016/j.lanepe.2021.100278.

255. Grasselli G, Greco M, Zanella A, et al. Risk factors associated with mortality among patients with COVID-19 in intensive care units in Lombardy, Italy. *JAMA Intern Med* 2020;180(10):1345–1355. doi: 10.1001/jamainternmed.2020.3539.

256. Grasselli G, Scaravilli V, Mangioni D, et al. Hospital-acquired infections in critically ill patients with COVID-19. *Chest* 2021;160(2):454–465. doi: 10.1016/j.chest.2021.04.002.

257. Greenhawt M, Abrams EM, Shaker M, et al. The risk of allergic reaction to SARS-CoV-2 vaccines and recommended evaluation and management: a systematic review, meta-analysis, GRADE Assessment, and International Consensus Approach. *J Allergy Clin Immunol Pract* 2021;9(10):3546–3567. doi: 10.1016/j.jaip.2021.06.006.

258. Grifoni A, Weiskopf D, Ramirez SI, et al. Targets of T cell responses to SARS-CoV-2 coronavirus in humans with COVID-19 disease and unexposed individuals. *Cell* 2020;181(7):1489–1501.e15. doi: 10.1016/j.cell.2020.05.015.

259. Grint DJ, Wing K, Houlihan C, et al. Severity of SARS-CoV-2 alpha variant (B.1.1.7) in England. *Clin Infect Dis* 2021:ciab754. doi: 10.1093/cid/ciab754.

260. Groß R, Conzelmann C, Müller JA, et al. Detection of SARS-CoV-2 in human breastmilk. *Lancet* 2020;395(10239):1757–1758. doi: 10.1016/s0140-6736(20)31181-8.

261. Groves LM, Usagawa L, Elm J, et al. Community transmission of SARS-CoV-2 at three fitness facilities—Hawaii, June-July 2020. *MMWR Morb Mortal Wkly Rep* 2021;70(9):316–320. doi: 10.15585/mmwr.mm7009e1.

262. Guan WJ, Liang WH, Zhao Y, et al. Comorbidity and its impact on 1590 patients with COVID-19 in China: a nationwide analysis. *Eur Respir J* 2020;55(5):2000547. doi: 10.1183/13993003.00547-2020.

263. Guan WJ, Ni ZY, Hu Y, et al. Clinical characteristics of coronavirus disease 2019 in China. *N Engl J Med* 2020;382(18):1708–1720. doi: 10.1056/NEJMoa2002032.

264. Guerrero JI, Barragán LA, Martínez JD, et al. Central and peripheral nervous system involvement by COVID-19: a systematic review of the pathophysiology, clinical manifestations, neuropathology, neuroimaging, electrophysiology, and cerebrospinal fluid findings. *BMC Infect Dis* 2021;21(1):515. doi: 10.1186/s12879-021-06185-6.

265. Guimarães PO, Quirk D, Furtado RH, et al. Tofacitinib in patients hospitalized with Covid-19 pneumonia. *N Engl J Med* 2021;385(5):406–415. doi: 10.1056/NEJMoa2101643.

266. Guney C, Akar F. Epithelial and endothelial expressions of ACE2: SARS-CoV-2 entry routes. *J Pharm Pharm Sci* 2021;24:84–93. doi: 10.18433/jpps31455.

267. Guo T, Fan Y, Chen M, et al. Cardiovascular implications of fatal outcomes of patients with coronavirus disease 2019 (COVID-19). *JAMA Cardiol* 2020;5(7):811–818. doi: 10.1001/jamacardio.2020.1017.

268. Guo X, Jie Y, Ye Y, et al. Upper respiratory tract viral ribonucleic acid load at hospital admission is associated with coronavirus disease 2019 disease severity. *Open Forum Infect Dis* 2020;7(7):ofaa282. doi: 10.1093/ofid/ofaa282.

269. Gupta A, Gonzalez-Rojas Y, Juarez E, et al. Early Covid-19 treatment with SARS-CoV-2 neutralizing antibody sotrovimab. *medRxiv* 2021:2021.05.27.21257096. doi: 10.1101/2021.05.27.21257096.

270. Gupta S, Coca SG, Chan L, et al. AKI treated with renal replacement therapy in critically ill patients with COVID-19. *J Am Soc Nephrol* 2021;32(1):161–176. doi: 10.1681/asn.2020060897.

271. Haas EJ, Angulo FJ, McLaughlin JM, et al. Impact and effectiveness of mRNA BNT162b2 vaccine against SARS-CoV-2 infections and COVID-19 cases, hospitalisations, and deaths following a nationwide vaccination campaign in Israel: an observational study using national surveillance data. *Lancet* 2021;397(10287):1819–1829. doi: 10.1016/S0140-6736(21)00947-8.

272. Hall VJ, Foulkes S, Charlett A, et al. SARS-CoV-2 infection rates of antibody-positive compared with antibody-negative health-care workers in England: a large, multicentre, prospective cohort study (SIREN). *Lancet* 2021;397(10283):1459–1469. doi: 10.1016/s0140-6736(21)00675-9.

273. Hamer SA, Ghai RR, Zecca IB, et al. SARS-CoV-2 B.1.1.7 variant of concern detected in a pet dog and cat after exposure to a person with COVID-19, USA. *Transbound Emerg Dis* 2021. May 6:10.1111/tbed.14122. doi: 10.1111/tbed.14122. Online ahead of print.

274. Hamer SA, Pauvolid-Corrêa A, Zecca IB, et al. SARS-CoV-2 infections and viral isolations among serially tested cats and dogs in households with infected owners in Texas, USA. *Viruses* 2021;13(5):938. doi: 10.3390/v13050938.

274a. Hammond J, Leister-Tebbe H, Gardner A, et al. Oral nirmatrelvir for high-risk, nonhospitalized adults with Covid-19. *N Engl J Med* 2022. doi: 10.1056/NEJMoa2118542.

275. Hamner L, Dubbel P, Capron I, et al. High SARS-CoV-2 attack rate following exposure at a choir practice—Skagit County, Washington, March 2020. *MMWR Morb Mortal Wkly Rep* 2020;69(19):606–610. doi: 10.15585/mmwr.mm6919e6.

276. Hampshire A, Trender W, Chamberlain SR, et al. Cognitive deficits in people who have recovered from COVID-19. *EClinicalMedicine* 2021;39:101044. doi: 10.1016/j.eclinm.2021.101044.

277. Hansen CH, Michlmayr D, Gubbels SM, et al. Assessment of protection against reinfection with SARS-CoV-2 among 4 million PCR-tested individuals in Denmark in 2020: a population-level observational study. *Lancet* 2021;397(10280):1204–1212. doi: 10.1016/s0140-6736(21)00575-4.

278. Hanson KE, Barker AP, Hillyard DR, et al. Self-collected anterior nasal and saliva specimens versus health care worker-collected nasopharyngeal swabs for the molecular detection of SARS-CoV-2. *J Clin Microbiol* 2020;58(11):e01824-20. doi: 10.1128/jcm.01824-20.

279. Harapan BN, Yoo HJ. Neurological symptoms, manifestations, and complications associated with severe acute respiratory syndrome coronavirus 2 (SARS-CoV-2) and coronavirus disease 19 (COVID-19). *J Neurol* 2021:1–13. doi: 10.1007/s00415-021-10406-y.

280. Harcourt J, Tamin A, Lu X, et al. Severe acute respiratory syndrome coronavirus 2 from patient with coronavirus disease, United States. *Emerg Infect Dis* 2020;26(6):1266–1273. doi: 10.3201/eid2606.200516.

281. Harrington D, Azim T, Rosmarin C, et al. Evaluation of 2 commercial anti-SARS-CoV-2 antibody assays in an immunocompetent and immunocompromised inpatient population with COVID-19. *Diagn Microbiol Infect Dis* 2021;101(2):115449. doi: 10.1016/j.diagmicrobio.2021.115449.

282. Hasan A, Al-Ozairi E, Al-Baqsumi Z, et al. Cellular and humoral immune responses in Covid-19 and immunotherapeutic approaches. *Immunotargets Ther* 2021;10:63–85. doi: 10.2147/itt.S280706.

283. Hasan SS, Capstick T, Ahmed R, et al. Mortality in COVID-19 patients with acute respiratory distress syndrome and corticosteroids use: a systematic review and meta-analysis. *Expert Rev Respir Med* 2020;14(11):1149–1163. doi: 10.1080/17476348.2020.1804365.

284. Hashemi SA, Safamanesh S, Ghasemzadeh-Moghaddam H, et al. High prevalence of SARS-CoV-2 and influenza A virus (H1N1) coinfection in dead patients in Northeastern Iran. *J Med Virol* 2021;93(2):1008–1012. doi: 10.1002/jmv.26364.

285. Haslak F, Barut K, Durak C, et al. Clinical features and outcomes of 76 patients with COVID-19-related multi-system inflammatory syndrome in children. *Clin Rheumatol* 2021;40(10):4167–4178. doi: 10.1007/s10067-021-05780-x.

286. Hause AM, Gee J, Baggs J, et al. COVID-19 vaccine safety in adolescents aged 12-17 years - United States, December 14, 2020-July 16, 2021. *MMWR Morb Mortal Wkly Rep* 2021;70(31):1053–1058. doi: 10.15585/mmwr.mm7031e1.

287. Havers FP, Whitaker M, Self JL, et al. Hospitalization of Adolescents Aged 12–17 Years with Laboratory-Confirmed COVID-19 - COVID-NET, 14 States, March 1, 2020-April 24, 2021. *MMWR Morb Mortal Wkly Rep* 2021;70(23):851–857. doi: 10.15585/mmwr.mm7023e1.

288. He X, Lau EHY, Wu P, et al. Temporal dynamics in viral shedding and transmissibility of COVID-19. *Nat Med* 2020;26(5):672–675. doi: 10.1038/s41591-020-0869-5.

289. Health. NIo. NIH Coronavirus Disease 2019 (COVID-19) Treatment Guidelines. https://www.covid19treatmentguidelines.nih.gov/. Accessed June 13, 2021.

290. Helms J, Tacquard C, Severac F, et al. High risk of thrombosis in patients with severe SARS-CoV-2 infection: a multicenter prospective cohort study. *Intensive Care Med* 2020;46(6):1089–1098. doi: 10.1007/s00134-020-06062-x.

291. Hermesch AC, Horve PF, Edelman A, et al. Severe Acute Respiratory Syndrome Coronavirus 2 (SARS-CoV-2) environmental contamination and childbirth. *Obstet Gynecol* 2020;136(4):827–829. doi: 10.1097/aog.0000000000004112.

292. Hermine O, Mariette X, Tharaux PL, et al. Effect of tocilizumab vs usual care in adults hospitalized with COVID-19 and moderate or severe pneumonia: a randomized clinical trial. *JAMA Intern Med* 2021;181(1):32–40. doi: 10.1001/jamainternmed.2020.6820.

293. Hinduja A, Nalleballe K, Onteddu S, et al. Impact of cerebral venous sinus thrombosis associated with COVID-19. *J Neurol Sci* 2021;425:117448. doi: 10.1016/j.jns.2021.117448.

294. Hoehl S, Rabenau H, Berger A, et al. Evidence of SARS-CoV-2 infection in returning travelers from Wuhan, China. *N Engl J Med* 2020;382(13):1278–1280. doi: 10.1056/NEJMc2001899.

295. Hogan CA, Stevens BA, Sahoo MK, et al. High frequency of SARS-CoV-2 RNAemia and association with severe disease. *Clin Infect Dis* 2021;72(9):e291–e295. doi: 10.1093/cid/ciaa1054.

296. Holshue ML, DeBolt C, Lindquist S, et al. First case of 2019 novel coronavirus in the United States. *N Engl J Med* 2020;382(10):929–936. doi: 10.1056/NEJMoa2001191.

297. Horby P, Lim WS, Emberson JR, et al. Dexamethasone in hospitalized patients with Covid-19. *N Engl J Med* 2021;384(8):693–704. doi: 10.1056/NEJMoa2021436.

298. Horby P, Mafham M, Linsell L, et al. Effect of hydroxychloroquine in hospitalized patients with Covid-19. *N Engl J Med* 2020;383(21):2030–2040. doi: 10.1056/NEJMoa2022926.

299. Hu S, Wang W, Wang Y, et al. Infectivity, susceptibility, and risk factors associated with SARS-CoV-2 transmission under intensive contact tracing in Hunan, China. *Nat Commun* 2021;12(1):1533. doi: 10.1038/s41467-021-21710-6.

300. Huang C, Huang L, Wang Y, et al. 6-month consequences of COVID-19 in patients discharged from hospital: a cohort study. *Lancet* 2021;397(10270):220–232. doi: 10.1016/s0140-6736(20)32656-8.

301. Huang C, Wang Y, Li X, et al. Clinical features of patients infected with 2019 novel coronavirus in Wuhan, China. *Lancet* 2020;395(10223):497–506. doi: 10.1016/s0140-6736(20)30183-5.

302. Huang CG, Lee KM, Hsiao MJ, et al. Culture-based virus isolation to evaluate potential infectivity of clinical specimens tested for COVID-19. *J Clin Microbiol* 2020;58(8):e01068-20. doi: 10.1128/jcm.01068-20.

303. Huang L, Yao Q, Gu X, et al. 1-year outcomes in hospital survivors with COVID-19: a longitudinal cohort study. *Lancet* 2021;398(10302):747–758. doi: 10.1016/s0140-6736(21)01755-4.

304. Hughes RAC, Swan AV, van Doorn PA. Intravenous immunoglobulin for Guillain-Barré syndrome. *Cochrane Database Syst Rev* 2014;(9):CD002063. doi: 10.1002/14651858.CD002063.pub6.

305. Hughes S, Troise O, Donaldson H, et al. Bacterial and fungal coinfection among hospitalized patients with COVID-19: a retrospective cohort study in a UK secondary-care setting. *Clin Microbiol Infect* 2020;26(10):1395–1399. doi: 10.1016/j.cmi.2020.06.025.

306. Hussain A, Via G, Melniker L, et al. Multi-organ point-of-care ultrasound for COVID-19 (PoCUS4COVID): international expert consensus. *Crit Care* 2020;24(1):702. doi: 10.1186/s13054-020-03369-5.

307. Iba T, Levy JH, Levi M, et al. Coagulopathy of coronavirus disease 2019. *Crit Care Med* 2020;48(9):1358–1364. doi: 10.1097/ccm.0000000000004458.

308. Inc. GS. VEKLURY® (remdesivir)—Highlights of Prescribing Information. June 13, 2021. https://www.gilead.com/-/media/files/pdfs/medicines/covid-19/veklury/veklury_pi.pdf

309. Inc. GS. Veklury® Global Marketing Authorization Status. June 12, 2021. https://www.gilead.com/Purpose/Advancing-Global-Health/COVID-19/Veklury-global-marketing-authorization

310. INSPIRATION Investigators. Effect of intermediate-dose vs standard-dose prophylactic anticoagulation on thrombotic events, extracorporeal membrane oxygenation treatment, or mortality among patients with COVID-19 admitted to the intensive care unit: the INSPIRATION randomized clinical trial. *JAMA* 2021;325(16):1620–1630. doi: 10.1001/jama.2021.4152.

311. Ippolito Bastidas H, Márquez-Pérez T, García-Salido A, et al. Cerebral venous sinus thrombosis in a pediatric patient with COVID-19. *Neurol Clin Pract* 2021;11(2):e208–e210. doi: 10.1212/cpj.0000000000000899.

312. Islam N, Lewington S, Kharbanda RK, et al. Sixty-day consequences of COVID-19 in patients discharged from hospital: an electronic health records study. *Eur J Public Health* 2021;31(2):280–282. doi: 10.1093/eurpub/ckab009.

312a. Iuliano AD, Brunkard JM, Boehmer TK, et al. Trends in disease severity and health care utilization during the early Omicron variant period compared with previous SARS-CoV-2 high transmission periods - United States, December 2020-January 2022. *MMWR Morb Mortal Wkly Rep* 2022;71(4):146–152. doi: 10.15585/mmwr.mm7104e4.

313. Iuliano AD, Chang HH, Patel NN, et al. Estimating under-recognized COVID-19 deaths, United States, March 2020-May 2021 using an excess mortality modelling approach. *Lancet Reg Health Am* 2021;1:100019. doi: 10.1016/j.lana.2021.100019.

314. Jacobi A, Chung M, Bernheim A, et al. Portable chest X-ray in coronavirus disease-19 (COVID-19): a pictorial review. *Clin Imaging* 2020;64:35–42. doi: 10.1016/j.clinimag.2020.04.001.

315. Jaiswal N, Puri M, Agarwal K, et al. COVID-19 as an independent risk factor for subclinical placental dysfunction. *Eur J Obstet Gynecol Reprod Biol* 2021;259:7–11. doi: 10.1016/j.ejogrb.2021.01.049.

316. JamaliMoghadamSiahkali S, Zarezade B, Koolaji S, et al. Safety and effectiveness of high-dose vitamin C in patients with COVID-19: a randomized open-label clinical trial. *Eur J Med Res* 2021;26(1):20. doi: 10.1186/s40001-021-00490-1.

317. Jang S, Han SH, Rhee JY. Cluster of coronavirus disease associated with fitness dance classes, South Korea. *Emerg Infect Dis* 2020;26(8):1917–1920. doi: 10.3201/eid2608.200633.

318. Janice Oh HL, Ken-En Gan S, Bertoletti A, et al. Understanding the T cell immune response in SARS coronavirus infection. *Emerg Microbes Infect* 2012;1(9):e23. doi: 10.1038/emi.2012.26.

319. Jassat W, Mudara C, Ozougwu L, et al. Difference in mortality among individuals admitted to hospital with COVID-19 during the first and second waves in South Africa: a cohort study. *Lancet Glob Health* 2021;9(9):e1216–e1225. doi: 10.1016/s2214-109x(21)00289-8.

319a. Jayk Bernal A, Gomes da Silva MM, Musungaie DB, et al. Molnupiravir for oral treatment of Covid-19 in nonhospitalized patients. *N Engl J Med* 2022;386(6):509–520. doi: 10.1056/NEJMoa2116044.

320. Jeong HW, Kim SM, Kim HS, et al. Viable SARS-CoV-2 in various specimens from COVID-19 patients. *Clin Microbiol Infect* 2020;26(11):1520–1524. doi: 10.1016/j.cmi.2020.07.020.

321. Jia JL, Kamceva M, Rao SA, et al. Cutaneous manifestations of COVID-19: a preliminary review. *J Am Acad Dermatol* 2020;83(2):687–690. doi: 10.1016/j.jaad.2020.05.059.
322. Jiménez D, García-Sanchez A, Rali P, et al. Incidence of VTE and bleeding among hospitalized patients with coronavirus disease 2019: a systematic review and meta-analysis. *Chest* 2021;159(3):1182–1196. doi: 10.1016/j.chest.2020.11.005.
323. Jin X, Lian JS, Hu JH, et al. Epidemiological, clinical and virological characteristics of 74 cases of coronavirus-infected disease 2019 (COVID-19) with gastrointestinal symptoms. *Gut* 2020;69(6):1002–1009. doi: 10.1136/gutjnl-2020-320926.
324. Johnson & Johnson. Johnson & Johnson Statement on COVID-19 Vaccine (7/12). Updated July 12, 2021. https://www.jnj.com/johnson-johnson-july-12-statement-on-covid-19-vaccine. Accessed July 17, 2021.
325. Johnson J. Johnson & Johnson Announces Real-World Evidence and Phase 3 Data Confirming Strong and Long-Lasting Protection of Single-Shot COVID-19 Vaccine in the U.S. https://www.jnj.com/johnson-johnson-announces-real-world-evidence-and-phase-3-data-confirming-strong-and-long-lasting-protection-of-single-shot-covid-19-vaccine-in-the-u-s. Accessed November 6, 2021.
326. Jones TC, Biele G, Mühlemann B, et al. Estimating infectiousness throughout SARS-CoV-2 infection course. *Science* 2021;373(6551):eabi5273. doi: 10.1126/science.abi5273.
327. Joyner MJ, Bruno KA, Klassen SA, et al. Safety update: COVID-19 convalescent plasma in 20,000 hospitalized patients. *Mayo Clin Proc* 2020;95(9):1888–1897. doi: 10.1016/j.mayocp.2020.06.028.
328. Kaafarani HMA, El Moheb M, Hwabejire JO, et al. Gastrointestinal complications in critically ill patients with COVID-19. *Ann Surg* 2020;272(2):e61–e62. doi: 10.1097/sla.0000000000004004.
329. Kadri SS, Sun J, Lawandi A, et al. Association between caseload surge and COVID-19 survival in 558 U.S. hospitals, march to august 2020. *Ann Intern Med* 2021;174(9):1240–1251. doi: 10.7326/m21-1213.
330. Kalil AC, Patterson TF, Mehta AK, et al. Baricitinib plus remdesivir for hospitalized adults with Covid-19. *N Engl J Med* 2021;384(9):795–807. doi: 10.1056/NEJMoa2031994.
331. Kang CR, Lee JY, Park Y, et al. Coronavirus disease exposure and spread from nightclubs, South Korea. *Emerg Infect Dis* 2020;26(10):2499–2501. doi: 10.3201/eid2610.202573.
332. Kang M, Wei J, Yuan J, et al. Probable evidence of fecal aerosol transmission of SARS-CoV-2 in a high-rise building. *Ann Intern Med* 2020;173(12):974–980. doi: 10.7326/m20-0928.
333. Kaptein FHJ, Stals MAM, Grootenboers M, et al. Incidence of thrombotic complications and overall survival in hospitalized patients with COVID-19 in the second and first wave. *Thromb Res* 2021;199:143–148. doi: 10.1016/j.thromres.2020.12.019.
334. Karaba SM, Jones G, Helsel T, et al. Prevalence of co-infection at the time of hospital admission in COVID-19 patients, a multicenter study. *Open Forum Infect Dis* 2021;8(1):ofaa578. doi: 10.1093/ofid/ofaa578.
335. Karami Z, Knoop BT, Dofferhoff ASM, et al. Few bacterial co-infections but frequent empiric antibiotic use in the early phase of hospitalized patients with COVID-19: results from a multicentre retrospective cohort study in The Netherlands. *Infect Dis (Lond)* 2021;53(2):102–110. doi: 10.1080/23744235.2020.1839672.
336. Karan A, Klompas M, Tucker R, et al. The risk of SARS-CoV-2 transmission from patients with undiagnosed Covid-19 to roommates in a large academic medical center. *Clin Infect Dis* 2021:ciab564. doi: 10.1093/cid/ciab564.
337. Kasper MR, Geibe JR, Sears CL, et al. An outbreak of Covid-19 on an aircraft carrier. *N Engl J Med* 2020;383(25):2417–2426. doi: 10.1056/NEJMoa2019375.
338. Katelaris AL, Wells J, Clark P, et al. Epidemiologic evidence for airborne transmission of sars-cov-2 during church singing, Australia, 2020. *Emerg Infect Dis* 2021;27(6):1677–1680. doi: 10.3201/eid2706.210465.
339. Kaufman AE, Naidu S, Ramachandran S, et al. Review of radiographic findings in COVID-19. *World J Radiol* 2020;12(8):142–155. doi: 10.4329/wjr.v12.i8.142.
340. Kenerly MJ, Shah P, Patel H, et al. Altered mental status is an independent predictor of mortality in hospitalized COVID-19 patients. *Ir J Med Sci* 2021:1–6. doi: 10.1007/s11845-021-02515-4.
341. Kennedy M, Helfand BKI, Gou RY, et al. Delirium in older patients with COVID-19 presenting to the emergency department. *JAMA Netw Open* 2020;3(11):e2029540. doi: 10.1001/jamanetworkopen.2020.29540.
342. Kermani-Alghoraishi M. A review of coronary artery thrombosis: a new challenging finding in COVID-19 patients and ST-elevation myocardial infarction. *Curr Probl Cardiol* 2021;46(3):100744. doi: 10.1016/j.cpcardiol.2020.100744.
343. Keyhanian K, Umeton RP, Mohit B, et al. SARS-CoV-2 and nervous system: from pathogenesis to clinical manifestation. *J Neuroimmunol* 2020;350:577436. doi: 10.1016/j.jneuroim.2020.577436.
344. Khalil BA, Elemam NM, Maghazachi AA. Chemokines and chemokine receptors during COVID-19 infection. *Comput Struct Biotechnol J* 2021;19:976–988. doi: 10.1016/j.csbj.2021.01.034.
345. Khalili M, Karamouzian M, Nasiri N, et al. Epidemiological characteristics of COVID-19: a systematic review and meta-analysis. *Epidemiol Infect* 2020;148:e130. doi: 10.1017/s0950268820001430.
346. Khan N, Mahmud N. Effectiveness of SARS-CoV-2 vaccination in a veterans affairs cohort of patients with inflammatory bowel disease with diverse exposure to immunosuppressive medications. *Gastroenterology* 2021;161(3):827–836. doi: 10.1053/j.gastro.2021.05.044.
347. Khanh NC, Thai PQ, Quach HL, et al. Transmission of SARS-CoV 2 during long-haul flight. *Emerg Infect Dis* 2020;26(11):2617–2624. doi: 10.3201/eid2611.203299.
348. Kharbanda EO, Haapala J, DeSilva M, et al. Spontaneous abortion following COVID-19 vaccination during pregnancy. *JAMA* 2021;326(16):1629–1631. doi: 10.1001/jama.2021.15494.
349. Khoury DS, Cromer D, Reynaldi A, et al. Neutralizing antibody levels are highly predictive of immune protection from symptomatic SARS-CoV-2 infection. *Nat Med* 2021;27(7):1205–1211. doi: 10.1038/s41591-021-01377-8.
350. Kim L, Garg S, O'Halloran A, et al. Risk factors for intensive care unit admission and in-hospital mortality among hospitalized adults identified through the U.S. coronavirus disease 2019 (COVID-19)-Associated Hospitalization Surveillance Network (COVID-NET). *Clin Infect Dis* 2021;72(9):e206–e214. doi: 10.1093/cid/ciaa1012.
351. Kim L, Whitaker M, O'Halloran A, et al. Hospitalization rates and characteristics of children aged <18 years hospitalized with laboratory-confirmed COVID-19 - COVID-NET, 14 States, March 1-July 25, 2020. *MMWR Morb Mortal Wkly Rep* 2020;69(32):1081–1088. doi: 10.15585/mmwr.mm6932e3.
352. Kirchdoerfer RN, Wang N, Pallesen J, et al. Stabilized coronavirus spikes are resistant to conformational changes induced by receptor recognition or proteolysis. *Sci Rep* 2018;8(1):15701–15701. doi: 10.1038/s41598-018-34171-7.
353. Klok FA, Kruip M, van der Meer NJM, et al. Incidence of thrombotic complications in critically ill ICU patients with COVID-19. *Thromb Res* 2020;191:145–147. doi: 10.1016/j.thromres.2020.04.013.
354. Kojima N, Turner F, Slepnev V, et al. Self-collected oral fluid and nasal swab specimens demonstrate comparable sensitivity to clinician-collected nasopharyngeal swab specimens for the detection of SARS-CoV-2. *Clin Infect Dis* 2021;73(9):e3106–e3109. doi: 10.1093/cid/ciaa1589.
355. Kolhe NV, Fluck RJ, Selby NM, et al. Acute kidney injury associated with COVID-19: a retrospective cohort study. *PLoS Med* 2020;17(10):e1003406. doi: 10.1371/journal.pmed.1003406.
356. Kollias A, Kyriakoulis KG, Lagou S, et al. Venous thromboembolism in COVID-19: a systematic review and meta-analysis. *Vasc Med* 2021;26(4):415–425. doi: 10.1177/1358863x21995566.
357. Kompaniyets L, Agathis NT, Nelson JM, et al. Underlying medical conditions associated with severe COVID-19 illness among children. *JAMA Netw Open* 2021;4(6):e2111182. doi: 10.1001/jamanetworkopen.2021.11182.
358. Kompaniyets L, Goodman AB, Belay B, et al. Body mass index and risk for COVID-19-related hospitalization, intensive care unit admission, invasive mechanical ventilation, and death—United States, March-December 2020. *MMWR Morb Mortal Wkly Rep* 2021;70(10):355–361. doi: 10.15585/mmwr.mm7010e4.
359. Kotlyar AM, Grechukhina O, Chen A, et al. Vertical transmission of coronavirus disease 2019: a systematic review and meta-analysis. *Am J Obstet Gynecol* 2021;224(1):35–53. doi: 10.1016/j.ajog.2020.07.049.
360. Krogstad P, Contreras D, Ng H, et al. No evidence of infectious SARS-CoV-2 in human milk: analysis of a cohort of 110 lactating women. *medRxiv* 2021:2021.04.05.21254897. doi: 10.1101/2021.04.05.21254897.
361. Kumar J, Meena J, Yadav A, et al. SARS-CoV-2 detection in human milk: a systematic review. *J Matern Fetal Neonatal Med* 2021:1–8. doi: 10.1080/14767058.2021.1882984.
362. Kwon KS, Park JI, Park YJ, et al. Evidence of long-distance droplet transmission of SARS-CoV-2 by direct air flow in a restaurant in Korea. *J Korean Med Sci* 2020;35(46):e415. doi: 10.3346/jkms.2020.35.e415.
363. Lacy JM, Brooks EG, Akers J, et al. COVID-19: postmortem diagnostic and biosafety considerations. *Am J Forensic Med Pathol* 2020;41(3):143–151. doi: 10.1097/paf.0000000000000567.
364. Lagunas-Rangel FA, Chávez-Valencia V. What do we know about the antibody responses to SARS-CoV-2? *Immunobiology* 2021;226(2):152054. doi: 10.1016/j.imbio.2021.152054.
365. Lai CC, Ko WC, Chen CJ, et al. COVID-19 vaccines and thrombosis with thrombocytopenia syndrome. *Expert Rev Vaccines* 2021;20(8):1027–1035. doi: 10.1080/14760584.2021.1949294.
366. Laing AG, Lorenc A, Del Molino Del Barrio I, et al. A dynamic COVID-19 immune signature includes associations with poor prognosis. *Nat Med* 2020;26(10):1623–1635. doi: 10.1038/s41591-020-1038-6.
367. Lala A, Johnson KW, Januzzi JL, et al. Prevalence and impact of myocardial injury in patients hospitalized with COVID-19 infection. *J Am Coll Cardiol* 2020;76(5):533–546. doi: 10.1016/j.jacc.2020.06.007.
368. Lamoth F, Lewis RE, Walsh TJ, et al. Navigating the uncertainties of COVID-19 associated aspergillosis (CAPA): a comparison with influenza associated aspergillosis (IAPA). *J Infect Dis* 2021:jiab163. doi: 10.1093/infdis/jiab163.
369. Langford BJ, So M, Raybardhan S, et al. Bacterial co-infection and secondary infection in patients with COVID-19: a living rapid review and meta-analysis. *Clin Microbiol Infect* 2020;26(12):1622–1629. doi: 10.1016/j.cmi.2020.07.016.
370. Lansbury L, Lim B, Baskaran V, et al. Co-infections in people with COVID-19: a systematic review and meta-analysis. *J Infect* 2020;81(2):266–275. doi: 10.1016/j.jinf.2020.05.046.
371. Lardaro T, Wang AZ, Bucca A, et al. Characteristics of COVID-19 patients with bacterial coinfection admitted to the hospital from the emergency department in a large regional healthcare system. *J Med Virol* 2021;93(5):2883–2889. doi: 10.1002/jmv.26795.
372. Larsen HD, Fonager J, Lomholt FK, et al. Preliminary report of an outbreak of SARS-CoV-2 in mink and mink farmers associated with community spread, Denmark, June to November 2020. *Euro Surveill* 2021;26(5):2100009. doi: 10.2807/1560-7917.Es.2021.26.5.210009.
373. Lau YL, Peiris JS. Pathogenesis of severe acute respiratory syndrome. *Curr Opin Immunol* 2005;17(4):404–410. doi: 10.1016/j.coi.2005.05.009.
374. Lauer SA, Grantz KH, Bi Q, et al. The incubation period of coronavirus disease 2019 (COVID-19) from publicly reported confirmed cases: estimation and application. *Ann Intern Med* 2020;172(9):577–582. doi: 10.7326/m20-0504.
374a. Lauring AS, Tenforde MW, Chappell JD, et al. Clinical severity of, and effectiveness of mRNA vaccines against, covid-19 from omicron, delta, and alpha SARS-CoV-2 variants in the United States: prospective observational study. *BMJ (Clinical Research Ed)* 2022;376:e069761. doi: 10.1136/bmj-2021-069761.
375. Lavery AM, Preston LE, Ko JY, et al. Characteristics of hospitalized COVID-19 patients discharged and experiencing same-hospital readmission—United States, March-August 2020. *MMWR Morb Mortal Wkly Rep* 2020;69(45):1695–1699. doi: 10.15585/mmwr.mm6945e2.
376. Lax SF, Skok K, Zechner P, et al. Pulmonary arterial thrombosis in COVID-19 with fatal outcome: results from a prospective, single-center, clinicopathologic case series. *Ann Intern Med* 2020;173(5):350–361. doi: 10.7326/m20-2566.
377. Le Bert N, Tan AT, Kunasegaran K, et al. SARS-CoV-2-specific T cell immunity in cases of COVID-19 and SARS, and uninfected controls. *Nature* 2020;584(7821):457–462. doi: 10.1038/s41586-020-2550-z.

378. Le Borgne P, Solis M, Severac F, et al. SARS-CoV-2 viral load in nasopharyngeal swabs in the emergency department does not predict COVID-19 severity and mortality. *Acad Emerg Med* 2021;28(3):306–313. doi: 10.1111/acem.14217.
379. Le Hingrat Q, Bouzid D, Choquet C, et al. Viral epidemiology and SARS-CoV-2 co-infections with other respiratory viruses during the first COVID-19 wave in Paris, France. *Influenza Other Respir Viruses* 2021;15(4):425–428. doi: 10.1111/irv.12853.
380. Lechien JR, Chiesa-Estomba CM, De Siati DR, et al. Olfactory and gustatory dysfunctions as a clinical presentation of mild-to-moderate forms of the coronavirus disease (COVID-19): a multicenter European study. *Eur Arch Otorhinolaryngol* 2020;277(8):2251–2261. doi: 10.1007/s00405-020-05965-1.
381. Lednicky JA, Lauzardo M, Fan ZH, et al. Viable SARS-CoV-2 in the air of a hospital room with COVID-19 patients. *Int J Infect Dis* 2020;100:476–482. doi: 10.1016/j.ijid.2020.09.025.
382. Lee N, Hui D, Wu A, et al. A major outbreak of severe acute respiratory syndrome in Hong Kong. *N Engl J Med* 2003;348(20):1986–1994. doi: 10.1056/NEJMoa030685.
383. Lee RA, Herigon JC, Benedetti A, et al. Performance of saliva, oropharyngeal swabs, and nasal swabs for SARS-CoV-2 molecular detection: a systematic review and meta-analysis. *J Clin Microbiol* 2021;59(5):e02881-20. doi: 10.1128/jcm.02881-20.
384. Lee WS, Wheatley AK, Kent SJ, et al. Antibody-dependent enhancement and SARS-CoV-2 vaccines and therapies. *Nat Microbiol* 2020;5(10):1185–1191. doi: 10.1038/s41564-020-00789-5.
385. Leentjens J, van Haaps TF, Wessels PF, et al. COVID-19-associated coagulopathy and antithrombotic agents lessons after 1 year. *Lancet Haematol* 2021;8(7):e524–e533. doi: 10.1016/s2352-3026(21)00105-8.
386. Lefrancq N, Paireau J, Hozé N, et al. Evolution of outcomes for patients hospitalised during the first 9 months of the SARS-CoV-2 pandemic in France: a retrospective national surveillance data analysis. *Lancet Reg Health Eur* 2021;5:100087. doi: 10.1016/j.lanepe.2021.100087.
387. Legros V, Denolly S, Vogrig M, et al. A longitudinal study of SARS-CoV-2-infected patients reveals a high correlation between neutralizing antibodies and COVID-19 severity. *Cell Mol Immunol* 2021;18(2):318–327. doi: 10.1038/s41423-020-00588-2.
388. Lehmann CJ, Pho MT, Pitrak D, et al. Community acquired co-infection in COVID-19: a retrospective observational experience. *Clin Infect Dis* 2021;72(8):1450–1452. doi: 10.1093/cid/ciaa902.
389. Lendacki FR, Teran RA, Gretsch S, et al. COVID-19 outbreak among attendees of an exercise facility—Chicago, Illinois, August-September 2020. *MMWR Morb Mortal Wkly Rep* 2021;70(9):321–325. doi: 10.15585/mmwr.mm7009e2.
390. Leonard WJ, O'Shea JJ. JAKS AND STATS: biological implications. *Annu Rev Immunol* 1998;16(1):293–322. doi: 10.1146/annurev.immunol.16.1.293.
391. Lester SN, Li K. Toll-like receptors in antiviral innate immunity. *J Mol Biol* 2014;426(6):1246–1264. doi: 10.1016/j.jmb.2013.11.024.
392. Levine-Tiefenbrun M, Yelin I, Alapi H, et al. Viral loads of Delta-variant SARS-CoV-2 breakthrough infections after vaccination and booster with BNT162b2. *Nat Med* 2021;27(12):2108–2110. doi: 10.1038/s41591-021-01575-4.
393. Lewnard JA, Liu VX, Jackson ML, et al. Incidence, clinical outcomes, and transmission dynamics of severe coronavirus disease 2019 in California and Washington: prospective cohort study. *BMJ* 2020;369:m1923. doi: 10.1136/bmj.m1923.
394. L'Huillier AG, Torriani G, Pigny F, et al. Culture-competent SARS-CoV-2 in nasopharynx of symptomatic neonates, children, and adolescents. *Emerg Infect Dis* 2020;26(10):2494–2497. doi: 10.3201/eid2610.202403.
395. Li B, Deng A, Li K, et al. Viral infection and transmission in a large, well-traced outbreak caused by the SARS-CoV-2 Delta variant. *medRxiv* 2021:2021.07.07.21260122. doi: 10.1101/2021.07.07.21260122.
396. Li C, Zhao H, Cheng L, et al. Anti-inflammation, immunomodulation and therapeutic repair in current clinical trials for the management of COVID-19. *Drug Des Devel Ther* 2021;15:1345–1356. doi: 10.2147/dddt.S301173.
397. Li D, Jin M, Bao P, et al. Clinical characteristics and results of semen tests among men with coronavirus disease 2019. *JAMA Netw Open* 2020;3(5):e208292. doi: 10.1001/jamanetworkopen.2020.8292.
398. Li J, Liao X, Zhou Y, et al. Comparison of associations between glucocorticoids treatment and mortality in COVID-19 patients and SARS patients: a systematic review and meta-analysis. *Shock* 2021;56(2):215–228. doi: 10.1097/shk.0000000000001738.
399. Li Q, Guan X, Wu P, et al. Early transmission dynamics in Wuhan, China, of novel coronavirus-infected pneumonia. *N Engl J Med* 2020;382(13):1199–1207. doi: 10.1056/NEJMoa2001316.
400. Li Y, Cai X, Mao Y, et al. Trends in racial and ethnic disparities in coronavirus disease 2019 (COVID-19) outcomes among nursing home residents. *Infect Control Hosp Epidemiol* 2021:1–7. doi: 10.1017/ice.2021.246.
401. Li Y, Qian H, Hang J, et al. Probable airborne transmission of SARS-CoV-2 in a poorly ventilated restaurant. *Build Environ* 2021;196:107788. doi: 10.1016/j.buildenv.2021.107788.
402. Lim ZJ, Subramaniam A, Ponnapa Reddy M, et al. Case fatality rates for patients with COVID-19 requiring invasive mechanical ventilation. A meta-analysis. *Am J Respir Crit Care Med* 2021;203(1):54–66. doi: 10.1164/rccm.202006-2405OC.
403. Lindner AK, Nikolai O, Kausch F, et al. Head-to-head comparison of SARS-CoV-2 antigen-detecting rapid test with self-collected nasal swab versus professional-collected nasopharyngeal swab. *Eur Respir J* 2021;57(4):2003961. doi: 10.1183/13993003.03961-2020.
404. Linschoten M, Peters S, van Smeden M, et al. Cardiac complications in patients hospitalised with COVID-19. *Eur Heart J Acute Cardiovasc Care* 2020;9(8):817–823. doi: 10.1177/2048872620974605.
405. Lisboa Bastos M, Tavaziva G, Abidi SK, et al. Diagnostic accuracy of serological tests for covid-19: systematic review and meta-analysis. *BMJ* 2020;370:m2516. doi: 10.1136/bmj.m2516.
406. Litmanovich DE, Chung M, Kirkbride RR, et al. Review of chest radiograph findings of COVID-19 pneumonia and suggested reporting language. *J Thorac Imaging* 2020;35(6):354–360. doi: 10.1097/rti.0000000000000541.
407. Liu J, Tu C, Zhu M, et al. The clinical course and prognostic factors of severe COVID-19 in Wuhan, China: a retrospective case-control study. *Medicine (Baltimore)* 2021;100(8):e23996. doi: 10.1097/md.0000000000023996.
408. Liu M, Lv F, Huang Y, et al. Follow-up study of the chest CT Characteristics of COVID-19 survivors seven months after recovery. *Front Med (Lausanne)* 2021;8:636298. doi: 10.3389/fmed.2021.636298.
409. Liu WD, Chang SY, Wang JT, et al. Prolonged virus shedding even after seroconversion in a patient with COVID-19. *J Infect* 2020;81(2):318–356. doi: 10.1016/j.jinf.2020.03.063.
410. Liu Y, Ning Z, Chen Y, et al. Aerodynamic analysis of SARS-CoV-2 in two Wuhan hospitals. *Nature* 2020;582(7813):557–560. doi: 10.1038/s41586-020-2271-3.
411. Lo MK, Feldmann F, Gary JM, et al. Remdesivir (GS-5734) protects African green monkeys from Nipah virus challenge. *Sci Transl Med* 2019;11(494):eaau9242. doi: 10.1126/scitranslmed.aau9242.
412. Lo MK, Jordan R, Arvey A, et al. GS-5734 and its parent nucleoside analog inhibit Filo-, Pneumo-, and Paramyxoviruses. *Sci Rep* 2017;7:43395. doi: 10.1038/srep43395.
413. Lodi L, Moriondo M, Pucci A, et al. Chronic asymptomatic SARS-CoV-2 infection in the immunocompromised patient: new challenges and urgent needs. *Clin Infect Dis* 2021;74(3):553.doi: 10.1093/cid/ciab538.
414. Lombardi CM, Carubelli V, Iorio A, et al. Association of troponin levels with mortality in Italian patients hospitalized with coronavirus disease 2019: results of a multicenter study. *JAMA Cardiol* 2020;5(11):1274–1280. doi: 10.1001/jamacardio.2020.3538.
415. Long B, Bridwell R, Gottlieb M. Thrombosis with thrombocytopenia syndrome associated with COVID-19 vaccines. *Am J Emerg Med* 2021;49:58–61. doi: 10.1016/j.ajem.2021.05.054.
416. Lopez Bernal J, Andrews N, Gower C, et al. Effectiveness of Covid-19 vaccines against the B.1.617.2 (Delta) variant. *N Engl J Med* 2021;385(7):585–594. doi: 10.1056/NEJMoa2108891.
417. Lopez Bernal J, Andrews N, Gower C, et al. Effectiveness of the Pfizer-BioNTech and Oxford-AstraZeneca vaccines on covid-19 related symptoms, hospital admissions, and mortality in older adults in England: test negative case-control study. *BMJ* 2021;373:n1088. doi: 10.1136/bmj.n1088.
418. Lu J, Gu J, Li K, et al. COVID-19 outbreak associated with air conditioning in restaurant, Guangzhou, China, 2020. *Emerg Infect Dis* 2020;26(7):1628–1631. doi: 10.3201/eid2607.200764.
419. Lu J, Yang Z. COVID-19 outbreak associated with air conditioning in restaurant, Guangzhou, China, 2020. *Emerg Infect Dis* 2020;26(11):2791–2793. doi: 10.3201/eid2611.203774.
420. Luke TC, Casadevall A, Watowich SJ, et al. Hark back: passive immunotherapy for influenza and other serious infections. *Crit Care Med* 2010;38(4 Suppl):e66–e73. doi: 10.1097/CCM.0b013e3181d44c1e.
421. Lundgren JD, Grund B, Barkauskas CE, et al. A neutralizing monoclonal antibody for hospitalized patients with Covid-19. *N Engl J Med* 2021;384(10):905–914. doi: 10.1056/NEJMoa2033130.
422. Luo S, Zhang X, Xu H. Don't overlook digestive symptoms in patients with 2019 novel coronavirus disease (COVID-19). *Clin Gastroenterol Hepatol* 2020;18(7):1636–1637. doi: 10.1016/j.cgh.2020.03.043.
423. Ma J, Qi X, Chen H, et al. COVID-19 patients in earlier stages exhaled millions of SARS-CoV-2 per hour. *Clin Infect Dis* 2021;72(10):e652–e654. doi: 10.1093/cid/ciaa1283.
424. Mackey K, Arkhipova-Jenkins I, Armstrong C, et al. *AHRQ Rapid Evidence Products Antibody Response Following SARS-CoV-2 Infection and Implications for Immunity: A Rapid Living Review*. Rockville, MD: Agency for Healthcare Research and Quality (US); 2021.
425. Mackey K, Ayers CK, Kondo KK, et al. Racial and ethnic disparities in COVID-19-related infections, hospitalizations, and deaths: a systematic review. *Ann Intern Med* 2021;174(3):362–373. doi: 10.7326/m20-6306.
426. MacNeil JR, Su JR, Broder KR, et al. Updated recommendations from the advisory committee on immunization practices for use of the Janssen (Johnson & Johnson) COVID-19 vaccine after reports of thrombosis with thrombocytopenia syndrome among vaccine recipients - United States, April 2021. *MMWR Morb Mortal Wkly Rep* 2021;70(17):651–656. doi: 10.15585/mmwr.mm7017e4.
427. Madewell ZJ, Yang Y, Longini IM Jr, et al. Factors associated with household transmission of SARS-CoV-2: an updated systematic review and meta-analysis. *JAMA Netw Open* 2021;4(8):e2122240. doi: 10.1001/jamanetworkopen.2021.22240.
428. Madewell ZJ, Yang Y, Longini IM Jr, et al. Household transmission of SARS-CoV-2: a systematic review and meta-analysis. *JAMA Netw Open* 2020;3(12):e2031756. doi: 10.1001/jamanetworkopen.2020.31756.
428a. Madhi SA, Kwatra G, Myers JE, et al. Population immunity and Covid-19 severity with Omicron variant in South Africa. *N Engl J Med* 2022;386(14):1314–1326. doi: 10.1056/NEJMoa2119658.
429. Maecker HT. Immune profiling of COVID-19: preliminary findings and implications for the pandemic. *J Immunother Cancer* 2021;9(5):e002550. doi: 10.1136/jitc-2021-002550.
430. Maes M, Higginson E, Pereira-Dias J, et al. Ventilator-associated pneumonia in critically ill patients with COVID-19. *Crit Care* 2021;25(1):25. doi: 10.1186/s13054-021-03460-5.
431. Maestre-Muñiz MM, Arias Á, Mata-Vázquez E, et al. Long-term outcomes of patients with coronavirus disease 2019 at one year after hospital discharge. *J Clin Med* 2021;10(13):2945. doi: 10.3390/jcm10132945.
432. Magleby R, Westblade LF, Trzebucki A, et al. Impact of SARS-CoV-2 viral load on risk of intubation and mortality among hospitalized patients with coronavirus disease 2019. *Clin Infect Dis* 2021;73(11):e4197–e4205. doi: 10.1093/cid/ciaa851.
433. Magro C, Mulvey JJ, Berlin D, et al. Complement associated microvascular injury and thrombosis in the pathogenesis of severe COVID-19 infection: a report of five cases. *Transl Res* 2020;220:1–13. doi: 10.1016/j.trsl.2020.04.007.
434. Mahat RK, Panda S, Rathore V, et al. The dynamics of inflammatory markers in coronavirus disease-2019 (COVID-19) patients: a systematic review and meta-analysis. *Clin Epidemiol Glob Health* 2021;11:100727. doi: 10.1016/j.cegh.2021.100727.
435. Mahdy MAA, Younis W, Ewaida Z. An overview of SARS-CoV-2 and animal infection. *Front Vet Sci* 2020;7:596391. doi: 10.3389/fvets.2020.596391.

436. Malik P, Patel U, Mehta D, et al. Biomarkers and outcomes of COVID-19 hospitalisations: systematic review and meta-analysis. *BMJ Evid Based Med* 2021;26(3):107–108. doi: 10.1136/bmjebm-2020-111536.
437. Mallett S, Allen AJ, Graziadio S, et al. At what times during infection is SARS-CoV-2 detectable and no longer detectable using RT-PCR-based tests? A systematic review of individual participant data. *BMC Med* 2020;18(1):346. doi: 10.1186/s12916-020-01810-8.
438. Maltezou HC, Raftopoulos V, Vorou R, et al. Association between upper respiratory tract viral load, comorbidities, disease severity, and outcome of patients with SARS-CoV-2 infection. *J Infect Dis* 2021;223(7):1132–1138. doi: 10.1093/infdis/jiaa804.
439. Marcenac P, Park GW, Duca LM, et al. Detection of SARS-CoV-2 on Surfaces in Households of Persons with COVID-19. *Int J Environ Res Public Health* 2021;18(15):8184.
440. Marconi VC, Ramanan AV, de Bono S, et al. Efficacy and safety of baricitinib in patients with COVID-19 infection: results from the randomised, double-blind, placebo-controlled, parallel-group COV-BARRIER phase 3 trial. *medRxiv* 2021:2021.04.30.21255934. doi: 10.1101/2021.04.30.21255934.
441. Marovich M, Mascola JR, Cohen MS. Monoclonal antibodies for prevention and treatment of COVID-19. *JAMA* 2020;324(2):131–132. doi: 10.1001/jama.2020.10245.
442. Martins MM, Prata-Barbosa A, da Cunha A. Update on SARS-CoV-2 infection in children. *Paediatr Int Child Health* 2021;41(1):56–64. doi: 10.1080/20469047.2021.1888026.
443. Marzano AV, Genovese G, Moltrasio C, et al. The clinical spectrum of COVID-19-associated cutaneous manifestations: an Italian multicenter study of 200 adult patients. *J Am Acad Dermatol* 2021;84(5):1356–1363. doi: 10.1016/j.jaad.2021.01.023.
444. Masters PS. The molecular biology of coronaviruses. *Adv Virus Res* 2006;66:193–292. doi: 10.1016/S0065-3527(06)66005-3.
445. Matar R, Alrahmani L, Monzer N, et al. clinical presentation and outcomes of pregnant women with coronavirus disease 2019: a systematic review and meta-analysis. *Clin Infect Dis* 2021;72(3):521–533. doi: 10.1093/cid/ciaa828.
446. Mathew D, Giles JR, Baxter AE, et al. Deep immune profiling of COVID-19 patients reveals distinct immunotypes with therapeutic implications. *Science* 2020;369(6508):eabc8511. doi: 10.1126/science.abc8511.
447. McAloon C, Collins Á, Hunt K, et al. Incubation period of COVID-19: a rapid systematic review and meta-analysis of observational research. *BMJ Open* 2020;10(8):e039652. doi: 10.1136/bmjopen-2020-039652.
448. McArdle AJ, Vito O, Patel H, et al. Treatment of multisystem inflammatory syndrome in children. *N Engl J Med* 2021;385(1):11–22. doi: 10.1056/NEJMoa2102968.
449. McCallum M, Bassi J, Marco AD, et al. SARS-CoV-2 immune evasion by variant B.1.427/B.1.429. *bioRxiv* 2021:2021.03.31.437925. doi: 10.1101/2021.03.31.437925.
450. McCormick DW, Richardson LC, Young PR, et al. Deaths in children and adolescents associated with COVID-19 and MIS-C in the United States. *Pediatrics* 2021;148(5):e2021052273. doi: 10.1542/peds.2021-052273.
451. McDonald SA, Miura F, Vos ERA, et al. Estimating the asymptomatic proportion of SARS-CoV-2 infection in the general population: analysis of nationwide serosurvey data in the Netherlands. *Eur J Epidemiol* 2021:1–5. doi: 10.1007/s10654-021-00768-y.
452. McMahan K, Yu J, Mercado NB, et al. Correlates of protection against SARS-CoV-2 in rhesus macaques. *Nature* 2021;590(7847):630–634. doi: 10.1038/s41586-020-03041-6.
453. Menezes MO, Takemoto MLS, Nakamura-Pereira M, et al. Risk factors for adverse outcomes among pregnant and postpartum women with acute respiratory distress syndrome due to COVID-19 in Brazil. *Int J Gynaecol Obstet* 2020;151(3):415–423. doi: 10.1002/ijgo.13407.
454. Meng H, Xiong R, He R, et al. CT imaging and clinical course of asymptomatic cases with COVID-19 pneumonia at admission in Wuhan, China. *J Infect* 2020;81(1):e33–e39. doi: 10.1016/j.jinf.2020.04.004.
455. Menter T, Haslbauer JD, Nienhold R, et al. Postmortem examination of COVID-19 patients reveals diffuse alveolar damage with severe capillary congestion and variegated findings in lungs and other organs suggesting vascular dysfunction. *Histopathology* 2020;77(2):198–209. doi: 10.1111/his.14134.
456. Mercado NB, Zahn R, Wegmann F, et al. Single-shot Ad26 vaccine protects against SARS-CoV-2 in rhesus macaques. *Nature* 2020;586(7830):583–588. doi: 10.1038/s41586-020-2607-z.
457. Merck. Merck and Ridgeback Biotherapeutics Provide Update on Progress of Clinical Development Program for Molnupiravir, an Investigational Oral Therapeutic for the Treatment of Mild-to-Moderate COVID-19. https://www.merck.com/news/merck-and-ridgeback-biotherapeutics-provide-update-on-progress-of-clinical-development-program-for-molnupiravir-an-investigational-oral-therapeutic-for-the-treatment-of-mild-to-moderate-covid-19/. Accessed October 30, 2021.
458. Mirsadraee S, Gorog DA, Mahon CF, et al. Prevalence of thrombotic complications in ICU-treated patients with coronavirus disease 2019 detected with systematic CT scanning. *Crit Care Med* 2021;49(5):804–815. doi: 10.1097/ccm.0000000000004890.
459. Mishra A, George AA, Sahu KK, et al. Tuberculosis and COVID-19 co-infection: an updated review. *Acta Biomed* 2020;92(1):e2021025. doi: 10.23750/abm.v92i1.10738.
460. Molteni E, Sudre CH, Canas LS, et al. Illness duration and symptom profile in symptomatic UK school-aged children tested for SARS-CoV-2. *Lancet Child Adolesc Health* 2021;5(10):708–718. doi: 10.1016/s2352-4642(21)00198-x.
461. Mondelli MU, Colaneri M, Seminari EM, et al. Low risk of SARS-CoV-2 transmission by fomites in real-life conditions. *Lancet Infect Dis* 2021;21(5):e112. doi: 10.1016/s1473-3099(20)30678-2.
462. Mondi A, Lorenzini P, Castilletti C, et al. Risk and predictive factors of prolonged viral RNA shedding in upper respiratory specimens in a large cohort of COVID-19 patients admitted to an Italian reference hospital. *Int J Infect Dis* 2021;105:532–539. doi: 10.1016/j.ijid.2021.02.117.
463. Monteiro RAA, Duarte-Neto AN, Silva L, et al. Ultrasound-guided minimally invasive autopsies: a protocol for the study of pulmonary and systemic involvement of COVID-19. *Clinics (Sao Paulo)* 2020;75:e1972. doi: 10.6061/clinics/2020/e1972.
464. Montenegro F, Unigarro L, Paredes G, et al. Acute respiratory distress syndrome (ARDS) caused by the novel coronavirus disease (COVID-19): a practical comprehensive literature review. *Expert Rev Respir Med* 2021;15(2):183–195. doi: 10.1080/17476348.2020.1820329.
465. Montgomery J, Ryan M, Engler R, et al. Myocarditis following immunization with mRNA COVID-19 vaccines in members of the US Military. *JAMA Cardiol* 2021;6(10):1202–1206. doi: 10.1001/jamacardio.2021.2833.
466. Moreira VM, Mascarenhas P, Machado V, et al. Diagnosis of SARS-Cov-2 infection by RT-PCR using specimens other than naso- and oropharyngeal swabs: a systematic review and meta-analysis. *Diagnostics (Basel)* 2021;11(2):363. doi: 10.3390/diagnostics11020363.
467. Morin L, Savale L, Pham T, et al. Four-month clinical status of a cohort of patients after hospitalization for COVID-19. *JAMA* 2021;325(15):1525–1534. doi: 10.1001/jama.2021.3331.
468. Morris SB, Schwartz NG, Patel P, et al. Case series of multisystem inflammatory syndrome in adults associated with SARS-CoV-2 infection - United Kingdom and United States, March-August 2020. *MMWR Morb Mortal Wkly Rep* 2020;69(40):1450–1456. doi: 10.15585/mmwr.mm6940e1.
469. Moustsen-Helms IR, Emborg H-D, Nielsen J, et al. Vaccine effectiveness after 1st and 2nd dose of the BNT162b2 mRNA Covid-19 Vaccine in long-term care facility residents and healthcare workers – a Danish cohort study. *medRxiv* 2021:2021.03.08.21252200. doi: 10.1101/2021.03.08.21252200.
470. Mozaffari E, Chandak A, Zhang Z, et al. Remdesivir treatment is associated with improved survival in hospitalized patients with COVID-19. Presented at: World Microbe Forum; 2021; Session WMF21-2970. https://www.abstractsonline.com/pp8/#!/9286/presentation/11269.
471. Mulangu S, Dodd LE, Davey RT, et al. A randomized, controlled trial of Ebola virus disease therapeutics. *N Engl J Med* 2019;381(24):2293–2303. doi: 10.1056/NEJMoa1910993.
472. Muller N, Kunze M, Steitz F, et al. Severe acute respiratory syndrome coronavirus 2 outbreak related to a nightclub, Germany, 2020. *Emerg Infect Dis* 2020;27(2):645–648. doi: 10.3201/eid2702.204443.
473. Mullins E, Hudak ML, Banerjee J, et al. Pregnancy and neonatal outcomes of COVID-19: coreporting of common outcomes from PAN-COVID and AAP-SONPM registries. *Ultrasound Obstet Gynecol* 2021;57(4):573–581. doi: 10.1002/uog.23619.
474. Munker D, Osterman A, Stubbe H, et al. Dynamics of SARS-CoV-2 shedding in the respiratory tract depends on the severity of disease in COVID-19 patients. *Eur Respir J* 2021;58(1):2002724. doi: 10.1183/13993003.02724-2020.
475. Murata T, Sakurai A, Suzuki M, et al. Shedding of viable virus in asymptomatic SARS-CoV-2 carriers. *mSphere* 2021;6(3). doi: 10.1128/mSphere.00019-21.
476. Mustafa Hellou M, Górska A, Mazzaferri F, et al. Nucleic acid amplification tests on respiratory samples for the diagnosis of coronavirus infections: a systematic review and meta-analysis. *Clin Microbiol Infect* 2021;27(3):341–351. doi: 10.1016/j.cmi.2020.11.002.
477. Nagashima M, Kumagai R, Yoshida I, et al. Characteristics of SARS-CoV-2 isolated from asymptomatic carriers in Tokyo. *Jpn J Infect Dis* 2020;73(4):320–322. doi: 10.7883/yoken.JJID.2020.137.
478. Nakajima Y, Ogai A, Furukawa K, et al. Prolonged viral shedding of SARS-CoV-2 in an immunocompromised patient. *J Infect Chemother* 2021;27(2):387–389. doi: 10.1016/j.jiac.2020.12.001.
479. Nalbandian A, Sehgal K, Gupta A, et al. Post-acute COVID-19 syndrome. *Nat Med* 2021;27(4):601–615. doi: 10.1038/s41591-021-01283-z.
480. Nanduri S, Pilishvili T, Derado G, et al. Effectiveness of Pfizer-BioNTech and Moderna vaccines in preventing SARS-CoV-2 infection among nursing home residents before and during widespread circulation of the SARS-CoV-2 B.1.617.2 (Delta) Variant - National Healthcare Safety Network, March 1-August 1, 2021. *MMWR Morb Mortal Wkly Rep* 2021;70(34):1163–1166. doi: 10.15585/mmwr.mm7034e3.
481. Nasreen S, Chung H, He S, et al. Effectiveness of COVID-19 vaccines against variants of concern in Ontario, Canada. *medRxiv* 2021:2021.06.28.21259420. doi: 10.1101/2021.06.28.21259420.
482. National Institute of Allergy and Infectious Diseases. NIH-Sponsored ACTIV-3 Clinical Trial Closes Enrollment into Two Sub-Studies. Updated March 4, 2021. https://www.nih.gov/news-events/news-releases/nih-sponsored-activ-3-clinical-trial-closes-enrollment-into-two-sub-studies
483. National Institute of Health COVID-19 Treatment Guidelines Panel. Coronavirus Disease 2019 (COVID-19) Treatment Guidelines. National Institutes of Health. 2021. https://www.covid19treatmentguidelines.nih.gov/. Accessed June 20, 2021.
484. Nehme M, Braillard O, Chappuis F, et al. Prevalence of symptoms more than seven months after diagnosis of symptomatic COVID-19 in an outpatient setting. *Ann Intern Med* 2021;174(9):1252–1260. doi: 10.7326/m21-0878.
485. Nie Y, Wang G, Shi X, et al. Neutralizing antibodies in patients with severe acute respiratory syndrome-associated coronavirus infection. *J Infect Dis* 2004;190(6):1119–1126. doi: 10.1086/423286.
486. Nissen K, Hagbom M, Krambrich J, et al. Presymptomatic viral shedding and infective ability of SARS-CoV-2; a case report. *Heliyon* 2021;7(2):e06328. doi: 10.1016/j.heliyon.2021.e06328.
487. Noh JY, Kwak JE, Yang JS, et al. Longitudinal assessment of anti-SARS-CoV-2 immune responses for six months based on the clinical severity of COVID-19. *J Infect Dis* 2021;224(5):754–763. doi: 10.1093/infdis/jiab124.
488. Nonaka CKV, Franco MM, Gräf T, et al. Genomic evidence of SARS-CoV-2 reinfection involving E484K spike mutation, Brazil. *Emerg Infect Dis* 2021;27(5):1522–1524. doi: 10.3201/eid2705.210191.
489. Nopp S, Moik F, Jilma B, et al. Risk of venous thromboembolism in patients with COVID-19: a systematic review and meta-analysis. *Res Pract Thromb Haemost* 2020;4(7):1178–1191. doi: 10.1002/rth2.12439.
490. Nordvig AS, Fong KT, Willey JZ, et al. Potential neurologic manifestations of COVID-19. *Neurol Clin Pract* 2021;11(2):e135–e146. doi: 10.1212/cpj.0000000000000897.
490a. Nyberg T, Ferguson NM, Nash SG, et al. Comparative analysis of the risks of hospitalisation and death associated with SARS-CoV-2 omicron (B.1.1.529) and delta (B.1.617.2) variants in England: a cohort study. *Lancet* 2022;399(10332):1303–1312. doi: 10.1016/s0140-6736(22)00462-7.
491. Nyberg T, Twohig KA, Harris RJ, et al. Risk of hospital admission for patients with SARS-CoV-2 variant B.1.1.7: cohort analysis. *BMJ* 2021;373:n1412. doi: 10.1136/bmj.n1412.
492. O Murchu E, Byrne P, Carty PG, et al. Quantifying the risk of SARS-CoV-2 reinfection over time. *Rev Med Virol* 2022;32(1):e2260. doi: 10.1002/rmv.2260.

493. Ojha V, Mani A, Pandey NN, et al. CT in coronavirus disease 2019 (COVID-19): a systematic review of chest CT findings in 4410 adult patients. *Eur Radiol* 2020;30(11):6129–6138. doi: 10.1007/s00330-020-06975-7.

494. Oliveira EA, Colosimo EA, Simões ESAC, et al. Clinical characteristics and risk factors for death among hospitalised children and adolescents with COVID-19 in Brazil: an analysis of a nationwide database. *Lancet Child Adolesc Health* 2021;5(8):559–568. doi: 10.1016/s2352-4642(21)00134-6.

495. Ong SWX, Chiew CJ, Ang LW, et al. Clinical and virological features of SARS-CoV-2 variants of concern: a retrospective cohort study comparing B.1.1.7 (Alpha), B.1.315 (Beta), and B.1.617.2 (Delta). *Clin Infect Dis* 2021:ciab721. doi: 10.1093/cid/ciab721.

496. Ong SWX, Fong SW, Young BE, et al. Persistent symptoms and association with inflammatory cytokine signatures in recovered coronavirus disease 2019 patients. *Open Forum Infect Dis* 2021;8(6):ofab156. doi: 10.1093/ofid/ofab156.

497. Ong SWX, Tan YK, Coleman KK, et al. Lack of viable severe acute respiratory coronavirus virus 2 (SARS-CoV-2) among PCR-positive air samples from hospital rooms and community isolation facilities. *Infect Control Hosp Epidemiol* 2021;42(11):1327–1332. doi: 10.1017/ice.2021.8.

498. Ortega-Paz L, Capodanno D, Montalescot G, et al. Coronavirus disease 2019-associated thrombosis and coagulopathy: review of the pathophysiological characteristics and implications for antithrombotic management. *J Am Heart Assoc* 2021;10(3):e019650. doi: 10.1161/jaha.120.019650.

499. Osmanov IM, Spiridonova E, Bobkova P, et al. Risk factors for long covid in previously hospitalised children using the ISARIC Global follow-up protocol: a prospective cohort study. *Eur Respir J* 2022;59(2):2101341. doi: 10.1183/13993003.01341-2021.

500. Osuchowski MF, Winkler MS, Skirecki T, et al. The COVID-19 puzzle: deciphering pathophysiology and phenotypes of a new disease entity. *Lancet Respir Med* 2021;9(6):622–642. doi: 10.1016/s2213-2600(21)00218-6.

501. Ou M, Zhu J, Ji P, et al. Risk factors of severe cases with COVID-19: a meta-analysis. *Epidemiol Infect* 2020;148:e175. doi: 10.1017/s095026882000179x.

502. Oude Munnink BB, Sikkema RS, Nieuwenhuijse DF, et al. Transmission of SARS-CoV-2 on mink farms between humans and mink and back to humans. *Science* 2021;371(6525):172–177. doi: 10.1126/science.abe5901.

503. Owen DR, Allerton CMN, Anderson AS, et al. An oral SARS-CoV-2 M^pro inhibitor clinical candidate for the treatment of COVID-19. *Science* 2021;374(6575):1586–1593. doi: 10.1126/science.abl4784.

504. Owusu D, Pomeroy MA, Lewis NM, et al. Persistent SARS-CoV-2 RNA shedding without evidence of infectiousness: a cohort study of individuals with COVID-19. *J Infect Dis* 2021;224(8):1362–1371. doi: 10.1093/infdis/jiab107.

504a. Pajon R, Doria-Rose NA, Shen X, et al. SARS-CoV-2 Omicron variant neutralization after mRNA-1273 booster vaccination. *N Engl J Med* 2022;386(11):1088–1091. doi: 10.1056/NEJMc2119912.

505. Pallesen J, Wang N, Corbett KS, et al. Immunogenicity and structures of a rationally designed prefusion MERS-CoV spike antigen. *Proc Natl Acad Sci U S A* 2017;114(35):E7348–E7357. doi: 10.1073/pnas.1707304114.

506. Pan F, Ye T, Sun P, et al. Time course of lung changes at chest CT during recovery from coronavirus disease 2019 (COVID-19). *Radiology* 2020;295(3):715–721. doi: 10.1148/radiol.2020200370.

507. Pan H, Peto R, Henao-Restrepo AM, et al. Repurposed antiviral drugs for Covid-19 - interim WHO solidarity trial results. *N Engl J Med* 2021;384(6):497–511. doi: 10.1056/NEJMoa2023184.

508. Pan L, Mu M, Yang P, et al. Clinical characteristics of COVID-19 patients with digestive symptoms in Hubei, China: a descriptive, cross-sectional, multicenter study. *Am J Gastroenterol* 2020;115(5):766–773. doi: 10.14309/ajg.0000000000000620.

509. Parasa S, Desai M, Thoguluva Chandrasekar V, et al. Prevalence of gastrointestinal symptoms and fecal viral shedding in patients with coronavirus disease 2019: a systematic review and meta-analysis. *JAMA Netw Open* 2020;3(6):e2011335. doi: 10.1001/jamanetworkopen.2020.11335.

510. Patberg ET, Adams T, Rekawek P, et al. Coronavirus disease 2019 infection and placental histopathology in women delivering at term. *Am J Obstet Gynecol* 2021;224(4):382.e1–382.e18. doi: 10.1016/j.ajog.2020.10.020.

511. Patel A, Agarwal R, Rudramurthy SM, et al. Multicenter epidemiologic study of coronavirus disease-associated mucormycosis, India. *Emerg Infect Dis* 2021;27(9):2349–2359. doi: 10.3201/eid2709.210934.

512. Patnaik UJ. Review article on COVID-19 and Guillain-Barré syndrome. *Front Biosci (Schol Ed)* 2021;13(1):97–104. doi: 10.52586/s555.

513. Patone M, Thomas K, Hatch R, et al. Mortality and critical care unit admission associated with the SARS-CoV-2 lineage B.1.1.7 in England: an observational cohort study. *Lancet Infect Dis* 2021;21(11):1518–1528. doi: 10.1016/s1473-3099(21)00318-2.

514. Pavord S, Scully M, Hunt BJ, et al. Clinical features of vaccine-induced immune thrombocytopenia and thrombosis. *N Engl J Med* 2021;385(18):1680–1689. doi: 10.1056/NEJMoa2109908.

515. Pawlowski C, Lenehan P, Puranik A, et al. FDA-authorized COVID-19 vaccines are effective per real-world evidence synthesized across a multi-state health system. *medRxiv* 2021:2021.02.15.21251623. doi: 10.1101/2021.02.15.21251623.

516. Payne AB, Gilani Z, Godfred-Cato S, et al. Incidence of multisystem inflammatory syndrome in children among US persons infected with SARS-CoV-2. *JAMA Netw Open* 2021;4(6):e2116420. doi: 10.1001/jamanetworkopen.2021.16420.

517. Peghin M, Palese A, Venturini M, et al. Post-COVID-19 symptoms 6 months after acute infection among hospitalized and non-hospitalized patients. *Clin Microbiol Infect* 2021;27(10):1507–1513. doi: 10.1016/j.cmi.2021.05.033.

518. Pegu A, O'Connell S, Schmidt SD, et al. Durability of mRNA-1273-induced antibodies against SARS-CoV-2 variants. *bioRxiv* 2021:2021.05.13.444010. doi: 10.1101/2021.05.13.444010.

519. Peiró Ó M, Carrasquer A, Sánchez-Gimenez R, et al. Biomarkers and short-term prognosis in COVID-19. *Biomarkers* 2021;26(2):119–126. doi: 10.1080/1354750x.2021.1874052.

520. Pelaia C, Tinello C, Vatrella A, et al. Lung under attack by COVID-19-induced cytokine storm: pathogenic mechanisms and therapeutic implications. *Ther Adv Respir Dis* 2020;14:1753466620933508. doi: 10.1177/1753466620933508.

521. Perera R, Tso E, Tsang OTY, et al. SARS-CoV-2 virus culture and subgenomic RNA for respiratory specimens from patients with mild coronavirus disease. *Emerg Infect Dis* 2020;26(11):2701–2704. doi: 10.3201/eid2611.203219.

522. Perna A, Passiatore M, Massaro A, et al. Skin manifestations in COVID-19 patients, state of the art. A systematic review. *Int J Dermatol* 2021;60(5):547–553. doi: 10.1111/ijd.15414.

523. Petrilli CM, Jones SA, Yang J, et al. Factors associated with hospital admission and critical illness among 5279 people with coronavirus disease 2019 in New York City: prospective cohort study. *BMJ* 2020;369:m1966. doi: 10.1136/bmj.m1966.

524. Pfizer. Pfizer's Novel COVID-19 Oral Antiviral Treatment Candidate Reduced Risk of Hospitalization or Death by 89% in Interim Analysis of Phase 2/3 EPIC-HR Study. https://www.pfizer.com/news/press-release/press-release-detail/pfizers-novel-covid-19-oral-antiviral-treatment-candidate. Accessed November 7, 2021.

525. Pijls BG, Jolani S, Atherley A, et al. Demographic risk factors for COVID-19 infection, severity, ICU admission and death: a meta-analysis of 59 studies. *BMJ Open* 2021;11(1):e044640. doi: 10.1136/bmjopen-2020-044640.

526. Pilishvili T, Fleming-Dutra KE, Farrar JL, et al. Interim estimates of vaccine effectiveness of Pfizer-BioNTech and Moderna COVID-19 vaccines among health care personnel - 33 U.S. Sites, January-March 2021. *MMWR Morb Mortal Wkly Rep* 2021;70(20):753–758. doi: 10.15585/mmwr.mm7020e2.

526a. Planas D, Saunders N, Maes P, et al. Considerable escape of SARS-CoV-2 Omicron to antibody neutralization. *Nature* 2022;602(7898):671–675. doi: 10.1038/s41586-021-04389-z.

527. Polack FP, Teng MN, Collins PL, et al. A role for immune complexes in enhanced respiratory syncytial virus disease. *J Exp Med* 2002;196(6):859–865. doi: 10.1084/jem.20020781.

528. Polack FP, Thomas SJ, Kitchin N, et al. Safety and efficacy of the BNT162b2 mRNA Covid-19 vaccine. *N Engl J Med* 2020;383(27):2603–2615. doi: 10.1056/NEJMoa2034577.

529. Potere N, Valeriani E, Candeloro M, et al. Acute complications and mortality in hospitalized patients with coronavirus disease 2019: a systematic review and meta-analysis. *Crit Care* 2020;24(1):389. doi: 10.1186/s13054-020-03022-1.

530. Pranata R, Lim MA, Yonas E, et al. Body mass index and outcome in patients with COVID-19: A dose-response meta-analysis. *Diabetes Metab* 2021;47(2):101178. doi: 10.1016/j.diabet.2020.07.005.

531. Prattes J, Wauters J, Giacobbe DR, et al. Risk factors and outcome of pulmonary aspergillosis in critically ill coronavirus disease 2019 patients- a multinational observational study by the European Confederation of Medical Mycology. *Clin Microbiol Infect* 2021:S1198-743X(21)00474-2. doi: 10.1016/j.cmi.2021.08.014.

532. Pray IW, Ford L, Cole D, et al. Performance of an antigen-based test for asymptomatic and symptomatic SARS-CoV-2 testing at two university campuses - Wisconsin, September-October 2020. *MMWR Morb Mortal Wkly Rep* 2021;69(5152):1642–1647. doi: 10.15585/mmwr.mm695152a3.

533. Prebensen C, Myhre PL, Jonassen C, et al. Severe acute respiratory syndrome coronavirus 2 RNA in plasma is associated with ICU admission and mortality in patients hospitalized with COVID-19. *Clin Infect Dis* 2021;73(3):e799–e802. doi: 10.1093/cid/ciaa1338.

533a. Price AM, Olson SM, Newhams MM, et al. BNT162b2 protection against the Omicron variant in children and adolescents. *N Engl J Med* 2022. doi: 10.1056/NEJMoa2202826.

534. Price-Haywood EG, Burton J, Fort D, et al. Hospitalization and mortality among black patients and white patients with Covid-19. *N Engl J Med* 2020;382(26):2534–2543. doi: 10.1056/NEJMsa2011686.

535. Prince-Guerra JL, Almendares O, Nolen LD, et al. Evaluation of Abbott BinaxNOW rapid antigen test for SARS-CoV-2 infection at two community-based testing sites - Pima County, Arizona, November 3–17, 2020. *MMWR Morb Mortal Wkly Rep* 2021;70(3):100–105. doi: 10.15585/mmwr.mm7003e3.

536. Pujadas E, Chaudhry F, McBride R, et al. SARS-CoV-2 viral load predicts COVID-19 mortality. *Lancet Respir Med* 2020;8(9):e70. doi: 10.1016/s2213-2600(20)30354-4.

537. Pulinx B, Kieffer D, Michiels I, et al. Vertical transmission of SARS-CoV-2 infection and preterm birth. *Eur J Clin Microbiol Infect Dis* 2020;39(12):2441–2445. doi: 10.1007/s10096-020-03964-y.

538. Pullen MF, Skipper CP, Hullsiek KH, et al. Symptoms of COVID-19 outpatients in the United States. *Open Forum Infect Dis* 2020;7(7):ofaa271. doi: 10.1093/ofid/ofaa271.

539. Qian G, Yang N, Ma AHY, et al. COVID-19 transmission within a family cluster by presymptomatic carriers in China. *Clin Infect Dis* 2020;71(15):861–862. doi: 10.1093/cid/ciaa316.

540. Qiu L, Liu X, Xiao M, et al. SARS-CoV-2 is not detectable in the vaginal fluid of women with severe COVID-19 infection. *Clin Infect Dis* 2020;71(15):813–817. doi: 10.1093/cid/ciaa375.

541. Rai B, Shukla A, Dwivedi LK. Estimates of serial interval for COVID-19: a systematic review and meta-analysis. *Clin Epidemiol Glob Health* 2021;9:157–161. doi: 10.1016/j.cegh.2020.08.007.

542. Ranzani OT, Bastos LSL, Gelli JGM, et al. Characterisation of the first 250,000 hospital admissions for COVID-19 in Brazil: a retrospective analysis of nationwide data. *Lancet Respir Med* 2021;9(4):407–418. doi: 10.1016/s2213-2600(20)30560-9.

543. Rao SN, Manissero D, Steele VR, et al. A systematic review of the clinical utility of cycle threshold values in the context of COVID-19. *Infect Dis Ther* 2020;9(3):573–586. doi: 10.1007/s40121-020-00324-3.

544. Raphaël JC, Chevret S, Hughes RAC, et al. Plasma exchange for Guillain-Barré syndrome. *Cochrane Database Syst Rev* 2012;(7):CD001798. doi: 10.1002/14651858.CD001798.pub2.

545. Raschetti R, Vivanti AJ, Vauloup-Fellous C, et al. Synthesis and systematic review of reported neonatal SARS-CoV-2 infections. *Nat Commun* 2020;11(1):5164. doi: 10.1038/s41467-020-18982-9.

546. Razazi K, Arrestier R, Haudebourg AF, et al. Risks of ventilator-associated pneumonia and invasive pulmonary aspergillosis in patients with viral acute respiratory distress syndrome related or not to Coronavirus 19 disease. *Crit Care* 2020;24(1):699. doi: 10.1186/s13054-020-03417-0.
547. RECOVERY Collaborative Group. Lopinavir-ritonavir in patients admitted to hospital with COVID-19 (RECOVERY): a randomised, controlled, open-label, platform trial. *Lancet* 2020;396(10259):1345–1352. doi: 10.1016/s0140-6736(20)32013-4.
548. RECOVERY Collaborative Group. Azithromycin in patients admitted to hospital with COVID-19 (RECOVERY): a randomised, controlled, open-label, platform trial. *Lancet* 2021;397(10274):605–612. doi: 10.1016/s0140-6736(21)00149-5.
549. RECOVERY Collaborative Group. Convalescent plasma in patients admitted to hospital with COVID-19 (RECOVERY): a randomised controlled, open-label, platform trial. *Lancet* 2021;397(10289):2049–2059. doi: 10.1016/s0140-6736(21)00897-7.
550. RECOVERY Collaborative Group. Tocilizumab in patients admitted to hospital with COVID-19 (RECOVERY): a randomised, controlled, open-label, platform trial. *Lancet* 2021;397(10285):1637–1645. doi: 10.1016/S0140-6736(21)00676-0.
551. RECOVERY Collaborative Group, Horby P, Lim WS, Emberson JR, et al. Dexamethasone in hospitalized patients with Covid-19. *N Engl J Med* 2020;384(8):693–704. doi: 10.1056/NEJMoa2021436.
552. RECOVERY Collaborative Group, Horby PW, Campbell M, et al. Colchicine in patients admitted to hospital with COVID-19 (RECOVERY): a randomised, controlled, open-label, platform trial. *medRxiv* 2021:2021.05.18.21257267. doi: 10.1101/2021.05.18.21257267.
553. RECOVERY Collaborative Group, Horby PW, Mafham M, et al. Casirivimab and imdevimab in patients admitted to hospital with COVID-19 (RECOVERY): a randomised, controlled, open-label, platform trial. *medRxiv* 2021:2021.06.15.21258542. doi: 10.1101/2021.06.15.21258542.
554. RECOVERY Collaborative Group, Horby PW, Pessoa-Amorim G, et al. Aspirin in patients admitted to hospital with COVID-19 (RECOVERY): a randomised, controlled, open-label, platform trial. *medRxiv* 2021:2021.06.08.21258132. doi: 10.1101/2021.06.08.21258132.
555. Redd WD, Zhou JC, Hathorn KE, et al. Prevalence and characteristics of gastrointestinal symptoms in patients with severe acute respiratory syndrome coronavirus 2 infection in the United States: a multicenter cohort study. *Gastroenterology* 2020;159(2):765–767.e2. doi: 10.1053/j.gastro.2020.04.045.
556. Regeneron. Phase 3 Prevention Trial Showed 81% Reduced Risk Of Symptomatic Sars-Cov-2 Infections With Subcutaneous Administration Of Regen-Cov™ (Casirivimab With Imdevimab). Updated April 12, 2021. https://investor.regeneron.com/news-releases/news-release-details/phase-3-prevention-trial-showed-81-reduced-risk-symptomatic-sars. Accessed July 31, 2021.
557. Regev-Yochay G, Amit S, Bergwerk M, et al. Decreased infectivity following BNT162b2 vaccination: a prospective cohort study in Israel. *Lancet Reg Health Eur* 2021;7:100150. doi: 10.1016/j.lanepe.2021.100150.
558. REMAP-CAP Investigators, Gordon AC, Mouncey PR, Al-Beidh F, et al. Interleukin-6 receptor antagonists in critically ill patients with Covid-19. *N Engl J Med* 2021;384(16):1491–1502. doi: 10.1056/NEJMoa2100433.
559. REMAP-CAP T, ACTIV-4a, ATTACC Investigators, Zarychanski R. Therapeutic anticoagulation in critically ill patients with Covid-19 – preliminary report. *medRxiv* 2021:2021.03.10.21252749. doi: 10.1101/2021.03.10.21252749.
560. Resende PC, Bezerra JF, Teixeira Vasconcelos RH, et al. Severe acute respiratory syndrome coronavirus 2 P.2 lineage associated with reinfection case, Brazil, June-October 2020. *Emerg Infect Dis* 2021;27(7):1789–1794. doi: 10.3201/eid2707.210401.
561. Rha MS, Shin EC. Activation or exhaustion of CD8(+) T cells in patients with COVID-19. *Cell Mol Immunol* 2021:1–9. doi: 10.1038/s41423-021-00750-4.
562. Richard M, Kok A, de Meulder D, et al. SARS-CoV-2 is transmitted via contact and via the air between ferrets. *Nat Commun* 2020;11(1):3496. doi: 10.1038/s41467-020-17367-2.
563. Rogers JP, Chesney E, Oliver D, et al. Psychiatric and neuropsychiatric presentations associated with severe coronavirus infections: a systematic review and meta-analysis with comparison to the COVID-19 pandemic. *Lancet Psychiatry* 2020;7(7):611–627. doi: 10.1016/s2215-0366(20)30203-0.
564. Rogers JP, Watson CJ, Badenoch J, et al. Neurology and neuropsychiatry of COVID-19: a systematic review and meta-analysis of the early literature reveals frequent CNS manifestations and key emerging narratives. *J Neurol Neurosurg Psychiatry* 2021;92(9):932–941.doi: 10.1136/jnnp-2021-326405.
565. Roman YM, Burela PA, Pasupuleti V, et al. Ivermectin for the treatment of COVID-19: A systematic review and meta-analysis of randomized controlled trials. *Clin Infect Dis* 2021:ciab591. doi: 10.1093/cid/ciab591.
566. Roncon L, Zuin M, Barco S, et al. Incidence of acute pulmonary embolism in COVID-19 patients: Systematic review and meta-analysis. *Eur J Intern Med* 2020;82:29–37. doi: 10.1016/j.ejim.2020.09.006.
567. Rosas IO, Bräu N, Waters M, et al. Tocilizumab in hospitalized patients with severe Covid-19 pneumonia. *N Engl J Med* 2021;384(16):1503–1516. doi: 10.1056/NEJMoa2028700.
568. Rosenberg ES, Holtgrave DR, Dorabawila V, et al. New COVID-19 cases and hospitalizations among adults, by vaccination status—New York, May 3-July 25, 2021. *MMWR Morb Mortal Wkly Rep* 2021;70(37):1306–1311. doi: 10.15585/mmwr.mm7037a7.
569. Rosenblum HG, Hadler SC, Moulia D, et al. Use of COVID-19 vaccines after reports of adverse events among adult recipients of Janssen (Johnson & Johnson) and mRNA COVID-19 vaccines (Pfizer-BioNTech and Moderna): update from the Advisory Committee on Immunization Practices - United States, July 2021. *MMWR Morb Mortal Wkly Rep* 2021;70(32):1094–1099. doi: 10.15585/mmwr.mm7032e4.
570. Rosenthal N, Cao Z, Gundrum J, et al. Risk factors associated with in-hospital mortality in a US national sample of patients with COVID-19. *JAMA Netw Open* 2020;3(12):e2029058. doi: 10.1001/jamanetworkopen.2020.29058.
571. Roshandel MR, Nateqi M, Lak R, et al. Diagnostic and methodological evaluation of studies on the urinary shedding of SARS-CoV-2, compared to stool and serum: a systematic review and meta-analysis. *Cell Mol Biol (Noisy-le-Grand)* 2020;66(6):148–156.
572. Rostad CA, Chahroudi A, Mantus G, et al. Quantitative SARS-CoV-2 serology in children with Multisystem Inflammatory Syndrome (MIS-C). *Pediatrics* 2020;146(6):e2020018242. doi: 10.1542/peds.2020-018242.
573. Roth GA, Emmons-Bell S, Alger HM, et al. Trends in patient characteristics and COVID-19 in-hospital mortality in the united states during the COVID-19 pandemic. *JAMA Netw Open* 2021;4(5):e218828. doi: 10.1001/jamanetworkopen.2021.8828.
574. Rothe K, Feihl S, Schneider J, et al. Rates of bacterial co-infections and antimicrobial use in COVID-19 patients: a retrospective cohort study in light of antibiotic stewardship. *Eur J Clin Microbiol Infect Dis* 2021;40(4):859–869. doi: 10.1007/s10096-020-04063-8.
575. Rouze A, Martin-Loeches I, Povoa P, et al. Early bacterial identification among intubated patients with COVID-19 or influenza pneumonia: a european multicenter comparative cohort study. *Am J Respir Crit Care Med* 2021;204(5):546–556. doi: 10.1164/rccm.202101-0030OC.
576. Rubin GD, Ryerson CJ, Haramati LB, et al. The role of chest imaging in patient management during the COVID-19 pandemic: a multinational consensus statement from the Fleischner Society. *Chest* 2020;158(1):106–116. doi: 10.1016/j.chest.2020.04.003.
577. Russell CD, Fairfield CJ, Drake TM, et al. Co-infections, secondary infections, and antimicrobial use in patients hospitalised with COVID-19 during the first pandemic wave from the ISARIC WHO CCP-UK study: a multicentre, prospective cohort study. *Lancet Microbe* 2021;2(8):e354–e365. doi: 10.1016/s2666-5247(21)00090-2.
578. Ryan DJ, Toomey S, Madden SF, et al. Use of exhaled breath condensate (EBC) in the diagnosis of SARS-COV-2 (COVID-19). *Thorax* 2021;76(1):86–88. doi: 10.1136/thoraxjnl-2020-215705.
579. Saatci D, Ranger TA, Garriga C, et al. Association between race and COVID-19 outcomes among 2.6 million children in England. *JAMA Pediatr* 2021;175(9):928–938. doi: 10.1001/jamapediatrics.2021.1685.
580. Saddique A, Rana MS, Alam MM, et al. Emergence of co-infection of COVID-19 and dengue: a serious public health threat. *J Infect* 2020;81(6):e16–e18. doi: 10.1016/j.jinf.2020.08.009.
581. Sadoff J, Gray G, Vandebosch A, et al. Safety and efficacy of single-dose Ad26.COV2.S vaccine against Covid-19. *N Engl J Med* 2021;384(23):2187–2201. doi: 10.1056/NEJMoa2101544.
582. Sahbudak Bal Z, Ozkul A, Bilen M, et al. The longest infectious virus shedding in a child infected with the G614 strain of SARS-CoV-2. *Pediatr Infect Dis J* 2021;40(7):e263–e265. doi: 10.1097/inf.0000000000003158.
583. Sakharkar M, Rappazzo CG, Wieland-Alter WF, et al. Prolonged evolution of the human B cell response to SARS-CoV-2 infection. *Sci Immunol* 2021;6(56):eabg6916. doi: 10.1126/sciimmunol.abg6916.
584. Salama C, Han J, Yau L, et al. Tocilizumab in patients hospitalized with Covid-19 pneumonia. *N Engl J Med* 2021;384(1):20–30. doi: 10.1056/NEJMoa2030340.
585. Salvarani C, Dolci G, Massari M, et al. Effect of tocilizumab vs standard care on clinical worsening in patients hospitalized with COVID-19 pneumonia: a randomized clinical trial. *JAMA Intern Med* 2021;181(1):24–31. doi: 10.1001/jamainternmed.2020.6615.
586. Sameni F, Hajikhani B, Yaslianifard S, et al. COVID-19 and skin manifestations: an overview of case reports/case series and meta-analysis of prevalence studies. *Front Med (Lausanne)* 2020;7:573188. doi: 10.3389/fmed.2020.573188.
587. Santarpia JL, Rivera DN, Herrera VL, et al. Aerosol and surface contamination of SARS-CoV-2 observed in quarantine and isolation care. *Sci Rep* 2020;10(1):12732. doi: 10.1038/s41598-020-69286-3.
588. Sardari A, Tabarsi P, Borhany H, et al. Myocarditis detected after COVID-19 recovery. *Eur Heart J Cardiovasc Imaging* 2021;22(1):131–132. doi: 10.1093/ehjci/jeaa166.
589. Scheschowitsch K, Leite JA, Assreuy J. New insights in glucocorticoid receptor signaling-more than just a ligand-binding receptor. *Front Endocrinol (Lausanne)* 2017;8:16. doi: 10.3389/fendo.2017.00016.
590. Schirmer P, Lucero-Obusan C, Sharma A, et al. Respiratory co-infections with COVID-19 in the Veterans Health Administration, 2020. *Diagn Microbiol Infect Dis* 2021;100(1):115312. doi: 10.1016/j.diagmicrobio.2021.115312.
591. Scorzolini L, Corpolongo A, Castilletti C, et al. Comment on the potential risks of sexual and vertical transmission of COVID-19. *Clin Infect Dis* 2020;71(16):2298. doi: 10.1093/cid/ciaa445.
592. Seeßle J, Waterboer T, Hippchen T, et al. Persistent symptoms in adult patients one year after COVID-19: a prospective cohort study. *Clin Infect Dis* 2021:ciab611. doi: 10.1093/cid/ciab611.
593. Sekhawat V, Green A, Mahadeva U. COVID-19 autopsies: conclusions from international studies. *Diagn Histopathol (Oxf)* 2021;27(3):103–107. doi: 10.1016/j.mpdhp.2020.11.008.
594. Sekine T, Perez-Potti A, Rivera-Ballesteros O, et al. Robust T cell immunity in convalescent individuals with asymptomatic or mild COVID-19. *Cell* 2020;183(1):158–168.e14. doi: 10.1016/j.cell.2020.08.017.
595. Seppälä E, Veneti L, Starrfelt J, et al. Vaccine effectiveness against infection with the Delta (B.1.617.2) variant, Norway, April to August 2021. *Euro Surveill* 2021;26(35):2100793. doi: 10.2807/1560-7917.Es.2021.26.35.2100793.
596. Sepulveda J, Westblade LF, Whittier S, et al. Bacteremia and Blood Culture Utilization during COVID-19 Surge in New York City. *J Clin Microbiol* 2020;58(8):e00875-20. doi: 10.1128/jcm.00875-20.
597. Sethuraman N, Jeremiah SS, Ryo A. Interpreting diagnostic tests for SARS-CoV-2. *JAMA* 2020;323(22):2249–2251. doi: 10.1001/jama.2020.8259.
598. Sevilla-Castillo F, Roque-Reyes OJ, Romero-Lechuga F, et al. Both chloroquine and lopinavir/ritonavir are ineffective for COVID-19 treatment and combined worsen the pathology: a single-center experience with severely ill patients. *Biomed Res Int* 2021;2021:8821318. doi: 10.1155/2021/8821318.
599. Shahjouei S, Tsivgoulis G, Farahmand G, et al. SARS-CoV-2 and stroke characteristics: a report from the multinational COVID-19 stroke study group. *Stroke* 2021;52(5):e117–e130. doi: 10.1161/strokeaha.120.032927.
600. Shahrizaila N, Lehmann HC, Kuwabara S. Guillain-Barré syndrome. *Lancet* 2021;397(10280):1214–1228. doi: 10.1016/s0140-6736(21)00517-1.

601. Shay DK, Gee J, Su JR, et al. Safety monitoring of the Janssen (Johnson & Johnson) COVID-19 vaccine - United States, March-April 2021. *MMWR Morb Mortal Wkly Rep* 2021;70(18):680–684. doi: 10.15585/mmwr.mm7018e2.

602. Sheahan TP, Sims AC, Graham RL, et al. Broad-spectrum antiviral GS-5734 inhibits both epidemic and zoonotic coronaviruses. *Sci Transl Med* 2017;9(396):eaal3653. doi: 10.1126/scitranslmed.aal3653.

603. Sheahan TP, Sims AC, Leist SR, et al. Comparative therapeutic efficacy of remdesivir and combination lopinavir, ritonavir, and interferon beta against MERS-CoV. *Nat Commun* 2020;11(1):222. doi: 10.1038/s41467-019-13940-6.

604. Sheikh A, McMenamin J, Taylor B, et al. SARS-CoV-2 Delta VOC in Scotland: demographics, risk of hospital admission, and vaccine effectiveness. *Lancet* 2021;397(10293):2461–2462. doi: 10.1016/S0140-6736(21)01358-1.

605. Shen C, Wang Z, Zhao F, et al. Treatment of 5 critically ill patients with COVID-19 with convalescent plasma. *JAMA* 2020;323(16):1582–1589. doi: 10.1001/jama.2020.4783.

606. Shi H, Han X, Jiang N, et al. Radiological findings from 81 patients with COVID-19 pneumonia in Wuhan, China: a descriptive study. *Lancet Infect Dis* 2020;20(4):425–434. doi: 10.1016/s1473-3099(20)30086-4.

607. Shi Q, Wang Z, Liu J, et al. Risk factors for poor prognosis in children and adolescents with COVID-19: a systematic review and meta-analysis. *EClinicalMedicine* 2021;41:101155. doi: 10.1016/j.eclinm.2021.101155.

608. Shi S, Qin M, Shen B, et al. Association of cardiac injury with mortality in hospitalized patients with COVID-19 in Wuhan, China. *JAMA Cardiol* 2020;5(7):802–810. doi: 10.1001/jamacardio.2020.0950.

609. Shimabukuro TT, Kim SY, Myers TR, et al. Preliminary findings of mRNA Covid-19 vaccine safety in pregnant persons. *N Engl J Med* 2021;384(24):2273–2282. doi: 10.1056/NEJMoa2104983.

610. Shin HS, Kim Y, Kim G, et al. Immune responses to middle east respiratory syndrome coronavirus during the acute and convalescent phases of human infection. *Clin Infect Dis* 2019;68(6):984–992. doi: 10.1093/cid/ciy595.

611. Siegel DA, Reses HE, Cool AJ, et al. Trends in COVID-19 cases, emergency department visits, and hospital admissions among children and adolescents aged 0–17 years - United States, August 2020-August 2021. *MMWR Morb Mortal Wkly Rep* 2021;70(36):1249–1254. doi: 10.15585/mmwr.mm7036e1.

612. Simonovich VA, Burgos Pratx LD, Scibona P, et al. A randomized trial of convalescent plasma in Covid-19 severe pneumonia. *N Engl J Med* 2021;384(7):619–629. doi: 10.1056/NEJMoa2031304.

613. Simpson S, Kay FU, Abbara S, et al. Radiological Society of North America Expert Consensus Statement on reporting chest CT findings related to COVID-19. Endorsed by the Society of Thoracic Radiology, the American College of Radiology, and RSNA - Secondary Publication. *J Thorac Imaging* 2020;35(4):219–227. doi: 10.1097/rti.0000000000000524.

614. Singanayagam A, Patel M, Charlett A, et al. Duration of infectiousness and correlation with RT-PCR cycle threshold values in cases of COVID-19, England, January to May 2020. *Euro Surveill* 2020;25(32):2001483. doi: 10.2807/1560-7917.Es.2020.25.32.2001483.

615. Sjoding MW, Dickson RP, Iwashyna TJ, et al. Racial bias in pulse oximetry measurement. *N Engl J Med* 2020;383(25):2477–2478. doi: 10.1056/NEJMc2029240.

616. Somekh I, Stein M, Karakis I, et al. Characteristics of SARS-CoV-2 infections in israeli children during the circulation of different SARS-CoV-2 variants. *JAMA Netw Open* 2021;4(9):e2124343. doi: 10.1001/jamanetworkopen.2021.24343.

617. Son MBF, Murray N, Friedman K, et al. Multisystem inflammatory syndrome in children - initial therapy and outcomes. *N Engl J Med* 2021;385(1):23–34. doi: 10.1056/NEJMoa2102605.

618. Song JW, Zhang C, Fan X, et al. Immunological and inflammatory profiles in mild and severe cases of COVID-19. *Nat Commun* 2020;11(1):3410. doi: 10.1038/s41467-020-17240-2.

619. Søraas A, Bø R, Kalleberg KT, et al. Self-reported memory problems 8 months after COVID-19 infection. *JAMA Netw Open* 2021;4(7):e2118717. doi: 10.1001/jamanetworkopen.2021.18717.

620. Spinner CD, Gottlieb RL, Criner GJ, et al. Effect of remdesivir vs standard care on clinical status at 11 days in patients with moderate COVID-19: a randomized clinical trial. *JAMA* 2020;324(11):1048–1057. doi: 10.1001/jama.2020.16349.

621. Stanoeva KR, van der Eijk AA, Meijer A, et al. Towards a sensitive and accurate interpretation of molecular testing for SARS-CoV-2: a rapid review of 264 studies. *Euro Surveill* 2021;26(10):2001134. doi: 10.2807/1560-7917.Es.2021.26.10.2001134.

622. Starr TN, Greaney AJ, Addetia A, et al. Prospective mapping of viral mutations that escape antibodies used to treat COVID-19. *Science* 2021;371(6531):850–854. doi: 10.1126/science.abf9302.

623. Staub T, Arendt V, Lasso de la Vega EC, et al. Case series of four re-infections with a SARS-CoV-2 B.1.351 variant, Luxembourg, February 2021. *Euro Surveill* 2021;26(18):2100423. doi: 10.2807/1560-7917.Es.2021.26.18.2100423.

624. Sterne JAC, Murthy S, Diaz JV, et al. Association between administration of systemic corticosteroids and mortality among critically ill patients with COVID-19: a meta-analysis. *JAMA* 2020;324(13):1330–1341. doi: 10.1001/jama.2020.17023.

625. Stierman B, Abrams JY, Godfred-Cato SE, et al. Racial and ethnic disparities in multisystem inflammatory syndrome in children in the United States, March 2020 to February 2021. *Pediatr Infect Dis J* 2021;40(11):e400–e406. doi: 10.1097/inf.0000000000003294.

626. Stokes AC, Lundberg DJ, Elo IT, et al. COVID-19 and excess mortality in the United States: a county-level analysis. *PLoS Med* 2021;18(5):e1003571. doi: 10.1371/journal.pmed.1003571.

627. Stone JH, Frigault MJ, Serling-Boyd NJ, et al. Efficacy of tocilizumab in patients hospitalized with Covid-19. *N Engl J Med* 2020;383(24):2333–2344. doi: 10.1056/NEJMoa2028836.

628. Stowe J, Tessier E, Zhao H, et al. Interactions between SARS-CoV-2 and influenza, and the impact of coinfection on disease severity: a test-negative design. *Int J Epidemiol* 2021;50(4):1124–1133. doi: 10.1093/ije/dyab081.

629. Strålin K, Wahlström E, Walther S, et al. Mortality trends among hospitalised COVID-19 patients in Sweden: a nationwide observational cohort study. *Lancet Reg Health Eur* 2021;4:100054. doi: 10.1016/j.lanepe.2021.100054.

630. Su H, Yang M, Wan C, et al. Renal histopathological analysis of 26 postmortem findings of patients with COVID-19 in China. *Kidney Int* 2020;98(1):219–227. doi: 10.1016/j.kint.2020.04.003.

631. Subbarao K, McAuliffe J, Vogel L, et al. Prior infection and passive transfer of neutralizing antibody prevent replication of severe acute respiratory syndrome coronavirus in the respiratory tract of mice. *J Virol* 2004;78(7):3572–3577. doi: 10.1128/jvi.78.7.3572-3577.2004.

632. Sudre CH, Murray B, Varsavsky T, et al. Attributes and predictors of long COVID. *Nat Med* 2021;27(4):626–631. doi: 10.1038/s41591-021-01292-y.

633. Sugano N, Ando W, Fukushima W. Cluster of severe acute respiratory syndrome coronavirus 2 infections linked to music clubs in Osaka, Japan. *J Infect Dis* 2020;222(10):1635–1640. doi: 10.1093/infdis/jiaa542.

634. Sun J, Patel RC, Zheng Q, et al. COVID-19 disease severity among people with HIV infection or solid organ transplant in the United States: a nationally-representative, multicenter, observational cohort study. *medRxiv* 2021:2021.07.26.21261028. doi: 10.1101/2021.07.26.21261028.

635. Sun J, Zhu A, Li H, et al. Isolation of infectious SARS-CoV-2 from urine of a COVID-19 patient. *Emerg Microbes Infect* 2020;9(1):991–993. doi: 10.1080/22221751.2020.1760144.

636. Sun J, Zhuang Z, Zheng J, et al. Generation of a broadly useful model for COVID-19 pathogenesis, vaccination, and treatment. *Cell* 2020;182(3):734–743 e5. doi: 10.1016/j.cell.2020.06.010.

637. Swift MD, Breeher LE, Tande AJ, et al. Effectiveness of mRNA COVID-19 vaccines against SARS-CoV-2 infection in a cohort of healthcare personnel. *Clin Infect Dis* 2021;73(6):e1376–e1379. doi: 10.1093/cid/ciab361.

638. Syangtan G, Bista S, Dawadi P, et al. Asymptomatic SARS-CoV-2 carriers: a systematic review and meta-analysis. *Front Public Health* 2020;8:587374. doi: 10.3389/fpubh.2020.587374.

639. Talasaz AH, Sadeghipour P, Kakavand H, et al. Antithrombotic therapy in COVID-19: systematic summary of ongoing or completed randomized trials. *medRxiv* 2021:2021.01.04.21249227. doi: 10.1101/2021.01.04.21249227.

640. Tammaro A, Adebanjo GAR, Del Nonno F, et al. Cutaneous endothelial dysfunction and complement deposition in COVID-19. *Am J Dermatopathol* 2021;43(3):237–238. doi: 10.1097/dad.0000000000001825.

641. Tamuzi JL, Ayele BT, Shumba CS, et al. Implications of COVID-19 in high burden countries for HIV/TB: a systematic review of evidence. *BMC Infect Dis* 2020;20(1):744. doi: 10.1186/s12879-020-05450-4.

642. Tan E, Song J, Deane AM, et al. Global impact of coronavirus disease 2019 infection requiring admission to the ICU: a systematic review and meta-analysis. *Chest* 2021;159(2):524–536. doi: 10.1016/j.chest.2020.10.014.

643. Tan YJ, Goh PY, Fielding BC, et al. Profiles of antibody responses against severe acute respiratory syndrome coronavirus recombinant proteins and their potential use as diagnostic markers. *Clin Diagn Lab Immunol* 2004;11(2):362–371. doi: 10.1128/cdli.11.2.362-371.2004.

644. Tande AJ, Pollock BD, Shah ND, et al. Impact of the COVID-19 vaccine on asymptomatic infection among patients undergoing pre-procedural COVID-19 molecular screening. *Clin Infect Dis* 2022;74(1):59–65. doi: 10.1093/cid/ciab229.

645. Tang N, Li D, Wang X, et al. Abnormal coagulation parameters are associated with poor prognosis in patients with novel coronavirus pneumonia. *J Thromb Haemost* 2020;18(4):844–847. doi: 10.1111/jth.14768.

646. Tang P, Hasan MR, Chemaitelly H, et al. BNT162b2 and mRNA-1273 COVID-19 vaccine effectiveness against the Delta (B.1.617.2) variant in Qatar. *medRxiv* 2021:2021.08.11.21261885. doi: 10.1101/2021.08.11.21261885.

647. Taquet M, Dercon Q, Luciano S, et al. Incidence, co-occurrence, and evolution of long-COVID features: a 6-month retrospective cohort study of 273,618 survivors of COVID-19. *PLoS Med* 2021;18(9):e1003773. doi: 10.1371/journal.pmed.1003773.

648. Tarhini H, Recoing A, Bridier-Nahmias A, et al. Long term SARS-CoV-2 infectiousness among three immunocompromised patients: from prolonged viral shedding to SARS-CoV-2 superinfection. *J Infect Dis* 2021;223(9):1522–1527. doi: 10.1093/infdis/jiab075.

649. Tartof SY, Qian L, Hong V, et al. Obesity and mortality among patients diagnosed with COVID-19: results from an integrated health care organization. *Ann Intern Med* 2020;173(10):773–781. doi: 10.7326/m20-3742.

650. Tay MZ, Poh CM, Renia L, et al. The trinity of COVID-19: immunity, inflammation and intervention. *Nat Rev Immunol* 2020;20(6):363–374. doi: 10.1038/s41577-020-0311-8.

651. Taylor CA, Patel K, Pham H, et al. Severity of disease among adults hospitalized with laboratory-confirmed COVID-19 before and during the period of SARS-CoV-2 B.1.617.2 (Delta) predominance—COVID-NET, 14 States, January-August 2021. *MMWR Morb Mortal Wkly Rep* 2021;70(43):1513–1519. doi: 10.15585/mmwr.mm7043e1.

651a. Taylor CA, Whitaker M, Anglin O, et al. COVID-19-associated hospitalizations among adults during SARS-CoV-2 Delta and Omicron variant predominance, by race/ethnicity and vaccination status - COVID-NET, 14 states, July 2021-January 2022. *MMWR Morb Mortal Wkly Rep* 2022;71(12):466–473. doi: 10.15585/mmwr.mm7112e2.

652. Tedim AP, Almansa R, Domínguez-Gil M, et al. Comparison of real-time and droplet digital PCR to detect and quantify SARS-CoV-2 RNA in plasma. *Eur J Clin Invest* 2021;51(6):e13501. doi: 10.1111/eci.13501.

653. Temperton NJ, Chan PK, Simmons G, et al. Longitudinally profiling neutralizing antibody response to SARS coronavirus with pseudotypes. *Emerg Infect Dis* 2005;11(3):411–416. doi: 10.3201/eid1103.040906.

654. Tenforde MW, Kim SS, Lindsell CJ, et al. Symptom duration and risk factors for delayed return to usual health among outpatients with COVID-19 in a multistate health care systems network—United States, March-June 2020. *MMWR Morb Mortal Wkly Rep* 2020;69(30):993–998. doi: 10.15585/mmwr.mm6930e1.

655. Tenforde MW, Olson SM, Self WH, et al. Effectiveness of Pfizer-BioNTech and Moderna vaccines against COVID-19 among hospitalized adults aged >/=65 years - United States, January-March 2021. *MMWR Morb Mortal Wkly Rep* 2021;70(18):674–679. doi: 10.15585/mmwr.mm7018e1.

655a. Tenforde MW, Self WH, Gaglani M, et al. Effectiveness of mRNA vaccination in preventing COVID-19-associated invasive mechanical ventilation and death - United States,

March 2021-January 2022. MMWR Morb Mortal Wkly Rep 2022;71(12):459–465. doi: 10.15585/mmwr.mm7112e1.
656. Tenforde MW, Patel MM, Ginde AA, et al. Effectiveness of SARS-CoV-2 mRNA vaccines for preventing Covid-19 hospitalizations in the United States. *medRxiv* 2021:2021.07.08.21259776. doi: 10.1101/2021.07.08.21259776.
657. The WHO Rapid Evidence Appraisal for COVID-19 Therapies (REACT) Working Group. Association between administration of IL-6 antagonists and mortality among patients hospitalized for COVID-19: a meta-analysis. *JAMA* 2021;326(6):499–518. doi: 10.1001/jama.2021.11330.
658. Thelen JM, Buenen AGN, van Apeldoorn M, et al. Community-acquired bacteraemia in COVID-19 in comparison to influenza A and influenza B: a retrospective cohort study. *BMC Infect Dis* 2021;21(1):199. doi: 10.1186/s12879-021-05902-5.
659. Thomas S, Patel D, Bittel B, et al. Effect of high-dose zinc and ascorbic acid supplementation vs usual care on symptom length and reduction among ambulatory patients with SARS-CoV-2 infection: the COVID A to Z randomized clinical trial. *JAMA Netw Open* 2021;4(2):e210369. doi: 10.1001/jamanetworkopen.2021.0369.
660. Thompson HA, Mousa A, Dighe A, et al. SARS-CoV-2 setting-specific transmission rates: a systematic review and meta-analysis. *Clin Infect Dis* 2021;73(3):e754–e764. doi: 10.1093/cid/ciab100.
661. Thompson MG, Burgess JL, Naleway AL, et al. Interim estimates of vaccine effectiveness of BNT162b2 and mRNA-1273 COVID-19 vaccines in preventing SARS-CoV-2 infection among health care personnel, first responders, and other essential and frontline workers — eight U.S. locations, December 2020–March 2021. *MMWR Morb Mortal Wkly Rep* 2021;70(13):495–500. doi: 10.15585/mmwr.mm7013e3.
661a. Thompson MG, Natarajan K, Irving SA, et al. Effectiveness of a third dose of mRNA vaccines against COVID-19-associated emergency department and urgent care encounters and hospitalizations among adults during periods of Delta and Omicron variant predominance - VISION network, 10 states, August 2021-January 2022. *MMWR Morb Mortal Wkly Rep* 2022;71(4):139–145. doi: 10.15585/mmwr.mm7104e3.
662. Tian S, Xiong Y, Liu H, et al. Pathological study of the 2019 novel coronavirus disease (COVID-19) through postmortem core biopsies. *Mod Pathol* 2020;33(6):1007–1014. doi: 10.1038/s41379-020-0536-x.
663. Toots M, Yoon J-J, Cox RM, et al. Characterization of orally efficacious influenza drug with high resistance barrier in ferrets and human airway epithelia. *Sci Transl Med* 2019;11(515):eaax5866. doi: 10.1126/scitranslmed.aax5866.
664. Torres-Machorro A, Anguiano-Álvarez VM, Grimaldo-Gómez FA, et al. Asymptomatic deep vein thrombosis in critically ill COVID-19 patients despite therapeutic levels of anti-Xa activity. *Thromb Res* 2020;196:268–271. doi: 10.1016/j.thromres.2020.08.043.
665. Toth AT, Tatem KS, Hosseinipour N, et al. Surge and mortality in ICUs in New York city's public healthcare system. *Crit Care Med* 2021;49(9):1439–1450. doi: 10.1097/ccm.0000000000004972.
666. Townsend L, Hughes G, Kerr C, et al. Bacterial pneumonia coinfection and antimicrobial therapy duration in SARS-CoV-2 (COVID-19) infection. *JAC Antimicrob Resist* 2020;2(3):dlaa071. doi: 10.1093/jacamr/dlaa071.
667. Trinité B, Tarrés-Freixas F, Rodon J, et al. SARS-CoV-2 infection elicits a rapid neutralizing antibody response that correlates with disease severity. *Sci Rep* 2021;11(1):2608. doi: 10.1038/s41598-021-81862-9.
668. Tsang NNY, So HC, Ng KY, et al. Diagnostic performance of different sampling approaches for SARS-CoV-2 RT-PCR testing: a systematic review and meta-analysis. *Lancet Infect Dis* 2021;21(9):1233–1245. doi: 10.1016/s1473-3099(21)00146-8.
669. Tseng CT, Sbrana E, Iwata-Yoshikawa N, et al. Immunization with SARS coronavirus vaccines leads to pulmonary immunopathology on challenge with the SARS virus. *PLoS One* 2012;7(4):e35421. doi: 10.1371/journal.pone.0035421.
670. Tu TM, Goh C, Tan YK, et al. Cerebral venous thrombosis in patients with COVID-19 infection: a case series and systematic review. *J Stroke Cerebrovasc Dis* 2020;29(12):105379. doi: 10.1016/j.jstrokecerebrovasdis.2020.105379.
671. Twohig KA, Nyberg T, Zaidi A, et al. Hospital admission and emergency care attendance risk for SARS-CoV-2 delta (B.1.617.2) compared with alpha (B.1.1.7) variants of concern: a cohort study. *Lancet Infect Dis* 2022;22(1):35–42. doi: 10.1016/s1473-3099(21)00475-8.
672. U.S. Department of Health & Human Services. COVID-19: Developing Drugs and Biological Products for Treatment or Prevention Guidance for Industry. February 2021.
673. U.S. Food and Drug Administration. Coronavirus (COVID-19) Update: FDA Takes Additional Actions on the Use of a Booster Dose for COVID-19 Vaccines. https://www.fda.gov/news-events/press-announcements/coronavirus-covid-19-update-fda-takes-additional-actions-use-booster-dose-covid-19-vaccines. Accessed November 5, 2021.
674. U.S. Food and Drug Administration. In Vitro Diagnostics EUAs. https://www.fda.gov/medical-devices/coronavirus-disease-2019-covid-19-emergency-use-authorizations-medical-devices/in-vitro-diagnostics-euas. Accessed May 31, 2021.
675. Update to living systematic review on prediction models for diagnosis and prognosis of covid-19. *BMJ* 2021;372:n236. doi: 10.1136/bmj.n236.
676. Vahidy FS, Pischel L, Tano ME, et al. Real world effectiveness of COVID-19 mRNA vaccines against hospitalizations and deaths in the United States. *medRxiv* 2021:2021.04.21.21255873. doi: 10.1101/2021.04.21.21255873.
677. van Doremalen N, Bushmaker T, Morris DH, et al. Aerosol and surface stability of SARS-CoV-2 as compared with SARS-CoV-1. *N Engl J Med* 2020;382(16):1564–1567. doi: 10.1056/NEJMc2004973.
678. van Griensven J, Edwards T, de Lamballerie X, et al. Evaluation of convalescent plasma for Ebola Virus disease in Guinea. *N Engl J Med* 2016;374(1):33–42. doi: 10.1056/NEJMoa1511812.
679. van Kampen JJA, van de Vijver D, Fraaij PLA, et al. Duration and key determinants of infectious virus shedding in hospitalized patients with coronavirus disease-2019 (COVID-19). *Nat Commun* 2021;12(1):267. doi: 10.1038/s41467-020-20568-4.
680. van Riel D, de Wit E. Next-generation vaccine platforms for COVID-19. *Nat Mater* 2020;19(8):810–812. doi: 10.1038/s41563-020-0746-0.
681. Varatharaj A, Thomas N, Ellul MA, et al. Neurological and neuropsychiatric complications of COVID-19 in 153 patients: a UK-wide surveillance study. *Lancet Psychiatry* 2020;7(10):875–882. doi: 10.1016/s2215-0366(20)30287-x.
682. Vaughn VM, Gandhi T, Petty LA, et al. Empiric antibacterial therapy and community-onset bacterial co-infection in patients hospitalized with COVID-19: a multi-hospital cohort study. *Clin Infect Dis* 2021;72(10):e533–e541. doi: 10.1093/cid/ciaa1239.
683. Venkatesan P. Repurposing drugs for treatment of COVID-19. *Lancet Respir Med* 2021;9(7):e63. doi: 10.1016/s2213-2600(21)00270-8.
684. Villar J, Ariff S, Gunier RB, et al. Maternal and neonatal morbidity and mortality among pregnant women with and without COVID-19 infection: the INTERCOVID Multinational Cohort Study. *JAMA Pediatr* 2021;175(8):817–826. doi: 10.1001/jamapediatrics.2021.1050.
685. Viner RM, Ward JL, Hudson LD, et al. Systematic review of reviews of symptoms and signs of COVID-19 in children and adolescents. *Arch Dis Child* 2020:archdischild-2020-320972. doi: 10.1136/archdischild-2020-320972.
686. Vivanti AJ, Vauloup-Fellous C, Prevot S, et al. Transplacental transmission of SARS-CoV-2 infection. *Nat Commun* 2020;11(1):3572. doi: 10.1038/s41467-020-17436-6.
687. Voysey M, Clemens SAC, Madhi SA, et al. Safety and efficacy of the ChAdOx1 nCoV-19 vaccine (AZD1222) against SARS-CoV-2: an interim analysis of four randomised controlled trials in Brazil, South Africa, and the UK. *Lancet* 2021;397(10269):99–111. doi: 10.1016/s0140-6736(20)32661-1.
688. W. H. O. Solidarity Trial Consortium, Pan H, Peto R, et al. Repurposed antiviral drugs for Covid-19 - interim WHO solidarity trial results. *N Engl J Med* 2021;384(6):497–511. doi: 10.1056/NEJMoa2023184.
689. Walker KF, O'Donoghue K, Grace N, et al. Maternal transmission of SARS-COV-2 to the neonate, and possible routes for such transmission: a systematic review and critical analysis. *BJOG* 2020;127(11):1324–1336. doi: 10.1111/1471-0528.16362.
690. Wang D, Hu B, Hu C, et al. Clinical characteristics of 138 hospitalized patients with 2019 novel coronavirus-infected pneumonia in Wuhan, China. *JAMA* 2020;323(11):1061–1069. doi: 10.1001/jama.2020.1585.
691. Wang K, Long QX, Deng HJ, et al. Longitudinal dynamics of the neutralizing antibody response to severe acute respiratory syndrome coronavirus 2 (SARS-CoV-2) infection. *Clin Infect Dis* 2021;73(3):e531–e539. doi: 10.1093/cid/ciaa1143.
692. Wang K, Zhang X, Sun J, et al. Differences of severe acute respiratory syndrome coronavirus 2 shedding duration in sputum and nasopharyngeal swab specimens among adult inpatients with coronavirus disease 2019. *Chest* 2020;158(5):1876–1884. doi: 10.1016/j.chest.2020.06.015.
693. Wang P, Nair MS, Liu L, et al. Antibody resistance of SARS-CoV-2 variants B.1.351 and B.1.1.7. *Nature* 2021;593(7857):130–135. doi: 10.1038/s41586-021-03398-2.
694. Wang W, Xu Y, Gao R, et al. Detection of SARS-CoV-2 in different types of clinical specimens. *JAMA* 2020;323(18):1843–1844. doi: 10.1001/jama.2020.3786.
695. Wang X, Che Q, Ji X, et al. Correlation between lung infection severity and clinical laboratory indicators in patients with COVID-19: a cross-sectional study based on machine learning. *BMC Infect Dis* 2021;21(1):192. doi: 10.1186/s12879-021-05839-9.
696. Wang Y, Dong C, Hu Y, et al. Temporal changes of CT findings in 90 patients with COVID-19 pneumonia: a longitudinal study. *Radiology* 2020;296(2):E55–E64. doi: 10.1148/radiol.2020200843.
697. Wang Y, Zhang D, Du G, et al. Remdesivir in adults with severe COVID-19: a randomised, double-blind, placebo-controlled, multicentre trial. *Lancet* 2020;395(10236):1569–1578. doi: 10.1016/S0140-6736(20)31022-9.
698. Wang Z, Muecksch F, Schaefer-Babajew D, et al. Naturally enhanced neutralizing breadth against SARS-CoV-2 one year after infection. *Nature* 2021;595(7867):426–431. doi: 10.1038/s41586-021-03696-9.
699. Warren TK, Jordan R, Lo MK, et al. Therapeutic efficacy of the small molecule GS-5734 against Ebola virus in rhesus monkeys. *Nature* 2016;531(7594):381–385. doi: 10.1038/nature17180.
700. Wassie GT, Azene AG, Bantie GM, et al. Incubation period of severe acute respiratory syndrome novel coronavirus 2 that causes coronavirus disease 2019: a systematic review and meta-analysis. *Curr Ther Res Clin Exp* 2020;93:100607. doi: 10.1016/j.curtheres.2020.100607.
701. Watson J, Whiting PF, Brush JE. Interpreting a covid-19 test result. *BMJ* 2020;369:m1808. doi: 10.1136/bmj.m1808.
702. Wee LE, Ko KKK, Ho WQ, et al. Community-acquired viral respiratory infections amongst hospitalized inpatients during a COVID-19 outbreak in Singapore: co-infection and clinical outcomes. *J Clin Virol* 2020;128:104436. doi: 10.1016/j.jcv.2020.104436.
703. Wei Q, Lin H, Wei R-G, et al. Tocilizumab treatment for COVID-19 patients: a systematic review and meta-analysis. *Infect Dis Poverty* 2021;10(1):71. doi: 10.1186/s40249-021-00857-w.
704. Wei SQ, Bilodeau-Bertrand M, Liu S, et al. The impact of COVID-19 on pregnancy outcomes: a systematic review and meta-analysis. *CMAJ* 2021;193(16):E540-e548. doi: 10.1503/cmaj.202604.
705. Weinreich DM, Sivapalasingam S, Norton T, et al. REGEN-COV antibody cocktail clinical outcomes study in Covid-19 outpatients. *medRxiv* 2021:2021.05.19.21257469. doi: 10.1101/2021.05.19.21257469.
706. Weinreich DM, Sivapalasingam S, Norton T, et al. REGN-COV2, a neutralizing antibody cocktail, in outpatients with Covid-19. *N Engl J Med* 2021;384(3):238–251. doi: 10.1056/NEJMoa2035002.
707. Western Cape Department of Health in collaboration with the National Institute for Communicable Diseases SA. Risk factors for coronavirus disease 2019 (COVID-19) death in a population cohort study from the Western Cape Province, South Africa. *Clin Infect Dis* 2021;73(7):e2005–e2015. doi: 10.1093/cid/ciaa1198.
708. White PL, Dhillon R, Cordey A, et al. A national strategy to diagnose coronavirus disease 2019–associated invasive fungal disease in the intensive care unit. *Clin Infect Dis* 2021;73(7):e1634–e1644. doi: 10.1093/cid/ciaa1298.
709. Wichmann D, Sperhake JP, Lütgehetmann M, et al. Autopsy findings and venous thromboembolism in patients with COVID-19: a prospective cohort study. *Ann Intern Med* 2020;173(4):268–277. doi: 10.7326/m20-2003.
710. Williamson EJ, Walker AJ, Bhaskaran K, et al. Factors associated with COVID-19-related death using OpenSAFELY. *Nature* 2020;584(7821):430–436. doi: 10.1038/s41586-020-2521-4.

711. Wölfel R, Corman VM, Guggemos W, et al. Virological assessment of hospitalized patients with COVID-2019. *Nature* 2020;581(7809):465–469. doi: 10.1038/s41586-020-2196-x.

712. Woloshin S, Patel N, Kesselheim AS. False negative tests for SARS-CoV-2 infection - challenges and implications. *N Engl J Med* 2020;383(6):e38. doi: 10.1056/NEJMp2015897.

713. Wongvibulsin S, Garibaldi BT, Antar AAR, et al. Development of Severe COVID-19 Adaptive Risk Predictor (SCARP), a calculator to predict severe disease or death in hospitalized patients with COVID-19. *Ann Intern Med* 2021;174(6):777–785. doi: 10.7326/m20-6754.

714. Woodruff RC, Campbell AP, Taylor CA, et al. Risk factors for severe COVID-19 in children. *Pediatrics* 2021:e2021053418. doi: 10.1542/peds.2021-053418.

715. World Health Organization. Classification of Omicron (B.1.1.529): SARS-CoV-2 Variant of Concern. https://www.who.int/news/item/26-11-2021-classification-of-omicron-(b.1.1.529)-sars-cov-2-variant-of-concern. Accessed December 4, 2021.

716. World Health Organization. COVID-19 Clinical Management: Living Guidance. https://www.who.int/publications/i/item/WHO-2019-nCoV-clinical-2021-1.

717. World Health Organization. The COVID-19 vaccine tracker and landscape compiles detailed information of each COVID-19 vaccine candidate in development by closely monitoring their progress through the pipeline. Updated October 29, 2021. https://www.who.int/publications/m/item/draft-landscape-of-covid-19-candidate-vaccinesAccessed October 30, 2021.

718. Wu C, Chen X, Cai Y, et al. Risk factors associated with acute respiratory distress syndrome and death in patients with coronavirus disease 2019 pneumonia in Wuhan, China. *JAMA Intern Med* 2020;180(7):934–943. doi: 10.1001/jamainternmed.2020.0994.

719. Wu HS, Hsieh YC, Su IJ, et al. Early detection of antibodies against various structural proteins of the SARS-associated coronavirus in SARS patients. *J Biomed Sci* 2004;11(1):117–126. doi: 10.1007/bf02256554.

720. Wu P, Liu F, Chang Z, et al. Assessing asymptomatic, presymptomatic, and symptomatic transmission risk of Severe Acute Respiratory Syndrome Coronavirus 2. *Clin Infect Dis* 2021;73(6):e1314–e1320. doi: 10.1093/cid/ciab271.

721. Wu X, Liu X, Zhou Y, et al. 3-month, 6-month, 9-month, and 12-month respiratory outcomes in patients following COVID-19-related hospitalisation: a prospective study. *Lancet Respir Med* 2021;9(7):747–754. doi: 10.1016/s2213-2600(21)00174-0.

722. Wu Z, McGoogan JM. Characteristics of and important lessons from the coronavirus disease 2019 (COVID-19) outbreak in China: summary of a report of 72 314 cases from the Chinese center for disease control and prevention. *JAMA* 2020;323(13):1239–1242. doi: 10.1001/jama.2020.2648.

723. Xiang T, Liang B, Fang Y, et al. Declining levels of neutralizing antibodies against SARS-CoV-2 in convalescent COVID-19 patients one year post symptom onset. *Front Immunol* 2021;12:708523. doi: 10.3389/fimmu.2021.708523.

724. Xiang X, Wang ZH, Ye LL, et al. Co-infection of SARS-COV-2 and influenza A virus: a case series and fast review. *Curr Med Sci* 2021;41(1):51–57. doi: 10.1007/s11596-021-2317-2.

725. Xiao F, Sun J, Xu Y, et al. Infectious SARS-CoV-2 in feces of patient with severe COVID-19. *Emerg Infect Dis* 2020;26(8):1920–1922. doi: 10.3201/eid2608.200681.

726. Xin H, Li Y, Wu P, et al. Estimating the latent period of coronavirus disease 2019 (COVID-19). *Clin Infect Dis* 2021;ciab746. doi: 10.1093/cid/ciab746.

727. Xu D, Zhou F, Sun W, et al. Relationship between serum SARS-CoV-2 nucleic acid(RNAemia) and organ damage in COVID-19 patients: a cohort study. *Clin Infect Dis* 2021;73(1):68–75. doi: 10.1093/cid/ciaa1085.

728. Xu K, Chen Y, Yuan J, et al. Factors associated with prolonged viral RNA shedding in patients with coronavirus disease 2019 (COVID-19). *Clin Infect Dis* 2020;71(15):799–806. doi: 10.1093/cid/ciaa351.

729. Xu X, Yu C, Qu J, et al. Imaging and clinical features of patients with 2019 novel coronavirus SARS-CoV-2. *Eur J Nucl Med Mol Imaging* 2020;47(5):1275–1280. doi: 10.1007/s00259-020-04735-9.

730. Xu Z, Tang Y, Huang Q, et al. Systematic review and subgroup analysis of the incidence of acute kidney injury (AKI) in patients with COVID-19. *BMC Nephrol* 2021;22(1):52. doi: 10.1186/s12882-021-02244-x.

731. Yan D, Liu XY, Zhu YN, et al. Factors associated with prolonged viral shedding and impact of lopinavir/ritonavir treatment in hospitalised non-critically ill patients with SARS-CoV-2 infection. *Eur Respir J* 2020;56(1):2000799. doi: 10.1183/13993003.00799-2020.

732. Yassin A, Nawaiseh M, Shaban A, et al. Neurological manifestations and complications of coronavirus disease 2019 (COVID-19): a systematic review and meta-analysis. *BMC Neurol* 2021;21(1):138. doi: 10.1186/s12883-021-02161-4.

733. Ye X, Xiao X, Li B, et al. Low humoral immune response and ineffective clearance of SARS-CoV-2 in a COVID-19 patient with CLL during a 69-day follow-up. *Front Oncol* 2020;10:1272. doi: 10.3389/fonc.2020.01272.

734. Yin X, Li Q, Hou S, et al. Demographic, signs and symptoms, imaging characteristics of 2126 patients with COVID-19 pneumonia in the whole quarantine of Wuhan, China. *Clin Imaging* 2021;77:169–174. doi: 10.1016/j.clinimag.2021.02.034.

735. Yomogida K, Zhu S, Rubino F, et al. Post-acute sequelae of SARS-CoV-2 infection among adults aged ≥18 years - long beach, California, April 1-December 10, 2020. *MMWR Morb Mortal Wkly Rep* 2021;70(37):1274–1277. doi: 10.15585/mmwr.mm7037a2.

736. Yoon SH, Kang JM, Ahn JG. Clinical outcomes of 201 neonates born to mothers with COVID-19: a systematic review. *Eur Rev Med Pharmacol Sci* 2020;24(14):7804–7815. doi: 10.26355/eurrev_202007_22285.

737. Young BE, Ong SWX, Ng LFP, et al. Viral dynamics and immune correlates of COVID-19 disease severity. *Clin Infect Dis* 2021;73(9):e2932–e2942. doi: 10.1093/cid/ciaa1280.

738. Yu J, Tostanoski LH, Peter L, et al. DNA vaccine protection against SARS-CoV-2 in rhesus macaques. *Science* 2020;369(6505):806–811. doi: 10.1126/science.abc6284.

739. Zachariah P, Johnson CL, Halabi KC, et al. Epidemiology, clinical features, and disease severity in patients with coronavirus disease 2019 (COVID-19) in a Children's Hospital in New York City, New York. *JAMA Pediatr* 2020;174(10):e202430. doi: 10.1001/jamapediatrics.2020.2430.

740. Zambrano LD, Ellington S, Strid P, et al. Update: characteristics of symptomatic women of reproductive age with laboratory-confirmed SARS-CoV-2 infection by pregnancy status - United States, January 22-October 3, 2020. *MMWR Morb Mortal Wkly Rep* 2020;69(44):1641–1647. doi: 10.15585/mmwr.mm6944e3.

741. Zauche LH, Wallace B, Smoots AN, et al. Receipt of mRNA Covid-19 vaccines and risk of spontaneous abortion. *N Engl J Med* 2021;385(16):1533–1535. doi: 10.1056/NEJMc2113891.

742. Zeng H, Ma Y, Zhou Z, et al. Spectrum and clinical characteristics of symptomatic and asymptomatic coronavirus disease 2019 (COVID-19) with and without pneumonia. *Front Med (Lausanne)* 2021;8:645651. doi: 10.3389/fmed.2021.645651.

743. Zhang C, Shen L, Le KJ, et al. Incidence of venous thromboembolism in hospitalized coronavirus disease 2019 patients: a systematic review and meta-analysis. *Front Cardiovasc Med* 2020;7:151. doi: 10.3389/fcvm.2020.00151.

744. Zhang J, Litvinova M, Wang W, et al. Evolving epidemiology and transmission dynamics of coronavirus disease 2019 outside Hubei province, China: a descriptive and modelling study. *Lancet Infect Dis* 2020;20(7):793–802. doi: 10.1016/s1473-3099(20)30230-9.

745. Zhang JJY, Lee KS, Ong CW, et al. Diagnostic performance of COVID-19 serological assays during early infection: a systematic review and meta-analysis of 11 516 samples. *Influenza Other Respir Viruses* 2021;15(4):529–538. doi: 10.1111/irv.12841.

746. Zhang L, Hou J, Ma FZ, et al. The common risk factors for progression and mortality in COVID-19 patients: a meta-analysis. *Arch Virol* 2021:1–17. doi: 10.1007/s00705-021-05012-2.

747. Zhang M XJ, Deng A, Zhang Y, et al. Transmission dynamics of an outbreak of the COVID-19 Delta Variant B.1.617.2 — Guangdong Province, China, May–June 2021. *China CDC Wkly* 2021;3(27):584–586. doi: 10.46234/ccdcw2021.148.

748. Zhang P, Wang T, Xie SX. Meta-analysis of several epidemic characteristics of COVID-19. *J Data Sci* 2020;18(3):536–549. doi: 10.6339/jds.202007_18(3).0019.

749. Zhang Y, Luo W, Li Q, et al. Risk factors for death among the first 80 543 COVID-19 cases in China: relationships between age, underlying disease, case severity, and region. *Clin Infect Dis* 2021:ciab493doi: 10.1093/cid/ciab493.

750. Zhao H, Zhu Q, Zhang C, et al. Tocilizumab combined with favipiravir in the treatment of COVID-19: a multicenter trial in a small sample size. *Biomed Pharmacother* 2021;133:110825. doi: https://doi.org/10.1016/j.biopha.2020.110825.

751. Zhao J, Yuan Q, Wang H, et al. Antibody responses to SARS-CoV-2 in patients with novel coronavirus disease 2019. *Clin Infect Dis* 2020;71(16):2027–2034. doi: 10.1093/cid/ciaa344.

752. Zhao J, Zhao J, Perlman S. T cell responses are required for protection from clinical disease and for virus clearance in severe acute respiratory syndrome coronavirus-infected mice. *J Virol* 2010;84(18):9318–9325. doi: 10.1128/JVI.01049-10.

753. Zhao W, Zhong Z, Xie X, et al. Relation between chest CT findings and clinical conditions of coronavirus disease (COVID-19) pneumonia: a multicenter study. *AJR Am J Roentgenol* 2020;214(5):1072–1077. doi: 10.2214/ajr.20.22976.

754. Zhao YH, Zhao L, Yang XC, et al. Cardiovascular complications of SARS-CoV-2 infection (COVID-19): a systematic review and meta-analysis. *Rev Cardiovasc Med* 2021;22(1):159–165. doi: 10.31083/j.rcm.2021.01.238.

755. Zheng L, Wang X, Zhou C, et al. Analysis of the infection status of healthcare workers in Wuhan during the COVID-19 outbreak: a cross-sectional study. *Clin Infect Dis* 2020;71(16):2109–2113. doi: 10.1093/cid/ciaa588.

756. Zheng S, Fan J, Yu F, et al. Viral load dynamics and disease severity in patients infected with SARS-CoV-2 in Zhejiang province, China, January-March 2020: retrospective cohort study. *BMJ* 2020;369:m1443. doi: 10.1136/bmj.m1443.

757. Zheng X, Wang H, Su Z, et al. Co-infection of SARS-CoV-2 and influenza virus in early stage of the COVID-19 epidemic in Wuhan, China. *J Infect* 2020;81(2):e128–e129. doi: 10.1016/j.jinf.2020.05.041.

758. Zhou C, Zhang T, Ren H, et al. Impact of age on duration of viral RNA shedding in patients with COVID-19. *Aging (Albany NY)* 2020;12(22):22399–22404. doi: 10.18632/aging.104114.

759. Zhou F, Yu T, Du R, et al. Clinical course and risk factors for mortality of adult inpatients with COVID-19 in Wuhan, China: a retrospective cohort study. *Lancet* 2020;395(10229):1054–1062. doi: 10.1016/s0140-6736(20)30566-3.

760. Zhou L, Yao M, Zhang X, et al. Breath-, air- and surface-borne SARS-CoV-2 in hospitals. *J Aerosol Sci* 2021;152:105693. doi: 10.1016/j.jaerosci.2020.105693.

761. Zhou W, Liu Y, Xu B, et al. Early identification of patients with severe COVID-19 at increased risk of in-hospital death: a multicenter case-control study in Wuhan. *J Thorac Dis* 2021;13(3):1380–1395. doi: 10.21037/jtd-20-2568.

762. Zhou X, Cheng Z, Luo L, et al. Incidence and impact of disseminated intravascular coagulation in COVID-19 a systematic review and meta-analysis. *Thromb Res* 2021;201:23–29. doi: 10.1016/j.thromres.2021.02.010.

763. Zhu L, She ZG, Cheng X, et al. Association of blood glucose control and outcomes in patients with COVID-19 and pre-existing type 2 diabetes. *Cell Metab* 2020;31(6):1068–1077.e3. doi: 10.1016/j.cmet.2020.04.021.

764. Zhu N, Zhang D, Wang W, et al. A novel coronavirus from patients with pneumonia in China, 2019. *N Engl J Med* 2020;382(8):727–733. doi: 10.1056/NEJMoa2001017.

Note: Page number followed by "*f*" and "*t*" indicates figure and table respectively.

A

Abacavir (ABC), 480
ACE2 usage, evolution of, 711
Acquired immunodeficiency syndrome (AIDS), 648
  in macaques, 666
  in monkeys, 665–666, 667*f*
Acute disease. *See specific types*
Acute disseminated encephalomyelitis (ADEM), 243*t*
  from measles, 242, 243*f*
Acute hepatitis A, in humans, clinical findings, 43, 44*f*
Acute necrotizing encephalopathy, reovirus, 351
Acute transforming retroviruses, 470*t*, 511–513, 512*f*
  gene variation in, 511
  genomes of, 511
  oncogenes in, host, acquisition by, 511–513, 512*f*
  Rous sarcoma virus in, 511
Acute transforming viruses, 470, 470*t*
Adeno-associated virus (AAV), 671–672
Adult rat model, for borna disease virus, 146–147
Adult T-cell leukemia (ATL)
  chromosomal instability, 537
  clinical features of, 527, 547*f*, 548*f*
  genomic instability, 537
  history of, 527
  pathogenesis of, 541–542
African horse sickness (AHS), 414
Allosteric IN inhibitors (ALLINIs), 578
Alpha variants, SARS-CoV-2/COVID-19, 744, 759
Alpharetroviruses, 466, 468*t*
  receptors for, virus, 474
Angiotensin converting enzyme 2 (ACE2), 743
Antibody-mediated neutralization, quasi-enveloped virions, 44–45, 45*f*
Antigenic drift, 182
Anti-inflammatory strategies, SARS-CoV-2/COVID-19, 761–763
Antiretroviral therapy (ART), for human immunodeficiency virus, 620*t*
  in acute (primary) HIV-1 infection, 635
  in chronic HIV-1 infection, 626
  drug resistance in, 633
  drug toxicity in, 628
  drugs in, 618–619
  principles of, 633–634
  targets of, 631–633
  treatment failure with, 636–637
  virologic and immunologic effects of, 635
Anti-SARS-CoV-2 monoclonal antibodies, 758, 758*f*
Antithrombotic prophylaxis, SARS-CoV-2/COVID-19, 763
AP-1, in human immunodeficiency virus, 581
APH-2, in HTLV, 535
APOBEC3
  in foamy viruses, 700
    Bet on, 696, 696*f*
APOBEC family
  functions of, 495
  in nonhuman lentiviruses, 651–657

retroviral DNA deamination by, 506
Vif and
  in human immunodeficiency virus, 602, 618
  in nonhuman lentiviruses, 651–654, 657
APOBEC3G
  functions of, 543
  in human immunodeficiency virus, 573, 619
    Vif and, 601–602, 601*f*, 619
  in nonhuman lentiviruses, 657
  retroviral DNA deamination by, 506
Apoptosis induction
  by lyssaviruses, 186
  by orthoreoviruses, 343–345
  by reoviruses, 343–345
  by vesicular stomatitis virus, 185–186
Aquareoviruses, pathogenicity of, 319
Arteriviridae (arteriviruses), 104–130
  cell and tissue tropism, 116–117
  classification of, 104–105
  clinical features
    in equine arteritis virus, 122
    in lactate dehydrogenase-elevating virus, 122
    in porcine reproductive and respiratory syndrome virus, 122
    in simian hemorrhage fever virus, 122
    Wobbly possum disease, 122–123
  clinical features of, 122–123
  epidemiology of
    in equine arteritis virus, 121
    in lactate dehydrogenase-elevating virus, 121
    in porcine reproductive and respiratory syndrome virus, 121
    in simian hemorrhage fever virus, 121–122
  genome structure and organization of, 106–108, 108*f*
  history of, 104–105
  immune responses to
    cell-mediated, 118
    humoral, 117–118
    and immune evasion, 118–119
    innate, 117
    overview of, 117
  pathogenesis and pathology of, 116–121
  persistence of, 120–121
  perspectives on, 124–125
  prevention and control of, 123–124
    diagnosis in, 123
    disease control in, 123
  primary replication site and spread of, 116–117
  release from host and transmission of, 119–120
  replication cycle of, 109–116
    assembly and release of, 114
    attachment and entry in, 109–110
    in cultured cells and host cell interactions, 109
    genome translation and replication in, 111
    proteases in, 110*f*
    proteins of, structural
      major, 115
      minor, 115–116

replicase processing in, posttranslational, 113
replicase proteins and replication complex in, 113–114
subgenomic mRNA synthesis and translation in, 111–113, 112*f*
structure of, virion, 105–106, 106*f*
vaccines in, 123–124
virulence of, 120
Arterivirus–host cell interactions, 116
Arthritis
  from caprine arthritis encephalitis virus, 469, 664
  from rubella, 94
Asialoglycoprotein receptor (ASGPR), 41–42
Asthma, human rhinovirus infection in, 11–12, 11*f*, 12*f*
Astroviridae (astroviruses, AstV), 59–74
  classification of, 60, 60*f*, 61*f*
  clinical features of, 70, 70*t*
  composition of virion in, 60–61, 61*f*
  diagnosis of, 70
  epidemiology of, 69–70
    genetic diversity of virus, 69–70
    origin and transmission in, 69
    prevalence and seroepidemiology, 69
  genome structure and organization in, 61–63, 61*f*
    general, 61–62
    ORF2 in, 62, 63*f*
    ORF1a and ORF1b in, 62, 62*f*
    ORF-X in, 62–63
    sgRNA synthesis promoter in, 62
  history of, 59, 60*f*
  immunity to, 68
  pathogenesis and pathology of, 66–69, 66*f*, 67*f*, 68*f*
  perspectives on, 71
  prevention and control of, 70–71
  replication stages of, 63–66, 63*f*
    assembly and release in, 66
    attachment and entry in, 64
    in nonstructural polyproteins, 64–65, 64*f*
    in structural polyproteins, 65, 65*f*
    transcription/replication in, 65–66
    translation in, 64–65
    uncoating in, 64
  structure of, virion, 60–61, 61*f*
att sites, retroviral, 485
Avastrovirus, 60, 61*f*
Avian bornavirus (ABV), 131–160
  clinical signs and seroprevalence, 145
  epidemiology of, 144–145
  genetic diversity of, 132
  geographic distribution, 144–145
  gross findings and histopathology, 145
  history of, 132
  host range, 144–145
  morphology and physical characteristics of, 132
  pathogenesis, 145
  route of infection and transmission, 145
Avian encephalomyocarditis virus, 24

Avian leukosis sarcoma viruses (ALSV)
    classification of, 466, 467*f*, 468*t*
    transformation by, 509
Avian leukosis virus (ALV)
    electron micrograph of, 467*f*
    types of, 470*t*

B

Back-fusion, in rhabdoviruses, 176
Bamlanivimab, SARS-CoV-2/COVID-19, 758–759
Baricitinib, SARS-CoV-2, 762
B-cell immunity, SARS-CoV-2/COVID-19, 744
B-cell lymphomas, ALV and *c-myc* activation in, 507
β1 intergrins, in reoviruses, 329–331
Bet protein, in foamy viruses, 686*f*, 696, 696*f*
Beta variants, SARS-CoV-2/COVID-19, 745, 759
Betaretroviruses, 467*f*, 468, 468*t*
    gene expression in, 494
    receptors for, virus, 475
Biliary atresia, reovirus, 351
Blue tongue virus (BTV), 414
    classification of, 414–415
    clinical signs and pathogenesis of, 436
    epidemiology of, 436–437
    genome structure and organization in, 420
    history of, 414
    host cell, effects of, 435–436
    immune response to, 437
    molecular genetics of, 420–422
    pathogenicity of, 319
    perspectives on, 439
    replication stages of, 422
    structure of, virion, 415–417
        core particle and proteins in, 415–417, 418*f*
        overview of, 418*f*, 419–420
        virion particle and outer capsid in, 415, 417*f*–418*f*
    vaccines for, 437–439
Blueberry muffin rash, 95, 95*t*
Bluetongue (BT) disease, 414
    vaccines, 437
Borna disease virus (BoDV). *See Bornaviridae* (bornaviruses)
Bornaviridae (bornaviruses), 131–160
    in avians
        clinical signs and seroprevalence, 145
        epidemiology, 144–145
        geographic distribution, 144–145
        gross findings and histopathology, 145
        host range, 144–145
        pathogenesis, 145
        route of infection and transmission, 145
    cell culture models, 145–146
    diagnosis of
        differential diagnoses, 149
        intra vitam diagnosis, 149
        postmortem diagnosis, 150, 152*f*–153*f*
    epidemiology of, 138–139
        in avian bornavirus, 144–145
        in borna disease virus, 138–139
    history of, 131–132
    in mammals, 146–149
        in adult rat, 146–147
        borna disease
            clinical signs and seroprevalence, 139
            epidemiology, 138–139
            geographic distribution, 138–139
            gross findings and histopathology, 139
            host range, 138–139
            pathogenesis, 139
            route of infection and transmission, 139
        human infections, 139–144, 140*t*–143*t*
        in mice, 148–149
        in neonatal rat, 147–148
        in nonhuman primates, 148

        in tree shrews, 148
    perspectives, 154
    public health considerations, 154
    taxonomy of, 132
    therapy and control
        therapeutics, 152–154
        vaccination, 150–152
    virus in, 132–137
        cycle of infection of
            assembly and release in, 138
            attachment and entry in, 137
            transcription, replication, and gene expression in, 137–138
        genetic diversity of, 132
        genome and coding strategy, 133–134, 133*f*–134*f*
        morphology and physical characteristics of, 132
        proteins in
            glycoprotein (G), 135*f*, 136
            matrix (M) protein, 135*f*, 136
            nucleocapsid (N) protein, 135*f*, 134–135
            phosphoprotein (P), 135*f*, 136
            RNA-dependent RNA polymerase, 135*f*, 136–137
            X protein, 135*f*, 135–136
Bottlenecks, genetic, in rhabdoviruses, 182
Bovine ephemeral fever (BEF), history of, 163
Bovine ephemeral fever virus (BEFV). *See also* Ephemeroviruses
    control of, 196
    diagnosis of, 194
    epidemiology of, 191
    history of, 163
    taxonomy of, 163–164, 167*f*
Bovine immunodeficiency virus (BIV)
    electron micrograph of, 467*f*
    history of, 648
Bovine leukemia virus (BLV), 468, 468*t*
    electron micrograph of, 467*f*
    receptors for, 475*t*, 476
Bovine rotavirus WC3 (Wistar calf) strain, 399
Bovine syncytial virus, 467*f*
Budding, in retroviruses, 467*f*

C

C protein, in measles virus, 231
Campaign jaundice, 22
Canine distemper virus (CDV), 244–245
Caprine arthritis–encephalitis virus (CAEV), 469, 649–650
Capsid, 83–87, 83*f*, 84*f*
    envelope glycoproteins E1 and E2, 87
    nonstructural roles of, 84–87, 86*f*
    in virus assembly, 84, 85*f*
Capsid (CA) protein
    in human immunodeficiency virus, 590*f*, 592–594, 593*f*
    in retroviruses, 502
        packing of, 498*f*, 504–505
    in rubella virus, 83–87, 83*f*, 84*f*
Cas-Br-E MLV, cytopathic effects of, 509
Casirivimab/imdevimab, SARS-CoV-2/COVID-19, 758–759
CCR5
    in human immunodeficiency virus, 562, 564
        as co-receptor, 562, 564
CD4, binding and coreceptor interactions, 566–568, 567*f*–568*f*
CD55, in measles virus, 239
CD46 receptor, in measles virus, 232–233, 233*f*
CD150 (SLAMF1) receptor, in measles virus, 232–233, 233*f*
Celiac disease, from orthoreoviruses, 352
Cell culture models, for borna disease virus, 145–146

Cell cycle arrest, HTLV Tax induction of, 537
Cell-mediated immune response, in HTLV, 543–544
Central nervous system infections. *See also specific types and viruses*
    with mumps virus, 213–214, 213*f*
    with orthoreoviruses, 351
Centrosome, HTLV Tax amplification of, 537
Chain terminators, 480
Chandipura virus (CHPV), 162
Charged multivesicular body protein 4B (CHMP4B), 33
Chemokines, in rhinovirus infection, 9
Children, SARS-CoV-2/COVID-19 in, 752–753
Ciprofloxacin, 458–459
cis-acting elements, in rubella virus, 80–82, 81*f*
Clathrin-dependent endocytosis, in reovirus, 329, 330*f*
2′-C-methylcytidine (2-CMC), 458–459
Cold, common, 1
Colorado tick fever virus, 319
Coltiviruses, 319
Common cold, 1
Community acquired infection
    with astrovirus, 69
    SARS-CoV-2/COVID-19, 750
Complementation, genetic, in orthoreoviruses, 327
Concerted integration, 576–577
Congenital infections, congenital rubella syndrome, 92, 95–97, 95*t*, 96*f*
Congenital rubella syndrome (CRS), 92, 95–97, 95*t*, 96*f*
    clinical consequences of, 95–96, 95*t*, 96*f*
    fetal immune response in, 96
    late-onset sequelae of
        delayed endocrine disease in, 96–97
        delayed neurologic disease in, 97
    pathogenesis of, 95
    teratogenesis in, 96
Constitutive transport elements (CTEs), in retroviruses, 491
Convalescent plasma, SARS-CoV-2/COVID-19, 763
Copy choice
    in retroviruses, 481–482
    in rhabdoviruses, 182
Core replicase/transcriptase complex proteins
    Nsp9, 725
    Nsp12, 722–724
    Nsp13, 725–726
    Nsp7 and Nsp8, 724
Co-receptors, in human immunodeficiency virus
    CCR5, 562, 564
    CXCR4, 562, 564
    HIV-1, 562
    interactions, 566–568
Coronavirus capping machinery proteins
    capping reactions, 726
    Nsp10, 726, 728*f*
    Nsp14, 727–729, 728*f*
    Nsp16, 729–730
Coronavirus life cycle, 711–716, 712*f*
Coronavirus S protein, 765
COVID-19. See SARS-CoV-2/COVID-19
3C^pro protease, in hepatoviruses, 31
Critical COVID-19, 747
CXCR4, in human immunodeficiency virus, as co-receptor, 564
Cyclophilin A, in HIV-1 virions, 499
Cytokines, RV-induced, 8, 8*t*
Cytorhabdoviruses. *See also Rhabdoviridae* (rhabdoviruses)
    taxonomy of, 163–164, 163*f*, 164*t*

D

DC-specific ICAM-3–grabbing nonintegrin (DC-SIGN)

in human T-cell leukemia viruses, 543
in measles virus, 234, 237, 241
Defective DNA repair, 537
Defective interfering (DI) particles
  internal deletion, 182
  in measles virus, 234, 238–239, 243
  panhandle or snap-back, 182
  in persistently infected cells, 91, 243
  in rhabdoviruses, 182
  in rubella virus, 91
Defective interfering (DI) RNAs
  in rhabdoviruses, 182
  in rubella virus, 91
Delta variants, SARS-CoV-2/COVID-19, 745, 759
Deltaretroviruses, 467f, 468, 468t
  gene expression in, 494
  receptors for, virus, 476
Deoxyuridine triphosphatase (dUTPase), in
        nonhuman lentiviruses, 654, 666
Deoxyuridine triphosphate (dUTP), in nonhuman
        lentiviruses, 654, 666
Dermatitis, infective, HTLV-1, 544
Dexamethasone, SARS-CoV-2, 761–762
Diffuse alveolar damage (DAD), 743
Dipeptidyl peptidase-4 (DPP4), 33
Direct biophysical analysis, 24–26
DNA polymerase, 479–480
  in reverse transcription, 480
DNA repair, HTLV Tax on, 537
Double-layered particle (DLP)
  in *Reoviridae*, 319
  in rotavirus
    liposome-mediated transfection of, 379
    in replication cycle, 374f
    schematic diagram of, 363f
    in virion structure, 364–366, 365f, 366f
Double-membrane vesicles (DMVs), in arterivirus-
        infected cells, 117
Double-stranded RNA (dsRNA) viruses
  classification of, 319
  genomes of, in reoviruses, 319
    as model, 319
  in orthoreoviruses, 319
    as model, 319
Drug resistance
  in adult T-cell leukemia, 550
  in human immunodeficiency virus
    with ART regimen, 563
    with PR inhibitors, 600
    principles of, 634
    reverse transcriptase of, 570–571, 571f
    treatment failure from, 636–637
  to reverse transcriptase, to *Retroviridae*, 481
Dynamic copy-choice model, in
        retroviruses, 572

E

E protein (glycoprotein), in arteriviruses, 117
E1 protein (glycoprotein), in rubella, 87, 88f
E2 protein/glycoprotein, in rubella, 87, 88f
Emtricitabine (FTC), 480
Encephalitis, from rubella, 95
Encephalopathy, from rubella, 95
Endocytosis
  clathrin-dependent, in reovirus, 329, 330f
  receptor-mediated, in reovirus, 331
Endocytosis, nHAV particle, 33–34
Endogenous viruses, in retroviruses
  in chickens, mice, and pigs, 513
  in humans, 513
Endosomal sorting complex required for transport
        (ESCRT) machinery, 590f, 596–598, 597f
Enterovirus 72, 24
env gene

expression of, 494
in nonhuman lentiviruses, 669
in retroviruses, expression of, 494
Env (envelope, E) protein/glycoprotein, in human
        immunodeficiency virus, 713f, 715. *See
        also specific viruses*
  in foamy viruses, 693–695, 693f–694f
  in human immunodeficiency virus
    viron incorporation of, 566f, 598
    in virus binding and entry, 566–569,
        567f–568f
  in rubella virus, 87, 88f
  in retroviruses, 470, 471f
Envelope (E) protein, 713f, 715
  in foamy viruses, 693–695, 693f–694f
  in human immunodeficiency virus
    viron incorporation of, 566f, 598
    in virus binding and entry, 566–569,
        567f–568f
  in rubella virus, 87, 88f
  in retroviruses, 470, 471f
Enzyme-linked immunosorbent (ELISA) assays, 50
Ephemeroviruses
  epidemiology of, 191
  history of, 163
  infection in
    clinical features of, 193
    diagnosis of, 194
    prevention and control of, 196
  taxonomy of, 163–164, 163f, 164t
Epidemic catarrhal jaundice, 22–23
Epizootic diarrhea of infant mice (EDIM), 362
Epsilonretroviruses, 467f, 468–469, 468t
  gene expression in, 494
Equine arteritis virus (EAV), 104
  clinical features of, 122
  epidemiology of, 121
  genome structure and organization of, 106–108
  history and classification of, 104–105
  immune response to, 117
  pathogenesis and pathology of, 116–121
  prevention and control of, 123–124
  release from host and transmission of, 119–120
  replication cycle of, 109–116
  structure of, virion, 105–106, 106f
  vaccine, 104
  virulence and persistence of, 117
Equine infectious anemia virus (EIAV), 662
  clinical and pathological features in, 664
  electron micrograph of, 467f
  history of, 648–649
Eradication, virus
  of human immunodeficiency virus, prospects for,
        638
  immunization for, 253
  of measles, prospects for, 253
  requirements for, for measles virus, 253
Etesevimab, SARS-CoV-2/COVID-19, 758–759
Extracellular hepatovirus virions, 31
Extrapulmonary complications, SARS-CoV-2/
        COVID-19, 749–750
Extrapulmonary dissemination through
        viremia, 746

F

F (fusion) protein/glycoprotein
  in human metapneumovirus, 271f, 273t, 274
  in human respiratory syncytial virus, 269f, 271f,
        273–274, 273t
  in measles virus, 231–232, 232f
  in mumps virus, 208t, 209
Favipiravir, 761
Feline acquired immunodeficiency syndrome
        (FAIDS), 509

Feline immunodeficiency virus (FIV), 650–651, 659,
        661, 664–665, 670
Feline leukemia viruses (FeLVs), 468
  receptors for, 475t, 476
  types of, 470t
Fetal infections, with congenital rubella syndrome, 95
Fish retroviruses, 510
Foamy virus (FV), 679–705
  apathogenicity of, 683
  cytopathic effect of, 679, 680f
  early phase, provirus establishment, 696–697, 698f
    attachment, 693f–694f, 696
    entry and intracellular trafficking, 696–697
    integration, 688f, 697
    uncoating, 697
  evolution of, 682
  genome structure and organization,
        686–687, 686f
  history of, 679
  isolation of, 679–680, 680f
  late phase, progeny viruses generation, 697–701,
        699f
    capsid assembly, 686f, 688f, 696f, 700
    membrane envelopment and release, 688f,
        700–701
    nuclear RNA export, 698–699
    transcription, 686f, 697–698
    translation, 686f, 699–700
  natural history and trans-species transmission of,
        680–682, 681f
  nucleic acids of, virion, 684–685
  perspectives on, 701
  proteins in, nonstructural, 695–696
    Bet, 686f, 696, 696f
    Tas, 686f, 695–696, 695f
  proteins in, virion-associated, 687–695
    Env, 693–695, 693f–694f
    Gag, 687–690, 688f
    Pol, 686f, 690–693, 691f, 692f
  replication of
    in natural host, *in vivo*, 683
    reverse transcription in, 685, 685f
    stages of, 696–701
    in vitro, 680f, 682
  RNA packaging in, 686f, 687
  RNA sequences in, *cis*-acting genomic, 686f, 687
  vectors
    cis-acting RNA sequences and RNA packaging
        in, 687
    concentration of, 685
    genome organization of, 686–687, 686f
    structure of, 684f
  virion structure, 683–685, 684f
Forced copy choice, in retroviruses, 481–482, 572
Förster resonance energy transfer (FRET) analyses,
        566–567
Full-site integration, 575
Fulminant Hepatitis A, 47
Fusion peptide
  back-fusion, in rhabdoviruses, 176
  in retrovirus transmembrane subunit TM, 504
  in rhabdoviruses, 176
Fusogenic orthoreoviruses, 321
Fv1, on retroviral infection, 505
Fv4, on retrovirus receptor, 505

G

G protein (glycoprotein)
  in bornaviruses, 135f, 136
  in human metapneumovirus, 270f, 271f, 273t, 275
  in human respiratory syncytial virus, 270f, 271f,
        274–276, 275f
  in rhabdovirus, 170, 172f
    assembly of, 179–180

gag gene, expression of, 491–492
Gag protein. *See also specific viruses*
    in foamy viruses, 687–690, 688*f*
    in human immunodeficiency virus, 589–598
        accessory proteins in, 561*f*, 600
            Nef, 560*f*, 605*f*, 605–606
            Vif, 601*f*, 601–602
            Vpr, 590*f*, 602*f*, 602–603
            Vpu, 603*f*, 604*f*, 603–605
            Vpx, 603
        capsid, Gag multimerization and capsid
            formation in, 590*f*, 592–594, 593*f*
        Env glycoprotein incorporation into virions in,
            566*f*, 598
        fundamentals of, 589–590, 591*f*–592*f*
        matrix, membrane binding, Gag targeting
            and Env incorporation in, 590*f*,
            591–592, 592*f*
        nucleocapsid, RNA encapsidation, Gag
            multimerization, and nucleic acid
            chaperone activity in, 561*f*, 590*f*,
            594–596, 594*f*, 595*f*
        p6, virus release and Vpr/Vpx incorporation in,
            590*f*, 596, 596*f*
        protease and virus maturation in, 591*f*–592*f*,
            598–600
    in retroviruses, 470, 471*f*
Gamma variants, SARS-CoV-2/COVID-19,
    745, 759
Gammaretroviruses, 467*f*, 468, 468*t*
    receptors for, virus, 475–476
Gastroenteritis, from astroviruses, 59, 60*f*, 67, 69–71.
    See also Astroviridae (astroviruses, AstV)
Gene delivery, via retroviruses, 466
Gene segments and nomenclature, in reovirus
    genome, 323*t*, 324
Gene therapy vectors, retrovirus, 514–515
Generalized maculopapular rash, 228, 229*f*
Genetic bottlenecks, in rhabdoviruses, 182
Genomic RNA modification, in reovirus genome, 324
Gibbon ape leukemia virus (GALV), 468
    receptors for, 475*t*, 476
GlaxoSmithKline, HEV vaccine, 460*t*
Glucose transporter 1 (GLUT-1), in HTLV-1 entry,
    538, 538*f*
GP2 protein, in arteriviruses, 115
GP3 protein, in arteriviruses, 115
GP4 protein, in arteriviruses, 107*t*
GP5 protein, in arteriviruses, 115
Guillain-Barré syndrome (GBS), vaccines, 766

H

HA (hemagglutinin) protein, in measles virus, 232,
    233*f*
HAV capsid, structure of, 31–32, 32*f*
HAV proteins
    nomenclature, 28–30, 29*f*
    P1 capsid proteins, 29*f*, 30
    P2 proteins, 30
    P3 proteins, 30–31
    replication cycle, 28–30, 29*f*
HBZ, in HTLV, 528
    functions of, 533–535
    HBZ gene transcription in, 533
    HBZ-Tax interplay in, 534*f*
    in T-cell proliferation, 527
Heat shock cognate protein 70 (hsc70), in rotaviruses,
    376
Helper-free particles, retrovirus, 514
Hepadnaviridae (hepadnaviruses), reverse
    transcription in, 685, 685*f*
Hepatitis A Virus (HAV). *See* Hepatoviruses
Hepatitis A virus cellular receptor 1 (HAVcr1), 33–34
Hepatitis A virus (HAV) vaccine
    inactivated, 51

live attenuated vaccine, 51
Hepatitis E virus (HEV), 443–464
    animal reservoirs and animal herpesviruses,
        445–446
    classification of, 443–446
    diagnosis of, 458
    epidemiology of, 456, 457*f*
    extrahepatic manifestations, 456
    genome structure and organization in, 447–451,
        448*f*
        ORF1, 447–450
        ORF2, 450
        ORF3, 450–451
        ORF4, 451
    global distribution by human-tropic genotypes,
        456–457, 457*f*
    Hepeviridae, phylogenetic tree of, 443, 444*f*
    histopathology of, 455–456, 455*f*
    history of, 443
    host range of, 443–445, 445*f*
    pathogenesis and
        disease progression of, 456–457, 457*f*
        pathology of, 454–456, 455*f*
    perspective on, 460
    during pregnancy, 456–457
    replication stages of, 451–454
        life cycle of, 452, 453*f*
        naked and and enveloped HEV attachment and
            entry, 451–452, 451*f*
        viral assembly, 452, 454*f*
        virion release, 452–454, 453*f*, 454*f*
    structure of, virion, 446, 446*f*, 447*f*
    treatment of, 458–459, 458*f*, 459*f*
    vaccination and prevention, 459–460, 460*t*
Hepatoviruses, 22–58
    classification and diversity, 24, 25*f*, 26*f*
    clinical manifestations, 49–50, 49*f*
    diagnosis, 50
    epidemiology
        global hepatitis A prevalence, 48, 48*f*
        globalization, 48–49, 48*f*
        incidence, 47–48, 48*f*
        transmission, 47
    genome structure
        3′ UTR structure and function, 28
        5′ UTR structure and function, 24–26, 27*f*
        genome organization, 23*f*, 24
        polyprotein-coding RNA, 26–28, 28*f*
    HAV proteins
        nomenclature, 28–30, 29*f*
        P1 capsid proteins, 29*f*, 30
        P2 proteins, 30
        P3 proteins, 30–31
        replication cycle, 28–30, 29*f*
    history of, 22–24
    versus human codon usage, 26–28, 28*f*
    management of, 50
    morphology and properties of
        infectious extracellular virions, 29*f*, 31
        naked nonenveloped virions (nHAV), 31–33
    organization of, 23*f*
    pathogenesis
        animal models, 39–41
        cell-intrinsic and innate immune host responses,
            42–43
        cellular immune responses, 45–46
        host range, 38
        humoral immune responses, 43–45
        immunity, 46
        mechanisms of liver injury, 46–47
        steps, 41–42
        tropism, 39
    perspectives, 51
    phylogeny
        and picornaviral species, 24, 25*f*

and sequence divergence, 24, 26*f*
    prevention and control of
        general measures, 50
        hepatitis A vaccines, 51
        passive immunoprophylaxis, 50–51
    replication cycle
        attachment, entry, and uncoating, 33–35
        capsid assembly, 37
        hepatovirus translation, 35–36
        polyprotein processing, 36
        quasi-envelopment and release, 37–38
        RNA packaging, 37
        RNA replication, 36–37
Histamine, in rhinovirus infection, 8
Histone acetyl transferases (HATs), 581
Histone deacetyl transferases (HDACs), 581
HN (hemagglutinin-neuraminidase) protein, in
    mumps virus, 208*t*, 209
Homologous serum jaundice, 22–23
HTLV-1 uveitis, 549
HTLV-1-associated myelopathy (HAM)
    clinical features of, 548–549
    history of, 527–528
HTLV-1-immortalized cells, 530–531
HTLV-1-transformed cells, 530
Human astroviruses (HAstV), 59–74. *See also
    Astroviridae* (astroviruses, AstV)
Human coronavirus (HCoV), history of, 706–707,
    707*f*
Human endogenous retroviruses (HERVs), 513
Human immunodeficiency virus (HIV), 618–639
    animal models of, HIV-1
        chimpanzees, 563
        humanized mouse model, 563–564
        SIV models in nonhuman primates, 563
    biology of infection in, 562–563
        of CD4, lymphocytes, HIV-1, 562
        of macrophages and dendritic cells, HIV-1, 562
        replication and tropism in, 562
        transmission, 562–563
    classification and origin of, 469*f*, 558–559, 559*f*,
        560*f*
        circulating recombinant forms, 559
        genetic heterogeneity in, 559
        genetic subtypes and distribution of, 559, 560*f*
        phylogenetic relationships in, 469*f*, 559, 560*f*
        quasispecies in, 559
    clinical features of, 626–629
        in advanced disease, 628
        CDC classification system in, 627*t*
        in chronic infection, 627–628
        complications in, non-AIDS, 628
        course of, 627*f*, 629
        disease progression in, determinants of,
            628–629
        in primary infection, 626–627
    diagnosis of
        differential, 629
        laboratory, 629–631, 630*f*
    epidemiology of, 558, 618–620
        early, 621–622
        global distribution of, current, 620
        origin of human immunodeficiency virus in,
            619–620
        transmission mechanisms in, 620, 620*t*
    epigenetic regulation of, 581–582
    eradication of, prospects for, 638
    genome organization of, 560–562, 560*f*, 561*f*
        cis-acting elements in, HIV-1, 561–562
        for progeny virion production, 560, 561*f*
        proteins encoded in, 560, 561*f*
        secondary structure in, 560–562, 561*f*
        simple and complex retroviruses, 560, 560*f*
    history of, 618
    host factors in infection with, 577–578

immunity to, host, 623
adaptive cellular immune responses in, 624
adaptive humoral immune responses in, 623
CD8 T-cell responses, 624
host genetics and viral control in, 625–626
immune failure in, 626
innate immune responses in, 623
recovery from viral infection and, 622
variable disease course in, 625
virus-specific CD4 T cells in, 624–625
infectious agent, 618
pathogenesis of
acute infection and CD4 cell depletion in,
621–622
latent viral reservoir establishment in, 622–623
perspectives on, 606
postexposure prophylaxis, 637
preexposure prophylaxis, 638
prevention of
and control, 631–639
other strategies in, 638–639
vaccines in, 638–639
recombination, in high rates of, 559
RNA splicing and nuclear export, 586, 587f
simian immunodeficiency virus origins of, 559,
619
transcription after integration, 579–581
AP-1, 581
LTR, 579f, 580
NFAT, 581
NF-κB, 581
phases, 579
regulation of, 580, 580f
Sp1, 581
treatment of, 631–637
antiretroviral therapy in
in acute (primary) HIV-1 infection, 621–622
in chronic HIV-1 infection, 623
drug resistance in, 637
drug toxicity in, 635–636
failure of, 636–637
principles of, 633–634
targets of, 631–633
virologic and immunologic effects of, 635
development of
mortality and, 618
as prevention, 631–639
Human immunodeficiency virus 1 (HIV-1)
classification of, 469, 558–559, 559f
coreceptors in, 562
cyclophilin A in virions of, 499
host proteins in virions of, 499
pathogenesis of, cytopathic effects in, 509–510
perspectives on, 606
receptors for, 475t, 476
Human immunodeficiency virus 2 (HIV-2),
classification of, 559, 560f
Human immunodeficiency virus (HIV) replication,
558–617
classification and origins of, 558–559, 559f, 560f
in infection biology, 562–563
molecular biology of, HIV-1, 564–606
accessory proteins in, 561f, 600
Nef, 560f, 605f, 605–606
Vif, 601f, 601–602
Vpr, 590f, 602f, 602–603
Vpu, 603f, 604f, 603–605
Vpx, 603
Env glycoprotein incorporation into virions in,
566f, 598
integration in, 575–579, 576f, 577f, 578f
nuclear import in, 572–573, 573f
overview of, 564, 565f
postentry blocks to lentiviral infection, 573–575
Mx2, 574–575

TRIM5α and TRIMCyp, 574f, 575f,
573–574
postentry trafficking of HIV capsid, 565f,
569–570
protease and virus maturation in, 591f–592f,
598–600
reverse transcription in, 561f, 570–572, 571f
SAMHD1 in, 562, 573, 603
viral gene expression in, 579–589
basal HIV transcription after integration,
579f, 580f, 579–581
epigenetic regulation, 581–582
HIV-1 and HIV-2 long terminal repeat,
579f, 579
HIV RNA splicing and nuclear export, 587f,
586
latency, 584–585
Rev, 588f, 586–589
Tat, 583f, 582f, 582–584
virus assembly and release in (Gag proteins),
589–598
capsid, Gag multimerization and capsid
formation in, 590f, 593f, 592–594
ESCRT machinery and virus release, 590f,
597f, 596–598
fundamentals of, 591f–592f, 589–590
matrix, membrane binding, Gag targeting
and Env incorporation in, 590f,
592f, 591–592
nucleocapsid, RNA encapsidation, Gag
multimerization, and nucleic
acid chaperone activity in, 590f,
594–596, 561f, 594f, 595f
p6, virus release and Vpr/Vpx incorporation
in, 590f, 596f, 596
virus binding and entry, Env glycoproteins,
566–569, 566f
CD4 binding and coreceptor interactions,
567f–568f, 566–568
membrane fusion, 566f, 568f, 569f, 568–569
perspectives on, 606
Human immunodeficiency virus (HIV) vaccine, 618
Human metapneumovirus (HMPV), 267–317
clinical features of, 297–298
diagnosis of, 298
epidemiology of, 294–297
in adults, 295
epidemics in, 296
in infants and young children, 295
in other high-risk populations, 295–296
history of, 267
immune response to, 287–293
antibodies in, 289–291
antigens in, 287–288
evasion of host immunity in, 292–293
innate immunity and inflammation in,
288–289
infectious agent in, 267–282
animal counterparts of, 273t, 280–281
antigenic subgroups and genotypes of, 273t,
281–282
classification of, 267–268
fusion F glycoprotein, 271f, 273t, 274
genetics and reverse genetics of, 280
propagation in vitro of, 279–280
proteins in, 273–278, 273t
pathogenesis and pathology of, 269f, 282–287
immunity in, host, 286
infectivity and tropism in, 282
persistence in, 286
spread of, 286
virus load and severity in, 286
perspectives on, 306–307
prevention of
infection control in, 300

vaccines in, 306
proteins of
glycoprotein G, 270f, 271f, 273t, 275
M2-2 protein, 270f, 273t, 278
matrix M protein, 270f, 273t, 276
nucleocapsid/polymerase proteins N, P, L, and
M2-1, 270f, 273t, 277
small hydrophobic SH protein, 271f, 273t, 276
replicative cycle of, 279
RNA in, 268–272, 270f
treatment of, 298–300
virion in, 268, 268f–269f
Human metapneumovirus (HMPV) vaccines, 306
Human respiratory syncytial virus (HRSV).
See Respiratory syncytial virus
Human rhinovirus (HRV), 1–21
Human rhinovirus A (HRV-A), 1–2, 2f
Human rhinovirus C (HRV-C), 1–2, 2f
Human T-cell leukemia virus (HTLV), 468,
527–557
acquired immune response, 543–544
clinical features of, 547–549
in adult T-cell leukemia, 547–548, 547f, 548f
in HTLV-1 uveitis, 549
in HTLV-1-associated myelopathy/tropical
spastic paresis, 548–549
in infective dermatitis, 549
natural course in, 547, 547f
diagnosis of, 550–551
epidemiology of, 546–547
evolution of, 530
history of, 527–528
infectious agent in, 544
APH-2 in, 535
genome in, 528, 528f–529f
HBZ-Tax interplay in, 534f
HTLV-1 gene regulation in, 529f
latent HTLV-1 infection in vivo in, 546
p30 transcriptional and posttranscriptional
regulation of cellular genes in, 532
p30 HBZ interplay in, 534f, 532
posttranscriptional viral RNA regulation by
p30 in, 532
posttranscriptional viral RNA regulation,
p30, 537
Rex-p30 interaction in, 537
Tax-dependent transcriptional activation
in, 531
p13 in, 536, 536f
p12/p8 in, 535–536, 535f
Tax3 and Tax 4 in, 537
Tax in, 537
genomic instability from, 537
HTLV-1 immortalization and persistent
infection from, 536
inflammation from, 546
innate immune response, 543
integration and clonality, 540–542
pathogenesis and persistence in vivo, 538–546
cell and tissue tropism in, 539–540
cell entry in, 538–539
host entry in, 538
of inflammatory diseases, 546
primary replication and spread of virus in, 529
provirus, in nonmalignant cells, 530
virological synapse, 539
prevention and control of
prevention in, 549–550
treatment in, 550–551
selection in vivo, 544–545
sequence variation and evolution, 529–530
site of replication and spread, 542
within-host evolution, 544
Human T-cell leukemia virus (HTLV) vaccines, 551
Hypervariable region (HVR), of HEV, 449

I

I (interaction) domain, in retroviruses, 496–497
I protein, in mumps virus, 208*t*, 210
ICAM-1, in rhinoviruses, 5
IFN-λ1-3, 458–459
IL-6 pathway inhibitors, SARS-CoV-2, 762–763
Immune reconstitution inflammatory syndrome
    (IRIS), 635
Immunization goals of, eradication or elimination
    in, 253
Immunocompromised, measles virus in, 243*f*,
    248–249
Immunodeficiency and HTLV-1-associated
    diseases, 544
Immunotherapy, for rotaviruses, 397
IN strand transfer inhibitors (INSTIs), 578–579
Indirect immunofluorescence assay (IFA)
    ABV-specific antibodies, 149, 150*f*
    BoDV-specific antibodies, 149, 149*f*
Ineffective therapies, SARS-CoV-2, 763
Infants
    epizootic diarrhea of infant mice in, 362
    human metapneumovirus in, 295
    human respiratory syncytial virus in, 286,
        294–295, 294*f*
    RVAs, diarrheal disease in infants, 362, 364
Infectious hematopoietic necrosis virus (IHNV)
    clinical features of, 193
    control of, 196
    diagnosis of, 194
    epidemiology of, 191–192
    history of, 163
    taxonomy of, 163–164, 167*f*
Infectious jaundice, 22–23
Infectious subvirion particles (ISVPs), in reoviruses,
    320*f*, 321–322, 322*f*, 330*f*,
    331–333, 346*f*
Infective dermatitis, HTLV-1, 549
Integrase (IN)
    in human immunodeficiency virus, 575–579,
        576*f*, 577*f*, 578*f*
    inhibition of, 578
    in retroviruses, 575–576, 576*f*, 578
    structure of, 485–486, 486*f*
Interferon (IFN)
    reovirus induction of, 349
        and viral replication, 341, 342*f*
Interferon-inducible transmembrane protein 3
    (IFITM3), 331
Interferon-stimulated genes (ISGs), in rhabdoviruses,
    184
Intermolecular template switches, in retroviruses, 572
Internal deletion DI particles, in rhabdoviruses, 182
Internal ribosome entry site (IRES)
    in hepatitis A virus, 26, 27*f*
    in retroviruses, 491
    in rhinovirus, 3–4, 3*f*–4*f*
Intracisternal A-type particles (IAPs), 466, 467*f*
Intramolecular jumps, in retroviruses, 572
Isfahan virus (ISFV), 162

J

φ, in reovirus pore formation, 333
JAK-STAT signaling pathway
    reoviruses on, 347
    in rhinoviruses, 9, 9*f*
jaunisse des camps, 22
Jembrana disease virus (JDV), 648
Jenner, Edward, 398–399
Jennerian vaccines, 398–399
Jeryl Lynn vaccine, 220*t*, 221
Junctional adhesion molecule-A (JAM-A), in
    reoviruses, 328–329, 330*f*

K

Kallikrein, in rhinovirus infection, 8
Kinins, in rhinovirus infection, 8, 8*t*

L

L (late) domain, in retroviruses, 497
L (large) protein
    in human metapneumovirus, 270*f*, 273*t*, 277
    in human respiratory syncytial virus, 270*f*, 273*t*,
        277
    in measles virus, 232
    in mumps virus, 208–209, 208*t*
    in reoviruses, 323*t*, 324
L1 protein, in reoviruses, 323*t*, 324
L2 protein, in reoviruses, 323*t*, 324
L3 protein, in reoviruses, 323*t*, 324
λ3, within reovirus core particles, 335*f*–336*f*, 337
Lactate dehydrogenase-elevating virus (LDV), 104
    clinical features of, 122
    epidemiology of, 121
    genome structure and organization of, 106–108
    history and classification of, 104–105
    immune response to, 117
    pathogenesis and pathology of, 116–121
    prevention and control of, 123–124
    release from host and transmission of, 119–120
    replication cycle of, 109–116
    structure of, virion, 105–106, 106*f*
    virulence and persistence of, 117
Lamivudine (3TC), 480
Large polymerase protein (L) protein, in
    rhabdoviruses, 170–174
Latency (latent infection)
    in human immunodeficiency virus, 626
    in human T-cell leukemia virus, 536–537
Latency reversing agents (LRAs), 672
LEDGF/p75, 577–578, 578*f*
Lentiviruses, 467*f*, 468*t*, 469
    gene expression in, 495
    genome organization and composition of, 562
    in human immunodeficiency virus
        Nef, 605–606
        Vif, 601
        Vpu, 603
        Vpx, 603
    morphology of, 558, 559*f*
    postentry blocks to infection in
        TRIM5α and TRIMCyp in, 573
    receptors for, virus, 476
Lentiviruses, nonhuman, 648–678
    classification, 650
    clinical and pathological features in
        caprine arthritis encephalitis virus, 664
        equine infectious anemia virus, 664
        feline immunodeficiency virus, 664–665
        maedi/visna virus, 664, 665*f*
        simian immunodeficiency virus,
            665–666, 667*f*
    diagnosis of, 670
    future perspectives, 672
    genome organization and composition, 650–654,
        651*t*–652*t*, 653*f*, 654*t*
        auxiliary genes in, 651–654, 654*t*
        dUTPase and dUTP in, 654
        nef gene in, 651–654, 654*t*
        phylogenetic relationships and gene products,
            649*f*–650*f*, 650–651, 651*t*
        pol gene sequence conservation in, 651
        rev gene and Rev response element in, 651–654,
            654*t*
        vif gene in, 651–654, 654*t*
        vpr and *vpu* genes in, 651–654, 654*t*
    historical perspective, 648–649

    individual genes and genetic elements in,
        666–669
        deoxyuridine triphosphatase, 654, 666
        env, 669
        nef, 668
        NF-κB and Sp1, 669
        Rev protein, 666
        S2 gene, 666
        Tat proteins, 666
        U3, 669
        vif, 668
        vpr, 668–669
        vpx, 669
    infectious agent, 649–650
    morphogenesis and morphology, 649–650, 652*f*
    nonprimate lentiviruses
        accessory genes of, 651–654, 654*t*
    pathogenesis and pathology of, 660–670
        CD4+ helper T cells destruction, 663
        cell and tissue tropism in, 661
        escape variants, 663
        genetic resistance in, 670
        immune responses and persistence in, 661–663,
            662*f*, 663*f*
        MHC class I down-regulation, 663
        portals of entry in, 660–661
        resistance to antibodies, 662
        virulence in, 663–664
    phylogeny of, 649*f*–650*f*
    prevention and control, 670
    primate lentiviruses
        accessory genes of, 651–654, 654*t*
        partial listing of, 649–650, 651*t*
        phylogeny of, 649–650, 650*f*
    propagation, 654–660
        and cell culture, 654, 655*t*
        germline integration in, 660, 660*t*
        host range in, 650*f*, 653*f*, 654–655, 656*f*
        receptor use in, 659–660
        restriction factors, 655–659
    properties of, 652*t*
    research on
        therapeutic regimens, 672
        vaccine development, 670–672
    species of, 649, 649*t*
Leukotrienes, in rhinovirus infection, 8, 8*t*
Lipid rafts
    definition of, 568
    in human immunodeficiency virus, 568, 592
    in human respiratory syncytial virus, 279
    in measles virus, 241–242
    in mumps virus, 209
    in orbiviruses, BTV protein interaction of,
        424–425
    in retroviruses, 492
    in rhabdoviruses, 180
    in rotaviruses, 374*f*, 376, 384
Liriope platyphylla, 458–459
Low-density lipoprotein receptor (LDLR)
    in rhinoviruses, 6–7
LTR. *See also specific viruses*
    in human immunodeficiency virus, 579*f*, 580
Lysimachia mauritiana, 458–459
Lysosome-associated membrane glycoprotein 1
    (LAMP1), 33
Lyssaviruses
    apoptosis induction by, 186
    epidemiology of, 189–191
    history of, 161–162
    infection in
        clinical features of, 192–193
        diagnosis of, 193–194, 194*f*
        prevention and control of
            in animals, 195–196

in humans, 194–195
mouse models of, immune response in, 189–191
taxonomy of, 163–164, 163f, 164t

M

M (membrane-binding) domain, in retroviruses, 496
M1 protein, in reoviruses, 323t, 324
M2 protein, in reoviruses, 323t, 324
M2-1 protein
  in human metapneumovirus, 270f, 273t, 277
  in human respiratory syncytial virus, 270f, 273t, 277
M2-2 protein
  in human metapneumovirus, 270f, 273t, 278
  in human respiratory syncytial virus, 270f, 273t, 277–278
M3 protein, in reoviruses, 323t, 324
M (matrix) protein
  in arteriviruses, 104–105, 105f
  in bornaviruses, 135f, 136
  in human metapneumovirus, 270f, 273t, 276
  in human respiratory syncytial virus, 270f, 273t, 276
  in measles virus, 231
  in mumps virus, 208t, 209
  in rhabdoviruses, 170, 171f
    assembly of, 180–181
M (medium) protein, in reoviruses, 323t, 324
MA (matrix) protein
  in human immunodeficiency virus, 590f, 591–592, 592f
  in retroviruses, 502
Macrophages
  functions of, 9
  in rhinovirus infection, 9
Macropinocytosis, in reoviruses, 331
Maedi/visna virus (MVV)
  clinical and pathological features of, 664, 665f
  history, 648
Malarial catarrhal fever, 414
Mammarovirus, 60, 61f
Mammals bornavirus infection, 146–149
  in adult rat, 146–147
  borna disease
    clinical signs and seroprevalence, 139
    epidemiology, 138–139
    geographic distribution, 138–139
    gross findings and histopathology, 139
    host range, 138–139
    pathogenesis, 139
    route of infection and transmission, 139
  human infections, 139–144, 140t–143t
  in mice, 148–149
  in neonatal rat, 147–148
  in nonhuman primates, 148
  in tree shrews, 148
Maraba virus (MARAV), 162
Mason-Pfizer monkey virus (MPMV)
  classification of, 468, 468t
  electron micrograph of, 467f
Measles inclusion body encephalitis (MIBE), 243t, 243f, 248–249
Measles, mumps, and rubella (MMR) vaccine, 220, 220t
Measles vaccine, 250, 250f–251f
  on epidemiology, 246–247
  eradication via, 253
Measles virus (MeV), 228–266
  clinical features of
    in atypical measles, 248
    in classic measles and its complications, 236f, 243f, 247–248
    in immunocompromised, 243f, 248–249
  diagnosis of, 249–250

epidemiology of, 246–247
  in classic measles, 246–247
  in subacute sclerosing panencephalitis, 247
  vaccination on, 246–247
eradication of, via vaccines, 253
genetic relations of, 228, 229f
geographic distribution of, 235, 235f
history of, 228–229
infectious agent in, 229–236
  budding in, 234–235
  cell culture propagation and assay, 229, 230f
  cell-to-cell spread, 235
  cytopathic effects in, 229, 230f, 234
  entry, 234
  evolution, antigenic composition, and strain
      variation in, 233f, 235–236, 235f
  hemagglutination, hemadsorption, and
      hemolysis in, 234
  as morbillivirus, 228, 229f
  proteins in, 230–232
    fusion protein, 232f, 231–232
    hemagglutinin protein, 233f, 232
    L protein, 232
    matrix protein, 231
    nucleocapsid protein, 230
    P, C, and V proteins, 231
  receptors in, cellular
    CD46/membrane cofactor protein, 233f, 232, 233
    nectin 4/poliovirus receptor–like 4, 233f, 233
    other receptors and cell surface interactions, 233–234
    SLAMF1, 233f, 232, 232–233
  replication, 234
neurologic complications of, 243t
pathogenesis and pathology of, 236–246
  in classic measles
    immune responses in, autoimmunity, 243f, 242
    release and transmission in, 242
    virulence in, 242–243
  experimental infection in animals in, 245–246
  in natural (wild type) measles, 236–243, 236f
    entry and primary replication sites in, 236
    immune responses in, 236f, 237f, 238f, 238f, 237–242
    immune responses in, cellular, 238f, 239–240
    immune responses in, durability, 240
    immune responses in, early innate, 238–239
    immune responses in, general, 237–242
    immune responses in, immune suppression, 240–242
    prodrome and onset of, 236f, 236
    spread of, 237f, 237
    target cells and tissues in, 237
  in persistent infection
    cells in culture in, 243
    other chronic diseases in, 244
    subacute sclerosing panencephalitis in, 243–244, 243t
  in veterinary correlates
    canine distemper in, 244–245
    morbillivirus infections of aquatic mammals
        in, 229f, 245
    peste des petits ruminants virus in, 245
    Rinderpest in, 245
phylogeny analysis, 228, 229f
prevention and control of, 250–253
  prospects for eradication in, 253
  treatment in, 250
Membrane (M) protein, 713f, 715
Metapneumovirus, 267–317
Mice, for borna disease virus, 148–149
Microdomain, in rhabdoviruses, 180

Minus-strand leader RNA, in rhabdoviruses, 183
Minus-strand trailer RNA, in rhabdoviruses, 183
Molnupiravir, 761
Moloney murine leukemia virus, 470t
Monoclonal antibodies, SARS-CoV-2/COVID-19, 757–758
Morbillivirus, 228, 229f
  aquatic mammal infections with, 229f, 245
Mouse mammary tumor virus (MMTV)
  electron micrograph of, 467f
  insertional activation by, 510
  pathogenicity of, host cell proliferation in, 509
  receptor for, 475, 475t
μ1 protein, in reoviruses, 332–333
μ1N, in reoviruses, 333
μ2, in reoviruses, 335f–336f, 337
Mucosa, genital, 538
Muller's ratchet, 182
Multisystem inflammatory syndrome in adults (MIS-A), 756
Multisystem-inflammatory syndrome in children
    (MIS-C), 755–756
Multivesicular bodies (MVBs)
  in human immunodeficiency virus, 596, 597f
  in rhabdoviruses, 176, 181
Mumps virus (MuV), 206–227
  clinical features of, 215, 215f
  diagnosis of
    clinical, 219
    differential, 219
    laboratory, 219
  epidemiology of, 216–219
    age in, 216
    epidemics in, 216–217
    morbidity and mortality in, 216
    new approaches to, 218–219, 218f
    prevalence and seroepidemiology of, 217–218, 217f
  history of, 206
  host cell infection by, 210–211, 211f
  immune responses to
    cell-mediated immunity in, 216
    humoral immunity in, 215–216
  infectious agent in, 206–211
    classification of, 206
    genomic organization in, 207–208, 208t
    virion morphology and structure in, 206–207, 207f
    virus proteins and replication in, 208–210
      I protein, 210, 208t
      matrix protein, 209, 208t
      N, P, and L proteins, 208–209, 208t
      SH protein, 210f, 208t
      surface glycoproteins, 209, 208t
      V protein, 209–210, 208t
  pathology and pathogenesis of, 211–215
    in central nervous system, 213–214, 213f
    deafness, 214
    in experimental animals, 211–212, 212f
    in fetus and newborn, 214
    in gonads, 214
    in heart and joint tissues, 214
    in humans, 212–214
    in kidneys, 214
    in pancreas, 214
    in parotid gland, 213
    virulence in, molecular basis of, 215
  phylogenetics of, 218–219, 218f
  treatment of, 219
Mumps virus (MuV) vaccine, 220–221, 220t
  adverse events with, 220–221, 220t
  use of, 221
Murine acquired immune deficiency syndrome
    (MAIDS) virus, 510

Murine leukemia virus (MuLV), 468, 470*t*
  Cas-Br-E, cytopathic effects of, 509
  disease pathogenesis by, 507
  electron micrograph of, 467*f*
  receptors for, 475, 475*t*
Murine models of human hepatitis A, 39–41, 41*f*
Murine sarcoma virus (MSV), 470*t*
Myocarditis
  from reoviruses, 352
  vaccines, 766
Myristyl switch, in retroviruses, 496
Myxovirus resistance (MX) proteins, 658

N

N (nucleocapsid, NC) protein
  in arteriviruses, 105, 106*f*
  in bornaviruses, 134–135, 135*f*
  in human immunodeficiency virus, 561*f*, 590*f*,
      594–596, 594*f*, 595*f*
  in human metapneumovirus, 270*f*, 273*t*, 277
  in human respiratory syncytial virus, 270*f*, 273*t*,
      276
  in measles virus, 230
  in mumps virus, 208–209, 208*t*
  in retroviruses, 503
  in rhabdoviruses, 166–168, 168*f*
Naked, nonenveloped virions (nHAV), 31–33
  endocytosis, 33–34
Naked virus entry, 33–34
Nebraska calf diarrhea virus (NCDV), 362
Nectin 4 receptor, in measles virus, 233, 233*f*
nef gene, in nonhuman lentiviruses, 651–654, 654*t*,
    668
Nef, in human immunodeficiency virus, 560*f*,
    605–606, 605*f*
Neonatal infections, rat, with borna disease virus,
    147–148
Neurons, reovirus infection of, 329
Neutrophils, in rhinovirus, 9
NF-κB
  activation of
    by HTLV Tax, 531–532, 532*f*
  in human immunodeficiency virus, 581
  in nonhuman lentiviruses, 669
  by reovirus, 343–345, 349
Nidovirales (nidoviruses), 124
Nogo-66 receptor 1 (NgR1), 329
Nonfusogenic orthoreoviruses, 320, 321*t*
Nonhuman primate models of infection, 39, 40*f*
Nonhuman primates
  for borna disease virus, 148
Nonnucleoside reverse transcriptase inhibitors
    (NNRTIs), 480–481, 636*f*
  for human immunodeficiency virus, 570–572, 578
Nonsevere COVID-19, 747
Non–sialic acid–binding reovirus strains, 326
Nonstructural proteins (NSPs) of SARS-CoV-2,
    716–730
Nonturreted viruses, 365–366
Novirhabdoviruses
  epidemiology of, 191–192
  history of, 163
  infection in
    clinical features of, 193
    diagnosis of, 194
  taxonomy of, 163–164, 163*f*, 164*t*
NS1, in orbiviruses, 420*t*, 425–427, 426*f*
NS2, in orbiviruses, 420*t*, 426–427, 427*f*
NS3, in orbiviruses, 420, 420*t*, 423–426, 433–434,
    433*f*
NS1 protein, in human respiratory syncytial virus,
    270*f*, 273*t*, 278

NS2 protein, in human respiratory syncytial virus,
    270*f*, 273*t*, 278
NS20 (NSP4), in rotaviruses, 368*t*–369*t*, 373*f*
NS26 (NSP5), in rotaviruses, 368*t*–369*t*, 373*f*
NS34 (NSP3), in rotaviruses, 368*t*–369*t*, 373*f*, 383*f*
NS35 (NSP2), in rotaviruses, 368*t*–369*t*, 373*f*
NS53 (NSP1), in rotaviruses, 368*t*–369*t*, 373*f*
NS3A, in orbiviruses, 420, 420*t*, 423–426
NSP1, in rotaviruses, 368*t*–369*t*, 373*f*
Nsp1, SARS-CoV-2, 716–718
nsp1a, in astroviruses, 62, 62*f*
nsp1ab, in astroviruses, 64, 64*f*
NSP2
  in rotavirus viroplasms, 380, 381*f*–383*f*
  in rotaviruses, 368*t*–369*t*, 380, 381*f*–383*f*, 382
Nsp2, SARS-CoV-2, 718
NSP3, in rotaviruses, 368*t*–369*t*, 373*f*, 379–380,
    383*f*
Nsp3, SARS-CoV-2, 718–720, 719*f*
Nsp4 proteins, 720–721
NSP4, in rotaviruses, 368*t*–369*t*, 373*f*, 374*f*, 380,
    382–383, 383*f*, 386*f*, 391
  as enterotoxin, 373, 385, 386*f*, 387, 391
Nsp5 proteins, 721–722, 721*f*
NSP5
  in rotavirus viroplasms, 380, 381*f*–383*f*
  in rotaviruses, 368*t*–369*t*, 380–381, 381*f*–383*f*
Nsp6 proteins, 720–721
NSP6, in rotaviruses, 368*t*–369*t*, 373*f*
Nsp7 and Nsp8, 724
Nsp7-Nsp16 replicase complex, 722–730, 723*f*
Nsp9, 725
Nsp10, 726, 728*f*
Nsp12, 722–724
Nsp13, 725–726
Nsp14, 727–729, 728*f*
Nsp16, 729–730
Nuclear factor of activated T cells (NFAT), in human
    immunodeficiency virus, 581
Nucleic acid amplification tests (NAATs), 756
Nucleocapsid (N) protein, 713*f*, 715–716
Nucleocapsid-M protein complexes, in rhabdoviruses,
    assembly of, 181
Nucleorhabdoviruses, 163–164, 163*f*, 164*t*
Nucleoside analogs (NUC), inhibitors of, 480
Nucleoside reverse transcriptase inhibitors (NRTIs),
    572, 632*t*
Nucleotide identity analysis, SARS-CoV-2,
    706–740:p0044, 710*f*
Nucleotide reverse transcriptase inhibitors (NtRTIs,
    NRTIs)
  for human immunodeficiency virus, 632*t*
  targets for, 623

O

Omicron variants, SARS-CoV-2/COVID-19, 745
Oncogenes, retroviruses, 466
Oncogenesis
  as multistep phenomenon, 507–509
  retrovirus insertional activation in, 466, 507–509,
      508*f*
Oncolytics, of reoviruses, 353
Open reading frame 1 (ORF1) protein, HEV genome
  cis-acting regulatory elements, 450
  helicase, 449–450
  hypervariable region, 449
  methyltransferase, 447
  putative papain-like cysteine protease, 447–449
  RNA-dependent RNA polymerase, 450
  sequence alignments, 447
  X/macro domain, 449
  Y-domain, of unknown function, 447

Orbiviruses, 414–415
  classification of, 414–415
  clinical signs and pathogenesis of, 421*f*, 436
  epidemiology of, 436–437
  genome structure and organization in, 420, 421*f*
  history of, 414
  host cells, effects of, 435–436
  immune response to, 437
  lytic release, 434
  molecular genetics of, 420–422
  nonlytic release, 434–435
  perspectives on, 439
  replication stages of, 422
    capsid assembly in, 428–432
      core and outer capsid proteins, 432*f*,
        431–432
      genomic RNA and packaging, 430–431
      overview of, 428
      VP7 assembly and core formation in, 431
      VP3 assembly and subcore formation in,
        428–430
    entry in, 422–423
    overview of, 422
    primary *vs.* secondary replication requirement of
        reverse genetic system in, 426–427
    protein synthesis and virus replication in
        NS1 and NS2, 426–427
      overview of, 425–426, 426
    trafficking, maturation, and egress of progeny
        virions in, 432–434
      NS3 in, 433–434
      raft interaction with BTV proteins in,
        432–433
    transcription and replication, 423–425
    transcription and replication in, 423–425
      largest protein VP1, RNA-dependent RNA
        polymerase in, 424–425
      minor protein VP6, helicase and RNA pack-
        aging enzyme, 425
      minor protein VP4, mRNA capping enzyme
        in, 425
      overall mechanisms of, 419–420
      VP4 helicase in, 419
  VIBs and virus assembly, 427–428
  virus entry, 422–423
  structure of, virion, 415–420
    core particle and proteins in, 415–417
      surface layer of core and VP7 trimers in,
        415, 420*t*
      VP3 molecule arrangement in inner layer of,
        422, 420*t*
    internal minor protein, structural arrangement
        in, 417–419, 418*f*
    overview of, 415–420, 423*f*
    RNA genome in x-ray of core structure in,
        419–420
    virion particle and outer capsid in, 415,
        417*f*–418*f*
  vaccines, 437–439
ORF3a protein, SARS-CoV-2, 731
ORF3b protein, SARS-CoV-2, 731
ORF6 encoded protein, SARS-CoV-2, 731
ORF7a, SARS-CoV-2, 731–732
ORF7b encoded protein, SARS-CoV-2, 732
ORF8, SARS-CoV-2, 732
ORF9b encoded protein, SARS-CoV-2, 732
Orthohepevirus A, 443–445
Orthohepevirus B, 445
Orthohepevirus C, 445
Orthohepevirus D, 445
Orthoreoviruses, 318–361
  basic features of, 318
  classification of, 319–321, 321*t*

dsRNA viruses, 319
family *Reoviridae*, 319, 320*f*
genus *Orthoreovirus* in, 320 321
    fusogenic, 321
    general features of, 320
    nonfusogenic, 320, 321*t*
clinical features of
    biliary atresia in, 351
    celiac disease, 352
    CNS disease in, 351
    general features of, 351
    myocarditis in, 352
    pneumonia in, 352
diagnosis of, 352
discovery of, 318–319
epidemiology of, 350–351
fusogenic, 321
genome structure and organization, 324–327
    genetics in
        directed mutagenesis ("reverse genetics") in, 326*f*, 326–327
        genetic complementation in, 327
        reassortment in, 325–326
        selection of mutants ("forward genetics") in, 326
    physical characteristics in, 323*t*, 324
    protein-coding strategies and nomenclature in, 323*t*, 325
    terminal nontranslated regions in, 325, 325*f*
historical background, 318–319
host cell responses to infection in, 341–345
    apoptosis induction and NF-κB activation in, 343–345
    cellular DNA synthesis inhibition and cell cycle progression in, 343
    cellular RNA and protein synthesis inhibition in, 342–343
    cellular stress response induction in, 342–343
    interferon induction and viral replication effects in, 341, 342*f*
host range of, 350–351
as model for dsRNA virus studies, 319
nonfusogenic mammalian, 320, 321*t*
oncolytics of, 353
pathogenesis and pathology in, 345–350
    adaptive immune responses in, 349–350
    cell and tissue tropism
        in central nervous system, 346*f*, 347
        general mechanisms of, 345–346
        in heart, 346*f*, 347–348
        in hepatobiliary system and diabetes, 348
        in lung, 346*f*, 348
        reovirus genetic determinants of, 346*f*, 348–349
    entry into host in, 345
    innate immune responses in, 349
    by organ system, 345, 346*f*
    site of primary replication, 345, 346*f*
    spread of virus in, 345
pathogenic, 319
perspectives on, 353–354
prevention and control of, 352–353
replication stages in, 327–341
    assembly, 336*f*, 340
    attachment, 327–329
        cleavage of σ1 by intestinal proteases in, 327*f*, 329
        JAM-A binding by σ1 in, 328–329
        neutralizing antibody response determinant in, 329
        nogo-66 receptor 1 and reovirus infection of neurons, 329
        reovirus attachment protein σ1 in, 320*f*, 327*f*, 327–328

sialic acid, as serotype-specific attachment factor, 322*f*, 328
entry and intracellular trafficking in
    β1 intergrins in entry and endocytic compartment sorting in, 329–331
    clathrin-dependent endocytosis, 330*f*, 329
    macropinocytosis to enter neurons, 331
    reovirus sorts to late endosomes for disassembly, 331
genome assortment and, 339–340
membrane penetration in
    host factors required for, 333–334
    ISVP formation, 333
    μ1 protein in, 332–333
    μ1N and φ in pore formation, 333
    other reovirus structural proteins, 333
release, 340–341
transcription in, 334–337
    cores as molecular machines in, 334
    enzymatic activities with, 335*f*–336*f*, 334–337
    fundamentals of, 334
    λ3 location within core particles in, 335*f*–336*f*, 337
    μ2 role in, 335*f*–336*f*, 337
    transcriptase activation in, 334
    transcriptional cycle in, 335*f*–336*f*, 334
translation and viral factory formation in, 337–339
    reovirus mRNAs, 336*f*, 337–338, 323*t*
    viral factories in, 336*f*, 338–339
uncoating, 331–332
    σ3 cleavage, 330*f*, 331–332
    σ1 conformational changes in, 322*f*, 327*f*, 332
virion structure, 321–324
    core particles in, 320*f*, 322–324, 322*f*
    infectious subvirion particles in, 320*f*, 322, 322*f*
    particle function, 320*f*, 321–322, 322*f*
    particles *in situ*, 324
    recombinant particles in, 324
    virions in, 322, 322*f*
Orthoretrovirinae, 679

P

P1 capsid proteins, in hepatoviruses, 29*f*, 30
P2 capsid proteins, in hepatoviruses, 30
P3 capsid proteins, in hepatoviruses, 30–31
p6, in human immunodeficiency virus, 590*f*, 596, 596*f*
p8, in HTLV, 535–536, 535*f*
p12, in HTLV, 535–536, 535*f*
p13, in HTLV, 536, 536*f*
p30, in HTLV
    posttranscriptional viral RNA regulation by, 536–537
    transcriptional and posttranscriptional regulation of cellular genes by, 537
p53, HTLV tax inactivation of, 537
p53, tumor suppressor, 537
p90, in rubella virus, 76*f*–77*f*, 82
p150, in rubella virus, 76*f*–77*f*, 82
P protein (phosphoprotein)
    in bornaviruses, 135*f*, 136
    in human metapneumovirus, 270*f*, 273*t*, 277
    in human respiratory syncytial virus, 270*f*, 273*t*, 276–277
    in measles virus, 231
    in mumps virus, 208–209, 208*t*
    in rhabdoviruses, 168–170, 169*f*
Packaging lines, retrovirus, 514–515
Panhandle DI particles, in rhabdoviruses, 182

Paramyxoviridae (paramyxoviruses), percent amino acid sequence identity in proteins in, 273*t*
Pasteur, Louis, rabies vaccine of, 162
Pathogen-recognition receptors (PRRs), in rhabdoviruses, 183
Pericarditis, vaccines, 766
Peste des petits ruminants virus (PPRV), 245
p30-*HBZ* interplay, in HTLV, 536–537
Phenotypic mixing, in rhabdoviruses, 180
PI3K/Akt pathway, HTLV Tax activation of, 532
Piscine retroviruses, 510
PMPA (*R*-9-2-phosphonylmethoxypropyl adenine), 672
Pneumonia, from orthoreoviruses, 352
pol gene
    conservation of, in lentiviruses, 651
    expression of, 492–494
Pol protein, in retroviruses, 470–471, 471*f*
Poliovirus receptor-like 4 receptor, in measles virus, 233, 233*f*
Porcine reproductive and respiratory syndrome virus (PRRSV), 104
    clinical features of, 122–123
    epidemiology of, 125
    genome structure and organization of, 106–108
    history and classification of, 104–105
    immune response to, 117
    pathogenesis and pathology of, 116–121
    prevention and control of, 123–124
    release from host and transmission of, 119–120
    replication cycle of, 109–116
    structure of, virion, 105–106, 106*f*
    virulence and persistence of, 117
Porcine reproductive and respiratory syndrome virus (PRRSV) vaccine, 104
Post-COVID conditions, 754–755
Postvaccination reactogenicity events, 766
PPT, in lentiviruses, 570
Pregenome, 685
Pregnancy, SARS-CoV-2/COVID-19 in, 759
Preintegration complex (PIC), in retroviruses, 486–487
pro gene expression, 492
Protease (PR)
    in arteriviruses, 108*f*, 113
    in astroviruses, 62, 62*f*
    in human immunodeficiency virus, 591*f*–592*f*, 598–600
    in reoviruses, 329
    in retroviruses
        activation of, 501–502
        inhibitors, 502
        structure and function of, 502
Protein kinase R (PKR), in rotaviruses, 380
Proto-oncogenes, insertional activation of, by retroviruses, 510
Prototype foamy virus (PFV), 469. *See also* Foamy virus (FV)
Proventricular dilation disease (PDD)
    in avians bornavirus, 144–145
    history of, 132
Proviral load, 542
Provirus DNA integration, in retroviruses, 483*f*, 484
Provirus-like elements, in retroviruses, 513–514
Pseudotypes, in rhabdoviruses, 180
Pulmonary complications, SARS-CoV-2/COVID-19, 749

Q

Quantitative viral outgrowth assay (QVOA), 585
Quasi-enveloped virions (eHAV), 24, 31, 33
    antibody-mediated neutralization of, 45*f*
    entry, 34–35

Quasispecies
  in human immunodeficiency virus, 559
  in rhabdoviruses, 181–182
Quasi-steady-state, in human immunodeficiency
    virus, 627

R

Rabbit endogenous lentivirus type K (RELIK), 660
Rabies. *See also* Lyssaviruses; *Rhabdoviridae*
    (rhabdoviruses)
  clinical features of, 192–193
  dumb, 192
  epidemiology of, 189–192
  furious, 192
  history of, 161–163
  prevention and control of infection in
    in animals, 195–196
    in humans, 162
  vaccine, 162
Rabies virus (RABV)
  clinical features of, 192–193
  diagnosis of, 193–194, 194f
  epidemiology of, 189–192
  history of, 161–163
  molecular genetics of, 181–183
  mouse models of, 186–189
  pathogenesis of, 183–186, 185f
  perspectives on, 196–197
  prevention and control of, 194–196
  replication stages of, 174–181
  structure of, virion, 164–165, 165f
  taxonomy of, 163–164, 167f
  virulence of, 189
Reactive oxygen species, HTLV Tax induction
    of, 530
Receptor binding motif (RBM) alignment,
    706–740:p0045, 710f
Receptor-binding domain (RBD), 765
  residues, 759
Receptor-mediated endocytosis, in reovirus, 331
Recombination, in human immunodeficiency virus,
    rates of, 559
Recovery, from viral infection, in human
    immunodeficiency virus, 628
Regdanvimab, SARS-CoV-2/COVID-19, 759
Reinfection with SARS-CoV-2, 754
RELIK (rabbit endogenous lentivirus type K), 660
Remdesivir, SARS-CoV-2/COVID-19, 759–761,
    760t, 760f
Reoviridae (reoviruses)
  basic features of, 318
  classification of, 319
    dsRNA viruses in, 319
    family characteristics in, 319, 320f
  discovery of, 318–319
  as model for dsRNA virus studies, 319
  oncolytics of, 353
  pathogenic, 319
Reovirus T3D, 353
Replicase complex
  Nsp7-Nsp16, 722–730, 723f
  RdRp and nucleotidyl transferase activities,
    706–740:p0096
Replication cycle
  HAV proteins, 28–30, 29f
  hepatoviruses
    attachment, entry, and uncoating, 33–35
    capsid assembly, 37
    hepatovirus translation, 35–36
    polyprotein processing, 36
    quasi-envelopment and release, 37–38
    RNA packaging, 37
    RNA replication, 36–37

Respiratory complications, SARS-CoV-2/COVID-
    19, 749
Respiratory syncytial virus, 267–317
  clinical features of, 297–298
  diagnosis of, 298
  epidemiology of, 294–297
    in adults, 295
    epidemics in, 296–297, 296f
    in infants and young children, 294–295, 294f
    in other high-risk populations, 295–296
  history of, 267, 294
  immune response to, 287–293
    antibodies in, 289–291, 290f
    antigens in, 287–288
    evasion of host immunity in, 292–293
    innate immunity and inflammation in, 285f,
      288–289
    T lymphocytes in, 291–292
  infectious agent in, 267–282
    animal counterparts of, 273t, 280–281
    classification of, 267–268
    genetics and reverse genetics of, 280
      antigenic subgroups and genotypes of,
        281–282, 273t
  pathogenesis and pathology of, 269f, 282–287
    disease manifestations in, 286
    histopathology in, 285f, 284
    immunity in, host, 286
    in infants, 286
    infectious agent in, 283f, 284
    persistence in, 286
    spread of, 286
    virus load and severity in, 275f, 286
  perspectives on, 306–307
  prevention of
    infection control in, 300
    passive immunoprophylaxis in, 300–301
    vaccines in, 301–302
  propagation in vitro of, 279–280
  proteins in, 273–278, 273t
    fusion F glycoprotein, 269f, 271f, 273–274,
      273t
    glycoprotein G, 270f, 271f, 275f, 274–275,
      275, 276
    M2-2 protein, 270f, 277–278, 273t
    matrix M protein, 270f, 276, 273t
    NS1 and NS2, 270f, 278, 273t
    nucleocapsid/polymerase proteins N, P, L, and
      M2-1, 270f, 276–277, 273t
    small hydrophobic SH protein, 270f, 271f, 276
  replicative cycle of, 278–279
  RNA in, 268–272, 270f
  treatment of, 298–300
  virion in, 268, 268f–269f
Retinoic acid-inducible gene I (RIG-I), in
    rhabdoviruses, 183
Retroviridae (retroviruses), 465–526. *See also specific*
    types
  acute transforming retroviruses in, 511–513, 512f
  assembly of, virion, 495–499
    B-type and D-type virions in, 496
    C-type virions in, 495–496
    Gag and virion assembly in, 496–497
    Gag precursor protein in, 495
    host proteins in, 499
    I domain in, 497
    incorporation of other proteins in, 498
    L domain in, 497
    M domain in, 496
    virion size in, 497
    in vitro, 497
  biochemistry of, 466
  budding of, 467f
  classification of, taxonomic, 466–470

    alpharetroviruses, 466, 467f, 468t
    betaretroviruses, 467f, 468, 468t
    deltaretroviruses, 467f, 468, 468t
    epsilonretroviruses, 467f, 468–469, 468t
    evolutionary relationships of, 469–470, 469f
    gammaretroviruses, 467f, 468, 468t
    genera, 466, 468t
    lentiviruses, 467f, 468t, 469
    spumaviruses, 467f, 468t, 469
    transforming viruses, 470, 470t
    virion core morphology in, 466, 467f
  as cytopathic viruses, 509–510
  diseases of, 507–511
    cytopathic viruses in, 509–510
    host cell proliferation in, stimulation of, 510
    host determinants of, 510–511
    oncogenesis by insertional activation in,
      507–509, 508f
    pathogenesis of, 507
    pathogenicity of, viral determinants of, 509
    from replication-competent retroviruses,
      507–510
  endogenous viruses and virus-like sequences in
    in chickens, 513
    in humans, 513
    in mice, 513
    in pigs, 513
    properties of, 513–514
    provirus-like elements in, 513–514
  evolutionary history markers in, 466
  expression in, viral RNA, 487–491
    beginning and ending the RNA in, 489–490
    RNA processing in, 490–491, 490f
    RNA synthesis overview in, 488–489, 488f
    transcription initiation in, 489
      trans-acting viral regulatory factors in, 489
      U3 negative regulatory elements in, 489
      U3 positive regulatory elements in, 489
  as gene delivery vectors, 466, 514–515
  genome packaging in, RNA, 499–501
    dimerization of genome in, 500–501
    GAG sequences in, 499
    RNA sequences in, 499–500
    tRNA primer incorporation in, 501
    tRNA primer placement in, 501
  genomes of, RNA
    changes in, 473, 473f
    organization of, 471–472, 472f
  life cycle of, 472–473, 472f
  oncogenic
    oncogene insertion activation of, 466
  packaging lines of, 514–515
  pathogenicity of, 466
  penetration and uncoating in, 476–477
  perspectives on, 515
  protein processing and virion maturation in,
    501–505
    cleaving in, 504
    Env precursor processing in
      surface subunit SU in, 474, 504
      transmembrane subunit TM in, 474, 504
    Gag precursor processing in, 502–503
      capsid protein CA in, 502
      matrix protein MA in, 502
      nucleocapsid protein NC in, 503
      other Gag products in, 503
    Gag-Pro-Pol precursor processing in, 493f, 503
    morphologic changes on virion maturation
      in, 504
    protease activation in, 501–502
    protease inhibitors and, 502
    protease structure and function in, 502
    virion core structure and CA packaging in, 498f,
      504–505

proviral DNA integration in, 482–487
  att sites in, viral, 485
  biochemistry of, 483f, 484–485
  entry into nucleus, 483f, 484
  host proteins and integration in, 487
  integrase structure in, 485–486, 486f
  integration site distribution in, 487
  overview of, 482
  preintegration complex in, 486–487
  provirus structure in, 483f, 484
  unintegrated DNA forms in, 482, 483f
receptors in, virus, 474–476, 475t
  alpharetrovirus, 474
  betaretrovirus, 475
  deltaretrovirus, 476
  gammaretrovirus, 475
  lentivirus, 476
recombination in, 481–482
resistance to infection with, host restriction factors
      in, 505–507
  APOBEC viral DNA deamination in, 506
  replication blocks mediated by endogenous
      retrovirus genes, 505
  SAMHD1 block of monocyte lineage cells in,
      506
  SERINC proteins, blocking envelope by, 507
  tetherin trapping of cell-surface virion particles
      in, 506–507
  TRIM5a infection block in, 505–506
  ZAP elimination of viral RNAs in, 506
reverse transcription in, 477–481, 478f, 685, 685f
structure of, virion
  component arrangement in, 471
  general, 470
  nomenclature for, 470–471, 471f
  virion proteins in, 470–471, 471f
transduction by, 466
translation and protein processing in, 491–495
  env gene expression in, 494
  gag gene expression in, 491–492
  ORF arrangements in, 491, 491f
  other viral gene products in
    in betaretroviruses, 494
    in deltaretroviruses, 494
    in epsilonretroviruses, 494
    in lentiviruses, 495
    in spumaviruses, 495
  pol gene expression in, 492–494
  pro gene expression in, 492
vectors, 514–515
Retrovirus vectors, 514–515
rev gene
  in nonhuman lentiviruses, 651–654, 654t, 666
  in human immunodeficiency virus, 586–589
    cofactors, 588–589
    nuclear export cycle, 589f, 589
    and Rev-responsive element, 588f, 587–588
    structure of, 588f, 586–587
Rev response element (RRE), 651–654
Reverse genetic experiments with alphacoronavirus
      HCoV-229E, 706–740:p0108
Reverse transcribing viruses, replication strategies of,
      685, 685f
Reverse transcriptase inhibitors, 480–481
  nonnucleoside, 480–481, 632, 632t
    for human immunodeficiency virus, 563,
        570–572
  nucleoside, 632, 632t
  nucleotide, 572
    anti-HIV, 631
    targets for, 631–633
Reverse transcriptase (RT)-SHIVs, 672
Reverse transcriptases (RTs)
  biochemistry and structure of, 479–481

crystal structures in, 480, 481f
  DNA polymerase in, 479–480
  RNase H in, 480
  subunit structures in, 480
inhibitors of, 480–481
Reverse transcription, 477–481, 478f, 685, 685f
  reverse transcriptases in, 479–481
  steps in, 478f
    completion of both strands in, 479
    first translocation in, 478
    long msDNA synthesis in, 478
    minus-strand strong-stop DNA in, 478
    plus-strand DNA synthesis initiation in, 478
    second translocation in, 479
    tRNA removal in, 478–479
Rex, in HTLV, posttranscriptional viral RNA
      regulation by, 532–533
Rex knockout HTLV-1 phenotypes, 528
Rex-p30 interaction in, 532
Rhabdoviridae (rhabdoviruses), 161–205
  clinical features of infection in, 192–193
    in ephemeroviruses, 193
    in lyssaviruses, 192–193
    in novirhabdoviruses, 193
    in vesiculoviruses, 193
  diagnosis of infection in, 193–194, 194f
    in ephemerovirus, 194
    in lyssaviruses, 193–194, 194f
    in novirhabdovirus, 194
    in vesiculovirus, 194
  epidemiology of, 189–192
    in ephemerovirus, 191
    in lyssaviruses, 189–191
    in novirhabdovirus, 191–192
    in vesiculoviruses, 191
  genome organization and encoded proteins
    genome in, 167f
    glycoprotein (G protein) in, 170, 172f
    large polymerase (L) protein in, 170–174, 173f
    matrix (M) protein in, 170, 171f
    nucleoprotein (N protein) in, 166–168, 168f
    phosphoprotein (P) protein in, 168–170,
        169f
  history of, 161–163
    ephemeroviruses in, 163
    lyssaviruses in, 161–162
    novirhabdoviruses in, 163
    sigma virus in, 163
    vesiculoviruses in, 162
  molecular genetics of, 181–183
    defective interfering particles in, 182
    genetic engineering in, 182–183
    quasispecies in, 181–182
    rapid evolution in, 181–182
  mouse models of, 186–189
    entry and site of initial replication in, 186–187,
        187f
    immune response in
      to lyssaviruses, 188–189
      recovery from, 187
      to vesiculoviruses, 187f, 187–188
    virulence determinants in, 189
    virus spread and tissue tropism in, 187
  pathogenesis of, molecular and cellular basis of,
      183–186
    cytopathic effects induction in, 185–186
      general mechanisms of, 185
      by lyssaviruses, 186
      by vesicular stomatitis virus, 185–186
    host antiviral response induction and
        suppression in, 183–185
      general mechanisms of, 183–184
      host gene expression inhibition by vesicular
          stomatitis virus in, 185f, 184–185

Interferon signaling suppression by rabies
      virus in, 184
  perspectives on, 196–197
  prevention and control of infection in, 194–196
    in ephemeroviruses, 196
    in lyssaviruses, 194–195
    in novirhabdoviruses, 196
    in vesiculoviruses, 196
  replication stages of, 174–181
    assembly of progeny virions in
      G protein, 179–180
      M protein, 180–181
    attachment in, 174–175
    genome replication in, 175f, 177f, 178–179
    overview of, 174, 175f
    penetration in, 167f, 176
    release of progeny virions in, 181
    secondary transcription in, 179
    uncoating and primary transcription in,
        176–178, 177f
  structure of, virion, 164–165, 165f
  taxonomy of, 163–164, 163f, 164t
Rhinoviruses, 1–21
  capsids in, 2–3, 4f
  clinical features of, 14–15
  in common cold, 1
  diagnosis of, 15–16, 15f
  discovery of, 1
  epidemiology of, 11–14
    age in, 11, 11f
    genetic diversity of virus in, 14
    morbidity in, 11–13, 11f, 12f, 13f
    origin and spread in, 13, 14f
    prevalence and seroepidemiology of, 14
  genome of, 3–4, 3f–4f
  infectious agent in, 1–4
    classification of, 1–2, 2f
    physical characteristics of, 2–4, 3f–4f
  pathogenesis and pathology in, 4–10
    cell and tissue tropism in, 6–7
    entry in, 4
    immune response to, 7–10
      airway epithelium in, 9f, 8–9
      antibody in, 10
      cellular, 9–10
      gene expression and metabolomics studies, 10
      immunohistochemistry in, 7
      inflammation mediators in, 8, 8t
    persistence in, 10
    primary replication site in, 5, 5f
    receptors in, 6–7, 6f
    species tropism in, 7
    spread of, 5–6, 5f
    transmission in, 10
    virulence in, 10
  perspectives on, 16–17
  prevention and control of, 16
RIG-I (retinoic acid-inducible gene I), in
      rhabdoviruses, 183
RIG-I receptors, in rhinovirus infection, 8–9, 9f
Rinderpest virus (RPV)
  genetic relations of, 228, 229f
  pathogenesis and pathology of, 245
RIT 4237 vaccine, 399
RNA
  packaging, 37
  replication, 36–37
RNA interference (RNAi, RNA silencing), in rubella
      virus, 86–87
RNA-dependent RNA polymerase (RdRp), 447,
      706–740:p0098
  in astroviruses, 60, 62, 62f, 65–66
RNase H, 480
Rotarix (RV1), 395, 400–402, 401t

RotaShield (RV4), 399–401
RotaTeq (RV5), 395, 399–402, 401*t*
Rotaviruses, 362–413
    classification of, 362–364
        capsid structural protein, serologic reactivity and
            genetic variability of, 363–364
        general characteristics in, 362–363, 363*t*
        nucleotide percentage identity in, 364, 364*t*
        Rotavirus Classification Working Group,
            363–364
        salient features, 363, 363*f*
        VP7 and VP4 capsid proteins, 364
    clinical symptoms, 394–396, 395*t*
    coding assignments in, 368*t*–369*t*, 371, 373*f*
    diagnosis of, 396–397
    electron micrograph of, 362, 363*f*
    epidemiology of, 387–389
        in adults, 388
        distribution in
            age, sex, race, and socioeconomic status in,
                389
            geographic, 389
            seasonal patterns of, 389
        incubation period in, 389
        molecular studies in, 389
        nosocomial infections in, 388
        serotypes in, 387–388
        transmission in, 388–389
    genome structure and organization in, 366*f*,
        367–371, 370*f*, 373*f*
        dsRNA in, 370, 373*f*
        major features of, 367–370, 370*f*
        rearranged genomes segments in,
            370–371, 373*f*
    history of, 362
    immunity in, 390–394
        adaptive, 390–392, 392*f*
        innate, 393–394, 393*f*
    morphologic and biochemical properties,
        362–363, 363*t*
    pathogenesis and pathology in, 385–387, 386*f*
    pathogenicity of, 319
    perspectives on, 402
    prevention and control of, 398–402
        passive immunization in, 402
    proteins in, 368*t*–369*t*, 371, 373*f*
    replication stages of, 371–384
        attachment in, 373–376, 374*f*, 375*f*
        genomic RNA encapsidation (packaging) and,
            381–382
        kinetics and cellular sites of transcription and
            replication in, 379–381,
            381*f*–383*f*
        overview of cycle of, 371–373, 374*f*
        penetration and uncoating of, 376–377, 376*f*
        reverse genetics, 384
        RNA synthesis in, 377–379, 378*f*
        virion maturation in, 382–384, 383*f*
        virus release in, 384
        virus–host interactions, 384
    structure of, virion, 364–367, 365*f*, 366*f*
        double- and triple-layered particles in, 365,
            365*f*, 366*f*
        proteins, 366–367, 368*t*–369*t*
        single-layered particles in, 365–366,
            365*f*, 366*f*
    treatment, 397–398
    vaccines
        attenuated rotavirus vaccines deployed on a
            national or restricted multinational
            basis, 401–402
        fundamentals of, 398
        initial monovalent animal rotavirus
            ("Jennerian") candidates in, 398–399

    other approaches to, 402
    quadrivalent RRV-based reassortant, 399–400
    Rotarix and RotaTeq postlicensure safety and
        efficacy studies in, 400–401, 401*t*
    two major currently licensed live, 400
Rough particles, in rotavirus, 364–365
Rous sarcoma virus (RSV), 511
RT-PCR cycle, SARS-CoV-2/COVID-19, 750–751
Rubella vaccines, 75, 76*f*, 98–99
    administration of, 98
    adverse reactions to, 98
    countries with strategies for, 75, 76*f*
    development of, 98
    new strategies for, 99
    pregnancy risk of, 98
Rubella virus (RUBV), 75–109
    clinical features of
        in acute rubella, 93–95, 93*f*–94*f*
        in congenital rubella syndrome, 95–97, 95*t*, 96*f*
    diagnosis of, 97–98
    epidemiology of
        age in, 92
        incidence in, 76*f*, 92
        molecular, 93
        origin and spread of epidemics in, 93
    history of, 75
    infectious agent in, 75–92
        animal models of, 91
        antigenic composition and determinants in, 92
            B-cell epitopes in, 92
            complement-fixing and hemagglutination
                antigens in, 92
            T-cell epitopes in, 92
        assembly and secretion, 90–91
        biological characteristics of
            host cell effects in, 79*f*–80*f*, 78–80
            host range in, 78
            phenotype variation in, 77*f*, 80
            replication kinetics in, 78
        genome structure and organization in, 75–77,
            76*f*–77*f*, 80–87
            cis-acting elements in, 81*f*, 80–82
            encapsulation signal in, 82
            envelope glycoproteins E1 and E2, 87
            nonstructural ORF and protein products in,
                76*f*–77*f*, 82
            structural ORF and protein products in,
                82–87
        morphology and physiochemical properties of,
            77–78, 77*f*–78*f*
        persistence in, 91
        replication strategy, 87–90
            attachment and internalization, 87
            entry in, 87
            replication complexes, 79*f*–80*f*, 89–90
            targeting of structural proteins to the bud-
                ding site, 90
    perspectives on, 99
    phylogenetic tree of, 75–77, 77*f*
    prevention and control of, vaccines in, 75, 76*f*,
        98–99
Rubini vaccine, 220

S

S (small) protein, in reoviruses, 323*t*, 324
S1 protein, in reoviruses, 323*t*, 324
S2 protein
    in nonhuman lentiviruses, 666
    in reoviruses, 323*t*, 324
S3 protein, in reoviruses, 323*t*, 324
S4 protein, in reoviruses, 323*t*, 324
SAMHD1
    in human immunodeficiency virus, 562, 573, 603

    retrovirus monocyte lineage cell block by, 506
SARS-CoV-2 Nsp1, 716–718
SARS-CoV-2 Nsp2, 718
SARS-CoV-2 Nsp3, 718–720, 719*f*
SARS-CoV-2 ORF8, 732
SARS-CoV-2 ORF6 encoded protein, 731
SARS-CoV-2 ORF7a, 731–732
SARS-CoV-2 ORF3a protein, 731
SARS-CoV-2 ORF3b protein, 731
SARS-CoV-2 ORF7b encoded protein, 732
SARS-CoV-2 ORF9b encoded protein, 732
SARS-CoV-2 reinfection, 754
SARS-CoV-2/COVID-19. *See also* Severe acute
        respiratory syndrome coronavirus 2
        (SARS-CoV-2)
    anti-inflammatory strategies, 761–763
    antithrombotic prophylaxis, 763
    antiviral agents, 759–761
    bamlanivimab, 758–759
    B-cell immunity, 744
    casirivimab/imdevimab, 758–759
    characterization, 742, 742*f*
    clinical disease, 747–749
        asymptomatic infection, 747
        clinical spectrum, 748–749
        critical illness, 747
        mild illness, 747
        moderate illness, 747
        severe illness, 747
        severity of, 747–748
    clinical issues after infection, 754–756
    clinical management, 757
    coagulation abnormalities, 742–743
    complications
        community-acquired invasive bacterial or fungal
            coinfection, 750
        extrapulmonary complications, 749–750
        laboratory biomarkers, 750
        pulmonary complications, 749
        respiratory complications, 749
        RT-PCR cycle, 750–751
    diagnostic testing, 756–757
    duration of infectiousness, 746–747
    epidemiologic parameters, 745–747
    etesevimab, 758–759
    genetic variants of, 744–745
    health inequities, 753
    immune responses, 743–744
    infection prevention and control, 764
    monoclonal antibodies, 757–758
    pathogenesis, 742–744
    pathophysiology, 742–743
    perspective, 769
    primary pathology, 743
    radiographic and computerized tomography, 751,
        751*f*
    regdanvimab, 759
    risk factors, 751–752
    serological assays, 757
    signs and symptoms, 752
        in children, 752–753
        in pregnancy, 753
    sotrovimab, 759
    T-cell immunity, 743–744
    transmission dynamics, 745–746
    transmission modes, 746
    treatment of, 763–764
        clinical care of hospitalized patients, 764
        clinical care of outpatients, 763–764
    vaccine, 765–769
    variants and monoclonal antibodies, 759
    vertical transmission, 753–754
    viral load and disease severity, 758, 758*f*
    viral tests, 756–757

Sedoreovirinae, 319
Septicemia, viral hemorrhagic, 193
Sequence variation and evolution, HTLV, 529–530
  causes, 529
  immune-mediated selection, 529
  significance of, 529–530
SERINC proteins, 606
Serine incorporator 3 (SERINC3), 658–659
Serine incorporator 5 (SERINC5), 658–659
Severe acute respiratory syndrome coronavirus 2
    (SARS-CoV-2). *See also* SARS-CoV-2/
    COVID-19
  accessory proteins, 730–732, 731*t*
  ACE2 usage, evolution of, 711
  assembly and release, 716
  beta and gamma variants, 706–740:p0132
  diversification of, 711
  evolution of, 707–709
  evolutionary history, 709–711
  nonstructural proteins, 716–730
  nucleotide identity analysis, 706–740:p0044, 710*f*
  origin and evolution, 709–711
  phylogenetic structure, 707–709, 708*f*
  recombinant viruses, 732
  replication and structural proteins, 711–716, 713*f*
  secondary transmission to wild and domestic
    animals, 733–734
  transmission and immune evasion, 732–733
  variants, 732–733
Severe COVID-19, 747
SFFV-A, pathogenicity of, 510
SH (small hydrophobic) protein
  in human metapneumovirus, 271*f*, 273*t*, 276
  in human respiratory syncytial virus, 270*f*, 271*f*,
    276
  in mumps virus, 208*t*, 210*f*
Sheep pulmonary adenomatosis (SPA), pathogenicity
    of, 510
Sialic acid, in orthoreoviruses, 328
σ1 attachment protein, reovirus, 327–328, 327*f*
  cleavage of, by intestinal proteases, 329
  conformational changes in, 322*f*, 327*f*, 332
  JAM-A binding by, 328–329
σ3 protein, reovirus, 330*f*, 331–332
Sigma virus, history of, 163
Simian agent 11 (SA11)
  coding assignments in, 371, 373*f*
  discovery of, 362
  genome structure and organization in, 367–371,
    370*f*, 373*f*
Simian foamy viruses (SFVs), 680
Simian hemorrhage fever virus (SHFV), 104
  clinical features of, 122
  epidemiology of, 121–122
  genome structure and organization of, 106–108
  history and classification of, 104–105
  immune response to, 118
  pathogenesis and pathology of, 116–121
  prevention and control of, 123–124
  release from host and transmission of, 119–120
  replication cycle of, 109–116
  structure of, virion, 105–106, 106*f*
  virulence and persistence of, 117
Simian immunodeficiency virus (SIV)
  accessory proteins in
    Nef, 604–606
    Vif, 601–602
    Vpr, 602
    Vpu, 603
    Vpx, 603
  classification of, 559, 560*f*
  clinical and pathological features, 665–666, 667*f*
  gp41 ectodomain residues of, trimeric structure of,
    568, 569*f*
  history, 648

human immunodeficiency virus from, 619
  models in nonhuman primates, 563
  receptors for, 475*t*, 476
  vaccine research on, 671
Simian rotavirus RRV strain (G3P(3)), 399
Simian sarcoma-associated virus (SSAV), 470*t*
  receptors for, 475*t*, 476
SIMPLE-Severe trial, 761
Single-layered particle (SLP), in rotavirus, 365–366,
    365*f*, 366*f*
SLAMF1 receptor, in measles virus, 232–233, 233*f*
Slow leukemia viruses, 507
Slow virus infections, 648
Small interfering RNA (siRNA) in echovirus control,
    in human T-cell leukemia viruses, 531
Snap-back DI particles, in rhabdoviruses, 182
Solid-phase ELISA assays, 34
Sotrovimab, SARS-CoV-2/COVID-19, 759
Sp1
  in human immunodeficiency virus, 581
  in nonhuman lentiviruses, 669
Spike (S) protein/glycoprotein, 712–715, 713*f*
  in astroviruses, 60–61, 61*f*
Spinareovirinae, 319
Spleen focus-forming virus (SFFV-P), 510
Sporadic catarrhal jaundice, 22–23
Spring viremia of carp virus (SVCV), 162
Spumaretrovirinae, 679
Spumaviruses, 467*f*, 468*t*, 469
STAT
  in mumps viruses, 209–210, 216
  in retroviruses, 489
  in rhinoviruses, 9
STAT1
  in arteriviruses, 119
  in measles viruses, 238–239, 242
  in *Rhabdoviridae*, 184, 187–189
  in rhinoviruses, 9
STAT2
  in measles viruses, 242
  in mumps viruses, 209–210
  in *Rhabdoviridae*, 184
STAT3, in mumps viruses, 209–210
Stavudine, 480
Stem-loop DNA, 533
Step-change, virus distribution, 436–437
Sterile alpha motif and histidine–aspartic acid
    domain–containing protein 1 (SAMHD1),
    658
Stress-associated RNA granules (stress granules)
  in human respiratory syncytial virus, 282–283
  in orthoreoviruses, 338, 342–343
Structural ORF and protein products in
  capsid in, 83–87, 83*f*, 84*f*
    envelope glycoproteins E1 and E2, 87
    nonstructural roles of, 84–87, 86*f*
    in virus assembly, 84, 85*f*
SU (surface) subunit, in retroviruses, 474, 504
Subacute sclerosing panencephalitis (SSPE)
  clinical features of, 249
  epidemiology of, 247
  from measles, 229, 243*f*
  pathogenesis and pathology of, 243–244, 243*t*
Switch (switching)
  myristyl, in retroviruses, 496
  template, in retroviruses, 572

T

T lymphocytes (T cells), nuclear factor of activated T
    cells (NFAT), in HIV, 580–581
Tas protein, in foamy viruses, 686*f*, 695–696, 695*f*
Tat, in human immunodeficiency virus, 582–584
  function in mice, 584
  vs. latency, 585

posttranslational modifications, 584
  P-TEFb, 582–583, 582*f*
  structure of, 582–584, 582*f*, 583*f*
  transactivation response region element, 582, 583*f*
tat, in nonhuman lentiviruses, 651–654, 654*t*, 666
Tax1, *in vitro* immortalizing and transforming
    activities of, 536
Tax (HTLV), 531
  apoptosis inhibition, 532
  in cell cycle arrest, 537
  cellular signaling pathways, 531–532
  centrosome amplification by, 537
  on DNA repair, 537
  expression and suppression by HBZ and Rex, 533
  genomic instability from, 537
  HBZ-Tax interplay in, 537
  in immortalization and persistent infection, 529*f*,
    530–531
  in inflammation, 546
  in microRNA deregulation, 537
  molecular mechanism, Tax-mediated
    transcriptional activation, 531
  NF-kB activation by, 531–532, 532*f*
  p53 inactivation by, 537
  physiological functions, 532
  PI3K/AKT pathway activation by, 532
  plus-strand transcription of the HTLV-1, 531
  in transcriptional activation, 531, 532*f*
T-cell immunity, SARS-CoV-2/COVID-19, 743–744
T-cell immunoglobulin mucin 1 (TIM-1), 45–46
T-cell responses, HAV infection
  in mice, 46
  in nonhuman primates, 45–46
Template switching, in retroviruses, 572
Tenofovir disoproxil fumarate (tenofovir), 480
Tetherin (BST2, CD317)
  cell surface trapping of virion particles by,
    506–507
  in foamy virus, 701
  in human immunodeficiency virus, 619
    Nef on, 606
    Vpu on, 603–605, 604*f*
    vpu on, 495, 619
  in nonhuman lentiviruses, 655–658
  Nef on, in simian immunodeficiency virus, 495,
    668
3AB, in hepatoviruses, 30
3D^pol polymerase, in hepatoviruses, 31
Thrombocytopenia, from rubella, 94–95
Thrombosis with thrombocytopenia syndrome
    (TTS), vaccines, 766
TM (transmembrane) subunit, in retroviruses, 474,
    504
TNF-related apoptosis-inducing ligand (TRAIL) in
    astrovirus, 66
Toll-like receptor (TLR)
  in rhabdoviruses, 183
  in rhinoviruses, 8–9, 9*f*
Transforming viruses, 470, 470*t*
  retroviruses as, 470, 470*t*
Transfusion, blood
  foamy virus from, 682
  hepatitis A virus hepatitis from, 47
  human immunodeficiency virus from, 558, 620
  human T-cell leukemia virus from, 538
Transmission dynamics, SARS-CoV-2/COVID-19,
    745–746
Transmission modes, SARS-CoV-2/COVID-19, 746
Tree shrews, for borna disease virus, 148
TRIM, 477
  in retroviruses, 477
TRIM protein, 573
TRIM5a
  on infection, 505–506
  in retroviruses, 505–506

TRIM5α, 657
  in HIV-1, 618
  in human immunodeficiency virus, 573–574, 574f, 575f, 593, 618
TRIM5-cyclophilin A (TRIM5-Cyp), in nonhuman lentiviruses, 657
TRIM28, in retroviruses, 489
TRIMCyp, 573–574, 574f, 575f
  in human immunodeficiency virus, 573–574, 574f, 575f
Tripartite motif-containing protein 5 (TRIM5)
  in nonhuman lentiviruses, 655–657, 670
Triple-layered particle (TLP), in rotavirus, 365, 365f, 366f
Tropical spastic paraparesis (TSP)
  clinical features of, 548–549
  history of, 527–528
Turreted viruses, 365–366
2B protein, in hepatoviruses, 30
2C protein, in hepatoviruses, 30

U

U3, in nonhuman lentiviruses, 669
Uveitis, HTLV-1, 549

V

Vaccination
  againsts hepatitis E virus, 459–460, 460t
  against smallpox, 398–399
  Bluetongue disease, 437
  borna disease virus, 150–152
  equine arteritis virus, 104
  hepatitis A virus, 51
    inactivated, 51
    live attenuated vaccine, 51
  human immunodeficiency virus, 638–639
  human T-cell leukemia virus, 551
  lentiviruses, nonhuman, 670–672
  measles virus
    attenuated live virus vaccines, 251–252
    eradication via, 253
    experimental, 252
    history of, 250, 250f–251f
    inactivated, 250–251
    on measles epidemiology, 246–247
  metapneumovirus, human, 306
  mumps virus, 220–221, 220t
  porcine reproductive and respiratory syndrome virus, 104
  rabies, 162
  respiratory syncytial virus, 301–302
  reverse genetics-based, 438–439
  rotavirus
    attenuated rotavirus vaccines deployed on a national or restricted multinational basis, 401–402
    fundamentals of, 398
    initial monovalent animal rotavirus ("Jennerian") candidates in, 398–399
    other approaches to, 402
    quadrivalent RRV-based reassortant, 399–400
    Rotarix and RotaTeq postlicensure safety and efficacy studies in, 400–401, 401t
    two major currently licensed live, 400
  rotaviruses, 398
  rubella, 75, 76f
    administration of, 98
    adverse reactions to, 98
    countries with strategies for, 75, 76f
    development of, 98
    new strategies for, 99
    pregnancy risk of, 98
  SARS-CoV-2/COVID-19, 765–769, 766t

adverse events, 766
booster, 768–769
effectiveness, 766
effectiveness against, 766, 767t–768t
efficacy, 765
immunocompromising conditions, 766–767
protein subunit vaccines, 765
simian immunodeficiency virus, 671
subunit/VLP, 437–438
Vaccine Adverse Events Reporting System (VAERS), 399
Vaccine booster, SARS-CoV-2/COVID-19, 768–769
Vaccine-induced neutralizing antibodies (nAbs), 765
Vaccines
  againsts hepatitis E virus, 459–460, 460t
  against smallpox, 398–399
  Bluetongue disease, 437
  borna disease virus, 150–152
  equine arteritis virus, 104
  hepatitis A virus, 51
    inactivated, 51
    live attenuated vaccine, 51
  human immunodeficiency virus, 638–639
  human T-cell leukemia virus, 551
  lentiviruses, nonhuman, 670–672
  measles virus
    attenuated live virus vaccines, 251–252
    eradication via, 253
    experimental, 252
    history of, 250, 250f–251f
    inactivated, 250–251
    on measles epidemiology, 246–247
  metapneumovirus, human, 306
  mumps virus, 220–221, 220t
  porcine reproductive and respiratory syndrome virus, 104
  rabies, 162
  respiratory syncytial virus, 301–302
  reverse genetics-based, 438–439
  rotavirus
    attenuated rotavirus vaccines deployed on a national or restricted multinational basis, 401–402
    fundamentals of, 398
    initial monovalent animal rotavirus ("Jennerian") candidates in, 398–399
    other approaches to, 402
    quadrivalent RRV-based reassortant, 399–400
    Rotarix and RotaTeq postlicensure safety and efficacy studies in, 400–401, 401t
    two major currently licensed live, 400
  rotaviruses, 398
  rubella, 75, 76f
    administration of, 98
    adverse reactions to, 98
    countries with strategies for, 75, 76f
    development of, 98
    new strategies for, 99
    pregnancy risk of, 98
  SARS-CoV-2/COVID-19, 765–769, 766t
    adverse events, 766
    booster, 768–769
    effectiveness, 766
    effectiveness against, 766, 767t–768t
    efficacy, 765
    immunocompromising conditions, 766–767
    protein subunit vaccines, 765
  simian immunodeficiency virus, 671
  subunit/VLP, 437–438
Variants of concern (VOC), SARS-CoV-2, 732–733
Vectors
  gene delivery, retroviruses as, 466
  for gene therapy, retrovirus, 514–515

retrovirus, 514–515
  for gene delivery, 466
Vesicular stomatitis Indiana virus (VSIV), 162
Vesicular stomatitis New Jersey virus (VSNJV), 162
Vesicular stomatitis virus (VSV)
  apoptosis induction by, 185–186
  clinical features of, 193
  control of infections with, 196
  diagnosis of, 194
  epidemiology of, 191
  genetic engineering of, 182–183
  history of, 162
  molecular genetics of, 182
  mouse models of, 186–189, 187f
  pathogenesis of, molecular and cellular basis of, 183–186
    cytopathic effects induction in, 185–186
    host antiviral response induction and suppression in, 183–185
    host gene expression inhibition in, 185f, 184–185
  perspectives on, 196–197
  replication stages of, 174–181
  structure of, virion, 164–165, 165f
  taxonomy of, 163–164, 163f, 164t
  virulence of, 189
Vesiculoviruses (VSIV)
  apoptosis induction by, 185–186
  epidemiology of, 191
  history of, 162
  immune response to, 187f, 188–189
    in recovery, 187
  infection in
    clinical features of, 193
    diagnosis of, 194, 194f
    prevention and control of, 196
  structure of, virion, 164–165, 165f
  taxonomy of, 163–164, 163f, 164t
vif gene, in nonhuman lentiviruses, 651–654, 654t, 668
Vif, in human immunodeficiency virus, 601–602, 601f
Viral hemorrhagic septicemia (VHS), 193
Viral hemorrhagic septicemia virus (VHSV)
  clinical features of, 193
  control of, 196–197
  diagnosis of, 194
  epidemiology of, 192
  taxonomy of, 163–164, 167f
  transmission of, 193
Viral inclusion bodies (VIBs), in reoviruses, 318, 336f, 338
Viral-like particles (VLPs), in hepatitis E virus, 446, 447f
Virological synapses, in HTLV-1 entry, 539
Viroplasms
  in orthoreoviruses, 318, 336f, 338
  in reoviruses, 318, 336f, 338
  in rotaviruses, 368t–369t, 373, 373f, 374f, 379–383, 386f
Virus inclusion bodies (VIBs), in orbiviruses, 427f
Virus-like particle (VLP)
  in foamy viruses, 700–701
  in human immunodeficiency virus, 589–590
  in human respiratory syncytial virus, 279
  in measles virus, 234–235
  in mumps virus, 209
  in orbiviruses, 428
  in retroviruses, 497
  in rotaviruses, 383–384, 390
  in rubella, 83–84
  in vaccines
    for rotaviruses, 402
Virus-like sequences, in retroviruses, 513–514
VP1

in hepatitis A virus, 28
in orbiviruses, 417–418, 419f, 420t
in rotaviruses, 365, 366f, 368t–369t, 373f
VP2
in hepatitis A virus, 28
in orbiviruses, 415, 418f, 420–422, 420t
in rotaviruses, 365–366, 366f, 368t–369t, 373f
VP3
in hepatitis A virus, 30
in orbiviruses, 417–418, 419f
in rotaviruses, 365, 366f, 368t–369t, 373f
VP4
in hepatitis A virus, 30
in orbiviruses, 417–419, 420t, 425
in rotaviruses, 363f, 366–367, 366f, 368t–369t, 373, 373f, 382–383
VP5, in orbiviruses, 418f, 420–422, 420t
VP5*, in rotaviruses, 366–367, 368t–369t, 375–377, 383
VP6
in orbiviruses, 419, 420t
in rotaviruses, 366–367, 366f, 368t–369t, 373f

VP6 helicase, in orbiviruses, 415, 420t
VP7
in orbiviruses, 415, 418f, 420t
in rotaviruses, 366–367, 366f, 368t–369t, 373f
VP8*, in rotaviruses, 366–367, 366f, 368t–369t, 371, 373–376, 375f
VP25, in astroviruses, 65, 65f
VP27, in astroviruses, 65, 65f
VP70, in astroviruses, 65–66, 65f
VP90, in astroviruses, 65–66, 65f
VPg (protein 3B)
in astroviruses, 62, 62f
in hepatitis A virus, 30
vpr gene, in nonhuman lentiviruses, 651–654, 654t, 668–669
Vpr, in human immunodeficiency virus, 590f, 602–603, 602f
V protein
in measles virus, 231
in mumps virus, 208t, 209–210
vpu gene, in nonhuman lentiviruses, 651–654, 654t

Vpu, in human immunodeficiency virus, 603–605, 603f, 604f
Vpx, in human immunodeficiency virus, 603
vpx, in human immunodeficiency virus, 651–654, 654t, 669

W
Walleye dermal sarcoma virus (WDSV), 468–469
Wheezing, from human rhinovirus infection, 11–12
Wooly monkey sarcoma virus, 470t

X
Xiamen Innovax , HEV vaccine, 460t
X protein, in bornaviruses, 135–136, 135f

Z
Zidovudine (azidothymidine, AZT), mechanisms of action of, 480
Zinc finger antiviral protein (ZAP), 659
retroviral RNA elimination by, 506